W9-CED-949

20th Anniversary Edition

Nursing2000

DRUG HANDBOOK®

NURSING2000 BOOKS™
SPRINGHOUSE CORPORATION
SPRINGHOUSE, PENNSYLVANIA

STAFF

Senior Vice President, Editorial
Patricia Dwyer Schull, RN, MSN

Publisher
Donna O. Carpenter, ELS

Editorial Director
William J. Kelly

Clinical Director
Ann M. Barrow, RN, MSN, CCRN

Art Director
John Hubbard

Managing Editor
Andrew T. McPhee, RN, BSN

Drug Information Editor
Lisa Truong, RPh, PharmD

Senior Editor
Naina Chohan

Editors
Rita M. Doyle, Peter H. Johnson

Clinical Editors
Eileen Cassin Gallen, RN, BSN; Christine M. Damico, RN, MSN, CPNP; Nancy Laplante, RN, BSN; Pamela S. Messer, RN, MSN; Lori Musolf Neri, RN, MSN, CCRN; Kimberly A. Zalewski, RN, MSN, CEN

Copy Editors
Karen C. Comerford (manager), Donna Birdsell, Colleen P. Coady, Leslie Dworkin, Pamela Wingrod

Designers
Arlene Putterman (associate art director), Elaine Kasmer Ezrow, Joseph John Clark, Don Knauss

Typographers
Diane Paluba (manager), Joyce Rossi Biletz

Manufacturing
Deborah Meiris (director), Patricia K. Dorshaw (manager), Otto Mezei (book production manager)

Editorial Assistants
Carrie R. Cameron, Carol A. Caputo

Indexer
Barbara Hodgson

The clinical procedures described and recommended in this publication are based on research and consultation with nursing, medical, pharmaceutical, and legal authorities. To the best of our knowledge, these procedures reflect currently accepted practice; nevertheless, they can't be considered absolute and universal recommendations. For individual application, all recommendations must be considered in light of the patient's clinical condition and, before the administration of new or infrequently used drugs, in light of the latest package-insert information. The authors and publisher disclaim responsibility for adverse effects resulting directly or indirectly from the suggested procedures, from undetected errors, or from the reader's misunderstanding of the text.

A member of the Reed Elsevier plc group

Visit our Web site at www.NDHnow.com

NDH-010799
ISSN 0273-320X
ISBN 0-87434-993-1

midazolam HCl	morphine sulfate	nalbuphine HCl	pentazocine lactate	pentobarbital Na	perphenazine	phenobarbital Na	prochlorperazine edisylate	promazine HCl	promethazine HCl	ranitidine HCl	scopolamine HBr	secobarbital Na	sodium bicarbonate	thiethylperazine maleate	thiopental Na	
Y	P	Y	P	P	Y		P	P	P	Y	P					atropine sulfate
Y	Y		Y	N	Y		Y		Y		Y			Y		butorphanol tartrate
Y	P		P	N	Y		P	P	P	N*	P				N	chlorpromazine HCl
Y	Y	Y	Y	N	Y		Y	Y	Y		Y	N				cimetidine HCl
																codeine phosphate
										Y						dexamethasone sodium phosphate
N	P		P	N	Y		N	N	N	Y	P				N	dimenhydrinate
Y	P	Y	P	N	Y		P	P	P	Y	P				N	diphenhydramine HCl
Y	P	Y	P	N	Y		P	P	P		P					droperidol
Y	P		P	N	Y		P	P	P	Y	P					fentanyl citrate
Y	Y	Y	N	N			Y	Y	Y	Y	Y	N	N		N	glycopyrrolate
	N*		N		P(5)			N								heparin Na
Y			Y	Y			N*		Y	Y	Y			Y		hydromorphone HCl
Y	P	Y	P	N	Y		P	P	P	N	P					hydroxyzine HCl
Y	N		P	N	Y		P	P	P	Y	P				N	meperidine HCl
Y	P		P		P		P	P	P	Y	P		N			metoclopramide HCl
	Y	Y		N	N		N	Y	Y	N	Y			Y		midazolam HCl
Y			P	N*	Y		P*	P	P*	Y	P				N	morphine sulfate
Y				N			Y		N*	Y	Y			Y		nalbuphine HCl
	P			N	Y		P	Y	Y	Y	P					pentazocine lactate
N	N*	N	N		N		N	N	N	N	P		Y		Y	pentobarbital Na
N	Y		Y	N			Y		Y	Y	Y		N			perphenazine
										N						phenobarbital Na
N	P*	Y	P	N	Y			P	P	Y	P				N	prochlorperazine edisylate
Y	P		Y	N			P		P		P					promazine HCl
Y	P*	N*	Y	N	Y		P	P		Y	P				N	promethazine HCl
N	Y	Y	Y	N	Y	N	Y		Y		Y			Y		ranitidine HCl
Y	P	Y	P	P	Y		P	P	P	Y					Y	scopolamine HBr
																secobarbital Na
			Y												N	sodium bicarbonate
Y		Y		N						Y						thiethylperazine maleate
	N			Y			N		N		Y		N			thiopental Na

CONTENTS

Autonomic Nervous System Drugs

Respiratory Tract Drugs

Gastrointestinal Tract Drugs

Photoguide to Tablets and Capsules

Hormonal Drugs

ADVISORS AND CLINICAL CONSULTANTS

At the time of publication, the advisors and clinical consultants held the following positions.

Advisors

Kathleen G. Andreoli, DSN, FAAN
Vice President, Nursing Affairs and the John L. and Helen Kellogg Dean of the College of Nursing of Rush University
Chicago

Lillian S. Brunner, RN, MSN, ScD, FAAN
Nurse-Author
Lancaster, Pa.

Kathleen A. Dracup, RN, DNSc, FAAN
Professor and L. W. Hassenplug Chair
University of California School of Nursing
Los Angeles

Stanley J. Dudrick, MD, FACS
Program Director
St. Mary's Hospital Department of Surgery
Waterbury, Conn.
Clinical Professor of Surgery
Yale University School of Medicine
New Haven, Conn.

Halbert E. Fillinger, MD
Forensic Pathologist and Coroner
Montgomery County, Pa.

M. Josephine Flaherty, RN, PhD
Consultant
Ottawa, Canada

Dennis E. Leavell, MD
Associate Professor
Mayo Medical Laboratories
Mayo Clinic
Rochester, Minn.

Ara G. Paul, PhD
Dean Emeritus and Professor of Pharmacognosy
College of Pharmacy
University of Michigan
Ann Arbor

Thomas E. Rubbert, JD, LLB, BSL
Attorney-at-Law
Pasadena, Calif.

Clinical Consultants

Steven R. Abel, PharmD, FASHP
Professor and Head - Department of Pharmacy Practice
Purdue University School of Pharmacy and Pharmacal Sciences
Indianapolis

Deborah Becker, MSN, CRNP, CCRN
Lecturer – Acute Care Nurse Practitioner Program
University of Pennsylvania School of Nursing
Philadelphia

Steven R. Benson, PharmD, BCPS
Pharmacotherapy Specialist
Express Scripts/ValueRx
Plymouth, Minn.

Jane Bliss-Holtz, DNSc, RN,C
Nurse Researcher
Ann May Center for Nursing – Meridian Health System
Neptune, N.J.

Rebecca E. Boehne, RN, PhD
Patient and Family Education Coordinator
Portland VA Medical Center
Portland, Ore.

Mary E. Bowen, RN, DNS, CNAA
Assistant Professor
Thomas Jefferson University
Philadelphia

Karen T. Bruchak, RN, MSN, MBA
Director of Nursing, Medical-Surgical/Specialty
Mercy Fitzgerald
Darby, Pa.

Lawrence Carey, RPh, PharmD
Clinical Pharmacist Coordinator
Jefferson Home Infusion Service
Philadelphia

Rachel Clark-Vetri, PharmD
Assistant Professor
Temple University
Philadelphia

Barbara Ann Costa, RN, MS
Retired Professor
Syracuse (N.Y.) University

Belle Erickson, RN, PhD
Assistant Professor of Nursing
Villanova (Pa.) University College of Nursing

Carmel A. Esposito, RN, MSN, EdD
Nurse Educator/Coordinator of Continuing Education
Trinity Health System School of Nursing
Steubenville, Ohio

Mary Jo Gerlach, RN, MSNEd
Assistant Professor, Adult Nursing
Medical College of Georgia, School of Nursing
Athens

Cynthia A. Gobin, PharmD
Clinical Assistant Professor
Temple University School of Pharmacy
Philadelphia

Mildred D. Gottwald, PharmD
Assistant Clinical Professor
University of California – Department of Clinical Pharmacy
San Francisco

Ronald L. Greenberg, PharmD, BCPS
Clinical Pharmacy Specialist
Fairview Ridges Hospital
Burnsville, Minn.

Barbara S. Kannewurf, PharmD
Clinical Pharmacist
Professional Consultants Ltd.
Stafford, Va.

James A. Koestner, BS-Pharm, PharmD
PharmD – Clinical Pharmacist – Trauma/Critical Care
Vanderbilt University Medical Center
Nashville, Tenn.

Jeanette M. Logan, PharmD
Fellow in Behavioral Health Science
University of California, San Francisco

Dawna Martich, RN, MSN
Manager, Member Care
Diabetes Treatment Centers of America
Pittsburgh

William O'Hara, PharmD
Clinical Pharmacy Specialist
Thomas Jefferson University Hospital
Philadelphia

Jeffrey B. Purcell, PharmD
Clinical Lead Pharmacist
Harborview Medical Center
Clinical Associate Professor
University of Washington School of Pharmacy
Seattle

Joseph F. Steiner, RPh, PharmD
Professor and Director of Pharmacy Practice
University of Wyoming, School of Pharmacy
Laramie

Eva M. Vasquez, PharmD, BCPS
Assistant Professor
University of Illinois at Chicago

Kenneth K. Wieland, PharmD
Independent Consultant
Lansdale, Pa.

Madeline D. Wiley, MSN, ARNP
Family Nurse Practitioner
Valley Medical Center Kent Primary Care
Kent, Wash.

Karriann Kyle Wood, RPh, PharmD
Clinical Pharmacist
Norton Suburban Hospital
Louisville, Ky.

How to use *Nursing2000 Drug Handbook*

Nursing2000 Drug Handbook was created by pharmacists and nurses to provide the nursing profession with drug information that zeroes in on precisely what nurses need to know. With that goal clearly in mind, *Nursing2000 Drug Handbook* emphasizes clinical aspects of drugs without attempting to replace detailed pharmacology texts. In addition, the book is designed to make the content readily accessible and applicable in any clinical setting.

Features in this edition
The 2000 edition contains several features to enhance nursing knowledge and skills:
• Charts that show the route, onset, peak, and duration of each drug.
• "Elderly" dosage and "Adjust-a-dose" categories detail possible dosage adjustments necessary in specific patient populations.
• New monographs on 76 new FDA approved drugs.
• An expanded Interactions section includes herbal agent interactions in addition to other drugs, foods, and lifestyle behaviors. (See "Interactions" later in this chapter for details.)
• Instructions for preparing and administering I.V. drugs are now highlighted in each appropriate entry.
• New appendices covering dialyzable drugs and therapeutic drug monitoring guidelines enhance the usefulness of this book.
• Free NDH*Plus!* CD-ROM (inside the back cover) lets the user take eight continuing education tests (and earn 28.5 contact hours), learn and perform dosage calculations, instantly identify common capsules and tablets by their drug imprint codes, and print out patient-teaching instructions for 200 commonly used drugs and herbs.
• NDH*Plus!* CD-ROM also links you directly to **www.NDHnow.com**, the *Nursing2000 Drug Handbook* Web site that provides drug updates and important drug news.

Introductory chapters
Chapter 2 explains, in a general way, how drugs work. It also tells about adverse reactions and gives general guidelines about drug use in pregnancy and the presence of drugs in breast milk. Chapters 3 and 4 discuss the unique problems of administering drugs to children and elderly patients and offer guidelines to minimize problems in these areas. Chapter 5 discusses drug therapy as it relates to the nursing process.

Therapeutic class chapters
In chapters 6 to 98, all drugs are classified according to their approved therapeutic uses. Drugs with multiple therapeutic uses are classified according to their most common use; they are also listed (with a cross-reference to the major drug entry) in drug groups that share their secondary applications. For example, nadolol, a beta-adrenergic blocker, is described in the chapter that covers antianginals because its major therapeutic application is the management of angina pectoris. Because the drug is less commonly used to treat hypertension, it is also listed among the generic drugs grouped as antihypertensives, with a cross-reference to Chapter 22, Antianginals.

Such classification by therapeutic use offers several advantages. It helps the reader identify an unknown drug by its clinical application alone. It also automatically identifies all other drugs that share the same use and provides easy comparison of their dosages and effects. In this way, it quickly identifies potential pharmacotherapeutic alternatives for patients who can't tolerate or who fail to respond to a particular drug.

Each chapter, representing a major therapeutic use, begins with an alphabetical list of the generic drugs described in that chapter. This is followed by a list of selected combination products in which these drugs are found. Specific information on each drug is arranged under the following headings: *Trade Name; Controlled Substance Schedule (where applicable); Pregnancy Risk Category; How Supplied; Action; Indications & Dosage; Adverse Reactions; Interactions; Effects on Diagnostic Tests; Contraindications; Nursing Considerations; I.V. Administration (where applicable); and Patient teaching.*

In each drug entry, the generic name is followed by an alphabetized list of its brand names. A brand name followed by an open diamond (◇) indicates a drug preparation that doesn't need a prescription. Brands that are specifically Canadian are designated with a dagger (†); those that are specifically Australian are followed by a double dagger (‡); and those that are specifically British are followed by a section mark (§). A brand name with no symbol is available in the United States, Canada, and possibly Australia and the U.K. The mention of a brand name in no way implies endorsement of that product or guarantees its legality.

Alcohol and tartrazine content

Many liquid drug preparations for oral use contain alcohol. Although the slight sedative effect that alcohol produces is not harmful in most patients—and can sometimes be beneficial—alcohol ingestion can be undesirable and even dangerous. Oral drugs that contain alcohol should be given cautiously, if at all, to patients who are:
• concomitantly taking potent CNS depressants such as barbiturates
• taking drugs that may produce a disulfiram-type reaction (such as chlorpropamide or metronidazole)
• taking disulfiram as part of a treatment program for their alcoholism. Such patients, upon ingestion of alcohol, will exhibit severe signs or symptoms that may include blurred vision, confusion, dyspnea, flushing, sweating, and tachycardia.

To help prevent inadvertent exposure to alcohol, the text signals alcohol content with a single asterisk (*) after each brand of a liquid preparation that may contain it. In many of the preparations so marked, the alcohol content is small. Nevertheless, these drugs should be avoided in patients

susceptible to adverse effects after exposure to alcohol.

Tartrazine dye, also known as FD&C Yellow No. 5, is a common coloring agent in some foods and drugs. Usually harmless, it can provoke a severe reaction in susceptible persons. For this reason, most drug manufacturers have begun to eliminate tartrazine from their products, but many drugs still contain it.

The incidence of tartrazine sensitivity is approximately 1 in 10,000 in the general population but somewhat higher in persons with asthma or sensitivity to aspirin. The reason for this is unknown. The most common signs and symptoms of tartrazine sensitivity are urticaria, rhinorrhea, asthma, and angioedema. Acutely sensitive persons may develop allergic vascular purpura, tachycardia, dyspnea, and chest pain. These allergic signs or symptoms typically subside spontaneously upon discontinuation of the drug but may require treatment with antihistamines or epinephrine.

Tartrazine may be present in yellow-colored drugs and those of many other colors, including turquoise, green, and maroon. This text signals tartrazine content with a double asterisk (**) after each brand that may contain it. If you suspect tartrazine sensitivity in a patient receiving such a drug, inform the doctor and contact the manufacturer to determine which dosage forms contain tartrazine.

Controlled substance schedules

If a drug is a controlled substance, that is indicated (example: Controlled Substance Schedule II). Drugs regulated under the jurisdiction of the Controlled Substances Act of 1970 are divided into the following groups, or schedules:
• Schedule I (C-I): High abuse potential and no accepted medical use—for example, heroin, marijuana, and LSD.
• Schedule II (C-II): High abuse potential with severe dependence liability—for example, narcotics, amphetamines, dronabinol, and some barbiturates.
• Schedule III (C-III): Less abuse potential than schedule II drugs and moderate dependence liability—for example, nonbarbiturate sedatives, nonamphetamine

stimulants, anabolic steroids, and limited amounts of certain narcotics.
• Schedule IV (C-IV): Less abuse potential than schedule III drugs and limited dependence liability—for example, some sedatives, antianxiety agents, and nonnarcotic analgesics.
• Schedule V (C-V): Limited abuse potential. Primarily small amounts of narcotics, such as codeine, used as antitussives or antidiarrheals. Under federal law, limited quantities of certain C-V drugs may be purchased without a prescription directly from a pharmacist if allowed under specific state statutes. The purchaser must be at least 18 years and must furnish suitable identification. All such transactions must be recorded by the dispensing pharmacist.

Pregnancy risk category
Each systemically absorbed drug has been assigned a pregnancy risk category based upon available clinical and preclinical information. The Pregnancy Risk Category parallels the five Pregnancy Categories (A, B, C, D, and X) assigned by the FDA to reflect a drug's potential to cause birth defects. Although drugs are best avoided during pregnancy, this rating system permits rapid assessment of the risk-benefit ratio should drug administration to a pregnant woman become necessary. Drugs in category A are generally considered safe to use in pregnancy; drugs in category X are generally contraindicated.
• A: Adequate studies in pregnant women have failed to show a risk to the fetus.
• B: Animal studies have not shown a risk to the fetus, but controlled studies have not been conducted in pregnant women; or animal studies have shown an adverse effect on the fetus, but adequate studies in pregnant women have not shown a risk to the fetus.
• C: Animal studies have shown an adverse effect on the fetus, but adequate studies have not been conducted in humans. The benefits from use in pregnant women may be acceptable despite potential risks.
• D: The drug may cause risk to the human fetus, but the potential benefits of use in pregnant women may be acceptable despite the risks (such as in a life-threatening situation or a serious disease for which safer drugs can't be used or are ineffective).
• X: Studies in animals or humans show fetal abnormalities, or adverse reaction reports indicate evidence of fetal risk. The risks involved clearly outweigh potential benefits.
• NR: Not rated.

How supplied
This section lists the preparations available for each drug (for example, tablets, capsules, solutions for injection), specifying available dosage forms and strengths. Dosage strengths that are specifically available in Canada are designated with a dagger (†), those available in Australia with a double dagger (‡), and those in the U.K. with a section mark (§). Preparations that do not require a prescription are marked with an open diamond (◇).

Action
This section succinctly describes the mechanism of action—that is, how the drug provides its therapeutic effect. For example, although all antihypertensives lower blood pressure, they don't all do so by the same pharmacologic process.
    Also included in chart form is the onset, peak (described in terms of effect or peak blood level), and duration of drug action for each route of administration, if data are available or applicable. Values listed are for patients with normal renal function, unless specified otherwise.

Indications & dosage
This section lists general dosage information for adults, children, and elderly patients, as applicable. Dosage instructions reflect current clinical trends in therapeutics and can't be considered as absolute or universal recommendations. For individual application, dosage instructions must be considered in light of the patient's clinical condition. The logo for "Adjust-a-dose" appears in this section.

Adverse reactions
This section lists adverse reactions to each drug by body system. The most

common adverse reactions (those experienced by at least 10% of people taking the drug in clinical trials) are in *italic* type; less common reactions are in roman type; life-threatening reactions are in ***bold italic*** type; and reactions that are common *and* life-threatening are in **BOLD CAPITAL LETTERS.**

Interactions

This section lists each drug's confirmed, *clinically significant* interactions with other drugs (additive effects, potentiated effects, and antagonistic effects); herbs (herbal preparations have the potential to significantly affect the anticipated action of a drug); foods, with specific suggestions for avoiding dangerous drug or food interactions (for example, by reducing doses or monitoring food intake); or lifestyle (such as alcohol use or smoking). Drug interactions are listed under the drug that is adversely affected. For example, magnesium trisilicate, an ingredient in antacids, interacts with tetracycline to cause decreased absorption of tetracycline. Therefore, this interaction is listed under tetracycline. To check on the possible effects of using two or more drugs simultaneously, refer to the interaction entry for each of the drugs in question.

Effects on diagnostic tests

This section lists significant interference with a diagnostic test or its result, either by a drug's direct effects on the test itself or by systemic effects that cause misleading test results.

Contraindications

This section lists any conditions, especially diseases, in which the use of the drug is undesirable.

Nursing considerations

This section lists recommendations for cautious use, followed by other useful information, such as monitoring techniques and suggestions for prevention and treatment of adverse reactions. Also included are suggestions for patient comfort and for preparing, administering, and storing each drug.

Guidelines for properly reconstituting and mixing I.V. drugs along with tips for added safety appear under the new "I.V. administration" subhead.

The "Patient teaching" section focuses on explaining the drug's purpose, promoting compliance, and ensuring proper use and storage of the drug. It also includes instructions for preventing or minimizing adverse reactions.

Photoguide to tablets and capsules

To make drug identification easier for nurses and to enhance patient safety, *Nursing2000 Drug Handbook* offers a full-color photoguide to the most commonly prescribed tablets and capsules. Shown in actual size, the drugs are arranged alphabetically for quick reference, along with their most common dosage strengths. Page references to the drugs appear in boldface type in the Index.

Common abbreviations

ACE	angiotensin-converting enzyme	LD	lactate dehydrogenase
ADH	antidiuretic hormone	M	molar
AIDS	acquired immunodeficiency syndrome	m^2	square meter
ALT	alanine transaminase	MAO	monoamine oxidase
AST	aspartate transaminase	mcg	microgram
AV	atrioventricular	mEq	milliequivalent
b.i.d.	twice daily	mg	milligram
BPH	benign prostatic hyperplasia	MI	myocardial infarction
BUN	blood urea nitrogen	ml	milliliter
cAMP	cyclic adenosine monophosphate	mm^3	cubic millimeter
CBC	complete blood count	Na	sodium
CK	creatine kinase	NaCl	sodium chloride
CMV	cytomegalovirus	NSAID	nonsteroidal anti-inflammatory drug
CNS	central nervous system	OTC	over-the-counter
COPD	chronic obstructive pulmonary disease	PABA	para-aminobenzoic acid
		PCA	patient-controlled analgesia
CSF	cerebrospinal fluid	P.O.	by mouth
CV	cardiovascular	P.R.	by rectum
CVA	cerebrovascular accident	p.r.n.	as needed
D_5W	dextrose 5% in water	PT	prothrombin time
DNA	deoxyribonucleic acid	PTT	partial thromboplastin time
ECG	electrocardiogram	PVC	premature ventricular contraction
EEG	electroencephalogram		
EENT	eyes, ears, nose, throat	q	every
FDA	Food and Drug Administration	q.i.d.	four times daily
		RBC	red blood cell
g	gram	RDA	recommended daily allowance
G	gauge		
GFR	glomerular filtration rate	REM	rapid eye movement
GGT	gamma-glutamyltransferase	RNA	ribonucleic acid
GI	gastrointestinal	RSV	respiratory syncytial virus
gtt	drops	SA	sinoatrial
GU	genitourinary	S.C.	subcutaneous
G6PD	glucose-6-phosphate dehydrogenase	SIADH	syndrome of inappropriate antidiuretic hormone
H_1	histamine$_1$	S.L.	sublingual
H_2	histamine$_2$	T_3	triiodothyronine
HIV	human immunodeficiency virus	T_4	thyroxine
		t.i.d.	three times daily
h.s.	at bedtime	U	units
I.D.	intradermal	USP	United States Pharmacopeia
I.M.	intramuscular	WBC	white blood cell
INR	international normalized ratio		
IPPB	intermittent positive-pressure breathing		
IU	international unit		
I.V.	intravenous		
kg	kilogram		

2

Drug actions, reactions, and interactions

Administration of any drug provokes a series of physicochemical events within the body. The first event, when a drug combines with cellular drug receptors, is known as the drug action. What follows as a result of this action is the drug effect. Depending on the number of different cellular drug receptors affected by a given drug, a drug effect can be local, systemic, or both. Obviously, a local effect follows application to the skin; however, transdermal absorption can produce systemic effects. Moreover, local effects can follow systemic absorption. For example, the antipeptic ulcer drug cimetidine acts solely by blocking histamine receptor cells in the parietal cells of the stomach. This is known as a local drug effect because the drug action is sharply limited to one area and does not spread to other parts of the body. On the other hand, diphenhydramine produces a systemic effect in that it blocks histamine receptors in widespread areas of the body. In other words, local drug effects are specific to a limited number of organ systems, whereas systemic drug effects are generalized and affect different and diverse organ systems.

Drug properties

Drug absorption, distribution, metabolism, and excretion make up a drug pharmacokinetic profile. This branch of pharmacology also describes a drug's onset of action, peak concentration level, duration of action, and bioavailability.

Absorption

Before a drug can act within the body, it must be absorbed into the bloodstream—usually after oral administration, the most commonly used route. Before a drug contained in a tablet or capsule can be absorbed, the dosage form must disintegrate—that is, break into smaller particles. Then these smaller particles can dissolve in gastric juices. Only after dissolving can a drug be absorbed. Most absorption of orally administered drugs occurs in the small intestine, where the mucosal villi provide extensive surface area. Once absorbed and circulated in the bloodstream, it is bioavailable, or ready to produce a drug effect. Whether such absorption is complete or partial depends on several factors: the drug's physicochemical effects, its dosage form, its route of administration, its interactions with other substances in the GI tract, and various patient characteristics. These same factors also determine the speed of absorption. Thus, oral solutions and elixirs, which bypass the need for disintegration and dissolution, are usually absorbed more rapidly. Some tablets have enteric coatings that prevent disintegration in the acidic environment of the stomach; others may have coatings of varying thickness that delay release of the drug.

Drugs administered I.M. must first be absorbed through the muscle into the bloodstream. Rectal suppositories must dissolve to be absorbed through the rectal mucosa. Drugs administered I.V., which are injected directly into the bloodstream, are completely and immediately bioavailable.

Distribution

After absorption, a drug moves from the bloodstream into various fluids and tissues within the body; this is distribution. Individual patient variations can greatly alter the amount of drug that is distributed throughout the body. For example, in an edematous patient, a given dose must be distributed to a larger volume than in a nonedematous patient; the amount of drug must sometimes be increased to account for this. Remember, the dose should be decreased when the edema is corrected. Conversely, in an extremely dehydrated patient, the drug will be distributed to a much smaller volume, so the dose must then be decreased. The total area to which a drug is distributed is known as volume of distribution. Patients who are particularly obese may present another problem when considering drug distribution. Some drugs—such as digoxin, gentamicin, and tobramycin—are not well distributed to fatty tissue. Therefore, dosing based on actual body weight may lead to overdose and serious toxicity. In some cases, dosing must be based on lean body weight, or adjusted body weight, which may be estimated from actuarial tables that give average weight range for height.

Metabolism

Most drugs are metabolized in the liver. Hepatic diseases may affect one or more of the metabolic functions of the liver. Therefore, in patients with hepatic disease, the metabolism of a drug may be increased, decreased, or unchanged. Clearly, all patients with hepatic disease must be monitored closely for drug effect and toxicity.

The rate at which a drug is metabolized varies with the individual. In some patients, drugs are metabolized so quickly that their blood and tissue levels prove therapeutically inadequate. In others, the rate of metabolism is so slow that ordinary doses can produce toxic results.

Excretion

The body eliminates drugs by metabolism (usually hepatic) and excretion (usually renal). Drug excretion refers to the movement of a drug or its metabolites from the tissues back into circulation and from the circulation into the organs of excretion where they are removed from the body. Although most drugs are excreted by the kidneys, some drugs can be eliminated via the lungs, exocrine glands (sweat, salivary, or mammary), liver, skin, and intestinal tract. Drugs may also be removed artificially by direct interventions, such as peritoneal dialysis or hemodialysis.

Other modifying factors

An important factor that influences a drug's action and effect is its *binding to plasma proteins,* especially albumin, and other tissue components. Because only a free, unbound drug can act in the body, such binding greatly influences effectiveness and duration of effect. Protein binding can be influenced by malnutrition, re-

nal failure, and other protein-bound drugs. When protein binding is altered, drug dosing may need to be modified.

The *patient's age* is another important factor. Elderly patients usually have decreased hepatic function, less muscle mass, diminished renal function, and decreased serum albumin. Consequently, they need lower doses and sometimes longer dosage intervals to avoid toxicity. With similar consequences, neonates have underdeveloped metabolic enzyme systems and inadequate renal function. They need highly individualized dosages and careful monitoring.

Underlying disease can also markedly affect drug action and effect. For example, acidosis may cause insulin resistance. Genetic diseases, such as G6PD deficiency and hepatic porphyria, may turn drugs into toxins with serious consequences. Patients with G6PD deficiency may develop hemolytic anemia when given sulfonamides or a number of other drugs. A genetically susceptible patient can develop an acute porphyria attack if given a barbiturate. Also, patients who have highly active hepatic enzyme systems (for example, rapid acetylators), when treated with isoniazid, can develop hepatitis from the rapid intrahepatic buildup of a toxic metabolite.

Drug administration issues

Factors related to the administration of a drug can also influence a drug's action within the body. The dosage form of a drug is important. Some tablets and capsules are too large to be easily swallowed by ill patients. Although an oral solution may be substituted, it produces higher drug blood levels than a tablet because the liquid is more easily and completely absorbed. When a potentially toxic drug (such as digoxin) is given, the increased amount absorbed could cause toxicity. Sometimes a change in dosage form requires a change in dosage itself.

Routes of administration are not therapeutically interchangeable. For example, diazepam is readily absorbed orally but is slowly and erratically absorbed I.M. On the other hand, gentamicin must be given parenterally because oral administration yields inadequate blood levels to treat systemic infections.

Improper storage can alter a drug's potency. Most drugs should be stored in tight containers protected from direct sunlight and extremes in temperature and humidity that can cause them to deteriorate. Some may require special storage conditions, such as refrigeration. Drugs should not be stored in the bathroom because of the constantly changing environment.

The timing of drug administration can be important. Sometimes, giving an oral drug during or shortly after mealtime decreases the amount of drug absorbed. This is not clinically significant with most drugs and may in fact be desirable with irritating drugs, such as aspirin. But penicillins and tetracyclines should not be scheduled for administration at mealtimes because certain foods can inactivate them. If in doubt about the effect of food on a certain drug, check with the pharmacist.

Consider the patient's age, height, and weight. The doctor will need this information when calculating the dosage for many drugs. It should be accurately recorded on the patient's chart. This chart should also include current laboratory data, especially renal and liver function studies, so the doctor can adjust the dosage as needed.

Watch for metabolic changes. Monitor for any physiologic change (depressed respiratory function, acidosis, or alkalosis) that might alter drug effect.

Know the patient's history. Whenever possible, obtain a comprehensive family history from the patient or his family. Ask about past reactions to drugs, possible genetic traits that might alter drug response, and the current use of other drugs. Multiple drug therapy can cause drug interactions that can dramatically change the effects of many drugs.

Drug interactions

When one drug administered in combination with or shortly after another drug alters the effect of one or both drugs, this is known as a drug interaction. Usually, the effect of one drug is increased or decreased. For instance, one drug may inhibit or stimulate the metabolism or excretion of the other, or it may release another from plasma protein-binding sites, freeing it for further action.

Combination therapy is based on drug interaction. One drug, for example, may be given to potentiate another. Probenecid, which blocks the excretion of penicillin, is sometimes given with penicillin to maintain adequate blood levels of penicillin for a longer period. In many cases, two drugs with similar actions are given together precisely because of the additive effect that results. For instance, aspirin and codeine, both analgesics, are commonly given in combination because together they provide greater pain relief than either alone.

Drug interactions are sometimes used to prevent or antagonize certain adverse reactions. Hydrochlorothiazide and spironolactone, both diuretics, are commonly administered in combination because the former is potassium depleting, whereas the latter is potassium sparing.

Not all drug interactions are beneficial. Multiple drugs can interact to produce effects that are undesirable and sometimes hazardous. Harmful drug interactions decrease efficacy or increase toxicity. For example, in a patient taking both diuretics and lithium, the diuretics may cause an increase in serum levels of lithium, resulting in lithium toxicity. Such a drug effect is known as antagonism. Drug combinations that produce these effects should be avoided if possible. Another kind of inhibiting effect occurs when a tetracycline drug is administered with calcium- or magnesium-containing drugs or foods (such as antacids or milk). These bind with tetracycline in the GI tract and cause inadequate absorption of tetracycline.

Adverse reactions

Any drug effect other than what is therapeutically intended can be called an adverse reaction. It may be expected and benign, or unexpected and potentially harmful. Mild, but *predictable,* adverse reactions are sometimes called adverse effects. Drowsiness caused by antihistamines is an example of this. During hay fever season, a patient may have to contend with this drowsiness to get relief from hay fever symptoms. In such a case, the dosage may be adjusted up or down to balance therapeutic effects with adverse effects.

An adverse reaction may be tolerated for a necessary therapeutic effect, or it may be hazardous and unacceptable and require discontinuation of the drug. Some adverse reactions subside with continued use. As an example, the drowsiness associated with paroxetine and the orthostatic hypotension associated with prazosin usually subside after several days, as the patient develops a tolerance to these effects. But many adverse reactions are dosage-related and lessen or disappear only if the dosage is reduced. Although most adverse reactions are not therapeutically desirable, an occasional one can be put to clinical use. An outstanding example of this is the drowsiness associated with diphenhydramine, which makes it clinically useful as a mild hypnotic.

Hypersensitivity, a term sometimes used interchangeably with drug allergy, is the result of an antigen-antibody immune reaction that occurs in the body when a drug is given to a susceptible patient. One of the most dangerous of all drug hypersensitivities is penicillin allergy. In its most severe form, penicillin anaphylaxis can rapidly become fatal.

Rarely, idiosyncratic reactions occur. These are highly unpredictable, individual, and unusual. Probably the best known idiosyncratic drug reaction is the aplastic anemia caused by the antibiotic chloramphenicol. This reaction appears in only 1 out of 40,000 patients, but when it does, it can be fatal. A more common idiosyncratic reaction is extreme sensitivity to very low doses of a drug, or insensitivity to higher-than-normal doses.

To deal with adverse reactions correctly, you need to be alert to even minor changes in the patient's clinical status. Such minor changes may be an early warning of pending toxicity. Listen to the patient's complaints about his reactions to a drug and consider each objectively. You may be able to reduce adverse reactions in several ways. Obviously, dosage reduction can help. But in many cases so does a simple rescheduling of the same dose. For example, pseudoephedrine may produce stimulation that will be no problem if it's given early in the day. Similarly, the drowsiness that occurs with antihistamines or tranquilizers can be totally harmless if the dose is given at bedtime. Most important, your patient needs to be told what adverse reactions to expect, so that he won't become worried or even stop taking the drug on his own. Of course, the patient should report any adverse reactions to the doctor.

Recognizing drug allergies or serious idiosyncratic reactions can sometimes be lifesaving. Ask each patient about drugs he is taking or has taken in the past and what, if any, unusual reactions he experienced from taking them. If a patient claims to be allergic to a drug, ask him to tell you exactly what happens when he takes it. He may be calling a harmless adverse effect such as upset stomach an allergic reaction, or he may have a true tendency toward anaphylaxis. In either case, you and the doctor need to know this. Of course, you must record and report any clinical changes throughout the patient's hospital stay. If you suspect a severe adverse reaction, withhold the drug until you can check with the pharmacist and the doctor.

Toxic reactions

Chronic drug toxicities are generally caused by the cumulative effect and resulting buildup of the drug in the body. These effects may be extensions of the desired therapeutic effect. For example, glyburide will normalize blood sugar when given in usual doses but can produce undesired hypoglycemia if given in larger doses.

Drug toxicities typically occur when drug blood levels rise due to impaired metabolism or excretion. For example, blood levels of theophylline rise when hepatic dysfunction impairs metabolism of the drug. Similarly, digoxin toxicity can follow impaired renal function because digoxin is eliminated from the body almost exclusively by the kidneys (via glomerular filtration). Of course, toxic blood levels also follow excessive dosage.

Tinnitus is usually a sign that the safe dose of aspirin has been exceeded.

Most drug toxicities are predictable and dosage-related; fortunately, most are also readily reversible once the dosage is adjusted. So be sure to monitor patients carefully for physiologic changes that might alter drug effect. Watch especially for impaired hepatic and renal function. Warn the patient about signs of pending toxicity, and tell him what to do if a toxic reaction occurs. Also, be sure to emphasize the importance of taking a drug exactly as prescribed. Warn the patient about serious problems that could arise if he changes the dose or the schedule for taking it.

Drugs and pregnancy

Ever since the thalidomide tragedy of the late 1950s—when thousands of malformed infants were born after their mothers used this mild sedative-hypnotic during pregnancy—use of drugs during pregnancy has been a source of serious medical concern and controversy. To identify drugs that may cause such teratogenic effects, preclinical drug studies always include tests on pregnant laboratory animals. These tests point out gross teratogenicity but do not clearly establish safety. Because different species react to drugs in different ways, animal studies do not rule out possible teratogenic effects in humans. For example, the preliminary studies on thalidomide gave no warning of teratogenic effects, and it was subsequently released for general use in Europe.

What about the placental barrier? Once thought to protect the fetus from drug effects, the placenta isn't much of a barrier at all. Except for drugs with exceptionally large molecular structure, almost every drug administered to a pregnant woman crosses the placenta and enters the fetal circulation. An example of a drug with a large molecular size is heparin, the injectable anticoagulant. Theoretically, then, heparin could be used in a pregnant woman without fear of harming the fetus—but even heparin carries a warning for cautious use in pregnancy. Conversely, just because a drug crosses the placenta

doesn't necessarily mean it's harmful to the fetus.

Actually, only one factor—stage of fetal development—seems clearly related to exaggerated risk during pregnancy. During two stages of pregnancy—the first and the third trimesters—the fetus is especially vulnerable to damage from maternal use of drugs. During these times, *all* drugs should be given with extreme caution.

The most sensitive period for drug-induced fetal malformation is the first trimester, when fetal organs are differentiating (organogenesis). During this time, *all* drugs, except those labeled as category A or B, should be withheld unless doing so would jeopardize the mother's health. Theoretically, during this sensitive time, even aspirin could harm the fetus. So, strongly advise your patient to avoid *all* self-prescribed drugs during early pregnancy. The other time of special fetal sensitivity to drugs is the last trimester. The reason? At birth, when separated from his mother, the neonate must rely on his own metabolism to eliminate any remaining drug. Because his detoxifying systems are not fully developed, any residual drug may take a long time to be metabolized—and thus may induce prolonged toxic reactions. Consequently, drugs should be used only when absolutely necessary during the last 3 months of pregnancy.

Of course, in many circumstances, pregnant women must continue to take certain drugs. For example, a woman with a seizure disorder that is well controlled with an anticonvulsant should continue to take the drug even during pregnancy. Similarly, a pregnant woman with a bacterial infection must receive antibiotics. In such cases, the potential risk to the fetus is outweighed by the mother's need. The relative risk to the fetus is expressed by the drug's pregnancy risk category (see Chapter 1, How to use *Nursing2000 Drug Handbook*).

Following these general guidelines can prevent indiscriminate and potentially harmful use of drugs in pregnancy:
• Before a drug is prescribed for a woman of childbearing age, she should be asked the date of her last menstrual period and

whether she may be pregnant. If a drug is a known teratogen (for example, isotretinoin), some manufacturers may recommend special precautions to ensure that the drug not be given to a female of childbearing age until pregnancy is ruled out and contraceptives are used throughout the course of therapy.

• Especially during the first and the third trimesters, a pregnant patient should avoid *all* drugs except those *essential* to maintain the pregnancy or maternal health.

• Topical drugs are not exempt from the warning against indiscriminate use during pregnancy. Many topically applied drugs can be absorbed in large enough amounts to be harmful to the fetus.

• When a pregnant patient needs *any* drug, the doctor should prescribe the *safest* possible drug in the *lowest* possible dose to minimize any harmful effect to the fetus.

• Every pregnant patient should check with her doctor before taking *any* drug.

Drugs and lactation

Most drugs a mother takes appear in breast milk. Drug levels in breast milk tend to be high when blood levels are high—generally, shortly after taking each dose. Therefore, the mother should be advised to breast-feed *before* taking medication, not *after.*

Nevertheless, with few exceptions, a mother who wishes to breast-feed may continue to do so with her doctor's permission. However, breast-feeding should be temporarily interrupted and replaced with bottle-feeding when the mother must take tetracyclines, chloramphenicol, sulfonamides (during first 2 weeks postpartum), oral anticoagulants, iodine-containing drugs, or antineoplastics.

To protect her infant, a breast-feeding mother should avoid taking drugs indiscriminately. If she needs to take a drug, she should first check with her doctor to be sure of taking the safest drug at the lowest dose.

Patient education

The following general guidelines will help to ensure that the patient gets maximal therapeutic benefits and avoids adverse reactions, accidental overdose, or potentially harmful changes in effectiveness:

• Tell the patient to store drugs in their original containers, at room temperature (unless directed otherwise), in places that are not accessible to children or exposed to sunlight. Avoid storage in the bathroom medicine cabinet, in the kitchen close to heat, or in the glove compartment or trunk of an automobile, where extremes of temperature and humidity will cause them to deteriorate.

• Instruct the patient to learn the trade name and generic name of all drugs he is taking and to inform his regular health care professionals about their use. Before taking a drug, tell him also to report unusual reactions experienced in the past, any allergies to foods and other substances, special medical problems, and medications taken over the last few weeks, including OTC or herbal drugs.

• Inform the patient to always read the label before taking a drug, to take it exactly as prescribed, and never to share prescription drugs.

• Instruct the patient to check the expiration date before taking the drug.

• Warn the patient not to change brands of a drug without medical approval to avoid potentially harmful changes in effectiveness. Certain generic preparations are not equivalent in effect to brand-name preparations of the same drug.

• Caution the patient never to mix different drugs in a single container, remove a drug from its original container, or remove the label. Relying on memory to identify a drug and specific directions for its use is hazardous.

• Instruct the patient to safely discard drugs that are outdated or no longer needed and to keep them away out of reach of children and pets.

• Advise the patient to inform the doctor about use of drugs before undergoing any surgery (including dental surgery).

• Stress the importance of informing the doctor about any adverse reactions experienced during drug therapy.

• Instruct the patient to call the doctor, poison control center, or pharmacist immediately if he or someone else has taken an overdose. Keep their phone numbers handy together with other emergency numbers. Also, have syrup of ipecac available at home to induce vomiting, but only if advised to do so by these professionals.

• Advise the patient to have all prescriptions filled at the same pharmacy so that the pharmacist can identify and warn against potentially harmful drug interactions. Also, tell the patient to inform the pharmacist and doctor of any OTC or herbal drugs being taken.

• Tell the patient to have a sufficient supply of drugs when traveling. He should carry them with him and not stow them in his luggage.

3

Drug therapy in children

Providing drug therapy to children and adolescents is challenging. Physiologic differences, including those in vital organ maturity and body composition, between children and adults can significantly influence a drug's effectiveness.

Physiologic changes affecting drug action

A child's absorption, distribution, metabolism, and excretion processes undergo profound changes that affect drug dosage. To ensure optimal drug effect and minimal toxicity, consider these factors when administering drugs to a child.

Absorption

Drug absorption in children depends on the form of the drug; its physical properties; other drugs or substances, such as food, taken simultaneously; physiologic changes; and concurrent disease.

The pH of neonatal gastric fluid is neutral or slightly acidic and becomes more acidic as the infant matures. This affects drug absorption. For example, nafcillin and penicillin G are better absorbed in an infant than in an adult because of low gastric acidity.

Various infant formulas or milk products may increase gastric pH and impede absorption of acidic drugs. If possible, give a child oral medications on an empty stomach.

Gastric emptying time and transit time through the small intestine—which is longer in children than in adults—can affect absorption. Also, intestinal hypermotility (as in diarrhea) can diminish the drug's absorption.

A child's comparatively thin epidermis allows increased absorption of topical drugs.

Distribution

As with absorption, changes in body weight and physiology during childhood can significantly influence a drug's distribution and effects. In a premature infant, body fluid makes up about 85% of total body weight; in a full-term infant, 55% to 70%; and in an adult, 50% to 55%. Extracellular fluid (mostly blood) constitutes 40% of a neonate's body weight, compared with 20% in an adult. Intracellular fluid remains fairly constant throughout life and has little effect on drug dosage.

Extracellular fluid volume influences a water-soluble drug's concentration and effect because most drugs travel through extracellular fluid to reach their receptors. Children have a larger proportion of fluid to solid body weight, so their distribution area is proportionately greater.

Because the proportion of fat to lean body mass increases with age, the distribution of fat-soluble drugs is more limited in children than adults. As a result, a drug's lipid or water solubility affects the dosage for a child.

Binding to plasma proteins

As the result of a decrease in albumin concentration or intermolecular attraction between drug and plasma protein, many drugs are less bound to plasma proteins in infants than in adults.

Furthermore, preparations that bind plasma proteins may displace endogenous compounds, such as bilirubin or free fatty acids. Conversely, an endogenous compound may displace a weakly bound drug. For example, displacement of bound bilirubin can cause a rise in unbound bilirubin, which can lead to increased risk of kernicterus at normal bilirubin levels.

Because only an unbound, or free, drug has a pharmacologic effect, any alteration in ratio of a protein-bound to an unbound active drug can greatly influence its effect.

Several diseases and disorders, such as nephrotic syndrome and malnutrition, can also decrease plasma protein and increase the concentration of an unbound drug, intensifying the drug's effect or producing toxicity.

Metabolism

A neonate's ability to metabolize a drug depends on the integrity of the hepatic enzyme system, the intrauterine exposure to the drug, and the nature of the drug itself.

Certain metabolic mechanisms are underdeveloped in neonates. Glucuronidation is a metabolic process that renders most drugs more water soluble, thereby facilitating renal excretion. This process is insufficiently developed to permit full pediatric doses until the infant is 1 month old. Because of this, the use of chloramphenicol in a neonate may cause gray baby syndrome, illustrating the infant's inability to metabolize the drug. Use of chloramphenicol in neonates, therefore, requires decreased dosage (25 mg/kg/day) and monitoring of blood levels.

Conversely, intrauterine exposure to drugs may induce precocious development of hepatic enzyme mechanisms, increasing the infant's capacity to metabolize potentially harmful substances.

Older children can metabolize some drugs (theophylline, for example) more rapidly than adults. This ability may come from their increased hepatic metabolic activity. Larger doses than those recommended for adults may be required.

Also, preparations given concurrently to a child may alter hepatic metabolism and induce production of hepatic enzymes. Phenobarbital, for example, can induce hepatic enzyme production and accelerate metabolism of drugs given concurrently.

Excretion

Renal excretion of a drug is the net effect of glomerular filtration, active tubular secretion, and passive tubular reabsorption. Because so many drugs are excreted in the urine, the degree of renal development or presence of renal disease can profoundly affect a child's dosage requirements.

If a child is unable to excrete a drug renally, drug accumulation and possible toxicity may result unless the dosage is reduced.

Physiologically, an infant's kidneys differ from an adult's in that they have a high resistance to blood flow and receive a smaller proportion of cardiac output; exhibit incomplete glomerular and tubular development and short, incomplete loops of Henle (a child's glomerular filtration reaches adult values between 2½ and 5 months; his tubular secretion may reach adult values between 7 and 12 months); have a low glomerular filtration rate (penicillins are eliminated by this route); demonstrate a decreased ability to concentrate urine or reabsorb various filtered compounds; and have a reduced ability of the proximal tubules to secrete organic acids.

Both children and adults have diurnal variations in urine pH that correlate with sleep-awake patterns.

Special administration considerations

Biochemically, a drug displays the same mechanisms of action in all individuals. However, the response of a drug can be affected by a child's age and size as well as the maturity of the target organ. To ensure optimal drug effect and minimal toxicity, consider the following factors when administering drugs to pediatric patients.

Adjusting dosages for children

When calculating children's dosages, don't use formulas that modify adult dosages: A child is not a scaled-down version of an adult. Pediatric dosages should be calculated on the basis of either body weight (mg/kg) or body surface area (mg/m²).

Reevaluate dosages at regular intervals to ensure necessary adjustments as the child develops. Although body surface area provides a useful standard for adults and older children, don't use it in premature or full-term infants. Use the body weight method instead. Don't exceed the maximum adult dosage when calculating amounts per kilogram of body weight (except with certain drugs, such as theophylline, if indicated).

Obtain an accurate maternal drug history—prescription and nonprescription drugs, vitamins, and herbs or other health foods taken during pregnancy. Drugs passed through breast milk can also have adverse effects on the breast-feeding infant. Before a drug is prescribed for a breast-feeding mother, the potential effects on the infant should be investigated.

For example, sulfonamides given to a breast-feeding mother for a urinary tract infection appear in breast milk and may cause kernicterus at lower-than-normal levels of unconjugated bilirubin. Also, high concentrations of isoniazid appear in breast milk. Because this drug is metabolized by the liver, an infant's immature hepatic enzyme mechanisms cannot metabolize the drug, and the infant may suffer CNS toxicity.

Administering oral medications
Consider the following when administering oral medications to a pediatric patient.

If the patient is an infant, administer it in liquid form if possible. For accuracy, measure and give the preparation by oral syringe; never use a vial or cup. Lift the patient's head to prevent aspiration of the medication, and press down on his chin to prevent choking. You may also place the drug in a nipple and allow the infant to suck the contents.

If the patient is a toddler, explain how you're going to give him the medication. If possible, have the parents enlist the child's cooperation. Don't mix medication with food or call it "candy," even if it has a pleasant taste. Let the child drink liquid medication from a calibrated medication cup rather than from a spoon: It's easier and more accurate. If the preparation is available only in tablet form, crush it and mix it with a compatible syrup. (Check with the pharmacist to verify that the tablet can be crushed without compromising its effectiveness.)

If the patient is an older child who can swallow a tablet or capsule by himself, have him place the medication on the back of his tongue and swallow it with water or fruit juice. Remember, milk or milk products may interfere with drug absorption.

Administering I.V. infusions
In infants, use a peripheral vein or a scalp vein in the temporal region for I.V. infusions. The scalp vein is safest in that the needle is not likely to be dislodged; however, the head must be shaved around the site. Temporary disfigurement may also result from the needle and infiltrated fluids. For these reasons, the scalp veins are not used as commonly today as they were in the past.

The extremities are the most accessible insertion sites; however, because patients tend to move about, take these precautions:
● Protect the insertion site to prevent catheter or needle dislodgment.
● Use a padded arm board to minimize dislodgment. Remove the arm board during range-of-motion exercises.
● Place the clamp out of the child's reach; if extension tubing is used to allow the child greater mobility, securely tape the connection.
● Provide a simple explanation to the child who must be restrained while asleep to allay anxiety and maintain trust.

During an I.V. infusion to a child, monitor flow rate and check the child's condition and insertion site at least hourly—more frequently if indicated.

Adjust the flow rate only while the patient is composed; crying and emotional upset can constrict blood vessels. Flow rate may vary if a pump isn't used. Flow should be adequate because some drugs (calcium, for example) can be irritating at low flow rates. Infants, small children, and children with compromised cardiopulmonary status are particularly vulnerable to fluid overload with I.V. medication administration. To prevent this problem and help ensure that a limited amount of fluid is infused in a controlled manner, use a volume-control set (a volume-control device in the I.V. tubing) and an infusion pump or a syringe. Do not place more than 2 hours worth of I.V. fluid at a time in the volume-control set.

Administering I.M. injections
I.M. injections are preferred when the drug cannot be given by other parenteral routes and rapid absorption is necessary.

The vastus lateralis muscle is the preferred injection site in children under 2 years; in older children, either the ventrogluteal area or the gluteus medius muscle can be used. To select the correct needle size, consider the patient's age, muscle mass, and nutritional status and the drug's viscosity; record and rotate injection sites. Explain to the patient that the injection will hurt, but that the medication will help him. Restrain him during the injection, if needed, and comfort him afterward.

Administering topical medications and inhalants

Consider the following when administering topical medications or inhalants.

Use eardrops warmed to room temperature; cold drops can cause considerable pain and possibly vertigo. To administer drops, turn the patient on his side, with the affected ear up. If he is under 3 years, pull the pinna down and back; if he is 3 years or over, pull the pinna up and back.

Avoid using inhalants in young children: obtaining their cooperation is difficult. Before attempting to administer medication through a metered-dose nebulizer to an older child, explain the inhaler to him.

Then have him hold the nebulizer upside down and close his lips around the mouthpiece. Have him exhale, pinch his nostrils shut and, when he starts to inhale, release one dose of medication into his mouth. Tell the patient to continue inhaling until his lungs feel full. Most inhaled agents are not useful if taken orally; therefore, if you doubt the patient's ability to use the inhalant correctly, don't use it.

Use topical corticosteroids with caution because chronic steroid use in children has been associated with delayed growth. When topical corticosteroids are used on the diaper area of infants, avoid covering this area with plastic or rubber pants, which will act as an occlusive dressing and enhance systemic absorption.

Administering parenteral nutrition

Administer I.V. nutrition to patients who can't or won't take adequate food orally and patients with hypermetabolic conditions who need supplementation. The latter group includes premature infants and children who have burns or other major trauma, intractable diarrhea, malabsorption syndromes, GI abnormalities, emo-

tional disorders (such as anorexia nervosa), and congenital abnormalities.

Before fat emulsions are administered to infants and children, however, potential benefits must be weighed against possible risks.

Fats—supplied as 10% or 20% emulsions—are administered both peripherally and centrally. Their use is limited by the child's ability to metabolize them. An infant or a child with a diseased liver cannot efficiently metabolize fats, for example.

Some fats, however, must be supplied both to prevent essential fatty acid deficiency and to permit normal growth and development. A minimum of calories (2% to 4%) must be supplied as linoleic acid—an essential fatty acid found in lipids. In infants, fats are essential for normal neurologic development.

Nevertheless, fat solutions may decrease oxygen perfusion and may adversely affect children with pulmonary disease. This risk can be minimized by supplying only the minimum fat needed for essential fatty acid requirements and not the usual intake of 40% to 50% of the child's total calories.

Fatty acids can also displace bilirubin bound to serum albumin, causing a rise in free, unconjugated bilirubin and an increased risk of kernicterus. However, fat solutions may interfere with some bilirubin assays and cause falsely elevated levels. To avoid this complication, a blood sample should be drawn 4 hours after infusion of the lipid emulsion; or if the emulsion is introduced over 24 hours, the blood sample should be centrifuged before the assay is performed.

Drug therapy in elderly patients

If you're administering drug therapy for elderly patients, you'll want to understand physiologic and pharmacokinetic changes that may alter appropriate drug dosage or cause common adverse reactions or compliance problems in elderly patients.

Physiologic changes affecting drug action

As a person ages, gradual physiologic changes occur. Some of these age-related changes may alter the therapeutic and toxic effects of medications.

Body composition

Proportions of fat, lean tissue, and water in the body change with age. Total body mass and lean body mass tend to decrease; the proportion of body fat tends to increase.

Varying from person to person, these changes in body composition affect the relationship between a drug's concentration and distribution in the body.

For example, a water-soluble drug, such as gentamicin, is not distributed to fat. Because there's relatively less lean tissue in an elderly person, more drug remains in the blood.

GI function

In elderly patients, decreases in gastric acid secretion and GI motility slow the emptying of stomach contents and the movement of intestinal contents through the entire tract. Furthermore, research suggests that elderly patients may have more difficulty absorbing medications. This is a particularly significant problem with drugs having a narrow therapeutic range, such as digoxin, in which any change in absorption can be crucial.

Hepatic function

The liver's ability to metabolize certain drugs decreases with age. This is caused by diminished blood flow to the liver, which results from the age-related decrease in cardiac output and from the diminished activity of certain liver enzymes. When an elderly patient takes certain sleep medications, such as flurazepam, the liver's reduced ability to metabolize the drug may produce a hangover effect the next morning.

Decreased hepatic function may cause more intense drug effects due to higher blood levels, longer-lasting drug effects due to prolonged blood concentrations, and a greater incidence of drug toxicity.

Renal function

Although an elderly person's renal function is usually sufficient to eliminate excess body fluid and waste, the ability to eliminate some medications may be reduced by 50% or more.

Many medications commonly used by elderly patients, such as digoxin, are excreted primarily through the kidneys. If the kidneys' ability to excrete the drug is decreased, high blood concentrations may result. Digoxin toxicity, therefore, is relatively common in elderly patients who are not receiving a reduced digoxin dosage that accommodates decreased renal function.

Drug dosages can be modified to compensate for age-related decreases in renal function. Aided by laboratory tests such as BUN and serum creatinine, doctors may adjust medication dosages so that the patient receives the expected therapeutic benefits without the risk of toxicity. Observe your patient for signs or symptoms of toxicity. A patient taking digoxin, for example, may experience anorexia, nausea, vomiting, or confusion.

Special administration considerations

Aging is usually accompanied by a decline in organ function that can profoundly affect drug distribution and clearance. This physiologic decline is likely to be exacerbated by a disease or chronic disorder. Together, these factors can significantly increase the risk of adverse reactions, drug toxicity, and noncompliance. Be aware of these changes when administering a drug to an elderly patient.

Adverse reactions

Compared with younger people, elderly patients experience twice as many adverse drug reactions relating to greater drug consumption, poor compliance, and physiologic changes.

Signs and symptoms of adverse drug reactions—confusion, weakness, and lethargy—are often mistakenly attributed to senility or disease. If the adverse reaction isn't identified, the patient may continue to receive the drug. Furthermore, he may receive unnecessary additional medication to treat complications caused by the original medication. This can sometimes result in a pattern of inappropriate and excessive medication use.

Although any medication can cause adverse reactions, most of the serious reactions in the elderly are caused by relatively few medications. Be particularly alert for toxicities resulting from diuretics, antihypertensives, digoxin, corticosteroids, sleeping aids, and nonprescription drugs.

Diuretic toxicity

Because total body water content decreases with age, normal dosages of potassium-wasting diuretics, such as hydrochlorothiazide and furosemide, may result in fluid loss and even dehydration in an elderly patient.

These diuretics may deplete serum potassium, causing weakness in the patient, and they may raise blood uric acid and glucose levels, complicating preexisting gout and diabetes mellitus.

Antihypertensive toxicity

Many elderly people experience lightheadedness or fainting when using antihypertensive medications, partly in response to atherosclerosis and decreased elasticity of the blood vessels. Antihypertensive drugs can lower blood pressure too rapidly, resulting in insufficient blood flow to the brain. This may cause dizziness, fainting, or even stroke.

Consequently, dosages of antihypertensive drugs must be carefully individualized. In elderly patients, too-aggressive treatment of high blood pressure may do more harm than good, so treatment goals should be reasonable. Although bringing blood pressure down to 135/90 mm Hg is appropriate, it needs to be done more slowly in elderly patients than in younger patients.

Digoxin toxicity

As the body's renal function and rate of excretion decline, digoxin concentrations in the blood may build to toxic levels, causing nausea, vomiting, diarrhea, and—most serious—cardiac arrhythmias. Try to prevent severe toxicity by monitoring serum levels and by observing your patient for early signs or symptoms, such as appetite loss, confusion, or depression.

Corticosteroid toxicity

Elderly patients on corticosteroids may experience short-term effects, including fluid retention and psychological manifestations ranging from mild euphoria to acute psychotic reactions. Long-term toxic effects, such as osteoporosis, can be especially severe in elderly patients who have been taking prednisone or related steroidal compounds for months or even years. To prevent serious toxicity, carefully monitor patients on long-term regimens. Observe them for subtle changes in appearance, mood, and mobility; signs of impaired healing; and fluid and electrolyte disturbances.

Anticoagulant effects

Elderly patients taking anticoagulants have an increased risk of bleeding, especially when they take NSAIDs at the same time (many do). Observe the INR carefully, and monitor the patient for bruising and other signs of bleeding.

Sleeping aid toxicity

Sedatives or sleeping aids, such as flurazepam, may cause excessive sedation or residual drowsiness. Keep in mind that ingestion of alcohol may exaggerate such depressant effects, even if the sleeping aid was taken the previous evening. These medications should be used sparingly in elderly patients.

OTC drug toxicity

When aspirin, aspirin-containing analgesics, and other OTC NSAIDs (such as ibuprofen, ketoprofen, naproxen) are used in moderation, toxicity is minimal, but prolonged ingestion may cause GI irritation—even ulcers—and gradual blood loss resulting in severe anemia. Prescription NSAIDs may cause similar problems, especially in the elderly. Although anemia from chronic aspirin consumption can affect all age-groups, elderly patients may be less able to compensate because of their already reduced iron stores.

Laxatives may cause diarrhea in elderly patients who are extremely sensitive to such drugs as bisacodyl. Chronic oral use of mineral oil as a lubricating laxative may result in lipid pneumonia from aspiration of small residual oil droplets in the patient's mouth.

Noncompliance

Poor compliance can be a problem with patients of any age. A significant number of hospitalizations are a result of noncompliance to medical regimen. However, in elderly patients, specific factors linked to aging—such as diminished visual acuity, hearing loss, forgetfulness, the common need for multiple drug therapy, and various socioeconomic factors—can combine to make compliance a special problem. Approximately one-third of elderly patients fail to comply with their prescribed drug therapy. They may fail to take prescribed doses or to follow the correct schedule, or they may take medications prescribed for previous disorders, discontinue medications prematurely, or indiscriminately use medications that are to be taken as needed. Elderly patients may also have multiple prescriptions for the same medication and, therefore, inadvertently take an overdose.

Review your patient's medication regimen with him. Make sure he understands the medication amount, the time and frequency of doses, and why he is taking the medication. Also, explain how he should take each medication—that is, with food or water or by itself.

Give your patient whatever help you can to avoid drug therapy problems. Suggest that he use drug calendars, pill "sorters," or other aids to help him comply, and refer him to the doctor or pharmacist if he needs further information.

Drug therapy and the nursing process

The nursing process guides nursing decisions about drug administration to ensure the patient's safety and meet medical and legal standards. This five-step process provides thorough assessment, appropriate nursing diagnosis, effective planning, correct interventions, and constant evaluation.

Assessment

During assessment, the nurse focuses on direct data collection by:
• obtaining a drug history from the patient, parent, spouse, or companion
• reviewing the patient's medical history
• performing a physical examination
• obtaining and interpreting relevant laboratory or diagnostic test results.

Drug history

Data collection begins at admission to the hospital or in an outpatient setting with specific questions about the patient's background, including allergies, medical history, habits, socioeconomic status, lifestyle and beliefs, and sensory deficits. These aspects of the patient's background can significantly influence drug therapy.

Allergies

The patient's allergy profile includes reactions to both drugs and food. Information about allergic reactions must specify the drug; a description of the reaction; its situation, time, and setting; and any contributing factors. Examples of contributing factors include concurrent use of stimulants, tobacco, alcohol, or illegal drugs, or a significant change in nutritional patterns. Asking the patient to describe his allergic reaction is especially important to help determine whether the patient reacts adversely or simply dislikes taking the drug.

Allergies to foods can also affect drug therapy. For example, allergies to shellfish can contraindicate use of drugs that contain iodine or are by-products of shellfish. Allergies to eggs are significant in

patients who are to receive vaccines, which are commonly derived from chick embryos.

Prescription drugs

The patient's drug history should explore the following:
• the reason for using the drug
• the patient's knowledge of the appropriate dosage
• the patient's knowledge about determining effectiveness of the drug (if appropriate), potential adverse effects, what to do about adverse effects, and when to contact the doctor
• route of administration
• the pattern of administration at home
• use of OTC drugs
• cognitive status.

Note any special monitoring the patient must perform, such as blood glucose monitoring before insulin administration or checking radial pulse rate before taking digoxin. Make sure the patient is performing such procedures correctly and that the results are within acceptable limits.

Discuss the effects of drug therapy with the patient and determine if new symptoms or unpredicted adverse reactions have developed. Noting the patient's pattern of administration may provide insight into why a particular drug regimen succeeds or fails.

OTC drugs

A comprehensive drug history should also list any OTC drugs the patient is taking. Many OTC drugs can inhibit or potentiate the effects of a prescribed drug. For example, aspirin potentiates the anticoagulant effects of warfarin.

OTC drugs include a wide range of products, from aspirin, nutritional supplements, herbal or natural products, and homeopathic remedies to various sprays and cleaning agents. The patient may not think of these as drugs, so the nurse may have to name types of products to get an accurate response.

Dosage and frequency of use are just as important as the type of OTC product. One aspirin tablet taken once a day may have no effect on concomitant drug therapy; however, a higher dosage (such as that used for arthritis) could profoundly influence therapy.

Ask open ended questions to allow the patient to provide information that may otherwise be missed.

Medical history

In gathering the medical history, note any chronic diseases or disorders the patient may have and record the following information for each:
- date of diagnosis
- initial prescribed treatment
- current treatment
- the doctor in charge.

Careful attention to this part of the medical history can uncover one of the most important problems with drug therapy—conflicting and incompatible drug regimens. The patient who does not have a family doctor to oversee and coordinate all care may seek the care of several specialists who may prescribe drug treatment without knowing what other drugs the patient is taking. Contacting the patient's pharmacist may be beneficial in obtaining a detailed list of medications. A carefully detailed medical history can uncover such problems. The nurse who identifies such conflicting or overlapping drug regimens must call them to the appropriate doctor's attention and then teach the patient about the importance of informing caregivers about all drugs he is taking.

Habits

Carefully consider dietary habits and the nontherapeutic use of drugs.

Certain foods can directly affect the effectiveness of many drugs. For example, a person who is taking the anticoagulant warfarin should not increase his intake of green leafy vegetables because they contain levels of vitamin K that can antagonize the drug's anticoagulant effect.

Nontherapeutic use of drugs can profoundly affect a patient's health and impair the effectiveness of drug therapy. Consider the possible use of alcohol, tobacco, caffeine, and illegal drugs, such as marijuana, cocaine, and heroin. For example, if the patient uses alcohol, note the frequency of use, the amount, and the type of alcohol consumed. Carefully document the intake of stimulants, such as caffeine, because they significantly affect a patient's CV status and nervous system. Record the type of stimulant, the frequency of intake, and the amount consumed.

For the patient who uses tobacco, document the following information:
- the number of years the patient has used tobacco
- the kind of tobacco the patient smokes (cigarettes, cigar, or pipe) or chews
- how many cigarettes or cigars the patient smokes per day or how much and how long he chews tobacco daily
- the brand of tobacco the patient smokes or chews.

Defining the patient's use of illegal drugs may be difficult. However, the nurse who suspects such use should encourage the patient to discuss it honestly, emphasizing that these drugs have profound effects that may cause serious drug interactions. If the patient admits using illegal drugs, document the drug, the amount and frequency of use, and the route of administration.

Socioeconomic status

Note the patient's age, educational level, occupation, and insurance coverage. These factors may be significant to compliance and to an effective plan of care. The patient's age, for example, can determine whom to include in the care (parents or other family members) and the level of information that is appropriate for teaching the patient.

Knowing the patient's educational background and occupation helps you select interventions at an appropriate level, plan a drug regimen that fits the patient's daily routine, and encourage compliance. Knowing the patient's insurance status may help you anticipate the need for financial assistance and counseling. Remember that noncompliance commonly results from inability to afford medications.

Lifestyle and beliefs

Support systems, marital status, child-bearing status, attitudes toward health and health care, use of the health care system, and daily patterns of activities all affect the plan of care and patient compliance. For example, an 18-year-old single parent who is a high-school dropout on medical assistance and has no family support will probably require more teaching and support to gain a commitment and compliance than a 40-year-old affluent professional who has family support, can understand why she needs the drug, and can readily pay for it.

Sensory deficits

Any sensory deficit can significantly shape an appropriate plan of care. For example, impaired vision, paralysis of one or more extremities, loss of a limb, or loss of sensation in an extremity can impair the patient's ability to administer a subcutaneous injection, break a scored tablet, or open a medication container. Color blindness may cause difficulty in distinguishing between two medications. Hearing impairment can complicate effective patient instruction. Any sensory deficit requires careful consideration in any plan of prescribed drug therapy.

Clinical status

Two other factors can profoundly influence drug therapy: the patient's cognitive status and the systemic effects of the prescribed drugs. A patient's intact cognitive abilities ensure that he can understand and implement the actions necessary for compliance. During the interview, note if the patient is alert and oriented, if he is able to interact appropriately with people, and if his conversation is appropriate. Consider whether the patient can think clearly and express his thoughts coherently. Finally, check both short- and long-term memory because the patient needs both to follow a specified drug regimen. If such evaluation identifies a cognitive deficit, determine the probable cause, which can range from a transient drug-related effect to permanent neurologic impairment, and then determine whether the patient can carry out the prescribed regi-

men. If not, the nurse must find another way to ensure that the patient receives the prescribed therapy.

After completing the drug history, perform a physical examination to assess those body systems that may be affected by a particular drug the patient is taking or that may be prescribed. Every drug has a desired effect on a body system, but it may have an undesired effect on another. For example, chemotherapeutic agents destroy cancerous cells, but they also affect normal cells and typically cause the patient to experience hair loss, diarrhea, or nausea. Therefore, examine the patient for expected drug effects; also, closely monitor the patient for potentially harmful adverse effects.

Nursing diagnosis

Using information gathered during assessment, define any potential or actual drug-related problems by formulating each in a relevant nursing diagnosis. The most common problem statements related to drug therapy are *Knowledge deficit, Noncompliance,* and *Altered health maintenance.*

Planning

Nursing diagnoses provide the framework for planning interventions and outcome criteria (patient goals).

Outcome criteria

Outcome criteria state the desired patient behaviors or responses that should result from nursing care. Such criteria should be measurable and objective, concise, realistic for the patient, and attainable by nursing management. They should also express patient behavior in terms of expectations and specify a time frame. If possible, include the patient when making the plan. Patients are more likely to adhere to regimens if they feel they are an active member of the decision-making team. A typical outcome statement is "Before discharge, the patient verbalizes major adverse effects related to his chemotherapy."

Intervention

After developing the outcome criteria, the nurse determines the interventions needed to help the patient reach the desired behavior or goals. Drug-related interventions may focus on patient teaching for a drug's action, adverse effects, scheduling, steps to avoid or treat a drug reaction, or drug administration techniques.

Appropriate interventions related to drug therapy will also include administration procedures and techniques, legal and ethical concerns, patient teaching, and any concerns related to special groups of patients (geriatric, pediatric, pregnant, or breast-feeding patients). Such interventions may be independent nursing actions, such as turning a bedridden patient every 2 hours, or may be nursing actions that require a doctor's order.

Evaluation

The final component of the nursing process, evaluation, is a formal and systematic process for determining the effectiveness of nursing care. This process enables the nurse to determine whether outcome criteria were met and thereby make informed decisions about subsequent interventions. For example, if the patient experienced relief of headache within 1 hour after the nurse administered an analgesic, as needed, the outcome criterion was met. If the headache was the same or worse, the outcome criterion was not met and requires a new assessment. This may result in a new plan of care, or may yield new data that invalidate the nursing diagnosis or suggest new nursing interventions that are more specific or more acceptable to the patient. This assessment could lead to a higher dosage, a different analgesic, or a reevaluation of the cause.

Evaluation enables the nurse to design and implement a revised plan of care, to continuously reevaluate outcome criteria, and to plan again until each nursing diagnosis is successfully completed.

6

Amebicides and antiprotozoals

atovaquone
chloroquine hydrochloride
(See Chapter 9, ANTIMALARIALS.)
chloroquine phosphate
(See Chapter 9, ANTIMALARIALS.)
metronidazole
metronidazole hydrochloride
pentamidine isethionate

COMBINATION PRODUCTS
None.

---

atovaquone
Mepron, Wellvone§

Pregnancy Risk Category: C

HOW SUPPLIED
Suspension: 750 mg/5 ml

ACTION
Unknown. Appears to interfere with electron transport in protozoal mitochondria, inhibiting enzymes needed for the synthesis of nucleic acids and adenosine triphosphate.

Route	Onset	Peak	Duration
PO	Unknown	1 hr-days	Unknown

INDICATIONS & DOSAGE
Acute, mild to moderate Pneumocystis carinii *pneumonia in patients who cannot tolerate co-trimoxazole*—
Adults: 750 mg P.O. b.i.d. with food for 21 days.

ADVERSE REACTIONS
CNS: *headache, insomnia,* asthenia, anxiety, dizziness.
EENT: *cough,* sinusitis, rhinitis, taste perversion.
GI: *nausea, diarrhea, vomiting,* constipation, *abdominal pain,* anorexia, dyspepsia.
Hematologic: anemia, *neutropenia.*
Hepatic: elevated liver function tests.
Skin: *rash,* pruritus, *diaphoresis.*

Other: *fever, oral* Candida, *pain,* hypoglycemia, hyponatremia, hypotension, sweating.

INTERACTIONS
Drug-drug. *Rifabutin, rifampin:* decreases atovaquone's steady-state concentration. Avoid concurrent use.

EFFECTS ON DIAGNOSTIC TESTS
None reported.

CONTRAINDICATIONS
Contraindicated in patients with hypersensitivity to drug.

NURSING CONSIDERATIONS
• Use cautiously in breast-feeding patients. In animal studies, drug was excreted in breast milk.
• Because drug is highly bound to plasma protein (over 99.9%), also use cautiously with other highly protein-bound drugs.
• Because of risk of other concurrent pulmonary infections, monitor patient closely during therapy.

✅ **Patient teaching**
• Instruct patient to take drug with meals because food enhances absorption significantly.

---

metronidazole
Apo-Metronidazole†, Flagyl,
Flagyl ER, Metizol, Metric-21,
Metrogyl‡, Metrozine‡, Novo-
Nidazol†, Protostat, Trikacide†

metronidazole hydrochloride
Flagyl I.V. RTU, Metro I.V.,
Novo-Nidazol†

Pregnancy Risk Category: B

HOW SUPPLIED
Tablets: 200 mg‡, 250 mg, 375 mg,
400 mg‡, 500 mg
Tablets (extended-release): 750 mg

Reactions may be *common,* uncommon, *life-threatening,* or COMMON AND LIFE-THREATENING.

Oral suspension (benzoyl metronidazole):
200 mg/5 ml‡
Injection: 500 mg/100 ml ready to use
Powder for injection: 500-mg single-dose
vials

ACTION
A direct-acting trichomonacide and amebicide that works at both intestinal and
extraintestinal sites. It is thought to enter
the cells of microorganisms that contain
nitroreductase. Unstable compounds are
then formed that bind to DNA and inhibit
synthesis, causing cell death.

Route	Onset	Peak	Duration
PO	Unknown	2 hr	Unknown
IV	Immediate	1 hr	Unknown

INDICATIONS & DOSAGE
Amoebic hepatic abscess—
Adults: 500 to 750 mg P.O. t.i.d. for 5 to
10 days.
Children: 30 to 50 mg/kg daily (in three
divided doses) for 10 days.
Intestinal amebiasis—
Adults: 750 mg P.O. t.i.d. for 5 to 10 days.
Children: 30 to 50 mg/kg daily (in three
divided doses) for 10 days.
Therapy for adults or children is fol-
lowed with oral iodoquinol.
Trichomoniasis—
Adults: 250 mg P.O. t.i.d. for 7 days or
2 g P.O. in single dose (may give the 2-g
dose in two 1-g doses, each on the same
day); 4 to 6 weeks should elapse between
courses of therapy.
Children: 5 mg/kg dose P.O. t.i.d. for 7
days.
Refractory trichomoniasis—
Adults: 250 mg P.O. b.i.d. for 10 days.
Alternatively, 500 mg P.O. b.i.d. for 7
days.
*Bacterial infections caused by anaerobic
microorganisms—*
Adults: loading dose is 15 mg/kg I.V. infused over 1 hour (approximately 1 g for a
70-kg [154-lb] adult). Maintenance dose
is 7.5 mg/kg I.V. or P.O. q 6 hours (approximately 500 mg for a 70-kg adult). First
maintenance dose should be given 6 hours
after loading dose. Maximum dosage not
to exceed 4 g daily.

*Prevention of postoperative infection in
contaminated or potentially contaminated
colorectal surgery—*
Adults: 15 mg/kg I.V. infused over 30 to
60 minutes and completed about 1 hour
before surgery. Then, 7.5 mg/kg I.V. infused over 30 to 60 minutes at 6 and 12
hours after initial dose.
Bacterial vaginosis—
Adults: 750 mg P.O. daily for 7 days.

ADVERSE REACTIONS
CNS: vertigo, *headache,* ataxia, dizziness, syncope, incoordination, confusion,
irritability, depression, weakness, insomnia, *seizures,* peripheral neuropathy.
CV: ECG change (flattened T wave), edema (with I.V. RTU preparation).
GI: abdominal cramping or pain, stomatitis, epigastric distress, *nausea,* vomiting,
anorexia, diarrhea, constipation, proctitis,
dry mouth.
GU: darkened urine, polyuria, dysuria,
cystitis, decreased libido, dyspareunia,
dryness of vagina and vulva, vaginal candidiasis, *vaginitis,* genital pruritus.
Hematologic: transient leukopenia, *neutropenia.*
Respiratory: upper respiratory infection,
rhinitis, sinusitis, pharyngitis.
Skin: flushing, rash.
Other: overgrowth of nonsusceptible organisms, especially *Candida* (glossitis,
furry tongue); metallic taste; fever;
thrombophlebitis after I.V. infusion; fleet-
ing joint pains, sometimes resembling
serum sickness.

INTERACTIONS
Drug-drug. *Cimetidine:* increased risk of
metronidazole toxicity because of inhibited hepatic metabolism. Monitor closely.
Disulfiram: acute psychoses and confu-
sional states. Do not use within 2 weeks
of last disulfiram dose.
Lithium: increased lithium levels resulting
in possible toxicity. Monitor serum lithium levels closely.
Oral anticoagulants: increased anticoagulant effects. Monitor closely.
Phenobarbital, phenytoin: decreased
metronidazole effectiveness. Total phenytoin clearance may be reduced. Monitor
closely.

Drug-lifestyle. *Alcohol use:* disulfiram-like reaction (nausea, vomiting, headache, cramps, flushing). Do not use together or for 3 days after completion of drug therapy.

EFFECTS ON DIAGNOSTIC TESTS

Metronidazole may interfere with the chemical analyses of aminotransferases and triglycerides, leading to falsely decreased values. It may flatten the T waves on an ECG or interfere with AST, ALT, LD, and glucose levels.

CONTRAINDICATIONS

Contraindicated in patients with hypersensitivity to drug or other nitroimidazole derivatives and during the first trimester of pregnancy.

NURSING CONSIDERATIONS

• Use cautiously in patients with history of blood dyscrasia or CNS disorder and in those with retinal or visual field changes. Use cautiously in patients with hepatic disease or alcoholism and in conjunction with hepatotoxic drugs.

• Monitor liver function tests carefully in elderly patients. If altered, metronidazole levels should be monitored closely to prevent toxicity.

• Know that the drug is contraindicated in the first trimester of pregnancy. However, if indicated during pregnancy for trichomoniasis, be aware that the 7-day regimen is preferred over the 2-g single-dose regimen.

• Give oral form with meals.

• Observe for edema, especially in patients receiving corticosteroids; Flagyl I.V. RTU may cause sodium retention.

• Record number and character of stools when used in the treatment of amebiasis. Metronidazole should be used only after *Trichomonas vaginalis* has been confirmed by wet smear or culture or *Entamoeba histolytica* has been identified. Asymptomatic sexual partners of patients being treated for *T. vaginalis* infection should be treated simultaneously to avoid reinfection.

🔲 I.V. administration

• No preparation is necessary for RTU (ready to use). To prepare lyophilized vials of metronidazole, add 4.4 ml of sterile water for injection, bacteriostatic water for injection, sterile 0.9% NaCl for injection, or bacteriostatic 0.9% NaCl for injection. The reconstituted drug contains 100 mg/ml. Add the contents of vial to 100 ml of D_5W, lactated Ringer's injection, or 0.9% NaCl for a final concentration of 5 mg/ml. The resulting highly acidic solution must be neutralized before administering. Carefully add 5 mEq sodium bicarbonate for each 500 mg metronidazole; carbon dioxide gas will form and may need to be vented.

Alert: Infuse drug over at least 1 hour. Do not give I.V. push.

• Do not refrigerate the neutralized diluted solution because precipitation may occur. If Flagyl I.V. RTU is refrigerated, crystals may form. These disappear after the solution warms to room temperature.

✅ Patient teaching

• Instruct patient to take oral form with food to minimize GI upset, although extended-release tablets should be taken at least 1 hour before or 2 hours after meals.

• Inform patient that sexual partners should be treated simultaneously to avoid reinfection.

• Instruct patient in proper hygiene.

• Tell patient to avoid alcohol or alcohol-containing medications during therapy and for at least 3 days after therapy is completed.

• Tell patient metallic taste and dark or red-brown urine may occur.

---

pentamidine isethionate
NebuPent, Pentacarinat, Pentam 300

Pregnancy Risk Category: C

HOW SUPPLIED

Injection: 300-mg vial
Aerosol: 300-mg vial

ACTION

Exact mechanism unknown, but is thought that drug interferes with biosynthesis of DNA, RNA, phospholipids, and proteins in susceptible organisms.

Route	Onset	Peak	Duration
IV	Unknown	1 hr	Unknown
IM, inhalation	Unknown	0.5 hr	Unknown

INDICATIONS & DOSAGE
Pneumocystis carinii pneumonia—
Adults and children: 3 to 4 mg/kg I.V. or I.M. once daily for 14 to 21 days.
Prevention of P. carinii *pneumonia in high-risk individuals—*
Adults: 300 mg by inhalation (using a Respirgard II nebulizer) once q 4 weeks.

ADVERSE REACTIONS
CNS: confusion, hallucinations, *fatigue, dizziness,* headache.
CV: *hypotension, ventricular tachycardia, chest pain.*
EENT: *burning in throat (with inhaled form), pharyngitis.*
GI: *nausea, metallic taste, decreased appetite, vomiting,* diarrhea, abdominal pain, anorexia, bad taste in mouth, pancreatitis.
GU: *elevated BUN and serum creatinine, acute renal failure.*
Hematologic: *leukopenia, thrombocytopenia,* anemia.
Hepatic: elevated AST and ALT.
Respiratory: *cough, bronchospasm, shortness of breath,* pneumothorax.
Skin: rash, *Stevens-Johnson syndrome.*
Other: *hypoglycemia,* hyperglycemia, hypocalcemia, *congestion, night sweats, chills,* edema, myalgia; *sterile abscess, pain, induration* (at injection site).

INTERACTIONS
Drug-drug. *Aminoglycosides, amphotericin B, capreomycin, cisplatin, colistin, methoxyflurane, polymyxin B, vancomycin:* increased risk of nephrotoxicity.
Antineoplastic agents: additive bone marrow suppression.

EFFECTS ON DIAGNOSTIC TESTS
None reported.

CONTRAINDICATIONS
Contraindicated in patients with a history of an anaphylactic reaction to drug.

NURSING CONSIDERATIONS
• Use cautiously in patients with hyper-

tension, hypotension, hypoglycemia, hypocalcemia, leukopenia, thrombocytopenia, anemia, diabetes, pancreatitis, Stevens-Johnson syndrome, or hepatic or renal dysfunction.
• Administer the aerosol form only by Respirgard II nebulizer. Dosage recommendations are based on the particle size and delivery rate of this device. To administer aerosol, mix the contents of one vial in 6 ml of sterile water for injection. *Do not use* 0.9% NaCl solution. Do not mix with other drugs.
• Do not use low-pressure (less than 20 psi) compressors. The flow rate should be 5 to 7 L/minute from a 40- to 50-psi air or oxygen source.
• For I.M. injection, reconstitute drug with 3 ml of sterile water for a solution containing 100 mg/ml; administer deeply. Expect pain and induration.
• Monitor blood glucose, serum calcium, serum creatinine, and BUN levels daily. After parenteral administration, blood glucose level may decrease initially; hypoglycemia may be severe in 5% to 10% of patients. This may be followed by hyperglycemia and insulin-dependent diabetes mellitus, which may be permanent due to pancreatic cell damage.
• In patients with AIDS, be aware that pentamidine may produce less severe adverse reactions than co-trimoxazole.

I.V. administration
• Reconstitute drug with 3 ml of sterile water for injection. Then dilute in 50 to 250 ml of D_5W. Inject over at least 60 minutes.
Alert: To minimize risk of hypotension when drug is given I.V., infuse drug slowly with patient lying down. Closely monitor blood pressure.

Patient teaching
• Instruct patient to use the aerosol device until the chamber is empty, which may take up to 45 minutes.
• Warn patient that I.M. injection is painful.
• Instruct patient to complete the full course of pentamidine therapy, even if feeling better.

Anthelmintics

mebendazole
pyrantel pamoate
thiabendazole

COMBINATION PRODUCTS
None.

---

mebendazole
Vermox

Pregnancy Risk Category: C

HOW SUPPLIED
Tablets (chewable): 100 mg

ACTION
Selectively and irreversibly inhibits uptake of glucose and other nutrients in susceptible helminths.

Route	Onset	Peak	Duration
PO	Unknown	2-4 hr	Variable

INDICATIONS & DOSAGE
Pinworm—
Adults and children over 2 years:
100 mg P.O. as a single dose; repeated if infection persists 2 to 3 weeks later.
Roundworm, whipworm, hookworm—
Adults and children over 2 years:
100 mg P.O. b.i.d. for 3 days; repeated if infection persists 3 weeks later.

ADVERSE REACTIONS
CNS: *seizures*
GI: occasional, transient abdominal pain and diarrhea in massive infection and expulsion of worms.
Other: fever, urticaria.

INTERACTIONS
Drug-drug. *Carbamazepine, hydantoins:* reduced plasma levels of mebendazole, potentially decreasing its effect. Monitor closely.
Cimetidine: increased plasma concentrations of mebendazole. Monitor closely.

EFFECTS ON DIAGNOSTIC TESTS
None reported.

CONTRAINDICATIONS
Contraindicated in patients with hypersensitivity to drug.

NURSING CONSIDERATIONS
• Be aware that tablets may be chewed, swallowed whole, or crushed and mixed with food.
• Administer drug to all family members, as prescribed, to decrease the risk of spreading the infection.
• Know that no dietary restrictions, laxatives, or enemas are necessary.
• Safe use in children under 2 years has not been established.

☑ **Patient teaching**
• Teach patient about personal hygiene, especially good hand-washing technique. Advise him to refrain from preparing food for others.
• To avoid reinfection, teach patient to wash perianal area daily, to change undergarments and bedclothes daily, and to wash hands and clean fingernails before meals and after bowel movements.

---

pyrantel pamoate
Antiminth, Combantrin†, Pin-Rid, Pin-X, Reese's Pinworm Medicine

Pregnancy Risk Category: C

HOW SUPPLIED
Tablets: 125 mg
Oral suspension: 50 mg/ml
Soft-gel capsules: 180 mg

ACTION
Blocks neuromuscular action, paralyzing the worm and causing its expulsion by normal peristalsis.

Route	Onset	Peak	Duration
PO	Variable	1-3 hr	Variable

Reactions may be *common*, uncommon, *life-threatening*, or COMMON AND LIFE-THREATENING.

INDICATIONS & DOSAGE
Roundworm and pinworm—
Adults and children over 2 years:
11 mg/kg P.O. as a single dose. Maximum dosage is 1 g. For pinworm, dosage should be repeated in 2 weeks.

ADVERSE REACTIONS
CNS: headache, dizziness, drowsiness, insomnia.
GI: anorexia, nausea, vomiting, gastralgia, abdominal cramps, diarrhea, tenesmus.
Hepatic: transient elevation of AST.
Skin: rash.
Other: fever, weakness.

INTERACTIONS
Drug-drug. *Piperazine salts:* possible antagonism. Don't give together.

EFFECTS ON DIAGNOSTIC TESTS
Pyrantel pamoate may cause transient elevations of liver function tests.

CONTRAINDICATIONS
Contraindicated in patients with hypersensitivity to drug.

NURSING CONSIDERATIONS
• Use cautiously in patients with severe malnutrition or anemia or in patients with hepatic dysfunction.
• Be aware that no diet restrictions, laxatives, or enemas are needed.
• Be aware that drug should be given to all family members.

☑**Patient teaching**
• Advise patient that pyrantel may be taken with food, milk, or fruit juices. Shake suspension well.
• Teach patient about personal hygiene, especially good hand-washing technique. To avoid reinfection, teach patient to wash perianal area daily, to change undergarments and bedclothes daily, and to wash hands and clean fingernails before meals and after bowel movements.
• Advise patient to refrain from preparing food for others.
• Advise patient to take entire dose as prescribed.

thiabendazole
Mintezol

Pregnancy Risk Category: C

HOW SUPPLIED
Tablets (chewable): 500 mg
Oral suspension: 500 mg/5 ml

ACTION
Unknown, but drug appears to inhibit the helminth-specific enzyme fumarate reductase.

Route	Onset	Peak	Duration
PO	Unknown	1-2 hr	Unknown

INDICATIONS & DOSAGE
Cutaneous infestations with larva migrans (creeping eruption)—
Adults and children: 25 mg/kg P.O. b.i.d. for 2 to 5 days. Maximum dosage is 3 g daily. If lesions persist 2 days after completion of a 2-day course of therapy, course is repeated.
Roundworm, threadworm, whipworm—
Adults and children: 25 mg/kg P.O. in two doses daily for 2 successive days.
Trichinosis—
Adults and children: 25 mg/kg P.O. in two doses daily for 2 to 4 successive days.

ADVERSE REACTIONS
CNS: impaired mental alertness, impaired coordination, numbness, *seizures, drowsiness, fatigue,* giddiness, *headache,* dizziness.
CV: hypotension.
EENT: tinnitus, blurry vision, dry mouth and eyes, xanthopsia.
GI: *anorexia, nausea, vomiting,* diarrhea, epigastric distress, cholestasis.
GU: hematuria, enuresis, crystalluria, malodorous urine.
Hematologic: *leukopenia.*
Hepatic: jaundice, *parenchymal liver damage.*
Skin: *rash, pruritus, erythema multiforme, Stevens-Johnson syndrome.*
Other: lymphadenopathy, fever, flushing, chills, *angioedema, anaphylaxis.*

INTERACTIONS
Drug-drug. *Theophylline:* may impair hepatic metabolism of theophylline, increasing risk of toxicity. Monitor patient closely.

EFFECTS ON DIAGNOSTIC TESTS
Transient elevations of AST levels have been reported.

CONTRAINDICATIONS
Contraindicated in patients with hypersensitivity to drug.

NURSING CONSIDERATIONS
• Use cautiously in patients with hepatic or renal dysfunction, severe malnutrition, and anemia, and in patients who are vomiting.
• Be aware that drug should be administered to all family members, as prescribed, to prevent risk of spreading infection.
• Be aware that no dietary restrictions, laxatives, or enemas are necessary. However, know that supportive therapy is indicated for anemic, dehydrated, or malnourished patients.

☑ Patient teaching
• Teach patient to take drug after meals. For oral suspension, shake before measuring dose. For tablets, advise patient to chew before swallowing.
• Advise patient to avoid hazardous activities, such as driving, because drug may cause drowsiness.
• Teach patient about personal hygiene, especially good hand-washing technique. To avoid reinfection, teach patient to wash perianal area daily, change undergarments and bedclothes daily, and wash hands and clean fingernails before meals and after bowel movements. Tell him not to prepare food for others during infestation.

---

amphotericin B
amphotericin B cholesteryl
sulfate complex
fluconazole
flucytosine
griseofulvin microsize
griseofulvin ultramicrosize
itraconazole
ketoconazole
miconazole
nystatin
terbinafine hydrochloride

COMBINATION PRODUCTS
None.

---

amphotericin B
Abelcet, AmbiSome, Amphocin,
Amphotec, Amphotericin B for
Injection, Fungilin‡, Fungizone
Intravenous

Pregnancy Risk Category: B

HOW SUPPLIED
Tablets: 100 mg‡
Oral suspension: 100 mg/ml‡
Lozenges: 10 mg‡
Injection: 50-mg lyophilized cake
Suspension for injection: 100 mg/20 ml

ACTION
Acts by binding to sterol in the fungal cell
membrane, altering cell permeability and
allowing leakage of intracellular components.

Route	Onset	Peak	Duration
PO	Unknown	Unknown	Unknown
IV	Immediate	Unknown	Unknown

INDICATIONS & DOSAGE
*Systemic fungal infections (histoplasmo-
sis, coccidioidomycosis, blastomycosis,
cryptococcosis, disseminated candidiasis,
aspergillosis, phycomycosis, zygomyco-
sis), meningitis—*
Adults: initially, a test dose of 1 mg in

20 ml of D_5W infused I.V. over 20 to 30
minutes may be recommended. If tolerated, daily dosage is then initiated as 0.25 to
0.3 mg/kg daily by slow I.V. infusion
(0.1 mg/ml) over 2 to 6 hours. Daily
dosage is gradually increased to maximum 1 mg/kg daily. If drug is discontinued for 1 week or more, drug is resumed
with initial dose and increased gradually.
Infections of the GI tract caused by Candida albicans—
Adults: 100 mg P.O. q.i.d. for 2 weeks.
Oral and perioral candidal infections—
Adults: 1 lozenge q.i.d. for 7 to 14 days.
Lozenge should dissolve slowly.

ADVERSE REACTIONS
CNS: *headache,* peripheral neuropathy,
seizures.
CV: hypotension, *arrhythmias, asystole,*
hypertension, tachycardia.
EENT: hearing loss, tinnitus, transient
vertigo, blurred vision, diplopia.
GI: *anorexia, weight loss, nausea, vomiting, dyspepsia, diarrhea, epigastric pain,
cramping, melena, steatorrhea, hemorrhagic gastroenteritis.*
GU: *abnormal renal function with hypokalemia, azotemia, hyposthenuria, renal tubular acidosis, nephrocalcinosis;
permanent renal impairment,* anuria,
oliguria, increased BUN and serum creatinine (with large doses).
Hematologic: *normochromic anemia,
normocytic anemia, thrombocytopenia,
leukopenia, agranulocytosis,* eosinophilia, leukocytosis.
Hepatic: hepatitis, jaundice, *acute liver
failure,* elevated alkaline phosphatase,
ALT, AST, GGT, LD, and bilirubin levels.
Metabolic: hypokalemia, hypoglycemia,
hyperglycemia, hyperuricemia, hypomagnesemia.
Respiratory: dyspnea, tachypnea, bronchospasm, wheezing.
Skin: maculopapular rash, pruritus (without rash).
Other: arthralgia, tissue damage (with
extravasation), myalgia, *fever, chills,*

---

*Liquid contains alcohol.   **May contain tartrazine.   †Canada   ‡Australia   §U.K.   ◇OTC

malaise, generalized pain, flushing, ***anaphylactoid reactions;*** *phlebitis, thrombophlebitis, pain* (at injection site).

INTERACTIONS
Drug-drug. *Antineoplastic agents (mechlorethamine):* may cause renal toxicity, bronchospasm, and hypotension. Use cautiously.
Cardiac glycosides: increased risk of digitalis toxicity in potassium-depleted patients. Monitor closely.
Corticosteroids: enhanced potassium depletion. Monitor serum potassium levels.
Flucytosine: synergistic effect; may cause increased toxicity of flucytosine. Monitor closely.
Other nephrotoxic drugs (such as antibiotics, pentamidine): may cause additive renal toxicity. Administer these drugs cautiously.
Thiazides: may intensify electrolyte depletion, especially potassium. Monitor for hypokalemia.
Drug-herb. *Gossypol:* enhanced or increased risk of renal toxicity when administered together. Avoid concomitant use.

EFFECTS ON DIAGNOSTIC TESTS
None reported.

CONTRAINDICATIONS
Contraindicated in patients with hypersensitivity to drug.

NURSING CONSIDERATIONS
• Use cautiously in patients with impaired renal function.
Alert: To reduce severe adverse reactions, be aware that the patient may receive premedication with antipyretics, antihistamines, antiemetics, or small doses of corticosteroids; and alternate-day schedule. For severe reactions, discontinue drug and notify doctor.
• Monitor fluid intake and output; report change in urine appearance or volume. Monitor BUN and serum creatinine (or creatinine clearance) at least weekly. Kidney damage is typically reversible if drug is stopped at first sign of dysfunction.
• Obtain liver and renal function studies weekly, if ordered. Drug may be stopped if alkaline phosphatase or bilirubin levels

increase. If BUN exceeds 40 mg/100 ml, or if serum creatinine exceeds 3 mg/100 ml, doctor may reduce or stop drug until renal function improves. Monitor CBC weekly.
• Monitor potassium levels closely, and report signs of hypokalemia. Check calcium and magnesium levels twice weekly, as ordered.

I.V. administration
• Be prepared to give initial test dose as prescribed. Monitor patient's pulse, respiratory rate, temperature, and blood pressure for at least 4 hours.
• Use an infusion pump and in-line filter with mean pore diameter larger than 1 micron. Rapid infusion may cause CV collapse.
• Choose I.V. sites in distal veins. If veins become thrombosed, alternate administration sites.
• Monitor vital signs every 30 minutes; fever, shaking chills, and hypotension may appear 1 to 2 hours after start of I.V. infusion and should subside within 4 hours of stopping drug.
• Give antibiotics separately; do not mix or piggyback them with amphotericin B.
• Know that amphotericin B seems to be compatible with limited amounts of heparin sodium, hydrocortisone sodium succinate, and methylprednisolone sodium succinate.
• Store the dry form at 35.6° to 46.4° F (2° to 8° C). Protect from light. Reconstitute with 10 ml of sterile water only. To avoid precipitation, do not mix with solutions containing sodium chloride, other electrolytes, or bacteriostatic agents (such as benzyl alcohol). Do not use if solution contains precipitate or foreign matter.
• Be aware that reconstituted solution is stable for 1 week under refrigeration or 24 hours at room temperature. It has 8-hour stability in room light.

✓ Patient teaching
• Warn patient of possible discomfort at I.V. site and of other potential adverse reactions. Instruct the patient to report signs and symptoms of hypersensitivity immediately.
• Inform patient that therapy may take

several months. Stress importance of compliance and recommended follow-up.

---

amphotericin B cholesteryl sulfate complex
Amphotec

Pregnancy Risk Category: B

HOW SUPPLIED
Injection: 50 mg/20 ml, 100 mg/50 ml

ACTION
Drug binds to sterols in cell membranes of sensitive fungi, resulting in leakage of intracellular contents and causing cell death due to changes in membrane permeability. The spectrum of activity includes *Aspergillus fumigatus, Candida albicans, Coccidioides immitis,* and *Cryptococcus neoformans.*

Route	Onset	Peak	Duration
IV	Unknown	3 hr	Unknown

INDICATIONS & DOSAGE
Invasive aspergillosis in patients in whom renal impairment or unacceptable toxicity precludes use of amphotericin B deoxycholate in effective doses and in those with invasive aspergillosis in whom prior amphotericin B deoxycholate therapy has failed—
Adults and children: 3 to 4 mg/kg/day I.V. Dilute in D_5W and administer by continuous infusion at 1 mg/kg/hour. Perform a test dose before commencing new courses of treatment; infuse a small amount of drug (10 ml of final preparation containing 1.6 to 8.3 mg of drug) over 15 to 30 minutes and monitor for next 30 minutes. Can shorten infusion time to 2 hours or lengthen infusion time based on patient tolerance.

ADVERSE REACTIONS
CNS: abnormal thinking, anxiety, agitation, confusion, depression, dizziness, hallucinations, headache, hypertonia, neuropathy, nervousness, paresthesia, psychosis, *seizures,* somnolence, speech disorder, stupor.
CV: *arrhythmias, atrial fibrillation,* *bradycardia, cardiac arrest, heart failure, hemorrhage,* hypertension, *hypotension,* phlebitis, postural hypotension, *shock, supraventricular tachycardia,* syncope, *tachycardia,* vasodilation, *ventricular extrasystoles.*
EENT: amblyopia, deafness, epistaxis, eye hemorrhage, pharyngitis, tinnitus.
GI: anorexia, GI disorder, GI hemorrhage, gingivitis, glossitis, hematemesis, melena, mouth ulceration, *nausea,* oral moniliasis, rectal disorder, stomatitis, *vomiting.*
GU: albuminuria, dysuria, glycosuria, *increased creatinine* and BUN, hematuria, oliguria, urinary incontinence or urine retention, *renal failure.*
Hematologic: anemia, coagulation disorders, ecchymosis, hypochromic anemia, leukocytosis, *leukopenia,* petechiae, prothrombin decreased, *thrombocytopenia.*
Hepatic: jaundice, *abnormal liver function test results, hepatic failure.*
Metabolic: acidosis, dehydration, *hypokalemia,* hypocalcemia, hypoglycemia, hypoproteinemia, hyperglycemia, hypervolemia, hypophosphatemia, hyponatremia, hyperkalemia, hyperlipemia, hypernatremia, *hyperbilirubinemia,* hypomagnesemia.
Musculoskeletal: arthralgia, myalgia.
Respiratory: *apnea,* asthma, dyspnea, hemoptysis, hyperventilation, hypoxia, increased cough, lung or respiratory disorders, pleural effusion, *pulmonary edema,* rhinitis, sinusitis.
Skin: acne, pruritus, rash, sweating, skin discoloration, nodule, ulcer, urticaria.
Other: *allergic reaction;* alopecia; *anaphylaxis;* asthenia; *chills;* edema; *fever;* abdominal, chest, neck, or back pain; peripheral or facial edema; infection; mucous membrane disorder; pain or reaction at injection site; *sepsis;* weight gain or loss.

INTERACTIONS
Drug-drug. *Antineoplastic agents:* may enhance renal toxicity, bronchospasm, and hypotension. Use cautiously.
Cardiac glycosides: can enhance potassium excretion and may potentiate digitalis toxicity. Monitor serum potassium closely.
Corticosteroids: enhanced potassium de-

pletion, which could predispose patient to cardiac dysfunction. Monitor electrolytes.

Cyclosporine, tacrolimus: may possibly increase serum creatinine levels. Monitor renal function.

Flucytosine: toxicity may be increased by amphotericin. Use together cautiously.

Imidazoles (clotrimazole, fluconazole, ketoconazole, miconazole): may antagonize effects of amphotericin, although their significance has not been determined. Monitor closely.

Nephrotoxic drugs (such as aminoglycosides, pentamidine): may enhance renal toxicity. Monitor renal function closely.

Skeletal muscle relaxants: amphotericin B–induced hypokalemia may enhance the effects of skeletal muscle relaxants. Monitor serum potassium closely.

EFFECTS ON DIAGNOSTIC TESTS
None reported.

CONTRAINDICATIONS
Contraindicated in patients with hypersensitivity to any component of drug unless the benefits outweigh risks.

NURSING CONSIDERATIONS
• It is unknown if drug is excreted in breast milk. Because of the potential for serious adverse reactions in breast-fed infants, a decision should be made to discontinue breast-feeding or to stop treatment, taking into account the importance of drug to the mother.
• Monitor intake and output; report changes in urine appearance or volume.
• Monitor renal and hepatic function tests, serum electrolytes (especially potassium, magnesium, and calcium), CBC, and PT.

I.V. administration
• Store unopened vials at room temperature. Reconstitute 50-mg vial with rapid addition of 10 ml of sterile water for injection, and 100-mg vial with rapid addition of 20 ml sterile water. Shake vial gently. Do not use diluent other than sterile water for injection. Reconstituted drug is clear or opalescent liquid and is stable for 24 hours refrigerated. Discard partially used vials. Do not administer undiluted drug.

• For infusion, add to bag of D_5W to final concentration of approximately 0.6 mg/ ml. Drug is incompatible with saline, electrolyte solutions, and bacteriostatic agents. Do not filter or use an in-line filter and do not freeze.
• Infuse drug over at least 2 hours. Do not mix with other drugs. If administered through an existing I.V. line, flush line with D_5W before infusion or use a separate line.

Alert: Monitor vital signs every 30 minutes during initial therapy. Acute infusion-related reactions (fever, chills, hypotension, nausea, tachycardia) usually occur 1 to 3 hours after starting I.V. infusion. These reactions are usually more severe after initial doses and usually diminish with subsequent doses. If severe respiratory distress occurs, stop infusion immediately and don't treat further with drug.
• Pretreatment with antihistamines and corticosteroids or reducing the rate of infusion (or both) may reduce the acute infusion-related reactions.

✓ **Patient teaching**
• Instruct patient to immediately report symptoms of hypersensitivity.
• Warn patient of possible discomfort at I.V. site.
• Advise patient of potential adverse effects such as fever, chills, nausea, and vomiting. Tell patient that these can be severe with initial treatment but usually subside with repeated doses.

---

fluconazole
Diflucan

Pregnancy Risk Category: C

HOW SUPPLIED
Tablets: 50 mg, 100 mg, 150 mg, 200 mg
Powder for oral suspension: 10 mg/ml, 40 mg/ml
Injection: 200 mg/100 ml, 400 mg/200 ml

ACTION
Inhibits fungal cytochrome P-450 (responsible for fungal sterol synthesis) and weakens fungal cell walls.

Reactions may be *common*, uncommon, *life-threatening*, or COMMON AND LIFE-THREATENING.

Route	Onset	Peak	Duration
PO	Unknown	1-2 hr	30 hr
IV	Immediate	Immediate	Unknown

INDICATIONS & DOSAGE

Oropharyngeal candidiasis—
Adults: 200 mg P.O. or I.V. on first day, followed by 100 mg once daily. Therapy should last at least 2 weeks.
Children: 6 mg/kg P.O. or I.V. on first day, followed by 3 mg/kg daily for 2 weeks.
Esophageal candidiasis—
Adults: 200 mg P.O. or I.V. on first day, followed by 100 mg once daily. Higher doses (up to 400 mg daily) have been used, depending on patient's condition and tolerance of treatment. Patients should receive drug for at least 3 weeks and for 2 weeks after symptoms resolve.
Children: 6 mg/kg P.O. or I.V. on first day followed by 3 mg/kg daily for at least 3 weeks, 2 weeks after symptoms resolve. Doses up to 12 mg/kg may be used based on clinical judgement.
Vulvovaginal candidiasis—
Adults: 150 mg P.O. for one dose only or 50 mg P.O. daily for 3 days.
Systemic candidiasis—
Adults: 400 mg P.O. or I.V. on first day, followed by 200 mg once daily. Treatment should continue for at least 4 weeks and for 2 weeks after symptoms resolve.
Children: 6 to 12 mg/kg/day P.O. or I.V.
Cryptococcal meningitis—
Adults: 400 mg P.O. or I.V. on first day, followed by 200 mg once daily. Higher doses (up to 400 mg daily) may be used. Treatment should continue for 10 to 12 weeks after CSF cultures are negative.
Children: 12 mg/kg/day P.O. or I.V. on first day, followed by 6 mg/kg daily for 10 to 12 weeks after CSF culture is negative.
Prevention of candidiasis in bone marrow transplant—
Adults: 400 mg P.O. or I.V. once daily. Start prophylaxis several days before anticipated agranulocytosis. Continue therapy for 7 days after neutrophil count rises above 1,000 cells/mm^3.
Suppression of relapse of cryptococcal meningitis in patients with AIDS—
Adults: 200 mg P.O. or I.V. daily.

Children: 3 to 6 mg/kg/day P.O. or I.V.
Adjust-a-dose: In renally impaired patients, if creatinine clearance is 11 to 50 ml/minute, dosage is reduced by 50%. Patients receiving regular hemodialysis treatment should receive the usual dose after each dialysis session.

ADVERSE REACTIONS
CNS: headache, dizziness.
GI: *nausea,* vomiting, abdominal pain, diarrhea, dyspepsia.
Hematologic: *leukopenia, thrombocytopenia.*
Hepatic: *hepatotoxicity* (rare), elevated liver enzymes.
Skin: rash, *Stevens-Johnson syndrome* (rare).
Other: *anaphylaxis,* taste perversion.

INTERACTIONS
Drug-drug. *Cyclosporine, phenytoin, theophylline:* may increase plasma concentrations of these drugs. Monitor serum cyclosporine or phenytoin levels.
Isoniazid, oral sulfonylureas, phenytoin, rifampin, valproic acid: increased incidence of elevated hepatic transaminases. Monitor closely.
Oral antidiabetic agents (glipizide, glyburide, tolbutamide): may increase plasma concentrations of these drugs. Monitor for enhanced hypoglycemic effect.
Rifampin: enhanced metabolism of fluconazole. Monitor for lack of response.
Warfarin: increased risk of bleeding. Monitor PT and INR.
Zidovudine: zidovudine activity may be increased. Monitor closely.
Drug-food. *Caffeine:* may increase caffeine plasma levels. Ofloxacin or lomefloxacin are alternative drugs.

EFFECTS ON DIAGNOSTIC TESTS
None reported.

CONTRAINDICATIONS
Contraindicated in patients with hypersensitivity to drug.

NURSING CONSIDERATIONS
• Use cautiously in patients with hypersensitivity to other antifungal azole com-

---

*Liquid contains alcohol.   **May contain tartrazine.   †Canada   ‡Australia   §U.K.   ◊OTC

pounds; no data exist regarding cross-sensitivity.
• Periodically monitor liver function during prolonged therapy, as ordered.
• If patient develops mild rash, monitor closely. Discontinue drug if lesions progress and notify doctor.
• Be aware that the incidence of adverse reactions appears to be greater in HIV-infected patients.

◖I.V. administration
• Do not remove protective overwrap from I.V. bags until just before use, to ensure product sterility. The plastic container may show some opacity from moisture absorbed during sterilization. This does not affect the drug and diminishes over time.
Alert: Administer by continuous infusion at a rate not to exceed 200 mg/hour. Use an infusion pump. To prevent air embolism, do not connect in series with other infusions. Do not add other drugs to the solution.

☑Patient teaching
• Instruct patient to take drug as directed, even after he feels better.
• Instruct patient to report adverse reactions promptly.

---

flucytosine (5-fluorocytosine, 5-FC)
Ancobon, Ancotil‡

Pregnancy Risk Category: C

HOW SUPPLIED
Capsules: 250 mg, 500 mg

ACTION
Unknown. Appears to penetrate fungal cells and cause defective protein synthesis.

Route	Onset	Peak	Duration
PO	Unknown	1-2 hr	Unknown

INDICATIONS & DOSAGE
Severe fungal infections caused by susceptible strains of Candida *(including septicemia, endocarditis, urinary tract and pulmonary infections) and* Cryptococcus *(meningitis, pulmonary infection, and possible urinary tract infection)—*
Adults and children weighing over 50 kg (110 lb): 50 to 150 mg/kg daily P.O. in four equally divided doses q 6 hours.
Adults and children weighing under 50 kg: 1.5 to 4.5 g/m^2/day P.O. in four divided doses.

ADVERSE REACTIONS
CNS: headache, vertigo, sedation, fatigue, weakness, confusion, hallucinations, psychosis, ataxia, hearing loss, paresthesia, parkinsonism, peripheral neuropathy.
CV: *cardiac arrest.*
GI: nausea, vomiting, diarrhea, abdominal pain, dry mouth, duodenal ulcer, *hemorrhage,* ulcerative colitis, anorexia.
GU: azotemia, elevated creatinine and BUN levels, crystalluria, *renal failure.*
Hematologic: anemia, *leukopenia, bone marrow suppression, thrombocytopenia,* eosinophilia, *agranulocytosis, aplastic anemia.*
Hepatic: elevated liver enzymes, elevated serum alkaline phosphatase, jaundice.
Respiratory: *respiratory arrest,* chest pain, dyspnea.
Skin: occasional rash, pruritus, urticaria, photosensitivity.
Other: hypoglycemia, hypokalemia.

INTERACTIONS
Drug-drug. *Amphotericin B:* synergistic effects and possibly enhanced toxicity when used together. Monitor closely.

EFFECTS ON DIAGNOSTIC TESTS
Flucytosine causes falsely elevated creatinine values on iminohydrolase enzymatic assay.

CONTRAINDICATIONS
Contraindicated in patients with hypersensitivity to drug.

NURSING CONSIDERATIONS
• Use with extreme caution in patients with impaired hepatic or renal function or bone marrow suppression.

• Administer capsules over 15 minutes to reduce adverse GI reactions.
• Monitor blood, liver, and renal function studies frequently during therapy; obtain susceptibility tests weekly, as ordered, to monitor drug resistance.
• If possible, regularly perform blood level assays of drug, as ordered, to maintain flucytosine at therapeutic level (25 to 120 mcg/ml). Higher blood levels may be toxic.
• Monitor fluid intake and output; report any marked change.

☑ **Patient teaching**
• Inform patient that therapeutic response may take weeks or months.
• Instruct patient to report adverse reactions promptly.

---

griseofulvin microsize
Fulcin‡, Fulvicin-U/F, Grifulvin V, Grisactin, Grisovin‡, Grisovin 500‡, Grisovin FP†

griseofulvin ultramicrosize
Fulvicin P/G, Grisactin Ultra, Griseostatin‡, Gris-PEG

Pregnancy Risk Category: C

HOW SUPPLIED
griseofulvin microsize
Tablets: 250 mg, 500 mg
Capsules: 125 mg, 250 mg
Oral suspension: 125 mg/5 ml
griseofulvin ultramicrosize
Tablets: 125 mg, 165 mg, 250 mg, 330 mg

ACTION
Arrests fungal cell activity by disrupting its mitotic spindle structure.

Route	Onset	Peak	Duration
PO	Unknown	4-8 hr	Unknown

INDICATIONS & DOSAGE
Ringworm infections of skin, hair, nails (tinea corporis, tinea capitis, tinea cruris) when caused by Trichophyton, Microsporum, *or* Epidermophyton—
Adults: 500 mg of microsize P.O. daily in

single or divided doses. Severe infections may require up to 1 g daily. Alternatively, 330 to 375 mg ultramicrosize P.O. daily in single or divided doses. Duration of therapy dependent upon place of infection, 2 to 8 weeks.
Tinea pedis and tinea unguium—
Adults: 0.75 to 1 g of microsize P.O. daily. Alternatively, 660 to 750 mg of ultramicrosize P.O. daily in divided doses. Duration of therapy is 4 weeks to 1 year.
Children: 11 mg/kg/day of microsize P.O. Alternatively, 7.3 mg/kg/day of ultramicrosize P.O.

ADVERSE REACTIONS
CNS: headache (in early stages of treatment), transient decrease in hearing, fatigue (with large doses), occasional mental confusion, impaired performance of routine activities, psychotic symptoms, dizziness, insomnia, paresthesia of hands and feet (after extended therapy).
GI: nausea, vomiting, flatulence, diarrhea, epigastric distress, *bleeding.*
GU: proteinuria.
Hematologic: leukopenia, *agranulocytosis* (requires discontinuation of drug), porphyria.
Hepatic: *hepatic toxicity.*
Skin: *rash, urticaria,* photosensitivity, angioedema.
Other: oral thrush, hypersensitivity reactions (rash), menstrual irregularities, lupus erythematosus.

INTERACTIONS
Drug-drug. *Coumarin anticoagulants:* decreased effectiveness. Monitor PT and INR when used concurrently.
Cyclosporine: decreased serum cyclosporine levels. Monitor closely.
Oral contraceptives: decreased effectiveness. Suggest alternative methods of contraception.
Phenobarbital: decreased griseofulvin blood levels due to decreased absorption or increased metabolism. Avoid using together or administer griseofulvin t.i.d.
Drug-food. *High-fat meals:* increased absorption. Administer together.
Drug-lifestyle. *Alcohol use:* may cause tachycardia, diaphoresis, and flushing. Avoid alcohol consumption.

EFFECTS ON DIAGNOSTIC TESTS
None reported.

CONTRAINDICATIONS
Contraindicated in patients with hypersensitivity to drug and in those with porphyria or hepatocellular failure. Also contraindicated in pregnant patients or women who intend to become pregnant during therapy.

NURSING CONSIDERATIONS
• Use cautiously in penicillin-sensitive patients.
Alert: Because of potential toxicity, know that drug is used only when topical treatment fails.
• Obtain laboratory tests as ordered to confirm diagnosis. Continue drug until clinical and laboratory examinations confirm eradication.
• Be aware that because griseofulvin ultramicrosize is dispersed in polyethylene glycol, it is absorbed more rapidly and completely than microsize preparations and is effective at one-half to two-thirds the usual griseofulvin dose.
• Administer after a high-fat meal to enhance absorption and minimize GI distress.
• Assess hematologic, renal, and hepatic function periodically during prolonged therapy, as ordered.
• Keep in mind that effective treatment of tinea pedis may require concomitant use of a topical agent.
• Safety in children under 2 years has not been established.

✅ **Patient teaching**
• Tell patient to take drug after a high-fat meal.
• Advise patient that prolonged treatment may be needed to control infection and prevent relapse, even if symptoms abate in first few days of therapy.
• Tell patient to keep skin clean and dry and to maintain good hygiene.
• Instruct patient to avoid intense sunlight.

itraconazole
Sporanox

Pregnancy Risk Category: C

HOW SUPPLIED
Capsules: 100 mg
Oral solution: 10 mg/ml

ACTION
Interferes with fungal cell-wall synthesis by inhibiting the formation of ergosterol and increasing cell-wall permeability that makes the fungus susceptible to osmotic instability.

Route	Onset	Peak	Duration
PO	Unknown	3-4 hr	Unknown

INDICATIONS & DOSAGE
Pulmonary and extrapulmonary blastomycosis; nonmeningeal histoplasmosis—
Adults: 200 mg P.O. daily. Dosage increased as needed and tolerated in 100-mg increments to a maximum of 400 mg daily. Dosages that exceed 200 mg daily should be given in two divided doses. Treatment should continue for a minimum of 3 months. In life-threatening illness, a loading dose of 200 mg t.i.d. is given for 3 days.
Aspergillosis—
Adults: 200 to 400 mg P.O. daily.
Onychomycosis (fungal nail disease) from dermatophytes of the toenail—
Adults: 200 mg P.O. once daily for 12 consecutive weeks.
Onychomycosis of the fingernail—
Adults: initially, 200 mg P.O. b.i.d. for 1 week; after 3 weeks, dosage is repeated.
Oropharyngeal candidiasis—
Adults: 200 mg swished in mouth vigorously and swallowed daily, for 1 to 2 weeks.
Oropharyngeal candidiasis in patients unresponsive to fluconazole tablets—
Adults: 100 mg swished in mouth vigorously and swallowed, b.i.d. for 2 to 4 weeks.
Esophageal candidiasis—
Adults: 100 to 200 mg swished in mouth vigorously and swallowed, daily for a minimum treatment of 3 weeks. Treat-

ment should continue for 2 weeks after symptoms resolve.

ADVERSE REACTIONS
CNS: headache, dizziness, somnolence.
CV: hypertension.
GI: *nausea,* vomiting, diarrhea, abdominal pain, anorexia.
GU: albuminuria.
Hepatic: impaired hepatic function.
Skin: rash, pruritus.
Other: edema, fatigue, fever, malaise, decreased libido, hypokalemia, impotence.

INTERACTIONS
Drug-drug. *Antacids, H_2-receptor antagonists, phenytoin, rifampin:* possible lowered itraconazole plasma levels. Avoid concomitant use.
Astemizole, cisapride: inhibited metabolism of these drugs, resulting in elevated blood levels and risk of serious cardiac toxicity. Never administer together.
Cyclosporine, digoxin, tacrolimus: possible increased plasma levels of these drugs. Monitor plasma levels closely.
Isoniazid: may decrease plasma levels of itraconazole. Monitor closely.
Oral anticoagulants: possible enhanced anticoagulant effects. Monitor PT and INR closely.
Oral antidiabetic agents: similar antifungals have caused hypoglycemia. Monitor blood glucose levels closely.

EFFECTS ON DIAGNOSTIC TESTS
None reported.

CONTRAINDICATIONS
Contraindicated in patients with hypersensitivity to drug; in those receiving astemizole, cisapride, triazolam, and midazolam (orally); and in breast-feeding patients because drug is excreted in breast milk.

NURSING CONSIDERATIONS
• Use cautiously in patients with hypochlorhydria; they may not absorb drug readily. Because hypochlorhydria can accompany HIV infection, use cautiously in HIV-infected patients.
• Use cautiously in patients receiving other highly bound medications because drug

and its metabolites are more than 99% bound to plasma proteins.
• Perform baseline liver function tests, as ordered, and monitor periodically.

☑**Patient teaching**
• Teach patient to recognize and report signs and symptoms of liver disease (anorexia, dark urine, pale stools, unusual fatigue, or jaundice).
• Tell patient to take drug with food to ensure maximal absorption.
• Instruct patient not to use interchangeably with itraconazole capsules.
• Tell patient that oral solution should be used 10 ml at a time.
• Advise patient to take solution without food.
• Inform patient to report all medications to doctor to avoid potential drug interactions.

ketoconazole
Nizoral

Pregnancy Risk Category: C

HOW SUPPLIED
Tablets: 200 mg
Oral suspension: 100 mg/5 ml†

ACTION
Inhibits purine transport and DNA, RNA, and protein synthesis; increases cell-wall permeability, making the fungus more susceptible to osmotic pressure.

Route	Onset	Peak	Duration
PO	Unknown	1-2 hr	Unknown

INDICATIONS & DOSAGE
Systemic candidiasis, chronic mucocandidiasis, oral thrush, candiduria, coccidioidomycosis, blastomycosis, histoplasmosis, chromomycosis, and paracoccidioidomycosis; severe cutaneous dermatophyte infections resistant to therapy with topical or oral griseofulvin—
Adults and children weighing over 40 kg (88 lb): initially, 200 mg P.O. daily in a single dose. Dosage may be increased to 400 mg once daily in patients who don't respond to lower dosage.

Children 2 years and over: 3.3 to 6.6 mg/kg P.O. daily as a single dose.

ADVERSE REACTIONS
CNS: headache, nervousness, dizziness, somnolence, photophobia, *suicidal tendencies,* severe depression.
GI: *nausea, vomiting,* abdominal pain, diarrhea.
Hematologic: *thrombocytopenia,* hemolytic anemia, leukopenia.
Hepatic: elevated liver enzymes or *fatal hepatotoxicity.*
Skin: pruritus.
Other: gynecomastia with tenderness, fever, chills, impotence, hyperlipidemia.

INTERACTIONS
Drug-drug. *Antacids, anticholinergics, H_2 blockers:* decreased absorption of ketoconazole. Wait at least 2 hours after ketoconazole dose before administering these drugs.
Anticoagulants: effects may be enhanced. Monitor INR, PT, and PTT and adjust as needed.
Astemizole: may increase plasma levels of these drugs, precipitating CV events. Avoid concomitant use.
Cisapride: may cause ventricular arrhythmias. Avoid concomitant use.
Cyclosporine: may increase cyclosporine plasma levels. Monitor serum levels.
Isoniazid, rifampin: increased ketoconazole metabolism. Monitor for decreased antifungal effect.
Paclitaxel: metabolism inhibited. Use together cautiously.
Theophylline: may decrease theophylline plasma levels. Monitor serum levels.
Drug-herb. *Yew:* inhibits ketoconazole metabolism. Avoid concomitant use.

EFFECTS ON DIAGNOSTIC TESTS
Ketoconazole has been reported to cause transient elevations of AST, ALT, and alkaline phosphatase levels. It has also been reported to cause transient alterations of serum cholesterol and triglyceride levels.

CONTRAINDICATIONS
Contraindicated in patients with hypersensitivity to drug and in those taking astemizole.

NURSING CONSIDERATIONS
• Use cautiously in patients with hepatic disease and in those who are taking other hepatotoxic drugs.
• Because of the potential for serious hepatotoxicity, be aware that ketoconazole should not be used for less serious conditions, such as fungus infections of the skin or nails.
• Monitor for elevated liver enzymes and nausea that does not subside as well as for unusual fatigue, jaundice, dark urine, or pale stool—all signs or symptoms of possible hepatotoxicity.
• Keep in mind that much larger doses (up to 800 mg/day) can be used to treat fungal meningitis and intracerebral fungal lesions.

☑ Patient teaching
• Instruct patient with achlorhydria to dissolve each tablet in 4 ml aqueous solution of 0.2 N hydrochloric acid, sip mixture through a glass or plastic straw (to avoid contact with teeth), and end procedure by drinking a glass of water because ketoconazole requires gastric acidity for dissolution and absorption.
• Make sure patient understands that treatment should be continued until all tests indicate that active fungal infection has subsided. If drug is discontinued too soon, infection will recur. Minimum treatment for candidiasis is 7 to 14 days; for other systemic fungal infections, 6 months; for resistant dermatophyte infections, at least 4 weeks.
• Reassure patient that nausea, common early in therapy, will subside. To minimize, divide daily dosage into two doses or take it with meals.

---

miconazole
Monistat i.v.

Pregnancy Risk Category: C

HOW SUPPLIED
Injection: 10 mg/ml

ACTION
Inhibits purine transport and DNA, RNA, and protein synthesis; increases cell-wall

permeability, making fungus more susceptible to osmotic pressure.

Route	Onset	Peak	Duration
IV	Immediate	Immediate	Unknown
Intrathecal	Unknown	Unknown	Unknown

INDICATIONS & DOSAGE

Systemic fungal infections (coccidioidomycosis, candidiasis, cryptococcosis, paracoccidioidomycosis), chronic mucocutaneous candidiasis—
Adults: 200 to 3,600 mg/day I.V. Dosages may vary with diagnosis and with infective agent. Daily dosage may be divided over 3 infusions, 200 to 1,200 mg per infusion. Dilute in at least 200 ml of 0.9% NaCl. Repeated courses may be needed because of relapse or reinfection.
Children 1 year and over: 20 to 40 mg/kg/day I.V. Do not exceed 15 mg/kg per infusion.
Children less than 1 year: 15 to 30 mg/kg/day I.V. Do not exceed 15 mg/kg per infusion.
Fungal meningitis—
Adults: 20 mg intrathecally as adjunct to I.V. administration q 1 to 2 days if S.C. ventricular reservoir is used or q 3 to 7 days if reservoir is not used.

ADVERSE REACTIONS

CNS: dizziness, drowsiness.
GI: *nausea,* vomiting, diarrhea.
Hematologic: transient decrease in hematocrit, *thrombocytopenia.*
Skin: *pruritic rash.*
Other: *anaphylactoid reactions,* fever, chills, transient decrease in serum sodium, *phlebitis at injection site.*

INTERACTIONS

Drug-drug. *Astemizole, cisapride:* may cause serious CV effects. Never administer together.
Oral anticoagulants: enhanced anticoagulant effect. Monitor closely.

EFFECTS ON DIAGNOSTIC TESTS

Miconazole may cause a transient decrease in hematocrit and an increase or decrease in platelet counts. It frequently causes erythrocyte aggregation. Miconazole also may cause hyponatremia, hyper-

lipidemia, and hypertriglyceridemia; abnormalities in lipoprotein and immunoelectrophoretic patterns are from the polyoxyl 35 castor oil vehicle.

CONTRAINDICATIONS

Contraindicated in patients with hypersensitivity to drug and in those taking astemizole or cisapride.

NURSING CONSIDERATIONS

• Use cautiously because drug is dissolved in a vehicle containing polyoxyl 35 castor oil, a substance known to cause anaphylactoid reactions. Give the first dose under continuous medical supervision with emergency resuscitative equipment immediately available. Subsequent doses may be administered on an outpatient basis in selected patients.
• To lessen adverse GI reactions, do not administer with meals.
• Know that premedication with antiemetic may lessen nausea and vomiting.
• For intrathecal use, administer drug undiluted using an S.C. intrathecal (Ommaya) reservoir. Alternatively, drug may be given by lumbar or cisternal puncture.
• Monitor levels of hemoglobin, hematocrit, electrolytes, and lipids regularly. Transient elevations in serum cholesterol and triglycerides may be caused by castor oil vehicle.
• In treatment of fungal meningitis and urinary bladder infections, assist with supplemental intrathecal administration and bladder irrigation, respectively.

I.V. administration

• Be aware that I.V. miconazole has been replaced largely by newer drugs that are better tolerated.
• Dilute infusion with at least 200 ml of 0.9% NaCl solution and infuse over 30 to 60 minutes.
Alert: Rapid I.V. injection of undiluted miconazole may produce arrhythmias.

Patient teaching

• Inform patient that pruritic rash, which may be controlled with diphenhydramine, may persist for weeks after drug is discontinued.
• Inform patient that adequate therapeutic

---

response may take weeks or months. Stress importance of compliance with drug therapy and follow-up.
• Instruct patient to report adverse reactions promptly.
• Advise patient to avoid performing hazardous activities if drowsiness or dizziness occurs.

nystatin
Mycostatin*, Nadostine†, Nilstat, Nystat-Rx, Nystex*

Pregnancy Risk Category: NR

HOW SUPPLIED
Tablets: 500,000 units
Oral suspension: 100,000 units/ml; 50, 150, or 500 million units; 1 or 2 billion units
Powder: 150, 250, or 500 million units; 1, 2, or 5 billion units
Troches: 200,000 units
Vaginal suppositories: 100,000 units

ACTION
Unknown. Probably acts by binding to sterols in fungal cell membrane, altering cell permeability and allowing leakage of intracellular components.

Route	Onset	Peak	Duration
PO, topical	Unknown	Unknown	Unknown

INDICATIONS & DOSAGE
GI infections—
Adults: 500,000 to 1 million units as oral tablets t.i.d.
Oral, vaginal, and intestinal infections caused by Candida albicans *(Monilia) and other* Candida *species—*
Adults: 400,000 to 600,000 units oral suspension q.i.d. for oral candidiasis.
Children and infants over 3 months: 250,000 to 500,000 units oral suspension q.i.d.
Neonates and premature infants: 100,000 units oral suspension q.i.d.
Vaginal infections—
Adults: 100,000 units, as vaginal tablets, inserted high into vagina, daily or b.i.d. for 14 days.

ADVERSE REACTIONS
GI: transient nausea, vomiting, diarrhea (usually with large oral dosage).

INTERACTIONS
None significant.

EFFECTS ON DIAGNOSTIC TESTS
None reported.

CONTRAINDICATIONS
Contraindicated in patients with hypersensitivity to drug.

NURSING CONSIDERATIONS
• Keep in mind that nystatin is not effective against systemic infections.
• Know that vaginal tablets can be used by pregnant patients up to 6 weeks before term to treat maternal infection that may cause thrush in neonates.
• For treatment of oral candidiasis (thrush): After the mouth is clean of food debris, have the patient hold suspension in mouth for several minutes before swallowing. When treating infants, swab medication on oral mucosa. Immunosuppressed patients are sometimes instructed by the doctor to suck on vaginal tablets (100,000 units) because this provides prolonged contact with oral mucosa.

☑ **Patient teaching**
• Advise patient to continue medication for at least 2 days after symptoms disappear. Consult doctor for exact length of therapy.
• Instruct patient to continue therapy during menstruation.
• Explain that predisposing factors of vaginal infection include use of antibiotics, oral contraceptives, and corticosteroids; diabetes; reinfection by sexual partner; and tight-fitting pantyhose. Encourage the patient to use cotton (not synthetic) underpants.
• Instruct patient in careful hygiene for affected areas, including cleaning perineal area from front to back after defecation.
• Advise patient to report redness, swelling, or irritation.
• Tell patient that overusing mouthwash or wearing poorly fitting dentures, especially in older patients, may promote infection.

Reactions may be *common*, uncommon, *life-threatening*, or COMMON AND LIFE-THREATENING.

terbinafine hydrochloride
Lamisil

Pregnancy Risk Category: B

HOW SUPPLIED
Tablets: 250 mg

ACTION
An antifungal agent that exerts its action by inhibiting squalene epoxidase, a key enzyme in sterol biosynthesis of fungi. This enzyme inhibition results in a deficiency of ergosterol and a corresponding accumulation of sterol within the fungal cell.

Route	Onset	Peak	Duration
PO	Unknown	2 hr	Unknown

INDICATIONS & DOSAGE
Treatment of fingernail onychomycosis due to dermatophytes (tinea unguium)—
Adults: 250 mg P.O. once daily for 6 weeks.
Treatment of toenail onychomycosis due to dermatophytes (tinea unguium)—
Adults: 250 mg P.O. once daily for 12 weeks.

ADVERSE REACTIONS
CNS: *headache.*
GI: diarrhea, dyspepsia, abdominal pain, nausea, flatulence.
Hepatic: hepatobiliary dysfunction (including cholestatic jaundice).
Hematologic: *neutropenia,* decrease in absolute lymphocyte counts.
Skin: rash, pruritus, urticaria, ***Stevens-Johnson syndrome, toxic epidermal necrolysis.***
Other: taste disturbances, visual disturbances, *hypersensitivity reactions, anaphylaxis.*

INTERACTIONS
Drug-drug. *Cimetidine:* decreases drug clearance by one-third. Avoid concomitant use.
Cyclosporine: drug increases clearance of cyclosporine. Monitor serum levels.
Rifampin: increases terbinafine clearance by 100%. Monitor patient.

Drug-food. *Caffeine:* I.V. caffeine clearance is decreased. Use cautiously together.

EFFECTS ON DIAGNOSTIC TESTS
None reported.

CONTRAINDICATIONS
Contraindicated in patients with hypersensitivity to drug.

NURSING CONSIDERATIONS
• Drug is not recommended in patients with preexisting liver disease or renal impairment (creatinine clearance below 50 ml/minute), during pregnancy, and in breast-feeding patients.
• Safety in children has not been established.

☑ Patient teaching
• Inform patient that successful treatment of nail infections may not be observed for 10 weeks for toenail infections and 4 weeks for fingernail infections.

9
Antimalarials

chloroquine hydrochloride
chloroquine phosphate
doxycycline
   (See Chapter 14, TETRACYCLINES.)
hydroxychloroquine sulfate
mefloquine hydrochloride
primaquine phosphate
pyrimethamine
pyrimethamine with sulfadoxine

COMBINATION PRODUCTS
None.

---

chloroquine hydrochloride
Aralen HCl, Chlorquin‡

chloroquine phosphate
Aralen Phosphate, Avloclor§,
Chlorquin‡

Pregnancy Risk Category: C

HOW SUPPLIED
chloroquine hydrochloride
Injection: 50 mg/ml (40-mg/ml base)
chloroquine phosphate
Tablets: 250 mg (150-mg base), 500 mg
(300-mg base)
Injection: 5 mg (200 mg base)

ACTION
Unknown. As an antimalarial, chloroquine may bind to and alter the properties
of DNA in susceptible parasites.

Route	Peak	Onset	Duration
PO	Unknown	1-3 hr	Unknown
IM	Unknown	0.5 hr	Unknown

INDICATIONS & DOSAGE
Acute malarial attacks caused by Plasmodium vivax, P. malariae, P. ovale, *and
susceptible strains of* P. falciparum—
Adults: initially, 600 mg (base) P.O., then
300 mg at 6, 24, and 48 hours. Or 160 to
200 mg (base) I.M. initially; repeated in 6
hours p.r.n. Switch patient to oral therapy
as soon as possible.

Children: initially, 10 mg (base)/kg P.O.,
then 5 mg (base)/kg at 6, 24, and 48 hours
(do not exceed adult dose). Or 5 mg
(base)/kg I.M. initially; repeated in 6
hours p.r.n. Do not exceed 10 mg (base)/
kg/24 hours. Switch patient to oral therapy as soon as possible.
Malaria prophylaxis—
Adults and children: 5 mg (base)/kg P.O.
(not to exceed 300 mg) weekly on the
same day (begun 2 weeks before probable
exposure and continued for 4 to 6 weeks
after leaving endemic area). If treatment
begins after exposure, the initial dose is
doubled (10 mg/kg) in two divided doses
P.O. 6 hours apart.
Extraintestinal amebiasis—
Adults: 1 g (600 mg base) chloroquine
phosphate P.O. daily for 2 days; then
500 mg (300 mg base) daily for 2 to 3
weeks. Treatment is usually combined
with an intestinal amebicide. When oral
therapy is unfeasible, administer 4 to 5 ml
chloroquine hydrochloride (200 to
250 mg; 160 to 200 mg base) I.M. daily
for 10 to 12 days. Resume oral therapy as
soon as possible.
Children: 16.7 mg/kg chloroquine phosphate (10 mg/kg base) P.O. once daily for
2 to 3 weeks. Maximum dosage is 500 mg
chloroquine phosphate (300 mg base)
daily.

ADVERSE REACTIONS
CNS: mild and transient headache, psychic stimulation, *seizures,* dizziness, neuropathy.
CV: hypotension, ECG-changes.
EENT: visual disturbances (blurred vision; difficulty in focusing; reversible
corneal changes; typically irreversible,
sometimes progressive or delayed retinal
changes, such as narrowing of arterioles;
macular lesions; pallor of optic disk; optic
atrophy; patchy retinal pigmentation, typically leading to blindness), ototoxicity
(nerve deafness, vertigo, tinnitus).
GI: anorexia, abdominal cramps, diarrhea, nausea, vomiting, stomatitis.

Reactions may be *common*, uncommon, **life-threatening**, or COMMON AND LIFE-THREATENING.

Hematologic: *agranulocytosis, aplastic anemia,* hemolytic anemia, *thrombocytopenia.*
Skin: pruritus, lichen planus eruptions, skin and mucosal pigmentary changes, pleomorphic skin eruptions.

INTERACTIONS
Drug-drug. *Cimetidine:* decreased hepatic metabolism of chloroquine. Monitor for toxicity.
Kaolin, magnesium and aluminum salts: decreased GI absorption. Separate administration times.
Drug-lifestyle. *Sun exposure:* may exacerbate drug-induced dermatoses. Tell patient to avoid excessive sun exposure.

EFFECTS ON DIAGNOSTIC TESTS
Chloroquine may cause inversion or depression of the T wave or widening of the QRS complex on ECG. Rarely, it may cause decreased WBC, RBC, or platelet counts.

CONTRAINDICATIONS
Contraindicated in patients with retinal or visual field changes, porphyria, or hypersensitivity to drug.

NURSING CONSIDERATIONS
• Use with extreme caution in patients with severe GI, neurologic, or blood disorders.
• Use cautiously in patients with hepatic disease or alcoholism because drug concentrates in liver, and in those with G6PD deficiency or psoriasis because drug may exacerbate these conditions.
• Ensure baseline and periodic ophthalmic examinations are performed. Check periodically for ocular muscle weakness after long-term use.
• Assist patient with obtaining audiometric examinations before, during, and after therapy, especially if long-term.
• Monitor CBCs and liver function studies periodically during long-term therapy as ordered; if a severe blood disorder not attributable to the disease develops, drug may need to be discontinued.
Alert: Monitor patient for possible overdose, which can quickly lead to toxic symptoms: headache, drowsiness, visual

disturbances, CV collapse, and seizures, followed by cardiopulmonary arrest. Children are extremely susceptible to toxicity; avoid long-term treatment.

✓Patient teaching
• To enhance compliance for prophylaxis, advise patient to take drug immediately before or after meals on same day each week.
• Instruct patient to avoid excessive sun exposure to prevent exacerbation of drug-induced dermatoses.
• Tell patient to report adverse reactions promptly, especially blurred vision, increased sensitivity to light, or muscle weakness.

hydroxychloroquine sulfate
Plaquenil Sulfate

Pregnancy Risk Category: C

HOW SUPPLIED
Tablets: 200 mg (155-mg base)

ACTION
Unknown. May bind to and alter the properties of DNA in susceptible organisms.

Route	Onset	Peak	Duration
PO	Unknown	2-4.5 hr	Unknown

INDICATIONS & DOSAGE
Suppressive prophylaxis of malaria attacks caused by Plasmodium vivax, P. malariae, P. ovale, *and susceptible strains of* P. falciparum—
Adults: 400 mg (310-mg base) P.O. weekly on same day of week (begin 2 weeks before entering endemic area and continue for 4 weeks after leaving endemic area). If not started before exposure, initial dose is doubled to 800 mg (620-mg base) in two divided doses.
Children: 5 mg/kg (base) P.O. weekly on same day of week (begin 2 weeks before entering endemic area and continue for 4 weeks after leaving endemic area). Do not exceed adult dose. If not started before exposure, initial dose is doubled to 10 mg/kg (base) in two divided doses.

Acute malarial attacks—
Adults: initially, 800 mg (sulfate) P.O., then 400 mg after 6 to 8 hours, then 400 mg daily for 2 days (total 2 g sulfate salt).
Children: 13 mg/kg (sulfate) P.O., then 6.5 mg/kg 6 hours later, then 6.5 mg/kg daily for 2 days.
Lupus erythematosus (chronic discoid and systemic)—
Adults: 400 mg (sulfate) P.O. daily or b.i.d., continued for several weeks or months, depending on response. For prolonged maintenance dosage, 200 to 400 mg (sulfate) daily.
Rheumatoid arthritis—
Adults: initially, 400 to 600 mg (sulfate) P.O. daily. When good response occurs (usually in 4 to 12 weeks), dosage is cut in half.

ADVERSE REACTIONS
CNS: irritability, nightmares, ataxia, *seizures,* psychosis, vertigo, nystagmus, dizziness, hypoactive deep tendon reflexes, ataxia, lassitude, skeletal muscle weakness, headache.
EENT: visual disturbances (blurred vision; difficulty in focusing; reversible corneal changes; typically irreversible, sometimes progressive or delayed retinal changes, such as narrowing of arterioles; macular lesions; pallor of optic disk; optic atrophy; visual field defects; patchy retinal pigmentation, commonly leading to blindness), ototoxicity (irreversible nerve deafness, tinnitus, labyrinthitis).
GI: anorexia, abdominal cramps, diarrhea, nausea, vomiting.
Hematologic: *agranulocytosis, leukopenia, thrombocytopenia, hemolysis in patients with G6PD deficiency, aplastic anemia.*
Skin: pruritus, lichen planus eruptions, skin and mucosal pigmentary changes, pleomorphic skin eruptions, worsened psoriasis.
Other: weight loss, alopecia, bleaching of hair.

INTERACTIONS
Drug-drug. *Cimetidine:* decreased hepatic metabolism of hydroxychloroquine. Monitor for toxicity.

Kaolin, magnesium and aluminum salts: decreased GI absorption. Separate administration times.

EFFECTS ON DIAGNOSTIC TESTS
Hydroxychloroquine sulfate may cause inversion or depression of the T wave or widening of the QRS complex on ECG. Rarely, it may cause decreased WBC, RBC, or platelet counts.

CONTRAINDICATIONS
Contraindicated in patients with retinal or visual field changes, porphyria, or hypersensitivity to drug and in long-term therapy for children.

NURSING CONSIDERATIONS
• Use with extreme caution in patients with severe GI, neurologic, or blood disorders.
• Use cautiously in patients with hepatic disease or alcoholism because drug concentrates in liver, and in those with G6PD deficiency or psoriasis because drug may exacerbate these conditions.
• Ensure baseline and periodic ophthalmic examinations are performed. Check periodically for ocular muscle weakness after long-term use.
• Assist patient with obtaining audiometric examinations before, during, and after therapy, especially if long-term.
• Monitor CBCs and liver function studies periodically during long-term therapy, as ordered; if severe blood disorder not attributable to disease develops, drug may need to be discontinued.
Alert: Monitor patient for possible overdose, which can quickly lead to toxic signs or symptoms: headache, drowsiness, visual disturbances, CV collapse, and seizures, followed by cardiopulmonary arrest. Children are extremely susceptible to toxicity; long-term treatment should be avoided.

☑ **Patient teaching**
• To enhance compliance for prophylaxis, advise patient to take hydroxychloroquine immediately before or after meals on same day each week.
• Instruct patient to report adverse reactions promptly.

Reactions may be *common,* uncommon, **life-threatening,** or COMMON AND LIFE-THREATENING.

mefloquine hydrochloride
Lariam

Pregnancy Risk Category: C

HOW SUPPLIED
Tablets: 250 mg

ACTION
Unknown. Antimalarial activity may be related to its ability to form complexes with hemin; may also act by raising intravesicular pH in parasite acid vesicles.

Route	Onset	Peak	Duration
PO	Unknown	7-24 hr	Unknown

INDICATIONS & DOSAGE
Acute malaria infections caused by mefloquine-sensitive strains of Plasmodium falciparum *or* P. vivax—
Adults: 1,250 mg P.O. as a single dose. Patients with *P. vivax* infections should receive subsequent therapy with primaquine or other 8-aminoquinolines to avoid relapse after treatment of the initial infection.
Malaria prophylaxis—
Adults: 250 mg P.O. once weekly. Prophylaxis should be initiated 1 week before entering endemic area and continued for 4 weeks after returning. If patient returns to an area without malaria after a prolonged stay in an endemic area, prophylaxis should end after three doses.

ADVERSE REACTIONS
CNS: dizziness, syncope, headache, psychotic manifestations, hallucinations, confusion, anxiety, fatigue, vertigo, depression, *seizures.*
EENT: tinnitus, visual disturbances.
GI: anorexia, vomiting, *nausea,* loose stools, diarrhea, abdominal discomfort or pain.
Skin: rash.
Other: fever, chills, myalgia.

INTERACTIONS
Drug-drug. *Beta-adrenergic blockers, quinidine, quinine:* ECG abnormalities and cardiac arrest may occur. Avoid concomitant use.

Chloroquine, quinine: increased risk of seizures. Avoid concomitant use.
Valproic acid: decreased valproic acid blood levels and loss of seizure control at start of mefloquine therapy. Monitor anticonvulsant blood levels.

EFFECTS ON DIAGNOSTIC TESTS
Drug may cause decreased hematocrit and transient elevations of transaminases, leukopenia, and thrombocytopenia.

CONTRAINDICATIONS
Contraindicated in patients with hypersensitivity to mefloquine or related compounds.

NURSING CONSIDERATIONS
• Use cautiously in patients with cardiac disease or seizure disorders.
• Because the health risks from concomitant administration of quinine and mefloquine are great, be aware that mefloquine therapy should not begin sooner than 12 hours after the last dose of quinine or quinidine.
• Keep in mind that patients with *P. vivax* infections are at high risk for relapse because the drug does not eliminate the hepatic phase (exoerythrocytic parasites). Follow-up therapy with primaquine is advisable.
• Monitor liver function tests periodically as ordered.
• In cases of suspected overdose, induce vomiting or perform gastric lavage as appropriate because of potential for cardiotoxicity. Animal studies reveal that mefloquine has cardiac actions similar to quinidine and quinine.

☑ **Patient teaching**
• Advise patient to take drug on the same day of the week when using it for prophylaxis.
• Tell patient not to take drug on an empty stomach and always to take it with a full glass (at least 8 oz [240 ml]) of water.
• Advise patient to use caution when performing activities that require alertness and coordination because dizziness, disturbed sense of balance, and neuropsychiatric reactions may occur.
• Instruct patient taking mefloquine pro-

---

*Liquid contains alcohol.   **May contain tartrazine.   †Canada   ‡Australia   §U.K.   ◊OTC

phylactically to discontinue drug if signs or symptoms of impending toxicity, such as unexplained anxiety, depression, confusion, or restlessness occur, and to notify doctor.
• Advise patient undergoing long-term therapy to have periodic ophthalmic examinations because ocular lesions have been noted in laboratory animals.

---

primaquine phosphate

Pregnancy Risk Category: C

HOW SUPPLIED
Tablets: 15 mg (base)

ACTION
Unknown. It may be effective because of drug's ability to bind to and alter the properties of DNA.

Route	Onset	Peak	Duration
PO	Unknown	1-3 hr	Unknown

INDICATIONS & DOSAGE
Radical cure of relapsing vivax malaria, eliminating symptoms and infection completely; prevention of relapse—
Adults: 15 mg (base) P.O. daily for 14 days. (A 26.3-mg tablet provides 15 mg of base.) Begin therapy during the last 2 weeks of, or following, a course of suppression with chloroquine or comparable agent.
Children: 0.5 mg/kg/day (0.3 mg base/kg/day; maximum 15 mg base/dose) P.O. for 14 days.

ADVERSE REACTIONS
GI: nausea, vomiting, epigastric distress, abdominal cramps.
Hematologic: *leukopenia, hemolytic anemia in G6PD deficiency*, methemoglobinemia in NADH methemoglobin reductase deficiency.

INTERACTIONS
Drug-drug. *Magnesium and aluminum salts:* decreased GI absorption. Separate administration times.
Quinacrine: enhanced toxicity of primaquine. Don't use together.

EFFECTS ON DIAGNOSTIC TESTS
Decreases or increases in WBC counts and decreases in RBC counts may occur during primaquine therapy. Methemoglobinemia may occur.

CONTRAINDICATIONS
Contraindicated in patients with systemic diseases in which agranulocytosis may develop (such as lupus erythematosus or rheumatoid arthritis) and in those taking bone marrow suppressants and potentially hemolytic drugs. Concomitant administration of quinicrine and primaquine is contraindicated.

NURSING CONSIDERATIONS
• Use cautiously in patients with previous idiosyncratic reaction (manifested by hemolytic anemia, methemoglobinemia, or leukopenia); in those with a family or personal history of favism; and in those with erythrocytic G6PD deficiency or NADH methemoglobin reductase deficiency.
• Administer drug with meals.
• Keep in mind that when administering drug, a fast-acting antimalarial (such as chloroquine) is used to reduce possibility of drug-resistant strains.
• Obtain frequent blood studies and urine examinations as ordered in light-skinned patients taking more than 30 mg (base) daily, dark-skinned patients taking more than 15 mg (base) daily, and patients with severe anemia or suspected sensitivity.
• Monitor patient for sudden fall in hemoglobin concentration, erythrocyte or leukocyte count, or marked darkening of the urine, which suggests impending hemolytic reactions. Discontinue drug immediately and notify doctor.

✅ Patient teaching
• Instruct patient to take drug with meals to minimize stomach upset. If stomach upset (nausea, vomiting, or stomach pain) persists, tell patient to notify doctor.
• Tell patient to stop drug therapy and notify doctor immediately if marked darkening of urine occurs.
• Stress importance of completing full course of therapy.

---

pyrimethamine
Daraprim

pyrimethamine with sulfadoxine
Fansidar

Pregnancy Risk Category: C

HOW SUPPLIED
pyrimethamine
Tablets: 25 mg
pyrimethamine with sulfadoxine
Tablets: pyrimethamine 25 mg, sulfadoxine 500 mg

ACTION
Inhibits the enzyme dihydrofolate reductase, thereby impeding reduction of dihydrofolic acid to tetrahydrofolic acid. Sulfadoxine competitively inhibits use of PABA.

Route	Onset	Peak	Duration
PO	Unknown	1.5-8 hr	2 wk

INDICATIONS & DOSAGE
Malaria prophylaxis and transmission control (pyrimethamine)—
Adults and children 10 years and older: 25 mg P.O. weekly.
Children 4 to 10 years: 12.5 mg P.O. weekly.
Children under 4 years: 6.25 mg P.O. weekly.

Needs to be continued in all age-groups 6 to 10 weeks after leaving endemic areas.
Acute attacks of malaria (Fansidar)—
Adults and children 14 years and older: 2 to 3 tablets as a single dose, either alone or in sequence with quinine or primaquine.
Children 9 to 14 years: 2 tablets.
Children 4 to 8 years: 1 tablet.
Children under 4 years: ½ tablet.
Malaria prophylaxis (Fansidar)—
Adults and children 14 years and older: 1 tablet weekly, or 2 tablets q 2 weeks.
Children 9 to 14 years: ¾ tablet weekly, or 1½ tablets q 2 weeks.
Children 4 to 8 years: ½ tablet weekly, or 1 tablet q 2 weeks.

Children under 4 years: ¼ tablet weekly, or ½ tablet q 2 weeks.
Acute attacks of malaria (pyrimethamine)—
Adults and children 15 years and older: 50 mg P.O. daily for 2 days, then once weekly dosed as described above.
Children under 15 years: 25 mg P.O. daily for 2 days, then once weekly dosed as described above.

Not recommended alone in nonimmune patients; should be used with faster-acting antimalarials, such as chloroquine, for 2 days to initiate transmission control and suppressive cure.
Toxoplasmosis (pyrimethamine)—
Adults: initially, 50 to 75 mg P.O. with 1 to 4 g sulfadiazine, continue for 1 to 3 weeks. Reduce after 3 weeks by half and continue for 4 to 5 weeks.
Children: initially, 1 mg/kg P.O. (not to exceed 100 mg) in two equally divided doses for 2 to 4 days, then 0.5 mg/kg daily for 4 weeks, along with 100 mg sulfadiazine/kg P.O. daily, divided q 6 hours.

ADVERSE REACTIONS
CNS: headache, peripheral neuritis, mental depression, *seizures*, ataxia, hallucinations, fatigue.
CV: *arrhythmias* (with large doses), allergic myocarditis.
EENT: photosensitivity, scleral irritation.
GI: anorexia, vomiting, atrophic glossitis.
Hematologic: *agranulocytosis, aplastic anemia,* megaloblastic anemia, *leukopenia, thrombocytopenia, pancytopenia*.
Skin: *Stevens-Johnson syndrome,* generalized skin eruptions, urticaria, pruritus, periorbital edema.

Note: Adverse drug reactions related to sulfadiazine are similar to sulfonamides.

INTERACTIONS
Drug-drug. *Co-trimoxazole, methotrexate, sulfonamides:* increased risk of bone marrow suppression. Do not use together.
Lorazepam: increased risk of hepatotoxicity. Avoid concomitant use.
PABA: decreased antitoxoplasmic effects. May require dosage adjustment.

EFFECTS ON DIAGNOSTIC TESTS
Pyrimethamine therapy may decrease WBC, RBC, and platelet counts.

CONTRAINDICATIONS
Pyrimethamine is contraindicated in patients with hypersensitivity to drug and in those with megaloblastic anemia caused by folic acid deficiency. Fansidar is contraindicated in patients with porphyria.

Repeated use of Fansidar is contraindicated in patients with severe renal insufficiency, marked parenchymal damage to the liver or blood dyscrasias, known hypersensitivity to pyrimethamine or sulfonamides, or documented megaloblastic anemia due to folate deficiency; in infants under 2 months; in pregnancy at term; and during breast-feeding.

NURSING CONSIDERATIONS
• Use cautiously in patients with impaired hepatic or renal function, severe allergy or bronchial asthma, G6PD deficiency, or seizure disorders (smaller doses may be needed), and after treatment with chloroquine.
• Obtain twice-weekly blood counts, including platelets, as ordered, for the patient with toxoplasmosis because dosages used approach toxic levels. If signs of folic acid or folinic acid deficiency develop, dosage should be reduced or discontinued while the patient receives parenteral folinic acid (leucovorin) until blood counts become normal.
• Keep in mind that, when used to treat toxoplasmosis in patients with AIDS, therapy may be lifelong.
• Know that Fansidar should be used only in areas where chloroquine-resistant malaria is prevalent and only if the traveler plans to stay longer than 3 weeks.

✅ **Patient teaching**
• Tell patient to take drug with meals.
• Inform patient with toxoplasmosis of importance of frequent laboratory studies and compliance with therapy. Tell patient of potential need for long-term therapy.
• Warn patient taking Fansidar to stop drug and notify doctor at first sign of rash.

• Tell patient to take first prophylactic dose 1 to 2 days before traveling.

10
Antituberculars and antileprotics

clofazimine
cycloserine
dapsone
ethambutol hydrochloride
isoniazid
pyrazinamide
rifabutin
rifampin
rifapentine
streptomycin sulfate
   (See Chapter 11, AMINOGLYCOSIDES.)

COMBINATION PRODUCTS
RIFAMATE: isoniazid 150 mg and rifampin 300 mg.
RIFATER: isoniazid 50 mg, rifampin 120 mg, and pyrazinamide 300 mg.
RIMACTANE/INH DUAL PACK: 30 300-mg isoniazid tablets and 60 300-mg rifampin capsules.

---

clofazimine
Lamprene

Pregnancy Risk Category: C

HOW SUPPLIED
Capsules: 50 mg

ACTION
Unknown. Thought to inhibit mycobacterial growth by binding preferentially to mycobacterial DNA. Also has anti-inflammatory effects that suppress skin reactions of erythema nodosum leprosum.

Route	Onset	Peak	Duration
PO	Unknown	1-6 hr	Unknown

INDICATIONS & DOSAGE
Dapsone-resistant leprosy (Hansen's disease)—
Adults: 100 mg P.O. daily in combination with other antileprotics for 3 years. Then, clofazimine *alone,* 100 mg daily.
Erythema nodosum leprosum—
Adults: 100 to 200 mg P.O. daily for up to 3 months; when prolonged, concomi-

tant corticosteroid therapy is necessary. Dosage is tapered to 100 mg daily as soon as possible. Dosages above 200 mg daily are not recommended.

ADVERSE REACTIONS
EENT: *conjunctival and corneal pigmentation, dryness, burning, itching, irritation.*
GI: *epigastric pain, diarrhea, nausea, vomiting, GI intolerance, **bowel obstruction, bleeding.***
Skin: *pink to brownish black pigmentation, ichthyosis and dryness,* rash, pruritus.
Other: *splenic infarction,* discolored body fluids and excrement.

INTERACTIONS
Drug-drug. *Dapsone:* impaired anti-inflammatory effects of clofazimine; no intervention appears necessary.
Isoniazid: may decrease skin levels and increase serum and urine levels of clofazimine. Monitor for decreased effectiveness.
Rifampin: decreased rifampin bioavailability. Monitor for decreased effectiveness.

EFFECTS ON DIAGNOSTIC TESTS
Clofazimine therapy can elevate blood glucose, albumin, serum bilirubin, and AST and can cause hypokalemia and eosinophilia.

CONTRAINDICATIONS
No known contraindications.

NURSING CONSIDERATIONS
• Use cautiously in patients with GI dysfunction, such as abdominal pain and diarrhea.
• Be aware that dosages exceeding 100 mg daily should be given for as short a period as possible and only under close medical supervision.
• If patient complains of colic, burning abdominal pain, or other GI symptoms,

---

*Liquid contains alcohol.   **May contain tartrazine.   †Canada   ‡Australia   §U.K.   ◇OTC

notify doctor, who may reduce dose or increase the interval between doses.

☑**Patient teaching**
• Advise patient to take drug with meals or milk.
• Warn patient that clofazimine may discolor skin, body fluids, and excrement. The color ranges from pink to brownish black. Reassure patient that the unsightly skin discoloration is reversible but may not disappear until several months or years after drug treatment ends.
• Tell patient to apply skin oil or cream to help reverse skin dryness or ichthyosis.

---

cycloserine
Seromycin

Pregnancy Risk Category: C

HOW SUPPLIED
Capsules: 250 mg

ACTION
Inhibits cell-wall biosynthesis by interfering with the bacterial use of amino acids. Action may be bacteriostatic or bactericidal, depending on the concentration of drug attained at the site of infection and the susceptibility of infecting organism.

Route	Onset	Peak	Duration
PO	Unknown	4-8 hr	Unknown

INDICATIONS & DOSAGE
Adjunctive treatment in pulmonary or extrapulmonary tuberculosis—
Adults: initially, 250 mg P.O. q 12 hours for 2 weeks; then, if blood levels are below 25 to 30 mcg/ml and no toxicity has developed, dose is increased to 250 mg q 8 hours for 2 weeks. If optimum blood levels are still not achieved and no toxicity has developed, then dose is increased to 250 mg q 6 hours. Maximum dosage is 1 g/day. If CNS toxicity occurs, drug is discontinued for 1 week, then resumed at 250 mg daily for 2 weeks. If no serious toxic effects occur, dosage is increased by 250-mg increments q 10 days until blood level of 25 to 30 mcg/ml is obtained.
Children: 10 to 20 mg/kg/day P.O. in two

divided doses (maximum of 0.75 to 1 g) has been recommended.

ADVERSE REACTIONS
CNS: *seizures,* drowsiness, somnolence, headache, tremor, dysarthria, vertigo, confusion, loss of memory, *possible suicidal tendencies,* psychosis, hyperirritability, paresthesia, paresis, hyperreflexia, *coma.*
CV: *sudden heart failure.*
Other: hypersensitivity reactions (allergic dermatitis), elevated transaminase level.

INTERACTIONS
Drug-drug. *Ethionamide:* increased risk of CNS toxicity (seizures). Monitor patient closely.
Isoniazid: CNS toxicity (dizziness or drowsiness). Monitor patient closely.
Drug-lifestyle. *Alcohol use:* increased risk of CNS toxicity (seizures). Monitor patient closely.

EFFECTS ON DIAGNOSTIC TESTS
Cycloserine may elevate serum transaminase levels, especially in patients with hepatic disease.

CONTRAINDICATIONS
Contraindicated in patients with hypersensitivity to drug and in those with seizure disorders, depression or severe anxiety, psychosis, severe renal insufficiency, or excessive concurrent use of alcohol.

NURSING CONSIDERATIONS
• Use cautiously in patients with impaired renal function; reduced dosage is required.
• Obtain specimen for culture and sensitivity tests before therapy begins and periodically thereafter to detect possible resistance.
• Know that cycloserine is considered a "second-line" drug in the treatment of tuberculosis and should always be administered with other antituberculars to prevent the development of resistant organisms.
• Monitor serum cycloserine levels periodically as ordered, especially in patients receiving high doses (more than 500 mg

---

daily) because toxic reactions may occur with blood levels above 30 mcg/ml.
• Monitor results of hematologic tests and renal and liver function studies.
• Observe for psychotic symptoms, hallucinations, and possible suicidal tendencies.
• Administer pyridoxine, anticonvulsants, tranquilizers, or sedatives, as ordered, to relieve adverse reactions.

✅ **Patient teaching**
• Warn patient to avoid alcohol, which may cause serious neurologic reactions.
• Advise patient not to perform hazardous activities if drowsiness occurs.
• Tell patient to report adverse reactions promptly because dosage adjustment may be necessary or other medications may be prescribed to relieve adverse reactions.

dapsone
Avlosulfon†, Dapsone 100‡

Pregnancy Risk Category: C

HOW SUPPLIED
Tablets: 25 mg, 100 mg

ACTION
Unknown. May inhibit folic acid biosynthesis in susceptible organisms.

Route	Onset	Peak	Duration
PO	Unknown	4-8 hr	Unknown

INDICATIONS & DOSAGE
All forms of leprosy (Hansen's disease)—
Adults: 100 mg P.O. daily, indefinitely; give with rifampin 600 mg P.O. daily for 6 months.
Children: 1 to 2 mg/kg P.O. daily for minimum of 3 years.
Dermatitis herpetiformis—
Adults: 50 mg P.O. daily; increased to 300 mg daily p.r.n.

ADVERSE REACTIONS
CNS: insomnia, psychosis, headache, paresthesia, peripheral neuropathy, vertigo.
EENT: tinnitus, blurred vision.
GI: anorexia, abdominal pain, nausea, vomiting.
GU: albuminuria, nephrotic syndrome, renal papillary necrosis.
Hematologic: *hemolytic anemia* (dose-related), *agranulocytosis, aplastic anemia.*
Skin: lupus erythematosus, phototoxicity, *exfoliative dermatitis, toxic erythema, erythema multiforme, toxic epidermal necrolysis,* morbilliform and scarlatiniform reactions, urticaria, *erythema nodosum.*
Other: fever, tachycardia, pancreatitis, male infertility, pulmonary eosinophilia, infectious mononucleosis-like syndrome, *sulfone syndrome* (fever, malaise, jaundice [with hepatic necrosis], lymphadenopathy, *methemoglobinemia, hemolytic anemia).*

INTERACTIONS
Drug-drug. *Activated charcoal:* may decrease dapsone's GI absorption and enterohepatic recycling. Monitor closely.
Didanosine: possible therapeutic failure of dapsone, leading to an increase in infection. Avoid concomitant use.
Folic acid antagonists (such as methotrexate): increased risk of adverse hematologic reactions. Avoid concomitant use.
PABA: may antagonize the effect of dapsone by interfering with the primary mechanism of action. Monitor for lack of efficacy.
Probenecid: reduces urinary excretion of dapsone metabolites, increasing plasma concentrations. Monitor closely.
Rifampin: increased hepatic metabolism of dapsone. Monitor for lack of efficacy.
Trimethoprim: increased serum levels of both drugs may occur, possibly increasing the pharmacologic and toxic effects of each drug. Monitor closely.

EFFECTS ON DIAGNOSTIC TESTS
None reported.

CONTRAINDICATIONS
Contraindicated in patients with hypersensitivity to drug. Also contraindicated while breast feeding due to potential for tumorigenicity.

---

*Liquid contains alcohol.   **May contain tartrazine.   †Canada   ‡Australia   §U.K.   ◊OTC

NURSING CONSIDERATIONS

• Use cautiously in patients with chronic renal, hepatic, or CV disease; refractory types of anemia; and G6PD deficiency.
• Obtain baseline CBC as ordered. Monitor CBC weekly for the first month, monthly for 6 months, and semiannually thereafter.
• Be prepared to reduce or temporarily discontinue dapsone if hemoglobin falls below 9 g/dl, WBC count falls below 5,000/mm^3, or RBC count falls below 2.5 million/mm^3 or remains low.
• If generalized, diffuse dermatitis occurs, notify doctor and prepare to interrupt therapy.
• Administer antihistamines, as ordered, to combat allergic dermatitis.
• Monitor for signs and symptoms of erythema nodosum reaction, which may occur during therapy as a result of *Mycobacterium leprae* bacilli (malaise, fever, painful inflammatory induration in the skin and mucosa, iritis, and neuritis). In severe cases, therapy should be stopped and glucocorticoids given cautiously.

☑ Patient teaching

Alert: Due to the potential for tumorigenicity shown in animal studies, breast-feeding should be discontinued while on medication. *Instruct breast-feeding patient to notify doctor of cyanosis in infant immediately.*
• Tell patient to avoid prolonged exposure to sunlight or sunlamps, as dapsone may cause photosensitivity.
• Inform of need for long-term therapy. Stress importance of compliance with drug therapy.

---

ethambutol hydrochloride
Etibi†, Myambutol

Pregnancy Risk Category: C

HOW SUPPLIED
Tablets: 100 mg, 400 mg

ACTION
Unknown. Appears to interfere with the synthesis of one or more metabolites of susceptible bacteria, altering cellular metabolism during cell division (bacteriostatic).

Route	Onset	Peak	Duration
PO	Unknown	2-4 hr	Unknown

INDICATIONS & DOSAGE
Adjunctive treatment in pulmonary tuberculosis—
Adults and children over 13 years: for patients who have not received previous antitubercular therapy, 15 mg/kg P.O. as a single dose daily.

Retreatment: 25 mg/kg P.O. daily as a single dose for 60 days (or until bacteriologic smears and cultures become negative) with at least one other antitubercular; then decreased to 15 mg/kg/day as a single dose.

ADVERSE REACTIONS
CNS: headache, dizziness, mental confusion, possible hallucinations, peripheral neuritis (numbness and tingling of extremities).
EENT: optic neuritis (related to dose and duration of treatment).
GI: anorexia, nausea, vomiting, abdominal pain, GI upset.
Skin: dermatitis, pruritus, *toxic epidermal necrolysis.*
Other: *anaphylactoid reactions,* fever, malaise, bloody sputum, *thrombocytopenia,* joint pain, elevated uric acid level, precipitation of acute gout, abnormal liver function test results.

INTERACTIONS
Drug-drug. *Aluminum salts:* may delay and reduce absorption of ethambutol. Separate administration times by several hours.

EFFECTS ON DIAGNOSTIC TESTS
Ethambutol may elevate serum urate levels and liver function test results.

CONTRAINDICATIONS
Contraindicated in patients with optic neuritis or hypersensitivity to drug and in children under 13 years.

NURSING CONSIDERATIONS
• Use cautiously in patients with impaired

---

renal function, cataracts, recurrent eye inflammations, gout, and diabetic retinopathy.
• Perform visual acuity and color discrimination tests before and during therapy.
• Obtain AST and ALT levels before therapy, and monitor these levels every 3 to 4 weeks, as ordered.
• Anticipate dosage reduction in patients with impaired renal function.
• Know that ethambutol should always be administered with other antituberculars to prevent the development of resistant organisms.
• Monitor serum uric acid level as ordered; observe patient for signs of gout.

✅ **Patient teaching**
• Reassure patient that visual disturbances will generally disappear several weeks to months after drug is stopped.
• Inform patient that drug is administered concurrently with other antituberculars.
• Stress importance of compliance with drug therapy.

---

isoniazid (isonicotinic acid hydrazide, INH)
Isotamine†, Laniazid, Nydrazid**, PMS-Isoniazid†

Pregnancy Risk Category: C

HOW SUPPLIED
Tablets: 50 mg, 100 mg, 300 mg
Oral solution: 50 mg/5 ml
Injection: 100 mg/ml

ACTION
Unknown. Appears to inhibit cell-wall biosynthesis by interfering with lipid and DNA synthesis (bactericidal).

Route	Onset	Peak	Duration
PO, IM	Unknown	1-2 hr	Unknown

INDICATIONS & DOSAGE
Actively growing tubercle bacilli—
Adults: 5 mg/kg P.O. or I.M. daily in a single dose, up to 300 mg/day, continued for 6 months to 2 years.
Infants and children: 10 to 20 mg/kg P.O. or I.M. daily in a single dose, up to

300 mg/day, continued long enough to prevent relapse. Concomitant administration of at least one other antitubercular is recommended.
Prevention of tubercle bacilli in those exposed to tuberculosis or those with positive skin test whose chest X-rays and bacteriologic studies are consistent with nonprogressive tuberculosis—
Adults: 300 mg P.O. daily in a single dose, continued for 6 months to 1 year.
Infants and children: 10 mg/kg P.O. daily in a single dose, up to 300 mg/day, continued for 1 year.

ADVERSE REACTIONS
CNS: *peripheral neuropathy* (dose-related and especially in patients who are malnourished, alcoholic, diabetic, or slow acetylators), usually preceded by paresthesia of hands and feet, *seizures,* toxic encephalopathy, optic neuritis and atrophy, memory impairment, toxic psychosis.
GI: nausea, vomiting, epigastric distress.
Hematologic: *agranulocytosis,* hemolytic anemia, *aplastic anemia,* eosinophilia, *thrombocytopenia,* sideroblastic anemia.
Hepatic: *hepatitis* (occasionally severe and sometimes fatal, especially in elderly patients), jaundice, *elevated serum transaminase levels,* bilirubinemia.
Other: rheumatic and lupus-like syndromes, *hypersensitivity reactions* (fever, rash, lymphadenopathy, vasculitis), hyperglycemia, metabolic acidosis, pyridoxine deficiency, hypocalcemia, hypophosphatemia, gynecomastia, irritation at I.M. injection site.

INTERACTIONS
Drug-drug. *Aluminum-containing antacids and laxatives:* may decrease the rate and amount of isoniazid absorbed. Give isoniazid at least 1 hour before antacid or laxative.
Benzodiazepines: isoniazid may inhibit the metabolic clearance of benzodiazepines that undergo oxidative metabolism (diazepam, triazolam), possibly increasing the activity of the benzodiazepine. Monitor closely.
Carbamazepine, halothane: increased risk of isoniazid hepatotoxicity. Use together cautiously.

---

*Liquid contains alcohol. **May contain tartrazine. †Canada ‡Australia §U.K. ◊OTC

Carbamazepine, phenytoin: increased plasma levels of these anticonvulsants. Monitor closely.

Cycloserine, meperidine: may increase CNS adverse reactions and hypotension (meperidine only). Institute safety precautions.

Disulfiram: may cause neurologic symptoms, including changes in behavior and coordination. Avoid concomitant use.

Enflurane: in rapid acetylators of isoniazid, high-output renal failure may occur due to nephrotoxic concentrations of inorganic fluoride. Monitor renal function.

Ketoconazole: serum concentrations of ketoconazole may be decreased. Monitor for lack of efficacy.

Oral anticoagulants: anticoagulant activity may be enhanced. Monitor patient closely.

Drug-food. *Tyramine-containing foods:* hypertensive crisis. Tell patient to avoid or eat in small quantities.

Drug-lifestyle. *Alcohol use:* may be associated with increased incidence of isoniazid-related hepatitis. Avoid concomitant use.

EFFECTS ON DIAGNOSTIC TESTS
Isoniazid alters results of urine glucose tests that use cupric sulfate method (Benedict's reagent or Diastix). Elevated liver function study results occur in about 15% of patients; most abnormalities are mild and transient, but some may persist throughout treatment.

CONTRAINDICATIONS
Contraindicated in patients with acute hepatic disease or isoniazid-associated liver damage.

NURSING CONSIDERATIONS
• Use cautiously in patients with chronic non-isoniazid-associated liver disease, seizure disorders (especially in those taking phenytoin), severe renal impairment, and chronic alcoholism and in elderly patients.

• Be aware that isoniazid should always be administered with other antituberculars to prevent the development of resistant organisms.

• Keep in mind that isoniazid pharmacokinetics may vary among patients because its metabolism occurs in the liver by genetically controlled acetylation. Fast acetylators metabolize the drug up to five times as fast as slow acetylators. About 50% of blacks and whites are slow acetylators; over 80% of Chinese, Japanese, and Inuits are fast acetylators.

• Monitor hepatic function closely for changes.

• Administer pyridoxine, as ordered, to prevent peripheral neuropathy, especially in malnourished patients.

☑ **Patient teaching**
• Instruct patient to take drug exactly as prescribed; warn against discontinuing drug without doctor's consent.

• Advise patient to take with food if GI irritation occurs.

• Tell patient to notify doctor immediately if symptoms of liver impairment occur (anorexia, fatigue, malaise, jaundice, dark urine).

• Advise patient to avoid alcoholic beverages while taking drug. Also tell him to avoid certain foods (fish, such as skipjack and tuna, and tyramine-containing products, such as aged cheese, beer, and chocolate) because drug has some MAO inhibitor activity.

• Encourage patient to comply fully with treatment, which may take months or years.

pyrazinamide
Pyrazinamide†, Tebrazid†, Zinamide‡

Pregnancy Risk Category: C

HOW SUPPLIED
Tablets: 500 mg

ACTION
Unknown.

Route	Onset	Peak	Duration
PO	Unknown	1-2 hr	Unknown

INDICATIONS & DOSAGE
Adjunctive treatment of tuberculosis (when primary and secondary antituberculars cannot be used or have failed)—

Reactions may be *common*, uncommon, *life-threatening*, or COMMON AND LIFE-THREATENING.

Adults: 15 to 30 mg/kg P.O. once daily. Maximum dosage is 2 g daily. Alternatively, when compliance is a problem, 50 to 70 mg/kg (based on lean body mass) P.O. twice weekly.

ADVERSE REACTIONS
GI: anorexia, nausea, vomiting.
GU: dysuria.
Hematologic: sideroblastic anemia, *thrombocytopenia.*
Hepatic: dose-related *hepatotoxicity*.
Skin: rash, urticaria, pruritus, photosensitivity.
Other: malaise, fever, porphyria, hyperuricemia and gout, interstitial nephritis, *arthralgia, myalgia, hepatitis.*

INTERACTIONS
None significant.

EFFECTS ON DIAGNOSTIC TESTS
Pyrazinamide may interfere with urine ketone determinations. Drug's systemic effects may temporarily decrease 17-ketosteroid levels; it may increase protein-bound iodine and urate levels and results of liver enzyme tests.

CONTRAINDICATIONS
Contraindicated in patients with severe hepatic disease, acute gout, or hypersensitivity to drug.

NURSING CONSIDERATIONS
• Use cautiously in patients with diabetes mellitus, renal failure, or gout.
• Be aware that pyrazinamide should always be administered with other antituberculars to prevent the development of resistant organisms.
• Know that drug is administered for the initial 2 months of a 6-month or longer treatment regimen for drug susceptible patients. Patients with concomitant HIV infection may require longer courses of therapy.
• Keep in mind that a reduced dosage is needed in patients with renal impairment because nearly 100% of the drug is excreted in urine.
• Question doses that exceed 35 mg/kg because they may cause liver damage.

• Monitor hematopoietic studies and serum uric acid levels, as ordered.
• Monitor liver function studies; assess for jaundice and liver tenderness or enlargement before and frequently during therapy.
• Watch closely for signs of gout and of liver impairment (anorexia, fatigue, malaise, jaundice, dark urine, and liver tenderness). Notify doctor at once.
• When used with surgical management of tuberculosis, pyrazinamide is started 1 to 2 weeks before surgery and continued for 4 to 6 weeks postoperatively.

☑ **Patient teaching**
• Inform patient that other antituberculars will be required concomitantly.
• Instruct patient to report adverse reactions promptly.
• Stress importance of compliance with drug therapy. If daily therapy poses a problem, tell patient to ask doctor about twice-weekly dosing.

rifabutin
Mycobutin

Pregnancy Risk Category: B

HOW SUPPLIED
Capsules: 150 mg

ACTION
Inhibits DNA-dependent RNA polymerase in susceptible bacteria, blocking bacterial protein synthesis.

Route	Onset	Peak	Duration
PO	Unknown	2-4 hr	Unknown

INDICATIONS & DOSAGE
Prevention of disseminated Mycobacterium avium *complex in patients with advanced HIV infection—*
Adults: 300 mg P.O. daily as a single dose or divided b.i.d.

ADVERSE REACTIONS
GI: dyspepsia, eructation, flatulence, diarrhea, nausea, vomiting, abdominal pain, anorexia, taste perversion.
GU: discolored urine.

Hematologic: NEUTROPENIA, LEUKOPENIA, *thrombocytopenia,* eosinophilia.
Hepatic: increased aminotransferases.
Skin: rash.
Other: fever, myalgia, headache.

INTERACTIONS
Drug-drug. *Oral contraceptives:* decreased effectiveness. Instruct patient to use nonhormonal forms of birth control. *Zidovudine, drugs metabolized by the liver:* may alter serum levels of these drugs. Dosage adjustments may be necessary.
Drug-food. *High-fat foods:* reduced rate but not extent of absorption. Avoid concurrent administration.

EFFECTS ON DIAGNOSTIC TESTS
None reported.

CONTRAINDICATIONS
Contraindicated in patients with hypersensitivity to drug or other rifamycin derivatives (such as rifampin). Also contraindicated in patients with active tuberculosis because single-agent therapy with rifabutin increases the risk of inducing bacterial resistance to both rifabutin and rifampin.

NURSING CONSIDERATIONS
• Use cautiously in patients with preexisting neutropenia and thrombocytopenia. Perform baseline hematologic studies and repeat periodically.
• Mix with soft foods, such as applesauce, for patients who have difficulty swallowing.
• Dose may be divided twice daily to decrease GI adverse effects.

☑**Patient teaching**
• Instruct patient to take drug for as long as prescribed, exactly as directed, even after feeling better.
• Tell patient that drug or its metabolites may discolor urine, feces, sputum, saliva, tears, and skin brownish-orange. Tell him to avoid wearing soft contact lenses because they may be permanently stained.
• Instruct patient to report photophobia, excessive lacrimation, or eye pain immediately; drug may cause uveitis (rare).

rifampin (rifampicin)
Rifadin, Rifadin IV, Rimactane, Rimycin‡, Rofact†

Pregnancy Risk Category: C

HOW SUPPLIED
Capsules: 150 mg, 300 mg
Injection: 600 mg

ACTION
Inhibits DNA-dependent RNA polymerase, thus impairing RNA synthesis (bactericidal).

Route	Onset	Peak	Duration
PO	Unknown	2-4 hr	Unknown
IV	Unknown	Unknown	Unknown

INDICATIONS & DOSAGE
Pulmonary tuberculosis—
Adults: 600 mg P.O. or I.V. daily in single dose 1 hour before or 2 hours after meals.
Children over 5 years: 10 to 20 mg/kg P.O. or I.V. daily in single dose 1 hour before or 2 hours after meals. Maximum dosage is 600 mg daily. Concomitant administration with other antituberculars is recommended.
Meningococcal carriers—
Adults: 600 mg P.O. or I.V. q 12 hours for 2 days, or 600 mg P.O. or I.V. once daily for 4 days.
Children 1 month to 12 years: 10 mg/kg P.O. or I.V. q 12 hours for 2 days, not to exceed 600 mg/day, or 10 to 20 mg/kg once daily for 4 days.
Neonates: 5 mg/kg P.O. or I.V. q 12 hours for 2 days.

ADVERSE REACTIONS
CNS: headache, fatigue, drowsiness, behavioral changes, dizziness, mental confusion, generalized numbness.
EENT: visual disturbances, exudative conjunctivitis.
GI: epigastric distress, anorexia, nausea, vomiting, abdominal pain, diarrhea, flatulence, sore mouth and tongue, pseudomembranous colitis, pancreatitis.
GU: hemoglobinuria, hematuria, and *acute renal failure.*
Hematologic: eosinophilia, *thrombocy-*

topenia, transient leukopenia, hemolytic anemia.

Hepatic: *hepatotoxicity, transient abnormalities in liver function tests.*

Skin: pruritus, urticaria, rash.

Other: flulike syndrome, discoloration of body fluids, hyperuricemia, shortness of breath, wheezing, *shock,* ataxia, osteomalacia, porphyria exacerbation, menstrual disturbances.

INTERACTIONS

Drug-drug. *Acetaminophen, analgesics, anticoagulants, anticonvulsants, barbiturates, beta-adrenergic blockers, clofibrate, chloramphenicol, corticosteroids, cyclosporine, cardiac glycosides, dapsone, diazepam, disopyramide, methadone, mexiletine, narcotics, oral contraceptives, progestins, quinidine, sulfonylureas, theophylline, verapamil:* reduced effectiveness of these drugs. Monitor closely.

Halothane: may increase risk of hepatotoxicity of both drugs. Monitor liver function closely.

Ketoconazole, para-aminosalicylate sodium: may interfere with absorption of rifampin. Give these drugs 8 to 12 hours apart.

Probenecid: may increase rifampin levels. Use cautiously.

Drug-lifestyle. *Alcohol use:* may increase risk of hepatotoxicity. Avoid use of alcohol during therapy.

EFFECTS ON DIAGNOSTIC TESTS

Rifampin alters standard serum folate and vitamin B_{12} assays. Drug's systemic effects may cause asymptomatic elevation of liver function tests (14%) and serum uric acid. Rifampin may cause temporary retention of sulfobromophthalein in the liver excretion test. It may also interfere with contrast material in gallbladder studies and urinalysis based on spectrophotometry.

CONTRAINDICATIONS

Contraindicated in patients with hypersensitivity to drug or related drugs.

NURSING CONSIDERATIONS

• Use cautiously in patients with liver disease.

• Be aware that concomitant treatment with at least one other antitubercular is recommended.

• Give 1 hour before or 2 hours after meals for optimal absorption; however, if GI irritation occurs, patient may take rifampin with meals.

• Monitor hepatic function, hematopoietic studies, and serum uric acid levels, as ordered.

• Watch closely for signs of hepatic impairment and, if present, report them to doctor.

• Drug may cause hemorrhage in neonates of rifampin-treated mothers.

I.V. administration

• Reconstitute vial with 10 ml of sterile water for injection to make a solution containing 60 mg/ml. Add to 100 ml of D_5W and infuse over 30 minutes, or add to 500 ml of D_5W and infuse over 3 hours. When dextrose is contraindicated, drug may be diluted with 0.9% NaCl for injection. Do not use other I.V. solutions.

Patient teaching

• Instruct patient who develops drug-induced GI upset to take drug with meals.

• Warn patient about drowsiness and possible red-orange discoloration of urine, feces, saliva, sweat, sputum, and tears. Soft contact lenses may be permanently stained.

• Advise patient to avoid alcoholic beverages while taking drug.

▼ *NEW DRUG*

rifapentine
Priftin

Pregnancy Risk Category: C

HOW SUPPLIED
Tablets (film-coated): 150 mg

ACTION
Rifapentine inhibits DNA-dependent RNA polymerase in susceptible strains of *Mycobacterium tuberculosis.* It has bacte-

ricidal activity against the organism both intra- and extracellularly. Rifapentine and rifampin share similar antimicrobial action.

Route	Onset	Peak	Duration
PO	Unknown	5-6 hr	Unknown

INDICATIONS & DOSAGE
Pulmonary tuberculosis, in conjunction with at least one other antitubercular agent to which the isolate is susceptible—
Adults: During the intensive phase of short-course therapy, 600 mg P.O. twice weekly for 2 months, with an interval between doses of not less than 3 days (72 hours).

During the continuation phase of short-course therapy, 600 mg P.O. once weekly for 4 months in combination with isoniazid or another agent to which the isolate is susceptible.

ADVERSE REACTIONS
CNS: headache, dizziness.
CV: hypertension.
GI: anorexia, nausea, vomiting, dyspepsia, diarrhea.
GU: pyuria, proteinuria, hematuria, urinary casts.
Hematologic: *neutropenia*, lymphopenia, anemia, *leukopenia*, thrombocytosis.
Hepatic: elevated AST and ALT.
Respiratory: hemoptysis.
Skin: rash, pruritus, acne, maculopapular rash.
Other: *hyperuricemia*, arthralgia, pain.

INTERACTIONS
Drug-drug. *Anticonvulsants (phenytoin), antiarrhythmics (disopyramide, mexiletine, quinidine, tocainide), antibiotics (chloramphenicol, clarithromycin, dapsone, doxycycline, fluoroquinolones), antifungals (fluconazole, itraconazole, ketoconazole), barbiturates, benzodiazepines (diazepam), beta blockers, calcium channel blockers (diltiazem, nifedipine, verapamil), cardiac glycosides, corticosteroids, clofibrate, haloperidol, HIV protease inhibitors (indinavir, nelfinavir, ritonavir, saquinavir), oral anticoagulants (warfarin), immunosuppressants (cyclosporine, tacrolimus), levothyroxine, narcotic analgesics (methadone), oral or other systemic hormonal contraceptives, oral hypoglycemics (sulfonylureas), progestins, quinine, reverse transcriptase inhibitors (delavirdine, zidovudine), sildenafil, theophylline, tricyclic antidepressants (amitriptyline, nortriptyline):* rifapentine induces metabolism of the hepatic cytochrome P-450 enzyme system, decreasing the activity of these medications. Dosage adjustments may be required.

EFFECTS ON DIAGNOSTIC TESTS
Serum assays for folate and vitamin B_{12} may be altered.

CONTRAINDICATIONS
Contraindicated in patients with history of hypersensitivity to a rifamycin (rifapentine, rifampin, or rifabutin).

NURSING CONSIDERATIONS
• Use drug cautiously and with frequent monitoring in patients with liver disease.
• Rifamycin antibiotics have been associated with hepatotoxicity. Monitor liver function test results before beginning drug therapy.
• Know that drug therapy may affect liver function test results, CBC, and platelet counts; monitor carefully.
• Concomitant administration of pyridoxine (vitamin B_6) is recommended in malnourished patients, in those predisposed to neuropathy (alcoholics, diabetics), and in adolescents.
Alert: Drug must be given with appropriate daily companion drugs. Compliance with all medications, especially with daily companion drugs on the days when rifapentine is not given, is crucial for early sputum conversion and protection from relapse of tuberculosis.
• Administration of drug during the last 2 weeks of pregnancy may lead to postnatal hemorrhage in the mother or infant. Monitor clotting parameters closely if drug is given.
• Be aware that rifapentine can turn body tissues and fluids red-orange. This can lead to permanent staining of contact lenses.
• Notify doctor of persistent or severe diarrhea.

Reactions may be *common*, uncommon, *life-threatening*, or COMMON AND LIFE-THREATENING.

✓Patient teaching

• Stress importance of strict compliance with drug and daily companion medications, as well as necessary follow-up visits and laboratory tests.

• Advise patient to use nonhormonal methods of birth control.

• Tell patient to take drug with food if nausea, vomiting, or GI upset occurs.

• Instruct patient to notify doctor if the following occur: fever, loss of appetite, malaise, nausea, vomiting, darkened urine, yellowish discoloration of the skin and eyes, pain or swelling of the joints, and excessive loose stools or diarrhea.

• Instruct patient to protect pills from excessive heat.

• Tell patient that rifapentine can turn body fluids red-orange. If patient wears contact lenses, these can become permanently stained.

11

Aminoglycosides

amikacin sulfate
gentamicin sulfate
neomycin sulfate
streptomycin sulfate
tobramycin sulfate

COMBINATION PRODUCTS
NEOSPORIN G.U. IRRIGANT: 40 mg neomycin sulfate and 200,000 units polymyxin B sulfate/ml.

---

amikacin sulfate
Amikin

Pregnancy Risk Category: D

HOW SUPPLIED
Injection: 50 mg/ml, 250 mg/ml

ACTION
Inhibits protein synthesis by binding directly to the 30S ribosomal subunit. Generally bactericidal.

Route	Onset	Peak	Duration
IV	Immediate	Immediate	8-12 hr
IM	Unknown	1 hr	8-12 hr

INDICATIONS & DOSAGE
Serious infections caused by sensitive strains of Pseudomonas aeruginosa, Escherichia coli, Proteus, Klebsiella, Serratia, Enterobacter, Acinetobacter, Providencia, Citrobacter, *and* Staphylococcus—
Adults and children: 15 mg/kg/day divided q 8 to 12 hours I.M. or I.V. infusion.
Neonates: initially, loading dose of 10 mg/kg I.V., followed by 7.5 mg/kg q 12 hours.
Uncomplicated urinary tract infection—
Adults: 250 mg I.M. or I.V. b.i.d.
Adjust-a-dose: In adult patients with impaired renal function, initially, 7.5 mg/kg. Subsequent doses and frequency determined by blood amikacin levels and renal function studies.

ADVERSE REACTIONS
CNS: *neuromuscular blockade.*
EENT: *ototoxicity.*
GU: *nephrotoxicity, azotemia.*
Other: arthralgia.
Respiratory: *apnea.*

INTERACTIONS
Drug-drug. *Cephalosporins:* increased nephrotoxicity. Use together cautiously.
Dimenhydrinate: may mask symptoms of ototoxicity. Use with caution.
General anesthetics, neuromuscular blockers: may potentiate neuromuscular blockade. Monitor closely.
Indomethacin: may increase serum trough and peak levels of amikacin. Monitor serum amikacin level closely.
I.V. loop diuretics (such as furosemide): increased ototoxicity. Use cautiously.
Other aminoglycosides, acyclovir, amphotericin B, cisplatin, methoxyflurane, vancomycin: increased nephrotoxicity. Use together cautiously.
Parenteral penicillins (such as ticarcillin): amikacin inactivation in vitro. Don't mix together.

EFFECTS ON DIAGNOSTIC TESTS
Drug-induced nephrotoxicity may elevate BUN, nonprotein nitrogen, or serum creatinine levels, and increase urinary excretion of casts.

CONTRAINDICATIONS
Contraindicated in patients with hypersensitivity to drug or other aminoglycosides.

NURSING CONSIDERATIONS
• Use cautiously in patients with impaired renal function or neuromuscular disorders, in neonates and infants, and in elderly patients.
• Obtain specimen for culture and sensitivity tests before giving first dose. Therapy may begin pending results.
• Evaluate patient's hearing before and during therapy. Notify doctor if patient

---

complains of tinnitus, vertigo, or hearing loss.

• Weigh patient and review renal function studies before therapy begins.

• Obtain blood for peak amikacin level 1 hour after I.M. injection and 30 minutes to 1 hour after infusion ends; for trough levels, draw blood just before next dose. Don't collect blood in a heparinized tube; heparin is incompatible with aminoglycosides.

• Be aware that peak blood levels above 35 mcg/ml and trough levels above 10 mcg/ml may be associated with a higher incidence of toxicity.

• Monitor renal function (output, specific gravity, urinalysis, BUN and creatinine levels, and creatinine clearance). Report decreasing renal function.

• Watch for superinfection (continued fever and other signs of new infection, especially of upper respiratory tract).

• Keep in mind that therapy is usually continued for 7 to 10 days. If no response occurs after 3 to 5 days, therapy may be stopped and new specimens obtained for culture and sensitivity testing.

🔵 I.V. administration

• Dilute I.V. drug in 100 to 200 ml of D_5W or 0.9% NaCl solution and infuse over 30 to 60 minutes.

• After I.V. infusion, flush line with 0.9% NaCl solution or D_5W.

✅ Patient teaching

• Instruct patient to report adverse reactions promptly.

• Encourage adequate fluid intake.

---

gentamicin sulfate
Cidomycin†, Garamycin, Gentamicin Sulfate ADD-Vantage, Genticin§, Jenamicin

Pregnancy Risk Category: D

HOW SUPPLIED

Injection: 40 mg/ml (adult), 10 mg/ml (pediatric), 2 mg/ml (intrathecal)
I.V. infusion (premixed): 40 mg, 60 mg, 70 mg, 80 mg, 90 mg, 100 mg, 120 mg, available in 0.9% NaCl solution

ACTION

Inhibits protein synthesis by binding directly to the 30S ribosomal subunit. Usually bactericidal.

Route	Onset	Peak	Duration
IV	Immediate	30-90 min	Unknown
IM	Unknown	30-90 min	Unknown
Intrathecal	Unknown	Unknown	Unknown

INDICATIONS & DOSAGE

Serious infections caused by sensitive strains of Pseudomonas aeruginosa, Escherichia coli, Proteus, Klebsiella, Serratia, Enterobacter, Citrobacter, *and* Staphylococcus—

Adults: 3 mg/kg daily in divided doses I.M. or I.V. infusion q 8 hours. For life-threatening infections, patient may receive up to 5 mg/kg daily in three to four divided doses; this dosage should be reduced to 3 mg/kg daily as soon as clinically indicated.

Children: 2 to 2.5 mg/kg q 8 hours I.M. or by I.V. infusion.

Neonates over 1 week or infants: 2.5 mg/kg q 8 hours I.M. or by I.V. infusion.

Neonates under 1 week and preterm infants: 2.5 mg/kg q 12 hours I.M. or by I.V. infusion.

Meningitis—

Adults: systemic therapy as above; or 4 to 8 mg intrathecally daily.

Children and infants over 3 months: systemic therapy as above; or 1 to 2 mg intrathecally daily.

Endocarditis prophylaxis for GI or GU procedure or surgery—

Adults: 1.5 mg/kg I.M. or I.V. 30 minutes before procedure or surgery. Maximum dosage is 80 mg. Given with ampicillin (vancomycin in penicillin-allergic patients).

Children: 2 mg/kg I.M. or I.V. 30 minutes before procedure or surgery. Maximum dosage is 80 mg. Given with ampicillin (vancomycin in penicillin-allergic patients).

After hemodialysis to maintain therapeutic blood levels—

Adults: 1 to 1.7 mg/kg I.M. or by I.V. infusion after each dialysis.

Children: 2 to 2.5 mg/kg I.M. or by I.V. infusion after each dialysis.
Adjust-a-dose: In adult patients with impaired renal function, doses and frequency are determined by serum gentamicin levels and renal function.

ADVERSE REACTIONS

CNS: headache, lethargy, encephalopathy, confusion, dizziness, *seizures,* numbness, peripheral neuropathy, vertigo, ataxia, tingling.
CV: hypotension.
EENT: *ototoxicity,* blurred vision, tinnitus.
GI: vomiting, nausea.
GU: *nephrotoxicity.*
Hematologic: anemia, eosinophilia, *leukopenia, thrombocytopenia, agranulocytosis.*
Hepatic: increased ALT, AST, bilirubin, LD.
Respiratory: apnea.
Skin: rash, urticaria, pruritus.
Other: fever, muscle twitching, myasthenia gravis–like syndrome, *anaphylaxis,* pain at injection site.

INTERACTIONS

Drug-drug. *Cephalosporins:* increased nephrotoxicity. Use together cautiously.
Dimenhydrinate: may mask symptoms of ototoxicity. Use with caution.
General anesthetics, neuromuscular blockers: may potentiate neuromuscular blockade. Monitor closely.
Indomethacin: may increase serum peak and trough levels of gentamicin. Monitor serum gentamicin levels closely.
I.V. loop diuretics (such as furosemide): increased ototoxicity. Use cautiously.
Other aminoglycosides, acyclovir, amphotericin B, cisplatin, methoxyflurane, vancomycin: increased ototoxicity and nephrotoxicity. Use together cautiously.
Parenteral penicillins (such as ampicillin and ticarcillin): gentamicin inactivation in vitro. Don't mix together.

EFFECTS ON DIAGNOSTIC TESTS

Gentamicin-induced nephrotoxicity may elevate levels of BUN, nonprotein nitrogen, or serum creatinine, and increase urinary excretion of casts.

CONTRAINDICATIONS

Contraindicated in hypersensitivity to drug or other aminoglycosides.

NURSING CONSIDERATIONS

• Use cautiously in neonates, infants, elderly patients, and patients with impaired renal function or neuromuscular disorders.
• Obtain specimen for culture and sensitivity tests before giving first dose.
• Evaluate patient's hearing before and during therapy. Notify doctor if patient complains of tinnitus, vertigo, or hearing loss.
• Weigh patient and review renal function studies before therapy begins.
Alert: Use preservative-free formulations of gentamicin when intrathecal route is ordered.
• Obtain blood for peak gentamicin level 1 hour after I.M. injection and 30 minutes to 1 hour after I.V. infusion; for trough levels, draw blood just before next dose. Don't collect blood in a heparinized tube; heparin is incompatible with aminoglycosides.
• Be aware that peak blood levels above 10 mcg/ml and trough levels above 2 mcg/ml may be associated with higher incidence of toxicity.
• Monitor urine output, specific gravity, urinalysis, BUN and creatinine levels, and creatinine clearance. Notify doctor of signs of decreasing renal function.
• Know that hemodialysis (8 hours) removes up to 50% of drug from blood.
• Watch for superinfection (continued fever and other signs of new infection, especially of upper respiratory tract).
• Know that therapy usually continues for 7 to 10 days. If no response occurs in 3 to 5 days, therapy may be stopped and new specimens obtained for culture and sensitivity testing.

⚕ I.V. administration

• When giving by intermittent I.V. infusion, dilute with 50 to 200 ml of D_5W or 0.9% NaCl injection and infuse over 30 minutes to 2 hours. After completing I.V. infusion, flush the line with 0.9% NaCl solution or D_5W.

Reactions may be *common*, uncommon, *life-threatening*, or COMMON AND LIFE-THREATENING.

☑**Patient teaching**
• Instruct patient to report adverse reactions promptly.
• Encourage adequate fluid intake.
• Caution patient not to perform hazardous activities if adverse CNS reactions occur.

---

neomycin sulfate
Mycifradin†, Neo-fradin, Neosulf‡, Neo-Tabs, Nivemycin§

Pregnancy Risk Category: D

HOW SUPPLIED
Tablets: 500 mg
Oral solution: 125 mg/5 ml

ACTION
Inhibits protein synthesis by binding directly to the 30S ribosomal subunit. Generally bactericidal.

Route	Onset	Peak	Duration
PO	Unknown	1-4 hr	8 hr

INDICATIONS & DOSAGE
Infectious diarrhea caused by enteropathogenic Escherichia coli—
Adults: 50 mg/kg daily P.O. in four divided doses for 2 to 3 days; maximum of 3 g daily is usually adequate.
Children: 50 to 100 mg/kg daily P.O. divided q 4 to 6 hours for 2 to 3 days.
Suppression of intestinal bacteria preoperatively—
Adults: 1 g P.O. q 1 hour for four doses, then 1 g q 4 hours for the balance of the 24 hours. A saline cathartic should precede therapy.
Children: 40 to 100 mg/kg daily P.O. divided q 4 to 6 hours. First dose should follow saline cathartic.
Adjunct treatment in hepatic coma—
Adults: 1 to 3 g P.O. q.i.d. for 5 to 6 days; or 200 ml of 1% solution or 100 ml of 2% solution as enema retained for 20 to 60 minutes q 6 hours.
Children: 50 to 100 mg/kg/day P.O. in divided doses for 5 to 6 days.

ADVERSE REACTIONS
EENT: *ototoxicity.*

GI: nausea, vomiting, diarrhea, malabsorption syndrome, *Clostridium difficile*–associated colitis.
GU: *nephrotoxicity.*

INTERACTIONS
Drug-drug. *Cephalosporins:* increased nephrotoxicity. Use together cautiously.
Digoxin: decreased digoxin absorption. Monitor closely.
Dimenhydrinate: may mask symptoms of ototoxicity. Use with caution.
I.V. loop diuretics (such as furosemide): increased ototoxicity. Use cautiously.
Oral anticoagulants: inhibited vitamin K–producing bacteria; may potentiate anticoagulant effect. Monitor PT or INR.
Other aminoglycosides, acyclovir, amphotericin B, cisplatin, methoxyflurane, vancomycin: increased nephrotoxicity. Use together cautiously.

EFFECTS ON DIAGNOSTIC TESTS
Neomycin-induced nephrotoxicity may elevate levels of BUN, nonprotein nitrogen, or serum creatinine; it may increase urinary excretion of casts if systemic absorption occurs.

CONTRAINDICATIONS
Contraindicated in patients with hypersensitivity to other aminoglycosides and in those with intestinal obstruction.

NURSING CONSIDERATIONS
• Use cautiously in patients with impaired renal function, neuromuscular disorders, or ulcerative bowel lesions and in elderly patients. Never administer parenterally.
• Monitor renal function (output, specific gravity, urinalysis, BUN and creatinine levels, and creatinine clearance). Notify doctor of signs of decreasing renal function.
• Evaluate patient's hearing before and during prolonged therapy. Notify doctor if patient complains of tinnitus, vertigo, or hearing loss. Onset of deafness may occur several weeks after drug is stopped.
• Watch for superinfection (fever or other signs of new infection).
• In adjunctive treatment of hepatic coma, decrease the patient's dietary protein, and

---

assess neurologic status frequently during therapy.
- For preoperative disinfection, provide a low-residue diet and a cathartic immediately before oral administration of neomycin, as ordered.
- Keep in mind that the ototoxic and nephrotoxic properties of neomycin limit its usefulness.
- Know that neomycin is nonabsorbable at the recommended dosage. However, more than 4 g/day may be systemically absorbed and lead to nephrotoxicity.
- Be aware that drug is available in combination with polymyxin B as a urinary bladder irrigant.

☑ **Patient teaching**
- Instruct patient to report adverse reactions promptly.
- Encourage adequate fluid intake.

streptomycin sulfate

Pregnancy Risk Category: D

HOW SUPPLIED
Injection: 1 g/2.5 ml ampules

ACTION
Inhibits protein synthesis by binding directly to the 30S ribosomal subunit. Generally bactericidal.

Route	Onset	Peak	Duration
IM	Unknown	1-2 hr	Unknown

INDICATIONS & DOSAGE
Streptococcal endocarditis—
Adults: 1 g q 12 hours I.M. for 1 week, then 500 mg I.M. q 12 hours for 1 week, given with penicillin.
Elderly: 500 mg I.M. q 12 hours for entire 2 weeks in conjunction with penicillin.
Primary and adjunctive treatment in tuberculosis—
Adults: 15 mg/kg (maximum of 1 g) I.M. daily for 2 to 3 months, then 1 g I.M. two or three times weekly.
Children: 20 to 40 mg/kg (maximum of 1 g) I.M. daily in divided doses injected deeply into large muscle mass. Given

concurrently with other antitubercular agents, but *not* with capreomycin; continued until sputum specimen becomes negative.
Enterococcal endocarditis—
Adults: 1 g I.M. q 12 hours for 2 weeks, then 500 mg I.M. q 12 hours for 4 weeks, given with penicillin.
Tularemia—
Adults: 1 to 2 g I.M. daily in divided doses injected deep into upper outer quadrant of buttocks; continued for 7 to 14 days or until patient is afebrile for 5 to 7 days.

ADVERSE REACTIONS
CNS: *neuromuscular blockade,* vertigo, paresthesia of the face.
EENT: *ototoxicity.*
GI: vomiting, nausea.
GU: some nephrotoxicity (not as frequently as with other aminoglycosides).
Hematologic: eosinophilia, *leukopenia, thrombocytopenia, hemolytic anemia.*
Respiratory: *apnea.*
Skin: *exfoliative dermatitis.*
Other: hypersensitivity reactions (rash, fever, urticaria, angioedema), *anaphylaxis.*

INTERACTIONS
Drug-drug. *Cephalosporins:* increased nephrotoxicity. Use together cautiously.
Dimenhydrinate: may mask symptoms of streptomycin-induced ototoxicity. Use together cautiously.
General anesthetics, neuromuscular blockers: may potentiate neuromuscular blockade. Monitor closely.
I.V. loop diuretics (such as furosemide): increased ototoxicity. Use together cautiously.
Other aminoglycosides, acyclovir, amphotericin B, cisplatin, methoxyflurane, vancomycin: increased nephrotoxicity. Use together cautiously.

EFFECTS ON DIAGNOSTIC TESTS
Streptomycin may cause a false-positive reaction in copper sulfate tests for urine glucose (Benedict's reagent or Diastix). Streptomycin-induced nephrotoxicity may elevate levels of BUN, nonprotein nitrogen, or serum creatinine, and increase urinary excretion of casts.

Reactions may be *common*, uncommon, *life-threatening*, or COMMON AND LIFE-THREATENING.

CONTRAINDICATIONS
Contraindicated in patients with hypersensitivity to drug or other aminoglycosides.

NURSING CONSIDERATIONS
• Use cautiously in patients with impaired renal function or neuromuscular disorders and in elderly patients.
• Evaluate patient's hearing before and during therapy. Notify doctor if patient complains of tinnitus, vertigo, or hearing loss.
Alert: Never administer streptomycin I.V.
• Obtain specimen for culture and sensitivity tests before giving first dose except when treating tuberculosis. Therapy may begin pending results.
• Evaluate patient's hearing before therapy and for 6 months afterward. Notify doctor if patient complains of hearing loss, roaring noises, or fullness in ears.
• Protect hands when preparing because drug is irritating.
• For I.M. administration, inject deeply into upper outer quadrant of buttocks. Rotate injection sites.
• Obtain blood for peak streptomycin level 1 to 2 hours after I.M. injection; for trough levels, draw blood just before next dose. Don't use a heparinized tube because heparin is incompatible with aminoglycosides.
• Watch for signs of superinfection (continued fever and other signs of new infection).
• Be aware that in primary treatment of tuberculosis, streptomycin is discontinued when sputum becomes negative.

☑ Patient teaching
• Instruct patient to report adverse reactions promptly.
• Encourage adequate fluid intake.
• Emphasize the need for blood tests to monitor streptomycin levels and determine the effectiveness of therapy.

tobramycin sulfate
Nebcin, TOBI

Pregnancy Risk Category: D

HOW SUPPLIED
Multidose vials: 80 mg/2 ml, 20 mg/2 ml (pediatric)
Premixed parenteral injection for I.V. infusion: 60 mg or 80 mg in 0.9% NaCl solution
Nebulizer solution (for inhalation): 300 mg/5 ml

ACTION
Inhibits protein synthesis by binding directly to the 30S ribosomal subunit. Generally bactericidal.

Route	Onset	Peak	Duration
IV	Immediate	Immediate	8 hr
IM	Unknown	30-90 min	8 hr
Inhalation	Unknown	Unknown	Unknown

INDICATIONS & DOSAGE
Serious infections caused by sensitive strains of Escherichia coli, Proteus, Klebsiella, Enterobacter, Serratia, Morganella morganii, Staphylococcus aureus, Pseudomonas, Citrobacter, *and* Providencia—
Adults: 3 mg/kg I.M. or I.V. daily in divided doses. Up to 5 mg/kg daily divided q 6 to 8 hours for life-threatening infections; this dosage should be reduced to 3 mg/kg daily as soon as clinically indicated.
Children: 6 to 7.5 mg/kg I.M. or I.V. daily in three or four divided doses.
Neonates under 1 week or premature infants: up to 4 mg/kg/day I.V. or I.M. in two equal doses q 12 hours.
Adjust-a-dose: For patients with renal impairment, loading dose is 1 mg/kg followed by decreased doses at 8 hour intervals or the same dose at prolonged intervals.
Management of cystic fibrosis patients with Pseudomonas aeruginosa—
Adults and children 6 years and older: 300 mg via nebulizer q 12 hours for 28 days (cycle of 28 days on drug and 28 days off drug).

ADVERSE REACTIONS
CNS: headache, lethargy, confusion, disorientation, *seizures*.
EENT: *ototoxicity*, hoarseness, *pharyngitis*.
GI: vomiting, nausea, diarrhea.

GU: *nephrotoxicity.*
Hematologic: anemia, eosinophilia, *leukopenia, thrombocytopenia, agranulocytosis.*
Musculoskeletal: muscle twitching.
Respiratory: bronchospasm.
Skin: fever, rash, urticaria, pruritus.
Other: electrolyte imbalances.

INTERACTIONS
Drug-drug. *Cephalosporins:* increased nephrotoxicity. Use together cautiously.
Dimenhydrinate: may mask symptoms of ototoxicity. Use with caution.
General anesthetics, neuromuscular blockers: may potentiate neuromuscular blockade. Monitor closely.
I.V. loop diuretics (such as furosemide): increased ototoxicity. Use together cautiously.
Other aminoglycosides, acyclovir, amphotericin B, cisplatin, methoxyflurane, vancomycin: increased nephrotoxicity. Use together cautiously.
Parenteral penicillins (such as ticarcillin): tobramycin inactivation in vitro. Don't mix together.

EFFECTS ON DIAGNOSTIC TESTS
Tobramycin may elevate BUN, nonprotein nitrogen, or serum creatinine levels and increase urinary excretion of casts.

CONTRAINDICATIONS
Contraindicated in patients with hypersensitivity to drug or other aminoglycosides.

NURSING CONSIDERATIONS
• Use cautiously in patients with impaired renal function or neuromuscular disorders and in elderly patients.
• Obtain specimen for culture and sensitivity tests before giving first dose. Therapy may begin pending results.
• Weigh patient and review renal function studies before therapy.
• Evaluate patient's hearing before and during therapy. Notify doctor if patient complains of tinnitus, vertigo, or hearing loss.
• Administer nebulizer solution over 10 to 15 minutes using hand-held Pari LC Plus reusable nebulizer with DeVilbiss Pulmo-Aide compressor.
• Do not dilute or mix TOBI with dornase alpha in the nebulizer.
• Obtain blood for peak level 1 hour after I.M. injection and ½ to 1 hour after infusion ends; draw blood for trough level just before next dose. Don't collect blood in a heparinized tube because heparin is incompatible with aminoglycosides.
Alert: Be aware that blood levels over 10 mcg/ml and trough levels above 2 mcg/ml may be associated with increased incidence of toxicity.
• Monitor renal function (output, specific gravity, urinalysis, creatinine clearance, and BUN and creatinine levels). Notify doctor of signs of decreasing renal function.
• Watch for signs of superinfection (continued fever and other signs of new infection).
• Be aware that if no response occurs in 3 to 5 days, therapy may be stopped and new specimens obtained for culture and sensitivity testing.

⬛ I.V. administration
• Dilute in 50 to 100 ml of 0.9% NaCl solution or D_5W for adults and in lesser volume for children. Infuse over 20 to 60 minutes. After I.V. infusion, flush line with 0.9% NaCl solution or D_5W.

☑ Patient teaching
• Instruct patient to report adverse reactions promptly.
• Caution patient not to perform hazardous activities if adverse CNS reactions occur.
• Encourage adequate fluid intake.
• Instruct patient on how to use and maintain nebulizer.
• Tell patient on multiple inhaled therapies to use TOBI last.
• Tell patient not to use TOBI if it is cloudy, if there are particles in the solution, or if it has been stored at room temperature for more than 28 days.

---

amoxicillin/clavulanate potassium
amoxicillin trihydrate
ampicillin
ampicillin sodium
ampicillin trihydrate
ampicillin sodium/sulbactam
  sodium
cloxacillin sodium
dicloxacillin sodium
mezlocillin sodium
nafcillin sodium
oxacillin sodium
penicillin G benzathine
penicillin G potassium
penicillin G procaine
penicillin G sodium
penicillin V
penicillin V potassium
piperacillin sodium
piperacillin sodium/tazobactam
  sodium
ticarcillin disodium
ticarcillin disodium/clavulanate
  potassium

COMBINATION PRODUCTS
AUGMENTIN, CLAVULIN†: amoxicillin
250 mg and clavulanate potassium
125 mg/tablet; amoxicillin 500 mg and
clavulanate potassium 125 mg/tablet;
amoxicillin 125 mg and clavulanate
potassium 31.25 mg/chewable tablet;
amoxicillin 250 mg and clavulanate
potassium 62.5 mg/chewable tablet;
amoxicillin 125 mg and clavulanate
potassium 31.25 mg/5 ml oral suspension;
amoxicillin 200 mg and clavulanate
potassium 28.5 mg/5 ml oral suspension;
amoxicillin 250 mg and clavulanate
potassium 62.5 mg/5 ml oral suspension;
amoxicillin 400 mg and clavulanate
potassium 57 mg/5 ml oral suspension.

amoxicillin/clavulanate potassium (amoxycillin/clavulanate potassium)
Augmentin, Clavulin†

Pregnancy Risk Category: B

HOW SUPPLIED
Tablets (chewable): 125 mg amoxicillin
trihydrate, 31.25 mg clavulanic acid;
200 mg amoxicillin trihydrate, 28.5 mg
clavulanic acid; 250 mg amoxicillin trihydrate, 62.5 mg clavulanic acid
Tablets (film-coated): 250 mg amoxicillin
trihydrate, 125 mg clavulanic acid;
500 mg amoxicillin trihydrate, 125 mg
clavulanic acid; 875 mg amoxicillin trihydrate, 125 mg clavulanic acid
Oral suspension: 125 mg amoxicillin trihydrate and 31.25 mg clavulanic acid/
5 ml (after reconstitution); 200 mg amoxicillin trihydrate and 28.5 mg clavulanic
acid/5 ml (after reconstitution); 250 mg
amoxicillin trihydrate and 62.5 mg clavulanic acid/5 ml (after reconstitution);
400 mg amoxicillin trihydrate and 57 mg
clavulanic acid/5 ml (after reconstitution)

ACTION
An aminopenicillin that prevents bacterial
cell-wall synthesis during replication.
Clavulanic acid increases amoxicillin effectiveness by inactivating beta lactamases, which destroy amoxicillin.

Route	Onset	Peak	Duration
PO	Unknown	1-2.5 hr	6-8 hr

INDICATIONS & DOSAGE
*Lower respiratory infections, otitis media,
sinusitis, skin and skin-structure infections, and urinary tract infections caused
by susceptible strains of gram-positive
and gram-negative organisms—*
**Adults and children weighing 40 kg
(88 lb) or over:** 250 mg (based on the
amoxicillin component) P.O. q 8 hours or
500 mg q 12 hours. For more severe in-

fections, 500 mg q 8 hours or 875 mg P.O. q 12 hours.

Children 3 months old or older weighing under 40 kg: 20 to 45 mg/kg (based on the amoxicillin component and severity of infection) P.O. daily in divided doses q 8 to 12 hours.

Children less than 3 months old: 30 mg/kg/day P.O. divided q 12 hours based on the amoxicillin component. Use of the 125 mg/5 ml oral suspension is recommended.

Adjust-a-dose: Do not give the 875-mg tablet to patients with renal impairment and creatinine clearance below 30 ml/minute. If creatinine clearance is 30 to 10 ml/minute, reduce dosage to 250 to 500 mg P.O. q 12 hours. If creatinine clearance is below 10 ml/minute, reduce dosage to 250 to 500 mg P.O. q 24 hours.

ADVERSE REACTIONS

CNS: agitation, anxiety, insomnia, confusion, behavioral changes, dizziness.
GI: *nausea,* vomiting, *diarrhea,* indigestion, gastritis, stomatitis, glossitis, black "hairy" tongue, enterocolitis, pseudomembranous colitis.
Hematologic: anemia, ***thrombocytopenia,*** thrombocytopenic purpura, eosinophilia, ***leukopenia, agranulocytosis.***
Other: hypersensitivity reactions (erythematous maculopapular rash, urticaria, ***anaphylaxis***), overgrowth of nonsusceptible organisms, vaginitis.

INTERACTIONS

Drug-drug. *Allopurinol:* increased incidence of rash. Monitor patient.
Oral contraceptives: efficacy of oral contraceptives may be decreased. Recommend additional form of contraception during penicillin therapy.
Probenecid: increased blood levels of amoxicillin and other penicillins. Probenecid may be used for this purpose.

EFFECTS ON DIAGNOSTIC TESTS

Amoxicillin/clavulanate potassium alters results of urine glucose tests that use cupric sulfate (Benedict's reagent or Clinitest). Make urine glucose determinations with glucose oxidase methods (Chemstrip uG). Positive Coombs' tests have been re-

ported with other clavulanate combinations. Amoxicillin may falsely decrease serum aminoglycoside concentrations.

CONTRAINDICATIONS

Contraindicated in patients with hypersensitivity to drug or other penicillins and in those with a previous history of amoxicillin-associated cholestatic jaundice or hepatic dysfunction.

NURSING CONSIDERATIONS

• Use cautiously in patients with other drug allergies, especially to cephalosporins (possible cross-sensitivity), and in those with mononucleosis (high incidence of maculopapular rash).
• Before giving, ask patient about allergic reactions to penicillin. However, not having a history of penicillin allergy is no guarantee against an allergic reaction.
• Obtain specimen for culture and sensitivity tests before giving first dose. Therapy may begin pending results.
• Give drug at least 1 hour before bacteriostatic antibiotics.
• Observe closely. With large doses and prolonged therapy, bacterial or fungal superinfection may occur, especially in elderly, debilitated, or immunosuppressed patients.
• Avoid use of 250-mg tablet in children weighing below 40 kg. Use chewable form instead.
Alert: Know that both 250-mg and 500-mg film-coated tablets contain the same amount of clavulanic acid (125 mg). Therefore, two 250 mg tablets are not equivalent to one 500 mg tablet.
• Be aware that this drug combination is particularly useful in clinical settings with a high prevalence of amoxicillin-resistant organisms.
• After reconstitution, refrigerate the oral suspension; discard after 10 days.

☑ Patient teaching

• Tell patient to take entire quantity of drug exactly as prescribed, even after feeling better.
• Instruct patient to take drug with food to prevent GI upset. If he is taking the oral suspension, tell him to keep drug refrigerated, to shake it well before administra-

---

tion, and to discard remaining drug after 10 days.
• Tell patient to call doctor if a rash occurs. A rash is a sign of an allergic reaction.

amoxicillin trihydrate (amoxycillin trihydrate)
Alphamox‡, Ampexin‡, Amoxil, Apo-Amoxi†, Cilamox‡, Moxacin‡, Novamoxin†, Nu-Amoxi†, Polymox, Trimox, Wymox

Pregnancy Risk Category: B

HOW SUPPLIED
Tablets (chewable): 125 mg, 250 mg
Capsules: 250 mg, 500 mg
Oral suspension: 50 mg/ml (pediatric drops), 125 mg/5 ml, 250 mg/5 ml (after reconstitution)

ACTION
An aminopenicillin that inhibits cell-wall synthesis during bacterial multiplication; bacteria resist amoxicillin by producing penicillinases—enzymes that hydrolyze amoxicillin.

Route	Onset	Peak	Duration
PO	Unknown	1-2 hr	6-8 hr

INDICATIONS & DOSAGE
Systemic infections, acute and chronic urinary tract infections caused by susceptible strains of gram-positive and gram-negative organisms—
Adults and children weighing 20 kg (44 lb) or over: 250 to 500 mg P.O. q 8 hours.
Children weighing under 20 kg: 20 mg/kg P.O. daily in divided doses q 8 hours; in severe infection, 40 mg/kg P.O. daily in divided doses q 8 hours or 500 mg to 1 g/m² P.O. in divided doses q 8 hours.
Uncomplicated gonorrhea—
Adults and children weighing over 45 kg (99 lb): 3 g P.O. with 1 g probenecid given as a single dose.
Children 2 years and older weighing under 45 kg: 50 mg/kg (maximum of 3 g) P.O. with 25 mg/kg (up to 1 g) of

probenecid as a single dose. Do not give probenecid to children under 2 years.
Endocarditis prophylaxis for dental procedures—
Adults: 2 g P.O. 1 hour before procedure.
Children: 50 mg/kg P.O. 1 hour before procedure.

ADVERSE REACTIONS
CNS: lethargy, hallucinations, *seizures,* anxiety, confusion, agitation, depression, dizziness, fatigue.
GI: *nausea,* vomiting, *diarrhea,* glossitis, stomatitis, gastritis, abdominal pain, enterocolitis, pseudomembranous colitis, black "hairy" tongue.
GU: interstitial nephritis, nephropathy.
Hematologic: anemia, *thrombocytopenia,* thrombocytopenic purpura, eosinophilia, *leukopenia,* hemolytic anemia, *agranulocytosis.*
Other: hypersensitivity reactions (erythematous maculopapular rash, urticaria, *anaphylaxis*), overgrowth of nonsusceptible organisms, vaginitis.

INTERACTIONS
Drug-drug. *Allopurinol:* increased incidence of rash. Monitor patient.
Oral contraceptives: efficacy of oral contraceptives may be decreased. Recommend additional form of contraception during penicillin therapy.
Probenecid: increased blood levels of amoxicillin and other penicillins. Probenecid may be used for this purpose.

EFFECTS ON DIAGNOSTIC TESTS
Amoxicillin may alter results of urine glucose tests that use cupric sulfate (Benedict's reagent or Clinitest). Make urine glucose determinations with glucose oxidase methods (Diastix or Chemstrip uG). Amoxicillin may falsely decrease serum aminoglycoside concentrations and cause a positive Coombs' test.

CONTRAINDICATIONS
Contraindicated in patients with hypersensitivity to drug or other penicillins.

NURSING CONSIDERATIONS
• Use cautiously in patients with other drug allergies, especially to cephalo-

---

*Liquid contains alcohol. **May contain tartrazine. †Canada ‡Australia §U.K. ◊OTC

sporins (possible cross-sensitivity), and in those with mononucleosis (high incidence of maculopapular rash).

• Before giving, ask patient about allergic reactions to penicillin. Not having a history of penicillin allergy is no guarantee against allergic reaction.

• Obtain specimen for culture and sensitivity tests before giving first dose. Therapy may begin pending results.

• Give amoxicillin at least 1 hour before bacteriostatic antibiotics.

• Observe closely. With large doses and prolonged therapy, superinfection may occur, especially in elderly, debilitated, or immunosuppressed patients.

• Store Trimox oral suspension at room temperature for up to 2 weeks. Be sure to check individual product labels for storage information.

• Keep in mind that amoxicillin generally causes diarrhea in fewer cases than ampicillin.

☑ Patient teaching
• Tell patient to take entire quantity of medication exactly as prescribed, even after he feels better.

• Instruct patient to take drug with food.

• Tell patient to notify doctor if rash, fever, or chills develop. A rash is the most common allergic reaction, especially if allopurinol is also being taken.

ampicillin
Apo-Ampi†, Novo Ampicillin†, Nu-Ampi†, Omnipen, Principen

ampicillin sodium
Ampicin†, Ampicyn‡, Omnipen-N, Penbritin†, Polycillin-N, Totacillin-N

ampicillin trihydrate
Omnipen, Penbritin†, Polycillin, Principen, Totacillin

Pregnancy Risk Category: B

HOW SUPPLIED
Capsules: 250 mg, 500 mg
Oral suspension: 100 mg/ml (pediatric drops), 125 mg/5 ml, 250 mg/5 ml, 500 mg/5 ml (after reconstitution)

Injection: 125 mg, 250 mg, 500 mg, 1 g, 2 g

ACTION
An aminopenicillin that inhibits cell-wall synthesis during microorganism multiplication; bacteria resist ampicillin by producing penicillinases—enzymes that hydrolyze ampicillin.

Route	Onset	Peak	Duration
PO	Unknown	2 hr	6-8 hr
IV	Immediate	Immediate	Unknown
IM	Unknown	1 hr	Unknown

INDICATIONS & DOSAGE
Systemic infections and acute and chronic urinary tract infections caused by susceptible strains of gram-positive and gram-negative organisms—
Adults and children weighing 40 kg (88 lb) or more: 250 to 500 mg P.O. q 6 hours, or 1 to 12 g I.M. or I.V. daily in divided doses q 4 to 6 hours.
Children weighing less than 40 kg: 25 to 100 mg/kg/day P.O. in equally divided doses q 6 hours, or 25 to 50 mg/kg/day I.M. or I.V. in divided doses q 6 to 8 hours. Pediatric dosages should not exceed recommended adult dosages.
Meningitis—
Adults: 150 to 200 mg/kg/day I.V. in divided doses q 3 to 4 hours. May be given I.M. after 3 days of I.V. therapy.
Children: 100 to 200 mg/kg I.V. daily in divided doses q 3 to 4 hours. Give I.V. for 3 days then give I.M.
Uncomplicated gonorrhea—
Adults and children weighing more than 45 kg (99 lb): 3.5 g P.O. with 1 g probenecid given as a single dose.
Endocarditis prophylaxis for dental procedures—
Adults: 2 g I.M. or I.V. within 30 minutes before procedure.
Children: 50 mg/kg I.M. or I.V. within 30 minutes before procedure.

ADVERSE REACTIONS
CNS: lethargy, hallucinations, *seizures,* anxiety, confusion, agitation, depression, dizziness, fatigue.
GI: *nausea,* vomiting, *diarrhea,* glossitis, stomatitis, gastritis, abdominal pain, ente-

rocolitis, pseudomembranous colitis, black "hairy" tongue.
GU: interstitial nephritis, nephropathy.
Hematologic: anemia, ***thrombocytopenia,*** thrombocytopenic purpura, eosinophilia, ***leukopenia,*** hemolytic anemia, ***agranulocytosis.***
Other: hypersensitivity reactions (erythematous maculopapular rash, urticaria, ***anaphylaxis***), overgrowth of nonsusceptible organisms, pain at injection site, vein irritation, thrombophlebitis, vaginitis.

INTERACTIONS
Drug-drug. *Allopurinol:* increased incidence of rash. Monitor patient.
Oral contraceptives: efficacy of oral contraceptives may be decreased. Recommend additional contraception during penicillin therapy.
Probenecid: increased blood levels of ampicillin and other penicillins. Probenecid may be used for this purpose.

EFFECTS ON DIAGNOSTIC TESTS
Drug alters results of urine glucose tests that use cupric sulfate (Benedict's reagent or Clinitest). Make urine glucose determinations with glucose oxidase methods (Diastix or Chemstrip uG). Ampicillin may falsely decrease serum aminoglycoside concentrations.

CONTRAINDICATIONS
Contraindicated in patients with hypersensitivity to drug or other penicillins.

NURSING CONSIDERATIONS
• Use cautiously in patients with other drug allergies, especially to cephalosporins (possible cross-sensitivity), or in those with mononucleosis (high incidence of maculopapular rash).
• Before giving, ask patient about allergic reactions to penicillin. However, not having a history of penicillin allergy is no guarantee against a future allergic reaction.
• Obtain specimen for culture and sensitivity tests before giving first dose. Therapy may begin pending results.
• Give drug I.M. or I.V. only if prescribed and the infection is severe or if patient can't take oral dose.

• Administer 1 to 2 hours before or 2 to 3 hours after meals. When given orally, drug may cause GI disturbances. Food may interfere with absorption.
• Give ampicillin at least 1 hour before bacteriostatic antibiotics.
• Observe closely. With large doses or prolonged therapy, bacterial or fungal superinfection may occur, especially in elderly, debilitated, or immunosuppressed patients.
• Know that dosage should be altered in patients with impaired renal function.
• Be aware that in pediatric meningitis, ampicillin may be given concurrently with parenteral chloramphenicol for 24 hours pending cultures.

🔳 I.V. administration
• For I.V. injection, reconstitute with bacteriostatic water for injection. Use 5 ml for the 125-mg, 250-mg, or 500-mg vials; 7.4 ml for the 1-g vials; or 14.8 ml for the 2-g vials. Give direct I.V. injections over 3 to 5 minutes for doses of 500 mg or less; over 10 to 15 minutes for larger doses. Do not exceed a rate of 100 mg/minute. Alternatively, dilute in 50 to 100 ml of 0.9% NaCl for injection and give by intermittent infusion over 15 to 30 minutes.
Alert: Do not mix with solutions containing dextrose or fructose because these promote rapid breakdown of ampicillin.
• Use initial dilution within 1 hour. Follow manufacturer's directions for stability data when ampicillin is further diluted for I.V. infusion.
• Give I.V. intermittently to prevent vein irritation. Change site every 48 hours.

✅ Patient teaching
• Tell patient to take entire quantity of medication exactly as prescribed, even after he feels better.
• Instruct patient to take oral form on an empty stomach 1 hour before or 2 hours after meals.
• Tell patient to notify doctor if rash, fever, or chills develop. A rash is the most common allergic reaction, especially if allopurinol is also being taken.
• Instruct patient to report discomfort at I.V. injection site.

---

ampicillin sodium/sulbactam sodium
Unasyn

Pregnancy Risk Category: B

HOW SUPPLIED
Injection: vials and piggyback vials containing 1.5 g (1 g ampicillin sodium with 0.5 g sulbactam sodium), 3 g (2 g ampicillin sodium with 1 g sulbactam sodium), and 10 g (10 g ampicillin sodium with 5 g sulbactam sodium).

ACTION
An aminopenicillin that inhibits cell-wall synthesis during microorganism multiplication; sulbactam inactivates bacterial beta-lactamase, which inactivates ampicillin and causes bacterial resistance to it.

Route	Peak	Onset	Duration
IV	15 min	Immediate	Unknown
IM	Unknown	Unknown	Unknown

INDICATIONS & DOSAGE
Intra-abdominal, gynecologic, and skin-structure infections caused by susceptible strains—
Adults and children weighing over 40 kg (88 lb): dosage expressed as total drug (each 1.5-g vial contains 1 g ampicillin sodium and 0.5 g sulbactam sodium)—1.5 to 3 g I.M. or I.V. q 6 hours. Maximum daily dosage is 4 g sulbactam and 8 g ampicillin (12 g of combined drugs).
Children 1 year and over weighing below 40 kg: 300 mg/kg/day (200 mg ampicillin/100 mg sulbactam) I.V. in divided doses q 6 hours. Do not exceed 4 g per day.
Adjust-a-dose: In renally impaired patients, if creatinine clearance is 15 to 29 ml/minute, give 1.5 to 3 g q 12 hours; if creatinine clearance is 5 to 14 ml/minute, give 1.5 to 3 g q 24 hours.

ADVERSE REACTIONS
CV: vein irritation, thrombophlebitis.
GI: *nausea,* vomiting, *diarrhea,* glossitis, stomatitis, gastritis, black "hairy" tongue, enterocolitis, pseudomembranous colitis.
GU: increased BUN, creatinine.
Hematologic: anemia, ***thrombocytopenia,*** thrombocytopenic purpura, eosinophilia, ***leukopenia, agranulocytosis.***
Hepatic: increased liver function tests.
Other: hypersensitivity reactions (erythematous maculopapular rash, urticaria, ***anaphylaxis***), ***overgrowth of nonsusceptible organisms,*** pain at injection site.

INTERACTIONS
Drug-drug. *Allopurinol:* increased incidence of rash. Monitor patient.
Oral contraceptives: efficacy of oral contraceptives may be decreased. Recommend additional form of contraception during penicillin therapy.
Probenecid: increased levels of ampicillin. Probenecid may be used for this purpose.

EFFECTS ON DIAGNOSTIC TESTS
Ampicillin alters results of urine glucose tests that use cupric sulfate (Benedict's reagent or Clinitest). Make urine glucose determinations with glucose oxidase methods (Diastix). In pregnant women, transient decreases in serum estradiol, conjugated estrone, conjugated estriol, and estriol glucuronide may occur.

CONTRAINDICATIONS
Contraindicated in patients with hypersensitivity to drug or other penicillins.

NURSING CONSIDERATIONS
• Use cautiously in patients with other drug allergies, especially to cephalosporins (possible cross-sensitivity), or in those with mononucleosis (high incidence of maculopapular rash).
• Before giving, ask patient about allergic reactions to penicillin. However, not having a history of penicillin allergy is no guarantee against a future allergic reaction.
• Obtain specimen for culture and sensitivity tests before giving first dose. Therapy may begin pending results.
• Monitor liver function tests during therapy, especially in patients with impaired liver function.
• Do not use I.M. route in children.
• For I.M. injection, reconstitute with

sterile water for injection or 0.5% or 2% lidocaine hydrochloride injection. Add 3.2 ml to a 1.5-g vial (or 6.4 ml to a 3-g vial) to yield a concentration of 375 mg/ml. Administer deeply.

• Observe closely. With large doses and prolonged therapy, bacterial or fungal superinfection may occur, especially in elderly, debilitated, or immunosuppressed patients.

• Know that dosage should be altered in patients with impaired renal function.

🖐 I.V. administration

• When preparing I.V. injection, reconstitute powder with the following diluents: 0.9% NaCl solution, sterile water for injection, D_5W, lactated Ringer's injection, 1/6 M sodium lactate, dextrose 5% and 0.45% NaCl for injection, and 10% invert sugar. Stability varies with diluent, temperature, and concentration of solution.

• After reconstitution, allow vials to stand for a few minutes for foam to dissipate. This will permit visual inspection of contents for particles.

• When giving I.V., don't add or mix with other drugs because they might prove incompatible.

• Give drug at least 1 hour before bacteriostatic antibiotics.

Alert: Give I.V. dose by slow injection (over 10 to 15 minutes), or dilute in 50 to 100 ml of a compatible diluent, and infuse over 15 to 30 minutes. If permitted, give intermittently to prevent vein irritation. Change site every 48 hours.

☑ Patient teaching

• Tell patient to report a rash, fever, or chills. A rash is the most common allergic reaction.

• Advise patient to report discomfort at I.V. insertion site.

• Warn patient that I.M. injection may cause pain at injection site.

cloxacillin sodium
Alclox‡, Apo-Cloxi†, Cloxapen, Novo-Cloxin†, Nu-Cloxi†, Orbenin†

Pregnancy Risk Category: B

HOW SUPPLIED
Capsules: 250 mg, 500 mg
Oral solution: 125 mg/5 ml (after reconstitution)

ACTION
A penicillinase-resistant penicillin that inhibits cell-wall synthesis during microorganism multiplication; bacteria resist penicillins by producing penicillinases—enzymes that convert penicillins to inactive penicillic acid. Cloxacillin resists these enzymes.

Route	Onset	Peak	Duration
PO	Unknown	2 hr	6 hr

INDICATIONS & DOSAGE
Systemic infections caused by penicillinase-producing staphylococci—
Adults and children weighing over 20 kg (44 lb): 250 to 500 mg P.O. q 6 hours.
Children weighing 20 kg or less: 50 to 100 mg/kg P.O. daily, in divided doses q 6 hours (maximum of 4 g daily).

ADVERSE REACTIONS
CNS: lethargy, hallucinations, *seizures,* anxiety, confusion, agitation, depression, dizziness, fatigue.
GI: nausea, vomiting, *epigastric distress, diarrhea,* enterocolitis, pseudomembranous colitis, black "hairy" tongue, abdominal pain.
GU: interstitial nephritis, nephropathy.
Hematologic: eosinophilia, anemia, *thrombocytopenia, leukopenia,* hemolytic anemia, *agranulocytosis.*
Other: hypersensitivity reactions (rash, urticaria, chills, fever, sneezing, wheezing, *anaphylaxis*), overgrowth of nonsusceptible organisms.

INTERACTIONS
Drug-drug. *Oral contraceptives:* efficacy

---

of oral contraceptives may be decreased. Recommend additional form of contraception during penicillin therapy.
Probenecid: increased blood levels of cloxacillin and other penicillins. Probenecid may be used for this purpose.
Drug-food. *Any food:* may interfere with absorption. Give 1 to 2 hours before or 2 to 3 hours after meals.
Carbonated beverages, fruit juice: inactivates drug. Do not give together.

EFFECTS ON DIAGNOSTIC TESTS

Drug alters test results for urine and serum proteins; it produces false-positive or elevated results in turbidimetric urine and serum protein tests using sulfosalicylic acid or trichloroacetic acid; it also reportedly produces false results on the Bradshaw screening test for Bence Jones protein.

Cloxacillin may cause transient elevations in liver function study results and transient reductions in RBC, WBC, and platelet counts. Elevated liver function test results may indicate drug-induced cholestasis or hepatitis. Cloxacillin may falsely decrease serum aminoglycoside levels.

CONTRAINDICATIONS

Contraindicated in patients with hypersensitivity to drug or other penicillins.

NURSING CONSIDERATIONS

• Use cautiously in patients with other drug allergies, especially to cephalosporins (possible cross-sensitivity), or in those with mononucleosis (high incidence of maculopapular rash).
• Before giving, ask patient about allergic reactions to penicillin. However, not having a history of penicillin allergy is no guarantee against a future allergic reaction.
• Obtain specimen for culture and sensitivity tests before giving first dose. Therapy may begin pending results.
• Give 1 to 2 hours before or 2 to 3 hours after meals. Drug may cause GI disturbances. Food may interfere with its absorption.
• Give cloxacillin at least 1 hour before bacteriostatic antibiotics.

• As ordered, periodically assess renal, hepatic, and hematopoietic function in patients receiving long-term therapy.
• Observe closely. With large doses and prolonged therapy, bacterial or fungal superinfection may occur, especially in elderly, debilitated, or immunosuppressed patients.

✓ Patient teaching
• Tell patient to take entire quantity of medication exactly as prescribed, even after he feels better.
• Instruct patient to take drug on an empty stomach.
Alert: Instruct patient to take each dose with full glass of water, not with fruit juice or carbonated beverage, because their acid will inactivate the drug.
• Tell patient to notify doctor if rash, fever, or chills develop. A rash is the most common allergic reaction.

---

dicloxacillin sodium
Diclocil‡, Dycill, Dynapen, Pathocil

Pregnancy Risk Category: B

HOW SUPPLIED
Capsules: 125 mg, 250 mg, 500 mg
Oral suspension: 62.5 mg/5 ml (after reconstitution)

ACTION
A penicillinase-resistant penicillin that inhibits cell-wall synthesis during microorganism multiplication; bacteria resist penicillins by producing penicillinases—enzymes that convert penicillins to inactive penicillic acid. Dicloxacillin resists these enzymes.

Route	Onset	Peak	Duration
PO	Unknown	2 hr	6 hr

INDICATIONS & DOSAGE
Systemic infections caused by penicillinase-producing staphylococci—
Adults and children weighing over 40 kg (88 lb): 125 to 250 mg P.O. q 6 hours.
Children weighing 40 kg or less: 12.5 to

25 mg/kg P.O. daily, in divided doses q 6 hours depending on severity.

ADVERSE REACTIONS

CNS: neuromuscular irritability, *seizures,* lethargy, hallucinations, anxiety, confusion, agitation, depression, dizziness, fatigue.
GI: *nausea,* vomiting, *epigastric distress,* flatulence, *diarrhea,* enterocolitis, pseudomembranous colitis, black "hairy" tongue, abdominal pain.
GU: interstitial nephritis, nephropathy.
Hematologic: eosinophilia, anemia, *thrombocytopenia,* eosinophilia, *leukopenia,* hemolytic anemia, *agranulocytosis.*
Other: hypersensitivity reactions (pruritus, urticaria, rash, *anaphylaxis*), overgrowth of nonsusceptible organisms.

INTERACTIONS

Drug-drug. *Oral contraceptives:* efficacy of oral contraceptives may be decreased. Recommend additional form of contraception during penicillin therapy.
Probenecid: increased blood levels of dicloxacillin and other penicillins. Probenecid may be used for this purpose.

EFFECTS ON DIAGNOSTIC TESTS

Drug alters test results for urine and serum proteins; it produces false-positive or elevated results in turbidimetric urine and serum protein tests using sulfosalicylic acid or trichloroacetic acid; it also reportedly produces false results on the Bradshaw screening test for Bence Jones protein.

Dicloxacillin may cause transient elevations in liver function study results and transient reductions in RBC, WBC, and platelet counts. Elevated liver function test results may indicate drug-induced cholestasis or hepatitis. Drug may falsely decrease serum aminoglycoside levels.

CONTRAINDICATIONS

Contraindicated in patients with hypersensitivity to drug or other penicillins. It is not recommended for use in newborns.

NURSING CONSIDERATIONS

• Use cautiously in patients with other drug allergies, especially to cephalosporins (possible cross-sensitivity), or in those with mononucleosis (high incidence of maculopapular rash).
• Before giving, ask patient about allergic reactions to penicillin. However, not having a history of penicillin allergy is no guarantee against a future allergic reaction.
• Obtain specimen for culture and sensitivity tests before giving first dose. Therapy may begin pending results.
• Give 1 to 2 hours before or 2 to 3 hours after meals. Drug may cause GI disturbances. Food may interfere with absorption.
• Give dicloxacillin at least 1 hour before bacteriostatic antibiotics.
• As ordered, periodically assess renal, hepatic, and hematopoietic function in patients receiving long-term therapy.
• Observe closely. With large doses and prolonged therapy, bacterial or fungal superinfection may occur, especially in elderly, debilitated, or immunosuppressed patients.

✓ Patient teaching

• Tell patient to take entire quantity of medication exactly as prescribed, even after he feels better.
• Instruct patient to take drug on an empty stomach.
• Tell patient to notify doctor if rash, fever, or chills develop. A rash is the most common allergic reaction.

---

mezlocillin sodium
Mezlin

Pregnancy Risk Category: B

HOW SUPPLIED
Injection: 1 g, 2 g, 3 g, 4 g

ACTION
An extended-spectrum penicillin that inhibits cell-wall synthesis during microorganism multiplication; bacteria resist mezlocillin by producing penicillinases—enzymes that hydrolyze mezlocillin.

Route	Onset	Peak	Duration
IV	Immediate	Immediate	Unknown
IM	Unknown	45-90 min	Unknown

INDICATIONS & DOSAGE

Systemic infections caused by susceptible strains of gram-positive and especially gram-negative organisms (including Proteus *and* Pseudomonas aeruginosa)—
Adults: 200 to 300 mg/kg daily I.V. or I.M. in four to six divided doses. Usual dose is 3 g q 4 hours or 4 g q 6 hours. For serious infections, up to 24 g daily may be administered.
Children 1 month to 12 years: 50 mg/kg q 4 hours I.V. or I.M.
Adjust-a-dose: In renally impaired patients, if creatinine clearance is below 30 mg/dl or serum creatinine exceeds 3 mg/dl, use reduced dosage.

ADVERSE REACTIONS

CNS: neuromuscular irritability, *seizures.*
GI: nausea, diarrhea, vomiting, abnormal taste sensation, pseudomembranous colitis.
GU: interstitial nephritis.
Hematologic: *bleeding* (with high doses), *neutropenia, thrombocytopenia*, eosinophilia, *leukopenia, hemolytic anemia*.
Other: hypersensitivity reactions (*anaphylaxis,* edema, fever, chills, rash, pruritus, urticaria), overgrowth of nonsusceptible organisms, *hypokalemia*, pain at injection site, vein irritation, phlebitis.

INTERACTIONS

Drug-drug. *Aminoglycoside antibiotics (such as amikacin, gentamicin, tobramycin):* chemically incompatible. Do not mix together in I.V. solution. Give 1 hour apart, especially in patients with renal insufficiency.
Oral contraceptives: efficacy of oral contraceptives may be decreased. Recommend additional form of contraception during penicillin therapy.
Probenecid: increased blood levels of mezlocillin. Probenecid may be used for this purpose.
Vecuronium: prolonged neuromuscular blockade. Use with caution.

EFFECTS ON DIAGNOSTIC TESTS

Drug alters tests for urine or serum proteins; it interferes with turbidimetric methods that use sulfosalicylic acid, trichloroacetic acid, acetic acid, or nitric acid. Mezlocillin does not interfere with tests using bromphenol blue (Albustix, Albutest, Multistix). Positive Coombs' tests have been reported in patients taking mezlocillin. Drug may prolong PT. It may also cause transient elevations in liver function test results and transient reductions in RBC, WBC, and platelet counts.

CONTRAINDICATIONS

Contraindicated in patients with hypersensitivity to drug or other penicillins.

NURSING CONSIDERATIONS

• Use cautiously in patients with other drug allergies, especially to cephalosporins (possible cross-sensitivity), or in those with bleeding tendencies, uremia, or hypokalemia.
• Before giving, ask patient about allergic reactions to penicillin. Not having a history of penicillin allergy, however, is no guarantee against future allergic reaction.
• Obtain specimen for culture and sensitivity tests before giving first dose. Therapy may begin pending results.
• When giving I.M., do not give more than 2 g per injection. Inject deeply and slowly (12 to 15 seconds) into the body of a large muscle.
• Check CBC and platelet counts frequently, as ordered. Drug may cause thrombocytopenia.
• Monitor serum potassium level.
Alert: Institute seizure precautions. Patients with high serum levels of drug may have seizures.
• Observe closely. With large doses and prolonged therapy, bacterial or fungal superinfection may occur, especially in elderly, debilitated, or immunosuppressed patients.
• Be aware that dosage should be altered in patients with impaired renal function.
• Be aware that drug is almost always used with another antibiotic, such as gentamicin.

◨ I.V. administration

• Reconstitute vials with at least 10 ml/g of drug using sterile water for injection, D_5W, or 0.9% NaCl for injection. Solutions with a concentration not exceeding 10% may be given by direct injection over

3 to 5 minutes. Alternatively, dilute in about 50 to 100 ml of suitable I.V. solution, and give by intermittent infusion over 30 minutes.
• Give I.V. intermittently to prevent vein irritation. Change site every 48 hours.
• Give mezlocillin at least 1 hour before bacteriostatic antibiotics.

☑ **Patient teaching**
• Instruct patient to report adverse reactions promptly.
• Tell patient to alert nurse if discomfort occurs at I.V. site.
• Caution patient to limit salt intake during mezlocillin therapy because of drug's high sodium content.

---

nafcillin sodium
Nafcil, Nallpen, Unipen

Pregnancy Risk Category: B

HOW SUPPLIED
Capsules: 250 mg
Tablets: 500 mg
Injection: 500 mg, 1 g, 2 g
I.V. infusion piggyback: 1 g, 2 g

ACTION
A penicillinase-resistant penicillin that inhibits cell-wall synthesis during microorganism multiplication; bacteria resist penicillins by producing penicillinases—enzymes that hydrolyze penicillins. Nafcillin resists these enzymes.

Route	Onset	Peak	Duration
PO	Unknown	0.5-2 hr	Unknown
IV	Immediate	Immediate	Unknown
IM	Unknown	0.5-1 hr	Unknown

INDICATIONS & DOSAGE
Systemic infections caused by penicillinase-producing staphylococci—
Adults: 250 to 500 mg P.O. q 4 to 6 hours (more severe infections may be treated with 1 g P.O. q 4 to 6 hours); or 500 mg I.M. q 4 to 6 hours or I.V. q 4 hours or (for more severe infections)1 g I.M. or I.V. q 4 hours.

Children older than 1 month and weighing below 40 kg (88 lb): 25 to 50 mg/kg P.O. daily, in divided doses q 6 hours; or 25 mg/kg I.M. b.i.d. or 100 to 200 mg/kg I.M. or I.V. daily in divided doses q 4 to 6 hours.
Neonates: 10 mg/kg I.M. b.i.d. or 10 mg/kg P.O. t.i.d. or q.i.d.

ADVERSE REACTIONS
GI: *nausea,* vomiting, diarrhea.
Hematologic: transient leukopenia, **neutropenia, agranulocytosis, thrombocytopenia** with high doses.
Other: hypersensitivity reactions (chills, fever, rash, pruritus, urticaria, **anaphylaxis**), vein irritation, thrombophlebitis.

INTERACTIONS
Drug-drug. *Aminoglycosides:* synergistic effect; monitor closely. Chemical and physical incompatibility. Do not mix together in same I.V. solution.
Oral contraceptives: efficacy of oral contraceptives may be decreased. Recommend additional form of contraception during penicillin therapy.
Probenecid: increased blood levels of nafcillin. Probenecid may be used for this purpose.
Rifampin: dose-dependent antagonism. Monitor closely.
Warfarin: increased risk of bleeding when used with I.V. nafcillin. Monitor PT and INR closely.

EFFECTS ON DIAGNOSTIC TESTS
Drug alters tests for urine and serum proteins; in many cases, turbidimetric urine and serum proteins are falsely positive or elevated in tests using sulfosalicylic acid or trichloroacetic acid. Nafcillin may cause transient reductions in RBC, WBC, and platelet counts. Abnormal urinalysis results may indicate drug-induced interstitial nephritis.

CONTRAINDICATIONS
Contraindicated in patients with hypersensitivity to drug or other penicillins.

NURSING CONSIDERATIONS
• Use cautiously in patients with other drug allergies, especially to cephalo-

---

sporins (possible cross-sensitivity), or in those with GI distress.

• Before giving, ask patient about allergic reactions to penicillin. However, not having a history of penicillin allergy is no guarantee against a future allergic reaction.

• Obtain specimen for culture and sensitivity tests before giving first dose. Therapy may begin pending results.

• Give 1 to 2 hours before or 2 to 3 hours after meals. When given orally, drug may cause GI disturbances. Food may interfere with absorption.

• Observe closely. With large doses and prolonged therapy, bacterial or fungal superinfection may occur, especially in elderly, debilitated, or immunosuppressed patients.

• Monitor serum sodium because each 1 g of nafcillin contains 2.9 mEq of sodium.

◖I.V. administration

• Reconstitute piggyback containers according to manufacturer's instructions. Reconstitute 500-mg, 1-g, or 2-g vials with sterile water for injection, D₅W, or 0.9% NaCl for injection. Add 1.7 ml for each 500 mg of drug. Reconstituted drug may be given I.M. Alternatively, dilute with 15 to 30 ml of sterile water for injection or 0.45% or 0.9% NaCl for injection, and give by direct injection into a vein or into the tubing of a free-flowing I.V. solution over 5 to 10 minutes. Or dilute drug to a concentration of 2 to 40 mg/ml, and give by intermittent I.V. infusion over 30 to 60 minutes.

• Avoid continuous I.V. infusions to prevent vein irritation. Change site every 48 hours.

• Give nafcillin at least 1 hour before bacteriostatic antibiotics.

☑Patient teaching

• Tell patient to take entire quantity of medication exactly as prescribed, even after he feels better.

• Instruct patient to take oral form of drug on an empty stomach.

• Tell patient to notify doctor if rash, fever, or chills develop. A rash is the most common allergic reaction.

oxacillin sodium
Bactocill

Pregnancy Risk Category: B

HOW SUPPLIED
Capsules: 250 mg, 500 mg
Oral solution: 250 mg/5 ml (after reconstitution)
Injection: 250 mg, 500 mg, 1 g, 2 g, 4 g
I.V. infusion: 1 g, 2 g, 4 g

ACTION
A penicillinase-resistant penicillin that inhibits cell-wall synthesis during microorganism multiplication; bacteria resist penicillins by producing penicillinases—enzymes that convert penicillins to inactive penicillic acid. Oxacillin resists these enzymes.

Route	Onset	Peak	Duration
PO	Unknown	0.5-2 hr	Unknown
IV	Immediate	Immediate	Unknown
IM	Unknown	0.5 hr	Unknown

INDICATIONS & DOSAGE
Systemic infections caused by penicillinase-producing staphylococci—
Adults and children weighing over 40 kg (88 lb): 500 mg to 1 g P.O. q 4 to 6 hours; or 250 mg to 1 g I.M. or I.V. every 4 to 6 hours.
Children older than 1 month and weighing 40 kg or less: 50 to 100 mg/kg P.O. daily, in divided doses q 6 hours; or 50 to 200 mg/kg I.M. or I.V. daily, in divided doses q 4 to 6 hours, depending on severity.

ADVERSE REACTIONS
CNS: neuropathy, neuromuscular irritability, *seizures,* lethargy, hallucinations, anxiety, confusion, agitation, depression, dizziness, fatigue.
GI: oral lesions, nausea, vomiting, diarrhea, enterocolitis, pseudomembranous colitis.
GU: interstitial nephritis, nephropathy.
Hematologic: *thrombocytopenia,* eosinophilia, *hemolytic anemia, neutropenia,* anemia, *agranulocytosis.*
Hepatic: elevated liver enzymes.

Other: hypersensitivity reactions (fever, chills, rash, urticaria, ***anaphylaxis***), overgrowth of nonsusceptible organisms, *thrombophlebitis*.

INTERACTIONS
Drug-drug. *Aminoglycosides:* possible synergistic effect. Monitor closely. Chemical and physical incompatibility. Do not mix together in same I.V. solution.
Oral contraceptives: efficacy of oral contraceptives may be decreased. Recommend additional form of contraception during penicillin therapy.
Probenecid: increased blood levels of oxacillin and other penicillins. Probenecid may be used for this purpose.
Rifampin: possible antagonism. Monitor closely.

EFFECTS ON DIAGNOSTIC TESTS
Drug alters tests for urine and serum proteins; in many cases, turbidimetric urine and serum proteins are falsely positive or elevated in tests using sulfosalicylic acid or trichloroacetic acid. Oxacillin may cause transient reductions in RBC, WBC, and platelet counts. Elevations in liver function test results may indicate drug-induced hepatitis or cholestasis. Abnormal urinalysis results may indicate drug-induced interstitial nephritis. Oxacillin may falsely decrease serum aminoglycoside concentrations.

CONTRAINDICATIONS
Contraindicated in patients with hypersensitivity to drug or other penicillins.

NURSING CONSIDERATIONS
• Use cautiously in patients with other drug allergies, especially to cephalosporins (possible cross-sensitivity); in neonates; and in infants.
• Before giving, ask patient about allergic reactions to penicillin. However, not having a history of penicillin allergy is no guarantee against a future allergic reaction.
• Obtain specimen for culture and sensitivity tests before giving first dose. Therapy may begin pending results.
• Give drug I.M. or I.V. only if ordered and the infection is severe or if the patient can't take oral dose.
• Give 1 to 2 hours before or 2 to 3 hours after meals. When given orally, drug may cause GI disturbances. Food may interfere with absorption.
• Give drug at least 1 hour before bacteriostatic antibiotics.
• Monitor periodic liver function studies; watch for elevated AST and ALT levels.
• Observe closely. With large doses and prolonged therapy, bacterial or fungal superinfection may occur, especially in elderly, debilitated, or immunosuppressed patients.

I.V. administration
• For direct I.V. injection, reconstitute vials with sterile water for injection or 0.9% NaCl for injection. Use 5 ml of diluent for a 250- or 500-mg vial, 10 ml of diluent for a 1-g vial, 20 ml of diluent for a 2-g vial, or 40 ml of diluent for a 4-g vial. When the solution is clear, withdraw the ordered dose and inject over 10 minutes. When giving by piggyback injection, reconstitute 1-g piggyback vial with 20 to 100 ml of diluent; reconstitute 2-g vial with 19 to 99 ml of diluent. For intermittent infusion, further dilute drug to a concentration of 5 to 40 mg/ml.
• To prevent vein irritation, avoid continuous infusions. Change site every 48 hours.

Patient teaching
• Tell patient to take entire quantity of medication exactly as prescribed, even after he feels better.
• Instruct patient to take drug on an empty stomach.
• Tell patient to notify doctor if rash, fever, or chills develop. A rash is the most common allergic reaction.

penicillin G benzathine (benzylpenicillin benzathine)
Bicillin L-A, Permapen

Pregnancy Risk Category: B

HOW SUPPLIED
Injection: 300,000 units/ml,

600,000 units/ml, 1,200,000 units/2 ml,
2,400,000 units/4 ml

ACTION

A natural penicillin that inhibits cell-wall
synthesis during microorganism multiplication; bacteria resist penicillins by producing penicillinases—enzymes that convert penicillins to inactive penicillic acid.

Route	Onset	Peak	Duration
IM	Unknown	13-24 hr	1-4 wk

INDICATIONS & DOSAGE

Congenital syphilis—
Children under 2 years: 50,000 units/kg
I.M. as a single dose.
*Group A streptococcal upper respiratory
infections—*
Adults: 1.2 million units I.M. as a single
injection.
Children weighing over 27 kg (59 lb):
900,000 units I.M. as a single injection.
Children weighing under 27 kg:
300,000 to 600,000 units I.M. as a single
injection.
*Prophylaxis of poststreptococcal
rheumatic fever—*
**Adults and children weighing over
27 kg:** 1.2 million units I.M. once month-
ly or 600,000 units q 2 weeks.
Children weighing 27 kg or less:
600,000 units I.M. once monthly.
Syphilis of less than 1 year's duration—
Adults: 2.4 million units I.M. as a single
dose.
Syphilis of more than 1 year's duration—
Adults: 2.4 million units I.M. weekly for
3 successive weeks.
Children: 50,000 units/kg I.M. weekly
for 3 successive weeks.

ADVERSE REACTIONS

CNS: neuropathy, *seizures* (with high
doses), lethargy, hallucinations, anxiety,
confusion, agitation, depression, dizziness, fatigue.
GI: nausea, vomiting, enterocolitis,
pseudomembranous colitis.
GU: interstitial nephritis, nephropathy.
Hematologic: eosinophilia, hemolytic
anemia, *thrombocytopenia, leukopenia,*
anemia, *agranulocytosis.*
Other: hypersensitivity reactions (macu-

lopapular and *exfoliative dermatitis,*
chills, fever, edema, *anaphylaxis*); pain,
sterile abscess (at injection site).

INTERACTIONS

Drug-drug. *Aminoglycosides:* physical
and chemical incompatibility. Administer
separately.
Colestipol: decreased serum concentrations of penicillin G benzathine. Administer penicillin G benzathine 1 hour before
or 4 hours after colestipol.
Oral contraceptives: efficacy of oral contraceptives may be decreased. Recommend additional form of contraception
during penicillin therapy.
Probenecid: increased blood levels of
penicillin. Probenecid may be used for
this purpose.
Tetracycline: may antagonize the effects.
Avoid concurrent use.

EFFECTS ON DIAGNOSTIC TESTS

Penicillin G alters test results for urine
and serum protein levels; it interferes with
turbidimetric methods using sulfosalicylic
acid, trichloracetic acid, acetic acid, and
nitric acid. Drug does not interfere with
tests using bromphenol blue (Albustix,
Albutest, Multistix). It alters urine glucose testing using cupric sulfate (Benedict's reagent); use Diastix or Chemstrip
uG instead. Penicillin G may cause falsely
elevated results of urine specific gravity
tests in patients with low urine output and
dehydration and falsely elevated Norymberski and Zimmerman tests results for
17-ketogenic steroids; it causes false-
positive CSF protein test results (Folin-
Ciocalteau method) and may cause positive Coombs' test results. Drug may falsely decrease serum aminoglycoside
concentrations. Adding beta-lactamase to
the sample inactivates the penicillin, rendering the assay more accurate. Alternatively, the sample can be spun down and
frozen immediately after collection.

CONTRAINDICATIONS

Contraindicated in patients with hypersensitivity to drug or other penicillins.

NURSING CONSIDERATIONS

• Use cautiously in patients with other

Reactions may be common, *uncommon,* **life-threatening,** *or* **COMMON AND LIFE-THREATENING.**

drug allergies, especially to cephalosporins (possible cross-sensitivity).

• Before giving, ask patient about allergic reactions to penicillin. However, not having a history of penicillin allergy is no guarantee against a future allergic reaction.

• Obtain specimen for culture and sensitivity tests before giving first dose. Therapy may begin pending results.

• Shake medication well before injection.
Alert: Never give I.V.—inadvertent I.V. administration has caused cardiac arrest and death.

• Inject deeply into upper outer quadrant of buttocks in adults; in midlateral thigh in infants and small children. Avoid injection into or near major nerves or blood vessels to prevent permanent neurovascular damage.

• Give penicillin G benzathine at least 1 hour before bacteriostatic antibiotics.

• Know that drug's extremely slow absorption time makes allergic reactions difficult to treat.

• Observe closely. With large doses and prolonged therapy, bacterial or fungal superinfection may occur, especially in elderly, debilitated, or immunosuppressed patients.

☑ **Patient teaching**
• Tell patient to report adverse reactions promptly.
• Inform patient that fever and eosinophilia are the most common reactions.
• Warn patient that I.M. injection may be painful but that ice applied to the site may ease discomfort.

penicillin G potassium
(benzylpenicillin potassium)
Megacillin†, Pfizerpen

Pregnancy Risk Category: B

HOW SUPPLIED
Tablets: 500,000 units†
Oral suspension: 250,000 units†, 500,000 units†
Injection: 1 million units, 5 million units, 10 million units, 20 million units

ACTION
A natural penicillin that inhibits cell-wall synthesis during microorganism multiplication; bacteria resist penicillins by producing penicillinases—enzymes that convert penicillins to inactive penicillic acid.

Route	Onset	Peak	Duration
PO	Unknown	30-60 min	Unknown
IV	Immediate	Immediate	Unknown
IM	Unknown	15-30 min	Unknown

INDICATIONS & DOSAGE
Moderate to severe systemic infection—
Adults and children 12 years and older: highly individualized; 1.6 to 3.2 million units P.O. daily in divided doses q 6 hours; 1.2 to 24 million units I.M. or I.V. daily in divided doses q 4 to 6 hours.
Children under 12 years: 25,000 to 100,000 units/kg P.O. daily in divided doses q 6 hours; or 25,000 to 400,000 units/kg I.M. or I.V. daily in divided doses q 4 to 6 hours.

ADVERSE REACTIONS
CNS: neuropathy, *seizures* (with high doses), lethargy, hallucinations, anxiety, confusion, agitation, depression, dizziness, fatigue.
GI: nausea, vomiting, enterocolitis, pseudomembranous colitis.
GU: interstitial nephritis, nephropathy.
Hematologic: hemolytic anemia, *leukopenia, thrombocytopenia,* anemia, eosinophilia, *agranulocytosis.*
Other: hypersensitivity reactions (rash, urticaria, maculopapular eruptions, *exfoliative dermatitis,* chills, fever, edema, *anaphylaxis*), overgrowth of nonsusceptible organisms, possible severe potassium poisoning with high doses (hyperreflexia, *seizures, coma*), thrombophlebitis, pain at injection site.

INTERACTIONS
Drug-drug. *Aminoglycosides:* physical and chemical incompatibility. Administer separately.
Colestipol: decreased serum concentrations of penicillin G potassium. Administer penicillin G potassium 1 hour before or 4 hours after colestipol.
Oral contraceptives: efficacy of oral con-

traceptives may be decreased. Recommend additional form of contraception during penicillin therapy.
Potassium-sparing diuretics: possible increased risk of hyperkalemia. Do not use together.
Probenecid: increased blood levels of penicillin. Probenecid may be used for this purpose.

EFFECTS ON DIAGNOSTIC TESTS

Penicillin G alters test results for urine and serum protein levels; it interferes with turbidimetric methods using sulfosalicylic acid, trichloroacetic acid, acetic acid, and nitric acid. It does not interfere with tests using bromphenol blue (Albustix, Albutest, Multistix). Drug alters urine glucose testing using cupric sulfate (Benedict's reagent); use Diastix or Chemstrip uG instead. Penicillin G may cause falsely elevated results of urine specific gravity tests in patients with low urine output and dehydration, and falsely elevated Norymberski and Zimmerman tests results for 17-ketogenic steroids; it causes false-positive CSF protein test results (Folin-Ciocalteau method) and may cause positive Coombs' test results. Drug may falsely decrease serum aminoglycoside concentrations. Adding beta-lactamase to the sample inactivates the penicillin, rendering the assay more accurate. Alternatively, the sample can be spun down and frozen immediately after collection.

CONTRAINDICATIONS

Contraindicated in patients with hypersensitivity to drug or other penicillins.

NURSING CONSIDERATIONS

• Use cautiously in patients with other drug allergies, especially to cephalosporins (possible cross-sensitivity).
• Before giving, ask patient about allergic reactions to penicillin. However, not having a history of penicillin allergy is no guarantee against a future allergic reaction.
• Obtain specimen for culture and sensitivity tests before giving first dose. Therapy may begin pending results.
• For I.M. injection, administer deeply

into large muscle; may be extremely painful.
• Give 1 to 2 hours before or 2 to 3 hours after meals. When given orally, drug may cause GI disturbances. Food may interfere with absorption.
• Monitor renal function closely. Patients with poor renal function are predisposed to high blood levels of drug.
• Monitor serum potassium and sodium levels closely in patients receiving more than 10 million units I.V. daily.
• Observe closely. With large doses and prolonged therapy, bacterial or fungal superinfection may occur, especially in elderly, debilitated, or immunosuppressed patients.
Alert: Institute seizure precautions. Patients with high blood levels of drug may develop seizures.

I.V. administration

• Reconstitute vials with sterile water for injection, D_5W, or 0.9% NaCl for injection. Volume of diluent varies with manufacturer.
• Give via intermittent I.V. infusion over 30 minutes to 2 hours.
• Give penicillin G potassium at least 1 hour before bacteriostatic antibiotics.

Patient teaching

• Tell patient taking oral form to take entire amount exactly as prescribed, even after he feels better.
• Instruct patient to take oral drug on empty stomach.
• Tell patient to notify doctor if rash, fever, or chills develop. A rash is the most common allergic reaction.
• Warn patient that I.M. injection may be painful but that ice applied to the site may alleviate discomfort.

---

penicillin G procaine (benzylpenicillin procaine)
Ayercillin†, Wycillin

Pregnancy Risk Category: B

HOW SUPPLIED
Injection: 300,000 units/ml, 500,000 units/ml, 600,000 units/ml

ACTION
A natural penicillin that inhibits cell-wall synthesis during microorganism multiplication; bacteria resist penicillins by producing penicillinases—enzymes that convert penicillins to inactive penicillic acid.

Route	Onset	Peak	Duration
IM	Unknown	1-4 hr	1-5 days

INDICATIONS & DOSAGE
Moderate to severe systemic infection—
Adults: 600,000 to 1.2 million units I.M. daily in a single dose.
Children over 1 month: 25,000 to 50,000 units/kg I.M. daily in a single dose.
Uncomplicated gonorrhea—
Adults and children weighing over 45 kg (99 lb): 1 g probenecid P.O.; after 30 minutes, 4.8 million units of penicillin G procaine I.M., divided between two injection sites as a single dose.
Pneumococcal pneumonia—
Adults and children over 12 years: 600,000 units to 1.2 million units I.M. daily for 7 to 10 days.

ADVERSE REACTIONS
CNS: *seizures,* lethargy, hallucinations, anxiety, confusion, agitation, depression, dizziness, fatigue.
GI: nausea, vomiting, enterocolitis, pseudomembranous colitis.
GU: interstitial nephritis, nephropathy.
Hematologic: *thrombocytopenia, hemolytic anemia, leukopenia,* anemia, eosinophilia, *agranulocytosis.*
Other: arthralgia, hypersensitivity reactions (rash, urticaria, chills, fever, edema, prostration, *anaphylaxis*), overgrowth of nonsusceptible organisms.

INTERACTIONS
Drug-drug. *Aminoglycosides:* physical and chemical incompatibility. Administer separately.
Colestipol: decreased serum concentrations of penicillin G procaine. Administer penicillin G procaine 1 hour before or 4 hours after colestipol.
Oral contraceptives: efficacy of oral contraceptives may be decreased. Recommend additional form of contraception during penicillin therapy.
Probenecid: increased blood levels of penicillin. Probenecid may be used for this purpose.

EFFECTS ON DIAGNOSTIC TESTS
Penicillin G alters test results for urine and serum protein levels. It interferes with turbidimetric methods using sulfosalicylic acid, trichloroacetic acid, acetic acid, and nitric acid. Drug does not interfere with tests using bromphenol blue (Albustix, Albutest, Multistix). Penicillin G alters urine glucose testing using cupric sulfate (Benedict's reagent); use Diastix instead. Penicillin G may cause falsely elevated results of urine specific gravity tests in patients with low urine output and dehydration, and falsely elevated Norymberski and Zimmerman tests results for 17-ketogenic steroids; it causes false-positive CSF protein test results (Folin-Ciocalteau method) and may cause positive Coombs' test results. Drug may falsely decrease serum aminoglycoside concentrations. Adding beta-lactamase to the sample inactivates the penicillin, rendering the assay more accurate. Alternatively, the sample can be spun down and frozen immediately after collection.

CONTRAINDICATIONS
Contraindicated in patients with hypersensitivity to drug or other penicillins.

NURSING CONSIDERATIONS
• Use cautiously in patients with other drug allergies, especially to cephalosporins (possible cross-sensitivity). Some formulations contain sulfites, which may cause allergic reactions in sensitive persons.
• Before giving, ask patient about allergic reactions to penicillin. However, not having a history of penicillin allergy is no guarantee against a future allergic reaction.
• Obtain specimen for culture and sensitivity tests before giving first dose. Therapy may begin pending results.
• Give deep I.M. in upper outer quadrant of buttocks in adults; in midlateral thigh in small children. Do not give S.C. Don't

---

*Liquid contains alcohol.   **May contain tartrazine.   †Canada   ‡Australia   §U.K.   ◇OTC

massage injection site. Avoid injection near major nerves or blood vessels to prevent permanent neurovascular damage.

Alert: Never give I.V.—inadvertent I.V. administration has caused death due to CNS toxicity caused by procaine.

• Give penicillin G procaine at least 1 hour before bacteriostatic antibiotics.

• Know that because of drug's slow absorption rate, allergic reactions are hard to treat.

• Monitor renal and hematopoietic function periodically, as ordered.

• Observe closely. With large doses and prolonged therapy, bacterial or fungal superinfection may occur, especially in elderly, debilitated, or immunosuppressed patients.

✓ Patient teaching

• Tell patient to report adverse reactions promptly. A rash is the most common allergic reaction.

• Warn patient that I.M. injection may be painful but that ice applied to the site may help alleviate discomfort.

---

penicillin G sodium (benzylpenicillin sodium)
Crystapen†

Pregnancy Risk Category: B

HOW SUPPLIED
Injection: 5 million-units vial

ACTION
A natural penicillin that inhibits cell-wall synthesis during active multiplication; bacteria resist penicillins by producing penicillinases—enzymes that convert penicillins to inactive penicillic acid.

Route	Onset	Peak	Duration
IV	Immediate	Immediate	Unknown
IM	Unknown	15-30 min	Unknown

INDICATIONS & DOSAGE
Moderate to severe systemic infection—
Adults and children 12 years and older: 1.2 to 24 million units daily I.M. or I.V. in divided doses q 4 to 6 hours.
Children under 12 years: 25,000 to 400,000 units/kg daily I.M. or I.V. in divided doses q 4 to 6 hours.

ADVERSE REACTIONS
CNS: neuropathy, *seizures,* lethargy, hallucinations, anxiety, confusion, agitation, depression, dizziness, fatigue.
CV: *heart failure* (with high doses).
GI: nausea, vomiting, enterocolitis, pseudomembranous colitis.
GU: interstitial colitis, nephropathy.
Hematologic: hemolytic anemia, *leukopenia, thrombocytopenia, agranulocytosis,* anemia, eosinophilia.
Other: arthralgia, hypersensitivity reactions (*exfoliative dermatitis,* urticaria, *anaphylaxis*), overgrowth of nonsusceptible organisms, vein irritation, pain at injection site, thrombophlebitis.

INTERACTIONS
Drug-drug. *Aminoglycosides:* physical and chemical incompatibility. Administer separately.
Colestipol: decreased serum concentrations of penicillin G sodium. Administer penicillin G sodium 1 hour before or 4 hours after colestipol.
Oral contraceptives: efficacy of oral contraceptives may be decreased. Recommend additional form of contraception during penicillin therapy.
Probenecid: increased blood levels of penicillin. Probenecid may be used for this purpose.

EFFECTS ON DIAGNOSTIC TESTS
Drug alters test results for urine and serum protein levels; it interferes with turbidimetric methods using sulfosalicylic acid, trichloroacetic acid, acetic acid, and nitric acid. Penicillin G does not interfere with tests using bromphenol blue (Albustix, Albutest, Multistix). Penicillin G alters urine glucose testing using cupric sulfate (Benedict's reagent); use Diastix instead. It may cause falsely elevated results of urine specific gravity tests in patients with low urine output and dehydration, and falsely elevated Norymberski and Zimmerman tests results for 17-ketogenic steroids; it causes false-positive CSF protein test results (Folin-Ciocalteau method) and may cause positive Coombs'

test results. Drug may falsely decrease serum aminoglycoside concentrations. Adding beta-lactamase to the sample inactivates the penicillin, rendering the assay more accurate. Alternatively, the sample can be spun down and frozen immediately after collection.

CONTRAINDICATIONS
Contraindicated in patients with hypersensitivity to drug or other penicillins and in patients on sodium-restricted diets.

NURSING CONSIDERATIONS
• Use cautiously in patients with other drug allergies, especially to cephalosporins (possible cross-allergenicity).
• Before giving, ask patient about allergic reactions to penicillin. However, not having a history of penicillin allergy is no guarantee against a future allergic reaction.
• Obtain specimen for culture and sensitivity tests before giving first dose. Therapy may begin pending results.
• In neonates and children, give divided doses over 15 to 30 minutes.
• Observe closely. With large doses and prolonged therapy, bacterial or fungal superinfection may occur, especially in elderly, debilitated, or immunosuppressed patients.
Alert: Institute seizure precautions. Patients with high blood levels of drug may develop seizures.

I.V. administration
• Reconstitute vials with sterile water for injection, 0.9% NaCl for injection, or D_5W. Check manufacturer's instructions for volume of diluent necessary to produce desired drug concentration.
• Give by intermittent I.V. infusion: Dilute drug in 50 to 100 ml, and give over 30 minutes to 2 hours q 4 to 6 hours.
• Give penicillin G sodium at least 1 hour before bacteriostatic antibiotics.

Patient teaching
• Tell patient to report adverse reactions promptly.
• Instruct patient to alert nurse if discomfort occurs at I.V. site.
• Warn patient receiving I.M. injection

that the injection may be painful but that ice applied to site may help alleviate discomfort.

penicillin V (phenoxymethylpenicillin)

penicillin V potassium (phenoxymethylpenicillin potassium)
Abbocillin VK‡, Apo-Pen VK†, Beepen-VK, Betapen-VK, Cilicaine VK‡, Ledercillin VK, Nadopen-V-200†, Nadopen-V-400†, Novo-Pen-VK†, Nu-Pen-VK†, Pen Vee†, Pen Vee K, PVF K†, PVK‡, V-Cillin K, Veetids**

Pregnancy Risk Category: B

HOW SUPPLIED
penicillin V
Tablets: 250 mg, 500 mg
Oral suspension: 125 mg/5 ml, 250 mg/5 ml (after reconstitution)
penicillin V potassium
Tablets: 125 mg, 250 mg, 500 mg
Tablets (film-coated): 250 mg, 500 mg
Capsules: 250 mg‡
Oral suspension: 125 mg/5 ml, 250 mg/5 ml (after reconstitution)

ACTION
A natural penicillin that inhibits cell-wall synthesis during microorganism multiplication; bacteria resist penicillins by producing penicillinases—enzymes that convert penicillins to inactive penicillic acid.

Route	Onset	Peak	Duration
PO	Unknown	0.5-1 hr	Unknown

INDICATIONS & DOSAGE
Mild to moderate systemic infections—
Adults and children 12 years and older: 125 to 500 mg (400,000 to 800,000 units) P.O. q 6 hours.
Children under 12 years: 15 to 62.5 mg/ kg (25,000 to 100,000 units/kg) P.O. daily, in divided doses q 6 to 8 hours.

ADVERSE REACTIONS
CNS: neuropathy.

GI: *epigastric distress,* vomiting, diarrhea, *nausea,* black "hairy" tongue.
GU: nephropathy.
Hematologic: eosinophilia, hemolytic anemia, *leukopenia, thrombocytopenia.*
Other: hypersensitivity reactions (rash, urticaria, fever, laryngeal edema, *anaphylaxis*), overgrowth of nonsusceptible organisms.

INTERACTIONS
Drug-drug. *Oral contraceptives:* efficacy of oral contraceptives may be decreased. Recommend additional form of contraception during penicillin therapy.
Probenecid: increased blood levels of penicillin. Probenecid may be used for this purpose.

EFFECTS ON DIAGNOSTIC TESTS
Drug alters test results for urine and serum protein levels; it interferes with turbidimetric methods using sulfosalicylic acid, trichloroacetic acid, acetic acid, and nitric acid. It does not interfere with tests using bromphenol blue (Albustix, Albutest, Multistix). Penicillin V may falsely decrease serum aminoglycoside levels.

CONTRAINDICATIONS
Contraindicated in patients with hypersensitivity to drug or other penicillins.

NURSING CONSIDERATIONS
• Use cautiously in patients with other drug allergies, especially to cephalosporins (possible cross-sensitivity), or in those with GI disturbances.
• Before giving, ask patient about allergic reactions to penicillins. However, not having a history of penicillin allergy is no guarantee against a future allergic reaction.
• Obtain specimen for culture and sensitivity tests before giving first dose. Therapy may begin pending results.
• Give penicillin V at least 1 hour before bacteriostatic antibiotics.
• As ordered, periodically assess renal and hematopoietic function in patients receiving long-term therapy.
• Observe closely. With large doses and prolonged therapy, bacterial or fungal superinfection may occur, especially in elderly, debilitated, or immunosuppressed patients.
• Be aware that The American Heart Association considers amoxicillin the preferred agent for endocarditis prophylaxis because GI absorption is better and serum levels are sustained longer. Penicillin V is considered an alternative agent.

☑ **Patient teaching**
• Instruct patient to take entire quantity of medication exactly as prescribed, even after he feels better.
• Tell patient to take drug with food if stomach upset occurs.
• Advise patient to notify doctor if rash, fever, or chills develop. A rash is the most common allergic reaction.

---

piperacillin sodium
Pipracil, Pipril‡

Pregnancy Risk Category: B

HOW SUPPLIED
Injection: 2 g, 3 g, 4 g

ACTION
Extended-spectrum penicillin that inhibits cell-wall synthesis during microorganism multiplication; bacteria resist penicillins by producing penicillinases—enzymes that convert penicillins to inactive penicillic acid.

Route	Onset	Peak	Duration
IV	Immediate	Immediate	Unknown
IM	Unknown	30-50 min	Unknown

INDICATIONS & DOSAGE
Systemic infections caused by susceptible strains of gram-positive and especially gram-negative organisms (including Proteus *and* Pseudomonas aeruginosa)—
Adults and children over 12 years: 100 to 300 mg/kg I.V. or I.M. daily in divided doses q 4 to 6 hours, not to exceed 24 g daily.
Prophylaxis of surgical infections—
Adults: 2 g I.V., given 30 to 60 minutes before surgery. Dose may be repeated during surgery and once or twice more after surgery.

Adjust-a-dose: Reduce dose in patients with a creatinine clearance less than 40 ml/minute.

ADVERSE REACTIONS
CNS: *seizures,* headache, dizziness, fatigue.
GI: nausea, diarrhea, vomiting, pseudomembranous colitis.
GU: interstitial nephritis.
Hematologic: *bleeding* (with high doses), *neutropenia,* eosinophilia, *leukopenia, thrombocytopenia,* prolonged PT and INR.
Hepatic: transient elevations in liver function tests.
Metabolic: *hypokalemia,* hypernatremia.
Other: hypersensitivity reactions (edema, fever, chills, rash, pruritus, urticaria, *anaphylaxis*), overgrowth of nonsusceptible organisms, pain at injection site, vein irritation, phlebitis, prolonged muscle relaxation.

INTERACTIONS
Drug-drug. *Oral contraceptives:* efficacy of oral contraceptives may be decreased. Recommend additional form of contraception during penicillin therapy.
Probenecid: increased blood levels of piperacillin. Probenecid may be used for this purpose.
Vecuronium: prolonged neuromuscular blockade: Do not use together.

EFFECTS ON DIAGNOSTIC TESTS
Drug may falsely decrease serum aminoglycoside levels. It may cause positive Coombs' tests.

CONTRAINDICATIONS
Contraindicated in patients with hypersensitivity to drug or other penicillins.

NURSING CONSIDERATIONS
• Use cautiously in patients with other drug allergies, especially to cephalosporins (possible cross-sensitivity), or in those with bleeding tendencies, uremia, and hypokalemia.
• Before giving, ask patient about allergic reactions to penicillin. However, not having a history of penicillin allergy is no guarantee against a future allergic reaction.
• Obtain specimen for culture and sensitivity tests before giving first dose. Therapy may begin pending results.
• For I.M. injection, reconstitute with sterile or bacteriostatic water for injection, 0.9% NaCl for injection (with or without preservative), or 0.5% to 1% lidocaine hydrochloride. Add 2 ml of diluent for each gram of drug. Final solution will contain 1 g/2.5 ml.
• Check CBC and platelet counts frequently, as ordered. Drug may cause thrombocytopenia.
• Monitor serum potassium and sodium levels.
• Monitor INR in patients receiving warfarin therapy as drug may prolong PT.
Alert: Institute seizure precautions. Patients with high serum levels of drug may have seizures.
• Observe closely. With large doses and prolonged therapy, bacterial or fungal superinfection may occur, especially in elderly, debilitated, or immunosuppressed patients.
• Be aware that patients with cystic fibrosis tend to be most susceptible to fever or rash.
• Be aware that drug may be better suited for patients on sodium-free diets than ticarcillin (piperacillin contains 1.85 mEq of sodium/g).
• Keep in mind that piperacillin is typically used with another antibiotic, such as gentamicin.

█ I.V. administration
• Reconstitute each gram of drug with 5 ml of diluent, such as sterile or bacteriostatic water for injection, 0.9% NaCl for injection (with or without preservative), D_5W, or dextrose 5% in 0.9% NaCl for injection. Shake until dissolved. Inject reconstituted solution directly into a vein or into the tubing of a free-flowing I.V. solution over 3 to 5 minutes. Alternatively, dilute with at least 50 ml of a compatible I.V. solution, and give by intermittent infusion over 30 minutes.
• Avoid continuous infusions to prevent vein irritation. Change site every 48 hours.

- Aminoglycoside antibiotics, such as gentamicin and tobramycin, are chemically incompatible with piperacillin. Do not mix in the same I.V. container.
- Give piperacillin at least 1 hour before bacteriostatic antibiotics.

✓**Patient teaching**
- Tell patient to report adverse reactions promptly.
- Instruct patient receiving drug I.V. to report discomfort at I.V. site.
- Advise patient to limit salt intake during therapy because drug contains 1.85 mEq of sodium/g.

piperacillin sodium/ tazobactam sodium
Zosyn

Pregnancy Risk Category: B

HOW SUPPLIED
Powder for injection: 2 g piperacillin and 0.25 g tazobactam per vial, 3 g piperacillin and 0.375 g tazobactam per vial, 4 g piperacillin and 0.5 g tazobactam per vial

ACTION
Piperacillin is an extended-spectrum penicillin that inhibits cell-wall synthesis during microorganism multiplication; tazobactam increases piperacillin's effectiveness by inactivating beta-lactamases, which destroy penicillins.

Route	Onset	Peak	Duration
IV	Immediate	Immediate	Unknown

INDICATIONS & DOSAGE
Appendicitis (complicated by rupture or abscess) and peritonitis caused by Escherichia coli, Bacteroides fragilis, B. ovatus, B. thetaiotaomicron, *or* B. vulgatus; *skin and skin-structure infections caused by* Staphylococcus aureus; *postpartum endometritis or pelvic inflammatory disease caused by* E. coli; *moderately severe community-acquired pneumonia caused by* Haemophilus influenzae—
Adults: 3 g piperacillin and 0.375 g tazobactam I.V. q 6 hours.
Adjust-a-dose: In renally impaired adult

patients, if creatinine clearance is 20 to 40 ml/minute, dosage is 2 g piperacillin and 0.25 g tazobactam I.V. q 6 hours; if it is below 20 ml/minute, 2 g piperacillin and 0.25 g tazobactam I.V. q 8 hours.
Nosocomial pneumonia (moderate to severe) caused by piperacillin-resistant, beta-lactamase-producing strains of S. aureus—
Adults: initially, 3.375 g I.V. over 30 minutes q 4 hours. Administer with an aminoglycoside.

ADVERSE REACTIONS
CNS: *headache, insomnia,* agitation, dizziness, anxiety.
CV: hypertension, tachycardia, chest pain, edema.
EENT: rhinitis.
GI: *diarrhea, nausea, constipation,* vomiting, dyspepsia, stool changes, abdominal pain.
GU: interstitial nephritis.
Hematologic: *leukopenia,* anemia, eosinophilia, *thrombocytopenia.*
Respiratory: dyspnea.
Skin: rash (including maculopapular, bullous, urticarial, and eczematoid), pruritus.
Other: fever; pain; candidiasis; inflammation, phlebitis at I.V. site; *anaphylaxis.*

INTERACTIONS
Drug-drug. *Oral anticoagulants:* prolonged effectiveness. Monitor PT or INR closely.
Oral contraceptives: efficacy of oral contraceptives may be decreased. Recommend additional form of contraception during penicillin therapy.
Probenecid: increased blood levels of piperacillin. Probenecid may be used for this purpose.
Vecuronium: prolonged neuromuscular blockade. Monitor closely.

EFFECTS ON DIAGNOSTIC TESTS
As with other penicillins, piperacillin/tazobactam may result in a false-positive reaction for urine glucose using a copper reduction method, such as Clinitest. Glucose tests based on enzymatic glucose oxidase reactions (such as Diastix) are recommended.

Reactions may be *common,* uncommon, *life-threatening,* or COMMON AND LIFE-THREATENING.

CONTRAINDICATIONS
Contraindicated in patients with hypersensitivity to drug or other penicillins.

NURSING CONSIDERATIONS
• Use cautiously in patients with other drug allergies, especially to cephalosporins (possible cross-sensitivity), or in those with bleeding tendencies, uremia, and hypokalemia.
• Obtain specimen for culture and sensitivity tests before giving first dose. Therapy may begin pending results.
• Because hemodialysis removes 6% of the piperacillin dose and 21% of the tazobactam dose, be aware that supplemental doses may be needed after hemodialysis.
• Observe closely. With large doses and prolonged therapy, bacterial and fungal superinfection may occur, especially in elderly, debilitated, or immunosuppressed patients.
• Drug contains 2.35 mEq sodium/g; monitor patient's sodium intake.
• There appears to be an increase of fever and rash in patients with cystic fibrosis. Monitor closely.

I.V. administration
• Reconstitute each gram of piperacillin with 5 ml of diluent, such as sterile or bacteriostatic water for injection, bacteriostatic 0.9% NaCl for injection, D_5W, dextrose 5% in 0.9% NaCl for injection, or dextran 6% in 0.9% NaCl for injection. Do not use lactated Ringer's injection. Shake until dissolved. Further dilute to a final volume of 50 ml before infusion.
• Infuse over at least 30 minutes. Discontinue any primary infusion during administration if possible. Do not mix with other drugs. Aminoglycoside antibiotics (such as amikacin, gentamicin and tobramycin) are chemically incompatible with this drug. Do not mix in the same I.V. container.
• Use drug immediately after reconstitution. Discard unused drug after 24 hours if stored at room temperature; 48 hours if refrigerated. Once diluted, drug is stable in I.V. bags for 24 hours at room temperature or 1 week if refrigerated.

• Change I.V. site every 48 hours.

✓ Patient teaching
• Tell patient to report adverse reactions promptly.
• Instruct patient to alert nurse if discomfort occurs at I.V. site.

---

ticarcillin disodium
Ticar, Ticillin‡

Pregnancy Risk Category: B

HOW SUPPLIED
Injection: 1 g, 3 g, 6 g
I.V. infusion: 3 g

ACTION
An extended-spectrum penicillin that inhibits cell-wall synthesis during microorganism multiplication; bacteria resist penicillins by producing penicillinases—enzymes that convert penicillins to inactive penicillic acid.

Route	Onset	Peak	Duration
IV	Immediate	Immediate	Unknown
IM	Unknown	30-75 min	Unknown

INDICATIONS & DOSAGE
Severe systemic infections caused by susceptible strains of gram-positive and especially gram-negative organisms (including Pseudomonas *and* Proteus)—
Adults: 200 to 300 mg/kg I.V. daily, in divided doses q 4 to 6 hours.
Children: 50 to 300 mg/kg I.V. daily, in divided doses q 4 to 6 hours.
Adjust-a-dose: Reduce dosage in patients with renal failure. If creatinine clearance is 30 to 60 ml/minute, dosage is 2 g I.V. q 4 hours; if it is 10 to 29 ml/minute, 2 g I.V. q 8 hours; and if it is less than 10 ml/minute, 2 g I.V. q 12 hours or 1 g I.M. q 6 hours.

ADVERSE REACTIONS
CNS: *seizures,* neuromuscular excitability.
GI: nausea, diarrhea, vomiting, pseudomembranous colitis.
Hematologic: *leukopenia, neutropenia,* eosinophilia, *thrombocytopenia,* hemolytic anemia.

Other: hypersensitivity reactions (rash, pruritus, urticaria, chills, fever, edema, *anaphylaxis*), overgrowth of nonsusceptible organisms, hypokalemia, pain at injection site, vein irritation, phlebitis.

INTERACTIONS
Drug-drug. *Lithium:* altered renal elimination of lithium. Monitor serum lithium levels closely.

Oral contraceptives: efficacy of oral contraceptives may be decreased. Recommend additional form of contraception during penicillin therapy.

Probenecid: increased blood levels of ticarcillin and other penicillins. Probenecid may be used for this purpose.

EFFECTS ON DIAGNOSTIC TESTS
Ticarcillin alters tests for urine or serum proteins; it interferes with turbidimetric methods that use sulfosalicylic acid, trichloroacetic acid, acetic acid, or nitric acid. Ticarcillin does not interfere with tests using bromphenol blue (Albustix, Albutest, Multistix). Ticarcillin may falsely decrease serum aminoglycoside concentrations. Systemic effects of ticarcillin may cause positive Coombs' test, hypokalemia and hypernatremia, and may prolong PT; it may also cause transient elevations in liver function studies and transient reductions in RBC, WBC, and platelet counts.

CONTRAINDICATIONS
Contraindicated in patients with hypersensitivity to drug or other penicillins.

NURSING CONSIDERATIONS
• Use cautiously in patients with other drug allergies, especially to cephalosporins (possible cross-sensitivity), or in those with impaired renal function, hemorrhagic conditions, hypokalemia, or sodium restrictions (contains 5.2 to 6.5 mEq sodium/g).

• Before giving, ask patient about allergic reactions to penicillin. However, not having a history of penicillin allergy is no guarantee against a future allergic reaction.

• Obtain specimen for culture and sensitivity tests before giving first dose. Therapy may begin pending results.

• For I.M. injection, reconstitute vials using sterile water for injection, 0.9% NaCl for injection, or lidocaine 1% (without epinephrine). Use 2 ml diluent for each gram of drug. Give deep I.M. into large muscle. Do not exceed 2 g per injection.

• Monitor serum potassium and sodium levels.

• Check CBC and platelet counts frequently, as ordered. Drug may cause thrombocytopenia.

Alert: Institute seizure precautions. Patients with high blood levels of ticarcillin may develop seizures.

• Be aware that ticarcillin is typically used with another antibiotic, such as gentamicin.

• Observe closely. With large doses and prolonged therapy, bacterial or fungal superinfection may occur, especially in elderly, debilitated, or immunosuppressed patients.

• Monitor INR in patients receiving warfarin therapy as drug may prolong PT.

I.V. administration
• Reconstitute vials using D_5W, 0.9% NaCl injection, sterile water for injection, or other compatible solution. Add 4 ml of diluent for each gram of drug. Further dilute to a maximum concentration of 50 mg/ml, and inject slowly directly into a vein or into the tubing of a free-flowing I.V. solution. Alternatively, dilute to a concentration of 10 to 100 mg/ml, and give by intermittent infusion over 30 to 120 minutes in adults or 10 to 20 minutes in neonates.

• Aminoglycoside antibiotics (such as amikacin, gentamicin, and tobramycin) are chemically incompatible with this drug. Do not mix in the same I.V. container.

• Avoid continuous infusion to prevent vein irritation. Change site every 48 hours.

• Give ticarcillin at least 1 hour before bacteriostatic antibiotics.

✓ Patient teaching
• Tell patient to report adverse reactions promptly.

• Instruct patient to alert nurse if discomfort occurs at I.V. insertion site.

ticarcillin disodium/clavulanate potassium
Timentin

Pregnancy Risk Category: B

HOW SUPPLIED
Injection: 3 g ticarcillin and 100 mg clavulanic acid

ACTION
Ticarcillin is an extended-spectrum penicillin that inhibits cell-wall synthesis during microorganism replication; clavulanic acid increases ticarcillin's effectiveness by inactivating beta lactamases, which destroy ticarcillin.

Route	Onset	Peak	Duration
IV	Immediate	Immediate	Unknown

INDICATIONS & DOSAGE
Lower respiratory tract, urinary tract, bone and joint, and skin and skin-structure infections and septicemia when caused by beta-lactamase-producing strains of bacteria or by ticarcillin-susceptible organisms—
Adults: 3.1 g (3 g ticarcillin and 100 mg clavulanic acid) administered by I.V. infusion q 4 to 6 hours.
Adjust-a-dose: Reduce dosage in patients with renal failure. If creatinine clearance is 30 to 60 ml/minute, dosage is 2 g I.V. q 4 hours; if it is 10 to 29 ml/ minute, 2 g I.V. q 8 hours; and if it is less than 10 ml/ minute, 2 g I.V. q 12 hours.

ADVERSE REACTIONS
CNS: *seizures,* neuromuscular excitability, headache, giddiness.
GI: nausea, diarrhea, stomatitis, vomiting, epigastric pain, flatulence, pseudomembranous colitis, taste and smell disturbances.
Hematologic: *leukopenia, neutropenia,* eosinophilia, *thrombocytopenia,* hemolytic anemia, anemia.
Other: hypersensitivity reactions (rash, pruritus, urticaria, chills, fever, edema, *anaphylaxis*), overgrowth of nonsusceptible organisms, hypokalemia, pain at injection site, vein irritation, phlebitis.

INTERACTIONS
Drug-drug. *Aminoglycoside antibiotics (such as amikacin, gentamicin, and tobramycin):* chemically incompatible. Do not mix in the same I.V. container.
Oral contraceptives: efficacy of oral contraceptives may be decreased. Recommend additional form of contraception during penicillin therapy.
Probenecid: increased blood levels of ticarcillin. Probenecid may be used for this purpose.

EFFECTS ON DIAGNOSTIC TESTS
Ticarcillin/clavulanate potassium alters tests for urine or serum proteins; it interferes with turbidimetric methods that use sulfosalicylic acid, trichloroacetic acid, acetic acid, or nitric acid. Drug does not interfere with tests using bromphenol blue (Albustix, Albutest, Multistix). Drug may falsely decrease serum aminoglycoside concentrations. Systemic effects of the drug may cause positive Coombs' test, hypokalemia and hypernatremia, and may prolong PT; it may also cause transient elevations in liver function studies and transient reductions in RBC, WBC, and platelet counts.

CONTRAINDICATIONS
Contraindicated in patients with hypersensitivity to drug or other penicillins.

NURSING CONSIDERATIONS
• Use cautiously in patients with other drug allergies, especially to cephalosporins (possible cross-sensitivity), and in those with impaired renal function, hemorrhagic conditions, hypokalemia, or sodium restrictions (contains 4.5 mEq sodium/g).
• Before giving, ask patient about allergic reactions to penicillin. However, not having a history of penicillin allergy is no guarantee against a future allergic reaction.
• Obtain specimen for culture and sensitivity tests before giving first dose. Therapy may begin pending results.

• Check CBC and platelet counts frequently, as ordered. Drug may cause thrombocytopenia.
• Monitor serum potassium.
• Observe closely. With large doses and prolonged therapy, bacterial or fungal superinfection may occur, especially in elderly, debilitated, or immunosuppressed patients.

I.V. administration
• Reconstitute drug with 13 ml of sterile water for injection or 0.9% NaCl for injection. Further dilute to a maximum of 10 to 100 mg/ml (based on ticarcillin component), and administer by I.V. infusion over 30 minutes. In fluid restricted patients, dilute to a maximum of 48 mg/ml if using D_5W, 43 mg/ml if using 0.9% NaCl for injection, or 86 mg/ml if using sterile water for injection.
• Give drug at least 1 hour before bacteriostatic antibiotics.

Patient teaching
• Tell patient to report adverse reactions promptly.
• Instruct patient to alert nurse if discomfort occurs at I.V. site.
• Advise patient to limit salt intake during drug therapy because of high sodium content.

13

Cephalosporins

cefaclor
cefadroxil monohydrate
cefazolin sodium
cefdinir
cefepime hydrochloride
cefixime
cefmetazole sodium
cefonicid sodium
cefoperazone sodium
cefotaxime sodium
cefotetan disodium
cefoxitin sodium
cefpodoxime proxetil
cefprozil
ceftazidime
ceftibuten
ceftizoxime sodium
ceftriaxone sodium
cefuroxime axetil
cefuroxime sodium
cephalexin hydrochloride
cephalexin monohydrate
cephradine
loracarbef

COMBINATION PRODUCTS
None.

---

cefaclor
Ceclor, Distaclor§, Distaclor MR§

Pregnancy Risk Category: B

HOW SUPPLIED
Capsules: 250 mg, 500 mg
Tablets (extended-release): 375 mg,
500 mg
Oral suspension: 125 mg/5 ml, 250 mg/
5 ml, 187 mg/5 ml, 375 mg/5 ml

ACTION
A second-generation cephalosporin that
inhibits cell-wall synthesis, promoting osmotic instability; usually bactericidal.

Route	Onset	Peak	Duration
PO	Unknown	0.5-1 hr	Unknown
PO (extended-release)	Unknown	1.5-2.5 hr	Unknown

INDICATIONS & DOSAGE
*Respiratory or urinary tract, skin, and
soft-tissue infections and otitis media
caused by* Haemophilus influenzae, Streptococcus pneumoniae, S. pyogenes, Escherichia coli, Proteus mirabilis, Klebsiella *species, and* staphylococci—
Adults: 250 to 500 mg P.O. q 8 hours. For
pharyngitis or otitis media, daily dosage
may be given in two equally divided doses
q 12 hours. For extended release forms,
500 mg P.O. q 12 hours for 7 days for
bronchitis; for pharyngitis or skin and
skin-structure infections, 375 mg P.O. q
12 hours for 10 days and 7 to 10 days, respectively.
Children: 20 mg/kg daily P.O. in divided
doses q 8 hours. For pharyngitis or otitis
media, daily dosage may be given in two
equally divided doses q 12 hours. In more
serious infections, 40 mg/kg daily are recommended, not to exceed 1 g daily.

ADVERSE REACTIONS
CNS: dizziness, headache, somnolence,
malaise.
GI: *nausea,* vomiting, *diarrhea,* anorexia,
dyspepsia, abdominal cramps,
pseudomembranous colitis, oral candidiasis.
GU: vaginal candidiasis, vaginitis.
Hematologic: *transient leukopenia,* anemia, eosinophilia, *thrombocytopenia,*
lymphocytosis.
Skin: *maculopapular rash,* dermatitis,
pruritus.
Other: hypersensitivity reactions (serum
sickness, *anaphylaxis*), fever, transient increases in liver enzymes.

INTERACTIONS
Drug-drug. *Antacids:* absorption of extended release cefaclor is decreased if

---

*Liquid contains alcohol.   **May contain tartrazine.   †Canada   ‡Australia   §U.K.   ◊OTC

taken within 1 hour. Separate administration by 1 hour.
Chloramphenicol: antagonistic effect. Do not use together.
Probenecid: may inhibit excretion and increase blood levels of cefaclor. Monitor patient.

EFFECTS ON DIAGNOSTIC TESTS
Drug may cause false-positive Coombs' test results. Cefaclor also causes false-positive results in urine glucose tests using cupric sulfate (Benedict's reagent or Clinitest); use glucose oxidase tests (Diastix or Chemstrip uG) instead. It causes false elevations in serum or urine creatinine levels in tests using Jaffé's reaction.

CONTRAINDICATIONS
Contraindicated in patients with hypersensitivity to other cephalosporins.

NURSING CONSIDERATIONS
• Use cautiously in patients with impaired renal function or a history of sensitivity to penicillin and in breast-feeding women.
• Obtain specimen for culture and sensitivity tests before giving first dose. Therapy may begin pending results.
• With large doses or prolonged therapy, monitor for superinfection, especially in high-risk patients.
• Store reconstituted suspension in refrigerator. Stable for 14 days if refrigerated. Shake well before using.

☑ Patient teaching
• Tell patient to take entire amount of medication exactly as prescribed, even after he feels better.
• Tell patient that drug may be taken with meals. If suspension is used, instruct him to shake container well before measuring dose and to keep the drug refrigerated.
• Advise patient to notify doctor if rash develops or signs of superinfection appear.
• Inform patient not to crush, cut or chew extended release tablets.

---

cefadroxil monohydrate
Duricef, Ultracef

Pregnancy Risk Category: B

HOW SUPPLIED
Tablets: 1 g
Capsules: 500 mg
Oral suspension: 125 mg/5 ml, 250 mg/5 ml, 500 mg/5 ml

ACTION
A first-generation cephalosporin that inhibits cell-wall synthesis, promoting osmotic instability; usually bactericidal.

Route	Onset	Peak	Duration
PO	Unknown	1-2 hr	Unknown

INDICATIONS & DOSAGE
Urinary tract infections caused by Escherichia coli, Proteus mirabilis, *and* Klebsiella *species; skin and soft-tissue infections caused by staphylococci and streptococci; and pharyngitis or tonsillitis caused by group A beta-hemolytic streptococci—*
Adults: 1 to 2 g P.O. daily, depending on infection being treated. Usually given once daily or b.i.d.
Children: 30 mg/kg P.O. daily in two divided doses q 12 hours.
Adjust-a-dose: In renally impaired patients, if creatinine clearance is 25 to 50 ml/minute, 1 g P.O. followed by 500 mg q 12 hours; between 10 and 24 ml/minute, 500 mg q 24 hours; and below 10 ml/minute, 500 mg q 36 hours.

ADVERSE REACTIONS
CNS: *seizures.*
GI: pseudomembranous colitis, *nausea,* vomiting, *diarrhea,* glossitis, abdominal cramps, oral candidiasis.
GU: genital pruritus, candidiasis, vaginitis, renal dysfunction.
Hematologic: *transient neutropenia,* eosinophilia, *leukopenia,* anemia, *agranulocytosis, thrombocytopenia.*
Skin: *maculopapular and erythematous rashes,* urticaria.
Other: hypersensitivity reactions (serum sickness, *anaphylaxis,* angioedema), tran-

---

Reactions may be *common,* uncommon, *life-threatening,* or COMMON AND LIFE-THREATENING.

sient increases in liver enzymes, dyspnea, fever.

INTERACTIONS

Drug-drug. *Probenecid:* may inhibit excretion and increase blood levels of cefadroxil. Use together cautiously.

EFFECTS ON DIAGNOSTIC TESTS

Cefadroxil causes false-positive results in urine glucose tests using cupric sulfate (Benedict's reagent or Clinitest); use glucose oxidase test (Diastix or Chemstrip uG) instead. It causes false elevations in serum or urine creatinine levels in tests using Jaffé's reaction. Positive Coombs' test results occur in about 3% of patients taking cephalosporins.

CONTRAINDICATIONS

Contraindicated in patients with hypersensitivity to drug or other cephalosporins.

NURSING CONSIDERATIONS

• Use cautiously in patients with a history of sensitivity to penicillin or in breast-feeding women. Also use cautiously in patients with impaired renal function; dosage adjustments may be necessary.
• Obtain specimen for culture and sensitivity tests before giving first dose. Therapy may begin pending results.
• Be aware that if creatinine clearance is below 50 ml/minute, dosage interval should be lengthened so drug doesn't accumulate. Monitor renal function in patients with renal dysfunction.
• With large doses or prolonged therapy, monitor for superinfection, especially in high-risk patients.

✅ Patient teaching
• Instruct patient to take drug with food or milk to lessen GI discomfort.
• Tell patient to take entire amount of medication exactly as prescribed, even after he feels better.
• Advise patient to notify doctor if rash develops or symptoms of superinfection appear.

cefazolin sodium
Ancef, Kefzol

Pregnancy Risk Category: B

HOW SUPPLIED
Injection (parenteral): 500 mg, 1 g
Infusion: 500 mg/50-ml vial, 1 g/50-ml vial

ACTION
A first-generation cephalosporin that inhibits cell-wall synthesis, promoting osmotic instability; usually bactericidal.

Route	Onset	Peak	Duration
IV	Immediate	Immediate	Unknown
IM	Unknown	1-2 hr	Unknown

INDICATIONS & DOSAGE
Perioperative prophylaxis in contaminated surgery—
Adults: 1 g I.M. or I.V. 30 to 60 minutes before surgery; then 0.5 to 1 g I.M. or I.V. q 6 to 8 hours for 24 hours. In long operations (over 2 hours), another 0.5- to 1-g I.M. or I.V. dose may be administered intraoperatively.
  Note: In cases where infection would be devastating, prophylaxis may be continued for 3 to 5 days.
Serious infections of respiratory, biliary, and GU tracts; skin, soft-tissue, bone, and joint infections; septicemia; and endocarditis caused by Escherichia coli, Enterobacteriaceae, *gonococci,* Haemophilus influenzae, Klebsiella, Proteus mirabilis, Staphylococcus aureus, Streptococcus pneumoniae, *and group A beta-hemolytic streptococci—*
Adults: 250 mg I.M. or I.V. q 8 hours to 1.5 g I.M. or I.V. q 6 hours. Maximum 12 g/day in life-threatening situations.
Children over 1 month: 25 to 50 mg/kg/day I.M. or I.V. in three or four divided doses. In severe infections, dosage may be increased to 100 mg/kg/day.
Adjust-a-dose: In patients with renal failure, if creatinine clearance is 35 to 54 ml/minute, give full dose q 8 hours; if clearance is 11 to 34 ml/minute, give 50% usual dose q 12 hours; and if clearance is less

than 10 ml/minute, give 50% of usual dose q 18 to 24 hours.

ADVERSE REACTIONS
GI: pseudomembranous colitis, nausea, anorexia, vomiting, *diarrhea,* glossitis, dyspepsia, abdominal cramps, anal pruritus, oral candidiasis.
GU: genital pruritus, candidiasis, vaginitis.
Hematologic: neutropenia, leukopenia, eosinophilia, thrombocytopenia.
Skin: *maculopapular and erythematous rashes, urticaria, pruritus.*
Other: hypersensitivity reactions (serum sickness, *anaphylaxis*); transient increases in liver enzymes; ***Stevens-Johnson syndrome; pain, induration, sterile abscesses, tissue sloughing*** (at injection site); *phlebitis, thrombophlebitis* (with I.V. injection).

INTERACTIONS
Drug-drug. *Probenecid:* may inhibit excretion and increase blood levels of cefazolin. Use cautiously.

EFFECTS ON DIAGNOSTIC TESTS
Cephalosporins cause false-positive results in urine glucose tests using cupric sulfate (Benedict's reagent or Clinitest); use glucose oxidase tests (Diastix or Chemstrip uG) instead. Drug causes false elevations in serum or urine creatinine levels in tests using Jaffé's reaction. It also causes positive Coombs' test results and may elevate liver function test results.

CONTRAINDICATIONS
Contraindicated in patients with hypersensitivity to other cephalosporins.

NURSING CONSIDERATIONS
• Use cautiously in patients with a history of sensitivity to penicillin and in breast-feeding women. Also use cautiously and with dosage adjustments in patients with renal failure.
• Obtain specimen for culture and sensitivity tests before giving first dose. Therapy may begin pending results.
• Be aware that dose and dosing interval will be adjusted if creatinine clearance is below 55 ml/minute.

• After reconstitution, inject drug I.M. without further dilution (this drug is not as painful as other cephalosporins). Administer injection deeply into a large muscle mass, such as the gluteus maximus or lateral aspect of the thigh.
• With large doses or prolonged therapy, monitor for superinfection, especially in high-risk patients.

I.V. administration
• Reconstitute with sterile water, bacteriostatic water, or 0.9% NaCl solution as follows: 2 ml to 500-mg vial; 2.5 ml to 1-g vial. Shake well until dissolved. Resultant concentration: 225 mg/ml or 330 mg/ml, respectively.
• Know that reconstituted cefazolin is stable for 24 hours at room temperature or 96 hours under refrigeration.
• For direct injection, further dilute Ancef with 5 ml, or Kefzol with 10 ml, of sterile water for injection. Inject into a large vein or into the tubing of a free-flowing I.V. solution over 3 to 5 minutes. For intermittent infusion, add reconstituted drug to 50 to 100 ml of compatible solution or use premixed solution. Commercially available frozen solutions of cefazolin in D_5W should be given only by intermittent or continuous I.V. infusion.
• Alternate injection sites if I.V. therapy lasts longer than 3 days. Use of small I.V. needles in larger available veins may be preferable.

Patient teaching
• Instruct patient to report adverse reactions promptly.
• Tell patient to alert nurse if discomfort occurs at I.V. injection site.

▼ *NEW DRUG*

cefdinir
Omnicef

Pregnancy Risk Category: B

HOW SUPPLIED
Capsules: 300 mg
Suspension: 125 mg/5 ml

ACTION
Cefdinir's bactericidal activity results from inhibition of cell-wall synthesis. Drug is stable in the presence of some beta-lactamase enzymes, causing some microorganisms resistant to penicillins and cephalosporins to be susceptible to cefdinir. Excluding *Pseudomonas, Enterobacter, Enterococcus,* and methicillin-resistant *Staphylococcus* species, cefdinir's spectrum of activity includes a broad range of gram-positive and gram-negative aerobic microorganisms.

Route	Onset	Peak	Duration
PO	Unknown	2-4 hr	Unknown

INDICATIONS & DOSAGE
Treatment of mild to moderate infections caused by susceptible strains of microorganisms for conditions of community-acquired pneumonia, acute exacerbations of chronic bronchitis, acute maxillary sinusitis, acute bacterial otitis media, and uncomplicated skin and skin-structure infections—
Adults and children 13 years and older: 300 mg P.O. q 12 hours or 600 mg P.O. q 24 hours for 10 days. (Use q-12-hour dosages for pneumonia and skin infections.)
Children 6 months to 12 years: 7 mg/kg P.O. q 12 hours or 14 mg/kg P.O. q 24 hours for 10 days, up to maximum dose of 600 mg daily. (Use q-12-hour dosages for skin infections.)
Treatment of pharyngitis and tonsillitis—
Adults and children 13 years and older: 300 mg P.O. q 12 hours for 5 to 10 days or 600 mg P.O. q 24 hours for 10 days.
Children 6 months to 12 years: 7 mg/kg P.O. q 12 hours for 5 to 10 days or 14 mg/kg P.O. q 24 hours for 10 days.
Adjust-a-dose: If creatinine clearance is below 30 ml/minute, reduce dosage to 300 mg P.O. once daily for adults and 7 mg/kg (up to 300 mg) P.O. once daily for children. In patients receiving chronic hemodialysis, 300 mg or 7 mg/kg P.O. at end of each dialysis session and subsequently every other day.

ADVERSE REACTIONS
CNS: headache.

GI: abdominal pain, *diarrhea,* nausea, vomiting.
GU: vaginal candidiasis, vaginitis, increased urine proteins and RBCs.
Skin: rash, cutaneous candidiasis.
Hepatic: elevated GGT and alkaline phosphatase.

INTERACTIONS
Drug-drug. *Antacids (magnesium- and aluminum-containing), iron supplements, and multivitamins containing iron:* decrease cefdinir's rate of absorption and bioavailability; administer such preparations 2 hours before or after cefdinir dose. *Probenecid:* inhibits the renal excretion of cefdinir. Monitor patient.

EFFECTS ON DIAGNOSTIC TESTS
False positive reaction for ketones (tests using nitroprusside only) and glucose (Clinitest, Benedict's solution or Fehling's solution) in urine may occur. Cephalosporins may occasionally induce a positive direct Coombs' test.

CONTRAINDICATIONS
Contraindicated in patients with known allergy to cephalosporin class of antibiotics.

NURSING CONSIDERATIONS
• Use cautiously in patients with known hypersensitivity to penicillin because of the possibility of cross-sensitivity with other beta-lactam antibiotics. Also, use with caution in patients with history of colitis and renal insufficiency.
• Prolonged drug treatment may result in possible emergence and overgrowth of resistant organisms. Monitor for symptoms of superinfection.
• Pseudomembranous colitis has been reported with cefdinir, and should be considered in patients with diarrhea subsequent to antibiotic therapy or in those with history of colitis.

☑ **Patient teaching**
• Instruct patient to take antacids and iron supplements 2 hours before or after a dose of cefdinir.
• Inform diabetic patient that each teaspoon of suspension contains 2.86 g of sucrose.

• Tell patient that drug may be taken without regard to meals.
• Advise patient to report severe diarrhea or diarrhea accompanied by abdominal pain.
• Tell patient to report adverse reactions or symptoms of superinfection promptly.

---

cefepime hydrochloride
Maxipime

Pregnancy Risk Category: B

HOW SUPPLIED
Injection: 500 mg/15 ml vial, 1 g/100 ml piggyback bottle, 1 g/ADD-Vantage vial, 1 g/15 ml vial, 2 g/100 ml piggyback bottle, 2 g/20 ml vial

ACTION
A fourth-generation cephalosporin that inhibits bacterial cell-wall synthesis, promotes osmotic instability, and destroys bacteria.

Route	Onset	Peak	Duration
IV, IM	0.5 hr	1-2 hr	Unknown

INDICATIONS & DOSAGE
Mild to moderate urinary tract infections caused by Escherichia coli, Klebsiella pneumoniae, *or* Proteus mirabilis, *including cases associated with concurrent bacteremia with these microorganisms*—
Adults and children 12 years and older: 0.5 to 1 g I.M. (I.M. route used only for infections caused by *E. coli*) or I.V. infused over 30 minutes q 12 hours for 7 to 10 days.
Severe urinary tract infections, including pyelonephritis, caused by E. coli *or* K. pneumoniae—
Adults and children 12 years and older: 2 g I.V. infused over 30 minutes q 12 hours for 10 days.
Moderate to severe pneumonia caused by Streptococcus pneumoniae, Pseudomonas aeruginosa, K. pneumoniae, *or* Enterobacter *species*—
Adults and children 12 years and older: 1 to 2 g I.V. infused over 30 minutes q 12 hours for 10 days.
Moderate to severe skin infections, un-complicated skin infections, and skin-structure infections caused by Staphylococcus aureus *(methicillin-susceptible strains only) or* Streptococcus pyogenes—
Adults and children 12 years and older: 2 g I.V. infused over 30 minutes q 12 hours for 10 days.
❋ *NEW INDICATION: Complicated intra-abdominal infections* (used in combination with metronidazole) *caused by* E. coli, *viridans group streptococci,* P. aeruginosa, K. pneumoniae, Enterobacter *species, or* B. fragilis—
Adults: 2 g I.V. infused over 30 minutes q 12 hours for 7 to 10 days.
Adjust-a-dose: In patients with renal failure, if creatinine clearance is 30 to 60 ml/minute, give full dose q 24 hours; if clearance is 11 to 29 ml/minute, give 50% usual dose q 24 hours; and if clearance is less than 11 ml/minute, give 25% of usual dose q 24 hours.

ADVERSE REACTIONS
CNS: headache.
GI: colitis, diarrhea, nausea, vomiting, oral candidiasis.
GU: vaginitis.
Skin: rash, pruritus, urticaria.
Other: phlebitis, pain, inflammation, fever.

INTERACTIONS
Drug-drug. *Aminoglycosides:* may increase risk of nephrotoxicity. Monitor renal function closely.
Potent diuretics (such as furosemide): may increase risk of nephrotoxicity. Monitor renal function closely.

EFFECTS ON DIAGNOSTIC TESTS
Cefepime may cause a false-positive reaction for glucose in the urine when using Clinitest tablets. Glucose tests based on enzymatic glucose oxidase reactions (such as Diastix or Chemstrip uG) should be used instead. A positive direct Coombs' test may occur during treatment with drug.

CONTRAINDICATIONS
Contraindicated in patients with hypersensitivity to drug, other cephalosporins,

---

Reactions may be *common*, uncommon, *life-threatening*, or COMMON AND LIFE-THREATENING.

penicillins, or other beta-lactam antibiotics.

NURSING CONSIDERATIONS
• Use cautiously in patients with renal impairment, poor nutrition, or history of GI disease (particularly colitis); in those receiving a protracted course of antimicrobial therapy; and in breast-feeding women.
• Safety of drug in children under 12 years has not been established.
• Obtain culture and sensitivity tests before giving first dose, if appropriate. Therapy may begin pending results.
• Dosage adjustment is necessary in patients with impaired renal function. Monitor renal function.
• For I.M. administration, constitute drug using sterile water for injection, 0.9% NaCl for injection, 5% dextrose injection, 0.5% or 1% lidocaine hydrochloride, or bacteriostatic water for injection with parabens or benzyl alcohol. Follow manufacturer's guidelines for quantity of diluent to use.
• Inspect solution for particulate matter before use. The powder and its solutions tend to darken, depending on storage conditions. Product potency is not adversely affected when stored as recommended.
• Monitor patient for superinfection. Drug may cause overgrowth of nonsusceptible bacteria or fungi.
• Be aware that many cephalosporins can reduce prothrombin activity. Patients at risk include those with renal or hepatic impairment or poor nutrition and those receiving prolonged cefepime therapy. Monitor PT and INR in these patients as ordered. Administer exogenous vitamin K as indicated and ordered.

I.V. administration
• Follow manufacturer's guidelines closely when reconstituting drug. Variations occur in constituting drug for administration, depending on concentration of drug ordered and how drug is packaged (piggyback vial, ADD-Vantage vial, or regular vial). Also be aware that the type of diluent used for constitution varies, depending on the product used. Use only solutions recommended by the manufactur-

er. The resulting solution should be administered over about 30 minutes.
• Intermittent I.V. infusion with a Y-type administration set can be accomplished with compatible solutions. However, during infusion of a solution containing cefepime, discontinuing the other solution is recommended.

✓ Patient teaching
• Warn patient receiving drug I.M. that pain may occur at injection site.
• Instruct patient to report signs and symptoms of superinfection or GI disturbance.

cefixime
Suprax

Pregnancy Risk Category: B

HOW SUPPLIED
Tablets: 200 mg, 400 mg
Oral suspension: 100 mg/5 ml (after reconstitution)

ACTION
A third-generation cephalosporin that inhibits cell-wall synthesis, promoting osmotic instability; usually bactericidal.

Route	Onset	Peak	Duration
PO	Unknown	3.1-4.4 hr	Unknown

INDICATIONS & DOSAGE
Uncomplicated urinary tract infections caused by Escherichia coli *and* Proteus mirabilis; *otitis media caused by* Haemophilus influenzae *(beta-lactamase positive and negative strains),* Moraxella (Branhamella) catarrhalis, *and* Streptococcus pyogenes; *pharyngitis and tonsillitis caused by* S. pyogenes; *acute bronchitis and acute exacerbations of chronic bronchitis caused by* S. pneumoniae *and* H. influenzae *(beta-lactamase positive and negative strains)—*
Adults and children over 12 years or weighing over 50 kg (110 lb):
400 mg/day P.O. as a single 400-mg tablet or 200 mg q 12 hours.
Children 12 years and younger or weighing 50 kg or less: 8 mg/kg/day sus-

pension P.O. as a single daily dose or 4 mg/kg q 12 hours.
Uncomplicated gonorrhea caused by Neisseria gonorrhoeae—
Adults: 400 mg P.O. as a single dose.
Adjust-a-dose: In patients with renal failure, if creatinine clearance is 21 to 60 ml/minute, give 75% of dose at usual intervals and if it is less than 20 ml/minute, give 50% of usual dose at usual intervals.

ADVERSE REACTIONS
CNS: headache, dizziness.
GI: *diarrhea,* loose stools, abdominal pain, nausea, vomiting, dyspepsia, flatulence, pseudomembranous colitis.
GU: genital pruritus, vaginitis, genital candidiasis, transient increases in BUN and serum creatinine levels.
Hematologic: *thrombocytopenia, leukopenia,* eosinophilia.
Skin: pruritus, rash, urticaria, *erythema multiforme, Stevens-Johnson syndrome.*
Other: drug fever, transient increases in liver enzymes, hypersensitivity reactions (serum sickness, *anaphylaxis*).

INTERACTIONS
Drug-drug. *Carbamazepine:* elevated carbamazepine levels reported when administered together. Avoid concomitant use.
Probenecid: may inhibit excretion and increase blood levels of cefixime. Use together cautiously.
Salicylates: may displace cefixime from plasma protein-binding sites. Clinical significance is unknown.

EFFECTS ON DIAGNOSTIC TESTS
Drug may cause false-positive results in urine glucose tests using cupric sulfate (Benedict's reagent or Clinitest); use glucose oxidase tests (Diastix or Chemstrip uG) instead. It may cause false-positive results in tests for urine ketones that utilize nitroprusside (but not nitroferricyanide). Positive direct Coombs' test results have been seen with other cephalosporins.

CONTRAINDICATIONS
Contraindicated in patients with hypersensitivity to drug or other cephalosporins.

NURSING CONSIDERATIONS
Alert: Use cautiously and with reduced dosage in patients with renal dysfunction. Monitor renal function.
● Use cautiously in patients with a history of sensitivity to penicillin and in breast-feeding women.
● Obtain specimen for culture and sensitivity tests before giving first dose. Therapy may begin pending results.
● To prepare oral suspension, add required amount of water to powder in two portions. Shake well after each addition. After mixing, suspension is stable for 14 days. No need to refrigerate, but keep tightly closed. Shake well before using.
● With large doses or prolonged therapy, monitor for superinfection, especially in high-risk patients.

☑ Patient teaching
● Tell patient to take all of the medication prescribed, even after he feels better.
● Instruct patient using oral suspension to shake container before measuring dose. Tell him suspension does not need to be refrigerated.
● Advise patient to notify doctor if rash or symptoms of superinfection develop.

---

cefmetazole sodium (cefmetazone)
Zefazone

Pregnancy Risk Category: B

HOW SUPPLIED
Injection: 1 g, 2 g

ACTION
A semisynthetic cephamycin antibiotic pharmacologically similar to second-generation cephalosporins that inhibits cell-wall synthesis, promoting osmotic instability; usually bactericidal.

Route	Onset	Peak	Duration
IV	Unknown	Immediate	Unknown

INDICATIONS & DOSAGE
Lower respiratory tract infections caused by Streptococcus pneumoniae, Staphylo-

coccus aureus *(penicillinase- and non-penicillinase-producing strains),* Escherichia coli, *and* Haemophilus influenzae *(non-penicillinase-producing strains); intra-abdominal infections caused by* E. coli *or* Bacteroides fragilis; *skin and skin-structure infections caused by* S. aureus *(penicillinase- and non-penicillinase-producing strains),* S. epidermidis, Streptococcus pyogenes, Streptococcus agalactiae, E. coli, Proteus mirabilis, Klebsiella pneumoniae, *and* B. fragilis—
Adults: 2 g I.V. q 6 to 12 hours for 5 to 14 days.
Urinary tract infections caused by E. coli—
Adults: 2 g I.V. q 12 hours.
Prophylaxis in patients undergoing vaginal hysterectomy—
Adults: 2 g I.V. 30 to 90 minutes before surgery as a single dose; or 1 g I.V. 30 to 90 minutes before surgery, repeated in 8 and 16 hours.
Prophylaxis in patients undergoing abdominal hysterectomy—
Adults: 1 g I.V. 30 to 90 minutes before surgery, repeated in 8 and 16 hours.
Prophylaxis in patients undergoing cesarean section—
Adults: 2 g I.V. as a single dose after clamping cord; or 1 g I.V. after clamping cord, repeated in 8 and 16 hours.
Prophylaxis in patients undergoing colorectal surgery—
Adults: 2 g I.V. as a single dose 30 to 90 minutes before surgery. Some clinicians follow with additional 2-g doses in 8 and 16 hours.
Prophylaxis in high-risk patients undergoing cholecystectomy—
Adults: 1 g I.V. 30 to 90 minutes before surgery, repeated in 8 and 16 hours.
Adjust-a-dose: In patients with renal failure, if creatinine clearance is 50 to 90 ml/minute, give 1 to 2 g q 12 hours; if clearance is 30 to 49 ml/minute, give 1 to 2 g q 16 hours; if clearance is 10 to 29 ml/minute, give 1 to 2 g q 24 hours; if clearance is less than 10 ml/minute, give 1 to 2 g q 48 hours (administered after hemodialysis).

ADVERSE REACTIONS
CNS: headache, hot flashes.

CV: *shock,* hypotension, phlebitis, thrombophlebitis.
EENT: epistaxis.
GI: nausea, vomiting, *diarrhea,* epigastric pain, pseudomembranous colitis, candidiasis, bleeding.
GU: vaginitis.
Hepatic: elevated liver function test results.
Respiratory: pleural effusion, dyspnea, respiratory distress.
Skin: rash, pruritus, generalized erythema.
Other: fever, bacterial or fungal superinfection, hypersensitivity reactions (serum sickness, *anaphylaxis*), altered color perception, pain at injection site, joint pain and inflammation.

INTERACTIONS
Drug-drug. *Aminoglycosides:* potential increased risk of nephrotoxicity. Monitor closely.
Probenecid: may inhibit excretion and increase blood levels of cefmetazole. May be used for this effect.
Drug-lifestyle. *Alcohol use:* possible disulfiram-like reaction. Avoid for 24 hours before and after administration of cefmetazole.

EFFECTS ON DIAGNOSTIC TESTS
Drug causes false-positive results of urine glucose tests that use cupric sulfate (Benedict's reagent or Clinitest) or glucose oxidase tests (Diastix or Chemstrip uG) instead. It may cause positive Coombs' test results.

CONTRAINDICATIONS
Contraindicated in patients with hypersensitivity to drug or other cephalosporins.

NURSING CONSIDERATIONS
• Use cautiously in patients with a history of sensitivity to penicillin and in breast-feeding women.
• Obtain specimen for culture and sensitivity tests before giving first dose. Therapy may begin pending results.
• Monitor patient for bacterial and fungal superinfections. Prolonged use may result

---

*Liquid contains alcohol.   **May contain tartrazine.   †Canada   ‡Australia   §U.K.   ◇OTC

in overgrowth of nonsusceptible organisms.
• Monitor INR in patients at risk (from renal or hepatic impairment, malnutrition, or prolonged therapy), as ordered. Drug's chemical structure includes the methylthiotetrazole side chain that has been associated with bleeding disorders. However, such bleeding has not been reported with drug.
• In patients undergoing hemodialysis, give dose at end of hemodialysis session.
• Monitor renal function.

⬤ I.V. administration
• Reconstitute with bacteriostatic water for injection, sterile water for injection, or 0.9% NaCl for injection. After reconstitution, drug may be further diluted to concentrations ranging from 1 to 20 mg/ml by adding it to 0.9% NaCl injection, D_5W, or lactated Ringer's injection. Reconstituted or dilute solutions are stable for 24 hours at room temperature (77° F [25° C]) or 1 week if refrigerated at 46° F (8° C).

☑ Patient teaching
• Tell patient to report adverse reactions promptly.
• Instruct patient to alert nurse if discomfort occurs at I.V. insertion site.

---

cefonicid sodium
Monocid

Pregnancy Risk Category: B

HOW SUPPLIED
Injection: 500 mg, 1 g
Infusion: 1 g/100 ml
Pharmacy bulk package: 10 g

ACTION
A second-generation cephalosporin that inhibits cell-wall synthesis, promoting osmotic instability; usually bactericidal.

Route	Onset	Peak	Duration
IV	Immediate	Immediate	Unknown
IM	Unknown	1-2 hr	Unknown

INDICATIONS & DOSAGE
Perioperative prophylaxis in contaminated surgery—
Adults: 1 g I.M. or I.V. 30 to 60 minutes before surgery; then 1 g I.M. or I.V. daily for 2 days after surgery. If used for prophylaxis in cesarean section, 1 g I.M. or I.V. after umbilical cord is clamped.
Serious infections of the lower respiratory and urinary tracts, skin and skin-structure infections, septicemia, bone and joint infections, and preoperative prophylaxis. Susceptible microorganisms include Streptococcus pneumoniae, Klebsiella pneumoniae, Escherichia coli, Haemophilus influenzae, Proteus mirabilis, Staphylococcus aureus, S. epidermidis, *and* Streptococcus pyogenes—
Adults: usual dosage is 1 g I.V. or I.M. q 24 hours; in life-threatening infections, 2 g q 24 hours.
Adjust-a-dose: In patients with renal failure, if creatinine clearance is 60 to 79 ml/minute, give 10 to 25 mg/kg q 24 hours; if clearance is 40 to 59 ml/minute, give 8 to 20 mg/kg q 24 hours; if clearance is 20 to 39 ml/minute, give 4 to 15 mg/kg q 24 hours; if clearance is 10 to 19 ml/minute, give 4 to 15 mg/kg q 48 hours; if clearance is 5 to 9 ml/minute, give 4 to 15 mg/kg q 3 to 5 days; if clearance is less than 5 ml/minute, give 3 to 4 mg/kg q 3 to 5 days.

ADVERSE REACTIONS
CNS: dizziness, headache, malaise, paresthesia.
GI: pseudomembranous colitis, diarrhea.
GU: *acute renal failure,* interstitial nephritis.
Hematologic: *neutropenia, leukopenia,* eosinophilia, anemia, thrombocytosis, *thrombocytopenia,* prolonged PT and INR.
Hepatic: elevated liver function test results.
Skin: *maculopapular and erythematous rashes, urticaria.*
Other: hypersensitivity reactions (serum sickness, *anaphylaxis*); *pain, induration, sterile abscesses, tissue sloughing* (at injection site); *phlebitis, thrombophlebitis,* fever, myalgia (with I.V. injection).

Reactions may be *common,* uncommon, *life-threatening,* or COMMON AND LIFE-THREATENING.

INTERACTIONS
Drug-drug. *Probenecid:* may inhibit excretion and increase blood levels of cefonicid. Use together cautiously.

EFFECTS ON DIAGNOSTIC TESTS
Drug causes positive Coombs' test results. It also causes false-positive results in urine glucose tests using cupric sulfate (Benedict's reagent or Clinitest); use glucose oxidase tests (Diastix or Chemstrip uG) instead. It causes false elevations in serum or urine creatinine levels in tests using Jaffé's reaction.

CONTRAINDICATIONS
Contraindicated in patients with hypersensitivity to drug or other cephalosporins.

NURSING CONSIDERATIONS
• Use cautiously in patients with a history of sensitivity to penicillin and in breast-feeding women. Also use cautiously and with dosage adjustments in patients with renal failure. Monitor renal function.
• Obtain specimen for culture and sensitivity tests before giving first dose. Therapy may begin pending results.
• Be aware that dosing interval will be adjusted for patients with renal impairment.
• For I.M. use, when administering 2-g I.M. doses once daily, divide the dose equally and inject deeply into large muscle masses, such as the gluteus maximus or the lateral aspect of the thigh.
• With large doses or prolonged therapy, monitor for superinfection, especially in high-risk patients.
• Be aware that the chemical structure of drug includes the methylthiotetrazole side chain that has been associated with bleeding disorders. However, such bleeding has not been reported with drug.

◻ I.V. administration
• Reconstitute 500-mg vial with 2 ml of sterile water for injection (yields a concentration of 220 mg/ml) and 1-g vial with 2.5 ml of sterile water for injection (yields a concentration of 325 mg/ml). Shake well. Reconstitute piggyback vials with 50 to 100 ml of sterile water for injection, bacteriostatic water for injection, or 0.9% NaCl solution.
• Infuse over 20 to 30 minutes.

☑ Patient teaching
• Tell patient to report adverse reactions or symptoms of superinfection promptly.
• Instruct patient to alert nurse if discomfort is felt at I.V. insertion site.

---

cefoperazone sodium
Cefobid

Pregnancy Risk Category: B

HOW SUPPLIED
Infusion: 1 g, 2 g piggyback
Parenteral: 1 g, 2 g
Pharmacy bulk package: 10-g vial

ACTION
A third-generation cephalosporin that inhibits cell-wall synthesis, promoting osmotic instability; usually bactericidal.

Route	Onset	Peak	Duration
IV	Immediate	Immediate	Unknown
IM	Unknown	1-2 hr	Unknown

INDICATIONS & DOSAGE
Serious infections of the respiratory tract; intra-abdominal, gynecologic, and skin infections; bacteremia; and septicemia. Susceptible microorganisms include Streptococcus pneumoniae *and* S. pyogenes; Staphylococcus aureus *(penicillinase- and non-penicillinase-producing) and* Staphylococcus epidermidis; *entero-cocci;* Escherichia coli; Klebsiella; Haemophilus influenzae; Enterobacter; Citrobacter; Proteus; *some* Pseudomonas, *including* P. aeruginosa; *and* Bacteroides fragilis—
Adults: usual dosage is 1 to 2 g q 12 hours I.M. or I.V. In severe infections or in infections caused by less sensitive organisms, total daily dosage or frequency may be increased up to 16 g/day.
Adjust-a-dose: In patients with hepatic or biliary obstruction, total daily dose should not exceed 4 g/day. In patients with hepatic and substantial renal impairment, do not exceed 2 g/day.

---

*Liquid contains alcohol.   **May contain tartrazine.   †Canada   ‡Australia   §U.K.   ◇OTC

ADVERSE REACTIONS

GI: pseudomembranous colitis, nausea, vomiting, *diarrhea.*

Hematologic: *transient neutropenia, eosinophilia,* anemia, hypoprothrombinemia, bleeding.

Skin: *maculopapular and erythematous rashes, urticaria.*

Other: mildly elevated liver enzymes; hypersensitivity reactions (serum sickness, *anaphylaxis*); *pain, induration, sterile abscesses, temperature elevation, tissue sloughing* (at I.M. injection site); *phlebitis, thrombophlebitis,* fever (with I.V. injection).

INTERACTIONS

Drug-drug. *Probenecid:* may inhibit excretion and increase blood levels of cefoperazone. Use together cautiously.

Drug-lifestyle. *Alcohol use:* possible disulfiram-like reaction. Warn patient not to drink alcohol for several days after discontinuing cefoperazone.

EFFECTS ON DIAGNOSTIC TESTS

Cephalosporins cause false-positive results in urine glucose tests using cupric sulfate (Benedict's reagent or Clinitest); use glucose oxidase (Diastix or Chemstrip uG) instead. Cefoperazone may cause positive Coombs' test results and elevated liver function test results and INR.

CONTRAINDICATIONS

Contraindicated in patients with hypersensitivity to drug or other cephalosporins.

NURSING CONSIDERATIONS

• Use cautiously in patients with impaired renal function or with a history of sensitivity to penicillin. Also use cautiously in breast-feeding women.

• Doses of 4 g/day should be given cautiously to patients with hepatic disease or biliary obstruction. Higher dosages require monitoring of serum levels.

• Periodically monitor liver and renal function and compare to baseline.

• Obtain specimen for culture and sensitivity tests before giving first dose. Therapy may begin pending results.

• To prepare drug for I.M. injection: using the 1-g vial, dissolve drug with 2 ml of sterile water for injection; then add 0.6 ml of 2% lidocaine hydrochloride for a final concentration of 333 mg/ml. Alternatively, dissolve drug with 2.8 ml of sterile water for injection; then add 1 ml of 2% lidocaine hydrochloride for a final concentration of 250 mg/ml. When using the 2-g vial, dissolve drug with 3.8 ml of sterile water for injection; then add 1.2 ml of 2% lidocaine hydrochloride for final concentration of 333 mg/ml. Alternatively, dissolve drug with 5.4 ml of sterile water for injection; then add 1.8 ml of 2% lidocaine hydrochloride for final concentration of 250 mg/ml.

• For I.M. administration, inject deeply into a large muscle mass, such as the gluteus maximus or the lateral aspect of the thigh.

• With large doses or prolonged therapy, monitor for superinfection, especially in high-risk patients.

• Monitor INR regularly. The drug's chemical structure includes the methylthiotetrazole side chain that has been associated with bleeding disorders. Vitamin K promptly reverses bleeding if it occurs.

☐ I.V. administration

• Reconstitute 1- or 2-g vial with a minimum of 2.8 ml of compatible I.V. solution; the manufacturer recommends using 5 ml/g. Give by direct injection into a large vein or into the tubing of a free-flowing I.V. solution over 3 to 5 minutes. When giving by intermittent infusion, add reconstituted drug to 20 to 40 ml of a compatible I.V. solution and infuse over 15 to 30 minutes.

✓ Patient teaching

• Tell patient to report adverse reactions and symptoms of superinfection promptly.

• Instruct patient to alert nurse if discomfort occurs at I.V. insertion site.

---

cefotaxime sodium
Claforan

Pregnancy Risk Category: B

HOW SUPPLIED
Injection: 500 mg, 1 g, 2 g
Infusion: 1 g, 2 g

ACTION
A third-generation cephalosporin that inhibits cell-wall synthesis, promoting osmotic instability; usually bactericidal.

Route	Onset	Peak	Duration
IV	Immediate	Immediate	Unknown
IM	Unknown	30 min	Unknown

INDICATIONS & DOSAGE
Perioperative prophylaxis in contaminated surgery—
Adults: 1 g I.M. or I.V. 30 to 60 minutes before surgery. Patients undergoing bowel surgery should receive preoperative mechanical bowel cleansing and a nonabsorbable anti-infective agent such as neomycin. Patients undergoing cesarean section should receive 1 g I.M. or I.V. as soon as the umbilical cord is clamped, then 1 g I.M. or I.V. 6 and 12 hours later.
Uncomplicated gonorrhea caused by penicillinase-producing strains of Neisseria gonorrhoeae *or non-penicillinase-producing strains of the organism—*
Adults and adolescents: 500 mg I.M. as a single dose.
Serious infections of the lower respiratory and urinary tracts, CNS, skin, bone, and joints; gynecologic and intra-abdominal infections; bacteremia; and septicemia. Susceptible microorganisms include streptococci, including Streptococcus pneumoniae *and* S. pyogenes; Staphylococcus aureus *(penicillinase- and non-penicillinase-producing) and* Staphylococcus epidermidis; Escherichia coli; Klebsiella; Haemophilus influenzae; Serratia marcescens; Pseudomonas *species, including* P. aeruginosa; Enterobacter; Proteus; *and* Peptostreptococcus—
Adults: usual dose is 1 g I.V. or I.M. q 6 to 8 hours. Up to 12 g daily can be given in life-threatening infections.
Children weighing 50 kg (110 lb) or more: the usual adult dose, but dosage should not exceed 12 g daily.
Children 1 month to 12 years weighing below 50 kg: 50 to 180 mg/kg/day I.M. or I.V. in four to six divided doses.

Neonates 1 to 4 weeks: 50 mg/kg I.V. q 8 hours.
Neonates to 1 week: 50 mg/kg I.V. q 12 hours.
Adjust-a-dose: In patients with renal failure, if creatinine clearance is below 20 ml/minute, give half usual dose at usual interval.

ADVERSE REACTIONS
CNS: headache.
GI: pseudomembranous colitis, nausea, vomiting, *diarrhea.*
GU: vaginitis, candidiasis, interstitial nephritis.
Hematologic: *transient neutropenia,* eosinophilia, hemolytic anemia, ***thrombocytopenia, agranulocytosis.***
Hepatic: elevated liver function tests.
Skin: *maculopapular and erythematous rashes, urticaria.*
Other: hypersensitivity reactions (serum sickness, *anaphylaxis*); transient increases in liver enzymes; elevated temperature; *pain, induration, sterile abscesses, temperature elevation, tissue sloughing* (at I.M. injection site); *phlebitis, thrombophlebitis* (with I.V. injection).

INTERACTIONS
Drug-drug. *Aminoglycosides:* may increase risk of nephrotoxicity. Monitor closely.
Probenecid: may inhibit excretion and increase blood levels of cefotaxime. Use together cautiously.

EFFECTS ON DIAGNOSTIC TESTS
Cefotaxime may cause positive Coombs' test results.

CONTRAINDICATIONS
Contraindicated in patients with hypersensitivity to drug or other cephalosporins.

NURSING CONSIDERATIONS
• Use cautiously in patients with a history of sensitivity to penicillin and in breast-feeding women. Also use cautiously and with dosage adjustments in patients who have renal failure. Monitor renal function.

• Obtain specimen for culture and sensitivity tests before giving first dose. Therapy may begin pending results.

• For I.M. administration, inject deeply into a large muscle mass, such as the gluteus maximus or the lateral aspect of the thigh.

• With large doses or prolonged therapy, monitor for superinfection, especially in high-risk patients.

I.V. administration

• For direct injection, reconstitute 500-mg, 1-g, or 2-g vials with 10 ml of sterile water for injection. Solutions containing 1 g/14 ml are isotonic. Inject drug into a large vein or into the tubing of a free-flowing I.V. solution over 3 to 5 minutes.

• For I.V. infusion, reconstitute infusion vials with 50 to 100 ml of D_5W or 0.9% NaCl solution. Infuse drug over 20 to 30 minutes. Interrupt flow of primary I.V. solution during infusion.

✓ Patient teaching

• Tell patient to report adverse reactions and symptoms of superinfection promptly.

• Instruct patient to alert nurse if discomfort occurs at I.V. insertion site.

---

cefotetan disodium
Cefotan

Pregnancy Risk Category: B

HOW SUPPLIED
Injection: 1 g, 2 g
Infusion: 1 g, 2 g piggyback

ACTION
A semisynthetic cephamycin antibiotic that is pharmacologically similar to the second-generation cephalosporins. Inhibits cell-wall synthesis, promoting osmotic instability; usually bactericidal.

Route	Onset	Peak	Duration
IV	Immediate	Immediate	Unknown
IM	Unknown	1.5-3 hr	Unknown

INDICATIONS & DOSAGE
Serious urinary tract and lower respiratory tract infections and gynecologic, skin and skin-structure, intra-abdominal, and bone and joint infections caused by susceptible streptococci, Staphylococcus aureus *(penicillinase- and non-penicillinase-producing) and* S. epidermidis, Escherichia coli, Klebsiella, Enterobacter, Proteus, Haemophilus influenzae, Neisseria gonorrhoeae, *and* Bacteroides, *including* B. fragilis—

Adults: 1 to 2 g I.V. or I.M. q 12 hours for 5 to 10 days. Up to 6 g daily in life-threatening infections.

Perioperative prophylaxis—

Adults: 1 to 2 g I.V. given once 30 to 60 minutes before surgery. In cesarean section, dose should be administered as soon as umbilical cord is clamped.

Adjust-a-dose: In patients with renal failure, if creatinine clearance is 10 to 30 ml/minute, give usual dose q 24 hours; if clearance is less than 10 ml/minute, give usual dose q 48 hours.

ADVERSE REACTIONS
GI: pseudomembranous colitis, nausea, *diarrhea.*
GU: *nephrotoxicity.*
Hematologic: *transient neutropenia,* eosinophilia, hemolytic anemia, hypoprothrombinemia, bleeding, thrombocytosis, *agranulocytosis, thrombocytopenia,* prolonged PT and INR.
Hepatic: elevated liver function test results.
Skin: *maculopapular and erythematous rashes, urticaria.*
Other: hypersensitivity reactions (serum sickness, *anaphylaxis*); transient increases in liver enzymes; elevated temperature; *pain, induration, sterile abscesses, tissue sloughing* (at injection site); *phlebitis, thrombophlebitis* (with I.V. injection).

INTERACTIONS
Drug-drug. *Aminoglycosides:* possible synergistic effect and possible increased risk of nephrotoxicity. Use with caution.
Probenecid: may inhibit excretion and increase blood levels of cefotetan. Sometimes used for this effect.

Drug-lifestyle. *Alcohol use:* possible disulfiram-like reaction. Warn patient not to drink alcohol for several days after discontinuing cefotetan.

EFFECTS ON DIAGNOSTIC TESTS
Drug causes false-positive results in urine glucose tests using cupric sulfate (Benedict's reagent or Clinitest); use glucose oxidase tests (Diastix or Chemstrip uG) instead. It causes false elevations in serum or urine creatinine levels in tests using Jaffé's reaction. It may cause positive Coombs' test results.

CONTRAINDICATIONS
Contraindicated in patients with hypersensitivity to drug or other cephalosporins.

NURSING CONSIDERATIONS
• Use cautiously in patients with history of sensitivity to penicillin and in breast-feeding women. Also use cautiously and with dosage adjustments in patients with renal failure. Monitor renal function.
• Obtain specimen for culture and sensitivity tests before giving first dose. Therapy may begin pending results.
• Reconstitute for I.M. injection with sterile water or bacteriostatic water for injection, 0.9% NaCl for injection, or 0.5% or 1% lidocaine hydrochloride. Shake to dissolve and let stand until clear.
• Know that reconstituted solution is stable for 24 hours at room temperature or 96 hours if refrigerated.
• With large doses or prolonged therapy, monitor for superinfection, especially in high-risk patients.
• Know that drug's chemical structure includes the methylthiotetrazole side chain that has been associated with bleeding disorders. However, such bleeding has not been reported with this drug.

I.V. administration
• Reconstitute with sterile water for injection. Then drug may be mixed with 50 to 100 ml of D₅W or 0.9% NaCl solution. Interrupt flow of primary I.V. solution during cefotetan infusion.
• Infuse over 20 to 60 minutes.

☑ Patient teaching
• Tell patient to report adverse reactions and symptoms of superinfection promptly.
• Instruct patient to alert nurse if discomfort occurs at I.V. site.
• Tell patient to notify doctor if loose stools or diarrhea occurs.

---

cefoxitin sodium
Mefoxin

Pregnancy Risk Category: B

HOW SUPPLIED
Injection: 1 g, 2 g
Infusion: 1 g, 2 g in 50-ml or 100-ml container

ACTION
A semisynthetic cephamycin antibiotic that is pharmacologically similar to the second-generation cephalosporins. Inhibits cell-wall synthesis, promoting osmotic instability; usually bactericidal.

Route	Onset	Peak	Duration
IV	Immediate	Immediate	Unknown
IM	Unknown	20-30 min	Unknown

INDICATIONS & DOSAGE
Serious infections of respiratory and GU tracts; skin; soft-tissue, bone, and joint infections; and bloodstream and intra-abdominal infections caused by susceptible Escherichia coli *and other coliform bacteria,* Staphylococcus aureus *(penicillinase- and non-penicillinase-producing) and* S. epidermidis, streptococci, Klebsiella, Haemophilus influenzae, *and* Bacteroides, *including* B. fragilis; *and perioperative prophylaxis—*
Adults: 1 to 2 g I.V. or I.M. q 6 to 8 hours for uncomplicated infections. Up to 12 g daily in life-threatening infections.
Children over 3 months: 80 to 160 mg/kg daily given in four to six equally divided doses. Maximum daily dose is 12 g.
Prophylactic use in surgery—
Adults: 2 g I.M. or I.V. 30 to 60 minutes before surgery, then 2 g I.M. or I.V. q 6

---

hours for 24 hours (72 hours after prosthetic arthroplasty).

Children 3 months or older: 30 to 40 mg/kg I.M. or I.V. 30 to 60 minutes before surgery, then 30 to 40 mg/kg q 6 hours for 24 hours (72 hours after prosthetic arthroplasty).

Adjust-a-dose: In patients with renal failure, if creatinine clearance is 30 to 50 ml/minute, give 1 to 2 g q 8 to 12 hours; if clearance is 10 to 29 ml/minute, give 1 to 2 g q 12 to 24 hours; and if clearance is below 10 ml/minute, give 500 mg q 24 to 48 hours.

ADVERSE REACTIONS
CV: hypotension.
GI: pseudomembranous colitis, nausea, vomiting, *diarrhea.*
GU: *acute renal failure.*
Hematologic: *transient neutropenia,* eosinophilia, hemolytic anemia, anemia, *thrombocytopenia.*
Hepatic: transient increases in liver enzymes.
Skin: *maculopapular and erythematous rashes, urticaria, exfoliative dermatitis.*
Other: hypersensitivity reactions (serum sickness, *anaphylaxis*); elevated temperature; *pain, induration, sterile abscesses, tissue sloughing* (at injection site); *phlebitis, thrombophlebitis,* dyspnea (with I.V. injection).

INTERACTIONS
Drug-drug. *Nephrotoxic agents:* possible increased risk of nephrotoxicity. Monitor closely.
Probenecid: may inhibit excretion and increase blood levels of cefoxitin. Sometimes used for this effect.

EFFECTS ON DIAGNOSTIC TESTS
Cefoxitin causes false-positive results in urine glucose tests using cupric sulfate (Benedict's reagent or Clinitest); use glucose oxidase tests (Diastix or Chemstrip uG) instead. It also causes false elevations in serum or urine creatinine levels in tests using Jaffé's reaction. Cefoxitin may cause positive Coombs' test results.

CONTRAINDICATIONS
Contraindicated in patients with hypersensitivity to drug or other cephalosporins.

NURSING CONSIDERATIONS
● Use cautiously in patients with a history of sensitivity to penicillin and in breast-feeding women. Also use cautiously and with dosage adjustments in patients with renal failure. Monitor renal function.
● Obtain specimen for culture and sensitivity tests before giving first dose. Therapy may begin pending results.
● For I.M. use, reconstitute each 1 g of drug with 2 ml of sterile water for injection or 0.5% or 1% lidocaine hydrochloride (without epinephrine) to minimize pain. Inject deeply into a large muscle mass, such as the gluteus maximus or the lateral aspect of the thigh.
● After reconstitution, store for 24 hours at room temperature or 1 week under refrigeration.
● With large doses or prolonged therapy, monitor for superinfection, especially in high-risk patients.

🔲 I.V. administration
● Reconstitute 1 g with at least 10 ml of sterile water for injection and 2 g with 10 to 20 ml of sterile water for injection. Solutions of D_5W and 0.9% NaCl for injection can also be used. For direct injection, inject drug into a large vein or into the tubing of a free-flowing I.V. solution over 3 to 5 minutes. For intermittent infusion, add reconstituted drug to 50 or 100 ml of D_5W or $D_{10}W$ or 0.9% NaCl injection. Interrupt flow of primary I.V. solution during infusion.
● Assess I.V. site frequently. Such use has been linked to development of thrombophlebitis.

✅ Patient teaching
● Tell patient to report adverse reactions and symptoms of superinfection promptly.
● Instruct patient to alert nurse if discomfort is felt at I.V. site.
● Instruct patient to notify doctor if loose stools or diarrhea occurs.

Reactions may be *common,* uncommon, *life-threatening,* or COMMON AND LIFE-THREATENING.

cefpodoxime proxetil
Vantin

Pregnancy Risk Category: B

HOW SUPPLIED
Tablets (film-coated): 100 mg, 200 mg
Oral suspension: 50 mg/5 ml, 100 mg/
5 ml in 100-ml bottles

ACTION
A third-generation cephalosporin that inhibits cell-wall synthesis, promoting osmotic instability; usually bactericidal.

Route	Onset	Peak	Duration
PO	Unknown	2-3 hr	Unknown

INDICATIONS & DOSAGE
Acute, community-acquired pneumonia caused by non-beta-lactamase-producing strains of Haemophilus influenzae *or* Streptococcus pneumoniae—
Adults and children 13 years and older: 200 mg P.O. q 12 hours for 14 days.
Acute bacterial exacerbation of chronic bronchitis caused by S. pneumoniae, H. influenzae *(non-beta-lactamase-producing strains only), or* Moraxella (Branhamella) catarrhalis—
Adults and children 13 years and older: 200 mg P.O. q 12 hours for 10 days.
Uncomplicated gonorrhea in men and women; rectal gonococcal infections in women—
Adults and children 13 years and older: 200 mg P.O. as a single dose. Follow with doxycycline 100 mg P.O. b.i.d. for 7 days.
Uncomplicated skin and skin-structure infections caused by Staphylococcus aureus *or* Streptococcus pyogenes—
Adults and children 13 years and older: 400 mg P.O. q 12 hours for 7 to 14 days.
Acute otitis media caused by S. pneumoniae, H. influenzae, *or* M. catarrhalis—
Children 6 months and older: 5 mg/kg (not to exceed 200 mg) P.O. q 12 hours or 10 mg/kg P.O. daily for 10 days.
Pharyngitis or tonsillitis caused by S. pyogenes—
Adults: 100 mg P.O. q 12 hours for 10 days.

Children 6 months and older: 5 mg/kg (not to exceed 100 mg) P.O. q 12 hours for 10 days.
Uncomplicated urinary tract infections caused by Escherichia coli, Klebsiella pneumoniae, Proteus mirabilis, *or* Staphylococcus saprophyticus—
Adults: 100 mg P.O. q 12 hours for 7 days.
Adjust-a-dose: In patients with renal failure, if creatinine clearance is below 30 ml/minute, dosage interval should be increased to q 24 hours. Dialysis patients should receive drug three times weekly after dialysis.

ADVERSE REACTIONS
CNS: headache.
GI: *diarrhea,* nausea, vomiting, abdominal pain.
GU: vaginal fungal infections.
Skin: rash.
Other: hypersensitivity reactions *(anaphylaxis).*

INTERACTIONS
Drug-drug. *Antacids,* H₂ *antagonists:* decreased absorption of cefpodoxime. Avoid concomitant use.
Probenecid: decreased excretion of cefpodoxime. Monitor for toxicity.
Drug-food. *Any food:* increased absorption. Give drug with food.

EFFECTS ON DIAGNOSTIC TESTS
Drug may induce a positive direct Coombs' test. Urine glucose determinations may be false-positive with copper sulfate tests (Clinitest); glucose enzymatic tests (Diastix or Chemstrip uG) are not affected.

CONTRAINDICATIONS
Contraindicated in patients with hypersensitivity to drug or other cephalosporins. Safety and efficacy in children under 6 months have not been established.

NURSING CONSIDERATIONS
• Use cautiously in patients with a history of penicillin hypersensitivity because of risk of cross-sensitivity and in patients receiving nephrotoxic drugs because other cephalosporins have been shown to have

nephrotoxic potential. Because drug is excreted in breast milk, also use cautiously in breast-feeding women.
• Monitor renal function and compare to baseline.
• Obtain specimen for culture and sensitivity tests before giving first dose. Therapy may begin pending results.
• Administer drug with food to enhance absorption. Shake suspension well before using.
• Store suspension in the refrigerator (36° to 46° F [2° to 8° C]). Discard unused portion after 14 days.
• Monitor for superinfection. Drug may cause overgrowth of nonsusceptible bacteria or fungi.

☑ **Patient teaching**
• Tell patient to take all of the medication as prescribed, even after he feels better.
• Instruct patient to take drug with food. If patient is using suspension, tell him to shake container before measuring dose and to keep it refrigerated.
• Tell patient to call doctor if rash or signs and symptoms of superinfection develop.
• Instruct patient to notify doctor if loose stools or diarrhea occurs.

---

cefprozil
Cefzil

Pregnancy Risk Category: B

HOW SUPPLIED
Tablets: 250 mg, 500 mg
Oral suspension: 125 mg/5 ml, 250 mg/5 ml

ACTION
A second-generation cephalosporin that interferes with cell-wall synthesis during microorganism replication, leading to osmotic instability and cell lysis (bactericidal).

Route	Onset	Peak	Duration
PO	Unknown	1.5 hr	Unknown

INDICATIONS & DOSAGE
Pharyngitis or tonsillitis caused by Streptococcus pyogenes—

Adults and children 13 years and older: 500 mg P.O. daily for at least 10 days.
Otitis media caused by S. pneumoniae, Haemophilus influenzae, *and* Moraxella (Branhamella) catarrhalis—
Infants and children 6 months to 12 years: 15 mg/kg P.O. q 12 hours for 10 days.
Secondary bacterial infections of acute bronchitis and acute bacterial exacerbation of chronic bronchitis caused by S. pneumoniae, H. influenzae, *and* M. catarrhalis—
Adults and children 13 years and older: 500 mg P.O. q 12 hours for 10 days.
Uncomplicated skin and skin-structure infections caused by Staphylococcus aureus *and* S. pyogenes—
Adults and children 13 years and older: 250 or 500 mg P.O. q 12 hours or 500 mg daily.
Acute sinusitis caused by S. pneumoniae, H. influenzae *(beta-lactamase positive and negative strains), and* M. catarrhalis *(including beta-lactamase-producing strains)—*
Adults and children 13 years and older: 250 mg P.O. q 12 hours for 10 days; for moderate to severe infection, 500 mg P.O. q 12 hours for 10 days.
Children 6 months to 12 years: 7.5 mg/kg P.O. q 12 hours for 10 days; for moderate to severe infections, 15 mg/kg P.O. q 12 hours for 10 days.
Adjust-a-dose: In patients with renal failure, if creatinine clearance is less than 30 ml/minute, 50% of usual dose.

ADVERSE REACTIONS
CNS: dizziness, hyperactivity, headache, nervousness, insomnia, confusion, somnolence.
GI: *diarrhea, nausea,* vomiting, abdominal pain.
GU: elevated BUN level, elevated serum creatinine level, genital pruritus, vaginitis.
Hematologic: decreased leukocyte count, eosinophilia.
Hepatic: elevated liver enzymes, cholestatic jaundice (rare).
Skin: rash, urticaria, diaper rash.
Other: superinfection, hypersensitivity reactions (serum sickness, ***anaphylaxis***).

Reactions may be *common,* uncommon, *life-threatening,* or COMMON AND LIFE-THREATENING.

INTERACTIONS

Drug-drug. *Aminoglycosides:* potential increased risk of nephrotoxicity. Monitor closely.

Probenecid: may inhibit excretion and increase blood levels of cefprozil. Use together cautiously.

EFFECTS ON DIAGNOSTIC TESTS

Cephalosporins may produce a false-positive result for urine glucose tests that use copper reduction method (Benedict's reagent, Fehling's solution, or Clinitest tablets); use enzymatic glucose oxidase methods instead. A false-negative reaction may occur in the ferricyanide test for blood glucose.

CONTRAINDICATIONS

Contraindicated in patients with hypersensitivity to drug or other cephalosporins.

NURSING CONSIDERATIONS

• Use cautiously in patients with history of sensitivity to penicillin and in breast-feeding women. Also use cautiously in patients with impaired hepatic or renal function.
• Monitor renal function and liver function tests.
• Obtain specimen for culture and sensitivity tests before giving first dose. Therapy may begin pending results.
• Administer after hemodialysis treatment is completed; drug is removed by hemodialysis.
• Monitor for superinfection. May cause overgrowth of nonsusceptible bacteria or fungi.

☑ Patient teaching

• Advise patient to take drug as prescribed, even after he feels better.
• Tell patient to shake suspension well before measuring dose.
• Inform patient that oral suspensions contain the drug in a bubble-gum-flavored form to improve palatability and promote compliance in children. Tell him to refrigerate reconstituted suspension and to discard unused drug after 14 days.
• Instruct patient to notify doctor if rash or symptoms of superinfection occur.

ceftazidime

Ceptaz, Fortaz, Fortum§,
Kefadim§, Tazicef, Tazidime

Pregnancy Risk Category: B

HOW SUPPLIED

Injection (with sodium carbonate):
500 mg, 1 g, 2 g, 6 g (pharmacy bulk package)
Injection (with arginine): 1 g, 2 g, 6 g, 10 g (pharmacy bulk package)
Infusion: 1 g, 2 g in 50-ml and 100-ml vials (premixed)

ACTION

A third-generation cephalosporin that inhibits cell-wall synthesis, promoting osmotic instability; usually bactericidal.

Route	Onset	Peak	Duration
IV	Immediate	Immediate	Unknown
IM	Unknown	1 hr	Unknown

INDICATIONS & DOSAGE

Serious infections of the lower respiratory and urinary tracts; gynecologic, intra-abdominal, CNS, and skin infections; bacteremia; and septicemia. Among susceptible microorganisms are streptococci, including Streptococcus pneumoniae *and* S. pyogenes; Staphylococcus aureus *(penicillinase- and non-penicillinase-producing);* Escherichia coli; Klebsiella; Proteus; Enterobacter; Haemophilus influenzae; Pseudomonas; *and some strains of* Bacteroides—
Adults and children 12 years and older: 1 g I.V. or I.M. q 8 to 12 hours; up to 6 g daily in life-threatening infections.
Children 1 month to 12 years: 25 to 50 mg/kg I.V. q 8 hours (sodium carbonate formulation).
Neonates up to 4 weeks: 30 mg/kg I.V. q 12 hours (sodium carbonate formulation).
Uncomplicated urinary tract infections—
Adults: 250 mg I.V. or I.M. q 12 hours.
Complicated urinary tract infections—
Adults and children 12 years and older: 500 mg to 1 g I.V. or I.M. q 8 hours.
Adjust-a-dose: In patients with renal failure, if creatinine clearance is 31 to 50 ml/minute, give 1 g q 12 hours; if clearance

is 16 to 30 ml/minute, give 1 g q 24 hours; if clearance is 6 to 15 ml/minute, give 500 mg q 24 hours; if clearance is less than 5 ml/minute, give 500 mg q 48 hours.

ADVERSE REACTIONS
CNS: headache, dizziness, paresthesia, *seizures.*
GI: pseudomembranous colitis, nausea, vomiting, diarrhea, candidiasis, abdominal cramps.
GU: vaginitis.
Hematologic: eosinophilia; thrombocytosis, *leukopenia,* hemolytic anemia, *agranulocytosis, thrombocytopenia.*
Hepatic: transient elevation in liver enzymes.
Skin: *maculopapular and erythematous rashes, urticaria.*
Other: hypersensitivity reactions (serum sickness, *anaphylaxis*); *pain, induration, sterile abscesses, tissue sloughing* (at injection site); *phlebitis, thrombophlebitis* (with I.V. injection).

INTERACTIONS
Drug-drug. *Aminoglycosides:* additive or synergistic effect against some strains of *Pseudomonas aeruginosa* and Enterobacteriaceae. Monitor for effects.
Chloramphenicol: antagonistic effect. Avoid concomitant use.
Probenecid: may inhibit excretion and increase levels. May be used as a therapeutic effect.

EFFECTS ON DIAGNOSTIC TESTS
Drug causes false-positive results in urine glucose tests using cupric sulfate (Benedict's reagent or Clinitest); use glucose oxidase (Diastix or Chemstrip uG) instead. Ceftazidime may cause positive Coombs' test results.

CONTRAINDICATIONS
Contraindicated in patients with hypersensitivity to drug or other cephalosporins.

NURSING CONSIDERATIONS
● Use cautiously in patients with a history of sensitivity to penicillin and in breast-feeding women. Also use cautiously and with dosage adjustments in patients with renal failure. Monitor renal function.
● Obtain specimen for culture and sensitivity tests before giving first dose. Therapy may begin pending results.
● For I.M. administration, inject deeply into a large muscle mass, such as the gluteus maximus or the lateral aspect of the thigh.
● With large doses or prolonged therapy, monitor for superinfection, especially in high-risk patients.
Alert: Keep in mind that commercially available preparations contain either sodium carbonate (Fortaz, Magnacef, Tazicef, Tazidime) or arginine (Ceptaz, Pentacef) to facilitate dissolution of drug. Safety and efficacy of arginine-containing solutions in children 12 years and under have not been established.
● Know that ceftazidime is removed by hemodialysis; a supplemental dose of drug is indicated after each dialysis period, as ordered.

⬗ I.V. administration
● Reconstitute sodium carbonate-containing solutions with sterile water for injection. Add 5 ml to a 500-mg vial; 10 ml to a 1-g or 2-g vial. Shake well to dissolve drug. Carbon dioxide is released during dissolution, and positive pressure will develop in the vial. Reconstitute arginine-containing solutions with 10 ml of sterile water for injection. This formulation won't release gas bubbles. Each brand of ceftazidime includes specific instructions for reconstitution. Read them carefully.
● Infuse over 15 to 30 minutes.

✓ Patient teaching
● Tell patient to report adverse reactions or symptoms of superinfection promptly.
● Instruct patient to alert nurse if discomfort is felt at I.V. insertion site.
● Advise patient to notify doctor if loose stools or diarrhea occurs.

---

ceftibuten
Cedax

Pregnancy Risk Category: B

HOW SUPPLIED
Capsules: 400 mg
Oral suspension: 90 mg/5 ml,
180 mg/5 ml

ACTION
Ceftibuten exerts its bacterial action by binding to essential target proteins of the bacterial cell wall, which leads to inhibition of cell-wall synthesis. It is a third-generation cephalosporin.

Route	Onset	Peak	Duration
PO	Unknown	2-4 hr	Unknown

INDICATIONS & DOSAGE
Acute bacterial exacerbation of chronic bronchitis due to Haemophilus influenzae, Moraxella catarrhalis, *or penicillin-susceptible strains of* Streptococcus pneumoniae—
Adults and children weighing over 45 kg (99 lb): 400 mg P.O. daily for 10 days.
Pharyngitis and tonsillitis due to Streptococcus pyogenes; *acute bacterial otitis media due to* H. influenzae, M. catarrhalis, *or* S. pyogenes—
Adults and children weighing over 45 kg: 400 mg P.O. daily for 10 days.
Children weighing under 45 kg: 9 mg/kg P.O. daily for 10 days.
Adjust-a-dose: In adult patients with renal impairment, if creatinine clearance is 30 to 49 ml/minute, give 4.5 mg/kg or 200 mg P.O. q 24 hours; if clearance is 5 to 29 ml/minute, give 2.25 mg/kg or 100 mg P.O. q 24 hours. In patients undergoing hemodialysis two or three times weekly, give single dose of 400 mg (capsule) or 9 mg/kg (suspension) P.O. after each hemodialysis session. Maximum dose is 400 mg.

ADVERSE REACTIONS
CNS: headache, dizziness, aphasia, psychosis.
GI: nausea, vomiting, diarrhea, dyspepsia, abdominal pain, loose stools, pseudomembranous colitis.
Hematologic: elevated levels of eosinophils, decreased hemoglobin levels, altered platelet count, *aplastic anemia,*

hemolytic anemia, *hemorrhage, neutropenia, agranulocytosis, pancytopenia.*
Hepatic: hepatic cholestasis, elevated liver enzymes and bilirubin.
Skin: *Stevens-Johnson syndrome.*
Other: elevated levels of BUN, toxic nephropathy, renal dysfunction, allergic reaction, *anaphylaxis,* drug fever.

INTERACTIONS
Drug-food. *Any food:* decreased bioavailability of drug, which slows its absorption. Administer drug 2 hours before or 1 hour after a meal.

EFFECTS ON DIAGNOSTIC TESTS
Although drug has not been known to affect the direct Coombs' test to date, other cephalosporins have caused a false-positive direct Coombs' test. Some cephalosporins may cause a false-positive test for urinary glucose.

CONTRAINDICATIONS
Contraindicated in patients with hypersensitivity to cephalosporin drugs.

NURSING CONSIDERATIONS
• Use cautiously if administering to patients with history of hypersensitivity to penicillin.
• Use cautiously in patients with impaired renal failure or GI disease, especially colitis. Monitor renal function.
• Use cautiously when administering to elderly patient.
• Safety and effectiveness in infants under 6 months have not been established.
• Drug should be used in pregnancy only if clearly needed. Not known if drug is excreted in breast milk; use cautiously in breast-feeding women.
Alert: If allergic reaction is suspected, drug should be discontinued. Emergency treatment may be required.
• Pseudomembranous colitis has been reported with nearly all antibacterial agents. Consider this diagnosis in patients who develop diarrhea secondary to therapy. Obtain specimens for *Clostridium difficile,* as ordered.
• Obtain specimen for culture and sensitivity tests before giving first dose. Therapy may begin pending test results.

• When preparing oral suspension, first tap the bottle to loosen powder. Follow chart supplied by manufacturer for amount of water to add to powder when mixing oral suspension form. Add water in two portions; shake well after each step. After mixing, suspension is stable for 14 days when refrigerated.
• Shake oral suspension well before administering.
• Drug may cause overgrowth of nonsusceptible bacteria or fungi. Monitor patient for superinfection.

☑ Patient teaching
• Instruct patient to take all of the medication prescribed, even if he feels better.
• Tell patient using oral suspension to take it at least 2 hours before or 1 hour after a meal.
• Instruct patient using oral suspension to shake bottle well before measuring.
• Inform patient to store oral suspension in the refrigerator, with lid tightly closed, and to discard any unused drug after 14 days.
• Caution breast-feeding woman that it is unknown whether ceftibuten is excreted in breast milk.
• Tell diabetic patient that suspension contains 1 g sucrose/teaspoon.
• Instruct patient to report adverse reactions or symptoms of superinfection.
• Tell patient to notify doctor if loose stools or diarrhea occurs.

---

ceftizoxime sodium
Cefizox

Pregnancy Risk Category: B

HOW SUPPLIED
Injection: 500 mg, 1 g, 2 g
Infusion: 1 g, 2 g in 100-ml vials or in 50 ml of D_5W

ACTION
A third-generation cephalosporin that inhibits cell-wall synthesis, promoting osmotic instability; usually bactericidal.

Route	Onset	Peak	Duration
IV	Immediate	Immediate	Unknown
IM	Unknown	0.5-1.5 hr	Unknown

INDICATIONS & DOSAGE
Serious infections of the lower respiratory and urinary tracts, gynecologic infections, bacteremia, septicemia, meningitis, intra-abdominal infections, bone and joint infections, and skin infections. Among susceptible microorganisms are streptococci, including Streptococcus pneumoniae *and* S. pyogenes; Staphylococcus aureus *and* Staphylococcus epidermidis; Escherichia coli; Klebsiella; Haemophilus influenzae; Enterobacter; Proteus; *some* Pseudomonas; *and* Peptostreptococcus—
Adults: usual dosage is 1 to 2 g I.V. or I.M. q 8 to 12 hours. In life-threatening infections, up to 2 g q 4 hours.
Children over 6 months: 33 to 50 mg/kg I.V. q 6 to 8 hours. Serious infections: up to 200 mg/kg/day in divided doses may be used. Don't exceed 12 g/day.
Adjust-a-dose: In patients with renal failure, if creatinine clearance is 50 to 79 ml/minute, give 500 mg to 1.5 g q 8 hours; if clearance is 5 to 49 ml/minute, give 250 mg to 1 g q 12 hours; if clearance is less than 5 ml/minute, give 500 mg to 1 g q 48 hours.

ADVERSE REACTIONS
GI: pseudomembranous colitis, nausea, anorexia, vomiting, *diarrhea.*
GU: vaginitis.
Hematologic: *transient neutropenia,* eosinophilia, hemolytic anemia, thrombocytosis, anemia, *thrombocytopenia.*
Hepatic: transient elevation in liver enzymes.
Skin: *maculopapular and erythematous rashes,* urticaria.
Other: hypersensitivity reactions (serum sickness, *anaphylaxis*); dyspnea; elevated temperature; *pain, induration, sterile abscesses, tissue sloughing* (at injection site); *phlebitis, thrombophlebitis* (with I.V. injection).

INTERACTIONS
Drug-drug. *Aminoglycosides:* potential increase in nephrotoxicity. Avoid use.
Probenecid: may inhibit excretion and increase blood levels of ceftizoxime. May be used for this effect.

EFFECTS ON DIAGNOSTIC TESTS

Drug causes false-positive results in urine glucose tests using cupric sulfate (Benedict's reagent or Clinitest); use glucose oxidase (Diastix or Chemstrip uG) instead. It also causes false elevations in urine creatinine levels using Jaffé's reaction. Ceftizoxime may cause positive Coombs' test results.

CONTRAINDICATIONS

Contraindicated in patients with hypersensitivity to drug or other cephalosporins.

NURSING CONSIDERATIONS

• Use cautiously in patients with history of sensitivity to penicillin and in breast-feeding women. Also use cautiously and with dosage adjustments in patients with renal failure. Monitor renal function.
• Obtain specimen for culture and sensitivity tests before giving first dose. Therapy may begin pending results.
• For I.M. administration, inject deeply into a large muscle mass, such as the gluteus maximus or the lateral aspect of the thigh. Larger doses (2 g) should be divided and administered at two separate sites.
• With large doses or prolonged therapy, monitor for superinfection, especially in high-risk patients.

I.V. administration

• To reconstitute powder, add 5 ml of sterile water to a 500-mg vial, 10 ml to a 1-g vial, or 20 ml to a 2-g vial.
• Inject directly into vein over 3 to 5 minutes or slowly into I.V. tubing with freely flowing compatible solution.
• Reconstitute piggyback vials with 50 to 100 ml of 0.9% NaCl solution or D₅W. Shake well.
• Infuse over 15 to 30 minutes.

Patient teaching

• Tell patient to report adverse reactions and symptoms of superinfection promptly.
• Instruct patient to alert nurse if discomfort is felt at I.V. site.
• Tell patient to notify doctor if loose stools or diarrhea occurs.

ceftriaxone sodium
Rocephin

Pregnancy Risk Category: B

HOW SUPPLIED

Injection: 250 mg, 500 mg, 1 g, 2 g
Infusion: 1 g, 2 g

ACTION

A third-generation cephalosporin that inhibits cell-wall synthesis, promoting osmotic instability; usually bactericidal.

Route	Onset	Peak	Duration
IV	Immediate	Immediate	Unknown
IM	Unknown	1.5-4 hr	Unknown

INDICATIONS & DOSAGE

Uncomplicated gonococcal vulvovaginitis—
Adults: 250 mg I.M. as a single dose, followed with 100 mg of doxycycline P.O. q 12 hours for 10 to 14 days.
Most infections caused by susceptible organisms; serious infections of the lower respiratory and urinary tracts; gynecologic, bone and joint, intra-abdominal, and skin infections; bacteremia; septicemia; and Lyme disease caused by such susceptible microorganisms as streptococci, including Streptococcus pneumoniae *and* S. pyogenes; Staphylococcus aureus *(penicillinase- and non-penicillinase-producing) and* Staphylococcus epidermidis; *Escherichia coli; Klebsiella; Haemophilus influenzae; Neisseria meningitidis; N. gonorrhoeae; Enterobacter; Proteus; Peptostreptococcus, Pseudomonas; and* Serratia marcescens—
Adults and children over 12 years: 1 to 2 g I.M. or I.V. daily or in equally divided doses q 12 hours. Total daily dosage should not exceed 4 g.
Children 12 years and under: 50 to 75 mg/kg I.M. or I.V., not to exceed 2 g/day, given in divided doses q 12 hours.
Meningitis—
Adults and children: initially, 100 mg/kg I.M. or I.V. (not to exceed 4 g); thereafter, 100 mg/kg I.M. or I.V., given once daily or in divided doses q 12 hours, not to exceed 4 g, for 7 to 14 days.

---

*Liquid contains alcohol.   **May contain tartrazine.   †Canada   ‡Australia   §U.K.   ◊OTC

Perioperative prophylaxis—
Adults: 1 g I.V. as a single dose ½ to 2 hours before surgery.
✳ *NEW INDICATION: Acute bacterial otitis media—*
Children: 50 mg/kg (not to exceed 1 g) I.M. as a single dose.

ADVERSE REACTIONS
CNS: headache, dizziness.
GI: pseudomembranous colitis, nausea, vomiting, diarrhea.
GU: genital pruritus, candidiasis, elevated BUN levels.
Hematologic: eosinophilia, thrombocytosis, *leukopenia.*
Hepatic: elevated liver function test results.
Skin: pain, induration, tenderness at injection site; phlebitis; *rash;* pruritus.
Other: hypersensitivity reactions (serum sickness, ***anaphylaxis***), elevated temperature, chills.

INTERACTIONS
Drug-drug. *Aminoglycosides:* additive or synergistic effect against some strains of *Pseudomonas aeruginosa* and Enterobacteriaceae. Monitor patient.
Probenecid: high doses (1 or 2 g/day) may enhance hepatic clearance of ceftriaxone and shorten its half-life. Avoid concomitant use.

EFFECTS ON DIAGNOSTIC TESTS
Drug causes false-positive results in urine glucose tests using cupric sulfate (Benedict's reagent or Clinitest); instead use glucose oxidase (Diastix or Chemstrip uG). It also causes false elevations in urine creatinine levels in tests using Jaffé's reaction. Ceftriaxone may cause positive Coombs' test results.

CONTRAINDICATIONS
Contraindicated in patients with hypersensitivity to drug or other cephalosporins.

NURSING CONSIDERATIONS
● Use cautiously in patients with a history of sensitivity to penicillin and in breast-feeding women.

● Obtain specimen for culture and sensitivity tests before giving first dose. Therapy may begin pending results.
● A commercially available intramuscular kit is available from the manufacturer containing 1% lidocaine as a diluent.
● For I.M. administration, inject deeply into a large muscle mass, such as the gluteus maximus or the lateral aspect of the thigh.
● With large doses or prolonged therapy, monitor for superinfection, especially in high-risk patients.
● Be aware that drug is commonly used in home antibiotic programs for outpatient treatment of serious infections, such as osteomyelitis.

🩸 I.V. administration
● Reconstitute with sterile water for injection, 0.9% NaCl injection, D_5W or $D_{10}W$ injection, or a combination of NaCl and dextrose injection and other compatible solutions. Reconstitute by adding 2.4 ml of diluent to the 250-mg vial, 4.8 ml to the 500-mg vial, 9.6 ml to the 1-g vial, and 19.2 ml to the 2-g vial. All reconstituted solutions yield a concentration that averages 100 mg/ml. After reconstitution, dilute further for intermittent infusion to desired concentration. I.V. dilutions are stable for 24 hours at room temperature.

✅ Patient teaching
● Tell patient to report adverse reactions promptly.
● Instruct patient to alert nurse if discomfort occurs at I.V. insertion site.
● Teach home care patient and family how to prepare and administer drug.
● If home care patient is a diabetic who is testing his urine for glucose, tell him drug may affect results of cupric sulfate tests; instead he should use an enzymatic test.
● Tell patient to notify doctor if loose stools or diarrhea occurs.

Reactions may be *common,* uncommon, *life-threatening,* or **COMMON AND LIFE-THREATENING.**

cefuroxime axetil
Ceftin, Zinnat§

cefuroxime sodium
Kefurox, Zinacef

Pregnancy Risk Category: B

HOW SUPPLIED
cefuroxime axetil
Tablets: 125 mg, 250 mg, 500 mg
Suspension: 125 mg/5 ml, 250 mg/5 ml
cefuroxime sodium
Injection: 750 mg, 1.5 g
Infusion: 750 mg, 1.5 g premixed,
frozen solution

ACTION
A second-generation cephalosporin that
inhibits cell-wall synthesis, promoting osmotic instability; usually bactericidal.

Route	Onset	Peak	Duration
PO	Unknown	15-60 min	Unknown
IV	Immediate	Immediate	Unknown
IM	Unknown	2 hr	Unknown

INDICATIONS & DOSAGE
*Injectable form is for serious infections of
the lower respiratory and urinary tracts;
skin and skin-structure infections; bone
and joint infections; septicemia; meningitis; and gonorrhea; and for perioperative
prophylaxis. Oral form is used to treat otitis media, pharyngitis, tonsillitis, infections of the urinary and lower respiratory
tracts, and skin and skin-structure infections. Among susceptible organisms are*
Streptococcus pneumoniae *and* S. pyogenes, Haemophilus influenzae, Klebsiella, Staphylococcus aureus, Escherichia
coli, Moraxella (Branhamella) catarrhalis
*(including beta-lactamase-producing
strains),* Enterobacter, *and* Neisseria gonorrhoeae—
Adults and children 12 years and older:
usual dosage of cefuroxime sodium is
750 mg to 1.5 g I.M. or I.V. q 8 hours for
5 to 10 days. For life-threatening infections and infections caused by less susceptible organisms, 1.5 g I.M. or I.V. q 6
hours; for bacterial meningitis, up to 3 g
I.V. q 8 hours.

Alternatively, administer 250 mg of cefuroxime axetil P.O. q 12 hours. For severe infections, dosage may be increased
to 500 mg q 12 hours.
Children and infants over 3 months: 50
to 100 mg/kg/day of cefuroxime sodium
I.M. or I.V. in equally divided doses q 6 to
8 hours. Higher dosage of 100 mg/kg/day
(not to exceed maximum adult dosage)
should be used for more severe or serious
infections. For bacterial meningitis, 200
to 240 mg/kg I.V. in divided doses q 6 to
8 hours. For other infections, 125 to
250 mg of cefuroxime axetil P.O. q 12
hours for a child who can swallow pills.
*Uncomplicated urinary tract infec-
tions—*
Adults: 125 to 250 mg P.O. q 12 hours.
Otitis media—
Children under 2 years: 125 mg P.O. q
12 hours.
Children 2 years and older: 250 mg
P.O. q 12 hours.
Perioperative prophylaxis—
Adults: 1.5 g I.V. 30 to 60 minutes before
surgery; in lengthy operations, 750 mg
I.V. or I.M. q 8 hours. For open-heart
surgery, 1.5 g I.V. at induction of anesthesia and then q 12 hours for a total dosage
of 6 g.
*Early Lyme disease (erythema migrans)
caused by* Borrelia burgdorferi—
**Adults and children 13 years and old-
er:** 500 mg P.O. b.i.d. for 20 days.
*Secondary bacterial infection of acute
bronchitis—*
Adults: 250 to 500 mg P.O. (tablets) b.i.d.
for 5 to 10 days.
Adjust-a-dose: For parenteral administration: In patients with renal failure, if creatinine clearance is 10 to 20 ml/minute,
give 750 mg I.M. or I.V. q 12 hours; if
clearance is less than 10 ml/minute, give
750 mg I.M. or I.V. q 24 hours.

ADVERSE REACTIONS
GI: pseudomembranous colitis, nausea,
anorexia, vomiting, *diarrhea.*
Hematologic: *transient neutropenia,*
eosinophilia, *hemolytic anemia, thrombocytopenia,* decreased hemoglobin and
hematocrit levels.
Hepatic: transient increases in liver enzymes.

Skin: *maculopapular and erythematous rashes, urticaria.*
Other: hypersensitivity reactions (serum sickness, ***anaphylaxis***); *pain, induration, sterile abscesses, temperature elevation, tissue sloughing* (at I.M. injection site); *phlebitis, thrombophlebitis* (with I.V. injection).

INTERACTIONS
Drug-drug. *Aminoglycosides:* Synergistic activity against some organisms; potential for increased nephrotoxicity. Monitor closely.
Diuretics: increased risk of adverse renal reactions. Monitor closely.
Probenecid: may inhibit excretion and increase blood levels of cefuroxime. Sometimes used for this effect.
Drug-food. *Any food:* increased absorption. Give drug with food.

EFFECTS ON DIAGNOSTIC TESTS
Drug causes false-positive results in urine glucose tests using cupric sulfate (Benedict's reagent or Clinitest); use glucose oxidase tests (Diastix or Chemstrip uG) instead. It also causes false elevations in serum or urine creatinine levels in tests using Jaffé's reaction. Cefuroxime may cause positive Coombs' test results.

CONTRAINDICATIONS
Contraindicated in patients with hypersensitivity to drug or other cephalosporins.

NURSING CONSIDERATIONS
• Use cautiously in patients with history of sensitivity to penicillin and in breast-feeding women. Also use cautiously and with reduced dosage in patients with impaired renal function. Monitor renal function.
• Obtain specimen for culture and sensitivity tests before giving first dose. Therapy may begin pending results.
• For I.M. administration, inject deeply into a large muscle mass, such as the gluteus maximus or the lateral aspect of the thigh.
• Know that absorption of cefuroxime axetil is enhanced by food.
• Keep in mind that cefuroxime axetil

tablets may be crushed for patients who cannot swallow tablets. Tablets may be allowed to dissolve in small amounts of apple, orange, or grape juice or chocolate milk. However, the drug has a bitter taste that is difficult to mask, even with food.
• Be aware that cefuroxime axetil film-coated tablet form and oral suspension are not bioequivalent and are not substitutable on a mg/mg basis.
• With large doses or prolonged therapy, monitor for superinfection, especially in high-risk patients.

◖ I.V. administration
• For each 750-mg vial of Kefurox, reconstitute with 9 ml of sterile water for injection. Withdraw 8 ml from the vial for the proper dose. For each 1.5-g vial of Kefurox, reconstitute with 16 ml of sterile water for injection; withdraw entire contents of vial for a dose. For each 750-mg vial of Zinacef, reconstitute with 8 ml of sterile water for injection; for each 1.5-g vial, reconstitute with 16 ml. In each case, withdraw entire contents of vial for a dose.
• To give by direct injection, inject into a large vein or into the tubing of a free-flowing I.V. solution over 3 to 5 minutes.
• For intermittent infusion, add reconstituted drug to 100 ml D_5W, 0.9% NaCl for injection, or other compatible I.V. solution. Infuse over 15 to 60 minutes.

✓ Patient teaching
• Tell patient to take all of the medication as prescribed, even after he feels better.
• Instruct patient to take oral form with food. If patient has difficulty swallowing tablets, tell him how to dissolve or crush tablets but warn him that the bitter taste that results is hard to mask, even with food. If suspension is being used, tell patient to shake container well before measuring dose.
• Tell patient to notify doctor if rash or symptoms of superinfection occur.
• Inform patient receiving drug I.V. to alert nurse if discomfort occurs at I.V. insertion site.
• Tell patient to notify doctor if loose stools or diarrhea occurs.

Reactions may be common, *uncommon,* **life-threatening,** *or* **COMMON AND LIFE-THREATENING.**

cephalexin hydrochloride
Keftab

cephalexin monohydrate
Apo-Cephalex†, Biocef, Cefanex, C-Lexin, Keflex, Novo-Lexin†, Nu-Cephalex†‡

Pregnancy Risk Category: B

HOW SUPPLIED
cephalexin hydrochloride
Tablets: 250 mg, 500 mg
cephalexin monohydrate
Tablets: 250 mg, 500 mg, 1 g
Capsules: 250 mg, 500 mg
Oral suspension: 100 mg/5 ml, 125 mg/5 ml, 250 mg/5 ml

ACTION
A first-generation cephalosporin that inhibits cell-wall synthesis, promoting osmotic instability; usually bactericidal.

Route	Onset	Peak	Duration
PO	Unknown	1 hr	Unknown

INDICATIONS & DOSAGE
Respiratory tract, GI tract, skin, soft-tissue, bone, and joint infections and otitis media caused by Escherichia coli *and other coliform bacteria, group A beta-hemolytic streptococci,* Klebsiella, Proteus mirabilis, Streptococcus pneumoniae, *and staphylococci—*
Adults: 250 mg to 1 g P.O. q 6 hours or 500 mg q 12 hours. Maximum 4 g daily.
Children: 6 to 12 mg/kg P.O. q 6 hours (monohydrate only). Maximum 25 mg/kg q 6 hours.
Adjust-a-dose: For adults with impaired renal function, the initial dose is the same. Recommended subsequent dosing is as follows: if creatinine clearance is below 5 ml/minute, give 250 mg P.O. q 12 to 24 hours; if clearance is 5 to 10 ml/minute, give 250 mg P.O. q 12 hours; if clearance is 11 to 40 ml/minute, give 500 mg P.O. q 8 to 12 hours.

ADVERSE REACTIONS
CNS: dizziness, headache, fatigue, agitation, confusion, hallucinations.
GI: pseudomembranous colitis, *nausea, anorexia,* vomiting, *diarrhea,* gastritis, glossitis, dyspepsia, abdominal pain, anal pruritus, tenesmus, oral candidiasis.
GU: genital pruritus, candidiasis, vaginitis, interstitial nephritis.
Hematologic: *neutropenia,* eosinophilia, anemia, *thrombocytopenia.*
Skin: *maculopapular and erythematous rashes,* urticaria.
Other: transient increases in liver enzymes, hypersensitivity reactions (serum sickness, *anaphylaxis*), arthritis, arthralgia, joint pain.

INTERACTIONS
Drug-drug. *Probenecid:* may increase blood levels of cephalosporins. May be used for this effect.

EFFECTS ON DIAGNOSTIC TESTS
Cephalexin causes false-positive results in urine glucose tests using cupric sulfate (Benedict's reagent or Clinitest); use glucose oxidase tests (Diastix or Chemstrip uG) instead. It also causes false elevations in serum or urine creatinine levels in tests using Jaffé's reaction. Positive Coombs' test results occur in about 3% of patients taking cephalexin.

CONTRAINDICATIONS
Contraindicated in patients with hypersensitivity to cephalosporins.

NURSING CONSIDERATIONS
• Use cautiously in breast-feeding women and in patients with impaired renal function or history of sensitivity to penicillin. Monitor renal function.
• Ask patient of past reaction to cephalosporin or penicillin therapy before giving first dose.
• Obtain specimen for culture and sensitivity tests before giving first dose. Therapy may begin pending results.
• To prepare oral suspension: Add required amount of water to powder in two portions. Shake well after each addition. After mixing, store in refrigerator. The mixture will remain stable for 14 days without significant loss of potency. Keep tightly closed and shake well before using.

• With large doses or prolonged therapy, monitor for superinfection, especially in high-risk patients.
• Know that group A beta-hemolytic streptococcal infections should be treated for a minimum of 10 days.

☑**Patient teaching**
• Tell patient to take all of the medication exactly as prescribed, even after he feels better.
• Instruct patient to take drug with food or milk to lessen GI discomfort. If patient is taking suspension form, instruct him to shake container well before measuring dose and to store in refrigerator.
• Tell patient to notify doctor if rash or symptoms of superinfection develop.

---

cephradine
Velosef**

Pregnancy Risk Category: B

HOW SUPPLIED
Capsules: 250 mg, 500 mg
Oral suspension: 125 mg/5 ml, 250 mg/5 ml

ACTION
First-generation cephalosporin that inhibits cell-wall synthesis, promoting osmotic instability; usually bactericidal.

Route	Onset	Peak	Duration
PO	Unknown	1 hr	Unknown

INDICATIONS & DOSAGE
Serious infections of respiratory, GU, or GI tract; skin and soft-tissue infections; bone and joint infections; septicemia; endocarditis; and otitis media caused by such susceptible organisms as Escherichia coli *and other coliform bacteria, group A beta-hemolytic streptococci,* Klebsiella, Proteus mirabilis, Staphylococcus aureus, Streptococcus pneumoniae, Streptococcus viridans, *and staphylococci; and perioperative prophylaxis*—
Adults: 250 to 500 mg P.O. q 6 hours or 500 mg to 1 g P.O. q 12 hours.
Children over 9 months: 25 to 50 mg/kg P.O. daily in divided doses q 6 to 12 hours.
Otitis media—
Children: 75 to 100 mg/kg P.O. daily in equally divided doses q 6 to 12 hours. Don't exceed 4 g daily.
All patients, regardless of age and weight, may be given larger doses (up to 1 g q.i.d.) for severe or chronic infections.

ADVERSE REACTIONS
CNS: dizziness, headache, malaise, paresthesia.
GI: pseudomembranous colitis, *nausea, anorexia,* vomiting, heartburn, abdominal cramps, *diarrhea,* oral candidiasis.
GU: genital pruritus, candidiasis, vaginitis.
Hematologic: *transient neutropenia,* eosinophilia, *thrombocytopenia.*
Hepatic: transient increases in liver enzymes.
Skin: *maculopapular and erythematous rashes,* urticaria.
Other: hypersensitivity reactions (serum sickness, *anaphylaxis*).

INTERACTIONS
Drug-drug. *Probenecid:* may increase blood levels of cephalosporins. Sometimes used for this effect.

EFFECTS ON DIAGNOSTIC TESTS
Drug causes false-positive results in urine glucose tests using cupric sulfate (Benedict's reagent or Clinitest); instead use glucose oxidase tests (Diastix or Chemstrip uG). It also causes false elevations in serum or urine creatinine levels in tests using Jaffé's reaction. Cephradine may cause positive Coombs' test results.

CONTRAINDICATIONS
Contraindicated in patients with hypersensitivity to drug and to other cephalosporins.

NURSING CONSIDERATIONS
• Use cautiously in patients with impaired renal function or with a history of sensitivity to penicillin. Also use cautiously in breast-feeding women.
• Monitor renal function.
• Obtain specimen for culture and sensi-

tivity tests before giving first dose. Therapy may begin pending results.
• Know that group A beta-hemolytic streptococcal infections should be treated for a minimum of 10 days.
• With large doses or prolonged therapy, monitor for superinfection, especially in high-risk patients.

☑ Patient teaching
• Instruct patient to take all of the medication as prescribed, even after he feels better.
• Inform patient to take drug with food or milk to lessen GI discomfort. If patient is taking suspension form, tell him to shake it well before measuring dose.
• Tell patient to notify doctor if rash or signs and symptoms of superinfection occur.
• Instruct patient to notify doctor if loose stools or diarrhea occurs.

---

loracarbef
Lorabid

Pregnancy Risk Category: B

HOW SUPPLIED
Pulvules: 200 mg, 400 mg
Powder for oral suspension: 100 mg/5 ml, 200 mg/5 ml in 50-ml and 100-ml bottles

ACTION
A synthetic beta-lactam antibiotic of the carbacephem class with actions similar to the second-generation cephalosporins. Inhibits cell-wall synthesis, promoting osmotic instability; usually bactericidal.

Route	Onset	Peak	Duration
PO	Unknown	0.5-1 hr	Unknown

INDICATIONS & DOSAGE
Secondary bacterial infections of acute bronchitis—
Adults: 200 to 400 mg P.O. q 12 hours for 7 days.
Acute bacterial exacerbations of chronic bronchitis—
Adults: 400 mg P.O. q 12 hours for 7 days.

Pneumonia—
Adults: 400 mg P.O. q 12 hours for 14 days.
Pharyngitis, sinusitis, or tonsillitis—
Adults: 200 to 400 mg P.O. q 12 hours for 10 days.
Children 6 months to 12 years: 15 mg/kg P.O. daily in divided doses q 12 hours for 10 days.
Acute otitis media—
Children 6 months to 12 years: 30 mg/kg (oral suspension) P.O. daily in divided doses q 12 hours for 10 days.
Uncomplicated skin and skin-structure infections—
Adults: 200 mg P.O. q 12 hours for 7 days.
Impetigo—
Children 6 months to 12 years: 15 mg/kg P.O. daily in divided doses q 12 hours for 7 days.
Uncomplicated cystitis—
Adults: 200 mg P.O. daily for 7 days.
Uncomplicated pyelonephritis—
Adults: 400 mg P.O. q 12 hours for 14 days.
Adjust-a-dose: Patients with creatinine clearance of 50 ml/minute or more don't require dose and interval changes. If creatinine clearance is 10 to 49 ml/minute, give half of usual dose at same interval and if it is below 10 ml/minute, give usual dose q 3 to 5 days. Hemodialysis patients require an additional dose after dialysis.

ADVERSE REACTIONS
CNS: headache, somnolence, nervousness, insomnia, dizziness.
CV: vasodilation.
GI: diarrhea, nausea, vomiting, abdominal pain, anorexia, pseudomembranous colitis.
GU: vaginal candidiasis, transient increases in BUN and creatinine levels.
Hematologic: *transient thrombocytopenia, leukopenia,* eosinophilia, increased PT and INR, pancytopenia, elevated LD level, *neutropenia.*
Hepatic: transient elevations in AST, ALT, and alkaline phosphatase levels.
Skin: rash, urticaria, pruritus, *erythema multiforme.*
Other: hypersensitivity reactions, including *anaphylaxis.*

INTERACTIONS

Drug-drug. *Probenecid:* decreased excretion of loracarbef, causing increased plasma levels. Monitor for toxicity.
Drug-food. *Any food:* decreased absorption. Have patent take drug on empty stomach at least 1 hour before or 2 hours after a meal.

EFFECTS ON DIAGNOSTIC TESTS

Drug can cause positive direct Coombs' test results.

CONTRAINDICATIONS

Contraindicated in patients with hypersensitivity to drug or other cephalosporins and in patients with diarrhea caused by pseudomembranous colitis.

NURSING CONSIDERATIONS

• Use cautiously in pregnant or breast-feeding women. Safety and efficacy of drug have not been established in infants under 6 months.
• Obtain specimen for culture and sensitivity tests before giving first dose. Therapy may begin pending results.
• To reconstitute powder for oral suspension, add 30 ml of water in two portions to the 50-ml bottle or 60 ml of water in two portions to the 100-ml bottle; shake after each addition.
• After reconstitution, store oral suspension for 14 days at room temperature (59° to 86° F [15° to 30° C]).
• Monitor for superinfection. May cause overgrowth of nonsusceptible bacteria or fungi.
• Monitor renal function.
Alert: Monitor patient for seizures. Beta-lactam antibiotics may trigger seizures in susceptible patients, especially when given without dosage modification to those with renal impairment. If seizures occur, discontinue drug and notify doctor. Administer anticonvulsants as ordered.
• For otitis media, remember that the more rapidly absorbed oral suspension produces higher peak plasma levels than do the capsules.

✓Patient teaching

• Instruct patient to take all of the medication prescribed, even after he feels better.
• Tell patient to take drug on an empty stomach, at least 1 hour before or 2 hours after meals. Tell him to shake container of suspension well before measuring dose.
• Advise patient to discard unused portion after 14 days.
• Instruct patient to notify doctor if rash or signs and symptoms of superinfection appears.
• Instruct patient to notify doctor if loose stools or diarrhea occurs.

demeclocycline hydrochloride
doxycycline calcium
doxycycline hyclate
doxycycline hydrochloride
doxycycline monohydrate
minocycline hydrochloride
tetracycline hydrochloride

COMBINATION PRODUCTS
UROBIOTIC-250: oxytetracycline hydrochloride 250 mg, sulfamethizole 250 mg, and phenazopyridine hydrochloride 50 mg.

---

demeclocycline hydrochloride
Declomycin, Ledermycin‡

Pregnancy Risk Category: D

HOW SUPPLIED
Tablets (film-coated): 150 mg, 300 mg
Capsules: 150 mg

ACTION
Unknown. Thought to exert bacteriostatic effect by binding to the 30S and possibly 50S ribosomal subunits of microorganisms, thus inhibiting protein synthesis. May also alter the cytoplasmic membrane of susceptible microorganisms.

Route	Onset	Peak	Duration
PO	Unknown	3-4 hr	Unknown

INDICATIONS & DOSAGE
Infections caused by susceptible gram-positive and gram-negative organisms (including Haemophilus ducreyi, Yersinia pestis, *and* Campylobacter fetus*),* Rickettsiae, Mycoplasma pneumoniae, Chlamydia trachomatis; *psittacosis; granuloma inguinale—*
Adults: 150 mg P.O. q 6 hours or 300 mg P.O. q 12 hours.
Children over 8 years: 6 to 13.2 mg/kg P.O. daily, in divided doses q 6 to 12 hours.

Gonorrhea—
Adults: initially, 600 mg P.O.; then 300 mg P.O. q 12 hours for 4 days (for a total of 3 g).

ADVERSE REACTIONS
CNS: *intracranial hypertension (pseudotumor cerebri),* dizziness.
CV: pericarditis.
EENT: dysphagia, glossitis, tinnitus, visual disturbances.
GI: anorexia, *nausea, vomiting, diarrhea,* enterocolitis, anogenital inflammation, pancreatitis.
GU: elevated serum BUN levels in patients with decreased renal function.
Hematologic: *neutropenia,* eosinophilia, *thrombocytopenia, hemolytic anemia.*
Skin: *maculopapular and erythematous rashes, photosensitivity,* increased pigmentation, urticaria.
Other: hypersensitivity reactions *(anaphylaxis),* elevated liver enzymes, diabetes insipidus syndrome (polyuria, polydipsia, weakness), permanent tooth discoloration or bone growth retardation if used in children under 9 years.

INTERACTIONS
Drug-drug. *Antacids (including sodium bicarbonate) and laxatives containing aluminum, magnesium, or calcium; antidiarrheals:* decreased antibiotic absorption. Give antibiotic 1 hour before or 2 hours after any of the above.
Ferrous sulfate, other iron products, zinc: decreased antibiotic absorption. Give antibiotic 3 hours after or 2 hours before iron administration.
Methoxyflurane: may cause nephrotoxicity with tetracyclines. Avoid concurrent use.
Oral anticoagulants: increased anticoagulant effect. Monitor PT and INR, and adjust dosage as ordered.
Oral contraceptives: decreased contraceptive effectiveness and increased risk of breakthrough bleeding. Use a nonhormonal birth control method.

---

*Liquid contains alcohol.   **May contain tartrazine.   †Canada   ‡Australia   §U.K.   ◇OTC

Penicillins: may interfere with bactericidal action of penicillins. Avoid use together.
Drug-food. *Milk, dairy products, other foods:* decreased antibiotic absorption. Give antibiotic 1 hour before or 2 hours after any of the above.
Drug-lifestyle. *Sun exposure:* photosensitivity reactions may occur. Take precautions.

EFFECTS ON DIAGNOSTIC TESTS

Drug causes false-negative results in urine glucose tests using glucose oxidase reagent (Diastix or Chemstrip uG). It also causes false elevations in fluorometric tests for urine catecholamines.

CONTRAINDICATIONS

Contraindicated in patients with hypersensitivity to drug or other tetracyclines.

NURSING CONSIDERATIONS

• Use cautiously in patients with impaired renal or hepatic function. Use of these drugs during last half of pregnancy and in children under 9 years may cause permanent discoloration of teeth, enamel defects, and bone growth retardation.
• Monitor renal and liver function test results.
• Monitor fluid balance and daily weights in patients with impaired kidney and liver function.
• Obtain specimen for culture and sensitivity tests before giving first dose. Therapy may begin pending test results.
Alert: Check expiration date. Outdated or deteriorated tetracyclines have been associated with reversible nephrotoxicity (Fanconi's syndrome).
• Don't expose drug to light or heat; store in tightly capped container.
• With large doses or prolonged therapy, monitor for superinfection, especially in high-risk patients.
• Check patient's tongue for signs of candidal infection. Stress good oral hygiene.

☑ **Patient teaching**
• Instruct patient to take entire amount of medication, exactly as prescribed, even after he feels better.
• Explain that drug's effectiveness is re-

duced when taken with milk or other dairy products, food, antacids, or iron products. Tell patient to take each dose with a full glass of water on an empty stomach, at least 1 hour before or 2 hours after meals. Also tell him to take drug at least 1 hour before bedtime to prevent esophageal irritation or ulceration.
• Warn patient to avoid direct sunlight and ultraviolet light, wear protective clothing, and use sunscreen. Photosensitivity reactions may occur within a few minutes to several hours after sun exposure. Photosensitivity persists for some time after discontinuation of drug.
• Instruct patient to report signs and symptoms of superinfection.

---

doxycycline calcium
Vibramycin

doxycycline hyclate
Apo-Doxy†, Doryx, Doxy Caps, Doxy 100, Doxy 200, Doxycin†, Monodox, Novo-Doxylin†, Vibramycin, Vibra-Tabs†

doxycycline hydrochloride
Doryx‡, Doxylin‡, Vibramycin‡, Vizam‡

doxycycline monohydrate
Monodox, Vibramycin

Pregnancy Risk Category: D

HOW SUPPLIED
doxycycline calcium
Oral suspension: 50 mg/5 ml
doxycycline hyclate
Tablets (film-coated): 100 mg
Capsules: 50 mg, 100 mg
Capsules (enteric-coated pellets): 100 mg
Injection: 100 mg, 200 mg
doxycycline hydrochloride
Tablets: 50 mg‡, 100 mg‡
Capsules: 50 mg‡, 100 mg‡, 250 mg‡
Injection: 100 mg‡
doxycycline monohydrate
Capsules: 50 mg, 100 mg
Oral suspension: 25 mg/5 ml

ACTION
Unknown. Thought to exert bacteriostatic effect by binding to the 30S and possibly 50S ribosomal subunits of microorganisms, thus inhibiting protein synthesis. May also alter the cytoplasmic membrane of susceptible microorganisms.

Route	Onset	Peak	Duration
PO	Unknown	1.5-4 hr	Unknown
IV	Immediate	Unknown	Unknown

INDICATIONS & DOSAGE
Infections caused by susceptible gram-positive and gram-negative organisms (including Haemophilus ducreyi, Yersinia pestis, and Campylobacter fetus), Rickettsiae, Mycoplasma pneumoniae, Chlamydia trachomatis, and Borrelia burgdorferi (Lyme disease); psittacosis; granuloma inguinale—
Adults and children over 8 years weighing 45 kg (99 lb) and over: 100 mg P.O. q 12 hours on first day, then 100 mg P.O. daily; or 200 mg I.V. on first day in one or two infusions, then 100 to 200 mg I.V. daily.
Children over 8 years weighing under 45 kg: 4.4 mg/kg P.O. or I.V. daily, in divided doses q 12 hours on first day; then 2.2 to 4.4 mg/kg daily in one or two divided doses.

Give I.V. infusion slowly (minimum 1 hour). Infusion must be completed within 12 hours (within 6 hours in lactated Ringer's solution or dextrose 5% in lactated Ringer's solution).
Gonorrhea in patients allergic to penicillin—
Adults: 100 mg P.O. b.i.d. for 7 days (10 days for epididymitis).
Primary or secondary syphilis in patients allergic to penicillin—
Adults: 300 mg P.O. daily in divided doses for at least 10 days.
Uncomplicated urethral, endocervical, or rectal infections caused by Chlamydia trachomatis or Ureaplasma urealyticum—
Adults: 100 mg P.O. b.i.d. for at least 7 days (10 days for epididymitis).
Prophylaxis of malaria—
Adults: 100 mg P.O. daily.
Children over 8 years: 2 mg/kg P.O.

once daily. Dosage should not exceed adult dose.
Note: Prophylaxis should begin 1 to 2 days before travel to endemic area and be continued during travel and for 4 weeks afterward.
Pelvic inflammatory disease—
Adults: 100 mg I.V. q 12 hours combined with cefoxitin or cefotetan and continued for at least 2 days after symptomatic improvement; thereafter, 100 mg P.O. q 12 hours for a total course of 14 days.

ADVERSE REACTIONS
CNS: *intracranial hypertension (pseudotumor cerebri).*
CV: pericarditis, thrombophlebitis.
EENT: glossitis, dysphagia.
GI: anorexia, *epigastric distress, nausea,* vomiting, *diarrhea,* oral candidiasis, enterocolitis, anogenital inflammation.
Hematologic: *neutropenia,* eosinophilia, ***thrombocytopenia,*** hemolytic anemia.
Skin: *maculopapular and erythematous rashes, photosensitivity, increased pigmentation, urticaria.*
Other: hypersensitivity reactions (***anaphylaxis***); elevated liver enzymes; permanent discoloration of teeth, enamel defects, and bone growth retardation if used in children under 9 years; superinfection.

INTERACTIONS
Drug-drug. *Antacids (including sodium bicarbonate) and laxatives containing aluminum, magnesium, or calcium; antidiarrheals:* decreased antibiotic absorption. Give antibiotic 1 hour before or 2 hours after any of the above.
Carbamazepine, phenobarbital: decreased antibiotic effect. Avoid if possible.
Ferrous sulfate, other iron products, zinc: decreased antibiotic absorption. Give drug 3 hours after or 2 hours before iron administration.
Methoxyflurane: may cause nephrotoxicity with tetracyclines. Monitor carefully.
Oral anticoagulants: increased anticoagulant effect. Monitor PT and INR, and adjust dosage as ordered.
Oral contraceptives: decreased contraceptive effectiveness and increased risk of

---

*Liquid contains alcohol.   **May contain tartrazine.   †Canada   ‡Australia   §U.K.   ◊OTC

breakthrough bleeding. Use a nonhormonal form of birth control.
Penicillins: may interfere with bactericidal action of penicillins. Avoid use together.
Drug-lifestyle. *Alcohol use:* decreased antibiotic effect. Avoid if possible.
Sun exposure: photosensitivity reactions may occur. Take precautions.

EFFECTS ON DIAGNOSTIC TESTS
Drug causes false-negative results in urine glucose tests using glucose oxidase reagent (Diastix or Chemstrip uG). Parenteral dosage form may cause false-positive Clinitest results. Drug also causes false elevations in fluorometric tests for urine catecholamines.

CONTRAINDICATIONS
Contraindicated in patients with hypersensitivity to drug or other tetracyclines.

NURSING CONSIDERATIONS
• Use cautiously in patients with impaired renal or hepatic function. Use of these drugs during last half of pregnancy and in children under 9 years may cause permanent discoloration of teeth, enamel defects, and bone growth retardation.
• Obtain specimen for culture and sensitivity tests before giving first dose. Therapy may begin pending test results.
Alert: Check expiration date. Outdated or deteriorated tetracyclines have been associated with reversible nephrotoxicity (Fanconi's syndrome).
• Administer drug with milk or food if adverse GI reactions develop.
• Know that reconstituted injectable solution is stable for 72 hours if refrigerated.
• With large doses or prolonged therapy, monitor for superinfection, especially in high-risk patients.
• Check patient's tongue for signs of fungal infection. Stress good oral hygiene.
• Know that drug is not indicated for the treatment of neurosyphilis.

I.V. administration
• Reconstitute powder for injection with sterile water for injection. Use 10 ml in 100-mg vial and 20 ml in 200-mg vial. Dilute solution to 100 to 1,000 ml for I.V. infusion. Avoid extravasation. Don't in-fuse solutions that are more concentrated than 1 mg/ml. Infusion time varies with dose, but usually ranges from 1 to 4 hours. Monitor I.V. infusion site for signs of thrombophlebitis, which may occur with I.V. administration.
• Don't expose drug to light or heat. Protect it from sunlight during infusion.

Patient teaching
• Tell patient to take entire amount of medication exactly as prescribed, even after he feels better.
• Instruct patient to report adverse reactions promptly. If drug is being administered I.V., tell patient to alert nurse if discomfort occurs at I.V site.
• Tell patient to take oral form of drug with food or milk if stomach upset occurs. Also advise patient not to take oral tablets or capsules within 1 hour of bedtime because of possible esophageal irritation or ulceration.
• Warn patient to avoid direct sunlight and ultraviolet light, wear protective clothing, and use sunscreen. Photosensitivity reactions may occur within a few minutes to several hours after exposure. Photosensitivity persists for some time after therapy ends.
• Tell patient to report signs and symptoms of superinfection to the doctor.

---

minocycline hydrochloride
Apo-Minocycline†, Dynacin, Minocin*, Minomycin‡, Minomycin IV‡

Pregnancy Risk Category: D

HOW SUPPLIED
Tablets (film-coated): 50 mg, 100 mg
Capsules (pellet-filled): 50 mg, 100 mg
Oral suspension: 50 mg/5 ml
Injection: 100 mg

ACTION
Unknown. Thought to exert bacteriostatic effect by binding to the 30S and possibly 50S ribosomal subunits of microorganisms, thus inhibiting protein synthesis. May also alter the cytoplasmic membrane of susceptible microorganisms.

Reactions may be *common*, uncommon, *life-threatening*, or COMMON AND LIFE-THREATENING.

Route	Onset	Peak	Duration
PO	Unknown	1-4 hr	Unknown
IV	Immediate	Immediate	Unknown

INDICATIONS & DOSAGE

Infections caused by susceptible gram-negative and gram-positive organisms (including Haemophilus ducreyi, Yersinia pestis, *and* Campylobacter fetus*),* Rickettsiae, Mycoplasma pneumoniae, *and* Chlamydia trachomatis; *psittacosis; granuloma inguinale—*
Adults: initially, 200 mg I.V.; then 100 mg I.V. q 12 hours. Not to exceed 400 mg/day. Alternatively, 200 mg P.O. initially; then 100 mg P.O. q 12 hours. Some clinicians use 100 or 200 mg P.O. initially, followed by 50 mg q.i.d.
Children over 8 years: initially, 4 mg/kg P.O. or I.V., followed by 2 mg/kg q 12 hours.

Given I.V. in 500- to 1,000-ml solution without calcium and administered over 6 hours.
Gonorrhea in patients allergic to penicillin—
Adults: initially, 200 mg P.O.; then 100 mg q 12 hours for at least 4 days.
Syphilis in patients allergic to penicillin—
Adults: initially, 200 mg P.O.; then 100 mg q 12 hours for 10 to 15 days.
Meningococcal carrier state—
Adults: 100 mg P.O. q 12 hours for 5 days.
Uncomplicated urethral, endocervical, or rectal infection caused by Chlamydia trachomatis *or* Ureaplasma urealyticum—
Adults: 100 mg P.O. b.i.d. for at least 7 days.
Uncomplicated gonococcal urethritis in men—
Adults: 100 mg P.O. b.i.d. for 5 days.

ADVERSE REACTIONS

CNS: headache, *intracranial hypertension (pseudotumor cerebri),* lightheadedness, dizziness, vertigo.
CV: pericarditis, *thrombophlebitis.*
EENT: dysphagia, glossitis.
GI: *anorexia,* epigastric distress, oral candidiasis, *nausea,* vomiting, *diarrhea,* enterocolitis, inflammatory lesions in anogenital region.

Hematologic: *neutropenia,* eosinophilia, *thrombocytopenia,* hemolytic anemia.
Skin: *maculopapular and erythematous rashes, photosensitivity, increased pigmentation,* urticaria.
Other: hypersensitivity reactions (*anaphylaxis*); elevated liver enzymes; increased BUN level; permanent discoloration of teeth, enamel defects, and bone growth retardation if used in children under 9 years; superinfection.

INTERACTIONS

Drug-drug. *Antacids (including sodium bicarbonate) and laxatives containing aluminum, magnesium, or calcium; antidiarrheals:* decreased antibiotic absorption. Give antibiotic 1 hour before or 2 hours after any of the above.
Ferrous sulfate, other iron products, zinc: decreased antibiotic absorption. Give drug 3 hours after or 2 hours before iron administration.
Methoxyflurane: may cause nephrotoxicity when given with tetracyclines. Monitor carefully.
Oral anticoagulants: increased anticoagulant effect. Monitor PT and INR, and adjust dosage as ordered.
Oral contraceptives: decreased contraceptive effectiveness and increased risk of breakthrough bleeding. Use a nonhormonal form of birth control.
Penicillins: may interfere with bactericidal action of penicillins. Avoid use together.
Drug-lifestyle. *Sun exposure:* photosensitivity reactions may occur. Take precautions.

EFFECTS ON DIAGNOSTIC TESTS

Drug causes false-negative results in urine glucose tests using glucose oxidase reagent (Diastix or Chemstrip uG). It also causes false elevations in fluorometric tests for urine catecholamines. Parenteral form may cause false-positive reading of copper sulfate tests (Clinitest).

CONTRAINDICATIONS

Contraindicated in patients with hypersensitivity to drug or other tetracyclines.

NURSING CONSIDERATIONS

• Use cautiously in patients with impaired

renal or hepatic function. Use of these drugs during last half of pregnancy and in children under 9 years may cause permanent discoloration of teeth, enamel defects, and bone growth retardation.

• Monitor renal and liver function test results.

• Obtain specimen for culture and sensitivity tests before first dose. Therapy may begin pending test results.

Alert: Check expiration date. Outdated or deteriorated tetracyclines have been associated with reversible nephrotoxicity (Fanconi's syndrome).

• Don't expose drug to light or heat. Keep cap tightly closed.

• With large doses or prolonged therapy, monitor for superinfection, especially in high-risk patients.

• Check patient's tongue for signs of candidal infection. Stress good oral hygiene.

• Be aware that drug may cause tooth discoloration in young adults. Observe for brown pigmentation, and notify doctor if it occurs.

• Know that drug is not indicated for the treatment of neurosyphilis.

🜂 I.V. administration
• Reconstitute 100 mg of powder with 5 ml of sterile water for injection, with further dilution to 500 to 1,000 ml for I.V. infusion. Although reconstituted solution is stable for 24 hours at room temperature, use as soon as possible. Infusions are usually over 6 hours.

• Be aware that patient may develop thrombophlebitis with I.V. administration of this drug. Avoid extravasation. Switch to oral therapy as soon as possible.

✓ Patient teaching
• Tell patient to take entire amount of medication exactly as prescribed, even after he feels better.

• Instruct patient to take oral form of drug with a full glass of water. Drug may be taken with food. Tell patient not to take within 1 hour of bedtime to avoid esophageal irritation or ulceration.

• Warn patient to avoid driving or other hazardous tasks due to possible adverse CNS effects.

• Caution patient to avoid direct sunlight and ultraviolet light, wear protective clothing, and use sunscreen. Photosensitivity reactions may occur within a few minutes to several hours after exposure. Photosensitivity persists for some time after discontinuation of therapy.

---

tetracycline hydrochloride
Achromycin V, Ala-Tet, Apo-Tetra†, Novo-Tetra†, Nu-Tetra†, Panmycin**, Robitet, Sumycin, Sustamycin§, Teline, Tetracap, Tetrachel§, Tetracyn, Tetralan, Tetram

Pregnancy Risk Category: D

HOW SUPPLIED
Tablets: 250 mg, 500 mg
Capsules: 100 mg, 250 mg, 500 mg
Oral suspension: 125 mg/5 ml

ACTION
Unknown. Thought to exert bacteriostatic effect by binding to the 30S and possibly 50S ribosomal subunits of microorganisms, thus inhibiting protein synthesis. May also alter the cytoplasmic membrane of susceptible microorganisms.

Route	Onset	Peak	Duration
PO	Unknown	1-4 hr	Unknown

INDICATIONS & DOSAGE
Infections caused by susceptible gram-negative and gram-positive organisms (including Haemophilus ducreyi, Yersinia pestis, *and* Campylobacter fetus), Rickettsia, Mycoplasma pneumoniae, *and* Chlamydia trachomatis; psittacosis; granuloma inguinale—
Adults: 250 to 500 mg P.O. q 6 hours.
Children over 8 years: 25 to 50 mg/kg P.O. daily, in divided doses q 6 hours.
Uncomplicated urethral, endocervical, or rectal infections caused by Chlamydia trachomatis—
Adults: 500 mg P.O. q.i.d. for at least 7 days, 10 days for epididymitis, and 21 days for lymphogranuloma venereum.
Brucellosis—
Adults: 500 mg P.O. q 6 hours for 3 weeks combined with 1 g of streptomycin

---

CVS PHARMACY

1233 N STATE ST   GREENFIELD, IN
PHARMACY: 462-7713   STORE: 467-2588

REG#12 TRAN#0939 CSHR#278985 STR#4633

1 RX ITEM 0074537602   .50N

```
TOTAL                     .50
CASH                     1.00
CHANGE                    .50
```

RECEIPT VALIDATION CODE
5463 3224 5093 9120

GET YOUR CVS EXTRACARE CARD

****

ENTER TO WIN
$10,000

BY TELLING US ABOUT
OUR SERVICE!
CALL TOLL FREE 1-888-308-6273

OFFER EXPIRES 12/31/2002
SEE RULES IN STORE

RECEIPT ID #: 246330
CUSTOMER #: 028 478 30
****

THANK YOU, SHOP ANYTIME AT CVS.COM!
SEPTEMBER 2, 2002   7:21 PM

RETURNS WITH RECEIPT THRU 11/01/02

I.M. q 12 hours for first week; once daily for second week.

Gonorrhea in patients allergic to penicillin—
Adults: initially, 1.5 g P.O.; then 500 mg q 6 hours for a total dose of 9 g; for epididymitis, 500 mg P.O. q 6 hours for 7 days.

Syphilis in patients allergic to penicillin—
Adults: total of 30 to 40 g P.O. in equally divided doses over 10 to 15 days.

Acne—
Adults and adolescents: initially, 250 mg P.O. q 6 hours; then 125 to 500 mg daily or every other day.

Helicobacter pylori *infection—*
Adults: 500 mg P.O. q 6 hours for 10 to 14 days with other agents, such as metronidazole, bismuth subsalicylate, amoxicillin, or omeprazole.

Cholera—
Adults: 500 mg P.O. q 6 hours for 48 to 72 hours.

Malaria caused by Plasmodium falciparum—
Adults: 250 to 500 mg P.O. daily for 7 days with quinine sulfate 650 mg P.O. q 8 hours for 3 to 7 days.

ADVERSE REACTIONS
CNS: dizziness, headache, *intracranial hypertension (pseudotumor cerebri).*
CV: pericarditis.
EENT: sore throat, glossitis, dysphagia.
GI: anorexia, *epigastric distress, nausea,* vomiting, *diarrhea,* esophagitis, oral candidiasis, stomatitis, enterocolitis, inflammatory lesions in anogenital region.
Hematologic: *neutropenia,* eosinophilia, *thrombocytopenia.*
Skin: *candidal superinfection, maculopapular and erythematous rash,* urticaria, *photosensitivity, increased pigmentation.*
Other: hypersensitivity reactions, elevated liver enzymes, *increased BUN levels, permanent discoloration of teeth, enamel defects, and bone growth retardation if used in children under 9 years.*

INTERACTIONS
Drug-drug. *Antacids (including sodium bicarbonate) and laxatives containing aluminum, magnesium, or calcium; antidiarrheals containing kaolin, pectin, or*

bismuth subsalicylate: decreased antibiotic absorption. Give antibiotic 1 hour before or 2 hours after any of the above.
Ferrous sulfate, other iron products, zinc: decreased antibiotic absorption. Give tetracyclines 3 hours after or 2 hours before iron administration.
Lithium carbonate: may alter serum lithium levels. Monitor levels.
Methoxyflurane: may cause severe nephrotoxicity with tetracyclines. Monitor carefully.
Oral anticoagulants: potentiated anticoagulant effects. Monitor PT and INR, and adjust anticoagulant dosage as ordered.
Oral contraceptives: decreased contraceptive effectiveness and increased risk of breakthrough bleeding. Use a nonhormonal form of birth control.
Penicillins: may interfere with bactericidal action of penicillins. Avoid use together.
Drug-food. *Milk, dairy products, other foods:* decreased antibiotic absorption. Give antibiotic 1 hour before or 2 hours after any of the above.
Drug-lifestyle. *Sun exposure:* photosensitivity reactions may occur. Take precautions.

EFFECTS ON DIAGNOSTIC TESTS
Drug causes false-negative results in urine glucose tests using glucose oxidase reagent (Diastix or Chemstrip uG), and false elevations in fluorometric tests for urine catecholamines. It may elevate BUN levels in patients with decreased renal function.

CONTRAINDICATIONS
Contraindicated in patients with hypersensitivity to tetracyclines.

NURSING CONSIDERATIONS
• Use with extreme caution in patients with impaired renal or hepatic function. Monitor renal and liver function test results. Also use with extreme caution (if at all) during last half of pregnancy and in children under 9 years because drug may cause permanent discoloration of teeth, enamel defects, and bone growth retardation.
• Obtain specimen for culture and sensi-

---

tivity tests before giving first dose. Therapy may begin pending test results.

Alert: Check expiration date. Outdated or deteriorated tetracyclines have been associated with reversible nephrotoxicity (Fanconi's syndrome).

• Don't expose drug to light or heat.

• With large doses or prolonged therapy, monitor for superinfection, especially in high-risk patients.

• Check patient's tongue for signs of candidal infection. Stress good oral hygiene.

• Know that drug is not indicated for the treatment of neurosyphilis.

☑ **Patient teaching**

• Tell patient to take drug exactly as prescribed, even after he feels better, and to take entire amount prescribed.

• Explain that effectiveness is reduced when taken with milk or other dairy products, food, antacids, or iron products. Tell patient to take each dose with a full glass of water on an empty stomach, at least 1 hour before or 2 hours after meals. Also tell him to take it at least 1 hour before bedtime to prevent esophageal irritation or ulceration.

• Warn patient to avoid direct sunlight and ultraviolet light, wear protective clothing, and use sunscreen. Photosensitivity reactions may occur within a few minutes to several hours after sun exposure. Photosensitivity persists after discontinuation of drug.

co-trimoxazole
sulfadiazine
sulfamethoxazole
sulfisoxazole
sulfisoxazole acetyl

COMBINATION PRODUCTS

AZO GANTANOL, AZO-SULFAMETHOX-AZOLE† tablets (film-coated): sulfamethoxazole 500 mg and phenazopyridine hydrochloride 100 mg.

AZO GANTRISIN, AZO-SULFISOXAZOLE tablets (film-coated): sulfisoxazole 500 mg and phenazopyridine hydrochloride 50 mg.

ERYZOLE, PEDIAZOLE, SULFIMYCIN suspension: sulfisoxazole 600 mg and erythromycin ethylsuccinate 200 mg/5 ml.

---

co-trimoxazole
(sulfamethoxazole-trimethoprim)

Apo-Sulfatrim†, Apo-Sulfatrim DS†, Bactrim*, Bactrim DS, Bactrim I.V., Novo-Trimel†, Novo-Trimel DS†, Nu-Cotrimox†, Pro-Trin†, Resprim‡, Roubac†, Septra*, Septra DS, Septra I.V., Septrin‡, SMZ-TMP, Sulfatrim

Pregnancy Risk Category: C
(contraindicated at term)

HOW SUPPLIED

Tablets: (single-strength) trimethoprim 80 mg and sulfamethoxazole 400 mg; *(double-strength)* trimethoprim 160 mg and sulfamethoxazole 800 mg
Oral suspension: trimethoprim 40 mg and sulfamethoxazole 200 mg/5 ml
Injection: trimethoprim 16 mg and sulfamethoxazole 80 mg/ml in 5-, 10-, 20-, and 30-ml vials

ACTION

Sulfamethoxazole inhibits formation of dihydrofolic acid from PABA; trimethoprim inhibits dihydrofolate reductase for-

mation. Both decrease bacterial folic acid synthesis; bactericidal.

Route	Onset	Peak	Duration
PO	Unknown	1-4 hr	Unknown
IV	Immediate	Immediate	Unknown

INDICATIONS & DOSAGE

Shigellosis or urinary tract infections (UTIs) caused by susceptible strains of Escherichia coli, Proteus *(indole positive or negative),* Klebsiella, *or* Enterobacter—

Adults: 160 mg trimethoprim/800 mg sulfamethoxazole (double-strength tablet) P.O. q 12 hours for 10 to 14 days in UTIs and for 5 days in shigellosis. For uncomplicated cystitis or acute urethral syndrome, one double-strength tablet q 12 hours for 3 days. If indicated, I.V. infusion is given: 8 to 10 mg/kg/day (based on trimethoprim component) in two to four divided doses q 6, 8, or 12 hours for up to 14 days for severe UTIs. Maximum daily dose is 960 mg trimethoprim.

Children 2 months and older: 8 mg/kg/day (based on trimethoprim component) P.O., in two divided doses q 12 hours (10 days for UTIs; 5 days for shigellosis). If indicated, I.V. infusion is given: 8 to 10 mg/kg/day (based on trimethoprim component) in two to four divided doses q 6, 8, or 12 hours. Adult dose should not be exceeded.

Otitis media in patients with penicillin allergy or penicillin-resistant infections—
Children 2 months and over: 8 mg/kg/day (based on trimethoprim component) P.O., in two divided doses q 12 hours for 10 to 14 days.

Chronic bronchitis and upper respiratory tract infections—
Adults: 160 mg trimethoprim/800 mg sulfamethoxazole P.O. q 12 hours for 10 to 14 days.

Traveler's diarrhea—
Adults: 160 mg trimethoprim/800 mg sulfamethoxazole P.O. b.i.d. for 3 to 5

---

*Liquid contains alcohol.   **May contain tartrazine.   †Canada   ‡Australia   §U.K.   ◊OTC

days. Some patients may require 2 days of therapy or less.

UTIs in men with prostatitis—
Adults: 160 mg trimethoprim/800 mg sulfamethoxazole P.O. b.i.d. for 3 to 6 months.

Prophylaxis for chronic UTIs—
Adults: 40 mg trimethoprim/200 mg sulfamethoxazole (½ tablet) or 80 mg trimethoprim/400 mg sulfamethoxazole P.O. daily or three times weekly for 3 to 6 months.

Prophylaxis for Pneumocystis carinii *pneumonia—*
Adults: 160 mg of trimethoprim/800 mg sulfamethoxazole P.O. daily.
Children 2 months and older: 150 mg/m² trimethoprim/750 mg/m² sulfamethoxazole P.O daily in two divided doses on 3 consecutive days each week.

Treatment of P. carinii *pneumonia—*
Adults and children over 2 months: 15 to 20 mg/kg/day (based on trimethoprim) I.V. or P.O. in three or four divided doses for 14 days.

Adjust-a-dose: In patients with renal failure, if creatinine clearance is 15 to 30 ml/minute, daily dose should be reduced by 50%. Drug is not recommended for patients with creatinine clearance below 15 ml/minute.

ADVERSE REACTIONS
CNS: headache, mental depression, aseptic meningitis, tinnitus, apathy, *seizures,* hallucinations, ataxia, nervousness, fatigue, muscle weakness, vertigo, insomnia.
GI: *nausea, vomiting, diarrhea,* abdominal pain, anorexia, stomatitis, pancreatitis, pseudomembranous colitis.
GU: *toxic nephrosis with oliguria and anuria,* crystalluria, hematuria, interstitial nephritis, increased BUN and serum creatinine concentrations.
Hematologic: *agranulocytosis, aplastic anemia,* megaloblastic anemia, *thrombocytopenia, leukopenia, hemolytic anemia.*
Hepatic: jaundice, *hepatic necrosis,* elevated liver function test results.
Respiratory: pulmonary infiltrates.
Skin: *erythema multiforme (Stevens-Johnson syndrome),* generalized skin eruption, *epidermal necrolysis, exfoliative dermatitis,* photosensitivity, urticaria, pruritus.
Other: hypersensitivity reactions (*serum sickness, drug fever, anaphylaxis*), thrombophlebitis, arthralgia, myalgia.

INTERACTIONS
Drug-drug. *Cyclosporine:* may decrease cyclosporine levels and increase nephrotoxicity risk. Avoid concomitant use.
Methotrexate: may increase methotrexate concentrations. Use together cautiously.
Oral anticoagulants: increased anticoagulant effect. Monitor for bleeding.
Oral antidiabetic agents: increased hypoglycemic effect. Monitor blood glucose levels.
Oral contraceptives: decreased contraceptive effectiveness and increased risk of breakthrough bleeding. Suggest a nonhormonal contraceptive.
Phenytoin: may inhibit hepatic metabolism of phenytoin. Monitor closely.
Drug-lifestyle. *Sun exposure:* photosensitivity reactions may occur. Take precautions.

EFFECTS ON DIAGNOSTIC TESTS
Trimethoprim can interfere with serum methotrexate assay as determined by the competitive binding protein technique. No interference occurs if radioimmunoassay is used.

CONTRAINDICATIONS
Contraindicated in patients with severe renal impairment (creatinine clearance below 15 ml/minute), porphyria, megaloblastic anemia caused by folate deficiency, or hypersensitivity to trimethoprim or sulfonamides; in pregnant women at term; in breast-feeding women; and in children under 2 months.

NURSING CONSIDERATIONS
• Use cautiously and in reduced dosages in patients with impaired hepatic or renal function (creatinine clearance, 15 to 30 ml/minute), severe allergy or bronchial asthma, G6PD deficiency, and blood dyscrasia.
• Monitor renal and liver function test results.

Reactions may be *common,* uncommon, **life-threatening,** or COMMON AND LIFE-THREATENING.

• Obtain specimen for culture and sensitivity tests before first dose. Therapy may begin pending results.
• Note that the "DS" product means "double strength."
• Never administer I.M.
• Promptly report complaints of rash, sore throat, fever, or mouth sores—early signs and symptoms of blood dyscrasia.
• Watch for superinfection (fever or other signs of new infection).
Alert: Be aware that adverse reactions, especially hypersensitivity reactions, rash, and fever, occur much more frequently in AIDS patients.

I.V. administration
• Dilute each 5 ml of concentrate for I.V. infusion in 75 to 125 ml of D_5W before administration. Don't mix with other drugs or solutions. Infuse slowly over 60 to 90 minutes. Don't give by rapid infusion or bolus injection. Don't refrigerate, and use within 6 hours.

Patient teaching
• Tell patient to take drug as prescribed, even if he feels better.
• Encourage adequate fluid intake.
• Tell patient to report adverse reactions promptly.
• Instruct patient receiving drug I.V. to alert nurse if discomfort occurs at I.V. insertion site.
• Advise patient to avoid prolonged sun exposure, wear protective clothing, and use sunscreen.
• Instruct patient to take oral medication with 8 oz (240 ml) of water on an empty stomach.

---

sulfadiazine
Coptin†

Pregnancy Risk Category: C (contraindicated at term)

HOW SUPPLIED
Tablets: 500 mg

ACTION
Inhibits formation of dihydrofolic acid from PABA, decreasing bacterial folic acid synthesis; bacteriostatic.

Route	Onset	Peak	Duration
PO	Unknown	4-6 hr	Unknown

INDICATIONS & DOSAGE
Asymptomatic meningococcal carriers—
Adults: 1 g P.O. q 12 hours for 2 days.
Children 1 to 12 years: 500 mg P.O. q 12 hours for 2 days.
Children 2 to 12 months: 500 mg P.O. daily for 2 days.
Rheumatic fever prophylaxis, as an alternative to penicillin—
Children weighing over 30 kg (66 lb): 1 g P.O. daily.
Children weighing under 30 kg: 500 mg P.O. daily.
Adjunct treatment in toxoplasmosis—
Adults: 2 to 8 g P.O. daily divided q 6 hours for 6 to 8 weeks or until improvement occurs. Usually given with pyrimethamine.
Children: 100 to 200 mg/kg P.O. daily divided q 6 hours (maximum 6 g daily) for 6 to 8 weeks or until improvement occurs. Usually given with pyrimethamine.
Malaria, treatment of chloroquine-resistant Plasmodium falciparum—
Adults: 500 mg P.O. q.i.d. for 5 days with quinine sulfate and pyrimethamine.
Children: 25 to 50 mg/kg P.O. q.i.d. (maximum 2 g daily) for 5 days with quinine sulfate and pyrimethamine.
Nocardiosis—
Adults: 4 to 8 g P.O. daily given in divided doses for a minimum of 6 weeks.

ADVERSE REACTIONS
CNS: headache, mental depression, *seizures,* hallucinations.
GI: *nausea, vomiting, diarrhea,* abdominal pain, anorexia, stomatitis.
GU: *toxic nephrosis with oliguria and anuria,* crystalluria, hematuria, elevated serum creatinine
Hematologic: *agranulocytosis, aplastic anemia,* megaloblastic anemia, *thrombocytopenia, leukopenia, hemolytic anemia.*
Hepatic: elevated liver function test results, jaundice.
Skin: *erythema multiforme (Stevens-*

Johnson syndrome), generalized skin eruption, **epidermal necrolysis, exfoliative dermatitis,** photosensitivity, urticaria, pruritus.
Other: hypersensitivity reactions (*serum sickness, drug fever,* **anaphylaxis**), local irritation, extravasation.

INTERACTIONS
Drug-drug. *Methotrexate:* may increase methotrexate levels. Use together cautiously.
Oral anticoagulants: increased anticoagulant effect. Monitor for bleeding.
Oral antidiabetic agents: increased hypoglycemic effect. Monitor blood glucose levels.
Oral contraceptives: decreased contraceptive effectiveness and increased risk of breakthrough bleeding. Suggest a nonhormonal contraceptive.
PABA-containing drugs: inhibited antibacterial action. Don't use together.
Drug-lifestyle. *Sun exposure:* photosensitivity reactions may occur. Take precautions.

EFFECTS ON DIAGNOSTIC TESTS
Drug alters urine glucose tests using cupric sulfate (Benedict's reagent or Clinitest).

CONTRAINDICATIONS
Contraindicated in patients with hypersensitivity to sulfonamides, in those with porphyria, in infants under 2 months (except in congenital toxoplasmosis), in pregnant women at term, and during breast-feeding.

NURSING CONSIDERATIONS
• Use cautiously and in reduced doses in patients with impaired hepatic or renal function, bronchial asthma, history of multiple allergies, G6PD deficiency, and blood dyscrasia.
• Monitor renal and liver function test results.
• Give drug on schedule to maintain constant blood level.
• Monitor for signs of blood dyscrasia (purpura, ecchymoses, sore throat, fever, and pallor). Report them immediately.
• Monitor urine cultures, CBCs, and uri-

nalyses before and during therapy, as ordered.
• Watch for superinfection (fever or other signs of new infection).
• Be aware that folic or folinic acid may be used during rest periods in toxoplasmosis therapy to reverse hematopoietic depression or anemia associated with pyrimethamine and sulfadiazine.
• Monitor fluid intake and output. Intake should be sufficient to produce output of 1,500 ml daily (between 3,000 and 4,000 ml daily for adults). If fluid intake is not adequate enough to prevent crystalluria, sodium bicarbonate may be administered to alkalinize urine, as ordered. Monitor urine pH daily.

☑ Patient teaching
• Tell patient to take drug as prescribed, even if he feels better.
• Tell patient to drink a glass of water with each dose and plenty of water each day to prevent crystalluria.
• Instruct patient to report adverse reactions promptly.
• Warn patient to avoid prolonged exposure to sunlight, wear protective clothing, and use sunscreen.

---

sulfamethoxazole (sulphamethoxazole)
Apo-Sulfamethoxazole†, Gantanol

Pregnancy Risk Category: C (contraindicated at term)

HOW SUPPLIED
Tablets: 500 mg
Oral suspension: 500 mg/5 ml

ACTION
Inhibits formation of dihydrofolic acid from PABA, decreasing bacterial folic acid synthesis; bacteriostatic.

Route	Onset	Peak	Duration
PO	Unknown	2 hr	Unknown

INDICATIONS & DOSAGE
Urinary tract and systemic infections—
Adults: initially, 2 g P.O., then 1 g P.O. b.i.d. up to t.i.d. for severe infections.

Chlamydia trachomatis *(lymphogranuloma venereum)*—
Adults: 1 g P.O. b.i.d. for 21 days.
Children and infants over 2 months: initially, 50 to 60 mg/kg P.O., then 25 to 30 mg/kg b.i.d. Maximum dosage should not exceed 75 mg/kg daily.

ADVERSE REACTIONS
CNS: headache, mental depression, *seizures,* hallucinations, aseptic meningitis, tinnitus, apathy.
GI: *nausea, vomiting, diarrhea,* abdominal pain, anorexia, stomatitis, pancreatitis, pseudomembranous colitis.
GU: *toxic nephrosis with oliguria and anuria,* crystalluria, hematuria, interstitial nephritis.
Hematologic: *agranulocytosis, aplastic anemia,* megaloblastic anemia, *thrombocytopenia, leukopenia, hemolytic anemia.*
Hepatic: elevated liver function test results, jaundice.
Skin: *erythema multiforme (Stevens-Johnson syndrome), generalized skin eruption, epidermal necrolysis, exfoliative dermatitis,* photosensitivity, urticaria, pruritus.
Other: hypersensitivity reactions (*serum sickness, drug fever, anaphylaxis*).

INTERACTIONS
Drug-drug. *Methotrexate:* may increase methotrexate levels. Use together cautiously.
Oral anticoagulants: increased anticoagulant effect. Monitor for bleeding.
Oral antidiabetic agents: increased hypoglycemic effect. Monitor blood glucose levels.
Oral contraceptives: decreased contraceptive effectiveness and increased risk of breakthrough bleeding. Suggest a nonhormonal contraceptive.
Phenytoin: may increase phenytoin effect. Monitor closely.
Drug-lifestyle. *Sun exposure:* may cause photosensitivity reactions. Use precautions.

EFFECTS ON DIAGNOSTIC TESTS
Drug alters results of urine glucose tests using cupric sulfate (Benedict's reagent or Clinitest).

CONTRAINDICATIONS
Contraindicated in patients with hypersensitivity to sulfonamides, in those with porphyria, in infants under 2 months (except in congenital toxoplasmosis), in pregnant women at term, and during breast-feeding.

NURSING CONSIDERATIONS
• Use cautiously and in reduced dosages in patients with impaired hepatic or renal function, severe allergy or bronchial asthma, G6PD deficiency, and blood dyscrasia.
• Monitor renal and liver function test results.
• Obtain specimen for culture and sensitivity tests before first dose. Therapy may begin pending results.
• Monitor urine cultures, CBCs, and urinalyses before and during therapy, as ordered.
• Watch for superinfection (fever or other signs of new infection).
• Monitor fluid intake and output. Intake should be sufficient to produce output of 1,500 ml daily (between 3,000 and 4,000 ml daily for adults). If fluid intake is not adequate enough to prevent crystalluria, sodium bicarbonate may be administered to alkalinize urine, as ordered. Monitor urine pH daily.

☑ **Patient teaching**
• Tell patient to take drug as prescribed, even if he feels better.
• Instruct patient to drink a glass of water with each dose and plenty of water each day to prevent crystalluria.
Alert: Tell patient to report early signs of blood dyscrasia (sore throat, fever, and pallor) to doctor.
• Warn patient to avoid prolonged exposure to sunlight, to wear protective clothing, and to use sunscreen.

---

*Liquid contains alcohol.   **May contain tartrazine.   †Canada   ‡Australia   §U.K.   ◊OTC

sulfisoxazole (sulfafurazole, sulphafurazole)
Azo-Sulfisoxazole, Gantrisin, Novo-Soxazole†

sulfisoxazole acetyl
Gantrisin Pediatric

Pregnancy Risk Category: C (contraindicated at term)

HOW SUPPLIED
sulfisoxazole
Tablets: 500 mg
sulfisoxazole acetyl
Liquid: 500 mg/5 ml

ACTION
Inhibits formation of dihydrofolic acid from PABA, decreasing bacterial folic acid synthesis; bacteriostatic.

Route	Onset	Peak	Duration
PO	Unknown	1-4 hr	Unknown

INDICATIONS & DOSAGE
Urinary tract and systemic infections—
Adults: initially, 2 to 4 g P.O., then 4 to 8 g daily divided in four to six doses.
Children over 2 months: initially, 75 mg/kg P.O. daily or 2 g/m² P.O., then 150 mg/kg or 4 g/m² P.O. daily in divided doses q 6 hours. Total daily dose should not exceed 6 g.
Chlamydia trachomatis *(lymphogranuloma venereum)—*
Adults: 500 mg to 1 g P.O. q.i.d. for 21 days.
Uncomplicated urethral, endocervical, or rectal infections caused by Chlamydia trachomatis—
Adults: 500 mg P.O. q.i.d. for 10 days.
*Adjust-a-dose:*In patients with renal failure, use normal dose at longer intervals. If creatinine clearance is 10 to 50 ml/minute, give q 8 to12 hours; if clearance is less than 10 ml/minute, give q 12 to 24 hours.

ADVERSE REACTIONS
CNS: headache, mental depression, *seizures,* hallucinations.
CV: tachycardia, palpitations, syncope, cyanosis.
GI: *nausea, vomiting, diarrhea,* abdominal pain, anorexia, stomatitis, pseudomembranous colitis.
GU: *toxic nephrosis with oliguria and anuria,* crystalluria, hematuria, *acute renal failure.*
Hematologic: *agranulocytosis, aplastic anemia,* megaloblastic anemia, *thrombocytopenia, leukopenia, hemolytic anemia.*
Hepatic: jaundice, elevated liver function test results, *hepatitis.*
Skin: *erythema multiforme,* generalized skin eruption, *epidermal necrolysis, exfoliative dermatitis,* photosensitivity, urticaria, pruritus.
Other: hypersensitivity reactions (*serum sickness, drug fever, anaphylaxis*).

INTERACTIONS
Drug-drug. *Methotrexate:* may increase methotrexate levels. Use together cautiously.
Oral anticoagulants: increased anticoagulant effect. Monitor for bleeding.
Oral antidiabetic agents: increased hypoglycemic effect. Monitor blood glucose levels.
Oral contraceptives: decreased contraceptive effectiveness, increased risk of breakthrough bleeding. Suggest a nonhormonal contraceptive.
Drug-lifestyle. *Sun exposure:* photosensitivity reactions may occur. Use precautions.

EFFECTS ON DIAGNOSTIC TESTS
Drug alters results of urine glucose tests using cupric sulfate (Benedict's reagent or Clinitest).

CONTRAINDICATIONS
Contraindicated in patients with hypersensitivity to sulfonamides, in infants under 2 months (except in congenital toxoplasmosis), in pregnant women at term, and during breast-feeding.

NURSING CONSIDERATIONS
• Use cautiously in patients with impaired hepatic or renal function, severe allergy or bronchial asthma, and G6PD deficiency.

• Monitor renal and liver function test results.

• Obtain specimen for culture and sensitivity tests before giving first dose. Therapy may begin pending results.

• Monitor urine cultures, CBCs, PT, and urinalyses before and during therapy, as ordered.

• Report moderate to severe diarrhea to health care provider.

• Watch for superinfection (fever or other signs of new infection).

• Monitor fluid intake and output. Maintain intake between 3,000 and 4,000 ml daily for adults to produce output of 1,500 ml daily. If fluid intake is not adequate enough to prevent crystalluria, sodium bicarbonate may be administered to alkalinize urine, as ordered. Monitor urine pH daily.

✅ Patient teaching

• Tell patient to take drug as prescribed, even if he feels better.

• Instruct patient to drink a glass of water with each dose and plenty of water each day to prevent crystalluria.

Alert: Tell patient to report early signs of blood dyscrasia (sore throat, fever, and pallor) and moderate to severe diarrhea to doctor.

• Warn patient to avoid sunlight and to wear protective clothing and use sunscreen.

16

Fluoroquinolones

alatrofloxacin mesylate
ciprofloxacin
enoxacin
grepafloxacin hydrochloride
levofloxacin
lomefloxacin hydrochloride
nalidixic acid
norfloxacin
ofloxacin
sparfloxacin
trovafloxacin mesylate

COMBINATION PRODUCTS
None.

---

ciprofloxacin
Cipro, Cipro I.V., Ciproxin‡

Pregnancy Risk Category: C

HOW SUPPLIED
Tablets (film-coated): 100 mg, 250 mg, 500 mg, 750 mg
Infusion (premixed): 200 mg in 100 ml D_5W, 400 mg in 200 ml D_5W
Injection: 200 mg, 400 mg

ACTION
Inhibits bacterial DNA synthesis, mainly by blocking DNA gyrase; bactericidal.

Route	Onset	Peak	Duration
PO	Unknown	0.5-2.3 hr	Unknown
IV	Unknown	Immediate	Unknown

INDICATIONS & DOSAGE
Mild to moderate urinary tract infections (UTIs) caused by Escherichia coli, Klebsiella pneumoniae, Enterobacter cloacae, Serratia marcescens, Proteus mirabilis, Providencia rettgeri, Morganella morganii, Citrobacter diversus, C. freundii, Pseudomonas aeruginosa, Staphylococcus epidermidis, *and* Enterococcus faecalis—
Adults: 250 mg P.O. or 200 mg I.V. q 12 hours.
Severe or complicated UTIs; mild to moderate bone and joint infections caused by E. cloacae, P. aeruginosa, *and* S. marcescens; *mild to moderate respiratory infections caused by* E. coli, K. pneumoniae, E. cloacae, P. mirabilis, P. aeruginosa, Haemophilus influenzae, *and* H. parainfluenzae; *mild to moderate skin and skin-structure infections caused by* E. coli, K. pneumoniae, E. cloacae, P. mirabilis, P. vulgaris, Providencia stuartii, M. morganii, C. freundii, Streptococcus pyogenes, P. aeruginosa, Staphylococcus aureus, *and* S. epidermidis; *infectious diarrhea caused by* E. coli, Campylobacter jejuni, Shigella flexneri, *and* S. sonnei; *typhoid fever*—
Adults: 500 mg P.O. or 400 mg I.V. q 12 hours.
Severe or complicated bone or joint infections; severe respiratory tract infections; severe skin and skin-structure infections—
Adults: 750 mg P.O. q 12 hours.
Chronic bacterial prostatitis caused by E. coli *or* P. mirabilis—
Adults: 500 mg P.O. q 12 hours for 28 days.
Complicated intra-abdominal infections (used with metronidazole) caused by E. coli, P. aeruginosa, P. mirabilis, K. pneumoniae, *or* Bacteroides fragilis—
Adults: 500 mg P.O. or 400 mg I.V. q 12 hours for 7 to 14 days.
Acute uncomplicated cystitis—
Adults: 100 mg P.O. q 12 hours for 3 days.
Mild to moderate acute sinusitis—
Adults: 500 mg P.O. q 12 hours for 10 days.
Adjust-a-dose: In patients with renal failure, if creatinine clearance is 30 to 50 ml/minute, give 250 to 500 mg P.O. q 12 hours or the usual I.V. dose; if clearance is 5 to 29 ml/minute, give 250 to 500 mg P.O. q 18 hours or 200 to 400 mg I.V. q 18 to 24 hours.

ADVERSE REACTIONS
CNS: headache, restlessness, tremor, dizziness, fatigue, drowsiness, insomnia,

depression, light-headedness, confusion, hallucinations, *seizures,* paresthesia.
GI: *nausea, diarrhea,* vomiting, abdominal pain or discomfort, oral candidiasis, pseudomembranous colitis, dyspepsia, flatulence, constipation.
GU: crystalluria, increased serum creatinine and BUN levels, interstitial nephritis.
Hematologic: eosinophilia, *leukopenia, neutropenia, thrombocytopenia.*
Musculoskeletal: arthralgia, arthropathy, joint or back pain, joint inflammation, joint stiffness, aching, neck or chest pain.
Skin: *rash,* photosensitivity, ***Stevens-Johnson syndrome, toxic epidermal necrolysis, exfoliative dermatitis.***
Other: elevated liver enzymes; hypersensitivity; thrombophlebitis, burning, pruritus, erythema, edema (with I.V. administration).

INTERACTIONS
Drug-drug. *Antacids containing magnesium hydroxide or aluminum hydroxide, sucralfate, iron supplements, zinc- or iron-containing multivitamins:* decreased ciprofloxacin absorption. Separate administration by at least 2 hours.
Probenecid: may elevate serum level of ciprofloxacin. Monitor for toxicity.
Theophylline: increased plasma theophylline concentrations and prolonged theophylline half-life. Monitor blood levels of theophylline and observe for adverse effects.
Drug-herb. *Yerba maté:* may decrease clearance of yerba maté's methylxanthines and cause toxicity. Use together cautiously.
Drug-food. *Caffeine:* increased effect of caffeine. Monitor closely.
Dairy products, other foods: delayed peak serum levels. Give drug on an empty stomach.
Drug-lifestyle. *Sun exposure:* photosensitivity reactions may occur. Take precautions.

EFFECTS ON DIAGNOSTIC TESTS
None reported.

CONTRAINDICATIONS
Contraindicated in patients sensitive to fluoroquinolone antibiotics.

NURSING CONSIDERATIONS
• Use cautiously in patients with CNS disorders, such as severe cerebral arteriosclerosis or seizure disorders, and in those at increased risk for seizures. Drug may cause CNS stimulation.
• Obtain specimen for culture and sensitivity tests before giving first dose. Therapy may begin pending results.
• Administer oral form 2 hours after a meal or 2 hours before or after taking antacids, sucralfate, or products that contain iron (such as vitamins with mineral supplements). Food does not affect absorption but may delay peak serum levels.
• Know that long-term therapy may result in overgrowth of organisms resistant to ciprofloxacin.
• Safety in children under 18 years has not been established. Erosion of cartilage in immature animals has been reported.
• Monitor patient's intake and output and observe for signs of crystalluria.

🔵 I.V. administration
• Dilute drug using D_5W or 0.9% NaCl for injection to a final concentration of 1 to 2 mg/ml before use. Infuse slowly (over 1 hour) into a large vein.

☑ Patient teaching
• Tell patient to take drug as prescribed, even after he feels better.
• Advise patient to drink plenty of fluids to reduce risk of crystalluria.
• Warn patient to avoid hazardous tasks that require alertness, such as driving, until CNS effects of drug are known.
• Instruct patient to avoid caffeine while taking drug because of potential for cumulative caffeine effects.
• Advise patient that hypersensitivity reactions may occur even after first dose. If a rash or other allergic reaction occurs, tell him to stop drug immediately and notify doctor.
• Tell patient to avoid excessive sunlight or artificial ultraviolet light during therapy and to stop drug and call the doctor if phototoxicity occurs.
• Inform patient to discontinue breast-feeding during treatment or ask to be treated with another drug. Drug is excreted in breast milk.

• Tell patient to take drug on an empty stomach.

---

enoxacin
Penetrex

Pregnancy Risk Category: C

HOW SUPPLIED
Tablets (film-coated): 200 mg, 400 mg

ACTION
Inhibits bacterial DNA synthesis, mainly by blocking DNA gyrase; bactericidal.

Route	Onset	Peak	Duration
PO	Unknown	1-3 hr	Unknown

INDICATIONS & DOSAGE
Uncomplicated urinary tract infections (UTIs) caused by susceptible strains of Escherichia coli, Staphylococcus epidermidis, *and* S. saprophyticus—
Adults 18 years and over: 200 mg P.O. q 12 hours for 7 days.
Severe or complicated UTIs caused by susceptible strains of E. coli, Proteus mirabilis, Pseudomonas aeruginosa, S. epidermidis, *and* Enterobacter cloacae—
Adults 18 years and over: 400 mg P.O. q 12 hours for 14 days.
Uncomplicated urethral or endocervical gonorrhea—
Adults: 400 mg P.O. as a single dose.
 Doxycycline therapy may follow to treat possible coexisting chlamydial infection.
Adjust-a-dose: In patients with renal failure, if creatinine clearance is 30 ml/minute or less, therapy is started with usual initial dose. Subsequent doses are decreased by 50%.

ADVERSE REACTIONS
CNS: headache, restlessness, tremor, light-headedness, confusion, hallucinations, *seizures.*
GI: *nausea, diarrhea,* vomiting, abdominal pain or discomfort, oral candidiasis.
GU: crystalluria.
Other: *rash,* photosensitivity, eosinophilia, dyspnea, cough, elevated liver enzymes, pruritus, hypersensitivity.

INTERACTIONS
Drug-drug. *Aminophylline, cyclosporine, theophylline:* increased levels of these drugs because of decreased metabolism. Use together cautiously.
Antacids containing magnesium hydroxide or aluminum hydroxide, oral iron supplements, sucralfate: decreased enoxacin absorption. Separate administration times by at least 2 hours.
Bismuth subsalicylate: bioavailability of enoxacin is decreased when given within 60 minutes of bismuth subsalicylate. Avoid concomitant use.
Digoxin: may increase digoxin serum levels. Monitor closely for toxicity.
Oral anticoagulants: increased anticoagulant effect. Use together cautiously.
Drug-food. *Any food:* affects absorption. Give drug on empty stomach.
Caffeine: increased effect of caffeine. Monitor closely.

EFFECTS ON DIAGNOSTIC TESTS
None reported.

CONTRAINDICATIONS
Contraindicated in patients with hypersensitivity to drug or other fluoroquinolone antibiotics.

NURSING CONSIDERATIONS
• Use cautiously in patients with CNS disorders, such as severe cerebral arteriosclerosis or seizure disorders, and in those at increased risk for seizures. Drug may cause CNS stimulation.
• Use cautiously and with dosage adjustments in patients with impaired renal or hepatic function. Monitor renal function tests and liver function tests.
• Obtain specimen for culture and sensitivity test before giving first dose. Therapy may begin pending results.
Alert: Patients being treated for gonorrhea should have an initial serologic test for syphilis before therapy starts. Drug has not been effective in treating syphilis and may mask signs and symptoms of infection. Have the serologic test repeated in 1 to 3 months.
• Administer 2 hours after a meal or 2 hours before or after antacids containing magnesium hydroxide or aluminum hy-

---

Reactions may be *common,* uncommon, *life-threatening,* or COMMON AND LIFE-THREATENING.

droxide, sucralfate, or products that contain iron (such as vitamins with mineral supplements).
• Monitor closely for superinfection.
• Safety in children under 18 years has not been established. Erosion of cartilage in immature animals has been reported.

☑ **Patient teaching**
• Tell patient to take drug as prescribed, even after he feels better.
• Instruct patient to take drug on an empty stomach.
• Advise patient to drink plenty of fluids to reduce risk of crystalluria.
• Warn patient to avoid hazardous tasks until adverse CNS effects of drug are known.
• Warn patient not to drink beverages containing caffeine. Enoxacin inhibits the metabolism of caffeine and can result in toxicity.
• Advise patient to avoid overexposure to direct sunlight and to use a sunblock and wear protective clothing while outdoors.
• Instruct patient to stop taking drug at first signs of an allergic reaction and to notify doctor.

grepafloxacin hydrochloride
Raxar

Pregnancy Risk Category: C

HOW SUPPLIED
Tablets: 200 mg (base)

ACTION
Exact mechanism is unknown, but bactericidal effects may result from drug inhibiting bacterial DNA gyrase and preventing replication in susceptible bacteria.

Route	Onset	Peak	Duration
PO	Unknown	2-3 hr	Unknown

INDICATIONS & DOSAGE
Acute bacterial exacerbations of chronic bronchitis caused by susceptible strains of Haemophilus influenzae, Streptococcus pneumoniae, *or* Moraxella catarrhalis—
Adults: 400 or 600 mg P.O. once daily for 10 days.

Community-acquired pneumonia caused by susceptible strains of H. influenzae, S. pneumoniae, M. catarrhalis, *or* Mycoplasma pneumoniae—
Adults: 600 mg P.O. once daily for 10 days.
Uncomplicated gonorrhea (urethral in males and endocervical and rectal in females) caused by Neisseria gonorrhoeae—
Adults: 400 mg P.O. as a single dose.
Nongonococcal urethritis and cervicitis caused by Chlamydia trachomatis—
Adults: 400 mg P.O. once daily for 7 days.

ADVERSE REACTIONS
CNS: asthenia, dizziness, headache, insomnia, pain, nervousness, somnolence, psychosis, confusion, hallucinations, *seizures,* tremor.
CV: QT_c prolongation.
GI: abdominal pain, anorexia, constipation, *nausea,* diarrhea, dry mouth, dyspepsia, *taste perversion*, vomiting, pseudomembranous colitis.
GU: leukorrhea, vaginitis, hyperuricemia, increased BUN and creatinine.
Hematologic: eosinophilia, leukocytosis, lymphocytosis.
Hepatic: increased alkaline phosphatase, GGT, AST, and ALT.
Metabolic: hyperglycemia, hypoglycemia, hyperlipidemia, hypernatremia.
Skin: pruritus, photosensitivity reactions, rash.
Other: infection, hypersensitivity, tendinitis, tendon rupture.

INTERACTIONS
Drug-drug. *Amiodarone, astemizole, bepridil, cisapride, cyclosporine, erythromycin, midazolam, pentamidine, phenothiazines, quinidine, sotalol, triazolam, tricyclic antidepressants:* possible QT prolongation. Do not use together.
Antacids, metal cations, multivitamins, sucralfate: chelates with antacids containing aluminum, magnesium, calcium, or sucralfate or multiple vitamins containing zinc to substantially interfere with absorption of grepafloxacin. Do not give these agents within 4 hours before or after grepafloxacin administration.

---

*Liquid contains alcohol. **May contain tartrazine. †Canada ‡Australia §U.K. ◇OTC

Antidiabetic agents: disturbances of blood glucose, including hyperglycemia and hypoglycemia, have been reported in patients treated concomitantly with grepafloxacin and an antidiabetic agent. Monitor serum glucose level closely.

NSAIDs: concomitant administration of NSAIDs with grepafloxacin may increase risk of CNS stimulation and seizures. Use with caution.

Theophylline: serum theophylline concentrations increase when grepafloxacin is initiated in patients maintained on theophylline. When initiating a multiday course of grepafloxacin in patients maintained on theophylline, half the maintenance dose of theophylline for the period of concurrent therapy. Monitor theophylline serum concentrations.

Warfarin: may enhance effects of warfarin. Monitor INR.

Drug-food. *Caffeine:* grepafloxacin interferes with metabolism of caffeine and may enhance its effects. Use together cautiously.

Dairy products: can decrease absorption of grepafloxacin. Do not give drug with dairy products.

Drug-lifestyle. *Sun exposure:* photosensitivity reactions may occur. Take precautions. Stop drug if reactions occur.

EFFECTS ON DIAGNOSTIC TESTS
None reported.

CONTRAINDICATIONS
Contraindicated in patients with hypersensitivity to drug or other quinolones, hepatic failure, or a known QT prolongation, and in those receiving concomitant therapy with medications known to produce an increase in the QT interval or torsades de pointes.

NURSING CONSIDERATIONS
• Use cautiously in patients with known or suspected CNS disorders that predispose patient to seizures. Drug is not recommended for patients with proarrhythmic conditions.
• Serious, sometimes fatal, reactions have occurred. Discontinue drug at first sign of a reaction.

• Safety and efficacy in children under 18 years have not been established.
• Safety in pregnant and breast-feeding patients has not been established.
• Drug therapy may start pending results of culture and sensitivity tests.
• Pseudomembranous colitis, which may range in severity from mild to life-threatening, has been reported.
• Test patients treated for gonorrhea for syphilis at time of diagnosis and for 3 months after treatment with grepafloxacin.
• Achilles and other tendon ruptures that required surgical repair have been reported. Grepafloxacin should be discontinued if patient experiences pain, inflammation, or rupture of a tendon.
• Phototoxicity reactions have been observed in patients who were exposed to direct sunlight or tanning booths. Excessive sunlight should be avoided. Therapy should be discontinued if phototoxicity occurs.

✔**Patient teaching**
• Inform patient that drug may be taken with or without meals.
• Tell patient to drink plenty of fluids.
• Inform patient that drug may increase the effects of caffeine.
• Advise patient that drug may be associated with hypersensitivity reactions. Tell him to stop drug at first sign of rash, hives, or other skin reactions, rapid heartbeat, or difficulty breathing or swallowing.
• Warn patient to avoid hazardous activities until the effects of drug are known. Grepafloxacin may cause dizziness or light-headedness.
• Tell patient to avoid excessive sunlight or artificial ultraviolet light during drug therapy, and to discontinue therapy if sunburn or skin eruptions occur.
• Instruct patient to stop drug, sit and rest, and notify doctor immediately if pain, inflammation, or rupture of tendon occurs.
• Advise patient not to take antacids, multivitamins, or sucralfate within 4 hours before or after taking drug.
• Instruct patient to notify doctor if loose stools or diarrhea occurs.

levofloxacin
Levaquin

Pregnancy Risk Category: C

HOW SUPPLIED
Tablets: 250 mg, 500 mg
Single-use vials: 500 mg
Infusion (premixed): 250 mg in 50 ml D_5W, 500 mg in 100 ml D_5W

ACTION
Inhibits bacterial DNA gyrase and prevents DNA replication, transcription, repair, and recombination in susceptible bacteria.

Route	Onset	Peak	Duration
PO, IV	Unknown	1-2 hr	Unknown

INDICATIONS & DOSAGE
Indicated for treatment of mild, moderate, and severe infections caused by susceptible microorganisms in adults 18 years and older.

Acute maxillary sinusitis caused by susceptible strains of Streptococcus pneumoniae, Moraxella catarrhalis, *or* Haemophilus influenzae—
Adults: 500 mg P.O. or I.V. daily for 10 to 14 days. (See *Adjust-a-dose* below.)

Acute bacterial exacerbation of chronic bronchitis caused by Staphylococcus aureus, S. pneumoniae, M. catarrhalis, H. influenzae, *or* H. parainfluenzae—
Adults: 500 mg P.O. or I.V. daily for 7 days. (See *Adjust-a-dose* below.)

Community-acquired pneumonia caused by S. aureus, S. pneumoniae, M. catarrhalis, H. influenzae, H. parainfluenzae, Klebsiella pneumoniae, Chlamydia pneumoniae, Legionella pneumophila, *or* Mycoplasma pneumoniae—
Adults: 500 mg P.O. or I.V. daily for 7 to 14 days. (See *Adjust-a-dose* below.)

Mild to moderate skin and skin-structure infections caused by S. aureus *or* Streptococcus pyogenes—
Adults: 500 mg P.O. or I.V. daily for 7 to 10 days. (See *Adjust-a-dose* below.)

Adjust-a-dose: If creatinine clearance is 20 to 49 ml/minute, subsequent dosages are half the initial dose. If it is 10 to 19 ml/minute, subsequent dosages are half the initial dose and the interval is increased to q 48 hours.

Urinary tract infections (mild to moderate) caused by Enterococcus faecalis, Enterobacter cloacae, Escherichia coli, K. pneumoniae, Proteus mirabilis, *or* Pseudomonas aeruginosa—
Adults: 250 mg P.O. or I.V. daily for 10 days. (See *Adjust-a-dose* below.)

Acute pyelonephritis (mild to moderate) caused by E. coli—
Adults: 250 mg P.O. or I.V. daily for 10 days. (See *Adjust-a-dose* below.)

Adjust-a-dose: If creatinine clearance is 10 to 19 ml/minute, dosage interval is increased to q 48 hours.

ADVERSE REACTIONS
CNS: headache, insomnia, dizziness, encephalopathy, paresthesia, *seizures*.
CV: chest pain, palpitations, vasodilation.
GI: nausea, diarrhea, constipation, vomiting, abdominal pain, dyspepsia, flatulence, *pseudomembranous colitis*.
Hematologic: eosinophilia, hemolytic anemia, lymphopenia.
Musculoskeletal: back pain, tendon rupture.
Respiratory: allergic pneumonitis.
Skin: rash, photosensitivity, pruritus, erythema multiforme, *Stevens-Johnson syndrome*.
Other: vaginitis, pain, hypoglycemia, hypersensitivity reactions, *anaphylaxis, multisystem organ failure*.

INTERACTIONS
Drug-drug. *Antacids containing aluminum or magnesium, iron salts, products containing zinc, sucralfate:* may interfere with the GI absorption of levofloxacin. Administer at least 2 hours apart.
Antidiabetic agents: may alter blood glucose levels. Monitor glucose levels closely.
NSAIDs: may increase CNS stimulation. Monitor for seizure activity.
Theophylline: decreased clearance of theophylline with some fluoroquinolones. Monitor theophylline levels.
Warfarin and derivatives: increased effect of oral anticoagulant with some fluoroquinolones. Monitor PT and INR.

Drug-lifestyle. *Sun exposure:* photosensitivity reactions may occur. Take precautions.

EFFECTS ON DIAGNOSTIC TESTS
Drug may cause an abnormal ECG.

CONTRAINDICATIONS
Contraindicated in patients with hypersensitivity to drug, its components, or other fluoroquinolones.

NURSING CONSIDERATIONS
• Know that the safety and efficacy of drug in children under 18 years and pregnant and breast-feeding women have not been established.
• Use cautiously in patients with history of seizure disorders or other CNS diseases, such as cerebral arteriosclerosis. If patient experiences symptoms of excessive CNS stimulation (restlessness, tremor, confusion, hallucinations), discontinue medication and notify doctor. Institute seizure precautions.
• Use cautiously and with dosage adjustment, as ordered, in patients with renal impairment.
• Know that acute hypersensitivity reactions may require treatment with epinephrine, oxygen, I.V. fluids, antihistamines, corticosteroids, pressor amines, and airway management.
• Be aware that most antibacterial agents can cause pseudomembranous colitis. Notify doctor if diarrhea occurs. Drug may be discontinued.
• Obtain specimen for culture and sensitivity before starting therapy and as needed to determine if bacterial resistance has occurred.
• Monitor blood glucose and renal, hepatic, and hematopoietic blood studies, as ordered.

I.V. administration
• Know that levofloxacin injection should be administered only by I.V. infusion. Dilute drug in single-use vials according to manufacturer's instructions, with D_5W or 0.9% NaCl injection to a final concentration of 5 mg/ml. Reconstituted solution should be clear, slightly yellow, and free of particulate matter. Reconstituted drug is stable for 72 hours at room temperature, for 14 days when refrigerated in plastic containers, and for 6 months when frozen. Thaw at room temperature or in refrigerator only. Do not mix drug with other medications. Infuse over 60 minutes.

☑ Patient teaching
• Tell patient to take drug as prescribed, even if symptoms disappear.
• Advise patient to take drug with plenty of fluids and to avoid antacids, sucralfate, and products containing iron or zinc for at least 2 hours before and after each dose.
• Warn patient to avoid hazardous tasks until adverse CNS effects of drug are known.
• Advise patient to use sunblock and wear protective clothing when exposed to excessive sunlight.
• Tell patient to stop drug and notify doctor if rash or other signs of hypersensitivity develop.
• Tell patient to notify doctor of pain or inflammation; tendon rupture can occur with drug.
• Instruct the diabetic patient to monitor blood glucose levels and notify doctor if a hypoglycemic reaction occurs.
• Instruct patient to notify doctor if loose stools or diarrhea occurs.

---

lomefloxacin hydrochloride
Maxaquin

Pregnancy Risk Category: C

HOW SUPPLIED
Tablets (film-coated): 400 mg

ACTION
Inhibits bacterial DNA gyrase, an enzyme necessary for bacterial replication; bactericidal.

Route	Onset	Peak	Duration
PO	Unknown	1.5 hr	Unknown

INDICATIONS & DOSAGE
Acute bacterial exacerbations of chronic bronchitis caused by Haemophilus in-

---

fluenzae *or* Moraxella (Branhamella) catarrhalis—
Adults: 400 mg P.O. daily for 10 days.
Uncomplicated urinary tract infections (cystitis) caused by Escherichia coli, Klebsiella pneumoniae, Proteus mirabilis, *or* Staphylococcus saprophyticus—
Adults: 400 mg P.O. daily for 10 days.
Complicated urinary tract infections caused by E. coli, K. pneumoniae, P. mirabilis, *or* Pseudomonas aeruginosa; *possibly effective against infections caused by* Citrobacter diversus *or* Enterobacter cloacae—
Adults: 400 mg P.O. daily for 14 days.
Adjust-a-dose: In patients with creatinine clearance of 10 to 40 ml/minute, give loading dose of 400 mg P.O. on first day followed by 200 mg daily for duration of therapy. Hemodialysis removes negligible amounts of drug.
Prophylaxis of infections after transurethral surgical procedures—
Adults: 400 mg P.O. as a single dose 2 to 6 hours before surgery.
Prophylaxis of urinary tract infections after transrectal prostate biopsy—
Adults: 400 mg P.O. as a single dose 1 to 6 hours before procedure.

ADVERSE REACTIONS
CNS: *dizziness, headache,* abnormal dreams, fatigue, malaise, asthenia, agitation, anorexia, anxiety, confusion, depersonalization, depression, increased appetite, insomnia, nervousness, somnolence, *seizures, coma,* hyperkinesis, tremor, vertigo, paresthesia, arthralgia, myalgia.
CV: flushing, hypotension, hypertension, edema, syncope, arrhythmia, tachycardia, bradycardia, extrasystoles, cyanosis, angina pectoris, *MI, cardiac failure, pulmonary embolism,* cerebrovascular disorder, cardiomyopathy, phlebitis.
EENT: epistaxis, abnormal vision, conjunctivitis, eye pain, earache, tinnitus, tongue discoloration, taste perversion.
GI: *diarrhea, nausea,* dry mouth, pseudomembranous colitis, abdominal pain, dyspepsia, vomiting, flatulence, constipation, inflammation, dysphagia, bleeding.
GU: dysuria, hematuria, anuria, epididymitis, orchitis, vaginitis, vaginal moniliasis, intermenstrual bleeding, perineal pain.
Hematologic: thrombocythemia, *thrombocytopenia.*
Respiratory: dyspnea, *bronchospasm,* respiratory disorder or infection, increased sputum, stridor.
Skin: pruritus, skin disorder, skin exfoliation, eczema, rash, urticaria, *photosensitivity.*
Other: *anaphylaxis,* increased diaphoresis, leg cramps, lymphadenopathy, thirst, chest or back pain, chills, allergic reaction, facial edema, flulike symptoms, decreased heat tolerance, hypoglycemia, elevated liver enzymes, gout.

INTERACTIONS
Drug-drug. *Antacids, sucralfate:* impaired absorption after binding with lomefloxacin in GI tract. Give no less than 4 hours before or 2 hours after a dose.
Cimetidine: increased half-life of other fluoroquinolones when administered to patients taking cimetidine; lomefloxacin has not been tested. Monitor for toxicity.
Cyclosporine, warfarin: increased effects or serum levels when combined with other fluoroquinolones; lomefloxacin has not been tested. Monitor for toxicity.
NSAIDs: possibility of increased CNS stimulation and seizures. Use cautiously.
Probenecid: decreased excretion of lomefloxacin. Monitor for toxicity.
Drug-lifestyle. *Sun exposure:* photosensitivity reactions may occur. Take precautions.

EFFECTS ON DIAGNOSTIC TESTS
None reported.

CONTRAINDICATIONS
Contraindicated in patients with hypersensitivity to drug or other fluoroquinolones.

NURSING CONSIDERATIONS
• Use cautiously in patients with known or suspected CNS disorders, such as seizure disorder or cerebral arteriosclerosis, that may predispose the patient to seizures.
• Obtain culture and sensitivity tests be-

fore giving first dose. Therapy may begin pending results.

• Be aware that although most fluoroquinolones exhibit photosensitizing effects, early studies suggest that photosensitization and phototoxicity are more common with lomefloxacin.

• Keep in mind that prolonged use may result in overgrowth of organisms resistant to lomefloxacin.

• Safety in children under 18 years has not been established. Erosion of cartilage in immature animals has been reported.

☑ Patient teaching

• Tell patient to take drug as prescribed, even after he feels better.

• Advise patient that hypersensitivity reactions may occur even after first dose. If rash or other allergic reaction occurs, patient should stop taking drug and notify doctor.

• Warn patient to avoid hazardous tasks until CNS effects of drug are known.

• Advise patient to wear protective clothing, use a sunscreen, and avoid prolonged exposure to sunlight during treatment and for a few days after therapy ends. If sunburn occurs, the patient should call doctor as soon as possible.

• Tell patient that drug may be taken with or without food.

• Instruct patient to notify doctor if loose stools or diarrhea occurs.

---

nalidixic acid
NegGram

Pregnancy Risk Category: B (safe use in first trimester unknown)

HOW SUPPLIED
Caplets: 250 mg, 500 mg, 1 g
Oral suspension: 250 mg/5 ml

ACTION
Inhibits microbial DNA synthesis.

Route	Onset	Peak	Duration
PO	Unknown	1-2 hr	Unknown

INDICATIONS & DOSAGE
Acute and chronic urinary tract infections
caused by susceptible gram-negative organisms (Proteus, Klebsiella, Enterobacter, *and* Escherichia coli)—
Adults: 1 g P.O. q.i.d. for 7 to 14 days; 2 g daily for long-term use.
Children over 3 months: 55 mg/kg P.O. daily divided q.i.d. for 7 to 14 days; 33 mg/kg daily for long-term use.

ADVERSE REACTIONS
CNS: drowsiness, weakness, headache, dizziness, vertigo, *seizures,* malaise, confusion, hallucinations, psychosis.
EENT: sensitivity to light, change in color perception, diplopia, blurred vision.
GI: *abdominal pain, nausea, vomiting,* diarrhea.
Hematologic: eosinophilia, *leukopenia, thrombocytopenia,* hemolytic anemia.
Skin: pruritus, photosensitivity, urticaria, rash.
Other: *angioedema, increased intracranial pressure and bulging fontanelles in infants and children,* arthralgia, joint stiffness, *anaphylactoid reaction.*

INTERACTIONS
Drug-drug. *Nitrofurantoin:* antagonizes effects of nalidixic acid. Monitor closely.
Oral anticoagulants: increased anticoagulant effect. Monitor for bleeding.
Drug-lifestyle. *Sun exposure:* photosensitivity reactions may occur. Take precautions.

EFFECTS ON DIAGNOSTIC TESTS
Drug may cause false-positive results in urine glucose tests using cupric sulfate (such as Benedict's reagent, Fehling's solution, and Clinitest). Urine 17-ketosteroid and urine 17-ketogenic steroid levels may be falsely elevated because nalidixic acid interacts with *M*-dinitrobenzene, used to measure these urine metabolites. Urine vanillylmandelic acid levels may also be falsely elevated.

CONTRAINDICATIONS
Contraindicated in patients with hypersensitivity to drug, in those with seizure disorders, and in infants under 3 months.

NURSING CONSIDERATIONS
• Use with extreme caution in prepubertal

---

children; erosion of cartilage in immature animals has been reported.

• Use cautiously in patients with impaired hepatic or renal function or with severe cerebral arteriosclerosis. Monitor renal and liver function test results.

• Obtain specimen for culture and sensitivity tests before starting therapy and repeat as needed. Therapy may begin pending results.

• Monitor CBC, renal, and liver function studies during long-term therapy, as ordered.

• Be aware that resistant bacteria may emerge in the first 48 hours of therapy.

✅**Patient teaching**
• Tell patient to take drug as prescribed, even after he feels better.

• Instruct patient to take drug with food to prevent GI upset.

• Tell patient to avoid exposure to sunlight, to wear protective clothing, and to use sunscreen.

• Tell patient to report visual disturbances or CNS symptoms immediately.

---

norfloxacin
Noroxin, Utinor§

Pregnancy Risk Category: C

HOW SUPPLIED
Tablets (film-coated): 400 mg

ACTION
Inhibits bacterial DNA synthesis, mainly by blocking DNA gyrase; bactericidal.

Route	Onset	Peak	Duration
PO	Unknown	0.5-2 hr	Unknown

INDICATIONS & DOSAGE
Complicated or uncomplicated urinary tract infections caused by susceptible strains of Enterococcus faecalis, Escherichia coli, Klebsiella pneumoniae, Enterobacter aerogenes, E. cloacae, Proteus mirabilis, P. vulgaris, Pseudomonas aeruginosa, Citrobacter freundii, Staphylococcus agalactiae, S. aureus, S. epidermidis, S. saprophyticus, *and* Serratia marcescens—

Adults: for uncomplicated infections, 400 mg P.O. q 12 hours for 7 to 10 days. For complicated infections, 400 mg P.O. q 12 hours for 10 to 21 days.
Cystitis caused by E. coli, K. pneumoniae, *or* P. mirabilis—
Adults: 400 mg P.O. q 12 hours for 3 days.
Acute, uncomplicated urethral and cervical gonorrhea—
Adults: 800 mg P.O. as a single dose, followed by doxycycline therapy to treat any coexisting chlamydial infection.
Adjust-a-dose: In adult patients with creatinine clearance of 30 ml/minute or less, 400 mg once daily for above indications.

ADVERSE REACTIONS
CNS: fatigue, somnolence, headache, dizziness, *seizures,* depression, insomnia.
GI: nausea, constipation, flatulence, heartburn, dry mouth, abdominal pain, diarrhea, vomiting, anorexia.
GU: increased serum creatinine and BUN levels, crystalluria.
Hematologic: eosinophilia.
Musculoskeletal: back pain.
Skin: rash, photosensitivity.
Other: hypersensitivity reactions (rash, *anaphylactoid reaction*), transient elevations of AST and ALT, fever, hyperhidrosis.

INTERACTIONS
Drug-drug. *Antacids, iron products, sucralfate:* may hinder absorption. Separate administration times by 2 hours.
Cyclosporine: increased serum concentrations of cyclosporine. Monitor serum levels.
Nitrofurantoin: antagonizes effects of norfloxacin. Monitor closely.
Oral anticoagulants: increased anticoagulant effect. Monitor closely.
Probenecid: may increase serum levels of norfloxacin by decreasing its excretion. Monitor for toxicity.
Theophylline: possibly impaired theophylline metabolism, resulting in increased plasma levels and risk of toxicity. Monitor closely.

EFFECTS ON DIAGNOSTIC TESTS
BUN, serum creatinine, ALT, AST, and al-

---

kaline phosphatase levels may increase; hematocrit may decrease; and eosinophilia and neutropenia may occur during norfloxacin therapy.

CONTRAINDICATIONS

Contraindicated in patients with hypersensitivity to fluoroquinolones.

NURSING CONSIDERATIONS

• Use cautiously in patients with conditions that may predispose them to seizure disorders, such as cerebral arteriosclerosis. Also use cautiously in those with renal impairment. Monitor renal function.
• Safety in children under 18 years has not been established. Erosion of cartilage in immature animals has been reported.
• Obtain culture and sensitivity before starting therapy.

☑ **Patient teaching**
• Tell patient to take drug as prescribed, even after he feels better.
• Advise patient to take drug 1 hour before or 2 hours after meals because food, antacids, iron products, and sucralfate may hinder absorption.
• Warn patient not to exceed the recommended dosages and to drink several glasses of water throughout the day to maintain hydration and adequate urine output.
• Warn patient to avoid hazardous tasks that require alertness until CNS effects of drug are known.
• Instruct patient to avoid exposure to sunlight and to wear protective clothing and use sunscreen.

---

ofloxacin
Floxin, Floxin I.V., Tarivid§

Pregnancy Risk Category: C

HOW SUPPLIED
Tablets (film-coated): 200 mg, 300 mg, 400 mg
Injection: 20 mg/ml, 40 mg/ml; 4 mg/ml premixed in D₅W

ACTION
Inhibits bacterial DNA synthesis by blocking DNA gyrase; bactericidal.

Route	Onset	Peak	Duration
PO	Unknown	0.5-2 hr	Unknown
IV	Unknown	Immediate	Unknown

INDICATIONS & DOSAGE
Lower respiratory tract infections caused by susceptible strains of Haemophilus influenzae *or* Streptococcus pneumoniae—
Adults: 400 mg I.V. or P.O. q 12 hours for 10 days.
Cervicitis or urethritis caused by Chlamydia trachomatis *or* Neisseria gonorrhoeae—
Adults: 300 mg I.V. or P.O. q 12 hours for 7 days.
Acute, uncomplicated gonorrhea—
Adults: 400 mg I.V. or P.O. as a single dose with doxycycline.
Mild to moderate skin and skin-structure infections caused by susceptible strains of Staphylococcus aureus, Streptococcus pyogenes, *or* Proteus mirabilis—
Adults: 400 mg I.V. or P.O. q 12 hours for 10 days.
Cystitis caused by Escherichia coli *or* Klebsiella pneumoniae—
Adults: 200 mg I.V. or P.O. q 12 hours for 3 days.
Urinary tract infections caused by susceptible strains of Citrobacter diversus, Enterobacter aerogenes, E. coli, P. mirabilis, *or* Pseudomonas aeruginosa—
Adults: 200 mg I.V. or P.O. q 12 hours for 7 days. Complicated infections may require therapy for 10 days.
Prostatitis caused by E. coli—
Adults: 300 mg I.V. or P.O. q 12 hours for 6 weeks.
Epididymitis—
Adults: 300 mg P.O. q 12 hours for 10 days.
Pelvic inflammatory disease (outpatient)—
Adults: 400 mg P.O. q 12 hours for 14 days in combination with clindamycin or metronidazole.
Adjust-a-dose: In renally impaired patients with creatinine clearance of 20 to 50 ml/minute, reduce dosage interval to once q 24 hours. If creatinine clearance is

---

below 20 ml/minute, give half the recommended dose q 24 hours.

ADVERSE REACTIONS

CNS: headache, dizziness, fatigue, lethargy, malaise, drowsiness, sleep disorders, nervousness, insomnia, visual disturbances, *seizures.*
CV: chest pain.
GI: *nausea,* anorexia, abdominal pain or discomfort, diarrhea, vomiting, constipation, dry mouth, flatulence, dysgeusia.
GU: vaginitis, vaginal discharge, genital pruritus.
Musculoskeletal: trunk pain.
Skin: rash, pruritus, photosensitivity.
Other: hypersensitivity reactions *(anaphylactoid reaction),* elevated liver enzymes, fever, phlebitis, hyperglycemia.

INTERACTIONS

Drug-drug. *Antacids containing aluminum or magnesium hydroxide, iron salts, sucralfate, products containing zinc:* may interfere with the GI absorption of ofloxacin. Separate administration by at least 2 hours.
Antidiabetic agents: may cause alterations in blood glucose levels. Monitor concentrations closely.
NSAIDs: possibility of increased CNS stimulation and seizures. Use cautiously.
Oral anticoagulants: increased effect. Monitor for bleeding and altered PT.
Theophylline: decreased clearance of theophylline with some fluoroquinolones. Monitor theophylline levels.
Drug-food. *Any food:* decreased absorption. Give drug on an empty stomach.
Drug-lifestyle. *Sun exposure:* photosensitivity reactions may occur. Take precautions.

EFFECTS ON DIAGNOSTIC TESTS
None reported.

CONTRAINDICATIONS
Contraindicated in patients with hypersensitivity to drug or other fluoroquinolones.

NURSING CONSIDERATIONS
• Use cautiously in patients with a history of seizure disorders or other CNS diseases, such as cerebral arteriosclerosis.
• Use cautiously and with dosage adjustment in patients with renal failure, as prescribed, because drug is mainly eliminated by renal excretion.
• Obtain culture and sensitivity prior to first dose.
• Monitor regular blood studies and hepatic and renal function tests during prolonged therapy, as ordered.
Alert: Know that patients treated for gonorrhea should have a serologic test for syphilis. Drug is not effective against syphilis, and treatment of gonorrhea may mask or delay symptoms of syphilis.
• Safe use in children under 18 years is unknown. Erosion of cartilage in immature animals has been reported.

I.V. administration
• Dilute concentrate for injection before use. Single-use vials containing 20 or 40 mg/ml must be diluted to a maximum concentration of 4 mg/ml with a compatible I.V. solution, such as D_5W, 0.9% NaCl for injection, D_5W in 0.9% NaCl for injection, or sterile water for injection. Infuse over at least 60 minutes.
• Because compatibility with other drugs is not known, don't mix ofloxacin with other drugs. If giving infusion at a Y-site, discontinue the flow of the other solution.

Patient teaching
• Tell patient to take drug as prescribed, even after he feels better.
• Advise patient to take drug with plenty of fluids, but not with meals, and to avoid antacids, sucralfate, and products containing iron or zinc for at least 2 hours before and after each dose.
• Warn patient to avoid hazardous tasks until adverse CNS effects of drug are known.
• Inform patient to use sunscreen and wear protective clothing.
• Tell patient to stop drug and notify doctor if rash or other signs of hypersensitivity develop.

---

*Liquid contains alcohol.   **May contain tartrazine.   †Canada   ‡Australia   §U.K.   ◇OTC

sparfloxacin
Zagam

Pregnancy Risk Category: C

HOW SUPPLIED
Tablets: 200 mg

ACTION
Inhibits bacterial DNA gyrase and prevents DNA replication, transcription, repair, and deactivation in susceptible bacteria.

Route	Onset	Peak	Duration
PO	Unknown	3-6 hr	Unknown

INDICATIONS & DOSAGE
Acute bacterial exacerbation of chronic bronchitis caused by Staphylococcus aureus, Streptococcus pneumoniae, Chlamydia pneumoniae, Enterobacter cloacae, Klebsiella pneumoniae, Moraxella catarrhalis, Haemophilus influenzae, *or* H. parainfluenzae—
Adults over 18 years: 400 mg P.O. on first day as a loading dose; then 200 mg daily for total of 10 days of therapy.
Community-acquired pneumonia caused by S. pneumoniae, M. catarrhalis, H. influenzae, H. parainfluenzae, C. pneumoniae, *or* Mycoplasma pneumoniae—
Adults over 18 years: 400 mg P.O. on first day as a loading dose; then 200 mg daily for total of 10 days of therapy.
Adjust-a-dose: In renally impaired patients with creatinine clearance below 50 ml/minute, give a loading dose of 400 mg P.O.; thereafter, 200 mg P.O. q 48 hours for total of 9 days of therapy.

ADVERSE REACTIONS
CNS: headache, dizziness, insomnia, asthenia, somnolence, *seizures.*
CV: QT interval prolongation, vasodilation.
EENT: dry mouth, taste perversion.
GI: nausea, diarrhea, vomiting, abdominal pain, dyspepsia, flatulence, *pseudomembranous colitis.*
GU: vaginal moniliasis.
Musculoskeletal: tendon rupture.
Skin: rash, photosensitivity, pruritus.

Other: elevated ALT and AST levels and WBC counts, hypersensitivity reactions, *anaphylaxis.*

INTERACTIONS
Drug-drug. *Antacids containing aluminum or magnesium, iron salts, zinc, sucralfate:* may interfere with GI absorption of levofloxacin. Administer at least 4 hours apart.
Drugs that prolong the QT interval or cause torsades de pointes (including amiodarone, astemizole, bepridil, cisapride, class Ia antiarrhythmics [such as quinidine and procainamide], class III drugs [such as sotalol], disopyramide, erythromycin, pentamidine, phenothiazines, tricyclic antidepressants): may cause torsades de pointes. Sparfloxacin is contraindicated in these patients.
Drug-lifestyle. *Sun exposure:* photosensitivity reactions may occur. Take precautions.

EFFECTS ON DIAGNOSTIC TESTS
Drug may produce false-negative culture results for *Mycobacterium tuberculosis.*

CONTRAINDICATIONS
Contraindicated in patients with history of hypersensitivity or photosensitivity reactions to drug and those who cannot stay out of the sun. Avoid concomitant administration with drugs known to prolong the QT interval or cause torsades de pointes. Drug is not recommended for patients with heart conditions that predispose them to arrhythmias.

NURSING CONSIDERATIONS
• Know that safety and efficacy of levofloxacin in pregnant and breast-feeding women and patients under 18 years have not been established.
• Use cautiously in patients with history of seizure disorder or other CNS diseases, such as cerebral arteriosclerosis. If patient experiences symptoms of excessive CNS stimulation (restlessness, tremor, confusion, hallucinations), discontinue medication and notify doctor. Then institute seizure precautions.
• Use cautiously and with dosage adjust-

ment in patients with renal impairment. Monitor renal function.

• Know that acute hypersensitivity reactions may require treatment with epinephrine, oxygen, I.V. fluids, antihistamines, corticosteroids, pressor amines, and airway management.

• Obtain specimen for culture and sensitivity before starting therapy and as needed and ordered to determine if bacterial resistance has occurred.

☑ **Patient teaching**
• Tell patient that drug may be taken with food, milk, or products that contain caffeine.

• Tell patient to take drug as prescribed, even if symptoms disappear.

• Advise patient to take drug with plenty of fluids and to avoid antacids, sucralfate, and products containing iron or zinc for at least 4 hours after each dose.

• Warn patient to avoid hazardous tasks until adverse CNS effects of drug are known.

Alert: Advise patient to avoid direct, indirect, and artificial ultraviolet light, even with sunscreen on, during treatment and for 5 days after treatment. Patient should stop taking drug and notify the doctor if signs or symptoms of phototoxicity (skin burning, redness, swelling, blisters, rash, itching) occur.

• Tell patient to stop drug and notify doctor if rash or other signs of hypersensitivity develop.

• Tell patient to discontinue drug and notify doctor of pain or inflammation; tendon rupture can occur with drug. He should rest and refrain from exercise until a diagnosis is made.

• Instruct patient to notify doctor if loose stools or diarrhea occurs.

▼ NEW DRUG

trovafloxacin mesylate
Trovan Tablets

alatrofloxacin mesylate
Trovan I.V.

Pregnancy Risk Category: C

HOW SUPPLIED
Tablets: 100 mg, 200 mg
Injection: 5 mg/ml in 40-ml (200 mg) and 60-ml (300 mg) vials

ACTION
Trovafloxacin is related to the fluoroquinolones with in vitro activity against a wide range of gram-positive and gram-negative aerobic and anaerobic microorganisms. Bactericidal action results from inhibition of DNA gyrase and topoisomerase IV, two enzymes involved in bacterial replication.

Route	Onset	Peak	Duration
PO, IV	Unknown	1 hr	Unknown

INDICATIONS & DOSAGE
Nosocomial pneumonia caused by Escherichia coli, Pseudomonas aeruginosa, Haemophilus influenzae, *or* Staphylococcus aureus; *gynecologic and pelvic infections caused by* E. coli, Bacteroides fragilis, *viridans group streptococci,* Enterococcus faecalis, Streptococcus agalactiae, Peptostreptococcus *species,* Prevotella *species, or* Gardnerella vaginalis; *complicated intra-abdominal infections including postsurgical infections caused by* E. coli, B. fragilis, *viridans group streptococci,* P. aeruginosa, Klebsiella pneumoniae, Peptostreptococcus *species, or* Prevotella *species*—
Adults: 300 mg I.V. daily followed by 200 mg P.O. daily for 7 to 14 days (10 to 14 days for pneumonia).
Community-acquired pneumonia caused by Streptococcus pneumoniae, H. influenzae, K. pneumoniae, S. aureus, Mycoplasma pneumoniae, Moraxella catarrhalis, Legionella pneumophila, *or* Chlamydia pneumoniae; *complicated skin and skin-structure infections including diabetic foot infections caused by* S. aureus, S. agalactiae, P. aeruginosa, E. faecalis, E. coli, *or* Proteus mirabilis *(not for treatment of osteomyelitis)*—
Adults: 200 mg P.O. or I.V. daily followed by 200 mg P.O. daily for 7 to 14 days (10 to 14 days for complicated skin and skin-structure infections).
Prophylaxis of infection associated with

elective colorectal surgery or vaginal and abdominal hysterectomy—
Adults: 200 mg P.O. or I.V as a single dose 30 minutes to 4 hours before surgery.
Acute sinusitis caused by H. influenzae, M. catarrhalis, *or* S. pneumoniae; *chronic prostatitis caused by* E. coli, E. faecalis, *or* Staphylococcus epidermis; *cervicitis caused by* Chlamydia trachomatis; *and pelvic inflammatory disease (mild to moderate) caused by* Neisseria gonorrhoeae *or* C. trachomatis—
Adults: 200 mg P.O. daily for 5 days (cervicitis), 10 days (acute sinusitis), 14 days (pelvic inflammatory disease), or 28 days (chronic prostatitis).
Uncomplicated urinary tract infections caused by E. coli; *uncomplicated skin and skin-structure infections caused by* S. aureus, Streptococcus pyogenes, *or* S. agalactiae; *acute bacterial exacerbation of chronic bronchitis caused by* H. influenzae, M. catarrhalis, S. pneumoniae, S. aureus, *or* Haemophilus parainfluenzae; *and uncomplicated gonorrhea caused by* N. gonorrhoeae—
Adults: 100 mg P.O. daily for 3 days (urinary tract infections), 7 to 10 days (skin and skin-structure infections, bronchitis) or single dose for treatment of gonorrhea.
Adjust-a-dose: For patients with mild to moderate cirrhosis (Child-Pugh Class A and B), reduce 300-mg I.V. dose to 200-mg I.V. and 200-mg I.V. or P.O. dose to 100-mg I.V. or P.O.; no reduction is needed for 100-mg P.O. dose.

ADVERSE REACTIONS
CNS: *dizziness,* light-headedness, headache, *seizures,* psychosis.
GI: diarrhea, nausea, vomiting, abdominal pain, pseudomembranous colitis.
GU: vaginitis, increased BUN and creatinine.
Hematologic: bone marrow aplasia (anemia, ***thrombocytopenia, leukopenia***), decreased hemoglobin and hematocrit, increased platelets.
Hepatic: increased ALT and AST.
Musculoskeletal: arthralgia, arthropathy, myalgia.
Skin: pruritus, rash, injection-site reaction (I.V.), photosensitivity.

INTERACTIONS
Drug-drug. *Antacids containing aluminum, magnesium, or citric acid buffered with sodium citrate (Bicitra), sucralfate, iron-containing preparations, and I.V. morphine:* bioavailability of trovafloxacin is significantly reduced following concomitant use with these agents. Give these agents 2 hours before or 2 hours after trovafloxacin. Avoid morphine I.V. for 4 hours if trovafloxacin is taken with food.
Drug-lifestyle. *Sun exposure:* photosensitivity reactions may occur. Take precautions.

EFFECTS ON DIAGNOSTIC TESTS
None reported.

CONTRAINDICATIONS
Contraindicated in patients with hypersensitivity to drug, alatrofloxacin, or other quinolone antimicrobials or any other components of these products.

NURSING CONSIDERATIONS
• Use cautiously in patients with CNS disorders (such as cerebral atherosclerosis or epilepsy) and in those at increased risk for seizures. As with other quinolones, drug may cause neurologic complications such as seizures, psychosis, or increased intracranial pressure may occur. Monitor patient with preexisting condition closely.
• Perform periodic assessment of liver function due to potential for increases in ALT, AST, and alkaline phosphatase levels.
• Drug can be given as a single daily dose without regard for food.
• Be aware that moderate to severe phototoxicity reactions have occurred in patients exposed to direct sunlight.
• Be aware that no dosage adjustment is necessary when switching from I.V. to oral form.
• Know that, if *P. aeruginosa* is the known or presumed pathogen, combination therapy with either an aminoglycoside or aztreonam may be indicated.

⬛I.V. administration
• Alatrofloxacin mesylate is supplied in single-use vials which must be further di-

luted with an appropriate solution (D_5W, 0.45% NaCl) before administration. Do not dilute drug with 0.9% NaCl or lactated Ringer's solution. Follow package insert for specific instructions regarding preparation of desired dosage.

• After dilution, administer alatrofloxacin mesylate by I.V. infusion over 60 minutes. Avoid rapid bolus or infusion. Do not administer drug with solutions containing multivalent cations (such as magnesium) through same I.V. line.

☑ **Patient teaching**

• Inform patient that drug may be taken without regard to meals; however, tell him to take products containing iron, aluminum, magnesium (vitamins, minerals, antacids), or sucralfate at least 2 hours before or 2 hours after a trovafloxacin dose.

• Advise patient to take drug with meals or at bedtime if light-headedness or dizziness occurs.

• Warn patient to avoid excessive sunlight or artificial ultraviolet light and to use an effective sunscreen to prevent burn.

• Instruct patient to discontinue treatment, refrain from exercise, and seek medical advice if pain, inflammation, or rupture of a tendon occurs.

• Advise patient to discontinue treatment at first sign of rash, hives, difficulty swallowing or breathing, or other symptoms suggesting an allergic reaction and to seek medical help immediately.

• Instruct patient to notify doctor if severe diarrhea occurs; this may indicate pseudomembranous colitis.

17

Antivirals

acyclovir sodium
amantadine hydrochloride
cidofovir
delavirdine mesylate
didanosine
efavirenz
famciclovir
fomivirsen sodium
foscarnet sodium
ganciclovir
indinavir sulfate
lamivudine
lamivudine/zidovudine
nelfinavir mesylate
nevirapine
ribavirin
rimantadine hydrochloride
ritonavir
saquinavir
saquinavir mesylate
stavudine
valacyclovir hydrochloride
zalcitabine
zidovudine

COMBINATION PRODUCTS
None.

---

acyclovir sodium
Avirax†, Zovirax

Pregnancy Risk Category: B

HOW SUPPLIED
Capsules: 200 mg
Tablets: 400 mg, 800 mg
Suspension: 200 mg/5 ml
Injection: 500 mg/vial, 1 g/vial

ACTION
Interferes with DNA synthesis and inhibits viral multiplication.

Route	Onset	Peak	Duration
PO	Unknown	2.5 hr	Unknown
IV	Immediate	Immediate	Unknown

INDICATIONS & DOSAGE
Initial and recurrent episodes of mucocutaneous herpes simplex virus (HSV-1 and HSV-2) infections in immunocompromised patients; severe initial episodes of genital herpes in patients who are not immunocompromised—
Adults and children 12 years and older: 5 mg/kg, given at a constant rate over 1 hour by I.V. q 8 hours for 7 to 14 days (5 to 7 days for severe initial episode of genital herpes).
Children under 12 years: 250 mg/m², given at a constant rate over 1 hour by I.V. q 8 hours for 7 days.
Initial genital herpes—
Adults: 200 mg P.O. q 4 hours while awake (total of five capsules daily); or 400 mg P.O. q 8 hours. Treatment should continue for 7 to 10 days for treatment of initial genital herpes episodes.
Intermittent therapy for recurrent genital herpes—
Adults: 200 mg P.O. q 4 hours while awake (total of five capsules daily). Treatment should continue for 5 days. Initiate therapy at the first sign of recurrence.
Chronic suppressive therapy for recurrent genital herpes—
Adults: 400 mg P.O. b.i.d. for up to 12 months. Alternatively, 200 mg P.O. three to five times daily for up to 12 months.
Treatment of varicella (chickenpox) infections in immunocompromised patients—
Adults and children 12 years and older: 10 mg/kg I.V. infused at a constant rate over 1 hour q 8 hours for 7 days. Dosage for obese patients is 10 mg/kg (based on ideal body weight) q 8 hours for 7 days. Do not exceed maximum dosage equivalent of 500 mg/m² q 8 hours.
Children under 12 years: 500 mg/m² I.V. infused at a constant rate over 1 hour q 8 hours for 7 to 10 days.
Varicella infection in immunocompetent patients—
Adults and children 2 years and older: 20 mg/kg (maximum 800 mg/dose) P.O. q.i.d. for 5 days. Start therapy as soon as

---

symptoms appear to achieve maximum efficacy.

Alternatively, in adults and children weighing over 40 kg (88 lb), 800 mg P.O. q.i.d. for 5 days. In children 2 years and older weighing 40 kg or less, 20 mg/kg P.O. q.i.d. for 5 days.

Acute herpes zoster infection in immuno-competent patients—

Adults and children 12 years and older: 800 mg P.O. q 4 hours five times daily for 7 to 10 days.

Herpes simplex encephalitis—

Adults and children over 6 months: 10 mg/kg I.V. infused at a constant rate over 1 hour q 8 hours for 10 days.

Alternatively, in children 6 months to 12 years, 500 mg/m² I.V. infused at a constant rate over 1 hour q 8 hours for 10 days.

Adjust-a-dose: In patients with renal failure, I.V. dosage for creatinine clearance over 50 ml/minute is 100% of dose q 8 hours; if 25 to 50 ml/minute, 100% dose q 12 hours; if 10 to 24 ml/minute, 100% dose q 24 hours; and if less than 10 ml/minute, 50% dose q 24 hours.

P.O. dosage: If normal dose is 200 mg q 4 hours five times daily and creatinine clearance is below 10 ml/minute, 200 mg P.O. q 12 hours. If normal dose is 400 mg q 12 hours and creatinine clearance is below 10 ml/minute, 200 mg q 12 hours. If normal dose is 800 mg q 4 hours five times daily and creatinine clearance is below 10 ml/minute, 800 mg q 12 hours; and if creatinine clearance is 10 to 25 ml/minute, 800 mg q 8 hours.

ADVERSE REACTIONS

CNS: *malaise, headache, encephalopathic changes (lethargy, obtundation, tremor, confusion, hallucinations, agitation, seizures, coma).*
GI: *nausea, vomiting,* diarrhea.
GU: *transient elevations of serum creatinine and BUN levels,* hematuria, *acute renal failure.*
Hematologic: *thrombocytopenia, leukopenia,* thrombocytosis.
Skin: rash, itching, urticaria.
Other: *inflammation, phlebitis* (at injection site).

INTERACTIONS

Drug-drug. *Interferon:* may have synergistic effect. Monitor closely.
Probenecid: increased acyclovir blood levels. Monitor for possible toxicity.
Zidovudine: may cause drowsiness or lethargy. Use together cautiously.

EFFECTS ON DIAGNOSTIC TESTS
None reported.

CONTRAINDICATIONS
Contraindicated in patients with hypersensitivity to drug.

NURSING CONSIDERATIONS
• Use cautiously in patients with underlying neurologic problems, renal disease, or dehydration and in those receiving other nephrotoxic drugs. Monitor renal function.
Alert: Don't administer I.M. or S.C.
• Know that encephalopathic changes are more likely to occur in patients with neurologic disorders or in those who have had neurologic reactions to cytotoxic drugs.
• Keep in mind that Glaxo-Wellcome, the manufacturer of Zovirax, maintains an ongoing registry of women exposed to the drug during pregnancy. Follow-up studies to date have not shown an increased risk for birth defects for infants born to patients exposed to the drug during pregnancy. Health care providers are encouraged to report such exposures to the registrar at 1-800-722-9292, ext. 39437.

I.V. administration
• Administer I.V. infusion over at least 1 hour to prevent renal tubular damage. Don't give by bolus injection. Bolus injection, dehydration (decreased urine output), preexisting renal disease, and concomitant use of other nephrotoxic drugs increase the risk of renal toxicity.
• Be aware that concentrated solutions (7 mg/ml or more) may be associated with a higher incidence of phlebitis.
• Encourage fluid intake because patient must be adequately hydrated during acyclovir infusion. Monitor intake and output especially within the first 2 hours post I.V. administration.

☑ **Patient teaching**
• Tell patient to take drug as prescribed, even after he feels better.
• Instruct patient that drug is effective in managing herpes infection but does not eliminate or cure it. Warn patient that acyclovir will not prevent spread of infection to others.
• Urge patient to recognize early symptoms of herpes infection (such as tingling, itching, or pain). He can then notify his doctor and get a prescription for acyclovir before the infection fully develops. Treatment started early is most effective.

---

amantadine hydrochloride
Symadine, Symmetrel

Pregnancy Risk Category: C

HOW SUPPLIED
Capsules: 100 mg
Syrup: 50 mg/5 ml

ACTION
Unknown. Possibly inhibits the uncoating of the virus.

Route	Onset	Peak	Duration
PO	Unknown	1-4 hr	Unknown

INDICATIONS & DOSAGE
Prophylaxis or symptomatic treatment of influenza type A virus, respiratory tract illnesses—
Adults up to 65 years with normal renal function: 200 mg P.O. daily in a single dose.
Children 9 to 12 years: 100 mg P.O. b.i.d.
Children 1 to 9 years or weighing below 45 kg (99 lb): 4.4 to 8.8 mg/kg P.O. as a total daily dose given once daily or divided equally b.i.d. Maximum dosage is 150 mg daily.
Elderly: 100 mg P.O. once daily in patients over 65 years with normal renal function.

Begin treatment within 24 to 48 hours after symptoms appear and continue for 24 to 48 hours after symptoms disappear (usually 2 to 7 days of therapy). Start prophylaxis as soon as possible after initial exposure and continue for at least 10 days after exposure. May continue prophylactic treatment up to 90 days for repeated or suspected exposures if influenza vaccine is unavailable. If used with influenza vaccine, continue dose for 2 to 3 weeks until antibody response to vaccine has developed.

Adjust-a-dose: In patients with renal failure, if creatinine clearance is 30 to 50 ml/minute, give 200 mg the first day and 100 mg thereafter; if clearance is 15 to 29 ml/minute, give 200 mg the first day followed by 100 mg on alternate days; if clearance is less than 15 ml/minute, give 200 mg q 7 days.

ADVERSE REACTIONS
CNS: depression, fatigue, confusion, *dizziness,* hallucinations, anxiety, *irritability,* ataxia, *insomnia,* headache, *lightheadedness.*
CV: peripheral edema, orthostatic hypotension, **heart failure.**
GI: anorexia, *nausea,* constipation, vomiting, dry mouth.
Skin: *livedo reticularis* (with prolonged use).

INTERACTIONS
Drug-drug. *Anticholinergics:* increased anticholinergic effects. Use together cautiously. Dosage of anticholinergic agent may be reduced prior to initiation of amantadine by some doctors.
CNS stimulants: additive CNS stimulation. Use together cautiously.
Drug-herb. *Jimson weed:* may adversely affect CV function. Avoid concomitant use.

EFFECTS ON DIAGNOSTIC TESTS
None reported.

CONTRAINDICATIONS
Contraindicated in patients with hypersensitivity to drug.

NURSING CONSIDERATIONS
• Use cautiously in those with seizure disorders, heart failure, peripheral edema, hepatic disease, mental illness, eczematoid rash, renal impairment, orthostatic hypotension, and CV disease and in elder-

ly patients. Monitor renal and liver function tests.

Alert: Be aware that elderly patients are more susceptible to adverse neurologic effects. Monitor for mental status changes.

☑ **Patient teaching**
• If insomnia occurs, tell patient to take drug several hours before bedtime.
• If orthostatic hypotension occurs, instruct patient not to stand or change positions too quickly.
• Instruct patient to notify doctor of adverse reactions, especially dizziness, depression, anxiety, nausea, and urine retention.

---

cidofovir
Vistide

Pregnancy Risk Category: C

HOW SUPPLIED
Injection: 75 mg/ml in 5-ml vial

ACTION
Suppresses CMV replication by selective inhibition of viral DNA synthesis.

Route	Onset	Peak	Duration
IV	Unknown	Unknown	Unknown

INDICATIONS & DOSAGE
CMV retinitis in patients with AIDS—
Adults: initially, 5 mg/kg I.V. infused over 1 hour once weekly for 2 consecutive weeks, followed by a maintenance dosage of 5 mg/kg I.V. infused over 1 hour once q 2 weeks. Administer probenecid and prehydration with 0.9% NaCl solution I.V. concomitantly; may reduce potential for nephrotoxicity.
Adjust-a-dose: In patients with renal failure, if serum creatinine increases 0.3 to 0.4 mg/dl above baseline, reduce dose to 3 mg/kg at same rate and frequency. If it increases 0.5 mg/dl or more above baseline, discontinue drug.

ADVERSE REACTIONS
CNS: *asthenia, headache,* amnesia, anxiety, confusion, **seizures,** depression, dizziness, abnormal gait, hallucinations, insomnia, neuropathy, paresthesia, somnolence.
CV: hypotension, orthostatic hypotension, pallor, syncope, tachycardia, vasodilation.
EENT: amblyopia, conjunctivitis, eye disorders, *ocular hypotony,* iritis, retinal detachment, uveitis, abnormal vision, taste perversion.
GI: *nausea, vomiting, diarrhea, anorexia, abdominal pain,* dry mouth, colitis, constipation, tongue discoloration, dyspepsia, dysphagia, flatulence, gastritis, melena, oral candidiasis, rectal disorders, stomatitis, aphthous stomatitis, mouth ulcerations.
GU: *elevated creatinine levels,* **nephrotoxicity, proteinuria,** decreased creatinine clearance levels, glycosuria, hematuria, urinary incontinence, urinary tract infection.
Hematologic: NEUTROPENIA, *anemia,* **thrombocytopenia.**
Hepatic: hepatomegaly, abnormal liver function test results, increased alkaline phosphatase levels.
Metabolic: fluid imbalance, hyperglycemia, hyperlipemia, hypocalcemia, hypokalemia, weight loss, decreased serum bicarbonate level.
Musculoskeletal: arthralgia, myasthenia, myalgia.
Respiratory: asthma, bronchitis, coughing, *dyspnea,* hiccups, increased sputum, lung disorders, pharyngitis, pneumonia, rhinitis, sinusitis.
Skin: *rash, alopecia,* acne, skin discoloration, dry skin, herpes simplex, pruritus, sweating, urticaria.
Other: *fever, infections, chills,* allergic reactions, facial edema, malaise, **sarcoma, sepsis,** pain in back, chest, or neck.

INTERACTIONS
Drug-drug. Nephrotoxic agents (such as amphotericin B, aminoglycosides, foscarnet, I.V. pentamidine): may increase nephrotoxicity. Avoid concomitant use.
Probenecid: known to interact with the metabolism or renal tubular excretion of many drugs. Monitor closely.

EFFECTS ON DIAGNOSTIC TESTS
None reported.

CONTRAINDICATIONS

Contraindicated in patients with hypersensitivity to drug or history of clinically severe hypersensitivity to probenecid or other sulfur-containing medication. Also contraindicated in patients receiving agents with nephrotoxic potential and in those with serum creatinine exceeding 1.5 mg/dl, a calculated creatinine clearance of 55 ml/minute or less, or a urine protein of 100 mg/dl or more (equivalent to 2+ proteinuria or more). Do not administer as a direct intraocular injection because it may be associated with significant decreases in intraocular pressure and vision impairment. Do not administer drug to breast-feeding women.

NURSING CONSIDERATIONS

• Use cautiously in patients with impaired renal function. Monitor renal function tests and patient's fluid balance.
• Administer 1 L 0.9% NaCl as ordered, usually over 1- to 2-hour period immediately before each cidofovir infusion.
• Administer probenecid, as ordered, with cidofovir.
• Monitor renal function (serum creatinine and urine protein) before each dose. Dosage may be modified by a doctor if changes in renal function occur.
• Be aware that drug should not be used in patients with baseline serum creatinine exceeding 1.5 mg/dl or calculated creatinine clearance of 55 ml/minute or less unless potential benefits outweigh potential risks.
• Know that Fanconi's syndrome and decreased serum bicarbonate levels associated with renal tubular damage have been reported in patients receiving cidofovir. Monitor patient closely.
• Monitor WBC counts with differential before each dose.
• Be aware that granulocytopenia has been observed with drug treatment. Monitor neutrophil counts during therapy.
• Be aware that intraocular pressure, visual acuity, and ocular symptoms should be monitored periodically.
• Know that cidofovir is indicated only for the treatment of CMV retinitis in patients with AIDS. Safety and efficacy of drug have not been established for treating other CMV infections, congenital or neonatal CMV disease, or CMV disease in patients not infected with HIV.
• Know that in animal studies, cidofovir was carcinogenic and teratogenic and caused hypospermia.
• Discontinue zidovudine therapy or reduce dosage by 50%, as ordered, on the days cidofovir is administered; probenecid reduces metabolic clearance of zidovudine.
• Know that dosage adjustment may be necessary in elderly patients with renal impairment.
• Safety and effectiveness in children have not been established.
• Be aware that it is unknown whether cidofovir is excreted in breast milk.

⬛ I.V. administration

• Because of the potential for increased nephrotoxicity, do not exceed recommended doses or frequency or rate of administration.
• To prepare cidofovir for infusion, extract the appropriate amount of cidofovir from the vial using a syringe and transfer the dose to an infusion bag containing 100 ml of 0.9% NaCl solution. Infuse the entire volume I.V. at a constant rate over a 1-hour period. Use a standard infusion pump for administration.
• Be aware that because of the mutagenic properties of cidofovir, drug should be prepared in a class II laminar flow biological safety cabinet. Personnel preparing drug should wear surgical gloves and a closed front surgical gown with knit cuffs.
• If drug contacts the skin, wash membranes and flush thoroughly with water. Excess drug and all other materials used in the admixture preparation and administration should be placed in a leakproof, puncture-proof container. Recommended method of disposal is high temperature incineration.
• Know that cidofovir infusion admixtures should be administered within 24 hours of preparation; refrigerator or freezer storage should not be used to extend this 24-hour period. If admixtures are not used immediately, they may be refrigerated at 36° to 46° F (2° to 8° C) for no more than 24 hours. Allow cidofovir to reach room temperature prior to use.

- Do not add other drugs or supplements to admixture for concurrent administration.
- Be aware that compatibility with Ringer's solution, lactated Ringer's solution, or bacteriostatic infusion fluids has not been evaluated.

☑Patient teaching
- Inform patient that drug is not a cure for CMV retinitis and that regular ophthalmologic follow-up examinations are necessary.
- Alert patients on zidovudine therapy that they'll need to obtain dosage guidelines on days cidofovir is administered.
- Tell patient that close monitoring of renal function will be needed and that abnormalities may require a change in cidofovir therapy.
- Stress importance of completing a full course of probenecid with each cidofovir dose. Tell patient to take probenecid after a meal to decrease nausea.
- Advise women of childbearing age to use effective contraception during and for 1 month following treatment with cidofovir.
- Advise men to practice barrier contraception during and for 3 months after treatment with the drug.
- Advise breast-feeding women that it is unknown whether cidofovir is excreted in breast milk.

---

delavirdine mesylate
Rescriptor

Pregnancy Risk Category: C

HOW SUPPLIED
Tablets: 100 mg

ACTION
Non-nucleoside reverse-transcriptase inhibitor of HIV-1. Drug binds directly to reverse transcriptase and blocks RNA- and DNA-dependent DNA polymerase activities.

Route	Onset	Peak	Duration
PO	Unknown	1 hr	Unknown

INDICATIONS & DOSAGE
Treatment of HIV-1 infection when therapy is warranted—
Adults: 400 mg P.O. t.i.d. in combination with other appropriate antiretroviral agents.

ADVERSE REACTIONS
CNS: abnormal coordination, agitation, amnesia, anxiety, change in dreams, cognitive impairment, confusion, depression, disorientation, dizziness, emotional lability, hallucinations, headache, hyperesthesia, hyperreflexia, hypesthesia, impaired concentration, insomnia, manic symptoms, migraine, nervousness, neuropathy, nightmares, pallor, paralysis, paranoid symptoms, paresthesia, restlessness, somnolence, tingling, tremor, vertigo, weakness.
CV: bradycardia, palpitation, orthostatic hypotension, syncope, tachycardia, vasodilation, chest pain.
EENT: blepharitis, conjunctivitis, diplopia, dry eyes, ear pain, epistaxis, nystagmus, pharyngitis, photophobia, rhinitis, sinusitis, taste perversion, tinnitus.
GI: abdominal cramps, distention, or pain (generalized or localized), anorexia, aphthous stomatitis, bloody stools, colitis, constipation, decreased appetite, diarrhea, diverticulitis, duodenitis, dry mouth, dyspepsia, dysphagia, enteritis, esophagitis, fecal incontinence, flatulence, gagging, gastritis, gastroesophageal reflux, GI bleeding, gingivitis, gum hemorrhage, increased thirst and appetite, increased saliva, mouth ulcer, *nausea,* nonspecific hepatitis, pancreatitis, rectal disorder, sialadenitis, stomatitis, tongue edema or ulceration, vomiting.
GU: epididymitis, hematuria, hemospermia, impotence, renal calculi, renal pain, metrorrhagia, nocturia, polyuria, proteinuria, vaginal candidiasis.
Hematologic: anemia, ecchymosis, eosinophilia, granulocytosis, *neutropenia, pancytopenia,* petechiae, prolonged PTT, purpura, spleen disorder, *thrombocytopenia.*
Hepatic: increased ALT and AST levels.
Metabolic: alcohol intolerance; bilirubinemia; hyperkalemia; hyperuricemia; hypocalcemia; hyponatremia; hypophos-

phatemia; increased gamma glutamyl transpeptidase, lipase, serum alkaline phosphatase, serum amylase, serum CK, and serum creatinine levels; peripheral edema; weight gain or loss.

Musculoskeletal: arthralgia or arthritis of single and multiple joints, asthenia, back pain, bone disorder, bone pain, leg cramps, muscle cramps, muscular weakness, myalgia, neck rigidity, tendon disorder, tenosynovitis.

Respiratory: bronchitis, chest congestion, cough, dyspnea, laryngismus, upper respiratory infection.

Skin: alopecia, angioedema, dermal leukocytoblastic vasculitis, dermatitis, desquamation, diaphoresis, dry skin, erythema, erythema multiforme, folliculitis, fungal dermatitis, maculopapular rash, nail disorder, petechial rash, pruritus, *rash*, seborrhea, skin nodule, **Stevens-Johnson syndrome,** urticaria, vesiculobullous rash.

Other: allergic reaction, breast enlargement, chills, decreased libido, edema (generalized or localized), epidermal cyst, fatigue, fever, flank pain, flu syndrome, lethargy, lip edema, malaise, pain (generalized or localized), sebaceous cyst, trauma, tetany.

INTERACTIONS

Drug-drug. *Amphetamines, astemizole, benzodiazepines, calcium channel blockers, cisapride, ergot alkaloid preparations, quinidine:* may result in potentially serious or life-threatening adverse events. Avoid concomitant use.

Antacids: reduced absorption of delavirdine. Separate doses by at least 1 hour.

Carbamazepine, phenobarbital, phenytoin, rifampin: substantially decreased plasma delavirdine levels. Avoid coadministration.

Clarithromycin: increased concentrations of both drugs. Monitor carefully.

Dapsone, warfarin: delavirdine increases plasma concentrations of these drugs. Monitor carefully.

Didanosine: coadministration with delavirdine results in a 20% decrease in absorption of both drugs. Separate administration by at least 1 hour.

Fluoxetine, ketoconazole: increased delavirdine trough levels. Monitor patient.

H2-receptor antagonists: may reduce absorption of delavirdine. Chronic use of these drugs with delavirdine is not recommended.

Indinavir: increased plasma concentrations of indinavir. A lower dose of indinavir should be considered.

Rifabutin: decreased delavirdine levels and increased rifabutin levels.

Saquinavir: five-fold increase in systemic levels of saquinavir. Monitor AST and ALT levels frequently when used together.

EFFECTS ON DIAGNOSTIC TESTS

None reported.

CONTRAINDICATIONS

Contraindicated in patients with hypersensitivity to drug's formulation.

NURSING CONSIDERATIONS

• Use cautiously in patients with impaired hepatic function.

• Drug-induced rash is more common in patients with lower CD4+ cell counts and usually occurs within first 3 weeks of treatment. It is typically diffuse, maculopapular, erythematous, and often pruritic. It occurs commonly and its incidence doesn't appear to be significantly reduced by titrated drug doses.

• Rash occurs mainly on the upper body and proximal arms. Using diphenhydramine, hydroxyzine, or topical corticosteroids may relieve symptoms.

• Because drug's effects in patients with hepatic or renal impairment have not been studied, monitor renal and liver function test results carefully.

• Drug has not been shown to reduce risk of transmission of HIV-1.

• Because resistance develops rapidly when used as monotherapy, always use drug in combination with appropriate antiretroviral therapy.

• Monitor patient's fluid balance and weight.

✓ Patient teaching

• Tell patient to discontinue drug and call doctor if severe rash or symptoms such as fever, blistering, oral lesions, conjunctivi-

tis, swelling or muscle or joint aches occur.
• Tell patient that drug is not a cure for HIV-1 infection and they may continue to acquire illnesses associated with HIV-1 infection, including opportunistic infections. Therapy has not been shown to reduce the incidence or frequency of such illnesses. Drug has not been shown to reduce the transmission of HIV.
• Advise patient to remain under medical supervision when taking drug because the long-term effects are not known.
• Tell patient to take drug as prescribed and not to alter doses without doctor's approval. If a dose is missed, tell patient to take the next dose as soon as possible; he should not double the next dose.
• Inform patient that drug may be dispersed in water before ingestion. Add tablets to at least 5 oz (148 ml) of water, allow to stand for a few minutes, and stir until a uniform dispersion occurs. Tell patient to drink dispersion promptly, rinse glass, and swallow the rinse to ensure that entire dose is consumed.
• Tell patient that drug may be taken without regard to food.
• Tell patient with achlorhydria to take drug with an acidic beverage such as orange or cranberry juice.
• Instruct patient to take drug and antacids at least 1 hour apart.
• Advise patient to report the use of other prescription or OTC medications.

didanosine (ddl)
Videx

Pregnancy Risk Category: B

HOW SUPPLIED
Tablets (buffered, chewable): 25 mg, 50 mg, 100 mg, 150 mg
Powder for oral solution (buffered): 100 mg/packet, 167 mg/packet, 250 mg/packet, 375 mg/packet
Powder for oral solution (pediatric): 4 oz, 8 oz glass bottles containing 2 g and 4 g of Videx, respectively

ACTION
Inhibits the enzyme HIV-RNA-dependent DNA polymerase (reverse transcriptase) and terminates DNA chain growth.

Route	Onset	Peak	Duration
PO	Unknown	0.5-1 hr	Unknown

INDICATIONS & DOSAGE
Treatment of HIV infection when antiretroviral therapy is warranted—
Adults weighing 60 kg (132 lb) and over: 200 mg (tablets) P.O. q 12 hours; or 250 mg buffered powder P.O. q 12 hours.
Adults weighing under 60 kg: 125 mg (tablets) P.O. q 12 hours; or 167 mg buffered powder P.O. q 12 hours.
Children: 120 mg/m² P.O. q 12 hours.
Adjust-a-dose: Patients on dialysis should receive 25% of usual dose.

ADVERSE REACTIONS
CNS: *headache, seizures,* confusion, anxiety, nervousness, abnormal thinking, twitching, depression, *peripheral neuropathy, dizziness,* insomnia.
CV: hypertension, edema, **heart failure.**
EENT: retinal changes, optic neuritis.
GI: *diarrhea, nausea, vomiting, abdominal pain, pancreatitis,* dry mouth, anorexia.
Hematologic: *leukopenia,* granulocytosis, ***thrombocytopenia,*** anemia.
Hepatic: *hepatic failure,* elevated liver enzymes.
Skin: rash, pruritus, alopecia.
Other: asthenia, pain, pneumonia, infection, sarcoma, dyspnea, allergic reactions, myopathy, increased serum uric acid levels, *chills, fever.*

INTERACTIONS
Drug-drug. *Antacids containing magnesium or aluminum hydroxides:* enhanced adverse effects of the antacid component (including diarrhea or constipation) when administered with didanosine tablets or pediatric suspension. Avoid concomitant use.
Dapsone, ketoconazole, drugs that require gastric acid for adequate absorption: decreased absorption from buffering action. Administer these drugs 2 hours before didanosine.
Fluoroquinolones, tetracyclines: decreased absorption from buffering agents

in didanosine tablets or antacids in pediatric suspension. Avoid concomitant use.
Itraconazole: decreased serum concentrations of itraconazole. Avoid concomitant use.

Drug-food. *Any food:* decreased rate of absorption. Give drug on an empty stomach at least 30 minutes before a meal.

EFFECTS ON DIAGNOSTIC TESTS
None reported.

CONTRAINDICATIONS
Contraindicated in patients with history of hypersensitivity to any component of the formulation.

NURSING CONSIDERATIONS
• Use cautiously in patients with history of pancreatitis; fatalities have occurred. Also use cautiously in patients with peripheral neuropathy, renal or hepatic impairment, or hyperuricemia. Monitor liver and renal function tests.
• Administer didanosine on an empty stomach, regardless of the dosage form used; administering drug with meals can decrease absorption by 50%.
• To administer single-dose packets containing buffered powder for oral solution, pour contents into 4 oz (120 ml) of water. Do not use fruit juice or other beverages that may be acidic. Stir for 2 or 3 minutes until the powder dissolves completely. Administer immediately.
• Keep in mind that in early clinical trials, the powder for oral solution was associated with a high incidence of diarrhea. The manufacturer suggests switching to the tablet formulation if diarrhea is a problem.
Alert: Know that the pediatric powder for oral solution must be prepared by a pharmacist before dispensing. It must be constituted with purified USP water and then diluted with an antacid (either Mylanta Double Strength Liquid or Maalox TC Suspension) to a final concentration of 10 mg/ml. The admixture is stable for 30 days if refrigerated (at 36° to 46° F [2° to 8° C]). Shake the solution well before measuring the dose.

☑ Patient teaching
• Instruct patient to take drug on an empty stomach.
• Because the tablets contain buffers that raise stomach pH to levels that prevent degradation of the active drug, instruct patient to chew tablets thoroughly before swallowing and drink at least 1 oz (30 ml) of water with each dose. Teach patient how to prepare crushed tablets or buffered powder form for ingestion, if appropriate.
• Inform patient receiving a sodium-restricted diet that each two-tablet dose of didanosine contains 529 mg of sodium; each single packet of buffered powder for oral solution contains 1.38 g of sodium.
• Tell patient to report symptoms of pancreatitis such as abdominal pain, nausea, vomiting, diarrhea.

▼ *NEW DRUG*

efavirenz
Sustiva

Pregnancy Risk Category: C

HOW SUPPLIED
Capsules: 50 mg, 100 mg, 200 mg

ACTION
A nonnucleoside, reverse transcriptase inhibitor (NNRTI) that inhibits the transcription of HIV-1 RNA to DNA, a critical step in the viral replication process. Therefore, drug lowers the amount of HIV in the blood (the viral load) and increases CD4 lymphocytes.

Route	Onset	Peak	Duration
PO	Unknown	3-5 hr	Unknown

INDICATIONS & DOSAGE
Treatment of HIV-1 infection—
Adults: 600 mg P.O. once daily in combination with a protease inhibitor or nucleoside analogue reverse transcriptase inhibitors.
Children 3 years and older weighing 40 kg (88 lb) or more: 600 mg P.O. once daily in combination with a protease inhibitor or nucleoside analogue reverse transcriptase inhibitors.

Children 3 years and older weighing 10 to under 40 kg (22 to under 88 lb):
Children weighing 10 to under 15 kg (22 to under 33 lb): 200 mg P.O. once daily.
Children weighing 15 to under 20 kg (33 to under 44 lb): 250 mg P.O. once daily.
Children weighing 20 to under 25 kg (44 to under 55 lb): 300 mg P.O. once daily.
Children weighing 25 to under 32.5 kg (55 to under 72 lb): 350 mg P.O. once daily.
Children weighing 32.5 to under 40 kg (72 to under 88 lb): 400 mg P.O. once daily.

Give above doses in combination with a protease inhibitor or nucleoside analogue reverse transcriptase inhibitors.

ADVERSE REACTIONS
CNS: abnormal dreams or thinking, agitation, amnesia, confusion, depersonalization, depression, *dizziness*, euphoria, fatigue, hallucinations, headache, hypoesthesia, impaired concentration, insomnia, somnolence, nervousness.
GI: abdominal pain, anorexia, *diarrhea,* dyspepsia, flatulence, *nausea,* vomiting.
GU: hematuria, kidney stones.
Hepatic: increased AST, ALT and total cholesterol.
Skin: increased sweating, ***erythema multiforme, Stevens-Johnson syndrome, toxic epidermal necrolysis,*** rash, pruritus.
Other: fever.

INTERACTIONS
Drug-drug. *Astemizole, cisapride, ergot derivatives, midazolam, triazolam:* competition for cytochrome P-450 enzyme system may result in inhibition of the metabolism of these drugs and cause serious or life-threatening adverse events (such as arrhythmias, prolonged sedation, or respiratory depression). Avoid concomitant use.
Clarithromycin, indinavir: decreased plasma concentrations. Consider alternative therapy or dosage adjustment.
Drugs that induce the cytochrome P-450 enzyme system (such as *phenobarbital, rifampin, rifabutin*): increased clearance of efavirenz resulting in lowered plasma concentrations. Avoid concomitant use.
Estrogens, ritonavir: increased plasma concentrations. Monitor patient.
Oral contraceptives: potential interaction

of efavirenz with oral contraceptive has not been determined. Advise use of a reliable method of barrier contraception in addition to oral contraceptives.
Psychoactive drugs: additive CNS effects. Avoid concomitant use.
Saquinavir: plasma concentrations of saquinavir decreased significantly. Do not use with saquinavir as sole protease inhibitor.
Warfarin: plasma concentrations and effects potentially increased or decreased. Monitor INR.
Drug-food. *High-fat meals:* increased absorption of drug. Instruct patient to maintain a proper low-fat diet.
Drug-lifestyle. *Alcohol:* enhanced CNS effects. Avoid concomitant use.

EFFECTS ON DIAGNOSTIC TESTS
Drug therapy may cause false-positive urine cannabinoid test results.

CONTRAINDICATIONS
Contraindicated in patients with hypersensitivity to drug or its components.

NURSING CONSIDERATIONS
• Use cautiously in patients with hepatic impairment or in those concurrently receiving hepatotoxic medications. Monitor liver function test results in patients with prior history of hepatitis B or C and in those also taking ritonavir.
• Monitor cholesterol levels.
Alert: Drug should be used in combination with other antiretroviral agents because resistant viruses emerge rapidly when used alone. Drug should not be used as monotherapy, or added on as a single agent to a failing regimen.
• Combination with ritonavir is associated with a higher frequency of adverse effects (such as dizziness, nausea, paresthesia) and laboratory abnormalities (elevated liver enzymes).
• Administer drug at bedtime to decrease noticeable CNS adverse effects.
• Be aware that pregnancy must be ruled out before starting therapy in female patients of childbearing age.
• Know that children may be more prone to adverse reactions, especially diarrhea, nausea, vomiting, and rash.

☑ **Patient teaching**
• Instruct patient to take drug with water, juice, milk or soda. It may be taken without regard to meals.
• Inform patient about need for scheduled blood tests to monitor liver function and cholesterol levels.
• Tell patient to use a reliable method of barrier contraception in addition to oral contraceptives and to notify doctor immediately if pregnancy is suspected.
• Inform patient that drug is not a cure for HIV infection and that it will not affect the development of opportunistic infections and other complications associated with HIV disease or transmission of HIV to others through sexual contact or blood contamination.
• Instruct patient to take drug at the same time daily and always in combination with other antiretroviral drugs.
• Tell patient to take drug exactly as prescribed and not to discontinue it without medical approval. Also instruct patient to report if adverse reactions occur.
• Inform patient that rash is the most common adverse effect. If this occurs, tell patient to report it immediately because it may be serious in rare cases.
• Advise patient to report use of other medications.
• Advise patient that dizziness, difficulty sleeping or concentrating, drowsiness, or unusual dreams may occur the first few days of therapy. Reassure him that these symptoms generally resolve after 2 to 4 weeks and may be less problematic if drug is taken at bedtime.
• Tell patient to avoid alcoholic beverages, driving, or operating machinery until the drug's effects are known.

---

famciclovir
Famvir

Pregnancy Risk Category: B

HOW SUPPLIED
Tablets: 125 mg, 250 mg, 500 mg

ACTION
A guanosine nucleoside that is converted to penciclovir, which enters viral cells and inhibits DNA polymerase and viral DNA synthesis.

Route	Onset	Peak	Duration
PO	Unknown	1 hr	Unknown

INDICATIONS & DOSAGE
Acute herpes zoster infection (shingles)—
Adults: 500 mg P.O. q 8 hours for 7 days.
Adjust-a-dose: In patients with reduced renal function, if creatinine clearance is 60 ml/minute or more, 500 mg P.O. q 8 hours; if clearance is 40 to 59 ml/minute, 500 mg P.O. q 12 hours; if 20 to 39 ml/minute, 500 mg P.O. q 24 hours; and if below 20 ml/minute, 250 mg P.O. q 48 hours.
   In hemodialysis patients, 250 mg P.O. after each hemodialysis.
Recurrent episodes of genital herpes—
Adults: 125 mg P.O. b.i.d. for 5 days. Therapy begins as soon as symptoms occur.
Adjust-a-dose: In patients with reduced renal function, if creatinine clearance is 40 ml/minute or more, 125 mg P.O. q 12 hours; if 20 to 39 ml/minute, 125 mg P.O. q 24 hours; if below 20 ml/minute, 125 mg P.O. q 48 hours.
   In hemodialysis patients, 125 mg P.O. after each hemodialysis session.
✱ *NEW INDICATION: Treatment of recurrent mucocutaneous herpes simplex infections in HIV-infected patients—*
Adults: 500 mg P.O. b.i.d. for 7 days.
Adjust-a-dose: In patients with reduced renal function, if creatinine clearance is 40 ml/minute or more, 500 mg P.O. q 12 hours; if 20 to 39 ml/minute, 500 mg P.O. q 24 hours; and if below 20 ml/minute, 250 mg P.O. q 24 hours.
   In hemodialysis patients, 250 mg P.O. after each hemodialysis session.

ADVERSE REACTIONS
CNS: *headache,* fatigue, dizziness, paresthesia, somnolence.
EENT: pharyngitis, sinusitis.
GI: diarrhea, *nausea,* vomiting, constipation, anorexia, abdominal pain.
Musculoskeletal: back pain, arthralgia.
Skin: pruritus; zoster-related signs, symptoms, and complications.
Other: fever.

Reactions may be *common,* uncommon, *life-threatening,* or **COMMON AND LIFE-THREATENING**.

INTERACTIONS
Drug-drug. *Probenecid:* may increase plasma concentrations of famciclovir. Monitor patient for increased adverse effects.

EFFECTS ON DIAGNOSTIC TESTS
None reported.

CONTRAINDICATIONS
Contraindicated in patients with hypersensitivity to drug.

NURSING CONSIDERATIONS
• Use cautiously in patients with renal or hepatic impairment. Know that dosage adjustment may be needed. Monitor renal and liver function tests.
• Drug may be taken without regard to meals.

☑**Patient teaching**
• Inform patient that drug is not a cure for genital herpes but can decrease the length and severity of symptoms.
• Teach patient how to prevent spread of infection to others.
• Urge patient to recognize the early symptoms of herpes infection, such as tingling, itching, or pain, and to report them. Treatment is more effective if therapy is started within 48 hours of rash onset.

▼ *NEW DRUG*

fomivirsen sodium
Vitravene

Pregnancy Risk Category: C

HOW SUPPLIED
Intravitreal injection: preservative-free, single-use vials containing 0.25 ml, 6.6 mg/ml

ACTION
A phosphorothioate oligonucleotide that inhibits human CMV replication by binding to the target mRNA and subsequently inhibiting virus replication.

Route	Onset	Peak	Duration
Intravitreal	Unknown	Unknown	Unknown

INDICATIONS & DOSAGE
Local treatment of CMV retinitis in patients with AIDS, who are intolerant of or have a contraindication to other treatment(s) or who were insufficiently responsive to previous treatment(s)—
Adults: induction dose is 330 mcg (0.05 ml) by intravitreal injection every other week for two doses. Subsequent maintenance dose is 330 mcg (0.05 ml) by intravitreal injection once q 4 weeks after induction.

ADVERSE REACTIONS
CNS: asthenia, headache, abnormal thinking, depression, dizziness, neuropathy, pain.
CV: chest pain.
EENT: abnormal or blurred vision, anterior chamber inflammation, cataract, conjunctival hemorrhage, decreased visual acuity, desaturation of color vision, eye pain, floaters, increased intraocular pressure, photophobia, retinal detachment, retinal edema, retinal hemorrhage, retinal pigment changes, *uveitis, vitritis,* application site reaction, conjunctival hyperemia, conjunctivitis, corneal edema, decreased peripheral vision, eye irritation, hypotony, keratic precipitates, optic neuritis, photopsia, retinal vascular disease, visual field defect, vitreous hemorrhage, vitreous opacity, sinusitis.
GI: abdominal pain, anorexia, diarrhea, nausea, vomiting, oral candidiasis, *pancreatitis.*
GU: catheter infection, *kidney failure.*
Hematologic: anemia, lymphoma-like reaction, *neutropenia, thrombocytopenia.*
Hepatic: abnormal liver function, increased GGT.
Metabolic: dehydration.
Musculoskeletal: back pain.
Respiratory: bronchitis, dyspnea, increased cough, pneumonia.
Skin: rash, sweating.
Other: allergic reactions, cachexia, decreased weight, fever, flulike syndrome, infection, *sepsis,* systemic CMV.

INTERACTIONS
None reported.

---

*Liquid contains alcohol.   **May contain tartrazine.   †Canada   ‡Australia   §U.K.   ◇OTC

EFFECTS ON DIAGNOSTIC TESTS
None reported.

CONTRAINDICATIONS
Contraindicated in patients with hypersensitivity to drug or its components or in those who have recently (within 2 to 4 weeks) been treated with either I.V. or intravitreal cidofovir because of an increased risk of exaggerated ocular inflammation.

NURSING CONSIDERATIONS
Alert: Drug is for ophthalmic use by intravitreal injection only.
• Drug provides localized therapy limited to the treated eye, and does not provide treatment for systemic CMV disease. Monitor patient for extraocular CMV disease or disease in the contralateral eye.
• Be aware that ocular inflammation (uveitis) is more common during induction dosing.
• Monitor light perception and optic nerve head perfusion postinjection.
• Monitor for intraocular pressure. This is usually transient and returns to normal without treatment or with temporary use of topical medications.

☑ Patient teaching
• Inform patient that drug is not a cure for CMV retinitis, and that some patients continue to experience progression of retinitis during and following treatment.
• Tell patient that drug treats only the eye(s) in which it has been injected, and that CMV may also exist in the body. Stress importance of follow-up visits to monitor progress and to check for additional infections.
• Instruct patient to also have regular ophthalmologic follow-up examinations.
• Advise HIV-infected patient to continue taking antiretroviral therapy as indicated.

**foscarnet sodium
(phosphonoformic acid)**
Foscavir

Pregnancy Risk Category: C

HOW SUPPLIED
Injection: 24 mg/ml in 250- and 500-ml bottles

ACTION
Inhibits all known herpesviruses in vitro by blocking the pyrophosphate binding site on DNA polymerases and reverse transcriptases.

Route	Onset	Peak	Duration
IV	Unknown	Immediate	Unknown

INDICATIONS & DOSAGE
CMV retinitis in patients with AIDS—
Adults: initially, 60 mg/kg I.V. as an induction treatment in patients with normal renal function. Administer q 8 hours for 2 to 3 weeks, depending on clinical response. Follow with a maintenance infusion of 90 to 120 mg/kg daily.
Adjust-a-dose: Refer to package insert for very specific dose adjustments. Dosage must be adjusted when creatinine clearance is below 1.5 ml/minute/kg. If creatinine clearance falls below 0.4 ml/minute/kg, discontinue drug.

ADVERSE REACTIONS
CNS: *headache, seizures, fatigue, malaise, asthenia, paresthesia, dizziness, hypoesthesia, neuropathy,* tremor, ataxia, generalized spasms, dementia, stupor, sensory disturbances, meningitis, aphasia, abnormal coordination, EEG abnormalities, depression, confusion, anxiety, insomnia, somnolence, nervousness, amnesia, agitation, aggressive reaction, hallucinations.
CV: *hypertension, palpitations, ECG abnormalities, sinus tachycardia,* cerebrovascular disorder, *first-degree AV block, hypotension, flushing,* edema.
EENT: visual disturbances, taste perversion, eye pain, conjunctivitis, sinusitis, pharyngitis, rhinitis.
GI: *nausea, diarrhea, vomiting, abdominal pain, anorexia,* constipation, dysphagia, rectal hemorrhage, dry mouth, dyspepsia, melena, flatulence, ulcerative stomatitis, *pancreatitis.*
GU: *abnormal renal function, decreased creatinine clearance and increased serum*

---

creatinine levels, albuminuria, dysuria, polyuria, urethral disorder, urine retention, urinary tract infections, **acute renal failure,** candidiasis.

Hematologic: anemia, granulocytopenia, **leukopenia, bone marrow suppression, thrombocytopenia,** platelet abnormalities, thrombocytosis, WBC count abnormalities, lymphadenopathy.

Hepatic: increased serum bilirubin, alkaline phosphatase, ALT, and AST.

Metabolic: hypokalemia, hypomagnesemia, hypophosphatemia or hyperphosphatemia, hypocalcemia, hyponatremia.

Musculoskeletal: leg cramps, arthralgia, myalgia.

Respiratory: cough, dyspnea, pneumonitis, respiratory insufficiency, pulmonary infiltration, stridor, pneumothorax, **bronchospasm,** hemoptysis, flulike symptoms.

Skin: rash, diaphoresis, pruritus, skin ulceration, erythematous rash, seborrhea, skin discoloration, facial edema.

Other: death, fever, pain, sepsis, rigors, inflammation and pain at infusion site, lymphoma-like disorder, sarcoma, back or chest pain, abnormal hepatic function, bacterial or fungal infections, abscess, increased liver enzymes.

INTERACTIONS
Drug-drug. Nephrotoxic drugs (such as amphotericin B, aminoglycosides): increased risk of nephrotoxicity. Avoid concomitant use.
Pentamidine: increased risk of nephrotoxicity; severe hypocalcemia has also been reported. Avoid concomitant use.
Zidovudine: possible increased incidence or severity of anemia. Monitor blood counts.

EFFECTS ON DIAGNOSTIC TESTS
None reported.

CONTRAINDICATIONS
Contraindicated in patients with hypersensitivity to drug.

NURSING CONSIDERATIONS
• Use cautiously and with reduced dosage in patients with abnormal renal function as ordered. Because drug is nephrotoxic, it can worsen renal impairment. Some degree of nephrotoxicity occurs in most patients treated with drug.
• Because drug is highly toxic and toxicity is probably dose-related, always use the lowest effective maintenance dose during therapy.
• Monitor creatinine clearance frequently during therapy because of drug's adverse effects on renal function. A baseline 24-hour creatinine clearance is recommended, followed by regular determinations two to three times weekly during induction and at least once every 1 to 2 weeks during maintenance.
• Because drug can alter serum electrolytes, monitor levels using a schedule similar to that established for creatinine clearance. Assess patient for tetany and seizures associated with abnormal electrolyte levels.
• Monitor patient's hemoglobin and hematocrit levels. Anemia is common (in up to 33% of patients treated with drug). It may be severe enough to require transfusions.
• Keep in mind that drug administration is associated with a dose-related transient decrease in ionized serum calcium, which may not always be reflected in the patient's laboratory values.

I.V. administration
• Use an infusion pump to administer foscarnet. To minimize renal toxicity, make sure patient is adequately hydrated before and during the infusion.
• Administer induction treatment over 1 hour; maintenance infusions over 2 hours.
Alert: Do not exceed the recommended dosage, infusion rate, or frequency of administration. All doses must be individualized according to patient's renal function.

Patient teaching
• Explain the importance of adequate hydration throughout therapy.
• Advise patient to report perioral tingling, numbness in the extremities, and paresthesia.
• Instruct patient to alert nurse if discomfort occurs at I.V. insertion site.

ganciclovir
Cymevene§, Cytovene

Pregnancy Risk Category: C

HOW SUPPLIED
Capsules: 250 mg
Injection: 500 mg/vial

ACTION
Inhibits binding of deoxyguanosine triphosphate to DNA polymerase, resulting in inhibition of DNA synthesis.

Route	Onset	Peak	Duration
PO	Unknown	1.8-3 hr	Unknown
IV	Unknown	Immediate	Unknown

INDICATIONS & DOSAGE
CMV retinitis in immunocompromised individuals, including patients with AIDS and normal renal function—
Adults and children over 3 months: induction treatment is 5 mg/kg I.V. q 12 hours for 14 to 21 days. Maintenance treatment is 5 mg/kg I.V. daily for 7 days weekly, or 6 mg/kg daily for 5 days weekly. Alternatively, 1,000 mg P.O. t.i.d. with food.
Adjust-a-dose: Refer to package insert for very specific dose adjustments. Dosage is adjusted for patients with impaired renal function and is based on creatinine clearance levels.
　　Dosage adjustment is necessary in patients with creatinine clearance below 70 ml/minute.
Prevention of CMV disease in patients with advanced HIV infection and normal renal function—
Adults: 1,000 mg P.O. t.i.d. with food.
Prevention of CMV disease in transplant recipients with normal renal function—
Adults: 5 mg/kg I.V. (given at a constant rate over 1 hour) q 12 hours for 7 to 14 days, then 5 mg/kg daily for 7 days weekly, or 6 mg/kg daily for 5 days weekly. Duration of therapy depends on degree of immunosuppression.

ADVERSE REACTIONS
CNS: altered dreams, confusion, ataxia, headache, *seizures, coma,* dizziness, somnolence, tremor, abnormal thinking, agitation, amnesia, anxiety, neuropathy, paresthesia, asthenia.
GI: *nausea, vomiting, diarrhea, anorexia, abdominal pain,* flatulence, dyspepsia, dry mouth.
GU: *increased serum creatinine levels.*
Hematologic: *agranulocytosis, thrombocytopenia, leukopenia, anemia.*
Other: retinal detachment in CMV retinitis patients; abnormal liver function test results; *fever;* infection; chills; sepsis; *rash; sweating;* pruritus; pneumonia; inflammation, pain, phlebitis (at injection site).

INTERACTIONS
Drug-drug. *Cytotoxic agents:* increased toxic effects, especially hematologic effects and stomatitis. Monitor closely.
Didanosine: increased plasma concentrations of didanosine when used concomitantly.
Imipenem/cilastatin: heightened seizure activity with concomitant use. Monitor closely.
Immunosuppressants (such as azathioprine, cyclosporine, corticosteroids): enhanced immune and bone marrow suppression. Use together cautiously.
Probenecid: increased ganciclovir blood levels. Monitor closely.
Zidovudine: increased incidence of agranulocytosis with concurrent use. Monitor closely.

EFFECTS ON DIAGNOSTIC TESTS
None reported.

CONTRAINDICATIONS
Contraindicated in patients with hypersensitivity to drug or acyclovir and in those with an absolute neutrophil count below 500 mm^3 or a platelet count below 25,000 mm^3.

NURSING CONSIDERATIONS
● Use cautiously and in reduced dosage in patients with renal dysfunction. Monitor renal function tests.
● Use caution when preparing ganciclovir solution, which is alkaline.
Alert: Do not administer S.C. or I.M.
● Because of the frequency of agranulocy-

tosis and thrombocytopenia, obtain neutrophil and platelet counts every 2 days during twice-daily ganciclovir dosing and at least weekly thereafter.

I.V. administration
• Administer infusion over at least 1 hour. Too-rapid infusions will result in increased toxicity. Use an infusion pump. Do not administer as an I.V. bolus.

Patient teaching
• Explain importance of adequate hydration during therapy.
• Instruct patient to report adverse reactions promptly.
• Tell patient to notify nurse if discomfort occurs at I.V. insertion site.
• Advise patient that drug causes birth defects. Instruct female patients to use effective birth control methods during treatment. Male patients should use barrier contraception during, and for at least 90 days following, treatment with ganciclovir.

---

indinavir sulfate
Crixivan

Pregnancy Risk Category: C

HOW SUPPLIED
Capsules: 200 mg, 400 mg

ACTION
Inhibits HIV protease, enzyme required for the proteolytic cleavage of viral polyprotein precursors into individual functional proteins found in infectious HIV. Indinavir binds to the protease active site and inhibits activity of the enzyme, preventing cleavage of the viral polyproteins and resulting in the formation of immature noninfectious viral particles.

Route	Onset	Peak	Duration
PO	Unknown	< 1 hr	Unknown

INDICATIONS & DOSAGE
Treatment of patients with HIV infection when antiretroviral therapy is warranted—
Adults: 800 mg P.O. q 8 hours.

Adjust-a-dose: In patients with mild to moderate hepatic insufficiency due to cirrhosis, reduce dosage to 600 mg P.O. q 8 hours.

ADVERSE REACTIONS
CNS: headache, insomnia, dizziness, somnolence, asthenia, fatigue.
CV: chest pain, palpitations.
EENT: blurred vision, eye pain or swelling.
GI: abdominal pain, *nausea,* diarrhea, vomiting, acid regurgitation, anorexia, dry mouth.
GU: nephrolithiasis, hematuria.
Hematologic: decreased hemoglobin, platelet, or neutrophil count.
Other: *hyperbilirubinemia,* hyperglycemia, flank pain, malaise, back pain, taste perversion, elevation in ALT, AST, and serum amylase levels.

INTERACTIONS
Drug-drug. *Astemizole, cisapride, midazolam, triazolam:* possible inhibition of the metabolism of these drugs as a result of competition for CYP3A4 by indinavir, creating potential for serious or life-threatening events, such as arrhythmias or prolonged sedation. Do not administer concurrently.
Clarithromycin: increased both drug levels. Monitor closely.
Didanosine: possible degradation of didanosine, formulated with buffering agents to increase pH. If administered concomitantly with indinavir, administer at least 1 hour apart on an empty stomach. Normal gastric pH (acidic) may be necessary for optimum absorption of indinavir but rapidly degrades didanosine.
Ketoconazole: increased plasma concentration of indinavir. Consider dosage reduction of indinavir to 600 mg P.O. q 8 hours when coadministered.
Rifabutin: increased plasma concentrations. Reduce dosage of rifabutin by 50% if administered concomitantly with indinavir.
Rifampin: markedly diminished plasma concentrations of indinavir. Avoid concomitant administration of indinavir and rifampin.

---

*Liquid contains alcohol. **May contain tartrazine. †Canada ‡Australia §U.K. ◊OTC

Ritonavir: increased indinavir levels. Monitor closely.

Drug-food. *Any food:* substantially decreased absorption of oral indinavir. Don't give together.

EFFECTS ON DIAGNOSTIC TESTS
None reported.

CONTRAINDICATIONS
Contraindicated in patients with hypersensitivity to any component of drug.

NURSING CONSIDERATIONS
• Use cautiously in patients with hepatic insufficiency due to cirrhosis.
• Know that drug must be taken at 8-hour intervals.
• Drug may cause nephrolithiasis. If signs and symptoms of nephrolithiasis occur, doctor may stop drug for 1 to 3 days during acute phases.
• Be aware that to prevent nephrolithiasis, patient should maintain adequate hydration (at least 48 oz or 1.5 L of fluids q 24 hours while on indinavir).
• Safety and effectiveness in children have not been established.

☑ Patient teaching
• Tell patient that drug is not a cure for HIV infection and that he may continue to develop opportunistic infections and other complications associated with HIV disease. Drug has not been shown to reduce the risk of HIV transmission.
• Instruct patient on use of barrier protection during sexual activity.
• Caution patient not to adjust dosage or discontinue indinavir therapy without first consulting his doctor.
• Advise patient that if a dose of indinavir is missed, he should take the next dose at the regular, scheduled time and should not double the dose.
• Instruct patient to take drug on an empty stomach with water 1 hour before or 2 hours after a meal. Alternatively, he may take it with other liquids (such as skim milk, juice, coffee, or tea) or a light meal.
• Inform patient that a meal high in fat, calories, and protein reduces absorption of drug.
• Instruct patient to store and use capsules

in the original container and to keep desiccant in the bottle; capsules are sensitive to moisture.
• Instruct patient to drink at least 48 oz (1.5 L) of fluid daily.
• Advise female patient to avoid breast-feeding because indinavir may be excreted in breast milk. In addition, an HIV-positive woman should not breast-feed to prevent transmitting the virus to the infant.

---

lamivudine
Epivir

Pregnancy Risk Category: C

HOW SUPPLIED
Tablets: 150 mg
Oral solution: 10 mg/ml

ACTION
A synthetic nucleoside analogue that inhibits HIV reverse transcription via viral DNA chain termination. RNA- and DNA-dependent DNA polymerase activities are also inhibited.

Route	Onset	Peak	Duration
PO	Unknown	1-3 hr	Unknown

INDICATIONS & DOSAGE
Treatment of HIV infection concomitantly with zidovudine—
Adults weighing 50 kg (110 lb) or more and children 12 years and older: 150 mg P.O. b.i.d.
Adults weighing less than 50 kg: 2 mg/kg P.O. b.i.d.
Children 3 months to 12 years: 4 mg/kg P.O. b.i.d. Maximum dosage is 150 mg b.i.d.
Adjust-a-dose: In patients with renal impairment, if creatinine clearance is 30 to 49 ml/minute, 150 mg P.O. daily. If clearance is 15 to 29 ml/minute, 150 mg P.O. on day 1, then 100 mg daily; if 5 to 14 ml/minute, 150 mg on day 1, then 50 mg daily; if less than 5 ml/minute, 50 mg on day 1, then 25 mg daily.

ADVERSE REACTIONS
Adverse reactions pertain to the combina-

tion therapy of lamivudine and zidovudine.

CNS: *headache, fatigue, neuropathy, dizziness, insomnia and other sleep disorders,* depressive disorders.
GI: *nausea, diarrhea, vomiting, anorexia,* abdominal pain, abdominal cramps, dyspepsia, pancreatitis (in children 3 months to 12 years).
EENT: *nasal symptoms.*
Hematologic: *neutropenia,* anemia, *thrombocytopenia.*
Respiratory: *cough.*
Skin: rash.
Other: *malaise, fever, chills, musculoskeletal pain,* myalgia, arthralgia, elevated liver enzymes and bilirubin.

INTERACTIONS
Drug-drug. *Trimethoprim/sulfamethoxazole:* may cause increased blood level of lamivudine because of decreased clearance of lamivudine. Monitor patient closely.
Zidovudine: increased serum zidovudine concentration. Monitor patient closely.

EFFECTS ON DIAGNOSTIC TESTS
None reported.

CONTRAINDICATIONS
Contraindicated in patients with hypersensitivity to drug.

NURSING CONSIDERATIONS
Alert: Know that drug should be used with extreme caution, if at all, in children with history of pancreatitis or other significant risk factors for development of pancreatitis. Stop lamivudine treatment immediately and notify doctor if clinical signs, symptoms, or laboratory abnormalities suggest pancreatitis. Monitor serum amylase.
• Use cautiously in patients with renal impairment.
• Breast-feeding should be discontinued if lamivudine is prescribed.
• Administer drug concomitantly with zidovudine. It is not currently indicated for use alone.
• Monitor patient's CBC, platelet count, renal and liver function studies, as ordered. Report abnormalities.

• Be aware that an Antiretroviral Pregnancy Registry has been established to monitor maternal-fetal outcomes of pregnant women exposed to lamivudine. To register a pregnant patient, the doctor can call 1-800-722-9292, ext. 39437.

☑ Patient teaching
• Inform patient that long-term effects of lamivudine are unknown.
• Stress importance of taking lamivudine exactly as prescribed.
• Teach parents the signs and symptoms of pancreatitis, and tell them to report them immediately.

▼ *NEW DRUG*

lamivudine/zidovudine
Combivir

Pregnancy Risk Category: C

HOW SUPPLIED
Tablets: 150 mg lamivudine and 300 mg zidovudine

ACTION
Lamivudine and zidovudine inhibit reverse transcriptase via DNA chain termination. Both drugs are also weak inhibitors of DNA polymerase. Together, they have synergistic antiretroviral activity. Combination therapy with lamivudine and zidovudine is targeted at suppressing or delaying the emergence of resistant strains that can occur with retroviral monotherapy, because dual resistance requires multiple mutations.

Route	Onset	Peak	Duration
PO	Unknown	Unknown	Unknown

INDICATIONS & DOSAGE
Treatment of HIV infection—
Adults and children 12 years and older weighing over 50 kg (110 lb): one tablet P.O. b.i.d.

ADVERSE REACTIONS
CNS: *headache, malaise, fatigue, insomnia, dizziness, neuropathy,* depression.
EENT: *nasal signs and symptoms.*
GI: *nausea, diarrhea, vomiting, anorexia,*

abdominal pain, abdominal cramps, dyspepsia.
Hematologic: *neutropenia,* anemia.
Hepatic: increased ALT, AST, amylase.
Musculoskeletal: *musculoskeletal pain,* myalgia, arthralgia.
Respiratory: *cough.*
Skin: rash.
Other: *fever, chills.*

INTERACTIONS
Drug-drug. *Ganciclovir, interferon-alpha, other bone marrow suppressive or cytotoxic agents* may increase zidovudine's hematologic toxicity. Monitor patient.

EFFECTS ON DIAGNOSTIC TESTS
None reported.

CONTRAINDICATIONS
Contraindicated in patients with known hypersensitivity to drug's components and in those requiring dosage adjustments, such as children under 12 years, those weighing under 50 kg, creatinine clearance below 50 ml/minute, or patients experiencing dose-limiting adverse effects.

NURSING CONSIDERATIONS
• Use combination cautiously in patients with bone marrow suppression as evidenced by granulocyte count below 1,000 cells/mm³ or hemoglobin below 9.5 g/dl.
• Lactic acidosis and severe hepatomegaly with steatosis have been reported in patients receiving lamivudine and zidovudine alone and in combination. Notify doctor if signs of lactic acidosis or hepatotoxicity develop (abdominal pain, jaundice).
• Monitor for bone marrow toxicity with frequent blood counts, particularly in patients with advanced HIV infection. Monitor patients for signs of lactic acidosis and hepatotoxicity.
• Assess patient's fine motor skills and peripheral sensation for evidence of peripheral neuropathies.
• Be aware that an Antiretroviral Pregnancy Registry has been established to monitor maternal-fetal outcomes of pregnant women exposed to Combivir. To register a pregnant patient, doctor can call 1-800-722-9292, ext. 39437.

☑ **Patient teaching**
• Advise patient that the lamivudine/zidovudine combination drug therapy is not a cure for HIV infection, and that he may continue to experience illness including opportunistic infections.
• Warn patient that HIV transmission can still occur with drug therapy.
• Educate patient to use protection when engaging in sexual activities to prevent disease transmission.
• Teach patient signs of neutropenia and anemia (fever, chills, infection, fatigue) and instruct him to report such occurrences.
• Tell patient to have blood counts followed closely while on medication, especially if he has advanced disease.
• Advise patient to consult doctor or pharmacist before taking other medications.
• Warn patient to report abdominal pain immediately.
• Instruct patient to report signs of myopathy or myositis (muscle inflammation, pain, weakness, decrease in muscle size).
• Stress importance of taking combination drug therapy exactly as prescribed to reduce the development of resistance.
• Tell patient he may take combination with or without food.
• Inform female patient that breast-feeding is contraindicated in HIV infection and during drug therapy.

---

nelfinavir mesylate
Viracept

Pregnancy Risk Category: B

HOW SUPPLIED
Tablet: 250 mg
Powder: 50 mg/g powder in 144-g bottle

ACTION
Nelfinavir is a HIV-1 protease inhibitor. Inhibition of the protease enzyme prevents cleavage of the viral polyprotein, resulting in the production of immature, noninfectious virus.

Route	Onset	Peak	Duration
PO	Unknown	2-4 hr	Unknown

INDICATIONS & DOSAGE
Treatment of HIV infection when anti-retroviral therapy is warranted—
Adults: 750 mg P.O. t.i.d. with meals or light snack.
Children 2 to 13 years: 20 to 30 mg/kg/dose P.O. t.i.d. with meals or light snack; do not to exceed 750 mg t.i.d.
Recommended children's dose given t.i.d. is shown below.

Body weight (kg)	Level 1-g scoops	Level teaspoons	Tablets
7 to < 8.5	4	1	-
8.5 to < 10.5	5	1.25	-
10.5 to < 12	6	1.5	-
12 to < 14	7	1.75	-
14 to < 16	8	2	-
16 to < 18	9	2.25	-
18 to < 23	10	2.5	2
23	15	3.75	3

ADVERSE REACTIONS
CNS: anxiety, depression, dizziness, emotional lability, hyperkinesia, insomnia, migraine, headache, paresthesia, *seizures,* sleep disorders, somnolence, **suicide ideation.**
EENT: iritis, eye disorder.
GI: nausea, *diarrhea,* flatulence, anorexia, dyspepsia, epigastric pain, GI bleeding, pancreatitis, mouth ulceration, vomiting.
GU: sexual dysfunction, renal calculus, urine abnormality.
Hematologic: anemia, *leukopenia,* **thrombocytopenia.**
Hepatic: *hepatitis,* elevated liver function test results.
Metabolic: dehydration, hyperglycemia, hyperlipidemia, hyperuricemia, hypoglycemia, increased amylase and creatinine phosphokinase levels.
Musculoskeletal: back pain, arthralgia, arthritis, cramps, myalgia, myasthenia, myopathy.
Respiratory: dyspnea, pharyngitis, rhinitis, sinusitis.
Skin: rash, dermatitis, folliculitis, fungal dermatitis, pruritus, sweating, urticaria.
Other: allergic reactions, fever, malaise.

INTERACTIONS
Drug-drug. *Amiodarone, astemizole, cisapride, ergot derivatives, midazolam, quinidine, triazolam:* nelfinavir may produce large increases in plasma levels of these drugs, which may increase risk for serious or life-threatening adverse events. Do not administer concurrently.
Anti-HIV protease inhibitors (indinavir, ritonavir): may increase nelfinavir plasma levels. Use together cautiously.
Carbamazepine, phenobarbital, phenytoin: may reduce the effectiveness of nelfinavir by decreasing nelfinavir plasma concentrations. Monitor closely.
Oral contraceptives (ethinyl estradiol, norethindrone): nelfinavir may decrease plasma levels. Suggest alternate or additional contraceptive measures during nelfinavir therapy.
Rifabutin: nelfinavir dramatically increases rifabutin plasma levels. Therefore, reduce dose of rifabutin to one-half the usual dose.
Rifampin: decreased nelfinavir plasma levels. Do not use together.

EFFECTS ON DIAGNOSTIC TESTS
None reported.

CONTRAINDICATIONS
Contraindicated in patients with hypersensitivity to any component of drug.

NURSING CONSIDERATIONS
• Use cautiously in patients with hepatic dysfunction or hemophilia types A and B. Monitor liver function test results.
• Drug dosage is same whether used alone or in combination with other antiretroviral agents.
• Administer oral powder in children unable to take tablets. May mix oral powder with small amount of water, milk, formula, soy formula, soy milk, or dietary supplements. Tell patient to consume entire contents.
• Do not reconstitute with water in its original container.
• Use reconstituted powder within 6 hours.
• Mixing with acidic foods or juice is not recommended due to bitter taste.
• It is not known if drug is excreted in

breast milk. Because safety has not been established, HIV-infected women should be advised not to breast-feed to avoid transmitting the virus to the infant.

☑ **Patient teaching**
• Advise patient to take drug with food.
• Inform patient that drug is not a cure for HIV infection.
• Tell patient that long-term effects of drug are currently unknown and that there are no supporting data that nelfinavir reduces risk of transmission of HIV.
• Advise patient to take drug daily as prescribed and not to alter dose or discontinue drug without medical approval.
• If patient misses a dose, tell him to take the dose as soon as possible and then return to his normal schedule. If a dose is skipped, advise patient not to double-dose.
• Tell patient that diarrhea is the most common adverse effect and that it can be controlled with loperamide if necessary.
• Instruct patient taking oral contraceptives to use alternate or additional contraceptive measures while on nelfinavir therapy.
• Warn patients with phenylketonuria that powder contains 11.2 mg phenylalanine per gram.
• Advise patient to report use of other prescribed or OTC drugs because of possible drug interactions.

---

nevirapine
Viramune

Pregnancy Risk Category: C

HOW SUPPLIED
Tablets: 200 mg

ACTION
Binds directly to reverse transcriptase and blocks RNA-dependent and DNA-dependent DNA polymerase activities by causing a disruption of the enzyme's catalytic site.

Route	Onset	Peak	Duration
PO	Unknown	4 hr	Unknown

INDICATIONS & DOSAGE
Adjunct treatment in patients with HIV-1 infection who have experienced clinical or immunologic deterioration—
Adults: 200 mg P.O. daily for the first 14 days, followed by 200 mg P.O. b.i.d. Used in combination with nucleoside analogue antiretroviral agents.

ADVERSE REACTIONS
CNS: headache, paresthesia.
GI: *nausea,* diarrhea, abdominal pain, ulcerative stomatitis.
Hematologic: *neutropenia,* decreased hemoglobin.
Hepatic: hepatitis, increased ALT, AST, gamma-glutamyl transpeptidase, and total bilirubin levels.
Skin: *rash, blistering, **Stevens-Johnson syndrome.***
Other: *fever,* myalgia.

INTERACTIONS
Drug-drug. *Drugs extensively metabolized by P-450 CYP3A:* may lower plasma concentration of these drugs, requiring dosage adjustment. Monitor closely.
Protease inhibitors, oral contraceptives, other hormonal contraceptives: may decrease plasma concentrations of these drugs. Do not administer concomitantly.
Rifabutin, rifampin: more data needed to assess whether dosage adjustments are necessary. When administering concurrently with nevirapine, monitor closely.

EFFECTS ON DIAGNOSTIC TESTS
None reported.

CONTRAINDICATIONS
Contraindicated in patients with hypersensitivity to drug.

NURSING CONSIDERATIONS
• Use cautiously in patients with impaired renal and hepatic function; pharmacokinetics have not been evaluated in those patients.
• Know that clinical chemistry tests, including renal and liver function tests, should be performed before initiating and regularly throughout therapy.
• Know that drug should be used in con-

---

junction with at least one additional anti-retroviral agent.

Alert: Monitor patient for blistering, oral lesions, conjunctivitis, muscle or joint aches, or general malaise. Be especially alert for a severe rash or rash accompanied by fever. Report such signs and symptoms to doctor. Patients who experience a rash during the initial 14 days of therapy should not have the dosage increased until the rash has resolved. Most rashes occur within the first 6 weeks of therapy.

• Know that moderate and severe liver function test abnormalities may warrant temporary discontinuance of therapy; drug may be restarted at half the previous dose level as ordered.

• Know that patients who have nevirapine therapy interrupted for more than 7 days should restart therapy as if receiving drug for the first time.

• Know that antiretroviral therapy may be changed if disease progression occurs while a patient is receiving nevirapine.

• Safety and effectiveness in children have not been established.

• Be aware that nevirapine is excreted in breast milk.

☑**Patient teaching**

• Inform patient that nevirapine is not a cure for HIV and that illnesses associated with advanced HIV-1 infection may still occur. Explain that drug does not reduce risk of HIV-1 transmission.

• Instruct patient to report rash immediately and to discontinue drug until told to resume.

• Stress importance of taking drug exactly as prescribed. If a dose is missed, tell patient to take the next dose as soon as possible. If a dose is skipped, patient should not double next dose.

• Tell patient not to use other medications unless approved by a doctor.

• Advise women of childbearing age that oral contraceptives and other hormonal methods of birth control should not be used with nevirapine.

• Advise women to avoid breast-feeding while taking drug to reduce risk of postnatal HIV transmission.

ribavirin
Virazole

Pregnancy Risk Category: X

HOW SUPPLIED
Powder to be reconstituted for inhalation: 6 g in 100-ml glass vial

ACTION
Inhibits viral activity by an unknown mechanism, possibly by inhibiting RNA and DNA synthesis by depleting intracellular nucleotide pools.

Route	Onset	Peak	Duration
Inhalation	Unknown	Unknown	Unknown

INDICATIONS & DOSAGE
Hospitalized infants and young children infected by respiratory syncytial virus (RSV)—
Infants and young children: solution in concentration of 20 mg/ml delivered via the Viratek Small Particle Aerosol Generator (SPAG-2) and mechanical ventilator or oxygen hood, face mask, or oxygen tent at a rate of about 12.5 L of mist per minute. Treatment is carried out for 12 to 18 hours/day for at least 3 days, and no more than 7 days.

ADVERSE REACTIONS
CV: *cardiac arrest,* hypotension, *bradycardia.*
EENT: conjunctivitis.
Hematologic: anemia, reticulocytosis.
Respiratory: worsening respiratory state, *apnea,* bacterial pneumonia, pneumothorax.
Other: rash or erythema of eyelids, elevated bilirubin, AST and ALT levels.

INTERACTIONS
None significant.

EFFECTS ON DIAGNOSTIC TESTS
None reported.

CONTRAINDICATIONS
Contraindicated in patients with hypersensitivity to drug. Although drug is used in children, manufacturer states that it's

also contraindicated in women who are or may become pregnant during treatment.

NURSING CONSIDERATIONS

• Administer ribavirin aerosol by the Viratek Small Particle Aerosol Generator (SPAG-2) only. Don't use any other aerosol-generating device.

• Use sterile USP water for injection, *not* bacteriostatic water. Water used to reconstitute this drug must not contain any antimicrobial agent.

• Discard solutions placed in the SPAG-2 unit at least every 24 hours before adding newly reconstituted solution.

• The most frequent adverse effects reported in health care personnel exposed to aerosolized ribavirin include eye irritation and headache. Pregnant personnel should be advised of these effects.

Alert: Monitor ventilator function frequently. Ribavirin may precipitate in ventilator apparatus, causing equipment malfunction with serious consequences.

• Store reconstituted solutions at room temperature for 24 hours.

• Keep in mind that ribavirin aerosol is indicated only for severe lower respiratory tract infection caused by RSV. Although treatment may begin while awaiting diagnostic test results, existence of RSV infection must eventually be documented.

• Be aware that most infants and children with RSV infection don't require treatment because the disease is commonly mild and self-limiting. Infants with underlying conditions, such as prematurity or cardiopulmonary disease, get RSV in its severest form and benefit most from treatment with ribavirin aerosol.

☑ Patient teaching

• Inform parents of need for drug and answer any questions.

• Encourage parents to report any subtle change in child immediately to nurse.

---

rimantadine hydrochloride
Flumadine

Pregnancy Risk Category: C

HOW SUPPLIED
Tablets (film-coated): 100 mg
Syrup: 50 mg/5 ml

ACTION
Unknown. Appears to prevent viral uncoating, an early step in virus reproductive cycle.

Route	Onset	Peak	Duration
PO	Unknown	6 hr	Unknown

INDICATIONS & DOSAGE
Prophylaxis of influenza A—
Adults and children over 10 years: 100 mg P.O. b.i.d.
Children under 10 years: 5 mg/kg (not to exceed 150 mg) P.O. once daily.
Elderly: 100 mg P.O. daily.
Adjust-a-dose: In patients with severe hepatic or renal dysfunction, or those experiencing adverse effects with normal dosage, 100 mg P.O. daily.

Prophylaxis should begin as soon as possible after initial exposure and should be continued through course of influenza A outbreak. Safety of prolonged therapy over 6 weeks has not been established. Can be used for prophylaxis in children up to 6 weeks after first dose of influenza vaccine or until 2 weeks after second dose of vaccine.

Treatment of influenza A—
Adults: 100 mg P.O. b.i.d. initiated within 24 to 48 hours after onset of symptoms and continued for 48 hours after symptoms disappear (usually 7-day total course).

ADVERSE REACTIONS
CNS: insomnia, headache, dizziness, nervousness, fatigue, asthenia.
GI: nausea, vomiting, anorexia, dry mouth, abdominal pain.

INTERACTIONS
Drug-drug. *Acetaminophen, aspirin:* reduced concentration of rimantadine. Monitor for decreased effectiveness of rimantadine.
Cimetidine: may decrease clearance of rimantadine. Monitor for adverse reactions.

EFFECTS ON DIAGNOSTIC TESTS
None reported.

CONTRAINDICATIONS
Contraindicated in patients with hypersensitivity to drug or amantadine.

NURSING CONSIDERATIONS
• Use cautiously in patients with renal or hepatic impairment and in patients with a history of seizures. Pregnant patients should consider the risks compared to the benefits before taking drug.
• Consider the risk to contacts of treated patients who may be subject to morbidity from influenza A. Influenza A-resistant strains can emerge during therapy. Patients taking the drug may still be able to spread the disease.

☑ Patient teaching
• Instruct patient to take drug several hours before bedtime to prevent insomnia.
• Inform patient that he may still be able to infect others with influenza A and to take infection-control precautions.

ritonavir
Norvir

Pregnancy Risk Category: B

HOW SUPPLIED
Capsules: 100 mg
Oral solution: 80 mg/ml

ACTION
An HIV protease inhibitor with activity against HIV-1 and HIV-2 proteases. HIV protease is an enzyme required for the proteolytic cleavage of viral polyprotein precursors into the individual functional proteins in infectious HIV. Ritonavir binds to the protease active site and inhibits activity of the enzyme, preventing cleavage of the viral polyproteins and resulting in the formation of immature noninfectious viral particles.

Route	Onset	Peak	Duration
PO	Unknown	2-4 hr	Unknown

INDICATIONS & DOSAGE
Treatment of HIV infection in combination with nucleoside analogues or as monotherapy when antiretroviral therapy is warranted—
Adults: 600 mg P.O. b.i.d with meals. If nausea occurs, gradually increasing dosage may provide some relief: 300 mg b.i.d. for 1 day, 400 mg b.i.d. for 2 days, 500 mg b.i.d. for 1 day, and then 600 mg b.i.d. thereafter.

ADVERSE REACTIONS
CNS: *asthenia,* headache, malaise, circumoral paresthesia, dizziness, insomnia, paresthesia, peripheral paresthesia, somnolence, thinking abnormality, migraine headache.
CV: vasodilation.
EENT: local throat irritation, blepharitis, diplopia, pharyngitis, photophobia, *taste perversion.*
GI: abdominal pain, anorexia, constipation, *diarrhea, nausea, vomiting,* dyspepsia, flatulence, cramping, jaundice.
GU: dysuria, hematuria, nocturia, polyuria, pyelonephritis, urethritis, hyperuricemia.
Hematologic: decreased hemoglobin and hematocrit levels, *leukopenia, thrombocytopenia,* decreased neutrophil and eosinophil levels.
Hepatic: elevated triglycerides, AST, ALT, GGT, alkaline phosphatase, total bilirubin, altered PT and INR.
Metabolic: hyperlipidemia, hyperglycemia, hyperkalemia.
Musculoskeletal: increased CK level, myalgia.
Skin: rash, sweating, urticaria.
Other: fever.

INTERACTIONS
Drug-drug. *Agents that increase CYP3A activity (such as carbamazepine, dexamethasone, phenobarbital, phenytoin, rifampin, rifabutin):* may increase clearance of ritonavir, resulting in decreased ritonavir plasma concentrations. Monitor patient closely.
Alprazolam, clorazepate, diazepam, dihydroergotamine, ergotamine, estazolam, flurazepam, midazolam, triazolam, zolpidem: significantly increased levels of

these drugs. Because of the potential for extreme sedation and respiratory depression, these agents should not be administered concurrently with ritonavir.

Amiodarone, astemizole, bupropion, cisapride, clozapine, encainide, flecainide, meperidine, piroxicam, propafenone, propoxyphene, quinidine, rifabutin: significantly increased plasma concentrations of these drugs, which increases patient's risk of arrhythmias, hematologic abnormalities, seizures, or other potentially serious adverse effects. Avoid concomitant use.

Clarithromycin: reduced creatinine clearance. Patients with impaired renal function receiving drug concomitantly with ritonavir require a 50% reduction in clarithromycin dose if creatinine clearance is 30 to 60 ml/minute and a 75% reduction if it is below 30 ml/minute.

Desipramine: increased overall serum concentrations of desipramine. Concomitant administration may require a dosage adjustment when administered with ritonavir. Monitor patient.

Directly glucuronidated agents: ritonavir may increase activity of glucoronosyl transferases with loss of therapeutic effects from these agents; may signify need for dosage alteration of these agents. Concomitant use should be accompanied by therapeutic drug concentration monitoring and increased monitoring of therapeutic and adverse effects, especially for agents with narrow therapeutic margins, such as oral anticoagulants and immunosuppressants. Dosage reduction greater than 50% may be required for agents extensively metabolized by CYP3A.

Disulfiram or other drugs that produce disulfiram-like reactions such as metronidazole: increased risk of disulfiram-like reactions. Ritonavir formulations contain alcohol that can produce reactions when co-administered. Monitor patient.

Oral contraceptives containing ethinyl estradiol: decreased overall serum concentrations of the contraceptive. Advise patient that concomitant therapy may require a dosage increase in the oral contraceptive or use of other contraceptive measures.

Saquinavir: inhibited metabolism of saquinavir, resulting in greatly increased

plasma levels. Safety of this combination has not been established.

Theophylline: decreased overall serum concentrations of theophylline. Increased dosage may be required when coadministered with ritonavir. Monitor level.

Drug-food. *Any food:* increased absorption. Give drug with food.

Drug-lifestyle. *Smoking:* decreased overall serum concentrations of ritonavir. Avoid use.

EFFECTS ON DIAGNOSTIC TESTS
None reported.

CONTRAINDICATIONS
Contraindicated in patients with hypersensitivity to any component of drug.

NURSING CONSIDERATIONS
• Use cautiously in patients with hepatic insufficiency.
• Know that drug may be administered alone or in combination with nucleoside analogs.
• Know that patients beginning combination regimens with ritonavir and nucleosides may improve GI tolerance by starting ritonavir alone and subsequently adding nucleosides before completing 2 weeks of ritonavir.
• Safety and effectiveness in children under 12 years have not been established.
• Be aware that it is not known whether ritonavir is excreted in breast milk.

☑ **Patient teaching**
• Inform patient that drug is not a cure for HIV infection. He may continue to develop opportunistic infections and other complications associated with HIV infection. Drug has not been shown to reduce the risk of transmitting HIV to others through sexual contact or blood contamination.
• Caution patient to take drug as prescribed and not to adjust dosage or discontinue therapy without first consulting the doctor.
• Tell patient he may improve the taste of ritonavir oral solution by mixing it with chocolate milk, Ensure, or Advera within 1 hour of the scheduled dose.

- Instruct patient to take drug with a meal to improve absorption.
- Tell patient that if a dose is missed, he should take the next dose as soon as possible. If a dose is skipped, he should not double the next dose.
- Advise patient to report use of other medications, including nonprescription drugs; ritonavir interacts with some drugs when taken together.
- Advise female patient not to breast-feed, to prevent transmission of infection.

saquinavir
Fortovase

saquinavir mesylate
Invirase

Pregnancy Risk Category: B

HOW SUPPLIED
saquinavir
Capsules (soft gelatin): 200 mg
saquinavir mesylate
Capsules (hard gelatin): 200 mg

ACTION
Inhibits the activity of HIV protease and prevents the cleavage of HIV polyproteins, which are essential for HIV maturation.

Route	Onset	Peak	Duration
PO	Unknown	Unknown	Unknown

INDICATIONS & DOSAGE
Adjunct treatment of advanced HIV infection in selected patients—
Adults: 600 mg (Invirase) or 1,200 mg (Fortovase) P.O. t.i.d. taken within 2 hours after a full meal and in combination with a nucleoside analogue, such as zalcitabine at a dosage of 0.75 mg P.O. t.i.d. or zidovudine at a dosage of 200 mg P.O. t.i.d.

ADVERSE REACTIONS
CNS: paresthesia, headache, dizziness, numbness.
CV: chest pain.
GI: diarrhea, ulcerated buccal mucosa, abdominal pain, nausea, dyspepsia, pancreatitis.
Hematologic: *pancytopenia, thrombocytopenia.*
Respiratory: bronchitis, cough.
Other: asthenia, rash, musculoskeletal pain.

INTERACTIONS
Drug-drug. *Astemizole, cisapride:* increased serum level of this drug, increased risk of arrhythmias, and sudden death. Avoid concomitant use.
Ketoconazole, ritonavir: increased serum saquinavir concentrations. Monitor patient closely.
Phenobarbital, phenytoin, rifabutin, rifampin: reduced steady state concentration of saquinavir. Use together cautiously.
Drug-food. *Any food:* increased absorption. Give drug with food.

EFFECTS ON DIAGNOSTIC TESTS
None reported.

CONTRAINDICATIONS
Contraindicated in patients with hypersensitivity to drug or to any component contained in the capsule.

NURSING CONSIDERATIONS
- Safety of drug is not established in pregnant or breast-feeding women or in children under 16 years.
- CBC, platelets, electrolytes, uric acid, liver enzymes, and bilirubin should be evaluated before therapy begins and at appropriate intervals throughout therapy, as ordered.
- Be aware that if serious toxicity occurs during treatment, drug should be discontinued until the etiology of the event is identified or the toxicity resolves. When drug is resumed, it may be done with no dosage modifications.
- Monitor patient's hydration if adverse GI reactions occur.
- Notify doctor if adverse reactions occur. Obtain an order for a mild analgesic if drug causes headache, an antiemetic if drug causes nausea, or an antidiarrheal agent if drug causes diarrhea.
- Be alert for adverse reactions associated with adjunct therapy (zidovudine or zalcitabine).

✓ Patient teaching
• Advise patient to take drug within 2 hours after a full meal.
• Inform patient that drug is usually administered with other AIDS-related antiviral agents.
• Instruct patient to take drug around the clock, not missing any doses, to decrease the risk of developing HIV resistance.
• Inform patient that any change from Invirase to Fortovase capsules should be made only under the supervision of a doctor.
• Tell patient to store Fortovase capsules in the refrigerator while Invirase capsules can be kept at room temperature.

---

stavudine (2,3 didehydro-3-deoxythymidine, d4T)
Zerit

Pregnancy Risk Category: C

HOW SUPPLIED
Capsules: 15 mg, 20 mg, 30 mg, 40 mg

ACTION
A thymidine nucleoside analogue that prevents replication of retroviruses, including HIV, by inhibiting the enzyme reverse transcriptase and causing termination of DNA chain growth.

Route	Onset	Peak	Duration
PO	Unknown	1 hr	Unknown

INDICATIONS & DOSAGE
Treatment of HIV-infected patients who have received prolonged prior zidovudine therapy—
Adults weighing 60 kg (132 lb) or more: 40 mg P.O. q 12 hours.
Adults weighing under 60 kg: 30 mg P.O. q 12 hours.
Children: 2 mg/kg/day P.O. in divided doses q 12 hours for children weighing under 30 kg (66 lb); adult dose should be used for children weighing 30 kg or more.
Adjust-a-dose: In patients with renal impairment, if creatinine clearance is 26 to 50 ml/minute, 20 mg (if weight exceeds 60 kg) or 15 mg (if weight is below 60 kg) P.O. q 12 hours; if creatinine clearance is 10 to 25 ml/minute, 20 mg (if weight exceeds 60 kg) or 15 mg (if weight is below 60 kg) P.O. q 24 hours.

ADVERSE REACTIONS
CNS: peripheral neuropathy, headache, malaise, insomnia, anxiety, depression, nervousness, dizziness.
CV: chest pain.
GI: *abdominal pain, diarrhea, nausea, vomiting, anorexia,* dyspepsia, constipation, weight loss, pancreatitis.
Hematologic: *neutropenia, thrombocytopenia,* anemia.
Skin: *rash, diaphoresis, pruritus,* maculopapular rash.
Other: *myalgia, **hepatotoxicity,** chills, fever, asthenia, back pain, arthralgia, dyspnea,* conjunctivitis.

INTERACTIONS
None reported.

EFFECTS ON DIAGNOSTIC TESTS
Stavudine may cause a mild to moderate increase in AST and ALT levels.

CONTRAINDICATIONS
Contraindicated in patients with hypersensitivity to drug.

NURSING CONSIDERATIONS
• Use cautiously in patients with renal impairment or history of peripheral neuropathy. Dosage adjustment is necessary for creatinine clearance below 50 ml/minute; dosage adjustment or discontinuation is necessary in onset of peripheral neuropathy. Also use cautiously in pregnant women.
Alert: Know that peripheral neuropathy appears to be the major dose-limiting adverse effect of stavudine. It may or may not resolve after drug is discontinued.
• Monitor CBC and serum levels of creatinine, AST, ALT, and alkaline phosphatase, as ordered.

✓ Patient teaching
• Tell patient that drug may be taken without regard to meals.
• Warn patient not to take other drugs for HIV or AIDS unless the doctor has approved them.

• Teach patient signs and symptoms of peripheral neuropathy—pain, burning, aching, weakness, or pins and needles in the extremities—and tell him to report these immediately.

• Tell patient to monitor weight patterns and report weight loss or gain.

---

valacyclovir hydrochloride
Valtrex

Pregnancy Risk Category: B

HOW SUPPLIED
Tablets: 500 mg

ACTION
Rapidly converts to acyclovir, which in turn becomes incorporated into viral DNA thereby terminating growth of the DNA chain and inhibits viral DNA polymerase, causing inhibition of viral replication.

Route	Onset	Peak	Duration
PO	30 min	Unknown	Unknown

INDICATIONS & DOSAGE
Herpes zoster infection (shingles)—
Adults: 1 g P.O. t.i.d. for 7 days.
Adjust-a-dose: In renally impaired patients with creatinine clearance of 50 ml/minute or more, use regular dose; if 30 to 49 ml/minute, 1 g P.O. q 12 hours; if 10 to 29 ml/minute, 1 g P.O. q 24 hours; if below 10 ml/minute, 500 mg P.O. q 24 hours.

In hemodialysis patients, 1 g P.O. after hemodialysis.
For initial episode of genital herpes—
Adults: 1 g P.O. b.i.d. for 10 days.
Adjust-a-dose: In renally impaired patients with creatinine clearance of 30 ml/minute or more, dosage is 1 g P.O. q 12 hours; if 10 to 29 ml/minute, 1 g P.O. q 24 hours; if below 10 ml/minute, 500 mg P.O. q 24 hours.

In hemodialysis patients, 1 g P.O. after hemodialysis.
Recurrent genital herpes—
Adults: 500 mg P.O. b.i.d. for 5 days, given at the first sign or symptom of an episode.

Adjust-a-dose: In renally impaired patients with creatinine clearance of 30 ml/minute or more, dosage is 500 mg P.O. q 12 hours; if 29 ml/minute or less, 500 mg P.O. q 24 hours.

In hemodialysis patients, 500 mg P.O. after hemodialysis.

ADVERSE REACTIONS
CNS: *headache,* dizziness.
GI: *nausea,* vomiting, diarrhea, constipation, abdominal pain, anorexia.
Other: asthenia.

INTERACTIONS
Drug-drug. *Cimetidine, probenecid:* reduced rate but not extent of conversion of valacyclovir to acyclovir and reduced renal clearance of acyclovir, thus increasing acyclovir blood levels. Monitor for possible toxicity.

EFFECTS ON DIAGNOSTIC TESTS
None reported.

CONTRAINDICATIONS
Contraindicated in patients with hypersensitivity or intolerance to valacyclovir, acyclovir, or any component of the formulation.

NURSING CONSIDERATIONS
• Know that valacyclovir is not recommended for use in patients with HIV or in bone marrow or renal transplant recipients. Thrombotic thrombocytopenic purpura and hemolytic uremic syndrome have occurred, resulting in death in some patients with advanced HIV disease and in bone marrow transplant and renal transplant recipients participating in clinical trials of valacyclovir at doses of 8 g/day.

• Use cautiously in patients with renal impairment, the elderly, and those receiving other nephrotoxic drugs. Monitor renal function test results.

• Safety and efficacy in children have not been established.

• Glaxo-Wellcome, the manufacturer, maintains an ongoing registry of women exposed to the drug during pregnancy. Use during pregnancy should only be considered if the benefits outweigh the

---

risks. Health care providers are encouraged to report such exposures to the registrar at 1-800-722-9292, ext 39437.
• Alert doctor if patient is breast-feeding; drug may need to be discontinued.
• Although there have been no reports of overdosage, precipitation of acyclovir in renal tubules may occur when solubility (2.5 mg/ml) is exceeded in the intratubular fluid. With acute renal failure and anuria, the patient may benefit from hemodialysis until renal function is restored.

☑ **Patient teaching**
• Inform patient that valacyclovir may be taken without regard to meals.
• Teach patient the signs and symptoms of herpes infection (rash, tingling, itching, and pain), and advise him to notify the doctor immediately if they occur. Treatment should be initiated as soon as possible after symptoms appear, preferably within 48 hours of the onset of zoster rash.
• Tell patient that valacyclovir is not a cure for herpes but may decrease the length and severity of symptoms.

---

zalcitabine (dideoxycytidine, ddC)
Hivid

Pregnancy Risk Category: C

HOW SUPPLIED
Tablets: 0.375 mg, 0.75 mg

ACTION
Inhibits replication of HIV by blocking viral DNA synthesis.

Route	Onset	Peak	Duration
PO	Unknown	1-2 hr	Unknown

INDICATIONS & DOSAGE
Monotherapy for treatment of advanced HIV disease in patients who either cannot tolerate zidovudine or who have disease progression while receiving zidovudine—
Adults and children 13 years or older: 0.75 mg P.O. q 8 hours.
Combination therapy with zidovudine for treatment of advanced HIV disease

(CD4+ cell count equal to or less than 300 cells/mm³)—
Adults and children 13 years or older: 0.75 mg P.O. q 8 hours administered concomitantly with zidovudine 200 mg P.O. q 8 hours.
Adjust-a-dose: In renally impaired patients with creatinine clearance of 10 to 40 ml/minute, dosage is 0.75 mg P.O. q 12 hours; if clearance below 10 ml/minute, 0.75 mg P.O. q 24 hours.
    If patient experiences moderate discomfort with signs and symptoms of peripheral neuropathy, discontinue drug temporarily. If symptoms improve after discontinuation of drug, it may be reintroduced at 0.375 mg P.O. q 8 hours.

ADVERSE REACTIONS
CNS: *peripheral neuropathy, headache, fatigue,* dizziness, confusion, *seizures,* impaired concentration, amnesia, insomnia, mental depression, tremor, hypertonia, anxiety.
CV: cardiomyopathy, *heart failure,* chest pain.
EENT: pharyngitis, cough, ocular pain, abnormal vision, ototoxicity, nasal discharge.
GI: nausea, vomiting, diarrhea, abdominal pain, anorexia, constipation, stomatitis, esophageal ulcer, glossitis, pancreatitis.
Hematologic: anemia, *neutropenia, leukopenia, thrombocytopenia.*
Hepatic: increased AST, ALT and alkaline phosphatase.
Skin: pruritus; night sweats; *erythematous, maculopapular, or follicular rash;* urticaria.
Other: myalgia, arthralgia, *fever,* hypoglycemia.

INTERACTIONS
Drug-drug. *Aminoglycosides, amphotericin B, foscarnet, other drugs that may impair renal function:* increased risk of nephrotoxicity. Avoid concomitant use when possible.
Antacids containing aluminum or magnesium: decreased bioavailability of zalcitabine. Do not use together.
Chloramphenicol, cisplatin, dapsone, didanosine, disulfiram, ethionamide,

---

Reactions may be *common,* uncommon, *life-threatening,* or COMMON AND LIFE-THREATENING.

glutethimide, gold salts, hydralazine, iodoquinol, isoniazid, metronidazole, nitrofurantoin, phenytoin, ribavirin, stavudine, vincristine, other drugs that can cause peripheral neuropathy: increased risk of peripheral neuropathy. Avoid concomitant use.

Cimetidine, probenecid: increased serum zalcitabine levels. Monitor patient carefully.

Pentamidine: increased risk of pancreatitis. Avoid concomitant use when possible.
Drug-food. *Any food:* decreased rate of absorption. Give drug on an empty stomach.

EFFECTS ON DIAGNOSTIC TESTS
None reported.

CONTRAINDICATIONS
Contraindicated in patients with hypersensitivity to drug or any component of the formulation.

NURSING CONSIDERATIONS
• Use with extreme caution in patients with preexisting peripheral neuropathy.
• Use cautiously in patients with hepatic failure, history of pancreatitis, baseline cardiomyopathy, or history of heart failure. Monitor liver function test results and pancreatic enzymes.
• Know that toxic effects of drug may cause abnormalities in several laboratory tests, including CBC, hemoglobin, leukocyte, reticulocyte, granulocyte, and platelet counts; and AST, ALT, and alkaline phosphatase levels.
• Do not administer drug with food because it decreases the rate and extent of absorption.
• Assess for signs of peripheral neuropathy, characterized by numbness and burning in the extremities, the drug's major toxic effects. If drug isn't withdrawn, peripheral neuropathy can progress to sharp shooting pain or severe continuous burning pain requiring opioid analgesics. It may or may not be reversible.

✓ **Patient teaching**
• Instruct patient to take drug on an empty stomach.
• Make sure patient understands that the

drug doesn't cure HIV infection and that opportunistic infections may still occur despite continued use. Review safe sex practices with the patient.
• Inform patient that peripheral neuropathy is the major toxicity associated with drug and that pancreatitis is the major life-threatening toxic reaction. Review the signs and symptoms of these adverse reactions, and instruct patient to call doctor promptly if any appear.
• Instruct patient of childbearing age to use an effective contraceptive while taking drug.

zidovudine (azidothymidine, AZT)
Apo-Zidovudine†, Novo-AZT†, Retrovir

Pregnancy Risk Category: C

HOW SUPPLIED
Capsules: 100 mg
Tablets: 300 mg
Syrup: 50 mg/5 ml
Injection: 10 mg/ml

ACTION
Inhibits replication of HIV by blocking DNA synthesis.

Route	Onset	Peak	Duration
PO, IV	Unknown	0.5-1.5 hr	Unknown

INDICATIONS & DOSAGE
Symptomatic HIV infection, including AIDS—
Adults and children 12 years and over: 100 mg P.O. q 4 hours around the clock, 300 mg (1 tablet) P.O. q 12 hours, 200 mg P.O. q 8 hours, or 1 mg/kg I.V. q 4 hours six times daily.
Children 3 months to 12 years: 180 mg/ m² P.O. q 6 hours (720 mg/m²/day), not to exceed 200 mg q 6 hours.
Asymptomatic HIV infection—
Adults and children 12 years and over: 100 mg P.O. q 4 hours while awake (500 mg daily). Or, 1 mg/kg I.V. q 4 hours while awake (5 mg/kg/day).
Children 3 months to 12 years: 180 mg/

m² P.O. q 6 hours (720 mg/m²/day), not to exceed 200 mg q 6 hours.

To reduce risk of transmission of HIV from infected mother with a baseline CD4+ lymphocyte count exceeding 200 cells/mm³ to the newborn—
Adults: 100 mg P.O. five times daily given initially between 14 and 34 weeks' gestation and continued throughout pregnancy. During labor, administer loading dose of 2 mg/kg I.V. over 1 hour followed by continuous I.V. infusion of 1 mg/kg/hour until umbilical cord is clamped.
Neonates: 2 mg/kg P.O. (syrup) q 6 hours for 6 weeks, beginning within 12 hours after birth. Or, 1.5 mg/kg I.V. q 6 hours.

Combination therapy with zalcitabine or other antiretroviral agents for treatment of advanced HIV disease—
Adults and children 13 years or older: 200 mg P.O. q 8 hours or 300 mg (1 tablet) P.O. q 12 hours administered concomitantly with zalcitabine 0.75 mg P.O. q 8 hours or other antiretroviral agents.
Adjust-a-dose: In end-stage renal disease on hemodialysis or peritoneal dialysis, 100 mg P.O. or 1 mg/kg I.V. q 6 to 8 hours.

ADVERSE REACTIONS
CNS: *headache,* **seizures,** *paresthesia, malaise,* insomnia, *dizziness,* somnolence.
GI: *nausea, anorexia, abdominal pain, vomiting,* constipation, *diarrhea,* dyspepsia.
Hematologic: *severe bone marrow suppression (resulting in anemia), agranulocytosis, thrombocytopenia.*
Skin: *rash.*
Other: myalgia, diaphoresis, *fever, asthenia,* taste perversion, increased liver enzymes, lactic acidosis, pancreatitis.

INTERACTIONS
Drug-drug: *Acetaminophen, aspirin, indomethacin:* may impair hepatic metabolism of zidovudine, increasing drug's toxicity. Monitor closely.
Acyclovir: possible seizures, lethargy, and fatigue. Use together cautiously.
Amphotericin B, dapsone, flucytosine, pentamidine: increased risk of nephrotoxicity and bone marrow suppression. Monitor closely.

Fluconazole, methadone, valproic acid: increased zidovudine concentration. Monitor for toxicity.
Ganciclovir, interferon-alpha: increased risk of hematologic toxicity. Monitor closely.
Other cytotoxic drugs: additive adverse effects on the bone marrow. Avoid concomitant use.
Probenecid: may decrease the renal clearance of zidovudine. Avoid concomitant use.
Ribavirin: antagonized antiviral activity of zidovudine against HIV. Avoid concomitant use.

EFFECTS ON DIAGNOSTIC TESTS
Drug may cause depression of formed elements (erythrocytes, leukocytes, and platelets) in peripheral blood.

CONTRAINDICATIONS
Contraindicated in patients with hypersensitivity to drug.

NURSING CONSIDERATIONS
• Use cautiously and with close monitoring in patients with advanced symptomatic HIV infection and in patients with severe bone marrow depression.
• Use with caution in patients with hepatomegaly, hepatitis, or other known risk factors for liver disease and in those with renal insufficiency. Monitor renal and liver function tests.
• Monitor blood studies every 2 weeks, as ordered, to detect anemia or agranulocytosis. Patients may require dosage reduction or temporary discontinuation of drug.
• Be aware that drug may temporarily decrease morbidity and mortality in certain patients with AIDS.

◪I.V. administration
• Dilute before administration. Remove the calculated dose from the vial; add to D_5W to achieve a concentration that does not exceed 4 mg/ml. Infuse drug over 1 hour at a constant rate. Avoid rapid infusion or bolus injection. Adding mixture to biological or colloidal fluids (for example, blood products, protein solutions) is not recommended. Protect undiluted vials from light.

Reactions may be *common,* uncommon, ***life-threatening,*** or COMMON AND LIFE-THREATENING.

☑ Patient teaching
• Tell patient to take drug exactly as directed and not to share it with others.
• Instruct patient to take drug on an empty stomach. To avoid esophageal irritation, tell patient to take drug while sitting upright and with adequate amount of fluids.
• Remind patient that he *must* comply with the dosage schedule. Suggest ways to avoid missing doses, perhaps by using an alarm clock.
• Advise patient that blood transfusions may be needed during treatment. Zidovudine frequently causes a low RBC count.
• Warn patient not to take other drugs for AIDS unless doctor has approved them.
• Advise pregnant, HIV-infected patient that drug therapy only *reduces* the risk of HIV transmission to her newborn. Long-term risks to infants are unknown.
• Advise health care worker who considers zidovudine prophylaxis after occupational exposure (following needle-stick injury, for example) that animal and human studies have not yet proved drug's safety or efficacy.

azithromycin
clarithromycin
dirithromycin
erythromycin base
erythromycin estolate
erythromycin ethylsuccinate
erythromycin lactobionate
erythromycin stearate

COMBINATION PRODUCTS
ERYZOLE, PEDIAZOLE, SULFIMYCIN: erythromycin (200 mg) and sulfisoxazole (600 mg)/5 ml.

---

azithromycin
Zithromax

Pregnancy Risk Category: B

HOW SUPPLIED
Capsules: 250 mg; Z-pak (contains 5 days of therapy)
Injection: 500 mg
Oral suspension: 100 mg/5 ml, 200 mg/5 ml
Single-dose powder for oral suspension: 1 g
Tablets: 250 mg, 600 mg

ACTION
Binds to the 50S subunit of bacterial ribosomes, blocking protein synthesis; bacteriostatic or bactericidal, depending on concentration.

Route	Onset	Peak	Duration
PO	Unknown	2.5-4.4 hr	Unknown
IV	Unknown	Unknown	Unknown

INDICATIONS & DOSAGE
Acute bacterial exacerbations of COPD caused by Haemophilus influenzae, Moraxella (Branhamella) catarrhalis, *or* Streptococcus pneumoniae; *uncomplicated skin and skin-structure infections caused by* Staphylococcus aureus, Streptococcus pyogenes, *or* Streptococcus agalactiae; *second-line therapy of pharyngitis or tonsillitis caused by* S. pyogenes—
Adults and adolescents 16 years and older: 500 mg P.O. as a single dose on day 1, followed by 250 mg daily on days 2 through 5. Total dose is 1.5 g.
Community-acquired pneumonia caused by Chlamydia pneumoniae, H. influenzae, Mycoplasma pneumoniae, S. pneumoniae; *I.V. form can also be used for* Legionella pneumophila, M. catarrhalis, *and* S. aureus—
Adults and adolescents 16 years and older: 500 mg P.O. as a single dose on day 1, followed by 250 mg P.O. daily on days 2 through 5. Total dose is 1.5 g. For patients requiring initial I.V. therapy, 500 mg I.V. as a single daily dose for 2 days, followed by 500 mg P.O. as a single daily dose to complete a 7-to 10-day course of therapy. Switch from I.V. to P.O. therapy should be done at the doctor's discretion and based on patient's clinical response.
Nongonococcal urethritis or cervicitis caused by Chlamydia trachomatis—
Adults and adolescents 16 years and older: 1 g P.O. as a single dose.
Prevention of disseminated Mycobacterium avium *complex disease in patients with advanced HIV infection—*
Adults: 1,200 mg P.O. once weekly, as indicated.
Urethritis and cervicitis due to Neisseria gonorrhoeae—
Adults: 2 g P.O. as a single dose.
Pelvic inflammatory disease caused by C. trachomatis, N. gonorrhoeae, *or* Mycoplasma hominis *in patients who require initial I.V. therapy—*
Adults: 500 mg I.V. as a single daily dose for 1 to 2 days, followed by 250 mg P.O. daily to complete a 7 day course of therapy. Switch from I.V. to P.O. therapy should be done at the doctor's discretion and based on patient's clinical response.
Genital ulcer disease in men due to Haemophilus ducreyi *(chancroid)—*
Adults: 1 g P.O. as a single dose.

Otitis media—
Children over 6 months: 10 mg/kg (maximum 500 mg) P.O. on day 1, followed by 5 mg/kg (maximum 250 mg) on days 2 to 5.
Pharyngitis, tonsillitis—
Children over 2 years: 12 mg/kg (maximum 500 mg) P.O. daily for 5 days.

ADVERSE REACTIONS
CNS: dizziness, vertigo, headache, fatigue, somnolence.
CV: palpitations, chest pain.
GI: *nausea, vomiting, diarrhea, abdominal pain,* dyspepsia, flatulence, melena, cholestatic jaundice, pseudomembranous colitis.
GU: candidiasis, vaginitis, nephritis.
Skin: rash, photosensitivity.
Other: *angioedema.*

INTERACTIONS
Drug-drug. *Aluminum- and magnesium-containing antacids:* lowered peak plasma levels of azithromycin. Separate administration times by at least 2 hours.
Astemizole, pimozide: prolongation of QT interval and ventricular tachycardia have been associated with other macrolide anti-infectives. Monitor patient closely.
Carbamazepine, cyclosporine, phenytoin: may increase levels of these drugs. Monitor closely.
Digoxin: may cause elevated digoxin levels. Monitor closely.
Ergotamine: acute ergotamine toxicity has occurred. Monitor closely.
Theophylline: may increase plasma theophylline levels with other macrolides; effect of azithromycin is unknown. Monitor theophylline levels carefully.
Triazolam: may decrease clearance of triazolam. Monitor closely.
Warfarin: may increase INR with other macrolides; effect of azithromycin is unknown. Monitor INR carefully.
Drug-food. *Any food:* decreased absorption. Take drug on an empty stomach.
Drug-lifestyle. *Sun exposure:* photosensitivity reactions may occur. Take precautions.

EFFECTS ON DIAGNOSTIC TESTS
None reported.

CONTRAINDICATIONS
Contraindicated in patients with hypersensitivity to erythromycin or other macrolides.

NURSING CONSIDERATIONS
• Use cautiously in patients with impaired hepatic function.
• Obtain specimen for culture and sensitivity tests before giving first dose. Therapy may begin pending results.
• Administer capsules and oral suspension 1 hour before or 2 hours after meals; do not administer with antacids. Tablets can be taken with or without food.
• Monitor for superinfection. May cause overgrowth of nonsusceptible bacteria or fungi.
• Single-dose 1-g packets for suspension should be reconstituted with 2 oz (60 ml) water, mixed, and administered to patient. Patient should rinse glass with additional 2 oz of water and drink to ensure he has consumed entire dose.

▶ I.V. administration
• Reconstitute 500 mg vial with 4.8 ml of sterile water for injection and shake well until all the drug is dissolved (yields a concentration of 100 mg/ml). Dilute this solution further in at least 250 ml of 0.9% NaCl, 0.45% NaCl, D₅W, or lactated Ringer's solution to yield a concentration range of 1 to 2 mg/ml.
Alert: Infuse a 500-mg dose of azithromycin I.V. over 1 hour or more. Never give it as a bolus or an I.M. injection.

✓ Patient teaching
• Tell patient to take drug as prescribed, even after he feels better.

---

clarithromycin
Biaxin, Klaricid§

Pregnancy Risk Category: C

HOW SUPPLIED
Tablets (film-coated): 250 mg, 500 mg
Suspension: 125 mg/5 ml, 250 mg/5 ml

ACTION
Binds to the 50S subunit of bacterial ribosomes, blocking protein synthesis; bacteriostatic or bactericidal, depending on concentration.

Route	Onset	Peak	Duration
PO	Unknown	2-4 hr	Unknown

INDICATIONS & DOSAGE
Pharyngitis or tonsillitis caused by Streptococcus pyogenes—
Adults: 250 mg P.O. q 12 hours for 10 days.
Children: 15 mg/kg/day P.O. in divided doses q 12 hours for 10 days.
Acute maxillary sinusitis caused by S. pneumoniae, Haemophilus influenzae, *or* Moraxella (Branhamella) catarrhalis—
Adults: 500 mg P.O. q 12 hours for 14 days.
Children: 15 mg/kg/day P.O. in divided doses q 12 hours for 10 days.
Acute exacerbations of chronic bronchitis caused by M. catarrhalis *or* S. pneumoniae; *pneumonia caused by* S. pneumoniae, Chlamydia pneumoniae, *or* Mycoplasma pneumoniae—
Adults: 250 mg P.O. q 12 hours for 7 to 14 days.
Acute exacerbations of chronic bronchitis caused by H. influenzae—
Adults: 500 mg P.O. q 12 hours for 7 to 14 days.
Uncomplicated skin and skin-structure infections caused by Staphylococcus aureus *or* S. pyogenes—
Adults: 250 mg P.O. q 12 hours for 7 to 14 days.
Children: 15 mg/kg/day P.O. in divided doses q 12 hours for 10 days.
Acute otitis media caused by H. influenzae, M. catarrhalis, *or* S. pneumoniae—
Children: 7.5 mg/kg P.O. q 12 hours for 10 days.
Mycobacterium avium *complex (MAC) disease in patients with HIV infection*—
Adults: 500 mg P.O. q 12 hours, in combination with other antimycobacterial drugs, for life.
Children: 7.5 mg/kg P.O. (maximum of 500 mg) q 12 hours, in combination with other antimycobacterial drugs, for life.

Prophylaxis against MAC disease in patients with advanced HIV infection—
Adults: 500 mg P.O. q 12 hours.
Children: 7.5 mg/kg P.O. (maximum of 500 mg) q 12 hours.
Active duodenal ulcer associated with Helicobacter pylori *infection*—
Adults: 500 mg P.O. t.i.d. for 14 days with omeprazole 40 mg P.O. each morning. Omeprazole therapy should continue at a dose of 20 mg P.O. each morning for days 15 to 28. Or, 500 mg P.O. t.i.d. for 14 days with ranitidine bismuth citrate 400 mg P.O. b.i.d. Ranitidine bismuth citrate therapy continues for days 15 to 28. Or, 500 mg P.O. b.i.d. plus lansoprazole 30 mg P.O. b.i.d. and amoxicillin 1 g P.O. b.i.d. for 14 days.

ADVERSE REACTIONS
CNS: headache.
CV: *ventricular arrhythmias.*
GI: *diarrhea, nausea, abnormal taste,* dyspepsia, abdominal pain or discomfort, elevated liver studies, pseudomembranous colitis.
GU: *increased BUN.*
Hematologic: *increased INR, **leukopenia, thrombocytopenia.***
Skin: rash, ***Stevens-Johnson syndrome,*** urticaria.

INTERACTIONS
Drug-drug. *Astemizole, cisapride, pimozide:* altered metabolism of these drugs, with prolongation of QT interval and ventricular tachycardia. Do not use these drugs with clarithromycin.
Carbamazepine: may increase serum levels of carbamazepine. Monitor blood levels.
Digoxin: may increase serum digoxin levels. Monitor for digitalis toxicity.
Fluconazole: increased clarithromycin levels. Monitor closely.
Theophylline: increased plasma theophylline levels possible with other macrolides; effect of clarithromycin is unknown. Monitor theophylline levels carefully.
Warfarin: increased INR possible with other macrolides; effect of clarithromycin is unknown. Monitor INR carefully.
Zidovudine: decreased zidovudine levels.

Monitor effectiveness of zidovudine closely.

EFFECTS ON DIAGNOSTIC TESTS
None reported.

CONTRAINDICATIONS
Contraindicated in patients with hypersensitivity to erythromycin or other macrolides and in those receiving astemizole, cisapride, and pimozide.

NURSING CONSIDERATIONS
• Use cautiously in patients with hepatic or renal impairment.
• Obtain specimen for culture and sensitivity tests before giving first dose. Therapy may begin pending results.
• Monitor patient for superinfection. Drug may cause overgrowth of nonsusceptible bacteria or fungi.

☑ **Patient teaching**
• Tell patient to take drug as prescribed, even after he feels better.
• Instruct patient to report persistent adverse reactions.
• Inform patient that drug may be taken with or without food. He should not refrigerate the suspension form. Discard unused portion after 10 days.

---

dirithromycin
Dynabac

Pregnancy Risk Category: C

HOW SUPPLIED
Tablets (enteric-coated): 250 mg

ACTION
Inhibits bacterial RNA-dependent protein synthesis by binding to the 50S subunit of the ribosome.

Route	Onset	Peak	Duration
PO	Unknown	4 hr	Unknown

INDICATIONS & DOSAGE
Acute bacterial exacerbations of chronic bronchitis due to Moraxella (Branhamella) catarrhalis *or* Streptococcus pneumoniae; *secondary bacterial infection of acute bronchitis due to* M. catarrhalis *or* S. pneumoniae; *uncomplicated skin and skin-structure infections due to* Staphylococcus aureus *(methicillin-susceptible strains)—*
Adults and children 12 years and older: 500 mg P.O. daily with food (or within 1 hour after eating) for 5 to 7 days.
Community-acquired pneumonia due to Legionella pneumophila, Mycoplasma pneumoniae, *or* S. pneumoniae—
Adults and children 12 years and older: 500 mg P.O. daily with food (or within 1 hour after eating) for 14 days.
Pharyngitis or tonsillitis due to Streptococcus pyogenes—
Adults and children 12 years and older: 500 mg P.O. daily with food (or within 1 hour after eating) for 10 days.
✳ *NEW INDICATION: Acute bacterial exacerbations of chronic bronchitis due to* Haemophilus influenzae; *uncomplicated skin and skin-structure infections due to* S. pyogenes—
Adults and children 12 years and older: 500 mg P.O. daily with food (or within 1 hour of a meal) for 5 to 7 days.

ADVERSE REACTIONS
CNS: headache, dizziness, vertigo, insomnia.
GI: abdominal pain, nausea, diarrhea, vomiting, dyspepsia, flatulence.
Hematologic: increased platelet, eosinophil, and neutrophil counts.
Respiratory: increased cough, dyspnea.
Skin: rash, pruritus, urticaria.
Other: pain (nonspecific), asthenia, hyperkalemia, decreased bicarbonate levels, increased CK and liver enzyme levels.

INTERACTIONS
Drug-drug. *Antacids, H_2 antagonists:* may slightly increase the absorption of dirithromycin when it is administered immediately after these drugs.
Theophylline: may alter steady-state plasma concentration of theophylline. Monitor theophylline plasma concentrations. Dosage adjustments may be needed.
Note: Alfentanil, oral anticoagulants, astemizole, bromocriptine, carbamazepine, cyclosporine, digoxin, disopyramide, ergotamine, hexobarbital, lova-

---

statin, phenytoin, triazolam, and valproate have been reported to interact with erythromycin products. It's unknown whether these same drugs interact with dirithromycin. Until further data are available, use caution during coadministration.
Drug-food. *Any food:* increased absorption. Administer drug with food.

EFFECTS ON DIAGNOSTIC TESTS
None reported.

CONTRAINDICATIONS
Contraindicated in patients with hypersensitivity to drug, erythromycin, or other macrolide antibiotics.

NURSING CONSIDERATIONS
• Use cautiously in patients with hepatic insufficiency and in breast-feeding women. Monitor liver function test results.
• Safety of drug in children under 12 years has not been established.
• Obtain culture and sensitivity results to ensure organism is sensitive to dirithromycin. Drug is not recommended for empiric use.
• Be aware that drug should not be used in patients with known, suspected, or potential bacteremias because serum levels are inadequate to provide antibacterial coverage of organisms within the bloodstream.
• Administer drug with food or within 1 hour of food intake.
• Monitor patient for superinfection. Drug may cause overgrowth of nonsusceptible bacteria or fungi.

☑ **Patient teaching**
• Tell patient to take drug as prescribed, even after he feels better.
• Instruct patient to take drug with food or within 1 hour after eating and not to cut, chew, or crush the tablet.

erythromycin base
Apo-Erythro†, EMU-V Tablets‡, E-Mycin, Eramycin, Erybid†, Eryc, Erythromid†, Erythromycin Base Filmtab, Erythromycin Delayed-Release, Novo-Rythro Encap†, PCE Dispertab, Robimycin

erythromycin estolate
Ilosone, Ilosone Pulvules, Novo-Rythro†

erythromycin ethylsuccinate
Apo-Erythro-ES†, E.E.S., EES-400‡, EES granules‡, Erymin§, EryPed, EryPed 200, EryPed 400, Erythroped§, Erythroped A§, Novo-Rythro†

erythromycin lactobionate
Erythrocin, Erythromycin Lactobionate

erythromycin stearate
Apo-Erythro-S†, Erythrocin Stearate, Novo-Rythro†

Pregnancy Risk Category: B

HOW SUPPLIED
erythromycin base
Tablets (enteric-coated): 250 mg, 333 mg, 500 mg
Tablets (filmtabs): 250 mg, 500 mg
Capsules (enteric-coated): 250 mg
erythromycin estolate
Tablets: 500 mg
Capsules: 250 mg
Oral suspension: 125 mg/5 ml, 250 mg/5 ml
erythromycin ethylsuccinate
Tablets (film-coated): 400 mg
Tablets (chewable): 200 mg
Oral suspension: 200 mg/5 ml, 400 mg/5 ml, 100 mg/2.5 ml
erythromycin lactobionate
Injection: 500-mg, 1-g vials
erythromycin stearate
Tablets (film-coated): 250 mg, 500 mg

ACTION
Inhibits bacterial protein synthesis by binding to the 50S subunit of the ribo-

some. Bacteriostatic or bactericidal, depending on concentration.

Route	Onset	Peak	Duration
PO	Unknown	1-4 hr	Unknown
IV	Unknown	Immediate	Unknown

INDICATIONS & DOSAGE

Acute pelvic inflammatory disease caused by Neisseria gonorrhoeae—
Adults: 500 mg I.V. (lactobionate) q 6 hours for 3 days, then 250 mg (base, estolate, stearate) or 400 mg (ethylsuccinate) P.O. q 6 hours for 7 days.
Endocarditis prophylaxis for dental procedures in patients allergic to penicillin—
Adults: initially, 1,600 mg (ethylsuccinate) or 1 g (base, estolate, stearate) P.O. 1½ to 2 hours before procedure; then 800 mg (ethylsuccinate) or 500 mg (base, estolate, stearate) P.O. 6 hours later.
Children: initially, 20 mg/kg (base, ethylsuccinate, stearate) P.O. 1½ to 2 hours before procedure; then half the initial dose 6 hours later.
Intestinal amebiasis due to Entamoeba histolytica—
Adults: 400 mg P.O. (ethylsuccinate) q.i.d. for 10 to 14 days. I.V. therapy not effective.
Children: 30 to 50 mg/kg (ethylsuccinate) P.O. daily, in divided doses, for 10 to 14 days. I.V. therapy not effective.
Erythrasma—
Adults: 250 mg P.O. (base, estolate, stearate) t.i.d. for 21 days.
Rheumatic fever prophylaxis—
Adults: 250 mg (base, estolate, stearate) P.O. q 12 hours.
Mild to moderately severe respiratory tract, skin, and soft-tissue infections caused by sensitive group A beta-hemolytic streptococci, Streptococcus pneumoniae, Mycoplasma pneumoniae, Corynebacterium diphtheriae, *or* Bordetella pertussis—
Adults: 250 to 500 mg (base, estolate, stearate) P.O. q 6 hours; or 400 to 800 mg (ethylsuccinate) P.O. q 6 hours; or 15 to 20 mg/kg I.V. daily, as continuous infusion or in divided doses q 6 hours for 10 days (3 weeks for *Mycoplasma* infection).
Children: 30 to 50 mg/kg (oral erythromycin salts) P.O. daily, in divided doses q

6 hours; or 15 to 20 mg/kg I.V. daily, in divided doses q 4 to 6 hours for 10 days (3 weeks for *Mycoplasma* infection).
Listeria monocytogenes *infection—*
Adults: 250 mg (base, estolate, stearate) P.O. q 6 hours or 500 mg P.O. q 12 hours.
Nongonococcal urethritis due to Ureaplasma urealyticum—
Adults: 500 mg (base, estolate, stearate) P.O. q 6 hours for at least 7 days.
Syphilis in patients allergic to penicillin—
Adults: 500 mg (base, estolate, stearate) P.O. q.i.d. for 10 days.
Legionnaires' disease—
Adults: 500 mg to 1 g I.V. or P.O. (base, estolate, stearate) or 800 to 1,600 mg (ethylsuccinate) q 6 hours for 21 days.
Uncomplicated urethral, endocervical, or rectal infections due to Chlamydia trachomatis *when tetracyclines are contraindicated—*
Adults: 500 mg (base, estolate, stearate) or 800 mg (ethylsuccinate) P.O. q.i.d. for 14 days.
Urogenital C. trachomatis *infections during pregnancy—*
Adults: 500 mg (base, estolate, stearate) P.O. q.i.d. for at least 7 days or 250 mg (base, estolate, stearate) or 400 mg (ethylsuccinate) P.O. q.i.d. for at least 14 days.
Conjunctivitis caused by C. trachomatis *in neonates—*
Neonates: 50 mg/kg (base, estolate, stearate) P.O. daily in four divided doses for 14 days.
Pneumonia in infants caused by C. trachomatis—
Infants: 50 mg/kg/day (base, estolate, stearate) P.O. in four divided doses for 10 to 14 days or 15 to 20 mg/kg/day (lactobionate) I.V. as a continuous infusion or in 4 divided doses

ADVERSE REACTIONS

CV: *ventricular arrhythmias.*
EENT: hearing loss (with high I.V. doses).
GI: *abdominal pain and cramping, nausea, vomiting, diarrhea.*
Hepatic: cholestatic jaundice (with erythromycin estolate).
Skin: urticaria, rash, eczema.
Other: overgrowth of nonsusceptible bac-

teria or fungi; *anaphylaxis;* fever; *vein irritation, thrombophlebitis* (after I.V. injection).

INTERACTIONS
Drug-drug. *Astemizole:* decreased metabolism, leading to increased levels of these antihistamines and cardiotoxicity. Avoid concomitant use.
Carbamazepine: increased carbamazepine blood levels and increased risk of toxicity. Monitor closely.
Cisapride: may increase cisapride concentrations leading to toxicity including arrhythmias.
Clindamycin, lincomycin: may be antagonistic. Don't use together.
Cyclosporine: increased concentrations of cyclosporine. Monitor closely.
Digoxin: increased serum digoxin levels. Monitor for digoxin toxicity.
Disopyramide: increased disopyramide plasma levels resulting, in some cases, in arrhythmias and increased QT intervals. Monitor ECG.
Midazolam, triazolam: increased effects of these drugs. Monitor closely.
Oral anticoagulants: increased anticoagulant effect. Monitor PT and INR closely.
Theophylline: decreased erythromycin blood level and increased theophylline toxicity. Use together cautiously.
Drug-herb. *Pill-bearing spurge:* may inhibit CYP3A enzymes affecting drug metabolism. Use together cautiously.

EFFECTS ON DIAGNOSTIC TESTS
Erythromycin may interfere with fluorometric determination of urine catecholamines. AST and ALT may become falsely elevated during erythromycin therapy (rare).

CONTRAINDICATIONS
Contraindicated in patients with hypersensitivity to drug or other macrolides. Erythromycin estolate is contraindicated in patients with hepatic disease.

NURSING CONSIDERATIONS
• Use erythromycin salts cautiously in patients with impaired hepatic function. Monitor liver function test results.
• Be aware that erythromycin estolate is not recommended during pregnancy because of the potential adverse effects on the mother and the fetus.
• Obtain urine specimen for culture and sensitivity tests before giving first dose. Therapy may begin pending results.
• When administering suspension, be sure to note the concentration.
• Monitor patient for superinfection. Drug may cause overgrowth of nonsusceptible bacteria or fungi.
• Monitor hepatic function (increased serum levels of alkaline phosphatase, ALT, AST, and bilirubin may occur). Erythromycin estolate may cause serious hepatotoxicity in adults (reversible cholestatic jaundice). Other erythromycin salts cause hepatotoxicity to a lesser degree.
• Keep in mind that drug may falsely elevate concentrations of urinary 17-hydroxycorticosteroids and 17-ketosteroids.
• Be aware that drug may interfere with colorimetric assays, resulting in falsely elevated AST and ALT levels.
• Keep in mind that coated tablets or encapsulated pellets have caused fewer instances of GI upset; they may be better tolerated by patients who cannot tolerate erythromycin.
• Know that drug is not indicated for the treatment of neurosyphilis.

◖ I.V. administration
• Reconstitute according to manufacturer's directions and dilute each 250 mg in at least 100 ml of 0.9% NaCl solution. Infuse over 1 hour.
Alert: Do not administer erythromycin lactobionate with other drugs.

✓ Patient teaching
• Tell patient to take drug as prescribed, even after he feels better.
• Instruct patient to take oral form of drug with full glass of water 1 hour before or 2 hours after meals for best absorption. Drug may be taken with food if GI upset occurs. Coated tablets may be taken with meals. Tell patient not to drink fruit juice with drug. Chewable erythromycin tablets should not be swallowed whole.
• Instruct patient to report adverse reactions, especially nausea, abdominal pain, and fever.

Reactions may be *common*, uncommon, *life-threatening*, or COMMON AND LIFE-THREATENING.

19
Miscellaneous anti-infectives

aztreonam
bacitracin
chloramphenicol sodium succinate
clindamycin hydrochloride
clindamycin palmitate
   hydrochloride
clindamycin phosphate
fosfomycin tromethamine
imipenem/cilastatin sodium
meropenem
nitrofurantoin macrocrystals
nitrofurantoin microcrystals
spectinomycin hydrochloride
trimethoprim
trimetrexate glucuronate
vancomycin hydrochloride

COMBINATION PRODUCTS
MACROBID: nitrofurantoin macrocrystals 25 mg and nitrofurantoin monohydrate 75 mg.

---

aztreonam
Azactam

Pregnancy Risk Category: B

HOW SUPPLIED
Injection: 500-mg vials, 1-g vials, 2-g vials

ACTION
Inhibits bacterial cell-wall synthesis, ultimately causing cell-wall destruction; bactericidal.

Route	Onset	Peak	Duration
IV	Unknown	Immediate	Unknown
IM	Unknown	< 1 hr	Unknown

INDICATIONS & DOSAGE
Urinary tract infections, lower respiratory tract infections, septicemia, skin and skin-structure infections, intra-abdominal infections, surgical infections, and gynecologic infections caused by susceptible strains of the following gram-negative aerobic organisms: Escherichia coli, Klebsiella pneumoniae, Proteus mirabilis, Pseudomonas aeruginosa, Enterobacter cloacae, Klebsiella oxytoca, *and* Citrobacter *species,* Serratia marcescens; *also respiratory infections caused by* Haemophilus influenzae—
Adults: 500 mg to 2 g I.V. or I.M. q 8 to 12 hours. For severe systemic or life-threatening infections, 2 g q 6 to 8 hours may be given. Maximum dosage is 8 g daily.
Children 9 months to 15 years: 30 mg/kg q 6 to 8 hours I.V. Maximum dose is 120 mg/kg/day.
Adjust-a-dose: In adults with renal impairment, if creatinine clearance is 10 to 30 ml/minute, dosage is 1 to 2 g, followed by 50% usual dose at the usual interval. If clearance is less than 10 ml/minute, 500 mg to 2 g followed by 25% usual dose at usual interval. For adults with alcoholic cirrhosis, decrease dose by 20% to 25%.

ADVERSE REACTIONS
CNS: *seizures,* headache, insomnia, confusion.
CV: hypotension.
GI: diarrhea, nausea, vomiting, pseudomembranous colitis.
GU: increased BUN and serum creatinine concentrations.
Hematologic: *neutropenia,* anemia, *pancytopenia, thrombocytopenia,* leukocytosis, thrombocytosis, prolonged PT, INR, and PTT.
Hepatic: transient elevation of ALT and AST.
Other: hypersensitivity reactions (rash, *anaphylaxis*), thrombophlebitis (at I.V. site), discomfort and swelling (at I.M. injection site), increased LD.

INTERACTIONS
Drug-drug. *Aminoglycosides, beta-lactam antibiotics, other anti-infectives:* synergistic effectiveness. Avoid concomitant use.
Cefoxitin, imipenem: possible antagonistic effect. Avoid concomitant use.
Probenecid: increased serum aztreonam levels. Avoid concomitant use.

---

*Liquid contains alcohol. **May contain tartrazine. †Canada ‡Australia §U.K. ◇OTC

EFFECTS ON DIAGNOSTIC TESTS
Drug therapy alters urine glucose determinations using cupric sulfate (Clinitest or Benedict's reagent). Coombs' test results may become positive during therapy.

CONTRAINDICATIONS
Contraindicated in patients with hypersensitivity to drug.

NURSING CONSIDERATIONS
• Use cautiously in elderly patients and in those with impaired renal function. Dosage adjustment may be necessary. Monitor renal function tests.
• Obtain culture and sensitivity tests before giving first dose. Therapy may begin pending results.
• Administer I.M. injections deep into a large muscle mass, such as the upper outer quadrant of the gluteus maximus or the lateral aspect of the thigh. Doses exceeding 1 g should be given I.V.
• Do not give I.M. injection to pediatric patients.
• Observe patient for signs of superinfection.
• Because drug is ineffective against gram-positive and anaerobic organisms, anticipate using it with other antibiotics for immediate treatment of life-threatening illnesses. Aztreonam is a narrow-spectrum antibiotic, effective only against gram-negative organisms.
• Be aware that patients who are allergic to penicillins or cephalosporins may not be allergic to aztreonam. However, close monitoring of those who have had an immediate hypersensitivity reaction to these antibiotics is recommended.

◖I.V. administration
• To administer a bolus of aztreonam, inject drug slowly (over 3 to 5 minutes) directly into a vein or I.V. tubing. Give infusions over 20 minutes to 1 hour.

✓Patient teaching
• Warn patient receiving I.M. drug that pain and swelling at the injection site may occur.
• Tell patient to alert nurse if discomfort occurs at I.V. insertion site.

• Instruct patient to report adverse reactions and signs of superinfection promptly.

---

bacitracin
Baciguent, BACI-IM, Bacitin†

Pregnancy Risk Category: C

HOW SUPPLIED
Injection: 50,000-unit vials

ACTION
Hinders bacterial cell-wall synthesis, damaging the bacterial plasma membrane and making the cell more vulnerable to osmotic pressure.

Route	Onset	Peak	Duration
IM	Unknown	1-2 hr	Unknown

INDICATIONS & DOSAGE
Pneumonia or empyema caused by susceptible staphylococci—
Infants weighing over 2.5 kg (5.5 lb): 1,000 units/kg I.M. daily, divided q 8 to 12 hours.
Infants weighing under 2.5 kg: 900 units/kg I.M. daily, divided q 8 to 12 hours.

ADVERSE REACTIONS
EENT: ototoxicity.
GI: nausea, vomiting.
GU: *nephrotoxicity (albuminuria,* cylindruria, oliguria, anuria, increased BUN, *tubular and glomerular necrosis*) increased BUN and serum creatinine.
Skin: urticaria, rash.
Other: pain (at injection site).

INTERACTIONS
Drug-drug. *Nephrotoxic drugs (such as aminoglycosides):* increased nephrotoxicity. Use together cautiously.
Neuromuscular blockers, inhalation anesthetics: prolonged muscle weakness. Monitor patient for excessive muscle weakness or respiratory distress.

EFFECTS ON DIAGNOSTIC TESTS
Urinary sediment tests may show increased protein and cast excretion.

CONTRAINDICATIONS

Contraindicated in patients with impaired renal function or hypersensitivity to drug. Because of significant risk of neurotoxicity, limit I.M. use to infants with staphylococcal pneumonia.

NURSING CONSIDERATIONS

• Use cautiously in patients with myasthenia gravis and neuromuscular disease.
• Obtain culture and sensitivity tests before giving first dose.
• Assess baseline renal function studies before and during therapy.
• Administer by deep I.M. injection only.
• Know that concentration of bacitracin should be between 5,000 and 10,000 units/ml. Reconstitute 50,000-unit vial with 9.8 ml of diluent. Store in refrigerator. Drug is inactivated if stored at room temperature.
• Maintain adequate fluid intake, and monitor urine output closely.
• Provide measures to keep urine pH above 6 to reduce risk of nephrotoxicity.
• Be aware that prolonged therapy may result in overgrowth of nonsusceptible organisms, especially *Candida albicans.*

☑ **Patient teaching**
• Warn patient that injection may be painful.
• Instruct patient to report adverse reactions promptly.

---

chloramphenicol sodium succinate
Chloromycetin Sodium Succinate, Kemicetine§, Pentamycetin†

Pregnancy Risk Category: C

HOW SUPPLIED
Injection: 1-g vial

ACTION
Inhibits bacterial protein synthesis by binding to the 50S subunit of the ribosome; bacteriostatic.

Route	Onset	Peak	Duration
IV	Unknown	1-3 hr	Unknown

INDICATIONS & DOSAGE
Haemophilus influenzae meningitis, acute Salmonella typhi *infection, and meningitis, bacteremia, or other severe infections caused by sensitive* Salmonella *species,* Rickettsia, *lymphogranuloma, psittacosis, or various sensitive gram-negative organisms—*
Adults: 50 to 100 mg/kg I.V. daily, divided q 6 hours. Maximum dosage is 100 mg/kg daily.
Full-term infants older than 2 weeks with normal metabolic processes: up to 50 mg/kg I.V. daily, divided q 6 hours.
Premature infants, neonates 2 weeks or younger, and children and infants with immature metabolic processes: 25 mg/kg I.V. once daily. I.V. route must be used to treat meningitis.

ADVERSE REACTIONS
CNS: headache, mild depression, confusion, delirium, peripheral neuropathy with prolonged therapy.
EENT: optic neuritis (in patients with cystic fibrosis), glossitis, decreased visual acuity.
GI: nausea, vomiting, stomatitis, diarrhea, enterocolitis.
Hematologic: *aplastic anemia, hypoplastic anemia, granulocytopenia, thrombocytopenia.*
Other: hypersensitivity reactions (fever, rash, urticaria, *anaphylaxis*), jaundice, *gray syndrome in neonates (abdominal distention, gray cyanosis, vasomotor collapse, respiratory distress, death within few hours of onset of symptoms).*

INTERACTIONS
Drug-drug. *Anticoagulants, barbiturates, hydantoins, iron salts, sulfonylureas:* increased blood levels of these agents possible. Monitor for toxicity.
Penicillins: synergistic effects may develop in the treatment of certain microorganisms, but antagonism may also occur. Monitor effectiveness closely.
Rifampin: may reduce chloramphenicol levels. Monitor for changes in effectiveness.
Vitamin B_{12}: may decrease response of vitamin B in patients with pernicious anemia. Monitor closely.

EFFECTS ON DIAGNOSTIC TESTS

False elevation of urine PABA levels will result if chloramphenicol is administered during a bentiromide test for pancreatic function. Treatment with chloramphenicol will cause false-positive results on tests for urine glucose using cupric sulfate (Clinitest). Erythrocyte, platelet, and leukocyte counts in the blood and possibly the bone marrow may decrease during chloramphenicol therapy (from reversible or irreversible bone marrow depression). Hemoglobinuria or lactic acidosis may also occur.

CONTRAINDICATIONS

Contraindicated in patients with hypersensitivity to drug.

NURSING CONSIDERATIONS

• Use cautiously in patients with impaired hepatic or renal function, acute intermittent porphyria, and G6PD deficiency and with other drugs that cause bone marrow suppression or blood disorders.
• Obtain specimen for culture and sensitivity tests before giving first dose. Therapy may begin pending results.
• Obtain plasma concentration levels. Therapeutic plasma concentrations are as follows: peak, 10 to 20 mcg/ml; trough, 5 to 10 mcg/ml.
• Monitor CBC, platelets, serum iron, and reticulocytes before and every 2 days during therapy, as ordered. Stop drug immediately if anemia, reticulocytopenia, leukopenia, or thrombocytopenia develops, and notify doctor.
• Monitor for evidence of superinfection.

◖ I.V. administration
• Give I.V. slowly over at least 1 minute. Check injection site daily for phlebitis and irritation.
• Reconstitute 1-g vial of powder for injection with 10 ml of sterile water for injection. Concentration will be 100 mg/ml. Stable for 30 days at room temperature, but refrigeration recommended. Do not use cloudy solutions.

☑ Patient teaching
• Instruct patient to notify doctor if adverse reactions occur, especially nausea, vomiting, diarrhea, fever, confusion, sore throat, or mouth sores.
• Tell patient receiving drug I.V. to alert nurse if discomfort occurs at I.V. insertion site.
• Instruct patient to report symptoms of superinfection.

---

clindamycin hydrochloride
Cleocin HCl, Dalacin C†‡

clindamycin palmitate hydrochloride
Cleocin Pediatric, Dalacin C Palmitate†‡

clindamycin phosphate
Cleocin Phosphate, Dalacin C†‡, Dalacin C Phosphate†‡

Pregnancy Risk Category: B

HOW SUPPLIED
clindamycin hydrochloride
Capsules: 75 mg, 150 mg, 300 mg
clindamycin palmitate hydrochloride
Granules for oral solution: 75 mg/5 ml
clindamycin phosphate
Injection: 150 mg base/ml, 300 mg base/2 ml, 600 mg base/4 ml, 900 mg base/6 ml, 9,000 mg base/60 ml
Injectable infusion (in 5% dextrose): 300 mg (50 ml), 600 mg (50 ml), 900 mg (50 ml)

ACTION
Inhibits bacterial protein synthesis by binding to the 50S subunit of the ribosome.

Route	Onset	Peak	Duration
PO	Unknown	45-60 min	Unknown
IV	Unknown	Immediate	Unknown
IM	Unknown	3 hr	Unknown

INDICATIONS & DOSAGE
Infections caused by sensitive staphylococci, streptococci, pneumococci, Bacteroides, Fusobacterium, Clostridium perfringens, *and other sensitive aerobic and anaerobic organisms*—
Adults: 150 to 450 mg P.O. q 6 hours; or

---

300 to 600 mg I.M. or I.V. q 6, 8, or 12 hours.

Children over 1 month: 8 to 20 mg/kg P.O. daily, in divided doses q 6 to 8 hours; or 15 to 40 mg/kg I.M. or I.V. daily, in divided doses q 6 or 8 hours.

Pelvic inflammatory disease—

Adults: 900 mg I.V. q 8 hours with gentamicin. Continue at least 48 hours after improvement in symptoms; then switch to oral clindamycin 450 mg 4 times daily for a total course of 10 to 14 days or doxycycline 100 mg P.O. q 12 hours for total of 10 to 14 days.

Pneumocystis carinii *pneumonia—*

Adults: 600 mg I.V. q 6 hours or 300 to 450 mg P.O. q 6 hours with primaquine.

ADVERSE REACTIONS

GI: *nausea,* vomiting, abdominal pain, *diarrhea, pseudomembranous colitis.*
Hematologic: *transient leukopenia,* eosinophilia, *thrombocytopenia.*
Hepatic: jaundice; transient increases in serum bilirubin, alkaline phosphatase, and AST.
Skin: maculopapular rash, urticaria.
Other: *anaphylaxis,* thrombophlebitis.

INTERACTIONS

Drug-drug. *Erythromycin:* may block access of clindamycin to its site of action. Avoid concomitant use.
Kaolin: decreased absorption of oral clindamycin. Separate administration times.
Neuromuscular blockers: potentiated neuromuscular blockade possible. Monitor closely.
Drug-food. *Diet foods with sodium cyclamate:* decreased serum concentration of drug. Do not use together.

EFFECTS ON DIAGNOSTIC TESTS
None reported.

CONTRAINDICATIONS
Contraindicated in patients with hypersensitivity to drug or lincomycin.

NURSING CONSIDERATIONS
• Use cautiously in neonates and patients with renal or hepatic disease, asthma, history of GI disease, or significant allergies.

• Know that drug does not penetrate blood-brain barrier.
• Obtain culture and sensitivity tests before giving first dose. Therapy may begin pending results.
• For I.M. administration, inject deeply. Rotate sites. Doses over 600 mg per injection are not recommended.
• Be aware that I.M. injection may raise CK in response to muscle irritation.
• Don't refrigerate reconstituted oral solution because it will thicken. Drug is stable for 2 weeks at room temperature.
• Monitor renal, hepatic, and hematopoietic functions during prolonged therapy, as ordered.
• Observe patient for signs of superinfection.
Alert: Don't give opioid antidiarrheals to treat drug-induced diarrhea. They may prolong and worsen diarrhea.

I.V. administration
• When giving I.V., check site daily for phlebitis and irritation. For I.V. infusion, dilute each 300 mg in 50 ml solution, and give no faster than 30 mg/minute (over 10 to 60 minutes). Never give undiluted as a bolus.

Patient teaching
• Advise patient taking the capsule form to take it with a full glass of water to prevent esophageal irritation.
• Warn patient that I.M. injection may be painful.
• Tell patient to alert nurse if discomfort occurs at I.V. insertion site.
• Instruct patient to report adverse reactions, especially diarrhea, to the doctor. Warn him not to treat such diarrhea himself.

fosfomycin tromethamine
Monurol

Pregnancy Risk Category: B

HOW SUPPLIED
Single-dose sachet: 3 g

ACTION
Bactericidal; inhibits bacterial cell-wall

synthesis. It is effective in the urinary tract because it reduces adherence of bacteria to uroepithelial cells.

Route	Onset	Peak	Duration
PO	Unknown	2 hr	Unknown

INDICATIONS & DOSAGE
Uncomplicated urinary tract infections (acute cystitis) caused by susceptible strains of Escherichia coli *and* Enterococcus faecalis *in women—*
Women over 18 years: 1 sachet P.O. mixed with cold water just before ingestion.

ADVERSE REACTIONS
CNS: headache, dizziness, asthenia.
GI: diarrhea, nausea, dyspepsia, abdominal pain.
GU: vaginitis, *dysmenorrhea.*
Other: rhinitis, *rash, back pain.*

INTERACTIONS
Drug-drug. *Metoclopramide:* reduced serum concentration of fosfomycin. Avoid concomitant use.

EFFECTS ON DIAGNOSTIC TESTS
None reported.

CONTRAINDICATIONS
Contraindicated in patients with known hypersensitivity to drug.

NURSING CONSIDERATIONS
• Use cautiously in patients with renal impairment.
• Know that fosfomycin should not be used during pregnancy unless clearly needed. Breast-feeding women should not take drug.
• Know that safety and effectiveness in children 12 years and less have not been established.
• Obtain urine specimens for culture and sensitivity before and after therapy has been completed.
• Know that using more than one single-dose sachet to treat a single episode of acute cystitis will not improve clinical success and may cause adverse reactions.

✅ Patient teaching
• Instruct patient about the proper way to take fosfomycin. Drug should not be taken in its dry form. The entire contents of a single-dose sachet should be mixed with 3 to 4 oz (½ cup) cold water. Stir to dissolve, and drink immediately.
• Tell patient to notify the doctor if symptoms have not improved in 2 to 3 days.

---

imipenem/cilastatin sodium
Primaxin IM, Primaxin IV

Pregnancy Risk Category: C

HOW SUPPLIED
Powder for injection: 250 mg, 500 mg, 750 mg

ACTION
Imipenem is bactericidal and inhibits bacterial cell-wall synthesis. Cilastatin inhibits the enzymatic breakdown of imipenem in the kidneys, thereby achieving adequate antibacterial levels of imipenem in the urine.

Route	Onset	Peak	Duration
IV	Unknown	Immediate	Unknown
IM	Unknown	1-2 hr	Unknown

INDICATIONS & DOSAGE
Serious infections of the lower respiratory and urinary tracts, intra-abdominal and gynecologic infections, bacterial septicemia, bone and joint infections, skin and soft-tissue infections, and endocarditis. Most known microorganisms are susceptible: Acinetobacter, Enterococcus, Staphylococcus, Streptococcus, Escherichia coli, Haemophilus, Klebsiella, Morganella, Proteus, Enterobacter, Pseudomonas aeruginosa, *and* Bacteroides, *including* B. fragilis—
Adults weighing over 70 kg (154 lb): 250 mg to 1 g by I.V. infusion q 6 to 8 hours. Maximum daily dosage is 50 mg/kg/day or 4 g/day, whichever is less. Alternatively, 500 to 750 mg I.M. q 12 hours. Maximum daily dosage is 1,500 mg/day.
Adjust-a-dose: In children over 12 years, patients weighing below 70 kg, or those

who are renally impaired, refer to package insert for dosage adjustments based on weight, creatinine clearance, and severity of infection.

ADVERSE REACTIONS
CNS: *seizures,* dizziness, somnolence.
CV: hypotension.
GI: nausea, vomiting, diarrhea, *pseudomembranous colitis.*
GU: increased BUN, or creatinine.
Hematologic: eosinophilia, *thrombocytopenia, leukopenia.*
Hepatic: transient increases in AST, ALT, alkaline phosphatase, and bilirubin.
Skin: rash, urticaria, pruritus.
Other: *hypersensitivity reactions (anaphylaxis),* fever; increased LD; thrombophlebitis, pain (at injection site).

INTERACTIONS
Drug-drug. *Aminoglycosides:* synergistic effect. Monitor closely.
Beta-lactam antibiotics: possible in vitro antagonism. Avoid concomitant use.
Ganciclovir: may cause seizures. Avoid concomitant use.
Probenecid: increased serum concentrations of cilastatin. Avoid concomitant use.

EFFECTS ON DIAGNOSTIC TESTS
Drug may interfere with glucose determination by Benedict's solution or Clinitest.

CONTRAINDICATIONS
Contraindicated in patients with hypersensitivity to drug.

NURSING CONSIDERATIONS
• Use cautiously in patients allergic to penicillins or cephalosporins because drug has similar properties.
• Also use cautiously in patients with history of seizure disorders, especially if they also have compromised renal function.
• Use with caution in children under 3 months.
• Obtain culture and sensitivity tests before giving first dose. Therapy may begin pending results.
• Adjust dosage for patients with a creatinine clearance below 70 ml/minute. Monitor renal function tests.

Alert: If seizures develop and persist despite anticonvulsant therapy, notify doctor; drug should then be discontinued.
• Monitor patient for bacterial or fungal superinfections and resistant infections during and after therapy.

I.V. administration
• Don't administer by direct I.V. bolus injection. Each 250- or 500-mg dose should be given by I.V. infusion over 20 to 30 minutes. Each 1-g dose should be infused over 40 to 60 minutes. If nausea occurs, the infusion may be slowed.
• When reconstituting powder, shake until the solution is clear. Solutions may range from colorless to yellow, and variations of color within this range do not affect drug's potency. After reconstitution, solution is stable for 10 hours at room temperature and for 48 hours when refrigerated.

✔ Patient teaching
• Instruct patient to report adverse reactions promptly.
• Tell patient to alert nurse if discomfort occurs at I.V. insertion site.
• Inform patient to notify doctor if loose stools or diarrhea occurs.

meropenem
Meronem§, Merrem IV

Pregnancy Risk Category: B

HOW SUPPLIED
Powder for injection: 500 mg/15 ml, 500 mg/20 ml, 500 mg/100 ml, 1 g/15 ml, 1 g/30 ml, 1 g/100 ml

ACTION
Meropenem inhibits cell-wall synthesis in bacteria. It readily penetrates cell wall of most gram-positive and gram-negative bacteria to reach penicillin-binding-protein targets.

Route	Onset	Peak	Duration
IV	Unknown	1 hr	Unknown

INDICATIONS & DOSAGE
Complicated appendicitis and peritonitis caused by viridans group streptococci,

Escherichia coli, Klebsiella pneumoniae, Pseudomonas aeruginosa, Bacteroides fragilis, Bacteroides thetaiotaomicron, *and* Peptostreptococcus *species; bacterial meningitis (pediatric patients only) caused by* Streptococcus pneumoniae, Haemophilus influenzae, *and* Neisseria meningitidis—

Adults: 1 g I.V. q 8 hours over 15 to 30 minutes as I.V. infusion or over 3 to 5 minutes as I.V. bolus injection (5 to 20 ml).

Children 3 months and older, weighing below 50 kg (110 lb): 20 mg/kg (intra-abdominal infection) or 40 mg/kg (bacterial meningitis) q 8 hours over 15 to 30 minutes as I.V. infusion or over 3 to 5 minutes as I.V. bolus injection (5 to 20 ml). Maximum dosage is 2 g I.V. q 8 hours.

Children weighing over 50 kg: 1 g I.V. q 8 hours for intra-abdominal infections and 2 g I.V. q 8 hours for meningitis.

Adjust-a-dose: In patients with renal insufficiency or renal failure with creatinine clearance of 26 to 50 ml/minute, usual dose q 12 hours; if clearance is 10 to 25 ml/minute, half the usual dose q 12 hours; and if it is less than 10 ml/minute, half the usual dose q 24 hours.

ADVERSE REACTIONS

CNS: *seizures,* headache.
GI: diarrhea, nausea, vomiting, constipation, pseudomembranous colitis, oral candidiasis, glossitis.
GU: increased creatinine or BUN levels, presence of RBCs in urine.
Hematologic: increased or decreased platelet count, increased eosinophil count, positive direct or indirect Coombs' test, decreased hemoglobin level or hematocrit, decreased WBC count, prolonged or shortened PT, INR, or PTT.
Hepatic: increased levels of ALT, AST, alkaline phosphatase, LD, and bilirubin.
Respiratory: *apnea,* dyspnea.
Skin: rash, pruritus.
Other: *hypersensitivity, anaphylactic reaction;* inflammation, phlebitis, thrombophlebitis (at injection site).

INTERACTIONS

Drug-drug. *Probenecid:* inhibited renal excretion of meropenem. Drug competes with meropenem for active tubular secretion, which significantly increases elimination half-life of drug and the extent of systemic exposure. Concomitant administration of probenecid with meropenem is not recommended.

EFFECTS ON DIAGNOSTIC TESTS
Drug may cause a positive direct or indirect Coombs' test.

CONTRAINDICATIONS
Contraindicated in patients with hypersensitivity to component of drug or other drugs in same class and in those who have demonstrated anaphylactic reactions to beta-lactams.

NURSING CONSIDERATIONS
• Use cautiously in the elderly and in patients with history of seizure disorders or impaired renal function.
• Know that safety and effectiveness of drug have not been established for patients under 3 months.
• Be aware that it is not known whether meropenem is excreted in breast milk. Use drug cautiously in breast-feeding women.
• Know that drug is not used to treat methicillin-resistant staphylococci.
• Obtain specimen for culture and sensitivity test before giving first dose. Therapy may begin pending test results.
Alert: Know that serious and occasionally fatal hypersensitivity reactions have been reported in patients receiving therapy with beta-lactams. Before therapy is initiated, determine whether previous hypersensitivity reactions to penicillins, cephalosporins, or other beta-lactams or to other allergens have occurred.
• Discontinue drug and notify doctor if an allergic reaction occurs. Serious anaphylactic reactions require immediate emergency treatment.
• Know that seizures and other CNS adverse reactions associated with meropenem therapy can occur in patients with CNS disorders, bacterial meningitis, and compromised renal function.
• If seizures occur during meropenem therapy, discontinue infusion and notify

doctor. Dosage adjustment may be ordered.

• Monitor patient for signs and symptoms of superinfection. Drug may cause overgrowth of nonsusceptible bacteria or fungi.
• Be aware that periodic assessment of organ system functions—including renal, hepatic, and hematopoietic function—is recommended during prolonged therapy.
• Monitor patient's fluid balance and weight carefully.

☐ I.V. administration
• For I.V. bolus administration, add 10 ml of sterile water for injection to 500 mg/20-ml vial size or 20 ml to 1 g/30-ml vial size. Shake to dissolve, and let stand until clear.
• For I.V. infusion, infusion vials (500 mg/100 ml and 1 g/100 ml) may be directly reconstituted with a compatible infusion fluid. Alternatively, an injection vial may be reconstituted, then the resulting solution added to an I.V. container and further diluted with an appropriate infusion fluid. Do not use ADD-Vantage vials for this purpose. For ADD-Vantage vials, constitute only with 0.45% NaCl injection, 0.9% NaCl injection, or 5% dextrose injection in 50-, 100-, or 250-ml Abbott ADD-Vantage flexible diluent containers. Follow manufacturer's guidelines closely when using ADD-Vantage vials.
• Do not mix or add meropenem to solutions containing other drugs.
• Use freshly prepared solutions of drug immediately whenever possible. Stability of drug varies with type of drug used (injection vial, infusion vial, or ADD-Vantage container). Consult manufacturer's literature for details.

☑ Patient teaching
• Advise breast-feeding patient of risk of transmitting drug to infant through breast milk.
• Instruct patient to report adverse reactions or symptoms of superinfection.

nitrofurantoin macrocrystals
Macrobid, Macrodantin

nitrofurantoin microcrystals
Apo-Nitrofurantoin†, Furadantin, Furalan, Macrodantin, Nephronex†, Novo-Furan†

Pregnancy Risk Category: B

HOW SUPPLIED
nitrofurantoin macrocrystals
Capsules: 25 mg, 50 mg, 100 mg
nitrofurantoin microcrystals
Oral suspension: 25 mg/5 ml

ACTION
Unknown. Appears to interfere with bacterial enzyme systems and possibly with bacterial cell-wall formation.

Route	Onset	Peak	Duration
PO	Unknown	Unknown	Unknown

INDICATIONS & DOSAGE
Urinary tract infections caused by susceptible Escherichia coli, Staphylococcus aureus, *enterococci; or certain strains of* Klebsiella *and* Enterobacter—
Adults and children over 12 years: 50 to 100 mg P.O. q.i.d. with meals and h.s.
Children 1 month to 12 years: 5 to 7 mg/kg P.O. daily, divided q.i.d.
Long-term suppression therapy—
Adults: 50 to 100 mg P.O. daily h.s.
Children: 1 mg/kg P.O. daily in a single dose h.s. or divided into two doses given q 12 hours.

ADVERSE REACTIONS
CNS: *peripheral neuropathy,* headache, dizziness, drowsiness, *ascending polyneuropathy with high doses or renal impairment.*
GI: *anorexia, nausea, vomiting,* abdominal pain, *diarrhea.*
Hematologic: *hemolysis in patients with G6PD deficiency* (reversed after stopping drug), *agranulocytosis, thrombocytopenia.*
Hepatic: *hepatitis, hepatic necrosis,* elevated bilirubin and alkaline phosphatase.
Respiratory: *pulmonary sensitivity reac-*

tions (cough, chest pain, fever, chills, dyspnea, pulmonary infiltration with consolidation or pleural effusion), *asthmatic attacks in patients with history of asthma.*
Skin: maculopapular, erythematous, or eczematous eruption; pruritus; urticaria; *exfoliative dermatitis; Stevens-Johnson syndrome.*
Other: hypersensitivity reactions *(anaphylaxis)*, transient alopecia, hypoglycemia, drug fever, overgrowth of nonsusceptible organisms in urinary tract.

INTERACTIONS
Drug-drug. *Magnesium-containing antacids:* decreased nitrofurantoin absorption. Separate administration times by 1 hour.
Probenecid, sulfinpyrazone: increased blood levels and decreased urine levels. May result in increased toxicity and lack of therapeutic effect. Don't use together.
Drug-food. *Any food:* increased absorption. Give drug with food.

EFFECTS ON DIAGNOSTIC TESTS
Nitrofurantoin may cause false-positive results in urine glucose tests using cupric sulfate (such as Benedict's reagent, Fehling's solution, or Clinitest) because it reacts with these agents.

CONTRAINDICATIONS
Contraindicated in children 1 month and under and in patients with moderate to severe renal impairment, anuria, oliguria, or creatinine clearance under 60 ml/minute. Contraindicated in pregnancy at term (38 to 42 weeks) and during labor and delivery.

NURSING CONSIDERATIONS
• Use cautiously in patients with renal impairment, anemia, diabetes mellitus, electrolyte abnormalities, vitamin B deficiency, debilitating disease, and G6PD deficiency.
• Obtain urine specimen for culture and sensitivity tests before starting therapy and repeat as needed. Therapy may begin pending results.
• Give with food or milk to minimize GI distress and improve absorption.

• Monitor fluid intake and output carefully. May turn urine brown or darker.
• Monitor CBC and pulmonary status regularly.
• Monitor the patient for signs of superinfection. Use of nitrofurantoin may result in growth of nonsusceptible organisms, especially *Pseudomonas.*
Alert: Know that hypersensitivity may develop when used for long-term therapy.
• Be aware that some patients may experience fewer adverse GI effects with nitrofurantoin macrocrystals.
• Know that dual-release capsules (25 mg nitrofurantoin macrocrystals combined with 75 mg nitrofurantoin monohydrate) enable patients to take drug only twice daily.
• Continue treatment for 3 days after sterile urine specimens have been obtained.
• Store drug in amber container. Keep away from metals other than stainless steel or aluminum to avoid precipitate formation.

✅ Patient teaching
• Instruct patient to take medication for as long as prescribed, exactly as directed, even after he feels better.
• Tell patient to take drug with food or milk to minimize stomach upset.
• Instruct patient to report adverse reactions.
• Alert patient that drug may turn urine a harmless dark yellow or brown color.
• Warn patient not to store drug in container made of metal other than stainless steel or aluminum.

spectinomycin hydrochloride
Trobicin

Pregnancy Risk Category: B

HOW SUPPLIED
Powder for injection: 2 g, 4 g

ACTION
Inhibits protein synthesis by binding to the 30S subunit of the ribosome.

Route	Onset	Peak	Duration
IM	Unknown	1-2 hr	Unknown

INDICATIONS & DOSAGE
Acute gonococcal urethritis and proctitis in men and cervicitis and proctitis in women. Alternative therapy for patient allergic to beta-lactam antibiotics—
Adults: 2 to 4 g I.M. single dose injected deeply into the upper outer quadrant of the buttock.
Disseminated gonococcal infection—
Adults: 2 g I.M. q 12 hours for 24 to 48 hours.

ADVERSE REACTIONS
CNS: insomnia, dizziness.
GI: nausea.
GU: decreased urine output and creatinine clearance, increased BUN.
Hematologic: decreased hemoglobin levels and hematocrit.
Hepatic: increased AST, serum alkaline phosphatase.
Skin: urticaria.
Other: *anaphylaxis*, fever, chills (may mask or delay symptoms of incubating syphilis), pain (at injection site).

INTERACTIONS
None significant.

EFFECTS ON DIAGNOSTIC TESTS
None reported.

CONTRAINDICATIONS
Contraindicated in patients with hypersensitivity to drug.

NURSING CONSIDERATIONS
● Spectinomycin isn't effective for pharyngeal gonorrhea.
● Shake vial vigorously after reconstitution and before withdrawing dose. Store at room temperature after reconstitution and use within 24 hours.
● Use 20G needle to administer drug. Divide the 4-g dose (10 ml) into two 5-ml injections—give one in each buttock.

☑ Patient teaching
● Inform patient that drug is not effective in the treatment of syphilis. Tell him that serologic test for syphilis should be done before therapy begins and for 3 months afterward.

● Tell patient to report adverse reactions promptly.
● Instruct patient to have all infection sites cultured 7 days posttreatment to confirm eradication of organism.

---

trimethoprim
Ipral§, Monotrim§, Proloprim, Trimopan§, Trimpex, Triprim‡

Pregnancy Risk Category: C

HOW SUPPLIED
Tablets: 100 mg, 200 mg

ACTION
Interferes with the action of dihydrofolate reductase, inhibiting bacterial synthesis of folic acid.

Route	Onset	Peak	Duration
PO	Unknown	1-4 hr	Unknown

INDICATIONS & DOSAGE
Uncomplicated urinary tract infections caused by susceptible strains of Escherichia coli, Proteus mirabilis, Klebsiella pneumoniae, Enterobacter *species, and coagulase-negative* Staphylococcus, *including* S. saprophyticus—
Adults: 200 mg P.O. daily as a single dose or in divided doses q 12 hours for 10 days.
Drug is not recommended for children under 12 years.
Adjust-a-dose: For patients with a creatinine clearance of 15 to 30 ml/minute, 50 mg P.O. q 12 hours; if clearance less than 15 ml/minute, do not use drug.

ADVERSE REACTIONS
GI: *epigastric distress, nausea, vomiting,* glossitis.
GU: increased BUN and serum creatinine.
Hematologic: *thrombocytopenia, leukopenia,* megaloblastic anemia, methemoglobinemia.
Hepatic: elevated liver function test results.
Skin: *rash, pruritus, exfoliative dermatitis.*
Other: fever.

INTERACTIONS
Drug-drug. *Phenytoin:* may decrease

phenytoin metabolism and increase its serum levels. Monitor for toxicity.

EFFECTS ON DIAGNOSTIC TESTS
Drug interferes with serum methotrexate assays.

CONTRAINDICATIONS
Contraindicated in patients with hypersensitivity to drug and in those with documented megaloblastic anemia caused by folate deficiency.

NURSING CONSIDERATIONS
• Use cautiously in patients with impaired hepatic or renal function. Dosage should be decreased in patients with severely impaired renal function. Also use cautiously in patients with possible folate deficiency. Monitor renal and liver function test results.
• Obtain urine specimen for culture and sensitivity tests before giving first dose. Therapy may begin pending results.
• Monitor CBC routinely. Clinical signs, such as sore throat, fever, pallor, or purpura, may be early indications of serious blood disorders.
• Monitor patient's fluid balance.
Alert: Prolonged use of trimethoprim at high doses may cause bone marrow suppression.
• Keep in mind that, because resistance to trimethoprim develops rapidly when administered alone, it is usually given in combination with other drugs.

☑ **Patient teaching**
• Instruct patient to take entire amount of drug, as prescribed, even after he feels better.
• Tell patient to report adverse reactions promptly, especially signs of infection or unusual bruising.
• Inform patient of the need for adequate hydration during therapy.

---

trimetrexate glucuronate
Neutrexin

Pregnancy Risk Category: D

HOW SUPPLIED
Injection: 25-mg vials, parenteral kit with leucovorin calcium, 50-mg vial

ACTION
Prevents reduction of folic acid to tetrahydrofolate by binding to dihydrofolate reductase.

Route	Onset	Peak	Duration
IV	Unknown	Unknown	Unknown

INDICATIONS & DOSAGE
Alternative treatment of moderate to severe Pneumocystis carinii *pneumonia in immunocompromised patients, including HIV-infected patients who are intolerant or refractory to co-trimoxazole—*
Adults: 45 mg/m^2 I.V. infusion over 60 minutes daily for 21 days, administered with 20 mg/m^2 of leucovorin I.V. or P.O. q 6 hours for 24 days.

ADVERSE REACTIONS
GI: nausea, vomiting, stomatitis.
Hematologic: *neutropenia, thrombocytopenia, anemia.*
Hepatic: *hepatotoxicity.*
Skin: rash.
Other: *increased creatinine, hyponatremia, hypocalcemia,* fever.

INTERACTIONS
Drug-drug. *Acetaminophen, cimetidine, clotrimazole, erythromycin, fluconazole, ketoconazole, miconazole, rifampin, rifabutin:* may interfere with trimetrexate metabolism and lead to toxicity. Monitor closely.
Chloride-containing solutions, leucovorin: precipitate will form if mixed with trimetrexate. Administer separately.
Hepatotoxic, myelosuppressive, or nephrotoxic drugs: enhanced toxicity. Use together cautiously and monitor closely.

EFFECTS ON DIAGNOSTIC TESTS
None reported.

CONTRAINDICATIONS
Contraindicated in patients with hypersensitivity to trimetrexate, methotrexate, or leucovorin.

Reactions may be *common,* uncommon, *__life-threatening,__* or COMMON AND LIFE-THREATENING.

NURSING CONSIDERATIONS
• Use cautiously in patients with impaired hematologic, renal, or hepatic function and in women of childbearing age because drug may cause fetal harm. Avoid using during pregnancy.
• Follow institutional policy when administering parenteral form of drug because this form is associated with carcinogenic, mutagenic, and teratogenic risks for personnel.
Alert: Know that leucovorin therapy must accompany trimetrexate treatments to avoid potentially life-threatening toxicity. Leucovorin therapy must extend for 3 days after trimetrexate therapy.
• Stop treatment if creatinine is over 2.5 mg/dl or transaminases or alkaline phosphatases exceed five times the upper limit.
• When calculating the oral dose of leucovorin, round dosage up to the next increment of 25 mg.
• Monitor patient closely. Many adverse effects may be decreased by adjusting the dosage of leucovorin.
• Avoid I.M. injections in patients with thrombocytopenia.
• Monitor CBC during therapy.

◖ I.V. administration
• Reconstitute 25-mg vial with 2 ml of D₅W or sterile water for injection to yield a solution of 12.5 mg/ml. Complete dissolution usually occurs within 30 seconds. Further dilute reconstituted solution with D₅W to yield a final concentration of 0.25 to 2 mg/ml. Infuse over 60 minutes. After reconstitution, drug is stable at room temperature or refrigerated for 24 hours.
• Use only D₅W for I.V. infusion. Drug is incompatible with chloride-containing solutions (including 0.9% NaCl solution) and leucovorin.
• Flush the I.V. line with at least 10 ml of D₅W immediately before and after the trimetrexate infusion.
• Administer leucovorin either before or after trimetrexate. When giving I.V., be sure to flush the I.V. line with D₅W because the two drugs are incompatible. Leucovorin calcium may be infused over 5 to 10 minutes.

☑ Patient teaching
• Instruct patient to alert nurse if discomfort occurs at I.V. site.
• Warn patient to watch for signs and symptoms of infection (fever, sore throat, fatigue) and bleeding (easy bruising, epistaxis, bleeding gums, melena) and instruct how to take infection control and bleeding precautions. Tell patients to take temperature daily.
• Advise female patient of childbearing age to avoid becoming pregnant during therapy. Also recommend consulting doctor before becoming pregnant.

---

vancomycin hydrochloride
Lyphocin, Vancocin, Vancoled

Pregnancy Risk Category: C

HOW SUPPLIED
Capsules: 125 mg, 250 mg
Powder for oral solution: 1-g bottles, 10-g bottles
Powder for injection: 500-mg vials, 1-g vials
I.V. infusion (frozen): 500 mg in 100 ml 5% D₅W

ACTION
Hinders bacterial cell-wall synthesis, damaging the bacterial plasma membrane and making the cell more vulnerable to osmotic pressure. Also interferes with RNA synthesis.

Route	Onset	Peak	Duration
PO	Unknown	Unknown	Unknown
IV	Unknown	Immediate	Unknown

INDICATIONS & DOSAGE
Serious or severe infections when other antibiotics are ineffective or contraindicated, including those caused by methicillin-resistant Staphylococcus aureus, Staphylococcus epidermidis, *and diphtheroid organisms—*
Adults: 1 to 1.5 g I.V. q 12 hours (dose based on weight and renal function; longer dosing intervals necessary in renal dysfunction).
Children: 10 mg/kg I.V. q 6 hours.
Neonates and young infants: 15 mg/kg

I.V. loading dose, followed by 10 mg/kg I.V. q 12 hours if less than 1 week of age or 10 mg/kg I.V. q 8 hours if older than 1 week but less than 1 month.
Antibiotic-associated pseudomembranous (Clostridium difficile) and staphylococcal enterocolitis—
Adults: 125 to 500 mg P.O. q 6 hours for 7 to 10 days.
Children: 40 mg/kg P.O. daily, in divided doses q 6 hours for 7 to 10 days. Maximum daily dosage is 2 g.
Endocarditis prophylaxis for dental procedures—
Adults: 1 g I.V. slowly over 1 hour, starting 1 hour before procedure.
Children: 20 mg/kg I.V. over 1 hour, starting 1 hour before procedure.

ADVERSE REACTIONS
EENT: tinnitus, ototoxicity.
GI: nausea, pseudomembranous colitis.
GU: *nephrotoxicity,* increased BUN and serum creatinine levels.
Hematologic: *neutropenia, leukopenia,* eosinophilia.
Skin: "red-neck" syndrome with rapid I.V. infusion (maculopapular rash on face, neck, trunk, and extremities; pruritus and hypotension associated with histamine release).
Other: chills; fever; *anaphylaxis;* superinfection; hypotension; wheezing; dyspnea; pain, thrombophlebitis (at injection site).

INTERACTIONS
Drug-drug. *Aminoglycosides, amphotericin B, cisplatin, pentamidine:* increased risk of nephrotoxicity and ototoxicity. Monitor closely.

EFFECTS ON DIAGNOSTIC TESTS
None reported.

CONTRAINDICATIONS
Contraindicated in patients with hypersensitivity to drug.

NURSING CONSIDERATIONS
• Use cautiously in patients receiving other neurotoxic, nephrotoxic, or ototoxic drugs; in patients over 60 years; and in those with impaired hepatic or renal func-

tion, preexisting hearing loss, or allergies to other antibiotics. Patients with renal dysfunction require dosage adjustment. Serum levels should be monitored to adjust I.V. dosage. Normal therapeutic levels of vancomycin are as follows: peak, 30 to 40 mg/L (drawn 1 hour after infusion ends); trough, 5 to 10 mg/L (drawn just before next dose is given).
• Monitor patient's fluid balance and observe for oliguria and cloudy urine.
• Obtain culture and sensitivity tests before giving first dose. Therapy may begin pending results.
• Obtain hearing evaluation and renal function studies before therapy.
• Monitor patient carefully for "red-neck" syndrome, which can occur if drug is infused too rapidly. If this reaction occurs, stop infusion and notify the doctor.
• Do not give drug I.M.
• Oral administration is ineffective for systemic infections, and I.V. administration is ineffective for pseudomembranous (*C. difficile*) diarrhea.
• Know that the oral preparation is stable for 2 weeks if refrigerated.
• Monitor renal function (BUN, serum creatinine, urinalysis, creatinine clearance, and urine output) during therapy. Also monitor for signs of superinfection.
• Have patient's hearing evaluated during prolonged therapy.
• Be aware that when using drug to treat staphylococcal endocarditis, it will be given for at least 4 weeks.

I.V. administration
• For I.V. infusion, dilute in 200 ml 0.9% NaCl injection or D_5W, and infuse over 60 to 90 minutes. Check site daily for phlebitis and irritation. Report pain at infusion site. Avoid extravasation; severe irritation and necrosis can result.
• Refrigerate I.V. solution after reconstitution and use within 96 hours.

Patient teaching
• Tell patient to take entire amount of medication exactly as directed, even after he feels better.
• Instruct patient receiving drug I.V. to alert nurse if discomfort occurs at I.V. insertion site.

---

amrinone lactate
digoxin
milrinone lactate

COMBINATION PRODUCTS
None.

---

amrinone lactate
Inocor

Pregnancy Risk Category: C

HOW SUPPLIED
Injection: 5 mg/ml in 20-ml ampules

ACTION
Unknown. Thought to produce inotropic action by increasing cellular levels of cAMP. Produces vasodilation through a direct relaxant effect on vascular smooth muscle.

Route	Onset	Peak	Duration
IV	2-5 min	10 min	0.5-2 hr

INDICATIONS & DOSAGE
Short-term management of heart failure—
Adults: initially, 0.75 mg/kg I.V. bolus over 2 to 3 minutes. Then begin maintenance infusion of 5 to 10 mcg/kg/minute. May give additional bolus of 0.75 mg/kg 30 minutes after starting therapy. Don't exceed total daily dosage of 10 mg/kg.

ADVERSE REACTIONS
CV: *arrhythmias,* hypotension.
GI: nausea, vomiting, anorexia, abdominal pain.
Hematologic: *thrombocytopenia* (depends on dose and duration of therapy).
Hepatic: elevated enzymes, hepatotoxicity (rare).
Other: burning at injection site, *hypersensitivity reactions* (pericarditis, ascites, myositis vasculitis, pleuritis), fever, chest pain.

INTERACTIONS
Drug-drug. *Cardiac glycosides:* enhanced inotropic effect. Beneficial drug interaction.
Disopyramide: excessive hypotension. Monitor patient.

EFFECTS ON DIAGNOSTIC TESTS
Drug may decrease serum potassium or increase serum hepatic enzymes.

CONTRAINDICATIONS
Contraindicated in patients with hypersensitivity to amrinone or bisulfites.

NURSING CONSIDERATIONS
• Know that amrinone should not be used in patients with severe aortic or pulmonic valvular disease in place of surgical correction of the obstruction or during acute phase of MI.
• Use cautiously in patients with hypertrophic cardiomyopathy.
• Be aware that amrinone is primarily prescribed for patients who have not responded to cardiac glycosides, diuretics, and vasodilators.
• Dosage depends on clinical response, including assessment of pulmonary artery wedge pressure and cardiac output.
• Anticipate that amrinone may be added to cardiac glycoside therapy in patients with atrial fibrillation and flutter because it slightly enhances AV conduction and increases ventricular response rate.
• Monitor platelet count. If it falls below 150,000/mm^3, decrease dosage as ordered.
• Patients with end-stage cardiac disease may receive home treatment with an amrinone drip while awaiting heart transplantation.

▢I.V. administration
• Administer drug with an infusion pump and use as supplied, or dilute in 0.45% or 0.9% NaCl solution to a concentration of 1 to 3 mg/ml. Use diluted solution within 24 hours.

• Don't dilute with solutions containing dextrose because a slow chemical reaction occurs over 24 hours. Amrinone can be injected into free-flowing dextrose infusions through a Y-connector or directly into tubing.

Alert: Don't administer furosemide and amrinone through the same I.V. line because precipitation occurs.

• Monitor blood pressure and heart rate throughout the infusion. If patient's blood pressure falls, slow or stop infusion and notify the doctor.

☑ **Patient teaching**
• Warn patient that burning may occur at the site of injection.
• Instruct home care patient and family on administration; tell them to report adverse reactions promptly.

---

digoxin
Digoxin, Lanoxicaps, Lanoxin*, Novo-Digoxin†

Pregnancy Risk Category: C

HOW SUPPLIED
Tablets: 0.125 mg, 0.25 mg, 0.5 mg
Capsules: 0.05 mg, 0.1 mg, 0.2 mg
Elixir: 0.05 mg/ml
Injection: 0.05 mg/ml†, 0.1 mg/ml (pediatric), 0.25 mg/ml

ACTION
Inhibits sodium-potassium activated adenosine triphosphatase, thereby promoting movement of calcium from extracellular to intracellular cytoplasm and strengthening myocardial contraction. Also acts on CNS to enhance vagal tone, slowing conduction through the SA and AV nodes and providing an antiarrhythmic effect.

Route	Onset	Peak	Duration
PO	1.5-2 hr	2-6 hr	3-4 days
IV	5-30 min	1-4 hr	3-4 days

INDICATIONS & DOSAGE
Heart failure, paroxysmal supraventricular tachycardia, atrial fibrillation and flutter—

Adults: loading dose is 0.5 to 1 mg I.V. or P.O. in divided doses over 24 hours; maintenance dosage is 0.125 to 0.5 mg I.V. or P.O. daily (average is 0.25 mg). Depending on response, larger doses may be needed for arrhythmias.
Elderly: in patients over 65 years, 0.125 mg P.O. daily as maintenance dose. Frail or underweight elderly patients may require only 0.0625 mg daily or 0.125 mg every other day.
Premature neonates: loading dose is 0.015 to 0.025 mg/kg I.V. in three divided doses over 24 hours; maintenance dosage is 0.01 mg/kg daily, divided q 12 hours.
Neonates: loading dose is 0.025 to 0.035 mg/kg P.O., divided q 8 hours over 24 hours; I.V. loading dose is 0.02 to 0.03 mg/kg; maintenance dosage is 0.01 mg/kg P.O. daily, divided q 12 hours.
Children 1 month to 2 years: loading dose is 0.035 to 0.06 mg/kg P.O. in three divided doses over 24 hours; I.V. loading dose is 0.03 to 0.05 mg/kg; maintenance dosage is 0.01 to 0.02 mg/kg P.O. daily, divided q 12 hours.
Children over 2 years: loading dose is 0.02 to 0.04 mg/kg P.O. daily, divided q 8 hours over 24 hours; I.V. loading dose is 0.015 to 0.035 mg/kg; maintenance dosage is 0.012 mg/kg P.O. daily, divided q 12 hours.
Adjust-a-dose: Smaller loading and maintenance doses are given to patients with impaired renal function.

ADVERSE REACTIONS
The following signs of toxicity may occur with all cardiac glycosides:
CNS: *fatigue, generalized muscle weakness, agitation, hallucinations,* headache, malaise, dizziness, vertigo, stupor, paresthesia.
CV: *arrhythmias* (most commonly, conduction disturbances with or without AV block, PVCs, and supraventricular arrhythmias); arrhythmias may lead to increased severity of heart failure and hypotension.
EENT: yellow-green halos around visual images, blurred vision, light flashes, photophobia, diplopia.
GI: *anorexia, nausea,* vomiting, diarrhea.

INTERACTIONS

Drug-drug. *Amiloride:* inhibited digoxin effect and increased digoxin excretion. Monitor for altered digoxin effect.

Amiodarone, diltiazem, nifedipine, quinidine, verapamil: increased digoxin blood levels. Monitor for toxicity.

Amphotericin B, carbenicillin, corticosteroids, diuretics (including loop diuretics, chlorthalidone, metolazone, thiazides), ticarcillin: hypokalemia, predisposing patient to digitalis toxicity. Monitor serum potassium levels.

Antacids, kaolin-pectin: decreased absorption of oral digoxin. Schedule doses as far as possible from oral digoxin administration.

Anticholinergics: may increase digoxin absorption of oral digoxin tablets. Monitor blood levels and observe for toxicity.

Cholestyramine, colestipol, metoclopramide: decreased absorption of oral digoxin. Monitor for decreased digitoxin effect and low blood levels. Space doses by giving digoxin 1½ hours before or 2 hours after other drugs.

Parenteral calcium, thiazides: hypercalcemia and hypomagnesemia, predisposing patient to digitalis toxicity. Monitor serum calcium and serum magnesium levels.

Drug-herb. *Betel palm, fumitory, lily-of-the-valley, goldenseal, motherwort, shepherd's purse, rue:* possible enhanced cardiac effects. Avoid concomitant use.

Licorice, oleander, Siberian ginseng, squill: possible enhanced toxicity. Monitor patient closely.

EFFECTS ON DIAGNOSTIC TESTS
None reported.

CONTRAINDICATIONS
Contraindicated in patients with digitalis-induced toxicity, ventricular fibrillation, ventricular tachycardia unless caused by heart failure, or hypersensitivity to drug.

NURSING CONSIDERATIONS
• Use with extreme caution in elderly patients and in those with acute MI, incomplete AV block, sinus bradycardia, PVCs, chronic constrictive pericarditis, hypertrophic cardiomyopathy, renal insufficiency, severe pulmonary disease, or hypothyroidism. Reduce dosage in patients with renal impairment.

• Be aware that hypothyroid patients are extremely sensitive to cardiac glycosides; hyperthyroid patients may need larger doses.

• Before administering the loading dose, obtain baseline data (heart rate and rhythm, blood pressure, and electrolytes) and question the patient about use of cardiac glycosides within the previous 2 to 3 weeks.

• Be aware that the loading dose is divided over the first 24 hours unless the situation indicates otherwise.

• Before giving, take apical-radial pulse for a full minute. Record and report to the doctor significant changes (sudden increase or decrease in pulse rate, pulse deficit, irregular beats and, particularly, regularization of a previously irregular rhythm). If any occur, check blood pressure and obtain a 12-lead ECG.

• Toxic effects on the heart may be life-threatening and require immediate attention.

• Absorption of digoxin from liquid-filled capsules is superior to absorption from tablets or elixir. Expect dosage reduction of 20% to 25% when changing from tablets or elixir to liquid-filled capsules or parenteral therapy.

• Monitor serum digoxin levels. Therapeutic levels range from 0.5 to 2 ng/ml. Obtain blood for digoxin levels 8 hours after last oral dose.

Alert: Excessive slowing of the pulse rate (60 beats/minute or less) may be a sign of digitalis toxicity. Withhold drug and notify doctor.

• Monitor serum potassium levels carefully. Take corrective action before hypokalemia occurs.

• Withhold drug for 1 to 2 days before elective cardioversion. Adjust dose after cardioversion.

I.V. administration
• Infuse drug slowly over at least 5 minutes.

Patient teaching
• Instruct patient and a responsible family

member about drug action, dosage regimen, how to take pulse, reportable signs, and follow-up care.
● Encourage patient to eat potassium-rich foods.
● Tell patient not to substitute one brand of digoxin for another.

milrinone lactate
Primacor

Pregnancy Risk Category: C

HOW SUPPLIED
Injection: 1 mg/ml
Injection (premixed): 200 mcg/ml in D_5W

ACTION
Produces inotropic action by increasing cellular levels of cAMP. Produces vasodilation by directly relaxing vascular smooth muscle.

Route	Onset	Peak	Duration
IV	5-15 min	1-2 hr	3-6 hr

INDICATIONS & DOSAGE
Short-term treatment of heart failure—
Adults: initial loading dose is 50 mcg/kg I.V., administered slowly over 10 minutes, followed by continuous I.V. infusion of 0.375 to 0.75 mcg/kg/minute. Adjust infusion dose according to clinical and hemodynamic responses, as ordered.
Adjust-a-dose: In patients with renal failure, if creatinine clearance is 50 ml/ minute or less, titrate dosage to maximum clinical effect; do not exceed 1.13 mg/kg/ day.

ADVERSE REACTIONS
CNS: headache.
CV: VENTRICULAR ARRHYTHMIAS, *ventricular ectopic activity,* nonsustained ventricular tachycardia, *sustained ventricular tachycardia, ventricular fibrillation.*

INTERACTIONS
None significant.

EFFECTS ON DIAGNOSTIC TESTS
None reported.

CONTRAINDICATIONS
Contraindicated in patients with hypersensitivity to drug.

NURSING CONSIDERATIONS
● Know that milrinone should not be used in patients with severe aortic or pulmonic valvular disease in place of surgical correction of the obstruction or during acute phase of MI.
● Use cautiously in patients with atrial flutter or fibrillation because drug slightly shortens AV node conduction time and may increase ventricular response rate. Administer a cardiac glycoside, if ordered, before beginning milrinone therapy.
● Be aware that drug is typically given with digoxin and diuretics.
● Be aware that inotropic agents may aggravate outflow tract obstruction in hypertrophic subaortic stenosis.
● Be aware that improved cardiac output may enhance urine output. Expect dosage reduction in patient's diuretic therapy as heart failure improves. Potassium loss may predispose patient to digitalis toxicity.
● Monitor fluid and electrolyte status, blood pressure, heart rate, and renal function during therapy. Excessive decrease in blood pressure requires discontinuing or slowing rate of infusion.

I.V. administration
● Prepare I.V. infusion solution using 0.45% or 0.9% NaCl or D_5W. Prepare the 100-mcg/ml solution by adding 180 ml of diluent per 20-mg (20-ml) vial, the 150-mcg/ml solution by adding 113 ml of diluent per 20-mg (20-ml) vial, and the 200-mcg/ml solution by adding 80 ml of diluent per 20-mg (20-ml) vial.
Alert: Administering furosemide into an I.V. line containing milrinone causes formation of a precipitate.

✓ Patient teaching
● Instruct patient to report adverse reactions promptly.
● Tell patient to alert the nurse if discomfort occurs at I.V. insertion site.

21

Antiarrhythmics

adenosine
amiodarone hydrochloride
atropine sulfate
bretylium tosylate
diltiazem hydrochloride
    (See Chapter 22, ANTIANGINALS.)
disopyramide
disopyramide phosphate
esmolol hydrochloride
flecainide acetate
ibutilide fumarate
lidocaine hydrochloride
mexiletine hydrochloride
moricizine hydrochloride
phenytoin
    (See Chapter 30, ANTICONVULSANTS.)
phenytoin sodium
    (See Chapter 30, ANTICONVULSANTS.)
procainamide hydrochloride
propafenone hydrochloride
propranolol hydrochloride
    (See Chapter 22, ANTIANGINALS.)
quinidine bisulfate
quinidine gluconate
quinidine polygalacturonate
quinidine sulfate
sotalol
tocainide hydrochloride
verapamil hydrochloride
    (See Chapter 22, ANTIANGINALS.)

COMBINATION PRODUCTS
None.

---

adenosine
Adenocard, Adenocor§

Pregnancy Risk Category: C

HOW SUPPLIED
Injection: 3 mg/ml in 2-ml and 5-ml vials

ACTION
A naturally occurring nucleoside that acts on the AV node to slow conduction and inhibit reentry pathways. Adenosine is also useful in treating paroxysmal supraventricular tachycardia (PSVT) associated with accessory bypass tracts (Wolff-Parkinson-White syndrome).

Route	Onset	Peak	Duration
IV	Immediate	Immediate	Unknown

INDICATIONS & DOSAGE
Conversion of PSVT to sinus rhythm—
Adults: 6 mg I.V. by rapid bolus injection over 1 to 2 seconds. If PSVT is not eliminated in 1 to 2 minutes, 12 mg by rapid I.V. push may be given and repeated if necessary. Single doses over 12 mg are not recommended.

ADVERSE REACTIONS
CNS: dizziness, light-headedness, numbness, tingling in arms.
CV: *facial flushing,* headache.
GI: nausea.
Respiratory: chest pressure, *dyspnea, shortness of breath.*

INTERACTIONS
Drug-drug. *Carbamazepine:* higher degrees of heart block may occur. Use with caution.
Digoxin, verapamil: potential for ventricular fibrillation. Monitor closely.
Dipyridamole: may potentiate adenosine's effects. Smaller doses may be necessary.
Methylxanthines: antagonism of adenosine's effects. Patients receiving theophylline may require higher doses or may not respond to adenosine therapy.
Drug-herb. *Guarana:* may decrease response. Monitor patient.
Drug-food. *Caffeine:* may antagonize adenosine's effects. Patient may require higher doses or not respond to adenosine therapy.

EFFECTS ON DIAGNOSTIC TESTS
None reported.

CONTRAINDICATIONS
Contraindicated in patients with hypersensitivity to drug and also in those with second- or third-degree heart block or si-

---

*Liquid contains alcohol.   **May contain tartrazine.   †Canada   ‡Australia   §U.K.   ◇OTC

nus node disease such as sick sinus syndrome or symptomatic bradycardia, unless an artificial pacemaker is present, because adenosine decreases conduction through the AV node and may produce first-, second-, or third-degree heart block. Patients who develop high level heart block after a single dose of adenosine should not receive additional doses.

NURSING CONSIDERATIONS
Alert: Monitor cardiac rhythm and be prepared to administer appropriate therapy due to the potential for new arrhythmias, including heart block or transient asystole.
• Use cautiously in patients with asthma because bronchoconstriction may occur.
• Crystals may form if solution is cold. If crystals are visible, gently warm solution to room temperature. Don't use solutions that aren't clear.
• Discard unused drug; adenosine lacks preservatives.

🔋 I.V. administration
• Rapid I.V. injection is necessary to ensure drug action. Administer directly into a vein if possible; when giving through an I.V. line, use the port closest to the patient, and flush immediately and rapidly with 0.9% NaCl solution to ensure that drug reaches the systemic circulation quickly.

☑ Patient teaching
• Instruct patient to report adverse reactions promptly.
• Tell patient to alert nurse if discomfort occurs at I.V. site.

---

amiodarone hydrochloride
Aratac‡, Cordarone,
Cordarone X‡

Pregnancy Risk Category: D

HOW SUPPLIED
Tablets: 100 mg‡, 200 mg
Injection: 50 mg/ml

ACTION
Unknown. Thought to prolong the refractory period and action potential duration.

Route	Onset	Peak	Duration
PO	2 days-3 wk	3-7 hr	Variable
IV	Unknown	Unknown	Variable

INDICATIONS & DOSAGE
Recurrent ventricular fibrillation or recurrent hemodynamically unstable ventricular tachycardia nonresponsive to adequate doses of other antiarrhythmics or when alternative agents cannot be tolerated—
Adults: give loading dose of 800 to 1,600 mg P.O. daily divided b.i.d. for 1 to 3 weeks until initial therapeutic response occurs, then 600 to 800 mg/day P.O. for 1 month, and then, for maintenance, 200 to 600 mg P.O. daily.
   Or, give loading dose of 150 mg I.V. over 10 minutes (15 mg/minute); then 360 mg I.V. over the next 6 hours (1 mg/minute); then 540 mg I.V. over the next 18 hours (0.5 mg/minute). After the first 24 hours, continue with a maintenance I.V. infusion of 720 mg/24 hours (0.5 mg/minute).

ADVERSE REACTIONS
CNS: peripheral neuropathy, ataxia, paresthesia, *tremor,* insomnia, sleep disturbances, headache, *malaise, fatigue.*
CV: bradycardia, hypotension, ***arrhythmias, heart failure, heart block, sinus arrest.***
EENT: *asymptomatic corneal microdeposits,* optic neuropathy or neuritis resulting in visual impairment, *visual disturbances.*
GI: anorexia, *nausea, vomiting,* constipation, abdominal pain.
Hepatic: *elevated liver enzymes,* hepatic dysfunction, ***hepatic failure.***
Respiratory: ***adult respiratory distress syndrome,*** SEVERE PULMONARY TOXICITY (PNEUMONITIS, ALVEOLITIS).
Skin: *photosensitivity,* solar dermatitis.
Other: abnormal taste and smell, *hypothyroidism,* hyperthyroidism, edema, ***coagulation abnormalities.***

Reactions may be *common,* uncommon, ***life-threatening,*** or COMMON AND LIFE-THREATENING.

INTERACTIONS

Drug-drug. *Antiarrhythmics:* amiodarone may reduce the hepatic or renal clearance of certain antiarrhythmics (especially flecainide, procainamide, quinidine); concomitant use of amiodarone with other antiarrhythmics (especially mexiletine, propafenone, quinidine, disopyramide, procainamide) may induce torsades de pointes. Avoid concomitant use.

Antihypertensives: increased hypotensive effect. Use together cautiously.

Beta blockers, calcium channel blockers: increased cardiac depressant effects; may potentiate slowing of SA node and AV conduction. Use together cautiously.

Digoxin: increased serum digoxin levels (average of 70% to 100%). Monitor digoxin levels closely and adjust dosage as ordered.

Phenytoin: may decrease phenytoin metabolism. Monitor serum phenytoin levels and adjust dosage as ordered.

Theophylline: increased theophylline levels with toxicity may occur. Monitor serum theophylline levels.

Warfarin: potentiation of anticoagulant response with the potential for serious or fatal bleeding. Decrease warfarin dosage 33% to 50% when amiodarone is initiated. Monitor patient closely.

Drug-herb. *Pennyroyal:* may change the rate of formation of toxic metabolites of pennyroyal. Avoid concurrent use.

Drug-lifestyle. *Sun exposure:* photosensitivity reaction may occur. Take precautions.

EFFECTS ON DIAGNOSTIC TESTS
None reported.

CONTRAINDICATIONS

Contraindicated in patients with cardiogenic shock, second- or third-degree AV block, severe SA node disease resulting in preexisting bradycardia unless an artificial pacemaker is present, or hypersensitivity to drug and in those in whom bradycardia has caused syncope.

NURSING CONSIDERATIONS

• Use with extreme caution in those receiving other antiarrhythmics.

• Use cautiously in patients with pulmonary, hepatic, or thyroid disease.

• Be aware of the high incidence of adverse reactions.

• Obtain baseline pulmonary, liver, and thyroid function tests.

• Administer loading doses in a hospital setting and with continuous ECG monitoring because of the slow onset of antiarrhythmic effect and risk of life-threatening arrhythmias.

• Divide oral loading dose into two equal doses and give with meals to decrease GI intolerance. Maintenance dosage may be given once daily, but may be divided into two doses taken with meals if GI intolerance occurs.

Alert: Amiodarone poses major management problems that could be life-threatening in a population at risk of sudden death and is only for use in patients with documented, life-threatening, recurrent ventricular arrhythmias when nonresponsive to documented adequate doses of other antiarrhythmics or when alternative agents could not be tolerated. Amiodarone has several potentially fatal toxicities including pulmonary toxicity and hepatic toxicity.

• Monitor carefully for pulmonary toxicity, which can be fatal. Incidence increases in patients receiving more than 400 mg/day.

• Monitor for symptoms of pneumonitis—exertional dyspnea, nonproductive cough, and pleuritic chest pain. Monitor pulmonary function tests and chest X-ray.

• Monitor liver and thyroid function tests and serum electrolytes, particularly potassium and magnesium levels.

• Instillation of methylcellulose ophthalmic solution is recommended during amiodarone therapy to minimize corneal microdeposits. Within 1 to 4 months after beginning amiodarone therapy, most patients show corneal microdeposits upon slit-lamp ophthalmic examination. However, only 2% to 3% have actual vision disturbances.

• Monitor blood pressure and heart rate and rhythm frequently. Perform continuous ECG monitoring during initiation and alteration of dosage. Notify doctor of significant change.

---

*Liquid contains alcohol.   **May contain tartrazine.   †Canada   ‡Australia   §U.K.   ◇OTC

I.V. administration

• Be aware that amiodarone may be given I.V. only in facilities where continuous ECG monitoring and electrophysiologic techniques are available. Mix initial dosage of 150 mg in 100 ml of D_5W solution. Mix infusions planned for administration over 30 minutes or more in glass bottles. Administer repeat doses through a central venous catheter.

• Administer I.V. amiodarone whenever possible via a central line dedicated to that purpose.

• Use an in-line filter with I.V. administration.

• Continuously monitor cardiac status of patient receiving drug I.V.

✓ Patient teaching

• Advise patient to use a sunscreen or protective clothing to prevent photosensitivity reaction. Monitor for burning or tingling skin followed by erythema and possible skin blistering. A blue-gray discoloration of the exposed skin may occur.

• Tell patient to take oral drug with food if GI reactions occur.

• Inform patient that amiodarone's adverse effects are more prevalent at high doses and become more frequent with treatment lasting more than 6 months but are generally reversible when drug is stopped. Resolution of adverse reactions may take up to 4 months.

---

atropine sulfate

Pregnancy Risk Category: C

HOW SUPPLIED

Tablets: 0.4 mg
Injection: 0.05 mg/ml, 0.1 mg/ml, 0.3 mg/ml, 0.4 mg/ml, 0.5 mg/ml, 0.8 mg/ml, 1 mg/ml

ACTION

An anticholinergic that inhibits acetylcholine at the parasympathetic neuroeffector junction, blocking vagal effects on the SA and AV nodes; this enhances conduction through the AV node and speeds heart rate.

Route	Onset	Peak	Duration
PO	0.5-2 hr	1-2 hr	4 hr
IV	Immediate	2-4 min	4 hr
IM	5-40 min	20-60 min	4 hr
SC	Unknown	Unknown	Unknown

INDICATIONS & DOSAGE

Symptomatic bradycardia, bradyarrhythmia (junctional or escape rhythm)—
Adults: usually 0.5 to 1 mg I.V. push, repeated q 3 to 5 minutes to maximum of 2 mg p.r.n. Lower doses (less than 0.5 mg) can cause bradycardia.
Children: 0.01 mg/kg I.V.; may repeat q 4 to 6 hours; maximum dose is 0.4 mg or 0.3 mg/m².
Antidote for anticholinesterase insecticide poisoning—
Adults: 2 to 3 mg I.V. repeated q 5 to 10 minutes until muscarinic symptoms disappear or signs of atropine toxicity appear. Severe poisoning may require up to 6 mg hourly.
Children: 0.05 mg/kg I.M. or I.V. repeated q 10 to 30 minutes until muscarinic signs and symptoms subside (may be repeated if they reappear) or until atropine toxicity occurs.
Preoperatively to diminish secretions and block cardiac vagal reflexes—
Adults and children weighing 20 kg (44 lb) or more: 0.4 to 0.6 mg I.M. or S.C. 30 to 60 minutes before anesthesia.
Children weighing less than 20 kg: 0.01 mg/kg I.M. or S.C. up to maximum dose of 0.4 mg 30 to 60 minutes before anesthesia.
Adjunct treatment of peptic ulcer disease; treatment of functional GI disorders such as irritable bowel syndrome—
Adults: 0.4 to 0.6 mg P.O. q 4 to 6 hours.
Children: 0.01 mg/kg or 0.3 mg/m² P.O. (not to exceed 0.4 mg) q 4 to 6 hours.

ADVERSE REACTIONS

CNS: *headache, restlessness,* ataxia, disorientation, hallucinations, delirium, *insomnia, dizziness,* excitement, agitation, confusion (especially in elderly patients).
CV: palpitations, bradycardia (with low doses); tachycardia (with higher doses).
EENT: photophobia, *blurred vision, mydriasis,* cycloplegia, increased intraocular pressure.

Reactions may be *common,* uncommon, *life-threatening,* or COMMON AND LIFE-THREATENING.

GI: *dry mouth,* thirst, *constipation,* nausea, vomiting.
GU: urine retention, impotence.
Other: severe allergic reactions, including ***anaphylaxis*** and urticaria.

INTERACTIONS
Drug-drug. *Antacids:* decreased absorption of anticholinergics. Separate administration times by at least 1 hour.
Anticholinergics, drugs with anticholinergic effects (such as amantadine, antiarrhythmics, antiparkinsonian agents, glutethimide, meperidine, phenothiazines, tricyclic antidepressants): additive anticholinergic effects. Use together cautiously.
Ketoconazole, levodopa: decreased absorption. Avoid concomitant use.
Methotrimeprazine: may produce extrapyramidal symptoms. Monitor patient carefully.
Potassium chloride wax-matrix tablets: increased risk of mucosal lesions. Use cautiously.
Drug-herb. *Jamborandi tree, pill-bearing spurge:* decreased effectiveness of drug. Avoid concomitant use.
Jimson weed: may adversely affect CV function. Avoid concomitant use.
Squaw vine: tannic acid may decrease metabolic breakdown. Monitor patient.

EFFECTS ON DIAGNOSTIC TESTS
None reported.

CONTRAINDICATIONS
Contraindicated in patients with acute angle-closure glaucoma, obstructive uropathy, obstructive disease of GI tract, paralytic ileus, toxic megacolon, intestinal atony, unstable CV status in acute hemorrhage, tachycardia, myocardial ischemia, asthma, myasthenia gravis, or hypersensitivity to drug.

NURSING CONSIDERATIONS
• Use cautiously in patients with Down syndrome because they may be more sensitive to drug.
• Be aware that many adverse reactions (such as dry mouth and constipation) vary with the dose.
• Monitor patients for paradoxical initial bradycardia, especially those receiving

small doses (0.4 to 0.6 mg). This usually disappears within 2 minutes.
Alert: Watch for tachycardia in cardiac patients because it may precipitate ventricular fibrillation.
• Monitor fluid intake and urine output. Drug causes urine retention and urinary hesitancy.

I.V. administration
• Administer via direct I.V. into a large vein or I.V. tubing over at least 1 minute.
• Be aware slow I.V. administration may cause paradoxical slowing of the heart rate.

Patient teaching
• Teach patient receiving oral form of drug how to handle distressing anticholinergic effects.
• Instruct patient to report serious or persistent adverse reactions promptly.
• Tell patient about potential for photophobia and suggest use of sunglasses.

---

bretylium tosylate
Bretylate†, Bretylol

Pregnancy Risk Category: C

HOW SUPPLIED
Injection: 50 mg/ml in 10-ml ampules, vials, and syringes and in 20-ml vials

ACTION
Unknown but considered a class III antiarrhythmic that initially exerts transient adrenergic stimulation through release of norepinephrine. Subsequent depletion of norepinephrine causes adrenergic blocking actions to predominate, prolonging repolarization and increasing the duration of action potential and an effective refractory period.

Route	Onset	Peak	Duration
IV	Immediate	Immediate	6-24 hr
IM	5-40 min	1 hr	6-24 hr

INDICATIONS & DOSAGE
Ventricular fibrillation or hemodynamically unstable ventricular tachycardia unresponsive to other antiarrhythmics—

Adults: 5 mg/kg by I.V. push over 1 minute. If necessary, dose increased to 10 mg/kg and repeated q 15 to 30 minutes until 30 to 35 mg/kg have been given. For continuous suppression, diluted solution administered at 1 to 2 mg/minute continuously or 5 to 10 mg/kg diluted over more than 8 minutes q 6 hours.

ADVERSE REACTIONS
CNS: *vertigo, dizziness, light-headedness, syncope* (usually secondary to hypotension).
CV: SEVERE HYPOTENSION (especially orthostatic), bradycardia, anginal pain, ***transient arrhythmias***, transient hypertension, increased PVC.
GI: severe nausea, vomiting (with rapid infusion).

INTERACTIONS
Drug-drug. *All antihypertensives:* may potentiate hypotension. Monitor blood pressure.
Other antiarrhythmics: additive or antagonistic antiarrhythmic effects. Monitor for additive toxicity.
Sympathomimetics: bretylium may potentiate effects of drugs given to correct hypotension. Monitor for effects.

EFFECTS ON DIAGNOSTIC TESTS
None reported.

CONTRAINDICATIONS
Contraindicated in digitalized patients unless arrhythmia is life-threatening, not caused by cardiac glycosides, and in those unresponsive to other antiarrhythmics.

NURSING CONSIDERATIONS
• Use with extreme caution in patients with fixed cardiac output (aortic stenosis and pulmonary hypertension) to avoid severe and sudden drop in blood pressure.
• Keep patient supine until tolerance to hypotension develops.
• Monitor patient closely. The initial release of norepinephrine caused by bretylium may induce transient hypertension and arrhythmias.
• Monitor blood pressure and heart rate and rhythm continuously. Immediately report significant change. If supine systolic blood pressure falls below 75 mm Hg, the doctor may order norepinephrine, dopamine, or volume expanders.
• Observe for increased anginal pain in susceptible patients.

▌I.V. administration
• When used for maintenance therapy, dilute using dextrose or NaCl for injection before administration. Follow manufacturer's guidelines for specific dilution guidelines (varies according to dosage). When administering as direct I.V. injection, use a 20G to 22G needle and inject over 1 minute into a vein or I.V. line containing a free-flowing, compatible solution.
• For intermittent I.V. administration, dilute and give over a period of 8 minutes or more to minimize nausea and vomiting.

☑Patient teaching
• Instruct patient to report adverse reactions immediately.
• Tell patient to alert nurse if discomfort occurs at I.V. insertion site.
• Inform patient to avoid sudden postural changes.

---

disopyramide
Dirythmin SA§, Rythmodan†‡

disopyramide phosphate
Norpace, Norpace CR,
Rythmodan Injection‡,
Rythmodan-LA†

Pregnancy Risk Category: C

HOW SUPPLIED
disopyramide
Capsules: 100 mg†, 150 mg†
disopyramide phosphate
Tablets (sustained-release): 250 mg†
Capsules: 100 mg, 150 mg
Capsules (controlled-release): 100 mg, 150 mg
Injection: 10 mg/ml‡

ACTION
Unknown, but drug is considered a class Ia antiarrhythmic that depresses phase O and prolongs the action potential. All

---

Reactions may be *common,* uncommon, *life-threatening,* or COMMON AND LIFE-THREATENING.

class I drugs have membrane-stabilizing effects.

Route	Onset	Peak	Duration
PO	0.5-3.5 hr	2-2.5 hr	1.5-8.5 hr
IV	Unknown	Unknown	Unknown

INDICATIONS & DOSAGE
Ventricular tachycardia and ventricular arrhythmias believed to be life-threatening—
P.O.—
Adults weighing over 50 kg (110 lb): 150 mg q 6 hours with conventional capsules or 300 mg q 12 hours with extended-release preparations.
Adults weighing 50 kg or less: highly individualized.
Children under 1 year: 10 to 30 mg/kg P.O. daily, divided into four doses (q 6 hours).
Children 1 to 4 years: 10 to 20 mg/kg P.O. daily, divided into four doses (q 6 hours).
Children 4 to 12 years: 10 to 15 mg/kg P.O. daily, divided into four doses (q 6 hours).
Children 12 to 18 years: 6 to 15 mg/kg P.O. daily, divided into four doses (q 6 hours).
Adjust-a-dose: In patients with advanced renal insufficiency, if creatinine clearance is 30 to 40 ml/minute, 100 mg q 8 hours; between 15 and 30 ml/minute, 100 mg q 12 hours; if it is less than 15 ml/minute, 100 mg q 24 hours.
I.V.—
Adults: for parenteral use, initially give 2 mg/kg I.V. slowly (over not less than 15 minutes). Administer until arrhythmias are eliminated or patient has received 150 mg. Repeat dosage if conversion is successful but arrhythmias return. Total I.V. dosage should not exceed 300 mg in first hour. Follow with I.V. infusion of 0.4 mg/kg/hour (usually 20 to 30 mg/hour) to maximum of 800 mg/day.

ADVERSE REACTIONS
CNS: dizziness, agitation, depression, fatigue, headache, nervousness, acute psychosis.
CV: *hypotension, heart failure, heart block,* edema, weight gain, *arrhythmias,* syncope, shortness of breath, chest pain.
EENT: blurred vision, dry eyes or nose, *dry mouth.*
GI: nausea, vomiting, anorexia, bloating, gas, abdominal pain, *constipation, diarrhea.*
GU: *urinary hesitancy.*
Hepatic: cholestatic jaundice.
Skin: rash, pruritus, dermatosis.
Other: aches, pain, muscle weakness, hypoglycemia (rare).

INTERACTIONS
Drug-drug. *Antiarrhythmics:* possible additive or antagonized antiarrhythmic effects. Monitor closely.
Erythromycin: increased disopyramide levels may occur. Monitor closely.
Phenytoin: increased metabolism of disopyramide. Monitor for decreased antiarrhythmic effect.
Rifampin: may decrease disopyramide levels. Monitor closely.
Drug-herb. *Jimson weed:* may adversely affect CV function. Avoid concomitant use.

EFFECTS ON DIAGNOSTIC TESTS
None reported.

CONTRAINDICATIONS
Contraindicated in patients with sick sinus syndrome, cardiogenic shock, second- or third-degree heart block in the absence of an artificial pacemaker, or hypersensitivity to drug.

NURSING CONSIDERATIONS
• Use with extreme caution and avoid, if possible, in patients with heart failure. Use cautiously in patients with underlying conduction abnormalities, urinary tract diseases (especially prostatic hyperplasia), hepatic or renal impairment, myasthenia gravis, or acute angle-closure glaucoma.
• Correct electrolyte abnormalities before therapy begins, as ordered.
• Check apical pulse before administering drug. Notify doctor if pulse rate is slower than 60 beats/minute or faster than 120 beats/minute.

• Know that sustained or controlled-release preparations should not be used for rapid control of ventricular arrhythmias, when therapeutic blood levels must be rapidly attained, in patients with cardiomyopathy or possible cardiac decompensation, or in those with severe renal impairment.

• For use in young children, pharmacist may prepare disopyramide suspension, using 100-mg capsules and cherry syrup. Suspension should be dispensed in amber glass bottles and protected from light.

• Watch for recurrence of arrhythmias and check for adverse reactions; notify doctor if these occur.

• Discontinue drug if heart block develops, if QRS complex widens by more than 25%, or if QT interval lengthens by more than 25% above baseline; also notify doctor.

• When transferring patient from immediate-release to sustained-release capsules, advise him to take the first sustained-release capsule 6 hours after taking the last immediate-release capsule.

⚡ **I.V. administration**
• Add 200 mg to 200 to 500 ml of a compatible solution, such as 0.9% NaCl or D_5W. Do not mix with other drugs; switch to oral therapy as soon as possible.

✅ **Patient teaching**
• Teach patient importance of taking drug on time and exactly as prescribed. This may require use of an alarm clock for overnight doses.

• If not contraindicated, advise patient to chew gum or hard candy to relieve dry mouth and to increase fiber and fluid intake to relieve constipation.

---

esmolol hydrochloride
Brevibloc

Pregnancy Risk Category: C

HOW SUPPLIED
Injection: 10 mg/ml in 10-ml vials, 250 mg/ml in 10-ml ampules

ACTION
A class II antiarrhythmic and ultrashort-acting selective beta$_1$-adrenergic blocker that decreases heart rate, contractility, and blood pressure.

Route	Onset	Peak	Duration
IV	Immediate	30 min	30 min after infusion

INDICATIONS & DOSAGE
Supraventricular tachycardia; to control ventricular rate in patients with atrial fibrillation or flutter in perioperative, postoperative, or other emergent circumstances; noncompensatory sinus tachycardia when heart rate requires specific interventions—
Adults: loading dose is 500 mcg/kg/minute by I.V. infusion over 1 minute, followed by 4-minute maintenance infusion of 50 mcg/kg/minute. If adequate response does not occur within 5 minutes, loading dose is repeated and followed by maintenance infusion of 100 mcg/kg/minute for 4 minutes. Loading dose is repeated and maintenance infusion is increased by 50-mcg/kg/minute increments. Maximum maintenance infusion for tachycardia is 200 mcg/kg/minute.
Perioperative and postoperative tachycardia or hypertension—
Adults: for perioperative treatment of tachycardia or hypertension, 80 mg (approximately 1 mg/kg) I.V. bolus over 30 seconds, followed by 150 mcg/kg/minute I.V. infusion, if needed. Adjust infusion rate p.r.n. up to maximum of 300 mcg/kg/minute; dosage for postoperative treatment of tachycardia and hypertension is same as for supraventricular tachycardia.

ADVERSE REACTIONS
CNS: anxiety, depression, dizziness, somnolence, headache, agitation, fatigue, confusion, *seizures.*
CV: HYPOTENSION (sometimes with diaphoresis), peripheral ischemia.
GI: *nausea,* vomiting.
Respiratory: *bronchospasm,* wheezing, dyspnea, nasal congestion.
Other: inflammation, induration (at infusion site).

Reactions may be *common,* uncommon, *life-threatening,* or COMMON AND LIFE-THREATENING.

INTERACTIONS

Drug-drug. *Digoxin:* serum digoxin levels may be increased by 10% to 20%. Monitor serum digoxin levels.
Morphine: may increase esmolol blood levels. Titrate esmolol carefully.
Reserpine (and other catecholamine-depleting drugs): may cause additive bradycardia and hypotension. Titrate esmolol carefully.
Succinylcholine: esmolol may prolong neuromuscular blockade.

EFFECTS ON DIAGNOSTIC TESTS
None reported.

CONTRAINDICATIONS
Contraindicated in patients with sinus bradycardia, heart block greater than first-degree, cardiogenic shock, or overt heart failure.

NURSING CONSIDERATIONS
• Use cautiously in patients with impaired renal function, diabetes, or bronchospasm.
• Remember that esmolol solutions are incompatible with diazepam, furosemide, sodium bicarbonate, and thiopental sodium.
Alert: Monitor ECG and blood pressure continuously during infusion. Up to 50% of all patients treated with esmolol develop hypotension. Monitor closely, especially if patient's pretreatment blood pressure was low.
• Hypotension can usually be reversed within 30 minutes by decreasing the dose or, if necessary, by stopping the infusion. Notify doctor if this becomes necessary.
• If a local reaction develops at the infusion site, change to another site. Avoid using butterfly needles.
• Be aware that esmolol is recommended only for short-term use, for no longer than 48 hours.
• When patient's heart rate becomes stable, esmolol will be replaced by alternative (longer-acting) antiarrhythmics, such as propranolol, digoxin, or verapamil. A half-hour after the first dose of the alternative agent is administered, reduce infusion rate by 50%. Monitor patient response and, if heart rate is controlled for 1 hour after administration of the second dose of the alternative drug, discontinue esmolol infusion.

◗ I.V. administration
• Don't give esmolol by I.V. push; use an infusion control device. The 10-mg/ml single-dose vials may be used without diluting, but the injection concentrate (250 mg/ml) must be diluted to a maximum concentration of 10 mg/ml before infusion. Remove 20 ml from 500 ml of D_5W, lactated Ringer's solution, or 0.45% or 0.9% NaCl solution and add two ampules of esmolol (final concentration 10 mg/ml).

☑ Patient teaching
• Instruct patient to report adverse reactions promptly.
• Tell patient to alert nurse if discomfort occurs at I.V. site.

---

flecainide acetate
Tambocor

Pregnancy Risk Category: C

HOW SUPPLIED
Tablets: 50 mg, 100 mg, 150 mg
Injection: 10 mg/ml‡

ACTION
A class Ic antiarrhythmic that decreases excitability, conduction velocity, and automaticity as a result of slowed atrial, AV node, His-Purkinje system, and intraventricular conduction and causes a slight but significant prolongation of refractory periods in these tissues.

Route	Onset	Peak	Duration
PO	Unknown	2-3 hr	Unknown
IV	Immediate	Immediate	Unknown

INDICATIONS & DOSAGE
Paroxysmal supraventricular tachycardia, paroxysmal atrial fibrillation or flutter in patients without structural heart disease; life-threatening ventricular arrhythmias such as sustained ventricular tachycardia—

Adults: for paroxysmal supraventricular tachycardia, 50 mg P.O. q 12 hours. Increased in increments of 50 mg b.i.d. q 4 days. Maximum dosage is 300 mg/day.

Adjust-a-dose: In patients with renal impairment (creatinine clearance of 35 ml/ minute or less), initial dosage is 100 mg once daily or 50 mg b.i.d.

For life-threatening ventricular arrhythmias, 100 mg P.O. q 12 hours. Increase in increments of 50 mg b.i.d. q 4 days until efficacy is achieved. Maximum dosage is 400 mg daily for most patients.

Initial dosage for patients with heart failure is 50 mg P.O. q 12 hours. Where available, flecainide may be given by I.V. injection‡—

Adults: 2 mg/kg I.V. push over not less than 10 minutes to maximum dose of 150 mg; or dilute the dose and administer as an infusion.

ADVERSE REACTIONS
CNS: *dizziness, headache,* fatigue, tremor, anxiety, insomnia, depression, malaise, paresthesia, ataxia, vertigo, *lightheadedness, syncope,* asthenia.
CV: *new or worsened arrhythmias,* chest pain, *heart failure, cardiac arrest,* palpitations.
EENT: eye pain, eye irritation, *blurred vision* and *other visual disturbances.*
GI: nausea, constipation, abdominal pain, dyspepsia, vomiting, diarrhea, anorexia.
Other: *dyspnea,* edema, skin rash, flushing, fever.

INTERACTIONS
Drug-drug. *Amiodarone, cimetidine:* altered pharmacokinetics. Monitor for toxicity.
Digoxin: flecainide may increase plasma digoxin levels by 15% to 25%. Monitor serum digoxin levels.
Disopyramide, verapamil: negative inotropic properties may be additive with flecainide; avoid concurrent administration.
Propranolol, other beta blockers: both flecainide and propranolol plasma levels increase by 20% to 30%. Monitor for propranolol and flecainide toxicity.
Urine acidifying and alkalinizing agents:

extremes of urine pH may substantially alter excretion of flecainide. Monitor for flecainide toxicity or decreased effectiveness.
Drug-lifestyle. *Smoking:* lowered flecainide serum concentrations. Monitor closely.

EFFECTS ON DIAGNOSTIC TESTS
None reported.

CONTRAINDICATIONS
Contraindicated in patients with preexisting second- or third-degree AV block or right bundle-branch block when associated with a left hemiblock (in the absence of an artificial pacemaker), recent MI, cardiogenic shock, or hypersensitivity to drug.

NURSING CONSIDERATIONS
• Use cautiously in patients with preexisting heart failure, cardiomyopathy, severe renal or hepatic disease, prolonged QT interval, sick sinus syndrome, or blood dyscrasia.
• Know that when used to prevent ventricular arrhythmias, drug should be reserved for patients with documented life-threatening arrhythmias.
• Check that pacing threshold was determined 1 week before and after initiating therapy in patients with pacemakers because flecainide can alter endocardial pacing thresholds.
• Correct hypokalemia or hyperkalemia as ordered before giving flecainide because these electrolyte disturbances may alter its effect.
• Know that most patients can be adequately maintained on an every-12-hour dosing schedule, but that some need to receive flecainide every 8 hours.
• Be aware that dosage adjustments should be made only once every 3 to 4 days.
• Monitor serum flecainide levels, especially in patients with renal failure or heart failure. Therapeutic serum levels of flecainide range from 0.2 to 1 mcg/ml. Incidence of adverse effects increases when trough blood levels exceed 1 mcg/ml.

Reactions may be *common,* uncommon, *life-threatening,* or COMMON AND LIFE-THREATENING.

🔋 I.V. administration
• When administering by I.V. push, give over at least 10 minutes. For I.V. infusion, mix only with D₅W.
• Because of flecainide's long half-life, its full therapeutic effect may take 3 to 5 days. Administer concomitant I.V. lidocaine, as ordered, for the first several days.

✅ Patient teaching
• Stress importance of taking drug exactly as prescribed.
• Instruct patient to report adverse reactions promptly and to limit fluid and sodium intake to minimize fluid retention.
• Tell patient receiving drug I.V. to alert nurse if discomfort occurs at the insertion site.

---

ibutilide fumarate
Corvert

Pregnancy Risk Category: C

HOW SUPPLIED
Injection: 0.1 mg/ml in 10-ml vials

ACTION
Prolongs action potential in isolated cardiac myocyte and increases atrial and ventricular refractoriness, namely class III electrophysiologic effects.

Route	Onset	Peak	Duration
IV	Unknown	Unknown	Unknown

INDICATIONS & DOSAGE
Rapid conversion of atrial fibrillation or atrial flutter of recent onset to sinus rhythm—
Adults weighing 60 kg (132 lb) or more: 1 mg I.V. over 10 minutes.
Adults weighing less than 60 kg: 0.01 mg/kg I.V. over 10 minutes.
Alert: Infusion should be stopped if arrhythmia is terminated or patient develops ventricular tachycardia (VT) or marked prolongation of QT or QTc. If arrhythmia is not terminated 10 minutes after infusion ends, may give a second 10-minute infusion of equal strength.

ADVERSE REACTIONS
CNS: headache.
CV: ventricular extrasystoles, nonsustained VT, hypotension, bundle-branch block, *sustained polymorphic VT,* AV block, *heart failure,* hypertension, QT-segment prolongation, bradycardia, palpitation, tachycardia.
GI: nausea.

INTERACTIONS
Drug-drug. *Class Ia antiarrhythmics (disopyramide, procainamide, quinidine), other class III drugs (amiodarone, sotalol):* increased potential for prolonged refractoriness. Don't give these drugs for at least 5 half-lives before and 4 hours after ibutilide dose.
Digoxin: supraventricular arrhythmias may mask cardiotoxicity associated with excessive digoxin levels. Use cautiously.
H₁-receptor antagonist antihistamines, phenothiazines, tetracyclic antidepressants, tricyclic antidepressants, other drugs that prolong QT interval: increased risk for proarrhythmia. Monitor closely.

EFFECTS ON DIAGNOSTIC TESTS
None reported.

CONTRAINDICATIONS
Contraindicated in patients with hypersensitivity to drug or its components.

NURSING CONSIDERATIONS
• Drug is not recommended for patients with history of polymorphic VT and in breast-feeding women.
• Use cautiously in patients with hepatic or renal dysfunction.
• Safety of drug has not been established in children.
• Drug should be given only by skilled personnel. Cardiac monitor, intracardiac pacing, cardioverter or defibrillator, and medication for sustained VT must be available.
• Before therapy, hypokalemia and hypomagnesemia should be corrected to reduce the potential for proarrhythmia. Patients with atrial fibrillation of more than 2 to 3 days' duration must be adequately anticoagulated, generally for at least 2 weeks.

• Monitor ECG continuously during administration and for at least 4 hours afterward or until QTc returns to baseline; drug can induce or worsen ventricular arrhythmias. Longer monitoring is required if ECG shows arrhythmia.

◖ I.V. administration
• Drug may be given undiluted or diluted in 50 ml of diluent; may be added to 0.9% NaCl injection or 5% dextrose injection before infusion. Contents of 10-ml vial (0.1 mg/ml) may be added to 50-ml infusion bag to form admixture of about 0.017 mg/ml ibutilide fumarate. Use aseptic technique. Drug can be used with polyvinyl chloride plastic bags or polyolefin bags.
• Admixtures with approved diluents are stable for 24 hours at room temperature; 48 hours if refrigerated.
• Inspect parenteral products for particulate matter and discoloration before administration.

☑ Patient teaching
• Tell patient to report adverse reactions promptly.
• Instruct patient to alert nurse of discomfort at injection site.

---

lidocaine hydrochloride (lignocaine hydrochloride)
LidoPen Auto-Injector, Xylocaine, Xylocard†‡

Pregnancy Risk Category: B

HOW SUPPLIED
Injection (for I.M. use): 300 mg/3 ml automatic injection device
Injection (for direct I.V. use): 1% (10 mg/ml), 2% (20 mg/ml)
Injection (for I.V. admixtures): 4% (40 mg/ml), 10% (100 mg/ml), 20% (200 mg/ml)
Infusion (premixed): 0.2% (2 mg/ml), 0.4% (4 mg/ml), 0.8% (8 mg/ml)

ACTION
Lidocaine, a class Ib antiarrhythmic, decreases the depolarization, automaticity, and excitability in the ventricles during the diastolic phase by direct action on the tissues, especially the Purkinje network.

Route	Onset	Peak	Duration
IV	Immediate	Immediate	10-20 min
IM	5-15 min	10 min	2 hr

INDICATIONS & DOSAGE
Ventricular arrhythmias resulting from MI, cardiac manipulation, or cardiac glycosides—
Adults: 50 to 100 mg (1 to 1.5 mg/kg) by I.V. bolus at 25 to 50 mg/minute. Bolus dose is repeated q 3 to 5 minutes until arrhythmias subside or adverse reactions develop. Don't exceed 300-mg total bolus during a 1-hour period. Simultaneously, constant infusion of 20 to 50 mcg/kg/minute (1 to 4 mg/minute) is begun. If single bolus has been given, smaller bolus dose may be repeated 15 to 20 minutes after start of infusion to maintain therapeutic serum level. Alternatively, 200 to 300 mg I.M., followed by second I.M. dose 60 to 90 minutes later, if needed.
Children: 0.5 to 1 mg/kg by I.V. bolus, followed by infusion of 10 to 50 mcg/kg/minute.
Elderly: reduce dosage and rate of infusion by 50%.
Adjust-a-dose: In patients with heart failure, renal or liver disease, or those weighing less than 50 kg (110 lb), use reduced dosage.

ADVERSE REACTIONS
CNS: *confusion, tremor,* lethargy, somnolence, *stupor, restlessness,* anxiety, hallucinations, nervousness, *light-headedness,* paresthesia, muscle twitching, **seizures.**
CV: *hypotension,* bradycardia, **new or worsened arrhythmias, cardiac arrest.**
EENT: *tinnitus, blurred or double vision.*
Other: **anaphylaxis, respiratory depression and arrest,** soreness at injection site, sensation of cold, vomiting.

INTERACTIONS
Drug-drug. *Beta blockers, cimetidine:* decreased metabolism of lidocaine. Monitor for toxicity.
Mexiletine, tocainide: additive pharmacologic effects. Avoid concomitant use.
Phenytoin, procainamide, propranolol,

---

quinidine: additive cardiac depressant effects. Monitor carefully.

Drug-herb. *Pareira:* may add to or potentiate the effects of neuromuscular blockade. Avoid concomitant use.

Drug-lifestyle. *Smoking:* may increase metabolism of lidocaine. Monitor closely.

EFFECTS ON DIAGNOSTIC TESTS

Because I.M. lidocaine therapy may increase CK levels, isoenzyme tests should be performed for differential diagnosis of acute MI.

CONTRAINDICATIONS

Contraindicated in patients with hypersensitivity to the amide-type local anesthetics; Adams-Stokes syndrome; Wolff-Parkinson-White syndrome; and severe degrees of SA, AV, or intraventricular block in absence of artificial pacemaker.

NURSING CONSIDERATIONS

● Use cautiously in patients with complete or second-degree heart block or sinus bradycardia, in elderly patients, in those with heart failure or renal or hepatic disease, and in those weighing under 50 kg. Use reduced dosage in these patients.

● Give I.M. injections in the deltoid muscle only.

● Monitor isoenzymes when using I.M. drug for suspected MI. A patient who has received I.M. lidocaine will show a sevenfold increase in serum CK level. Such an increase originates in the skeletal muscle, not the heart.

● Monitor serum levels as ordered. Therapeutic levels are 2 to 5 mcg/ml.

Alert: Monitor patient for toxicity. In many severely ill patients, seizures may be the first clinical sign of toxicity. However, severe reactions usually are preceded by somnolence, confusion, and paresthesia.

● If signs of toxicity (such as dizziness) occur, stop drug at once and notify doctor. Continuing could lead to seizures and coma. Give oxygen via nasal cannula if not contraindicated. Keep oxygen and cardiopulmonary resuscitation equipment available.

● Monitor patient's response, especially blood pressure and serum electrolytes, BUN, and creatinine levels, as ordered. Notify doctor promptly if abnormalities develop.

● Discontinue infusion and notify doctor if arrhythmias worsen or ECG changes, such as widening QRS complex or substantially prolonged PR interval, are evident.

☐ I.V. administration

● Patients receiving infusions must be on a cardiac monitor and must be attended at all times. Use an infusion control device for administering infusion precisely. Do not exceed rate of 4 mg/minute; faster rate greatly increases risk of toxicity.

☑ Patient teaching

● Inform patient receiving drug I.M. that drug may cause soreness at injection site. Instruct patient receiving drug I.V. to alert nurse if discomfort occurs at the insertion site.

● Tell patient to report adverse reactions promptly because toxicity can occur.

---

mexiletine hydrochloride
Mexitil

Pregnancy Risk Category: C

HOW SUPPLIED

Capsules: 50 mg‡, 100 mg†, 150 mg, 200 mg, 250 mg
Injection: 250 mg/10 ml‡

ACTION

A class Ib antiarrhythmic that blocks the fast sodium channel in cardiac tissues, especially the Purkinje network, without involving the autonomic nervous system. Reduces the rate of rise and amplitude of the action potential and decreases automaticity in the Purkinje fibers. Shortens the duration of the action potential and, to a lesser extent, decreases the effective refractory period in the Purkinje fibers.

Route	Onset	Peak	Duration
PO	0.5-2 hr	2-3 hr	Unknown
IV	Immediate	Immediate	Unknown

INDICATIONS & DOSAGE

Refractory life-threatening ventricular arrhythmias, including ventricular tachycardia and PVC—
Adults: 200 to 400 mg P.O. followed by 200 mg q 8 hours. Dose increased q 2 to 3 days to 400 mg q 8 hours if satisfactory control is not obtained. Patients who respond well to an q-12-hour schedule may be given up to 450 mg q 12 hours.
Where available, mexiletine may be given I.V.‡—
Adults: loading dose is 100 to 250 mg I.V. at a rate of 25 mg/minute. Then prepare an infusion solution of 250 mg mexiletine in 500 ml of D₅W, and administer the first 120 ml (60 mg) over 1 hour. If clinical response is inadequate, give another bolus of 200 mg over 10 to 20 minutes. Maintenance dosage is 0.5 mg/minute (1 ml/minute of prepared solution).

ADVERSE REACTIONS

CNS: *tremor, dizziness,* blurred vision, diplopia, confusion, *light-headedness, incoordination,* changes in sleep habits, paresthesia, weakness, fatigue, speech difficulties, tinnitus, depression, *nervousness,* headache.
CV: **new or worsened arrhythmias,** palpitations, chest pain, nonspecific edema, angina.
GI: *nausea, vomiting, upper GI distress, heartburn,* diarrhea, constipation, dry mouth, changes in appetite, abdominal pain.
Skin: rash.

INTERACTIONS

Drug-drug. *Antacids, atropine, narcotics:* slowed mexiletine absorption. Monitor patient.
Cimetidine: increased or decreased mexiletine blood levels. Monitor carefully.
Methylxanthines (such as caffeine, theophylline): reduced clearance of methylxanthines, possibly resulting in toxicity. Monitor carefully.
Metoclopramide: mexiletine absorption may be accelerated. Monitor for toxicity.
Phenobarbital, phenytoin, rifampin, urine acidifiers: decreased mexiletine blood levels. Monitor carefully.

Urine alkalinizers: increased mexiletine blood levels. Monitor carefully.

EFFECTS ON DIAGNOSTIC TESTS

Liver function test results may be transiently altered during drug therapy.

CONTRAINDICATIONS

Contraindicated in patients with cardiogenic shock or preexisting second- or third-degree AV block in the absence of an artificial pacemaker.

NURSING CONSIDERATIONS

• Use cautiously in patients with preexisting first-degree heart block, a ventricular pacemaker, preexisting sinus node dysfunction, intraventricular conduction disturbances, hypotension, severe heart failure, or seizure disorder.
• When changing from lidocaine to mexiletine, stop the lidocaine infusion when the first mexiletine dose is given. Keep the infusion line open, however, until the arrhythmia appears to be satisfactorily controlled.
• Administer oral dose with meals to lessen GI distress.
• If you feel patient may be a good candidate for every 12-hour therapy, notify doctor. Twice-daily dosage enhances compliance.
• Monitor therapeutic levels, as ordered. Levels range from 0.5 to 2 mcg/ml.
• Monitor patient for toxicity. An early sign of mexiletine toxicity is tremor, usually a fine tremor of the hands. This progresses to dizziness and later to ataxia and nystagmus as the drug's blood level increases. Question patients about these symptoms.
• Monitor blood pressure and heart rate and rhythm frequently. Notify doctor of significant change.

I.V. administration
• Mexiletine injection is compatible with 0.9% NaCl, D₅W, 5% sodium bicarbonate, 1/6 M sodium lactate, and 10% fructose (levulose) solutions.

Patient teaching
• Tell patient to take drug exactly as pre-

---

scribed and to take with food or antacids if GI reactions occur.
● Instruct patient to report adverse reactions promptly.
● Tell patient receiving drug I.V. to report discomfort at insertion site.

moricizine hydrochloride
Ethmozine

Pregnancy Risk Category: B

HOW SUPPLIED
Tablets: 200 mg, 250 mg, 300 mg

ACTION
A class I antiarrhythmic that reduces the fast inward current carried by sodium ions across myocardial cell membranes. Has potent local anesthetic activity and membrane-stabilizing effect.

Route	Onset	Peak	Duration
PO	2 hr	0.5-2 hr	10-24 hr

INDICATIONS & DOSAGE
Life-threatening ventricular arrhythmias—
Adults: individualized dosage is based on clinical response and patient tolerance. Therapy should begin in the hospital. Most patients respond to 600 to 900 mg P.O. daily in divided doses q 8 hours. Daily dosage increased q 3 days by 150 mg until desired clinical effect is seen.
Adjust-a-dose: In patients with hepatic or renal impairment, 600 mg or less P.O. daily.

ADVERSE REACTIONS
CNS: *dizziness,* headache, fatigue, hyperesthesias, anxiety, asthenia, depression, nervousness, paresthesia, sleep disorders.
CV: *proarrhythmic events (ventricular tachycardia, PVC, supraventricular arrhythmias), ECG abnormalities (including conduction defects, sinus pause, junctional rhythm, and AV block), heart failure,* palpitations, chest pain, *cardiac death,* hypotension, hypertension, vasodilation, cerebrovascular events.
EENT: blurred vision.

GI: nausea, vomiting, abdominal pain, dyspepsia, diarrhea, dry mouth.
GU: urine retention, urinary frequency, dysuria.
Hepatic: elevated liver function test results.
Respiratory: dyspnea.
Skin: rash.
Other: drug-induced fever, diaphoresis, musculoskeletal pain, thrombophlebitis.

INTERACTIONS
Drug-drug. *Cimetidine:* increased plasma levels and decreased clearance of moricizine. Begin moricizine therapy at low dosage (not more than 600 mg daily), and monitor plasma levels and therapeutic effect closely.
Digoxin, propranolol: additive prolongation of PR interval. Monitor closely.
Theophylline: increased clearance and reduced plasma levels of theophylline. Monitor plasma levels and therapeutic response; adjust theophylline dosage as needed.

EFFECTS ON DIAGNOSTIC TESTS
None reported.

CONTRAINDICATIONS
Contraindicated in patients with preexisting second- or third-degree AV block or right bundle-branch block when associated with left hemiblock (bifascicular block) unless an artificial pacemaker is present, cardiogenic shock, or hypersensitivity to drug.

NURSING CONSIDERATIONS
● Know that, because drug has been detected in breast milk, a decision should be made to discontinue breast-feeding or discontinue drug, depending on its potential benefit to mother.
● Use with extreme caution in patients with sick sinus syndrome because drug may cause sinus bradycardia or sinus arrest. Also use with extreme caution in patients with coronary artery disease and left ventricular dysfunction because these patients may be at risk for sudden death when treated with the drug.
● Patients with hepatic or renal dysfunction will have decreased moricizine clear-

ance. Administer drug cautiously and monitor effects closely.

• Know that when substituting moricizine for another antiarrhythmic, previous drug should be withdrawn for one to two of the drug's half-lives before moricizine is started. Patients who have shown a tendency to develop life-threatening arrhythmias after withdrawal of previous antiarrhythmic drug therapy should be hospitalized during withdrawal and adjustment to moricizine. Guidelines doctors use for when to start moricizine therapy are as follows:

–disopyramide, 6 to 12 hours after the last dose.
–flecainide, 12 to 24 hours after last dose.
–mexiletine, 8 to 12 hours after last dose.
–procainamide, 3 to 6 hours after last dose.
–propafenone, 8 to 12 hours after last dose.
–quinidine, 6 to 12 hours after last dose.
–tocainide, 8 to 12 hours after last dose.

• Determine electrolyte status and correct imbalances before therapy as ordered. Hypokalemia, hyperkalemia, and hypomagnesemia may alter the effects of drug.

✅**Patient teaching**
• Instruct patient to take drug exactly as prescribed and not to abruptly discontinue use.
• Tell patient to avoid hazardous activities if adverse CNS reactions or blurred vision occurs.
• Instruct patient to report persistent or serious adverse reactions promptly.

---

procainamide hydrochloride
Procanbid, Promine, Pronestyl**,
Pronestyl-SR

Pregnancy Risk Category: C

HOW SUPPLIED
Tablets: 250 mg, 375 mg, 500 mg
Tablets (extended-release): 250 mg, 500 mg, 750 mg, 1,000 mg
Capsules: 250 mg, 375 mg, 500 mg
Injection: 100 mg/ml, 500 mg/ml

ACTION
A class Ia antiarrhythmic that decreases excitability, conduction velocity, automaticity, and membrane responsiveness with prolonged refractory period. Larger than usual doses may induce AV block.

Route	Onset	Peak	Duration
PO	1-2 hr	0.5-1.5 hr	Unknown
IV	Immediate	Immediate	Unknown
IM	10-30 min	15-60 min	Unknown

INDICATIONS & DOSAGE
Life-threatening ventricular arrhythmias—
Adults: 100 mg by slow I.V. push q 5 minutes, no faster than 25 to 50 mg/minute until arrhythmias disappear, adverse reactions develop, or 1 g has been given. Usual effective dose is 500 to 600 mg. When arrhythmias disappear, give continuous infusion of 1 to 6 mg/minute. If arrhythmias recur, repeat bolus as above and increase infusion rate. Alternatively, give 0.5 to 1 g I.M. q 4 to 8 hours until oral therapy begins.

For oral therapy, give 50 mg/kg daily in divided doses q 3 hours (average is 250 to 500 mg q 3 hours); for extended-release tablets, give 50 mg/kg daily in divided doses q 6 hours. For Procanbid extended-release tablets, 50 mg/kg daily P.O. in equally divided doses q 12 hours.
Adjust-a-dose: In patients with renal or hepatic dysfunction, decreased dosages or longer dosing intervals may be needed.

ADVERSE REACTIONS
CNS: hallucinations, confusion, *seizures,* depression, dizziness.
CV: *hypotension,* bradycardia, AV block, *ventricular fibrillation* (after parenteral use), *ventricular asystole.*
GI: abdominal pain, nausea, vomiting, anorexia, diarrhea, bitter taste.
Hematologic: *thrombocytopenia, neutropenia, agranulocytosis, hemolytic anemia.*
Hepatic: increased bilirubin, alkaline phosphatase, ALT, and AST.
Skin: *maculopapular rash, urticaria, pruritus, flushing, angioneurotic edema.*
Other: *fever, lupus-like syndrome* (espe-

---

cially after prolonged administration), elevated LD.

INTERACTIONS
Drug-drug. *Amiodarone:* increased procainamide levels and toxicity; additive effects on QT interval and QRS complex. Avoid concomitant use.
Anticholinergics: additive anticholinergic effects. Monitor closely.
Anticholinesterase agents: may decrease effect of anticholinesterase agents. Anticholinesterase dosage may need to be increased.
Beta blockers, cimetidine, ranitidine, trimethoprim: may increase procainamide blood levels. Monitor for toxicity.
Neuromuscular blockers: increased skeletal muscle relaxant effects. Monitor patient closely.
Drug-herb. *Jimson weed:* may adversely affect CV function. Avoid concomitant use.
Licorice: may prolong the QT interval and be potentially additive. Use cautiously.
Drug-lifestyle. *Alcohol use:* reduced drug levels. Avoid use.

EFFECTS ON DIAGNOSTIC TESTS
Drug will invalidate bentiromide test results; discontinue at least 3 days before bentiromide test. Procainamide may alter edrophonium test results; positive antinuclear antibody (ANA) titers; positive direct antiglobulin (Coombs') tests, and ECG changes may be seen.

CONTRAINDICATIONS
Contraindicated in patients with complete, second-, or third-degree heart block in the absence of an artificial pacemaker; myasthenia gravis; systemic lupus erythematosus; atypical ventricular tachycardia (torsades de pointes) because procainamide may aggravate this condition; or hypersensitivity to procaine and related drugs.

NURSING CONSIDERATIONS
• Use with extreme caution when treating patients with ventricular tachycardia during coronary occlusion.
• Use cautiously in patients with heart failure or other conduction disturbances,
such as bundle-branch heart block, sinus bradycardia, or digitalis intoxication, or with hepatic or renal insufficiency. Also use cautiously in those with preexisting blood dyscrasias or bone marrow suppression.
• Monitor plasma levels of procainamide and its active metabolite NAPA. To suppress ventricular arrhythmias, therapeutic serum concentrations of procainamide are 4 to 8 mcg/ml; therapeutic levels of NAPA are 10 to 30 mcg/ml.
• Monitor QT interval closely in patients with renal failure.
• Hypokalemia predisposes patients to arrhythmias; therefore, monitor serum electrolytes, especially potassium level.
• Elderly patients may be more likely to develop hypotension. Monitor blood pressure carefully.
• Monitor CBC frequently during first 3 months of therapy.
• Be aware that positive ANA titer is common in about 60% of patients who don't have symptoms of lupus-like syndrome. This response seems to be related to prolonged use, not dosage. May progress to systemic lupus erythematosus if drug is not discontinued.

I.V. administration
Alert: Monitor blood pressure and ECG continuously during I.V. administration. Watch for prolonged QT intervals and QRS complexes, heart block, or increased arrhythmias. If these occur, withhold drug, obtain rhythm strip, and notify doctor immediately.
• Attend patient receiving infusions *at all times*. Use an infusion control device to administer the infusion precisely.
• Note that the vials for I.V. injection contain 1 g of drug: 100 mg/ml (10 ml) or 500 mg/ml (2 ml).
• Keep patient in supine position during I.V. administration. If drug is given too rapidly, hypotension can occur. Watch closely for adverse reactions during infusion, and notify doctor if they occur.

Patient teaching
• Stress importance of taking drug exactly as prescribed. This may require use of an alarm clock for nighttime doses.

---

*Liquid contains alcohol.   **May contain tartrazine.   †Canada   ‡Australia   §U.K.   ◇ OTC

• Instruct patient to report fever, rash, muscle pain, diarrhea, bleeding, bruises, or pleuritic chest pain.
• Tell patient not to crush or break sustained-release tablets.
• Reassure patient who is taking the extended-release form that a wax-matrix "ghost" from the tablet may be passed in stools. Drug is completely absorbed before this occurs.

---

propafenone hydrochloride
Arythmol§, Rythmol

Pregnancy Risk Category: C

HOW SUPPLIED
Tablets: 150 mg, 225 mg, 300 mg

ACTION
A class Ic antiarrhythmic that reduces inward sodium current in Purkinje and myocardial cells. Decreases excitability, conduction velocity, and automaticity in AV nodal, His-Purkinje, and intraventricular tissue; causes slight but significant prolongation of refractory period in AV nodal tissue.

Route	Onset	Peak	Duration
PO	Unknown	3.5 hr	Unknown

INDICATIONS & DOSAGE
Suppression of life-threatening ventricular arrhythmias such as sustained ventricular tachycardia—
Adults: initially, 150 mg P.O. q 8 hours. May increase dosage at 3- to 4-day intervals to 225 mg q 8 hours; if necessary, increase dosage to 300 mg q 8 hours. Maximum daily dosage is 900 mg.

ADVERSE REACTIONS
CNS: anxiety, ataxia, *dizziness,* drowsiness, fatigue, headache, insomnia, syncope, tremor.
CV: atrial fibrillation, bradycardia, bundle-branch block, *heart failure,* angina, chest pain, edema, first-degree AV block, hypotension, increased QRS duration, intraventricular conduction delay, palpitations, *proarrhythmic events (ventricular tachycardia, PVC, ventricular fibrillation).*
EENT: blurred vision.
GI: abdominal pain or cramps, constipation, diarrhea, dyspepsia, anorexia, flatulence, *nausea, vomiting,* dry mouth, unusual taste.
Respiratory: dyspnea.
Skin: rash.
Other: diaphoresis, joint pain.

INTERACTIONS
Drug-drug. *Antiarrhythmics:* increased risk of heart failure. Monitor closely.
Cardiac glycosides, cyclosporine, oral anticoagulants: propafenone may increase serum levels of these agents by 35% to 85%, resulting in toxicity. Monitor closely.
Cimetidine: decreased metabolism of propafenone. Monitor closely.
Local anesthetics: increased risk of CNS toxicity. Monitor closely.
Metoprolol, propranolol: propafenone slows the metabolism of these agents. Adjust dosage as ordered.
Quinidine: slowed metabolism of propafenone. Avoid concomitant use.
Rifampin: increased clearance of propafenone. Monitor closely.

EFFECTS ON DIAGNOSTIC TESTS
Although drug may slow conduction and increase PR interval and QRS duration, ECG changes alone cannot be used to predict plasma concentration or drug efficacy.

CONTRAINDICATIONS
Contraindicated in patients with severe or uncontrolled heart failure; cardiogenic shock; SA, AV, or intraventricular disorders of impulse conduction in the absence of a pacemaker; bradycardia; marked hypotension; bronchospastic disorders; electrolyte imbalance; or hypersensitivity to drug.

NURSING CONSIDERATIONS
• Use cautiously in patients with heart failure because propafenone can exert a negative inotropic effect on the heart. Also use cautiously in patients taking oth-

er cardiac depressant drugs and in those with hepatic or renal failure.

• To minimize adverse GI reactions, administer drug with food.

• Continuous cardiac monitoring is recommended during initiation of therapy and during dosage adjustments. If PR interval or QRS complex increases by more than 25%, a reduction in dosage may be necessary.

• During concomitant use with digoxin, frequently monitor ECG and serum digoxin levels.

✓Patient teaching
• Stress importance of taking drug exactly as prescribed.
• Tell patient to report adverse reactions promptly.

---

quinidine bisulfate
(66.4% quinidine base) Biquin Durules†, Kinidin Durules‡

quinidine gluconate
(62% quinidine base) Quinaglute Dura-Tabs, Quinate†

quinidine polygalacturonate
(60.5% quinidine base) Cardioquin

quinidine sulfate
(83% quinidine base) Apo-Quinidine†, Cin-Quin, Novoquinidin†, Quinidex Extentabs, Quinora

Pregnancy Risk Category: C

HOW SUPPLIED
quinidine bisulfate
Tablets (extended-release): 250 mg†‡
quinidine gluconate
Tablets (extended-release): 324 mg, 325 mg†, 330 mg
Injection: 80 mg/ml
quinidine polygalacturonate
Tablets: 275 mg
quinidine sulfate
Tablets: 200 mg, 300 mg
Tablets (extended-release): 300 mg
Capsules: 200 mg, 300 mg
Injection: 200 mg/ml†

ACTION
A class Ia antiarrhythmic, quinidine has both direct and indirect (anticholinergic) effects on cardiac tissue. Automaticity, conduction velocity, and membrane responsiveness are decreased. The effective refractory period is prolonged. The anticholinergic action reduces vagal tone.

Route	Onset	Peak	Duration
PO	1-3 hr	1-6 hr	6-8 hr
IV	Immediate	Immediate	Unknown
IM	0.5-1.5 min	Unknown	Unknown

INDICATIONS & DOSAGE
Atrial flutter or fibrillation—
Adults: 200 mg quinidine sulfate or equivalent base P.O. q 2 to 3 hours for five to eight doses, with subsequent daily increases until sinus rhythm is restored or toxic effects develop. Administer quinidine only after AV node has been blocked with a beta blocker, digoxin, or a calcium channel blocker to avoid increasing AV conduction. Maximum dosage is 3 to 4 g daily.
Paroxysmal supraventricular tachycardia—
Adults: 400 to 600 mg P.O. gluconate q 2 to 3 hours until toxic adverse reactions develop or arrhythmia subsides.
Premature atrial and ventricular contractions; paroxysmal AV junctional rhythm; paroxysmal atrial tachycardia; paroxysmal ventricular tachycardia; maintenance after cardioversion of atrial fibrillation or flutter—
Adults: test dose is 200 mg P.O. or I.M. Quinidine sulfate or equivalent base 200 to 400 mg P.O. q 4 to 6 hours; or initially, quinidine gluconate 600 mg I.M., then up to 400 mg q 2 hours, p.r.n.; or quinidine gluconate 800 mg (10 ml of the commercially available solution) added to 40 ml of D_5W, infused I.V. at 16 mg (1 ml)/minute.
Children: 30 mg/kg/24 hours or 900 mg/m^2/24 hours P.O. in five divided doses.
Severe Plasmodium falciparum malaria—
Adults: 10 mg/kg gluconate I.V. diluted in 250 ml of 0.9% NaCl solution and infused over 1 to 2 hours, followed by a continuous maintenance infusion of

0.02 mg/kg/minute for 72 hours or until parasitemia is reduced to less than 1%.
Adjust-a-dose: Use reduced dosage in patients with impaired hepatic function or heart failure.

ADVERSE REACTIONS
CNS: *vertigo, headache, light-headedness,* confusion, ataxia, depression, dementia.
CV: *PVC; ventricular tachycardia; atypical ventricular tachycardia (torsades de pointes); hypotension; complete AV block,* tachycardia; *aggravated heart failure; ECG changes (particularly widening of QRS complex, widened QT and PR intervals).*
EENT: *tinnitus,* excessive salivation, blurred vision, diplopia, photophobia.
GI: *diarrhea, nausea, vomiting,* anorexia, abdominal pain.
Hematologic: *hemolytic anemia, thrombocytopenia, agranulocytosis.*
Hepatic: *hepatotoxicity.*
Respiratory: acute asthmatic attack, *respiratory arrest.*
Skin: rash, petechial hemorrhage of buccal mucosa, pruritus, urticaria, lupus erythematosus, photosensitivity.
Other: *angioedema, fever, cinchonism.*

INTERACTIONS
Drug-drug. *Acetazolamide, antacids, sodium bicarbonate, thiazide diuretics:* may increase quinidine blood levels because of alkaline urine. Monitor for increased effect.
Amiodarone, cimetidine: increased serum quinidine levels. Monitor for increased effect.
Barbiturates, phenytoin, rifampin: may lower blood levels of quinidine. Monitor for decreased effect.
Digoxin: increased serum digoxin levels after initiating quinidine therapy. Monitor closely.
Nifedipine: may decrease quinidine blood levels. Monitor carefully.
Other antiarrhythmics (such as lidocaine, procainamide, propranolol): increased risk of toxicity. Use together cautiously.
Phenytoin: decreased effectiveness of quinidine. May require dosage adjustments.

Tricyclic antidepressants: increased blood levels with increased effect. Monitor closely.
Verapamil: may result in hypotension, bradycardia, or AV block. Monitor blood pressure and heart rate.
Warfarin: increased anticoagulant effect. Monitor closely.
Drug-herb. *Jimson weed:* may adversely affect CV function. Avoid concomitant use.
Licorice: may prolong the QT interval and be potentially additive. Use together cautiously.

EFFECTS ON DIAGNOSTIC TESTS
None reported.

CONTRAINDICATIONS
Contraindicated in patients with idiosyncrasy or hypersensitivity to quinidine or related cinchona derivatives, and in those with myasthenia gravis, intraventricular conduction defects, digitalis toxicity when AV conduction is grossly impaired, abnormal rhythms due to escape mechanisms, and history of prolonged QT syndrome.

NURSING CONSIDERATIONS
• Use cautiously in patients with asthma, muscle weakness, or infection accompanied by fever because hypersensitivity reactions to drug may be masked.
• Also use cautiously in patients with hepatic or renal impairment because systemic accumulation may occur.
• Check apical pulse rate and blood pressure before therapy. If extremes in pulse rate are detected, withhold drug and notify doctor at once.
• Know that anticoagulant therapy is commonly advised before quinidine therapy in long-standing atrial fibrillation because restoration of normal sinus rhythm may result in thromboembolism caused by dislodgment of thrombi from atrial wall.
• When changing route of administration or oral salt form, be aware that dosage needs to be altered to compensate for variations in quinidine base content.
• Never use discolored (brownish) quinidine solution.
• Do not crush extended-release tablets.

Reactions may be *common,* uncommon, *life-threatening,* or COMMON AND LIFE-THREATENING.

Alert: In the treatment of severe malaria, patients should be hospitalized in an intensive-care setting. Continuous monitoring is necessary. Decrease infusion rate if plasma quinidine level exceeds 6 mcg/ml, uncorrected QT interval exceeds 0.6 second, or QRS complex widening exceeds 25% of baseline.

• Monitor liver function test results during first 4 to 8 weeks of therapy.
• Monitor serum quinidine levels as ordered. Therapeutic plasma levels for antiarrhythmic effects are 2 to 5 mcg/ml.
• Monitor patient response carefully. If adverse GI reactions occur, especially diarrhea, notify doctor. Check quinidine blood levels, which are toxic when greater than 8 mcg/ml. GI symptoms may be decreased by giving drug with meals or aluminum hydroxide antacids.
• Store drug away from heat and direct light.

◖ I.V. administration
• Dilute drug for infusion in appropriate solutions. Discard diluted solutions after 24 hours.
• During infusion, continuously monitor patient's blood pressure and ECG.

☑ Patient teaching
• Stress importance of taking drug exactly as prescribed and to take it with food if adverse GI reactions occur.
• Tell patient not to crush or chew extended-release tablets.
• Tell patient to report persistent or serious adverse reactions promptly, especially signs and symptoms of quinidine toxicity.

sotalol
Beta-Cardone§, Betapace, Sotacor†‡

Pregnancy Risk Category: B

HOW SUPPLIED
Tablets: 80 mg, 120 mg, 160 mg, 240 mg

ACTION
A nonselective beta-adrenergic blocker that depresses sinus heart rate, slows AV conduction, decreases cardiac output, and lowers systolic and diastolic blood pressure.

Route	Onset	Peak	Duration
PO	Unknown	2.5-4 hr	Unknown

INDICATIONS & DOSAGE
Documented, life-threatening ventricular arrhythmias—
Adults: initially, 80 mg P.O. b.i.d. Dosage is increased q 2 to 3 days as needed and tolerated; most patients respond to daily dosage of 160 to 320 mg. A few patients with refractory arrhythmias have received as much as 640 mg daily.
Adjust-a-dose: In patients with renal failure, if creatinine clearance is above 60 ml/minute, no adjustment in dosage interval is needed. If creatinine clearance is 30 to 60 ml/minute, dosage interval is increased to q 24 hours; between 10 and 30 ml/minute, q 36 to 48 hours; and if it is less than 10 ml/minute, dosage must be individualized.

ADVERSE REACTIONS
CNS: *asthenia, headache, dizziness, weakness, fatigue,* sleep problems, *lightheadedness.*
CV: *bradycardia,* **arrhythmias, heart failure, AV block, proarrhythmic events (polymorphic ventricular tachycardia, PVC, ventricular fibrillation),** edema, *palpitations, chest pain,* ECG abnormalities, hypotension.
GI: *nausea, vomiting,* diarrhea, dyspepsia.
Respiratory: *dyspnea, bronchospasm.*

INTERACTIONS
Drug-drug. *Antiarrhythmics:* additive effects. Avoid concomitant use.
Antihypertensives, catecholamine-depleting drugs (such as guanethidine, reserpine): enhanced hypotensive effects. Monitor closely.
Calcium channel blockers: enhanced myocardial depression. Avoid concomitant use.
Clonidine: beta blockers may enhance rebound effect after withdrawal of clonidine. Discontinue sotalol several days before withdrawing clonidine.

General anesthetics: may cause additional myocardial depression. Monitor closely.
Insulin, oral antidiabetic agents: may cause hyperglycemia. Adjust dosage. May mask symptoms of hypoglycemia.
Drug-food. *Any food:* decreased absorption by 20%. Give drug on empty stomach.

EFFECTS ON DIAGNOSTIC TESTS
Drug may increase blood glucose and liver enzyme levels. It may result in a false-positive catecholamine level.

CONTRAINDICATIONS
Contraindicated in patients with severe sinus node dysfunction, sinus bradycardia, second- and third-degree AV block in the absence of an artificial pacemaker, congenital or acquired long QT syndrome, cardiogenic shock, uncontrolled heart failure, bronchial asthma, or hypersensitivity to drug.

NURSING CONSIDERATIONS
• Use cautiously in patients with renal impairment or diabetes mellitus. Beta blockers may mask signs and symptoms of hypoglycemia.
• Because proarrhythmic events may occur at start of therapy and during dosage adjustments, patient should be hospitalized. Facilities and personnel should be available for cardiac rhythm monitoring and interpretation of ECG.
• Note that although patients receiving I.V. lidocaine have started sotalol therapy without ill effect, other antiarrhythmic drugs should be withdrawn before therapy with sotalol. Sotalol therapy typically is delayed until two or three half-lives of the withdrawn drug have elapsed. After withdrawal of amiodarone, sotalol shouldn't be administered until the QT interval normalizes.
• Be aware that dosage should be adjusted slowly, allowing 2 to 3 days between dosage increments for adequate monitoring of QT intervals and for plasma levels of drug to reach a steady-state level.
• Monitor serum electrolytes regularly, especially if patient is receiving diuretics. Electrolyte imbalances, such as hypokalemia or hypomagnesemia, may enhance

QT-interval prolongation and increase the risk of serious arrhythmias, such as torsades de pointes.

✓ Patient teaching
• Explain importance of taking drug as prescribed, even when the patient is feeling well. Caution against suddenly discontinuing drug.
• Caution against taking OTC cold medications and decongestants while taking drug.
• Because food can interfere with absorption, tell patient to take drug on an empty stomach, 1 hour before or 2 hours after meals.

---

tocainide hydrochloride
Tonocard

Pregnancy Risk Category: C

HOW SUPPLIED
Tablets: 400 mg, 600 mg

ACTION
A class Ib antiarrhythmic that blocks the fast sodium channel in cardiac tissues, especially the Purkinje network, without involvement of the autonomic nervous system. It reduces the rate of rise and amplitude of the action potential and decreases automaticity in the Purkinje fibers. It shortens the duration of action potential and, to a lesser extent, decreases the effective refractory period in the Purkinje fibers.

Route	Onset	Peak	Duration
PO	Unknown	0.5-2 hr	8 hr

INDICATIONS & DOSAGE
Suppression of symptomatic life-threatening ventricular arrhythmias—
Adults: initially, 400 mg P.O. q 8 hours. Usual dosage is between 1,200 and 1,800 mg daily in three divided doses.
Adjust-a-dose: In patients with renal or hepatic impairment, dosage of less than 1,200 mg daily may be adequate.

ADVERSE REACTIONS
CNS: ataxia, *light-headedness, tremor,*

paresthesia, *dizziness, vertigo,* drowsiness, fatigue, confusion, headache.
CV: hypotension, ***new or worsened arrhythmias, heart failure,*** bradycardia, palpitations.
EENT: blurred vision, tinnitus.
GI: *nausea, vomiting,* diarrhea, anorexia.
Hematologic: *blood dyscrasias.*
Hepatic: hepatitis, abnormal liver function test results.
Respiratory: ***respiratory arrest,*** pulmonary fibrosis, pneumonitis, ***pulmonary edema.***
Skin: rash, diaphoresis.

INTERACTIONS
Drug-drug. *Beta blockers:* decreased myocardial contractility; increased CNS toxicity. Monitor closely.
Cimetidine: may decrease tocainide peak concentration. Monitor closely.
Disopyramide, lidocaine, mexiletine, phenytoin, procainamide, quinidine: additive pharmacologic effect and CV and CNS toxicity. Monitor patient.
Rifampin: increased clearance of tocainide. Monitor efficacy of tocainide.

EFFECTS ON DIAGNOSTIC TESTS
None reported.

CONTRAINDICATIONS
Contraindicated in patients with hypersensitivity to lidocaine or other amide-type local anesthetics and in those with second- or third-degree AV block in the absence of an artificial pacemaker.

NURSING CONSIDERATIONS
• Use cautiously in patients with heart failure or diminished cardiac reserve and in those with hepatic or renal impairment. These patients often may be treated effectively with a lower dose.
• Be aware that drug may ease transition from I.V. lidocaine to oral antiarrhythmic. Monitor patient carefully.
• Correct potassium deficits, as ordered; drug may be ineffective in hypokalemia.
• Monitor patient for tremor, which may indicate that maximum dosage has been reached.
• Monitor blood levels as ordered. Therapeutic range is 4 to 10 mcg/ml.

☑ **Patient teaching**
• Instruct patient to report immediately unusual bruising or bleeding or signs of infection. Agranulocytosis and bone marrow suppression have been reported in patients taking usual doses of drug, typically within first 12 weeks of therapy.
• Advise patient to report sudden onset of pulmonary symptoms, such as coughing, wheezing, or exertional dyspnea. Drug has been associated with serious pulmonary toxicity.
• Tell elderly patient to take safety precautions because dizziness and falling may occur.

22

Antianginals

amlodipine besylate
amyl nitrite
bepridil hydrochloride
diltiazem hydrochloride
isosorbide dinitrate
isosorbide mononitrate
nadolol
nicardipine hydrochloride
nifedipine
nitroglycerin
propranolol hydrochloride
verapamil
verapamil hydrochloride

COMBINATION PRODUCTS
None.

---

amlodipine besylate
Istin§, Norvasc

Pregnancy Risk Category: C

HOW SUPPLIED
Tablets: 2.5 mg, 5 mg, 10 mg

ACTION
Inhibits calcium ion influx across cardiac and smooth-muscle cells, thus decreasing myocardial contractility and oxygen demand. Also dilates coronary arteries and arterioles.

Route	Onset	Peak	Duration
PO	Unknown	6-12 hr	24 hr

INDICATIONS & DOSAGE
Chronic stable angina; vasospastic angina (Prinzmetal's or variant angina)—
Adults: initially, 5 to 10 mg P.O. daily. Most patients require 10 mg daily.
Elderly: initially, 5 mg P.O. daily.
Adjust-a-dose: In small, frail patients or those with hepatic insufficiency, initially 5 mg P.O. daily.
Hypertension—
Adults: initially, 2.5 to 5 mg P.O. daily. Dosage adjusted according to patient response and tolerance. Maximum daily dosage is 10 mg.
Elderly: initially, 2.5 mg P.O. daily.
Adjust-a-dose: In small, frail, patients; those currently receiving other antihypertensives; or those with hepatic insufficiency, initially 2.5 mg P.O. daily.

ADVERSE REACTIONS
CNS: *headache,* somnolence, fatigue, dizziness, light-headedness, paresthesia.
CV: *edema,* flushing, palpitations.
GI: nausea, abdominal pain.
Other: dyspnea, muscle pain, rash, pruritus.

INTERACTIONS
None significant.

EFFECTS ON DIAGNOSTIC TESTS
None reported.

CONTRAINDICATIONS
Contraindicated in patients with hypersensitivity to drug.

NURSING CONSIDERATIONS
• Use cautiously in patients receiving other peripheral vasodilators, especially those with severe aortic stenosis, and in those with heart failure. Because drug is metabolized by the liver, use cautiously and in reduced dosage in patients with severe hepatic disease.
Alert: Monitor patient carefully. Some patients, especially those with severe obstructive coronary artery disease, have developed increased frequency, duration, or severity of angina or even acute MI after initiation of calcium channel blocker therapy or at time of dosage increase.
• Monitor blood pressure frequently during initiation of therapy. Because drug-induced vasodilation has a gradual onset, acute hypotension is rare.
• Notify doctor if signs of heart failure occur, such as swelling of hands and feet or shortness of breath.

Reactions may be *common*, uncommon, *life-threatening*, or COMMON AND LIFE-THREATENING.

• Caution patient to continue taking drug, even when feeling better.
• Tell patient S.L. nitroglycerin may be taken as needed when anginal symptoms are acute. If patient continues nitrate therapy during titration of amlodipine dosage, urge continued compliance.

amyl nitrite

Pregnancy Risk Category: X

HOW SUPPLIED
Ampules (crushable): 0.3 ml

ACTION
Antianginal action unknown. Thought to be the result of dilation of both arterial and venous beds. The net effect is a reduction in myocardial oxygen demand, improving perfusion to the ischemic myocardium. Converts hemoglobin to methemoglobin (which binds cyanide) to treat cyanide poisoning.

Route	Onset	Peak	Duration
Inhalation	30 sec	Unknown	3-5 min

INDICATIONS & DOSAGE
Relief of angina pectoris—
Adults and children: 0.3 ml by inhalation (one glass ampule), p.r.n.
Antidote for cyanide poisoning—
Adults and children: 0.3 ml by inhalation for 15 to 60 seconds q 5 minutes until conscious.

ADVERSE REACTIONS
CNS: *headache, sometimes with throbbing;* dizziness; weakness.
CV: *orthostatic hypotension, tachycardia,* flushing, palpitations, syncope.
GI: nausea, vomiting.
Hematologic: methemoglobinemia.
Skin: cutaneous vasodilation, rash.
Other: *hypersensitivity reactions.*

INTERACTIONS
Drug-drug. *Calcium channel blockers:* increased risk of symptomatic orthostatic hypotension. Monitor closely.
Drug-lifestyle. *Alcohol use:* severe hypotension and CV collapse may occur. Monitor patient.

EFFECTS ON DIAGNOSTIC TESTS
Drug alters the Zlatkis-Zak color reaction, causing a false decrease in serum cholesterol levels.

CONTRAINDICATIONS
Contraindicated in patients with severe anemia, angle-closure glaucoma, orthostatic hypotension, early MI, increased intracranial pressure, or hypersensitivity to nitrates and in pregnant patients.

NURSING CONSIDERATIONS
• Use cautiously in patients with glaucoma (except angle-closure type, which is a contraindication), volume depletion, or hypotension.
• Extinguish all cigarettes before use, or ampule may ignite.
• Wrap ampule in cloth and crush. Hold near patient's nose and mouth so vapor is inhaled.
• Watch for orthostatic hypotension.
• Store away from light.
• Be aware that drug is claimed to have aphrodisiac benefits and is often abused. Street name is "Amy."

• Instruct patient how to administer drug. Stress importance of extinguishing all cigarettes before use.
• Tell patient to sit and avoid position changes while inhaling drug to prevent orthostatic hypotension.
• Advise patient to take a mild analgesic for drug-induced headache.

bepridil hydrochloride
Vascor

Pregnancy Risk Category: C

HOW SUPPLIED
Tablets: 200 mg, 300 mg, 400 mg

ACTION
A calcium channel blocker that inhibits calcium ion influx across cardiac and smooth-muscle cells. This action dilates

---

coronary arteries as well as peripheral arteries and arterioles; it may reduce heart rate, decrease myocardial contractility, and slow AV node conduction.

Route	Onset	Peak	Duration
PO	1 hr	2-3 hr	24 hr

INDICATIONS & DOSAGE
Chronic stable angina in patients who cannot tolerate or who fail to respond to other agents—
Adults: initially, 200 mg P.O. daily. After 10 days, dosage increased based on response. Maintenance daily dosage in most patients is 300 mg; maximum daily dosage is 400 mg.

ADVERSE REACTIONS
CNS: *dizziness,* drowsiness, *nervousness, headache,* insomnia, paresthesia, *asthenia,* tremor.
CV: edema, flushing, palpitations, tachycardia, *ventricular arrhythmias, including torsades de pointes, ventricular tachycardia, ventricular fibrillation.*
EENT: tinnitus.
GI: *nausea, diarrhea,* constipation, abdominal discomfort, dry mouth, anorexia.
Respiratory: dyspnea, shortness of breath.
Skin: rash.
Other: flu syndrome.

INTERACTIONS
Drug-drug. *Antiarrhythmics, cardiac glycosides, drugs that increase QT interval:* may exaggerate prolongation of the QT interval or depression of AV node with bepridil. Monitor closely.
Digoxin: serum digoxin levels may be increased. Monitor combined use.
Fentanyl: may cause severe hypotension. Monitor patient.

EFFECTS ON DIAGNOSTIC TESTS
Increased ALT levels and abnormal liver function test results have been observed.

CONTRAINDICATIONS
Contraindicated in patients with hypersensitivity to drug; uncompensated cardiac insufficiency; sick sinus syndrome or second- or third-degree AV block unless pacemaker is present; hypotension (below 90 mm Hg systolic); congenital QT-interval prolongation; or history of serious ventricular arrhythmias. Also contraindicated in those receiving other drugs that prolong the QT interval.

NURSING CONSIDERATIONS
• Use cautiously in patients with left bundle-branch block, sinus bradycardia, impaired renal or hepatic function, or heart failure.
• Monitor patient for adverse reactions. Bepridil has been associated with severe ventricular arrhythmias, including torsades de pointes.
• Know that dosage should not be adjusted more frequently than every 10 to 14 days because of bepridil's long half-life and the time it takes to reach steady-state blood levels.

☑**Patient teaching**
• Instruct patient to take drug exactly as directed.
• Tell patient to protect drug from light.

---

diltiazem hydrochloride
Adizem-60§, Adizem-SR§ , Adizem-XL§ , Angitil SR§ , Apo-Diltiaz†, Calcicard CR§, Cardizem, Cardizem CD, Cardizem SR, Dilacor XR, Dilzem SR§, Dilzem XL§, Slozem§, Tiazac, Tildiem§, Tildiem LA§, Tildiem Retard§, Viazem XL§, Zemtard 300XL§

Pregnancy Risk Category: C

HOW SUPPLIED
Tablets: 30 mg, 60 mg, 90 mg, 120 mg
Capsules (extended-release; Cardizem CD, Dilacor XR, Tiazac): 120 mg, 180 mg, 240 mg, 300 mg, 360 mg (Tiazac)
Capsules (sustained-release; Cardizem SR): 60 mg, 90 mg, 120 mg, 180 mg, 240 mg
Injection: 5 mg/ml

ACTION
A calcium channel blocker that inhibits

calcium ion influx across cardiac and smooth-muscle cells, decreasing myocardial contractility and oxygen demand. Also dilates coronary arteries and arterioles.

Route	Onset	Peak	Duration
PO	0.5-1 hr	2-3 hr	6-8 hr
PO (extended, sustained)	2-3 hr	10-14 hr	12-24 hr
IV	3 min	Immediate	1-10 hr

INDICATIONS & DOSAGE

Vasospastic angina (Prinzmetal's or variant angina) and classic chronic stable angina pectoris—
Adults: 30 mg P.O. t.i.d. or q.i.d. before meals and h.s. Dosage increased gradually to maximum of 360 mg daily in divided doses. Alternatively, 120 or 180 mg (extended-release). Titrated as needed and tolerated to maximum of 480 mg daily.
Hypertension—
Adults: 60 to 120 mg P.O. b.i.d. (sustained-release). Titrated to effect. Maximum recommended dosage is 360 mg daily. Alternatively, initially 180 to 240 mg daily (extended-release). Dosage adjusted p.r.n.
Atrial fibrillation or flutter; paroxysmal supraventricular tachycardia—
Adults: 0.25 mg/kg as an I.V. bolus injection over 2 minutes. If response is inadequate, 0.35 mg/kg I.V. after 15 minutes followed with a continuous infusion of 10 mg/hour. Some patients respond well to rates of 5 mg/hour; maximum dose is 15 mg/hour.

ADVERSE REACTIONS

CNS: *headache,* dizziness, asthenia, somnolence.
CV: *edema,* **arrhythmias,** flushing, bradycardia, hypotension, conduction abnormalities, **heart failure,** AV block, abnormal ECG.
GI: *nausea, constipation,* abdominal discomfort.
Hepatic: acute hepatic injury.
Skin: *rash.*

INTERACTIONS

Drug-drug. *Anesthetics:* effects may be potentiated. Monitor patient.
Cimetidine: may inhibit diltiazem metabolism. Monitor for toxicity, additive AV node conduction slowing.
Cyclosporine: diltiazem may increase serum cyclosporine levels, possibly by decreasing its metabolism, leading to increased risk of cyclosporine toxicity. If used concurrently, monitor cyclosporine levels.
Digoxin: diltiazem may increase serum levels of digoxin. Monitor for toxicity.
Furosemide: forms a precipitate when mixed with diltiazem injection. Administer through separate I.V. lines.
Propranolol, other beta blockers: may precipitate heart failure or prolong conduction time. Use together cautiously.

EFFECTS ON DIAGNOSTIC TESTS
None reported.

CONTRAINDICATIONS
Contraindicated in patients with sick sinus syndrome or second- or third-degree AV block in the absence of an artificial pacemaker, systolic blood pressure below 90 mm Hg, acute MI, pulmonary congestion (documented by X-ray), or hypersensitivity to drug.

NURSING CONSIDERATIONS
• Use cautiously in elderly patients and in those with heart failure or impaired hepatic or renal function.
• Monitor blood pressure and heart rate during initiation of therapy and dosage adjustments.
• If systolic blood pressure is below 90 mm Hg or heart rate is below 60 beats/minute, withhold dose and notify doctor.

I.V. administration
• Infusions lasting longer than 24 hours are not recommended.

Patient teaching
• Advise patient to avoid hazardous activities during initiation of therapy.
• If nitrate therapy is prescribed during titration of diltiazem dosage, urge patient compliance. Tell patient that S.L. nitro-

glycerin, especially, may be taken concomitantly as needed when anginal symptoms are acute.
• Tell patient to swallow Dilacor XR whole, not to open, crush, or chew it.

---

isosorbide dinitrate
Apo-ISDN†, Cedocard Retard§, Cedocard SR†, Coradur†, Coronex†, Dilatrate-SR, Isoket Retard§, Isonate, Isorbid, Isordil, Isordil Tembids, Isordil Titradose, Isotrate, Novosorbide†, Sorbid SA§, Sorbichew§, Sorbitrate

isosorbide mononitrate
Elantan§, Imdur, Isib 60XL§, ISMO, Isotrate§, Modisal XL§, Monit§, Mono-Cedocard§, Monoket, Monosorb XL 60§

Pregnancy Risk Category: C

HOW SUPPLIED
isosorbide dinitrate
Tablets: 5 mg, 10 mg, 20 mg, 30 mg, 40 mg
Tablets (S.L.): 2.5 mg, 5 mg, 10 mg
Tablets (chewable): 5 mg, 10 mg
Tablets (sustained-release): 40 mg
Capsules: 40 mg
Capsules (sustained-release): 40 mg
isosorbide mononitrate
Tablets: 10 mg, 20 mg
Tablets (extended-release): 30 mg, 60 mg, 120 mg

ACTION
Not completely known. Thought to reduce cardiac oxygen demand by decreasing preload and afterload. Drug also may increase blood flow through the collateral coronary vessels.

Route	Onset	Peak	Duration
PO	15-40 min	Unknown	4-6 hr
PO (SL)	2-5 min	Unknown	1.5 hr
PO (chewable)	2-5 min	Unknown	2-2.5 hr
PO (extended)	0.5-4 hr	Unknown	12 hr

INDICATIONS & DOSAGE
Acute anginal attacks (S.L. and chewable tablets of isosorbide dinitrate only); prophylaxis in situations likely to cause anginal attacks—
Adults: *S.L. form*—2.5 to 5 mg S.L. for prompt relief of anginal pain, repeated q 5 to 10 minutes (maximum of three doses for each 30-minute period). For prophylaxis, 2.5 to 10 mg q 2 to 3 hours.
Chewable form—5 to 10 mg p.r.n. for acute attack or q 2 to 3 hours for prophylaxis, but only after initial test dose of 5 mg to determine risk of severe hypotension.
Oral form (isosorbide dinitrate)—5 to 30 mg P.O. t.i.d. or q.i.d. for prophylaxis only (use smallest effective dose); 20 to 40 mg P.O. (sustained-release) q 6 to 12 hours.
Oral form (isosorbide mononitrate using Imdur)—30 to 60 mg P.O. once daily upon arising; increased to 120 mg once daily after several days, if needed.
Oral form (isosorbide mononitrate using ISMO or Monoket)—20 mg b.i.d. with the two doses given 7 hours apart.

ADVERSE REACTIONS
CNS: *headache* (sometimes with throbbing); dizziness; weakness.
CV: *orthostatic hypotension, tachycardia, palpitations, ankle edema,* fainting.
GI: nausea, vomiting.
Skin: cutaneous vasodilation, *flushing,* rash.
Other: hypersensitivity reactions, sublingual burning.

INTERACTIONS
Drug-drug. *Antihypertensives:* may increase hypotensive effects. Monitor closely during initial therapy.
Drug-lifestyle. *Alcohol use:* may increase hypotension. Avoid concomitant use.

EFFECTS ON DIAGNOSTIC TESTS
May interfere with serum cholesterol determination tests using the Zlatkis-Zak color reaction, causing a falsely decreased value.

CONTRAINDICATIONS
Contraindicated in patients with severe

---

hypotension, angle-closure glaucoma, increased intracranial pressure, shock, acute MI with low left ventricular filling pressure, and hypersensitivity or idiosyncrasy to nitrates.

NURSING CONSIDERATIONS
• Use cautiously in patients with blood volume depletion (such as from diuretic therapy) or mild hypotension.
• To prevent development of tolerance, a nitrate-free interval of 8 to 12 hours/day has been recommended. The regimen for isosorbide mononitrate (one tablet upon awakening with the second dose in 7 hours, or one extended-release tablet daily) is intended to minimize nitrate tolerance by providing a substantial nitrate-free interval.
• Monitor blood pressure and intensity and duration of drug response.
• Drug may cause headaches, especially at beginning of therapy. Dosage may be reduced temporarily, but tolerance usually develops. Treat headache with aspirin or acetaminophen.

☑ Patient teaching
• Caution patient to take medication regularly, as prescribed, and to keep it accessible at all times.
Alert: Advise patient that abrupt discontinuation of drug may cause coronary vasospasm with increased anginal symptoms and potential risk of MI.
• Tell patient to take S.L. tablet at first sign of attack. The tablet should be wet with saliva and placed under the tongue until absorbed; the patient should sit down and rest. Dose may be repeated every 10 to 15 minutes for a maximum of three doses. If drug doesn't provide relief, tell patient to seek medical help promptly.
• Advise patient who complains of tingling sensation with S.L. drug to try holding tablet in buccal pouch.
• Warn patient not to confuse S.L. with oral form.
• Advise patient taking oral form of isosorbide dinitrate to take oral tablet on an empty stomach, either 30 minutes before or 1 to 2 hours after meals; to swallow oral tablets whole; and to chew chewable tablets thoroughly before swallowing.
• Tell patient to minimize orthostatic hypotension by changing to upright position slowly. Advise him to go up and down stairs carefully and to lie down at first sign of dizziness.
• Inform patient to store drug in a cool place, in a tightly closed container, away from light.

---

nadolol
Corgard

Pregnancy Risk Category: C

HOW SUPPLIED
Tablets: 20 mg, 40 mg, 80 mg, 120 mg, 160 mg

ACTION
A beta-adrenergic blocker that reduces cardiac oxygen demand by blocking catecholamine-induced increases in heart rate, blood pressure, and force of myocardial contraction. Depresses renin secretion.

Route	Onset	Peak	Duration
PO	Unknown	2-4 hr	Unknown

INDICATIONS & DOSAGE
Angina pectoris—
Adults: 40 mg P.O. once daily. Dosage increased in 40- to 80-mg increments at 3- to 7-day intervals until optimum response occurs. Usual maintenance dosage is 40 to 80 mg once daily; up to 240 mg once daily may be needed.
Hypertension—
Adults: 40 mg P.O. once daily. Dosage increased in 40- to 80-mg increments until optimum response occurs. Usual maintenance dosage is 40 to 80 mg once daily. Doses of 320 mg may be needed.

ADVERSE REACTIONS
CNS: fatigue, dizziness.
CV: *bradycardia, hypotension, **heart failure,*** peripheral vascular disease, rhythm and conduction disturbances.
GI: nausea, vomiting, diarrhea, abdominal pain, constipation, anorexia.

Respiratory: *increased airway resistance.*
Skin: rash.
Other: fever.

INTERACTIONS

Drug-drug. *Antihypertensives:* enhanced antihypertensive effect. Monitor closely.
Cardiac glycosides: excessive bradycardia and additive effects on AV conduction. Use together cautiously.
Epinephrine: severe vasoconstriction and reflex bradycardia. Monitor blood pressure carefully.
Phenothiazines: can result in additive hypotensive effects. Monitor closely.
Insulin, oral antidiabetic agents: can alter dosage requirements in previously stabilized diabetic patients. Observe patient carefully.
NSAIDs: decreased antihypertensive effect. Monitor blood pressure and adjust dosage.

EFFECTS ON DIAGNOSTIC TESTS

None reported.

CONTRAINDICATIONS

Contraindicated in patients with bronchial asthma, sinus bradycardia and greater than first-degree heart block, and cardiogenic shock.

NURSING CONSIDERATIONS

• Use cautiously in patients with heart failure, chronic bronchitis, emphysema, or renal or hepatic impairment and in patients undergoing major surgery involving general anesthesia. Also use cautiously in diabetic patients because beta-adrenergic blockers may mask certain signs and symptoms of hypoglycemia.
• Check apical pulse before giving drug. If slower than 60 beats/minute, withhold drug and call doctor.
• Monitor blood pressure frequently. If patient develops severe hypotension, administer a vasopressor, as prescribed.
Alert: Know that abrupt discontinuation can exacerbate angina and precipitate MI. Dosage should be reduced gradually over 1 to 2 weeks.
• Be aware that nadolol masks signs of shock and hyperthyroidism.

✓ **Patient teaching**
• Explain importance of taking drug as prescribed, even when patient is feeling well.
• Teach patient how to check pulse rate and to do so before each dose. If pulse rate is below 60 beats/minute, tell patient to notify doctor.
• Caution patient not to discontinue drug suddenly.

---

nicardipine hydrochloride
Cardene, Cardene IV,
Cardene SR

Pregnancy Risk Category: C

HOW SUPPLIED

Capsules (immediate-release): 20 mg, 30 mg
Capsules (sustained-release): 30 mg, 45 mg, 60 mg
Injection: 2.5 mg/ml

ACTION

A calcium channel blocker that inhibits calcium ion influx across cardiac and smooth-muscle cells, decreasing myocardial contractility and oxygen demand. Also dilates coronary arteries and arterioles.

Route	Onset	Peak	Duration
PO (immediate)	0.5-1.5 min	Unknown	Unknown
PO (sustained)	20 min	1-4 hr	12 hr
IV	Immediate	Immediate	Unknown

INDICATIONS & DOSAGE

Chronic stable angina (used alone or in combination with other antianginal agents)—
Adults: initially, 20 mg P.O. t.i.d. (immediate-release only). Dosage titrated based on patient response q 3 days. Usual dosage range is 20 to 40 mg t.i.d.
Hypertension—
Adults: initially, 20 mg P.O. t.i.d. (immediate-release); range, 20 to 40 mg t.i.d. Or, 30 mg b.i.d. (sustained-release); range, 30 to 60 mg b.i.d. Dosage increased based on patient response. Alter-

natively, for patients unable to take oral nicardipine, 50 ml/hour (5 mg/hour) I.V. infusion initially; then increased by 25 ml/hour (2.5 mg/hour) q 15 minutes up to maximum of 150 ml/hour (15 mg/ hour).

ADVERSE REACTIONS
CNS: *dizziness, light-headedness, headache, asthenia.*
CV: *peripheral edema, palpitations,* angina, tachycardia.
GI: nausea, abdominal discomfort, dry mouth.
Skin: rash, *flushing.*

INTERACTIONS
Drug-drug. *Antihypertensives:* enhanced antihypertensive effect. Monitor closely.
Beta blockers: may increase cardiac depressant effects. Monitor closely.
Cimetidine: may decrease metabolism of calcium channel blockers. Monitor for increased pharmacologic effect.
Cyclosporine: nicardipine may increase plasma levels of cyclosporine. Monitor for toxicity.
Theophylline: pharmacologic effects of theophylline may be enhanced. Monitor for toxicity.

EFFECTS ON DIAGNOSTIC TESTS
None reported.

CONTRAINDICATIONS
Contraindicated in patients with advanced aortic stenosis or hypersensitivity to drug.

NURSING CONSIDERATIONS
• Use cautiously in patients with hypotension, heart failure, and impaired hepatic and renal function.
• Measure blood pressure frequently during initial therapy. Maximum blood pressure response occurs about 1 hour after dosing with the immediate-release form and 2 to 4 hours with the sustained-release form. Check for potential orthostatic hypotension. Because large swings in blood pressure may occur based on blood level of drug, assess adequacy of antihypertensive effect 8 hours after dosing.

■ I.V. administration
• Adjust infusion rate if hypotension or tachycardia occurs, as ordered.
• When switching to oral therapy other than nicardipine, initiate therapy upon discontinuation of the infusion. If oral nicardipine is to be used, administer first dose of t.i.d. regimen 1 hour before discontinuing infusion.

☑ Patient teaching
• Tell patient to take oral form of drug exactly as prescribed.
• Advise patient to report chest pain immediately. Some patients may experience increased frequency, severity, or duration of chest pain at beginning of therapy or during dosage adjustments.

---

nifedipine
Adalat, Adalat CC, Adalat FT†, Adalat PA†, Adipine MR§, Apo-Nifed†, Cardilate MR§, Coracten§, Hypolar Retard 20§, Nifedotard 20 MR§, Nifelease§, Nifensar XL§, Novo-Nifedin†, Nu-Nifed†, Procardia, Procardia XL, Tensipine MR§, Unipine XL§

Pregnancy Risk Category: C

HOW SUPPLIED
Tablets (extended-release): 30 mg, 60 mg, 90 mg
Capsules: 10 mg, 20 mg

ACTION
Unknown. Thought to inhibit calcium ion influx across cardiac and smooth-muscle cells, decreasing contractility and oxygen demand. Also may dilate coronary arteries and arterioles.

Route	Onset	Peak	Duration
PO	20 min	0.5-1 hr	4-8 hr
PO (extended)	20 min	6 hr	24 hr

INDICATIONS & DOSAGE
Vasospastic angina (also called Prinzmetal's or variant angina) and classic chronic stable angina pectoris—

Adults: initially 10 mg P.O. t.i.d. Usual effective dose range is 10 to 20 mg t.i.d. Some patients may require up to 30 mg q.i.d. Maximum daily dosage is 180 mg.
Hypertension—
Adults: 30 or 60 mg P.O. (extended-release form) once daily. Titrated over 7 to 14 days. Doses larger than 90 mg (for Adalat CC) and 120 mg (for Procardia XL) are not recommended.

ADVERSE REACTIONS
CNS: *dizziness, light-headedness, flushing, headache, weakness,* syncope, nervousness.
CV: *peripheral edema,* hypotension, palpitations, heart failure, *MI,* pulmonary edema.
EENT: nasal congestion.
GI: *nausea,* diarrhea, constipation, abdominal discomfort.
Respiratory: dyspnea, cough.
Skin: rash, pruritus.
Other: muscle cramps, hypokalemia.

INTERACTIONS
Drug-drug. *Cimetidine, ranitidine:* decreased nifedipine metabolism. Dose may be adjusted.
Fentanyl: severe hypotension may occur. Monitor closely.
Phenytoin: may reduce phenytoin metabolism. Monitor closely.
Propranolol, other beta blockers: may cause hypotension and heart failure. Use together cautiously.
Drug-food. *Grapefruit juice:* increased bioavailability of nifedipine. Monitor closely if given together.

EFFECTS ON DIAGNOSTIC TESTS
Mild to moderate increase in serum concentrations of alkaline phosphate, LD, AST, and ALT have been noted.

CONTRAINDICATIONS
Contraindicated in patients with hypersensitivity to drug.

NURSING CONSIDERATIONS
• Use cautiously in patients with heart failure or hypotension and in elderly patients. Use extended-release tablets cautiously in patients with severe GI narrowing.
• When a rapid response to drug is desired, have patient bite and swallow the capsule. If he can't chew capsules, the liquid can be withdrawn by puncturing the capsule with a needle and squeezing the contents into the mouth. When these methods are used, continuous blood pressure and ECG monitoring is recommended. This method is not recommended for the treatment of hypertension.
• Despite widespread S.L. use of nifedipine capsules, this route of administration should be avoided. Peak serum levels are lower and take longer to occur than when capsules are bitten and swallowed.
• Monitor blood pressure regularly, especially in patients who are taking beta blockers or antihypertensives.
• Be aware that although rebound effect hasn't been observed when drug is stopped, dosage should be reduced slowly under doctor's supervision.

☑**Patient teaching**
• If patient is kept on nitrate therapy while nifedipine dosage is being titrated, urge continued compliance. S.L. nitroglycerin, especially, may be taken as needed when anginal symptoms are acute.
• Tell patient he may briefly develop anginal exacerbation when beginning drug therapy or when dosage is increased.
• Instruct patient to swallow extended-release tablets without breaking, crushing, or chewing.
• Reassure patient who is taking the extended-release form that a wax-matrix "ghost" from the tablet may be passed in the stools. Drug is completely absorbed before this occurs.
• Warn patient not to switch brands. Procardia XL and Adalat CC are not therapeutically equivalent because of major differences in their pharmacokinetics.
• Tell patient to protect capsules from direct light and moisture and to store at room temperature.

---

nitroglycerin
(glyceryl trinitrate)
Anginine‡, Deponit, Minitran,
Nitradisc‡, Nitro-Bid, Nitro-Bid I.V.,
Nitrocine, Nitrodisc, Nitro-Dur,
Nitrogard, Nitrogard SR†,
Nitroglyn, Nitrol, Nitrolingual,
Nitrong, Nitrostat, Nitro-Time,
NTS, Transderm-Nitro,
Transiderm-Nitro‡, Tridil

Pregnancy Risk Category: C

HOW SUPPLIED
Tablets (buccal): 1 mg, 2 mg, 3 mg
Tablets (S.L.): 0.15 mg (1/400 gr), 0.3 mg
(1/200 gr), 0.4 mg (1/150 gr), 0.6 mg
(1/100 gr)
Tablets (sustained-release): 2.6 mg,
6.5 mg, 9 mg, 13 mg
Capsules (sustained-release): 2.5 mg,
6.5 mg, 9 mg, 13 mg
Aerosol (translingual): 0.4 mg metered
spray
Topical: 2% ointment
Transdermal: 0.1 mg, 0.2 mg, 0.3 mg,
0.4 mg, 0.6 mg, 0.8 mg per hour release
rate
Injection: 0.5 mg/ml, 5 mg/ml

ACTION
A nitrate that reduces cardiac oxygen demand by decreasing left ventricular end-
diastolic pressure (preload) and, to a lesser extent, systemic vascular resistance
(afterload). Also increases blood flow
through the collateral coronary vessels.

Route	Onset	Peak	Duration
PO	20-45 min	Unknown	3-8 hr
PO (buccal)	3 min	Unknown	3-5 hr
PO (SL)	1-3 min	Unknown	0.5-1 hr
IV	Immediate	Immediate	3-5 min
Trans-lingual	2-4 min	Unknown	0.5-1 hr
Topical	30 min	Unknown	2-12 hr
Trans-dermal	30 min	Unknown	24 hr

INDICATIONS & DOSAGE
*Prophylaxis against chronic anginal at-
tacks—*
Adults: 2.5 or 2.6 mg sustained-release
capsule or tablet q 8 to 12 hours, titrated
upward to an effective dose in 2.5- or 2.6-
mg increments b.i.d. to q.i.d. Or, use 2%
ointment: Start dosage with ½″ ointment,
increasing by ½″ increments until desired
results are achieved. Range of dosage
with ointment is ½″ to 5″. Usual dose is 1″
to 2″. Alternatively, transdermal disc or
pad (Nitrodisc, Nitro-Dur, or Transderm-
Nitro) 0.2 to 0.4 mg/hour once daily.
*Acute angina pectoris, prophylaxis to pre-
vent or minimize anginal attacks before
stressful events—*
Adults: 1 S.L. tablet (gr 1/400, 1/200,
1/150, 1/100) dissolved under the tongue
or in the buccal pouch as soon as angina
begins. Repeat q 5 minutes, if needed, for
15 minutes. Or, using Nitrolingual spray,
one or two sprays into mouth, preferably
onto or under the tongue. Repeat q 3 to 5
minutes, if needed, to a maximum of three
doses within a 15-minute period. Or, 1 to
3 mg transmucosally q 3 to 5 hours during waking hours.
*Hypertension associated with surgery;
heart failure associated with MI; angina
pectoris in acute situations; to produce
controlled hypotension during surgery (by
I.V. infusion)—*
Adults: initial infusion rate is 5 mcg/
minute, increased p.r.n. by 5 mcg/minute
q 3 to 5 minutes until response occurs. If
a 20 mcg/minute rate doesn't produce a
response, may increase dosage by as
much as 20 mcg/minute q 3 to 5 minutes.
Up to 100 mcg/minute may be needed.

ADVERSE REACTIONS
CNS: *headache, sometimes with throb-
bing; dizziness;* weakness.
CV: *orthostatic hypotension, tachycardia,
flushing, palpitations,* fainting.
GI: nausea, vomiting.
Skin: cutaneous vasodilation, contact der-
matitis (patch), rash.
Other: hypersensitivity reactions, sublin-
gual burning.

INTERACTIONS
Drug-drug. *Antihypertensives:* possible
enhanced hypotensive effect. Monitor
closely.
Heparin: I.V. nitroglycerin interferes with

anticoagulant effect of heparin in some patients. Monitor PTT.

Drug-lifestyle. *Alcohol use:* possible increased hypotension. Avoid alcohol intake.

EFFECTS ON DIAGNOSTIC TESTS
Nitroglycerin may interfere with serum cholesterol determination tests using the Zlatkis-Zak color reaction, resulting in falsely decreased values.

CONTRAINDICATIONS
Contraindicated in patients with early MI, severe anemia, increased intracranial pressure, angle-closure glaucoma, orthostatic hypotension, allergy to adhesives (transdermal), or hypersensitivity to nitrates. I.V. nitroglycerin is contraindicated in patients with cardiac tamponade, restrictive cardiomyopathy, constrictive pericarditis, or hypersensitivity to I.V. form.

NURSING CONSIDERATIONS
• Use cautiously in patients with hypotension or volume depletion.
• Closely monitor vital signs during infusion. Be particularly aware of blood pressure, especially in a patient with an MI. Excessive hypotension may worsen the MI.
• To apply ointment, measure the prescribed amount on the application paper; then place the paper on any nonhairy area. Do not rub in. Cover with plastic film to aid absorption and to protect clothing. Remove all excess ointment from previous site before applying the next dose. Avoid getting ointment on fingers.
• Know that transdermal dosage forms can be applied to any nonhairy part of the skin except distal parts of the arms or legs (absorption will not be maximal at distal sites).
• Remove transdermal patch before defibrillation. Because of its aluminum backing, the electric current may cause arcing that can result in damage to paddles and burns to the patient.
• When stopping transdermal treatment of angina, gradually reduce the dose and frequency of application over 4 to 6 weeks, as ordered.

• Monitor blood pressure and intensity and duration of drug response.
• Drug may cause headaches, especially at beginning of therapy. Dosage may be reduced temporarily, but tolerance usually develops. Treat headache with aspirin or acetaminophen.
• Tolerance to drug can be minimized with a 10- to 12-hour nitrate-free interval. To achieve this, remove the transdermal system in the early evening and apply a new system the next morning or omit the last daily dose of a buccal, sustained-release, or ointment form. Check with the doctor for alterations in dosage regimen if tolerance is suspected.

🔵 **I.V. administration**
• Dilute with D_5W or 0.9% NaCl for injection. Concentration should not exceed 400 mcg/ml. Always administer with an infusion control device and titrate to desired response. Also, always mix in glass bottles and avoid use of I.V. filters because drug binds to plastic. Regular polyvinyl chloride tubing can bind up to 80% of drug, making it necessary to infuse higher dosages. A special nonabsorbent polyvinyl chloride tubing is available from the manufacturer; patients receive more drug when these infusion sets are used. Always use the same type of infusion set when changing I.V. lines.
• When changing the concentration of infusion, flush the I.V. administration set with 15 to 20 ml of the new concentration before use. This will clear the line of the old drug solution.

✅ **Patient teaching**
• Caution patient to take nitroglycerin regularly, as prescribed, and to have it accessible at all times.
Alert: Advise patient that abrupt discontinuation of drug causes coronary vasospasms.
• Teach patient how to administer the prescribed form of nitroglycerin.
• Tell patient to take S.L. tablet at first sign of attack. The tablet should be wet with saliva and placed under the tongue until absorbed, and the patient should sit down and rest. Dose may be repeated every 5 minutes for a maximum of three

---

doses. If drug doesn't provide relief, medical help should be obtained promptly.
- Advise patient who complains of a tingling sensation with S.L. drug to try holding tablet in buccal pouch.
- Tell patient to take oral tablets on an empty stomach, either 30 minutes before or 1 to 2 hours after meals; to swallow oral tablets whole; and not to chew tablets.
- Remind patient using translingual aerosol form that he should *not* inhale the spray, but should release it onto or under the tongue. Also tell him to wait about 10 seconds or so before swallowing.
- Tell patient to place the buccal tablet between the lip and gum above the incisors or between the cheek and gum. Tablets should not be swallowed or chewed.
- Tell patient to take an additional dose before anticipated stress or at bedtime if angina is nocturnal.
- Instruct patient to use caution when wearing transdermal patch near microwave oven. Leaking radiation may heat patch's metallic backing and cause burns.
- Advise patient to avoid alcohol.
- To minimize orthostatic hypotension, tell patient to change to upright position slowly. Advise him to go up and down stairs carefully and to lie down at the first sign of dizziness.
- Tell patient to store drug in cool, dark place in a tightly closed container. Remove cotton from container because it absorbs drug.
- Tell patient to store S.L. tablets in original container or other container specifically approved for this use and to carry the container in a jacket pocket or purse, not in a pocket close to the body.

---

propranolol hydrochloride
Apo-Propranolol†, Deralin‡, Inderal, Inderal LA, Novopranol†, pms Propranolol†

Pregnancy Risk Category: C

HOW SUPPLIED
Tablets: 10 mg, 20 mg, 40 mg, 60 mg, 80 mg, 90 mg

Capsules (extended-release): 60 mg, 80 mg, 120 mg, 160 mg
Oral solution: 4 mg/ml, 8 mg/ml, 80 mg/ml (concentrate)
Injection: 1 mg/ml

ACTION
Reduces cardiac oxygen demand by blocking catecholamine-induced increases in heart rate, blood pressure, and force of myocardial contraction. Depresses renin secretion and prevents vasodilation of cerebral arteries.

Route	Onset	Peak	Duration
PO	30 min	1-1.5 hr	12 hr
IV	1 min	Immediate	5 min

INDICATIONS & DOSAGE
Angina pectoris—
Adults: total daily doses of 80 to 320 mg P.O. when given b.i.d., t.i.d., or q.i.d. Or, one 80-mg extended-release capsule daily. Dosage increased at 3- to 7-day intervals.
Mortality reduction after MI—
Adults: 180 to 240 mg P.O. daily in divided doses beginning 5 to 21 days after MI has occurred. Usually administered t.i.d. or q.i.d.
Supraventricular, ventricular, and atrial arrhythmias; tachyarrhythmias caused by excessive catecholamine action during anesthesia, hyperthyroidism, or pheochromocytoma—
Adults: 0.5 to 3 mg by slow I.V. push, not to exceed 1 mg/minute. After 3 mg have been given, another dose may be given in 2 minutes; subsequent doses, no sooner than q 4 hours. May be diluted and infused slowly. Usual maintenance dosage is 10 to 30 mg P.O. t.i.d. or q.i.d.
Hypertension—
Adults: initially, 80 mg P.O. daily in two to four divided doses or extended-release form once daily. Increased at 3- to 7-day intervals to maximum daily dosage of 640 mg. Usual maintenance dosage is 160 to 480 mg daily.
Prevention of frequent, severe, uncontrollable, or disabling migraine or vascular headache—
Adults: initially, 80 mg P.O. daily in divided doses or one extended-release cap-

sule daily. Usual maintenance dosage is 160 to 240 mg daily, t.i.d. or q.i.d.
Essential tremor—
Adults: 40 mg (tablets, oral solution) P.O. b.i.d. Usual maintenance dosage is 120 to 320 mg daily in three divided doses.
Hypertrophic subaortic stenosis—
Adults: 20 to 40 mg P.O. t.i.d. or q.i.d., or 80 to 160 mg extended-release capsules once daily.
Adjunct therapy in pheochromocytoma—
Adults: 60 mg P.O. daily in divided doses with an alpha-adrenergic blocker 3 days before surgery.

ADVERSE REACTIONS
CNS: *fatigue, lethargy,* vivid dreams, hallucinations, mental depression, lightheadedness, insomnia.
CV: *bradycardia, hypotension,* **heart failure,** intermittent claudication, intensification of AV block.
GI: abdominal cramping, constipation, diarrhea, nausea, vomiting.
Respiratory: bronchospasm.
Skin: rash.
Other: *agranulocytosis,* fever.

INTERACTIONS
Drug-drug. *Aminophylline:* antagonized beta-blocking effects of propranolol. Use together cautiously.
Cardiac glycosides, diltiazem, verapamil: hypotension, bradycardia, and increased depressant effect on myocardium. Use together cautiously.
Cimetidine: inhibited metabolism of propranolol. Monitor for increased beta-blocking effect.
Epinephrine: severe vasoconstriction. Monitor blood pressure and observe patient carefully.
Glucagon, isoproterenol: antagonized propranolol effect. May be used therapeutically and in emergencies.
Haloperidol: cardiac arrest has occurred with concomitant therapy. Avoid use together.
Insulin, oral antidiabetic agents: can alter requirements for these drugs in previously stabilized diabetics. Monitor for hypoglycemia.
Phenothiazines, reserpine: additive effect. Use cautiously.

Drug-herb. *Betel palm:* decreased temperature elevating effects and enhanced CNS effects. Avoid concomitant use.
Drug-lifestyle. *Cocaine use:* increased angina-inducing potential of cocaine. Monitor patient carefully.

EFFECTS ON DIAGNOSTIC TESTS
Propranolol may elevate serum transaminase, alkaline phosphatase, and LD levels, and may elevate BUN levels in patients with severe heart disease.

CONTRAINDICATIONS
Contraindicated in patients with bronchial asthma, sinus bradycardia and heart block greater than first-degree, cardiogenic shock, and heart failure (unless failure is secondary to a tachyarrhythmia that can be treated with propranolol).

NURSING CONSIDERATIONS
• Use cautiously in patients with renal impairment, nonallergic bronchospastic diseases, or hepatic disease and in those taking other antihypertensives. Because drug blocks some symptoms of hypoglycemia, use with caution in patients with diabetes mellitus. Also use cautiously in patients with thyrotoxicosis because drug may mask some signs of that disorder. Elderly patients may experience enhanced adverse reactions and may need dosage adjustment.
• Always check patient's apical pulse before giving drug. If you detect extremes in pulse rates, withhold drug and call the doctor immediately.
• Give consistently with meals. Food may increase absorption of propranolol.
• Be aware that drug masks common signs of shock and hypoglycemia.
• *Don't discontinue drug before surgery for pheochromocytoma.* Before any surgical procedure, tell anesthesiologist that patient is receiving propranolol.
• Compliance may be improved by administering drug twice-daily or as extended-release capsule. Check with doctor.

◖ I.V. administration
• Give by direct injection into a large vessel or into the tubing of a free-flowing, compatible I.V. solution; continuous I.V.

infusion generally is not recommended. Alternatively, dilute drug with 0.9% NaCl and give by intermittent infusion over 10 to 15 minutes in 0.1- to 0.2-mg increments. Drug is compatible with D_5W and 0.45% and 0.9% NaCl and lactated Ringer's solutions.

• Double-check dose and route. I.V. doses are much smaller than oral doses.

• Monitor blood pressure, ECG, and heart rate and rhythm frequently, especially during I.V. administration. If the patient develops severe hypotension, notify the doctor; a vasopressor may be prescribed.

• For overdose, give I.V. isoproterenol, I.V. atropine, or glucagon; refractory cases may require a pacemaker.

☑ **Patient teaching**
• Caution patient to continue taking this drug as prescribed, even when he is feeling well.

• Instruct patient to take drug with food.

Alert: Tell patient not to discontinue drug suddenly because this can exacerbate angina and precipitate MI.

---

verapamil
Apo-Verap†, Calan, Isoptin, Novo-Veramil†, Nu-Verap†

verapamil hydrochloride
Anpec‡, Calan, Calan SR, Cordilox‡, Cordilox SR‡, Half Securon SR§, Isoptin, Isoptin SR, Novo-Veramil†, Securon§, Securon SR§, Univer§, Veracaps SR‡, Verapress MR§, Verelan

Pregnancy Risk Category: C

HOW SUPPLIED
verapamil
Tablets: 40 mg, 80 mg, 120 mg
verapamil hydrochloride
Tablets: 40 mg, 80 mg, 120 mg, 160 mg‡
Tablets (extended-release): 120 mg, 180 mg, 240 mg, 360 mg
Capsules (extended-release): 120 mg, 160 mg‡, 180 mg, 240 mg, 360 mg
Injection: 2.5 mg/ml

ACTION
Not clearly defined. Verapamil is a calcium channel blocker that inhibits calcium ion influx across cardiac and smooth-muscle cells, thus decreasing myocardial contractility and oxygen demand; it also dilates coronary arteries and arterioles.

Route	Onset	Peak	Duration
PO	0.5 hr	1-2 hr	8-10 hr
PO (extended)	0.5 hr	5-9 hr	24 hr
IV	1-5 min	Immediate	1-6 hr

INDICATIONS & DOSAGE
Vasospastic angina (also called Prinzmetal's or variant angina) and classic chronic, stable angina pectoris; chronic atrial fibrillation—
Adults: starting dose is 80 to 120 mg P.O. t.i.d. Dosage increased at weekly intervals p.r.n. Some patients may require up to 480 mg daily.
Supraventricular arrhythmias—
Adults: 0.075 to 0.15 mg/kg (5 to 10 mg) by I.V. push over 2 minutes with ECG and blood pressure monitoring. Repeat dose in 30 minutes if no response occurs.
Children under 1 year: 0.1 to 0.2 mg/kg as I.V. bolus over 2 minutes with continuous ECG monitoring. Repeat dose in 30 minutes if no response occurs.
Children 1 to 15 years: 0.1 to 0.3 mg/kg as I.V. bolus over 2 minutes; not to exceed 5 mg.
Hypertension—
Adults: 240 mg extended-release tablet P.O. once daily in the morning. If response is not adequate, give an additional 120 mg in the evening or 240 mg q 12 hours or an 80-mg immediate-release tablet t.i.d.

ADVERSE REACTIONS
CNS: dizziness, headache, asthenia.
CV: *transient hypotension,* **heart failure,** pulmonary edema, bradycardia, AV block, **ventricular asystole, ventricular fibrillation,** peripheral edema.
GI: *constipation,* nausea.
Hepatic: elevated liver enzymes.
Skin: rash.

INTERACTIONS

Drug-drug. *Antihypertensives, quinidine:* may result in hypotension. Monitor blood pressure.

Carbamazepine, cardiac glycosides: may increase serum levels of these drugs. Monitor for toxicity.

Cyclosporine: may increase cyclosporine serum levels. Monitor cyclosporine levels.

Disopyramide, flecainide, propranolol (other beta blockers, including ophthalmic timolol): may cause heart failure. Use together cautiously.

Lithium: may decrease or increase serum lithium levels. Monitor closely.

Rifampin: may decrease oral bioavailability of verapamil. Monitor the patient for lack of effect.

Drug-herb. *Black catechu:* additive effects. Avoid concomitant use.

Yerba maté: may decrease clearance of yerba maté methylxanthines and cause toxicity. Use together cautiously.

Drug-food. *Any food:* increased absorption. Take drug with food.

Drug-lifestyle. *Alcohol use:* verapamil may enhance the effects of alcohol. Avoid use.

EFFECTS ON DIAGNOSTIC TESTS

None reported.

CONTRAINDICATIONS

Contraindicated in patients with hypersensitivity to drug; severe left ventricular dysfunction; cardiogenic shock; second- or third-degree AV block or sick sinus syndrome except in presence of functioning pacemaker; atrial flutter or fibrillation and accessory bypass tract syndrome; severe heart failure (unless secondary to verapamil therapy); and severe hypotension. I.V. verapamil is contraindicated in patients receiving I.V. beta-adrenergic blocking agents and in those with ventricular tachycardia.

NURSING CONSIDERATIONS

● Use cautiously in elderly patients, in patients with increased intracranial pressure, and in patients with hepatic or renal disease.

● Although drug should be taken with food, be aware that taking extended-release tablets with food may decrease rate and extent of absorption but allows smaller fluctuations of peak and trough blood levels.

● Patients with severely compromised cardiac function or those receiving beta blockers should receive lower doses of verapamil. Monitor these patients closely.

● Be aware that if verapamil is being used to terminate supraventricular tachycardia, doctor may have the patient perform vagal maneuvers after receiving drug.

● Monitor blood pressure at the start of therapy and during dosage adjustments. Assist patient with ambulation because dizziness may occur.

● Notify doctor if signs of heart failure, such as swelling of hands and feet or shortness of breath, occur.

● Monitor liver function during prolonged treatment, as ordered.

I.V. administration

● Give by direct injection into a vein or into the tubing of a free-flowing, compatible I.V. solution. Compatible solutions include D_5W and 0.45%, 0.9% NaCl, Ringer's, and lactated Ringer's solutions. Administer I.V. doses over at least 3 minutes to minimize the risk of adverse reactions.

● Monitor ECG and blood pressure continuously in patient receiving I.V. verapamil.

Patient teaching

● Instruct patient to take oral form of drug exactly as prescribed.

● Tell patient to take drug with food.

● Caution patient against abruptly discontinuing the drug.

● If patient is kept on nitrate therapy during titration of oral verapamil dosage, urge continued compliance. S.L. nitroglycerin, especially, may be taken as needed when anginal symptoms are acute.

● Encourage patient to increase fluid and fiber intake to combat constipation. Administer a stool softener as ordered.

Reactions may be *common*, uncommon, **life-threatening**, or COMMON AND LIFE-THREATENING.

23

Antihypertensives

acebutolol
acebutolol hydrochloride
amlodipine besylate
(See Chapter 22, ANTIANGINALS.)
atenolol
benazepril hydrochloride
betaxolol hydrochloride
bisoprolol fumarate
candesartan cilexetil
captopril
carteolol
carvedilol
clonidine
clonidine hydrochloride
diazoxide
diltiazem hydrochloride
(See Chapter 22, ANTIANGINALS.)
doxazosin mesylate
enalaprilat
enalapril maleate
felodipine
fenoldopam mesylate
fosinopril sodium
guanabenz acetate
guanadrel sulfate
guanethidine monosulfate
guanfacine hydrochloride
hydralazine hydrochloride
irbesartan
isradipine
labetalol hydrochloride
lisinopril
losartan potassium
methyldopa
methyldopate hydrochloride
metoprolol succinate
metoprolol tartrate
minoxidil
moexipril hydrochloride
nadolol
(See Chapter 22, ANTIANGINALS.)
nicardipine hydrochloride
(See Chapter 22, ANTIANGINALS.)
nifedipine
(See Chapter 22, ANTIANGINALS.)
nisoldipine
nitroprusside sodium
penbutolol sulfate
phentolamine mesylate

pindolol
prazosin hydrochloride
propranolol hydrochloride
(See Chapter 22, ANTIANGINALS.)
quinapril hydrochloride
ramipril
telmisartan
terazosin hydrochloride
timolol maleate
trandolapril
valsartan
verapamil hydrochloride
(See Chapter 22, ANTIANGINALS.)

COMBINATION PRODUCTS

ALDOCLOR-150: chlorothiazide 150 mg and methyldopa 250 mg.
ALDOCLOR-250: chlorothiazide 250 mg and methyldopa 250 mg.
ALDORIL-15: hydrochlorothiazide 15 mg and methyldopa 250 mg.
ALDORIL-25: hydrochlorothiazide 25 mg and methyldopa 250 mg.
ALDORIL D30: hydrochlorothiazide 30 mg and methyldopa 500 mg.
ALDORIL D50: hydrochlorothiazide 50 mg and methyldopa 500 mg.
APRESAZIDE 25/25: hydrochlorothiazide 25 mg and hydralazine hydrochloride 25 mg.
APRESAZIDE 50/50: hydrochlorothiazide 50 mg and hydralazine hydrochloride 50 mg.
APRESAZIDE 100/50: hydrochlorothiazide 50 mg and hydralazine hydrochloride 100 mg.
APRESOLINE-ESIDRIX: hydrochlorothiazide 15 mg and hydralazine hydrochloride 25 mg.
CAM-AP-ES: hydrochlorothiazide 15 mg, hydralazine hydrochloride 25 mg, and reserpine 0.1 mg.
CAPOZIDE 25/15: hydrochlorothiazide 15 mg and captopril 25 mg.
CAPOZIDE 25/25: hydrochlorothiazide 25 mg and captopril 25 mg.
CAPOZIDE 50/15: hydrochlorothiazide 15 mg and captopril 50 mg.

CAPOZIDE 50/25: hydrochlorothiazide 25 mg and captopril 50 mg.

CHERAPAS: hydrochlorothiazide 15mg, hydralazine hydrochloride 25 mg, and reserpine 0.1 mg.

COMBIPRES 0.1: chlorthalidone 15 mg and clonidine hydrochloride 0.1 mg.

COMBIPRES 0.2: chlorthalidone 15 mg and clonidine hydrochloride 0.2 mg.

CORZIDE: nadolol 40 mg or 80 mg and bendroflumethiazide 5 mg.

DEMI-REGROTON: chlorthalidone 25 mg and reserpine 0.125 mg.

DIUPRES-250: chlorothiazide 250 mg and reserpine 0.125 mg.

DIUPRES-500: chlorothiazide 500 mg and reserpine 0.125 mg.

DIURESE-R: trichlormethiazide 4 mg and reserpine 0.1 mg.

DIURIGEN WITH RESERPINE: chlorothiazide 250 mg and reserpine 0.125 mg.

DIUTENSEN-R: methyclothiazide 2.5 mg and reserpine 0.1 mg.

ENDURONYL: methyclothiazide 5.0 mg and deserpidine 0.25 mg.

ENDURONYL FORTE: methyclothiazide 5.0 mg and deserpidine 0.5 mg.

ESIMIL: hydrochlorothiazide 25 mg and guanethidine monosulfate 10 mg.

HYDROPINE: hydroflumethiazide 25 mg and reserpine 0.125 mg.

HYDROPINE H.P.: hydroflumethiazide 50 mg and reserpine 0.125 mg.

HYDROPRES-25: hydrochlorothiazide 25 mg and reserpine 0.125 mg.

HYDRO-SERP: hydrochlorothiazide 25 or 50 mg and reserpine 0.125 mg.

HYDROSERPINE: hydrochlorothiazide 25 or 50 mg and reserpine 0.125 mg.

HYDROTENSIN-25 tablets: hydrochlorothiazide 25 mg and reserpine 0.125 mg.

HYZAAR: losartan 50 mg and hydrochlorothiazide12.5 mg.

INDERIDE 40/25: propranolol hydrochloride 40 mg and hydrochlorothiazide 25 mg.

INDERIDE 80/25: propranolol hydrochloride 80 mg and hydrochlorothiazide 25 mg.

INDERIDE LA 80/50: propranolol hydrochloride 80 mg and hydrochlorothiazide 50 mg.

INDERIDE LA 120/50: propranolol hydrochloride 120 mg and hydrochlorothiazide 50 mg.

INDERIDE LA 160/50: propranolol hydrochloride 160 mg and hydrochlorothiazide 50 mg.

LOPRESSOR HCT 50/25: metoprolol tartrate 50 mg and hydrochlorothiazide 25 mg.

LOPRESSOR HCT 100/25: metoprolol tartrate 100 mg and hydrochlorothiazide 25 mg.

LOPRESSOR HCT 100/50: metoprolol tartrate 100 mg and hydrochlorothiazide 50 mg.

MAXZIDE: triamterene 75 mg and hydrochlorothiazide 50 mg.

MINIZIDE 1: polythiazide 0.5 mg and prazosin hydrochloride 1 mg.

MINIZIDE 2: polythiazide 0.5 mg and prazosin hydrochloride 2 mg.

MINIZIDE 5: polythiazide 0.5 mg and prazosin hydrochloride 5 mg.

NAQUIVAL: trichlormethiazide 4 mg and reserpine 0.1 mg.

PRINZIDE 12.5: lisinopril 20 mg and hydrochlorothiazide 12.5 mg.

PRINZIDE 25: lisinopril 20 mg and hydrochlorothiazide 25 mg.

RAUZIDE**: bendroflumethiazide 4 mg and powdered rauwolfia serpentina 50 mg.

REGROTON: chlorthalidone 50 mg and reserpine 0.25 mg.

RENESE-R: polythiazide 2 mg and reserpine 0.25 mg.

R-HCTZ-H: hydrochlorothiazide 15 mg, hydralazine hydrochloride 25 mg, and reserpine 0.1 mg.

SALUTENSIN: hydroflumethiazide 50 mg and reserpine 0.125 mg.

SALUTENSIN-DEMI: hydroflumethiazide 25 mg and reserpine 0.125 mg.

SER-A-GEN: hydrochlorothiazide 15 mg, hydralazine hydrochloride 25 mg, and reserpine 0.1 mg.

SERALAZIDE: hydrochlorothiazide 15 mg, hydralazine hydrochloride 25 mg, and reserpine 0.1 mg.

SER-AP-ES: hydrochlorothiazide 15 mg, reserpine 0.1 mg, and hydralazine hydrochloride 25 mg.

SERPAZIDE: hydrochlorothiazide 15 mg, hydralazine hydrochloride 25 mg, and reserpine 0.1 mg.

Reactions may be *common*, uncommon, *life-threatening*, or COMMON AND LIFE-THREATENING.

TENORETIC 50: atenolol 50 mg and chlorthalidone 25 mg.
TENORETIC 100: atenolol 100 mg and chlorthalidone 25 mg.
TIMOLIDE 10/25: timolol maleate 10 mg and hydrochlorothiazide 25 mg.
TRI-HYDROSERPINE: hydrochlorothiazide 15 mg, hydralazine hydrochloride 25 mg, and reserpine 0.1 mg.
UNIPRES: hydrochlorothiazide 15 mg, reserpine 0.1 mg, and hydralazine hydrochloride 25 mg.
VASERETIC: enalapril maleate 10 mg and hydrochlorothiazide 25 mg.
ZESTORETIC 20-12.5: lisinopril 20 mg and hydrochlorothiazide 12.5 mg.
ZESTORETIC 20-25: lisinopril and hydrochlorothiazide 25 mg.
ZIAC: bisoprolol fumarate 2.5 mg, 5 mg, or 10 mg and hydrochlorothiazide 6.5 mg.

acebutolol
Sectral

acebutolol hydrochloride
Monitan†

Pregnancy Risk Category: B

HOW SUPPLIED
Capsules: 200 mg, 400 mg

ACTION
Antihypertensive action is unknown. Possible mechanisms include reduced cardiac output, decreased sympathetic outflow to peripheral vasculature, and inhibition of renin release. Drug decreases myocardial contractility and heart rate. Drug has mild intrinsic sympathomimetic activity.

Route	Onset	Peak	Duration
PO	1-1.5 hr	2.5 hr	24 hr

INDICATIONS & DOSAGE
Hypertension—
Adults: 400 mg P.O. either as a single daily dose or in divided doses b.i.d. Maximum dosage is 1,200 mg daily.
Ventricular arrhythmias—
Adults: 400 mg P.O. daily divided b.i.d. Dosage increased to provide an adequate

clinical response. Usual dosage is 600 to 1,200 mg daily.
Elderly: may require lower dosage; dosage should not exceed 800 mg daily.
Adjust-a-dose: In renally impaired patients with creatinine clearance of 50 to 25 ml/minute, reduce dosage by 50%; if clearance is less than 25 ml/minute, reduce dosage by 75%.

ADVERSE REACTIONS
CNS: *fatigue,* headache, dizziness, insomnia, depression.
CV: chest pain, edema, bradycardia, *heart failure,* hypotension.
GI: nausea, constipation, diarrhea, dyspepsia, flatulence, vomiting.
Respiratory: dyspnea, *bronchospasm,* cough.
Skin: rash.
GU: dysuria, impotence, nocturia, urinary frequency.
Other: arthralgia, myalgia.

INTERACTIONS
Drug-drug. *Cardiac glycosides, diltiazem, verapamil:* excessive bradycardia and increased depressant effect on myocardium. Use together cautiously.
Catecholamine-depleting drugs (such as reserpine): effects may be additive. Monitor closely.
Diuretics, other antihypertensive agents: increased hypotensive effect. Use together cautiously.
Insulin, oral antidiabetic agents: can alter dosage requirements in previously stabilized diabetic patients. Observe patient carefully.
NSAIDs: decreased antihypertensive effect. Monitor blood pressure and adjust dosage.
Sympathomimetic agents: effects antagonized by acebutolol. Greater than usual dosages of beta-adrenergic agonist bronchodilators may be required.

EFFECTS ON DIAGNOSTIC TESTS
Acebutolol may cause positive antinuclear antibody titers.

CONTRAINDICATIONS
Contraindicated in patients with persistent severe bradycardia, second- and third-

degree heart block, overt cardiac failure, and cardiogenic shock.

NURSING CONSIDERATIONS
• Use cautiously in those with cardiac failure, peripheral vascular disease, bronchospastic disease, and diabetes.
• Check apical pulse before giving drug; if slower than 60 beats/minute, withhold drug and call doctor. Also monitor blood pressure.
• Before surgery, tell anesthesiologist that patient is taking drug.
• Be aware that acebutolol may mask signs of hyperthyroidism.

☑ Patient teaching
• Instruct patient to take drug exactly as prescribed.
• Instruct patient to avoid taking OTC oral cold preparations or topical nasal decongestants, due to the potential for severe hypertensive reaction.
• Warn patient not to discontinue drug suddenly, and to notify doctor promptly of unpleasant adverse reactions.
• Teach patient how to take his pulse and instruct him to withhold the dose and notify doctor if pulse rate is below 60 beats/minute.

---

atenolol
Anselol‡, Apo-Atenol†, Noten‡, Nu-Atenol†, Tenormin, Tensig‡

Pregnancy Risk Category: D

HOW SUPPLIED
Tablets: 25 mg, 50 mg, 100 mg
Injection: 5 mg/10 ml

ACTION
A beta-adrenergic blocker that selectively blocks beta$_1$-adrenergic receptors; decreases cardiac output, peripheral resistance, and cardiac oxygen consumption; and depresses renin secretion.

Route	Onset	Peak	Duration
PO	1 hr	2-4 hr	24 hr
IV	5 min	5 min	12 hr

INDICATIONS & DOSAGE
Hypertension—
Adults: initially, 50 mg P.O. daily as a single dose, increased to 100 mg once daily after 7 to 14 days. Dosages over 100 mg are unlikely to produce further benefit.
Angina pectoris—
Adults: 50 mg P.O. once daily, increased p.r.n. to 100 mg daily after 7 days for optimal effect. Maximum dosage is 200 mg daily.
To reduce CV mortality and risk of re-infarction in patients with acute MI—
Adults: 5 mg I.V. over 5 minutes, followed by another 5 mg 10 minutes later. After an additional 10 minutes, 50 mg P.O., followed by 50 mg P.O. in 12 hours. Thereafter, 100 mg P.O. daily (as a single dose or 50 mg b.i.d.) for at least 7 days.
Adjust-a-dose: In renally impaired patients with creatinine clearance of 15 to 35 ml/minute, maximum dosage is 50 mg/day; if it is less than 15 ml/minute, maximum dosage is 25 mg/day.

Hemodialysis patients require 25 to 50 mg after each dialysis session; monitor closely because of risk of hypotension.

ADVERSE REACTIONS
CNS: *fatigue,* lethargy, vertigo, drowsiness, *dizziness.*
CV: *bradycardia, hypotension,* **heart failure,** intermittent claudication.
GI: nausea, diarrhea.
GU: elevated BUN and creatinine.
Hematologic: elevated platelet count.
Hepatic: elevated transaminase, alkaline phosphatase, LD levels.
Metabolic: elevated serum levels of potassium, uric acid; increased or decreased serum glucose levels in diabetic patients.
Respiratory: dyspnea, **bronchospasm.**
Skin: rash.
Other: fever, leg pain.

INTERACTIONS
Drug-drug. *Antihypertensives:* enhanced hypotensive effect. Use together cautiously.
Cardiac glycosides, diltiazem, verapamil: excessive bradycardia and increased de-

---

pressant effect on myocardium. Use together cautiously.

Insulin, oral antidiabetic agents: can alter dosage requirements in previously stabilized diabetic patients. Observe patient carefully.

Reserpine: may cause hypotension. Use with caution.

EFFECTS ON DIAGNOSTIC TESTS
Atenolol also may cause changes in exercise tolerance and ECG.

CONTRAINDICATIONS
Contraindicated in patients with sinus bradycardia, greater than first-degree heart block, overt cardiac failure, or cardiogenic shock.

NURSING CONSIDERATIONS
• Use cautiously in patients at risk for heart failure and in patients with bronchospastic disease, diabetes, hyperthyroidism, and impaired renal or hepatic function.
• Check apical pulse before giving drug; if slower than 60 beats/minute, withhold drug and call doctor.
• Monitor patient's blood pressure.
Alert: Know that drug should be withdrawn gradually over 2 weeks to avoid serious adverse reactions.

🔳 I.V. administration
• Give by slow I.V. injection, not exceeding 1 mg/minute. I.V. doses may be mixed with D_5W, 0.9% NaCl, or dextrose and NaCl solutions. Solution is stable for 48 hours after mixing.

☑ Patient teaching
• Instruct patient to take drug exactly as prescribed, at the same time every day.
• Caution patient not to stop drug suddenly, but to call doctor if unpleasant adverse reactions occur.
• Teach patient how to take his pulse. Tell him to withhold drug and call doctor if pulse rate is below 60 beats/minute.
• Tell female patient to notify doctor if pregnancy occurs. Drug will need to be discontinued.

benazepril hydrochloride
Lotensin

Pregnancy Risk Category: C
(D in second and third trimesters)

HOW SUPPLIED
Tablets: 5 mg, 10 mg, 20 mg, 40 mg

ACTION
Benazepril and its active metabolite, benazeprilat, inhibit ACE, preventing conversion of angiotensin I to angiotensin II, a potent vasoconstrictor. Reduced formation of angiotensin II decreases peripheral arterial resistance, thus decreasing aldosterone secretion. This reduces sodium and water retention and lowers blood pressure. Benazepril also has antihypertensive activity in patients with low-renin hypertension.

Route	Onset	Peak	Duration
PO	1 hr	2-4 hr	24 hr

INDICATIONS & DOSAGE
Hypertension—
Adults: in patients not receiving a diuretic, 10 mg P.O. daily initially. Dosage titrated as needed and tolerated; most patients take 20 to 40 mg daily in one or two doses. In patients receiving a diuretic, 5 mg P.O. daily.
Adjust-a-dose: In renally impaired patients with creatinine clearance below 30 ml/minute, 5 mg P.O. daily. Dosage may be adjusted up to 40 mg/day.

ADVERSE REACTIONS
CNS: headache, dizziness, drowsiness, fatigue, somnolence.
CV: symptomatic hypotension.
GI: nausea.
Respiratory: dry, persistent, nonproductive cough.
Skin: hypersensitivity reactions (rash, pruritus).
Other: *angioedema,* arthralgia, arthritis, impotence, increased diaphoresis, myalgia, hyperkalemia.

INTERACTIONS
Drug-drug. *Diuretics, other antihyper-*

tensives: risk of excessive hypotension. Discontinue diuretic or lower dose of benazepril as needed.
Lithium: increased serum lithium levels and lithium toxicity. Coadminister with caution; monitor serum lithium levels.
Potassium-sparing diuretics, potassium supplements: risk of hyperkalemia. Monitor closely.
Drug-food. *Salt substitutes containing potassium:* risk of hyperkalemia. Monitor closely.

EFFECTS ON DIAGNOSTIC TESTS
ACE inhibitors may cause agranulocytosis and bone marrow depression; however, available data are insufficient to show that benazepril does not affect the CBC in the same way. Benazepril may increase serum creatinine and BUN levels. Elevations of liver enzymes, serum bilirubin, uric acid, and blood glucose have been reported, along with scattered incidents of hyponatremia, ECG changes, leukopenia, eosinophilia, and proteinuria.

CONTRAINDICATIONS
Contraindicated in patients with hypersensitivity to ACE inhibitors.

NURSING CONSIDERATIONS
• Use cautiously in patients with impaired hepatic or renal function.
• Monitor for hypotension. Excessive hypotension can occur when drug is given with diuretics. If possible, diuretic therapy should be discontinued 2 to 3 days before starting benazepril to decrease potential for excessive hypotensive response. If benazepril does not adequately control blood pressure, diuretic may be reinstituted with care.
• Measure blood pressure when drug levels are at peak (2 to 6 hours after administration) and at trough (just before a dose) to verify adequate blood pressure control.
• Assess renal and hepatic function before and periodically throughout therapy. Monitor serum potassium levels, as ordered.
• Know that other ACE inhibitors have been associated with agranulocytosis and neutropenia. Monitor CBC with differen-

tial counts before therapy and periodically thereafter.

☑ Patient teaching
• Instruct patient to avoid salt substitutes; these products may contain potassium, which can cause hyperkalemia in patients taking drug.
• Light-headedness can occur, especially during the first few days of therapy. Tell patient to rise slowly to minimize this effect and to report symptoms to doctor. If syncope occurs, patient should stop taking drug and call doctor immediately.
• Warn patient to use caution in hot weather and during exercise. Inadequate fluid intake, vomiting, diarrhea, and excessive perspiration can lead to light-headedness and syncope.
• Advise patient to report signs of infection, such as fever and sore throat. Tell him to call doctor if the following signs or symptoms occur: easy bruising or bleeding; swelling of tongue, lips, face, eyes, mucous membranes, or extremities; difficulty swallowing or breathing; or hoarseness.
• Tell female patient to notify doctor if pregnancy occurs. Drug will need to be discontinued.

betaxolol hydrochloride
Kerlone

Pregnancy Risk Category: C

HOW SUPPLIED
Tablets: 10 mg, 20 mg

ACTION
Unknown. A selective beta$_1$-adrenergic blocker that decreases blood pressure, possibly by slowing heart rate and decreasing cardiac output.

Route	Onset	Peak	Duration
PO	3 hr	2-4 hr	24-48 hr

INDICATIONS & DOSAGE
Hypertension (used alone or with other antihypertensives)—
Adults: initially, 10 mg P.O. once daily; if necessary, 20 mg P.O. once daily if de-

sired response is not achieved in 7 to 14 days.

ADVERSE REACTIONS
CNS: dizziness, fatigue, headache, insomnia, lethargy, anxiety.
CV: bradycardia, chest pain, *heart failure,* edema.
GI: nausea, diarrhea, dyspepsia.
Respiratory: dyspnea, pharyngitis, *bronchospasm.*
Skin: rash.
Other: impotence, arthralgia.

INTERACTIONS
Drug-drug. *Calcium channel blockers:* increased risk of hypotension, left ventricular failure, and AV conduction disturbances. Use I.V. calcium channel blockers with caution.
Catecholamine-depleting drugs, reserpine: may have an additive effect. Monitor closely.
General anesthetics: increased hypotensive effects. Observe carefully for excessive hypotension or bradycardia or orthostatic hypotension.
Lidocaine: may increase lidocaine's effects. Monitor patient.

EFFECTS ON DIAGNOSTIC TESTS
Oral beta blockers have been reported to decrease serum glucose levels from blockage of normal glycogen release after hypoglycemia. Oral beta blockers may alter the results of glucose tolerance tests.

CONTRAINDICATIONS
Contraindicated in patients with severe bradycardia, greater than first-degree heart block, cardiogenic shock, uncontrolled heart failure, or hypersensitivity to drug.

NURSING CONSIDERATIONS
• Use cautiously in patients with heart failure controlled by cardiac glycosides and diuretics because these patients may exhibit signs of cardiac decompensation with beta-blocker therapy.
• When discontinuing drug, withdraw over 2 weeks.
• Monitor blood pressure closely.
• Monitor blood glucose levels regularly

in patients with diabetes. Beta blockade may inhibit glycogenolysis as well as the signs and symptoms of hypoglycemia (such as tachycardia and blood pressure changes).
• Know that withdrawal of beta-blocker therapy before surgery is controversial. Some clinicians advocate withdrawal to prevent impairment of cardiac responsiveness to reflex stimuli and decreased responsiveness to administration of catecholamines. Advise anesthesiologist that patient is receiving a beta blocker so that isoproterenol or dobutamine is made readily available for reversal of drug's cardiac effects.
• Beta blockers may mask tachycardia associated with hyperthyroidism. In patients with suspected thyrotoxicosis, withdraw beta blocker gradually, as ordered, to avoid thyroid storm.

☑ **Patient teaching**
• Instruct patient to take drug exactly as prescribed.
Alert: Advise patient that abrupt discontinuation may precipitate angina pectoris in patients with unrecognized coronary artery disease.
• Emphasize importance of promptly reporting signs of heart failure, including shortness of breath or difficulty breathing, unusually fast heartbeat, cough, or fatigue with exertion.

---

bisoprolol fumarate
Emcor§, Monocor§, Zebeta

Pregnancy Risk Category: C

HOW SUPPLIED
Tablets: 5 mg, 10 mg

ACTION
Not completely defined. Bisoprolol is a beta₁-selective blocker that decreases myocardial contractility, heart rate, and cardiac output; lowers blood pressure; and reduces myocardial oxygen consumption.

Route	Onset	Peak	Duration
PO	Unknown	1-4 hr	24 hr

INDICATIONS & DOSAGE

Hypertension (used alone or in combination with other antihypertensives)—
Adults: initially, 5 mg P.O. once daily. If response is inadequate, increase to 10 mg once daily or to 20 mg P.O. daily if needed. Maximum recommended dosage is 20 mg daily.
Adjust-a-dose: In patients with renal or hepatic impairment, 2.5 mg P.O. daily initially. Titrate subsequent dosage cautiously.

ADVERSE REACTIONS

CNS: asthenia, fatigue, dizziness, *headache,* hypoesthesia, vivid dreams, depression, insomnia.
CV: bradycardia, peripheral edema, chest pain, **heart failure.**
EENT: pharyngitis, rhinitis, sinusitis.
GI: nausea, vomiting, diarrhea, dry mouth.
Respiratory: cough, dyspnea.
Other: arthralgia.

INTERACTIONS

Drug-drug: *Calcium channel blockers:* can cause myocardial depression and AV conduction inhibition. Monitor closely.
Guanethidine, reserpine: can cause hypotension. Monitor closely.
NSAIDs: decreased antihypertensive effect. Monitor blood pressure and adjust dosage.

EFFECTS ON DIAGNOSTIC TESTS

Drug may produce hypoglycemia and interfere with glucose or insulin tolerance tests.

CONTRAINDICATIONS

Contraindicated in patients with cardiogenic shock, overt cardiac failure, marked sinus bradycardia, second- or third-degree AV block, or hypersensitivity to drug.

NURSING CONSIDERATIONS

• Use cautiously in patients with bronchospastic disease. In general, these patients should avoid beta-adrenergic blockers because blockade of pulmonary beta$_2$-receptors may result in worsening of symptoms. For patients who cannot tolerate or do not respond to other antihypertensives, bisoprolol is given in low doses,

starting with 2.5 mg P.O. daily. Know that bisoprolol blocks beta$_2$-receptors in higher doses (20 mg daily or more).
• Also use cautiously in patients with diabetes, peripheral vascular disease, or thyroid disease and in those with a history of heart failure.
• Monitor blood pressure frequently.
• Monitor blood glucose levels in diabetic patients closely. Beta blockers may mask some manifestations of hypoglycemia, such as tachycardia.
• Know that drug must be withdrawn gradually over 1 to 2 weeks.

✅ Patient teaching

• Explain importance of taking drug as prescribed, even when patient is feeling well.
• Advise patient not to stop drug suddenly but to call the doctor if unpleasant adverse reactions occur.
• Tell patient to check with doctor or pharmacist before taking OTC medications.

▼ *NEW DRUG*

candesartan cilexetil
Atacand

Pregnancy Risk Category: C
(D in second and third trimesters)

HOW SUPPLIED

Tablets: 4 mg, 8 mg, 16 mg, 32 mg

ACTION

Inhibits the vasoconstrictive action of angiotensin II by blocking the angiotensin II receptor on the surface of vascular smooth muscle and other tissue cells.

Route	Onset	Peak	Duration
PO	Unknown	3-4 hr	24 hr

INDICATIONS & DOSAGE

Treatment of hypertension (used alone or in combination with other antihypertensive agents)—
Adults: initially, 16 mg P.O. once daily when used as monotherapy; usual dosage range is 8 to 32 mg P.O. daily as a single dose or divided b.i.d.

ADVERSE REACTIONS
CNS: dizziness, fatigue, headache.
CV: chest pain, peripheral edema.
EENT: pharyngitis, rhinitis, sinusitis.
GI: abdominal pain, diarrhea, nausea, vomiting.
GU: albuminuria.
Musculoskeletal: arthralgia, back pain.
Respiratory: coughing, bronchitis, upper respiratory tract infection.

INTERACTIONS
None reported.

EFFECTS ON DIAGNOSTIC TESTS
None reported.

CONTRAINDICATIONS
Contraindicated in patients with hypersensitivity to drug or its ingredients.

NURSING CONSIDERATIONS
• Use cautiously in patients whose renal function depends on the renin-angiotensin-aldosterone system (such as patients with heart failure) due to the potential for oliguria and progressive azotemia with acute renal failure or death.
• Use cautiously in patients who are volume- or salt-depleted due to potential for symptomatic hypotension. Start therapy with a lower dosage range, as ordered, and monitor blood pressure carefully.
• Know that drugs that act directly on the renin-angiotensin system (such as candesartan) can cause fetal and neonatal morbidity and death when administered to pregnant women. These problems have not been detected when exposure has been limited to first trimester. If pregnancy is suspected, notify doctor because drug should be discontinued.
• If hypotension occurs after a dose of candesartan, place patient in the supine position and, if necessary, give an I.V. infusion of normal saline, as ordered.
• Most of the antihypertensive effect is present within 2 weeks. Maximal antihypertensive effect is obtained within 4 to 6 weeks. Diuretic may be added if blood pressure is not controlled by drug alone.
• Carefully monitor therapeutic response and the occurrence of adverse reactions in the elderly and in those with renal disease.

☑ **Patient teaching**
• Inform female patient of childbearing age of the consequences of second and third trimester exposure to drug. Advise her to notify doctor immediately if pregnancy is suspected.
• Advise breast-feeding patient about risk for adverse drug effects on infant and need to either stop breast-feeding or discontinue drug.
• Instruct patient to store medication at room temperature and to keep container tightly sealed.
• Inform patient to report adverse reactions without delay.
• Inform patient that drug may be taken without regards to meals.

captopril
Acenorm‡, Capoten, Enzace‡,
Novo-Captoril†

*Pregnancy Risk Category: C
(D in second and third trimesters)*

HOW SUPPLIED
Tablets: 12.5 mg, 25 mg, 50 mg, 100 mg

ACTION
Not clearly defined. Thought to inhibit ACE, preventing conversion of angiotensin I to angiotensin II, a potent vasoconstrictor. Reduced formation of angiotensin II decreases peripheral arterial resistance, thus decreasing aldosterone secretion. This reduces sodium and water retention and lowers blood pressure.

Route	Onset	Peak	Duration
PO	0.25-1 hr	1-1.5 hr	6-12 hr

INDICATIONS & DOSAGE
Hypertension—
Adults: 25 mg P.O. b.i.d. or t.i.d. initially. If blood pressure isn't satisfactorily controlled in 1 to 2 weeks, increase dosage to 50 mg b.i.d. or t.i.d. If not satisfactorily controlled after another 1 to 2 weeks, expect a diuretic to be added. If further blood pressure reduction is necessary,

dosage may be raised to 150 mg t.i.d. while continuing the diuretic. Maximum dosage is 450 mg daily.
Heart failure; to reduce risk of death and to slow development of heart failure after MI—
Adults: 6.25 to 12.5 mg P.O. t.i.d. initially. Gradually increased to 50 mg t.i.d. p.r.n. Maximum daily dosage is 450 mg.
Diabetic nephropathy—
Adults: 25 mg P.O. t.i.d.

ADVERSE REACTIONS
CNS: dizziness, fainting, headache, malaise, fatigue.
CV: *tachycardia, hypotension,* angina pectoris.
GI: abdominal pain, anorexia, constipation, diarrhea, dry mouth, dysgeusia, nausea, vomiting.
Hematologic: *leukopenia, agranulocytosis, pancytopenia,* anemia, *thrombocytopenia.*
Hepatic: transient increase in hepatic enzymes.
Respiratory: *dry, persistent, nonproductive cough,* dyspnea.
Skin: *urticarial rash, maculopapular rash,* pruritus, alopecia.
Other: fever, *angioedema of face and extremities,* hyperkalemia.

INTERACTIONS
Drug-drug. *Antacids:* decreased captopril effect. Separate administration times.
Digoxin: may increase serum digoxin concentration by 15% to 30%. Monitor closely.
Diuretics, other antihypertensives: risk of excessive hypotension. Diuretic may need to be discontinued or captopril dosage lowered.
Insulin, oral antidiabetic agents: risk of hypoglycemia when captopril therapy is initiated. Monitor closely.
Lithium: increased lithium levels and symptoms of toxicity may occur. Monitor patient closely.
NSAIDs: may reduce antihypertensive effect. Monitor blood pressure.
Potassium-sparing diuretics, potassium supplements: increased risk of hyperkalemia. Avoid these agents unless hypokalemic blood levels are confirmed.

Drug-herb. *Black catechu:* additional hypotensive effect. Avoid concomitant use.

EFFECTS ON DIAGNOSTIC TESTS
Drug may cause false-positive results for urinary acetone.

CONTRAINDICATIONS
Contraindicated in patients with hypersensitivity to drug or other ACE inhibitors.

NURSING CONSIDERATIONS
• Use cautiously in patients with impaired renal function or serious autoimmune disease (particularly systemic lupus erythematosus) or in patients who have been exposed to other drugs known to affect WBC counts or immune response.
• Monitor patient's blood pressure and pulse rate frequently.
Alert: Be aware that elderly patients may be more sensitive to drug's hypotensive effects.
• In patients with impaired renal function or collagen vascular disease, monitor WBC and differential counts before starting treatment, every 2 weeks for the first 3 months of therapy, and periodically thereafter.

☑**Patient teaching**
• Instruct patient to take drug 1 hour before meals; food in the GI tract may reduce absorption.
• Inform patient that light-headedness can occur, especially during first few days of therapy. Tell him to rise slowly to minimize this effect and to report symptoms to doctor. If syncope occurs, he should stop drug and call doctor immediately.
• Tell patient to use caution in hot weather and during exercise. Inadequate fluid intake, vomiting, diarrhea, and excessive perspiration can lead to light-headedness and syncope.
• Advise patient to report signs of infection, such as fever and sore throat.
• Tell female patient to notify doctor if pregnancy occurs. Drug will need to be discontinued.

Reactions may be *common,* uncommon, *life-threatening,* or COMMON AND LIFE-THREATENING.

carteolol
Cartrol

Pregnancy Risk Category: C

HOW SUPPLIED
Tablets: 2.5 mg, 5 mg

ACTION
Unknown. Carteolol is a nonselective beta-adrenergic blocker with intrinsic sympathomimetic activity. Its antihypertensive effects are probably caused by decreased sympathetic outflow from the brain and decreased cardiac output. Carteolol does not have a consistent effect on renin output.

Route	Onset	Peak	Duration
PO	Unknown	1-3 hr	24 hr

INDICATIONS & DOSAGE
Hypertension—
Adults: initially, 2.5 mg P.O. as a single daily dose; gradually increased to 5 or 10 mg as a single daily dose, p.r.n. Dosages that exceed 10 mg daily do not produce a greater response and may actually decrease it.
Adjust-a-dose: In patients with substantial renal failure, if creatinine clearance is over 60 ml/minute, dosage interval is 24 hours; between 20 and 60 ml/minute, dosage interval is 48 hours; and if less than 20 ml/minute, dosage interval is 72 hours.

ADVERSE REACTIONS
CNS: lassitude, fatigue, somnolence, *asthenia*, paresthesia.
CV: conduction disturbances, bradycardia.
GI: diarrhea, nausea, abdominal pain.
Other: *muscle cramps,* arthralgia, nasal congestion, rash, sweating.

INTERACTIONS
Drug-drug. *Calcium channel blockers:* increased risk of hypotension, left ventricular failure, and AV conduction disturbances. Use I.V. calcium channel blockers with caution.
Cardiac glycosides: may produce additive effects on slowing AV node conduction. Avoid concomitant use.

Catecholamine-depleting drugs, reserpine: may have an additive effect. Monitor closely.
General anesthetics: increased hypotensive effects. Observe carefully for excessive hypotension or bradycardia or orthostatic hypotension.
Insulin, oral antidiabetic agents: may alter hypoglycemic response. Adjust dosage as necessary.

EFFECTS ON DIAGNOSTIC TESTS
None reported.

CONTRAINDICATIONS
Contraindicated in patients with bronchial asthma, severe bradycardia, greater than first-degree heart block, cardiogenic shock, or uncontrolled heart failure.

NURSING CONSIDERATIONS
• Use cautiously in patients with heart failure controlled by cardiac glycosides and diuretics because these patients may exhibit signs of cardiac decompensation with beta-blocker therapy.
• Monitor blood pressure frequently.
• Know that beta blockade may inhibit glycogenolysis and the signs and symptoms of hypoglycemia (such as tachycardia and blood pressure changes). It may also attenuate insulin release. Monitor blood glucose levels frequently.
• Know that withdrawal of beta-blocker therapy before surgery is controversial. Some clinicians advocate withdrawal to prevent impairment of cardiac responsiveness to reflex stimuli and decreased responsiveness to administration of catecholamines. However, the beta-blocking effects of carteolol may persist for weeks, and discontinuing drug before surgery may be impractical. Advise anesthesiologist that patient is receiving a beta blocker so that isoproterenol or dobutamine is made readily available for reversal of drug's cardiac effects.
• Beta blockers may mask tachycardia associated with hyperthyroidism. In patients with suspected thyrotoxicosis, gradually withdraw beta-blocker therapy, as ordered, to avoid thyroid storm.
Alert: Be aware that patients with unrecognized coronary artery disease may ex-

---

*Liquid contains alcohol.   **May contain tartrazine.   †Canada   ‡Australia   §U.K.   ◊OTC

hibit signs of angina pectoris on withdrawal of drug. Monitor closely.

✔ **Patient teaching**
• Instruct patient to take drug exactly as prescribed.
• Tell patient not to stop drug suddenly but to call doctor and discuss unpleasant adverse reactions.
• Emphasize importance of reporting signs of heart failure, including shortness of breath or difficulty breathing, unusually fast heartbeat, cough, or fatigue with exertion.

---

carvedilol
Coreg, Eucardic§,

Pregnancy Risk Category: C

HOW SUPPLIED
Tablets: 3.125 mg, 6.25 mg, 12.5 mg, 25 mg

ACTION
Nonselective beta-adrenergic blocking agent with alpha$_1$-blocking activity.

Route	Onset	Peak	Duration
PO	Unknown	1-2 hr	7-10 hr

INDICATIONS & DOSAGE
Hypertension—
Adults: dosage highly individualized. Initially, 6.25 mg P.O. b.i.d. Obtain a standing blood pressure 1 hour after initial dose. If tolerated, continue dosage for 7 to 14 days. May increase to 12.5 mg P.O. b.i.d. for 7 to 14 days, following blood pressure monitoring protocol noted above. Maximum dosage is 25 mg P.O. b.i.d. as tolerated.
Heart failure—
Adults: dosage highly individualized. Initially, 3.125 mg P.O. b.i.d. for 2 weeks; if tolerated, can increase to 6.25 mg P.O. b.i.d. Dosage may be doubled q 2 weeks as tolerated. Maximum dosage for patients weighing under 85 kg (187 lb) is 25 mg P.O. b.i.d.; for those weighing over 85 kg, dosage is 50 mg P.O. b.i.d.
Adjust-a-dose: If patient experiences bradycardia with pulse rate below 55 beats/minute, use reduced dosage.

ADVERSE REACTIONS
CNS: *dizziness, fatigue,* headache, hypoesthesia, insomnia, pain, paresthesia, somnolence, vertigo.
CV: aggravated angina pectoris, *AV block, bradycardia,* chest pain, fluid overload, hypertension, hypotension, orthostatic hypotension, syncope.
EENT: abnormal vision.
GI: abdominal pain, *diarrhea,* melena, nausea, periodontitis, vomiting.
GU: abnormal renal function, albuminuria, hematuria, impotence, urinary tract infection, elevated BUN levels.
Hematologic: purpura, *thrombocytopenia, decreased PT.*
Hepatic: increased serum alkaline phosphatase, BUN, ALT, and AST levels.
Metabolic: dehydration, glycosuria, gout, hypercholesterolemia, *hyperglycemia,* hypertriglyceridemia, hypervolemia, hypovolemia, hyperuricemia, hypoglycemia, hyponatremia, weight gain.
Respiratory: bronchitis, dyspnea, pharyngitis, rhinitis, sinusitis, *upper respiratory tract infection.*
Other: allergy, arthralgia, back pain, edema, fever, malaise, myalgia, peripheral edema, *sudden death,* viral infection.

INTERACTIONS
Drug-drug. *Calcium channel blockers:* can cause isolated conduction disturbances. Monitor patient's heart rhythm and blood pressure.
Catecholamine-depleting agents (such as MAO inhibitors, reserpine): may cause bradycardia or severe hypotension. Monitor patient closely.
Cimetidine: increased bioavailability of carvedilol. Monitor vital signs carefully.
Clonidine: may potentiate blood pressure and heart-rate-lowering effects. Monitor vital signs closely.
Digoxin: increased concentrations of digoxin by about 15% while on concurrent therapy. Monitor digoxin levels.
Insulin, oral antidiabetic agents: concomitant use may enhance hypoglycemic properties. Monitor blood glucose levels.
Rifampin: reduced plasma concentrations of carvedilol by 70%. Monitor vital signs closely.
Drug-food. *Any food:* delayed rate of ab-

Reactions may be *common,* uncommon, **life-threatening,** or COMMON AND LIFE-THREATENING.

sorption of carvedilol but does not alter extent of bioavailability. Advise patient to take drug with food to minimize orthostatic effects.

EFFECTS ON DIAGNOSTIC TESTS
None reported.

CONTRAINDICATIONS
Contraindicated in patients with New York Heart Association (NYHA) class IV decompensated cardiac failure requiring I.V. inotropic therapy, bronchial asthma or related bronchospastic conditions, second- or third-degree AV block, sick sinus syndrome (unless a permanent pacemaker is in place), cardiogenic shock, severe bradycardia, symptomatic hepatic impairment, or hypersensitivity to drug.

NURSING CONSIDERATIONS
● Use cautiously in hypertensive patients with left ventricular failure, perioperative patients who receive anesthetics that depress myocardial function (ether, cyclopropane, trichloroethylene, others), or diabetic patients receiving insulin or oral antidiabetic agents and in those subject to spontaneous hypoglycemia. Also use with caution in patients with thyroid disease (may mask hyperthyroidism; withdrawal may precipitate thyroid storm or exacerbation of hyperthyroidism), pheochromocytoma, Prinzmetal's or variant angina, bronchospastic disease, or peripheral vascular disease (may precipitate or aggravate symptoms of arterial insufficiency). Also use cautiously in breast-feeding women.
Alert: Patients on beta blocker therapy with history of severe anaphylactic reaction to several allergens may be more reactive to repeated challenge (accidental, diagnostic, or therapeutic). They may be unresponsive to dosages of epinephrine typically used to treat allergic reactions.
● Mild hepatocellular injury may occur during therapy. At first sign of hepatic dysfunction, perform tests for hepatic injury or jaundice; if present, stop drug.
● If patient needs to be taken off drug, discontinue it gradually over 1 to 2 weeks.
● Monitor patient with heart failure for worsened condition, renal dysfunction, or

fluid retention; diuretics may need to be increased.
● Monitor diabetic patient closely; drug may mask signs of hypoglycemia, or hyperglycemia may be worsened.
● Observe patient for dizziness or lightheadedness for 1 hour after administration of each new dosage.
● Be aware that prior to initiation of carvedilol, dosages of digoxin, diuretics, or ACE inhibitors should be stabilized.
● Safety and efficacy in patients under 18 years have not been established.
● Monitor elderly patients carefully; plasma levels are about 50% higher in elderly patients compared with younger ones.

☑ **Patient teaching**
● Tell patient not to interrupt or discontinue drug without medical approval.
● Inform patient that improvement of heart failure symptoms might take several weeks of carvedilol therapy.
● Advise patient with heart failure to call doctor if weight gain or shortness of breath occurs.
● Inform patient that he may experience low blood pressure when standing. If dizziness or fainting (rare) occur, advise him to sit or lie down.
● Caution patient against performing hazardous tasks during initiation of therapy. If dizziness or fatigue occur, tell him to call for an adjustment in dosage.
● Advise diabetic patient to report changes in blood glucose promptly.
● Inform patient who wears contact lenses that decreased lacrimation may occur.

---

clonidine
Catapres-TTS

clonidine hydrochloride
Catapres, Dixarit††‡

Pregnancy Risk Category: C

HOW SUPPLIED
clonidine
Transdermal: TTS-1 (releases 0.1 mg/24 hours), TTS-2 (releases 0.2 mg/24 hours), TTS-3 (releases 0.3 mg/24 hours)

---

clonidine hydrochloride
Tablets: 0.025 mg†‡, 0.1 mg, 0.2 mg,
0.3 mg

ACTION

Unknown. Thought to stimulate alpha$_2$-
adrenergic receptors centrally and inhibit
the central vasomotor centers, thereby decreasing sympathetic outflow to the heart,
kidneys, and peripheral vasculature; this
results in decreased peripheral vascular
resistance, decreased systolic and diastolic blood pressure, and decreased heart
rate.

Route	Onset	Peak	Duration
PO	0.5-1 hr	2-4 hr	12-24 hr
Trans-dermal	2-3 days	2-3 days	7-8 days

INDICATIONS & DOSAGE

Essential and renal hypertension—
Adults: initially, 0.1 mg P.O. b.i.d. Then
increased by 0.1 or 0.2 mg daily on a
weekly basis. Usual dosage range is 0.2 to
0.6 mg daily in divided doses; infrequently, dosages as high as 2.4 mg daily are
used.
   Or, a transdermal patch is applied to
a nonhairy area of intact skin on upper
arm or torso once q 7 days, starting with
0.1-mg system and titrated with another
0.1-mg system or larger system.
Children: 50 to 400 mcg P.O. b.i.d.

ADVERSE REACTIONS

CNS: *drowsiness, dizziness,* fatigue, *sedation, weakness,* malaise, agitation, depression.
CV: orthostatic hypotension, bradycardia,
severe rebound hypertension.
GI: *constipation, dry mouth,* nausea,
vomiting, anorexia.
GU: urine retention, impotence, loss of libido.
Skin: *pruritus, dermatitis* (with transdermal patch), rash.
Other: weight gain.

INTERACTIONS

Drug-drug. *CNS depressants:* enhanced
CNS depression. Use together cautiously.
Diuretics, other antihypertensive agents:
increased hypotensive effect. Monitor
closely.
Levodopa: may reduce effectiveness of
levodopa. Monitor patient.
*MAO inhibitors, prazosin, tricyclic anti-
depressants:* may decrease antihypertensive effect. Use together cautiously.
Propranolol, other beta blockers: paradoxical hypertensive response. Monitor
carefully.
Verapamil: may cause AV block and severe hypotension.
Drug-herb. *Capsicum:* may reduce antihypertensive effectiveness. Avoid concomitant use.

EFFECTS ON DIAGNOSTIC TESTS

Clonidine may decrease urinary excretion
of vanillylmandelic acid and catecholamines; it may slightly increase blood or
serum glucose levels and may cause a
weakly positive Coombs' test.

CONTRAINDICATIONS

Contraindicated in patients with hypersensitivity to drug. Transdermal form is
contraindicated in patients with hypersensitivity to any component of the adhesive
layer of transdermal system.

NURSING CONSIDERATIONS

• Use cautiously in patients with severe
coronary insufficiency, recent MI, cerebrovascular disease, chronic renal failure,
or impaired liver function.
• Know that clonidine may be given to
rapidly lower blood pressure in some hypertensive emergencies.
• Monitor blood pressure and pulse rate
frequently. Dosage is usually adjusted to
patient's blood pressure and tolerance.
• Elderly patients may be more sensitive
to drug's hypotensive effects.
• Observe patient for tolerance to drug's
therapeutic effects, which may require increased dosage.
• Antihypertensive effects of transdermal
clonidine may take 2 to 3 days to become
apparent. Oral antihypertensive therapy
may have to be continued in the interim.
Alert: Remove transdermal patch before
defibrillation to prevent arcing.
• When stopping therapy in patients receiving both clonidine and a beta blocker,

gradually withdraw the beta blocker first to minimize adverse reactions, as ordered.
• Be aware that discontinuation for surgery is not recommended.

☑ **Patient teaching**
• Instruct patient to take drug exactly as prescribed.
• Advise patient that abrupt discontinuation of drug may cause severe rebound hypertension. Tell him dosage must be reduced gradually over 2 to 4 days as instructed by doctor.
• Tell patient to take the last dose immediately before retiring.
• Reassure patient that the transdermal patch usually adheres despite showering and other routine daily activities. Instruct him on the use of the adhesive "overlay" to provide additional skin adherence if necessary. Also tell patient to place the patch at a different site each week.
• Caution patient that drug may cause drowsiness but that this adverse effect will usually diminish over 4 to 6 weeks.
• Inform patient that orthostatic hypotension can be minimized by rising slowly and avoiding sudden position changes.

---

diazoxide
Eudemine§, Hyperstat IV

Pregnancy Risk Category: C

HOW SUPPLIED
Injection: 300 mg/20 ml, 15 mg/ml

ACTION
Exact antihypertensive action unknown. Directly relaxes arteriolar smooth muscle and decreases peripheral vascular resistance.

Route	Onset	Peak	Duration
IV	1 min	2-5 min	2-12 hr

INDICATIONS & DOSAGE
Hypertensive crisis—
Adults and children: 1 to 3 mg/kg by I.V. bolus (up to maximum of 150 mg) q 5 to 15 minutes until adequate response is seen. Repeat at 4- to 24-hour intervals, p.r.n.

ADVERSE REACTIONS
CNS: *headache,* dizziness, light-headedness, weakness, ***seizures, paralysis,*** euphoria, ***cerebral ischemia.***
CV: *sodium and water retention,* orthostatic hypotension, diaphoresis, flushing, warmth, angina, myocardial ischemia, ***arrhythmias,*** ECG changes, ***shock, MI.***
GI: *nausea, vomiting,* abdominal discomfort, dry mouth, constipation, diarrhea.
Other: inflammation and pain resulting from extravasation, *hyperglycemia,* hyperuricemia, optic nerve infarction.

INTERACTIONS
Drug-drug. *Antihypertensives (such as hydralazine):* may cause severe hypotension. Use together cautiously.
Hydantoins: may decrease levels of hydantoins, resulting in decreased anticonvulsant action. Monitor closely.
Sulfonylureas: may cause hyperglycemia. Monitor serum glucose levels.
Thiazide diuretics: may increase diazoxide's effects. Use together cautiously.

EFFECTS ON DIAGNOSTIC TESTS
Drug inhibits glucose-stimulated insulin release and may cause false-negative insulin response to glucagon. Prolonged use of oral diazoxide may decrease hemoglobin and hematocrit levels.

CONTRAINDICATIONS
Contraindicated in patients with hypersensitivity to drug, other thiazides, or other sulfonamide-derived drugs. Also contraindicated in the treatment of compensatory hypertension (such as that associated with coarctation of the aorta or arteriovenous shunt).

NURSING CONSIDERATIONS
• Use cautiously in patients with impaired cerebral or cardiac function or uremia.
• Check patient's standing blood pressure before discontinuing close monitoring for hypotension.
• Monitor patient's fluid intake and output carefully. If fluid or sodium retention develops, the doctor may order diuretics.
• Weigh patient daily and notify doctor of weight increase.
• Diazoxide may alter requirements for

---

insulin, diet, or oral antidiabetic agents in previously controlled diabetic patients. Monitor blood glucose daily; watch for signs of severe hyperglycemia or hyperosmolar nonketotic syndrome. Insulin may be needed.
• Check uric acid levels frequently and report abnormalities to doctor.

🔲 I.V. administration
• Monitor blood pressure and ECG continuously. Place patient in supine position or in Trendelenburg's position during and for 1 hour after infusion. Notify doctor immediately if severe hypotension develops. Keep norepinephrine available.
• Protect I.V. solutions from light. Darkened I.V. solutions of diazoxide are subpotent and should not be used.
• Take care to avoid extravasation.

✅ Patient teaching
• Inform patient that orthostatic hypotension can be minimized by rising slowly and avoiding sudden position changes. Instruct patient to remain in the supine position for 60 minutes after injection.
• Tell patient to alert nurse if discomfort occurs at I.V. insertion site.

---

doxazosin mesylate
Cardura, Carduran‡

Pregnancy Risk Category: C

HOW SUPPLIED
Tablets: 1 mg, 2 mg, 4 mg, 8 mg

ACTION
An alpha₁-adrenergic blocker that acts on the peripheral vasculature to reduce peripheral vascular resistance and produce vasodilation.

Route	Onset	Peak	Duration
PO	1-2 hr	2-3 hr	24 hr

INDICATIONS & DOSAGE
Essential hypertension—
Adults: initially, 1 mg P.O. daily and determine effect on standing and supine blood pressure at 2 to 6 hours and 24 hours after dosing. If necessary, dose is increased to 2 mg daily. To minimize adverse reactions, dosage is titrated slowly (dosage typically increased only q 2 weeks). If necessary, dose increased to 4 mg daily, then 8 mg. Maximum daily dosage is 16 mg, but dosage that exceeds 4 mg daily is associated with a greater incidence of adverse reactions.
Benign prostatic hyperplasia—
Adults: initially, 1 mg P.O. once daily in the morning or evening; may be increased to 2 mg and, thereafter, 4 mg and 8 mg once daily, p.r.n. Recommended titration interval is 1 to 2 weeks.

ADVERSE REACTIONS
CNS: *dizziness,* vertigo, somnolence, drowsiness, *asthenia, headache.*
CV: *orthostatic hypotension,* hypotension, edema, palpitations, ***arrhythmias,*** tachycardia.
GI: nausea, vomiting, diarrhea, constipation.
Skin: rash, pruritus.
Other: rhinitis, arthralgia, myalgia, pain, dyspnea, pharyngitis, abnormal vision.

INTERACTIONS
Drug-herb. *Butcher's broom:* possible diminished effect of doxazosin. Avoid concomitant use.

EFFECTS ON DIAGNOSTIC TESTS
Mean WBC and neutrophil counts may be decreased.

CONTRAINDICATIONS
Contraindicated in patients with hypersensitivity to drug and quinazoline derivatives (including prazosin and terazosin).

NURSING CONSIDERATIONS
• Use cautiously in patients with impaired hepatic function.
• Monitor blood pressure closely.
• If syncope occurs, place patient in a recumbent position and treat supportively. A transient hypotensive response is not considered a contraindication to continued therapy.

✅ Patient teaching
• Instruct patient to take drug exactly as prescribed.

Alert: Advise patient that he is susceptible to a "first-dose" effect similar to that produced by other alpha-adrenergic blockers—marked orthostatic hypotension accompanied by dizziness or syncope. Orthostatic hypotension is most common after first dose but also can occur during dosage adjustment or interruption of therapy. Warn patient that dizziness or fainting may occur. Advise him to avoid driving and other hazardous activities until drug's CNS effects are known.

---

enalaprilat
Innovace§, Vasotec I.V.

enalapril maleate
Amprace‡, Renitec‡, Vasotec

Pregnancy Risk Category: C
(D in second and third trimesters)

HOW SUPPLIED
enalaprilat
Injection: 1.25 mg/ml
enalapril maleate
Tablets: 2.5 mg, 5 mg, 10 mg, 20 mg

ACTION
Unknown, but does inhibit ACE, preventing conversion of angiotensin I to angiotensin II, a potent vasoconstrictor. Reduced formation of angiotensin II decreases peripheral arterial resistance, thus decreasing aldosterone secretion.

Route	Onset	Peak	Duration
PO	1 hr	4-6 hr	24 hr
IV	15 min	1-4 hr	6 hr

INDICATIONS & DOSAGE
Hypertension—
Adults: in patient not receiving diuretics, initially 5 mg P.O. once daily, then adjusted according to response. Usual dosage range is 10 to 40 mg daily as a single dose or two divided doses. Alternatively, 1.25 mg I.V. infusion q 6 hours over 5 minutes.
Adjust-a-dose: In patient on diuretics, initially 2.5 mg P.O. once daily. Alternatively, 0.625 mg I.V. over 5 minutes, repeated in 1 hour if needed, then followed by 1.25 mg I.V. q 6 hours.

To convert from I.V. therapy to oral therapy—
Adults: initially, 2.5 mg P.O. once daily; if patient was receiving 0.625 mg I.V. q 6 hours, then 2.5 mg P.O. once daily. Dosage is adjusted to response.
To convert from oral therapy to I.V. therapy—
Adults: 1.25 mg I.V. over 5 minutes q 6 hours. Higher doses have not demonstrated greater efficacy.
Adjust-a-dose: In patients with renal impairment or hyponatremia, if serum creatinine is above 1.6 mg/dl or serum sodium is below 130 mEq/L, dosage is initiated at 2.5 mg P.O. daily and titrated slowly.

ADVERSE REACTIONS
CNS: headache, dizziness, fatigue, vertigo, asthenia, syncope.
CV: *hypotension,* chest pain, angina.
GI: diarrhea, nausea, abdominal pain, vomiting.
GU: decreased renal function (in patients with bilateral renal artery stenosis or heart failure), increased BUN and creatinine levels.
Hematologic: *neutropenia, thrombocytopenia, agranulocytosis,* decreased hemoglobin and hematocrit, bone marrow depression.
Hepatic: increased liver function test results and bilirubin.
Respiratory: *dry, persistent, tickling, nonproductive cough,* dyspnea.
Skin: rash.
Other: *angioedema.*

INTERACTIONS
Drug-drug. *Diuretics:* excessive reduction of blood pressure. Use together cautiously.
Insulin, oral antidiabetic agents: risk of hypoglycemia, especially at initiation of enalapril therapy. Monitor closely.
Lithium: lithium toxicity can occur. Monitor lithium levels.
NSAIDs: may reduce antihypertensive effect. Monitor blood pressure.
Potassium-sparing diuretics, potassium supplements: increased risk of hyperkalemia. Avoid these drugs unless hypokalemic blood levels are confirmed.

EFFECTS ON DIAGNOSTIC TESTS
None reported.

CONTRAINDICATIONS
Contraindicated in patients with hypersensitivity to drug or history of angioedema related to previous treatment with an ACE inhibitor.

NURSING CONSIDERATIONS
• Use cautiously in renally impaired patients.
• Monitor blood pressure response to drug closely.
• Monitor CBC with differential counts before and during therapy.
• Diabetic patients, those with impaired renal function or heart failure, and those receiving drugs that can increase serum potassium may develop hyperkalemia. Monitor potassium intake and serum potassium level.

I.V. administration
• Inject drug slowly over at least 5 minutes, or dilute in 50 ml of a compatible solution and infuse over 15 minutes. Compatible solutions include D_5W, 0.9% NaCl injection, dextrose 5% in lactated Ringer's injection, and dextrose 5% in 0.9% NaCl injection.

Patient teaching
• Instruct patient to report breathing difficulty or swelling of face, eyes, lips, or tongue. Angioedema (including laryngeal edema) may occur, especially after the first dose.
• Advise patient to report signs of infection, such as fever and sore throat.
• Inform patient that light-headedness can occur, especially during first few days of therapy. Tell him to rise slowly to minimize this effect and to notify doctor if symptoms develop. If syncope occurs, he should stop taking drug and call doctor immediately.
• Tell patient to use caution in hot weather and during exercise. Inadequate fluid intake, vomiting, diarrhea, and excessive perspiration can lead to light-headedness and syncope.
• Advise patient to avoid salt substitutes; these products may contain potassium,

which can cause hyperkalemia in patients taking this drug.
• Tell female patient to notify doctor if pregnancy occurs. Drug will need to be discontinued.

---

felodipine
Agon SR‡, Plendil, Plendil ER‡, Renedil†

Pregnancy Risk Category: C

HOW SUPPLIED
Tablets (extended-release): 2.5 mg, 5 mg, 10 mg

ACTION
Unknown. A dihydropyridine-derivative calcium channel blocker that prevents the entry of calcium ions into vascular smooth-muscle and cardiac cells; shows some selectivity for smooth muscle as compared with cardiac muscle.

Route	Onset	Peak	Duration
PO	2-5 hr	2.5-5 hr	24 hr

INDICATIONS & DOSAGE
Hypertension—
Adults: initially, 5 mg P.O. daily. Dosage is adjusted based on patient response, generally at intervals not less than 2 weeks. Usual dose is 5 to 10 mg daily; maximum recommended dosage is 10 mg daily.
Elderly: 5 mg P.O. daily; dosage is adjusted as for adults. Maximum recommended dosage is 10 mg daily.
Adjust-a-dose: In patients with impaired hepatic function, 5 mg P.O. daily; dosage adjusted as for adults. Maximum recommended dosage is 10 mg daily.

ADVERSE REACTIONS
CNS: *headache,* dizziness, paresthesia, asthenia.
CV: *peripheral edema,* chest pain, palpitations.
EENT: rhinorrhea, pharyngitis.
GI: abdominal pain, nausea, constipation, diarrhea.
Respiratory: upper respiratory infection, cough.

Reactions may be *common,* uncommon, *life-threatening,* or COMMON AND LIFE-THREATENING.

Skin: rash, flushing.
Other: muscle cramps, back pain.

INTERACTIONS
Drug-drug. *Anticonvulsants:* decreased plasma concentration of felodipine. Avoid concomitant use.
Cimetidine: decreased clearance of felodipine. Use lower doses of felodipine.
Metoprolol: may alter pharmacokinetics of metoprolol. No dosage adjustment appears necessary; monitor for adverse effects.
Theophylline: may slightly decrease theophylline levels. Monitor patient's response closely.
Drug-food. *Grapefruit juice:* increased bioavailability and effect when taken together. Monitor closely.

EFFECTS ON DIAGNOSTIC TESTS
None reported.

CONTRAINDICATIONS
Contraindicated in patients with hypersensitivity to drug.

NURSING CONSIDERATIONS
• Use cautiously in patients with heart failure, particularly those receiving beta-adrenergic blockers, and in patients with impaired hepatic function.
• Monitor blood pressure for response.
• Monitor patient for peripheral edema. Peripheral edema appears to be both dose- and age-related: it's more common in patients taking higher doses, especially those over 60 years.

☑ Patient teaching
• Tell patient to swallow tablets whole and not to crush or chew them.
• Teach patient to continue taking drug even when he feels better; to watch his diet; and to check with the doctor or pharmacist before taking other medications, including OTC drugs.
• Advise patient to observe good oral hygiene and to see a dentist regularly; use of drug has been associated with mild gingival hyperplasia.

fenoldopam mesylate
Corlopam

Pregnancy Risk Category: B

HOW SUPPLIED
Ampules: 10 mg/ml in single-dose ampules of 5 ml

ACTION
Rapid-acting vasodilator. Drug is an agonist for D_1-like dopamine receptors and binds with moderate affinity to $alpha_2$ adrenoceptors.

Route	Onset	Peak	Duration
IV	15 min	20 min	Unknown

INDICATIONS & DOSAGE
Short-term (up to 48 hours) hospital management of severe hypertension when rapid but quickly reversible reduction of blood pressure is indicated, including malignant hypertension with deteriorating end-organ function—
Adults: administer by continuous I.V. infusion. Initiate infusion rates at 0.025 to 0.3 mcg/kg/minute and titrate upward or downward to achieve desired blood pressure no more frequently than q 15 minutes. Recommended increments for titration are 0.05 to 0.1 mcg/kg/minute.

ADVERSE REACTIONS
CNS: dizziness, headache, insomnia.
CV: hypotension, palpitations, bradycardia, tachycardia, angina, *MI*, T-wave inversion.
GI: nausea, vomiting, abdominal pain, constipation, diarrhea.
GU: oliguria.
Hematologic: leukocytosis, bleeding.
Metabolic: hypokalemia, increased BUN, glucose, LD, and transaminases.
Musculoskeletal: limb cramp, back pain.
Respiratory: dyspnea.
Skin: flushing.
Other: nasal congestion, pyrexia, nonspecific chest pain.

INTERACTIONS
Drug-drug. *Beta blockers:* may cause hypotension. Avoid concurrent use.

EFFECTS ON DIAGNOSTIC TESTS
None reported.

CONTRAINDICATIONS
No known contraindications.

NURSING CONSIDERATIONS
• Use with caution in patients with glaucoma or ocular hypertension as it can cause dose-dependent increases in intraocular pressure. Drug may cause symptomatic hypotension; use particular caution when administering to patients who have sustained an acute cerebral infarction or hemorrhage. Use during pregnancy only if clearly needed. Drug may be excreted in milk; use caution in administering to breast-feeding women.
• Safety and effectiveness in children have not been established.
• Drug causes a dose-related tachycardia which diminishes over time but remains substantial at higher doses.
Alert: Drug contains sodium metabisulfite, which may cause allergic-type reactions (including anaphylactic symptoms and severe asthmatic episodes in susceptible individuals). Sulfite sensitivity is more frequent in asthmatic than in nonasthmatic people.
• Monitor serum electrolytes and watch for hypokalemia.

I.V. administration
• Follow manufacturer's instructions for diluting drug. Diluted solution is stable at room temperature for at least 24 hours.
• Infuse drug with a calibrated mechanical infusion pump.
• A bolus dose should *not* be used.
• May abruptly discontinue or gradually taper infusion. Oral antihypertensive agents can be added once blood pressure is stable during infusion or after its discontinuation.
• Monitor blood pressure frequently during infusions. Check blood pressure and heart rate every 15 minutes until patient is stable.

✓ Patient teaching
• Tell patient that drug causes dose-related decreases in blood pressure and increases in heart rate. Advise patient to change positions slowly to avoid orthostatic symptoms.
• Encourage patient to report adverse reactions promptly.

---

fosinopril sodium
Monopril, Staril§

Pregnancy Risk Category: C
(D in second and third trimesters)

HOW SUPPLIED
Tablets: 10 mg, 20 mg

ACTION
Antihypertensive action not clearly defined. Inhibits ACE, preventing conversion of angiotensin I to angiotensin II, a potent vasoconstrictor. Reduced formation of angiotensin II decreases peripheral arterial resistance, thus decreasing aldosterone secretion.

Route	Onset	Peak	Duration
PO	1 hr	3 hr	24 hr

INDICATIONS & DOSAGE
Hypertension—
Adults: initially, 10 mg P.O. daily. Dosage is adjusted based on blood pressure response at peak and trough levels. Usual dosage is 20 to 40 mg, up to 80 mg daily. Dosage is divided if needed.
Heart failure—
Adults: initially, 10 mg P.O. once daily. Dosage increased over several weeks to a maximum dosage of 40 mg P.O. daily, if needed.
Adjust-a-dose: In patients with moderate to severe renal failure or vigorous diuresis, initially, 5 mg P.O. once daily.

ADVERSE REACTIONS
CNS: *CVA,* headache, dizziness, fatigue, syncope, paresthesia, sleep disturbance.
CV: chest pain, angina, *MI,* rhythm disturbances, palpitations, hypotension, orthostatic hypotension.
EENT: tinnitus, sinusitis.
GI: nausea, vomiting, diarrhea, pancreatitis, hepatitis, dry mouth, abdominal distention, abdominal pain, constipation.

Reactions may be *common,* uncommon, *life-threatening,* or COMMON AND LIFE-THREATENING.

GU: sexual dysfunction, decreased libido, renal insufficiency.
Respiratory: *dry, persistent, tickling, nonproductive cough;* **bronchospasm.**
Skin: urticaria, rash, photosensitivity, pruritus.
Other: *angioedema,* arthralgia, musculoskeletal pain, myalgia, gout, hyperkalemia.

INTERACTIONS
Drug-drug. *Antacids:* may impair absorption. Separate administration times by at least 2 hours.
Diuretics, other antihypertensives: risk of excessive hypotension. Diuretic may need to be discontinued or fosinopril dosage lowered.
Lithium: increased serum lithium levels and lithium toxicity. Monitor serum lithium levels.
Potassium-sparing diuretics, potassium supplements: risk of hyperkalemia. Monitor closely during concomitant use.
Drug-food. *Salt substitutes containing potassium:* risk of hyperkalemia. Monitor closely during concomitant use.

EFFECTS ON DIAGNOSTIC TESTS
False low measurements of digoxin levels may result with the Digi-Tab radioimmunoassay kit for digoxin; other kits may be used. Transient elevations of BUN, serum creatinine levels, and liver function test results and decreases in hematocrit or hemoglobin may also occur.

CONTRAINDICATIONS
Contraindicated in patients with hypersensitivity to drug or other ACE inhibitors and in breast-feeding patients.

NURSING CONSIDERATIONS
• Use cautiously in patients with impaired renal or hepatic function.
• Monitor blood pressure for effect.
• Monitor potassium intake and serum potassium level. Diabetic patients, those with impaired renal function, and those receiving drugs that can increase serum potassium may develop hyperkalemia.
• Other ACE inhibitors have been associated with agranulocytosis and neutropenia. Monitor CBC with differential

counts, as ordered, before therapy and periodically thereafter.
• Assess renal and hepatic function before and periodically throughout therapy.

☑ **Patient teaching**
• Tell patient to avoid salt substitutes; these products may contain potassium, which can cause hyperkalemia in patients taking this drug.
• Advise patient to report signs of infection, such as fever and sore throat.
• Instruct patient to call doctor if the following signs or symptoms occur: easy bruising or bleeding; swelling of tongue, lips, face, eyes, mucous membranes, or extremities; difficulty swallowing or breathing; and hoarseness.
• Tell patient to use caution in hot weather and during exercise. Inadequate fluid intake, vomiting, diarrhea, and excessive perspiration can lead to light-headedness and syncope.
• Tell female patient to notify doctor if pregnancy occurs. Drug will need to be discontinued.

guanabenz acetate
Wytensin

Pregnancy Risk Category: C

HOW SUPPLIED
Tablets: 4 mg, 8 mg

ACTION
Unknown. A centrally acting antihypertensive, its action is thought to be due to central alpha-adrenergic stimulation, which results in decreased sympathetic outflow to the heart, kidneys, and peripheral vasculature.

Route	Onset	Peak	Duration
PO	1 hr	2-5 hr	12 hr

INDICATIONS & DOSAGE
Hypertension—
Adults: initially, 4 mg P.O. b.i.d. Dosage increased in increments of 4 to 8 mg/day q 1 to 2 weeks. Maximum daily dosage is 32 mg b.i.d. To ensure adequate overnight blood pressure control, give last dose h.s.

ADVERSE REACTIONS
CNS: *drowsiness, sedation, dizziness, weakness,* headache.
CV: *rebound hypertension.*
GI: *dry mouth.*

INTERACTIONS
Drug-drug. *CNS depressants:* may cause increased sedation. Use together cautiously.
Diuretics, other antihypertensive agents: increased risk of excessive hypotension.
MAO inhibitors, tricyclic antidepressants: may decrease antihypertensive effect. Monitor closely.

EFFECTS ON DIAGNOSTIC TESTS
Drug may reduce serum cholesterol and total triglyceride levels slightly, but it does not alter high-density lipoprotein fraction; drug may cause nonprogressive elevations in liver enzyme levels.

Chronic use of guanabenz decreases plasma norepinephrine, dopamine, beta-hydroxylase, and plasma renin activity.

CONTRAINDICATIONS
Contraindicated in patients with hypersensitivity to drug.

NURSING CONSIDERATIONS
• Use cautiously in patients with severe coronary insufficiency, recent MI, cerebrovascular disease, or severe hepatic or renal failure. Also use cautiously in elderly patients.
• Monitor blood pressure for effects. Elderly patients may be more sensitive to drug's hypotensive effects.
• Store drug in light resistant container.

☑ **Patient teaching**
• Caution patient that abrupt discontinuation of drug may cause rebound hypertension.
• Advise patient to avoid hazardous tasks that require alertness until drug's CNS effects are known.
• Inform patient that orthostatic hypotension can be minimized by rising slowly and avoiding sudden position changes. Dry mouth can be relieved with chewing gum, sour hard candy, or ice chips.
• Warn patient that tolerance to alcohol or other CNS depressants may be diminished.

---

guanadrel sulfate
Hylorel

Pregnancy Risk Category: B

HOW SUPPLIED
Tablets: 10 mg, 25 mg

ACTION
Acts peripherally, inhibiting norepinephrine release and depleting norepinephrine stores in adrenergic nerve endings.

Route	Onset	Peak	Duration
PO	2 hr	4-6 hr	4-14 hr

INDICATIONS & DOSAGE
Hypertension—
Adults: initially, 5 mg P.O. b.i.d. Dosage adjusted until blood pressure is controlled. Most patients require dosages of 20 to 75 mg/day, usually given b.i.d.; however, tolerance to hypotensive effect may necessitate upward titration to 100 to 400 mg daily in three to four divided doses.
Adjust-a-dose: In patients with renal impairment, dosage is reduced to 5 mg P.O. once daily if creatinine clearance is 30 to 60 ml/minute; if creatinine clearance is below 30 ml/minute, dosage interval increased to 48 hours. Dosage is adjusted q 7 to 14 days.

ADVERSE REACTIONS
CNS: depression, *fatigue, drowsiness, faintness, headache, confusion, paresthesia.*
CV: *palpitations, chest pain, peripheral edema, orthostatic hypotension.*
GI: *diarrhea,* dry mouth, *indigestion, constipation, anorexia,* nausea, vomiting, abdominal pain.
GU: impotence, *ejaculation disturbances, nocturia, urination frequency.*
Respiratory: *shortness of breath, cough.*
Other: *weight gain, aching limbs, leg cramps, visual disturbances,* glossitis.

INTERACTIONS
Drug-drug. *Amphetamines, ephedrine,*

methylphenidate, norepinephrine, phenothiazines, tricyclic antidepressants: may inhibit guanadrel's antihypertensive effect. Adjust dose accordingly.
Diuretics, other antihypertensives: hypotensive effect of guanadrel increased. Monitor blood pressure closely.
MAO inhibitors: antagonized hypotensive effects of guanadrel. Don't give guanadrel concurrently or within 1 week of MAO inhibitor therapy.

EFFECTS ON DIAGNOSTIC TESTS
None reported.

CONTRAINDICATIONS
Contraindicated in patients with known or suspected pheochromocytoma, frank heart failure, or hypersensitivity to drug. Avoid concurrent use with or within 1 week of MAO inhibitor therapy.

NURSING CONSIDERATIONS
• Use cautiously in patients with regional vascular disease, bronchial asthma, or history of peptic ulcer disease.
• Monitor both supine and standing blood pressure, especially during dosage adjustment periods.
• Be aware that elderly patients may be more sensitive to drug's hypotensive effects.
• Know that guanadrel should be discontinued 48 to 72 hours before surgery to minimize risk of vascular collapse during anesthesia.

☑ **Patient teaching**
• Inform patient that orthostatic hypotension can be minimized by rising slowly from a supine position and by avoiding sudden position changes. Dry mouth can be relieved with chewing gum, sour hard candy, or ice chips.
• Warn patient to avoid strenuous exercise and hot showers; these may cause a hypotensive reaction. An ambient temperature that is too hot also may potentiate the hypotensive effects of guanadrel as can alcohol ingestion.
• Tell patient to check with doctor or pharmacist before taking cold, cough, or allergy preparations.

guanethidine monosulfate
Apo-Guanethidine†, Ismelin

Pregnancy Risk Category: C

HOW SUPPLIED
Tablets: 10 mg, 25 mg

ACTION
An adrenergic neuron blocker that acts peripherally, inhibiting norepinephrine release and depleting norepinephrine stores in adrenergic nerve endings. This reduces arteriolar vasoconstriction.

Route	Onset	Peak	Duration
PO	Unknown	8 hr	3-4 days

INDICATIONS & DOSAGE
Moderate to severe hypertension and renal hypertension (in outpatients)—
Adults: initially, 10 mg P.O. daily. Increase by 10 mg at weekly to monthly intervals p.r.n. Usual dosage is 25 to 50 mg daily. Some patients may require up to 300 mg daily.
Children: initially 0.2 mg/kg/day. Increase at 0.2-mg increments q 7 to 10 days. Maximum dosage is 3 mg/kg/24 hours.
Adjust-a-dose: In adult hospitalized patients, initially, 25 to 50 mg P.O. daily. Increase by 25 to 50 mg daily or every other day.

ADVERSE REACTIONS
CNS: *syncope, fatigue, headache, drowsiness, paresthesia, confusion.*
CV: *palpitations, chest pain, orthostatic hypotension, peripheral edema, bradycardia,* **heart failure.**
EENT: *visual disturbances,* glossitis.
GI: *diarrhea, indigestion, constipation, anorexia, nausea, vomiting.*
GU: *nocturia, urination frequency, ejaculation disturbances,* impotence.
Respiratory: shortness of breath, cough.
Other: *weight gain, aching limbs, leg cramps.*

INTERACTIONS
Drug-drug. *Amphetamines, ephedrine, MAO inhibitors, methylphenidate, norepi-*

nephrine, phenothiazines, tricyclic antidepressants: may inhibit guanethidine's antihypertensive effect. Adjust dose accordingly. Discontinue MAO inhibitor therapy 1 week before starting guanethidine.
Antihypertensives, diuretics, levodopa: may increase hypotensive effect of guanethidine. Use together cautiously.
Digoxin: may note increased slowing of heart rate. Monitor patient closely.
Reserpine: may cause excessive orthostatic hypotension, bradycardia, and depression. Use cautiously.
Drug-lifestyle. *Alcohol use:* may increase hypotensive effect of guanethidine. Use together cautiously.

EFFECTS ON DIAGNOSTIC TESTS
None reported.

CONTRAINDICATIONS
Contraindicated in patients with pheochromocytoma, frank heart failure, or hypersensitivity to drug and in those receiving MAO inhibitor therapy.

NURSING CONSIDERATIONS
• Use cautiously in patients with severe cardiac disease, recent MI, cerebrovascular disease, peptic ulceration, impaired renal function, or bronchial asthma and in those taking other antihypertensives.
• Monitor blood pressure for effects, especially after dosage adjustments.
• Elderly patients may be more sensitive to drug's hypotensive effects.
• Know that drug should be discontinued 2 to 3 weeks before elective surgery to reduce the possibility of vascular collapse and cardiac arrest during anesthesia.
• Know that if patient develops diarrhea, the doctor may prescribe atropine or paregoric.

☑ **Patient teaching**
• Inform patient that orthostatic hypotension can be minimized by rising slowly and avoiding sudden position changes. Dry mouth can be relieved with chewing gum, sour hard candy, or ice chips.
• Give patient instructions about a low-salt diet. Tell him to report possible weight gain and edema.
• Warn patient to avoid strenuous exercise

and hot showers; these may cause a hypotensive reaction. An ambient temperature that is too hot also may potentiate the hypotensive effects of guanethidine.
• Instruct patient to inform doctor of OTC medications being taken.

---

guanfacine hydrochloride
Tenex

Pregnancy Risk Category: B

HOW SUPPLIED
Tablets: 1 mg, 2 mg

ACTION
Unknown. Thought to be due to inhibition of the central vasomotor center, thereby decreasing sympathetic outflow to the heart, kidneys, and peripheral vasculature. This decreases blood pressure.

Route	Onset	Peak	Duration
PO	Unknown	1-4 hr	24 hr

INDICATIONS & DOSAGE
Hypertension—
Adults: initially, 1 mg P.O. daily h.s. Dosage may be increased to 2 mg P.O. h.s. after 3 to 4 weeks, p.r.n. Dosage may be further increased to 3 mg P.O. h.s. after an additional 3 to 4 weeks, p.r.n. Average dosage is 1 to 3 mg daily.

ADVERSE REACTIONS
CNS: *dizziness,* fatigue, headache, insomnia, *somnolence,* asthenia.
CV: bradycardia.
GI: *constipation,* diarrhea, nausea, *dry mouth.*
Skin: dermatitis, pruritus.

INTERACTIONS
Drug-drug. *CNS depressants:* may potentially increase sedation. Use together cautiously.
Tricyclic antidepressants: may inhibit antihypertensive effects. Avoid concurrent use.

EFFECTS ON DIAGNOSTIC TESTS
Drug alters urinary catecholamine concentrations and urinary vanillylmandelic

---

acid excretion (may be decreased during therapy but may increase on abrupt withdrawal). Plasma growth hormone levels may be increased after a single dose; chronic elevation does not follow long-term use.

CONTRAINDICATIONS
Contraindicated in patients with hypersensitivity to drug.

NURSING CONSIDERATIONS
• Use cautiously in patients with severe coronary insufficiency, recent MI, cerebrovascular disease, or chronic renal or hepatic insufficiency.
• Monitor blood pressure frequently.
• Be aware that the incidence and severity of adverse reactions increase with higher dosages.
• Know that guanfacine may be used alone or with a diuretic.

☑ **Patient teaching**
• Tell patient not to discontinue therapy abruptly. Rebound hypertension is less common than with similar drugs but may occur.
• Advise patient to avoid activities that require alertness until response to drug is established; drowsiness may occur.

---

hydralazine hydrochloride
Alphapress‡, Apresoline**,
Novo-Hylazin†, Suprest†

Pregnancy Risk Category: C

HOW SUPPLIED
Tablets: 10 mg, 25 mg, 50 mg, 100 mg
Injection: 20 mg/ml

ACTION
Unknown. A direct-acting vasodilator, its predominant effect relaxes arteriolar smooth muscle.

Route	Onset	Peak	Duration
PO	20-30 min	1-2 hr	2-4 hr
IV	5-20 min	10-80 min	2-6 hr
IM	10-30 min	1 hr	2-6 hr

INDICATIONS & DOSAGE
Essential hypertension (orally, alone, or in combination with other antihypertensives); severe essential hypertension (parenterally, to lower blood pressure quickly)—
Adults: *P.O.*—initially, 10 mg P.O. q.i.d.; gradually increased to 50 mg q.i.d. p.r.n. Maximum recommended dosage is 200 mg daily, but some patients may require 300 to 400 mg daily.
I.V.—10 to 20 mg given slowly and repeated as necessary, switching to oral antihypertensives as soon as possible.
I.M.—10 to 50 mg, repeated as necessary, switching to oral form as soon as possible.
Children: *P.O.*—initially, 0.75 mg/kg/day P.O. divided into four doses; gradually increased over 3 to 4 weeks to a maximum of 7.5 mg/kg or 200 mg daily. Maximum initial P.O. dose is 25 mg.
I.V.—0.1 to 0.2 mg/kg I.V. q 4 to 6 hours p.r.n. Maximum initial parenteral dose is 20 mg.

ADVERSE REACTIONS
CNS: peripheral neuritis, *headache, dizziness.*
CV: orthostatic hypotension, *tachycardia,* edema, *angina, palpitations.*
GI: *nausea, vomiting, diarrhea, anorexia,* constipation.
Hematologic: neutropenia, leukopenia, ***agranulocytopenia, agranulocytosis, thrombocytopenia*** with or without purpura; decreased hemoglobin and RBC count.
Skin: rash.
Other: *lupus-like syndrome* (especially with high doses), nasal congestion.

INTERACTIONS
Drug-drug. *Diazoxide, MAO inhibitors:* may cause severe hypotension. Use together cautiously.
Indomethacin: may decrease effects of hydralazine. Monitor blood pressure.

EFFECTS ON DIAGNOSTIC TESTS
Hydralazine may cause positive antinuclear antibody titer and positive lupus erythematosus cell preparation.

---

*Liquid contains alcohol. **May contain tartrazine. †Canada ‡Australia §U.K. ◊OTC

CONTRAINDICATIONS
Contraindicated in patients with coronary artery disease, mitral valvular rheumatic heart disease, or hypersensitivity to drug.

NURSING CONSIDERATIONS
• Use cautiously in patients with suspected cardiac disease, CVA, or severe renal impairment and in those taking other antihypertensives.
• Monitor patient's blood pressure, pulse rate, and body weight frequently. Some doctors combine hydralazine therapy with diuretics and beta-adrenergic blockers to decrease sodium retention and tachycardia and to prevent anginal attacks.
• Be aware that elderly patients may be more sensitive to drug's hypotensive effects.
• Monitor CBC, lupus erythematosus cell preparation, and antinuclear antibody titer determination before therapy and periodically during long-term therapy, as ordered.
Alert: Watch patient closely for signs of lupus-like syndrome (sore throat, fever, muscle and joint aches, and rash). Notify doctor immediately if these develop.
• Compliance may be improved by administering drug b.i.d. Check with doctor.

◖I.V. administration
• Give slowly and repeat as necessary, generally q 4 to 6 hours. Hydralazine will undergo color changes in most infusion solutions; these color changes do not indicate loss of potency. Compatible with 0.9% NaCl, Ringer's, and lactated Ringer's solutions, and several other common I.V. solutions. Drug may undergo a reaction with dextrose. The manufacturer does not recommend mixing drug in infusion solutions. Check with the pharmacist for additional compatibility information.

☑Patient teaching
• Instruct patient to take oral form with meals to increase absorption.
• Inform patient that orthostatic hypotension can be minimized by rising slowly and avoiding sudden position changes.
• Tell female patient to notify doctor if she suspects pregnancy; drug should be stopped.

irbesartan
Aprovel§, Avapro

Pregnancy Risk Category: C
(D in second and third trimesters)

HOW SUPPLIED
Tablets: 75 mg, 150 mg, 300 mg

ACTION
Produces antihypertensive effect by competitive antagonist activity at the angiotensin II receptor.

Route	Onset	Peak	Duration
PO	Unknown	1.5-2 hr	24 hr

INDICATIONS & DOSAGE
Hypertension–
Adults: initially 150 mg P.O. daily, increased to maximum of 300 mg daily if necessary.
Adjust-a-dose: In volume- and salt-depleted patients, initially 75 mg P.O. daily.

ADVERSE REACTIONS
CNS: fatigue, anxiety, dizziness, headache.
CV: chest pain, edema, tachycardia.
EENT: pharyngitis, rhinitis, sinus abnormality.
GI: diarrhea, dyspepsia, abdominal pain, nausea, vomiting.
GU: urinary tract infection.
Musculoskeletal: musculoskeletal trauma or pain.
Respiratory: upper respiratory infection.
Skin: rash.

INTERACTIONS
None reported.

EFFECTS ON DIAGNOSTIC TESTS
None reported.

CONTRAINDICATIONS
Contraindicated in patients with hypersensitivity to drug or its ingredients.

NURSING CONSIDERATIONS
• Use in pregnancy can cause injury and death to the developing fetus. When preg-

---

Reactions may be *common*, uncommon, *life-threatening*, or COMMON AND LIFE-THREATENING.

nancy is detected, discontinue drug as soon as possible.

• Use with caution in patients with impaired renal function, heart failure, and renal artery stenosis and in breast-feeding women.

• Drug may be administered with a diuretic or other antihypertensive if necessary for control of hypertension.

• Symptomatic hypotension may occur in volume- or salt-depleted patients (vigorous diuretic use or dialysis). The cause of volume depletion should be corrected prior to administration or a lower dose employed.

• If hypotension occurs, place patient in a supine position and give an I.V. infusion of 0.9% NaCl solution if needed. Once blood pressure has stabilized after a transient hypotensive episode, may continue drug without problems.

☑**Patient teaching**
• Warn female patient of childbearing age of consequences of drug exposure to fetus. Tell her to call doctor immediately if pregnancy is suspected.

• Tell patient that drug may be taken once daily with or without food.

---

isradipine
DynaCirc, Prescal§

Pregnancy Risk Category: C

HOW SUPPLIED
Capsules: 2.5 mg, 5 mg

ACTION
Unknown. A calcium channel blocker that inhibits calcium ion influx across cardiac and smooth-muscle cells and is thought to decrease arteriolar resistance and blood pressure.

Route	Onset	Peak	Duration
P.O.	2 hr	1.5 hr	12 hr

INDICATIONS & DOSAGE
Essential hypertension—
Adults: initially, 2.5 mg P.O. b.i.d., alone or with a thiazide diuretic. Dosage increased by gradual titration. If response is inadequate after first 2 to 4 weeks, dosage increased by 5-mg daily increments q 2 to 4 weeks to maximum of 20 mg daily.

ADVERSE REACTIONS
CNS: dizziness, *headache,* fatigue.
CV: edema, flushing, syncope, angina, tachycardia.
GI: nausea, diarrhea, abdominal discomfort, vomiting.
Respiratory: dyspnea.
Skin: rash.

INTERACTIONS
Drug-drug. *Cimetidine:* increases levels of isradipine. Monitor for increased effects.
Fentanyl anesthesia: severe hypotension has been reported with concomitant use of a beta blocker and a calcium channel blocker. Avoid concomitant use.
Rifampin: reduced isradipine effects. Monitor closely.

EFFECTS ON DIAGNOSTIC TESTS
None reported.

CONTRAINDICATIONS
Contraindicated in patients with hypersensitivity to drug.

NURSING CONSIDERATIONS
• Use cautiously in patients with heart failure, especially if combined with a beta blocker.

• Monitor patient for adverse reactions. Like other calcium channel blockers, isradipine is known to cause symptomatic hypotension. Most adverse reactions are mild and transient and related to vasodilation (dizziness, edema, flushing, palpitations, and tachycardia).

• Monitor blood pressure closely.

• Before surgery, inform the anesthesiologist that patient is taking a calcium channel blocker.

☑**Patient teaching**
• Tell patient that drug has some diuretic activity. He may note an increased need to void.

• Advise patient to avoid hazardous tasks if adverse CNS reactions occur.

---

labetalol hydrochloride
Normodyne, Presolol‡, Trandate

Pregnancy Risk Category: C

HOW SUPPLIED
Tablets: 100 mg, 200 mg, 300 mg
Injection: 5 mg/ml

ACTION
Unknown. May be related to reduced peripheral vascular resistance mainly as a result of beta-adrenergic blockade and also alpha blockade.

Route	Onset	Peak	Duration
PO	20 min	2-4 hr	8-12 hr
IV	2-5 min	5 min	2-4 hr

INDICATIONS & DOSAGE
Hypertension—
Adults: 100 mg P.O. b.i.d. with or without a diuretic. If needed, dosage is increased to 200 mg b.i.d. after 2 days. Further increases may be made q 2 to 3 days until optimum response is reached. Usual maintenance dosage is 200 to 400 mg b.i.d.
Severe hypertension and hypertensive emergencies—
Adults: 200 mg diluted in 160 ml of D$_5$W, infused at 2 mg/minute until satisfactory response is obtained; then infusion is stopped. May be repeated q 6 to 12 hours.
  Alternatively, administered by repeated I.V. injection: initially, 20 mg I.V. slowly over 2 minutes. Then repeat injections of 40 to 80 mg q 10 minutes until maximum dosage of 300 mg is reached, p.r.n.

ADVERSE REACTIONS
CNS: vivid dreams, fatigue, headache, paresthesia, syncope, transient scalp tingling.
CV: *orthostatic hypotension, dizziness,* **ventricular arrhythmias.**
EENT: nasal stuffiness.
GI: nausea, vomiting.
GU: sexual dysfunction, urine retention.
Respiratory: dyspnea, bronchospasm.
Skin: rash.

INTERACTIONS
Drug-drug. *Beta-adrenergic agonists:* may blunt bronchodilator effect of these drugs in patients with bronchospasm. Therefore, greater than normal doses of these agents may be required.
Cimetidine: may enhance labetalol's effect. Give together cautiously.
Halothane: additive hypotensive effect. Monitor blood pressure closely.
Insulin, oral antidiabetic agents: can alter dosage requirements in previously stabilized diabetic patients. Observe patient carefully.

EFFECTS ON DIAGNOSTIC TESTS
Labetalol therapy may cause a false-positive increase of urine free and total catecholamine levels when measured by a nonspecific trihydroxindole fluorometric method. Causes increases in serum transaminases and blood urea.

CONTRAINDICATIONS
Contraindicated in patients with bronchial asthma, overt cardiac failure, greater than first-degree heart block, cardiogenic shock, severe bradycardia, other conditions associated with severe and prolonged hypotension, and hypersensitivity to drug.

NURSING CONSIDERATIONS
• Use cautiously in patients with heart failure, hepatic failure, chronic bronchitis, emphysema, preexisting peripheral vascular disease, and pheochromocytoma.
• Monitor blood pressure frequently. Know that drug masks common signs of shock.
• If dizziness occurs, ask doctor if patient may take a dose at bedtime or take smaller doses t.i.d. to help minimize this adverse reaction.
• Monitor blood glucose levels in diabetic patients closely because beta blockers may mask certain signs and symptoms of hypoglycemia.

⬙ I.V. administration
• Administer labetalol injection with an infusion control device. Monitor blood pressure closely: every 5 minutes for 30 minutes, then every 30 minutes for 2

---

hours, then hourly for 6 hours. Patient should remain in a supine position for 3 hours after infusion.

• Be aware that when administered I.V. for hypertensive emergencies, labetalol produces a rapid, predictable fall in blood pressure within 5 to 10 minutes.

Alert: Be aware that sodium bicarbonate injection is incompatible with I.V. labetalol.

☑ **Patient teaching**
• Tell patient that abrupt discontinuation of therapy can exacerbate angina and precipitate MI.

• Advise patient that dizziness is the most troublesome adverse reaction and tends to occur in early stages of treatment, in patients also receiving diuretics, and in those receiving higher dosages. Inform patient that this can be minimized by rising slowly and avoiding sudden position changes.

• Warn patient that transient scalp tingling may occur, especially at beginning of therapy, but is harmless.

---

lisinopril
Carace§, Prinivil, Zestril

*Pregnancy Risk Category: C
(D in second and third trimesters)*

HOW SUPPLIED
Tablets: 2.5 mg, 5 mg, 10 mg, 20 mg, 40 mg

ACTION
Unknown. Thought to result primarily from suppression of the renin-angiotensin-aldosterone system.

Route	Onset	Peak	Duration
PO	1 hr	7 hr	24 hr

INDICATIONS & DOSAGE
Hypertension—
Adults: initially, 10 mg P.O. daily for patients not receiving a diuretic. Most patients are well controlled on 20 to 40 mg daily as a single dose.
Adjust-a-dose: In patients receiving a diuretic, 5 mg P.O. daily.

Treatment adjunct in heart failure (with diuretics and cardiac glycosides)—
Adults: initially, 5 mg P.O. daily; increased as warranted to maximum of 20 mg P.O. daily.
Adjust-a-dose: In patients with serum sodium less than 130 mEq/L or a creatinine clearance below 30 ml/minute, initiate dose at 2.5 mg daily.
Treatment of hemodynamically stable patients within 24 hours of acute MI to improve survival—
Adults: initially 5 mg P.O., followed by 5 mg after 24 hours, 10 mg after 48 hours, and then 10 mg once daily for 6 weeks.
Adjust-a-dose: In patients with low systolic blood pressure (120 mm Hg or less) when treatment is started or during the first 3 days after an infarct, dose should be decreased to 2.5 mg P.O. If hypotension occurs (systolic blood pressure 100 mm Hg or less), daily maintenance dose of 5 mg may be reduced to 2.5 mg if needed. If prolonged hypotension occurs (systolic blood pressure below 90 mm Hg for over 1 hour), drug should be withdrawn.

ADVERSE REACTIONS
CNS: *dizziness,* headache, fatigue, paresthesia.
CV: hypotension, *orthostatic hypotension,* chest pain.
EENT: *nasal congestion.*
GI: *diarrhea,* nausea, dyspepsia.
GU: impaired renal function, impotence, increased BUN and creatinine.
Hematologic: neutropenia, *agranulocytopenia.*
Hepatic: increased liver enzymes and serum bilirubin.
Respiratory: dry, persistent, tickling, nonproductive cough, dyspnea.
Skin: rash.
Other: *angioedema,* hyperkalemia.

INTERACTIONS
Drug-drug. *Allopurinol:* increased risk of hypersensitivity reaction. Use with caution.
Capsaicin: may increase risk of ACE inhibitor induced cough. Monitor patient.
Diuretics, thiazide diuretics: excessive

---

hypotension with diuretics. Monitor closely.

Indomethacin, phenothiazines: attenuated hypotensive effect. Monitor closely.

Insulin, oral antidiabetic agents: risk of hypoglycemia, especially at initiation of lisinopril therapy. Monitor closely.

Potassium-sparing diuretics, potassium supplements: possible hyperkalemia. Monitor closely.

Drug-food. *Potassium-containing salt substitutes:* possible hyperkalemia. Monitor closely.

EFFECTS ON DIAGNOSTIC TESTS
None reported.

CONTRAINDICATIONS
Contraindicated in patients with hypersensitivity to ACE inhibitors or history of angioedema related to previous treatment with ACE inhibitor.

NURSING CONSIDERATIONS
• Use cautiously in patients with impaired renal function; dosage adjustment is required. Also use cautiously in patients at risk for hyperkalemia.
• When used in acute MI, patient should receive, as appropriate, the standard recommended treatment, such as thrombolytics, aspirin, and beta blockers.
• Monitor blood pressure often. Know that if drug does not adequately control blood pressure, diuretics may be added.
• Monitor WBC with differential counts before therapy, every 2 weeks for first 3 months of therapy, and periodically thereafter.

☑ **Patient teaching**
Alert: Angioedema (including laryngeal edema) may occur, especially after first dose. Advise patient to report signs or symptoms, such as swelling of face, eyes, lips, or tongue or breathing difficulty.
• Inform patient that light-headedness can occur, especially during the first few days of therapy. Tell him to rise slowly to minimize this effect and to report symptoms to the doctor. Patients who experience syncope should stop taking drug and call the doctor immediately.
• Tell patient not to discontinue drug suddenly, but to call the doctor if unpleasant adverse reactions occur.
• Advise patient to report signs of infection, such as fever and sore throat.
• Tell female patient to notify doctor if pregnancy occurs. Drug will need to be discontinued.
• Instruct patient not to use salt substitutes that contain potassium without consulting doctor first.

losartan potassium
Cozaar

Pregnancy Risk Category: C
(D in second and third trimesters)

HOW SUPPLIED
Tablets: 25 mg, 50 mg

ACTION
An angiotensin II receptor antagonist that inhibits the vasoconstricting and aldosterone-secreting effects of angiotensin II by selectively blocking the binding of angiotensin II to its receptor sites that are found in many tissues, including vascular smooth muscle and adrenal glands.

Route	Onset	Peak	Duration
PO	Unknown	1 hr	Unknown

INDICATIONS & DOSAGE
Hypertension—
Adults: initially, 25 to 50 mg P.O. daily. Maximum daily dosage is 100 mg in one or two divided doses.
Adjust-a-dose: In patients with impaired hepatic function and in those who are intravascularly volume-depleted (such as those receiving diuretics), use lowest dosage (25 mg) initially.

ADVERSE REACTIONS
CNS: dizziness, insomnia.
GI: diarrhea, dyspepsia.
Musculoskeletal: muscle cramps, myalgia, back or leg pain.
Respiratory: nasal congestion, cough, upper respiratory tract infection, sinusitis.

INTERACTIONS
None significant.

Reactions may be *common*, uncommon, *life-threatening*, or COMMON AND LIFE-THREATENING.

EFFECTS ON DIAGNOSTIC TESTS
None reported.

CONTRAINDICATIONS
Contraindicated in patients with hypersensitivity to drug.

NURSING CONSIDERATIONS
• Know that breast-feeding is not recommended during losartan therapy.
• Use cautiously in patients with impaired renal or hepatic function.
• Know that drugs that act directly on the renin-angiotensin system (such as losartan) can cause fetal and neonatal morbidity and death when administered to pregnant women. These problems have not been detected when exposure has been limited to the first trimester. If pregnancy is suspected, notify doctor because drug should be discontinued.
• Be aware that losartan can be used alone or with other antihypertensives.
• Be aware that if the antihypertensive effect measured by the serum trough level of drug, using once-daily dosing, is inadequate, a twice-daily regimen using the same total daily dosage or an increase in dosage may give a more satisfactory response.
• Monitor patient's blood pressure closely to evaluate effectiveness of therapy. Know that when losartan is used alone, the effect on blood pressure is notably less in black patients than in patients of other races.
• Monitor patients who also are taking diuretics for symptomatic hypotension.
• Regularly assess the patient's renal function (via serum creatinine and BUN levels), as ordered.
• Be aware that patients with severe heart failure whose renal function depends on the angiotensin-aldosterone system have experienced acute renal failure during ACE inhibitor therapy. Manufacturer of losartan states that drug would be expected to do the same. Closely monitor patient, especially during the first few weeks of therapy.

☑ **Patient teaching**
• Tell patient to avoid salt substitutes; these products may contain potassium, which can cause hyperkalemia in patients taking losartan.
• Inform female patient of childbearing age about the consequences of second- and third-trimester exposure to losartan, and instruct her to notify doctor immediately if pregnancy is suspected.

methyldopa
Aldomet, Apo-Methyldopa†, Aldopren‡, Dopamet††, Hydopa‡, Novo-Medopa†, Nu-Medopa†

methyldopate hydrochloride
Aldomet

Pregnancy Risk Category: B (P.O.); C (I.V.)

HOW SUPPLIED
methyldopa
Tablets: 125 mg, 250 mg, 500 mg
Oral suspension: 250 mg/5 ml
methyldopate hydrochloride
Injection: 250 mg/5 ml

ACTION
Unknown. Thought to involve inhibition of the central vasomotor centers, thereby decreasing sympathetic outflow to the heart, kidneys, and peripheral vasculature.

Route	Onset	Peak	Duration
PO	Unknown	4-6 hr	12-48 hr
IV	Unknown	4-6 hr	10-16 hr

INDICATIONS & DOSAGE
Hypertension, hypertensive crisis—
Adults: *P.O.*—initially, 250 mg P.O. b.i.d. to t.i.d. in first 48 hours. Then increased p.r.n. q 2 days. May give entire daily dosage in the evening or h.s. Adjust dosages if other antihypertensives are added to or deleted from therapy. Maintenance dosage is 500 mg to 2 g daily in two to four divided doses. Maximum recommended daily dosage is 3 g.
I.V.—250 to 500 mg q 6 hours. Maximum dosage is 1 g q 6 hours. Switch to oral antihypertensives as soon as possible.
Children: initially, 10 mg/kg P.O. daily in two to four divided doses; or 20 to 40 mg/kg I.V. daily in four divided doses. In-

crease dose daily until desired response occurs. Maximum daily dosage is 65 mg/kg or 3 g, whichever is less.

ADVERSE REACTIONS
CNS: *sedation,* headache, weakness, dizziness, *decreased mental acuity,* paresthesia, parkinsonism, involuntary choreoathetoid movements, psychic disturbances, depression, nightmares.
CV: bradycardia, *orthostatic hypotension,* aggravated angina, *myocarditis, edema.*
EENT: *nasal congestion.*
GI: nausea, vomiting, diarrhea, pancreatitis, *dry mouth,* constipation.
Hematologic: *hemolytic anemia, thrombocytopenia,* leukopenia, bone marrow depression.
Hepatic: *hepatic necrosis,* abnormal liver function tests, hepatitis.
Skin: rash.
Other: arthralgia, gynecomastia, galactorrhea, drug-induced fever.

INTERACTIONS
Drug-drug. *Amphetamines, nonselective beta blockers, norepinephrine, phenothiazines, tricyclic antidepressants:* possible hypertensive effects. Monitor carefully.
Anesthetics: may require lower doses of anesthetics while on methyldopa therapy. Use together cautiously.
Barbiturates: may decrease actions of methyldopa. Monitor closely.
Haloperidol: adverse mental symptoms and increased sedation when used concomitantly with methyldopa. Use together cautiously.
Levodopa: additive hypotensive effects may increase adverse CNS reactions. Monitor closely.
Lithium: may increase lithium levels. Monitor for increased lithium levels.
Tolbutamide: Metabolism of tolbutamide may be impaired. Monitor for hypoglycemic effect.
Drug-herb. *Capsicum:* may reduce antihypertensive effectiveness. Avoid concomitant use.

EFFECTS ON DIAGNOSTIC TESTS
Drug alters urinary uric acid, serum creatinine, and AST levels; it may also cause falsely high levels of urinary catecholamines, interfering with the diagnosis of pheochromocytoma. A positive direct antiglobulin (Coombs') test may also occur.

CONTRAINDICATIONS
Contraindicated in patients with active hepatic disease (such as acute hepatitis), active cirrhosis, or hypersensitivity to drug. Also contraindicated if previous methyldopa therapy has been associated with liver disorders.

NURSING CONSIDERATIONS
• Use cautiously in patients with history of impaired hepatic function or sulfite sensitivity, and in breast-feeding patients.
• Monitor patient's blood pressure regularly. Be aware that elderly patients are more likely to experience hypotension and sedation.
• After dialysis, monitor patient for hypertension and notify doctor if necessary. Patient may need an extra dose of methyldopa.
• Monitor CBC with differential counts before therapy and periodically thereafter.
• Patients who require blood transfusions should have direct and indirect Coombs' tests to prevent crossmatching problems.
• Monitor patient's Coombs' test results. In patients who have received this drug for several months, positive reaction to direct Coombs' test indicates hemolytic anemia.
• Observe for and report involuntary choreoathetoid movements. The doctor may discontinue drug if this occurs.

⬛I.V. administration
• Dilute appropriate dose in 100 ml D_5W and infuse slowly over 30 to 60 minutes.

✅Patient teaching
• Tell patient not to suddenly stop taking drug, but to notify doctor if unpleasant adverse reactions occur.
• Instruct patient to report signs of infection.
• Tell patient to check his weight daily and to notify doctor of weight gain over 2 kg (5 lb). Sodium and water retention may occur but can be relieved with diuretics.

Reactions may be *common,* uncommon, ***life-threatening,*** or **COMMON AND LIFE-THREATENING.**

- Warn patient that drug may impair ability to perform tasks that require mental alertness, particularly at start of therapy. A once-daily dosage at bedtime will minimize daytime drowsiness.
- Inform patient that orthostatic hypotension can be minimized by rising slowly and avoiding sudden position changes. Dry mouth can be relieved with chewing gum, sour hard candy, or ice chips.
- Tell patient that urine may turn dark if left standing in toilet bowls or in toilet bowls treated with bleach.

---

metoprolol succinate
Toprol XL

metoprolol tartrate
Apo-Metoprolol†, Apo-Metoprolol (Type L)†, Betaloc†‡, Betaloc Durules†, Lopresor†, Lopresor SR†, Lopressor, Minax‡, Novo-Metoprol†, Nu-Metop†

Pregnancy Risk Category: C

HOW SUPPLIED
metoprolol succinate
Tablets (extended-release): 50 mg, 100 mg, 200 mg
metoprolol tartrate
Tablets: 50 mg, 100 mg
Tablets (extended-release): 100 mg†, 200 mg†
Injection: 1 mg/ml in 5-ml ampules

ACTION
Unknown for antihypertensive action. A beta$_1$-selective blocking agent that decreases myocardial contractility, heart rate, cardiac output, and blood pressure and reduces myocardial oxygen use. Also depresses renin secretion.

Route	Onset	Peak	Duration
PO	15 min	1 hr	6-12 hr
PO (extended)	15 min	6-12 hr	24 hr
IV	5 min	20 min	5-8 hr

INDICATIONS & DOSAGE
Hypertension—
Adults: initially, 50 mg P.O. b.i.d. or 100 mg P.O. once daily, then up to 100 to 450 mg daily in two or three divided doses. Alternatively, 50 to 100 mg of extended-release tablets (tartrate equivalent) once daily. Dosage is adjusted as needed and tolerated at intervals of not less than 1 week to maximum of 400 mg daily.
Early intervention in acute MI (metoprolol tartrate)—
Adults: three 5-mg I.V. boluses q 2 minutes. Then, beginning 15 minutes after last dose, 25 to 50 mg P.O. q 6 hours for 48 hours. Maintenance dosage is 100 mg P.O. b.i.d. for 3 months to 3 years.
Angina pectoris—
Adults: initially, 100 mg P.O. daily as a single dose or in two equally divided doses; increased at weekly intervals until an adequate response or a pronounced decrease in heart rate is seen. Daily dosage beyond 400 mg has not been studied. Alternatively, give 100 mg of extended-release tablets (tartrate equivalent) once daily. Dosage adjusted as needed and tolerated at intervals of not less than 1 week to maximum of 400 mg daily.

ADVERSE REACTIONS
CNS: *fatigue, dizziness,* depression.
CV: *bradycardia,* hypotension, ***heart failure, AV block.***
GI: nausea, diarrhea.
Hepatic: elevated serum transaminase, alkaline phosphatase
Respiratory: dyspnea, ***bronchospasm.***
Skin: rash.
Other: elevated LD and uric acid levels.

INTERACTIONS
Drug-drug. *Barbiturates, rifampin:* increased metabolism of metoprolol. Monitor for decreased effect.
Cardiac glycosides, diltiazem, verapamil: excessive bradycardia and increased depressant effect on myocardium. Use together cautiously.
Catecholamine-depleting drugs (such as reserpine), H$_2$ antagonists, MAO inhibitors: may have additive effect when given with beta blockers. Monitor for hypotension and bradycardia.
Chlorpromazine, cimetidine, verapamil: decreased hepatic clearance. Monitor for greater beta-blocking effect.

---

*Liquid contains alcohol.   **May contain tartrazine.   †Canada   ‡Australia   §U.K.   ◇OTC

Indomethacin: decreased antihypertensive effect. Monitor blood pressure and adjust dosage.

Insulin, oral antidiabetic agents: can alter dosage requirements in previously stabilized diabetic patients. Observe patient carefully.

Propafenone: may increase metoprolol serum levels. Monitor vital signs.

Terbutaline: may antagonize the bronchodilatory effects of terbutaline. Monitor patient.

Drug-food. *Any food:* may increase absorption. Give drug with food.

EFFECTS ON DIAGNOSTIC TESTS
None reported.

CONTRAINDICATIONS
Contraindicated in patients with hypersensitivity to drug or other beta blockers. Also contraindicated in patients with sinus bradycardia, heart block greater than first-degree, cardiogenic shock, or overt cardiac failure when used to treat hypertension or angina. When used to treat MI, drug is contraindicated in patients with heart rate less than 45 beats/minute, second- or third-degree heart block, PR interval of 0.24 seconds or longer with first-degree heart block, systolic blood pressure less than 100 mm Hg, or moderate to severe cardiac failure.

NURSING CONSIDERATIONS
• Use cautiously in patients with heart failure, diabetes, or respiratory or hepatic disease.
• Always check patient's apical pulse rate before giving drug. If it's slower than 60 beats/minute, withhold drug and call the doctor immediately.
• Monitor blood glucose levels closely in diabetic patients because drug masks common signs of hypoglycemia.
• Monitor blood pressure frequently. Know that metoprolol masks common signs of shock.
• Store drug at room temperature and protect from light. Discard solution if it's discolored or contains particles.

I.V. administration
• Give undiluted by direct injection. Although mixing with other drugs should be avoided, studies have shown that metoprolol is compatible when mixed with meperidine hydrochloride or morphine sulfate or when administered with alteplase infusion at a Y-site connection.

✓ Patient teaching
• Instruct patient to take drug exactly as prescribed and to take it with meals.
• Tell patient not to stop drug suddenly but to notify doctor about unpleasant adverse reactions. Inform him that drug must be withdrawn gradually over 1 to 2 weeks.

---

minoxidil
Loniten

Pregnancy Risk Category: C

HOW SUPPLIED
Tablets: 2.5 mg, 10 mg

ACTION
Unknown. Predominant effect produces direct arteriolar vasodilation.

Route	Onset	Peak	Duration
PO	0.5 hr	2-3 hr	2-5 days

INDICATIONS & DOSAGE
Severe hypertension—
Adults: initially, 5 mg P.O. as a single dose. Effective dosage range is usually 10 to 40 mg daily. Maximum dosage is 100 mg daily.
Children under 12 years: 0.2 mg/kg P.O. (maximum 5 mg) as a single daily dose. Effective dosage range usually is 0.25 to 1 mg/kg daily. Maximum dosage is 50 mg.

ADVERSE REACTIONS
CV: *edema, tachycardia, pericardial effusion and tamponade,* **heart failure,** ECG changes, rebound hypertension.
GI: nausea, vomiting.
GU: elevated BUN and serum creatinine levels.
Hematologic: transiently decreased hemoglobin and hematocrit levels.

Reactions may be *common,* uncommon, *life-threatening,* or COMMON AND LIFE-THREATENING.

Hepatic: elevated serum alkaline phosphatase.
Skin: rash, *Stevens-Johnson syndrome.*
Other: *hypertrichosis* (elongation, thickening, and enhanced pigmentation of fine body hair), breast tenderness, weight gain.

INTERACTIONS
Drug-drug. *Guanethidine:* severe orthostatic hypotension. Advise patient to stand up slowly.

EFFECTS ON DIAGNOSTIC TESTS
Minoxidil may also alter direction and magnitude of T waves on ECG and elevate antinuclear antibody titers.

CONTRAINDICATIONS
Contraindicated in patients with pheochromocytoma or hypersensitivity to drug.

NURSING CONSIDERATIONS
• Use cautiously in those with impaired renal function and after acute MI.
• Closely monitor blood pressure and pulse at beginning of therapy.
• Know that elderly patients may be more sensitive to drug's hypotensive effects.
• Drug is removed by hemodialysis. Be sure to administer dose after dialysis.
• Monitor fluid intake and urine output. Check for weight gain and edema.

☑ **Patient teaching**
• Make sure patient receives and reads the manufacturer's package insert that describes in layman's terms the drug and its adverse reactions. Also provide an oral explanation.
• Tell patient not to suddenly stop taking drug, but to call doctor if unpleasant adverse effects occur.
• Make sure patient understands the importance of compliance with total treatment regimen. Minoxidil usually is prescribed with a beta blocker to control tachycardia and a diuretic to counteract fluid retention.
• Teach patient how to take his own pulse and to notify doctor of increases over 20 beats/minute.
• Tell patient to weigh himself at least

weekly and to report weight gain of over 2 kg (5 lb).
• About 8 of 10 patients will experience hypertrichosis within 3 to 6 weeks of beginning treatment. Unwanted hair can be controlled with a depilatory or shaving. Assure patient that extra hair will disappear within 1 to 6 months of stopping minoxidil. Advise patient, however, not to discontinue drug without doctor's approval.

---

moexipril hydrochloride
Perdix§, Univasc

Pregnancy Risk Category: C
(D in second and third trimesters)

HOW SUPPLIED
Tablets: 7.5 mg, 15 mg

ACTION
Unknown. Thought to result primarily from suppression of renin-angiotensin-aldosterone system.

Route	Onset	Peak	Duration
PO	1 hr	1.5 hr	24 hr

INDICATIONS & DOSAGE
Hypertension—
Adults: initially, 7.5 mg (3.75 mg if patient is receiving a diuretic) P.O. once daily 1 hour before meal. If control is inadequate, dose may be increased or divided. Recommended maintenance dosage is 7.5 mg to 30 mg daily, in one or two divided doses 1 hour before meal. Subsequent dosage depends on response.
Adjust-a-dose: In renally impaired patients with creatinine clearance less than 40 ml/minute, initial dose is 3.75 mg/day and titrate to maximum of 15 mg/day.

ADVERSE REACTIONS
CNS: dizziness, headache, fatigue.
CV: peripheral edema, hypotension, orthostatic hypotension, chest pain, flushing.
EENT: pharyngitis, rhinitis, sinusitis.
GI: diarrhea, dyspepsia, nausea.
GU: urinary frequency.
Hematologic: neutropenia.

Respiratory: persistent nonproductive cough, upper respiratory infection.
Skin: rash.
Other: myalgia, *anaphylactoid reactions, angioedema,* hyperkalemia, flu syndrome, pain.

INTERACTIONS
Drug-drug. *Diuretics:* risk of excessive hypotension. Expect diuretic to be discontinued or moexipril dose lowered.
Lithium: increased serum lithium level and lithium toxicity. Use together cautiously and monitor serum lithium levels frequently.
Potassium-sparing diuretics, potassium supplements: risk of hyperkalemia. Monitor serum potassium level closely.
Drug-food. *Salt substitutes containing potassium:* risk of hyperkalemia. Monitor serum potassium level closely.

EFFECTS ON DIAGNOSTIC TESTS
Drug may cause minor elevations in creatinine and BUN levels. Elevations of liver enzymes and uric acid may also occur.

CONTRAINDICATIONS
Contraindicated in patients with hypersensitivity to drug or history of angioedema related to treatment with ACE inhibitor.

NURSING CONSIDERATIONS
• Know that safety of drug is not established in children.
• Use cautiously in patients with impaired renal function, heart failure, or renal artery stenosis and in breast-feeding women.
• Monitor for excessive hypotension.
• Measure blood pressure at trough (just before dose) to verify blood pressure control.
• Assess renal function before and during therapy. Monitor serum potassium level, as ordered.
• Know that other ACE inhibitors have been associated with agranulocytosis and neutropenia. Monitor CBC with differential before therapy, especially in patients who have collagen-vascular disease with impaired renal function.
• Because angioedema associated with

the tongue, glottis, or larynx can cause a fatal airway obstruction, be prepared with appropriate therapy, such as S.C. epinephrine 1:1,000 (0.3 to 0.5 ml), and equipment to ensure a patent airway.

☑ **Patient teaching**
• Tell patient to take drug on an empty stomach at least 1 hour before a meal to avoid impaired absorption.
• Advise patient to avoid salt substitutes with potassium, which can cause hyperkalemia in patients taking drug.
• Tell patient to use caution in hot weather and during exercise. Inadequate fluid intake, vomiting, diarrhea, and excessive perspiration can lead to light-headedness and syncope.
• Urge patient to rise slowly to minimize light-headedness. Tell him to stop taking drug and to notify doctor immediately if syncope occurs.
• Advise patient to report fever; sore throat; easy bruising or bleeding; swelling of tongue, lips, face, eyes, mucous membranes, or extremities; difficulty swallowing or breathing; or hoarseness.
• Tell female patient to notify doctor if pregnancy occurs. Drug must be discontinued.

---

nisoldipine
Sular, Syscor MR§

Pregnancy Risk Category: C

HOW SUPPLIED
Tablets (extended-release): 10 mg, 20 mg, 30 mg, 40 mg

ACTION
Prevents calcium ions from entering vascular smooth-muscle cells, thereby causing dilation of arterioles, which in turn decreases peripheral vascular resistance.

Route	Onset	Peak	Duration
PO	Unknown	6-12 hr	24 hr

INDICATIONS & DOSAGE
Hypertension—
Adults: initially, 20 mg P.O. once daily; increased by 10 mg/week or at longer in-

tervals, p.r.n. Usual maintenance dosage is 20 to 40 mg/day. Dosages over 60 mg/day are not recommended.
Elderly: initially, 10 mg P.O. once daily; dosage is adjusted as for adults.
Adjust-a-dose: In patients with impaired liver function, initially 10 mg P.O. once daily; dosage is adjusted as for adults.

ADVERSE REACTIONS
CNS: *headache,* dizziness.
CV: vasodilation, palpitation, chest pain.
EENT: sinusitis.
GI: nausea.
Respiratory: pharyngitis.
Skin: rash.
Other: *peripheral edema.*

INTERACTIONS
Drug-drug. *Cimetidine:* increased bioavailability and peak concentration of nisoldipine. Monitor blood pressure closely.
Quinidine: decreased bioavailability of nisoldipine. Adjust dosage accordingly.
Drug-food. *Grapefruit juice:* increased bioavailability and concentration of drug. Monitor blood pressure closely.
High-fat meal: increased peak drug concentration. Monitor blood pressure closely.

EFFECTS ON DIAGNOSTIC TESTS
None reported.

CONTRAINDICATIONS
Contraindicated in patients with hypersensitivity to dihydropyridine calcium channel blockers.

NURSING CONSIDERATIONS
• Use cautiously in patients with heart failure or compromised ventricular function, particularly in those receiving beta blockers and in patients with severe hepatic dysfunction.
• Know that drug should not be used in breast-feeding women.
• Monitor patient carefully. Some patients, especially those with severe obstructive coronary artery disease, have developed increased frequency, duration, or severity of angina or even acute MI after starting calcium channel blocker therapy or at time of dosage increase.

• Monitor blood pressure regularly, especially during the initial administration and titration of drug.

☑ **Patient teaching**
• Tell patient to take drug as prescribed, even if he feels better.
• Advise patient to swallow tablet whole and not to chew, divide, or crush it.
• Remind patient not to take drug with a high-fat meal or with grapefruit products. Both may increase the amount of drug in the body over the intended amount.

---

nitroprusside sodium
Nipride†, Nitropress

Pregnancy Risk Category: C

HOW SUPPLIED
Injection: 50 mg/vial in 2-ml, 5-ml vials

ACTION
Relaxes both arteriolar and venous smooth muscle.

Route	Onset	Peak	Duration
IV	1-2 min	Immediate	10 min

INDICATIONS & DOSAGE
To lower blood pressure quickly in hypertensive emergencies; to produce controlled hypotension during anesthesia; to reduce preload and afterload in cardiac pump failure or cardiogenic shock (may be used with or without dopamine)—
Adults: 50 mg vial diluted with 2 to 3 ml of D_5W and then added to 250, 500, or 1,000 ml of D_5W; infused at 0.3 to 10 mcg/kg/minute. Average dose is 3 mcg/kg/minute. Maximum infusion rate is 10 mcg/kg/minute.
Adjust-a-dose: Patients taking other antihypertensives together with nitroprusside are extremely sensitive to nitroprusside. Adjust dosage accordingly. Use with caution in patients with renal failure; reduce dose as much as possible.

ADVERSE REACTIONS
CNS: *headache, dizziness,* loss of consciousness, apprehension, ***increased in-***

tracranial pressure, restlessness, muscle twitching, diaphoresis.
CV: bradycardia, hypotension, tachycardia, palpitations, ECG changes.
GI: *nausea, abdominal pain,* ileus.
GU: increased serum creatinine.
Skin: pink color, flushing, rash.
Other: acidosis, *thiocyanate toxicity, methemoglobinemia, cyanide toxicity,* venous streaking, irritation at infusion site, hypothyroidism.

INTERACTIONS
Drug-drug. *Antihypertensives:* may cause sensitivity to nitroprusside. Adjust dosage as ordered.
Ganglionic blocking agents, general anesthetics, negative inotropic agents, other antihypertensives: additive effects. Monitor blood pressure closely.

EFFECTS ON DIAGNOSTIC TESTS
None reported.

CONTRAINDICATIONS
Contraindicated in patients with compensatory hypertension (such as in arteriovenous shunt or coarctation of the aorta), inadequate cerebral circulation, acute heart failure associated with reduced peripheral vascular resistance, congenital optic atrophy, tobacco-induced amblyopia, or hypersensitivity to drug.

NURSING CONSIDERATIONS
• Use with extreme caution in patients with increased intracranial pressure. Use cautiously in patients with hypothyroidism, hepatic or renal disease, hyponatremia, or low vitamin B_{12} concentration.
• Obtain baseline vital signs before giving drug, and find out what parameters the doctor wants to achieve.
• Keep patient in the supine position when initiating or titrating nitroprusside therapy.

I.V. administration
• Don't use bacteriostatic water for injection or sterile NaCl solution for reconstitution.
• Because drug is sensitive to light, wrap I.V. solution in foil; it's not necessary to wrap the tubing. Fresh solution should

have faint brownish tint. Discard after 24 hours.
• Infuse with an infusion pump. Drug is best given via piggyback through a peripheral line with no other medication. Don't adjust rate of main I.V. line while drug is being infused. Even a small bolus of nitroprusside can cause severe hypotension.
• Check blood pressure every 5 minutes at start of infusion and every 15 minutes thereafter. If severe hypotension occurs, discontinue nitroprusside infusion—effects of drug quickly reverse. Notify doctor. If possible, start an arterial pressure line. Regulate drug flow to specified level.
Alert: Excessive doses or rapid infusion greater than 10 mcg/kg/minute can cause cyanide toxicity; therefore, if these factors are present check serum thiocyanate levels q 72 hours. Levels above 100 mcg/ml are associated with toxicity. Watch for profound hypotension, metabolic acidosis, dyspnea, headache, loss of consciousness, ataxia, and vomiting. If these occur, discontinue drug immediately and notify doctor.

Patient teaching
• Instruct patient to report adverse reactions promptly.
• Tell patient to alert nurse if discomfort occurs at I.V. insertion site.

---

penbutolol sulfate
Levatol

Pregnancy Risk Category: C

HOW SUPPLIED
Tablets: 20 mg

ACTION
Unknown.

Route	Onset	Peak	Duration
PO	1 hr	1.5-3 hr	24 hr

INDICATIONS & DOSAGE
Mild to moderate hypertension—
Adults: 20 mg P.O. once daily. Usually given with other antihypertensives, such

as thiazide diuretics. Maximum 80 mg/
day.

ADVERSE REACTIONS
CNS: *dizziness,* headache, fatigue, in-
somnia, asthenia.
CV: chest pain, ***heart failure.***
GI: nausea, diarrhea, dyspepsia.
GU: impotence.
Respiratory: cough, dyspnea, upper res-
piratory infection.
Skin: excessive diaphoresis.

INTERACTIONS
Drug-drug. *Clonidine:* may cause paradoxical hypertension. Also, beta blockers
may enhance rebound hypertension when
clonidine is withdrawn.
Digoxin, diltiazem, verapamil: may produce additive depressant effects on AV
node conduction. Monitor closely.
Insulin, oral antidiabetic agents: hypoglycemic response to these drugs may be
altered. Monitor patient closely.
Lidocaine: volume of distribution affected. May need higher loading doses of lidocaine.
NSAIDs: may decrease antihypertensive
effects. Monitor closely.
Prazosin, terazosin: "first-dose" orthostatic hypotension seen with these drugs may
be enhanced. Use together cautiously.
*Sympathomimetics, including dobuta-
mine, dopamine, isoproterenol, norepinephrine:* decreased hypotensive response. Monitor closely.
Theophylline: may decrease bronchodilator effect. Monitor patient closely.

EFFECTS ON DIAGNOSTIC TESTS
Drug may interfere with glucose or insulin tolerance tests.

CONTRAINDICATIONS
Contraindicated in patients with sinus
bradycardia, cardiogenic shock, overt cardiac failure, greater than first-degree
heart block, bronchial asthma, and hypersensitivity to drug or other beta blockers.

NURSING CONSIDERATIONS
• Use cautiously in patients with heart
failure controlled by drug therapy and in
those with a history of bronchospastic

disease. Also use cautiously in diabetic
patients because beta-adrenergic blockers
may mask certain signs and symptoms of
hypoglycemia.
• Always check patient's apical pulse before giving drug. If you detect extremes in
pulse rates, withhold drug and call doctor
immediately.
• Monitor blood pressure, ECG, and heart
rate and rhythm frequently.

☑**Patient teaching**
• Instruct patient to take drug exactly as
prescribed.
• Tell patient not to stop drug suddenly
but to notify doctor about unpleasant adverse reactions.
• Teach patient the signs and symptoms of
heart failure (edema and pulmonary congestion). Advise him to notify doctor if
these occur.

phentolamine mesylate
Regitine, Rogitine†

Pregnancy Risk Category: C

HOW SUPPLIED
Injection: 5 mg/ml in 1-ml vials,
10 mg/ml‡

ACTION
An alpha-adrenergic blocker that competitively blocks the effects of catecholamines on alpha-adrenergic receptors.

Route	Onset	Peak	Duration
IV, IM	Unknown	Unknown	Unknown

INDICATIONS & DOSAGE
*To aid in diagnosis of pheochromocy-
toma; to control or prevent hypertension
before or during pheochromocytomec-
tomy—*
Adults: I.V. diagnostic dose is 2.5 mg
with close monitoring of blood pressure.
Before surgical removal of tumor, 5 mg
I.M. or I.V. During surgery, patient may
need 5 mg I.V.
Children: I.V. diagnostic dose is 1 mg
with close monitoring of blood pressure.
Before surgical removal of tumor, 1 mg

I.V. or I.M. During surgery, patient may need 1 mg I.V.

Dermal necrosis and sloughing after I.V. extravasation of norepinephrine—
Adults and children: infiltrate area with 5 to 10 mg phentolamine in 10 ml of 0.9% NaCl solution, or give half the dosage through the infiltrated I.V. and the other half around the site. Must be done within 12 hours.

ADVERSE REACTIONS
CNS: *dizziness, weakness, flushing,* **cerebrovascular occlusion,** cerebrovascular spasm.
CV: *hypotension,* **shock,** *arrhythmias, tachycardia,* **MI.**
EENT: *nasal congestion.*
GI: *diarrhea, nausea, vomiting.*

INTERACTIONS
Drug-drug. *Ephedrine, epinephrine:* excessive hypotension. Don't use together.

EFFECTS ON DIAGNOSTIC TESTS
None reported.

CONTRAINDICATIONS
Contraindicated in patients with angina, coronary artery disease, MI or history of MI, or hypersensitivity to drug.

NURSING CONSIDERATIONS
• Use cautiously in patients with gastritis or peptic ulcer.
• When drug is given as a diagnostic test for pheochromocytoma, take the patient's blood pressure first; also monitor blood pressure frequently during administration.
Alert: Don't administer epinephrine to treat phentolamine-induced hypotension because it may cause additional fall in blood pressure ("epinephrine reversal"). Use norepinephrine instead, as ordered.

🔲 I.V. administration
• For pheochromocytoma diagnosis, inject drug rapidly. Test is positive if severe hypotension results.

☑ Patient teaching
• Explain use and administration of drug.
• Tell patient to report adverse reactions promptly.

pindolol
Apo-Pindol†, Barbloc‡, Novo-Pindol†, Syn-Pindolol†, Visken

Pregnancy Risk Category: B

HOW SUPPLIED
Tablets: 5 mg, 10 mg, 15 mg‡

ACTION
Unknown. A nonselective beta-adrenergic blocker that has intrinsic sympathomimetic activity. Possible mechanisms include reduced cardiac output, decreased sympathetic outflow to peripheral vasculature, and inhibition of renin release by the kidneys.

Route	Onset	Peak	Duration
PO	Unknown	1-2 hr	24 hr

INDICATIONS & DOSAGE
Hypertension—
Adults: initially, 5 mg P.O. b.i.d. Dosage increased as needed and tolerated to maximum of 60 mg daily.

ADVERSE REACTIONS
CNS: *insomnia, fatigue, dizziness, nervousness,* vivid dreams, weakness, paresthesia.
CV: *edema,* bradycardia, **heart failure,** chest pain.
GI: *nausea,* abdominal discomfort.
Respiratory: *increased airway resistance,* dyspnea.
Skin: rash, pruritus.
Other: *muscle pain, joint pain.*

INTERACTIONS
Drug-drug. *Cardiac glycosides, diltiazem, verapamil:* excessive bradycardia and additive depression of AV node. Use together cautiously.
Catecholamine-depleting drugs (such as reserpine): may have additive effects. Monitor for hypotension and bradycardia.
Epinephrine: severe vasoconstriction. Monitor blood pressure and observe patient carefully.
Indomethacin: decreased antihypertensive

effect. Monitor blood pressure and adjust dosage.

Insulin, oral antidiabetic agents: can alter requirements for these drugs in previously stabilized diabetic patients. Monitor patient for hypoglycemia.

EFFECTS ON DIAGNOSTIC TESTS
Pindolol may elevate serum transaminase, alkaline phosphatase, LD, and uric acid levels.

CONTRAINDICATIONS
Contraindicated in patients with bronchial asthma, severe bradycardia, heart block greater than first degree, cardiogenic shock, overt cardiac failure, or hypersensitivity to drug.

NURSING CONSIDERATIONS
• Use cautiously in patients with heart failure, nonallergic bronchospastic disease, diabetes, hyperthyroidism, and impaired renal or hepatic function.
• Always check patient's apical pulse rate before giving drug. If you detect extremes in pulse rates, withhold medication and call doctor immediately.
• Monitor blood pressure frequently and notify the doctor if severe hypotension occurs. A vasopressor may be required.
• Withdraw drug over 1 to 2 weeks after long-term therapy, as ordered.
• Monitor blood glucose levels in diabetic patients closely because drug masks certain signs and symptoms of hypoglycemia.

✅ Patient teaching
• Tell patient to take drug exactly as prescribed.
• Tell patient not to stop drug suddenly but to call doctor to discuss unpleasant adverse drug reactions.

---

prazosin hydrochloride
Hypovase§, Minipress

Pregnancy Risk Category: C

HOW SUPPLIED
Capsules: 1 mg, 2 mg, 5 mg

ACTION
Unknown. Its alpha-adrenergic blocking activity is thought to account primarily for its effects.

Route	Onset	Peak	Duration
PO	0.5-1.5 hr	2-4 hr	7-10 hr

INDICATIONS & DOSAGE
Mild to moderate hypertension, alone or in combination with a diuretic or other antihypertensive—
Adults: oral test dose is 1 mg h.s. to prevent "first-dose syncope." Initial dose is 1 mg P.O. b.i.d. or t.i.d. Dosage increased slowly. Maximum daily dosage is 20 mg. Maintenance dosage is 6 to 15 mg daily in three divided doses. Some patients need dosages larger than this (up to 40 mg daily). If other antihypertensives or diuretics are added to this drug, prazosin is decreased to 1 to 2 mg t.i.d. and retitrated.

ADVERSE REACTIONS
CNS: *dizziness,* headache, drowsiness, nervousness, paresthesia, weakness, *"first-dose syncope,"* depression.
CV: orthostatic hypotension, *palpitations.*
EENT: blurred vision, tinnitus, conjunctivitis.
GI: vomiting, diarrhea, abdominal cramps, *nausea,* elevated serum uric acid and BUN levels.
GU: priapism, impotence, urinary frequency, incontinence.
Hematologic: *leukopenia* (transient).
Respiratory: dyspnea, nasal congestion, epistaxis.
Other: arthralgia, myalgia, pruritus, edema, fever.

INTERACTIONS
Drug-drug. *Propranolol, other beta blockers:* increased frequency of syncope with loss of consciousness. Advise patient to sit or lie down if dizziness occurs.
Verapamil: increased serum prazosin levels. Monitor closely.
Drug-herb. *Butcher's broom:* possible diminished effect. Avoid concomitant use.

EFFECTS ON DIAGNOSTIC TESTS
Drug alters results of screening tests for pheochromocytoma and causes increases

---

in levels of the urinary metabolite of nor-epinephrine and vanillylmandelic acid; it may cause positive antinuclear antibody titer and liver function test abnormalities.

CONTRAINDICATIONS
Contraindicated in patients hypersensitive to drug or other alpha$_1$ blockers.

NURSING CONSIDERATIONS
• Use cautiously in patients receiving other antihypertensives.
• Monitor patient's blood pressure and pulse rate frequently.
• Know that elderly patients may be more sensitive to drug's hypotensive effects.
• Compliance *might* be improved with twice-daily dosing. Suggest this dosing change with doctor if you suspect compliance problems.
Alert: Be aware that if initial dose is greater than 1 mg, severe syncope with loss of consciousness may occur ("first-dose syncope").

☑ **Patient teaching**
• Warn patient that dizziness may occur with first dose. If he experiences dizziness, tell him to sit or lie down. Reassure him that this effect disappears with continued dosing.
• Tell patient not to suddenly stop taking drug but to call doctor if unpleasant adverse reactions occur.
• Advise patient to minimize orthostatic hypotension by rising slowly and avoiding sudden position changes. Dry mouth can be relieved with chewing gum, sour hard candy, or ice chips.

---

quinapril hydrochloride
Accupril, Accupro§, Asig‡

*Pregnancy Risk Category: C
(D in second and third trimesters)*

HOW SUPPLIED
Tablets: 5 mg, 10 mg, 20 mg, 40 mg

ACTION
Unknown, but thought to be related to inhibition of angiotensin I to angiotensin II, a potent vasoconstrictor. Reduced formation of angiotensin II decreases peripheral arterial resistance, thus decreasing aldosterone secretion.

Route	Onset	Peak	Duration
PO	1 hr	2-6 hr	24 hr

INDICATIONS & DOSAGE
Hypertension—
Adults: initially, 10 mg P.O. daily. Dosage adjusted based on patient response at intervals of about 2 weeks. Most patients are controlled at 20, 40, or 80 mg daily as a single dose or in two divided doses. If patient is taking a diuretic, initiate therapy with 5 mg daily.
Heart failure—
Adults: initially, 5 mg P.O. b.i.d. if patient is receiving a diuretic and 10 to 20 mg P.O. b.i.d. if patient is not receiving a diuretic. Dosage increased at weekly intervals. Usual effective dose is 20 to 40 mg b.i.d. in equally divided doses.
Adjust-a-dose: In renally impaired patients, use a lower initial dose.

ADVERSE REACTIONS
CNS: somnolence, vertigo, nervousness, headache, dizziness, fatigue, depression.
CV: palpitations, tachycardia, angina, hypertensive crisis, orthostatic hypotension, rhythm disturbances.
GI: dry mouth, abdominal pain, constipation, vomiting, nausea, hemorrhage.
Hepatic: elevated liver enzymes.
Respiratory: *dry, persistent, tickling, nonproductive cough.*
Skin: pruritus, *exfoliative dermatitis,* photosensitivity, diaphoresis.
Other: *angioedema,* hyperkalemia.

INTERACTIONS
Drug-drug. *Diuretics, other antihypertensives:* risk of excessive hypotension. Discontinue diuretic or lower dose of quinapril as needed.
Lithium: increased serum lithium levels and lithium toxicity. Monitor serum lithium levels.
Potassium-sparing diuretics, potassium supplements: risk of hyperkalemia. Monitor closely during concomitant use.
Tetracycline: absorption decreased with

Reactions may be *common,* uncommon, ***life-threatening,*** or COMMON AND LIFE-THREATENING.

administration of quinapril. Avoid concomitant use.

Drug-food. *Salt substitutes containing potassium:* risk of hyperkalemia. Monitor closely during concomitant use.

EFFECTS ON DIAGNOSTIC TESTS
None reported.

CONTRAINDICATIONS
Contraindicated in patients with hypersensitivity to ACE inhibitors or history of angioedema related to treatment with an ACE inhibitor.

NURSING CONSIDERATIONS
• Use cautiously in patients with impaired renal function.
• Assess renal and hepatic function before and periodically throughout therapy.
• Monitor blood pressure for effectiveness of therapy.
• Monitor serum potassium levels as ordered. Be aware that risk factors for the development of hyperkalemia include renal insufficiency, diabetes, and concomitant use of drugs that raise potassium level.
• Other ACE inhibitors have been associated with agranulocytosis and neutropenia. Monitor CBC with differential counts before therapy and periodically thereafter, as ordered.

☑ **Patient teaching**
• Advise patient to report signs of infection, such as fever and sore throat.
Alert: Angioedema (including laryngeal edema) may occur, especially after the first dose. Advise patient to report signs or symptoms, such as swelling of face, eyes, lips, or tongue or breathing difficulty.
• Light-headedness can occur, especially during the first few days of therapy. Tell patient to rise slowly to minimize effect and to report symptoms to doctor. If syncope occurs, patient should stop taking drug and call doctor immediately.
• Inform patient that inadequate fluid intake, vomiting, diarrhea, and excessive perspiration can lead to light-headedness and syncope. Tell him to use caution in hot weather and during exercise.

• Tell patient to avoid salt substitutes; these products may contain potassium, which can cause hyperkalemia in patients taking quinapril.
• Tell female patient to notify doctor if pregnancy occurs. Drug will need to be discontinued.

ramipril
Altace, Ramace‡, Tritace‡

*Pregnancy Risk Category: C
(D in second and third trimesters)*

HOW SUPPLIED
Capsules: 1.25 mg, 2.5 mg, 5 mg, 10 mg

ACTION
Unknown, but thought to be related to inhibition of angiotensin I to angiotensin II, a potent vasoconstrictor. Reduced formation of angiotensin II decreases peripheral arterial resistance, thus decreasing aldosterone secretion.

Route	Onset	Peak	Duration
PO	1-2 hr	1-3 hr	24 hr

INDICATIONS & DOSAGE
Hypertension—
Adults: initially, 2.5 mg P.O. once daily for patients not receiving a diuretic, and 1.25 mg P.O. once daily for patients receiving a diuretic. Dosage increased p.r.n. based on patient response. Maintenance dosage is 2.5 to 20 mg daily as a single dose or in divided doses.
Adjust-a-dose: In renally impaired patients with creatinine clearance less than 40 ml/minute, 1.25 mg P.O. daily. Dosage is titrated gradually according to response. Maximum daily dosage is 5 mg.
Heart failure—
Adults: initially, 2.5 mg P.O. b.i.d. If hypotension occurs, dosage decreased to 1.25 mg P.O. b.i.d. Dosage may be gradually increased to maximum of 5 mg P.O. b.i.d., p.r.n.
Adjust-a-dose: In renally impaired patients with creatinine clearance less than 40 ml/minute, 1.25 mg P.O. daily. Dosage is titrated gradually according to re-

sponse. Maximum daily dosage is 2.5 mg b.i.d.

ADVERSE REACTIONS
CNS: headache, dizziness, fatigue, asthenia, malaise, light-headedness, anxiety, amnesia, *seizures,* depression, insomnia, nervousness, neuralgia, neuropathy, paresthesia, somnolence, tremor, vertigo.
CV: heart failure, orthostatic hypotension, syncope, angina, *arrhythmias,* chest pain, palpitations, *MI.*
EENT: epistaxis, tinnitus.
GI: nausea, vomiting, abdominal pain, anorexia, constipation, diarrhea, dyspepsia, dry mouth, gastroenteritis.
GU: impotence, elevated BUN and creatinine levels.
Hematologic: decrease in hemoglobin and hematocrit.
Hepatic: elevated liver enzymes and bilirubin.
Respiratory: *dry, persistent, tickling, nonproductive cough;* dyspnea.
Skin: hypersensitivity reactions, rash, dermatitis, pruritus, photosensitivity.
Other: *angioedema,* edema, elevated uric acid levels, hyperglycemia, hyperkalemia, increased diaphoresis, weight gain, arthralgia, arthritis, myalgia.

INTERACTIONS
Drug-drug. *Diuretics:* excessive hypotension, especially at the start of therapy. Discontinue diuretic at least 3 days before therapy begins, increase sodium intake, or reduce starting dose of ramipril.
Insulin, oral antidiabetic agents: risk of hypoglycemia, especially at initiation of ramipril therapy. Monitor closely.
Lithium: increased serum lithium levels. Use together cautiously and monitor serum lithium levels.
Potassium-sparing diuretics, potassium supplements: increased risk of hyperkalemia because ramipril attenuates potassium loss. Monitor plasma potassium levels closely.
Drug-food. *Salt substitutes containing potassium:* increased risk of hyperkalemia because ramipril attenuates potassium loss. Monitor plasma potassium levels closely.

EFFECTS ON DIAGNOSTIC TESTS
None reported.

CONTRAINDICATIONS
Contraindicated in patients with hypersensitivity to ACE inhibitors or history of angioedema related to treatment with an ACE inhibitor.

NURSING CONSIDERATIONS
• Use cautiously in patients with renal impairment.
• Monitor blood pressure regularly for drug effectiveness.
• Closely assess renal function in patients during first few weeks of therapy. Regular assessment of renal function (serum creatinine and BUN levels) is advisable. Patients with severe heart failure whose renal function depends on the angiotensin-aldosterone system have experienced acute renal failure during ACE inhibitor therapy. Hypertensive patients with renal artery stenosis also may show signs of worsening renal function at start of therapy.
• Monitor CBC with differential counts before therapy and periodically thereafter. These effects may occur especially in patients with impaired renal function or collagen vascular diseases (systemic lupus erythematosus or scleroderma).
• Monitor serum potassium levels. Risk factors for the development of hyperkalemia include renal insufficiency, diabetes, and concomitant use of agents that raise potassium levels.

☑ **Patient teaching**
• Tell patient to avoid abrupt discontinuation of therapy but to call doctor to discuss unpleasant adverse reactions.
Alert: Angioedema (including laryngeal edema) may occur, especially after the first dose. Advise patient to report signs or symptoms, such as swelling of face, eyes, lips, or tongue or breathing difficulty.
• Inform patient that light-headedness can occur, especially during the first few days of therapy. Tell him to rise slowly to minimize this effect and to report symptoms to the doctor. If syncope occurs, patient should stop taking drug and call doctor immediately.

Reactions may be *common*, uncommon, *life-threatening*, or COMMON AND LIFE-THREATENING.

• Tell patient if he has difficulty swallowing capsules, ramipril can be opened and contents sprinkled on a small amount of applesauce.

• Advise patient to report signs of infection, such as fever and sore throat.

• Tell patient to avoid salt substitutes; these products may contain potassium, which can cause hyperkalemia in patients taking ramipril.

• Tell female patient to notify doctor if pregnancy occurs. Drug will need to be discontinued.

▼ *NEW DRUG*

telmisartan
Micardis

Pregnancy Risk Category: C
(D in second and third trimesters)

HOW SUPPLIED
Tablets: 40 mg, 80 mg

ACTION
Blocks the vasoconstricting and aldosterone-secreting effects of angiotensin II by selectively blocking the binding of angiotensin II to the AT_1 receptor in many tissues, such as vascular smooth muscle and the adrenal gland.

Route	Onset	Peak	Duration
PO	Unknown	0.5-1 hr	24 hr

INDICATIONS & DOSAGE
Treatment of hypertension (used alone or in combination with other antihypertensives)—
Adults: 40 mg P.O. daily. Blood pressure response is dose-related over range of 20 to 80 mg daily.

ADVERSE REACTIONS
CNS: dizziness, pain, fatigue, headache.
CV: chest pain, hypertension, peripheral edema.
EENT: pharyngitis, sinusitis.
GI: abdominal pain, diarrhea, dyspepsia, nausea.
GU: urinary tract infection.
Hepatic: elevated liver enzymes.
Musculoskeletal: back pain, myalgia.

Respiratory: cough, upper respiratory tract infection.
Other: flulike symptoms.

INTERACTIONS
Drug-drug. *Digoxin:* increased digoxin plasma concentrations. Monitor digoxin levels closely.
Warfarin: slightly decreased plasma warfarin concentrations. Monitor INR.

EFFECTS ON DIAGNOSTIC TESTS
None reported.

CONTRAINDICATIONS
Contraindicated in patients hypersensitive to drug or its components.

NURSING CONSIDERATIONS
• Use cautiously in patients with biliary obstruction disorders or renal and hepatic insufficiency and in those with an activated renin-angiotensin system, such as volume- or salt-depleted patients (for example, those being treated with high doses of diuretics).

• Know that drugs that act on the renin-angiotensin system (such as telmisartan) can cause fetal and neonatal morbidity and death when administered to pregnant women. These problems have not been detected when exposure has been limited to the first trimester. If preganancy is suspected, notify doctor because drug should be discontinued.

• Monitor for hypotension following initiation of drug. Place patient in supine position if hypotension occurs and administer I.V. normal saline if necessary, as ordered.

• Most of the antihypertensive effect is present within 2 weeks. Maximal blood pressure reduction is generally attained after 4 weeks. Diuretic may be added if blood pressure is not controlled by drug alone.

• Know that in patients whose renal function may depend on the activity of the renin-angiotensin-aldosterone system (such as patients with severe heart failure), treatment with ACE inhibitors and angiotensin receptor antagonists has been associated with oliguria or progressive azotemia and (rarely) with acute renal failure or death.

● Drug is not removed by hemodialysis. Patients undergoing dialysis may develop orthostatic hypotension. Closely monitor blood pressure.

☑ Patient teaching
● Instruct patient to report suspected pregnancy to doctor immediately.
● Inform female patient of childbearing age of the consequences of second and third trimester exposure to drug.
● Advise breast-feeding patient about risk for adverse drug effects on infant and the need to discontinue drug or breast-feeding.
● Tell patient that transient hypotension may occur. Instruct him to lie down if feeling dizzy and to rise slowly from a lying to standing position or when climbing stairs.
● Tell patient that drug may be taken without regard to meals.
● Tell patient that drug should not be removed from blister-sealed packet until immediately before use.

---

terazosin hydrochloride
Hytrin

Pregnancy Risk Category: C

HOW SUPPLIED
Tablets: 1 mg, 2 mg, 5 mg, 10 mg
Capsules: 1 mg, 2 mg, 5 mg, 10 mg

ACTION
Decreases blood pressure by vasodilation produced in response to blockade of alpha$_1$-adrenergic receptors. Improves urine flow in patients with BPH by blocking alpha$_1$-adrenergic receptors in the smooth muscle of the bladder neck and prostate, thus relieving urethral pressure and reestablishing urine flow.

Route	Onset	Peak	Duration
PO	15 min	2-3 hr	24 hr

INDICATIONS & DOSAGE
Hypertension—
Adults: initially, 1 mg P.O. h.s. Dosage increased gradually based on patient response. Usual dosage range is 1 to 5 mg daily. Maximum recommended dosage is 20 mg daily.
Symptomatic BPH—
Adults: initially, 1 mg P.O. h.s. Dosage increased in a stepwise fashion to 2, 5, or 10 mg once daily to achieve optimal response. Most patients require 10 mg daily for optimal response.

ADVERSE REACTIONS
CNS: asthenia, dizziness, headache, nervousness, paresthesia, somnolence.
CV: palpitations, orthostatic hypotension, tachycardia, *peripheral edema.*
EENT: *nasal congestion,* sinusitis, blurred vision.
GI: nausea.
GU: impotence.
Hematologic: decreases in hematocrit, hemoglobin, WBCs, total protein, and albumin.
Respiratory: dyspnea.
Other: back pain, muscle pain.

INTERACTIONS
Drug-drug. *Antihypertensives:* excessive hypotension. Use together cautiously.
Clonidine: clonidine's antihypertensive effect may be decreased. Monitor patient.
Drug-herb. *Butcher's broom:* possible diminished effect. Avoid concomitant use.

EFFECTS ON DIAGNOSTIC TESTS
None reported.

CONTRAINDICATIONS
Contraindicated in patients with hypersensitivity to drug.

NURSING CONSIDERATIONS
● Monitor blood pressure frequently.
Alert: Know that if terazosin is discontinued for several days, patient will need to be retitrated using initial dosing regimen (1 mg P.O. h.s.).

☑ Patient teaching
● Tell patient not to discontinue drug suddenly, but to call doctor if adverse reactions occur.
● Warn patient to avoid hazardous activities that require mental alertness, such as

---

driving or operating heavy machinery, for 12 hours after the first dose.

timolol maleate
Apo-Timol†, Betim§, Blocadren

Pregnancy Risk Category: C

HOW SUPPLIED
Tablets: 5 mg, 10 mg, 20 mg

ACTION
Mechanism of antihypertensive action unknown. In MI, may decrease myocardial oxygen requirements. Prevents arterial dilation through beta blockade for migraine headache prophylaxis.

Route	Onset	Peak	Duration
PO	15-30 min	1-2 hr	6-12 hr

INDICATIONS & DOSAGE
Hypertension—
Adults: initially, 10 mg P.O. b.i.d. Usual daily maintenance dosage is 20 to 40 mg. Maximum daily dosage is 60 mg. Allow at least 7 days to elapse between increases in dosage.
MI (long-term prophylaxis in patients who have survived acute phase)—
Adults: 10 mg P.O. b.i.d.
Migraine headache prophylaxis—
Adults: initially, 10 mg P.O. b.i.d. Increase dosage as needed and tolerated to maximum of 30 mg daily divided dose. Discontinue treatment if no response occurs after 6 to 8 weeks of therapy at maximum dosage.

ADVERSE REACTIONS
CNS: fatigue, lethargy, dizziness.
CV: *bradycardia, hypotension,* **heart failure,** peripheral vascular disease, arrhythmias, pulmonary edema.
GI: nausea, vomiting, diarrhea.
GU: slightly increased BUN levels.
Hematologic: decreased hemoglobin and hematocrit levels.
Respiratory: dyspnea, *bronchospasm, increased airway resistance.*
Skin: pruritus.
Other: increased serum potassium, uric acid, and blood glucose levels.

INTERACTIONS
Drug-drug. *Cardiac glycosides, diltiazem, verapamil:* excessive bradycardia and increased depressant effect on myocardium. Use together cautiously.
Catecholamine-depleting drugs (such as reserpine): may have additive effect when given with beta blockers. Monitor for hypotension and bradycardia.
Indomethacin: decreased antihypertensive effect. Monitor blood pressure and adjust dosage.
Insulin, oral antidiabetic agents: can alter requirements for these drugs in previously stabilized diabetic patients. Monitor patient for hypoglycemia.

EFFECTS ON DIAGNOSTIC TESTS
None reported.

CONTRAINDICATIONS
Contraindicated in patients with bronchial asthma, severe COPD, sinus bradycardia and heart block greater than first-degree, cardiogenic shock, heart failure, or hypersensitivity to drug.

NURSING CONSIDERATIONS
• Use cautiously in patients with heart failure; hepatic, renal, or respiratory disease; diabetes; and hyperthyroidism.
• Check patient's apical pulse rate before giving drug. If you detect extremes in pulse rates, withhold drug and call the doctor immediately.
• Monitor blood pressure frequently.
• Monitor blood glucose levels in diabetic patients; drug can mask signs and symptoms of hypoglycemia.

☑ Patient teaching
• Tell patient to take drug exactly as prescribed.
• Instruct patient not to discontinue drug suddenly but to call doctor to discuss unpleasant adverse reactions. Tell him dosage should be reduced gradually over 1 to 2 weeks.

trandolapril
Gopten§, Odrik§, Mavik

Pregnancy Risk Category: C
(D in second and third trimesters)

HOW SUPPLIED
Tablets: 1 mg, 2 mg, 4 mg

ACTION
Unknown. Thought to result primarily from the inhibition of circulating and tissue ACE activity, thereby reducing angiotensin II formation, decreasing vasoconstriction, decreasing aldosterone secretion, and increasing plasma renin. Decreased aldosterone secretion leads to diuresis, natriuresis, and a small increase in serum potassium. Trandolapril is converted in the liver to the prodrug, trandolaprilat.

Route	Onset	Peak	Duration
PO	Unknown	1-10 hr	24 hr

INDICATIONS & DOSAGE
Hypertension—
Adults: for patient not receiving a diuretic, initially 1 mg for a nonblack patient and 2 mg for a black patient P.O. once daily. If control is not adequate, dosage can be increased at intervals of at least 1 week. Maintenance dosages range from 2 to 4 mg daily for most patients. Some patients receiving once-daily doses of 4 mg may need b.i.d. doses. For a patient receiving a concurrent diuretic, the initial dose of trandolapril should be 0.5 mg P.O. once daily. Subsequent dosage adjustment is made according to blood pressure response.
Post-MI: heart failure or ventricular dysfunction—
Adults: initially 1 mg P.O. daily, titrated to 4 mg P.O. daily. If patient cannot tolerate 4 mg, continue at highest tolerated dose.
Adjust-a-dose: In patients with hepatic disease or renal failure who have a creatinine clearance less than 30 ml/minute, initial dose is 0.5 mg daily.

ADVERSE REACTIONS
CNS: dizziness, headache, fatigue, drowsiness, insomnia, paresthesia, vertigo, anxiety.
CV: chest pain, first-degree AV block, bradycardia, edema, flushing, hypotension, palpitations.
EENT: epistaxis, throat irritation, upper respiratory tract infection.
GI: diarrhea, dyspepsia, abdominal distention, abdominal pain or cramps, constipation, vomiting, pancreatitis.
GU: elevated BUN and creatinine levels, urinary frequency, impotence, decreased libido.
Hematologic: neutropenia, leukopenia.
Hepatic: elevated liver enzymes.
Respiratory: persistent, nonproductive cough; dyspnea.
Skin: rash, pruritus, pemphigus.
Other: *anaphylactic reactions, angioedema,* hyperkalemia, hyponatremia.

INTERACTIONS
Drug-drug. *Diuretics:* increased risk of excessive hypotension. Diuretic may be discontinued or treatment initiated with a lower dose of trandolapril, as ordered.
Lithium: increased serum lithium levels and lithium toxicity. Avoid concomitant use. Monitor serum lithium levels.
Potassium-sparing diuretics, potassium supplements: increased risk of hyperkalemia. Monitor serum potassium closely.
Drug-food. *Salt substitutes containing potassium:* increased risk of hyperkalemia. Monitor serum potassium closely.

EFFECTS ON DIAGNOSTIC TESTS
None reported.

CONTRAINDICATIONS
Contraindicated in patients with hypersensitivity to drug or history of angioedema related to previous treatment with an ACE inhibitor. Drug is not recommended for use during pregnancy.

NURSING CONSIDERATIONS
• Use cautiously in patients with impaired renal function, heart failure, or renal artery stenosis.
• Monitor serum potassium levels closely.
• Monitor for hypotension. Excessive hy-

---

potension can occur when drug is given with diuretics. If possible, diuretic therapy should be discontinued 2 to 3 days before starting trandolapril to decrease potential for excessive hypotension response. If trandolapril does not adequately control blood pressure, diuretic therapy may be reinstituted cautiously, as ordered.

● Assess patient's renal function before and periodically throughout therapy.

● Know that other ACE inhibitors have been associated with agranulocytosis and neutropenia. Monitor CBC with differential before therapy, especially in patients with collagen vascular disease with impaired renal function.

Alert: Be aware that angioedema associated with involvement of the tongue, glottis, or larynx may be fatal because of airway obstruction. Appropriate therapy should be ordered, including epinephrine 1:1,000 (0.3 to 0.5 ml) S.C., and resuscitation equipment for maintaining a patent airway should be readily available.

● If patient develops jaundice, discontinue drug under doctor's advice because, although rare, ACE inhibitors have been associated with a syndrome of cholestatic jaundice, fulminant hepatic necrosis, and death.

● Safety and effectiveness in children have not been established.

● Be aware that it is unknown whether trandolapril is excreted in breast milk. Drug should not be given to breast-feeding women.

✔ Patient teaching

● Instruct patient to report jaundice.

● Advise patient to report signs of infection, such as fever and sore throat, and if the following signs or symptoms occur: easy bruising or bleeding; swelling of the tongue, lips, face, eyes, mucous membranes, or extremities; difficulty swallowing or breathing; hoarseness; and nonproductive, persistent cough.

● Tell patient to avoid salt substitutes during drug therapy; these products may contain potassium, which can cause hyperkalemia.

● Tell patient that light-headedness can occur, especially during first few days of therapy. Tell patient to rise slowly to minimize this effect and report it immediately.

● Advise patient to use caution in hot weather and during exercise. Inadequate fluid intake, vomiting, diarrhea, and excessive perspiration can lead to lightheadedness and syncope.

● Tell female patient to report suspected pregnancy immediately. Drug will need to be discontinued.

● Advise patient planning to undergo surgery or anesthesia to inform doctor that he is taking this drug.

valsartan
Diovan

Pregnancy Risk Category: C (D in second and third trimesters)

HOW SUPPLIED
Capsules: 80 mg, 160 mg

ACTION
Blocks the binding of angiotensin II to receptor sites in vascular smooth muscle and the adrenal gland, which inhibits the pressor effects of the renin-angiotensin system.

Route	Onset	Peak	Duration
PO	2 hr	2-4 hr	24 hr

INDICATIONS & DOSAGE
Hypertension, used alone or in combination with other antihypertensives—
Adults: initially, 80 mg P.O. once daily. Expect to see a reduction in blood pressure in 2 to 4 weeks. If additional antihypertensive effect is needed, dosage may be increased to 160 or 320 mg daily, or a diuretic may be added. (Addition of a diuretic has a greater effect than dosage increases beyond 80 mg.) Usual dosage range is 80 to 320 mg daily.

ADVERSE REACTIONS
CNS: dizziness, headache, insomnia.
CV: edema, hyperkalemia.
GI: abdominal pain, diarrhea, nausea.
Hematologic: neutropenia.
Musculoskeletal: arthralgia.

Respiratory: upper respiratory infection, cough, rhinitis, sinusitis, pharyngitis.
Other: viral infection, fatigue.

INTERACTIONS
Drug-drug. *Diuretics:* risk of excessive hypotension. Assess fluid status before starting concomitant therapy. Monitor closely.
Drug-food. *Any food:* decreased peak levels. Give drug on an empty stomach.

EFFECTS ON DIAGNOSTIC TESTS
None reported.

CONTRAINDICATIONS
Contraindicated in patients with known hypersensitivity to drug.

NURSING CONSIDERATIONS
• Use cautiously in patients with renal or hepatic disease.
• Know that drug can cause fetal or neonatal morbidity and death if administered to a pregnant woman in the second or third trimester. Breast-feeding women should not take drug.
• Be aware that safety and effectiveness in children have not been established.
• Monitor for hypotension. Excessive hypotension can occur when drug is given with high doses of diuretics. Correct volume and salt depletions as ordered before starting drug.

☑**Patient teaching**
• Tell female patient to notify doctor if pregnancy occurs; drug will need to be discontinued.
• Tell patient drug may be taken with or without food.

24

Antilipemics

atorvastatin calcium
cerivastatin sodium
cholestyramine
colestipol hydrochloride
fenofibrate (micronized)
fluvastatin sodium
gemfibrozil
lovastatin
niacin
   (See Chapter 90, VITAMINS AND
   MINERALS.)
pravastatin sodium
simvastatin

COMBINATION PRODUCTS
None.

---

atorvastatin calcium
Lipitor

Pregnancy Risk Category: X

HOW SUPPLIED
Tablets: 10 mg, 20 mg, 40 mg

ACTION
Inhibits 3-hydroxy-3-methylglutaryl-
coenzyme A reductase, an early (and rate-
limiting) step in cholesterol biosynthesis.

Route	Onset	Peak	Duration
PO	Unknown	1-2 hr	Unknown

INDICATIONS & DOSAGE
*Adjunct to diet to reduce low-density
lipoprotein (LDL), total cholesterol, apo
B, and triglyceride levels in patients with
primary hypercholesterolemia and mixed
dyslipidemia (Fredrickson Types IIa and
IIb)—*
Adults: initially, 10 mg P.O. once daily.
Dosage increased p.r.n. to maximum of
80 mg daily as a single dose. Dosage
based on blood lipid levels drawn within
2 to 4 weeks after starting therapy.
*Alone or as an adjunct to lipid-lowering
treatments such as LDL apheresis in patients with homozygous familial hypercholesterolemia—*
Adults: 10 to 80 mg P.O. once daily.
✳ *NEW INDICATION: Adjunctive therapy to
diet for the treatment of patients with elevated serum triglyceride levels (Fredrickson Type IV)—*
Adults: initially, 10 mg P.O. once daily.
Dosage increased p.r.n. to maximum of
80 mg daily as a single dose. Dosage
based on blood lipid levels drawn within
2 to 4 weeks after starting therapy.
✳ *NEW INDICATION: Treatment of patients
with primary dysbetalipoproteinemia
(Fredrickson Type III) who do not respond
adequately to diet—*
Adults: initially, 10 mg P.O. once daily.
Dosage increased p.r.n. to maximum of
80 mg daily as a single dose. Dosage
based on blood lipid levels drawn within
2 to 4 weeks after starting therapy.

ADVERSE REACTIONS
CNS: *headache,* asthenia, insomnia.
GI: abdominal pain, dyspepsia, flatu-
lence, nausea.
Hepatic: increased liver function tests.
Musculoskeletal: arthritis, arthralgia,
myalgia.
Respiratory: bronchitis, rhinitis.
Skin: rash.
Other: infection, accidental injury, flulike
syndrome, allergic reaction, urinary tract
infection, peripheral edema.

INTERACTIONS
Drug-drug. *Azole antifungals, cyclosporine, erythromycin, fibric acid derivatives, niacin:* possible risk of rhabdomyolysis. Avoid concomitant use.
Digoxin: may increase plasma digoxin
levels. Monitor serum digoxin levels.
Erythromycin: will increase plasma concentration of drug. Monitor patient.
Oral contraceptives: increased levels of
hormones. Consider when selecting an
oral contraceptive.

EFFECTS ON DIAGNOSTIC TESTS
None reported.

CONTRAINDICATIONS
Contraindicated in patients hypersensitive to drug or with active liver disease or conditions associated with unexplained persistent elevations of serum transaminase levels. Also contraindicated in pregnant and breast-feeding patients and in female patients of childbearing age (except those not at risk for becoming pregnant).

NURSING CONSIDERATIONS
• Use cautiously in patients with history of liver disease or heavy alcohol use.
• Know that drug should be withheld or discontinued in patients with serious, acute conditions that suggest myopathy or those at risk for renal failure secondary to rhabdomyolysis as a result of trauma; major surgery; severe metabolic, endocrine, and electrolyte disorders; severe acute infection; hypotension; or uncontrolled seizures.
• Know that experience in children has been limited to those over 9 years with homozygous familial hypercholesterolemia.
• Initiate drug therapy only after diet and other nonpharmacologic treatments prove ineffective. Patient should follow a standard low-cholesterol diet before and during therapy.
• Before initiating treatment, secondary causes for hypercholesterolemia should be excluded and a baseline lipid profile done. Obtain periodic liver function test results and lipid levels, as ordered, before starting treatment, at 6 and 12 weeks after initiation, or after an increase in dosage and periodically thereafter.
• Know that drug may be given as a single dose at any time of day, with or without food.
• Watch for signs of myositis.

☑ Patient teaching
• Teach patient about proper dietary management, weight control, and exercise. Explain their importance in controlling elevated serum lipid levels.
• Warn patient to avoid alcohol.
• Tell patient to inform doctor of adverse reactions, such as muscle pain, malaise, and fever.
Alert: Inform female patient that drug is contraindicated during pregnancy because of the potential of danger to the fetus. Advise her to notify doctor immediately if pregnancy occurs.

---

cerivastatin sodium
Baycol, Lipobay§

Pregnancy Risk Category: X

HOW SUPPLIED
Tablets: 0.2 mg, 0.3 mg

ACTION
Competitive inhibitor of 3-hydroxy-3-methylglutaryl-coenzyme A (HMG-CoA) reductase that is responsible for the conversion of HMG-CoA, a precursor of cholesterol. The end result is a reduction in the plasma cholesterol concentration.

Route	Onset	Peak	Duration
PO	1 wk	4 wk	Unknown

INDICATIONS & DOSAGE
Adjunct to diet, to reduce total and low-density cholesterol levels in patients with primary hypercholesterolemia or mixed dyslipidemia when diet and other nonpharmacologic measures have been inadequate—
Adults: 0.3 mg P.O. daily in the evening.
Adjust-a-dose: In patients with moderate or severe renal dysfunction (creatinine clearance 60 ml/minute or less), starting dose is 0.2 mg P.O. daily.

ADVERSE REACTIONS
CNS: dizziness, *headache,* insomnia.
CV: chest pain, peripheral edema.
EENT: *pharyngitis, rhinitis,* sinusitis.
GI: constipation, diarrhea, dyspepsia, flatulence, nausea.
GU: urinary tract infection.
Musculoskeletal: arthralgia, back or leg pain, myalgia.
Respiratory: increased cough.
Skin: rash.
Other: flulike syndrome.

Reactions may be *common,* uncommon, *life-threatening,* or COMMON AND LIFE-THREATENING.

INTERACTIONS

Drug-drug. *Azole antifungals, cyclosporine, erythromycin, fibric acid derivatives, niacin:* may increase the incidence of myopathy. Use cautiously together.
Cholestyramine: decreased absorption and decreased peak plasma levels of cerivastatin when given within 4 hours of drug. Use cautiously together.
Erythromycin: may decrease hepatic metabolism of drug and has resulted in increases of cerivastatin of up to 50%. Use cautiously together.

EFFECTS ON DIAGNOSTIC TESTS

Drug may elevate transaminases, CK, alkaline phosphatase, GGT, and bilirubin levels. Thyroid function abnormalities have also been reported.

CONTRAINDICATIONS

Contraindicated in patients with active liver disease, unexplained persistent elevations of serum transaminases, or hypersensitivity to drug and during pregnancy or breast-feeding.

NURSING CONSIDERATIONS

● Use cautiously in patients with history of liver disease or heavy alcohol use.
● Safety and efficacy in children have not been established.
● Drug should be given to women of childbearing age only if conception is highly unlikely and they have been warned of potential risks to fetus.
● Know that therapy with lipid-lowering drugs should be started after appropriate diet, exercise, and weight reduction programs are unsuccessful in controlling cholesterol levels.
● Perform liver function tests before starting treatment, at 6 and 12 weeks after initiation of therapy, and periodically thereafter.
● Withhold drug temporarily in patients experiencing an acute or serious condition predisposing them to renal failure secondary to rhabdomyolysis. Rare cases of rhabdomyolysis have been reported with other HMG-CoA reductase inhibitors.

☑ **Patient teaching**
● Tell patient to take drug at bedtime and allow at least 1 hour before or 4 hours after cholestyramine or colestipol.
● Inform patient that it may take up to 4 weeks for full therapeutic effect to occur.
● Caution patient to stop drug if pregnancy occurs or is suspected.
● Advise breast-feeding patient to avoid use of drug.
● Tell patient to notify doctor if an unexplained muscle pain, tenderness, or weakness (particularly if accompanied by fever or malaise) occurs.

---

cholestyramine
LoCholest, Prevalite, Questran**,
Questran Light, Questran Lite‡

Pregnancy Risk Category: NR

HOW SUPPLIED

Powder: 378-g cans, 9-g single-dose packets. Each scoop of powder or single-dose packet contains 4 g of cholestyramine resin.
Tablets: 1 g

ACTION

A bile-acid sequestrant that combines with bile acid to form an insoluble compound that is excreted. The liver must synthesize new bile acid from cholesterol, which reduces low-density-lipoprotein cholesterol levels.

Route	Onset	Peak	Duration
PO	Unknown	Unknown	2-4 wk

INDICATIONS & DOSAGE

Primary hyperlipidemia or pruritus caused by partial bile obstruction; adjunct for reduction of elevated serum cholesterol in patients with primary hypercholesterolemia—
Adults: 4 g once or twice daily. Maintenance dosage is 8 to 16 g daily divided into two doses. Maximum daily dosage is 24 g.

ADVERSE REACTIONS

CNS: headache, anxiety, vertigo, dizziness, insomnia, fatigue, syncope, tinnitus.
GI: *constipation, fecal impaction,* hemorrhoids, *abdominal discomfort,* flatulence,

---

nausea, vomiting, steatorrhea, GI bleeding, diarrhea, anorexia.
GU: hematuria, dysuria.
Hematologic: anemia, bleeding tendencies, ecchymoses.
Hepatic: increased serum alkaline phosphatase.
Musculoskeletal: backache, muscle and joint pains, osteoporosis.
Skin: *rash;* irritation of skin, tongue, and perianal area.
Other: *vitamin A, D, E, and K deficiencies from decreased absorption;* hyperchloremic acidosis (with long-term use or very high dosage).

INTERACTIONS
Drug-drug. *Acetaminophen, beta-adrenergic blockers, cardiac glycosides, corticosteroids, fat-soluble vitamins (A, D, E, and K), iron preparations, niacin, thiazide diuretics, thyroid hormones, warfarin and other coumarin derivatives:* absorption may be substantially decreased by cholestyramine. Administer other drugs 1 hour before or 4 to 6 hours after cholestyramine.

EFFECTS ON DIAGNOSTIC TESTS
Cholecystography using iopanoic acid will yield abnormal results because iopanoic acid is also bound by cholestyramine.

CONTRAINDICATIONS
Contraindicated in patients with complete biliary obstruction or hypersensitivity to bile-acid sequestering resins.

NURSING CONSIDERATIONS
• Use cautiously in patients predisposed to constipation and in those with conditions aggravated by constipation, such as severe, symptomatic coronary artery disease.
• Monitor serum cholesterol and triglyceride levels regularly during therapy.
• Monitor serum levels of cardiac glycosides in patients receiving cardiac glycosides and cholestyramine concurrently. If cholestyramine therapy is discontinued, adjust dosage of cardiac glycosides as ordered to avoid toxicity.

• Monitor bowel habits. Encourage a diet high in fiber and fluids. If severe constipation develops, decrease dosage, add a stool softener, or discontinue drug, as ordered.
• Be aware that long-term use may be associated with deficiencies of vitamins A, D, E, and K and folic acid.

✓ **Patient teaching**
Alert: Tell patient never to take drug in its dry form; esophageal irritation or severe constipation may result.
• Instruct patient to mix powder as follows: Using a large glass, patient should sprinkle the powder on the surface of preferred beverage; let mixture stand a few minutes; then stir thoroughly. The best diluents are water, milk, and juice (especially pulpy fruit juice). Mixing with carbonated beverages may result in excessive foaming. After drinking this preparation, patient should swirl a small additional amount of liquid in the same glass and then drink it to ensure ingestion of the entire dose.
• Advise patient to take all other drugs at least 1 hour before or 4 to 6 hours after cholestyramine to avoid blocking their absorption.
• Teach patient about proper dietary management of serum lipids. When appropriate, recommend weight-control, exercise, and smoking-cessation programs.

---

colestipol hydrochloride
Colestid

Pregnancy Risk Category: NR

HOW SUPPLIED
Granules: 300-g and 500-g bottles, 5-g packets
Tablets: 1 g

ACTION
Combines with bile acid to form an insoluble compound that is excreted in feces. The liver must synthesize new bile acid from cholesterol; this leads to re-

---

duced low-density-lipoprotein cholesterol levels.

Route	Onset	Peak	Duration
PO	1 mo	Unknown	1 mo

INDICATIONS & DOSAGE
Primary hypercholesterolemia—
Adults: 5 to 30 g (granules) P.O. once daily or in divided doses. Or, 2 to 16 g (tablets) P.O. daily given once or in divided doses.

ADVERSE REACTIONS
CNS: headache, dizziness, anxiety, vertigo, insomnia, fatigue, syncope, tinnitus.
CV: angina, chest pain.
GI: *constipation, fecal impaction,* hemorrhoids, abdominal discomfort, flatulence, nausea, vomiting, steatorrhea, GI bleeding, diarrhea, anorexia.
GU: dysuria, hematuria.
Hepatic: increased serum levels of alkaline phosphatase, ALT, AST.
Musculoskeletal: backache, muscle and joint pain, osteoporosis.
Skin: rash, irritation of tongue and perianal area.
Other: vitamin A, D, E, and K deficiencies from decreased absorption; hyperchloremic acidosis (with long-term use or high dosage), anemia, ecchymoses, bleeding tendencies.

INTERACTIONS
Drug-drug. *Oral antidiabetic agents:* may antagonize response to colestipol. Monitor serum lipids.
Orally administered drugs: colestipol may decrease absorption. Separate administration times; give other drugs at least 1 hour before or 4 hours after colestipol.

EFFECTS ON DIAGNOSTIC TESTS
None reported.

CONTRAINDICATIONS
Contraindicated in patients with hypersensitivity reactions to bile-acid sequestering resins.

NURSING CONSIDERATIONS
● Use cautiously in patients predisposed to constipation and in those with condi-

tions aggravated by constipation, such as severe, symptomatic coronary artery disease.
● Monitor serum cholesterol and triglyceride levels regularly during therapy.
● Monitor bowel habits; if severe constipation develops, decrease dosage or add stool softener as ordered. Encourage a diet high in fiber and fluids.
● Monitor serum levels of cardiac glycosides in patients receiving cardiac glycosides and colestipol concurrently. If colestipol therapy is discontinued, adjust dosage of cardiac glycosides to avoid toxicity, as ordered.

☑**Patient teaching**
Alert: Tell patient never to take drug in its dry form; esophageal irritation or severe constipation may result.
● To prepare, instruct patient to use a large glass containing water, milk, or juice (especially pulpy fruit juice). He should sprinkle the powder on the surface of the preferred beverage; let the mixture stand a few minutes; then stir thoroughly to obtain a uniform suspension. After drinking this preparation, patient should swirl a small additional amount of liquid in the same glass and then drink it to ensure ingestion of the entire dose.
● To enhance palatability, tell patient to mix and refrigerate the next daily dose the previous evening.
● Instruct patient taking tablet form to swallow tablets whole and not to crush, cut, or chew them.
● Advise patient to take all other drugs at least 1 hour before or 4 to 6 hours after colestipol to avoid blocking their absorption.
● Teach patient about proper dietary management of serum lipids. When appropriate, recommend weight-control, exercise, and smoking-cessation programs.
● Inform patient that long-term use may be associated with deficiencies of vitamins A, D, E, and K and folic acid. Instruct patient to report unusual signs and symptoms.

▼ *NEW DRUG*

fenofibrate (micronized)
Tricor

Pregnancy Risk Category: C

HOW SUPPLIED
Capsules: 67 mg

ACTION
Exact mechanism not known. Fenofibrate is thought to lower triglyceride levels by inhibiting triglyceride synthesis, resulting in a decrease in the amount of very-low-density lipoproteins (VLDL) released into the circulation. Fenofibrate may stimulate the breakdown of triglyceride-rich protein.

Route	Onset	Peak	Duration
PO	Unknown	6-8 hr	Unknown

INDICATIONS & DOSAGE
Adjunctive therapy to diet for treatment of patients with very high serum triglyceride levels (type IV and V hyperlipidemia) who are at risk of pancreatitis and who do not respond adequately to a determined dietary effort—
Adults: initially, 67 mg P.O. daily. Dosage may be increased following repeat serum triglyceride estimations at 4- to 8-week intervals to maximum dosage of three capsules daily (201 mg).
Adjust-a-dose: Minimize dose in patients with severe renal impairment. Initiate therapy at a dose of 67 mg/day and increase only after effects on renal function and triglyceride levels have been evaluated at this dose. No modification is needed for patients with moderate renal impairment.

ADVERSE REACTIONS
CNS: dizziness, localized pain, asthenia, fatigue, paresthesia, insomnia, increased appetite, headache, decreased libido.
CV: *arrhythmias.*
EENT: eye irritation, eye floaters, earache, conjunctivitis, blurred vision, rhinitis, sinusitis.
GI: dyspepsia, eructation, flatulence,

nausea, vomiting, abdominal pain, constipation, diarrhea.
GU: increased BUN and creatinine levels, polyuria, vaginitis.
Hepatic: increased ALT, AST levels.
Musculoskeletal: arthralgia.
Respiratory: cough
Skin: pruritus, rash.
Other: decreased hemoglobin and uric acid levels, hypersensitivity reaction, *infection,* flu syndrome.

INTERACTIONS
Drug-drug. *Bile acid sequestrants:* may bind and inhibit absorption of fenofibrate. Give drug 1 hour before or 4 to 6 hours after bile acid sequestrants.
Coumarin-type anticoagulants: potentiation of anticoagulant effect, prolonged PT. Monitor PT and INR closely. Dosage of anticoagulant may need to be reduced.
Cyclosporine, immunosuppressants, nephrotoxic agents: induced renal dysfunction may compromise the elimination of fenofibrate. Use together cautiously.
3-Hydroxy-3-methylglutaryl coenzyme A (HMG-CoA) reductase inhibitors: no data are available on concomitant use with fenofibrate. Because of risk of myopathy, rhabdomyolysis, and acute renal failure reported with combined use of HMG-CoA reductase inhibitors with gemfibrozil (another fibrate derivative), do not give these drugs together.
Drug-food: *Any food:* absorption of fenofibrate is increased when administered with food. Give drug with meals.
Drug-lifestyle: *Alcohol use:* may elevate triglycerides. Avoid concomitant use.

EFFECTS ON DIAGNOSTIC TESTS
None reported.

CONTRAINDICATIONS
Contraindicated in patients with preexisting gallbladder disease, hepatic dysfunction, primary biliary cirrhosis, severe renal dysfunction, unexplained persistent liver function abnormalities, or hypersensitivity to drug.

NURSING CONSIDERATIONS
• Use cautiously in patients with a history of pancreatitis.

Reactions may be *common,* uncommon, ***life-threatening***, or COMMON AND LIFE-THREATENING.

• Obtain baseline lipid levels and liver function tests before starting therapy. Perform periodic monitoring of liver function for duration of drug therapy. Discontinue therapy if enzyme levels persist above three times normal limit.

• Monitor for symptoms of pancreatitis, myositis, rhabdomyolysis, cholelithiasis, and renal failure. Be alert to occurrence of myalgia, muscle tenderness, or weakness, especially in the presence of malaise or fever.

• Be aware that, if an adequate response has not been obtained after 2 months of treatment with the maximum daily dosage, therapy must be discontinued.

• Know that drug lowers serum uric acid levels in patients with or without hyperuricemia by increasing uric acid excretion.

• Be aware that beta-adrenergic blocking agents, estrogens, and thiazide diuretics use may increase plasma triglyceride levels; the continued use of these agents should be evaluated.

• Mild to moderate decreases in hemoglobin, hematocrit, and WBC count may occur on initiation of therapy but stabilize on long-term administration.

☑ **Patient teaching**

• Inform patient that drug therapy does not reduce the importance of adhering to triglyceride-lowering diet.

• Advise patient to promptly report symptoms of unexplained muscle weakness, pain, or tenderness, especially if it is accompanied by malaise or fever.

• Inform patient to take drug with meals to optimize drug absorption.

• Advise patient to continue weight-control measures, including diet and exercise, and to reduce alcohol intake before starting drug therapy.

• Instruct patients who are also taking bile acid resins to take fenofibrate 1 hour before or 4 to 6 hours after taking bile acid resin.

• Advise breast-feeding patient about potential for tumor growth and instruct her that a decision must be made to either discontinue breast-feeding or drug therapy.

fluvastatin sodium
Lescol

Pregnancy Risk Category: X

HOW SUPPLIED
Capsules: 20 mg, 40 mg

ACTION
Inhibits 3-hydroxy-3-methylglutaryl coenzyme A reductase. This enzyme is an early (and rate-limiting) step in the synthetic pathway of cholesterol.

Route	Onset	Peak	Duration
PO	Unknown	1 hr	Unknown

INDICATIONS & DOSAGE
Reduction of low-density lipoprotein and total cholesterol levels in patients with primary hypercholesterolemia (types IIa and IIb)—
Adults: initially, 20 to 40 mg P.O. h.s. Increase dosage p.r.n. to maximum of 80 mg daily (in divided doses).
To slow progression of coronary atherosclerosis in patients with coronary artery disease—
Adults: initially, 20 to 40 mg P.O. h.s. Increase dosage p.r.n. to maximum of 80 mg daily (in divided doses).

ADVERSE REACTIONS
CNS: headache, fatigue, dizziness, insomnia.
GI: dyspepsia, diarrhea, nausea, vomiting, abdominal pain, constipation, flatulence, tooth disorder.
Hematologic: *thrombocytopenia, hemolytic anemia, leukopenia.*
Hepatic: increased liver enzymes.
Respiratory: sinusitis, *upper respiratory infection,* rhinitis, cough, pharyngitis, bronchitis.
Other: arthropathy, muscle pain, hypersensitivity reactions (rash, pruritus), elevated CK, abnormal thyroid function tests.

INTERACTIONS
Drug-drug. *Cholestyramine, colestipol:* may bind with fluvastatin in the GI tract

and decrease absorption. Separate administration times by at least 4 hours.
Cimetidine, omeprazole, ranitidine: decreased fluvastatin metabolism. Monitor for enhanced effects.
Cyclosporine and other immunosuppressants, erythromycin, gemfibrozil, niacin: possible increased risk of polymyositis and rhabdomyolysis. Avoid concomitant use.
Digoxin: may alter digoxin pharmacokinetics. Monitor serum digoxin levels carefully.
Rifampin: enhanced fluvastatin metabolism and decreased plasma levels. Monitor for lack of effect.
Warfarin: increased anticoagulant effect with bleeding. Monitor patient.
Drug-lifestyle. *Alcohol use:* increased risk of hepatotoxicity. Avoid concomitant use.

EFFECTS ON DIAGNOSTIC TESTS
None reported.

CONTRAINDICATIONS
Contraindicated in patients hypersensitive to drug; in those with active liver disease or conditions associated with unexplained persistent elevations of serum transaminase levels; in pregnant and breast-feeding women; and in women of childbearing age unless there is no risk of pregnancy.

NURSING CONSIDERATIONS
• Use cautiously in patients with severe renal impairment and history of liver disease or heavy alcohol use.
• Know that fluvastatin should be initiated only after diet and other nonpharmacologic therapies prove ineffective. Patient should be on a standard low-cholesterol diet during therapy.
• Be aware that liver function tests should be performed at the start of therapy and periodically thereafter.
• Watch for signs of myositis.

☑ **Patient teaching**
• Tell patient that drug may be taken without regard to meals; however, efficacy is enhanced if drug is taken in the evening.
• Teach patient about proper dietary management, weight control, and exercise.

Explain their importance in controlling elevated serum lipid levels.
• Warn patient to avoid alcohol.
• Tell patient to notify doctor of adverse reactions, particularly muscle aches and pains.
Alert: Inform female patient that drug is contraindicated during pregnancy. Advise her to notify doctor immediately if pregnancy occurs.

gemfibrozil
Apo-Gemfibrozil†, Lopid

Pregnancy Risk Category: C

HOW SUPPLIED
Tablets: 600 mg
Capsules: 300 mg

ACTION
Inhibits peripheral lipolysis and also reduces triglyceride synthesis in the liver. Lowers serum triglyceride levels and increases high-density-lipoprotein cholesterol levels.

Route	Onset	Peak	Duration
PO	2-5 days	4 wk	Unknown

INDICATIONS & DOSAGE
Types IV and V hyperlipidemia unresponsive to diet and other drugs; reduction of risk of coronary heart disease in patients with type IIb hyperlipidemia who cannot tolerate or who are refractory to treatment with bile acid sequestrants or niacin—
Adults: 1,200 mg P.O. daily in two divided doses, 30 minutes before morning and evening meals.

ADVERSE REACTIONS
CNS: headache, fatigue, vertigo.
CV: atrial fibrillation.
GI: *abdominal and epigastric pain,* diarrhea, nausea, vomiting, *dyspepsia,* constipation, acute appendicitis.
Hematologic: *anemia, leukopenia,* eosinophilia, *thrombocytopenia.*
Hepatic: bile duct obstruction, elevated liver enzymes.
Skin: rash, dermatitis, pruritus, eczema.

Reactions may be *common,* uncommon, *life-threatening,* or COMMON AND LIFE-THREATENING.

INTERACTIONS

Drug-drug. *Lovastatin, simvastatin:* myopathy with rhabdomyolysis has been reported. Do not use together.
Oral anticoagulants: gemfibrozil may enhance the clinical effects of oral anticoagulants. Monitor closely.

EFFECTS ON DIAGNOSTIC TESTS

Drug therapy may elevate serum levels of creatinine phosphokinase, ALT, AST, alkaline phosphatase, and LD; it may also decrease serum potassium, hematocrit, hemoglobin, and leukocyte counts.

CONTRAINDICATIONS

Contraindicated in patients with hepatic or severe renal dysfunction (including primary biliary cirrhosis), preexisting gallbladder disease, or hypersensitivity to drug.

NURSING CONSIDERATIONS

• Know that periodic CBCs and liver function tests should be performed during the first 12 months of therapy.
• If drug has no beneficial effects after 3 months of therapy, expect doctor to discontinue it.

☑**Patient teaching**
• Instruct patient to take drug 30 minutes before breakfast and dinner.
• Teach patient about proper dietary management of serum lipids. When appropriate, recommend weight-control, exercise, and smoking-cessation programs.
• Because of possible dizziness and blurred vision, advise patient to avoid driving or other potentially hazardous activities until CNS effects of drug are known.
• Tell patient to observe bowel movements and to report evidence of steatorrhea or other signs of bile duct obstruction.

---

lovastatin (mevinolin)
Mevacor

Pregnancy Risk Category: X

HOW SUPPLIED
Tablets: 10 mg, 20 mg, 40 mg

ACTION

Inhibits 3-hydroxy-3-methylglutaryl coenzyme A reductase. This enzyme is an early (and rate-limiting) step in the synthetic pathway of cholesterol.

Route	Onset	Peak	Duration
PO	Unknown	2 hr	Unknown

INDICATIONS & DOSAGE

Reduction of low-density lipoprotein and total cholesterol levels in patients with primary hypercholesterolemia (types IIa and IIb)—
Adults: initially, 20 mg P.O. once daily with evening meal. Recommended daily dosage range is 10 to 80 mg in a single or two divided doses.

ADVERSE REACTIONS

CNS: headache, dizziness, peripheral neuropathy, insomnia.
EENT: blurred vision.
GI: constipation, diarrhea, dyspepsia, flatulence, abdominal pain or cramps, heartburn, nausea, vomiting.
Skin: rash, pruritus, alopecia.
Other: muscle cramps, myalgia, myositis, *rhabdomyolysis*, abnormal liver test results, chest pain.

INTERACTIONS

Drug-drug. *Cyclosporine or other immunosuppressants, erythromycin, gemfibrozil, niacin:* possible increased risk of polymyositis and rhabdomyolysis (maximum recommended lovastatin dosage is 20 mg daily); monitor patient closely.
Oral anticoagulants: lovastatin may enhance the clinical effects of oral anticoagulants. Monitor patient closely.
Drug-lifestyle. *Alcohol use:* increased risk of hepatotoxicity. Avoid concomitant use.

EFFECTS ON DIAGNOSTIC TESTS

Drug may elevate serum CK or serum transaminase levels.

CONTRAINDICATIONS

Contraindicated in patients with hypersensitivity to drug; in those with active liver disease or conditions associated with unexplained persistent elevations of

---

serum transaminase levels; in pregnant and breast-feeding patients; and in women of childbearing age unless there is no risk of pregnancy.

NURSING CONSIDERATIONS
• Use cautiously in patients who consume substantial quantities of alcohol or have a past history of liver disease.
• Know that lovastatin should be initiated only after diet and other nonpharmacologic therapies prove ineffective. Patient should be on a standard low-cholesterol diet during therapy.
• Be aware that liver function tests should be performed at the start of therapy and periodically thereafter.

☑ **Patient teaching**
• Instruct patient to take drug with the evening meal, when absorption is enhanced and cholesterol biosynthesis is greater.
• Teach patient about proper dietary management of serum lipids. When appropriate, recommend weight-control, exercise, and smoking-cessation programs.
• Advise patient to have periodic eye examinations; related compounds have caused cataracts in laboratory animals.
• Inform patient to store tablets at room temperature in a light-resistant container.
• Advise patient to promptly report unexplained muscle pain, tenderness or weakness, particularly when accompanied by malaise or fever.
Alert: Inform female patient that drug is contraindicated during pregnancy. Advise her to notify doctor immediately if pregnancy occurs.

pravastatin sodium (eptastatin)
Lipostat§, Pravachol

Pregnancy Risk Category: X

HOW SUPPLIED
Tablets: 10 mg, 20 mg, 40 mg

ACTION
Inhibits 3-hydroxy-3-methylglutaryl coenzyme A reductase. This enzyme is an early (and rate-limiting) step in the synthetic pathway of cholesterol.

Route	Onset	Peak	Duration
PO	Unknown	1-1.5 hr	Unknown

INDICATIONS & DOSAGE
Adjunct to diet to reduce low-density lipoprotein, total cholesterol, and triglyceride levels in patients with primary hypercholesterolemia and mixed dyslipidemia (Fredrickson Types IIa and IIb); primary prevention of coronary events in hypercholesterolemic patients without clinical evidence of heart disease—
Adults: initially, 10 or 20 mg P.O. h.s. Dosage adjusted q 4 weeks based on patient tolerance and response; maximum daily dosage is 40 mg.
Elderly: initially, 10 mg P.O. h.s. Most respond to daily dosage of 20 mg or less.
Reduction of risk of acute coronary events or slowing progression of coronary atherosclerosis in hypercholesterolemic patients with clinical evidence of coronary artery diseae, including prior MI; reduction of risk of undergoing myocardial revascularization procedure, recurrent MI, stroke, or transient ischemic attacks in post-MI patients with normal cholesterol levels—
Adults: initially, 10 or 20 mg P.O. h.s. Dosage adjusted q 4 weeks based on patient tolerance and response; maximum daily dosage is 40 mg.
Elderly: initially, 10 mg P.O. h.s. Most respond to daily dosage of 20 mg or less.

ADVERSE REACTIONS
CNS: headache, dizziness, fatigue.
CV: chest pain.
EENT: rhinitis.
GI: vomiting, diarrhea, heartburn, abdominal pain, constipation, flatulence, nausea.
GU: renal failure secondary to myoglobinuria, urinary abnormality.
Respiratory: cough, influenza, common cold.
Skin: rash.
Other: flulike symptoms, myositis, myopathy, *localized muscle pain,* myalgia, ***rhabdomyolysis.***

Reactions may be *common,* uncommon, *life-threatening,* or COMMON AND LIFE-THREATENING.

INTERACTIONS
Drug-drug. *Cholestyramine, colestipol:* concomitant administration decreases plasma levels of pravastatin. Administer pravastatin 1 hour before or 4 hours after these drugs.
Drugs that decrease levels or activity of endogenous steroids (such as cimetidine, ketoconazole, spironolactone): may increase risk of developing endocrine dysfunction. No intervention appears necessary; take complete drug history in patients who develop endocrine dysfunction.
Erythromycin, fibric acid derivatives (such as clofibrate, gemfibrozil), immunosuppressants (such as cyclosporine), high doses (1 g or more daily) of niacin (nicotinic acid): may increase the risk of rhabdomyolysis. Monitor patient closely if concomitant use cannot be avoided.
Gemfibrozil: decreases protein-binding and urinary clearance of pravastatin. Avoid concomitant use.
Hepatotoxic drugs: increased risk of hepatotoxicity. Avoid concomitant use.
Drug-lifestyle. *Alcohol use:* increased risk of hepatotoxicity. Avoid concomitant use.

EFFECTS ON DIAGNOSTIC TESTS
Serum ALT, AST, CK, alkaline phosphatase, and bilirubin levels are increased; thyroid function test is abnormal.

CONTRAINDICATIONS
Contraindicated in patients hypersensitive to drug; in those with active liver disease or conditions that cause unexplained, persistent elevations of serum transaminase levels; in pregnant and breast-feeding patients; and in women of childbearing age unless there is no risk of pregnancy.

NURSING CONSIDERATIONS
• Use cautiously in patients who consume large quantities of alcohol or have history of liver disease.
• Know that pravastatin should be initiated only after diet and other nonpharmacologic therapies prove ineffective. Patients should be on a standard low-cholesterol diet during therapy.
• Know that liver function tests should be performed at the start of therapy and periodically thereafter. A liver biopsy may be performed if liver enzyme elevations persist.

☑**Patient teaching**
• Instruct patient to take the recommended dosage in the evening, preferably at bedtime.
• Teach patient about proper dietary management of serum lipids. When appropriate, recommend weight-control, exercise, and smoking-cessation programs.
*Alert:*Inform female patient that drug is contraindicated during pregnancy. Advise her to notify doctor immediately if pregnancy occurs.

---

simvastatin (synvinolin)
Lipex‡, Zocor

Pregnancy Risk Category: X

HOW SUPPLIED
Tablets: 5 mg, 10 mg, 20 mg, 40 mg

ACTION
Inhibits 3-hydroxy-3-methylglutaryl coenzyme A reductase. This enzyme is an early (and rate-limiting) step in the synthetic pathway of cholesterol.

Route	Onset	Peak	Duration
PO	Unknown	1.3-2.4 hr	Unknown

INDICATIONS & DOSAGE
Reduction of low-density lipoprotein (LDL) and total cholesterol levels in patients with primary hypercholesterolemia (types IIa and IIb)—
Adults: initially, 5 to 10 mg P.O. daily in the evening. Dosage adjusted q 4 weeks based on patient tolerance and response; maximum daily dosage is 40 mg.
Elderly: initially, 5 mg P.O. daily in the evening. Maximum daily dosage is 20 mg.

ADVERSE REACTIONS
CNS: headache, asthenia.
GI: abdominal pain, constipation, diarrhea, dyspepsia, flatulence, nausea, vomiting.
Hepatic: elevated liver enzymes.

Respiratory: upper respiratory tract infection.

INTERACTIONS

Drug-drug. *Digoxin:* simvastatin may elevate digoxin levels slightly. Closely monitor plasma digoxin levels at initiation of simvastatin therapy.

Drugs that decrease levels or activity of endogenous steroids (such as cimetidine, ketoconazole, spironolactone): may increase risk of developing endocrine dysfunction. No intervention appears necessary; take complete drug history in patients who develop endocrine dysfunction.

Erythromycin, fibric acid derivatives (such as clofibrate, gemfibrozil), immunosuppressants (such as cyclosporine), high doses (1 g or more daily) of niacin (nicotinic acid): may increase risk of rhabdomyolysis. Monitor patient closely if concomitant use cannot be avoided. Limit daily dosage of simvastatin to 10 mg if the patient must take cyclosporine.

Hepatotoxic drugs: increased risk of hepatotoxicity. Avoid concomitant use.

Warfarin: anticoagulant effect may be slightly enhanced. Monitor INR at start of therapy and during dosage adjustments.

Drug-lifestyle. *Alcohol use:* increased risk of hepatotoxicity. Avoid concomitant use.

EFFECTS ON DIAGNOSTIC TESTS

As expected, simvastatin will reduce total plasma cholesterol, very-low-density lipoprotein, and LDL and may variably increase high-density lipoprotein (HDL). The ratios of total cholesterol to HDL, total cholesterol to LDL, and LDL to HDL are reduced. Modest decreases in triglycerides may also occur.

Toxic effects of drug may be evident by marked, persistent elevations of serum transaminases. During clinical trials, about 5% of patients had asymptomatic marked elevations in the noncardiac fraction of CK.

CONTRAINDICATIONS

Contraindicated in patients hypersensitive to drug; in those with active liver disease or conditions that cause unexplained persistent elevations of serum transaminase; in pregnant and breast-feeding patients; and in women of childbearing age unless there is no risk of pregnancy.

NURSING CONSIDERATIONS

• Use cautiously in patients who consume substantial quantities of alcohol or have a history of liver disease.

• Know that drug is initiated only after diet and other nonpharmacologic therapies prove ineffective. Patient should be on a standard low-cholesterol diet during therapy.

• Know that liver function tests should be performed at the start of therapy and periodically thereafter. A liver biopsy may be performed if enzyme elevations persist.

☑ **Patient teaching**

• Instruct patient to take drug with the evening meal; absorption is enhanced and cholesterol biosynthesis is greater.

• Teach patient about proper dietary management of serum lipids. When appropriate, recommend weight-control, exercise, and smoking-cessation programs.

• Tell patient to inform doctor if adverse reactions occur, particularly muscle aches and pains.

Alert: Inform female patient that drug is contraindicated during pregnancy. Advise her to notify doctor immediately if pregnancy occurs.

---

abciximab
alprostadil
arbutamine hydrochloride
clopidogrel bisulfate
dipyridamole
eptifibatide
midodrine hydrochloride
pentoxifylline
ticlopidine hydrochloride
tirofiban hydrochloride
tolazoline hydrochloride

COMBINATION PRODUCTS
None.

---

abciximab
ReoPro

Pregnancy Risk Category: C

HOW SUPPLIED
Injection: 2 mg/ml

ACTION
Binds to the glycoprotein IIb/IIIa (GPIIb/IIIa) receptor of human platelets and inhibits platelet aggregation.

Route	Onset	Peak	Duration
IV	Immediate	Immediate	48 hr

INDICATIONS & DOSAGE
Adjunct to percutaneous transluminal coronary angioplasty (PTCA) or atherectomy for the prevention of acute cardiac ischemic complications in patients at high risk for abrupt closure of the treated coronary vessel—
Adults: 0.25 mg/kg as an I.V. bolus administered 10 to 60 minutes before start of PTCA or atherectomy, followed by a continuous I.V. infusion of 10 mcg/minute for 12 hours.
Patients with unstable angina not responding to conventional medical therapy who are to undergo percutaneous coronary intervention within 24 hours—
Adults: 0.25 mg/kg as an I.V. bolus fol-

lowed by an 18- to 24-hour infusion of 10 mcg/minute, concluding 1 hour after percutaneous coronary intervention.

ADVERSE REACTIONS
CNS: hyperesthesia, hypoesthesia, confusion.
CV: *hypotension,* bradycardia, peripheral edema.
EENT: abnormal vision.
GI: *nausea, vomiting.*
Hematologic: *bleeding, **thrombocytopenia,*** anemia, leukocytosis.
Respiratory: pleural effusion, pleurisy, pneumonia.
Other: pain.

INTERACTIONS
Drug-drug. *Antiplatelet agents, dipyridamole, heparin, NSAIDs, other anticoagulants, thrombolytics, ticlopidine:* increased risk of bleeding. Monitor patient closely.

EFFECTS ON DIAGNOSTIC TESTS
None reported.

CONTRAINDICATIONS
Contraindicated in patients hypersensitive to drug, its ingredients, or murine proteins; in those with active internal bleeding, recent (within 6 weeks) GI or GU bleeding of clinical significance, history of CVA within past 2 years or CVA with significant residual neurologic deficit, bleeding diathesis, thrombocytopenia (under 100,000/mm^3), recent (within 6 weeks) major surgery or trauma, intracranial neoplasm, intracranial arteriovenous malformation, intracranial aneurysm, severe uncontrolled hypertension, or history of vasculitis; when oral anticoagulants have been administered within past 7 days unless PT is 1.2 times control or less; or with use of I.V. dextran before PTCA or intent to use it during PTCA.

NURSING CONSIDERATIONS
• Use with caution in patients at increased

risk for bleeding. Patients at risk include those weighing under 75 kg (165 lb), are over 65 years, have history of GI disease, or are receiving thrombolytic agents. Conditions that also increase patient's risk of bleeding include PTCA within 12 hours of onset of symptoms for acute MI, prolonged PTCA (lasting more than 70 minutes), or failed PTCA. Heparin used in conjunction with drug also may contribute to the risk of bleeding.

• Consider patients undergoing PTCA and with one or more of the following conditions candidates for drug therapy: unstable angina or a non–Q-wave MI, acute Q-wave MI within 12 hours of onset of symptoms, presence of two type B lesions in the artery to be dilated, presence of one type B lesion in the artery to be dilated in female patients over 65 years or in diabetic patients, presence of one type C lesion in the artery to be dilated, or angioplasty of an infarct-related lesion within 7 days of MI.

• Review and monitor concomitant medications, drug is intended for use with aspirin and heparin.

*Alert:*Keep epinephrine, dopamine, theophylline, antihistamines, and corticosteroids readily available in case anaphylaxis occurs.

• Monitor patient closely for bleeding. Bleeding associated with therapy falls into two broad categories: that observed at the arterial access site used for cardiac catheterization and internal bleeding involving the GI or GU tract, or retroperitoneal sites.

• Institute bleeding precautions. Maintain patient on bedrest for 6 to 8 hours following sheath removal or discontinuation of drug infusion, whichever is later. Minimize or avoid, if possible, arterial and venous punctures; I.M. injections; use of urinary catheters, nasogastric tubes, or automatic blood pressure cuffs; and nasotracheal intubation.

◖I.V. administration
• Inspect solution for particulate matter before administration. If visibly opaque particles occur, discard solution and obtain new vial. Withdraw necessary amount of drug for I.V. bolus injection through a sterile, nonpyrogenic, low-protein-binding 0.2- or 0.22-micron filter into a syringe. Administer I.V. bolus 10 to 60 minutes before procedure.

• Withdraw 4.5 ml of drug for continuous I.V. infusion through a sterile, nonpyrogenic, low-protein-binding 0.2- or 0.22-micron filter into a syringe. Inject into 250 ml of sterile 0.9% NaCl solution or D_5W, and infuse at a rate of 10 mcg/minute for 12 hours via a continuous infusion pump equipped with an in-line filter. Discard unused portion at end of 12-hour infusion.

• Administer drug in a separate I.V. line; no other medication should be added to the infusion solution.

☑Patient teaching
• Explain use and administration of drug to patient and family.
• Instruct patient to report adverse reactions immediately.

---

alprostadil
Prostin VR Pediatric

Pregnancy Risk Category: NR

HOW SUPPLIED
Injection: 500 mcg/ml

ACTION
A prostaglandin derivative that relaxes the smooth muscle of the ductus arteriosus.

Route	Onset	Peak	Duration
IV	20 min	1-2 hr	Length of infusion

INDICATIONS & DOSAGE
Palliative therapy for temporary maintenance of patency of ductus arteriosus until surgery can be performed—
Infants: 0.05 to 0.1 mcg/kg/minute by I.V. infusion. When therapeutic response is achieved, infusion rate reduced to lowest dosage that will maintain response. Maximum dosage is 0.4 mcg/kg/minute. Or, drug can be administered through umbilical artery catheter placed at ductal opening.

Reactions may be *common,* uncommon, *life-threatening,* or COMMON AND LIFE-THREATENING.

ADVERSE REACTIONS
CNS: *seizures.*
CV: bradycardia, hypotension, tachycardia, *cardiac arrest,* edema.
GI: diarrhea.
Hematologic: disseminated intravascular coagulation.
Other: APNEA, *flushing, fever, sepsis,* hypokalemia.

INTERACTIONS
None significant.

EFFECTS ON DIAGNOSTIC TESTS
None reported.

CONTRAINDICATIONS
No known contraindications.

NURSING CONSIDERATIONS
• Know that a differential diagnosis should be made between respiratory distress syndrome and cyanotic heart disease before drug is administered. Drug should not be used in neonates with respiratory distress syndrome.
• Use cautiously in neonates with bleeding tendencies because drug inhibits platelet aggregation.
• Keep respiratory support available.
• In infants with restricted pulmonary blood flow, measure drug's effectiveness by monitoring blood oxygenation. In infants with restricted systemic blood flow, measure drug's effectiveness by monitoring systemic blood pressure and blood pH.
• Monitor arterial pressure by umbilical artery catheter, auscultation, or Doppler transducer. Slow rate of infusion if arterial pressure falls significantly.
Alert: If apnea and bradycardia (may reflect drug overdose) occur, stop infusion immediately.
• Keep in mind that CV and CNS adverse reactions are more frequent in infants weighing under 2 kg (4.5 lb) and in those receiving infusions for longer than 48 hours.

🔲 I.V. administration
• Dilute drug before administering. Prepare fresh solution daily; discard solution after 24 hours.

• Do not use diluents that contain benzyl alcohol. Fatal toxic syndrome may occur.
• Reduce infusion rate if fever or significant hypotension occurs.
• Know that drug is not recommended for direct injection or intermittent infusion. Administer by continuous infusion using a constant-rate pump. Infuse through a large peripheral or central vein or through an umbilical artery catheter placed at the level of the ductus arteriosus. If flushing occurs from peripheral vasodilation, reposition catheter.

✅ Patient teaching
• Inform parents of the need for drug and explain its use.
• Encourage parents to ask questions and express concerns.

▼ *NEW DRUG*

arbutamine hydrochloride
GenESA

Pregnancy Risk Category: B

HOW SUPPLIED
Injection: 20-ml prefilled syringe containing 1 mg (0.05 mg/ml)

ACTION
A sympathomimetic that increases cardiac workload through both positive inotropic and chronotropic actions.

Route	Onset	Peak	Duration
IV	1 min	Unknown	Variable

INDICATIONS & DOSAGE
Single-dose diagnostic aid in patients with suspected coronary artery disease (CAD) who cannot exercise adequately (stress induction with arbutamine is indicated as an aid in diagnosing the presence or absence of CAD)—
Adults: 0.1 mcg/kg/minute for 1 minute via GenESA I.V. infusion system. The device adjusts dose until the maximal heart rate limit (set by user) is achieved or a maximum infusion rate of 0.8 mcg/kg/minute (maximum total dosage, 10 mcg/kg).

ADVERSE REACTIONS
CNS: anxiety, dizziness, fatigue, headache, hypoesthesia, pain, paresthesia, *tremor.*
CV: *angina pectoris,* ARRHYTHMIAS, chest pain, flushing, hypotension, hot flashes, palpitation, vasodilation.
EENT: dry mouth, taste perversion.
GI: nausea.
Respiratory: dyspnea.
Skin: increased sweating.

INTERACTIONS
Drug-drug. *Beta-blocking agents:* may attenuate arbutamine's effects. Discontinue drug at least 48 hours before administration of arbutamine.

EFFECTS ON DIAGNOSTIC TESTS
None reported.

CONTRAINDICATIONS
Contraindicated in patients with idiopathic hypertrophic subaortic stenosis, a history of recurrent sustained ventricular tachycardia, heart failure (New York Heart Association class III or IV), or with known hypersensitivity to drug. Also contraindicated in patients who have an implanted cardiac pacemaker or automated cardioverter or defibrillator, and in those receiving digoxin, atropine, other anticholinergic drugs, or tricyclic antidepressants.

NURSING CONSIDERATIONS
• Use cautiously in patients with a known sulfite allergy. Arbutamine contains sodium metabisulfite, a sulfite that may produce an allergic response in susceptible patients.
• Avoid use in patients with unstable angina, mechanical left ventricular outflow obstruction (such as severe valvular aortic stenosis), uncontrolled systemic hypertension, cardiac transplant, history of cerebrovascular disease, peripheral vascular disorder resulting in cerebral or aortic aneurysm, narrow-angle glaucoma, supraventricular tachyarrhythmias or ventricular arrhythmias, or uncontrolled hyperthyroidism, or in patients receiving class I antiarrhythmic agents such as quinidine, lidocaine, or flecainide.

• Safety and efficacy of arbutamine in patients with a recent history (within 30 days) of MI have not been evaluated; do not use in these patients.
• Do not administer atropine to enhance drug-induced chronotropic response; coadministration may lead to tachyarrhythmias.
Alert: Before using the GenESA system, it is essential to read and understand the manufacturer's directions for use.
• Monitor blood pressure, heart rate, and a diagnostic quality ECG continuously throughout drug infusion.
• A crash cart should be available by the bedside during drug administration.
• Transient prolongation of the corrected QT interval, as measured from a surface ECG, occurs with administration.
• Transient reductions in serum potassium concentrations may occur but rarely to hypokalemic levels.

⬛**I.V. administration**
• Drug is manufactured in a prefilled glass syringe and plunger rod.
Alert: Do not dilute before administration. Arbutamine should only be administered via the prefilled syringe using the GenESA system (a closed-loop, computer-controlled, I.V. infusion device). Syringe should be inspected before administration for evidence of particulate matter or discoloration.

☑**Patient teaching**
• Instruct patient on need to discontinue beta-blocking agents at least 48 hours before undergoing cardiac stress testing with arbutamine as ordered by doctor.
• Inform patient that drug will temporarily increase heart rate, but that he will be closely monitored.
• Inform patient of potential adverse events.

clopidogrel bisulfate
Plavix

Pregnancy Risk Category: B

HOW SUPPLIED
Tablets: 75 mg

ACTION

Inhibits platelet aggregation by inhibiting the binding of adenosine diphosphate (ADP) to its platelet receptor inhibiting ADP-mediated activation and subsequent platelet aggregation. Because clopidogrel acts by irreversibly modifying the platelet ADP receptor, platelets exposed to the drug are affected for their life span.

Route	Onset	Peak	Duration
PO	2 hr	Unknown	5 days

INDICATIONS & DOSAGE

To reduce atherosclerotic events in patients with atherosclerosis documented by recent CVA, MI, or peripheral arterial disease—
Adults: 75 mg P.O. daily.

ADVERSE REACTIONS

CNS: headache, dizziness, fatigue, depression.
CV: edema, hypertension.
EENT: rhinitis.
GI: *hemorrhage,* abdominal pain, dyspepsia, gastritis, constipation, diarrhea, ulcers.
GU: urinary tract infection.
Hematologic: purpura, epistaxis.
Respiratory: bronchitis, coughing, dyspnea, upper respiratory infection.
Skin: *rash,* pruritus.
Other: arthralgia, flu symptoms, pain.

INTERACTIONS

Drug-drug. *Aspirin, NSAIDs:* may increase risk for GI bleeding. Use cautiously.
Heparin, warfarin: safety has not been established. Use together cautiously.
Drug-herb. *Red clover:* possible increased risk of bleeding. Use together cautiously.

EFFECTS ON DIAGNOSTIC TESTS

None reported.

CONTRAINDICATIONS

Contraindicated in patients with pathologic bleeding (such as peptic ulcer or intracranial hemorrhage) and hypersensitivity to drug or its components.

NURSING CONSIDERATIONS

• Use with caution in patients at risk for increased bleeding from trauma, surgery, or other pathologic conditions and in patients with hepatic impairment.
• Be aware that platelet aggregation will not return to normal for at least 5 days after clopidogrel has been discontinued.
• Be aware that drug is usually used in patients who are hypersensitive or intolerant to aspirin or after stent placement.

☑ **Patient teaching**
• Inform patient it may take longer than usual to stop bleeding. Tell him to refrain from activities in which trauma and bleeding may occur and encourage him to wear a seatbelt when in a car.
• Instruct patient to notify doctor if unusual bleeding or bruising occurs.
• Tell patient to inform doctor or dentist that he is taking drug before having surgery or starting new drug therapy.
• Inform patient that drug may be taken without regard to meals.

---

dipyridamole
Apo-Dipyridamole†,
I.V. Persantine, Novo-Dipiradol†,
Persantin‡, Persantine**

Pregnancy Risk Category: B

HOW SUPPLIED
Tablets: 25 mg, 50 mg, 75 mg
Injection: 10 mg/2 ml

ACTION
Unknown, but may involve its ability to increase adenosine, which is a coronary vasodilator and platelet aggregation inhibitor.

Route	Onset	Peak	Duration
PO	Unknown	75 min	Unknown
IV	Unknown	2 min	Unknown

INDICATIONS & DOSAGE
Inhibition of platelet adhesion in prosthetic heart valves (in combination with warfarin or aspirin)—
Adults: 75 to 100 mg P.O. q.i.d.
Alternative to exercise in evaluation of

coronary artery disease during thallium myocardial perfusion scintigraphy—
Adults: 0.57 mg/kg as an I.V. infusion at a constant rate over 4 minutes (0.142 mg/kg/minute).
Acute coronary insufficiency—
Adults: 10 mg I.V. or I.M.

ADVERSE REACTIONS
CNS: *headache, dizziness.*
CV: flushing, syncope, hypotension; angina, chest pain, ***ECG abnormalities,*** blood pressure lability, hypertension (with I.V. infusion).
GI: *nausea,* vomiting, diarrhea, abdominal distress.
Skin: rash, irritation (with undiluted injection), pruritus.

INTERACTIONS
Drug-drug. *Heparin:* may increase risk of bleeding. Monitor closely.
Theophylline: may prevent the coronary vasodilation by I.V. dipyridamole; could lead to a false-negative thallium imaging result. Avoid concomitant use.

EFFECTS ON DIAGNOSTIC TESTS
Drug's physiologic effects on platelet aggregation will cause an increase in bleeding time.

CONTRAINDICATIONS
Contraindicated in patients with hypersensitivity to drug.

NURSING CONSIDERATIONS
• Use cautiously in patients with hypotension.
• If patient develops GI distress, administer drug 1 hour before meals or with meals.
• Observe for adverse reactions, especially with large doses. Monitor blood pressure.
• Observe for signs of bleeding; note prolonged bleeding time (especially with large doses or long-term therapy).
• Know that dipyridamole's value as part of an antithrombotic regimen is controversial; using it may not provide significantly better results than using aspirin alone.

⚕ I.V. administration
• If administering as a diagnostic agent, dilute in 0.45% or 0.9% NaCl or D_5W in at least a 1:2 ratio for a total volume of 20 to 50 ml. Inject ^{201}Tl within 5 minutes after completing the 4-minute dipyridamole infusion.

☑ Patient teaching
• Instruct patient to take drug exactly as prescribed.
• Tell patient to report adverse reactions promptly.
• Tell patient receiving drug I.V. to alert nurse if discomfort occurs at insertion site.

▼ *NEW DRUG*

eptifibatide
Integrilin

Pregnancy Risk Category: B

HOW SUPPLIED
Injection: 10-ml (2 mg/ml), 100-ml (0.75 mg/ml) vials

ACTION
Reversibly binds to the glycoprotein IIb/IIIa (GP IIb/IIIa) receptor on human platelets and inhibits platelet aggregation.

Route	Onset	Peak	Duration
IV	Immediate	Immediate	4-6 hr after end of infusion

INDICATIONS & DOSAGE
Treatment of patients with acute coronary syndrome (unstable angina or non-Q-wave MI), including patients who are to be managed medically and those undergoing percutaneous coronary intervention—
Adults: I.V. bolus of 180 mcg/kg (up to maximum dose of 22.6 mg) as soon as possible following diagnosis, followed by a continuous I.V. infusion of 2 mcg/kg/minute (up to maximum infusion rate of 15 mg/hour) for up to 72 hours. Infusion rate may be decreased to 0.5 mcg/kg/minute during percutaneous coronary intervention. Infusion should then be con-

tinued for an additional 20 to 24 hours after the procedure for up to 96 hours of therapy.
Treatment of patients not presenting with an acute coronary syndrome who are undergoing percutaneous coronary intervention—
Adults: I.V. bolus of 135 mcg/kg administered immediately before procedure, followed by a continuous infusion of 0.5 mcg/kg/minute for 20 to 24 hours.

ADVERSE REACTIONS
CV: hypotension.
GU: hematuria.
Hematologic: *bleeding,* ***thrombocytopenia.***
Other: bleeding at femoral artery access site.

INTERACTIONS
Drug-drug. *Clopidogrel, dipyridamole, NSAIDs, oral anticoagulants (warfarin), thrombolytics, ticlopidine:* increased risk of bleeding. Monitor patient closely.
Other inhibitors of platelet receptor IIb/IIIa: potential for serious bleeding. Do not administer together.

EFFECTS ON DIAGNOSTIC TESTS
None reported.

CONTRAINDICATIONS
Contraindicated in patients with known hypersensitivity to drug or its ingredients; history of bleeding diathesis or evidence of active abnormal bleeding within previous 30 days; severe hypertension (systolic blood pressure exceeding 200 mm Hg or diastolic blood pressure over 110 mm Hg) not adequately controlled on antihypertensive therapy; major surgery within previous 6 weeks; history of stroke within 30 days or history of hemorrhagic stroke; current or planned use of another parenteral GP IIb/IIIa inhibitor; platelet count below 100,000/mm^3; in patients whose serum creatinine is 2 mg/dl or higher (for the 180 mcg/kg bolus and 2 mcg/kg/minute infusion) or 4 mg/dl or higher (for the 135 mcg/kg bolus and 0.5 mcg/kg/minute infusion); or patients who are dependent on renal dialysis.

NURSING CONSIDERATIONS
• Use cautiously in patients at increased risk of bleeding and patients weighing over 143 kg (315 lb).
• Know that drug is intended for use with heparin and aspirin.
• Discontinue eptifibatide and heparin and achieve sheath hemostasis by standard compressive techniques at least 4 hours before hospital discharge.
• If patient is to undergo coronary artery bypass graft surgery, infusion should be stopped before surgery.
• Minimize use of arterial and venous punctures, I.M. injections, and the use of urinary catheters, nasotracheal tubes, and nasogastric tubes.
• When obtaining I.V. access, avoid use of noncompressible sites (such as subclavian or jugular veins).
• Monitor patient for bleeding.
• If patient's platelet count is below 100,000/mm^3, discontinue eptifibatide and heparin.
• Perform baseline laboratory tests before start of drug therapy; hematocrit, hemoglobin, and platelet count, serum creatinine level, PT, INR, and aPTT.
• Store vials in refrigerator at 36° to 46° F (2° to 8° C). Protect from light until administration.

◖ I.V. administration
• Withdraw bolus dose from 10-ml vial into a syringe and administer by I.V. push over 1 to 2 minutes. Administer I.V. infusion undiluted directly from 100-ml vial using an infusion pump.
• Inspect solution for particulate before administration. If visible particles occur, then the sterility is suspect; discard solution.
• Drug may be administered in same I.V. line as alteplase, atropine, dobutamine, heparin, lidocaine, meperidine, metoprolol, midazolam, morphine, nitroglycerin, or verapamil.
• Do not administer drug in same I.V. line as furosemide.
• Drug may be administered in same I.V. line with normal saline or 0.9% NaCl and 5% dextrose and may also contain up to 60 mEq/L of potassium chloride.

☑**Patient teaching**
• Explain that drug is a blood thinner used to prevent chest pain and heart attack.
• Explain that risk of serious bleeding is far outweighed by the benefits of drug.
• Instruct patient to report chest discomfort or other adverse events immediately.
• Caution patient to avoid activities that might cause bleeding or bruising.

---

midodrine hydrochloride
ProAmatine

Pregnancy Risk Category: C

HOW SUPPLIED
Tablets: 2.5 mg, 5 mg

ACTION
Midodrine forms an active metabolite, desglymidodrine, which is an alpha$_1$-agonist. It increases blood pressure by activating alpha-adrenergic receptors in arteriolar and venous vasculature.

Route	Onset	Peak	Duration
PO	Unknown	1-2 hr	Unknown

INDICATIONS & DOSAGE
Treatment of symptomatic orthostatic hypotension unresponsive to standard clinical care—
Adults: 10 mg P.O. t.i.d. Suggested dosing schedule: Dose 1 shortly before or upon arising in the morning; dose 2 at midday; and dose 3 in late afternoon but no later than 6 p.m.
Adjust-a-dose: In patients with abnormal renal function, initial dose of 2.5 mg is recommended.

ADVERSE REACTIONS
CNS: *paresthesia,* headache, confusion, anxiety.
CV: *supine hypertension, vasodilation.*
GU: urine retention, frequency, and urgency; *dysuria.*
Skin: *piloerection (goose bumps), pruritus,* rash.
Other: pain, chills, dry mouth.

INTERACTIONS
Drug-drug. *Alpha-adrenergic blockers:* may antagonize drug effects. Avoid concomitant use.
Alpha-adrenergics: enhanced vasopressor effects. Monitor blood pressure closely.
Beta blockers, cardiac glycosides, psychopharmacologic agents: may enhance or cause bradycardia, AV block, or arrhythmias. Avoid concomitant use.
Fludrocortisone acetate: may increase risk of supine hypertension. May also lead to increased intraocular pressure and worsened glaucoma. Monitor closely.

EFFECTS ON DIAGNOSTIC TESTS
None reported.

CONTRAINDICATIONS
Contraindicated in patients with severe organic heart disease, persistent and excessive supine hypertension, acute renal disease, urine retention, pheochromocytoma, or thyrotoxicosis.

NURSING CONSIDERATIONS
• Use cautiously in patients with history of urine retention, visual problems, diabetes, or renal or hepatic impairment and in breast-feeding women.
• Know that drug should be used in pregnancy only if the benefit justifies the potential risk to the fetus.
• Know that safety and effectiveness in children have not been established.
• Monitor supine and sitting blood pressures closely, and notify doctor if supine blood pressure increases excessively.
• Know that drug should be taken during the day when patient can be upright and performing activities of daily living. Space doses at least 3 hours apart. Midodrine should not be given after the evening meal or within 4 hours before bedtime, to reduce potential for supine hypertension during sleep.
• Be aware that midodrine should be continued only if patient experiences symptomatic improvement during initial therapy.
• Perform renal and hepatic tests before and during drug therapy as ordered.

☑**Patient teaching**
• Instruct patient about proper dosing intervals and to take last dose of the day 4 hours before bedtime.

Reactions may be *common,* uncommon, *life-threatening,* or COMMON AND LIFE-THREATENING.

• Tell patient to report symptoms of supine hypertension (cardiac awareness, pounding in ears, headache, blurred vision) immediately to doctor and to stop drug.
• Tell patient to consult doctor before taking OTC medications.

pentoxifylline
Trental

Pregnancy Risk Category: C

HOW SUPPLIED
Tablets (extended-release): 400 mg

ACTION
Unknown. Improves capillary blood flow probably by increasing RBC flexibility and lowering blood viscosity.

Route	Onset	Peak	Duration
PO	Unknown	1 hr	Unknown

INDICATIONS & DOSAGE
Intermittent claudication caused by chronic occlusive vascular disease—
Adults: 400 mg P.O. t.i.d. with meals. May decrease to 400 mg b.i.d. if GI and CNS adverse effects occur.

ADVERSE REACTIONS
CNS: headache, dizziness.
GI: dyspepsia, nausea, vomiting.

INTERACTIONS
Drug-drug. *Anticoagulants:* increased anticoagulant effect. Adjust anticoagulant dosage as ordered.
Antihypertensives: increased hypotensive effect. Dosage adjustments may be necessary.
Theophylline: may cause increase of theophylline level. Monitor closely.
Drug-lifestyle. *Smoking:* vasoconstriction may result. Advise patient to avoid smoking; it may worsen his condition.

EFFECTS ON DIAGNOSTIC TESTS
None reported.

CONTRAINDICATIONS
Contraindicated in patients who are intol-

erant to methylxanthines, such as caffeine, theophylline, and theobromine, and in those with recent cerebral or retinal hemorrhage.

NURSING CONSIDERATIONS
• Know that drug is useful in patients who are not good surgical candidates.
• Be aware that elderly patients may be more sensitive to drug's effects.

☑Patient teaching
• Advise patient to take with meals to minimize GI upset.
• Instruct patient to swallow medication whole, without breaking, crushing, or chewing.
• Tell patient to report GI or CNS adverse reactions; doctor may reduce the dosage.
• Inform patient not to discontinue drug during the first 8 weeks of therapy unless directed by doctor.

ticlopidine hydrochloride
Ticlid

Pregnancy Risk Category: B

HOW SUPPLIED
Tablets: 250 mg

ACTION
Unknown. An antiplatelet agent that probably blocks adenosine diphosphate-induced platelet-to-fibrinogen and platelet-to-platelet binding.

Route	Onset	Peak	Duration
PO	Unknown	2 hr	Unknown

INDICATIONS & DOSAGE
To reduce risk of thrombotic stroke in patients with history of stroke or who have experienced stroke precursors—
Adults: 250 mg P.O. b.i.d. with meals.

ADVERSE REACTIONS
CNS: dizziness, peripheral neuropathy.
CV: vasculitis.
EENT: conjunctival hemorrhage.
GI: *diarrhea,* nausea, dyspepsia, abdominal pain, anorexia, vomiting, flatulence, bleeding.

GU: hematuria, *nephrotic syndrome,* dark-colored urine.

Hematologic: *neutropenia, pancytopenia, agranulocytosis, immune thrombocytopenia.*

Hepatic: hepatitis, cholestatic jaundice, abnormal liver function tests.

Respiratory: *allergic pneumonitis.*

Skin: rash, pruritus, ecchymoses, maculopapular rash, urticaria, *thrombocytopenic purpura.*

Other: hypersensitivity reactions, postoperative bleeding, systemic lupus erythematosus, *serum sickness,* arthropathy, myositis, *hyponatremia.*

INTERACTIONS

Drug-drug. *Antacids:* decreased plasma ticlopidine levels. Separate administration times by at least 2 hours.

Aspirin: effects of aspirin on platelets potentiated. Avoid concomitant use.

Cimetidine: decreased clearance of ticlopidine and increased risk of toxicity. Avoid concomitant use.

Digoxin: slight decrease in serum digoxin levels. Monitor serum digoxin levels.

Theophylline: decreased theophylline clearance and risk of toxicity. Monitor closely and adjust theophylline dosage as ordered.

Drug-herb. *Red clover:* possible increased risk of bleeding. Use together cautiously.

EFFECTS ON DIAGNOSTIC TESTS

Pharmacologic effects of drug result in prolonged bleeding time. Toxic effects are evident in a decreased neutrophil or platelet count and elevated liver function tests. A positive antinuclear antibody titer has been reported rarely.

CONTRAINDICATIONS

Contraindicated in patients with severe hepatic impairment, hematopoietic disorders, active pathologic bleeding from peptic ulceration, active intracranial bleeding, or hypersensitivity to drug.

NURSING CONSIDERATIONS

• Use cautiously and with close monitoring of CBC and WBC differentials. Moderate to severe neutropenia and agranulocytosis have occurred in patients taking ticlopidine.

• Monitor baseline liver function tests before therapy.

• Determine CBC and WBC differentials at second week of therapy and repeat every 2 weeks until end of third month, as ordered.

• Monitor liver function tests and repeat if dysfunction is suspected.

• Know that thrombocytopenia has occurred rarely. Discontinue drug in patients with platelet count of 80,000/mm³ or less. If necessary, give methylprednisolone 20 mg I.V. to normalize bleeding time within 2 hours, as ordered.

• Know that when used preoperatively, ticlopidine may decrease incidence of graft occlusion in patients receiving coronary artery bypass grafts and reduce severity of drop in platelet count in patients receiving extracorporeal hemoperfusion during open heart surgery.

✓ Patient teaching

• Tell patient to take drug with meals.

• Warn patient to avoid aspirin and aspirin-containing products and to check with doctor or pharmacist before taking OTC medications.

• Explain that drug will prolong bleeding time and that unusual or prolonged bleeding should be reported. Advise patient to tell dentists and other doctors that he is taking ticlopidine.

• Stress importance of regular blood tests. Because neutropenia can result from increased risk of infection, tell patient to immediately report signs of infection, such as fever, chills, or sore throat.

• If ticlopidine is being substituted for a fibrinolytic or anticoagulant, tell patient to discontinue those drugs before starting ticlopidine therapy as ordered.

• Advise patient to discontinue drug 10 to 14 days before undergoing elective surgery, as ordered. Also tell patient to immediately report yellow skin or sclera, severe or persistent diarrhea, rashes, S.C. bleeding, light-colored stools, or dark urine.

Reactions may be *common,* uncommon, *life-threatening,* or COMMON AND LIFE-THREATENING.

▼ NEW DRUG

tirofiban hydrochloride
Aggrastat

Pregnancy Risk Category: B

HOW SUPPLIED
Injection: 50-ml vials (250 mcg/ml),
500-ml premixed vials (50 mcg/ml)

ACTION
Reversibly binds to the glycoprotein IIb/
IIIa (GP IIb/IIIa) receptor on human
platelets and inhibits platelet aggregation.

Route	Onset	Peak	Duration
IV	Immediate	Immediate	4-8 hr after end of infusion

INDICATIONS & DOSAGE
*Treatment of acute coronary syndrome, in
combination with heparin, including patients who are to be managed medically
and those undergoing percutaneous transluminal coronary angioplasty (PTCA) or
atherectomy—*
Adults: I.V. loading dose of 0.4 mcg/kg/
minute for 30 minutes followed by a continuous I.V. infusion of 0.1 mcg/kg/
minute. Continue infusion through angiography and for 12 to 24 hours after angioplasty or atherectomy.
Adjust-a-dose: In patients with renal insufficiency (creatinine clearance below
30 ml/minute), use a loading dose of
0.2 mcg/kg/minute for 30 minutes followed by a continuous infusion of
0.05 mcg/kg/minute. Continue infusion
through angiography and for 12 to 24
hours after angioplasty or atherectomy.

ADVERSE REACTIONS
CNS: dizziness, fever, headache.
CV: *bradycardia*, *coronary artery dissec-
tion,* edema.
GI: nausea, *occult bleeding.*
Hematologic: *bleeding, thrombocytope-
nia,* decreased hemoglobin and hemat-
ocrit.
Skin: sweating.
Other: bleeding at arterial access site,
pelvic pain, vasovagal reaction, leg pain.

INTERACTIONS
Drug-drug. *Clopidogrel, dipyridamole,
NSAIDs, oral anticoagulants (warfarin),
thrombolytics, ticlopidine:* increased risk
of bleeding. Monitor patient closely.
Levothyroxine, omeprazole: increased renal clearance of tirofiban. Monitor patient.

CONTRAINDICATIONS
Contraindicated in patients with known
hypersensitivity to drug or its ingredients;
in those with active internal bleeding or
history of bleeding diathesis within the
previous 30 days; history of intracranial
hemorrhage, intracranial neoplasm, arteriovenous malformation, or aneurysm; history of thrombocytopenia following prior
exposure to tirofiban; history of stroke
within 30 days or history of hemorrhagic
stroke; history, symptoms, or findings
suggestive of aortic dissection; severe hypertension (systolic blood pressure over
180 mm Hg or diastolic blood pressure
over 110 mm Hg); acute pericarditis; major surgical procedure or severe physical
trauma within previous month; or concomitant use of another parenteral GP
IIb/IIIa inhibitor.

NURSING CONSIDERATIONS
• Use cautiously in patients with increased risk of bleeding, including those
with hemorrhagic retinopathy or platelet
count below 150,000/mm³.
• Monitor hemoglobin and hematocrit and
platelet counts before starting therapy, 6
hours following loading dose, and at least
daily during therapy.
• Monitor patient for bleeding.
• Minimize injection and avoid noncom-
patible I.V. sites.
• Administer drug with concomitant aspirin and heparin.
• Know that safety and effectiveness have
not been studied in patients under 18
years.
• Notify doctor if thrombocytopenia occurs.
• Be aware that the most common adverse
effect is bleeding at the arterial access site
for cardiac catheterization.
• Store drug at room temperature. Protect
from light.

I.V. administration
• Dilute 50-ml injection vials (250 mcg/ml) to same strength as 500-ml premixed vials (50 mcg/ml) as follows: withdraw and discard 100 ml from a 500-ml bag of sterile 0.9% NaCl or D₅W and replace this volume with 100 ml of tirofiban injection (from two 50-ml vials) or withdraw 50 ml from a 250-ml bag of sterile 0.9% NaCl or D₅W and replace this volume with 50 ml of tirofiban injection, to achieve a concentration of 50 mcg/ml.
• Inspect solution for particulate matter before administration, and check for leaks by squeezing the inner bag firmly. If visible particles are present or if leaks occur, discard solution.
• Discard unused solution 24 hours following the start of infusion.
• Heparin and tirofiban can be administered through same I.V. catheter.

Patient teaching
• Explain that drug is a blood thinner that is used to prevent chest pain and heart attacks.
• Explain that risk of serious bleeding is far outweighed by the benefits of drug.
• Instruct patient to report chest discomfort or other adverse events immediately.
• Inform patient that frequent blood sampling may be needed to evaluate therapy.

---

tolazoline hydrochloride
Priscoline

Pregnancy Risk Category: C

HOW SUPPLIED
Injection: 25 mg/ml in 4-ml ampules

ACTION
Direct-acting vasodilator. May have some alpha-receptor blocking effects.

Route	Onset	Peak	Duration
IV	0.5 hr	Unknown	Unknown

INDICATIONS & DOSAGE
Persistent pulmonary hypertension in neonates—
Neonates: initially, 1 to 2 mg/kg I.V. over 10 minutes, followed by infusion of 1 to 2 mg/kg/hour.

ADVERSE REACTIONS
CV: *arrhythmias,* pain, *hypertension, flushing,* tachycardia, *hypotension.*
GI: nausea, vomiting, diarrhea, *GI hemorrhage.*
GU: edema, oliguria, hematuria.
Hematologic: leukopenia, *thrombocytopenia.*
Respiratory: *pulmonary hemorrhage.*
Skin: increased pilomotor activity with tingling and chilliness, rash.

INTERACTIONS
Drug-drug. *Vasopressors (epinephrine, norepinephrine):* may cause paradoxical fall in blood pressure. Monitor patient closely.

EFFECTS ON DIAGNOSTIC TESTS
None reported.

CONTRAINDICATIONS
Contraindicated in neonates with hypersensitivity to drug.

NURSING CONSIDERATIONS
• Use cautiously in patients with known or suspected mitral stenosis.
• Place patient in the supine position during infusion.
• Keep patient warm during parenteral administration.
Alert: Appearance of flushing usually indicates maximum tolerable dose.
• Monitor vital signs for blood pressure changes and arrhythmias.

I.V. administration
• Know that response should be evident within 30 minutes. Little information exists regarding infusions lasting longer than 48 hours.

Patient teaching
• Inform parents of need for drug and explain its use.
• Encourage parents to ask questions and express concerns.

26

Nonnarcotic analgesics and antipyretics

acetaminophen
aspirin
choline magnesium trisalicylate
    (choline salicylate and
    magnesium salicylate)
diflunisal
magnesium salicylate

COMBINATION PRODUCTS
ALLEREST NO-DROWSINESS TABLETS ◇,
COLDRINE, ORNEX NO DROWSINESS
CAPLETS ◇, SINUS-RELIEF TABLETS, SIN-
UTAB NO DROWSINESS ◇: acetaminophen
325 mg and pseudoephedrine hydrochlo-
ride 30 mg.
AMAPHEN, ANOQUAN, BUTACE, ENDOLOR,
ESGIC, FEMCET, FIORICET, ISOPAP, MEDI-
GESIC, REPAN, TENCET, TRIAD, TWO-DYNE:
acetaminophen 325 mg, caffeine 40 mg,
and butalbital 50 mg.
ASCRIPTIN, MAGNAPRIN: aspirin 325 mg,
magnesium hydroxide 50 mg, aluminum
hydroxide 50 mg, and calcium carbonate
50 mg ◇.
ASCRIPTIN A/D, MAGNAPRIN ARTHRITIS
STRENGTH: aspirin 325 mg, magnesium
hydroxide 75 mg, aluminum hydroxide
75 mg, and calcium carbonate 75 mg ◇.
BUFFERIN AF NITE TIME ◇, EXCEDRIN
P.M. ◇: acetaminophen 500 mg and
diphenhydramine citrate 38 mg.
CAMA ARTHRITIS PAIN RELIEVER: aspirin
500 mg, magnesium oxide 150 mg, and
aluminum hydroxide 150 mg.
DOAN'S P.M. EXTRA STRENGTH ◇: magnesium salicylate 500 mg and diphenhydramine 25 mg.
EXCEDRIN EXTRA STRENGTH ◇: aspirin
250 mg, acetaminophen 250 mg, and caffeine 65 mg.
FIORGEN, FIORINAL, ISOLLYL, LANORINAL,
MARNAL: aspirin 325 mg, caffeine 40 mg,
and butalbital 50 mg.
MIDRIN: isometheptene mucate 65 mg,
dichloralphenazone 100 mg, and acetaminophen 325 mg.
P-A-C TABLETS ◇: aspirin 400 mg and
caffeine 32 mg.

PHRENILIN: acetaminophen 325 mg and
butalbital 50 mg.
PHRENILIN FORTE: acetaminophen 650 mg
and butalbital 50 mg.
SINUS EXCEDRIN EXTRA STRENGTH ◇:
acetaminophen 500 mg and pseudoephedrine hydrochloride 30 mg.
SINUTAB ◇: acetaminophen 325 mg,
chlorpheniramine 2 mg, and pseudoephedrine hydrochloride 30 mg.
SINUTAB MAXIMUM STRENGTH ◇: acetaminophen 500 mg, pseudoephedrine hydrochloride 30 mg, and chlorpheniramine
maleate, 2 mg.
TECNAL†: aspirin 330 mg, caffeine 40 mg,
and butalbital 50 mg.
VANQUISH ◇: aspirin 227 mg, acetaminophen 194 mg, caffeine 33 mg, aluminum
hydroxide 25 mg, and magnesium hydroxide 50 mg.

acetaminophen (APAP, paracetamol)
Abenol† ◇; Aceta Elixir* ◇;
Acetaminophen Uniserts ◇; Aceta
Tablets ◇; Actamin ◇; Actamin
Extra ◇; Actimol† ◇; Aminofen ◇;
Aminofen Max ◇; Anacin-3 ◇;
Anacin-3 Extra Strength ◇; Apacet
Capsules ◇; Apacet Elixir* ◇;
Apacet Extra Strength Caplets ◇;
Apacet Extra Strength Tablets ◇;
Apacet, Infants' ◇; Apacet Regular
Strength Tablets ◇; Apo-
Acetaminophen† ◇; Arthritis Pain
Formula Aspirin Free ◇; Atasol
Caplets† ◇; Atasol Drops† ◇;
Atasol Forte Caplets† ◇; Atasol
Forte Tablets† ◇; Atasol Tablets† ◇;
Banesin ◇; Dapa ◇; Dapa X-S ◇;
Datril Extra-Strength; Dymadon‡ ◇;
Dymadon P‡ ◇; Exdol† ◇; Exdol
Strong† ◇; Feverall, Children's;
Feverall Junior Strength; Feverall
Sprinkle Caps, Children's; Feverall
Sprinkle Caps Junior Strength;
Genapap Children's Elixir ◇;

Genapap Children's Tablets ◊ ;
Genapap Extra Strength Caplets ◊ ;
Genapap Extra Strength Tablets ◊ ;
Genapap, Infants' ◊ ; Genapap
Regular Strength Tablets ◊ ;
Genebs Extra Strength Caplets ◊ ;
Genebs Regular Strength
Tablets ◊ ; Genebs X-Tra ◊ ; Halenol
Children's* ◊ ; Liquiprin Infants'
Drops ◊ ; Mapap, Children's* ◊ ;
Mapap, Infant Drops ◊ ; Meda
Cap ◊ ; Neopap ◊ ; Oraphen-PD ◊ ;
Panadol ◊ ; Panadol, Children's ◊ ;
Panadol Extra Strength ◊ ; Panadol,
Infants' ◊ ; Panadol Junior Strength
Caplets ◊ ; Panadol Maximum
Strength Caplets ◊ ; Panadol
Maximum Strength Tablets ◊ ;
Panamax‡ ◊ ; Paralgin‡ ◊ ;
Redutemp ◊ ; Robigesic† ◊ ;
Rounox† ◊ ; Snaplets-FR ◊ ; St.
Joseph Aspirin-Free Fever Reducer
for Children ◊ ; Suppap-120 ◊ ;
Suppap-325 ◊ ; Suppap-650 ◊ ;
Tapanol Extra Strength Caplets ◊ ;
Tapanol Extra Strength Tablets ◊ ;
Tempra ◊ ; Tempra Caplets ◊ ;
Tempra Chewable Tablets ◊ ;
Tempra Drops ◊ ; Tempra D.S. ◊ ;
Tempra, Infants' ◊ ; Tempra
Syrup ◊ ; Tylenol Caplets ◊ ; Tylenol
Children's Chewable Tablets ◊ ;
Tylenol Children's Elixir ◊ ; Tylenol
Children's Tablets ◊ ; Tylenol
Children's Drops ◊ ; Tylenol Elixir* ◊ ; Tylenol
Extended Relief ◊ ; Tylenol Extra
Strength Adult Liquid Pain
Reliever ◊ ; Tylenol Extra Strength
Caplets ◊ ; Tylenol Extra Strength
Gelcaps ◊ ; Tylenol Extra Strength
Tablets ◊ ; Tylenol, Infants' Drops;
Tylenol Infants' Suspension
Drops ◊ ; Tylenol Junior Strength
Caplets ◊ ; Tylenol Junior Strength
Tablets ◊ ; Tylenol Regular Strength
Caplets ◊ ; Tylenol Regular Strength
Tablets ◊ ; Tylenol Tablets ◊ ;
Valorin ◊ ; Valorin Extra ◊

Pregnancy Risk Category: B

HOW SUPPLIED
Tablets: 160 mg ◊ , 325 mg ◊ , 500 mg ◊ ,
650 mg ◊

Tablets (chewable): 80 mg ◊
Caplets: 160 mg, 500 mg ◊
Caplets (extended-release): 650 mg
Capsules: 500 mg ◊ , 325 mg ◊
Gelcaps: 500 mg ◊
Oral liquid: 160 mg/5 ml ◊ ,
500 mg/15 ml ◊
Oral solution: 48 mg/ml ◊ , 100 mg/ml ◊
Oral suspension: 120 mg/5 ml‡ ,
160 mg/5 ml ◊ , 80 mg/ml
Oral syrup: 16 mg/ml ◊
Elixir: 120 mg/5 ml, 160 mg/5 ml* ◊ ,
325 mg/5 ml* ◊ , 80 mg/5 ml
Sprinkles: 80 mg/capsule, 160 mg/
capsule
Suppositories: 80 mg ◊ , 120 mg ◊ ,
125 mg ◊ , 300 mg ◊ , 325 mg ◊ ,
650 mg ◊

ACTION
Unknown. Thought to produce analgesia
by blocking generation of pain impulses,
probably by inhibiting prostaglandin synthesis in the CNS or the synthesis or action of other substances that sensitize pain
receptors to mechanical or chemical stimulation. It is thought to relieve fever by
central action in the hypothalamic heat-
regulating center.

Route	Onset	Peak	Duration
PO, PR	Unknown	1-3 hr	3-4 hr

INDICATIONS & DOSAGE
Mild pain or fever—
Adults: 325 to 650 mg P.O. q 4 to 6
hours; or 1 g P.O. t.i.d. or q.i.d., p.r.n. Alternatively, two extended-release caplets
P.O. q 8 hours. Or, 650 mg P.R. q 4 to 6
hours, p.r.n. Maximum dosage should not
exceed 4 g daily. Dosage for long-term
therapy should not exceed 2.6 g daily.
Children over 14 years: 650 mg P.O. q 4
to 6 hours.
Children 12 to 14 years: 640 mg P.O. q 4
to 6 hours.
Children 11 years: 480 mg P.O. q 4 to 6
hours.
Children 9 to 10 years: 400 mg P.O. q 4
to 6 hours.
Children 6 to 8 years: 320 mg P.O. q 4 to
6 hours.
Children 4 to 5 years: 240 mg P.O. q 4 to
6 hours.

Children 2 to 3 years: 160 mg P.O. q 4 to 6 hours.

Children 12 to 23 months: 120 mg P.O. q 4 to 6 hours.

Children 4 to 11 months: 80 mg P.O. q 4 to 6 hours.

Children up to 3 months: 40 mg P.O. q 4 to 6 hours.

Children 6 to 12 years: 325 mg P.R. q 4 to 6 hours.

Children 3 to 6 years: 120 to 125 mg P.R. q 4 to 6 hours.

Children 1 to 3 years: 80 mg P.R. q 4 to 6 hours.

Children 3 to 11 months: 80 mg P.R. q 6 hours.

ADVERSE REACTIONS

Hematologic: hemolytic anemia, neutropenia, leukopenia, *pancytopenia, thrombocytopenia* (rare).

Hepatic: *severe liver damage* (with toxic doses), jaundice.

Skin: rash, urticaria.

Other: hypoglycemia.

INTERACTIONS

Drug-drug. *Barbiturates, carbamazepine, hydantoins, rifampin, sulfinpyrazone:* high doses or long-term use of these drugs may reduce therapeutic effects and enhance hepatotoxic effects of acetaminophen. Avoid concomitant use.

Warfarin: may increase hypoprothrombinemic effects with long-term use with high doses of acetaminophen. Monitor INR closely.

Zidovudine: may increase incidence of bone marrow suppression because of impaired zidovudine metabolism. Monitor patient closely.

Drug-herb. *Watercress:* may inhibit oxidative metabolism of acetaminophen. Avoid concomitant use.

Drug-food. *Caffeine:* may enhance analgesic effects of acetaminophen. Avoid concomitant use.

Drug-lifestyle. *Alcohol use:* increased risk of hepatic damage. Avoid concomitant use.

EFFECTS ON DIAGNOSTIC TESTS

Drug may cause a false-positive test result for urinary 5-hydroxyindoleacetic acid or interfere with home glucose testing.

CONTRAINDICATIONS

Contraindicated in patients with hypersensitivity to acetaminophen.

NURSING CONSIDERATIONS

● Use cautiously in patients with history of chronic alcohol use because hepatotoxicity has occurred after therapeutic doses.

● Many OTC products contain acetaminophen; be aware of this when calculating total daily dosage.

● Liquid form is recommended for children and for all patients who have difficulty swallowing.

● Know that acetaminophen may produce false-positive decreases in blood glucose levels in home monitoring systems.

☑**Patient teaching**

● Tell parents to consult doctor before giving drug to children under 2 years.

● Tell patient that drug is only for short-term use and to consult doctor if administering to children for more than 5 days or adults for more than 10 days.

● Tell patient not to use for self-medication of marked fever (over 103.1° F [39.5° C]), fever persisting longer than 3 days, or recurrent fever unless directed by doctor.

Alert: Warn patient that high doses or unsupervised long-term use can cause hepatic damage. Excessive ingestion of alcoholic beverages may increase the risk of hepatotoxicity.

● Tell breast-feeding patient that acetaminophen is found in breast milk in low concentrations (less than 1% of dose). Such patients may use it safely if therapy is short-term and does not exceed recommended doses.

---

aspirin (acetylsalicylic acid)
Artria S.R. ◇, ASA ◇,
Aspergum ◇, Aspro‡, Astrint† ◇,
Bayer Aspirin ◇, Bex‡,
Coryphen† ◇, Easprin ◇,
Ecotrin ◇, Empirin ◇,
Entrophen† ◇, Halfprin, Norwich
Extra Strength ◇, Novasen† ◇,
Solprin‡, Vincent's Powders‡,
Winsprin Capsules‡, ZORprin ◇

*Pregnancy Risk Category: C
(D in 3rd trimester)*

Route	Onset	Peak	Duration
PO (tablet)	5-30 min	25-40 min	1-4 hr
PO (buffered)	5-30 min	1-2 hr	1-4 hr
PO (extended)	5-30 min	1-4 hr	1-4 hr
PO (enteric-coated)	5-30 min	4-8 hr	1-4 hr
PO (solution)	5-30 min	15-40 min	1-4 hr
PR	Unknown	3-4 hr	1-4 hr

HOW SUPPLIED
Tablets: 325 mg ◇, 500 mg ◇
Tablets (chewable): 81 mg ◇
Tablets (enteric-coated): 165 mg,
325 mg ◇, 500 mg ◇, 650 mg ◇,
975 mg
Tablets (controlled-release): 800 mg
Tablets (timed-release): 650 mg ◇
Chewing gum: 227.5 mg ◇
Suppositories: 120 mg ◇, 200 mg ◇,
300 mg ◇, 600 mg ◇

ACTION
Produces analgesia by blocking prostaglandin synthesis (peripheral action). Aspirin and other salicylates may prevent the lowering of the pain threshold that occurs when prostaglandins sensitize pain receptors to mechanical and chemical stimulation. Exerts its anti-inflammatory effect by inhibiting prostaglandin synthesis; also may inhibit the synthesis or action of other mediators of the inflammatory response. Relieves fever by acting on the hypothalamic heat-regulating center to cause peripheral vasodilation. This increases peripheral blood supply and promotes sweating, which leads to heat loss and to cooling by evaporation. In low doses, aspirin also appears to impede clotting by blocking prostaglandin synthesis, which prevents formation of the platelet-aggregating substance thromboxane A_2.

INDICATIONS & DOSAGE
Rheumatoid arthritis, osteoarthritis, or other polyarthritic or inflammatory conditions—
Adults: initially, 2.4 to 3.6 g P.O. daily in divided doses. Maintenance dosage is 3.2 to 6 g P.O. daily in divided doses.
Juvenile rheumatoid arthritis—
Children: 60 to 110 mg/kg/day P.O. divided q 6 to 8 hours.
Mild pain or fever—
Adults and children over 11 years: 325 to 650 mg P.O. or P.R. q 4 hours, p.r.n.
Children 2 to 11 years: 10 to 15 mg/kg/dose P.O. or P.R. q 4 hours up to 80 mg/kg/day.
Prevention of thrombosis—
Adults: 1.3 g P.O. daily in two to four divided doses.
Reduction of risk of heart attack in patients with previous MI or unstable angina—
Adults: 160 to 325 mg P.O. daily.
Kawasaki syndrome (mucocutaneous lymph node syndrome)—
Adults: 80 to 180 mg/kg P.O. daily in four divided doses during the febrile phase. When fever subsides, dosage decreased to 10 mg/kg once daily, adjusted according to serum salicylate concentration.
Acute rheumatic fever—
Adults: 5 to 8 g daily.
Children: 100 mg/kg/day for 2 weeks, then 75 mg/kg/day for 4 to 6 weeks.

ADVERSE REACTIONS
EENT: *tinnitus, hearing loss.*
GI: *nausea,* GI distress, occult bleeding, dyspepsia, ***GI bleeding.***

Reactions may be *common,* uncommon, ***life-threatening,*** or COMMON AND LIFE-THREATENING.

Hematologic: leukopenia, *thrombocytopenia, prolonged bleeding time.*
Hepatic: abnormal liver function studies, *hepatitis.*
Skin: *rash,* bruising, urticaria.
Other: angioedema, hypersensitivity reactions, (*anaphylaxis,* asthma), *Reye's syndrome.*

INTERACTIONS
Drug-drug. *ACE inhibitors:* may decrease antihypertensive effects. Monitor blood pressure closely.
Ammonium chloride, other urine acidifiers: increased blood levels of aspirin products. Monitor for aspirin toxicity.
Antacids in high doses (and other urine alkalinizers): decreased levels of aspirin products. Monitor for decreased aspirin effect.
Anticoagulants: increased risk of bleeding. Avoid using together if possible.
Beta blockers: decreased antihypertensive effect. Avoid long-term aspirin use if patient is taking antihypertensives.
Corticosteroids: enhanced salicylate elimination. Monitor for decreased salicylate effect.
Methotrexate: increased risk of methotrexate toxicity. Avoid concomitant use.
Nizatidine: may increase risk of salicylate toxicity in patients receiving high doses of aspirin. Monitor closely.
NSAIDs, including diflunisal, fenoprofen, ibuprofen, indomethacin, meclofenamate, naproxen, piroxicam: altered pharmacokinetics of these agents, leading to lowered serum levels and decreased effectiveness. Avoid concomitant use.
NSAIDs, steroids: increased risk of GI bleeding. Avoid concomitant use.
Oral antidiabetic agents: increased hypoglycemic effect. Monitor closely.
Probenecid, sulfinpyrazone: decreased uricosuric effect. Avoid aspirin during therapy with these agents.
Valproic acid: may increase serum valproic acid concentrations. Avoid concomitant use.
Drug-herb. *Horse chestnut, kelpware, red clover:* increased risk of bleeding. Monitor patient closely for increased effects.

Drug-food. *Caffeine:* may increase the absorption of aspirin. Monitor for increased effects.
Drug-lifestyle. *Alcohol use:* increased risk of GI bleeding. Avoid concomitant use.

EFFECTS ON DIAGNOSTIC TESTS
Aspirin will cause an increased bleeding time. It interferes with urinary glucose analysis performed with Diastix, Chemstrip uG, Clinitest, and Benedict's solution, and with urinary 5-hydroxyindoleacetic acid and vanillylmandelic acid tests. Serum uric acid levels may be falsely increased. Aspirin may also interfere with the Gerhardt's test for urine acetoacetic acid.

CONTRAINDICATIONS
Contraindicated in patients with G6PD deficiency; bleeding disorders, such as hemophilia, von Willebrand's disease, or telangiectasia; NSAID-induced sensitivity reactions; or hypersensitivity to drug.

NURSING CONSIDERATIONS
• Use cautiously in patients with GI lesions, impaired renal function, hypoprothrombinemia, vitamin K deficiency, thrombocytopenia, thrombotic thrombocytopenic purpura, or severe hepatic impairment.
Alert: Because of epidemiologic association with Reye's syndrome, the Centers for Disease Control and Prevention recommends not giving salicylates to children or teenagers with chickenpox or flu-like illness.
• Be aware that for inflammatory conditions, rheumatic fever, and thrombosis, aspirin is administered on a scheduled, rather than as-needed basis.
• Know that because enteric-coated and sustained-release tablets are slowly absorbed, they are not suitable for rapid relief of acute pain, fever, or inflammation. They do cause less GI bleeding and may be more suited for long-term therapy, such as for the treatment of arthritis.
• For patient with swallowing difficulties, crush nonenteric-coated aspirin and dissolve in soft food or liquid. Administer

liquid immediately after mixing because drug will break down rapidly.
• For patients who cannot tolerate oral medications, ask doctor about the possibility of using aspirin rectal suppositories. Watch for rectal mucosal irritation or bleeding.
• Be aware that febrile, dehydrated children can develop toxicity rapidly.
• Monitor elderly patients closely because they may be more susceptible to aspirin's toxic effects.
• Monitor blood salicylate levels as indicated and ordered. Therapeutic blood salicylate level in arthritis is 10 to 30 mg/100 ml. Tinnitus may occur at plasma levels of 30 mg/100 ml and above, but this is not a reliable indicator of toxicity, especially in very young patients and those over age 60. With chronic therapy, mild toxicity may occur at plasma levels of 20 mg/100 ml.
• During prolonged therapy, hematocrit, hemoglobin level, PT, INR, and renal function should be assessed periodically as ordered.
• Know that aspirin irreversibly inhibits platelet aggregation. It should be discontinued 5 to 7 days before elective surgery as ordered to allow time for the production and release of new platelets.

☑**Patient teaching**
• Tell patient who is allergic to tartrazine dye to avoid aspirin.
• Advise patient on sodium-restricted diets that 1 tablet of buffered aspirin contains 553 mg of sodium.
• Advise patient to take with food, milk, antacid, or large glass of water to reduce adverse GI reactions.
• Tell patient that sustained-release or enteric-coated preparations should not be crushed or chewed but swallowed whole.
• Instruct patient to discard aspirin tablets with a strong vinegar-like odor.
• Tell patient to consult doctor if administering to children for more than 5 days or adults for more than 10 days.
• Advise patient receiving prolonged treatment with large doses of aspirin to watch for petechiae, bleeding gums, and signs of GI bleeding, and to maintain adequate fluid intake. Encourage use of a soft-bristled toothbrush.
• Because of the many possible drug interactions involving aspirin, warn patient taking prescription drugs to check with doctor or pharmacist before taking aspirin or OTC combination products containing aspirin.
• Inform female patient to avoid aspirin during last trimester of pregnancy unless specifically directed by doctor.
• Caution parents to keep out of reach of children—aspirin is one of the leading causes of poisoning in children. Encourage the use of child-resistant containers.

choline magnesium trisalicylate (choline salicylate and magnesium salicylate)
Trilisate

Pregnancy Risk Category: C

HOW SUPPLIED
Tablets: 500 mg, 750 mg, 1,000 mg of salicylate
Solution: 500 mg of salicylate/5 ml

ACTION
Produces analgesia by blocking prostaglandin synthesis (peripheral action). Salicylates may prevent the lowering of the pain threshold that occurs when prostaglandins sensitize pain receptors to mechanical and chemical stimulation. Exerts its anti-inflammatory effect by inhibiting prostaglandin synthesis. Relieves fever by acting on the hypothalamic heat-regulating center to produce peripheral vasodilation. This increases peripheral blood supply and promotes sweating, which leads to heat loss and to cooling by evaporation.

Route	Onset	Peak	Duration
PO	Unknown	1-2 hr	Unknown

INDICATIONS & DOSAGE
Rheumatoid arthritis and osteoarthritis or other polyarthritic or inflammatory conditions—

Adults: initially, 1.5 to 2.5 g P.O. daily as a single dose or in two or three divided doses. Dosage is adjusted according to patient response. Maintenance dosage range is 1 to 4.5 g daily.
Juvenile rheumatoid arthritis—
Children: 60 to 110 mg/kg/day P.O. in divided doses (q 6 to 8 hours).
Mild to moderate pain and fever—
Adults: 2 to 3 g P.O. daily in divided doses q 4 to 6 hours.
Children: for children weighing 37 kg (82 lb) or less, 50 mg/kg/day P.O. in divided doses b.i.d.; for those weighing over 37 kg, 2,250 mg/day.

ADVERSE REACTIONS
EENT: tinnitus, hearing loss.
GI: GI distress, nausea, vomiting.
Skin: rash.
Other: hypersensitivity reactions *(anaphylaxis), Reye's syndrome.*

INTERACTIONS
Drug-drug. *ACE inhibitors, beta blockers, diuretics:* effects of these agents may be decreased. Monitor patient closely.
Ammonium chloride, other urine acidifiers: increased blood levels of salicylates. Monitor for salicylate toxicity.
Antacids in high doses, other urine alkalinizers: decreased levels of salicylates. Monitor for decreased salicylate effect.
Corticosteroids: enhanced salicylate elimination. Monitor for decreased salicylate effect.
Methotrexate: increased risk of methotrexate toxicity. Avoid concomitant use.
Oral anticoagulants: increased risk of bleeding. Use together cautiously.
Steroids, other NSAIDs: enhanced risk of adverse GI effects. Avoid concomitant use.
Uricosuric agents: decreased uricosuric effect. Avoid concomitant use.
Drug-lifestyle. *Alcohol use:* enhanced risk of adverse GI effects. Avoid concomitant use.

EFFECTS ON DIAGNOSTIC TESTS
Choline salicylates may interfere with urinary glucose analysis performed via Diastix, Chemstrip uG, Clinitest, and Bene-

dict's solution. These drugs also interfere with urinary 5-hydroxyindoleacetic acid and vanillylmandelic acid.

CONTRAINDICATIONS
Contraindicated in patients with hemophilia, bleeding ulcers, hemorrhagic states, or hypersensitivity to drug.

NURSING CONSIDERATIONS
● Use cautiously in patients with renal insufficiency, hepatic impairment, peptic ulcer disease, and gastritis.
Alert: Because of epidemiologic association with Reye's syndrome, the Centers for Disease Control and Prevention recommends not giving salicylates to children or teenagers with chickenpox or flu-like illness.
● Be aware that febrile, dehydrated children can develop toxicity rapidly.
● Monitor serum salicylate levels in long-term therapy. Therapeutic blood salicylate level in arthritis is 15 to 30 mg/100 ml. Tinnitus may occur at plasma levels of 30 mg/100 ml and above, but this is not a reliable indicator of toxicity, especially in the very young and those over 60 years. In chronic therapy, mild toxicity may occur at plasma levels of 20 mg/100 ml.
● Periodically monitor hemoglobin level, PT, and INR in patients receiving long-term treatment with large doses.
● Know that drug causes less GI distress than aspirin. If an antacid is needed, give it 2 hours after meals and choline magnesium trisalicylate before meals.

☑ **Patient teaching**
● Tell patient to take tablets with food and to take solution with a full glass of water. Solution may be mixed with fruit juice, but not antacids.
● Warn patient not to take drug longer than prescribed or to increase dosage without consulting doctor.

diflunisal
Dolobid

Pregnancy Risk Category: C

HOW SUPPLIED
Tablets: 250 mg, 500 mg

ACTION
Unknown. Probably related to inhibition of prostaglandin synthesis.

Route	Onset	Peak	Duration
PO	1 hr	2-3 hr	8-12 hr

INDICATIONS & DOSAGE
Osteoarthritis and rheumatoid arthritis—
Adults: 500 to 1,000 mg P.O. daily in two divided doses, usually q 12 hours. Maximum dosage is 1,500 mg daily.
Elderly: in patients over 65 years, one-half usual adult dose.
Mild to moderate pain—
Adults: 1 g P.O. followed by 500 mg q 8 to 12 hours. A lower dose of 500 mg P.O. followed by 250 mg q 8 to 12 hours may be appropriate.

ADVERSE REACTIONS
CNS: dizziness, somnolence, insomnia, *headache*, fatigue.
EENT: tinnitus, visual disturbances (rare).
GI: nausea, dyspepsia, GI pain, diarrhea, vomiting, constipation, flatulence.
GU: renal impairment, hematuria, ***interstitial nephritis.***
Skin: rash, pruritus, sweating, stomatitis, erythema multiforme, ***Stevens-Johnson syndrome.***

INTERACTIONS
Drug-drug. *Acetaminophen, hydrochlorothiazide, indomethacin:* diflunisal may substantially increase blood levels, increasing the risk of toxicity. Avoid concomitant use.
Antacids, aspirin: decreased diflunisal blood levels. Monitor for possible decreased therapeutic effect.
Anticoagulants, thrombolytic agents: diflunisal may enhance pharmacologic effects of these agents. Use together cautiously.
Cyclosporine: diflunisal may enhance the nephrotoxicity of cyclosporine. Avoid concomitant use.
Methotrexate: diflunisal may enhance the toxicity of methotrexate. Avoid concomitant use.
Sulindac: diflunisal decreases blood levels of sulindac's active metabolite. Monitor for reduced effect.

EFFECTS ON DIAGNOSTIC TESTS
Physiologic effects of the drug may prolong bleeding time; increase serum BUN, creatinine, and potassium levels; decrease serum uric acid; and increase liver function tests.

CONTRAINDICATIONS
Contraindicated in patients with hypersensitivity to drug or for whom acute asthmatic attacks, urticaria, or rhinitis are precipitated by aspirin or other NSAIDs.

NURSING CONSIDERATIONS
• Use cautiously in GI bleeding, history of peptic ulcer disease, renal impairment, and compromised cardiac function, hypertension, or other conditions predisposing patient to fluid retention.
Alert: Because of the epidemiologic association with Reye's syndrome, the Centers for Disease Control and Prevention recommends not giving salicylates to children and teenagers with chickenpox or flulike illness.

✓Patient teaching
• Advise patient to take with water, milk, or meals.
• Tell patient that tablets must be swallowed whole.
• Instruct patient to avoid aspirin or acetaminophen while using diflunisal unless ordered.
• Inform breast-feeding patient that drug is excreted in breast milk and that a decision should be made to discontinue either breast-feeding or drug.

Reactions may be *common*, uncommon, *life-threatening*, or COMMON AND LIFE-THREATENING.

magnesium salicylate
Doan's, Doan's P.M.
Extra-Strength† ◊, Magan ◊,
Mobidin ◊

Pregnancy Risk Category: C

HOW SUPPLIED
Tablets: 545 mg, 600 mg
Caplets: 325 mg ◊, 500 mg ◊

ACTION
Produces analgesia by blocking prostaglandin synthesis (peripheral action). Salicylates may prevent the lowering of the
pain threshold that occurs when prostaglandins sensitize pain receptors to mechanical and chemical stimulation. Exerts
its anti-inflammatory effect by inhibiting
prostaglandin synthesis. Relieves fever by
acting on the hypothalamic heat-regulating center to produce peripheral vasodilation. This increases peripheral blood supply and promotes sweating, which leads
to heat loss and to cooling by evaporation.

Route	Onset	Peak	Duration
PO	Unknown	1.5-2 hr	Unknown

INDICATIONS & DOSAGE
Arthritis—
Adults: 545 mg to 1.2 g P.O. t.i.d. or
q.i.d.
Mild pain or fever—
Adults and children over 11 years: 300
to 600 mg P.O. q 4 hours, not to exceed
3.5 g daily.

ADVERSE REACTIONS
EENT: tinnitus, hearing loss.
GI: nausea, vomiting, *GI distress.*
Hepatic: abnormal liver function studies,
hepatitis.
Skin: rash, bruising.
Other: hypersensitivity reactions (*ana-
phylaxis,* asthma), *Reye's syndrome.*

INTERACTIONS
Drug-drug. *ACE inhibitors, beta blockers, diuretics, uricosuric agents:* effects of
these drugs may be decreased. Monitor
patient closely.
Ammonium chloride, other urine acidi-
fiers: increased blood levels of salicylates. Monitor for salicylate toxicity.
*Antacids in high doses, other urine alka-
linizers:* decreased levels of salicylates.
Monitor for decreased salicylate effect.
Anticoagulants: increased risk of bleeding. Avoid using together.
Corticosteroids: enhanced salicylate elimination. Monitor for decreased salicylate
effect.
Methotrexate: increased risk of methotrexate toxicity. Avoid concomitant use.
Other NSAIDs, steroids: increased risk of
GI bleeding. Avoid concomitant use.
Drug-lifestyle. *Alcohol use:* increased
risk of GI bleeding. Avoid concomitant
use.

EFFECTS ON DIAGNOSTIC TESTS
In high doses, drug may cause false-
positive urine glucose test results using
copper sulfate method; it may cause false-
negative urine glucose test results using
glucose enzymatic method. False increases or decreases have been seen in urine
vanillylmandelic acid tests; false increases in serum uric acid have been seen.
Magnesium salicylate may interfere with
the Gerhardt's test for urine acetoacetic
acid. Magnesium salicylate may increase
serum levels of AST, ALT, alkaline phosphatase, and bilirubin.

CONTRAINDICATIONS
Contraindicated in patients with bleeding
disorders, severe chronic renal insufficiency because of risk of magnesium toxicity, or hypersensitivity to drug or aspirin.

NURSING CONSIDERATIONS
• Use cautiously in hypoprothrombinemia
and vitamin K deficiency.
Alert: Because of epidemiologic association with Reye's syndrome, the Centers
for Disease Control and Prevention recommends not giving salicylates to children or teenagers with chickenpox or flulike illness.
• Know that febrile, dehydrated children
can develop toxicity rapidly.
• Monitor serum salicylate levels when
drug is used long term, as ordered. Therapeutic blood salicylate level in arthritis is

10 to 30 mg/100 ml. Tinnitus may occur at plasma levels of 30 mg/100 ml and above, but this is not a reliable indicator of toxicity, especially in very young patients and those over 60 years. With chronic therapy, mild toxicity may occur at plasma levels of 20 mg/100 ml.

• Monitor hemoglobin level, PT, and INR in long-term treatment with large doses.

☑ **Patient teaching**

• Advise patient that the risk of GI irritation can be reduced by taking the drug with food, milk, antacid, or a large glass of water.

• Instruct patients not to crush or cut tablets and caplets.

27
Nonsteroidal anti-inflammatory drugs

diclofenac sodium
diclofenac potassium
etodolac
fenoprofen calcium
flurbiprofen
ibuprofen
indomethacin
indomethacin sodium trihydrate
ketoprofen
ketorolac tromethamine
nabumetone
naproxen
naproxen sodium
oxaprozin
piroxicam
sulindac

COMBINATION PRODUCTS

ADVIL COLD AND SINUS CAPLETS ◊,
DIMETAPP SINUS CAPLETS, DRISTAN SINUS
CAPLETS ◊, MOTRIN IB SINUS, SINE-AID
IB CAPLETS: pseudoephedrine hydrochloride 30 mg and ibuprofen 200 mg.

---

diclofenac sodium
Diclomax Retard§, Fenac‡,
Voltaren, Voltaren XR, Voltaren
Rapide†, Voltaren SR†, Voltarol§

diclofenac potassium
Cataflam

Pregnancy Risk Category: B

HOW SUPPLIED
Tablets: 50 mg
Tablets (enteric-coated): 25 mg, 50 mg,
75 mg
Tablets (extended-release): 100 mg
Suppositories: 50 mg†, 100 mg†

ACTION
Unknown. Produces anti-inflammatory,
analgesic, and antipyretic effects, possibly
by inhibiting prostaglandin synthesis.

Route	Onset	Peak	Duration
PO, PR	10 min	1 hr	8 hr
PO (enteric)	30 min	2-3 hr	8 hr

INDICATIONS & DOSAGE
Ankylosing spondylitis—
Adults: 25 mg P.O. q.i.d. (and h.s., p.r.n.)
Osteoarthritis—
Adults: 50 mg P.O. b.i.d. or t.i.d., or
75 mg P.O. b.i.d. (diclofenac sodium
only).
Rheumatoid arthritis—
Adults: 50 mg P.O. t.i.d. or q.i.d. Alternatively, 75 mg P.O. b.i.d. (diclofenac sodium only) or 50 to 100 mg P.R. (where
available) h.s. as substitute for last oral
dose of the day. Not to exceed 225 mg
daily.
Analgesia and primary dysmenorrhea—
Adults: 50 mg P.O. t.i.d. (diclofenac
potassium only).

ADVERSE REACTIONS
CNS: anxiety, depression, dizziness,
drowsiness, insomnia, irritability,
headache.
CV: *heart failure,* hypertension, edema,
fluid retention.
EENT: tinnitus, *laryngeal edema,*
swelling of the lips and tongue, blurred
vision, eye pain, night blindness, epistaxis, taste disorder, reversible hearing
loss.
GI: abdominal pain or cramps, constipation, diarrhea, indigestion, nausea, abdominal distention, flatulence, peptic ulceration, *bleeding,* melena, bloody diarrhea, appetite change, colitis.
GU: proteinuria, *acute renal failure,*
oliguria, interstitial nephritis, papillary
necrosis, *nephrotic syndrome,* fluid retention.
Hepatic: elevated liver enzymes, jaundice, *hepatitis, hepatotoxicity.*
Respiratory: asthma.
Skin: rash, pruritus, urticaria, eczema,
dermatitis, alopecia, photosensitivity, bul-

---

lous eruption, *Stevens-Johnson syndrome* (rare), allergic purpura.
Other: *anaphylaxis; anaphylactoid reactions;* angioedema; back, leg, or joint pain; hypoglycemia; hyperglycemia.

INTERACTIONS
Drug-drug. *Anticoagulants (including warfarin):* possible increased incidence of bleeding. Monitor patient closely.
Aspirin: may decrease effectiveness of diclofenac. May increase GI toxicity. Concomitant use not recommended by manufacturer.
Beta blockers: antihypertensive effects may be blunted. Monitor closely.
Cyclosporine, lithium, methotrexate: diclofenac may reduce renal clearance of these drugs and increase risk of toxicity. Monitor patient closely.
Diuretics: decreased effectiveness of diuretics. Avoid concomitant use.
Insulin, oral antidiabetic agents: diclofenac may alter requirements for antidiabetic agents. Monitor patient closely.
Phenytoin: increased serum levels. Monitor for toxicity.
Potassium-sparing diuretics: enhanced potassium retention and increased serum potassium levels. Monitor serum potassium level.
Drug-lifestyle. *Sun exposure:* may cause photosensitivity reactions. Take precautions.

EFFECTS ON DIAGNOSTIC TESTS
Drug increases plasma aggregation time but does not alter bleeding time, plasma thrombin clotting time, INR, plasma fibrinogen, or factors V and VII to XII.

CONTRAINDICATIONS
Contraindicated in patients with hepatic porphyria; history of asthma, urticaria, or other allergic reactions after taking aspirin or other NSAIDs; and hypersensitivity to drug. Drug is not recommended for use during late pregnancy or breast-feeding.

NURSING CONSIDERATIONS
• Use cautiously in patients with history of peptic ulcer disease, hepatic dysfunction, cardiac disease, hypertension, conditions associated with fluid retention, or impaired renal function.
• Because NSAIDs impair the synthesis of renal prostaglandins, they can decrease renal blood flow and lead to reversible renal impairment, especially in patients with preexisting renal failure, liver dysfunction, or heart failure; in elderly patients; and in those taking diuretics. Monitor these patients closely.
• Elevations of liver tests may occur during therapy. Monitor serum transaminase, especially ALT levels, periodically in patients undergoing long-term therapy as ordered. Know that the first serum transaminase measurement should be no later than 8 weeks after initiation of therapy.
• Be aware that because of their antipyretic and anti-inflammatory actions, NSAIDs may mask the signs and symptoms of infection.

☑**Patient teaching**
• Tell patient to take drug with milk or meals to minimize GI distress.
• Instruct patient not to crush, break, or chew enteric-coated tablets.
• Serious GI toxicity, including peptic ulceration and bleeding, can occur in patients taking NSAIDs despite the absence of GI symptoms. Teach patient signs and symptoms of GI bleeding, and tell him to contact doctor immediately if these occur.
• Teach patient the signs and symptoms of hepatotoxicity, including nausea, fatigue, lethargy, pruritus, jaundice, right upper quadrant tenderness, and flulike symptoms. Tell him to contact doctor immediately if these symptoms appear.
• Advise patient to avoid consumption of alcoholic beverages or aspirin while taking diclofenac.
• Tell patient to wear sunscreen or protective clothing because drug may cause photosensitivity reactions.
• Warn patient to avoid hazardous activities that require alertness until adverse CNS effects of drug are known.
• Tell patient to avoid use during last trimester of pregnancy.

Reactions may be *common*, uncommon, *life-threatening*, or COMMON AND LIFE-THREATENING.

etodolac
Lodine, Lodine XL

Pregnancy Risk Category: C

HOW SUPPLIED
Capsules: 200 mg, 300 mg
Tablets: 400 mg, 500 mg
Tablets (extended-release): 400 mg, 500 mg, 600 mg

ACTION
Unknown, but believed related to inhibition of prostaglandin biosynthesis.

Route	Onset	Peak	Duration
PO	30 min	1-2 hr	4-12 hr
PO (extended)	Unknown	3-12 hr	6-12 hr

INDICATIONS & DOSAGE
Acute and chronic management of osteoarthritis, rheumatoid arthritis, and pain—
Adults: 200 to 400 mg P.O. q 6 to 8 hours, p.r.n., not to exceed 1,200 mg daily. For patients weighing 60 kg (132 lb) or less, don't exceed total daily dose of 20 mg/kg.

ADVERSE REACTIONS
CNS: asthenia, malaise, dizziness, depression, drowsiness, nervousness, insomnia.
CV: hypertension, *heart failure,* syncope, flushing, palpitations, edema, fluid retention.
EENT: blurred vision, tinnitus, photophobia, dry mouth.
GI: *dyspepsia,* flatulence, abdominal pain, diarrhea, nausea, constipation, gastritis, melena, vomiting, anorexia, peptic ulceration with or without *GI bleeding* or *perforation,* ulcerative stomatitis, thirst.
GU: dysuria, urinary frequency, *renal failure.*
Hematologic: anemia (rare), leukopenia, *thrombocytopenia,* hemolytic anemia, *agranulocytosis.*
Hepatic: hepatitis.
Respiratory: asthma.
Skin: pruritus, rash, *Stevens-Johnson syndrome.*

Other: chills, fever, weight gain.

INTERACTIONS
Drug-drug. *Antacids:* may decrease peak levels of drug. Monitor for decreased effect of etodolac.
Aspirin: reduced protein-binding of etodolac without altering its clearance. Clinical significance unknown. May increase GI toxicity. Avoid concomitant use.
Beta blockers, diuretics: effects may be blunted. Monitor closely.
Cyclosporine: impaired elimination and increased risk of nephrotoxicity. Avoid concomitant use.
Digoxin, lithium, methotrexate: etodolac may impair elimination of these drugs, resulting in increased levels and risk of toxicity. Monitor blood levels.
Phenytoin: increased serum levels of phenytoin. Monitor for toxicity.
Warfarin: etodolac decreases the protein-binding of warfarin but does not change its clearance. Although no dosage adjustment is necessary, monitor INR closely and watch for bleeding.
Drug-lifestyle. *Alcohol use:* increased chance of adverse effects. Avoid use.
Sun exposure: photosensitivity reactions may occur; take precautions.

EFFECTS ON DIAGNOSTIC TESTS
A false-positive test for urinary bilirubin may be caused by phenolic metabolites. Decreased serum uric acid levels and borderline elevations of one or more liver test results may occur.

CONTRAINDICATIONS
Contraindicated in patients with hypersensitivity to drug and in those with history of aspirin- or NSAID-induced asthma, rhinitis, urticaria, or other allergic reactions.

NURSING CONSIDERATIONS
• Use cautiously in patients with history of GI bleeding, ulceration, and perforation and renal or hepatic impairment.
• Because NSAIDs impair the synthesis of renal prostaglandins, they can decrease renal blood flow and lead to reversible renal impairment, especially in patients with preexisting renal failure, liver dys-

function, or heart failure; in elderly patients; and in those taking diuretics. Monitor these patients closely during therapy.
Alert: Know that drug appears to cause fewer GI problems than most NSAIDs. Minimal GI blood loss has been reported at dosages up to 1,200 mg daily.

☑ **Patient teaching**
• Tell patient to take drug with milk or meals to minimize GI discomfort.
• Serious GI toxicity, including peptic ulceration and bleeding, can occur in patient taking NSAIDs despite the absence of GI symptoms. Teach patient signs and symptoms of GI bleeding, and tell him to contact doctor immediately if they occur.
• Advise patient to avoid consumption of alcoholic beverages or aspirin while taking drug.
• Warn patient to avoid hazardous activities that require alertness until adverse CNS effects of drug are known.
• Advise patient to use a sunblock, wear protective clothing, and avoid prolonged exposure to sunlight to avoid photosensitivity reactions.
• Tell patient to avoid use during last trimester of pregnancy.

---

fenoprofen calcium
Fenopron§, Nalfon

Pregnancy Risk Category: NR

HOW SUPPLIED
Tablets: 600 mg
Capsules: 200 mg, 300 mg

ACTION
Unknown. Produces anti-inflammatory, analgesic, and antipyretic effects, possibly by inhibiting prostaglandin synthesis.

Route	Onset	Peak	Duration
PO	15-30 min	2 hr	4-6 hr

INDICATIONS & DOSAGE
Rheumatoid arthritis and osteoarthritis—
Adults: 300 to 600 mg P.O. t.i.d. or q.i.d. Maximum dosage is 3.2 g daily.
Mild to moderate pain—
Adults: 200 mg P.O. q 4 to 6 hours, p.r.n.

ADVERSE REACTIONS
CNS: *headache,* dizziness, *somnolence,* fatigue, nervousness, asthenia, tremor, confusion.
CV: peripheral edema, palpitations.
EENT: tinnitus, blurred vision, decreased hearing.
GI: epigastric distress, nausea, *GI bleeding,* vomiting, occult blood loss, peptic ulceration, constipation, anorexia, dyspepsia, flatulence.
GU: oliguria, interstitial nephritis, proteinuria, *reversible renal failure, papillary necrosis,* cystitis, hematuria.
Hematologic: prolonged bleeding time, anemia, *aplastic anemia, agranulocytosis, thrombocytopenia, hemorrhage,* bruising, hemolytic anemia.
Hepatic: elevated enzymes, hepatitis.
Respiratory: dyspnea, upper respiratory tract infections, nasopharyngitis.
Skin: pruritus, rash, urticaria, *anaphylaxis,* increased diaphoresis.
Other: *angioedema.*

INTERACTIONS
Drug-drug. *Aspirin:* decreased fenoprofen half-life; may increase GI toxicity. Avoid concomitant use.
Corticosteroids: increased risk of adverse GI reactions. Avoid concomitant use.
Diuretics: decreased diuretic effectiveness. Monitor patient closely.
Oral anticoagulants, sulfonylureas: fenoprofen enhances pharmacologic effects of these drugs. Use together cautiously.
Phenobarbital: enhanced metabolism of fenoprofen. Monitor for lack of fenoprofen effectiveness.
Drug-lifestyle. *Alcohol use:* increased risk of adverse GI reactions. Avoid concomitant use.

EFFECTS ON DIAGNOSTIC TESTS
Physiologic effects of drug may increase bleeding time, BUN, serum creatinine, potassium, alkaline phosphatase, LD, and transaminase levels. Fenoprofen or its metabolite may cross-react with the antibody used in the Amerlex-M assay. Limited data suggest that drug may alter free and total T_3 concentrations determined by the Corning method. Drug may cause false elevations in both free and total

---

Reactions may be *common*, uncommon, *life-threatening*, or COMMON AND LIFE-THREATENING.

serum T_3, but thyroid-stimulating hormone and thyroxine are unaffected.

CONTRAINDICATIONS
Contraindicated in patients with history of aspirin- or NSAID-induced asthma or rhinitis, significantly impaired renal function, or hypersensitivity to drug and during pregnancy.

NURSING CONSIDERATIONS
• Use cautiously in elderly patients; in patients with history of serious GI events or peptic ulcer disease, compromised cardiac function or hypertension.
• Be aware that safety has not been established for pregnancy. Use during pregnancy is not recommended.
• Because NSAIDs impair the synthesis of renal prostaglandins, they can decrease renal blood flow and lead to reversible renal impairment, especially in patients with preexisting renal failure, liver dysfunction, or heart failure; in elderly patients; and in those taking diuretics. Monitor these patients closely during therapy.
• Know that because of their antipyretic and anti-inflammatory actions, NSAIDs may mask the signs and symptoms of infection.
• Be aware that renal, hepatic, ocular, and auditory function should be checked periodically in long-term therapy. Drug should be stopped if abnormalities occur.
• Know that drug is not recommended for use in children.

☑ **Patient teaching**
• Tell patient that full therapeutic effect for arthritis may be delayed for 2 to 3 weeks.
• Tell patient to take drug 30 minutes before or 2 hours after meals. If adverse GI reactions occur, drug may be taken with milk or meals.
• Serious GI toxicity, including peptic ulceration and bleeding, can occur in patients taking NSAIDs despite the absence of GI symptoms. Teach patient the signs and symptoms of GI bleeding, and tell him to contact doctor immediately if they occur.
• Advise patient to avoid consumption of alcoholic beverages or aspirin while taking drug.

• Warn patient to avoid hazardous activities that require alertness until adverse CNS effects of drug are known.

---

flurbiprofen
Ansaid, Apo-Flurbiprofen†, Froben†, Froben SR†

Pregnancy Risk Category: B

HOW SUPPLIED
Tablets: 50 mg, 100 mg
Capsules (extended-release): 200 mg†

ACTION
Unknown. Possibly inhibits prostaglandin synthesis.

Route	Onset	Peak	Duration
PO	Unknown	1.5 hr	Unknown

INDICATIONS & DOSAGE
Rheumatoid arthritis and osteoarthritis—
Adults: 200 to 300 mg P.O. daily, divided b.i.d. to q.i.d. Where available, patients maintained on 200 mg daily may switch to one 200-mg extended-release capsule P.O. daily, taken in the evening after food. Doses over 300 mg/day are not recommended.
Elderly: may require lower dosage. Monitor closely.
Adjust-a-dose: In debilitated patients and those with hepatic or renal dysfunction, reduced dosage may be needed. Monitor closely.

ADVERSE REACTIONS
CNS: headache, anxiety, insomnia, dizziness, increased reflexes, tremors, amnesia, asthenia, drowsiness, malaise, depression.
CV: edema, *heart failure,* hypertension, vasodilation.
EENT: rhinitis, tinnitus, visual changes, epistaxis.
GI: dyspepsia, diarrhea, abdominal pain, nausea, constipation, *bleeding,* flatulence, vomiting.
GU: symptoms suggesting urinary tract infection, hematuria, interstitial nephritis, *renal failure.*

Hematologic: *thrombocytopenia,* neutropenia, anemia, *aplastic anemia.*
Hepatic: elevated liver enzymes, jaundice.
Respiratory: asthma.
Skin: rash, photosensitivity, urticaria, angioedema.
Other: weight changes.

INTERACTIONS
Drug-drug. *Anticoagulants:* increased risk of bleeding. Monitor patient closely.
Aspirin: decreased flurbiprofen levels. May increase GI toxicity. Avoid concomitant use.
Beta-adrenergic blockers: antihypertensive effect of beta blockers may be impaired. Monitor blood pressure.
Cyclosporine: increased risk of nephrotoxicity. Avoid concomitant use.
Diuretics: possible decreased diuretic effect. Monitor patient closely.
Lithium: serum lithium levels may be increased. Avoid use together.
Methotrexate: increased risk of methotrexate toxicity. Monitor patient closely.
Drug-lifestyle. *Alcohol use:* increased risk of adverse GI reactions. Avoid concomitant use.
Sun exposure: photosensitivity reactions may occur. Take precautions.

EFFECTS ON DIAGNOSTIC TESTS
None reported.

CONTRAINDICATIONS
Contraindicated in patients with hypersensitivity to drug and history of aspirin- or NSAID-induced asthma, urticaria, or other allergic-type reactions.

NURSING CONSIDERATIONS
• Use cautiously in patients with history of peptic ulcer disease, hepatic dysfunction, cardiac disease, or other conditions associated with fluid retention or impaired renal function.
• Safety and effectiveness of drug use in children have not been established.
• Know that drug use is not recommended during last trimester of pregnancy.
• Be aware that elderly or debilitated patients and those patients with hepatic or renal dysfunction may be at risk for renal

toxicity, jaundice, or toxic hepatitis. Periodically monitor renal and hepatic function as ordered.
• Because NSAIDs impair the synthesis of renal prostaglandins, they can decrease renal blood flow and lead to reversible renal impairment, especially in patients with preexisting renal failure, liver dysfunction, or heart failure; in elderly patients; and in those taking diuretics. Monitor these patients closely during therapy.
• Know that patients receiving long-term therapy should have periodic liver function studies, eye examinations, and hematocrit determinations.

✓ **Patient teaching**
• Instruct patient to take drug with food, milk, or antacid if GI upset occurs.
• Tell patient taking extended-release capsules to swallow them whole; do not crush, chew, or break open the capsules.
• Serious GI toxicity, including peptic ulceration and bleeding, can occur in patients taking NSAIDs despite the absence of GI symptoms. Teach patient the signs and symptoms of GI bleeding, and tell him to notify doctor immediately if they occur.
• Advise patients to avoid consumption of alcoholic beverages or aspirin while taking drug.
• Warn patient to avoid hazardous activities that require mental alertness until CNS effects are known.

ibuprofen
ACT-3‡, Actiprofen‡, Advil◇, Apo-Ibuprofen†, Bayer Select Pain Relief Formula, Brufen‡, Children's Advil, Children's Motrin◇, Excedrin IB◇, Excedrin IB Caplets◇, Genpril Caplets◇, Genpril Tablets◇, Haltran◇, Ibuprin◇, Ibuprohm Caplets◇, Ibuprohm◇, Ibu-Tab◇, Junifen Sugar Free§, Medipren◇, Medipren Caplets◇, Menadol, Midol IB, Motrin, Motrin-IB Caplets◇, Motrin-IB Tablets◇, Novo-Profen†, Nuprin◇, Nuprin Caplets◇, Nurofen‡, Nurofen Junior‡, Pamprin-IB, Pedia Profen,

Rafen‡, Rufen, Saleto-200,
Saleto-400, Saleto-600,
Saleto-800, Trendar◇

Pregnancy Risk Category: NR

HOW SUPPLIED
Tablets: 100 mg, 200 mg ◇, 300 mg,
400 mg, 600 mg, 800 mg
Tablets (chewable): 50 mg, 100 mg
Oral suspension: 100 mg/5 ml
Oral drops: 40 mg/ml

ACTION
Unknown. Produces anti-inflammatory,
analgesic, and antipyretic effects, possibly
by inhibiting prostaglandin synthesis.

Route	Onset	Peak	Duration
PO	Variable	1-2 hr	4-6 hr

INDICATIONS & DOSAGE
*Rheumatoid arthritis, osteoarthritis,
arthritis—*
Adults: 300 to 800 mg P.O. t.i.d. or q.i.d.
not to exceed 3.2 g daily.
Mild to moderate pain, dysmenorrhea—
Adults: 400 mg P.O. q 4 to 6 hours, p.r.n.
Fever—
Adults: 200 to 400 mg P.O. q 4 to 6
hours. Do not exceed 1.2 g daily or give
longer than 3 days.
Children 6 months to 12 years: if fever
is below 102.5° F (39.2° C), the recommended dose is 5 mg/kg P.O. q 6 to 8
hours. Treat higher fevers with 10 mg/kg
q 6 to 8 hours. Do not exceed 40 mg/kg
daily.
Juvenile arthritis—
Children: 30 to 70 mg/kg/day P.O. in
three or four divided doses.

ADVERSE REACTIONS
CNS: headache, dizziness, nervousness,
aseptic meningitis.
CV: peripheral edema, fluid retention,
edema.
EENT: tinnitus.
GI: epigastric distress, nausea, occult
blood loss, peptic ulceration, diarrhea,
constipation, dyspepsia, flatulence, heartburn, decreased appetite.
GU: acute renal failure, azotemia, cystitis, hematuria.

Hematologic: prolonged bleeding time,
anemia, neutropenia, pancytopenia,
thrombocytopenia, aplastic anemia,
leukopenia, ***agranulocytosis.***
Hepatic: elevated enzymes.
Respiratory: *bronchospasm.*
Skin: pruritus, rash, urticaria, ***Stevens-
Johnson syndrome.***

INTERACTIONS
Drug-drug. *Antihypertensives, furosemide, thiazide diuretics:* ibuprofen may
decrease the effectiveness of diuretics or
antihypertensives. Monitor patient closely.
Aspirin: may decrease serum levels of
ibuprofen. Avoid concomitant use.
Aspirin, corticosteroids: increased risk of
adverse GI reactions. Avoid concomitant
use.
Cyclosporine: nephrotoxicity of both
agents may be increased. Avoid concomitant use.
Digoxin, lithium, oral anticoagulants: ibuprofen may increase plasma levels or effects of these drugs. Monitor for toxicity.
Methotrexate: decreased methotrexate
clearance and increased toxicity. Use together cautiously.
Drug-lifestyle. *Alcohol use:* increased
risk of adverse GI reactions. Avoid concomitant use.
Sun exposure: may cause photosensitivity
reactions. Take precautions.

EFFECTS ON DIAGNOSTIC TESTS
Physiologic effects of drug may prolong
INR, bleeding time; decrease blood glucose concentrations (note that each ml of
suspension contains 0.3 g sucrose); increase BUN and serum creatinine and
potassium levels; decrease serum uric
acid, hemoglobin, and hematocrit levels;
increase PT; and increase serum alkaline
phosphatase, LD, and transaminase levels.

CONTRAINDICATIONS
Contraindicated in patients with angioedema, syndrome of nasal polyps, bronchospastic reaction to aspirin or other
NSAIDs, or hypersensitivity to drug.

NURSING CONSIDERATIONS
• Use cautiously in patients with GI disorders, history of peptic ulcer disease, he-

patic or renal disease, cardiac decompensation, hypertension, or known intrinsic coagulation defects.
• Know that use during pregnancy is not recommended.
• Check renal and hepatic function periodically in patients on long-term therapy. Stop drug if abnormalities occur and notify doctor.
• Be aware that because of their antipyretic and anti-inflammatory actions, NSAIDs may mask the signs and symptoms of infection.
• Know that blurred or diminished vision and changes in color vision have occurred.
• Know that it may take 1 to 2 weeks before full anti-inflammatory effects occur.

☑ **Patient teaching**
• Tell patient to take with meals or milk to reduce adverse GI reactions.
Alert: Drug is available OTC in several brands (200 mg). Instruct patient not to exceed 1.2 g daily, give to children under 12 years, or self-medicate for extended periods without consulting doctor.
• Tell patient that full therapeutic effect for arthritis may be delayed for 2 to 4 weeks. Although analgesic effect occurs at low dosage levels, anti-inflammatory effect does not occur at dosages below 400 mg q.i.d.
• Caution patient that concomitant use with aspirin, alcohol, or corticosteroids may increase the risk of GI adverse reactions.
• Serious GI toxicity, including peptic ulceration and bleeding, can occur in patients taking NSAIDs despite the absence of GI symptoms. Teach patient the signs and symptoms of GI bleeding, and tell him to notify doctor immediately if they occur.
• Warn patient to avoid hazardous activities that require mental alertness until CNS effects are known.
• Advise patient to wear sunscreen to avoid photosensitivity reactions.

indomethacin
Apo-Indomethacin†, Arthrexin‡, Indochron E-R, Indocid†‡, Indocid SR†, Indocin, Indocin SR, Novo-Methacin†

indomethacin sodium trihydrate
Apo-Indomethacin†, Indocid PDA, Indocin I.V., Novo-Methacin†

Pregnancy Risk Category: NR

HOW SUPPLIED
indomethacin
Capsules: 25 mg, 50 mg
Capsules (sustained-release): 75 mg
Oral suspension: 25 mg/5 ml
Suppositories: 50 mg
indomethacin sodium trihydrate
Injection: 1-mg vials

ACTION
Unknown. Produces anti-inflammatory, analgesic, and antipyretic effects, possibly by inhibiting prostaglandin synthesis.

Route	Onset	Peak	Duration
PO	0.5 hr	1-4 hr	4-6 hr
IV	Immediate	Immediate	4-6 hr
PR	Unknown	Unknown	4-6 hr

INDICATIONS & DOSAGE
Moderate to severe rheumatoid arthritis or osteoarthritis, ankylosing spondylitis—
Adults: 25 mg P.O. or P.R. b.i.d. or t.i.d. with food or antacids; increase daily dosage by 25 or 50 mg q 7 days, up to 200 mg daily. Or, sustained-release capsules (75 mg): 75 mg P.O. to start, in the morning or h.s., followed, if necessary, by 75 mg b.i.d.
Acute gouty arthritis—
Adults: 50 mg P.O. t.i.d. Dose reduced as soon as possible; then discontinued. Sustained-release capsules shouldn't be used for this condition.
Acute painful shoulders (bursitis or tendinitis)—
Adults: 75 to 150 mg P.O. daily in divided doses t.i.d. or q.i.d. for 7 to 14 days.
To close a hemodynamically significant

patent ductus arteriosus in premature infants (I.V. form only)—

Neonates under 48 hours: 0.2 mg/kg I.V. followed by two doses of 0.1 mg/kg at 12- to 24-hour intervals.

Neonates 2 to 7 days: 0.2 mg/kg I.V. followed by two doses of 0.2 mg/kg at 12- to 24-hour intervals.

Neonates over 7 days: 0.2 mg/kg I.V. followed by two doses of 0.25 mg/kg at 12- to 24-hour intervals.

ADVERSE REACTIONS
P.O. and P.R. forms—

CNS: *headache,* dizziness, depression, drowsiness, confusion, somnolence, fatigue, peripheral neuropathy, *seizures,* psychic disturbances, syncope, *vertigo.*

CV: hypertension, edema, *heart failure.*

EENT: blurred vision, corneal and retinal damage, hearing loss, tinnitus.

GI: nausea, anorexia, diarrhea, peptic ulceration, *GI bleeding,* constipation, dyspepsia, pancreatitis.

GU: hematuria, *acute renal failure.*

Hematologic: *hemolytic anemia, aplastic anemia, agranulocytosis,* leukopenia, *thrombocytopenic purpura,* iron deficiency anemia.

Skin: pruritus, urticaria, *Stevens-Johnson syndrome.*

Other: hypersensitivity (rash, respiratory distress, *anaphylaxis, angioedema*), hyperkalemia.

I.V. form—

GU: *renal failure,* hematuria, proteinuria, interstitial nephritis.

INTERACTIONS
Drug-drug. *Aminoglycosides, cyclosporine, methotrexate:* indomethacin may enhance the toxicity of these agents. Avoid concomitant use.

Anticoagulants: increased risk of bleeding. Monitor patient closely.

Antihypertensives: reduced antihypertensive effect. Monitor patient closely.

Aspirin: decreased blood levels of indomethacin. Avoid concomitant use.

Aspirin, corticosteroids: increased risk of GI toxicity. Do not use together.

Diflunisal, probenecid: decreased indomethacin excretion. Watch for increased incidence of indomethacin adverse reactions.

Digoxin: indomethacin may prolong the half-life of digoxin. Use together cautiously.

Dipyridamole: enhanced fluid retention. Avoid concomitant use.

Furosemide, thiazide diuretics, antihypertensive agents: impaired response to both drugs. Avoid using together if possible.

Lithium: increased plasma lithium levels. Monitor for toxicity.

Penicillamine: may increase bioavailability of penicillamine. Monitor closely.

Phenytoin: increased serum phenytoin levels may occur. Monitor closely.

Triamterene: possible nephrotoxicity. Monitor patient closely.

Drug-herb. *Senna:* blocked diarrheal effects. Avoid concomitant use.

Drug-lifestyle. *Alcohol use:* increased risk of GI toxicity. Don't use together.

EFFECTS ON DIAGNOSTIC TESTS
Drug may interfere with results of the dexamethasone suppression test. It may also interfere with urinary 5-hydroxy-indoleacetic acid determinations.

CONTRAINDICATIONS
Contraindicated in patients with hypersensitivity to drug or history of aspirin- or NSAID-induced asthma, rhinitis, or urticaria and in pregnant or breast-feeding patients. Also contraindicated in infants with untreated infection, active bleeding, coagulation defects or thrombocytopenia, congenital heart disease in whom patency of the ductus arteriosus is necessary, necrotizing enterocolitis, or impaired renal function. Suppositories are contraindicated in patients with history of proctitis or recent rectal bleeding.

NURSING CONSIDERATIONS
• Use cautiously in patients with epilepsy, parkinsonism, hepatic or renal disease, CV disease, infection, and mental illness or depression. Also use cautiously in elderly patients and patients with history of GI disease.

• Be aware that because of its high incidence of adverse effects during chronic

use, indomethacin should not be used routinely as an analgesic or antipyretic.
• Know that use during pregnancy is not recommended.
• Administer oral dosage with food, milk, or antacid to prevent GI upset.
• Be aware that if ductus arteriosus reopens, a second course of one to three doses may be given. If ineffective, surgery may be necessary.
• Monitor for bleeding in patients receiving anticoagulants, patients with coagulation defects, and neonates.
• Because NSAIDs impair the synthesis of renal prostaglandins, they can decrease renal blood flow and lead to reversible renal impairment, especially in patients with preexisting renal failure, liver dysfunction, or heart failure; in elderly patients; and in those taking diuretics. Monitor these patients closely during therapy.
• Drug causes sodium retention; monitor for weight gain (especially in elderly patients) and increased blood pressure in patients with hypertension.
• Know that because of their antipyretic and anti-inflammatory actions, NSAIDs may mask the signs and symptoms of infection.

◑ I.V. administration
• Reconstitute powder for injection with sterile water or 0.9% NaCl for injection or 0.9% NaCl. For each 1-mg vial, add 1 ml of diluent for a solution containing 1 mg/ml.
Alert: Use only preservative-free sterile NaCl or sterile water to prepare I.V. injection. Never use diluents containing benzyl alcohol because this has been associated with toxicity in newborns. Because the injection contains no preservatives, reconstitute immediately before administration, and discard unused solution.
• Hold administration of second or third scheduled I.V. dose if anuria or marked oliguria is evident; notify doctor.
• Monitor carefully for bleeding and for reduced urine output with I.V. administration.

☑ Patient teaching
• Tell patient to take oral form with food, milk, or antacid to prevent GI upset.

• Alert patient that concomitant use of oral form with aspirin, alcohol, or corticosteroids may increase the risk of adverse GI reactions.
• Serious GI toxicity, including peptic ulceration and bleeding, can occur in patients taking oral NSAIDs despite the absence of GI symptoms. Teach patient signs and symptoms of GI bleeding, and tell him to notify doctor immediately if they occur.
• Warn patient to avoid hazardous activities that require mental alertness until CNS effects are known.
• Tell patient to notify doctor immediately if visual or hearing changes occur. Patient on long-term oral therapy should have regular eye examinations, hearing tests, CBC, and renal function tests to monitor for toxicity.

---

ketoprofen
Actron, Apo-Keto†, Apo-Keto-E†, Novo-Keto-EC†, Orudis, Orudis E†, Orudis KT, Orudis SR†‡, Oruvail, Rhodis†, Rhodis-EC†

Pregnancy Risk Category: B

HOW SUPPLIED
Tablets: 12.5 mg ◇
Tablets (extended-release): 200 mg†
Tablets (enteric-coated): 50 mg†, 100 mg†
Capsules (extended-release): 100 mg, 150 mg, 200 mg
Capsules: 25 mg, 50 mg, 75 mg
Suppositories: 100 mg†

ACTION
Unknown. Produces anti-inflammatory, analgesic, and antipyretic effects, possibly by inhibiting prostaglandin synthesis.

Route	Onset	Peak	Duration
PO, PR	1-2 hr	0.5-2 hr	3-4 hr

INDICATIONS & DOSAGE
Rheumatoid arthritis and osteoarthritis—
Adults: 75 mg t.i.d. or 50 mg q.i.d. or 200 mg as an extended-release tablet once daily. Maximum dosage is 300 mg daily. Alternatively, where suppository is avail-

---

able, 100 mg P.R. b.i.d.; or 1 suppository h.s. (in conjunction with oral ketoprofen during the day).
Elderly: reduce initial dose to between one-third and one-half of normal initial dose.
Mild to moderate pain; dysmenorrhea—
Adults: 25 to 50 mg P.O. q 6 to 8 hours, p.r.n.
Elderly: reduce initial dose to between one-third and one-half of normal initial dose.
Minor aches and pain or fever—
Adults: 12.5 mg q 4 to 6 hours. Do not exceed 25 mg in a 4- to 6-hour period or 75 mg in 24 hours.
Elderly: reduce initial dose to between one-third and one-half of normal initial dose.
Adjust-a-dose: For patients with impaired renal function, reduce initial dose to between one-third and one-half of normal initial dose.

ADVERSE REACTIONS
CNS: headache, dizziness, CNS excitation or depression.
EENT: tinnitus, visual disturbances.
GI: nausea, abdominal pain, diarrhea, constipation, flatulence, *peptic ulceration, dyspepsia,* anorexia, vomiting, stomatitis.
GU: *nephrotoxicity,* elevated BUN.
Hematologic: prolonged bleeding time, *thrombocytopenia, agranulocytosis.*
Hepatic: elevated liver enzymes.
Respiratory: dyspnea, *bronchospasm, laryngeal edema.*
Skin: rash, photosensitivity, *exfoliative dermatitis.*
Other: peripheral edema.

INTERACTIONS
Drug-drug. *Antihypertensives:* reduced antihypertensive effect. Don't use together.
Aspirin, corticosteroids: increased risk of adverse GI reactions. Avoid concomitant use.
Aspirin, probenecid: increased plasma levels of ketoprofen. Avoid concomitant use.
Cyclosporine: increased nephrotoxicity. Avoid use together.

Hydrochlorothiazide, other diuretics: decreased diuretic effectiveness. Monitor for lack of effect.
Lithium, methotrexate, phenytoin: increased levels of these drugs, leading to toxicity. Monitor patient closely.
Warfarin: increased risk of bleeding. Monitor patient closely.
Drug-lifestyle. *Alcohol use:* increased risk of GI toxicity. Don't use together.
Sun exposure: may cause photosensitivity reactions. Take precautions.

EFFECTS ON DIAGNOSTIC TESTS
In vitro interactions with glucose determinations have been reported with glucose oxidase and peroxidase methods. Drug may interfere with serum iron determinations (false increases or decreases depending on method used) and produce false increases in serum bilirubin levels. These interactions were reported with drug concentrations above those seen clinically (60 mg/ml).

CONTRAINDICATIONS
Contraindicated in patients with hypersensitivity to drug and history of aspirin- or NSAID-induced asthma, urticaria, or other allergic-type reactions.

NURSING CONSIDERATIONS
• Use cautiously in patients with history of peptic ulcer disease, renal dysfunction, hypertension, heart failure, or fluid retention.
• Avoid use during last trimester of pregnancy.
• Know that the sustained-release dosage form is not recommended for patients in acute pain.
• Because NSAIDs impair the synthesis of renal prostaglandins, they can decrease renal blood flow and lead to reversible renal impairment, especially in patients with preexisting renal failure, liver dysfunction, or heart failure; in elderly patients; and in those taking diuretics. Monitor these patients closely during therapy.
• Check renal and hepatic function every 6 months or as indicated.
• Be aware that NSAIDs may mask the signs and symptoms of infection because

of their antipyretic and anti-inflammatory actions.
- Know that drug is not recommended for use in children.

☑ Patient teaching
Alert: Drug is available OTC. Instruct patient not to exceed dosage of 75 mg/day.
- Tell patient to take drug 30 minutes before or 2 hours after meals. If adverse GI reactions occur, patient may take drug with milk or meals.
- Tell patient that full therapeutic effect may be delayed for 2 to 4 weeks.
- Serious GI toxicity, including peptic ulceration and bleeding, can occur in patient taking NSAIDs despite the absence of GI symptoms. Teach patient the signs and symptoms of GI bleeding, and tell him to notify doctor immediately if they occur.
- Alert patient that concomitant use with aspirin, alcohol, or corticosteroids may increase the risk of adverse GI reactions.
- Warn patient to avoid hazardous activities that require mental alertness until CNS effects are known.
- Advise patient to use a sunblock, wear protective clothing, and avoid prolonged exposure to sunlight. Drug has been associated with photosensitivity reactions.
- Instruct patient to report visual or auditory adverse reactions immediately.

ketorolac tromethamine
Toradol

Pregnancy Risk Category: C

HOW SUPPLIED
Tablets: 10 mg
Injection: 15 mg/ml, 30 mg/ml

ACTION
Unknown. Thought to inhibit prostaglandin synthesis.

Route	Onset	Peak	Duration
PO	0.5-1 hr	0.5-1 hr	6-8 hr
IV	Immediate	Immediate	6-8 hr
IM	10 min	0.5-1 hr	6-8 hr

INDICATIONS & DOSAGE
Short-term management of moderately severe, acute pain for single-dose treatment—
Adults: in patients under 65 years, 60 mg I.M. or 30 mg I.V.
Elderly: in patients 65 years or older, 30 mg I.M. or 15 mg I.V.
Adjust-a-dose: In renally impaired patients or those weighing below 50 kg (110 lb), 30 mg I.M. or 15 mg I.V.
Short-term management of moderately severe, acute pain for multiple-dose treatment—
Adults: in patients under 65 years, 30 mg I.M. or I.V. q 6 hours. Maximum daily dose is 120 mg.
Elderly: in patients 65 years or older, 15 mg I.M. or I.V. q 6 hours. Maximum daily dose is 60 mg.
Adjust-a-dose: In renally impaired patients or those weighing below 50 kg (110 lb), 15 mg I.M. or I.V. q 6 hours. Maximum daily dose is 60 mg.
Short-term management of moderately severe, acute pain when switching from parenteral to oral administration (oral therapy is indicated only as continuation of parenterally administered drug and should never be given without patient first having received parenteral therapy)—
Adults: in patients under 65 years, 20 mg P.O. as single dose followed by 10 mg P.O. q 4 to 6 hours. Maximum daily dose is 40 mg.
Elderly: in patients 65 years or older, 10 mg P.O. as single dose followed by 10 mg P.O. q 4 to 6 hours. Maximum daily dose is 40 mg.
Adjust-a-dose: In renally impaired patients or those weighing below 50 kg (110 lb), 10 mg P.O. as single dose followed by 10 mg P.O. q 4 to 6 hours. Maximum daily dose is 40 mg.

ADVERSE REACTIONS
CNS: *drowsiness, sedation,* dizziness, *headache.*
CV: edema, hypertension, palpitations, arrhythmias.
GI: *nausea, dyspepsia, GI pain,* diarrhea, **peptic ulceration,** vomiting, constipation, flatulence, stomatitis.
GU: *acute renal failure.*

Reactions may be *common,* uncommon, *life-threatening,* or COMMON AND LIFE-THREATENING.

Hematologic: decreased platelet adhesion, purpura, *thrombocytopenia.*
Other: pain at injection site, pruritus, rash, diaphoresis, *bronchospasm.*

INTERACTIONS
Drug-drug. *ACE inhibitors:* may increase risk of renal impairment, particularly in volume-depleted patients. Do not use together in volume-depleted patients.
Anticoagulants, salicylates: ketorolac may increase the levels of free (unbound) salicylates or anticoagulants in the blood. Use with extreme caution and monitor patient closely.
Antihypertensives, diuretics: decreased effectiveness. Monitor patient closely.
Lithium: increased lithium levels. Monitor patient closely.
Methotrexate: decreased methotrexate clearance and increased toxicity. Do not use together.

EFFECTS ON DIAGNOSTIC TESTS
Like other NSAIDs, ketorolac has been associated with borderline elevations of one or more liver function test results. Meaningful elevations of AST or ALT—three times the upper limit—occur in less than 1% of patients. Because drug inhibits platelet aggregation, it can prolong bleeding time.

CONTRAINDICATIONS
Contraindicated in patients hypersensitive to drug and in those with active peptic ulcer disease, recent GI bleeding or perforation, advanced renal impairment, risk for renal impairment due to volume depletion, suspected or confirmed cerebrovascular bleeding, hemorrhagic diathesis, incomplete hemostasis, or high risk of bleeding. Also contraindicated in patients with history of peptic ulcer disease or GI bleeding, past allergic manifestations to aspirin or other NSAIDs, and during labor and delivery or breast-feeding. Also contraindicated as prophylactic analgesic before major surgery or intraoperatively when hemostasis is critical; and in patients currently receiving aspirin, an NSAID, or probenecid. Do not administer drug epidurally or intrathecally because of alcohol content.

NURSING CONSIDERATIONS
● Use of ketorolac is not recommended in children.
● Use cautiously in patients with hepatic or renal impairment.
Alert: The maximum combined duration of therapy (parenteral and oral) must be limited to 5 days.
● I.M. administration may cause pain at the injection site. Holding pressure over the site for 15 to 30 seconds after the injection may minimize local effects. Give deep I.M.
● Carefully observe patients with coagulopathies and those who are taking anticoagulants. Ketorolac inhibits platelet aggregation and can prolong bleeding time. This effect will disappear within 48 hours of discontinuing the drug. It will not alter platelet count, INR, PTT, or PT.
● Be aware that NSAIDs may mask the signs and symptoms of infection because of their antipyretic and anti-inflammatory actions.

🔋 I.V. administration
● Do not mix with morphine sulfate, meperidine hydrochloride, promethazine hydrochloride, or hydroxyzine hydrochloride. Ketorolac tromethamine will precipitate out in solution.
● Give I.V. injection in no less than 15 seconds.

☑ Patient teaching
● Warn patient receiving drug I.M. that pain may occur at injection site.
● Serious GI toxicity, including peptic ulceration and bleeding, can occur in patient taking NSAIDs despite the absence of GI symptoms. Teach patient the signs and symptoms of GI bleeding, and tell him to notify doctor immediately if they occur.

---

nabumetone
Relafen, Relifex§

Pregnancy Risk Category: C

HOW SUPPLIED
Tablets: 500 mg, 750 mg

ACTION

Unknown. Probably acts by inhibiting prostaglandin synthesis.

Route	Onset	Peak	Duration
PO	Unknown	2-4 hr	Unknown

INDICATIONS & DOSAGE

Rheumatoid arthritis or osteoarthritis—
Adults: initially, 1,000 mg P.O. daily as a single dose or in divided doses b.i.d. Maximum daily dosage is 2,000 mg.

ADVERSE REACTIONS

CNS: dizziness, headache, fatigue, insomnia, nervousness, somnolence.
CV: vasculitis, edema.
EENT: tinnitus.
GI: *diarrhea, dyspepsia, abdominal pain,* constipation, flatulence, nausea, dry mouth, gastritis, stomatitis, anorexia, vomiting, ***bleeding,*** ulceration.
Respiratory: dyspnea, pneumonitis.
Skin: pruritus, rash, increased diaphoresis.

INTERACTIONS

Drug-drug. *Diuretics:* NSAIDs may decrease diuretic effectiveness. Monitor patients closely during therapy.
Warfarin, other highly protein-bound drugs: increased risk of adverse effects from displacement of drugs by nabumetone. Use together cautiously.
Drug-food. *Any food:* increased absorption. Give drug with food.
Drug-lifestyle. *Alcohol use:* associated with an increased risk of additive GI toxicity. Avoid concomitant use.

EFFECTS ON DIAGNOSTIC TESTS

None reported.

CONTRAINDICATIONS

Contraindicated in patients with hypersensitivity reactions and history of aspirin- or NSAID-induced asthma, urticaria, or other allergic-type reactions.

NURSING CONSIDERATIONS

• Use cautiously in patients with renal or hepatic impairment; heart failure, hypertension, or other conditions that may predispose patient to fluid retention; and in patients with history of peptic ulcer disease.
• Know that use is not recommended during third trimester of pregnancy.
• Because NSAIDs impair the synthesis of renal prostaglandins, they can decrease renal blood flow and lead to reversible renal impairment, especially in patients with preexisting renal failure, liver dysfunction, or heart failure; in elderly patients; and in those taking diuretics. Monitor these patients closely during therapy.
• During long-term therapy, periodically monitor renal and liver function, CBC, and hematocrit as ordered; assess patients for signs and symptoms of GI bleeding.
• Know that drug is not recommended for use in children.

✓ **Patient teaching**
• Instruct patient to take drug with food, milk, or antacids. Drug is absorbed more rapidly when taken with food or milk.
• Advise patient to limit alcohol intake because of additive GI toxicity risk.
• Serious GI toxicity, including peptic ulceration and bleeding, can occur in patient taking NSAIDs despite the absence of GI symptoms. Teach patient signs and symptoms of GI bleeding and tell him to notify doctor immediately if they occur.
• Warn patient against hazardous activities that require mental alertness until CNS effects are known.

naproxen

Apo-Naproxen†, EC-Naprosyn, Naprosyn, Naprosyn-E†, Naprosyn-SR, Naxen†, Novo-Naprox†, Nu-Naprox†, Nycopren§

naproxen sodium

Aleve ◊ , Anaprox, Anaprox DS, Apo-Napro-Na†, Naprelan, Naprogesic‡, Novo-Naprox Sodium†, Synflex†

Pregnancy Risk Category: B

HOW SUPPLIED

naproxen
Tablets: 250 mg, 375 mg, 500 mg

Tablets (delayed-release): 375 mg, 500 mg
Tablets (extended-release): 750 mg, 1,000 mg
Oral suspension: 125 mg/5 ml
Suppositories: 500 mg‡
naproxen sodium
Tablets (controlled-release): 421.5 mg, 550 mg
Tablets (film-coated): 220 mg ◊ , 275 mg, 550 mg
   Note: 275 mg of naproxen sodium contains 250 mg of naproxen.

ACTION

Unknown. Produces anti-inflammatory, analgesic, and antipyretic effects, possibly by inhibiting prostaglandin synthesis.

Route	Onset	Peak	Duration
PO	1 hr	2-4 hr	7 hr
PR	Unknown	Unknown	Unknown

INDICATIONS & DOSAGE

Rheumatoid arthritis, osteoarthritis, ankylosing spondylitis, pain, dysmenorrhea, tendinitis, bursitis—
Adults: 250 to 500 mg (naproxen) b.i.d.; maximum is 1.5 g daily for a limited time. Or, 375 to 500 mg delayed-release (EC-Naprosyn) b.i.d.; or 750 to 1,000 mg controlled-release (Naprelan) daily; or 275 to 550 mg naproxen sodium b.i.d.
Juvenile arthritis—
Children: 10 mg/kg P.O. in two divided doses.
Acute gout—
Adults: 750 mg (naproxen) P.O., followed by 250 mg q 8 hours until attack subsides. Or, 825 mg naproxen sodium, followed by 275 mg q 8 hours until attack subsides; or 1,000 to 1,500 mg/day controlled-release (Naprelan) on first day, followed by 1,000 mg daily until attack subsides.
Mild to moderate pain, primary dysmenorrhea—
Adults: 500 mg (naproxen) P.O., followed by 250 mg q 6 to 8 hours up to 1.25 g/day. Or, 550 mg naproxen sodium, followed by 275 mg q 6 to 8 hours up to 1,375 mg/day; or 1,000 mg controlled-release (Naprelan) once daily.
Elderly: in patients over 65 years, do not exceed 400 mg/day.

ADVERSE REACTIONS

CNS: headache, drowsiness, dizziness, vertigo.
CV: edema, palpitations.
EENT: visual disturbances, *tinnitus,* auditory disturbances.
GI: epigastric distress, occult blood loss, nausea, *peptic ulceration,* constipation, dyspepsia, heartburn, diarrhea, stomatitis, thirst.
GU: *acute renal failure.*
Hematologic: *thrombocytopenia,* eosinophilia, *agranulocytosis,* neutropenia.
Hepatic: elevated liver enzyme levels.
Respiratory: dyspnea.
Skin: pruritus, rash, urticaria, ecchymosis, diaphoresis, purpura.

INTERACTIONS

Drug-drug: *ACE inhibitors:* may increase risk of renal impairment. Use together cautiously.
Antihypertensives, diuretics: decreased effect of these drugs. Monitor patient closely.
Aspirin, corticosteroids: increased risk of adverse GI reactions. Avoid concomitant use.
Methotrexate: increased risk of toxicity. Monitor patient closely.
Oral anticoagulants, sulfonylureas, other highly protein-bound drugs: increased risk of toxicity. Monitor patient closely.
Probenecid: decreased elimination of naproxen. Monitor for toxicity.
Drug-lifestyle. *Alcohol use:* increased risk of adverse GI reactions. Avoid concomitant use.

EFFECTS ON DIAGNOSTIC TESTS

Drug and its metabolite may interfere with urinary 5-hydroxyindoleacetic acid and 17-hydroxycorticosteroid determinations. The physiologic effects of naproxen may lead to an increase in bleeding time (may persist for 4 days after withdrawal of drug); serum creatinine and potassium, BUN, and serum transaminase levels may also increase.

CONTRAINDICATIONS

Contraindicated in patients with hyper-

---

*Liquid contains alcohol.   **May contain tartrazine.   †Canada   ‡Australia   §U.K.   ◊ OTC

sensitivity to drug or with the syndrome of asthma, rhinitis, and nasal polyps.

NURSING CONSIDERATIONS
• Use cautiously in elderly patients and in patients with renal disease, CV disease, GI disorders, hepatic disease, or a history of peptic ulcer disease.
• Know that use should be avoided during last trimester of pregnancy.
• Because NSAIDs impair the synthesis of renal prostaglandins, they can decrease renal blood flow and lead to reversible renal impairment, especially in patients with preexisting renal failure, liver dysfunction, or heart failure; in elderly patients; and in those taking diuretics. Monitor these patients closely during therapy.
• Monitor CBC and renal and hepatic function every 4 to 6 months or as indicated and ordered during long-term therapy.
• Be aware that because of their antipyretic and anti-inflammatory actions, NSAIDs may mask the signs and symptoms of infection.

☑ **Patient teaching**
Alert: Drug is available OTC (naproxen sodium, 200 mg). Instruct patient not to exceed 600 mg in 24 hours. Dosage in patient over 65 years should not exceed 400 mg/day.
• Advise patient to take drug with food or milk to minimize GI upset. A full glass of water or other liquid should be taken with each dose.
• Tell patient taking prescription doses of naproxen for arthritis that full therapeutic effect may be delayed 2 to 4 weeks.
• Warn patient against taking both naproxen and naproxen sodium at the same time because both circulate in the blood as the naproxen anion.
• Serious GI toxicity, including peptic ulceration and bleeding, can occur in patient taking NSAIDs despite the absence of GI symptoms. Teach patient signs and symptoms of GI bleeding and tell him to notify doctor immediately if they occur.
• Caution patient that concomitant use with aspirin, alcohol, or corticosteroids may increase the risk of adverse GI reactions.
• Warn patient against hazardous activities that require mental alertness until CNS effects are known.

oxaprozin
Daypro

Pregnancy Risk Category: C

HOW SUPPLIED
Caplets: 600 mg

ACTION
Unknown. Produces anti-inflammatory, analgesic, and antipyretic effects, possibly by inhibiting prostaglandin synthesis.

Route	Onset	Peak	Duration
PO	Unknown	3-5 hr	Unknown

INDICATIONS & DOSAGE
Osteoarthritis or rheumatoid arthritis—
Adults: initially, 1,200 mg P.O. daily. Then, individualized to smallest effective dosage to minimize adverse reactions. Smaller patients or those with mild symptoms may require only 600 mg daily. Maximum is 1,800 mg or 26 mg/kg, whichever is lower, in divided doses.

ADVERSE REACTIONS
CNS: depression, sedation, somnolence, confusion, sleep disturbances.
EENT: tinnitus, blurred vision.
GI: nausea, dyspepsia, diarrhea, constipation, abdominal pain or distress, anorexia, flatulence, vomiting, *hemorrhage,* stomatitis.
GU: dysuria, urinary frequency.
Hepatic: elevated liver function test results (with chronic use); severe hepatic dysfunction (rare).
Skin: *rash,* photosensitivity.

INTERACTIONS
Drug-drug. *Antihypertensives, diuretics:* decreased effect. Monitor patient closely and adjust dosage, as ordered.
Aspirin: oxaprozin displaces salicylates from plasma protein-binding sites, increasing risk of salicylate toxicity. Avoid concomitant use.
Aspirin, corticosteroids: increased risk of

---

adverse GI reactions. Avoid concomitant use.

Cyclosporine: nephrotoxicity may be increased. Avoid use together.

Methotrexate: increased risk of methotrexate toxicity. Avoid concomitant use.

Oral anticoagulants: although problems haven't been reported, there is an increased risk of bleeding. Use together cautiously.

Phenytoin, lithium: serum levels of these drugs may be increased. Avoid concomitant use.

Drug-lifestyle. *Alcohol use:* increased risk of adverse GI reactions. Avoid concomitant use.

Sun exposure: photosensitivity reactions may occur. Take precautions.

EFFECTS ON DIAGNOSTIC TESTS
Drug can alter platelet aggregation and prolong bleeding time. It also may decrease hemoglobin levels, causing anemia, and elevate liver function studies.

CONTRAINDICATIONS
Contraindicated in patients with hypersensitivity to drug or with the syndrome of nasal polyps, angioedema, and bronchospastic reaction to aspirin or other NSAIDs.

NURSING CONSIDERATIONS
• Use cautiously in patients with history of peptic ulcer disease, hepatic or renal dysfunction, hypertension, CV disease, or conditions predisposing patient to fluid retention.

• Because renal prostaglandins play a role in the maintenance of renal perfusion, patients with preexisting conditions leading to a reduction in renal blood flow may experience renal toxicity with NSAID therapy. Patients at greatest risk are the elderly, those taking diuretics, and those with impaired renal, hepatic, or cardiac function. Closely monitor renal function in these patients, and discontinue NSAID therapy if problems develop.

• Elevations of liver function tests can occur after chronic use. These abnormal findings may persist, worsen, or resolve with continued therapy. Rarely, patients may progress to severe hepatic dysfunction. Periodically monitor liver function

tests in patients receiving long-term therapy, and closely monitor patients with abnormal test results.

• Be aware that because of their antipyretic and anti-inflammatory actions, NSAIDs may mask the signs and symptoms of infection.

☑ Patient teaching
• Tell patient to take drug 30 minutes before or 2 hours after meals. If adverse GI reactions occur, drug may be taken with milk or meals.

• Inform patient that full therapeutic effects may be delayed for 2 to 4 weeks.

• Serious GI toxicity, including peptic ulceration and bleeding, can occur in patient taking NSAIDs despite the absence of GI symptoms. Teach patient signs and symptoms of GI bleeding and tell him to notify doctor immediately if they occur.

• Tell patient to report adverse visual or auditory reactions immediately.

• Warn patient against hazardous activities that require mental alertness until CNS effects are known.

• Advise patient to use a sunblock, wear protective clothing, and avoid prolonged exposure to sunlight. Drug has been associated with photosensitivity reactions.

piroxicam
Apo-Piroxicam†, Feldene,
Novo-Pirocam†, Pirox‡

*Pregnancy Risk Category: B
(D in third trimester or near delivery)*

HOW SUPPLIED
Capsules: 10 mg, 20 mg

ACTION
Unknown. Produces anti-inflammatory, analgesic, and antipyretic effects, possibly by inhibiting prostaglandin synthesis.

Route	Onset	Peak	Duration
PO	1 hr	3-5 hr	48-72 hr

INDICATIONS & DOSAGE
Osteoarthritis and rheumatoid arthritis—
Adults: 20 mg P.O. daily. If desired, dosage may be divided b.i.d.

ADVERSE REACTIONS

CNS: headache, drowsiness, dizziness, somnolence, vertigo.
CV: peripheral edema.
EENT: auditory disturbances.
GI: epigastric distress, nausea, occult blood loss, *peptic ulceration, severe GI bleeding,* diarrhea, constipation, abdominal pain, dyspepsia, flatulence, anorexia, stomatitis.
GU: *nephrotoxicity,* elevated BUN level.
Hematologic: prolonged bleeding time, anemia, leukopenia, *aplastic anemia, agranulocytosis,* eosinophilia, *thrombocytopenia.*
Hepatic: elevated liver enzymes.
Respiratory: *bronchospasm.*
Skin: pruritus, rash, urticaria, *photosensitivity.*

INTERACTIONS

Drug-drug. *Antihypertensives, diuretics:* decreased effects. Avoid use together.
Aspirin, corticosteroids: increased risk of GI toxicity. Decreased plasma levels of piroxicam. Avoid concomitant use.
Cyclosporine, methotrexate: increased toxicity. Monitor patient closely.
Lithium: increased plasma lithium levels. Monitor for toxicity.
Oral anticoagulants, other highly protein-bound drugs: increased risk of toxicity. Monitor patient closely.
Oral antidiabetic agents: enhanced antidiabetic effects. Monitor patient closely.
Drug-lifestyle. *Alcohol use:* increased risk of GI toxicity. Decreased plasma levels of piroxicam. Avoid concomitant use.
Sun exposure: photosensitivity reactions may occur. Take precautions.

EFFECTS ON DIAGNOSTIC TESTS

Physiologic effects of drug may prolong bleeding time (may persist for 2 weeks after discontinuing drug); increase BUN, creatinine, and potassium levels, INR or PT; decrease serum glucose (in diabetic patients), hemoglobin, hematocrit, or uric acid levels; and increase liver function test results (alkaline phosphatase, LD, or transaminase levels).

CONTRAINDICATIONS

Contraindicated in patients hypersensitive to drug; in those with bronchospasm or angioedema precipitated by aspirin or NSAIDs; and in pregnant or breast-feeding women.

NURSING CONSIDERATIONS

• Use cautiously in elderly patients and in patients with GI disorders, history of renal or peptic ulcer disease, cardiac disease, hypertension, or conditions predisposing to fluid retention.
• Because NSAIDs impair the synthesis of renal prostaglandins, they can decrease renal blood flow and lead to reversible renal impairment, especially in the elderly; patients with preexisting renal failure, liver dysfunction, or heart failure; and in those taking diuretics. Monitor closely.
• Check renal, hepatic, and auditory function and CBC periodically during prolonged therapy. Discontinue drug if abnormalities occur and notify doctor.
• Be aware that NSAIDs may mask the signs and symptoms of infection because of their antipyretic and anti-inflammatory actions.

☑ **Patient teaching**
• Tell patient to take drug with milk, antacids, or meals if GI adverse reactions occur.
• Inform patient that full therapeutic effects may be delayed for 2 to 4 weeks.
• Serious GI toxicity, including peptic ulceration and bleeding, can occur in patient taking NSAIDs despite the absence of GI symptoms. Teach patient what signs and symptoms of GI bleeding to look for and when to report them.
• Warn patient against hazardous activities that require mental alertness until CNS effects are known.
• Advise patient to use a sunblock, wear protective clothing, and avoid prolonged exposure to sunlight. Causes adverse skin reactions more often than other drugs in its class. Photosensitivity reactions are the most common.

Reactions may be *common,* uncommon, *life-threatening*, or COMMON AND LIFE-THREATENING.

sulindac
Aclin‡, Apo-Sulin†, Clinoril,
Novo-Sundac†, Saldac‡

Pregnancy Risk Category: NR

HOW SUPPLIED
Tablets: 100 mg‡, 150 mg, 200 mg

ACTION
Produces anti-inflammatory, analgesic,
and antipyretic effects, possibly by inhibiting prostaglandin synthesis.

Route	Onset	Peak	Duration
PO	Unknown	2-4 hr	Unknown

INDICATIONS & DOSAGE
*Osteoarthritis, rheumatoid arthritis,
ankylosing spondylitis—*
Adults: initially, 150 mg P.O. b.i.d.; increased to 200 mg b.i.d., p.r.n. Maximum
dosage is 400 mg daily.
*Acute subacromial bursitis or supraspina-
tus tendinitis, acute gouty arthritis—*
Adults: 200 mg P.O. b.i.d. for 7 to 14
days. Dose reduced as symptoms subside.
Maximum dosage is 400 mg daily.

ADVERSE REACTIONS
CNS: dizziness, headache, nervousness,
psychosis.
CV: hypertension, *heart failure,* palpitations.
EENT: tinnitus, transient visual disturbances.
GI: *epigastric distress, peptic ulceration,
pancreatitis,* occult blood loss, nausea,
constipation, dyspepsia, flatulence,
anorexia, *GI bleeding.*
GU: interstitial nephritis, *nephrotic syndrome, renal failure.*
Hematologic: prolonged bleeding time,
aplastic anemia, thrombocytopenia, neutropenia, *agranulocytosis,* hemolytic anemia.
Skin: rash, pruritus.
Other: edema, drug fever, *anaphylaxis,*
angioedema, *hypersensitivity syndrome.*

INTERACTIONS
Drug-drug. *Anticoagulants:* increased
risk of bleeding. Monitor PT closely.

Aspirin: decreased sulindac plasma concentration and increased risk of GI adverse reactions. Do not use together.
Cyclosporine: increased nephrotoxicity of
cyclosporine. Avoid concomitant use.
Diflunisal, dimethyl sulfoxide: decreased
metabolism of sulindac to its active
metabolite, reducing its effectiveness. Do
not use together.
Methotrexate: increased methotrexate
toxicity. Avoid concomitant use.
Probenecid: increased plasma levels of
sulindac and its active metabolite. Monitor for toxicity.
*Sulfonamides, sulfonylureas, other highly
protein-bound drugs:* possible displacement of these drugs from plasma protein-
binding sites, leading to increased toxicity. Monitor closely.

EFFECTS ON DIAGNOSTIC TESTS
Physiologic effects of the drug may result
in increased bleeding time; increased
BUN and serum creatinine and potassium
levels; and increased serum alkaline phosphatase and transaminase concentrations.

CONTRAINDICATIONS
Contraindicated in patients with hypersensitivity to drug or in whom acute asthmatic attacks, urticaria, or rhinitis is precipitated by aspirin or NSAIDs.

NURSING CONSIDERATIONS
● Use cautiously in patients with a history
of ulcers and GI bleeding, renal dysfunction, compromised cardiac function, hypertension, or conditions predisposing to
fluid retention.
● Know that use during pregnancy is not
recommended.
● Periodically monitor hepatic and renal
function and CBC in patients receiving
long-term therapy as ordered.
● Be aware that NSAIDs may mask the
signs and symptoms of infection.

☑ Patient teaching
● Tell patient to take drug with food, milk,
or antacids.
● Serious GI toxicity, including peptic ulceration and bleeding, can occur in patient taking NSAIDs despite the absence
of GI symptoms. Teach patient signs and

symptoms of GI bleeding and tell him to
contact the doctor immediately if they occur.
Alert: Tell patient to notify doctor immediately if easy bruising or prolonged
bleeding occurs.
• Advise patient to avoid hazardous activities that require mental alertness until
CNS effects are known.
• Instruct patient to report edema and
have blood pressure checked monthly.
Drug causes sodium retention but is
thought to have less effect on the kidneys
than other NSAIDs.
• Advise patient to notify doctor and have
complete eye examinations if visual disturbances occur.

28
Narcotic and opioid analgesics

alfentanil hydrochloride
buprenorphine hydrochloride
butorphanol tartrate
codeine phosphate
codeine sulfate
fentanyl citrate
fentanyl transdermal system
fentanyl transmucosal
hydromorphone hydrochloride
meperidine hydrochloride
methadone hydrochloride
morphine hydrochloride
morphine sulfate
morphine tartrate
nalbuphine hydrochloride
oxycodone hydrochloride
oxycodone pectinate
oxymorphone hydrochloride
pentazocine hydrochloride
pentazocine hydrochloride and
     naloxone hydrochloride
pentazocine lactate
propoxyphene hydrochloride
propoxyphene napsylate
remifentanil hydrochloride
sufentanil citrate
tramadol hydrochloride

COMBINATION PRODUCTS

222†: aspirin 375 mg, codeine phosphate 8 mg, and caffeine citrate 30 mg.

282†: aspirin 375 mg, codeine phosphate 15 mg, and caffeine citrate 30 mg.

292†: aspirin 375 mg, codeine phosphate 30 mg, and caffeine citrate 30 mg.

293†: aspirin 375 mg, codeine phosphate 30 mg, codeine phosphate (slow-release) 30 mg, and caffeine citrate 30 mg.

692†: aspirin 375 mg, propoxyphene hydrochloride 65 mg, and caffeine 30 mg.

A.C. & C.†: aspirin 375 mg, codeine phosphate 8 mg, and caffeine 30 mg.

ACETA WITH CODEINE, EMPRACET-30†, EMTEC-30†: acetaminophen 300 mg and codeine phosphate 30 mg.

ANACIN WITH CODEINE†: aspirin 325 mg, codeine phosphate 8 mg, and caffeine 32 mg.

ANCASAL 8†, C2 WITH CODEINE†: aspirin 375 mg, codeine phosphate 8 mg, and caffeine 15 mg.

ANCASAL 15†: aspirin 375 mg, codeine phosphate 15 mg, and caffeine 15 mg.

ANCASAL 30†: aspirin 375 mg, codeine phosphate 30 mg, and caffeine 15 mg.

ANEXSIA 5/500: hydrocodone bitartrate 5 mg, acetaminophen 500 mg.

CAPITAL WITH CODEINE, TYLENOL WITH CODEINE ELIXIR*: acetaminophen 120 mg and codeine phosphate 12 mg/5 ml.

DARVOCET-N 50: acetaminophen 325 mg and propoxyphene napsylate 50 mg.

DARVOCET-N 100, PROPACET 100: acetaminophen 650 mg and propoxyphene napsylate 100 mg.

DARVON COMPOUND†: aspirin 325 mg, propoxyphene hydrochloride 32 mg, and caffeine 32.4 mg.

DARVON COMPOUND-65†: aspirin 389 mg, propoxyphene hydrochloride 65 mg, and caffeine 32.4 mg.

DARVON-N COMPOUND†: aspirin 375 mg, propoxyphene napsylate 100 mg, and caffeine 30 mg.

DARVON-N WITH A.S.A.†: aspirin 325 mg and propoxyphene napsylate 100 mg.

DARVON WITH A.S.A.†: aspirin 325 mg and propoxyphene hydrochloride 65 mg.

E-LOR, WYGESIC: acetaminophen 650 mg and propoxyphene hydrochloride 65 mg.

EMPIRIN WITH CODEINE NO. 3, PHENAPHEN WITH CODEINE NO. 3: aspirin 325 mg and codeine phosphate 30 mg.

EMPIRIN WITH CODEINE NO. 4, PHENAPHEN WITH CODEINE NO. 4: aspirin 325 mg and codeine phosphate 60 mg.

EMPRACET-60†: acetaminophen 300 mg and codeine phosphate 60 mg.

ENDOCET, OXYCOCET†, PERCOCET, ROXI-CET: acetaminophen 325 mg and oxycodone hydrochloride 5 mg.

ENDODAN†, OXYCODAN†, PERCODAN†: aspirin 325 mg and oxycodone hydrochloride 5 mg.

FIORICET WITH CODEINE: acetaminophen 325 mg, butalbital 50 mg, caffeine 40 mg, and codeine phosphate 30 mg.

FIORINAL WITH CODEINE: aspirin 325 mg,

butalbital 50 mg, caffeine 40 mg, and codeine 30 mg.

INNOVAR: droperidol 2.5 mg and fentanyl citrate 0.05 mg/ml.

LENOLTEC WITH CODEINE NO. 1†, LORCET 10/650: acetaminophen 650 mg and hydrocodone bitartrate 10 mg.

LORCET PLUS: acetaminophen 650 mg, hydrocodone bitartrate 7.5 mg

LORTAB 2.5/500: acetaminophen 500 mg and hydrocodone bitartrate 2.5 mg.

LORTAB 5/500: acetaminophen 500 mg and hydrocodone bitartrate 5 mg.

LORTAB 7.5/500: acetaminophen 500 mg and hydrocodone bitartrate 7.5 mg.

NOVO-GESIC C8†: acetaminophen 300 mg, codeine phosphate 8 mg, and caffeine 15 mg.

PERCODAN-DEMI: aspirin 325 mg, oxycodone hydrochloride 2.25 mg, and oxycodone terephthalate 0.19 mg.

PERCODAN-DEMI†: aspirin 325 mg and oxycodone hydrochloride 2.5 mg.

PERCODAN, ROXIPRIN: aspirin 325 mg, oxycodone hydrochloride 4.5 mg, and oxycodone terephthalate 0.38 mg.

ROUNOX AND CODEINE 15†: acetaminophen 325 mg and codeine phosphate 15 mg.

ROUNOX AND CODEINE 30†: acetaminophen 325 mg and codeine phosphate 30 mg.

ROUNOX AND CODEINE 60†: acetaminophen 325 mg and codeine phosphate 60 mg.

ROXICET 5/500, TYLOX: acetaminophen 500 mg and oxycodone hydrochloride 5 mg.

ROXICET ORAL SOLUTION*: acetaminophen 325 mg and oxycodone hydrochloride 5 mg/5 ml.

TALACEN: acetaminophen 650 mg and pentazocine hydrochloride 25 mg.

TALWIN COMPOUND: aspirin 325 mg and pentazocine hydrochloride 12.5 mg.

TYLENOL WITH CODEINE NO. 1: acetaminophen 300 mg and codeine phosphate 7.5 mg.

TYLENOL WITH CODEINE NO. 2: acetaminophen 300 mg and codeine phosphate 15 mg.

TYLENOL WITH CODEINE NO. 3: acetaminophen 300 mg and codeine phosphate 30 mg.

TYLENOL WITH CODEINE NO. 4: acetaminophen 300 mg and codeine phosphate 60 mg.

VICODIN: acetaminophen 500 mg and hydrocodone bitartrate 5 mg.

VICODIN ES: acetaminophen 750 mg and hydrocodone bitartrate 7.5 mg.

alfentanil hydrochloride
Alfenta, CD Rapifen§

Controlled Substance Schedule II
Pregnancy Risk Category: C

HOW SUPPLIED
Injection: 500 mcg/ml

ACTION
Binds with opiate receptors in the CNS, altering both perception of and emotional response to pain through an unknown mechanism.

Route	Onset	Peak	Duration
IV	1 min	1.5-2 min	5-10 min

INDICATIONS & DOSAGE
Adjunct to general anesthetic—
Adults: initially, 8 to 50 mcg/kg I.V.; then increments of 3 to 15 mcg/kg I.V. q 5 to 20 minutes.
As a primary anesthetic—
Adults: initially, 130 to 245 mcg/kg I.V.; then 0.5 to 1.5 mcg/kg/minute I.V.
Monitored anesthesia care—
Adults: initially, 3 to 8 mcg/kg I.V.; then 3 to 5 mcg/kg I.V. q 5 to 20 minutes or 0.25 to 1 mcg/kg/minute I.V. Total dose is 3 to 40 mcg/kg I.V.
Elderly: dosage should be reduced.
Adjust-a-dose: In debilitated patients, dosage should be reduced. In obese patients, dosage is based on lean body weight.

ADVERSE REACTIONS
CNS: anxiety, headache, confusion, dizziness, sleepiness, sedation.
CV: *hypotension, hypertension,* BRADYCARDIA, *tachycardia,* ARRHYTHMIAS.
EENT: blurred vision.
GI: *nausea, vomiting.*

Reactions may be *common,* uncommon, *life-threatening,* or COMMON AND LIFE-THREATENING.

Musculoskeletal: skeletal muscle movements.
Respiratory: *chest wall rigidity, **bronchospasm, respiratory depression,*** hypercapnia, ***respiratory arrest,*** laryngospasm.
Skin: pruritus, urticaria.

INTERACTIONS
Drug-drug. *Cimetidine:* CNS toxicity. Monitor closely.
CNS depressants: additive effects. Use together cautiously.
Diazepam: CV depression and decreased blood pressure with high doses of alfentanil. Monitor closely.
Drug-lifestyle. *Alcohol use:* additive effects. Use together cautiously.

EFFECTS ON DIAGNOSTIC TESTS
Drug may increase biliary tract pressure with resultant increases in amylase and lipase plasma levels.

CONTRAINDICATIONS
Contraindicated in patients with hypersensitivity to drug.

NURSING CONSIDERATIONS
• Use cautiously in patients with head injury, pulmonary disease, decreased respiratory reserve, or hepatic or renal impairment.
Alert: To administer small volumes of alfentanil accurately, use a tuberculin syringe.
• Accidental skin contact should be treated by rinsing the area with water.
• Periodically monitor postoperative vital signs and bladder function. Because drug decreases both rate and depth of respirations, monitoring of arterial oxygen saturation may aid in assessing respiratory depression.

◖I.V. administration
• Compatible with D_5W, D_5W in lactated Ringer's solution, and 0.9% NaCl solution. Most clinicians use infusions containing 25 to 80 mcg/ml.
• Discontinue infusion at least 10 to 15 minutes before the end of surgery.
• Be aware drug should be administered only by persons specifically trained in the use of I.V. anesthetics.

• Keep narcotic antagonist (naloxone) and resuscitation equipment available when giving drug I.V.

☑ Patient teaching
• Explain the anesthetic effect of alfentanil as well as preoperative and postoperative care measures.
• Inform patient that another analgesic will be available to relieve pain after effects of alfentanil have worn off.

---

buprenorphine hydrochloride
Buprenex, Temgesic Injection‡

Controlled Substance Schedule V
Pregnancy Risk Category: C

HOW SUPPLIED
Injection: 0.324 mg (equivalent to 0.3 mg base/ml)

ACTION
Binds with opiate receptors in the CNS, altering both perception of and emotional response to pain through an unknown mechanism.

Route	Onset	Peak	Duration
IV	Immediate	2 min	6 hr
IM	15 min	1 hr	6 hr

INDICATIONS & DOSAGE
Moderate to severe pain—
Adults and children 13 years and over: 0.3 mg I.M. or slow I.V. q 6 hours, p.r.n. or around the clock; dosage repeated (up to 0.3 mg), if required, 30 to 60 minutes after initial dose.
Children 2 to 12 years: 2 to 6 mcg/kg I.M. or I.V. q 4 to 6 hours.
Elderly: reduce dose by one-half.
Adjust-a-dose: Reduce dose by one-half in high-risk patients, such as debilitated patients.

ADVERSE REACTIONS
CNS: *dizziness, sedation,* headache, confusion, nervousness, euphoria, *vertigo, increased intracranial pressure.*
CV: hypotension, bradycardia, tachycardia, hypertension.
EENT: *miosis,* blurred vision.

GI: *nausea,* vomiting, constipation, dry mouth.
GU: urine retention.
Respiratory: *respiratory depression,* hypoventilation, dyspnea.
Skin: pruritus, diaphoresis.

INTERACTIONS
Drug-drug. *CNS depressants, MAO inhibitors:* additive effects. Use together cautiously.
Drug-lifestyle. *Alcohol use:* additive effects. Use together cautiously.

EFFECTS ON DIAGNOSTIC TESTS
None reported.

CONTRAINDICATIONS
Contraindicated in patients with hypersensitivity to drug.

NURSING CONSIDERATIONS
• Use cautiously in elderly or debilitated patients or patients with head injury, intracranial lesions, and increased intracranial pressure; severe respiratory, liver, or kidney impairment; CNS depression or coma; thyroid irregularities; adrenal insufficiency; and prostatic hyperplasia, urethral stricture, acute alcoholism, delirium tremens, or kyphoscoliosis.
• S.C. administration is not recommended.
• Be aware that buprenorphine 0.3 mg is equal to 10 mg of morphine and 75 mg of meperidine in analgesic potency. It has longer duration of action than morphine or meperidine.
Alert: Know that naloxone will not completely reverse the respiratory depression caused by buprenorphine overdose; an overdose may necessitate mechanical ventilation. Larger than customary doses of naloxone (more than 0.4 mg) and doxapram also may be ordered.
• Accidental skin exposure should be treated by removing exposed clothing and rinsing skin with water.
• Be aware that drug's narcotic antagonist properties may precipitate withdrawal syndrome in narcotic-dependent patients.
• Know that if dependence occurs, withdrawal symptoms may appear up to 14 days after drug is stopped.

I.V. administration
• Give by direct I.V. injection, slowly into a vein or through the tubing of a free-flowing, compatible I.V. solution over not less than 2 minutes.

Patient teaching
• Caution ambulatory patient about getting out of bed or walking.
• When drug is used postoperatively, encourage patient to turn, cough, and deep-breathe to prevent atelectasis.

butorphanol tartrate
Stadol, Stadol NS

Controlled Substance Schedule IV
Pregnancy Risk Category: C

HOW SUPPLIED
Injection: 1 mg/ml, 2 mg/ml
Nasal spray: 10 mg/ml

ACTION
Binds with opiate receptors in the CNS, altering both perception of and emotional response to pain through an unknown mechanism.

Route	Onset	Peak	Duration
IV	2-3 min	30-60 min	3-4 hr
IM	10-15 min	30-60 min	3-4 hr
Nasal	15 min	1-2 hr	4-5 hr

INDICATIONS & DOSAGE
Moderate to severe pain—
Adults: 1 to 4 mg I.M. q 3 to 4 hours, p.r.n. or around the clock; or 0.5 to 2 mg I.V. q 3 to 4 hours, p.r.n. or around the clock. Not to exceed 4 mg per dose. Alternatively, 1 mg by nasal spray q 3 to 4 hours (1 spray in one nostril); repeated in 60 to 90 minutes if pain relief is inadequate.
Elderly: use one-half of usual dose at twice the interval for I.V. use; for nasal use, allow 1.5 to 2 hours to elapse before repeating dose.
Labor for patients at full term and in early labor—
Adults: 1 to 2 mg I.V. or I.M., repeated after 4 hours, p.r.n.

Preoperative anesthesia or preanesthesia—
Adults: 2 mg. I.M. 60 to 90 minutes before surgery.
Adjunct to balanced anesthesia—
Adults: 2 mg I.V. shortly before induction or 0.5 to 1.0 mg I.V. in increments during anesthesia
Elderly: use one-half of usual dose at twice the interval for I.V. use.
Adjust-a-dose: In patients with renal or hepatic impairment, increase dosage interval to 6 to 8 hours.

ADVERSE REACTIONS
CNS: confusion, nervousness, lethargy, headache, *somnolence, dizziness,* insomnia, anxiety, paresthesia, euphoria, hallucinations, flushing, increased intracranial pressure.
CV: palpitations, vasodilation, hypotension.
EENT: blurred vision, *nasal congestion* (with nasal spray), tinnitus, unpleasant taste.
GI: *nausea, vomiting,* constipation, anorexia.
Respiratory: *respiratory depression.*
Skin: rash, hives, clamminess, excessive diaphoresis.
Other: sensation of heat.

INTERACTIONS
Drug-drug. *CNS depressants:* additive effects. Use together cautiously.
Drug-lifestyle. *Alcohol use:* additive effects. Use together cautiously.

EFFECTS ON DIAGNOSTIC TESTS
None reported.

CONTRAINDICATIONS
Contraindicated in patients with narcotic addiction; may precipitate withdrawal syndrome. Also contraindicated in patients with hypersensitivity to drug or to preservative, benzethonium chloride.

NURSING CONSIDERATIONS
• Use cautiously in patients with head injury, increased intracranial pressure, acute MI, ventricular dysfunction, coronary insufficiency, respiratory disease or depression, and renal or hepatic dysfunction.

Also administer cautiously to patients who have recently received repeated doses of narcotic analgesic medication.
• S.C. route is not recommended.
• Know that respiratory depression apparently does not increase with larger dosage.
• Be aware that psychological and physical addiction may occur.
• Periodically monitor postoperative vital signs and bladder function. Because drug decreases both rate and depth of respirations, monitoring of arterial oxygen saturation may aid in assessing respiratory depression.

◖ I.V. administration
• Give by direct injection into a vein or into the tubing of a free-flowing I.V. solution. Compatible solutions include D_5W and 0.9% NaCl.

☑ Patient teaching
• Caution ambulatory patient about getting out of bed or walking. Warn outpatient to avoid driving and other potentially hazardous activities that require mental alertness until drug's CNS effects are known.
• Inform patient about administration technique for and storage of nasal spray, if applicable.
• Instruct patient to avoid alcohol.

codeine phosphate
Paveral†

codeine sulfate

Controlled Substance Schedule II
Pregnancy Risk Category: C

HOW SUPPLIED
codeine phosphate
Oral solution: 15 mg/5 ml, 10 mg/ml†
Injection: 30 mg/ml, 60 mg/ml
Tablets (soluble): 30 mg, 60 mg
codeine sulfate
Tablets: 15 mg, 30 mg, 60 mg
Tablets (soluble): 15 mg, 30 mg, 60 mg

ACTION
Binds with opiate receptors in the CNS,

altering both perception of and emotional response to pain through an unknown mechanism. Also suppresses the cough reflex by direct action on the cough center in the medulla.

Route	Onset	Peak	Duration
PO	30-45 min	1-2 hr	4-6 hr
IV	Immediate	Immediate	4-6 hr
IM	10-30 min	0.5-1 hr	4-6 hr
SC	10-30 min	Unknown	4-6 hr

INDICATIONS & DOSAGE

Mild to moderate pain—
Adults: 15 to 60 mg P.O. or 15 to 60 mg (phosphate) S.C., I.M., or I.V. q 4 to 6 hours, p.r.n. Maximum dosage is 360 mg/day.
Children over 1 year: 0.5 mg/kg P.O., S.C., or I.M. q 4 hours, p.r.n. *Do not use I.V. in children.*
Nonproductive cough—
Adults: 10 to 20 mg P.O. q 4 to 6 hours. Maximum dosage is 120 mg/day.
Children 6 to 12 years: 5 to 10 mg P.O. q 4 to 6 hours. Maximum dosage is 60 mg/day.
Children 2 to 6 years: 2.5 to 5 mg P.O. q 4 to 6 hours. Do not exceed 30 mg/day.

ADVERSE REACTIONS

CNS: *sedation, clouded sensorium,* euphoria, dizziness, light-headedness.
CV: hypotension, bradycardia.
GI: nausea, vomiting, *constipation,* dry mouth, ileus.
GU: urine retention.
Respiratory: *respiratory depression.*
Skin: pruritus, flushing, *diaphoresis.*
Other: physical dependence.

INTERACTIONS

Drug-drug. *CNS depressants, general anesthetics, hypnotics, MAO inhibitors, other narcotic analgesics, sedatives, tranquilizers, tricyclic antidepressants:* additive effects. Use together with extreme caution. Monitor patient response.
Drug-lifestyle. *Alcohol use:* additive effects. Use together cautiously.

EFFECTS ON DIAGNOSTIC TESTS

Codeine may increase plasma amylase and lipase levels, delay gastric emptying, increase biliary tract pressure resulting from contraction of the sphincter of Oddi, and may interfere with hepatobiliary imaging studies.

CONTRAINDICATIONS

Contraindicated in patients with hypersensitivity to drug.

NURSING CONSIDERATIONS

• Use with extreme caution in patients with head injury, increased intracranial pressure, increased CSF pressure, hepatic or renal disease, hypothyroidism, Addison's disease, acute alcoholism, seizures, severe CNS depression, bronchial asthma, COPD, respiratory depression, and shock. Also use with extreme caution in elderly or debilitated patients.
Alert: Do not mix with other solutions because codeine phosphate is incompatible with many drugs.
• Do not administer discolored solution.
• Know that codeine and aspirin or acetaminophen are often prescribed together to provide enhanced pain relief.
• For full analgesic effect, administer drug before patient has intense pain.
• Be aware that drug is an antitussive and should not be used when cough is a valuable diagnostic sign or is beneficial (as after thoracic surgery).
• Monitor cough type and frequency.
• Monitor respiratory and circulatory status.
• Opiates may cause constipation. Assess bowel function and need for stool softeners or laxatives.

🛢 I.V. administration
• Give by direct injection into a large vein. Administer very slowly.

☑ Patient teaching
• Advise patient that GI distress caused by oral administration can be minimized by taking with milk or meals.
• Instruct patient to ask for or to take drug before pain is intense.
• Caution ambulatory patient about getting out of bed or walking. Warn outpatient to avoid driving and other potentially hazardous activities that require mental

alertness until drug's CNS effects are known.
● Advise patient to avoid alcohol.

---

fentanyl citrate
Sublimaze

fentanyl transdermal system
Duragesic-25, Duragesic-50, Duragesic-75, Duragesic-100

fentanyl transmucosal
Fentanyl Oralet

Controlled Substance Schedule II
Pregnancy Risk Category: C

HOW SUPPLIED
Injection: 50 mcg/ml
Transdermal system: patches designed to release 25 mcg, 50 mcg, 75 mcg, or 100 mcg of fentanyl per hour
Transmucosal: 100 mcg, 200 mcg, 300 mcg, 400 mcg

ACTION
Unknown. Binds with opiate receptors in the CNS, altering both perception of and emotional response to pain through an unknown mechanism.

Route	Onset	Peak	Duration
IV	1-2 min	3-5 min	0.5-1 hr
IM	7-15 min	20-30 min	1-2 hr
Trans-dermal	12-24 hr	1-3 days	Variable
Trans-mucosal	5-15 min	20-30 min	Unknown

INDICATIONS & DOSAGE
Adjunct to general anesthetic—
Adults: for low-dose therapy, 2 mcg/kg I.V. For moderate-dose therapy, 2 to 20 mcg/kg I.V.; then 25 to 100 mcg I.V., p.r.n. For high-dose therapy, 20 to 50 mcg/kg I.V.; then 25 mcg to one-half the initial loading dose I.V., p.r.n.
Adjunct to regional anesthesia—
Adults: 50 to 100 mcg I.M. or slowly I.V. over 1 to 2 minutes, p.r.n.
Induction and maintenance of anesthesia—
Children 2 to 12 years: 2 to 3 mcg/kg I.V.

Postoperatively—
Adults: 50 to 100 mcg I.M. q 1 to 2 hours, p.r.n.
Preoperatively—
Adults: 50 to 100 mcg I.M. 30 to 60 minutes before surgery. Alternatively, 5 mcg/kg dispensed as oralet unit, 20 to 40 minutes prior to need of desired effects.
Management of chronic pain—
Adults: one transdermal system applied to a portion of the upper torso on an area of skin that is not irritated and has not been irradiated. Therapy initiated with the 25-mcg/hour system; dosage adjusted as needed and tolerated. Each system may be worn for 72 hours, although some patients may require systems to be applied q 48 hours. Upward titration may be done q 3 days after initial dose; then 6 days thereafter.

ADVERSE REACTIONS
CNS: *sedation, somnolence, clouded sensorium, euphoria,* dizziness, headache, *confusion, asthenia,* nervousness, hallucinations, anxiety, depression, *seizures.*
CV: hypotension, hypertension, *arrhythmias,* chest pain.
GI: nausea, vomiting, constipation, ileus, abdominal pain, dry mouth, anorexia, diarrhea, dyspepsia.
GU: urine retention.
Respiratory: *respiratory depression,* hypoventilation, dyspnea, apnea.
Skin: reaction at application site (erythema, papules, edema), *pruritus, diaphoresis.*
Other: physical dependence.

INTERACTIONS
Drug-drug. *CNS depressants, general anesthetics, hypnotics, MAO inhibitors, other narcotic analgesics, sedatives, tricyclic antidepressants:* additive effects. Use together with extreme caution. Fentanyl dose should be reduced by one-quarter to one-third. Also give above drugs in reduced dosages.
Diazepam: CV depression when given with high doses of fentanyl. Monitor closely.
Droperidol: hypotension and decreased pulmonary arterial pressure. Use together cautiously.

Drug-lifestyle. *Alcohol use:* additive effects. Use together cautiously.

EFFECTS ON DIAGNOSTIC TESTS
Fentanyl increases plasma amylase and lipase levels.

CONTRAINDICATIONS
Contraindicated in patients with known intolerance of drug.

NURSING CONSIDERATIONS
• Use with caution in patients with head injury, increased CSF pressure, COPD, decreased respiratory reserve, potentially compromised respirations, hepatic or renal disease, and cardiac bradyarrhythmias. Also use with caution in elderly or debilitated patients.
• For better analgesic effect, administer drug before patient has intense pain.
Alert: Be aware that high doses can produce muscle rigidity, which can be reversed with neuromuscular blockers; however, patient must be artificially ventilated.
• Monitor circulatory and respiratory status and urinary function carefully. Drug may cause respiratory depression, hypotension, urine retention, nausea, vomiting, ileus, or altered level of consciousness without regard to route of administration.
• Periodically monitor postoperative vital signs and bladder function. Because drug decreases both rate and depth of respirations, monitoring of arterial oxygen saturation (SaO_2) may help assess respiratory depression. Immediately report respiratory rate below 12 breaths/minute, decreased respiratory volume, or decreased SaO_2.
Transdermal form
• Know that transdermal fentanyl is not recommended for postoperative pain.
• Dosage equivalent charts are available to calculate the fentanyl transdermal dose based on the daily morphine intake—for example, for every 90 mg of oral morphine or 15 mg of I.M. morphine per 24 hours, 25 mcg/hour of transdermal fentanyl is required.
• Be aware that dosage adjustments in patients using the transdermal system

should be made gradually. Reaching steady-state levels of a new dosage may take up to 6 days; delay dosage adjustment until after at least two applications.
• Monitor patients who develop adverse reactions to the transdermal system for at least 12 hours after removal. Serum levels of fentanyl drop gradually and may take as long as 17 hours to decline by 50%.
• Most patients experience good control of pain for 3 days while wearing the transdermal system, but a few may need a new application after 48 hours.
• Because serum fentanyl concentration rises for the first 24 hours after application, analgesic effect cannot be evaluated on the first day. Be sure patient has adequate supplemental analgesic to prevent breakthrough pain.
• When reducing opiate therapy or switching to a different analgesic, know the transdermal system should be withdrawn gradually. Because fentanyl's serum level drops gradually after removal, give half of the equianalgesic dose of the new analgesic 12 to 18 hours after removal as ordered.
Transmucosal form
• Remove foil overwrap of fentanyl oralet just prior to administration.
• Have patient place the fentanyl oralet in mouth and suck (not chew or swallow) it.
• Remove fentanyl oralet unit, using the handle, after it has been consumed, patient shows adequate effect, or patient shows signs of respiratory depression. Place any remaining portion in the plastic overwrap provided, and dispose accordingly for Schedule II drugs.

◖I.V. administration
• Know that only staff trained in administration of I.V. anesthetics and management of their potential adverse effects should administer I.V. fentanyl.
• Be aware that drug is often used I.V. with droperidol to produce neuroleptanalgesia.
• Keep narcotic antagonist (naloxone) and resuscitation equipment available when giving drug I.V.

Reactions may be *common*, uncommon, *life-threatening*, or COMMON AND LIFE-THREATENING.

☑ Patient teaching
• When used for pain control, instruct patient to ask for drug before pain becomes intense.
• When drug is used postoperatively, encourage patient to turn, cough, and deep-breathe to prevent atelectasis.
• Instruct patient to avoid performing hazardous activities until CNS effects subside.
• Tell home care patient to avoid drinking alcohol or taking other CNS-type drugs while receiving fentanyl because additive effects can occur.
• Teach patient about the proper application of the prescribed transdermal patch. Tell patient to clip hair at application site, but not to use a razor, which may irritate the skin. Wash area with clear water if necessary, but not with soaps, oils, lotions, alcohol, or other substances that may irritate the skin or prevent adhesion. Dry the area completely before application.
• Tell patient to remove the transdermal system from the package just before applying, hold in place for 30 seconds, and be sure the edges of the patch adhere to the skin.
• Teach patient to dispose of the transdermal patch by folding so the adhesive side adheres to itself and then flushing it down the toilet.
• Tell patient that, if another patch is needed after 48 to 72 hours, to apply it to a new site.
• Inform patient that heat from fever or environment, such as from heating pads, electric blankets, heat lamps, hot tubs, or water beds, may increase transdermal delivery and cause toxicity requiring dosage adjustment. Instruct patient to notify doctor if fever occurs or if he'll be spending time in a hot climate.

hydromorphone hydrochloride (dihydromorphinone hydrochloride)
CD Palladone§,
CD Palladone SR§, Dilaudid,
Dilaudid-5, Dilaudid HP

Controlled Substance Schedule II
Pregnancy Risk Category: C

HOW SUPPLIED
Tablets: 1 mg, 2 mg, 3 mg, 4 mg, 8 mg
Injection: 1 mg/ml, 2 mg/ml, 3 mg/ml, 4 mg/ml, 10 mg/ml
Suppositories: 3 mg
Syrup: 1 mg/5 ml
Liquid: 5 mg/5 ml

ACTION
Binds with opiate receptors in the CNS, altering both perception of and emotional response to pain through an unknown mechanism. Also suppresses the cough reflex by direct action on the cough center in the medulla.

Route	Onset	Peak	Duration
PO	30 min	1.5-2 hr	4 hr
IV	10-15 min	15-30 min	2-3 hr
IM	15 min	0.5-1 hr	4-5 hr
SC	15 min	0.5-1.5 hr	4 hr
PR	Unknown	Unknown	4 hr

INDICATIONS & DOSAGE
Moderate to severe pain—
Adults: 2 to 4 mg P.O. q 4 to 6 hours, p.r.n.; or 1 to 4 mg I.M., S.C., or I.V. (slowly over at least 2 to 5 minutes) q 4 to 6 hours, p.r.n.; or 3 mg P.R. suppository q 6 to 8 hours, p.r.n.
Cough—
Adults and children over 12 years: 1 teaspoon (5 ml) P.O. q 3 to 4 hours, p.r.n.

ADVERSE REACTIONS
CNS: *sedation, somnolence, clouded sensorium,* dizziness, *euphoria.*
CV: hypotension, bradycardia.
EENT: blurred vision, diplopia, nystagmus.
GI: nausea, vomiting, constipation, ileus.
GU: urine retention.

---

*Liquid contains alcohol.   **May contain tartrazine.   †Canada   ‡Australia   §U.K.   ◇OTC

Respiratory: *respiratory depression, bronchospasm.*
Other: induration with repeated S.C. injections, physical dependence.

INTERACTIONS
Drug-drug. *CNS depressants, general anesthetics, hypnotics, MAO inhibitors, other narcotic analgesics, sedatives, tranquilizers, tricyclic antidepressants:* additive effects. Use together with extreme caution. Reduce hydromorphone dose and monitor patient response.
Drug-lifestyle. *Alcohol use:* additive effects. Use together cautiously.

EFFECTS ON DIAGNOSTIC TESTS
Drug increases plasma amylase and lipase levels. It may delay gastric emptying; increased biliary tract pressure resulting from contraction of the sphincter of Oddi may interfere with hepatobiliary imaging studies.

CONTRAINDICATIONS
Contraindicated in patients hypersensitive to drug, in those with intracranial lesions associated with increased intracranial pressure, and whenever ventilator function is depressed, such as in status asthmaticus, COPD, cor pulmonale, emphysema, and kyphoscoliosis.

NURSING CONSIDERATIONS
• Use with extreme caution in patients with hepatic or renal disease, hypothyroidism, Addison's disease, prostatic hyperplasia, or urethral stricture. Also use with caution in elderly or debilitated patients.
• For better analgesic effect, give drug before patient has intense pain.
• Dilaudid-HP, a highly concentrated form (10 mg/ml), may be administered in smaller volumes to prevent the discomfort associated with large-volume I.M. or S.C. injections. Check dosage carefully.
• Rotate injection sites to avoid induration with S.C. injection.
• Monitor respiratory and circulatory status and bowel function.
• Keep narcotic antagonist (naloxone) available.

• Be aware that drug may worsen or mask gallbladder pain.
• Be aware that drug is a commonly abused narcotic.

◖I.V. administration
• Give by direct injection over no less than 2 minutes. For infusion, drug may be mixed in D_5W, 0.9% NaCl, dextrose 5% in 0.9% NaCl, dextrose 5% in 0.45% NaCl, or Ringer's or lactated Ringer's solutions.
• Respiratory depression and hypotension can occur with I.V. administration. Give very slowly and monitor patient constantly. Keep resuscitation equipment available.

☑ Patient teaching
• Instruct patient to ask for or take drug before pain becomes intense.
• Tell patient to store suppositories in refrigerator.
• Tell patient to take drug with food if GI upset occurs.
• When drug is used postoperatively, encourage patient to turn, cough, and breathe deeply to avoid atelectasis.
• Caution ambulatory patient about getting out of bed or walking. Warn outpatient to avoid hazardous activities that require mental alertness until drug's CNS effects are known.
• Advise patient to avoid alcohol.

---

meperidine hydrochloride (pethidine hydrochloride)
CD Pamergan P100§,
CD Pethidine§, Demerol

Controlled Substance Schedule II
Pregnancy Risk Category: B
(D if used for prolonged periods or in high doses at term)

HOW SUPPLIED
Tablets: 50 mg, 100 mg
Syrup: 50 mg/5 ml
Injection: 10 mg/ml, 25 mg/ml, 50 mg/ml, 75 mg/ml, 100 mg/ml

ACTION
Binds with opiate receptors in the CNS,

altering both perception of and emotional response to pain through an unknown mechanism.

Route	Onset	Peak	Duration
PO	15 min	1-1.5 hr	2-4 hr
IV	1 min	5-7 min	2-4 hr
IM	10-15 min	30-50 min	2-4 hr
SC	10-15 min	40-60 min	2-4 hr

INDICATIONS & DOSAGE
Moderate to severe pain—
Adults: 50 to 150 mg P.O., I.M., or S.C. q 3 to 4 hours, p.r.n.
Children: 1.1 to 1.8 mg/kg P.O., I.M., or S.C. q 3 to 4 hours. Maximum dosage is 100 mg q 4 hours, p.r.n.
Preoperatively—
Adults: 50 to 100 mg I.M. or S.C. 30 to 90 minutes before surgery.
Children: 1 to 2 mg/kg I.M. or S.C. up to the adult dose 30 to 90 minutes before surgery.
Adjunct to anesthesia—
Adults: repeated slow I.V. injections of fractional doses (10 mg/ml); alternatively, continuous I.V. infusion of a more dilute solution (1 mg/ml) titrated to patient's needs.
Obstetric analgesia—
Adults: 50 to 100 mg I.M. or S.C. when pain becomes regular, repeated at 1- to 3-hour intervals.

ADVERSE REACTIONS
CNS: *sedation, somnolence, clouded sensorium, euphoria,* paradoxical excitement, tremor, *dizziness, seizures* (with large doses), headache, hallucinations, syncope, *light-headedness.*
CV: hypotension, bradycardia, tachycardia, *cardiac arrest, shock.*
GI: constipation, ileus, dry mouth, *nausea, vomiting,* biliary tract spasms.
GU: urine retention.
Respiratory: *respiratory depression,* respiratory arrest.
Skin: pruritus, urticaria, *diaphoresis.*
Other: physical dependence, muscle twitching, phlebitis after I.V. delivery, pain at injection site; local tissue irritation, induration (after S.C. injection).

INTERACTIONS
Drug-drug. *Aminophylline, barbiturates, heparin, methicillin, morphine sulfate, phenytoin, sodium bicarbonate, sulfonamides:* incompatible when mixed in the same I.V. container. Don't use together.
CNS depressants, general anesthetics, hypnotics, other narcotic analgesics, phenothiazines, sedatives, tricyclic antidepressants: possible respiratory depression, hypotension, profound sedation, or coma. Use together with extreme caution. Reduce meperidine dosage.
MAO inhibitors: increased CNS excitation or depression that can be severe or fatal. Do not use together.
Phenytoin: decreased blood levels of meperidine. Monitor for decreased analgesia.
Drug-herb. *Parsley:* may promote or produce serotonin syndrome. Avoid concomitant use.
Drug-lifestyle. *Alcohol use:* additive effects. Use together cautiously.

EFFECTS ON DIAGNOSTIC TESTS
Drug increases plasma amylase and lipase levels through increased biliary tract pressure; levels may be unreliable for 24 hours after meperidine administration.

CONTRAINDICATIONS
Contraindicated in patients with hypersensitivity to drug and in those who have received MAO inhibitors within past 14 days.

NURSING CONSIDERATIONS
• Use with extreme caution in patients with increased intracranial pressure, head injury, asthma, and other respiratory conditions; supraventricular tachycardias, seizures, acute abdominal conditions, hepatic or renal disease, hypothyroidism, Addison's disease, urethral stricture, and prostatic hyperplasia; and in elderly or debilitated patients.
• Drug may be used in some patients allergic to morphine.
• S.C. injection is not recommended because it is very painful. However, it may be suitable for occasional use.
*Alert:*Oral dose is less than half as effective as parenteral dose. Give I.M. if possi-

ble. When changing from parenteral to oral route, know that dosage should be increased.
• Syrup has local anesthetic effect. Give with full glass of water.
• Drug and its active metabolite normeperidine accumulate in the body. Monitor for increased toxic effect, especially in patients with impaired renal function.
• Because drug toxicity often appears after several days of treatment, this drug is not recommended for treatment of chronic pain.
• Monitor respirations of neonates exposed to drug during labor. Have resuscitation equipment and naloxone available.
• Monitor respiratory and CV status carefully. Don't give if respirations are below 12 breaths/minute, if respiratory rate or depth is decreased, or if change in pupils is noted.
• Watch for withdrawal symptoms if drug is discontinued abruptly after long-term use.
• Monitor bladder function in postoperative patients.
• Monitor bowel function. Patient may need a laxative or stool softener.

◻ I.V. administration
• Give slowly by direct I.V. injection. Meperidine also may be given by slow continuous I.V. infusion. Drug is compatible with most I.V. solutions, including D_5W, 0.9% NaCl, and Ringer's or lactated Ringer's solutions.
• Keep narcotic antagonist (naloxone) available when giving this drug I.V.

☑ Patient teaching
• When drug is used postoperatively, encourage patient to turn, cough, and breathe deeply and to use an incentive spirometer to prevent atelectasis.
• Caution ambulatory patient about getting out of bed or walking. Warn outpatient to avoid driving and other potentially hazardous activities that require mental alertness until drug's CNS effects are known.
• Advise patient to avoid alcohol.

methadone hydrochloride
Dolophine, Methadose, Physeptone‡

Controlled Substance Schedule II
Pregnancy Risk Category: C

HOW SUPPLIED
Tablets: 5 mg, 10 mg
Dispersible tablets (for methadone maintenance therapy): 40 mg
Oral solution: 5 mg/5 ml, 10 mg/5 ml, 10 mg/10 ml, 10 mg/ml (concentrate)
Injection: 10 mg/ml

ACTION
Binds with opiate receptors at many sites in the CNS (brain, brain stem, and spinal cord), altering both perception of and emotional response to pain through an unknown mechanism.

Route	Onset	Peak	Duration
PO	0.5-1 hr	1.5-2 hr	4-6 hr
IV	Immediate	15-30 min	4-6 hr
IM	10-20 min	1-2 hr	4-5 hr

INDICATIONS & DOSAGE
Severe pain—
Adults: 2.5 to 10 mg P.O., I.M., or S.C. q 3 to 4 hours, p.r.n.
Narcotic withdrawal syndrome—
Adults: 15 to 40 mg P.O. daily (highly individualized). Maintenance dosage is 20 to 120 mg P.O. daily. Dosage adjusted p.r.n. Daily dosages greater than 120 mg require special state and federal approval.

ADVERSE REACTIONS
CNS: *sedation, somnolence, clouded sensorium,* euphoria, *dizziness,* choreic movements, *seizures* (with large doses), headache, insomnia, agitation, *lightheadedness,* syncope.
CV: hypotension, bradycardia, ***shock, cardiac arrest,*** palpitations.
EENT: visual disturbances.
GI: *nausea, vomiting,* constipation, ileus, dry mouth, anorexia, biliary tract spasm.
GU: urine retention, decreased libido.
Respiratory: *respiratory depression, respiratory arrest.*

Reactions may be *common,* uncommon, *life-threatening,* or COMMON AND LIFE-THREATENING.

Skin: diaphoresis, pruritus, urticaria, edema.
Other: physical dependence; pain at injection site; tissue irritation, induration (following S.C. injection).

INTERACTIONS

Drug-drug. *Ammonium chloride, other urine acidifiers, phenytoin:* may reduce methadone effect. Monitor for decreased pain control.
CNS depressants, general anesthetics, hypnotics, MAO inhibitors, sedatives, tranquilizers, tricyclic antidepressants: possible respiratory depression, hypotension, profound sedation, or coma. Use together with extreme caution. Monitor patient response.
Rifampin: withdrawal symptoms; reduced blood levels of methadone. Use together cautiously.
Drug-lifestyle. *Alcohol use:* additive effects. Use together cautiously.

EFFECTS ON DIAGNOSTIC TESTS

Drug increases plasma amylase levels.

CONTRAINDICATIONS

Contraindicated in patients with hypersensitivity to drug.

NURSING CONSIDERATIONS

● Use with extreme caution in patients with acute abdominal conditions, severe hepatic or renal impairment, hypothyroidism, Addison's disease, prostatic hyperplasia, urethral stricture, head injury, increased intracranial pressure, asthma, and other respiratory conditions. Also use with caution in elderly or debilitated patients.
● Oral liquid form legally required in maintenance programs. Completely dissolve tablets in 120 ml (½ cup) of orange juice or powdered citrus drink.
● For parenteral use, I.M. injection is preferred. Rotate injection sites.
● Know that oral dose is half as potent as injected dose.
● Know that an around-the-clock regimen is necessary to manage severe, chronic pain.
● Be aware that patient treated for narcotic withdrawal syndrome usually will require

an additional analgesic if pain control is necessary.
● Monitor patient closely because drug has cumulative effect; marked sedation can occur after repeated doses.
● Monitor circulatory and respiratory status and bladder and bowel function. Patient may need a laxative.
● Be aware that when used as an adjunct in the treatment of narcotic addiction (maintenance), withdrawal usually will be delayed and mild.

🔌 I.V. administration

● Dilute to a maximum concentration of 10 mg/ml using 0.9% NaCl. Give slowly by direct injection. Alternatively, dilute to 1 mg/ml and give as a slow I.V. infusion (15 to 35 mg/hour).

☑ Patient teaching

● Caution ambulatory patient about getting out of bed or walking. Warn outpatient to avoid hazardous activities that require mental alertness until drug's CNS effects are known.
● Instruct patient to increase fluid and fiber in diet, if not contraindicated, to combat constipation.
● Advise patient to avoid alcohol.

---

morphine hydrochloride
Morphitec†, M.O.S.†, M.O.S.-S.R.†

morphine sulfate
Anamorph‡, Astramorph PF, CD Morcap SR§, CD MST Continus§, CD Sevredol§, CD Zomorph§, Duramorph, Epimorph†, Infumorph 200, Infumorph 500, Morphine HP†, MS Contin, MSIR, MS/L, OMS Concentrate, Oramorph SR, RMS Uniserts, Roxanol, Roxanol 100, Roxanol Rescudose, Roxanol SR, Roxanol UD, Statex

morphine tartrate‡

Controlled Substance Schedule II
Pregnancy Risk Category: C

HOW SUPPLIED
morphine hydrochloride
Tablets: 10 mg†, 20 mg†, 40 mg†,
60 mg†
Tablets (extended-release): 30 mg†,
60 mg†
Oral solution: 1 mg/ml†, 5 mg/ml†,
10 mg/ml†, 20 mg/ml†, 50 mg/ml†
Syrup: 1 mg/ml†, 5 mg/ml†, 10 mg/ml†,
20 mg/ml†, 50 mg/ml†
Suppositories: 10 mg†, 20 mg†, 30 mg†
morphine sulfate
Tablets: 15 mg, 30 mg
Tablets (extended-release): 15 mg, 30 mg,
60 mg, 100 mg, 200 mg
Soluble tablets: 10 mg, 15 mg, 30 mg
Oral solution: 10 mg/5 ml, 20 mg/5 ml,
20 mg/ml (concentrate), 100 mg/5 ml
Syrup: 1 mg/ml, 5 mg/ml
Injection (with preservative): 0.5 mg/ml,
1 mg/ml, 2 mg/ml, 3 mg/ml, 4 mg/ml,
5 mg/ml, 8 mg/ml, 10 mg/ml, 15 mg/ml,
25 mg/ml, 50 mg/ml
Injection (without preservative): 0.5 mg/
ml, 1 mg/ml, 10 mg/ml, 25 mg/ml
Suppositories: 5 mg, 10 mg, 20 mg,
30 mg
morphine tartrate
Injection: 80 mg/ml‡

ACTION
Binds with opiate receptors in the CNS,
altering both perception of and emotional
response to pain through an unknown
mechanism.

Route	Onset	Peak	Duration
PO	1 hr	1-2 hr	4-12 hr
IV	5 min	20 min	4-5 hr
IM	10-30 min	30-60 min	4-5 hr
SC	10-30 min	50-90 min	4-5 hr
PR	20-30 min	20-60 min	4-5 hr
Epidural	15-60 min	15-60 min	24 hr
Intrathecal	15-60 min	30-60 min	24 hr

INDICATIONS & DOSAGE
Severe pain—
Adults: 5 to 20 mg S.C. or I.M. or 2.5 to
15 mg I.V. q 4 hours, p.r.n.; or 10 to 30 mg
P.O. or 10 to 20 mg P.R. q 4 hours, p.r.n.
When given by continuous I.V. infusion, a
loading dose of 15 mg I.V. may be followed by a continuous infusion of 0.8 to
10 mg/hour. 15 to 30 mg extended-release

tablets P.O. q 8 to 12 hours may also be
administered. As an epidural injection,
5 mg by epidural catheter; then, if adequate pain relief not obtained within 1
hour, additional doses of 1 to 2 mg given
at intervals sufficient to assess efficacy.
Maximum total epidural dosage should
not exceed 10 mg/24 hours. As an intrathecal injection, a single dose of
0.2 mg to 1 mg may provide pain relief
for 24 hours (only in the lumbar area).
Repeat injections not recommended.
Children: 0.1 to 0.2 mg/kg S.C. or I.M.
q 4 hours. Maximum single dose is
15 mg.

ADVERSE REACTIONS
CNS: *sedation, somnolence, clouded sensorium, euphoria,* **seizures** *(with large
doses), dizziness, nightmares (with long-
acting oral forms), light-headedness,* hallucinations, nervousness, depression, syncope.
CV: hypotension, **bradycardia, shock,
cardiac arrest,** tachycardia, hypertension.
GI: *nausea, vomiting, constipation,* ileus,
dry mouth, biliary tract spasms, anorexia.
GU: urine retention, decreased libido.
Hematologic: **thrombocytopenia.**
Respiratory: **respiratory depression, apnea, respiratory arrest.**
Skin: pruritus and skin flushing (with
epidural administration), diaphoresis, edema.
Other: physical dependence.

INTERACTIONS
Drug-drug. *CNS depressants, general
anesthetics, hypnotics, MAO inhibitors,
other narcotic analgesics, sedatives, tranquilizers, tricyclic antidepressants:* possible respiratory depression, hypotension,
profound sedation, or coma. Use together
with extreme caution. Reduce morphine
dosage and monitor patient response.
Drug-lifestyle. *Alcohol use:* additive effects. Use together cautiously.

EFFECTS ON DIAGNOSTIC TESTS
Drug increases plasma amylase levels.

CONTRAINDICATIONS
Contraindicated in patients with hypersensitivity to drug or conditions that

would preclude administration of opioids by I.V. route (acute bronchial asthma or upper airway obstruction).

NURSING CONSIDERATIONS
• Use with extreme caution in patients with head injury, increased intracranial pressure, seizures, chronic pulmonary disease, prostatic hyperplasia, severe hepatic or renal disease, acute abdominal conditions, hypothyroidism, Addison's disease, and urethral stricture. Also use with extreme caution in elderly or debilitated patients.
• Keep narcotic antagonist (naloxone) and resuscitation equipment available.
• Oral solutions of various concentrations as well as an intensified oral solution (20 mg/ml) are available. Carefully note the strength administered.
• Do not crush, break, or chew extended-release tablets.
• Oral capsules may be carefully opened and the entire beaded contents poured into cool, soft foods, such as water, orange juice, applesauce, or pudding; mixture should be consumed immediately.
• S.L. administration may be ordered. Measure oral solution with tuberculin syringe. Administer dose a few drops at a time to allow maximal S.L. absorption and minimize swallowing.
• Refrigeration of rectal suppository is not necessary. In some patients, rectal and oral absorption may not be equivalent.
• Preservative-free preparations are available for epidural and intrathecal administration.
• When given epidurally, monitor closely for respiratory depression up to 24 hours after the injection. Check respiratory rate and depth every 30 to 60 minutes for 24 hours.
• Know that morphine is the drug of choice in relieving MI pain. May cause transient decrease in blood pressure.
• Be aware that an around-the-clock regimen best manages severe, chronic pain.
• Be aware that morphine may worsen or mask gallbladder pain.
• Monitor circulatory, respiratory, bladder, and bowel functions carefully. Drug may cause respiratory depression, hypotension, urine retention, nausea, vomiting,

ileus, or altered level of consciousness regardless of the route used. Withhold dose and notify doctor if respirations are below 12 breaths/minute.
• Constipation is often severe with maintenance dosage. Ensure that stool softener or other laxative is ordered.

I.V. administration
• When given by direct injection, 2.5 to 15 mg may be diluted in 4 or 5 ml of sterile water for injection and given over 4 to 5 minutes. Alternatively, drug may be mixed with D_5W to a concentration of 0.1 to 1 mg/ml and administered by a continuous infusion device. Morphine sulfate is compatible with most common I.V. solutions.

✓ Patient teaching
• When drug is used postoperatively, encourage patient to turn, cough, and breathe deeply and to use incentive spirometer to prevent atelectasis.
• Caution ambulatory patient about getting out of bed or walking. Warn outpatient to avoid driving and other potentially hazardous activities that require mental alertness until drug's adverse CNS effects are known.
• Advise patient to avoid alcohol.

nalbuphine hydrochloride
Nubain

Pregnancy Risk Category: B

HOW SUPPLIED
Injection: 10 mg/ml, 20 mg/ml

ACTION
Binds with opiate receptors in the CNS, altering both perception of and emotional response to pain through an unknown mechanism.

Route	Onset	Peak	Duration
IV	2-3 min	30 min	3-6 hr
IM	15 min	1 hr	3-6 hr
SC	15 min	Unknown	3-6 hr

INDICATIONS & DOSAGE
Moderate to severe pain—
Adults: for an average (70-kg [154-lb]) person, 10 to 20 mg S.C., I.M., or I.V. q 3 to 6 hours, p.r.n. Maximum daily dosage is 160 mg.
Adjunct to balanced anesthesia—
Adults: 0.3 mg/kg to 3.0 mg/kg I.V. over 10 to 15 minutes followed by maintenance doses of 0.25 to 0.50 mg/kg in single I.V. dose, p.r.n.

ADVERSE REACTIONS
CNS: *headache, sedation, dizziness, vertigo,* nervousness, depression, restlessness, crying, euphoria, hostility, unusual dreams, confusion, hallucinations, speech difficulty, delusions.
CV: hypertension, hypotension, tachycardia, bradycardia.
EENT: blurred vision, dry mouth.
GI: cramps, dyspepsia, bitter taste, nausea, vomiting, constipation, biliary tract spasms.
GU: urinary urgency.
Respiratory: *respiratory depression,* dyspnea, asthma, *pulmonary edema.*
Skin: pruritus, burning, urticaria, clamminess.

INTERACTIONS
Drug-drug. *CNS depressants, general anesthetics, hypnotics, MAO inhibitors, sedatives, tranquilizers, tricyclic antidepressants:* possible respiratory depression, hypertension, profound sedation, or coma. Use together with extreme caution. Monitor patient response.
Narcotic analgesics: possible decreased analgesic effect. Avoid concomitant use.
Drug-lifestyle. *Alcohol use:* additive effects. Use together cautiously.

EFFECTS ON DIAGNOSTIC TESTS
None reported.

CONTRAINDICATIONS
Contraindicated in patients with hypersensitivity to drug.

NURSING CONSIDERATIONS
• Use cautiously in patients with history of drug abuse or in patients with emotional instability, head injury, increased intracranial pressure, impaired ventilation, MI accompanied by nausea and vomiting, upcoming biliary surgery, and hepatic or renal disease.
• Know that drug acts as a narcotic antagonist; may precipitate withdrawal syndrome. For patients who have chronically received opiates, administer 25% of the usual dose initially as ordered. Observe for signs of withdrawal.
Alert: Be aware that drug causes respiratory depression, which at 10 mg is equal to the respiratory depression produced by 10 mg of morphine.
• Monitor circulatory and respiratory status and bladder and bowel function. Withhold dose and notify doctor if respirations are shallow or rate is below 12 breaths/minute.
• Constipation is often severe with maintenance therapy. Make sure stool softener or other laxative is ordered.
• Know that psychological and physical dependence may occur with prolonged use.

I.V. administration
• Inject slowly over at least 2 to 3 minutes into a vein or into an I.V. line containing a compatible, free-flowing I.V. solution, such as D_5W, 0.9% NaCl, or lactated Ringer's solution.
• Respiratory depression can be reversed with naloxone. Keep resuscitation equipment available, particularly when administering I.V.

Patient teaching
• Caution ambulatory patient about getting out of bed or walking. Warn outpatient to avoid driving and other potentially hazardous activities that require mental alertness until drug's CNS effects are known.
• Instruct patient on how to manage troublesome adverse effects such as constipation.

Reactions may be *common*, uncommon, *life-threatening*, or COMMON AND LIFE-THREATENING.

oxycodone hydrochloride
Endone‡, OxyContin, Oxy IR, Roxicodone, Roxicodone Intensol, Supeudol†

oxycodone pectinate
Proladone‡

Controlled Substance Schedule II
Pregnancy Risk Category: C

HOW SUPPLIED
oxycodone hydrochloride
Capsules: 5 mg
Tablets: 5 mg
Tablets (controlled-release): 10 mg, 20 mg, 40 mg, 80 mg
Oral solution: 5 mg/5 ml, 20 mg/ml (concentrate)
Suppositories: 10 mg†, 20 mg†
oxycodone pectinate
Suppositories: 30 mg‡

ACTION
Binds with opiate receptors in the CNS, altering both perception of and emotional response to pain through an unknown mechanism.

Route	Onset	Peak	Duration
PO	10-15 min	1 hr	3-6 hr
PR	Unknown	Unknown	Unknown

INDICATIONS & DOSAGE
Moderate to severe pain—
Adults: 5 mg P.O. q 6 hours, p.r.n. Alternatively, 1 to 3 suppositories P.R. daily, p.r.n.

ADVERSE REACTIONS
CNS: *sedation, somnolence, clouded sensorium,* euphoria, *dizziness, light-headedness.*
CV: *hypotension,* bradycardia.
GI: *nausea, vomiting,* constipation, ileus.
GU: urine retention.
Respiratory: *respiratory depression.*
Skin: diaphoresis, pruritus.
Other: physical dependence.

INTERACTIONS
Drug-drug. *Anticoagulants:* oxycodone hydrochloride products containing aspirin may increase anticoagulant effect. Monitor clotting times. Use together cautiously.
CNS depressants, general anesthetics, hypnotics, MAO inhibitors, other narcotic analgesics, sedatives, tranquilizers, tricyclic antidepressants: additive effects. Use together with extreme caution. Reduce oxycodone dose and monitor patient response.
Drug-lifestyle. *Alcohol use:* additive effects. Use together cautiously.

EFFECTS ON DIAGNOSTIC TESTS
Oxycodone increases plasma amylase, lipase, and liver enzyme levels.

CONTRAINDICATIONS
Contraindicated in patients with hypersensitivity to drug.

NURSING CONSIDERATIONS
• Use with extreme caution in patients with head injury, increased intracranial pressure, seizures, asthma, COPD, prostatic hyperplasia, severe hepatic or renal disease, acute abdominal conditions, urethral stricture, hypothyroidism, Addison's disease, and arrhythmias. Also use with extreme caution in elderly or debilitated patients.
• For full analgesic effect, administer drug before patient has intense pain.
• To minimize GI upset, administer drug after meals or with milk.
• Be aware that single-agent oxycodone solution or tablets are especially useful for patients who shouldn't take aspirin or acetaminophen.
• Monitor circulatory and respiratory status. Withhold dose and notify doctor if respirations are shallow or if respiratory rate falls below 12 breaths/minute.
• Monitor patient's bladder and bowel patterns. Patient may require a laxative because drug has a constipating effect.

☑ **Patient teaching**
• Instruct patient to ask for drug before pain is intense.
• Tell patient to take drug with milk or after eating.
• Caution ambulatory patient about getting out of bed or walking. Warn outpatient to avoid driving and other potentially

hazardous activities that require mental alertness until drug's CNS effects are known.
• Advise patient to avoid alcohol.

---

oxymorphone hydrochloride
Numorphan, Numorphan H.P.

*Controlled Substance Schedule II
Pregnancy Risk Category: B
(D if used for prolonged periods or
high doses at term)*

HOW SUPPLIED
Injection: 1 mg/ml, 1.5 mg/ml
Suppositories: 5 mg

ACTION
Binds with opiate receptors in the CNS, altering both perception of and emotional response to pain through an unknown mechanism.

Route	Onset	Peak	Duration
IV	5-10 min	15-30 min	3-4 hr
IM	10-15 min	0.5-1.5 hr	3-6 hr
SC	10-20 min	1-1.5 hr	3-6 hr
PR	15-30 min	2 hr	3-6 hr

INDICATIONS & DOSAGE
Moderate to severe pain—
Adults: 1 to 1.5 mg I.M. or S.C. q 4 to 6 hours, p.r.n.; or 0.5 mg I.V. q 4 to 6 hours, p.r.n.; or 5 mg P.R. q 4 to 6 hours, p.r.n.
Analgesia during labor—
Adults: 0.5 to 1 mg I.M.

ADVERSE REACTIONS
CNS: *sedation, somnolence, clouded sensorium, euphoria,* dizziness, **seizures** (with large doses), light-headedness, headache.
CV: *hypotension,* bradycardia.
GI: *nausea, vomiting, constipation,* ileus.
GU: *urine retention.*
Respiratory: *respiratory depression.*
Skin: pruritus.
Other: physical dependence.

INTERACTIONS
Drug-drug. *CNS depressant, general anesthetics, MAO inhibitors, tricyclic an-* *tidepressants:* additive effects. Use together with extreme caution.
Drug-lifestyle. *Alcohol use:* additive effects. Use together cautiously.

EFFECTS ON DIAGNOSTIC TESTS
Drug increases plasma amylase levels.

CONTRAINDICATIONS
Contraindicated in patients with hypersensitivity to drug.

NURSING CONSIDERATIONS
• Use with extreme caution in patients with head injury, increased intracranial pressure, seizures, asthma, COPD, acute abdominal conditions, prostatic hyperplasia, severe hepatic or renal disease, urethral stricture, respiratory depression, hypothyroidism, Addison's disease, and arrhythmias. Also use with extreme caution in elderly or debilitated patients.
• Keep narcotic antagonist (naloxone) and resuscitation equipment available.
• Drug is not for mild pain. May worsen gallbladder pain.
• For better effect, administer drug before patient has intense pain.
• Monitor CV and respiratory status. Withhold dose and notify doctor if respirations decrease or rate is below 12 breaths/minute.
• Monitor patient's bladder and bowel function. Patient may need laxative.

I.V. administration
• Give by direct I.V. injection. If necessary, drug may be diluted in 0.9% NaCl solution.

Patient teaching
• Instruct patient to ask for drug before pain is intense.
• When drug is used postoperatively, encourage patient to turn, cough, and breathe deeply and to use incentive spirometer to avoid atelectasis.
• Caution ambulatory patient about getting out of bed or walking. Warn outpatient to avoid driving and other potentially hazardous activities that require mental alertness until drug's CNS effects are known.

Reactions may be *common,* uncommon, *life-threatening,* or COMMON AND LIFE-THREATENING.

- Instruct patient to store suppositories in refrigerator.
- Advise patient to avoid alcohol.

pentazocine hydrochloride
Fortral†‡, Talwin†

pentazocine hydrochloride and naloxone hydrochloride
Talwin Nx

pentazocine lactate
Fortral‡, Talwin

Controlled Substance Schedule IV
Pregnancy Risk Category: C

HOW SUPPLIED
pentazocine hydrochloride
Tablets: 25 mg‡, 50 mg†‡
pentazocine hydrochloride and naloxone hydrochloride
Tablets: 50 mg pentazocine hydrochloride and 500 mcg naloxone hydrochloride
pentazocine lactate
Injection: 30 mg/ml

ACTION
Binds with opiate receptors at many sites in the CNS, altering both perception of and emotional response to pain through an unknown mechanism.

Route	Onset	Peak	Duration
PO	15-30 min	1-3 hr	2-3 hr
IV	2-3 min	15-30 min	2-3 hr
IM, SC	10-20 min	30-60 min	2-3 hr

INDICATIONS & DOSAGE
Moderate to severe pain—
Adults: 50 to 100 mg P.O. q 3 to 4 hours, p.r.n. Maximum oral dosage is 600 mg/day. Alternatively, 30 mg I.M., I.V., or S.C. q 3 to 4 hours, p.r.n. Maximum parenteral dosage is 360 mg/day. Single doses above 30 mg I.V. or 60 mg I.M. or S.C. are not recommended.
Labor—
Adults: 30 mg I.M. or 20 mg I.V. q 2 to 3 hours when contractions become regular.

ADVERSE REACTIONS
CNS: *sedation,* visual disturbances, hal-lucinations, drowsiness, *dizziness, light-headedness,* confusion, *euphoria,* headache, psychotomimetic effects.
CV: circulatory depression, **shock,** hypertension.
EENT: dry mouth.
GI: *nausea, vomiting,* constipation.
GU: urine retention.
Respiratory: *respiratory depression,* dyspnea, **apnea.**
Skin: induration, nodules, sloughing, sclerosis (at injection site); diaphoresis; pruritus.
Other: hypersensitivity reactions *(ana-phylaxis),* physical and psychological dependence.

INTERACTIONS
Drug-drug. *CNS depressants:* additive effects. Use together cautiously.
Narcotic analgesics: possible decreased analgesic effect. Avoid concomitant use.
Drug-lifestyle. *Alcohol use:* additive effects. Use together cautiously.
Smoking: may increase requirements for pentazocine. Monitor drug's effectiveness.

EFFECTS ON DIAGNOSTIC TESTS
Drug may interfere with certain laboratory tests for urinary 17-hydroxycorticosteroids.

CONTRAINDICATIONS
Contraindicated in patients with hypersensitivity to drug or its components. It is not recommended for children under 12 years.

NURSING CONSIDERATIONS
- Use cautiously in patients with hepatic or renal disease, acute MI, head injury, increased intracranial pressure, and respiratory depression.
- Have naloxone readily available. Respiratory depression can be reversed with naloxone.
- *Alert:* When giving by S.C. or I.M. injection, rotate injection sites to minimize tissue irritation. If possible, avoid giving by S.C. route.
- Know that drug possesses narcotic antagonist properties. May precipitate withdrawal syndrome in narcotic-dependent patients.

• Psychological and physical dependence may occur with prolonged use.
• Know that pentazocine may interfere with certain laboratory tests for urinary 17-hydroxycorticosteroids.

🔋 I.V. administration
• Give by direct I.V. injection slowly. Do not mix in syringe with aminophylline, barbiturates, or other alkaline substances.
• Know that Talwin Nx, the oral pentazocine available in the United States, contains the narcotic antagonist naloxone. This prevents illicit I.V. use.

☑ Patient teaching
• Instruct patient to ask for drug before pain is intense.
• Caution ambulatory patient about getting out of bed or walking. Warn outpatient to avoid driving and other potentially hazardous activities that require mental alertness until drug's CNS effects are known.
• Advise patient to avoid alcohol.
• Instruct patient or family to report skin rash, disorientation, or confusion to doctor.

---

propoxyphene hydrochloride (dextropropoxyphene hydrochloride)
Darvon, Dolene, Novo-Propoxyn†, 642†

propoxyphene napsylate (dextropropoxyphene napsylate)
Darvon-N, Doloxene‡

Controlled Substance Schedule IV
Pregnancy Risk Category: C

HOW SUPPLIED
propoxyphene hydrochloride
Capsules: 32 mg, 65 mg
propoxyphene napsylate
Tablets: 100 mg
Oral suspension: 10 mg/ml

ACTION
Binds with opiate receptors in the CNS, altering both perception of and emotional

response to pain through an unknown mechanism.

Route	Onset	Peak	Duration
PO	15-60 min	2-2.5 hr	4-6 hr

INDICATIONS & DOSAGE
Mild to moderate pain—
Adults: 65 mg (hydrochloride) P.O. q 4 hours, p.r.n. Maximum dosage is 390 mg/day.
Mild to moderate pain—
Adults: 100 mg (napsylate) P.O. q 4 hours, p.r.n. Maximum dosage is 600 mg/day.
Adjust-a-dose: In patients with hepatic or renal dysfunction, reduce dose.

ADVERSE REACTIONS
CNS: *dizziness,* headache, *sedation,* euphoria, light-headedness, weakness, hallucinations.
GI: *nausea, vomiting,* constipation, abdominal pain.
Respiratory: *respiratory depression.*
Other: psychological and physical dependence, abnormal liver function tests.

INTERACTIONS
Drug-drug. *Carbamazepine:* may increase carbamazepine levels. Monitor closely.
CNS depressants: additive effects. Use together cautiously.
Warfarin: may increase anticoagulant effect. Monitor PT and INR.
Drug-lifestyle. *Alcohol use:* additive effects. Use together cautiously.
Smoking: increased metabolism of propoxyphene. Monitor closely.

EFFECTS ON DIAGNOSTIC TESTS
Drug may cause false decreases in tests for urinary steroid excretion.

CONTRAINDICATIONS
Contraindicated in patients with hypersensitivity to drug.

NURSING CONSIDERATIONS
• Use cautiously in hepatic or renal disease, emotional instability, or history of drug or alcohol abuse.
• Remember that 65 mg of propoxyphene

hydrochloride equals 100 mg of propoxyphene napsylate.

• Be aware that drug is considered a mild narcotic analgesic, but pain relief is equivalent to that provided by aspirin. Tolerance and physical dependence may occur. Used with aspirin or acetaminophen to maximize analgesia.

• Know that smokers may need increased dosage because smoking may induce liver enzymes responsible for the metabolism of the drug, thereby decreasing its efficacy.

☑ **Patient teaching**

• To minimize GI upset, advise patient to take drug with food or milk.

• Warn patient not to exceed recommended dosage. Respiratory depression, hypotension, profound sedation, and coma may result if used in excessive doses or with other CNS depressants. Advise patient to avoid alcohol intake or use of other CNS-type drugs when taking propoxyphene.

• Caution ambulatory patient about getting out of bed or walking. Warn outpatient to avoid driving and other hazardous activities that require mental alertness until drug's CNS effects are known.

---

remifentanil hydrochloride
Ultiva

Controlled Substance Schedule II
Pregnancy Risk Category: C

HOW SUPPLIED
Injection (vials): 1 mg/3 ml, 2 mg/5 ml, 5 mg/10 ml

ACTION
Binds with μ-opiate receptors throughout CNS, resulting in analgesia and anesthesia.

Route	Onset	Peak	Duration
IV	Immediate	Unknown	5-10 min

INDICATIONS & DOSAGE
Induction of anesthesia through intubation—
Adults: 0.5 to 1 mcg/kg/minute with hypnotic or volatile agent; may load with 1 mcg/kg over 30 to 60 seconds if endotracheal intubation is to occur less than 8 minutes after start of remifentanil infusion.
Maintenance of anesthesia—
Adults: 0.25 to 0.4 mcg/kg/minute, dependent on concurrent anesthetic modalities (nitrous oxide, isoflurane, propofol). Increase doses by 25% to 100% and decrease by 25% to 50% q 2 to 5 minutes, p.r.n. If rate exceeds 1 mcg/kg/minute, consider increases in concomitant anesthetic agents. May supplement with 1 mcg/kg boluses over 30 to 60 seconds q 2 to 5 minutes, p.r.n.
Continuation as analgesic immediately postoperatively—
Adults: initially, 0.1 mcg/kg/minute. Adjust rate by 0.025 mcg/kg/minute increments q 5 minutes, p.r.n. Rates over 0.2 mcg/kg/minute are associated with respiratory depression (under 8 breaths/minute).
Monitored anesthesia care—
Adults: as single I.V. dose: 0.5 to 1 mcg/kg over 30 to 60 seconds starting 90 seconds before placement of local or regional anesthetic. As continuous I.V. infusion: 0.1 mcg/kg/minute beginning 5 minutes before giving local anesthetic; after placement of local anesthetic, adjust rate to 0.05 mcg/kg/minute. Adjust rate by 0.025 mcg/kg/minute q 5 minutes, p.r.n. Rates over 0.2 mcg/kg/minute are associated with respiratory depression (less than 8 breaths/minute). Decrease dose by 50% if given with 2 mg midazolam. Bolus doses administered simultaneously with continuously infusing remifentanil to spontaneously breathing patients are not recommended.
Elderly: decrease initial dose by 50%.
Adjust-a-dose: In obese patients (more than 30% over ideal body weight), base starting dose on ideal body weight.

ADVERSE REACTIONS
CNS: agitation, dizziness, headache.
CV: bradycardia, hypertension, *hypotension*, tachycardia.
EENT: visual disturbances.
GI: *nausea, vomiting.*
Musculoskeletal: *muscle rigidity.*

Respiratory: *apnea, hypoxia, respiratory depression.*
Skin: flushing, pain at injection site, pruritus.
Other: chills, fever, postoperative pain, shivering, sweating, warm sensation.

INTERACTIONS

Drug-drug. *Benzodiazepine, hypnotics, inhaled anesthetics:* produce a synergistic effect. Monitor patient closely.

EFFECTS ON DIAGNOSTIC TESTS

None reported.

CONTRAINDICATIONS

Contraindicated in patients with known hypersensitivity to fentanyl analogues. Do not use via epidural or intrathecal routes because of presence of glycine in preparation.

NURSING CONSIDERATIONS

• Use cautiously in breast-feeding patients because fentanyl analogues are excreted in breast milk.
• Monitor vital signs and oxygenation continually throughout drug administration.
• Do not use as a single agent in general anesthesia.
• Manage respiratory depression in spontaneously breathing patients by decreasing infusion rate by 50% or by temporarily discontinuing infusion.
• Skeletal muscle rigidity may occur. To treat, either stop or decrease the rate of infusion in spontaneously breathing patients.
• Effects of long-term (over 16 hours) use in intensive care settings are not known.
• Bradycardia has been reported and responds to ephedrine, atropine, and glycopyrrolate.
• Interruption of drug infusion results in rapid reversal (no residual opioid effects within 5 to 10 minutes of infusion discontinuation) of effects; adequate postoperative anesthesia should first be established.
• Drug should not be used outside the monitored anesthesia care setting. Keep narcotic antagonist (naloxone) and resuscitation equipment available. Naloxone

may be used to manage severe respiratory depression.
• Drug is incompatible with blood products.
• Obtain history from patient regarding previous adverse anesthesia reactions in patient or patient's family.

▣ I.V. administration

• To reconstitute solution, add 1 ml of diluent per mg of drug. Shake well to dissolve. Reconstituted solution contains 1 mg/ml and should be clear and colorless. Further dilute to concentration of 25, 50, or 250 mcg/ml before administration. Drug is stable at room temperature for 24 hours when in final concentration in D_5W, D_5W in 0.9% NaCl, 0.9% NaCl, 0.45% NaCl, or D_5W in lactated Ringer's solution. Drug is stable for 4 hours when mixed in lactated Ringer's solution. Continuous infusion of drug must be administered by infusion device. Upon discontinuation of drug, I.V. tubing should be cleared to avoid inadvertent administration of drug at a later time.
• Hypotension may occur and can be treated by decreasing rate of infusion or administering I.V. fluids or catecholamine.
• I.V. bolus administration should be used only during maintenance of general anesthesia. In nonintubated patients, single doses should be administered over 30 to 60 seconds.

☑ Patient teaching

• Reassure patient that appropriate monitoring will occur during anesthesia administration.

sufentanil citrate
Sufenta

Controlled Substance Schedule II
Pregnancy Risk Category: C

HOW SUPPLIED
Injection: 50 mcg/ml

ACTION
Binds with opiate receptors in the CNS, altering both perception of and emotional

response to pain through an unknown mechanism.

Route	Onset	Peak	Duration
IV	1 min	1 min	5 min

INDICATIONS & DOSAGE
Adjunct to general anesthetic—
Adults: 1 to 8 mcg/kg I.V. administered with nitrous oxide and oxygen; additional 10 to 25 mcg I.V. may be administered, p.r.n., when movement or changes in vital signs indicate surgical stress or lightening of analgesia.
As a primary anesthetic—
Adults: 8 to 30 mcg/kg I.V. administered with 100% oxygen and a muscle relaxant; additional 25 to 50 mcg I.V. may be administered, p.r.n., when movement or changes in vital signs indicate surgical stress or lightening of analgesia.
Children under 12 years undergoing CV surgery: 10 to 25 mcg/kg I.V. administered with 100% oxygen and a muscle relaxant. Additional doses up to 50 mcg may be given p.r.n.
Elderly: reduced dosage is required.
Adjust-a-dose: Use reduced dosage in debilitated patients. For obese patients who exceed 20% of their ideal body weight, base dosage calculations on an estimate of ideal weight.

ADVERSE REACTIONS
CNS: chills, somnolence.
CV: *hypotension,* hypertension, arrhythmias, *bradycardia,* tachycardia.
GI: nausea, vomiting.
Respiratory: *chest wall rigidity, apnea, bronchospasm.*
Skin: *pruritus,* erythema.
Other: intraoperative muscle movement.

INTERACTIONS
Drug-drug. *CNS depressants:* additive effects. Use together cautiously.
Drug-lifestyle. *Alcohol use:* additive effects. Use together cautiously.

EFFECTS ON DIAGNOSTIC TESTS
Sufentanil may increase plasma amylase, lipase, and serum prolactin levels.

CONTRAINDICATIONS
Contraindicated in patients with hypersensitivity to drug.

NURSING CONSIDERATIONS
• Use with extreme caution in head injury; in pulmonary, hepatic, or renal disease; in decreased respiratory reserve; and in elderly or debilitated patients.
• When used at doses over 8 mcg/kg, postoperative mechanical ventilation and observation are essential because of prolonged respiratory depression.
• Keep narcotic antagonist (naloxone) and resuscitation equipment available.
• Because drug decreases both rate and depth of respirations, monitoring of arterial oxygen saturation may aid in assessing respiratory depression. Notify doctor if respirations decrease or rate falls below 12 breaths/minute.
• Monitor respirations of neonates exposed to the drug during labor.
Alert: Know that high doses can produce muscle rigidity reversible by neuromuscular blockers; however, patient must be artificially ventilated.
• Monitor postoperative vital signs frequently, including circulatory and respiratory status and urinary function. Drug may cause respiratory depression, hypotension, urine retention, nausea, vomiting, ileus, or altered level of consciousness.

I.V. administration
• Drug should be administered only by persons trained in the use of I.V. anesthetics.
• Give by direct I.V. injection. Drug has been given by intermittent I.V. infusion, but drug compatibility and stability in I.V. solutions have not been fully investigated.

Patient teaching
• Inform patient and family of need for drug and answer any questions.
• Encourage turning, coughing, and deep breathing postoperatively to prevent atelectasis.

tramadol hydrochloride
Ultram, Zamadol§, Zydol§

Pregnancy Risk Category: C

HOW SUPPLIED
Tablets: 50 mg

ACTION
Unknown. A centrally acting synthetic analgesic compound not chemically related to opiates. Thought to bind to opioid receptors and inhibit reuptake of norepinephrine and serotonin.

Route	Onset	Peak	Duration
PO	Unknown	2 hr	Unknown

INDICATIONS & DOSAGE
Moderate to moderately severe pain—
Adults: 50 to 100 mg P.O. q 4 to 6 hours, p.r.n. Maximum dosage is 400 mg daily.
Elderly: in patients over 75 years, maximum dosage is 300 mg/day in divided doses.
Adjust-a-dose: In renally impaired patients with creatinine clearance below 30 ml/minute, increase dose interval to q 12 hours; maximum daily dosage is 200 mg. In patients with cirrhosis, 50 mg q 12 hours.

ADVERSE REACTIONS
CNS: *dizziness, vertigo, headache, somnolence, CNS stimulation, asthenia,* anxiety, confusion, coordination disturbance, euphoria, nervousness, sleep disorder, *seizures.*
CV: vasodilation.
EENT: visual disturbances.
GI: *nausea, constipation, vomiting,* dyspepsia, dry mouth, diarrhea, abdominal pain, anorexia, flatulence.
GU: urine retention, urinary frequency, menopausal symptoms.
Respiratory: *respiratory depression.*
Skin: *pruritus,* diaphoresis, rash.
Other: malaise, hypertonia.

INTERACTIONS
Drug-drug. *Carbamazepine:* increased tramadol metabolism. Patients receiving chronic carbamazepine therapy at a dosage of up to 800 mg daily may require up to twice the recommended dose of tramadol.
CNS depressants: additive effects. Use together with caution. Dosage of tramadol may need to be reduced.
MAO inhibitors, neuroleptics: increased risk of seizures. Monitor patient closely.

EFFECTS ON DIAGNOSTIC TESTS
Tramadol may increase creatinine clearance and liver enzyme levels, decrease hemoglobin levels, and cause proteinuria.

CONTRAINDICATIONS
Contraindicated in patients with hypersensitivity to drug or with acute intoxication from alcohol, hypnotics, centrally acting analgesics, opioids, or psychotropic drugs.

NURSING CONSIDERATIONS
• Use cautiously in patients at risk for seizures or respiratory depression; in increased intracranial pressure or head injury, acute abdominal conditions, or renal or hepatic impairment; and in physical dependence on opioids.
• Monitor CV and respiratory status. Withhold dose and notify doctor if respirations decrease or rate is below 12 breaths/minute.
• Monitor bowel and bladder function. Anticipate the need for a laxative.
• For better analgesic effect, give drug before onset of intense pain.
• Monitor patients at risk for seizures. Drug may reduce seizure threshold.
• Monitor patient for drug dependence. Drug can produce dependence similar to that of codeine or dextropropoxyphene and thus has potential for abuse.

☑ **Patient teaching**
• Tell patient to take drug as prescribed and not to increase dosage or dosage interval unless ordered by doctor.
• Caution ambulatory patient to be careful when rising and walking. Warn outpatient to avoid driving and other potentially hazardous activities that require mental alertness until drug's CNS effects are known.
• Advise patient to check with doctor before taking OTC medications; drug interactions can occur.

Reactions may be *common*, uncommon, *life-threatening*, or COMMON AND LIFE-THREATENING.

29
Sedative-hypnotics

butabarbital sodium
chloral hydrate
estazolam
flurazepam hydrochloride
pentobarbital
pentobarbital sodium
phenobarbital sodium
   (See Chapter 30, ANTICONVULSANTS.)
secobarbital sodium
temazepam
triazolam
zolpidem tartrate

COMBINATION PRODUCTS
TUINAL 100 mg PULVULES: amobarbital
sodium 50 mg and secobarbital sodium
50 mg.
TUINAL 200 mg PULVULES: amobarbital
sodium 100 mg and secobarbital sodium
100 mg.

---

butabarbital sodium
(butabarbitone sodium)
Butisol*†**

Controlled Substance Schedule III
Pregnancy Risk Category: D

HOW SUPPLIED
Tablets: 15 mg, 30 mg, 50 mg, 100 mg
Elixir: 30 mg/5 ml

ACTION
Unknown. A barbiturate that probably interferes with transmission of impulses
from the thalamus to the cortex of the
brain.

Route	Onset	Peak	Duration
PO	45-60 min	3 hr	6-8 hr

INDICATIONS & DOSAGE
Sedation—
Adults: 15 to 30 mg P.O. t.i.d. or q.i.d.
Children: 6 mg/kg or 180 mg/m² P.O. di-
vided t.i.d. Dosage range is 7.5 to 30 mg
P.O. t.i.d.

Preoperatively—
Adults: 50 to 100 mg P.O. 60 to 90 min-
utes before surgery.
Children: 2 to 6 mg/kg P.O. (not to ex-
ceed 100 mg) 60 to 90 minutes before
surgery.
Insomnia—
Adults: 50 to 100 mg P.O., h.s.
Elderly: use reduced doses.
Adjust-a-dose: In patients with hepatic or
renal failure, use reduced doses.

ADVERSE REACTIONS
CNS: drowsiness, lethargy, hangover,
paradoxical excitement (in elderly pa-
tients), somnolence.
GI: nausea, vomiting.
Hematologic: exacerbation of porphyria.
Respiratory: respiratory depression, ap-
nea.
Skin: rash, urticaria, Stevens-Johnson
syndrome.
Other: angioedema, physical and psy-
chological dependence.

INTERACTIONS
Drug-drug. Chloramphenicol, MAO inhibitors, valproic acid: inhibits metabolism of barbiturates; may cause prolonged
CNS depression. Reduce barbiturate
dosage.
CNS depressants, including narcotic
analgesics: excessive CNS and respiratory depression. Use together cautiously.
Corticosteroids, digitoxin, doxycycline,
estrogens and oral contraceptives, oral
anticoagulants, theophylline, tricyclic antidepressants, verapamil: barbiturates
may enhance the metabolism of these
drugs. Monitor for decreased effectiveness.
Griseofulvin: decreased absorption of
griseofulvin. Monitor effectiveness of
griseofulvin.
Rifampin: may decrease barbiturate levels. Monitor for decreased effect.
Drug-lifestyle. Alcohol use: excessive
CNS and respiratory depression. Use together cautiously.

---

*Liquid contains alcohol.   **May contain tartrazine.   †Canada   ‡Australia   §U.K.   ◇OTC

EFFECTS ON DIAGNOSTIC TESTS
Drug may cause a false-positive phentolamine test. The physiologic effects of drug may impair the absorption of cyanocobalamin ^{57}Co; it may decrease serum bilirubin concentrations in neonates, epileptic patients, and patients with congenital nonhemolytic unconjugated hyperbilirubinemia. EEG patterns are altered, with a change in low-voltage, fast activity; changes persist for a time after discontinuation of therapy. Barbiturates may increase sulfobromophthalein retention.

CONTRAINDICATIONS
Contraindicated in patients with bronchopneumonia or other severe pulmonary insufficiency, porphyria, or hypersensitivity to barbiturates.

NURSING CONSIDERATIONS
• Use cautiously in patients with acute or chronic pain, depression, suicidal tendencies, history of drug abuse, or hepatic or renal impairment.
• Know that elderly patients are more sensitive to drug's adverse CNS reactions. Assess mental status before and after initiating therapy.
• Take precautions to prevent hoarding or self-overdosing by patients who are depressed, suicidal, or drug-dependent or who have a history of drug abuse.
• Watch for signs of barbiturate toxicity: coma, pupillary constriction, cyanosis, clammy skin, and hypotension. Overdose can be fatal.
• Discontinue drug when skin reactions occur because skin eruptions may precede potentially fatal reactions to barbiturate therapy. In some patients, high fever, stomatitis, headache, or rhinitis may precede skin reactions.
• Be aware that long-term use is not recommended; drug loses its efficacy in promoting sleep after 14 days. A drug-free interval of at least 1 week is advised if continued treatment is appropriate. Long-term high dosage may cause drug dependence, and patients may experience withdrawal symptoms if drug is suddenly stopped. Withdraw barbiturates gradually.

☑ Patient teaching
• Tell patient that morning "hangover" is common after hypnotic dose. Hypnotic doses suppress REM sleep. Patients may experience increased dreaming after drug is discontinued.
• Tell patient to avoid alcohol use while taking drug.
• Caution patient about performing activities that require mental alertness or physical coordination.
• Instruct patient who uses oral contraceptives that she should consider alternative birth control methods because drug may enhance contraceptive hormone metabolism and decrease its effect.

---

chloral hydrate
Aquachloral Supprettes, Noctec, Novo-Chlorhydrate†

Controlled Substance Schedule IV
Pregnancy Risk Category: C

HOW SUPPLIED
Capsules: 250 mg, 500 mg
Syrup: 250 mg/5 ml, 500 mg/5 ml
Suppositories: 324 mg, 500 mg, 648 mg

ACTION
Unknown. Sedative effects may be caused by its primary metabolite, trichloroethanol.

Route	Onset	Peak	Duration
PO	0.5 hr	Unknown	4-8 hr
PR	Unknown	Unknown	4-8 hr

INDICATIONS & DOSAGE
Sedation—
Adults: 250 mg P.O. or P.R. t.i.d. after meals.
Children: 25 mg/kg /day P.O. or P.R. Maximum daily dosage is 500 mg per single dose; doses may be divided.
Insomnia—
Adults: 500 mg to 1 g P.O. or P.R. 15 to 30 minutes before bedtime.
Children: 50 mg/kg P.O. or P.R. 15 to 30 minutes before bedtime. Maximum single dose is 1 g.

Reactions may be *common*, uncommon, *life-threatening*, or COMMON AND LIFE-THREATENING.

Preoperatively—
Adults: 500 mg to 1 g P.O. or P.R. 30 minutes before surgery.
Premedication for EEG—
Children: 20 to 25 mg/kg P.O. or P.R.

ADVERSE REACTIONS

CNS: drowsiness, nightmares, dizziness, ataxia, paradoxical excitement, hangover, somnolence, disorientation, delirium, light-headedness, hallucinations, confusion, vertigo, malaise.
GI: *nausea, vomiting, diarrhea,* flatulence.
Hematologic: eosinophilia, leukopenia.
Skin: hypersensitivity reactions (rash, urticaria).
Other: physical and psychological dependence.

INTERACTIONS

Drug-drug. *Alkaline solutions:* incompatible with aqueous solutions of chloral hydrate. Don't mix together.
CNS depressants, including narcotic analgesics: excessive CNS depression or vasodilation reaction. Use together cautiously.
Furosemide I.V.: causes sweating, flushes, variable blood pressure, nausea, and uneasiness. Use together cautiously or use a different hypnotic drug.
Oral anticoagulants: increased risk of bleeding. Monitor patient closely.
Phenytoin: decreased phenytoin levels. Monitor closely.
Drug-lifestyle. *Alcohol use:* excessive CNS and respiratory depression. Use together cautiously.

EFFECTS ON DIAGNOSTIC TESTS

Drug therapy may produce false-positive results for urine glucose with tests using cupric sulfate, such as Benedict's reagent. It does not interfere with Diastix or Chemstrip uG results. It will interfere with fluorometric tests for urine catecholamines; do not use drug for 48 hours before the test. Drug may interfere with Reddy-Jenkins-Thorn test for urinary 17-hydroxycorticosteroids. It may also cause a false-positive phentolamine test.

CONTRAINDICATIONS

Contraindicated in patients with hepatic or renal impairment, severe cardiac disease, or hypersensitivity to chloral hydrate. Oral administration contraindicated in patients with gastric disorders.

NURSING CONSIDERATIONS

● Use with extreme caution in patients with severe cardiac disease. Use cautiously in patients with mental depression, suicidal tendencies, or history of drug abuse.
Alert: Note two strengths of oral liquid form. Double-check dose, especially when administering to children. Fatal overdoses have occurred.
● To minimize unpleasant taste and stomach irritation, dilute or administer with liquid. Drug should be taken after meals.
● Take precautions to prevent hoarding or self-overdosing by patients who are depressed, suicidal, or drug-dependent or who have a history of drug abuse.
● Be aware that long-term use is not recommended; drug loses its efficacy in promoting sleep after 14 days of continued use. Long-term use may cause drug dependence, and patient may experience withdrawal symptoms if drug is suddenly stopped.
● Do not administer drug for 48 hours before fluorometric test, as ordered.
● Monitor BUN levels as ordered; large dosage may raise BUN levels.

☑ Patient teaching

● Instruct patient to take capsules with a full glass of water or juice and to swallow the capsule whole.
● Tell patient to avoid alcohol use while taking drug.
● Caution patient about performing activities that require mental alertness or physical coordination.
● Inform patient to store drug in dark container; store suppositories in refrigerator.

estazolam
ProSom

Controlled Substance Schedule IV
Pregnancy Risk Category: X

HOW SUPPLIED
Tablets: 1 mg, 2 mg

ACTION
Unknown. Thought to act on the limbic system and thalamus of the CNS by binding to specific benzodiazepine receptors.

Route	Onset	Peak	Duration
PO	Unknown	1-3 hr	Unknown

INDICATIONS & DOSAGE
Insomnia—
Adults: 1 mg P.O. h.s. Some patients may require 2 mg.
Elderly: 1 mg P.O. h.s. Use higher doses with extreme care. Frail elderly or debilitated patients may take 0.5 mg, but this low dose may be only marginally effective.

ADVERSE REACTIONS
CNS: fatigue, dizziness, daytime drowsiness, *somnolence, asthenia,* hypokinesia, abnormal thinking.
GI: dyspepsia, abdominal pain.
Other: back pain, stiffness.

INTERACTIONS
Drug-drug. *Cimetidine, disulfiram, isoniazid, oral contraceptives:* may impair the metabolism and clearance of benzodiazepines and prolong their plasma half-life. Monitor for increased CNS depression.
CNS depressants, including antihistamines, opiate analgesics, and other benzodiazepines: increased CNS depression. Avoid concomitant use.
Digoxin: Digoxin serum levels may increase, resulting in toxicity. Monitor closely.
Phenytoin: possible increase in phenytoin levels, resulting in toxicity. Monitor closely.
Rifampin: may increase metabolism and clearance and decrease plasma half-life. Monitor for decreased effectiveness.
Theophylline: pharmacologic antagonism. Monitor for decreased effectiveness of estazolam.
Drug-lifestyle. *Alcohol use:* excessive CNS and respiratory depression. Use together cautiously.
Smoking: may increase metabolism and clearance and decrease plasma half-life. Monitor for decreased effectiveness.

EFFECTS ON DIAGNOSTIC TESTS
AST levels may be increased.

CONTRAINDICATIONS
Contraindicated in patients with hypersensitivity to drug and during pregnancy.

NURSING CONSIDERATIONS
• Use cautiously in patients with hepatic, renal, or pulmonary disease; depression; or suicidal tendencies.
• Be aware that liver and renal function and CBC should be checked before and periodically during long-term therapy as ordered.
• Take precautions to prevent hoarding by depressed, suicidal, or drug-dependent patients or those who have a history of drug abuse.
• Be aware that patients who receive prolonged treatment with benzodiazepines may experience withdrawal symptoms if the drug is suddenly discontinued (possibly after 6 weeks of continuous therapy).

☑ **Patient teaching**
• Advise patient to inform doctor if pregnancy is suspected or is being planned during therapy.
• Tell patient not to increase drug dosage but to inform doctor if he thinks that drug is no longer effective.
• Caution patient about performing activities that require mental alertness or physical coordination.
• Warn patient that additive depressant effects can occur if alcohol is consumed while taking this drug or within 24 hours after taking drug.

flurazepam hydrochloride
Apo-Flurazepam†, Dalmane, Novo-Flupam†

Controlled Substance Schedule IV
Pregnancy Risk Category: NR

HOW SUPPLIED
Capsules: 15 mg, 30 mg

Reactions may be *common,* uncommon, *life-threatening,* or COMMON AND LIFE-THREATENING.

ACTION
Unknown. A benzodiazepine that is thought to act on the limbic system, thalamus, and hypothalamus of the CNS to produce hypnotic effects.

Route	Onset	Peak	Duration
PO	Unknown	0.5-1 hr	Unknown

INDICATIONS & DOSAGE
Insomnia—
Adults: 15 to 30 mg P.O. h.s. Dose repeated once, p.r.n.
Elderly: initiate with 15-mg dose until response determined.

ADVERSE REACTIONS
CNS: *daytime sedation, dizziness, drowsiness, disturbed coordination,* lethargy, confusion, *headache,* light-headedness, nervousness, hallucinations, staggering, ataxia, disorientation, ***coma.***
GI: nausea, vomiting, heartburn, diarrhea, abdominal pain.
Hepatic: elevated liver enzymes.
Other: physical or psychological dependence.

INTERACTIONS
Drug-drug. *Cimetidine:* increased sedation. Monitor carefully.
CNS depressants, including narcotic analgesics: excessive CNS depression. Use together cautiously.
Digoxin: Digoxin serum levels may increase, resulting in toxicity. Monitor closely.
Disulfiram, isoniazid, oral contraceptives: decreased metabolism of benzodiazepines, leading to toxicity. Monitor closely.
Phenytoin: increased phenytoin levels. Monitor for toxicity.
Rifampin: enhanced metabolism of benzodiazepines. Monitor for decreased effectiveness.
Theophylline: antagonist with flurazepam. Monitor for decreased effectiveness.
Drug-lifestyle. *Alcohol use:* excessive CNS and respiratory depression. Use together cautiously.
Smoking: may increase metabolism and clearance and decrease plasma half-life. Monitor for decreased effectiveness.

EFFECTS ON DIAGNOSTIC TESTS
Minor changes in EEG patterns (usually low-voltage, fast activity) may occur during and after flurazepam therapy.

CONTRAINDICATIONS
Contraindicated in patients with hypersensitivity to drug and during pregnancy.

NURSING CONSIDERATIONS
• Use cautiously in patients with impaired hepatic or renal function, chronic pulmonary insufficiency, mental depression, suicidal tendencies, or history of drug abuse.
• Check hepatic and renal function and CBC before and periodically during long-term therapy. May cause elevations in certain liver function tests (AST, ALT, total and direct bilirubin, and alkaline phosphatase).
• Assess mental status before initiating therapy. Elderly patients are more sensitive to drug's adverse CNS reactions.
• Take precautions to prevent hoarding or self-overdosing by patients who are depressed, suicidal, or drug-dependent or who have a history of drug abuse.
• Be aware that physical and psychological dependence is possible with long-term use.

☑ **Patient teaching**
• Inform patient that drug is more effective on second, third, and fourth nights because active metabolite accumulates.
• Warn patient not to abruptly discontinue use after taking for 1 month or more.
• Tell patient to avoid alcohol use while taking drug.
• Caution patient about performing activities that require mental alertness or physical coordination.

pentobarbital
(pentobarbitone)
Nembutal*†**

pentobarbital sodium
Nembutal Sodium*, Nova Rectal†,
Novo-Pentobarb†

*Controlled Substance Schedule II
(III for suppositories)
Pregnancy Risk Category: D*

HOW SUPPLIED
pentobarbital
Elixir: 18.2 mg/5 ml
pentobarbital sodium
Capsules: 50 mg, 100 mg
Injection: 50 mg/ml
Suppositories: 30 mg, 60 mg, 120 mg,
200 mg

ACTION
Unknown. Probably interferes with transmission of impulses from the thalamus to
the cortex of the brain. A barbiturate.

Route	Onset	Peak	Duration
PO	20 min	0.5-1 hr	1-4 hr
IV	Immediate	Immediate	15 min
IM	10-25 min	Unknown	Unknown
PR	20 min	Unknown	1-4 hr

INDICATIONS & DOSAGE
Sedation—
Adults: 20 mg P.O. t.i.d. or q.i.d.
Children: 2 to 6 mg/kg daily P.O. in three
divided doses. Maximum daily dosage is
100 mg.
Insomnia—
Adults: 100 to 200 mg P.O. h.s. or 150 to
200 mg deep I.M.; 100 mg initially I.V.;
then additional doses up to 500 mg; 120
or 200 mg P.R.
Children: 2 to 6 mg/kg or 125 mg/m^2
I.M. Maximum dosage is 100 mg. P.R.
dose for child 2 months to 1 year is
30 mg; 1 to 4 years, 30 or 60 mg; 5 to 11
years, 60 mg; 12 to 14 years, 60 or
120 mg.
Preoperative sedation—
Adults: 150 to 200 mg I.M.
Children: 5 mg/kg P.O. or I.M. if 10
years or older; 5 mg/kg I.M. or P.R. if
younger than 10 years.

ADVERSE REACTIONS
CNS: *drowsiness, lethargy, hangover,*
paradoxical excitement in elderly patients,
somnolence.
GI: nausea, vomiting.
Hematologic: exacerbation of porphyria.
Respiratory: *respiratory depression.*
Skin: rash, urticaria, ***Stevens-Johnson
syndrome.***
Other: ***angioedema,*** physical and psy-
chological dependence.

INTERACTIONS
Drug-drug. *CNS depressants, including
narcotic analgesics:* excessive CNS and
respiratory depression. Use together cautiously.
*Corticosteroids, digitoxin, doxycycline,
estrogens and oral contraceptives, oral
anticoagulants, theophylline, verapamil:*
pentobarbital may enhance the metabolism of these drugs. Monitor for decreased effect.
Griseofulvin: decreased absorption of
griseofulvin. Monitor effectiveness of
griseofulvin.
MAO inhibitors: inhibited metabolism of
barbiturates; may cause prolonged CNS
depression. Reduce barbiturate dosage.
Rifampin: may decrease barbiturate levels. Monitor for decreased effect.
Drug-herb. *Kava:* may cause additive effects. Avoid concomitant use.
Drug-lifestyle. *Alcohol use:* excessive
CNS and respiratory depression. Use together cautiously.

EFFECTS ON DIAGNOSTIC TESTS
Drug may cause a false-positive phentolamine test. The physiologic effects of
drug may impair the absorption of
cyanocobalamin ^{57}Co; it may decrease
serum bilirubin concentrations in neonates, epileptic patients, and patients with
congenital nonhemolytic unconjugated
hyperbilirubinemia. EEG patterns show a
change in low-voltage, fast activity;
changes persist for a time after discontinuation of therapy.

CONTRAINDICATIONS

Contraindicated in patients with porphyria or hypersensitivity to barbiturates.

NURSING CONSIDERATIONS

• Use cautiously in patients with acute or chronic pain, mental depression, suicidal tendencies, history of drug abuse, or hepatic impairment. Also administer cautiously to elderly or debilitated patients.

• Assess mental status before initiating therapy and use reduced doses as ordered. Elderly patients are more sensitive to the drug's adverse CNS effects.

Alert: Administer I.M. injection deeply. Superficial injection may cause pain, sterile abscess, and sloughing.

• To ensure accurate dosage, don't divide suppositories.

• Take precautions to prevent hoarding or self-overdosing by patients who are depressed, suicidal, or drug-dependent or who have a history of drug abuse.

• Watch for signs of barbiturate toxicity: coma, pupillary constriction, cyanosis, clammy skin, and hypotension. Overdose can be fatal.

• Inspect patient's skin. Skin eruptions may precede potentially fatal reactions to barbiturate therapy. Discontinue drug when skin reactions occur and call doctor. In some patients, high fever, stomatitis, headache, or rhinitis may precede skin reactions.

• Know that pentobarbital has no analgesic effect and may cause restlessness or delirium in patients with pain.

• Be aware that long-term use is not recommended; drug loses its efficacy in promoting sleep after 14 days of continued use. Long-term high dosage may cause drug dependence, and patient may experience withdrawal symptoms if drug is suddenly discontinued. Withdraw barbiturates gradually.

I.V. administration

• Know that I.V. administration of barbiturates may cause severe respiratory depression, laryngospasm, or hypotension. Have emergency resuscitation equipment available.

• To minimize deterioration, use I.V injection solution within 30 minutes after opening container. Do not use cloudy solution.

• Reserve I.V. injection for emergency treatment, which should be given under close supervision. Administer slowly at a rate not exceeding 50 mg/minute.

• Know that parenteral solution is alkaline. Local tissue reactions and injection site pain have followed I.V. use. Avoid extravasation. Assess patency of I.V. site before and during administration.

• Do not mix in syringe or in I.V. solutions or lines with other drugs.

✓ Patient teaching

• Inform patient that morning "hangover" is common after hypnotic dose, which suppresses REM sleep. Patient may experience increased dreaming after drug is discontinued.

• Caution patient about performing activities that require mental alertness or physical coordination.

• Tell patient to avoid alcohol use while taking drug.

• Instruct patient who uses oral contraceptives that she should consider alternative birth control methods because drug may decrease oral contraceptive's effect.

secobarbital sodium
Novo-Secobarb†, Seconal Sodium

Controlled Substance Schedule II
Pregnancy Risk Category: D

HOW SUPPLIED
Capsules: 100 mg
Injection: 50 mg/ml

ACTION
Unknown. Probably interferes with transmission of impulses from the thalamus to the cortex of the brain. A barbiturate.

Route	Onset	Peak	Duration
PO	15 min	15-30 min	1-4 hr
IV	Immediate	1-3 min	15 min
IM	Unknown	7-10 min	Unknown

INDICATIONS & DOSAGE
Preoperative sedation—
Adults: 200 to 300 mg P.O. 1 to 2 hours

before surgery, or 1 mg/kg I.M. 10 to 15 minutes before surgery.
Children: 2 to 6 mg/kg P.O. 1 to 2 hours before surgery. Maximum single dose is 100 mg P.O., or 4 to 5 mg/kg I.M. as a single dose.
Insomnia—
Adults: 100 to 200 mg P.O. or I.M. or 50 to 250 mg I.V.
Children: 3 to 5 mg/kg I.M. or 125 mg/m^2, not to exceed 100 mg, with no more than 5 ml injected in any one site.
Acute tetanus seizure—
Adults and children: 5.5 mg/kg I.M. or slow I.V., repeated q 3 to 4 hours, if needed; I.V. injection rate not to exceed 50 mg/15 seconds.
Status epilepticus—
Children: 15 to 20 mg/kg I.V. over 15 minutes.

ADVERSE REACTIONS
CNS: *drowsiness, lethargy, hangover,* paradoxical excitement (in elderly patients), somnolence.
CV: hypotension (with I.V. use).
GI: nausea, vomiting.
Hematologic: exacerbation of porphyria.
Respiratory: *respiratory depression.*
Skin: rash, urticaria, *Stevens-Johnson syndrome,* tissue reactions, injection-site pain.
Other: *angioedema,* physical and psychological dependence.

INTERACTIONS
Drug-drug. *Chloramphenicol, MAO inhibitors, valproic acid:* inhibited metabolism of barbiturates; may cause prolonged CNS depression. Reduce barbiturate dosage.
CNS depressants, including narcotic analgesics: excessive CNS and respiratory depression. Use together cautiously.
Corticosteroids, digitoxin, doxycycline, estrogens and oral contraceptives, oral anticoagulants, theophylline, tricyclic antidepressants, verapamil: secobarbital may enhance the metabolism of these drugs. Monitor for decreased effect.
Griseofulvin: decreased absorption of griseofulvin. Monitor effectiveness of griseofulvin.

Rifampin: may decrease barbiturate levels. Monitor for decreased effect.
Drug-lifestyle. *Alcohol use:* excessive CNS and respiratory depression. Use together cautiously.

EFFECTS ON DIAGNOSTIC TESTS
Drug may cause a false-positive phentolamine test. The physiologic effects of drug may impair the absorption of cyanocobalamin ^{57}Co; it may decrease serum bilirubin concentrations in neonates, epileptic patients, and patients with congenital nonhemolytic unconjugated hyperbilirubinemia. EEG patterns are altered, with a change in low-voltage, fast activity; changes persist for a time after discontinuation of therapy.

CONTRAINDICATIONS
Contraindicated in patients with marked liver impairment, respiratory disease in which dyspnea or obstruction is evident, porphyria, or hypersensitivity to barbiturates.

NURSING CONSIDERATIONS
• Use cautiously in patients with acute or chronic pain, depression, suicidal tendencies, history of drug abuse, hepatic or renal impairment or who are elderly or debilitated.
• Assess mental status before initiating therapy. Elderly patients are more sensitive to the drug's adverse CNS effects.
• Know that secobarbital sodium injection is not compatible with lactated Ringer's solution, but is compatible with Ringer's solution, sterile water for injection, and 0.9% NaCl. Don't mix with acidic solutions.
• Use injection solution within 30 minutes after opening container to minimize deterioration. Do not use if cloudy solution.
Alert: Give I.M. injection deeply. Superficial injection may cause pain, sterile abscess, and sloughing.
• Take precautions to prevent hoarding or self-overdosing by patients who are depressed, suicidal, or drug-dependent or who have a history of drug abuse.
• Watch for signs of barbiturate toxicity: coma, pupillary constriction, cyanosis, clammy skin, and hypotension. Overdose can be fatal.

Reactions may be *common*, uncommon, *life-threatening*, or COMMON AND LIFE-THREATENING.

• Inspect patient's skin. Skin eruptions may precede potentially fatal reactions to barbiturate therapy. Discontinue drug when skin reactions occur and notify doctor. In some patients, high fever, stomatitis, headache, or rhinitis may precede skin reactions.

• Be aware that long-term use is not recommended; drug loses its efficacy in promoting sleep after 14 days of continued use.

⚫ I.V. administration

• Know that I.V. injection is reserved for emergency treatment and given under close supervision by direct injection and administered slowly at a rate not exceeding 50 mg/15 seconds. May be administered as supplied or diluted.

• Be aware that local tissue reactions and injection-site pain have been noted with I.V. use. Assess patency of I.V. site before and during administration.

• Know that I.V. administration of barbiturates may cause severe respiratory depression, laryngospasm, or hypotension. Have emergency resuscitation equipment readily available.

✅ Patient teaching

• Tell patient that morning "hangover" is common after hypnotic dose, which suppresses REM sleep. Patient may experience increased dreaming after drug is discontinued.

• Tell patient to avoid alcohol use while taking drug.

• Caution patient about performing activities that require mental alertness or physical coordination.

• Instruct patient who uses oral contraceptives that she should consider alternative birth control methods.

---

temazepam
Euhypnos 10‡, Euhypnos 20‡, Nomapam‡, Normison‡, Restoril, Temaze‡, Temtabs‡

Controlled Substance Schedule IV
Pregnancy Risk Category: X

HOW SUPPLIED
Capsules: 10 mg‡, 15 mg, 20 mg‡, 30 mg

ACTION
Unknown. A benzodiazepine that probably acts on the limbic system, thalamus, and hypothalamus of the CNS to produce hypnotic effects.

Route	Onset	Peak	Duration
PO	Unknown	1-2 hr	Unknown

INDICATIONS & DOSAGE
Insomnia—
Adults: 15 to 30 mg P.O. h.s.
Elderly: in patients over 65 years, 15 mg P.O. h.s.

ADVERSE REACTIONS
CNS: drowsiness, dizziness, lethargy, disturbed coordination, daytime sedation, confusion, nightmares, vertigo, euphoria, weakness, headache, fatigue, nervousness, anxiety, depression.
EENT: blurred vision.
GI: diarrhea, nausea, dry mouth.
Other: physical and psychological dependence.

INTERACTIONS
Drug-drug. *CNS depressants:* increased CNS depression. Use together cautiously.
Drug-lifestyle. *Alcohol use:* increased CNS depression. Use together cautiously.

EFFECTS ON DIAGNOSTIC TESTS
Drug therapy may increase liver function test results. Minor changes in EEG patterns (usually low-voltage, fast activity) may occur during and after therapy.

CONTRAINDICATIONS
Contraindicated in patients with hypersensitivity to drug or other benzodiazepines and during pregnancy.

NURSING CONSIDERATIONS
• Use cautiously in patients with chronic pulmonary insufficiency, impaired hepatic or renal function, severe or latent mental depression, suicidal tendencies, and history of drug abuse.
• Assess mental status before initiating

---

therapy. Elderly patients are more sensitive to the drug's adverse CNS effects.
• Take precautions to prevent hoarding or self-overdosing by patients who are depressed, suicidal, or drug-dependent or who have a history of drug abuse.

☑Patient teaching
• Tell patient to avoid alcohol use while taking drug.
• Caution patient about performing activities that require mental alertness or physical coordination.
• Warn patient not to discontinue drug abruptly if taken for 1 month or longer.
• Tell patient that onset of drug's effects may take as long as 2 to 2½ hours.

---

triazolam
Apo-Triazo†, Halcion,
Novo-Triolam†, Nu-Triazo†

Controlled Substance Schedule IV
Pregnancy Risk Category: X

HOW SUPPLIED
Tablets: 0.125 mg, 0.25 mg

ACTION
Unknown. A benzodiazepine that probably acts on the limbic system, thalamus, and hypothalamus of the CNS to produce hypnotic effects.

Route	Onset	Peak	Duration
PO	Unknown	1-2 hr	Unknown

INDICATIONS & DOSAGE
Insomnia—
Adults: 0.125 to 0.5 mg P.O. h.s.
Elderly: 0.125 mg P.O. h.s.; increased, p.r.n., to 0.25 mg P.O. h.s.

ADVERSE REACTIONS
CNS: *drowsiness,* dizziness, headache, rebound insomnia, amnesia, lack of coordination, mental confusion, depression, nervousness, ataxia.
GI: nausea, vomiting.
Other: physical or psychological dependence.

INTERACTIONS
Drug-drug. *Cimetidine, erythromycin:* may cause prolonged triazolam blood levels. Monitor for increased sedation.
CNS depressants: excessive CNS depression. Use together cautiously.
Drug-lifestyle. *Alcohol use:* excessive CNS depression. Use together cautiously.

EFFECTS ON DIAGNOSTIC TESTS
Drug therapy may increase liver function test results. Minor changes in EEG patterns (usually low-voltage, fast activity) may occur during and after therapy.

CONTRAINDICATIONS
Contraindicated in patients with hypersensitivity to benzodiazepines and during pregnancy.

NURSING CONSIDERATIONS
• Use cautiously in breast-feeding patients and those with impaired hepatic or renal function, chronic pulmonary insufficiency, sleep apnea, mental depression, suicidal tendencies, or history of drug abuse.
• Assess mental status before initiating therapy. Elderly patients are more sensitive to the drug's CNS effects.
• Take precautions to prevent hoarding or self-overdosing by patients who are depressed, suicidal, or drug-dependent or who have a history of drug abuse.

☑Patient teaching
• Warn patient not to take more than the prescribed amount; overdose can occur at a total daily dosage of 2 mg (or four times highest recommended amount).
• Tell patient to avoid alcohol use while taking drug.
• Warn patient not to discontinue drug abruptly if taken for 2 weeks or longer.
• Caution patient about performing activities that require mental alertness or physical coordination.
• Inform patient that drug tends not to cause morning drowsiness.
• Tell patient that rebound insomnia may develop for 1 or 2 nights after stopping therapy.

Reactions may be *common,* uncommon, *life-threatening,* or COMMON AND LIFE-THREATENING.

zolpidem tartrate
Ambien, Stilnoct§

Controlled Substance Schedule IV
Pregnancy Risk Category: B

HOW SUPPLIED
Tablets: 5 mg, 10 mg

ACTION
Although zolpidem interacts with one of three identified gamma-aminobutyric acid-benzodiazepine receptor complexes, it's not a benzodiazepine. It exhibits hypnotic activity, but no muscle relaxant or anticonvulsant properties.

Route	Onset	Peak	Duration
PO	Rapid	0.5-2 hr	Unknown

INDICATIONS & DOSAGE
Short-term management of insomnia—
Adults: 10 mg P.O. immediately before bedtime.
Elderly: 5 mg P.O. immediately before bedtime. Maximum daily dosage is 10 mg.
Adjust-a-dose: In debilitated patients and in those with hepatic insufficiency, 5 mg P.O. immediately before bedtime. Maximum daily dosage is 10 mg.

ADVERSE REACTIONS
CNS: daytime drowsiness, light-headedness, abnormal dreams, amnesia, dizziness, *headache,* hangover, sleep disorder, lethargy, depression.
CV: palpitations.
EENT: sinusitis, pharyngitis, dry mouth.
GI: nausea, vomiting, diarrhea, dyspepsia, constipation, abdominal pain.
Skin: rash.
Other: back or chest pain, flulike symptoms, hypersensitivity reactions, myalgia, arthralgia.

INTERACTIONS
Drug-drug. *CNS depressants:* excessive CNS depression. Use together cautiously.
Drug-lifestyle. *Alcohol use:* excessive CNS depression. Use together cautiously.

EFFECTS ON DIAGNOSTIC TESTS
None reported.

CONTRAINDICATIONS
No known contraindications.

NURSING CONSIDERATIONS
● Use cautiously in patients with compromised respiratory status.
● Be aware that hypnotics should be used only for short-term management of insomnia, usually 7 to 10 days.
● Know that the smallest effective dose should be used in all patients.
● Take precautions to prevent hoarding or self-overdosing by patients who are depressed, suicidal, or drug-dependent or who have a history of drug abuse.

☑**Patient teaching**
● For rapid sleep onset, instruct patient not to take drug with or immediately after meals.
● Tell patient to avoid alcohol.
● Caution patient about performing activities that require mental alertness or physical coordination.

30

Anticonvulsants

acetazolamide sodium
(See Chapter 62, DIURETICS.)
carbamazepine
clonazepam
clorazepate dipotassium
(See Chapter 32, ANTIANXIETY DRUGS.)
diazepam
(See Chapter 32, ANTIANXIETY DRUGS.)
divalproex sodium
ethosuximide
fosphenytoin sodium
gabapentin
lamotrigine
magnesium sulfate
phenobarbital
phenobarbital sodium
phenytoin
phenytoin sodium
phenytoin sodium (extended)
primidone
tiagabine hydrochloride
topiramate
valproate sodium
valproic acid

COMBINATION PRODUCTS
None.

---

carbamazepine
Apo-Carbamazepine†, Atretol,
Carbatrol, Epitol, Mazepine†,
Novo-Carbamaz†,
PMS-Carbamazepine†, Tegretol,
Tegretol CR†, Tegretol-XR, Teril‡

Pregnancy Risk Category: C

HOW SUPPLIED
Tablets: 200 mg
Tablets (chewable): 100 mg
Tablets (extended-release)†: 100 mg,
200 mg, 400 mg
Capsules (extended-release):
200 mg, 300 mg
Oral suspension: 100 mg/5 ml

ACTION
Unknown. Thought to stabilize neuronal membranes and limit seizure activity by either increasing efflux or decreasing influx of sodium ions across cell membranes in the motor cortex during generation of nerve impulses.

Route	Onset	Peak	Duration
PO	Unknown	1.5-12 hr	Unknown

INDICATIONS & DOSAGE
Generalized tonic-clonic and complex partial seizures, mixed seizure patterns—
Adults and children over 12 years: initially, 200 mg P.O. b.i.d. for tablets or 1 tsp of suspension P.O. q.i.d. May be increased at weekly intervals by 200 mg P.O. daily, in divided doses at 6- to 8-hour intervals. Adjusted to minimum effective level. Maximum daily dosage is 1 g/day in children 12 to 15 years, or 1.2 g/day in patients over 15 years.
Children 6 to 12 years: initially, 100 mg P.O. b.i.d. or ½ tsp of suspension P.O. q.i.d. Increased at weekly intervals by 100 mg P.O. daily. Maximum daily dosage is 1 g/day.
Trigeminal neuralgia—
Adults: initially, 100 mg P.O. b.i.d. or ½ tsp of suspension q.i.d. with meals. Increased by 100 mg q 12 hours for tablets or ½ tsp of suspension q.i.d. until pain is relieved. Maximum daily dosage is 1.2 g/day. Maintenance dosage is 200 to 400 mg P.O. b.i.d.

ADVERSE REACTIONS
CNS: *dizziness, vertigo, drowsiness,* fatigue, *ataxia,* **worsening of seizures** (usually in patients with mixed seizure disorders, including atypical absence seizures), confusion, headache, syncope.
CV: *heart failure,* hypertension, hypotension, aggravation of coronary artery disease, **arrhythmias, AV block.**
EENT: conjunctivitis, dry mouth and pharynx, blurred vision, diplopia, nystagmus.
GI: *nausea, vomiting,* abdominal pain, diarrhea, anorexia, stomatitis, glossitis.

Reactions may be *common,* uncommon, *life-threatening,* or COMMON AND LIFE-THREATENING.

GU: urinary frequency, urine retention, impotence, albuminuria, glycosuria, elevated BUN.

Hematologic: *aplastic anemia, agranulocytosis,* eosinophilia, leukocytosis, *thrombocytopenia.*

Hepatic: elevated liver function test results, *hepatitis.*

Respiratory: pulmonary hypersensitivity.

Skin: rash, urticaria, erythema multiforme, *Stevens-Johnson syndrome.*

Other: excessive diaphoresis, fever, chills, SIADH, decreased thyroid function tests.

INTERACTIONS

Drug-drug. *Cimetidine, danazol, diltiazem, fluoxetine, fluvoxamine, isoniazid, macrolides (such as erythromycin), propoxyphene, valproic acid, verapamil:* may increase carbamazepine blood levels. Use cautiously.

Doxycycline, felbamate, haloperidol, oral contraceptives, phenytoin, theophylline, warfarin: carbamazepine may decrease blood levels of these drugs. Monitor for decreased effect.

Lithium: increased CNS toxicity of lithium. Avoid concomitant use.

MAO inhibitors: increased depressant and anticholinergic effects. Do not use together.

Phenobarbital, phenytoin, primidone: may decrease carbamazepine levels. Monitor for decreased effect.

Drug-herb. *Plantains:* psyllium seed has been reported to inhibit GI absorption. Avoid concomitant use.

EFFECTS ON DIAGNOSTIC TESTS
None reported.

CONTRAINDICATIONS
Contraindicated in patients with history of previous bone marrow suppression or hypersensitivity to carbamazepine or tricyclic antidepressants and in those who have taken an MAO inhibitor within 14 days of therapy.

NURSING CONSIDERATIONS
● Use cautiously in patients with mixed seizure disorders because they may experience an increased incidence of seizures.

● Obtain baseline determinations of urinalysis, BUN level, liver function, CBC, platelet and reticulocyte counts, and serum iron level as ordered. Monitor periodically thereafter.

● Shake oral suspension well before measuring dose.

● When administering by nasogastric tube, mix dose with an equal volume of water, 0.9% NaCl solution, or D_5W. Flush tube with 100 ml of diluent after administering dose.

● Never discontinue drug suddenly when treating seizures. Notify doctor immediately if adverse reactions occur.

● Know that adverse reactions may be minimized by increasing dosage gradually.

● Be aware that therapeutic carbamazepine blood level is 4 to 12 mcg/ml. Monitor blood levels and effects closely. Ask patient when last dose of medication was taken to better evaluate blood levels.

● When managing seizures, institute appropriate precautions.

Alert: Observe for signs of anorexia or subtle appetite changes, which may indicate excessive blood levels.

☑ Patient teaching
● Tell patient to take drug with food to minimize GI distress. Tell patient who takes suspension form to shake container well before measuring dose.

● Tell patient to keep tablets in the original container, tightly closed, and away from moisture. Some formulations may harden when exposed to excessive moisture, resulting in decreased bioavailability and loss of seizure control.

● Inform patient that, when drug is used for trigeminal neuralgia, an attempt to decrease dosage or withdraw drug is usually done every 3 months.

● Tell patient to notify doctor immediately if fever, sore throat, mouth ulcers, or easy bruising or bleeding occurs.

● Tell patient that drug may cause mild to moderate dizziness and drowsiness when first taken. Advise him to avoid hazardous activities until effects disappear, usually within 3 to 4 days.

● Advise patient that periodic eye examinations are recommended.

clonazepam
Klonopin, Paxam‡, Rivotril†

Controlled Substance Schedule IV
Pregnancy Risk Category: D

HOW SUPPLIED
Tablets: 0.5 mg, 1 mg, 2 mg
Drops: 2.5 mg/ml‡
Injection: 1 mg/ml‡

ACTION
Unknown. A benzodiazepine that probably acts by facilitating the effects of the inhibitory neurotransmitter gamma-aminobutyric acid.

Route	Onset	Peak	Duration
PO	Unknown	1-2 hr	Unknown
IV	Unknown	Unknown	Unknown

INDICATIONS & DOSAGE
✳ *NEW INDICATION: Lennox-Gastaut syndrome; atypical absence seizures; akinetic and myoclonic seizures—*
Adults: initially, not to exceed 1.5 mg P.O. daily in three divided doses. May be increased by 0.5 to 1 mg q 3 days until seizures are controlled. If given in unequal doses, largest dose given h.s. Maximum recommended daily dosage is 20 mg.
Children up to 10 years or 30 kg (66 lb): initially, 0.01 to 0.03 mg/kg P.O. daily (not to exceed 0.05 mg/kg daily), in two or three divided doses. Increased by 0.25 to 0.5 mg q third day to maximum maintenance dosage of 0.1 to 0.2 mg/kg daily, p.r.n.
Status epilepticus (where parenteral form is available)—
Adults: 1 mg by slow I.V. infusion.
Children: 0.5 mg by slow I.V. infusion.
Panic disorder—
Adults: initially, 0.25 mg P.O. b.i.d.; increase to target dose of 1 mg/day after 3 days. Some may benefit from doses up to maximum of 4 mg/day. To achieve 4 mg/day, increase dosage in increments of 0.125 to 0.25 mg b.i.d. q 3 days as tolerated until panic disorder is controlled. Discontinue drug gradually with decrease of 0.125 mg b.i.d. q 3 days until drug stopped.

ADVERSE REACTIONS
CNS: *drowsiness,* ataxia, behavioral disturbances (especially in children), slurred speech, tremor, confusion, psychosis, agitation.
CV: palpitations.
EENT: nystagmus, abnormal eye movements, sore gums.
GI: constipation, gastritis, change in appetite, nausea, anorexia, diarrhea.
GU: dysuria, enuresis, nocturia, urine retention.
Hematologic: *leukopenia, thrombocytopenia,* eosinophilia.
Respiratory: *respiratory depression,* chest congestion, shortness of breath.
Skin: rash.

INTERACTIONS
Drug-drug. *Carbamazepine, phenobarbital, phenytoin:* lowered plasma clonazepam levels. Monitor closely.
CNS depressants: increased CNS depression. Avoid concomitant use.
Drug-lifestyle. *Alcohol use:* increased CNS depression. Avoid concomitant use.

EFFECTS ON DIAGNOSTIC TESTS
Drug may elevate liver function test results.

CONTRAINDICATIONS
Contraindicated in patients with significant hepatic disease, acute angle-closure glaucoma, or sensitivity to benzodiazepines.

NURSING CONSIDERATIONS
• Use cautiously in patients with mixed type of seizure because drug may precipitate generalized tonic-clonic seizures. Also use cautiously in children and in patients with chronic respiratory disease or open-angle glaucoma.
• Never withdraw suddenly because seizures may worsen. Call doctor at once if adverse reactions develop.
• Monitor blood levels. Therapeutic blood level is 20 to 80 ng/ml.
• Assess elderly patient's response closely.

Reactions may be *common,* uncommon, *life-threatening,* or COMMON AND LIFE-THREATENING.

Elderly patients are more sensitive to the drug's CNS effects.
- Monitor patient for oversedation.
- Monitor CBCs and liver function tests as ordered.
- Know that withdrawal symptoms are similar to those of barbiturates.
- To reduce the inconvenience of somnolence when used for panic disorder, administration of one dose at bedtime may be desirable.

I.V. administration
- Mix solutions in glass bottles because the drug binds to polyvinyl chloride plastic. If polyvinyl chloride infusion bags are used, administer immediately and infuse at a rate of 60 ml/hour or faster.
- Give slowly by direct injection or by slow I.V. infusion. Drug may be diluted with D₅W, dextrose 2.5% in water, or 0.9% NaCl or 0.45% NaCl solution.

Patient teaching
- Advise patient to avoid driving and other potentially hazardous activities that require mental alertness until drug's CNS effects are known.
- Instruct parent to monitor child's school performance because clonazepam may interfere with attentiveness in school.
- Instruct patient and parents never to stop drug abruptly because seizures may occur.

ethosuximide
Emeside§, Zarontin

Pregnancy Risk Category: C

HOW SUPPLIED
Capsules: 250 mg
Syrup: 250 mg/5 ml

ACTION
Not clearly defined. A succinimide derivative that probably increases seizure threshold. Reduces the paroxysmal spike-and-wave pattern of absence seizures by depressing nerve transmission in the motor cortex.

Route	Onset	Peak	Duration
PO	Unknown	3-7 hr	Unknown

INDICATIONS & DOSAGE
Absence seizures—
Adults and children 6 years and older: 500 mg P.O. daily. Optimal dose is 20 mg/kg/day.
Children 3 to 6 years: 250 mg P.O. daily. Adjust dosage until control is achieved. Optimal dose is 20 mg/kg/day.
Alert: Dosages exceeding 1.5 g daily require administration under doctor's strict supervision.

ADVERSE REACTIONS
CNS: drowsiness, headache, fatigue, dizziness, ataxia, irritability, hiccups, euphoria, lethargy, depression, psychosis.
EENT: myopia, tongue swelling, gingival hyperplasia.
GI: nausea, vomiting, diarrhea, weight loss, cramps, anorexia, epigastric and abdominal pain.
GU: vaginal bleeding, urinary frequency.
Hematologic: *leukopenia,* eosinophilia, *agranulocytosis, pancytopenia.*
Skin: urticaria, pruritic and erythematous rashes, hirsutism.

INTERACTIONS
Drug-drug. *Phenytoin:* serum phenytoin levels may be increased. Monitor levels closely.
Valproic acid: may increase or decrease serum levels of ethosuximide. Monitor levels closely.
Drug-lifestyle. *Alcohol use:* increased CNS depression. Avoid concomitant use.

EFFECTS ON DIAGNOSTIC TESTS
Drug may elevate liver enzyme levels and may cause false-positive Coombs' test results. It may also cause abnormal results of renal function tests.

CONTRAINDICATIONS
Contraindicated in patients with hypersensitivity to succinimide derivatives.

NURSING CONSIDERATIONS
- Use with extreme caution in patients with hepatic or renal disease.
- Be aware that ethosuximide is currently drug of choice for treating absence seizures.
- Never withdraw drug suddenly. Call

doctor immediately if adverse reactions develop.
• Monitor blood levels. Therapeutic blood levels are 40 to 100 mcg/ml.
• Obtain CBC every 3 to 6 months as ordered.

Alert: Know that drug may increase frequency of generalized tonic-clonic seizures when used alone in patients who have mixed types of seizures.

☑ **Patient teaching**
• Advise patient to take drug with food to minimize GI distress.
• Advise patient to avoid hazardous activities that require mental alertness until drug's CNS effects are known.
• Tell patient to notify doctor if rash, joint pain, fever, sore throat, or bruising occurs.
• Warn patient and parents not to stop drug abruptly.

---

fosphenytoin sodium
Cerebyx

Pregnancy Risk Category: D

HOW SUPPLIED
Injection: 2 ml (150 mg fosphenytoin sodium equivalent to 100 mg phenytoin sodium), 10 ml (750 mg fosphenytoin sodium equivalent to 500 mg phenytoin sodium)

ACTION
Fosphenytoin is a prodrug of phenytoin, so its anticonvulsant action is that of phenytoin. Phenytoin is thought to stabilize neuronal membranes and limit seizure activity by modulation of voltage-dependent sodium channels of neurons, inhibition of calcium flux across neuronal membranes, modulation of voltage-dependent calcium channels of neurons, and enhancement of sodium-potassium ATPase activity of neurons and glial cells.

Route	Onset	Peak	Duration
IV	Unknown	End of infusion	Unknown
IM	Unknown	30 min	Unknown

INDICATIONS & DOSAGE
Status epilepticus—
Adults: 15 to 20 mg phenytoin sodium equivalent (PE)/kg I.V. at 100 to 150 mg PE/minute as loading dose; then 4 to 6 mg PE/kg/day I.V. as maintenance dose. (Phenytoin may be used instead of fosphenytoin as maintenance, using the appropriate dose.)

Prevention and treatment of seizures during neurosurgery (nonemergent loading or maintenance dosing)—
Adults: loading dose of 10 to 20 mg PE/kg I.M. or I.V. at infusion rate not exceeding 150 mg PE/minute. Maintenance dose is 4 to 6 mg PE/kg/day I.V. or I.M.

Short-term substitution for oral phenytoin therapy—
Adults: same total daily dosage equivalent as oral phenytoin sodium therapy given as a single daily dose I.M. or I.V. at infusion rate not exceeding 150 mg PE/minute. Some patients may require more frequent dosing.

Elderly: phenytoin clearance is decreased slightly in elderly patients; lower or less frequent dosing may be required.

ADVERSE REACTIONS
CNS: increased or decreased reflexes, speech disorders, dysarthria, asthenia, *intracranial hypertension*, thinking abnormalities, nervousness, hypesthesia, extrapyramidal syndrome, brain edema, headache, *nystagmus, dizziness, somnolence, ataxia,* stupor, incoordination, paresthesia, tremor, agitation, vertigo.
CV: hypertension, vasodilation, tachycardia, hypotension.
GI: constipation, taste perversion.
Hematologic: *thrombocytopenia, leukopenia, agranulocytosis, granulocytopenia, pancytopenia.*
Respiratory: pneumonia.
Skin: rash, ecchymosis, *pruritus.*
Other: lymphadenopathy, hypokalemia, hyperglycemia, pelvic pain, back pain, accidental injury, myasthenia, injection site reaction and pain, infection, chills.

INTERACTIONS
Most significant drug interactions expected to occur are those that are commonly seen with phenytoin.

Reactions may be *common,* uncommon, *life-threatening,* or COMMON AND LIFE-THREATENING.

Drug-drug. *Amiodarone, chloramphenicol, chlordiazepoxide, cimetidine, diazepam, dicumarol, disulfiram, estrogens, ethosuximide, fluoxetine, H_2 antagonists, halothane, isoniazid, methylphenidate, phenothiazines, phenylbutazone, salicylates, succinimides, sulfonamides, tolbutamide, trazodone:* may increase plasma phenytoin concentrations and thus its therapeutic effects. Use together cautiously.

Carbamazepine, reserpine: may decrease plasma phenytoin levels. Monitor patient.

Coumarin, corticosteroids, digitoxin, doxycycline, estrogens, furosemide, oral contraceptives, quinidine, rifampin, theophylline, vitamin D: efficacy may be decreased by phenytoin as a result of increased hepatic metabolism. Monitor closely.

Phenobarbital, valproate sodium, valproic acid: may increase or decrease plasma phenytoin levels. Similarly, the effects of phenytoin on the concentrations of these drugs is unpredictable. Monitor patient.

Tricyclic antidepressants: may lower seizure threshold and require adjustments in phenytoin dosage. Use cautiously.

Drug-lifestyle. *Acute alcohol use:* may increase plasma phenytoin concentration and thus its therapeutic effects. Use cautiously.

Chronic alcohol use: may decrease plasma phenytoin levels. Monitor patient.

EFFECTS ON DIAGNOSTIC TESTS
Drug may decrease serum concentrations of T_4. It may also produce artificially low results in dexamethasone or metyrapone tests. Phenytoin may cause increased serum concentrations of glucose, alkaline phosphatase, and gamma glutamyl transpeptidase. Can lower serum folate levels.

CONTRAINDICATIONS
Contraindicated in patients with sinus bradycardia, SA block, second- or third-degree AV block, Adams-Stokes syndrome, or hypersensitivity to drug or its components, phenytoin, or other hydantoins.

NURSING CONSIDERATIONS
• Use cautiously in patients with porphyria and in those with history of hypersensitivity to similarly structured drugs, such as barbiturates, oxazolidinediones, and succinimides.

Alert: Know that fosphenytoin should always be prescribed and dispensed in phenytoin sodium equivalent units (PE). Do not make adjustments in the recommended doses when substituting fosphenytoin for phenytoin, and vice versa.

• Be aware that phosphate load provided by fosphenytoin (0.0037 mmol phosphate/mg PE fosphenytoin) must be taken into consideration when treating patients who require phosphate restriction, such as those with severe renal impairment. Monitor laboratory values.

• Discontinue drug and notify doctor if rash appears. If rash is exfoliative, purpuric, or bullous or if lupus erythematosus, Stevens-Johnson syndrome, or toxic epidermal necrolysis is suspected, drug should be discontinued and alternative therapy considered. If rash is mild (measlelike or scarlatiniform), therapy may be resumed after rash disappears. If rash recurs on reinstitution of therapy, further fosphenytoin or phenytoin administration is contraindicated. Document that patient is allergic to drug.

• Know that drug should be stopped in patients with acute hepatotoxicity.

• Know that I.M. administration generates systemic phenytoin concentrations similar enough to oral phenytoin sodium to allow essentially interchangeable use when ordered.

• Keep in mind that following fosphenytoin administration, phenytoin concentrations should not be monitored until conversion to phenytoin is essentially complete—about 2 hours after the end of an I.V. infusion or 4 hours after I.M. administration.

• Interpret total phenytoin plasma concentration levels cautiously in patients with renal or hepatic disease or with hypoalbuminemia due to an increased fraction in unbound phenytoin. Unbound phenytoin concentrations may be more useful in these patients. When giving drug I.V., monitor patients with renal and hepatic

disease because they are at increased risk for more frequent and severe adverse reactions.
• Know that abrupt withdrawal of drug may precipitate status epilepticus.

I.V. administration
• Before I.V. infusion, dilute fosphenytoin in 5% D₅W or 0.9% NaCl solution for injection to a concentration ranging from 1.5 to 25 mg PE/ml. Do not administer at a rate exceeding 150 mg PE/minute.
• Administer dose of I.V. fosphenytoin used to treat status epilepticus at a maximum rate of 150 mg PE/minute. Typical infusion to a 50-kg (110-lb) patient takes 5 to 7 minutes. (An infusion of an identical molar dose of phenytoin cannot be accomplished in less than 15 to 20 minutes because of adverse CV effects that accompany direct I.V. administration of phenytoin at rates above 50 mg/minute.) Do not use fosphenytoin I.M. for status epilepticus because therapeutic phenytoin concentrations may not be reached as rapidly as with I.V. administration.
• Know that patients receiving 20 mg PE/kg of drug infused at a rate of 150 mg PE/minute are expected to experience sensory discomfort, most often in the groin. Occurrence and intensity of discomfort can be lessened by slowing or temporarily stopping infusion.
• Know that, if rapid phenytoin loading is a primary goal, I.V. administration of drug is preferred because it takes longer to achieve therapeutic plasma phenytoin concentrations after I.M. injection than after I.V. infusion.
• Monitor patient's ECG, blood pressure, and respiration continuously throughout the period during which maximal serum phenytoin concentrations occur—about 10 to 20 minutes after the end of fosphenytoin infusions. Severe CV complications are most commonly encountered in elderly or gravely ill patients. Reducing the rate of administration or discontinuing the drug may be necessary.

Patient teaching
• Warn patient that sensory disturbances may occur with I.V. administration.

• Instruct patient to immediately report adverse reactions, especially rash.
• Warn patient never to stop drug abruptly or adjust dosage without discussing with his doctor.
• Inform female patient that breast-feeding is not recommended.

---

gabapentin
Neurontin

Pregnancy Risk Category: C

HOW SUPPLIED
Capsules: 100 mg, 300 mg, 400 mg

ACTION
Unknown. Although structurally related to gamma-aminobutyric acid (GABA), the drug doesn't interact with GABA receptors and isn't converted metabolically into GABA or a GABA agonist.

Route	Onset	Peak	Duration
PO	Unknown	Unknown	Unknown

INDICATIONS & DOSAGE
Adjunctive treatment of partial seizures with and without secondary generalization in adults with epilepsy—
Adults: initially, 300 mg P.O. h.s. on day 1; 300 mg P.O. b.i.d. on day 2; then 300 mg P.O. t.i.d. on day 3. Dosage increased as needed and tolerated to 1,800 mg daily in divided doses. Dosages up to 3,600 mg daily have been well tolerated.
Adjust-a-dose: In patients with renal failure with creatinine clearance over 60 ml/minute, 400 mg P.O. t.i.d.; if creatinine clearance is between 30 and 60 ml/minute, 300 mg P.O. b.i.d.; between 15 and 30 ml/minute, 300 mg P.O. daily; and if creatinine clearance is under 15 ml/minute, 300 mg P.O. every other day. Patients on dialysis should receive a loading dose of 300 to 400 mg P.O.; then 200 to 300 mg P.O. q 4 hours while on hemodialysis.

ADVERSE REACTIONS
CNS: *fatigue, somnolence, dizziness, ataxia,* nystagmus, tremor, nervousness,

---

dysarthria, amnesia, depression, abnormal thinking, twitching, incoordination.
CV: peripheral edema, vasodilation.
EENT: diplopia, rhinitis, pharyngitis, dry throat, coughing, amblyopia.
GI: nausea, vomiting, dyspepsia, dry mouth, constipation.
GU: impotence.
Hematologic: *leukopenia,* decreased WBC count.
Skin: pruritus, abrasion.
Other: dental abnormalities, increased appetite, weight gain, back pain, myalgia, fractures.

INTERACTIONS
Drug-drug. *Antacids:* decreased absorption of gabapentin. Separate administration times by at least 2 hours.

EFFECTS ON DIAGNOSTIC TESTS
Drug causes false-positive results with the Ames-N-Multistix SG dipstick test for urinary protein when added to other antiepileptic drugs. The more specific sulfosalicylic acid precipitation procedure is recommended to determine the presence of urine protein.

CONTRAINDICATIONS
Contraindicated in patients hypersensitive to drug.

NURSING CONSIDERATIONS
• Know that first dose should be given at bedtime to minimize drowsiness, dizziness, fatigue, and ataxia.
• If drug therapy is discontinued or alternative medication is substituted, do so gradually over at least 1 week, as ordered, to minimize risk of precipitating seizures.
Alert: Do not suddenly withdraw other anticonvulsants in patients starting gabapentin therapy.
• Know that routine monitoring of plasma drug levels is not necessary. Drug does not appear to alter plasma levels of other anticonvulsants.

☑ Patient teaching
• Instruct patient to take first dose at bedtime to minimize adverse reactions.
• Warn patient to avoid driving and operating heavy machinery until drug's CNS effects are known.

lamotrigine
Lamictal

Pregnancy Risk Category: C

HOW SUPPLIED
Tablets: 25 mg, 100 mg, 150 mg, 200 mg
Tablets (chewable dispersible): 5 mg, 25 mg

ACTION
Unknown. May cause inhibited release of glutamate and aspartate (excitatory neurotransmitters) in the brain. This may occur by way of an action at voltage-sensitive sodium channels.

Route	Onset	Peak	Duration
PO	Unknown	1.4-4.8 hr	Unknown

INDICATIONS & DOSAGE
Adjunct therapy in treatment of partial seizures caused by epilepsy—
Adults and children over 16 years: for patients taking valproic acid in combination with other enzyme-inducing antiepileptics, 25 mg P.O. every other day for 2 weeks, followed by 25 mg P.O. daily for 2 weeks. Thereafter, no more than 150 mg P.O. daily in two divided doses.

In patients receiving enzyme-inducing antiepileptics, but not valproic acid, 50 mg P.O. daily for 2 weeks, followed by 100 mg P.O. daily in two divided doses for 2 weeks. Thereafter, usual maintenance dosage is 300 to 500 mg P.O. daily in two divided doses.
Adjust-a-dose: Use lower maintenance dosage in patients with severe renal impairment.
❋ *NEW INDICATION: Adjunctive treatment of the generalized seizures of Lennox-Gastaut syndrome—*
Adults and children over 12 years: for patients on an antiepileptic drug regimen with valproic acid, 25 mg P.O. every other day for 2 weeks, followed by 25 mg P.O. daily for 2 weeks. Thereafter, usual maintenance dosage is 100 to 400 mg P.O. daily in one or two divided doses. For pa-

tients taking enzyme-inducing antiepileptics, but not valproic acid, 50 mg P.O. daily for 2 weeks, followed by 100 mg P.O. daily in two divided doses for 2 weeks. Thereafter, usual maintenance dosage is 300 to 500 mg P.O. daily in two divided doses.

Children 2 to 12 years weighing over 17 kg (37 lb): in patients on an antiepileptic drug regimen with valproic acid, 0.15 mg/kg/day P.O. in one or two divided doses (rounded down to nearest 5 mg) for 2 weeks. If calculated daily dose of lamotrigine is 2.5 to 5 mg, then 5 mg of lamotrigine should be taken on alternate days. Then 0.3 mg/kg/day P.O. in one or two doses rounded down to nearest 5 mg for 2 weeks. Thereafter, usual maintenance dosage is 1 to 5 mg/kg/day (maximum dosage 200 mg/day in one to two divided doses). For patients on an antiepileptic drug regimen without valproic acid, 0.6 mg/kg/day P.O. in two divided doses rounded down to nearest 5 mg for 2 weeks, followed by 1.2 mg/kg/day P.O. in two divided doses rounded down to nearest 5 mg for 2 weeks. Thereafter, usual maintenance dosage is 5 to 15 mg/kg/day (maximum dosage is 400 mg/day in two divided doses).

ADVERSE REACTIONS
CNS: *dizziness, headache, ataxia, somnolence,* incoordination, insomnia, tremor, depression, anxiety, *seizures,* irritability, speech disorder, decreased memory, aggravated reaction, concentration disturbance, sleep disorder, emotional lability, vertigo, mind racing.
EENT: *diplopia, blurred vision,* vision abnormality, nystagmus, *rhinitis,* pharyngitis.
GI: *nausea, vomiting,* diarrhea, dyspepsia, abdominal pain, constipation, tooth disorder, anorexia, dry mouth.
GU: dysmenorrhea, vaginitis, amenorrhea.
Respiratory: cough, dyspnea.
Skin: *rash, Stevens-Johnson syndrome, toxic epidermal necrolysis,* pruritus, hot flashes, alopecia, acne.
Other: palpitations, dysarthria, muscle spasm, flulike syndrome, fever, infection, neck pain, malaise, chills.

INTERACTIONS
Drug-drug. *Acetaminophen:* may decrease therapeutic effects. Monitor patient.
Carbamazepine, phenobarbital, phenytoin, primidone: decreased lamotrigine's steady-state concentrations. Monitor patient closely.
Folate inhibitors (such as co-trimoxazole, methotrexate): lamotrigine inhibits dihydrofolate reductase, an enzyme involved in folic acid synthesis. May have an additive effect. Monitor patient.
Valproic acid: decreased clearance of lamotrigine, which increases the drug's steady-state concentrations. Also decreases valproic acid concentrations. Monitor patient closely for toxicity.
Drug-lifestyle. *Sun exposure:* photosensitivity reactions may occur. Take precautions.

EFFECTS ON DIAGNOSTIC TESTS
None reported.

CONTRAINDICATIONS
Contraindicated in patients with hypersensitivity to drug or its ingredients.

NURSING CONSIDERATIONS
• Use cautiously in patients with renal, hepatic, or cardiac impairment.
• Know that drug should not be discontinued abruptly because of possibility of increased seizure frequency. Instead, drug should be tapered over at least 2 weeks.
Alert: Know that drug should be stopped at first sign of rash unless rash is not drug-related.
• Be aware that lamotrigine dosage should be lowered if drug is added to a multidrug regimen that includes valproic acid.
• Know that chewable dispersible tablets may be swallowed whole, chewed, or dispersed in water or diluted fruit juice. If tablets are chewed, a small amount of water or diluted fruit juice should be given to aid in swallowing.
• Be aware that safety and effectiveness in children under 16 years other than those with Lennox-Gastaut syndrome have not been established. Children weighing below 17 kg (37 lb) should not receive drug because therapy cannot be initiated using

dosing guidelines and currently available tablet strength.
• Be aware that patients should be evaluated for changes in seizure activity. Adjunct anticonvulsant's serum levels should be checked, as ordered.

☑ **Patient teaching**
• Inform patient that drug may cause rash. Combination therapy of valproic acid and lamotrigine may cause a serious rash. Tell patient to report rash or signs or symptoms of hypersensitivity promptly to the doctor because they may warrant drug discontinuation.
• Warn patient not to engage in hazardous activity until drug's CNS effects are known.
• Warn patient that photosensitivity reactions may occur and to take precautions until tolerance is determined.

magnesium sulfate

Pregnancy Risk Category: A

HOW SUPPLIED
Injection: 4%, 8%, 10%, 12.5%, 25%, 50%
Injection solution: 1% in 5% dextrose, 2% in 5% dextrose

ACTION
May decrease acetylcholine released by nerve impulses, but its anticonvulsant mechanism is unknown.

Route	Onset	Peak	Duration
IV	1-2 min	Rapid	30 min
IM	1 hr	Unknown	3-4 hr

INDICATIONS & DOSAGE
Prevention or control of seizures in pre-eclampsia or eclampsia—
Women: initially, 4 g I.V. in 250 ml D₅W and 4 to 5 g deep I.M. into each buttock; then 4 to 5 g deep I.M. into alternate buttock q 4 hours, p.r.n. Alternatively, 4 g I.V. loading dose, followed by 1 to 2 g hourly as I.V. infusion. Total dosage should not exceed 30 to 40 g daily.
Hypomagnesemia—
Adults: for mild deficiency, 1 g I.M. q 6

hours for four doses; for severe deficiency, 5 g in 1,000 ml D₅W or 0.9% NaCl infused over 3 hours.
Seizures, hypertension, and encephalopathy associated with acute nephritis in children—
Children: 0.2 ml/kg of 50% solution I.M. q 4 to 6 hours, p.r.n. For severe symptoms, 100 to 200 mg/kg I.V. slowly over 1 hour with 50% of dose administered in first 15 to 20 minutes. Dosage titrated according to blood magnesium levels and seizure response.
Management of paroxysmal atrial tachycardia—
Adults: 3 to 4 g I.V. over 30 seconds.
Management of life-threatening ventricular arrhythmias, such as sustained ventricular tachycardia or torsades de pointes—
Adults: 2 to 6 g I.V. over several minutes, followed by a continuous I.V. infusion of 3 to 20 mg/minute for 5 to 48 hours. Dosage and duration of therapy based on patient response and serum magnesium levels.

ADVERSE REACTIONS
CNS: drowsiness, *depressed reflexes, flaccid paralysis, hypothermia.*
CV: *hypotension, flushing,* **circulatory collapse,** depressed cardiac function.
Other: diaphoresis, ***respiratory paralysis,*** hypocalcemia.

INTERACTIONS
Drug-drug. *Anesthetics, CNS depressants:* may cause additive CNS depression. Use cautiously.
Cardiac glycosides: concomitant use may exacerbate arrhythmias. Use together cautiously.
Neuromuscular blockers: may cause increased neuromuscular blockade. Use cautiously.

EFFECTS ON DIAGNOSTIC TESTS
None reported.

CONTRAINDICATIONS
Parenteral administration of drug contraindicated in patients with heart block or myocardial damage. Do not give in

toxemia of pregnancy during 2 hours preceding delivery.

NURSING CONSIDERATIONS
• Use cautiously in patients with impaired renal function. Also use cautiously in women who are in labor.
• If used to treat seizures, institute appropriate seizure precautions.
Alert: Watch for respiratory depression and signs of heart block.
• Keep I.V. calcium gluconate available to reverse magnesium intoxication; however, use cautiously in patients undergoing digitalization because of danger of arrhythmias.
• Check blood magnesium levels after repeated doses. Disappearance of knee-jerk and patellar reflexes is a sign of impending magnesium toxicity.
• Signs of hypermagnesemia begin to appear at blood levels of 4 mEq/L.
• Monitor fluid intake and output. Urine output should be 100 ml or more in 4-hour period before each dose.
• Observe neonates for signs of magnesium toxicity, including neuromuscular or respiratory depression, when giving I.V. form of drug to toxemic mothers within 24 hours before delivery.

I.V. administration
• If necessary, dilute to a maximum concentration of 20%. Infuse no faster than 150 mg/minute (1.5 ml/minute of a 10% solution or 0.75 ml/minute of a 20% solution). Drug is compatible with D₅W.
• Maximum infusion rate is 150 mg/minute. Too-rapid infusion will induce uncomfortable feeling of heat.
• Monitor vital signs every 15 minutes when giving drug I.V.

Patient teaching
• Inform patient of short-term need for drug, and answer any questions and address concerns.
• Review potential adverse reactions and instruct patient to promptly report any occurrences. Reassure patient that, although adverse reactions can occur, frequent monitoring of vital signs, reflexes, and blood levels will be made to ensure safety.

phenobarbital (phenobarbitone)
Ancalixir†, Barbita, Solfoton

phenobarbital sodium (phenobarbitone sodium)
Luminal Sodium

Controlled Substance Schedule IV
Pregnancy Risk Category: D

HOW SUPPLIED
Tablets: 15 mg, 16 mg, 30 mg, 60 mg, 100 mg
Capsules: 16 mg
Elixir*: 15 mg/5 ml, 20 mg/5 ml
Injection: 30 mg/ml, 60 mg/ml, 65 mg/ml, 130 mg/ml

ACTION
Unknown. A barbiturate that probably depresses monosynaptic and polysynaptic transmission in CNS and increases threshold for seizure activity in motor cortex. As a sedative, probably interferes with transmission of impulses from thalamus to cortex of brain.

Route	Onset	Peak	Duration
PO	1 hr	8-12 hr	10-12 hr
IV	5 min	30 min	4-10 hr
IM	> 5 min	> 30 min	4-10 hr

INDICATIONS & DOSAGE
All forms of epilepsy, febrile seizures—
Adults: 60 to 200 mg P.O. daily in divided dose t.i.d. or as single dose h.s.
Children: 3 to 6 mg/kg P.O. daily, usually divided q 12 hours. It can be administered once daily, usually h.s.
Status epilepticus—
Adults: 200 to 600 mg I.V.
Children: 100 to 400 mg I.V. Do not exceed 50 mg/minute.
Sedation—
Adults: 30 to 120 mg P.O. daily in two or three divided doses.
Children: 3 to 5 mg/kg P.O. daily in divided doses t.i.d.
Insomnia—
Adults: 100 to 200 mg P.O. or I.M. h.s.
Preoperative sedation—

Reactions may be *common*, uncommon, *life-threatening*, or COMMON AND LIFE-THREATENING.

Adults: 100 to 200 mg I.M. 60 to 90 minutes before surgery.
Children: 16 to 100 mg I.M. or 1 to 3 mg/kg I.V., I.M., or P.O. 60 to 90 minutes before surgery.

ADVERSE REACTIONS
CNS: *drowsiness, lethargy, hangover,* paradoxical excitement (in elderly patients), somnolence.
CV: bradycardia, hypotension.
GI: nausea, vomiting.
Hematologic: exacerbation of porphyria.
Respiratory: *respiratory depression,* apnea.
Skin: rash, *erythema multiforme, Stevens-Johnson syndrome,* urticaria, pain, swelling, thrombophlebitis, necrosis, nerve injury (at injection site).
Other: *angioedema,* physical and psychological dependence.

INTERACTIONS
Drug-drug. *Chloramphenicol, MAO inhibitors, valproic acid:* potentiated barbiturate effect. Monitor patient for increased CNS and respiratory depression.
CNS depressants, including narcotic analgesics: excessive CNS depression. Monitor closely.
Corticosteroids, digitoxin, doxycycline, estrogens and oral contraceptives, oral anticoagulants, tricyclic antidepressants: phenobarbital may enhance the metabolism of these drugs. Monitor for decreased effect.
Diazepam: increased effects of both drugs. Use together cautiously.
Griseofulvin: decreased absorption of griseofulvin. Monitor effectiveness of griseofulvin.
Mephobarbital, primidone: excessive phenobarbital blood levels. Monitor closely.
Rifampin: may decrease barbiturate levels. Monitor for decreased effect.
Valproic acid: increased phenobarbital levels. Monitor for toxicity.
Drug-lifestyle. *Alcohol use:* excessive CNS depression. Avoid concomitant use.

EFFECTS ON DIAGNOSTIC TESTS
Drug may cause a false-positive phentolamine test. The physiologic effects of drug may impair the absorption of cyanocobalamin ^{57}Co. It may decrease serum bilirubin concentrations in neonates, epileptics, and in patients with congenital nonhemolytic unconjugated hyperbilirubinemia. Barbiturates may increase sulfobromophthalein retention. EEG patterns show a change in low-voltage, fast activity. Changes persist for a time after discontinuation of therapy.

CONTRAINDICATIONS
Contraindicated in patients with barbiturate hypersensitivity or history of manifest or latent porphyria, hepatic dysfunction, respiratory disease with dyspnea or obstruction, and nephritis.

NURSING CONSIDERATIONS
• Use cautiously in patients with acute or chronic pain, depression, suicidal tendencies, history of drug abuse, blood pressure alterations, CV disease, shock, or uremia, and in elderly or debilitated patients.
• Do not use injectable solution if it contains a precipitate.
• Give I.M. injection deeply. Superficial injection may cause pain, sterile abscess, and tissue sloughing.
• Know that elderly patients are more sensitive to drug's effects.
Alert: Watch for signs of barbiturate toxicity: coma, asthmatic breathing, cyanosis, clammy skin, and hypotension. Overdose can be fatal.
• Therapeutic blood levels are 15 to 40 mcg/ml.
• Don't stop drug abruptly because seizures may worsen. Call doctor immediately if adverse reactions develop.

I.V. administration
• Know that I.V. injection is reserved for emergency treatment. Give slowly under close supervision. Monitor respirations closely. When administering, do not give more than 60 mg/minute. Have resuscitation equipment available.
• Do not mix parenteral form with acidic solutions; precipitation may result.

Patient teaching
• Make sure that patient is aware that phenobarbital is available in different mil-

ligram strengths and sizes. Advise him to check prescription and refills closely.
• Inform patient that full therapeutic effects are not seen for 2 to 3 weeks, except when loading dose is used.
• Advise patient to avoid driving and other potentially hazardous activities that require mental alertness until drug's CNS effects are known.
• Warn patient and parents not to discontinue drug abruptly.
• Tell female patient who uses oral contraceptives that she should consider another birth-control method because drug may decrease effect of contraceptive.

---

phenytoin (diphenylhydantoin)
Dilantin-125, Dilantin Infatab, Epanutin§

phenytoin sodium
Dilantin, Phenytex

phenytoin sodium (extended)
Dilantin Kapseals

Pregnancy Risk Category: D

HOW SUPPLIED
phenytoin
Tablets (chewable): 50 mg
Oral suspension: 125 mg/5 ml
phenytoin sodium
Capsules: 100 mg (92-mg base)
Injection: 50 mg/ml (46-mg base)
phenytoin sodium (extended)
Capsules: 30 mg (27.6-mg base), 100 mg (92-mg base)

ACTION
Unknown. A hydantoin derivative that probably stabilizes neuronal membranes and limits seizure activity by either increasing efflux or decreasing influx of sodium ions across cell membranes in the motor cortex during generation of nerve impulses.

Route	Onset	Peak	Duration
PO	Unknown	1.5-12 hr	Unknown
IV	Immediate	1-2 hr	Unknown
IM	Unknown	Unknown	Unknown

INDICATIONS & DOSAGE
Control of tonic-clonic (grand mal) and complex partial (temporal lobe) seizures—
Adults: highly individualized. Initially, 100 mg P.O. t.i.d., increased in increments of 100 mg P.O. q 2 to 4 weeks until desired response is obtained. Usual range is 300 to 600 mg daily. If patient is stabilized with extended-release capsules, once-daily dosing with 300-mg extended-release capsules possible as an alternative.
Children: 5 mg/kg or 250 mg/m^2 P.O. divided b.i.d. or t.i.d. Maximum daily dosage is 300 mg.
For patient requiring a loading dose—
Adults: initially, 1 g P.O. daily divided into three doses and administered at 2-hour intervals. Alternatively, 10 to 15 mg/kg I.V. at a rate not exceeding 50 mg/minute. Normal maintenance dosage instituted 24 hours later.
Children: 5 mg/kg/day P.O. in two or three equally divided doses with subsequent dosage individualized to maximum of 300 mg daily.
Prevention and treatment of seizures occurring during neurosurgery—
Adults: 100 to 200 mg I.M. q 4 hours during surgery and continued during postoperative period.
Status epilepticus—
Adults: loading dose of 10 to 15 mg/kg I.V. (1 to 1.5 g may be needed) at a rate not exceeding 50 mg/minute, followed by maintenance doses of 100 mg P.O. or I.V. q 6 to 8 hours.
Elderly: may require lower dosages.
Children: loading dose of 15 to 20 mg/kg I.V., at a rate not exceeding 1 to 3 mg/kg/minute, followed by highly individualized maintenance dosages.

ADVERSE REACTIONS
CNS: *ataxia, slurred speech,* dizziness, insomnia, nervousness, twitching, headache, *mental confusion, decreased coordination.*
CV: periarteritis nodosa.
EENT: *nystagmus, diplopia,* blurred vision, *gingival hyperplasia* (especially in children).
GI: *nausea, vomiting,* constipation.
Hematologic: *thrombocytopenia,*

Reactions may be *common,* uncommon, *__life-threatening__,* or COMMON AND LIFE-THREATENING.

leukopenia, agranulocytosis, pancytopenia, macrocythemia, megaloblastic anemia.
Hepatic: *toxic hepatitis.*
Skin: scarlatiniform or morbilliform rash; bullous, *exfoliative,* or purpuric dermatitis; *Stevens-Johnson syndrome;* lupus erythematosus; *hirsutism; toxic epidermal necrolysis;* photosensitivity; pain, necrosis, inflammation (at injection site); discoloration of skin ("purple-glove syndrome") if given by I.V. push in back of hand.
Other: lymphadenopathy, hyperglycemia, osteomalacia, hypertrichosis.

INTERACTIONS

Drug-drug. *Amiodarone, antihistamines, chloramphenicol, cimetidine, cycloserine, diazepam, disulfiram, isoniazid, phenylbutazone, salicylates, sulfamethizole, valproate:* may increase phenytoin activity and toxicity. Monitor patient.
Barbiturates, carbamazepine, dexamethasone, diazoxide, folic acid, rifampin: decreased phenytoin activity. Monitor levels.
Carbamazepine, cardiac glycosides, oral contraceptives, quinidine, theophylline, valproic acid: effects may be decreased by phenytoin. Monitor patient.
Drug-food. *Oral tube feedings with Osmolite or Isocal:* may interfere with absorption of oral phenytoin. Stop enteral feedings for 2 hours before and 2 hours after phenytoin administration.
Drug-lifestyle. *Chronic alcohol use:* decreased phenytoin activity. Inform patient that heavy alcohol use may diminish drug's benefits.

EFFECTS ON DIAGNOSTIC TESTS

Drug may raise blood glucose levels by inhibiting pancreatic insulin release; it may also cause reduced serum protein-bound iodine and free thyroxine levels without clinical signs of hypothyroidism; a slight decrease in urinary 17-hydroxysteroid and 17-ketosteroid levels; increased urine 6-b hydroxycortisol excretion and serum levels of alkaline phosphatase or gamma-glutamyltransferase; and decreased values for dexamethasone suppression or metyrapone tests.

CONTRAINDICATIONS

Contraindicated in patients with hydantoin hypersensitivity, sinus bradycardia, SA block, second- or third-degree AV block, or Adams-Stokes syndrome.

NURSING CONSIDERATIONS

• Use cautiously in patients with hepatic dysfunction, hypotension, myocardial insufficiency, diabetes, and respiratory depression; in elderly or debilitated patients; and in patients receiving other hydantoin derivatives.
• Be aware that elderly patients tend to metabolize phenytoin slowly and may require lower dosages.
• Know that phenytoin requirements usually increase during pregnancy.
• Use only clear solution for injection. A slight yellow color is acceptable. Don't refrigerate.
• Do not give I.M. unless dosage adjustments are made; drug may precipitate at injection site, cause pain, and be absorbed erratically.
• Divided doses given with or after meals may decrease adverse GI reactions.
• Be aware that drug should be discontinued if rash appears. If rash is scarlatiniform or morbilliform, drug may be resumed after rash clears. If rash reappears, therapy should be discontinued. If rash is exfoliative, purpuric, or bullous, drug will not be resumed.
• Don't withdraw drug suddenly because seizures may worsen. Call doctor at once if adverse reactions develop.
• Monitor blood levels as ordered. Therapeutic phenytoin blood level is 10 to 20 mcg/ml.
• Monitor CBC and serum calcium level every 6 months, and periodically monitor hepatic function as ordered. If megaloblastic anemia is evident, doctor may order folic acid and vitamin B_{12}.
• If using to treat seizures, take appropriate safety precautions.
• Mononucleosis may decrease phenytoin levels. Monitor for increased seizure activity.

▌ I.V. administration

• Administer slowly (50 mg/minute) as I.V. bolus. If giving as an infusion, don't

---

mix drug with D_5W because it will precipitate. Clear I.V. tubing first with 0.9% NaCl solution. Never use cloudy solution. May mix with 0.9% NaCl solution if necessary and give as an infusion over 30 minutes to 1 hour, when possible. Infusion must begin within 1 hour after preparation and should run through an in-line filter. Discard 4 hours after preparation.
Alert: Check patency of I.V. catheter before administering. Extravasation has caused severe local tissue damage.
• Avoid administering phenytoin by I.V. push into veins on the back of the hand to avoid discoloration known as purple-glove syndrome. Inject into larger veins or central venous catheter if available.
• Check vital signs, blood pressure, and ECG during I.V. administration.

☑ **Patient teaching**
• Advise patient to avoid driving and other potentially hazardous activities that require mental alertness until drug's CNS effects are known.
• Advise patient not to change brands or dosage forms once he's stabilized on therapy.
• Dilantin capsules are the only oral form that can be given once daily. Toxic levels may result if any other brand or form is given once daily. Dilantin brand tablets and oral suspension should never be taken once daily.
• Warn patient and parents not to stop drug abruptly.
• Stress importance of good oral hygiene and regular dental examinations. Gingivectomy may be necessary periodically if dental hygiene is poor.
• Caution patient that drug may color urine pink, red, or reddish brown.

---

primidone
Apo-Primidone†, Mysoline, PMS Primidone†, Sertan†

Pregnancy Risk Category: NR

HOW SUPPLIED
Tablets: 50 mg, 250 mg
Oral suspension: 250 mg/5 ml

ACTION
Unknown, but some activity may be caused by phenylethylmalonamide and phenobarbital, which are active metabolites.

Route	Onset	Peak	Duration
PO	Unknown	3-4 hr	Unknown

INDICATIONS & DOSAGE
Tonic-clonic, complex partial, and simple partial seizures—
Adults and children 8 years and over: initially, 100 to 125 mg P.O. h.s. on days 1 to 3; then 100 to 125 mg P.O. b.i.d. on days 4 to 6; then 100 to 125 mg P.O. t.i.d. on days 7 to 9, followed by maintenance dosage of 250 mg P.O. t.i.d. Maintenance dosage increased to 250 mg q.i.d., if needed. Dosage may be increased to maximum of 2 g daily in divided doses.
Children under 8 years: initially, 50 mg P.O. h.s. for 3 days; then 50 mg P.O. b.i.d. for days 4 to 6; then 100 mg P.O. b.i.d. for days 7 to 9, followed by maintenance dosage of 125 to 250 mg P.O. t.i.d.

ADVERSE REACTIONS
CNS: *drowsiness, ataxia,* emotional disturbances, vertigo, hyperirritability, fatigue, paranoia.
EENT: *diplopia,* nystagmus.
GI: anorexia, *nausea, vomiting.*
GU: impotence, polyuria.
Hematologic: megaloblastic anemia, ***thrombocytopenia.***
Skin: morbilliform rash.

INTERACTIONS
Drug-drug. *Acetazolamide, succinimide:* may decrease primidone concentrations. Monitor levels.
Carbamazepine: increased carbamazepine levels and decreased primidone and phenobarbital levels. Observe for toxicity.
Isoniazid: increased primidone concentration. Monitor levels.
Phenytoin: stimulated conversion of primidone to phenobarbital. Observe for increased phenobarbital effect.

EFFECTS ON DIAGNOSTIC TESTS
Primidone may cause abnormalities in liver function test results.

CONTRAINDICATIONS
Contraindicated in patients with phenobarbital hypersensitivity or porphyria.

NURSING CONSIDERATIONS
• Shake liquid suspension well.
• Don't withdraw drug suddenly because seizures may worsen. Notify doctor immediately if adverse reactions develop.
• Be aware that therapeutic blood level of primidone is 5 to 12 mcg/ml. Therapeutic blood level of phenobarbital is 15 to 40 mcg/ml.
• Monitor CBC and routine blood chemistry every 6 months.
• Know that brand interchange is not recommended because of documented bioequivalence problems for primidone products marketed by different manufacturers.

☑ **Patient teaching**
• Advise patient to avoid driving and other potentially hazardous activities that require mental alertness until drug's CNS effects are known.
• Warn patient and parents not to stop drug therapy suddenly.
• Tell patient that full therapeutic response may take 2 weeks or more.

---

tiagabine hydrochloride
Gabitril

Pregnancy Risk Category: C

HOW SUPPLIED
Tablets: 4 mg, 12 mg, 16 mg, 20 mg

ACTION
Unknown, but tiagabine may act by enhancing the activity of gamma aminobutyric acid (GABA), the major inhibitory neurotransmitter in the central nervous system. It binds to recognition sites associated with the GABA uptake carrier and may thus permit more GABA to be available for binding to receptors on postsynaptic cells.

Route	Onset	Peak	Duration
PO	Rapid	45 min	7-9 hr

INDICATIONS & DOSAGE
Adjunctive therapy in the treatment of partial seizures—
Adults: initially, 4 mg P.O. once daily. Total daily dosage may be increased by 4 to 8 mg at weekly intervals until clinical response or up to 56 mg/day. Total daily dosage should be given in divided doses b.i.d. to q.i.d.
Children 12 to 18 years: initially, 4 mg P.O. once daily. Total daily dosage may be increased by 4 mg at the beginning of week 2 and thereafter by 4 to 8 mg/week until clinical response or up to 32 mg/day. Total daily dosage should be given in divided doses b.i.d. to q.i.d.
Adjust-a-dose: In patients with impaired liver function, reduced initial and maintenance doses or longer dosing intervals may be required.

ADVERSE REACTIONS
CNS: *dizziness, asthenia, somnolence, nervousness,* tremor, difficulty with concentration and attention, insomnia, ataxia, confusion, speech disorder, difficulty with memory, paresthesia, depression, emotional lability, abnormal gait, hostility, language problems, agitation.
CV: vasodilation.
EENT: nystagmus, pharyngitis.
GI: abdominal pain, *nausea,* diarrhea, vomiting, increased appetite, mouth ulceration.
Respiratory: increased cough.
Skin: rash, pruritus.
Other: generalized weakness, pain, myasthenia.

INTERACTIONS
Drug-drug. *Carbamazepine, phenobarbital, phenytoin:* increased tiagabine clearance. Monitor closely.
CNS depressants: enhanced CNS effects. Use cautiously.
Drug-lifestyle. *Alcohol use:* enhanced CNS effects. Use cautiously.

EFFECTS ON DIAGNOSTIC TESTS
None reported.

CONTRAINDICATIONS
Contraindicated in patients with hypersensitivity to drug or its ingredients.

NURSING CONSIDERATIONS
• Use cautiously in breast-feeding patients.
• Never withdraw drug suddenly because seizure frequency may increase. Withdraw tiagabine gradually unless safety concerns require a more rapid withdrawal.
Alert: Status epilepticus and sudden unexpected death in epilepsy have occurred in patients receiving antiepilepsy drugs, including tiagabine.
• Know that patients who are *not* receiving at least one concomitant enzyme-inducing antiepilepsy drug at the time of tiagabine initiation may require lower doses or a slower dose titration.
• Be aware that moderately severe to incapacitating generalized weakness has occurred in patients receiving tiagabine. The weakness resolved after a dose reduction or discontinuation of tiagabine.

☑ **Patient teaching**
• Advise patient to take drug only as prescribed.
• Tell patient to take drug with food.
• Warn patient that drug may cause dizziness, somnolence, and other symptoms and signs of CNS depression. Advise patient to avoid driving and other potentially hazardous activities that require mental alertness until drug's CNS effects are known.
• Tell female patient to call doctor if she becomes pregnant or plans to become pregnant during therapy.
• Instruct female patient to notify doctor if planning to breast-feed because tiagabine may be excreted in breast milk.

---

topiramate
Topamax

Pregnancy Risk Category: C

HOW SUPPLIED
Tablets: 25 mg, 100 mg, 200 mg

ACTION
Unknown. Thought to block action potential, suggestive of a sodium channel blocking action. Drug may also potentiate the activity of gamma-aminobutyrate (GABA) and antagonize the ability of kainate to activate the kainate/alpha-amino-3-hydroxy-5-methylisoxazole-4-proprionic acid subtype of excitatory amino acid (glutamate) receptor. Drug also has weak carbonic anhydrase inhibitor activity, which is unrelated to its antiepileptic properties.

Route	Onset	Peak	Duration
PO	Unknown	2 hr	Unknown

INDICATIONS & DOSAGE
Adjunctive therapy for adults with partial onset seizures—
Adults: titrate up to maximum daily dose of 400 mg P.O. in divided doses b.i.d. Titration schedule is as follows: Week 1: 50 mg P.O. in evening; week 2, 50 mg P.O. b.i.d.; week 3, 50 mg P.O. in morning and 100 mg P.O. in evening; week 4, 100 mg P.O. b.i.d.; week 5, 100 mg P.O. in morning and 150 mg P.O. in evening; week 6, 150 mg P.O. b.i.d.; week 7, 150 mg P.O. in morning and 200 mg P.O. in evening; week 8, 200 mg P.O. b.i.d.
Adjust-a-dose: In renally impaired patients with creatinine clearance below 70 ml/minute, reduce dosage by 50%. For hemodialysis patients, supplemental doses may be required to avoid rapid drops in drug levels during prolonged dialysis treatment.

ADVERSE REACTIONS
CNS: abnormal coordination; aggressive reaction; agitation; apathy; asthenia; *ataxia; confusion;* depression; depersonalization; difficulty with concentration, attention, language, or *memory; dizziness;* emotional lability; euphoria; *generalized tonic-clonic seizures;* hallucination; hyperkinesia; hypertonia; hypoesthesia; hypokinesia; insomnia; mood problems; *nervousness; nystagmus; paresthesia;* personality disorder; *psychomotor slowing;* psychosis; *somnolence; speech disorders;* stupor; *suicide attempts; tremor;* vertigo.
CV: chest pain, palpitations, vasodilation.
EENT: *abnormal vision,* conjunctivitis, *diplopia,* eye pain, hearing problems, taste perversion, tinnitus, pharyngitis, sinusitis.

Reactions may be *common,* uncommon, *life-threatening,* or COMMON AND LIFE-THREATENING.

GI: abdominal pain, anorexia, constipation, diarrhea, dry mouth, dyspepsia, flatulence, gastroenteritis, gingivitis, *nausea,* vomiting.

GU: amenorrhea, decreased libido, dysuria, dysmenorrhea, hematuria, impotence, intermenstrual bleeding, menstrual disorder, menorrhagia, micturition frequency, renal calculus, urinary incontinence, urinary tract infection, vaginitis.

Hematologic: anemia, epistaxis, *leukopenia,* lymphadenopathy.

Metabolic: increased or decreased weight.

Musculoskeletal: arthralgia, back or leg pain, muscle weakness, myalgia, rigors.

Respiratory: bronchitis, coughing, dyspnea, *upper respiratory infection.*

Skin: acne, alopecia, increased sweating, pruritus, rash.

Other: breast pain, body odor, edema, *fatigue,* fever, flulike symptoms, hot flashes, leukorrhea, malaise.

INTERACTIONS

Drug-drug. *Carbamazepine:* decreased topiramate concentrations. Monitor patient.

Carbonic anhydrase inhibitors (acetazolamide, dichlorphenamide): increased risk of renal calculus formation. Avoid concomitant use.

CNS depressants: possible topiramate-induced CNS depression as well as other adverse cognitive and neuropsychiatric events. Use with caution.

Oral contraceptives: decreased efficacy. Report changes in bleeding patterns.

Phenytoin: decreased topiramate concentrations and increased phenytoin concentrations. Monitor levels.

Valproic acid: decrease in valproic acid and topiramate levels. Monitor patient.

Drug-lifestyle. *Alcohol use:* possible topiramate-induced CNS depression as well as other adverse cognitive and neuropsychiatric events. Use with caution.

EFFECTS ON DIAGNOSTIC TESTS
Drug may cause elevated liver enzymes.

CONTRAINDICATIONS
Contraindicated in patients with hypersensitivity to drug or its ingredients.

NURSING CONSIDERATIONS
● Use with caution in breast-feeding or pregnant patients and in those with hepatic impairment.
● If necessary, withdraw antiepileptic drugs (including topiramate) gradually to minimize risk of increased seizure activity.
● Know that monitoring plasma levels of topiramate is not necessary.
● Be aware that drug is rapidly cleared by dialysis. A prolonged period of dialysis may result in low drug levels and seizures. A supplemental dose may be required.

☑ **Patient teaching**
● Tell patient to maintain adequate fluid intake during therapy to minimize risk of forming renal calculi.
● Advise patient not to drive or operate hazardous machinery until CNS effects of drug are known because drug can cause somnolence, dizziness, confusion, and difficulty concentrating.
● Tell patient that drug may decrease effectiveness of oral contraceptives. Advise patient taking oral contraceptives to report any change in her bleeding patterns.
● Tell patient to avoid crushing or breaking tablets because of bitter taste.
● Inform patient that drug can be taken without regard to food.

---

valproate sodium
Depakene, Depacon, Epilim‡, Valpro‡

valproic acid
Convulex§, Depakene

divalproex sodium
Depakote, Depakote Sprinkle, Epival†

Pregnancy Risk Category: D

HOW SUPPLIED
valproate sodium
Syrup: 250 mg/5ml
valproic acid
Tablets (enteric-coated): 200 mg‡, 500 mg‡
Tablets (crushable): 100 mg‡

Capsules: 250 mg
Syrup: 200 mg/5 ml‡
divalproex sodium
Capsules (delayed-release): 125 mg
Tablets (enteric-coated): 125 mg, 250 mg, 500 mg
Injection: 500-mg vial

ACTION
Unknown. Probably increases brain levels of gamma-aminobutyric acid, which transmits inhibitory nerve impulses in the CNS.

Route	Onset	Peak	Duration
PO	Unknown	15 min-4 hr	Unknown
IV	Unknown	1 hr	Unknown

INDICATIONS & DOSAGE
Simple and complex absence seizures, mixed seizure types (including absence seizures)—
Adults and children: initially, 15 mg/kg P.O. or I.V. daily; then increase by 5 to 10 mg/kg daily at weekly intervals up to maximum of 60 mg/kg daily.
Mania (divalproex sodium only)—
Adults and children: initially, 750 mg daily in divided doses. Adjust dosage according to patient's response; maximum dosage is 60 mg/kg/day.
Prophylaxis for migraine headache (divalproex sodium only)—
Adults: initially, 250 mg P.O. b.i.d. Some patients may require up to 1,000 mg/day.
Complex partial seizures—
Adults and children 10 years and older: 10 to 15 mg/kg P.O. or I.V. daily; then increase by 5 to 10 mg/kg daily at weekly intervals, up to 60 mg/kg/day.
Elderly: reduce initial dose.

ADVERSE REACTIONS
Because drug usually is used in combination with other anticonvulsants, adverse reactions reported may not be caused by valproic acid alone.
CNS: asthenia, *sedation,* emotional upset, depression, psychosis, aggressiveness, hyperactivity, behavioral deterioration, muscle weakness, tremor, ataxia, *headache, dizziness,* incoordination.
EENT: nystagmus, *diplopia.*
GI: *nausea, vomiting, indigestion, diarrhea,* abdominal cramps, constipation, increased appetite and weight gain, anorexia, ***pancreatitis.*** (*Note:* Lower incidence of GI effects occurs with divalproex sodium.)
Hematologic: *thrombocytopenia,* increased bleeding time, petechiae, bruising, eosinophilia, ***hemorrhage, leukopenia, bone marrow suppression.***
Hepatic: *elevated liver enzymes,* ***toxic hepatitis.***
Skin: rash, alopecia, pruritus, photosensitivity, erythema multiforme.

INTERACTIONS
Drug-drug. *Aspirin, chlorpromazine, cimetidine, erythromycin, felbamate:* may cause valproic acid toxicity. Use together cautiously and monitor blood levels. Monitor patient closely.
Benzodiazepines, other CNS depressants: excessive CNS depression. Avoid concomitant use.
Lamotrigine: increased lamotrigine levels, decreased valproate levels. Monitor levels closely.
Phenobarbital: increased phenobarbital levels. Monitor patient closely.
Phenytoin: increased or decreased phenytoin levels, decreased valproate levels. Monitor patient closely.
Rifampin: may decrease valproate levels. Monitor levels.
Warfarin: valproic acid may displace warfarin from binding sites. Monitor PT and INR.
Drug-lifestyle: *Alcohol use:* excessive CNS depression. Avoid concomitant use.

EFFECTS ON DIAGNOSTIC TESTS
Drug may produce false-positive results for urine ketones; it may also cause abnormalities in liver function test results. Valproic acid reportedly alters thyroid function tests, but clinical importance of this is not known.

CONTRAINDICATIONS
Contraindicated in patients with hepatic disease, significant hepatic dysfunction, or hypersensitivity to drug.

NURSING CONSIDERATIONS
• Monitor liver function studies, platelet

Reactions may be *common,* uncommon, **life-threatening**, or COMMON AND LIFE-THREATENING.

counts, and PT before starting drug and periodically thereafter, as ordered.
• Don't administer syrup to patients who need sodium restriction. Check with doctor.
• Never withdraw drug suddenly because sudden withdrawal may worsen seizures. Call doctor at once if adverse reactions develop.
Alert: Be aware that serious or fatal hepatotoxicity may follow nonspecific symptoms, such as malaise, fever, and lethargy. Notify doctor at once because drug will need to be discontinued in the presence of suspected or apparent substantial hepatic dysfunction.
• Know that patients at high risk for hepatotoxicity include those with congenital metabolic disorders, mental retardation, or presence of organic brain disease; those taking multiple anticonvulsants; and children under 2 years.
• Notify doctor if tremors occur (a dosage reduction may be necessary).
• Monitor blood levels, as ordered. Therapeutic blood level is 50 to 100 mcg/ml.
• Use caution when converting patients to a generic product because breakthrough seizures have been reported in patients converted from brand name to generic.

I.V. administration
• I.V. use in only indicated in patients who are unable to take drug orally. Switch patient to oral form as soon as clinically feasible; use of I.V. dosage for more than 14 days has not been studied.
• Dilute valproate sodium injection with at least 50 ml of a compatible diluent. It is physically compatible and chemically stable in D_5W, 0.9% NaCl, and lactated Ringer's solution for 24 hours.
• Administer drug as a 60-minute I.V. infusion (but not more than 20 mg/minute) with the same frequency as oral dosage.
• Know that monitoring of plasma concentrations and dosage adjustment may be needed.

Patient teaching
• Tell patient to take drug with food or milk to reduce adverse GI effects.
• Advise patient not to chew capsules; irritation of mouth and throat may result.
• Tell patient and parents that syrup shouldn't be mixed with carbonated beverages; may be irritating to mouth and throat.
• Tell patient and parents to keep drug out of children's reach.
• Warn patient and parents not to stop drug therapy abruptly.
• Advise patient to avoid driving and other potentially hazardous activities that require mental alertness until drug's CNS effects are known.

31

Antidepressants

amitriptyline hydrochloride
amitriptyline pamoate
amoxapine
bupropion hydrochloride
citalopram hydrobromide
clomipramine hydrochloride
desipramine hydrochloride
doxepin hydrochloride
fluoxetine hydrochloride
imipramine hydrochloride
imipramine pamoate
mirtazapine
nefazodone hydrochloride
nortriptyline hydrochloride
paroxetine hydrochloride
phenelzine sulfate
sertraline hydrochloride
tranylcypromine sulfate
trazodone hydrochloride
trimipramine maleate
venlafaxine hydrochloride

COMBINATION PRODUCTS
ETRAFON: perphenazine 2 mg and
amitriptyline hydrochloride 25 mg.
ETRAFON 2-10: perphenazine 2 mg and
amitriptyline hydrochloride 10 mg.
ETRAFON-A: perphenazine 4 mg and
amitriptyline hydrochloride 10 mg.
ETRAFON-FORTE: perphenazine 4 mg and
amitriptyline hydrochloride 25 mg.
LIMBITROL DS: chlordiazepoxide 10 mg
and amitriptyline hydrochloride 25 mg.
TRIAVIL 2-10, TRIAVIL 4-10, TRIAVIL 2-25,
TRIAVIL 4-25 are products identical to the
Etrafon products listed above. Triavil is
also available as TRIAVIL 4-50 (perphenazine 4 mg and amitriptyline hydrochloride 50 mg).

amitriptyline hydrochloride
Apo-Amitriptyline†, Elavil, Endep,
Levate†, Novo-Triptyn†,
Tryptanol‡, Tryptine‡

amitriptyline pamoate
Elavil†

Pregnancy Risk Category: NR

HOW SUPPLIED
amitriptyline hydrochloride
Tablets: 10 mg, 25 mg, 50 mg, 75 mg,
100 mg, 150 mg
Injection: 10 mg/ml
amitriptyline pamoate†
Syrup: 10 mg/5 ml*†

ACTION
Unknown, but a tricyclic antidepressant
(TCA) that increases the amount of nor-
epinephrine, serotonin, or both in the
CNS by blocking their reuptake by the
presynaptic neurons.

Route	Onset	Peak	Duration
PO, IM	Unknown	2-12 hr	Unknown

INDICATIONS & DOSAGE
Depression—
Adults: initially, 50 to 100 mg P.O. h.s.,
increasing to 150 mg daily; maximum
dosage is 300 mg daily, if needed. Maintenance dose is 50 to 100 mg/day. Or 20
to 30 mg I.M. q.i.d.
Elderly and adolescents: 10 mg P.O.
t.i.d. and 20 mg h.s. daily.

ADVERSE REACTIONS
CNS: *coma, seizures,* hallucinations,
delusions, disorientation, ataxia, tremor,
peripheral neuropathy, anxiety, insomnia,
restlessness, drowsiness, dizziness, weakness, fatigue, headache, extrapyramidal
reactions.
CV: *MI, stroke, arrhythmias,* heart block,
orthostatic hypotension, tachycardia,
ECG changes, hypertension.

EENT: blurred vision, tinnitus, mydriasis, increased intraocular pressure.
GI: *dry mouth,* nausea, vomiting, anorexia, epigastric distress, diarrhea, constipation, paralytic ileus.
GU: urine retention.
Hematologic: *agranulocytosis, thrombocytopenia, leukopenia,* eosinophilia.
Skin: rash, urticaria, photosensitivity.
Other: diaphoresis, *hypersensitivity reaction,* edema.
After abrupt withdrawal of long-term therapy: nausea, headache, malaise (does not indicate addiction).

INTERACTIONS

Drug-drug. *Barbiturates, CNS depressants:* enhanced CNS depression. Avoid concomitant use.
Cimetidine, fluoxetine, fluvoxamine, oral contraceptives, paroxetine, sertraline: increased TCA blood levels. Monitor for increased antidepressant adverse effects.
Clonidine: may cause hypertensive crisis. Avoid coadministration.
Epinephrine, norepinephrine: increased hypertensive effect. Use with caution.
MAO inhibitors: may cause severe excitation, hyperpyrexia, or seizures, usually with high dosage. Avoid concomitant use.
Drug-lifestyle. *Alcohol use:* enhanced CNS depression. Avoid concomitant use.
Smoking: may lower plasma concentrations of drug. Monitor for lack of effect.
Sun exposure: increased risk of photosensitivity reactions. Avoid unprotected or prolonged exposure to sun.

EFFECTS ON DIAGNOSTIC TESTS

Drug may prolong conduction time (elongation of QT and PR intervals, flattened T waves on ECG); it also may elevate liver function test results, decrease WBC counts, and decrease or increase serum glucose levels.

CONTRAINDICATIONS

Contraindicated during acute recovery phase of MI, in patients with hypersensitivity to drug, and in those who have received an MAO inhibitor within the past 14 days.

NURSING CONSIDERATIONS

● Use cautiously in patients with history of seizures, urine retention, angle-closure glaucoma, or increased intraocular pressure; in those with hyperthyroidism, CV disease, diabetes, or impaired liver function; and in those receiving thyroid medications.
Alert: Know that parenteral form of drug is for I.M. administration only. Drug should not be given I.V.
● Amitriptyline has strong anticholinergic effects and is one of the most sedating TCAs. Be aware that anticholinergic effects have a rapid onset even though therapeutic effect is delayed for weeks.
● If signs of psychosis occur or increase, expect doctor to reduce dosage. Record mood changes. Monitor patient for suicidal tendencies, and allow only a minimum supply of drug.
● Because hypertensive episodes have occurred during surgery in patients receiving TCAs, be aware that drug should be gradually discontinued several days before surgery.
● Do not withdraw drug abruptly.

✓ Patient teaching

● Advise patient to take full dose at bedtime, but warn him of possible morning orthostatic hypotension.
● Tell patient to avoid alcohol while taking this drug.
● Advise patient to consult doctor before taking other medications.
● Warn patient to avoid activities that require alertness and good psychomotor coordination until CNS effects of drug are known. Drowsiness and dizziness usually subside after a few weeks.
● Inform patient that dry mouth may be relieved with sugarless hard candy or gum. Saliva substitutes may be needed.
● To prevent photosensitivity reactions, advise patient to use a sunblock, wear protective clothing, and avoid prolonged exposure to strong sunlight.
● Warn patient not to stop drug therapy abruptly.

---

amoxapine
Asendin

Pregnancy Risk Category: C

HOW SUPPLIED
Tablets: 25 mg, 50 mg, 100 mg, 150 mg

ACTION
Unknown, but a tricyclic antidepressant (TCA) that increases the amount of norepinephrine, serotonin, or both in the CNS by blocking their reuptake by the presynaptic neurons.

Route	Onset	Peak	Duration
PO	Unknown	1.5 hr	Unknown

INDICATIONS & DOSAGE
Depression—
Adults: initially, 50 mg P.O. b.i.d. or t.i.d. Increased to 100 mg b.i.d. or t.i.d. by the end of week 1 of therapy if tolerated. Increases above 300 mg daily are made only if 300 mg daily has been ineffective during a trial period of at least 2 weeks. Maximum recommended dosage for outpatients is 400 mg daily. When effective dosage is established, entire dosage (not to exceed 300 mg) may be given h.s.
Elderly: initially, 25 mg P.O. b.i.d. or t.i.d. If tolerated by end of week 1, increase to 50 mg b.i.d. or t.i.d. Carefully increase up to 300 mg daily.

ADVERSE REACTIONS
CNS: *drowsiness, dizziness,* excitation, tremor, weakness, confusion, anxiety, insomnia, restlessness, nightmares, ataxia, fatigue, headache, nervousness, tardive dyskinesia, EEG changes, **seizures,** extrapyramidal reactions (rare), **neuroleptic malignant syndrome** (high fever, tachycardia, tachypnea, profuse diaphoresis).
CV: *orthostatic hypotension, tachycardia,* hypertension, palpitations.
EENT: blurred vision.
GI: *dry mouth,* constipation, nausea, excessive appetite.
GU: urine retention, **acute renal failure** (with overdose).
Skin: rash, edema, diaphoresis.
After abrupt withdrawal of long-term

therapy: nausea, headache, malaise (does not indicate addiction).

INTERACTIONS
Drug-drug. *Barbiturates:* decreased TCA blood levels. Monitor for decreased antidepressant effect.
Cimetidine, fluoxetine, fluvoxamine, paroxetine, sertraline: may increase amoxapine serum levels. Monitor for increased adverse effects.
Clonidine, epinephrine, norepinephrine: increased hypertensive effect. Use with caution.
CNS depressants: enhanced CNS depression. Avoid concomitant use.
MAO inhibitors: may cause severe excitation, hyperpyrexia, or seizures, usually with high dosage. Avoid concomitant use.
Drug-lifestyle. *Alcohol use:* enhanced CNS depression. Avoid concomitant use.
Sun exposure: increased risk of photosensitivity. Avoid unprotected or prolonged exposure to sun.

EFFECTS ON DIAGNOSTIC TESTS
Drug may prolong conduction time (elongation of QT and PR intervals, flattened T waves on ECG); it also may elevate liver function tests, decrease WBC counts, and decrease or increase serum glucose levels.

CONTRAINDICATIONS
Contraindicated in patients with hypersensitivity to drug, during acute recovery phase of MI, and in those who have received an MAO inhibitor within the past 14 days.

NURSING CONSIDERATIONS
• Use cautiously in patients with history of urine retention, angle-closure glaucoma, or increased intraocular pressure as well as in patients with CV disease. Use with extreme caution in patients with history of seizure disorders.
• Know that safe use of drug in children under 16 years has not been determined.
• Do not withdraw drug abruptly.
• Because hypertensive episodes have occurred during surgery in patients receiving TCAs, be aware that drug should be gradually discontinued several days before surgery.

Reactions may be *common,* uncommon, *life-threatening,* or COMMON AND LIFE-THREATENING.

• Expect delay of 2 weeks or more before noticeable effect. Full effect may take 4 weeks or more. However, know that adverse anticholinergic effects can occur rapidly.
• If signs of psychosis occur or increase, expect doctor to reduce dosage. Record mood changes. Monitor patient for suicidal tendencies, and allow only a minimum supply of drug.
• Monitor for signs and symptoms of tardive dyskinesia, especially in elderly women.
• Amoxapine therapy has been associated with neuroleptic malignant syndrome, a rare but life-threatening syndrome usually seen with phenothiazines. Discontinue drug immediately and institute appropriate therapy if symptoms occur.
• Relieve dry mouth with sugarless hard candy or gum. Saliva substitutes may be necessary.

☑ Patient teaching
• Whenever possible, tell patient to take full dose at bedtime.
• Warn patient not to stop drug therapy abruptly.
• Warn patient to avoid activities that require alertness and good psychomotor coordination until CNS effects of the drug are known. Drowsiness and dizziness usually subside after a few weeks.
• To prevent photosensitivity reactions, advise patient to use sunblock, wear protective clothing, and avoid prolonged exposure to strong sunlight.

bupropion hydrochloride
Wellbutrin, Wellbutrin SR

Pregnancy Risk Category: B

HOW SUPPLIED
Tablets: 75 mg, 100 mg
Tablets (sustained-release): 100 mg, 150 mg

ACTION
Unknown. Bupropion is not a tricyclic antidepressant (TCA), does not inhibit MAO, and is a weak inhibitor of norepinephrine, dopamine, and serotonin reuptake.

Route	Onset	Peak	Duration
PO	Unknown	2 hr	Unknown
PO (sustained)	Unknown	3 hr	Unknown

INDICATIONS & DOSAGE
Depression—
Adults: initially, 100 mg P.O. b.i.d., increased after 3 days to 100 mg P.O. t.i.d. if needed. If no response occurs after several weeks of therapy, dosage increased to 150 mg t.i.d. No single dose should exceed 150 mg. For sustained-release tablets, initially, 150 mg P.O. q morning; increased to target dose of 150 mg P.O. b.i.d. as tolerated as early as day 4 of dosing. Maximum dosage is 400 mg/day.

ADVERSE REACTIONS
CNS: *headache, seizures,* anxiety, confusion, delusions, euphoria, hostility, impaired sleep quality, *insomnia, sedation, tremor,* akinesia, akathisia, *agitation, dizziness,* fatigue.
CV: *arrhythmias,* hypertension, hypotension, palpitations, syncope, *tachycardia.*
EENT: *auditory disturbances,* blurred vision.
GI: *dry mouth,* taste disturbance, increased appetite, *constipation,* dyspepsia, *nausea, vomiting, weight loss, anorexia, weight gain,* diarrhea.
GU: impotence, menstrual complaints, urinary frequency, decreased libido, urine retention.
Skin: pruritus, rash, cutaneous temperature disturbance, *excessive diaphoresis.*
Other: arthritis, fever and chills.

INTERACTIONS
Drug-drug. *Levodopa, phenothiazines, TCAs; recent and rapid withdrawal of benzodiazepines:* increased risk of adverse reactions, including seizures. Monitor patient closely.
MAO inhibitors: altered seizure threshold. Avoid concomitant use.
Drug-lifestyle. *Alcohol use:* altered seizure threshold. Avoid concomitant use.

EFFECTS ON DIAGNOSTIC TESTS
None reported.

CONTRAINDICATIONS
Contraindicated in patients with seizure disorders, hypersensitivity to drug, or history of bulimia or anorexia nervosa because of a higher incidence of seizures and in those who have taken MAO inhibitors within the previous 14 days. Do not use with Zyban or other medications containing bupropion used for smoking cessation.

NURSING CONSIDERATIONS
• Use cautiously in patients with recent history of MI or unstable heart disease, as well as renal or hepatic impairment.
• Know that many patients experience a period of increased restlessness, especially at initiation of therapy. This may include agitation, insomnia, and anxiety.
Alert: Risk of seizure may be minimized by not exceeding 450 mg/day and by administering daily dosage in three to four equally divided doses. Be aware that patients who experience seizures often have predisposing factors, including history of head trauma, prior seizures, or CNS tumors, or they may be taking a drug that lowers the seizure threshold.
• Monitor patient with history of bipolar disorders closely. Antidepressants can cause manic episodes during the depressed phase of bipolar disorder.

☑ Patient teaching
• Advise patient to take drug as scheduled and to take each day's dosage in three divided doses to minimize the risk of seizures.
• Advise patient to consult doctor before taking other prescription or OTC medications.
• Tell patient to avoid alcohol while taking drug because it may contribute to the development of seizures.
• Advise patient to avoid hazardous activities that require alertness and good psychomotor coordination until CNS effects of drug are known.

▼ NEW DRUG

citalopram hydrobromide
Celexa

Pregnancy Risk Category: C

HOW SUPPLIED
Tablets: 20 mg, 40 mg

ACTION
A selective serotonin reuptake inhibitor (SSRI) whose action is presumed to be linked to potentiation of serotonergic activity in the central nervous system resulting from inhibition of neuronal reuptake of serotonin.

Route	Onset	Peak	Duration
PO	Unknown	4 hr	Unknown

INDICATIONS & DOSAGE
Depression—
Adults: initially, 20 mg P.O. once daily, increasing to 40 mg daily after no less than 1 week. Maximum recommended dose is 40 mg daily.
Elderly: 20 mg/day P.O. with titration to 40 mg/day only for nonresponding patients.
Adjust-a-dose: For patients with hepatic impairment, use 20 mg/day P.O. with titration to 40 mg/day only for nonresponding patients.

ADVERSE REACTIONS
CNS: tremor, *somnolence, insomnia,* anxiety, agitation, dizziness, paresthesia, migraine, impaired concentration, amnesia, depression, apathy, ***suicide attempt,*** confusion, decreased libido, fatigue.
CV: tachycardia, orthostatic hypotension, hypotension.
EENT: rhinitis, sinusitis, abnormal accommodation.
GI: *dry mouth, nausea,* diarrhea, anorexia, dyspepsia, vomiting, abdominal pain, taste perversion, increased saliva, flatulence, decreased and increased weight, increased appetite.
GU: dysmenorrhea, amenorrhea, ejaculation disorder, impotence, polyuria.
Musculoskeletal: arthralgia, myalgia.

Reactions may be *common,* uncommon, *life-threatening,* or COMMON AND LIFE-THREATENING.

Respiratory: upper respiratory tract infection, coughing.
Skin: rash, pruritus.
Other: *increased sweating,* fever, yawning.

INTERACTIONS
Drug-drug. *Carbamazepine:* may increase citalopram clearance. Monitor for effects.
CNS drugs: additive effects. Use together cautiously.
Drugs that inhibit cytochrome P-450 isoenzymes 3A4 and 2C19: decreased clearance of citalopram. Monitor closely.
Imipramine, other tricyclic antidepressants: concentration of imipramine metabolite desipramine increased by approximately 50%. Use together cautiously.
MAO inhibitors: serious, sometimes fatal, reactions may occur. Do not use drug within 14 days of MAO inhibitor use.
Lithium: may enhance serotonergic effect of citalopram. Use with caution, and monitor lithium levels.
Warfarin: prothrombin time increased by 5%. Monitor closely.
Drug-lifestyle. *Alcohol use:* may increase CNS effects. Avoid concomitant use.

EFFECTS ON DIAGNOSTIC TESTS
None reported.

CONTRAINDICATIONS
Contraindicated in patients also taking MAO inhibitors or within 14 days of stopping MAO inhibitor therapy and in those with hypersensitivity to drug or its inactive ingredients.

NURSING CONSIDERATIONS
• Use cautiously in patients with history of mania, seizures, suicidal ideation, or hepatic or renal impairment.
• Safety and effectiveness have not been established in children.
• Be aware that, although drug has not been shown to impair psychomotor performance, any psychoactive drug has the potential to impair judgment, thinking, or motor skills.
• Be aware that the possibility of a suicide attempt is inherent in depression and may persist until significant remission occurs.

Closely supervise high-risk patients at the start of drug therapy. Reduce risk of overdose by limiting the amount of drug available per refill.
• Know that at least 14 days should elapse between MAO inhibitor therapy and citalopram therapy.

☑ **Patient teaching**
• Inform patient that although improvement may occur within 1 to 4 weeks, he should continue therapy as prescribed.
• Instruct patient to exercise caution when operating hazardous machinery, including automobiles, because of the potential of psychoactive drugs to impair judgment, thinking, and motor skills.
• Advise patient to consult doctor before taking other prescription or OTC medications or breast-feeding an infant.
• Warn patient to avoid concomitant use of alcohol.
• Instruct female patient of childbearing age to use birth control during drug therapy and to notify doctor immediately if pregnancy is suspected.
• Caution patient against use of MAO inhibitors while taking citalopram.
• Tell patient that drug may be taken in the morning or evening without regard to meals.

---

clomipramine hydrochloride
Anafranil, Placil‡

Pregnancy Risk Category: C

HOW SUPPLIED
Capsules: 25 mg, 50 mg, 75 mg

ACTION
Unknown, but a tricyclic antidepressant (TCA) that selectively inhibits reuptake of serotonin.

Route	Onset	Peak	Duration
PO	≥ 2 wk	2-6 hr	Unknown

INDICATIONS & DOSAGE
Obsessive-compulsive disorder—
Adults: initially, 25 mg P.O. daily with meals, gradually increased to 100 mg daily in divided doses during first 2 weeks.

Thereafter, increased to maximum dosage of 250 mg daily in divided doses with meals, p.r.n. After titration, total daily dosage may be given h.s.

Children and adolescents: initially, 25 mg P.O. daily with meals, gradually increased over first 2 weeks to daily maximum of 3 mg/kg or 100 mg P.O. in divided doses, whichever is smaller. Maximum daily dosage is 3 mg/kg or 200 mg, whichever is smaller; may be given h.s. after titration. Periodic reassessment and adjustment necessary.

ADVERSE REACTIONS
CNS: *somnolence, tremor, dizziness, headache, insomnia, nervousness, myoclonus, fatigue,* EEG changes, **seizures.**
CV: *orthostatic hypotension, palpitations,* tachycardia.
EENT: *pharyngitis, rhinitis, visual changes.*
GI: *dry mouth, constipation, nausea, dyspepsia, increased appetite,* diarrhea, *anorexia, abdominal pain.*
GU: *urinary hesitancy,* urinary tract infection, *dysmenorrhea, ejaculation failure, impotence, altered libido.*
Hematologic: purpura.
Skin: *diaphoresis,* rash, pruritus, dry skin.
Other: *myalgia, weight gain.*

INTERACTIONS
Drug-drug. *Barbiturates:* decreased TCA blood levels. Monitor for decreased antidepressant effect.
Cimetidine, fluoxetine, fluvoxamine, sertraline: increased TCA blood levels. Monitor for enhanced antidepressant effect.
Clonidine, epinephrine, norepinephrine: increased hypertensive effect. Use with caution.
CNS depressants: enhanced CNS depression. Avoid concomitant use.
MAO inhibitors: may cause hyperpyretic crisis, seizures, coma, or death. Avoid concomitant use.
Drug-lifestyle. *Alcohol use:* enhanced CNS depression. Avoid concomitant use.
Sun exposure: increased risk of photosensitivity. Avoid unprotected or prolonged exposure to sun.

EFFECTS ON DIAGNOSTIC TESTS
None reported.

CONTRAINDICATIONS
Contraindicated in patients with hypersensitivity to drug or other TCAs, in those who have taken MAO inhibitors within the previous 14 days, and in patients during acute recovery period after MI.

NURSING CONSIDERATIONS
● Use cautiously in patients with history of seizure disorders or with brain damage of varying etiology; in patients receiving other seizure threshold-lowering drugs; in patients at risk for suicide; in patients with history of urine retention or angle-closure glaucoma, increased intraocular pressure, CV disease, impaired hepatic or renal function, or hyperthyroidism; in patients with tumors of the adrenal medulla; in patients receiving thyroid medication or electroconvulsive therapy; and in those undergoing elective surgery.
● Know that total daily dose may be taken at bedtime after titration. During titration, dosage may be divided.
● Do not withdraw drug abruptly.
● Because hypertensive episodes have occurred during surgery in patients receiving TCAs, know that drug should be gradually discontinued several days before surgery.
● Relieve dry mouth with sugarless candy or gum. Saliva substitutes may be necessary.

☑ **Patient teaching**
● Warn patient to avoid hazardous activities requiring alertness and good psychomotor coordination, especially during titration. Daytime sedation and dizziness may occur.
● Tell patient to avoid alcohol while taking drug.
● Warn patient not to withdraw drug suddenly.
● Advise patient to use sunblock, wear protective clothing, and avoid prolonged exposure to strong sunlight to prevent photosensitivity reactions.

Reactions may be *common*, uncommon, ***life-threatening***, or COMMON AND LIFE-THREATENING.

desipramine hydrochloride
Norpramin**, Pertofran‡,
Pertofrane†

Pregnancy Risk Category: NR

HOW SUPPLIED
Tablets: 10 mg, 25 mg, 50 mg, 75 mg,
100 mg, 150 mg
Capsules: 25 mg, 50 mg

ACTION
Unknown, but a tricyclic antidepressant
(TCA) that increases the amount of nor-
epinephrine, serotonin, or both in the
CNS by blocking their reuptake by the
presynaptic neurons.

Route	Onset	Peak	Duration
PO	Unknown	4-6 hr	Unknown

INDICATIONS & DOSAGE
Depression—
Adults: 100 to 200 mg P.O. daily in divided doses, increased to maximum of
300 mg daily. Alternatively, entire dosage
can be given h.s.
Elderly and adolescents: 25 to 100 mg
P.O. daily in divided doses, increased
gradually to maximum of 150 mg daily if
needed.

ADVERSE REACTIONS
CNS: *drowsiness, dizziness,* excitation,
tremor, weakness, confusion, anxiety,
restlessness, agitation, headache, nervous-
ness, EEG changes, *seizures,* extrapyra-
midal reactions.
CV: orthostatic hypotension, *tachycardia,*
ECG changes, hypertension.
EENT: *blurred vision,* tinnitus, mydriasis.
GI: *dry mouth,* constipation, nausea,
vomiting, anorexia, paralytic ileus.
GU: urine retention.
Skin: rash, urticaria, photosensitivity.
Other: diaphoresis, *hypersensitivity reaction, sudden death* (in children).
**After abrupt withdrawal of long-term
therapy:** nausea, headache, malaise (does
not indicate addiction).

INTERACTIONS
Drug-drug. *Barbiturates, CNS depres-*
sants: enhanced CNS depression. Avoid
concomitant use.
*Cimetidine, fluvoxamine, fluoxetine, par-
oxetine, sertraline:* may increase serum
desipramine levels. Monitor for adverse
reactions.
Clonidine, epinephrine, norepinephrine:
increased hypertensive effect. Use with
caution.
MAO inhibitors: may cause severe excitation, hyperpyrexia, or seizures, usually
with high dosage. Avoid concomitant use.
Drug-lifestyle. *Alcohol use:* enhanced
CNS depression. Avoid concomitant use.
Smoking: may lower plasma desipramine
levels. Monitor for lack of effect.
Sun exposure: increased risk of photosensitivity. Avoid unprotected or prolonged
sun exposure.

EFFECTS ON DIAGNOSTIC TESTS
Drug may prolong conduction time (elongation of QT and PR intervals, flattened T
waves on ECG); it also may elevate liver
function test results, decrease WBC
counts, and decrease or increase serum
glucose levels.

CONTRAINDICATIONS
Contraindicated in patients hypersensitive
to drug, in those who have taken MAO inhibitors within the previous 14 days, and
during acute recovery phase of MI.

NURSING CONSIDERATIONS
• Use with extreme caution in patients
with CV disease, history of urine retention, glaucoma, or thyroid disease, in
those taking thyroid medication, and in
patients with history of seizure disorders.
• Do not withdraw drug abruptly.
• Because hypertensive episodes have occurred during surgery in patients receiving TCAs, know that drug should be gradually discontinued several days before
surgery.
• If signs of psychosis occur or increase,
expect doctor to reduce dosage. Record
mood changes. Monitor patient for suicidal tendencies, and allow only a minimum
supply of drug.
• Know that because desipramine produces fewer anticholinergic effects than

---

other TCAs, it is often prescribed for cardiac patients.
• Relieve dry mouth with sugarless hard candy or gum. Saliva substitutes may be necessary.

☑ **Patient teaching**
• Advise patient to take full dose at bedtime.
• Warn patient to avoid hazardous activities that require alertness and good psychomotor coordination until CNS effects of the drug are known. Drowsiness and dizziness usually subside after a few weeks.
• Tell patient to avoid alcohol while taking this drug because it may antagonize effects of desipramine.
• Tell patient to consult doctor before taking other prescription or OTC medications.
• Warn patient not to stop drug therapy suddenly.
• To prevent photosensitivity reactions, advise patient to use sunblock, wear protective clothing, and avoid prolonged exposure to strong sunlight.

---

doxepin hydrochloride
Deptran‡, Novo-Doxepin†,
Sinequan, Triadapin†

Pregnancy Risk Category: NR

HOW SUPPLIED
Capsules: 10 mg, 25 mg, 50 mg, 75 mg, 100 mg, 150 mg
Oral concentrate: 10 mg/ml

ACTION
Unknown, but a tricyclic antidepressant (TCA) that increases the amount of norepinephrine, serotonin, or both in the CNS by blocking their reuptake by the presynaptic neurons.

Route	Onset	Peak	Duration
PO	Unknown	2 hr	Unknown

INDICATIONS & DOSAGE
Depression or anxiety—
Adults: initially, 25 to 75 mg P.O. daily in divided doses to maximum of 300 mg

daily. Alternatively, entire maintenance dosage may be given once daily with a maximum dose of 150 mg.

ADVERSE REACTIONS
CNS: *drowsiness, dizziness,* confusion, numbness, hallucinations, paresthesia, ataxia, weakness, headache, ***seizures,*** extrapyramidal reactions.
CV: *orthostatic hypotension, tachycardia.*
EENT: *blurred vision,* tinnitus.
GI: *dry mouth, constipation,* nausea, vomiting, anorexia.
GU: urine retention.
Skin: rash, urticaria, photosensitivity, *diaphoresis.*
Other: *hypersensitivity reaction.*
After abrupt withdrawal of long-term therapy: nausea, headache, malaise (does not indicate addiction).

INTERACTIONS
Drug-drug. *Barbiturates, CNS depressants:* enhanced CNS depression. Avoid concomitant use.
Cimetidine, fluoxetine, sertraline: may increase serum doxepin levels. Monitor for increased adverse reactions.
Clonidine, epinephrine, norepinephrine: increased hypertensive effect. Use with caution.
MAO inhibitors: may cause severe excitation, hyperpyrexia, or seizures, usually with high dosage. Avoid concomitant use.
Drug-lifestyle. *Alcohol use:* enhanced CNS depression. Avoid concomitant use.
Sun exposure: increased risk of photosensitivity reactions. Avoid unprotected or prolonged exposure to sun.

EFFECTS ON DIAGNOSTIC TESTS
Drug may prolong conduction time (elongation of QT and PR intervals, flattened T waves on ECG); it also may elevate liver function test results, decrease WBC counts, and decrease or increase serum glucose levels.

CONTRAINDICATIONS
Contraindicated in patients with glaucoma, tendency to urine retention, or hypersensitivity to drug; in those who have received an MAO inhibitor within the past

---

Reactions may be *common,* uncommon, ***life-threatening,*** or COMMON AND LIFE-THREATENING.

14 days; or during acute recovery phase of an MI.

NURSING CONSIDERATIONS
• Do not withdraw drug abruptly.
Alert: Because hypertensive episodes have occurred during surgery in patients receiving TCAs, be aware that drug should be gradually discontinued several days before surgery.
• If signs of psychosis occur or increase, expect doctor to reduce dosage. Record mood changes. Monitor patient for suicidal tendencies, and allow only a minimum supply of drug.
• Doxepin has strong anticholinergic effects; it is one of the most sedating TCAs. Adverse anticholinergic effects can occur rapidly.
• Relieve dry mouth with sugarless hard candy or gum. Saliva substitutes may be necessary.

☑ **Patient teaching**
• Tell patient to dilute oral concentrate with 4 oz (120 ml) of water, milk, or juice (orange, grapefruit, tomato, prune, or pineapple, but not grape juice); preparation is incompatible with carbonated beverages.
• Inform patient to take full dose at bedtime but warn him of possible morning orthostatic hypotension.
• Advise patient to consult doctor before taking other prescription or OTC medications.
• Warn patient to avoid hazardous activities that require alertness and good psychomotor coordination until CNS effects of drug are known. Drowsiness and dizziness usually subside after a few weeks.
• Tell patient to avoid alcohol while taking drug.
• Tell patient that the maximum antidepressant effect may not be evident for 2 to 3 weeks.
• Warn patient not to stop drug therapy suddenly.
• To prevent photosensitivity reactions, advise patient to use sunblock, wear protective clothing, and avoid prolonged exposure to strong sunlight.

fluoxetine hydrochloride
Prozac, Prozac-20‡, Erocap‡, Lovan‡, Zactin‡

Pregnancy Risk Category: B

HOW SUPPLIED
Pulvules: 10 mg, 20 mg
Oral solution: 20 mg/5 ml

ACTION
Unknown, but presumed to be linked to its inhibition of CNS neuronal uptake of serotonin.

Route	Onset	Peak	Duration
PO	Unknown	6-8 hr	Unknown

INDICATIONS & DOSAGE
Depression; obsessive-compulsive disorder—
Adults: initially, 20 mg P.O. in the morning; dosage increased according to patient response. May be given b.i.d. in the morning and at noon. Maximum dosage is 80 mg/day.
Adjust-a-dose: In patients with renal or hepatic impairment, a lower or less frequent dosage should be used.
Treatment of binge-eating and vomiting behavior in patients with moderate to severe bulimia nervosa—
Adults: 60 mg P.O. in the morning.

ADVERSE REACTIONS
CNS: *nervousness, anxiety, insomnia, headache, drowsiness,* fatigue, *tremor, dizziness, asthenia.*
CV: palpitations, hot flashes.
EENT: nasal congestion, pharyngitis, cough, sinusitis.
GI: *nausea, diarrhea, dry mouth, anorexia,* dyspepsia, constipation, abdominal pain, vomiting, flatulence, increased appetite.
GU: sexual dysfunction.
Respiratory: upper respiratory infection, respiratory distress.
Skin: rash, pruritus, diaphoresis.
Other: flulike syndrome, muscle pain, weight loss, fever.

INTERACTIONS
Drug-drug. *Carbamazepine, flecainide, vinblastine:* increased serum levels of these drugs. Monitor serum levels and the patient for adverse effects.
Cyproheptadine: may reverse or decrease pharmacologic effect. Monitor patient closely.
Insulin, oral antidiabetic agents: altered blood glucose levels and possible altered requirements for antidiabetic medication. Adjust dosage, as ordered.
Lithium, tricyclic antidepressants: risk of increased adverse CNS effects. Avoid concomitant use.
Phenytoin: increased plasma phenytoin levels and risk of toxicity. Monitor serum phenytoin levels and adjust dosage, as ordered.
Tryptophan: increased agitation, restlessness, GI problems. Use with caution.
Warfarin, other highly protein-bound agents: may increase plasma levels of fluoxetine or other highly protein-bound drugs. Monitor patient closely.
Drug-lifestyle. *Alcohol use:* increased CNS depression. Avoid concomitant use.

EFFECTS ON DIAGNOSTIC TESTS
None reported.

CONTRAINDICATIONS
Contraindicated in patients hypersensitive to drug and in those taking MAO inhibitors within 14 days of starting therapy. MAO inhibitors should not be started within 5 weeks of stopping fluoxetine therapy.

NURSING CONSIDERATIONS
• Use cautiously in patients at high risk for suicide and in patients with history of hepatic, renal, or CV disease; diabetes mellitus; or history of seizures.
• Use antihistamines or topical corticosteroids as ordered to treat rashes or pruritus.

☑ Patient teaching
• Tell patient to avoid taking drug in the afternoon because fluoxetine commonly causes nervousness and insomnia.
• Drug may cause dizziness or drowsiness in some patients. Warn patient to avoid driving and other hazardous activities that require alertness and good psychomotor coordination until CNS effects of drug are known.
• Tell patient to consult doctor before taking other prescription or OTC medications.
• Warn patient to avoid food high in tryptophan, including meats, poultry, fish, liver, kidney, eggs, nuts, peanut butter, broad beans, and wheat germ.

imipramine hydrochloride
Apo-Imipramine†, Impril†, Melipramine‡, Norfranil, Novo-Pramine†, Tipramine, Tofranil**

imipramine pamoate
Tofranil-PM**

Pregnancy Risk Category: D

HOW SUPPLIED
imipramine hydrochloride
Tablets: 10 mg, 25 mg, 50 mg
Injection: 12.5 mg/ml
imipramine pamoate
Capsules: 75 mg, 100 mg, 125 mg, 150 mg

ACTION
Unknown, but a tricyclic antidepressant (TCA) that increases the amount of norepinephrine, serotonin, or both in the CNS by blocking their reuptake by the presynaptic neurons.

Route	Onset	Peak	Duration
PO	Unknown	1-2 hr	Unknown
IM	Unknown	30 min	Unknown

INDICATIONS & DOSAGE
Depression—
Adults: 75 to 100 mg P.O. or I.M. daily in divided doses, increased in 25- to 50-mg increments. Maximum dosage for outpatients is 200 mg daily; 300 mg daily may be used for hospitalized patients. Entire dosage may be given h.s.
Elderly and adolescents: initially, 30 to 40 mg daily; usually not necessary to exceed 100 mg daily.

Childhood enuresis—
Children 5 years and older: 25 mg P.O.
1 hour before bedtime. If no response
within 1 week, increased to 50 mg if child
is under 12 years; increased to 75 mg for
children 12 years and over. In either case,
maximum dosage is 2.5 mg/kg/day.

ADVERSE REACTIONS

CNS: *drowsiness, dizziness,* excitation,
tremor, confusion, hallucinations, anxiety,
ataxia, paresthesia, nervousness, EEG
changes, *seizures,* extrapyramidal reactions.
CV: *orthostatic hypotension, tachycardia,
ECG changes,* hypertension, *MI, stroke,
arrhythmias, heart block,* precipitation of
heart failure.
EENT: *blurred vision,* tinnitus, mydriasis.
GI: *dry mouth, constipation,* nausea,
vomiting, anorexia, paralytic ileus, abdominal cramps.
GU: *urine retention.*
Skin: rash, urticaria, photosensitivity,
pruritus.
Other: diaphoresis, *hypersensitivity reaction.*
**After abrupt withdrawal of long-term
therapy:** nausea, headache, malaise (does
not indicate addiction).

INTERACTIONS

Drug-drug. *Barbiturates, CNS depressants:* enhanced CNS depression. Avoid
concomitant use.
Cimetidine, fluoxetine, sertraline: may increase serum imipramine levels. Monitor
for adverse reactions.
Clonidine, epinephrine, norepinephrine:
increased hypertensive effect. Use with
caution.
MAO inhibitors: may cause hyperpyretic
crisis, severe seizures, and death. Avoid
concomitant use.
Drug-lifestyle. *Alcohol use:* enhanced
CNS depression. Avoid concomitant use.
Smoking: may lower plasma concentrations of imipramine. Monitor for lack of
effect.
Sun exposure: increased risk of photosensitivity. Avoid unprotected or prolonged
exposure to sun.

EFFECTS ON DIAGNOSTIC TESTS

Drug may prolong conduction time (elongation of QT and PR intervals, flattened T
waves on ECG); it also may elevate liver
function test results, decrease WBC
counts, and decrease or increase serum
glucose levels.

CONTRAINDICATIONS

Contraindicated during acute recovery
phase of MI, in patients with hypersensitivity to drug, and in those receiving
MAO inhibitors.

NURSING CONSIDERATIONS

● Use with extreme caution in patients at
risk for suicide; in patients with history of
urine retention or angle-closure glaucoma, increased intraocular pressure, CV
disease, impaired hepatic function, hyperthyroidism, history of seizure disorders,
impaired renal function; and in patients
receiving thyroid medications. Injectable
form contains sulfites, which may cause
allergic reactions in hypersensitive patients.
● Do not withdraw drug abruptly.
● Because of hypertensive episodes during surgery in patients receiving TCAs, be
aware that drug should be gradually discontinued several days before surgery.
● If signs of psychosis occur or increase,
expect doctor to reduce dosage. Record
mood changes. Monitor patient for suicidal tendencies, and allow only a minimum
supply of drug.
● To prevent relapse in children receiving
drug for enuresis, be aware that drug
should be withdrawn gradually.
● Relieve dry mouth with sugarless hard
candy or gum. Saliva substitutes may be
necessary.

☑Patient teaching
● Advise patient to take full dose at bedtime but warn him of possible morning
orthostatic hypotension.
● If child is an "early night" bedwetter,
tell parents it may be more effective to divide dosage and administer the first dose
earlier in the day.
● Tell patient to avoid alcohol while taking this drug.
● Advise patient to consult doctor before

---

taking other prescription or OTC medications.
• Warn patient to avoid hazardous activities that require alertness and good psychomotor coordination until CNS effects of the drug are known. Drowsiness and dizziness usually subside after a few weeks.
• Warn patient not to stop drug suddenly.
• To prevent photosensitivity reactions, advise patient to use sunblock, wear protective clothing, and avoid prolonged exposure to strong sunlight.

mirtazapine
Remeron, Zispin§

Pregnancy Risk Category: C

HOW SUPPLIED
Tablets: 15 mg, 30 mg

ACTION
Antidepressant action is thought to be due to enhancement of central noradrenergic and serotonergic activity.

Route	Onset	Peak	Duration
PO	Unknown	2 hr	Unknown

INDICATIONS & DOSAGE
Depression—
Adults: initially, 15 mg P.O. h.s. Maintenance dosage ranges from 15 to 45 mg daily. Dosage adjustments should be made at intervals of no less than 1 to 2 weeks.

ADVERSE REACTIONS
CNS: *somnolence,* dizziness, asthenia, abnormal dreams, abnormal thinking, tremors, confusion.
GI: nausea, *increased appetite, dry mouth, constipation.*
GU: urinary frequency.
Hematologic: *agranulocytosis* (rare).
Respiratory: dyspnea.
Other: *weight gain,* back pain, flu syndrome, edema, peripheral edema, myalgia.

INTERACTIONS
Drug-drug. *Diazepam, other CNS depressants:* possible additive CNS effects. Avoid concomitant use.

MAO inhibitors: sometimes fatal reactions. Avoid concomitant use.
Drug-lifestyle. *Alcohol use:* possible additive CNS effects. Avoid concomitant use.

EFFECTS ON DIAGNOSTIC TESTS
Drug may increase cholesterol, triglyceride, and ALT levels.

CONTRAINDICATIONS
Contraindicated in patients with hypersensitivity to drug. Drug should not be used with MAO inhibitor or within 14 days of initiating or discontinuing therapy with MAO inhibitor. At least 14 days should elapse after stopping mirtazapine before starting an MAO inhibitor.

NURSING CONSIDERATIONS
• Use cautiously in patients with CV or cerebrovascular disease, seizure disorders, suicidal ideations, impaired hepatic or renal function, or history of mania or hypomania.
• Use cautiously in patients with conditions that predispose them to hypotension, such as dehydration, hypovolemia, or treatment with antihypertensive medication.
• Know that although incidence of agranulocytosis is rare, discontinue drug and monitor patient closely if he develops a sore throat, fever, stomatitis, or other signs of infection together with a low WBC count.
• Monitor patient closely for signs of dependence; it is not known whether mirtazapine causes physical or psychological dependence.
• Administer drug cautiously to elderly patients; pharmacokinetic studies reveal decreased clearance in the elderly.

☑ Patient teaching
• Caution patient not to perform hazardous activities if somnolence occurs.
• Tell patient to report signs and symptoms of infection, such as fever, chills, sore throat, mucous membrane ulceration, or flulike symptoms.
• Instruct patient not to use alcohol or other CNS depressants while taking drug.
• Stress importance of compliance with therapy.

Reactions may be *common,* uncommon, *life-threatening,* or COMMON AND LIFE-THREATENING.

• Instruct patient not to take concomitant medications without doctor's approval.
• Tell female patient of childbearing age to report suspected pregnancy immediately and to notify doctor if she is breast-feeding.

nefazodone hydrochloride
Dutonin§, Serzone

Pregnancy Risk Category: C

HOW SUPPLIED
Tablets: 100 mg, 150 mg, 200 mg, 250 mg

ACTION
Not precisely defined. Drug inhibits neuronal uptake of serotonin ($5-HT_2$) and norepinephrine; it also occupies serotonin and alpha$_1$-adrenergic receptors in the CNS.

Route	Onset	Peak	Duration
PO	Unknown	1 hr	Unknown

INDICATIONS & DOSAGE
Depression—
Adults: initially, 200 mg/day P.O. in two divided doses. Dosage increased in increments of 100 to 200 mg/day at intervals of no less than 1 week, p.r.n. Usual dosage range is 300 to 600 mg/day.
Elderly: initially, 100 mg/day P.O. in two divided doses.
Adjust-a-dose: In debilitated patients, initially 100 mg/day P.O. in two divided doses.

ADVERSE REACTIONS
CNS: *headache, somnolence, dizziness, asthenia, insomnia, light-headedness, confusion,* memory impairment, paresthesia, vasodilation, abnormal dreams, decreased concentration, ataxia, incoordination, psychomotor retardation, tremor, hypertonia.
CV: orthostatic hypotension, hypotension, peripheral edema.
EENT: blurred vision, abnormal vision, tinnitus, visual field defect.
GI: *dry mouth, nausea, constipation,* taste perversion, dyspepsia, diarrhea, increased appetite, vomiting.
GU: urinary frequency, urinary tract infection, urine retention, vaginitis.
Respiratory: pharyngitis, cough.
Skin: pruritus, rash.
Other: infection, flulike syndrome, chills, fever, neck rigidity, breast pain, thirst, arthralgia.

INTERACTIONS
Drug-drug. *Alprazolam, triazolam:* coadministration with nefazodone potentiates the effects of these drugs. Do not administer concurrently. However, if necessary, dosage of alprazolam and triazolam may need to be reduced greatly.
Astemizole: may cause decreased metabolism, leading to increased antihistamine level and cardiotoxicity. Avoid concomitant use.
CNS drugs: may alter CNS activity. Use together cautiously.
Digoxin: may increase digoxin level. Use together cautiously and monitor digoxin levels.
MAO inhibitors: may cause severe excitation, hyperpyrexia, seizures, delirium, or coma. Avoid concomitant use.
Other highly protein-bound drugs: may increase incidence and severity of adverse reactions. Monitor patient closely.
Drug-lifestyle. *Alcohol use:* enhanced CNS depression. Avoid concomitant use.

EFFECTS ON DIAGNOSTIC TESTS
None reported.

CONTRAINDICATIONS
Contraindicated in patients with hypersensitivity to drug or other phenylpiperazine antidepressants. Also contraindicated within 14 days of MAO inhibitor therapy and in coadministration with astemizole.

NURSING CONSIDERATIONS
• Use cautiously in patients with CV or cerebrovascular disease that could be exacerbated by hypotension (such as history of MI, angina, or CVA) and conditions that would predispose patients to hypotension (such as dehydration, hypovolemia, and treatment with antihypertensives).

Also use cautiously in patients with a history of mania.
- Know that at least 1 week should elapse between stopping nefazodone and starting MAO inhibitor therapy, and that at least 14 days should elapse before a patient begins taking nefazodone after MAO inhibitor therapy has been discontinued.
- Record mood changes. Monitor patient for suicidal tendencies, and allow only a minimum supply of drug.

☑ **Patient teaching**
- Warn patient not to engage in hazardous activity until CNS effects of drug are known.
Alert: Instruct men who experience prolonged or inappropriate erections to stop drug immediately and notify doctor.
- Instruct female patient to notify doctor if she becomes pregnant or intends to become pregnant during therapy.
- Tell patient to notify doctor if rash, hives, or related allergic reactions occur.
- Instruct patient to avoid alcoholic beverages during therapy.
- Tell patient to notify doctor before taking OTC drugs.
- Inform patient that several weeks of therapy will be required to obtain full antidepressant effect. Once improvement occurs, advise patient not to discontinue drug until directed by doctor.

---

nortriptyline hydrochloride
Allegron‡, Aventyl*, Pamelor*

Pregnancy Risk Category: NR

HOW SUPPLIED
Tablets: 10 mg‡, 25 mg‡
Capsules: 10 mg, 25 mg, 50 mg, 75 mg
Oral solution: 10 mg/5 ml (4% alcohol)

ACTION
Unknown, but a tricyclic antidepressant (TCA) that increases the amount of norepinephrine, serotonin, or both in the CNS by blocking their reuptake by the presynaptic neurons.

Route	Onset	Peak	Duration
PO	Unknown	7-8.5 hr	Unknown

INDICATIONS & DOSAGE
Depression—
Adults: 25 mg P.O. t.i.d. or q.i.d., gradually increased to maximum of 150 mg daily. Entire dosage may be given h.s. Monitor plasma levels when doses above 100 mg/day are given.
Elderly and adolescents: 30 to 50 mg daily given once or in divided doses.

ADVERSE REACTIONS
CNS: *drowsiness, dizziness, seizures,* tremor, weakness, confusion, headache, nervousness, EEG changes, extrapyramidal reactions, insomnia, nightmares, hallucinations, paresthesia, ataxia, agitation.
CV: ECG changes, *tachycardia,* hypertension, hypotension, *MI, heart block, stroke.*
EENT: *blurred vision,* tinnitus, mydriasis.
GI: dry mouth, *constipation,* nausea, vomiting, anorexia, paralytic ileus.
GU: *urine retention.*
Hematologic: bone marrow depression, *agranulocytosis,* eosinophilia, *thrombocytopenia.*
Skin: rash, urticaria, photosensitivity.
Other: diaphoresis, *hypersensitivity reaction.*
After abrupt withdrawal of long-term therapy: nausea, headache, malaise (does not indicate addiction).

INTERACTIONS
Drug-drug. *Barbiturates, CNS depressants:* enhanced CNS depression. Avoid concomitant use.
Cimetidine, fluoxetine, sertraline: may increase nortriptyline serum levels. Monitor for adverse reactions.
Clonidine, epinephrine, norepinephrine: increased hypertensive effect. Use with caution.
MAO inhibitors: may cause severe excitation, hyperpyrexia, or seizures, usually with high dosage. Avoid concomitant use.
Drug-lifestyle. *Alcohol use:* enhanced CNS depression. Avoid concomitant use.
Smoking: may lower plasma concentrations of nortriptyline. Monitor for lack of clinical effect.
Sun exposure: increased risk of photosensitivity reaction. Avoid unprotected or prolonged exposure to sun.

Reactions may be *common,* uncommon, *life-threatening,* or COMMON AND LIFE-THREATENING.

EFFECTS ON DIAGNOSTIC TESTS
Drug may prolong conduction time (elongation of QT and PR intervals, flattened T waves on ECG); it also may elevate liver function test results, decrease WBC counts, and decrease or increase serum glucose levels.

CONTRAINDICATIONS
Contraindicated during acute recovery phase of MI and in patients with hypersensitivity to drug or MAO therapy within past 14 days.

NURSING CONSIDERATIONS
• Use with extreme caution in patients with glaucoma, suicidal tendency, history of urine retention or seizures, CV disease, or hyperthyroidism and in those receiving thyroid medication.
• Do not withdraw drug abruptly.
• Because hypertensive episodes have occurred during surgery in patients receiving TCAs, know that dosage should be gradually discontinued several days before surgery.
• If signs of psychosis occur or increase, expect doctor to reduce dosage. Record mood changes. Monitor patient for suicidal tendencies, and allow him only a minimum supply of drug.
• Relieve dry mouth with sugarless hard candy or gum. Saliva substitutes may be necessary.

☑ Patient teaching
• Whenever possible, advise patient to take full dose at bedtime to reduce the risk of orthostatic hypotension.
• Warn patient to avoid activities that require alertness and good psychomotor coordination until CNS effects of drug are known. Drowsiness and dizziness usually subside after a few weeks.
• Tell patient to consult doctor before taking other prescription or OTC medications.
• Warn patient not to stop drug suddenly.
• To prevent photosensitivity reactions, advise patient to use sunblock, wear protective clothing, and avoid prolonged exposure to strong sunlight.

paroxetine hydrochloride
Paxil, Aropax‡, Seroxat§

Pregnancy Risk Category: C

HOW SUPPLIED
Tablets: 10 mg, 20 mg, 30 mg, 40 mg

ACTION
Unknown, but presumed to be linked to its inhibition of CNS neuronal uptake of serotonin.

Route	Onset	Peak	Duration
PO	Unknown	2-8 hr	Unknown

INDICATIONS & DOSAGE
Depression—
Adults: initially, 20 mg P.O. daily, preferably in the morning as indicated. If patient does not respond after full antidepressant effect has occurred, dosage may be increased in 10-mg/day increments at weekly intervals, to maximum of 50 mg daily.
Elderly: initially, 10 mg P.O. daily, preferably in the morning as indicated. If patient does not respond after full antidepressant effect has occurred, dosage may be increased in 10-mg/day increments at weekly intervals, to maximum of 40 mg daily.
Adjust-a-dose: In debilitated patients or those with renal or hepatic failure, initially, 10 mg P.O. daily, preferably in the morning. If patient does not respond after full antidepressant effect has occurred, dosage may be increased in 10-mg/day increments at weekly intervals to maximum of 40 mg daily.
Panic disorder—
Adults: initially, 10 mg/day. Dosage may be increased in 10-mg/week increments and at weekly intervals. Maximum dosage should not exceed 60 mg/day.

ADVERSE REACTIONS
CNS: *somnolence, dizziness, insomnia, tremor, nervousness,* anxiety, paresthesia, confusion, *headache,* agitation.
CV: palpitations, vasodilation, orthostatic hypotension.
EENT: lump or tightness in throat.

GI: *dry mouth, nausea, constipation, diarrhea,* flatulence, vomiting, dyspepsia, dysgeusia, increased appetite, abdominal pain.
GU: decreased libido, ejaculatory disturbances, male genital disorders (including anorgasmy, erectile difficulties, delayed ejaculation or orgasm, impotence, and sexual dysfunction), urinary frequency, other urinary disorders, female genital disorders (including anorgasmy, difficulty with orgasm).
Skin: rash, pruritus.
Other: *asthenia, diaphoresis,* myopathy, myalgia, myasthenia, yawning.

INTERACTIONS
Drug-drug. *Cimetidine:* decreased hepatic metabolism of paroxetine, leading to risk of toxicity. Dosage adjustments may be necessary.
Digoxin: may decrease digoxin levels. Monitor closely.
MAO inhibitors: may increase risk of serious, sometimes fatal, adverse reactions. Avoid concomitant use.
Phenobarbital, phenytoin: may alter pharmacokinetics of both drugs. Dosage adjustments may be necessary.
Procyclidine: may increase procyclidine levels. Monitor for excessive anticholinergic effects.
Tryptophan: may increase incidence of adverse reactions, such as diaphoresis, headache, nausea, and dizziness. Avoid concomitant use.
Theophylline: decreased clearance. Dose reductions are necessary.
Warfarin: increased risk of bleeding. Use concomitantly with caution.
Drug-herb. *St. John's wort:* may result in sedative-hypnotic intoxication. Avoid concurrent use.
Drug-lifestyle. *Alcohol use:* may alter psychomotor function. Limit intake.

EFFECTS ON DIAGNOSTIC TESTS
None reported.

CONTRAINDICATIONS
Contraindicated in patients taking MAO inhibitors or within 14 days of discontinuing MAO inhibitor therapy and in those hypersensitive to drug.

NURSING CONSIDERATIONS
• Use cautiously in patients with a history of seizure disorders or mania and in those with severe, concomitant systemic illness.
• Use cautiously in patients at risk for volume depletion, and monitor appropriately.
• If signs of psychosis occur or increase, expect doctor to reduce dosage. Record mood changes. Monitor patient for suicidal tendencies, and allow only a minimum supply of drug.

☑**Patient teaching**
• Warn patient to avoid activities that require alertness and good psychomotor coordination until CNS effects of drug are known.
• Tell patient to avoid alcohol and to consult doctor before taking other prescription or OTC medications.

---

phenelzine sulfate
Nardil

Pregnancy Risk Category: C

HOW SUPPLIED
Tablets: 15 mg

ACTION
Unknown. An MAO inhibitor that probably promotes accumulation of neurotransmitters by inhibiting their metabolism.

Route	Onset	Peak	Duration
PO	Unknown	2-4 hr	≤ 10 days

INDICATIONS & DOSAGE
Depression—
Adults: 15 mg P.O. t.i.d., increased rapidly to 60 mg daily. Maximum dosage is 90 mg daily. Then dosage can usually be reduced to 15 mg daily.

ADVERSE REACTIONS
CNS: *dizziness, vertigo, headache,* hyperreflexia, tremor, muscle twitching, *insomnia,* drowsiness, weakness, fatigue.
CV: *postural hypotension,* edema.
GI: dry mouth, *anorexia,* nausea, *constipation.*
Other: diaphoresis, weight gain.

INTERACTIONS
Drug-drug. *Amphetamines, antihistamines, buspirone, ephedrine, levodopa, meperidine, metaraminol, methylphenidate, phenylephrine, phenylpropanolamine, sympathomimetics:* enhanced pressor effects. Avoid concomitant use.

Antihypertensives containing thiazide diuretics, barbiturates, dextromethorphan, methotrimeprazine, narcotics, other sedatives, serotonin reuptake inhibitors, spinal anesthetics, tricyclic antidepressants: unpredictable interaction. Use these agents with caution and in reduced dosage.

Insulin, oral antidiabetic agents: increased risk of hypoglycemia. Use with caution and in reduced dosages.

Drug-herb. *Cacao tree:* potential vasopressor effects. Avoid concomitant use.

Ginseng: may cause headache, tremors, mania. Avoid concomitant use.

Drug-food. *Foods high in tryptophan, tyramine, caffeine:* may precipitate hypertensive crisis. Avoid concomitant use. Watch for adverse effects.

Drug-lifestyle. *Alcohol use:* may precipitate hypertensive crisis. Avoid concomitant use.

EFFECTS ON DIAGNOSTIC TESTS
Drug therapy elevates liver function test results and urinary catecholamine levels and may elevate WBC count.

CONTRAINDICATIONS
Contraindicated in patients with hypersensitivity to drug, heart failure, pheochromocytoma, hypertension, significant renal impairment, cerebrovascular defect, liver disease, and CV disease. Also contraindicated during therapy with other MAO inhibitors (isocarboxazid, tranylcypromine) or within 10 days of such therapy or within 10 days of elective surgery requiring general anesthesia, cocaine use, or local anesthesia containing sympathomimetic vasoconstrictors.

NURSING CONSIDERATIONS
● Use cautiously with antihypertensives containing thiazide diuretics, with spinal anesthetics, and in patients at risk for suicide, diabetes, or seizure disorders.

● Obtain baseline blood pressure, heart rate, CBC, and liver function test results before therapy, and continue to monitor throughout treatment.

● In most patients, discontinue MAO inhibitors 14 days before elective surgery as ordered to avoid drug interactions that may occur during anesthesia.

● Monitor patient closely for suicidal tendencies, and allow only a minimum supply of drug.

● If patient develops symptoms of overdose (severe hypotension, palpitations, or frequent headaches), withhold dose and notify doctor.

Alert: Have phentolamine available to combat severe hypertension.

● Continue precautions 14 days after stopping drug because it has long-lasting effects.

☑ Patient teaching
● Advise patient to consult doctor before taking other prescription or OTC medications. Severe adverse effects can occur if MAO inhibitors are taken with OTC cold, hay-fever, or diet preparations.

● Warn patient about the probability of orthostatic hypotension. Supervise walking. Tell patient to get out of bed slowly, sitting up first for 1 minute.

● Because MAO inhibitors may suppress chest pain in patients with angina, warn such patients to engage in moderate activities and to avoid overexertion.

● Advise patient to avoid the following foods: pickled herring, liver, dry sausage, broad bean pods, sauerkraut, cheese, yogurt, yeast extract, meat extract, and pickled, fermented, or smoked foods.

---

sertraline hydrochloride
Lustral§, Zoloft

Pregnancy Risk Category: B

HOW SUPPLIED
Tablets: 50 mg, 100 mg
Capsules†: 25 mg, 50 mg, 100 mg

ACTION
Unknown, but presumed to be linked to

---

its inhibition of neuronal uptake of serotonin in the CNS.

Route	Onset	Peak	Duration
PO	Unknown	4.5-8.5 hr	Unknown

INDICATIONS & DOSAGE
Depression—
Adults: 50 mg P.O. daily. Dosage adjusted as needed and tolerated; clinical trials involved dosage of 50 to 200 mg daily. Dosage adjustments should be made at intervals of no less than 1 week.
Obsessive-compulsive disorder—
Adults: 50 mg P.O. once daily. If no response, dose may be increased to maximum of 200 mg/day. Dosage adjustments should be made at intervals of no less than 1 week.
Children 6 to 17 years: initially 25 mg P.O. daily in children 6 to 12 years, or 50 mg P.O. daily in children 13 to 17 years. May increase dosage p.r.n. up to 200 mg/day at intervals of no less than 1 week.
Panic disorder—
Adults: initially, 25 mg P.O. daily. After one week, increase dose to 50 mg P.O. daily. If no response, dose may be increased to maximum of 200 mg/day. Dosage adjustments should be made at intervals of no less than 1 week.
Adjust-a-dose: In patients with hepatic disease, lower or less frequent doses should be used.

ADVERSE REACTIONS
CNS: *headache, tremor, dizziness, insomnia, somnolence,* paresthesia, hypoesthesia, *fatigue,* nervousness, anxiety, agitation, hypertonia, twitching, confusion.
CV: palpitations, chest pain, hot flashes.
GI: *dry mouth, nausea, diarrhea, loose stools, dyspepsia,* vomiting, constipation, thirst, flatulence, anorexia, abdominal pain, increased appetite.
GU: *male sexual dysfunction.*
Skin: rash, pruritus.
Other: diaphoresis, myalgia.

INTERACTIONS
Drug-drug. *Benzodiazepines, tolbutamide:* decreased clearance of these drugs. Clinical significance unknown; however, monitor patients for increased drug effects.
Cimetidine: decreased clearance of sertraline. Monitor closely.
MAO inhibitors: may cause serious, sometimes fatal, reactions including myoclonus rigidity, mental status changes, hyperthermia, autonomic nervous system instability, rapid fluctuations of vital signs, delirium, coma, and death. Avoid concomitant use.
Warfarin, other highly protein-bound drugs: may increase plasma levels of sertraline or other highly bound drug. Small (8%) increases in PT or INR have been seen with concomitant use of warfarin. Monitor closely.

EFFECTS ON DIAGNOSTIC TESTS
Minor changes in several laboratory values have occurred. Elevated serum AST and ALT levels have occurred, usually within the first 9 weeks of therapy; values returned to normal after discontinuing drug. Minor increases in serum cholesterol and triglycerides and minor decreases in uric acid have also been seen. Clinical significance is unknown.

CONTRAINDICATIONS
Contraindicated in patients taking MAO inhibitors or within 14 days of discontinuing MAO inhibitor therapy.

NURSING CONSIDERATIONS
• Use cautiously in patients at risk for suicide, and in those with seizure disorder, major affective disorder, or diseases or conditions that affect metabolism or hemodynamic responses.
• Administer sertraline once daily, either in the morning or evening. May be given with or without food.
• Record mood changes. Monitor patient for suicidal tendencies, and allow only a minimum supply of drug.

☑**Patient teaching**
• Advise patient to use caution when performing hazardous tasks that require alertness.
• Tell patient to avoid alcohol and to consult doctor before taking OTC medications.

Reactions may be *common*, uncommon, *life-threatening*, or COMMON AND LIFE-THREATENING.

tranylcypromine sulfate
Parnate

Pregnancy Risk Category: C

HOW SUPPLIED
Tablets: 10 mg

ACTION
Unknown. An MAO inhibitor that probably promotes accumulation of neurotransmitters by inhibiting MAO.

Route	Onset	Peak	Duration
PO	Unknown	1-3.5 hr	≤ 10 days

INDICATIONS & DOSAGE
Depression—
Adults: 10 mg P.O. t.i.d. Increased by 10 mg P.O. daily at 1- to 3-week intervals to maximum of 60 mg daily, if necessary, after 2 weeks of therapy.

ADVERSE REACTIONS
CNS: *dizziness, headache,* anxiety, agitation, paresthesia, drowsiness, weakness, numbness, tremor, jitters, confusion, *vertigo.*
CV: *orthostatic hypotension, tachycardia,* paradoxical hypertension, palpitations.
EENT: blurred vision, tinnitus.
GI: dry mouth, *anorexia,* nausea, diarrhea, constipation, abdominal pain.
GU: impotence, SIADH, urine retention, impaired ejaculation.
Hematologic: anemia, *leukopenia, agranulocytosis, thrombocytopenia.*
Skin: rash.
Other: *edema,* hepatitis, muscle spasm, myoclonic jerks, chills.

INTERACTIONS
Drug-drug. *Amphetamines, antihistamines, antihypertensives, diuretics, ephedrine, levodopa, meperidine, metaraminol, methylphenidate, phenylephrine, phenylpropanolamine, sympathomimetics:* enhanced pressor effects of these drugs. Avoid concomitant use.
Antiparkinsonian drugs, barbiturates, dextromethorphan, methotrimeprazine, narcotics, other sedatives, selective serotonin reuptake inhibitors, spinal anesthetics, tricyclic antidepressants: enhanced adverse CNS effects. Avoid concomitant use. If necessary, use with caution and in reduced dosage.
Buspirone: may elevate blood pressure. Monitor patient closely.
Insulin, oral antidiabetic agents: increased risk of hypoglycemia. Use with caution and in reduced dosages.
Drug-herb. *Cacao tree:* potential vasopressor effects. Avoid concomitant use.
Ginseng: may cause headache, tremors, mania. Monitor for effects.
Drug-food. *Foods high in caffeine, tyramine, tryptophan:* may cause hypertensive crisis. Avoid concomitant use.
Drug-lifestyle. *Alcohol use:* enhanced CNS effects. Avoid concomitant use.

EFFECTS ON DIAGNOSTIC TESTS
Drug therapy elevates liver function tests and urinary catecholamine levels.

CONTRAINDICATIONS
Contraindicated in patients receiving MAO inhibitors or dibenzazepine derivatives; sympathomimetics (including amphetamines); some CNS depressants (including narcotics and alcohol); antihypertensive, diuretic, antihistaminic, sedative or anesthetic drugs; bupropion hydrochloride, buspirone hydrochloride, dextromethorphan, meperidine; cheese or other foods with a high tyramine or tryptophan content; or excessive quantities of caffeine.

Also contraindicated in patients with a confirmed or suspected cerebrovascular defect, hypersensitivity to drug, pheochromocytoma, heart failure, CV disease, hypertension, hepatic disease, significant renal impairment, or history of headache, and in those undergoing elective surgery.

NURSING CONSIDERATIONS
• Use cautiously in patients with renal disease, diabetes, seizure disorder, Parkinson's disease, or hyperthyroidism, and in those at risk for suicide.
• Obtain baseline blood pressure, heart rate, CBC, and liver function test results before beginning therapy, and continue to monitor throughout treatment.

- Know that dosage usually is reduced to maintenance level as soon as possible.
- Do not withdraw drug abruptly.
- In most patients, discontinue MAO inhibitors 14 days before elective surgery as ordered to avoid drug interactions that may occur during anesthesia.
- Monitor patient for suicidal tendencies and allow only a minimum supply of drug.
- If patient develops symptoms of overdose (palpitations, severe hypotension, or frequent headaches), withhold dose and notify doctor.

Alert: Have phentolamine available to combat severe hypertension.

- Continue precautions for 10 days after stopping drug because it has long-lasting effects.

☑ **Patient teaching**
- Warn patient to avoid foods high in tyramine or tryptophan and large amounts of caffeine. Tranylcypromine is the MAO inhibitor most often reported to cause hypertensive crisis with ingestion of tyramine-rich foods, including aged cheese, Chianti wine, beer, avocados, chicken livers, chocolate, bananas, soy sauce, meat tenderizers, salami, and bologna.
- Tell patient to avoid alcohol and to consult doctor before taking other prescription or OTC medications.
- To prevent dizziness resulting from orthostatic hypotension, tell patient to get out of bed slowly, sitting up for 1 minute first.
- Because MAO inhibitors may suppress anginal pain, warn patient to moderate activities and to avoid overexertion.
- Warn patient not to stop drug suddenly.
- Advise patient to avoid the following: cheese, sour cream, pickled herring, anchovies, caviar, liver, canned figs, raisins, bananas, avocados, chocolate, soy sauce, sauerkraut, broad beans, yeast extracts, yogurt, meat extracts, meat prepared with tenderizers.

trazodone hydrochloride
Desyrel, Molipaxin§, Trazon, Trialodine

Pregnancy Risk Category: C

HOW SUPPLIED
Tablets: 50 mg, 100 mg, 150 mg, 300 mg

ACTION
Unknown, although it inhibits serotonin uptake in the brain. Not a tricyclic derivative.

Route	Onset	Peak	Duration
PO	Unknown	1-2 hr	Unknown

INDICATIONS & DOSAGE
Depression—
Adults: initial dosage, 150 mg P.O. daily in divided doses; increased by 50 mg daily q 3 to 4 days, p.r.n. Average dosage ranges from 150 mg to 400 mg daily. Maximum daily dosage is 600 mg for inpatients and 400 mg for outpatients.

ADVERSE REACTIONS
CNS: *drowsiness, dizziness,* nervousness, fatigue, confusion, tremor, weakness, hostility, anger, nightmares, vivid dreams, headache, insomnia.
CV: orthostatic hypotension, tachycardia, hypertension, syncope, shortness of breath.
EENT: blurred vision, tinnitus, nasal congestion.
GI: dry mouth, dysgeusia, constipation, nausea, vomiting, anorexia.
GU: urine retention; priapism, possibly leading to impotence; decreased libido; hematuria.
Hematologic: anemia.
Skin: rash, urticaria.
Other: diaphoresis.

INTERACTIONS
Drug-drug. *Antihypertensives:* increased hypotensive effect of trazodone. Antihypertensive dosage may have to be decreased.
Clonidine, CNS depressants: enhanced CNS depression. Avoid concomitant use.

Reactions may be *common,* uncommon, *life-threatening,* or COMMON AND LIFE-THREATENING.

Digoxin, phenytoin: may increase serum levels of these drugs. Monitor for toxicity.
MAO inhibitors: effects unknown. Use together with extreme caution.
Drug-herb. *St. John's wort:* serotonin syndrome may result. Avoid concomitant use.
Drug-lifestyle. *Alcohol use:* enhanced CNS depression. Avoid concomitant use.

EFFECTS ON DIAGNOSTIC TESTS
Drug may prolong conduction time (elongation of QT and PR intervals, flattened T waves on ECG); it also may elevate liver function tests, and decrease WBC counts.

CONTRAINDICATIONS
Contraindicated in patients with hypersensitivity to drug.

NURSING CONSIDERATIONS
• Use cautiously in patients with cardiac disease, during initial recovery phase of MI, and in patients at risk for suicide.
• Administer after meals or a light snack for optimal absorption and to decrease incidence of dizziness.
• Record mood changes. Monitor patient for suicidal tendencies, and allow only minimum supply of drug.

☑ **Patient teaching**
Alert: Inform male patient that priapism is a potential problem in men taking trazodone and to report its presence immediately; it may require surgical intervention.
• Warn patient to avoid activities that require alertness and good psychomotor coordination until CNS effects of the drug are known. Drowsiness and dizziness usually subside after the first few weeks.
• Teach caregivers how to recognize signs of suicidal tendency or suicidal ideation.

---

trimipramine maleate
Apo-Trimip†, Novo-Tripramine†, Rhotrimine†, Surmontil

Pregnancy Risk Category: C

HOW SUPPLIED
Tablets: 25 mg‡
Capsules: 25 mg, 50 mg, 100 mg

ACTION
Unknown, but a tricyclic antidepressant (TCA) that increases the amount of norepinephrine, serotonin, or both in the CNS by blocking their reuptake by the presynaptic neurons.

Route	Onset	Peak	Duration
PO	Unknown	2 hr	Unknown

INDICATIONS & DOSAGE
Depression—
Adults: 75 to 100 mg P.O. daily in divided doses, increased to 200 to 300 mg daily. Dosages over 300 mg daily not recommended in hospitalized patients; not over 200 mg in outpatients. Total dosage requirement may be given h.s.
Elderly and adolescents: initially, 50 mg/day, gradually increased to 100 mg/day.

ADVERSE REACTIONS
CNS: *drowsiness, dizziness,* paresthesia, ataxia, hallucinations, delusions, anxiety, agitation, insomnia, tremor, weakness, confusion, headache, EEG changes, *seizures,* extrapyramidal reactions.
CV: *orthostatic hypotension, tachycardia,* hypertension, ***arrhythmias, heart block, MI, stroke.***
EENT: *blurred vision,* tinnitus, mydriasis.
GI: *dry mouth, constipation,* nausea, vomiting, anorexia, paralytic ileus.
GU: *urine retention.*
Skin: rash, urticaria, photosensitivity.
Other: *diaphoresis,* ***hypersensitivity reaction.***
After abrupt withdrawal of long-term therapy: nausea, headache, malaise (does not indicate addiction).

INTERACTIONS
Drug-drug. *Barbiturates:* decreased TCA blood levels. Monitor for decreased antidepressant effect.
Cimetidine, fluoxetine, sertraline: may increase serum trimipramine levels. Monitor for increased adverse reactions.
Clonidine, epinephrine, norepinephrine: increased hypertensive effect. Use with caution.
CNS depressants: enhanced CNS depression. Avoid concomitant use.

MAO inhibitors: may cause severe excitation, hyperpyrexia, or seizures, usually with high dosage. Avoid concomitant use.
Drug-lifestyle. *Alcohol use:* enhanced CNS depression. Avoid concomitant use.
Sun exposure: increased risk of photosensitivity reactions. Avoid unprotected or prolonged sun exposure.

EFFECTS ON DIAGNOSTIC TESTS
Drug may prolong conduction time (elongation of QT and PR intervals, flattened T waves of ECG); it also may elevate liver function test levels, decrease WBC counts, and alter serum glucose levels. Trimipramine may alter prothrombin time.

CONTRAINDICATIONS
Contraindicated during acute recovery phase of MI and in patients with hypersensitivity to drug or receiving MAO inhibitor therapy within 14 days.

NURSING CONSIDERATIONS
• Use with extreme caution in patients with CV disease, history of urine retention or angle-closure glaucoma, increased intraocular pressure, hyperthyroidism, impaired hepatic function, or history of seizures and in those receiving thyroid medications, guanethidine, or similar agents.
• Do not withdraw drug abruptly.
Alert: Because hypertensive episodes have occurred during surgery in patients receiving TCAs, be aware that dosage should be gradually discontinued several days before surgery.
• If signs of psychosis occur or increase, expect doctor to reduce dosage. Record mood changes. Monitor patient for suicidal tendencies, and allow only a minimum supply of drug.
• Relieve dry mouth with sugarless hard candy or gum. Saliva substitutes may be necessary.

☑ **Patient teaching**
• Tell patient to take full dose at bedtime to avoid daytime sedation. Warn him about possible morning orthostatic hypotension.
• Tell patient to avoid alcohol and to con-

sult doctor before taking other prescription or OTC medications.
• Warn patient to avoid hazardous activities that require alertness and good psychomotor coordination until CNS effects of the drug are known. Drowsiness and dizziness usually subside after a few weeks.
• Warn patient not to stop drug suddenly.
• To prevent photosensitivity reactions, advise patient to use sunblock, wear protective clothing, and avoid prolonged exposure to strong sunlight.

venlafaxine hydrochloride
Efexor‡, Effexor, Effexor XR

Pregnancy Risk Category: C

HOW SUPPLIED
Capsules (extended-release): 37.5 mg, 75 mg, 150 mg
Tablets: 25 mg, 37.5 mg, 50 mg, 75 mg, 100 mg

ACTION
Blocks reuptake of norepinephrine and serotonin into neurons in the CNS.

Route	Onset	Peak	Duration
PO	Unknown	Unknown	Unknown

INDICATIONS & DOSAGE
Depression—
Adults: initially, 75 mg P.O. daily, in two or three divided doses with food. Dosage increased as tolerated and needed in increments of 75 mg/day at intervals of no less than 4 days. For moderately depressed outpatients, usual maximum dosage is 225 mg/day; in certain severely depressed patients, dosage may be as high as 375 mg/day. For extended-release capsules, 75 mg P.O. daily, in a single dose. For some patients it may be desirable to start at 37.5 mg P.O. daily for 4 to 7 days before increasing to 75 mg daily. Dosage may be increased at increments of 75 mg/day q 4 days to maximum of 225 mg/day.
Adjust-a-dose: For renally impaired patients, reduce total daily dosage by 25%. In patients undergoing hemodialysis, reduce total daily dosage by 50% and with-

hold dose until dialysis is completed. For patients with hepatic impairment, reduce total daily dosage by 50%.

ADVERSE REACTIONS
CNS: *headache, somnolence, dizziness, nervousness, insomnia,* anxiety, tremor, abnormal dreams, paresthesia, agitation.
CV: hypertension.
EENT: blurred vision.
GI: *nausea, constipation,* vomiting, *dry mouth, anorexia,* diarrhea, dyspepsia, flatulence.
GU: *abnormal ejaculation,* impotence, urinary frequency, impaired urination.
Other: *diaphoresis, asthenia,* weight loss, rash, yawning, chills, infection.

INTERACTIONS
Drug-drug. *MAO inhibitors:* may precipitate a syndrome similar to neuroleptic malignant syndrome (myoclonus, hyperthermia, seizures, and death). Avoid concomitant use.
Drug-herb. *Yohimbe:* additive stimulation. Use together cautiously.

EFFECTS ON DIAGNOSTIC TESTS
None reported.

CONTRAINDICATIONS
Contraindicated in patients with hypersensitivity to drug or within 14 days of MAO inhibitor therapy.

NURSING CONSIDERATIONS
• Use cautiously in patients with renal impairment, diseases or conditions that could affect hemodynamic responses or metabolism, and in those with history of mania or seizures.
• Carefully monitor blood pressure. Venlafaxine therapy is associated with sustained, dose-dependent increases in blood pressure. Greatest increases (averaging about 7 mm Hg above baseline) occur in patients taking 375 mg daily.

☑ **Patient teaching**
• Inform patient who has received drug for 6 weeks or more that drug should be gradually discontinued by tapering dosage over a 2-week period as instructed by doctor.

• Warn patient to avoid hazardous activities that require alertness and good psychomotor coordination until CNS effects of drug are known.
• Tell patient to avoid alcohol and to consult doctor before taking other prescription or OTC medications.

32

Antianxiety drugs

alprazolam
buspirone hydrochloride
chlordiazepoxide
chlordiazepoxide hydrochloride
clorazepate dipotassium
diazepam
doxepin hydrochloride
   (See Chapter 31, ANTIDEPRESSANTS.)
hydroxyzine embonate
hydroxyzine hydrochloride
hydroxyzine pamoate
lorazepam
meprobamate
midazolam hydrochloride
oxazepam

COMBINATION PRODUCTS
EQUAGESIC: meprobamate 200 mg and aspirin 325 mg.
LIBRAX: chlordiazepoxide hydrochloride 5 mg and clidinium bromide 2.5 mg.
LIMBITROL DS: chlordiazepoxide 10 mg and amitriptyline hydrochloride 25 mg.

---

alprazolam
Apo-Alpraz†, Kalma‡,
Novo-Alprazol†, Nu-Alpraz†,
Ralozam‡, Xanax

Controlled Substance Schedule IV
Pregnancy Risk Category: D

HOW SUPPLIED
Tablets: 0.25 mg, 0.5 mg, 1 mg, 2 mg
Oral solution: 0.5 mg/5 ml, 1 mg/ml
(concentrate)

ACTION
Unknown. A benzodiazepine that probably potentiates the effects of gamma-aminobutyric acid, an inhibitory neurotransmitter, and depresses the CNS at the limbic and subcortical levels of the brain.

Route	Onset	Peak	Duration
PO	Unknown	1-2 hr	Unknown

INDICATIONS & DOSAGE
Anxiety—
Adults: usual initial dose, 0.25 to 0.5 mg P.O. t.i.d. Maximum dosage is 4 mg daily in divided doses.
Elderly: usual initial dose, 0.25 mg P.O. b.i.d. or t.i.d. Maximum dosage is 4 mg daily in divided doses.
Panic disorders—
Adults: 0.5 mg P.O. t.i.d., increased at intervals of 3 to 4 days in increments of no more than 1 mg. Maximum dosage is 10 mg daily in divided doses.
Adjust-a-dose: In debilitated patients or those with advanced hepatic disease, usual initial dose is 0.25 mg P.O. b.i.d. or t.i.d. Maximum dosage is 4 mg daily in divided doses.

ADVERSE REACTIONS
CNS: *drowsiness, light-headedness,* headache, confusion, tremor, dizziness, syncope, *depression,* insomnia, memory impairment, nervousness.
CV: hypotension, tachycardia.
EENT: blurred vision, nasal congestion.
GI: *dry mouth,* nausea, vomiting, *diarrhea, constipation,* increased salivation.
Skin: dermatitis.
Other: muscle rigidity, weight gain or loss.

INTERACTIONS
Drug-drug. *Cimetidine:* decreased alprazolam clearance with potential for increased adverse reactions. Monitor patient carefully.
CNS depressants: increased CNS depression. Avoid concomitant use.
Digoxin: may increase serum digoxin levels, increasing toxicity. Monitor patient closely.
Tricyclic antidepressants (TCAs): increased plasma levels of TCAs. Monitor for toxicity.
Drug-herb. *Kava:* may cause coma. Avoid concomitant use.
Drug-lifestyle. *Alcohol use:* increased CNS depression. Avoid concomitant use.

Reactions may be *common,* uncommon, *life-threatening,* or COMMON AND LIFE-THREATENING.

Smoking: decreased effectiveness of benzodiazepines. Monitor patient closely.

EFFECTS ON DIAGNOSTIC TESTS
Drug therapy may elevate liver function test results. Minor changes in EEG patterns, usually low-voltage, fast activity, may occur during and after alprazolam therapy.

CONTRAINDICATIONS
Contraindicated in patients with acute angle-closure glaucoma or hypersensitivity to drug or other benzodiazepines.

NURSING CONSIDERATIONS
• Use cautiously in patients with hepatic, renal, or pulmonary disease.
• Know that drug should not be prescribed for daily stress or for long-term use (more than 4 months).
• Know that drug should not be withdrawn abruptly after long-term use; withdrawal symptoms, including seizures, may occur. Abuse or addiction is possible.
• Monitor liver, renal, and hematopoietic function studies periodically in patients receiving repeated or prolonged therapy, as ordered.

☑ **Patient teaching**
• Warn patient to avoid hazardous activities that require alertness and good psychomotor coordination until CNS effects of drug are known.
• Tell patient to avoid alcohol while taking drug.
• Notify patient that smoking may decrease effectiveness of drug.
• Warn patient not to abruptly stop using drug because withdrawal symptoms or seizures may occur.

buspirone hydrochloride
BuSpar

Pregnancy Risk Category: B

HOW SUPPLIED
Tablets: 5 mg, 10 mg, 15 mg

ACTION
Unknown. May inhibit neuronal firing and reduce serotonin turnover in cortical, amygdaloid, and septohippocampal tissue.

Route	Onset	Peak	Duration
PO	Unknown	40-90 min	Unknown

INDICATIONS & DOSAGE
Anxiety disorders; short-term relief of anxiety—
Adults: initially, 5 mg P.O. t.i.d. Dosage increased at 3-day intervals in 5-mg increments. Usual maintenance dosage is 20 to 30 mg daily in divided doses. Do not exceed 60 mg daily.

ADVERSE REACTIONS
CNS: *dizziness, drowsiness,* nervousness, insomnia, headache, light-headedness, fatigue, numbness.
EENT: blurred vision.
GI: dry mouth, nausea, diarrhea, abdominal distress.

INTERACTIONS
Drug-drug. *CNS depressants:* increased CNS depression. Avoid concomitant use.
MAO inhibitors: may elevate blood pressure. Avoid concomitant use.
Drug-lifestyle. *Alcohol use:* increased CNS depression. Avoid concomitant use.

EFFECTS ON DIAGNOSTIC TESTS
None reported.

CONTRAINDICATIONS
Contraindicated in patients hypersensitive to drug or within 14 days of therapy with an MAO inhibitor.

NURSING CONSIDERATIONS
• Use cautiously in patients with hepatic or renal failure.
• Monitor patient closely for adverse CNS reactions. Buspirone is less sedating than other antianxiety agents. However, CNS effects in individual patients may be unpredictable.
Alert: Before initiating buspirone therapy in patient already being treated with benzodiazepines, warn him against stopping the benzodiazepine abruptly; withdrawal reaction may occur.
• Be aware that drug has shown no potential for abuse and has not been classified

---

*Liquid contains alcohol.   **May contain tartrazine.   †Canada   ‡Australia   §U.K.   ◇OTC

as a controlled substance. However, it is not recommended for relief of daily stress.

☑ Patient teaching
• Warn patient to avoid hazardous activities that require alertness and good psychomotor coordination until CNS effects of drug are known.
• Notify patient that drug's effects may not be seen for several weeks.
• Warn patients receiving benzodiazepine therapy not to abruptly withdraw the benzodiazepine due to risk of withdrawal symptoms.
• Tell patient to avoid alcohol during therapy.

chlordiazepoxide
Libritabs

chlordiazepoxide hydrochloride
Apo-Chlordiazepoxide†, Librium, Novo-Poxide†, Solium†

Controlled Substance Schedule IV
Pregnancy Risk Category: NR

HOW SUPPLIED
chlordiazepoxide
Tablets: 5 mg, 10 mg, 25 mg
chlordiazepoxide hydrochloride
Capsules: 5 mg, 10 mg, 25 mg
Powder for injection: 100-mg ampule

ACTION
Unknown. A benzodiazepine that probably potentiates the effects of gamma-aminobutyric acid, an inhibitory neurotransmitter, and depresses the CNS at the limbic and subcortical levels of the brain. Suppresses spread of seizure activity produced by epileptogenic foci in the cortex, thalamus, and limbic structures.

Route	Onset	Peak	Duration
PO	Unknown	0.5-4 hr	Unknown
IV	1-5 min	Unknown	15-60 min
IM	Unknown	Unknown	Unknown

INDICATIONS & DOSAGE
Mild to moderate anxiety—
Adults: 5 to 10 mg P.O. t.i.d. or q.i.d.

Children over 6 years: 5 mg P.O. b.i.d. to q.i.d. Maximum dosage is 10 mg P.O. b.i.d. or t.i.d.
Severe anxiety—
Adults: 20 to 25 mg P.O. t.i.d. or q.i.d.
Elderly: 5 mg P.O. b.i.d. to q.i.d.
Adjust-a-dose: In debilitated patients, 5 mg P.O. b.i.d. to q.i.d.
Withdrawal symptoms of acute alcoholism—
Adults: 50 to 100 mg P.O., I.M., or I.V. Repeated in 2 to 4 hours, p.r.n. Maximum dosage is 300 mg daily.
Preoperative apprehension and anxiety—
Adults: 5 to 10 mg P.O. t.i.d. or q.i.d. on day preceding surgery; or 50 to 100 mg I.M. 1 hour before surgery.
    Note: Parenteral form not recommended in children under 12 years.

ADVERSE REACTIONS
CNS: *drowsiness, lethargy,* ataxia, confusion, extrapyramidal symptoms.
GI: nausea, constipation.
GU: increased or decreased libido, menstrual irregularities.
Hematologic: *agranulocytosis.*
Hepatic: jaundice.
Skin: *swelling, pain at injection site,* skin eruptions, edema.

INTERACTIONS
Drug-drug. *Cimetidine:* decreased chlordiazepoxide clearance, with potential for increased adverse reactions. Monitor patient carefully.
CNS depressants: increased CNS depression. Avoid concomitant use.
Digoxin: increased serum digoxin levels and risk of toxicity. Monitor patient closely.
Drug-lifestyle. *Alcohol use:* increased CNS depression. Avoid concomitant use.
Smoking: decreased effectiveness of benzodiazepines. Monitor patient closely.

EFFECTS ON DIAGNOSTIC TESTS
Drug therapy may elevate results of liver function tests. Minor changes in EEG patterns, usually low-voltage, fast activity, may occur during and after therapy. Drug may cause a false-positive pregnancy test, depending on method used. It may also alter urinary 17-ketosteroids (Zimmerman

---

Reactions may be *common,* uncommon, **life-threatening**, or COMMON AND LIFE-THREATENING.

reaction), urine alkaloid determination (Frings thin layer chromatography method), and urinary glucose determinations (with Chemstrip uG and Diastix).

CONTRAINDICATIONS
Contraindicated in patients hypersensitive to drug.

NURSING CONSIDERATIONS
• Use cautiously in patients with mental depression, porphyria, or hepatic or renal disease.
• Know that drug should be avoided during pregnancy, especially during first trimester.
• Know that drug should not be prescribed regularly for daily stress.
• Injectable form (as hydrochloride) comes in two types of ampules—as diluent and as powdered drug. Read directions carefully.
• Keep powder away from light and refrigerate; mix just before use and discard remainder.
• For I.M. use, add 2 ml of diluent to powder and agitate gently until clear. Use immediately. I.M. form may be absorbed erratically.
• Monitor liver, renal, and hematopoietic function studies periodically in patients receiving repeated or prolonged therapy, as ordered.
• Possibility of abuse and addiction exists. Drug should not be withdrawn abruptly after long-term administration; withdrawal symptoms may occur.
Alert: Recommended for I.M. use only, but may be given I.V.

I.V. administration
• Use 5 ml of 0.9% NaCl solution or sterile water for injection as diluent; do not give packaged diluent I.V. Administer over 1 minute.
• When giving drug I.V., be sure equipment and personnel needed for emergency airway management are available. Monitor respirations every 5 to 15 minutes and before each repeated I.V. dose.

✓Patient teaching
• Warn patient to avoid hazardous activities that require alertness and good psy-

chomotor coordination until CNS effects of drug are known.
• Tell patient to avoid alcohol while taking drug.
• Notify patient that smoking may decrease the effectiveness of drug.
• Warn patient not to abruptly stop using the drug, because withdrawal symptoms may occur.
• Caution patient to avoid use during pregnancy.

clorazepate dipotassium
Apo-Clorazepate†, Gen-XENE, Novo-Clopate†, Tranxene, Tranxene-SD, Tranxene T-TAB

Controlled Substance Schedule IV
Pregnancy Risk Category: D

HOW SUPPLIED
Tablets: 3.75 mg, 7.5 mg, 11.25 mg, 15 mg, 22.5 mg
Capsules: 3.75 mg, 7.5 mg, 15 mg

ACTION
Unknown. A benzodiazepine that may exert its anxiolytic effects by facilitating the action of the inhibitory neurotransmitter gamma-aminobutyric acid. Depresses the CNS at the limbic and subcortical levels of the brain and suppresses the spread of seizure activity produced by epileptogenic foci in the cortex, thalamus, and limbic structures.

Route	Onset	Peak	Duration
PO	Unknown	0.5-2 hr	Unknown

INDICATIONS & DOSAGE
Acute alcohol withdrawal—
Adults: day 1—30 mg P.O. initially, followed by 30 to 60 mg P.O. in divided doses; day 2—45 to 90 mg P.O. in divided doses; day 3—22.5 to 45 mg P.O. in divided doses; day 4—15 to 30 mg P.O. in divided doses; then gradually reduce dosage to 7.5 to 15 mg daily. Maximum recommended daily dosage is 90 mg.
Anxiety—
Adults: 15 to 60 mg P.O. daily.
Elderly: initially, 7.5 to 15 mg daily in divided doses or as a single dose h.s.

Adjust-a-dose: In debilitated patients, initially, 7.5 to 15 mg daily in divided doses or as a single dose h.s.

Adjunct in partial seizure disorder—
Adults and children over 12 years:
Maximum recommended initial dosage is 7.5 mg P.O. t.i.d. Dosage increases should not exceed 7.5 mg weekly. Maximum dosage should not exceed 90 mg daily.
Children 9 to 12 years: Maximum recommended initial dosage is 7.5 mg P.O. b.i.d. Dosage increases should not exceed 7.5 mg weekly. Maximum dosage should not exceed 60 mg daily.

ADVERSE REACTIONS
CNS: *drowsiness,* dizziness, nervousness, confusion, headache, insomnia, depression, irritability, tremor.
CV: hypotension.
EENT: blurred vision, diplopia.
GI: nausea, vomiting, abdominal discomfort, dry mouth.
GU: urine retention, incontinence.
Skin: rash.

INTERACTIONS
Drug-drug. *Cimetidine:* decreased clorazepate clearance, with increased potential for adverse reactions. Monitor patient carefully.
CNS depressants: increased CNS depression. Avoid concomitant use.
Digoxin: may increase serum digoxin levels and risk of toxicity. Monitor patient closely.
Drug-lifestyle. *Alcohol use:* increased CNS depression. Avoid concomitant use.
Smoking: decreased effectiveness of benzodiazepines. Monitor patient closely.

EFFECTS ON DIAGNOSTIC TESTS
Drug may elevate liver function test results. Minor changes in EEG patterns, usually low-voltage, fast activity, may occur during and after drug therapy.

CONTRAINDICATIONS
Contraindicated in patients with acute angle-closure glaucoma or hypersensitivity to drug.

NURSING CONSIDERATIONS
• Know that drug should be avoided during pregnancy, especially the first trimester.
• Use cautiously in patients with suicidal tendencies, renal or hepatic impairment, pulmonary disease, or history of drug abuse.
• Monitor liver, renal, and hematopoietic function studies periodically in patients receiving repeated or prolonged therapy as ordered.
• Know that possibility of abuse and addiction exists. Do not withdraw drug abruptly after prolonged use because withdrawal symptoms may occur.
• Know that drug is not recommended for use in children under 9 years.

☑ **Patient teaching**
• Warn patient to avoid activities that require alertness and good psychomotor coordination until CNS effects of drug are known.
• Tell patient to avoid alcohol while taking drug.
• Notify patient that smoking may decrease effectiveness of drug.
• Warn patient not to abruptly stop using drug because withdrawal symptoms may occur.
• Caution patient to avoid use during pregnancy.
• Inform patient that sugarless chewing gum or hard candy can relieve dry mouth.

diazepam
Antenex‡, Apo-Diazepam†, Diazemuls†‡, Diazepam Intensol, Ducene‡, Novo-Dipam†, PMS-Diazepam†, Valium, Valrelease, Vivol†, Zetran

Controlled Substance Schedule IV
Pregnancy Risk Category: D

HOW SUPPLIED
Tablets: 2 mg, 5 mg, 10 mg
Capsules (extended-release): 15 mg
Oral solution: 5 mg/5 ml, 5 mg/ml
Injection: 5 mg/ml
Sterile emulsion for injection: 5 mg/ml

ACTION
Unknown. A benzodiazepine that proba-

bly potentiates the effects of gamma-aminobutyric acid, an inhibitory neurotransmitter, and depresses the CNS at the limbic and subcortical levels of the brain. Suppresses spread of seizure activity produced by epileptogenic foci in the cortex, thalamus, and limbic structures.

Route	Onset	Peak	Duration
PO	0.5 hr	2 hr	3-8 hr
IV	1-5 min	Immediate	15-60 min
IM	Unknown	2 hr	Unknown

INDICATIONS & DOSAGE

Anxiety—

Adults: depending on severity, 2 to 10 mg P.O. b.i.d. to q.i.d. or 15 to 30 mg extended-release capsules P.O. once daily. Alternatively, 2 to 10 mg I.M. or I.V. q 3 to 4 hours, p.r.n.

Children 6 months and older: 1 to 2.5 mg P.O. t.i.d. or q.i.d., increased gradually, as needed and tolerated.

Elderly: initially, 2 to 2.5 mg once or twice daily; increased gradually.

Acute alcohol withdrawal—

Adults: 10 mg P.O. t.i.d. or q.i.d. first 24 hours, reduced to 5 mg P.O. t.i.d. or q.i.d., p.r.n. Alternatively, initially, 10 mg I.M. or I.V., then 5 to 10 mg I.M. or I.V. q 3 to 4 hours, p.r.n.

Before endoscopic procedures—

Adults: I.V. dose titrated to desired sedative response (up to 20 mg). Alternatively, 5 to 10 mg I.M. 30 minutes before procedure.

Muscle spasm—

Adults: 2 to 10 mg P.O. b.i.d. to q.i.d. or 15 to 30 mg extended-release capsules once daily. Alternatively, 5 to 10 mg I.M. or I.V. initially, then 5 to 10 mg I.M. or I.V. q 3 to 4 hours, p.r.n. For tetanus, larger doses may be required.

Children over 30 days to 5 years: 1 to 2 mg I.M. or I.V. slowly, repeated q 3 to 4 hours, p.r.n.

Children 5 years and older: 5 to 10 mg I.M. or I.V. q 3 to 4 hours, p.r.n.

Preoperative sedation—

Adults: 10 mg I.M. (preferred) or I.V. before surgery.

Cardioversion—

Adults: 5 to 15 mg I.V. within 5 to 10 minutes before procedure.

Adjunct in seizure disorders—

Adults: 2 to 10 mg P.O. b.i.d. to q.i.d.

Children 6 months and older: 1 to 2.5 mg P.O. t.i.d. or q.i.d. initially; increased as needed and tolerated.

Status epilepticus and severe recurrent seizures—

Adults: 5 to 10 mg I.V. (preferred) or I.M. initially. Repeated q 10 to 15 minutes, p.r.n., up to maximum dose of 30 mg. Repeated q 2 to 4 hours, if necessary.

Children over 30 days to 5 years: 0.2 to 0.5 mg I.V. slowly q 2 to 5 minutes up to maximum of 5 mg. Repeated q 2 to 4 hours, if necessary.

Children 5 years and older: 1 mg I.V. q 2 to 5 minutes up to maximum of 10 mg. Repeated q 2 to 4 hours, if necessary.

ADVERSE REACTIONS

CNS: *drowsiness,* dysarthria, slurred speech, tremor, transient amnesia, fatigue, ataxia, headache, insomnia, paradoxical anxiety, hallucinations.

CV: hypotension, *CV collapse, bradycardia.*

EENT: diplopia, blurred vision, nystagmus.

GI: nausea, constipation.

GU: incontinence, urine retention, altered libido.

Hematologic: *neutropenia.*

Respiratory: *respiratory depression.*

Skin: rash.

Other: physical or psychological dependence, *acute withdrawal syndrome* (after sudden discontinuation in physically dependent persons), jaundice; *pain, phlebitis* (at injection site).

INTERACTIONS

Drug-drug. *Cimetidine:* decreased clearance of diazepam, with increased potential for adverse effects. Monitor patient carefully.

CNS depressants: increased CNS depression. Avoid concomitant use.

Digoxin: may increase serum digoxin levels and risk of toxicity. Monitor patient closely.

Phenobarbital: increased effects of both drugs. Use together cautiously.

---

*Liquid contains alcohol. **May contain tartrazine. †Canada ‡Australia §U.K. ◇OTC

Drug-lifestyle. *Alcohol use:* increased CNS depression. Avoid concomitant use. *Smoking:* decreased effectiveness of benzodiazepines. Monitor patient closely.

EFFECTS ON DIAGNOSTIC TESTS
Drug may elevate liver function test results. Minor changes in EEG patterns, usually low-voltage, fast activity, may occur during and after drug therapy.

CONTRAINDICATIONS
Contraindicated in patients with hypersensitivity to drug or soy protein; in patients experiencing shock, coma, or acute alcohol intoxication (parenteral form); and in children under 6 months (oral form).

NURSING CONSIDERATIONS
• Know that drug should be avoided during pregnancy, especially the first trimester.
• Use cautiously in patients with liver or renal impairment, depression, or chronic open-angle glaucoma; and in elderly and debilitated patients.
• Do not mix injectable diazepam with other drugs; also, do not store parenteral solution in plastic syringes.
• When oral concentrate solution is used, dilute the dose just before administering.
• Parenteral emulsion—a stabilized oil-in-water emulsion—should appear milky white and uniform. Avoid mixing with any other drugs or solutions, and avoid infusion sets or containers made from polyvinyl chloride. If dilution is necessary, drug may be mixed with I.V. fat emulsion. Use admixture within 6 hours.
• Monitor periodic liver, renal, and hematopoietic function studies in patients receiving repeated or prolonged therapy, as ordered.
• Possibility of abuse and addiction exists. Do not withdraw drug abruptly after long-term use; withdrawal symptoms may occur.

◖ I.V. administration
• I.V. route is the most reliable parenteral route; I.M. administration is not recommended because absorption is variable and injection is painful.

• Give I.V. at rate not exceeding 5 mg/minute. When injecting, administer directly into the vein. If this is impossible, inject slowly through infusion tubing as near to the vein insertion site as possible. Watch daily for phlebitis at injection site.
• Avoid extravasation. Do not inject into small veins.
Alert: Monitor respirations every 5 to 15 minutes and before each repeated I.V. dose. Have emergency resuscitation equipment and oxygen at bedside.

☑ Patient teaching
• Warn patient to avoid activities that require alertness and good psychomotor coordination until CNS effects of drug are known.
• Tell patient to avoid alcohol while taking drug.
• Notify patient that smoking may decrease effectiveness of drug.
• Warn patient not to abruptly stop using drug because withdrawal symptoms may occur.
• Caution patient to avoid use during pregnancy.

---

hydroxyzine embonate‡
Atarax

hydroxyzine hydrochloride
Anxanil, Apo-Hydroxyzine†, Atarax*, Hydroxacen, Hyzine-50, Multipax†, Novo-Hydroxyzin†, Quiess, Ucerax§, Vistacon-50, Vistaject-25, Vistaject-50, Vistaril, Vistazine 50

hydroxyzine pamoate
Vistaril

Pregnancy Risk Category: NR

HOW SUPPLIED
hydroxyzine embonate‡
Capsules: 25 mg, 50 mg
hydroxyzine hydrochloride
Tablets: 10 mg, 25 mg, 50 mg, 100 mg
Capsules: 10 mg†‡, 25 mg†‡, 50 mg†‡
Syrup: 10 mg/5 ml
Injection: 25 mg/ml, 50 mg/ml

---

hydroxyzine pamoate
Capsules: 25 mg, 50 mg, 100 mg
Oral suspension: 25 mg/5 ml

ACTION
Unknown. A piperazine antihistamine whose action may be due to a suppression of activity in certain key regions of the subcortical area of the CNS.

Route	Onset	Peak	Duration
PO	15-30 min	2 hr	4-6 hr
IM	Unknown	Unknown	4-6 hr

INDICATIONS & DOSAGE
Anxiety—
Adults: 50 to 100 mg P.O. q.i.d.
Children under 6 years: 50 mg P.O. daily in divided doses.
Children 6 years and older: 50 to 100 mg P.O. daily in divided doses.
Preoperative and postoperative adjunctive therapy—
Adults: 25 to 100 mg I.M. q 4 to 6 hours.
Children: 1.1 mg/kg I.M. q 4 to 6 hours.
Pruritus due to allergies—
Adults: 25 mg P.O. t.i.d. or q.i.d.
Children under 6 years: 50 mg P.O. daily in divided doses.
Children 6 years and older: 50 to 100 mg P.O. daily in divided doses.
Psychiatric and emotional emergencies, including acute alcoholism—
Adults: 50 to 100 mg I.M. q 4 to 6 hours, p.r.n.
Nausea and vomiting (excluding nausea and vomiting of pregnancy)—
Adults: 25 to 100 mg I.M.
Children: 1.1 mg/kg I.M.
Antepartum and postpartum adjunctive therapy—
Adults: 25 to 100 mg I.M.

ADVERSE REACTIONS
CNS: *drowsiness,* involuntary motor activity.
GI: *dry mouth.*
Other: marked discomfort at I.M. injection site, ***hypersensitivity reactions*** (wheezing, dyspnea, chest tightness).

INTERACTIONS
Drug-drug. *CNS depressants:* increased CNS depression. Avoid concomitant use.

Drug-lifestyle. *Alcohol use:* increased CNS depression. Avoid concomitant use.

EFFECTS ON DIAGNOSTIC TESTS
Drug therapy causes falsely elevated urinary 17-hydroxycorticosteroid levels. It also may cause false-negative skin allergen tests by attenuating or inhibiting the cutaneous response to histamine.

CONTRAINDICATIONS
Contraindicated in patients hypersensitive to drug, during early pregnancy, and in breast-feeding patients.

NURSING CONSIDERATIONS
● Parenteral form (hydroxyzine hydrochloride) for I.M. use only; never administer I.V. or S.C. The Z-track injection method is preferred.
● Aspirate I.M. injection carefully to prevent inadvertent intravascular injection. Inject deeply into a large muscle mass.
● If patient is taking other CNS drugs, observe for oversedation.

✅ Patient teaching
● Warn patient to avoid hazardous activities that require alertness and good psychomotor coordination until CNS effects of drug are known.
● Tell patient to avoid alcohol while taking drug.
● Advise patient to use sugarless hard candy or gum to relieve dry mouth.
● Warn patient to avoid use of drug during pregnancy and breast feeding.

---

lorazepam
Apo-Lorazepam†, Ativan, Lorazepam Intensol, Novo-Lorazem†, Nu-Loraz†

Controlled Substance Schedule IV
Pregnancy Risk Category: D

HOW SUPPLIED
Tablets: 0.5 mg, 1 mg, 2 mg
Tablets (S.L.): 0.5 mg†, 1 mg†, 2 mg
Oral solution (concentrated): 2 mg/ml
Injection: 2 mg/ml, 4 mg/ml

ACTION
Unknown. A benzodiazepine that probably potentiates the effects of gamma-aminobutyric acid, an inhibitory neurotransmitter, and depresses the CNS at the limbic and subcortical levels of the brain.

Route	Onset	Peak	Duration
PO	1 hr	2 hr	12-24 hr
IV	5 min	1-1.5 hr	6-8 hr
IM	15-30 min	1-1.5 hr	6-8 hr

INDICATIONS & DOSAGE
Anxiety—
Adults: 2 to 6 mg P.O. daily in divided doses. Maximum dosage is 10 mg daily.
Elderly: initially, 1 to 2 mg daily.
Insomnia due to anxiety—
Adults: 2 to 4 mg P.O. h.s.
Preoperative sedation—
Adults: 0.05 mg/kg I.M. 2 hours before procedure. Total dosage should not exceed 4 mg. Alternatively, 2 mg I.V. total or 0.044 mg/kg I.V., whichever is smaller. Larger doses up to 0.05 mg/kg I.V., up to total of 4 mg, may be required.

ADVERSE REACTIONS
CNS: *drowsiness,* amnesia, insomnia, agitation, *sedation,* dizziness, weakness, unsteadiness, disorientation, depression, headache.
CV: hypotension.
EENT: visual disturbances.
GI: abdominal discomfort, nausea, change in appetite.
Other: *acute withdrawal syndrome* (following sudden discontinuation in physically dependent persons).

INTERACTIONS
Drug-drug. *CNS depressants:* increased CNS depression. Avoid concomitant use.
Digoxin: may increase serum digoxin levels and risk of toxicity. Monitor patient closely.
Drug-lifestyle. *Alcohol use:* increased CNS depression. Avoid concomitant use.
Smoking: decreased effectiveness of benzodiazepines. Monitor patient closely.

EFFECTS ON DIAGNOSTIC TESTS
Lorazepam therapy may increase the results of liver function tests.

CONTRAINDICATIONS
Contraindicated in patients with acute angle-closure glaucoma or hypersensitivity to drug, other benzodiazepines, or its vehicle (used in parenteral dosage form).

NURSING CONSIDERATIONS
• Know that drug should be avoided during pregnancy, especially the first trimester.
• Use cautiously in patients with pulmonary, renal, or hepatic impairment. Also use cautiously in elderly, acutely ill, or debilitated patients.
• For I.M. administration, inject deeply into a muscle mass. Don't dilute.
• Refrigerate parenteral form to prolong shelf life.
• Monitor liver, renal, and hematopoietic function studies periodically in patients receiving repeated or prolonged therapy, as ordered.
• Know that possibility of abuse and addiction exists. Do not withdraw drug abruptly after long-term use because withdrawal symptoms may occur.

I.V. administration
• Give slowly, at rate not exceeding 2 mg/minute. Dilute with an equal volume of sterile water for injection, 0.9% NaCl for injection, or dextrose 5% injection.
Alert: Monitor respirations every 5 to 15 minutes and before each repeated I.V. dose. Have emergency resuscitation equipment and oxygen available.

☑ Patient teaching
• Know that, as a premedication before surgery, lorazepam provides substantial preoperative amnesia. Patient teaching requires extra care to ensure adequate recall. Provide written materials or inform a family member, if possible.
• Warn patient to avoid hazardous activities that require alertness or good psychomotor coordination until CNS effects of drug are known.
• Tell patient to avoid alcohol while taking drug.
• Notify patient that smoking may decrease effectiveness of drug.
• Warn patient not to abruptly stop using

Reactions may be *common,* uncommon, *life-threatening,* or COMMON AND LIFE-THREATENING.

drug because withdrawal symptoms may occur.
● Caution patient to avoid use during pregnancy.

---

meprobamate
Apo-Meprobamate†, Equanil**, Meprospan 200, Meprospan-400, Miltown-200, Miltown-400, Miltown-600, Neuramate, Probate, Trancot

Controlled Substance Schedule IV
Pregnancy Risk Category: D

HOW SUPPLIED
Tablets: 200 mg, 400 mg, 600 mg
Capsules (sustained-release): 200 mg, 400 mg

ACTION
Unknown. It appears to act at multiple sites in the CNS.

Route	Onset	Peak	Duration
PO	Unknown	Unknown	Unknown

INDICATIONS & DOSAGE
Anxiety—
Adults: 1.2 to 1.6 g P.O. daily in three or four equally divided doses. Maximum dosage is 2.4 g daily. Alternatively, 400 to 800 mg sustained-release capsule P.O. b.i.d.
Children 6 to 12 years: 200 to 600 mg P.O. in two or three divided doses. Or, 200 mg sustained-release capsule P.O. b.i.d. Not recommended for children under 6 years.

ADVERSE REACTIONS
CNS: *drowsiness,* ataxia, dizziness, slurred speech, headache, vertigo, *seizures.*
CV: palpitations, tachycardia, hypotension, *arrhythmias,* syncope.
GI: nausea, vomiting, diarrhea.
Hematologic: *aplastic anemia, thrombocytopenia, agranulocytosis.*
Skin: pruritus, urticaria, erythematous maculopapular rash, *hypersensitivity reactions.*
Alert: After abrupt withdrawal of long-term therapy, severe generalized tonic-clonic seizures may occur.

INTERACTIONS
Drug-drug. *CNS depressants:* increased CNS depression. Avoid concomitant use.
Drug-lifestyle. *Alcohol use:* increased CNS depression. Avoid concomitant use.

EFFECTS ON DIAGNOSTIC TESTS
Drug therapy may falsely elevate urinary 17-ketosteroids, 17-ketogenic steroids (as determined by the Zimmerman reaction), and 17-hydroxycorticosteroid levels (as determined by the Glenn-Nelson technique).

CONTRAINDICATIONS
Contraindicated in patients with porphyria or hypersensitive to drug or related compounds (such as carisoprodol, mebutamate, tybamate, and carbromal).

NURSING CONSIDERATIONS
● Know that drug should be avoided during pregnancy, especially the first trimester.
● Use cautiously in patients with impaired hepatic or renal function, seizure disorders, or suicidal tendencies.
● Know that Miltown-600 is not recommended for use in children.
● Give drug with meals to reduce GI distress.
● Know that possibility of abuse and addiction exists with long-term use. Withdraw drug gradually over 2 weeks to avoid withdrawal symptoms.
● Periodically monitor CBC and renal and liver function tests in patients receiving high doses, as ordered.

☑ Patient teaching
● Advise patient to take drug with meals and not to crush or chew sustained-release capsules but to swallow them whole.
● Warn patient to avoid hazardous activities that require alertness and good psychomotor coordination until CNS effects of drug are known.
● Tell patient to avoid alcohol while taking drug.
● Advise patient to report unusual bruising or bleeding, fever, or sore throat.

These symptoms may indicate serious hematologic toxicity.
• Warn patient not to abruptly stop using drug because withdrawal symptoms may occur.
• Caution patient to avoid use during pregnancy.

---

midazolam hydrochloride
Hypnovel‡, Versed

Controlled Substance Schedule IV
Pregnancy Risk Category: D

HOW SUPPLIED
Injection: 1 mg/ml, 5 mg/ml

ACTION
Unknown. Thought to depress CNS at the limbic and subcortical levels of the brain by potentiating the effects of gamma-aminobutyric acid.

Route	Onset	Peak	Duration
IV	1.5-5 min	Rapid	2-6 hr
IM	15 min	15-60 min	2-6 hr

INDICATIONS & DOSAGE
Preoperative sedation (to induce sleepiness or drowsiness and relieve apprehension)—
Adults: 0.07 mg to 0.08 mg/kg I.M. approximately 1 hour before surgery.
Conscious sedation before short diagnostic or endoscopic procedures—
Adults under 60 years: initially, small dose not to exceed 2.5 mg I.V. administered slowly; repeated in 2 minutes, if needed, in small increments of initial dose over at least 2 minutes to achieve desired effect. Total dose of up to 5 mg may be used. For maintenance, additional doses to maintain desired level of sedation may be given by slow titration in increments of 25% of dose used to first reach the sedative endpoint.
Elderly: 1.5 mg or less over at least 2 minutes. If additional titration is needed, give at rate not exceeding 1 mg over 2 minutes. Total doses exceeding 3.5 mg are not usually necessary.
To induce sleepiness and amnesia and to relieve apprehension before anesthesia or

before or during procedures in pediatric patients—
I.M.—
Children: 0.1 to 0.15 mg/kg I.M. Doses up to 0.5 mg/kg can be used for more anxious patients.
I.V.—
Children 6 months to 5 years: 0.05 to 0.1 mg/kg I.V. over 2 to 3 minutes. Additional doses may be given in small increments after 2 to 3 minutes. A total dose of up to 0.6 mg/kg, not to exceed 6 mg, may be used.
Children 6 to 12 years: 0.025 to 0.05 mg/kg I.V. over 2 to 3 minutes. Additional doses may be given in small increments after 2 to 3 minutes. A total dose up to 0.4 mg/kg, not to exceed 10 mg, may be used.
Children 12 to 16 years: dose as adults, with total dose not to exceed 10 mg.
Adjust-a-dose: In obese children, base dose on ideal body weight; high risk or debilitated children and children receiving other sedatives require lower doses.
Induction of general anesthesia—
Adults over 55 years: 0.3 mg/kg I.V. over 20 to 30 seconds if patient has not received premedication, or 0.2 mg/kg I.V. over 20 to 30 seconds if patient has received sedative or narcotic premedication. Additional increments of 25% of initial dose may be needed to complete induction.
Adults under 55 years: 0.3 to 0.35 mg/kg I.V. over 20 to 30 seconds if patient has not received premedication, or 0.25 mg/kg I.V. over 20 to 30 seconds if patient has received sedative or narcotic premedication. Additional increments of 25% of initial dose may be needed to complete induction.
Adjust-a-dose: In debilitated patients, initially, 0.2 to 0.25 mg/kg. As little as 0.15 mg/kg may be needed.
Continuous infusion for sedation of intubated patients in the critical care setting—
Adults: initially, 0.01 to 0.05 mg/kg may be given I.V. over several minutes, repeated at 10 to 15 minute intervals until adequate sedation is achieved. For maintenance of sedation, usual initial infusion rate is 0.02 to 0.10 mg/kg/hour. Higher

---

loading dose or infusion rates may be required in some patients. Use the lowest effective rate.

Children: initially, 0.05 to 0.2 mg/kg may be given I.V. over at least 2 to 3 minutes, followed by continuous infusion at rate of 0.06 to 0.12 mg/kg/hour. Increase or decrease infusion to maintain desired effect.

Neonates under 32 weeks: initially, 0.03 mg/kg/hour. Adjust rate p.r.n., using lowest possible rate.

Neonates over 32 weeks: initially, 0.06 mg/kg/hour. Adjust rate p.r.n., using lowest possible rate.

ADVERSE REACTIONS

CNS: headache, oversedation, drowsiness, amnesia, involuntary movements, nystagmus, paradoxical behavior or excitement.

CV: variations in blood pressure and pulse rate.

GI: *nausea,* vomiting, *hiccups.*

Respiratory: *decreased respiratory rate,* APNEA.

Other: *pain at injection site.*

INTERACTIONS

Drug-drug. *CNS depressants:* may increase the risk of apnea. Avoid concomitant use. Prepare to adjust dosage of midazolam if used with opiates or other CNS depressants.

Erythromycin: may alter the metabolism of midazolam. Use with caution.

Oral contraceptives: prolonged half-life of midazolam. Use with caution.

Theophylline: sedative effects of midazolam may be antagonized by theophylline. Use with caution.

Drug-lifestyle. *Alcohol use:* may increase the risk of apnea. Avoid concomitant use.

EFFECTS ON DIAGNOSTIC TESTS

None reported.

CONTRAINDICATIONS

Contraindicated in patients with acute angle-closure glaucoma, shock, coma, acute alcohol intoxication or hypersensitivity to drug.

NURSING CONSIDERATIONS

● Use cautiously in patients with uncompensated acute illness and in elderly or debilitated patients.

Alert: Before administering, have oxygen and resuscitation equipment available in case of severe respiratory depression. Excessive dosage or rapid infusion has been associated with respiratory arrest.

● May be mixed in the same syringe with morphine sulfate, meperidine, atropine sulfate, or scopolamine.

● When injecting I.M., give deep into a large muscle mass.

● Monitor blood pressure, heart rate and rhythm, respirations, airway integrity, and arterial oxygen saturation during procedure.

I.V. administration

● Administer slowly over at least 2 minutes, and wait at least 2 minutes when titrating doses to effect. When mixing infusion, use 5 mg/ml vial, dilute to a concentration of 0.5 mg/ml with D_5W or 0.9% NaCl.

● When administering I.V., take care to avoid extravasation.

Patient teaching

● Because drug's beneficial amnesic effect diminishes patient's recall of perioperative events, provide written information, family member instruction, and follow-up contact to ensure that patient has adequate information.

● Warn patient to avoid hazardous activities that require alertness or good psychomotor coordination until CNS effects of drug are known.

● Tell patient to avoid alcohol while taking drug.

---

oxazepam

Alepam‡, Apo-Oxazepam†, Murelax‡, Novo-Oxapam†, Oxpam†, Serax**, Serepax‡, Zapex†

Controlled Substance Schedule IV
Pregnancy Risk Category: D

HOW SUPPLIED

Tablets, capsules: 10 mg, 15 mg, 30 mg

ACTION
Unknown. Believed to stimulate gamma-aminobutyric acid receptors in the ascending reticular activating system.

Route	Onset	Peak	Duration
PO	Unknown	3 hr	Unknown

INDICATIONS & DOSAGE
Alcohol withdrawal, severe anxiety—
Adults: 15 to 30 mg P.O. t.i.d. or q.i.d.
Mild to moderate anxiety—
Adults: 10 to 15 mg P.O. t.i.d. or q.i.d.
Elderly: initially, 10 mg t.i.d.; increased to 15 mg t.i.d. to q.i.d.

ADVERSE REACTIONS
CNS: *drowsiness, lethargy,* dizziness, vertigo, headache, syncope, tremor, slurred speech.
CV: edema.
GI: nausea.
Hematologic: *leukopenia* (rare).
Hepatic: *hepatic dysfunction.*
Skin: rash.
Other: altered libido.

INTERACTIONS
Drug-drug. *CNS depressants:* increased CNS depression. Avoid concomitant use.
Digoxin: may increase serum digoxin levels and risk of toxicity. Monitor patient closely.
Drug-lifestyle. *Alcohol use:* increased CNS depression. Avoid concomitant use.
Smoking: decreased effectiveness of benzodiazepines. Monitor patient closely.

EFFECTS ON DIAGNOSTIC TESTS
Drug therapy may increase liver function test results. Changes in EEG patterns, usually low-voltage, fast activity, may occur during and after drug therapy.

CONTRAINDICATIONS
Contraindicated in patients with psychoses or hypersensitivity to drug.

NURSING CONSIDERATIONS
• Know that drug should be avoided during pregnancy, especially the first trimester.
• Use cautiously in elderly patients and in patients with history of drug abuse or in whom a drop in blood pressure might lead to cardiac problems.
• Monitor liver, renal, and hematopoietic function studies periodically in patients receiving repeated or prolonged therapy as ordered.
• Know that the possibility of abuse and addiction exists. Do not stop drug abruptly because withdrawal symptoms may occur.

✔ **Patient teaching**
• Warn patient to avoid hazardous activities that require alertness or good psychomotor coordination until CNS effects of drug are known.
• Tell patient to avoid alcohol while taking drug.
• Notify patient that smoking may decrease effectiveness of drug.
• Warn patient not to abruptly stop using drug because withdrawal symptoms may occur.
• Caution patient to avoid use during pregnancy.

33
Antipsychotics

chlorpromazine hydrochloride
clozapine
fluphenazine decanoate
fluphenazine enanthate
fluphenazine hydrochloride
haloperidol
haloperidol decanoate
haloperidol lactate
loxapine hydrochloride
loxapine succinate
mesoridazine besylate
molindone hydrochloride
olanzapine
perphenazine
pimozide
prochlorperazine
  (See Chapter 51, ANTIEMETICS.)
quetiapine fumarate
risperidone
thioridazine hydrochloride
thiothixene
thiothixene hydrochloride
trifluoperazine hydrochloride

COMBINATION PRODUCTS
ETRAFON 2-10: perphenazine 2 mg and
amitriptyline hydrochloride 10 mg.
ETRAFON-A: perphenazine 2 mg and
amitriptyline hydrochloride 25 mg.
ETRAFON-FORTE: perphenazine 4 mg and
amitriptyline hydrochloride 25 mg.
TRIAVIL 2-10, TRIAVIL 4-10, TRIAVIL 2-25
are identical to Etrafon products above.
Triavil also is available as TRIAVIL 4-25
(perphenazine 4 mg and amitriptyline hydrochloride 25 mg) and TRIAVIL 4-50
(perphenazine 4 mg and amitriptyline hydrochloride 50 mg).

---

chlorpromazine hydrochloride
Chlorpromanyl-5†,
Chlorpromanyl-20†,
Chlorpromanyl-40†, Largactil†‡,
Novo-Chlorpromazine†,
Ormazine, Thorazine, Thor-Prom

Pregnancy Risk Category: C

HOW SUPPLIED
Tablets: 10 mg, 25 mg, 50 mg, 100 mg,
200 mg
Capsules (extended-release): 30 mg,
75 mg, 150 mg, 200 mg, 300 mg
Oral concentrate: 30 mg/ml, 100 mg/ml
Syrup: 10 mg/5 ml
Injection: 25 mg/ml
Suppositories: 25 mg, 100 mg

ACTION
Unknown. An aliphatic phenothiazine that
probably blocks postsynaptic dopamine
and alpha-adrenergic receptors in the
brain and inhibits the medullary chemoreceptor trigger zone.

Route	Onset	Peak	Duration
PO	0.5-1 hr	Unknown	4-6 hr
PO (extended)	0.5-1 hr	Unknown	10-12 hr
IV, IM	Unknown	Unknown	Unknown
PR	> 1 hr	Unknown	3-4 hr

INDICATIONS & DOSAGE
Psychosis—
Adults: 25 to 75 mg P.O. daily in two to
four divided doses. Dosage increased by
20 to 50 mg twice weekly until symptoms
are controlled. Up to 800 mg daily may be
required in some patients. Or, 25 to 50 mg
I.M. q 1 to 4 hours, p.r.n. Subsequent I.M.
doses should be gradually increased over
several days to maximum of 400 mg q 4
to 6 hours. Switch to oral therapy as soon
as possible.
Children 6 months and older: 0.55 mg/
kg P.O. q 4 to 6 hours or I.M. q 6 to 8
hours; or 1.1 mg/kg P.R. q 6 to 8 hours.
Maximum I.M. dosage in children under
5 years or weighing below 22.7 kg (50 lb)
is 40 mg. Maximum I.M. dosage in children 5 to 12 years or weighing 22.7 to
45.5 kg (50 to 100 lb) is 75 mg.
Nausea and vomiting—
Adults: 10 to 25 mg P.O. q 4 to 6 hours,
p.r.n.; or 50 to 100 mg P.R. q 6 to 8 hours,
p.r.n.; or 25 mg I.M. initially. If no hypotension occurs, 25 to 50 mg I.M. q 3 to 4

---

hours, may be given p.r.n., until vomiting stops.

Children 6 months and older: 0.55 mg/kg P.O. q 4 to 6 hours or I.M. q 6 to 8 hours; or 1.1 mg/kg P.R. q 6 to 8 hours. Maximum I.M. dosage in children under 5 years or weighing below 22.7 kg is 40 mg. Maximum I.M. dosage in children 5 to 12 years or weighing 22.7 to 45.5 kg is 75 mg.

Intractable hiccups, acute intermittent porphyria—
Adults: 25 to 50 mg P.O. t.i.d. or q.i.d. If symptoms persist for 2 to 3 days, 25 to 50 mg I.M. For hiccups, if symptoms still persist, 25 to 50 mg diluted in 500 to 1,000 ml of 0.9% NaCl solution and infused slowly with patient in supine position.

Tetanus—
Adults: 25 to 50 mg I.V. or I.M. t.i.d. or q.i.d.

Children 6 months and older: 0.55 mg/kg I.M. or I.V. q 6 to 8 hours. Maximum parenteral dosage in children weighing below 22.7 kg is 40 mg daily; for children weighing 22.7 to 45.5 kg, 75 mg, except in severe cases.

Surgery—
Adults: preoperatively, 25 to 50 mg P.O. 2 to 3 hours before surgery or 12.5 to 25 mg I.M. 1 to 2 hours before surgery; during surgery, 12.5 mg I.M., repeated in 30 minutes if needed, or fractional 2-mg doses I.V. at 2-minute intervals up to maximum dose of 25 mg; postoperatively, 10 to 25 mg P.O. q 4 to 6 hours or 12.5 to 25 mg I.M., repeated in 1 hour, if needed.

Children 6 months and older: preoperatively, 0.55 mg/kg P.O. 2 to 3 hours before surgery or I.M. 1 to 2 hours before surgery; during surgery, 0.275 mg/kg I.M., repeated in 30 minutes if needed, or fractional 1-mg doses I.V. at 2-minute intervals up to total of 0.275 mg/kg; may repeat fractional I.V. regimen in 30 minutes if needed; postoperatively, 0.55 mg/kg P.O. or I.M. q 4 to 6 hours (oral dose) or 1 hour (I.M. dose), if needed, and hypotension does not occur.

Elderly: lower dosages are sufficient; dosage increments should be more gradual than in adults.

ADVERSE REACTIONS
CNS: *extrapyramidal reactions,* drowsiness, *sedation,* **seizures,** *tardive dyskinesia,* pseudoparkinsonism, dizziness.
CV: *orthostatic hypotension,* tachycardia, ECG changes.
EENT: ocular changes, blurred vision, nasal congestion.
GI: *dry mouth, constipation,* nausea.
GU: *urine retention,* menstrual irregularities, gynecomastia, inhibited ejaculation, lactation, priapism.
Hematologic: *leukopenia, agranulocytosis,* eosinophilia, hemolytic anemia, *aplastic anemia, thrombocytopenia.*
Hepatic: jaundice, abnormal liver function test results.
Skin: *mild photosensitivity,* allergic reactions, *pain at I.M. injection site,* sterile abscess, skin pigmentation.
Other: *neuroleptic malignant syndrome.*
After abrupt withdrawal of long-term therapy: gastritis, nausea, vomiting, dizziness, tremor.

INTERACTIONS
Drug-drug. *Antacids:* inhibited absorption of oral phenothiazines. Separate antacid and phenothiazine doses by at least 2 hours.
Anticholinergics including antidepressants, antiparkinsonian agents: increased anticholinergic activity, aggravated parkinsonian symptoms. Use with caution.
Anticonvulsants: may lower seizure threshold. Monitor patient closely.
Barbiturates, lithium: may decrease phenothiazine effect. Observe patient.
Centrally acting antihypertensives: decreased antihypertensive effect. Monitor blood pressure.
CNS depressants: increased CNS depression. Avoid concomitant use.
Electroconvulsive therapy, insulin: may precipitate severe reactions. Monitor patient closely.
Propranolol: increased levels of both propranolol and chlorpromazine. Monitor patient closely.
Warfarin: decreased effect of oral anticoagulants. Monitor PT and INR.
Drug-lifestyle. *Alcohol use:* increased CNS depression. Avoid concomitant use.

Reactions may be *common,* uncommon, **life-threatening**, or COMMON AND LIFE-THREATENING.

Sun exposure: photosensitivity reactions may occur. Take precautions.

EFFECTS ON DIAGNOSTIC TESTS
Drug causes false-positive test results for urinary porphyrins, urobilinogen, amylase, and 5-hydroxyindoleacetic acid because of darkening of urine by metabolites; it also causes false-positive results in urine pregnancy tests using human chorionic gonadotropin. Chlorpromazine elevates tests for liver function and protein-bound iodine and causes quinidine-like ECG effects.

CONTRAINDICATIONS
Contraindicated in patients with hypersensitivity to drug or in those experiencing CNS depression, bone marrow suppression, subcortical damage, or coma.

NURSING CONSIDERATIONS
• Use cautiously in elderly or debilitated patients and in patients with hepatic or renal disease, severe CV disease (may cause sudden drop in blood pressure), exposure to extreme heat or cold (including antipyretic therapy) or organophosphate insecticides, respiratory disorders, hypocalcemia, glaucoma, or prostatic hyperplasia.
• Use cautiously in acutely ill or dehydrated children.
• Obtain baseline measures of blood pressure before starting therapy and monitor regularly. Watch for orthostatic hypotension, especially with parenteral administration. Monitor blood pressure before and after I.M. administration. Keep patient supine for 1 hour afterward and have him get up slowly.
• Know that slight yellowing of injection or concentrate is common and does not affect potency. Discard markedly discolored solutions.
• Give deep I.M. only in upper outer quadrant of buttocks. Massage slowly afterward to prevent sterile abscess. Injection stings.
• Wear gloves when preparing solutions, and prevent any contact with skin and clothing. Oral liquid and parenteral forms can cause contact dermatitis.
• Protect liquid concentrate from light.

Dilute with fruit juice, milk, or semisolid food just before administration.
• Monitor patient for tardive dyskinesia, which may occur after prolonged use. It may not appear until months or years later and may disappear spontaneously or persist for life, despite discontinuation of drug.
• Watch for symptoms of neuroleptic malignant syndrome (extrapyramidal effects, hyperthermia, autonomic disturbance). It is rare, but frequently fatal. It is not necessarily related to length of drug use or type of neuroleptic, but over 60% of affected patients are men.
• Monitor therapy with weekly bilirubin tests during 1st month, periodic blood tests (CBC and liver function), and ophthalmic tests (long-term use) as ordered.
• Do not withdraw drug abruptly unless required by severe adverse reactions.
• Withhold dose and notify doctor if patient develops jaundice, symptoms of blood dyscrasia (fever, sore throat, infection, cellulitis, weakness), persistent extrapyramidal reactions (longer than a few hours), or any such reaction in pregnant patients or in children.

⚠ I.V. administration
• For direct injection, drug may be diluted with 0.9% NaCl for injection and administered into a large vein or through the tubing of a free-flowing I.V. solution. Do not exceed 1 mg/minute for adults or 0.5 mg/minute for children. Drug also may be given as an intermittent I.V. infusion; dilute with 50 or 100 ml of a compatible solution and infuse over 30 minutes. Chlorpromazine is compatible with most common I.V. solutions, including D_5W, Ringer's injection, lactated Ringer's injection, and 0.9% NaCl for injection.

☑ Patient teaching
• Warn patient to avoid activities that require alertness or good psychomotor coordination until CNS effects of drug are known. Drowsiness and dizziness usually subside after first few weeks.
• Tell patient to avoid alcohol while taking drug.
• Have patient report urine retention or constipation.

*Liquid contains alcohol.   **May contain tartrazine.   †Canada   ‡Australia   §U.K.   ◇OTC

• Tell patient to use sunblock and to wear protective clothing to avoid photosensitivity reactions. Chlorpromazine causes higher incidence of photosensitivity than any other drug in its class.

• Tell patient to relieve dry mouth with sugarless gum or hard candy.

• Advise patient receiving drug parenterally to remain supine for 1 hour after receiving drug and to rise slowly.

---

clozapine
Clozaril

Pregnancy Risk Category: B

HOW SUPPLIED
Tablets: 25 mg, 100 mg

ACTION
Unknown. Binds to dopaminergic receptors (both D-1 and D-2) within the limbic system of the CNS and may interfere with adrenergic, cholinergic, histaminergic, and serotoninergic receptors.

Route	Onset	Peak	Duration
PO	Unknown	2.5 hr	4-12 hr

INDICATIONS & DOSAGE
Schizophrenia in severely ill patients unresponsive to other therapies—
Adults: initially, 12.5 mg P.O. once daily or b.i.d., titrated upward at 25 to 50 mg daily (if tolerated) to 300 to 450 mg daily by end of 2 weeks. Individual dosage is based on clinical response, patient tolerance, and adverse reactions. Subsequent dosage should not be increased more than once or twice weekly, and should not exceed 100 mg. Many patients respond to dosages of 300 to 600 mg daily, but some may require as much as 900 mg daily. Do not exceed 900 mg daily.

ADVERSE REACTIONS
CNS: *drowsiness, sedation,* **seizures,** *dizziness,* syncope, *vertigo,* headache, tremor, disturbed sleep or nightmares, restlessness, hypokinesia or akinesia, agitation, rigidity, akathisia, confusion, fatigue, insomnia, hyperkinesia, weakness, lethargy, ataxia, slurred speech, depression, myoclonus, anxiety.
CV: *tachycardia, hypotension,* hypertension, chest pain, ECG changes, orthostatic hypotension.
GI: dry mouth, *constipation,* nausea, vomiting, *excessive salivation,* heartburn, diarrhea.
GU: urinary abnormalities (urinary frequency or urgency, urine retention), incontinence, abnormal ejaculation.
Hematologic: *leukopenia, agranulocytosis.*
Skin: rash.
Other: fever, muscle pain or spasm, muscle weakness, weight gain, visual disturbances, diaphoresis.
After abrupt withdrawal of long-term therapy: possible abrupt recurrence of psychotic symptoms.

INTERACTIONS
Drug-drug. *Anticholinergics:* may potentiate anticholinergic effects of clozapine. Avoid concomitant use. Monitor blood pressure.
Antihypertensives: may potentiate hypotensive effects. Monitor blood pressure.
Bone marrow suppressants: may increase bone marrow toxicity. Don't use together.
Digoxin, warfarin, other highly protein-bound drugs: may increase serum levels of these drugs. Monitor closely for adverse reactions.
Psychoactive drugs: may produce additive effects. Use together cautiously.
Drug-herb. *Nutmeg:* may reduce effectiveness of drug therapy. Avoid concomitant use.
Drug-food. *Caffeine-containing beverages:* may inhibit antipsychotic effects of clozapine. Monitor closely.
Drug-lifestyle. *Alcohol use:* increased CNS depression. Use cautiously.

EFFECTS ON DIAGNOSTIC TESTS
Toxic effects of drug may be evidenced by depressed blood counts.

CONTRAINDICATIONS
Contraindicated in patients with uncontrolled epilepsy, history of clozapine-induced agranulocytosis, WBC count below 3,500/mm³, severe CNS depression

---

Reactions may be *common*, uncommon, *life-threatening*, or COMMON AND LIFE-THREATENING.

or coma, and myelosuppressive disorders. Also contraindicated in patients taking other drugs that suppress bone marrow function.

NURSING CONSIDERATIONS

• Use cautiously in patients with prostatic hyperplasia or angle-closure glaucoma because clozapine has potent anticholinergic effects; also use cautiously in patients with hepatic, renal, or cardiac disease or those receiving general anesthesia. *Alert:* Clozapine carries significant risk of agranulocytosis. If possible, patients should receive at least two trials of drug therapy with a standard antipsychotic before clozapine therapy is initiated. Baseline WBC and differential counts are required before therapy. Monitor WBC counts weekly for at least 4 weeks after clozapine therapy is discontinued, as ordered.

• When administering clozapine, ensure that WBC counts and blood tests are performed weekly and that no more than a 1-week supply of drug is dispensed for first 6 months of therapy. If WBC count is maintained at 3,000/mm^3 or more and an absolute neutrophil count at 1,500/mm^3 or more during first 6 months of continuous therapy, may reduce frequency of monitoring blood counts to every other week.

• If WBC count drops below 3,500/mm^3 after therapy is initiated or if it exhibits a substantial drop from baseline, monitor patient closely for signs of infection. If WBC count is 3,000 to 3,500/mm^3 and granulocyte count is above 1,500/mm^3, perform WBC and differential count twice weekly. If WBC count drops below 3,000/mm^3 and granulocyte count drops below 1,500/mm^3, interrupt therapy, notify doctor, and monitor patient for signs of infection. Be aware that therapy may be restarted cautiously if WBC count returns to above 3,000/mm^3 and granulocyte count returns to above 1,500/mm^3. Continue monitoring WBC and differential counts twice weekly until WBC count exceeds 3,500/mm^3, as ordered.

• If WBC count drops below 2,000/mm^3 and granulocyte count drops below 1,000/mm^3, patient may require protective isolation. If patient develops infection, prepare cultures according to institutional policy and administer antibiotics, as ordered. Some doctors may perform bone marrow aspiration to assess bone marrow function. Know that future clozapine therapy is contraindicated in such patients.

• Be aware that seizures may occur, especially in patients receiving high doses.

• Some patients experience transient fevers (temperature over 100.4° F [38° C]), especially in the first 3 weeks of therapy. Monitor patients closely.

• If clozapine therapy must be discontinued, withdraw drug gradually (over 1- to 2-week period). However, changes in patient's medical condition (including development of leukopenia) may require abrupt discontinuation of drug. Monitor closely for recurrence of psychotic symptoms.

• If therapy is reinstated in patients withdrawn from drug, follow usual guidelines for dosage increase. However, reexposure of patient to drug may increase severity and risk of adverse reactions. If therapy was terminated because WBC counts were below 2,000/mm^3 or granulocyte counts were below 1,000/mm^3, do not expect drug to be continued.

☑ Patient teaching

• Warn patient about the risk of agranulocytosis. Tell patient about need for weekly blood tests to monitor for agranulocytosis. Advise him to report flulike symptoms, fever, sore throat, lethargy, malaise, or other signs of infection.

• Warn patient to avoid hazardous activities that require alertness and good psychomotor coordination while taking drug.

• Tell patient to check with doctor before taking OTC medications or alcohol.

• Tell patient to rise slowly to avoid orthostatic hypotension.

• Inform patient that ice chips or sugarless candy or gum may help relieve dry mouth.

fluphenazine decanoate
Modecate†‡, Modecate Concentrate†, Prolixin Decanoate

fluphenazine enanthate
Moditen Enanthate†, Prolixin Enanthate

fluphenazine hydrochloride
Anatensol‡*, Apo-Fluphenazine†, Moditen HCl†, Moditen HCl-H.P.†, Permitil*†**, Permitil Concentrate, Prolixin*†**, Prolixin Concentrate

Pregnancy Risk Category: C

HOW SUPPLIED
fluphenazine decanoate
Depot injection: 25 mg/ml
fluphenazine enanthate
Depot injection: 25 mg/ml
fluphenazine hydrochloride
Tablets: 1 mg, 2.5 mg, 5 mg, 10 mg
Oral concentrate: 5 mg/ml (contains 1% alcohol)
Elixir: 2.5 mg/5 ml (with 14% alcohol)
I.M. injection: 2.5 mg/ml

ACTION
Unknown. A piperazine phenothiazine that probably blocks postsynaptic dopamine, alpha-adrenergic, and cholinergic receptors in the brain.

Route	Onset	Peak	Duration
PO	< 1 hr	0.5 hr	6-8 hr
IM (HCl)	< 1 hr	1.5-2 hr	6-8 hr
IM	24-72 hr	Unknown	1-6 wk
SC	Unknown	Unknown	Unknown

INDICATIONS & DOSAGE
Psychotic disorders—
Adults: initially, 0.5 to 10 mg hydrochloride P.O. daily in divided doses q 6 to 8 hours; may increase cautiously to 20 mg. Higher doses (50 to 100 mg) have been given. Maintenance dosage is 1 to 5 mg P.O. daily. I.M. doses are one-third to one-half of oral doses. Usual I.M. dose is 1.25 mg. Use dosages above 10 mg/day with caution.

Alternatively, 12.5 to 25 mg of long-acting esters (decanoate or enanthate) I.M. or S.C. q 1 to 6 weeks; maintenance dosage is 25 to 100 mg, p.r.n.
Elderly: use lower dosages for elderly patients (1 to 2.5 mg daily).

ADVERSE REACTIONS
CNS: *extrapyramidal reactions, tardive dyskinesia,* sedation, pseudoparkinsonism, EEG changes, drowsiness, *seizures,* dizziness.
CV: orthostatic hypotension, tachycardia, ECG changes.
EENT: ocular changes, *blurred vision,* nasal congestion.
GI: *dry mouth, constipation.*
GU: *urine retention,* dark urine, menstrual irregularities, gynecomastia, inhibited ejaculation.
Hematologic: *leukopenia, agranulocytosis,* eosinophilia, hemolytic anemia, *aplastic anemia, thrombocytopenia.*
Hepatic: cholestatic jaundice, abnormal liver function test results.
Skin: *mild photosensitivity,* allergic reactions.
Other: weight gain; increased appetite; rarely, *neuroleptic malignant syndrome.*
After abrupt withdrawal of long-term therapy: gastritis, nausea, vomiting, dizziness, tremor, feeling of warmth or cold, diaphoresis, tachycardia, headache, insomnia.

INTERACTIONS
Drug-drug. *Antacids:* inhibited absorption of oral phenothiazines. Separate antacid and phenothiazine doses by at least 2 hours.
Anticholinergics: increased anticholinergic effects. Avoid concomitant use.
Barbiturates, lithium: may decrease phenothiazine effect. Observe patient.
Centrally acting antihypertensives: decreased antihypertensive effect. Monitor blood pressure.
CNS depressants: increased CNS depression. Avoid concomitant use.
Drug-lifestyle. *Alcohol use:* increased CNS depression. Avoid concomitant use.
Sun exposure: photosensitivity reactions may occur. Take precautions.

Reactions may be *common,* uncommon, *life-threatening,* or COMMON AND LIFE-THREATENING.

EFFECTS ON DIAGNOSTIC TESTS

Drug causes false-positive test results for urinary porphyrins, urobilinogen, amylase, and 5-hydroxyindoleacetic acid because of darkening of urine by metabolites; it also causes false-positive urine pregnancy test results using human chorionic gonadotropin. Fluphenazine elevates test results for liver enzymes and protein-bound iodine and causes quinidine-like ECG effects.

CONTRAINDICATIONS

Contraindicated in patients with hypersensitivity to drug or in those experiencing coma, CNS depression, bone marrow suppression or other blood dyscrasia, subcortical damage, or liver damage.

NURSING CONSIDERATIONS

• Use cautiously in elderly or debilitated patients and in those with pheochromocytoma, severe CV disease (may cause sudden drop in blood pressure), peptic ulcer, exposure to extreme heat or cold (including antipyretic therapy) or phosphorus insecticides, respiratory disorder, hypocalcemia, seizure disorder (may lower seizure threshold), severe reactions to insulin or electroconvulsive therapy, mitral insufficiency, glaucoma, or prostatic hyperplasia. Use parenteral form cautiously in asthmatic patients and patients allergic to sulfites.

• Know that Prolixin Concentrate and Permitil Concentrate are 10 times more concentrated than Prolixin elixir (5 mg/ml versus 0.5 mg/ml). Check dosage order carefully.

• Dilute liquid concentrate with water, fruit juice, milk, or semisolid food just before administration.

• For long-acting forms (decanoate and enanthate), which are oil preparations, use a dry needle of at least 21G. Allow 24 to 96 hours for onset of action. Note and report adverse reactions in patients taking these drug forms.

• Be aware that oral liquid and parenteral forms can cause contact dermatitis. Wear gloves when preparing solutions, and prevent contact with skin and clothing.

• Protect medication from light. Slight yellowing of injection or concentrate is common and does not affect potency. Discard markedly discolored solutions.

• Monitor patient for tardive dyskinesia, which may occur after prolonged use. It may not appear until months or years later and disappear spontaneously or persist for life, despite discontinuation of drug.

• Watch patient for neuroleptic malignant syndrome (extrapyramidal effects, hyperthermia, autonomic disturbance). It is rare, but frequently fatal. It is not necessarily related to length of drug use or type of neuroleptic, but over 60% of affected patients are men.

• Monitor therapy with weekly bilirubin tests during 1st month, periodic blood tests (CBC and liver function), and periodic renal function and ophthalmic tests (long-term use) as ordered.

• Do not withdraw drug abruptly unless serious adverse reactions occur.

• Withhold dose and notify doctor if patient develops symptoms of blood dyscrasia (fever, sore throat, infection, cellulitis, weakness) or persistent extrapyramidal reactions (longer than a few hours), especially in pregnant patients or in children.

✔ Patient teaching

• Warn patient to avoid activities that require alertness and good psychomotor coordination until CNS effects of drug are known. Drowsiness and dizziness usually subside after first few weeks.

• Warn patient to avoid alcohol while taking drug.

• Tell patient to relieve dry mouth with sugarless gum or hard candy.

• Have patient report urine retention or constipation.

• Advise patient to use sunblock and to wear protective clothing to avoid photosensitivity reactions.

• Tell patient that drug may discolor urine.

haloperidol
Apo-Haloperidol†, Dozic§,
Haldol**, Novo-Peridol†, Peridol†,
Serenace§‡

haloperidol decanoate
Haldol Decanoate, Haldol LA†

haloperidol lactate
Haldol, Haldol Concentrate,
Haloperidol Injection, Haloperidol
Intensol

Pregnancy Risk Category: C

HOW SUPPLIED
haloperidol
Tablets: 0.5 mg, 1 mg, 2 mg, 5 mg,
10 mg, 20 mg
haloperidol decanoate
Injection: 50 mg/ml, 100 mg/ml
haloperidol lactate
Oral concentrate: 2 mg/ml
Injection: 5 mg/ml

ACTION
Unknown. A butyrophenone that probably
exerts its antipsychotic effects by blocking postsynaptic dopamine receptors in
the brain.

Route	Onset	Peak	Duration
PO	Unknown	3-6 hr	Unknown
IM (decanoate)	Unknown	3-9 days	Unknown
IM (lactate)	Unknown	10-20 min	Unknown

INDICATIONS & DOSAGE
Psychotic disorders—
Adults and children 12 and older:
dosage varies for each patient. Initial
range, 0.5 to 5 mg P.O. b.i.d. or t.i.d.; or 2
to 5 mg I.M. q 4 to 8 hours, although
hourly administration may be needed until
control obtained. Maximum dosage is
100 mg P.O. daily.
Children 3 to 12 years: 0.05 mg/kg to
0.15 mg/kg P.O. daily. Severely disturbed
children may require higher dosages.
*Chronic psychotic patients who require
prolonged therapy—*

Adults: 50 to 100 mg I.M. haloperidol
decanoate q 4 weeks.
Nonpsychotic behavior disorders—
Children 3 to 12 years: 0.05 mg/kg P.O.
daily. Maximum daily dosage is 6 mg.
Tourette syndrome—
Adults: 0.5 to 5 mg P.O. b.i.d. or t.i.d., or
p.r.n.
Children 3 to 12 years: 0.05 to 0.075 mg/
kg P.O. daily in two or three divided doses.
Elderly: 0.5 to 2 mg P.O. b.i.d. or t.i.d.,
increased gradually p.r.n.
Adjust-a-dose: In debilitated patients, use
0.5 to 2 mg P.O. b.i.d. or t.i.d., increased
gradually p.r.n.

ADVERSE REACTIONS
CNS: *severe extrapyramidal reactions,
tardive dyskinesia,* sedation, drowsiness,
lethargy, headache, insomnia, confusion,
vertigo, *seizures.*
CV: tachycardia, hypotension, hypertension, ECG changes.
EENT: blurred vision.
GI: dry mouth, anorexia, constipation, diarrhea, nausea, vomiting, dyspepsia.
GU: urine retention, menstrual irregularities, gynecomastia, priapism.
Hematologic: *leukopenia,* leukocytosis.
Skin: rash, other skin reactions, diaphoresis.
Other: *neuroleptic malignant syndrome,*
altered liver function tests, jaundice.

INTERACTIONS
Drug-drug. *Anticholinergics:* increased
anticholinergic effects, glaucoma. Avoid
concomitant use.
CNS depressants: increased CNS depres-
sion. Avoid concomitant use.
Lithium: lethargy and confusion after
high doses. Monitor patient.
Drug-herb. *Nutmeg:* may reduce effec-
tiveness or interfere with drug therapy.
Avoid concomitant use.
Drug-lifestyle. *Alcohol use:* increased
CNS depression. Avoid concomitant use.

EFFECTS ON DIAGNOSTIC TESTS
None reported.

CONTRAINDICATIONS
Contraindicated in patients with hyper-

sensitivity to drug or in those experiencing parkinsonism, coma, or CNS depression.

NURSING CONSIDERATIONS
• Use cautiously in elderly and debilitated patients; in patients with history of seizures or EEG abnormalities, severe CV disorders, allergies, glaucoma, or urine retention; and in conjunction with anticonvulsant, anticoagulant, antiparkinsonian, or lithium medications.
Alert: Do not administer decanoate form I.V.
• When changing from tablets to decanoate injection, know that patient should be given 10 to 15 times the oral dose once a month (maximum 100 mg).
• Protect drug from light. Slight yellowing of injection or concentrate is common and does not affect potency. Discard markedly discolored solutions.
• Do not withdraw drug abruptly unless required by severe adverse reactions.
• Monitor patient for tardive dyskinesia, which may occur after prolonged use. It may not appear until months or years later and disappear spontaneously or persist for life, despite discontinuation of drug.
• Watch patient for neuroleptic malignant syndrome (extrapyramidal effects, hyperthermia, autonomic disturbance). It is rare, but frequently fatal. It is not necessarily related to length of drug use or type of neuroleptic, but over 60% of affected patients are men.
• Dilute dose with water or a beverage, such as orange juice, apple juice, tomato juice, or cola, immediately before administration.

☑ Patient teaching
• Although drug is the least sedating of the antipsychotics, warn patient to avoid activities that require alertness and good psychomotor coordination until CNS effects of drug are known. Drowsiness and dizziness usually subside after a few weeks.
• Warn patient to avoid alcohol while taking drug.
• Advise patient to relieve dry mouth with sugarless gum or hard candy.

loxapine hydrochloride
Loxapac†, Loxitane C, Loxitane IM

loxapine succinate
Loxapac†, Loxitane

Pregnancy Risk Category: NR

HOW SUPPLIED
loxapine hydrochloride
Oral concentrate: 25 mg/ml
Injection: 50 mg/ml
loxapine succinate
Capsules: 5 mg, 10 mg, 25 mg, 50 mg
Tablets: 5 mg†, 10 mg†, 25 mg†, 50 mg†

ACTION
Unknown. A dibenzoxazepine that probably exerts its antipsychotic effects by blocking postsynaptic dopamine receptors in the brain.

Route	Onset	Peak	Duration
PO, IM	30 min	1.5-3 hr	12 hr

INDICATIONS & DOSAGE
Psychotic disorders—
Adults: 10 mg P.O. b.i.d. to q.i.d., rapidly increasing to 60 to 100 mg P.O. daily for most patients; dosage varies among patients. If patient is unable to take oral dose, 12.5 to 50 mg I.M. q 4 to 6 hours or longer, both dosage and interval depending on patient response. Dosages exceeding 250 mg/day are not recommended.
Elderly: initially, 3 to 5 mg P.O. b.i.d.

ADVERSE REACTIONS
CNS: *extrapyramidal reactions, sedation,* drowsiness, *seizures,* numbness, confusion, syncope, *tardive dyskinesia,* pseudoparkinsonism, EEG changes, dizziness.
CV: orthostatic hypotension, tachycardia, ECG changes, hypertension.
EENT: *blurred vision,* nasal congestion.
GI: *dry mouth, constipation,* nausea, vomiting, paralytic ileus.
GU: *urine retention,* menstrual irregularities, gynecomastia.
Hematologic: *leukopenia, agranulocytosis, thrombocytopenia.*
Skin: *mild photosensitivity,* allergic reactions, rash, pruritus.

Other: weight gain, *neuroleptic malignant syndrome,* jaundice.

INTERACTIONS
Drug-drug. *CNS depressants:* increased CNS depression. Avoid concomitant use.
Drug-lifestyle. *Alcohol use:* increased CNS depression. Avoid concomitant use.

EFFECTS ON DIAGNOSTIC TESTS
Loxapine causes false-positive test results for urinary porphyrins, urobilinogen, amylase, and 5-hydroxyindoleacetic acid because of darkening of urine by metabolites; it also causes false-positive urine pregnancy test results using human chorionic gonadotropin. Drug elevates test results for liver enzymes and protein-bound iodine and causes quinidine-like effects on the ECG.

CONTRAINDICATIONS
Contraindicated in patients with hypersensitivity to dibenzoxazepines and in those experiencing coma, severe CNS depression, or drug-induced depressed states.

NURSING CONSIDERATIONS
• Use with extreme caution in patients with seizure disorder, CV disorder, glaucoma, and history of urine retention.
• Obtain baseline measures of blood pressure before starting therapy, and monitor regularly.
• Dilute liquid concentrate with orange or grapefruit juice just before giving.
• Monitor patient for tardive dyskinesia, which may occur after prolonged use. It may not appear until months or years later and disappear spontaneously or persist for life, despite discontinuation of drug.
• Monitor patient for neuroleptic malignant syndrome (extrapyramidal effects, hyperthermia, autonomic disturbance). It is rare, but frequently fatal. It is not necessarily related to length of drug use or type of neuroleptic, but over 60% of affected patients are men.

☑ **Patient teaching**
• Warn patient to avoid activities that require alertness and good psychomotor coordination until CNS effects of drug are known. Drowsiness and dizziness usually subside after first few weeks.
• Advise patient to report bruising, fever, or sore throat immediately.
• Tell patient to avoid alcohol while taking drug.
• Advise patient to get up slowly to avoid orthostatic hypotension.
• Tell patient to relieve dry mouth with sugarless gum or hard candy.
• Inform patient that periodic eye examinations are recommended.

---

mesoridazine besylate
Serentil*, Serentil Concentrate

Pregnancy Risk Category: NR

HOW SUPPLIED
Tablets: 10 mg, 25 mg, 50 mg, 100 mg
Oral concentrate: 25 mg/ml (0.6% alcohol)
Injection: 25 mg/ml

ACTION
Unknown. A piperidine phenothiazine and the major sulfoxide metabolite of thioridazine that probably exerts its antipsychotic effects by blocking postsynaptic dopamine receptors in the brain.

Route	Onset	Peak	Duration
PO, IM	Unknown	Unknown	Unknown

INDICATIONS & DOSAGE
Alcoholism—
Adults and children over 12 years: 25 mg P.O. b.i.d. up to maximum of 200 mg daily.
Behavior problems associated with chronic organic mental syndrome—
Adults and children over 12 years: 25 mg P.O. t.i.d. up to maximum of 300 mg daily.
Psychoneurotic manifestations (anxiety)—
Adults and children over 12 years: 10 mg P.O. t.i.d. up to maximum of 150 mg daily.
Schizophrenia—
Adults and children over 12 years: initially, 50 mg P.O. t.i.d. or 25 mg I.M. repeated in 30 to 60 minutes, p.r.n. Maxi-

---

mum oral dosage is 400 mg daily; maximum I.M. dosage is 200 mg.

ADVERSE REACTIONS
CNS: *extrapyramidal reactions, tardive dyskinesia, sedation,* drowsiness, tremor, rigidity, weakness, EEG changes, dizziness.
CV: *hypotension,* tachycardia, ECG changes.
EENT: *ocular changes, blurred vision,* retinitis pigmentosa, nasal congestion.
GI: *dry mouth, constipation,* nausea, vomiting.
GU: *urine retention,* menstrual irregularities, gynecomastia, inhibited ejaculation.
Hematologic: *leukopenia, agranulocytosis, aplastic anemia,* eosinophilia, *thrombocytopenia.*
Hepatic: jaundice, abnormal liver function test results.
Skin: *mild photosensitivity,* allergic reactions, pain at I.M. injection site, sterile abscess, rash.
Other: weight gain, *neuroleptic malignant syndrome.*
After abrupt withdrawal of long-term therapy: gastritis, nausea, vomiting, dizziness, tremor, feeling of warmth or cold, diaphoresis, tachycardia, headache, insomnia.

INTERACTIONS
Drug-drug. *Antacids:* inhibited absorption of oral phenothiazines. Separate antacid and phenothiazine doses by at least 2 hours.
Anticholinergics: may increase anticholinergic effects. Use together cautiously.
Barbiturates: may decrease phenothiazine effect. Observe patient.
CNS depressants: increased CNS depression. Use together cautiously.
Drug-lifestyle. *Alcohol use:* increased CNS depression. Avoid concomitant use.
Sun exposure: photosensitivity reactions may occur. Take precautions.

EFFECTS ON DIAGNOSTIC TESTS
Drug causes false-positive test results for urinary porphyrins, urobilinogen, amylase, and 5-hydroxyindoleacetic acid because of darkening of urine by metabolites; it also causes false-positive urine

pregnancy test results using human chorionic gonadotropin. Mesoridazine elevates tests for liver function and protein-bound iodine and causes quinidine-like effects on the ECG.

CONTRAINDICATIONS
Contraindicated in patients with hypersensitivity to drug or in those experiencing severe CNS depression or in comatose states.

NURSING CONSIDERATIONS
● Obtain baseline measures of blood pressure before starting therapy and monitor regularly. Watch for orthostatic hypotension, especially with parenteral administration.
● Oral liquid and parenteral forms may cause contact dermatitis. Wear gloves when preparing solutions, and prevent contact with skin and clothing.
● Give deep I.M. only in upper outer quadrant of buttocks. Massage slowly afterward to prevent sterile abscess. Injection may sting.
● Protect drug from light. Slight yellowing of injection or concentrate is common and does not affect potency. Discard markedly discolored solutions.
● Monitor patient for tardive dyskinesia, which may occur after prolonged use. It may not appear until months or years later and disappear spontaneously or persist for life, despite discontinuation of drug.
● Assess patient for neuroleptic malignant syndrome (extrapyramidal effects, hyperthermia, autonomic disturbance). It is rare, but frequently fatal. It is not necessarily related to length of drug use or type of neuroleptic, but over 60% of affected patients are men.
● Withhold dose and notify doctor if patient develops jaundice, symptoms of blood dyscrasia (fever, sore throat, infection, cellulitis, weakness), or persistent extrapyramidal reactions (longer than a few hours), especially in pregnant patients or in children.
● Monitor therapy with weekly bilirubin tests during 1st month, periodic blood tests (CBC and liver function), and ophthalmic tests (long-term use), as ordered.

• Do not withdraw drug abruptly unless required by severe adverse reactions.

☑ **Patient teaching**
• Warn patient to avoid activities that require alertness and good psychomotor coordination until CNS effects of drug are known. Drowsiness and dizziness usually subside after a few weeks.
• Advise patient to change position slowly.
• Warn patient to avoid alcohol while taking drug.
• Have patient report urine retention or constipation.
• Tell patient that drug may discolor urine.
• Instruct patient to relieve dry mouth with sugarless gum or hard candy.
• Advise patient to use sunblock and to wear protective clothing to avoid photosensitivity reactions.

molindone hydrochloride
Moban

Pregnancy Risk Category: C

HOW SUPPLIED
Tablets: 5 mg, 10 mg, 25 mg, 50 mg, 100 mg
Oral solution: 20 mg/ml

ACTION
Unknown. A dihydroindolone that probably blocks postsynaptic dopamine receptors in the brain.

Route	Onset	Peak	Duration
PO	Unknown	1.5 hr	24-36 hr

INDICATIONS & DOSAGE
Psychotic disorders—
Adults: initially, 50 to 75 mg P.O. daily; then increased to 100 to 225 mg/day in 3 or 4 days. Maintenance dosage as follows: mild severity—5 to 15 mg P.O. t.i.d. to q.i.d.; moderate severity—10 to 25 mg P.O. t.i.d. or q.i.d.; acute severity—225 mg/day P.O.

ADVERSE REACTIONS
CNS: *extrapyramidal reactions, tardive dyskinesia, sedation,* drowsiness, depression, euphoria, pseudoparkinsonism, EEG changes, dizziness.
CV: *orthostatic hypotension,* tachycardia, ECG changes.
EENT: *blurred vision.*
GI: *dry mouth, constipation,* nausea.
GU: *urine retention,* menstrual irregularities, gynecomastia, inhibited ejaculation.
Hematologic: *leukopenia,* leukocytosis.
Hepatic: jaundice, abnormal liver function test results.
Skin: *mild photosensitivity,* allergic reactions.
Other: *neuroleptic malignant syndrome.*

INTERACTIONS
Drug-drug. *CNS depressants:* increased CNS depression. Avoid concomitant use.
Drug-lifestyle. *Alcohol use:* increased CNS depression. Avoid concomitant use.

EFFECTS ON DIAGNOSTIC TESTS
Drug causes false-positive results in urine pregnancy tests using human chorionic gonadotropin and additive potential for causing seizures with metrizamide myelography. Molindone elevates levels of liver enzymes (AST, ALT), free fatty acids, and BUN; drug may alter WBC counts and may increase or decrease serum glucose levels.

CONTRAINDICATIONS
Contraindicated in patients with hypersensitivity to drug or in those experiencing coma or severe CNS depression.

NURSING CONSIDERATIONS
• Use cautiously when increased physical activity would be harmful because this agent may cause hyperactivity. Also use cautiously in patients subject to seizures (may lower seizure threshold).
• Monitor patient for tardive dyskinesia, which may occur after prolonged use. It may not appear until months or years later and may disappear spontaneously or persist for life, despite discontinuation of drug.
• Assess patient for neuroleptic malignant syndrome (extrapyramidal effects, hyperthermia, autonomic disturbance). It is rare, but frequently fatal. It is not necessarily related to length of drug use or type

of neuroleptic, but over 60% of affected patients are men.

☑ **Patient teaching**
• Warn patient to avoid activities that require alertness or good psychomotor coordination until CNS effects of drug are known. Drowsiness and dizziness usually subside after first few weeks.
• Tell patient to avoid alcohol while taking drug.
• Advise patient to relieve dry mouth with sugarless gum or hard candy.

olanzapine
Zyprexa

Pregnancy Risk Category: C

HOW SUPPLIED
Tablets: 5 mg, 7.5 mg, 10 mg

ACTION
Unknown. Binds to dopamine and serotonin receptors; may interfere with adrenergic, cholinergic, and histaminergic receptors.

Route	Onset	Peak	Duration
PO	Unknown	6 hr	Unknown

INDICATIONS & DOSAGE
Psychotic disorders—
Adults: initially, 5 to 10 mg P.O. once daily. Dosage adjustments in 5-mg daily increments should occur at intervals of not less than 1 week. Most patients respond to dosages of 10 mg/day. Do not exceed 20 mg/day.
Adjust-a-dose: In patients who are debilitated, predisposed to hypotension, or have an alteration in metabolism due to smoking status, gender, or age, or who are pharmacologically sensitive to drug, 5 mg initially.

ADVERSE REACTIONS
CNS: *somnolence, agitation, insomnia, headache, nervousness, hostility,* parkinsonism, *dizziness,* anxiety, personality disorder, akathisia, hypertonia, tremor, amnesia, articulation impairment, euphoria, stuttering, tardive dyskinesia.

CV: orthostatic hypotension, tachycardia, chest pain, hypotension, edema.
EENT: amblyopia, blepharitis, corneal lesion, *rhinitis,* pharyngitis.
GI: constipation, dry mouth, abdominal pain, increased appetite, increased salivation, nausea, vomiting, thirst.
GU: premenstrual syndrome, hematuria, metrorrhagia, urinary incontinence, urinary tract infection.
Musculoskeletal: joint pain, extremity pain, back pain, neck rigidity, twitching.
Respiratory: increased cough, dyspnea.
Skin: vesiculobullous rash.
Other: weight gain or loss, fever, intentional injury.

INTERACTIONS
Drug-drug. *Antihypertensives:* may potentiate hypotensive effects. Monitor blood pressure closely.
Carbamazepine, omeprazole, rifampin: increased clearance of olanzapine. Monitor patient.
Diazepam: increased CNS effects. Monitor closely.
Dopamine agonists, levodopa: antagonized activity of these agents. Monitor patient.
Drug-herb. *Nutmeg:* may reduce effectiveness or interfere with drug therapy. Avoid concomitant use.
Drug-lifestyle. *Alcohol use:* increased CNS effects. Avoid concomitant use.

EFFECTS ON DIAGNOSTIC TESTS
Drug may cause asymptomatic increases in AST, ALT, GGT, CK, serum prolactin, and eosinophil count.

CONTRAINDICATIONS
Contraindicated in patients with known hypersensitivity to drug.

NURSING CONSIDERATIONS
• Use cautiously in patients with heart disease, cerebrovascular disease, conditions that predispose patient to hypotension, history of seizures or conditions that might lower the seizure threshold, and hepatic impairment. Also use cautiously in elderly patients, those with a history of paralytic ileus, and those at risk for aspi-

ration pneumonia, prostatic hypertrophy, or narrow-angle glaucoma.
• Know that drug should be used in pregnancy only if the benefit justifies the potential risk to the fetus. Women taking drug should not breast-feed.
• Know that safety and effectiveness in patients under 18 years have not been established.
• Monitor patient for signs of neuroleptic malignant syndrome (hyperpyrexia, muscle rigidity, altered mental status, autonomic instability)—a rare but frequently fatal adverse reaction that can occur with the administration of antipsychotic drugs. Drug should be stopped immediately and patient monitored and treated as required.
• Monitor patient for tardive dyskinesia, which may occur after prolonged use. It may not appear until months or years later and may disappear spontaneously or persist for life, despite discontinuation of drug.
• Obtain baseline and periodic liver function tests, as ordered.

☑ **Patient teaching**
• Warn patient to avoid hazardous tasks until adverse CNS effects of drug are known.
• Warn patient against exposure to extreme heat; drug may impair the body's ability to reduce core temperature.
• Tell patient to avoid alcohol.
• Tell patient to rise slowly to avoid orthostatic hypotension.
• Instruct patient to relieve dry mouth with ice chips or sugarless candy or gum.
• Advise female patient to notify doctor if she becomes pregnant or intends to become pregnant during drug therapy. Advise her not to breast-feed during therapy.

---

perphenazine
Apo-Perphenazine†, Fentazin§, PMS Perphenazine†, Trilafon, Trilafon Concentrate

Pregnancy Risk Category: NR

HOW SUPPLIED
Tablets: 2 mg, 4 mg, 8 mg, 16 mg
Oral concentrate: 16 mg/5 ml

Syrup: 2 mg/5 ml†
Injection: 5 mg/ml

ACTION
Unknown. Probably exerts its antipsychotic effects by blocking postsynaptic dopamine receptors in the brain and inhibits the medullary chemoreceptor trigger zone.

Route	Onset	Peak	Duration
PO, IM, IV	Unknown	Unknown	Unknown

INDICATIONS & DOSAGE
Psychosis in nonhospitalized patients—
Adults: initially, 4 to 8 mg P.O. t.i.d., reduced as soon as possible to minimum effective dosage.
Children over 12 years: lowest adult dosage.
Psychosis in hospitalized patients—
Adults: initially, 8 to 16 mg P.O. b.i.d., t.i.d., or q.i.d., increased to 64 mg daily, p.r.n. Alternatively, 5 to 10 mg I.M. q 6 hours, p.r.n. Maximum dosage is 30 mg.
Children over 12 years: lowest limit of adult dosage.
Severe nausea and vomiting—
Adults: 8 to 16 mg P.O. daily in divided doses up to maximum of 24 mg. Alternatively, 5 to 10 mg I.M., p.r.n. May be given I.V., diluted to 0.5 mg/ml with saline solution. Dosage should not exceed 5 mg.

ADVERSE REACTIONS
CNS: *extrapyramidal reactions, tardive dyskinesia,* sedation, pseudoparkinsonism, dizziness, **seizures,** drowsiness.
CV: *orthostatic hypotension,* tachycardia, ECG changes.
EENT: ocular changes, *blurred vision,* nasal congestion.
GI: *dry mouth, constipation,* nausea, vomiting, diarrhea.
GU: *urine retention,* dark urine, menstrual irregularities, gynecomastia, inhibited ejaculation.
Hematologic: **leukopenia, agranulocytosis,** eosinophilia, **hemolytic anemia, thrombocytopenia.**
Hepatic: jaundice.
Skin: *mild photosensitivity,* allergic reactions, pain at I.M. injection site, sterile abscess.

Reactions may be *common,* uncommon, *life-threatening*, or COMMON AND LIFE-THREATENING.

Other: weight gain, *neuroleptic malignant syndrome.*
After abrupt withdrawal of long-term therapy: gastritis, nausea, vomiting, dizziness, tremor, feeling of warmth or cold, diaphoresis, tachycardia, headache, insomnia.

INTERACTIONS
Drug-drug. *Antacids:* inhibited absorption of oral phenothiazines. Separate antacid and phenothiazine doses by at least 2 hours.
Barbiturates: may decrease phenothiazine effect. Observe patient.
CNS depressants: increased CNS depression. Avoid concomitant use.
Drug-lifestyle. *Alcohol use:* increased CNS depression. Avoid concomitant use.
Sun exposure: photosensitivity reactions may occur. Take precautions.

EFFECTS ON DIAGNOSTIC TESTS
Drug causes false-positive test results for urinary porphyrins, urobilinogen, amylase, and 5-hydroxyindoleacetic acid because of darkening of urine by metabolites; it also causes false-positive urine pregnancy test results using human chorionic gonadotropin. Drug elevates test results for liver enzymes and protein-bound iodine and causes quinidine-like effects on the ECG.

CONTRAINDICATIONS
Contraindicated in patients with CNS depression, blood dyscrasia, bone marrow depression, liver damage, subcortical damage, or hypersensitivity to drug; in patients experiencing coma; and in those receiving large doses of CNS depressants.

NURSING CONSIDERATIONS
● Use cautiously with other CNS depressants or anticholinergics, and in elderly or debilitated patients.
● Use cautiously in patients with alcohol withdrawal, psychic depression, suicidal tendency, severe adverse reactions to other phenothiazines, impaired renal function, CV disease, and respiratory disorders.
● Obtain baseline measures of blood pressure before starting therapy and monitor

regularly. Watch for orthostatic hypotension, especially with parenteral administration. Keep patient supine for 1 hour after administration of drug; tell him to change positions slowly.
● Prevent contact dermatitis by keeping drug away from skin and clothes. Wear gloves when preparing liquid forms.
● Dilute liquid concentrate with fruit juice, milk, carbonated beverage, or semisolid food just before giving. Exceptions: Oral concentrate causes turbidity or precipitation in colas, black coffee, grape or apple juice, or tea. Do not mix with these liquids.
● Protect drug from light. Slight yellowing of injection or concentrate is common and does not affect potency. Discard markedly discolored solutions.
● Give deep I.M. only in upper outer quadrant of buttocks. Massage slowly afterward to prevent sterile abscess. Injection may sting.
● Monitor patient for tardive dyskinesia, which may occur after prolonged use. It may not appear until months or years later and disappear spontaneously or persist for life, despite discontinuation of drug.
● Assess patient for neuroleptic malignant syndrome (extrapyramidal effects, hyperthermia, autonomic disturbance). It is rare, but frequently fatal. It is not necessarily related to length of drug use or type of neuroleptic, but over 60% of affected patients are men.
● Monitor therapy with weekly bilirubin tests during 1st month, periodic blood tests (CBC and liver function), and ophthalmic tests (long-term use), as ordered.
● Do not withdraw drug abruptly unless required by severe adverse reactions.
● Withhold dose and notify doctor if patient develops jaundice, symptoms of blood dyscrasia (fever, sore throat, infection, cellulitis, weakness), or persistent extrapyramidal reactions (longer than a few hours).

☑ Patient teaching
● Tell patient what beverages to use to dilute oral concentrate.
● Warn patient to avoid activities that require alertness or good psychomotor coordination until CNS effects of drug are

known. Drowsiness and dizziness usually subside after a few weeks.
• Tell patient to avoid alcohol while taking drug.
• Advise patient to report urine retention or constipation.
• Tell patient to use sunblock and to wear protective clothing to avoid photosensitivity reactions.
• Advise patient to relieve dry mouth with sugarless gum or hard candy.

---

pimozide
Orap

Pregnancy Risk Category: C

HOW SUPPLIED
Tablets: 2 mg, 4 mg†, 10 mg

ACTION
Unknown. Thought to block dopamine nonselectively at both the presynaptic and postsynaptic receptors on neurons in the CNS.

Route	Onset	Peak	Duration
PO	Unknown	4-12 hr	Unknown

INDICATIONS & DOSAGE
Suppression of motor and phonic tics in patients with Tourette syndrome refractory to first-line therapy—
Adults and children over 12 years: initially, 1 to 2 mg P.O. daily in divided doses; then increased every other day, p.r.n. Maintenance dose: under 0.2 mg/kg/day or 10 mg/day, whichever is less. Maximum dosage is 10 mg daily.

ADVERSE REACTIONS
CNS: *parkinsonian-like symptoms,* drowsiness, headache, insomnia, other extrapyramidal symptoms (dystonia, akathisia, hyperreflexia, opisthotonos, oculogyric crisis), *tardive dyskinesia, sedation.*
CV: *ECG changes (prolonged QT interval),* hypotension, hypertension, tachycardia.
EENT: visual disturbances.
GI: *dry mouth, constipation.*
GU: impotence, urinary frequency.
Skin: rash, diaphoresis.

Other: *neuroleptic malignant syndrome,* muscle rigidity.

INTERACTIONS
Drug-drug. *Antiarrhythmics, phenothiazines, tricyclic antidepressants:* increased incidence of ECG abnormalities. Monitor patient closely.
CNS depressants: increased CNS depression. Avoid concomitant use.
Drug-lifestyle. *Alcohol use:* increased CNS depression. Avoid concomitant use.

EFFECTS ON DIAGNOSTIC TESTS
Drug causes quinidine-like ECG effects (including prolongation of QT interval and flattened T waves).

CONTRAINDICATIONS
Contraindicated in patients with hypersensitivity to drug, in the treatment of simple tics or tics other than those associated with Tourette syndrome, and in concurrent drug therapy known to cause motor and phonic tics. Also contraindicated in patients with congenital long QT syndrome or history of arrhythmias, severe toxic CNS depression, and in those experiencing coma.

NURSING CONSIDERATIONS
• Use cautiously in patients with hepatic or renal dysfunction, glaucoma, prostatic hyperplasia, seizure disorder, or EEG abnormalities.
Alert: Perform an ECG before treatment begins and periodically thereafter as ordered. Monitor for prolonged QT interval.
• Know that concurrent administration of other drugs that prolong the QT interval, such as antiarrhythmics, should be avoided.
• Monitor patient for tardive dyskinesia, which may occur after prolonged use. It may not appear until months or years later and may disappear spontaneously or persist for life, despite discontinuation of drug.
• Assess patient for neuroleptic malignant syndrome (extrapyramidal effects, hyperthermia, autonomic disturbance). It is rare, but frequently fatal. It is not necessarily related to length of drug use or type

---

Reactions may be *common,* uncommon, *life-threatening,* or COMMON AND LIFE-THREATENING.

of neuroleptic, but over 60% of affected patients are men.
• Monitor patients who also are taking anticonvulsants for increased seizure activity. Pimozide may lower the seizure threshold.

☑ Patient teaching
• Warn patient not to stop taking drug abruptly and not to exceed prescribed dosage.
• Tell patient to avoid alcohol while taking drug.
• Advise patient to use sugarless hard candy, gum, and liquids to relieve dry mouth.

---

quetiapine fumarate
Seroquel

Pregnancy Risk Category: C

HOW SUPPLIED
Tablets: 25 mg, 100 mg, 200 mg

ACTION
Unknown. A dibenzoxazepine that may block dopamine D-2 receptors and serotonin 5-HT$_2$ receptors in the brain and may also act as H$_1$ receptors and adrenergic-alpha$_1$ receptors.

Route	Onset	Peak	Duration
PO	Unknown	1.5 hr	Unknown

INDICATIONS & DOSAGE
Management of the manifestations of psychotic disorders—
Adults: initially, 25 mg b.i.d., with increases in increments of 25 to 50 mg b.i.d. or t.i.d. on days 2 and 3, as tolerated. Target dosage range of 300 to 400 mg daily, divided into two or three doses, by day 4. Further dosage adjustments, if indicated, should generally occur at intervals of not less than 2 days. Dosages can be increased or decreased by 25 to 50 mg b.i.d. Antipsychotic efficacy is generally in the dosage range of 150 to 750 mg/day. Safety of dosages above 800 mg/day has not been evaluated.
Elderly: lower doses, slower titration, and

careful monitoring in the initial dosing period.
Adjust-a-dose: In patients with hepatic impairment or hypotension or in debilitated patients, consider lower doses and slower titration.

ADVERSE REACTIONS
CNS: *dizziness, headache, somnolence,* hypertonia, dysarthria.
CV: orthostatic hypotension, tachycardia, palpitations, peripheral edema.
EENT: ear pain, pharyngitis, rhinitis.
GI: dry mouth, dyspepsia, abdominal pain, constipation, anorexia.
Hematologic: *leukopenia.*
Metabolic: *weight gain.*
Respiratory: increased cough, dyspnea.
Skin: rash, diaphoresis.
Other: asthenia, back pain, fever, flulike syndrome.

INTERACTIONS
Drug-drug. *Antihypertensive agents:* increased effects. Monitor blood pressure.
Carbamazepine, glucocorticoids, phenobarbital, phenytoin, rifampin: increased quetiapine clearance. Adjust quetiapine dose as needed.
CNS depressants: increased CNS effects. Use cautiously.
Erythromycin, fluconazole, itraconazole, ketoconazole: decreased quetiapine clearance. Use cautiously.
Lorazepam: reduced clearance of lorazepam. Monitor patient.
Drug-lifestyle. *Alcohol use:* increased CNS effects. Use cautiously.

EFFECTS ON DIAGNOSTIC TESTS
Asymptomatic increases in ALT and increases in both total cholesterol and triglycerides have occurred. Decreases in T$_4$ and thyroid-stimulating hormone levels have been observed.

CONTRAINDICATIONS
Contraindicated in patients hypersensitive to drug or its ingredients.

NURSING CONSIDERATIONS
• Use with caution in patients with CV or cerebrovascular disease or conditions that predispose patients to hypotension, in

---

those with a history of seizures or conditions that lower the seizure threshold, and in patients who will be experiencing conditions in which the core body temperature may be elevated.

• Watch for symptoms of neuroleptic malignant syndrome (extrapyramidal effects, hyperthermia, autonomic disturbance). It is rare, but frequently fatal. It is not necessarily related to length of drug use or type of neuroleptic, but over 60% of affected patients are men.

• Monitor patient for tardive dyskinesia, which may occur after prolonged use. It may not appear until months or years later and may disappear spontaneously or persist for life, despite discontinuation of drug.

• Dispense the lowest appropriate quantity of drug to reduce risk of overdose.

☑ **Patient teaching**

• Advise patient of risk of orthostatic hypotension. The risk is greatest during the 3- to 5-day period of initial dose titration, when reinitiating treatment, or when increasing dosages.

• Tell patient to avoid becoming overheated or dehydrated.

• During the initial dose titration period or dosage increases, warn patient to avoid activities that require mental alertness, such as driving a car or operating hazardous machinery, until CNS effects of drug are known.

• Remind patient to have an initial eye examination at the beginning of quetiapine therapy and every 6 months while on drug to monitor for possibility of cataract formation.

• Tell patient to notify doctor of other medications (prescription or OTC) he is taking or plans to take.

• Tell female patient to notify doctor if she becomes pregnant or intends to become pregnant during drug therapy. Advise her not to breast-feed during therapy.

• Advise patient to avoid alcohol while taking drug.

---

risperidone
Risperdal

Pregnancy Risk Category: C

HOW SUPPLIED
Tablets: 1 mg, 2 mg, 3 mg, 4 mg

ACTION
Blocks dopamine and serotonin receptors; also blocks alpha$_1$, alpha$_2$, and H$_1$ receptors in the CNS.

Route	Onset	Peak	Duration
PO	Unknown	1 hr	Unknown

INDICATIONS & DOSAGE
Psychosis—
Adults: initially, 1 mg P.O. b.i.d. Increased in increments of 1 mg b.i.d. on days 2 and 3 of treatment to a target dosage of 3 mg b.i.d. At least 1 week must pass before dosage is adjusted further. Safety of dosages exceeding 16 mg/day has not been evaluated.
Elderly: initially, 0.5 mg P.O. b.i.d. Increased in increments of 0.5 mg b.i.d. on days 2 and 3 of treatment to a target dosage of 1.5 mg P.O. b.i.d. At least 1 week must pass before dosage is increased further.
Adjust-a-dose: In patients with severe renal or hepatic impairment or hypotension or in debilitated patients, initially, 0.5 mg P.O. b.i.d. Increased in increments of 0.5 mg b.i.d. on days 2 and 3 of treatment to a target dosage of 1.5 mg P.O. b.i.d. At least 1 week must pass before dosage is increased further.

ADVERSE REACTIONS
CNS: *somnolence, extrapyramidal symptoms,* headache, *insomnia, agitation, anxiety,* tardive dyskinesia, aggressiveness.
CV: tachycardia, chest pain, orthostatic hypotension, ***prolonged QT interval.***
EENT: *rhinitis,* coughing, upper respiratory infection, sinusitis, pharyngitis, abnormal vision.
GI: *constipation, nausea, vomiting, dyspepsia.*
Skin: rash, dry skin, photosensitivity.

Reactions may be *common,* uncommon, *life-threatening*, or COMMON AND LIFE-THREATENING.

Other: arthralgia; back pain; fever; rarely, *neuroleptic malignant syndrome.*

INTERACTIONS
Drug-drug. *Carbamazepine:* increased clearance of risperidone, leading to decreased effectiveness. Monitor patient closely.
Clozapine: decreased clearance of risperidone, increasing toxicity. Monitor patient closely.
CNS depressants: additive CNS depression. Avoid concomitant use.
Levodopa: antagonized effects. Avoid concomitant use.
Drug-lifestyle. *Alcohol use:* additive CNS depression. Avoid concomitant use.
Sun exposure: photosensitivity reactions may occur. Take precautions.

EFFECTS ON DIAGNOSTIC TESTS
Drug may increase serum prolactin levels.

CONTRAINDICATIONS
Contraindicated in patients hypersensitive to drug and in breast-feeding patients.

NURSING CONSIDERATIONS
• Use cautiously in patients with prolonged QT interval, CV disease, cerebrovascular disease, dehydration, hypovolemia, history of seizures, exposure to extreme heat, or conditions that could affect metabolism or hemodynamic responses.
Alert: Obtain baseline measures of blood pressure before starting therapy, and monitor regularly. Watch for orthostatic hypotension, especially during initial dosage titration.
• Monitor patient for tardive dyskinesia, which may occur after prolonged use. It may not appear until months or years later and disappear spontaneously or persist for life, despite discontinuation of drug.
• Assess for neuroleptic malignant syndrome (extrapyramidal effects, hyperthermia, autonomic disturbance). It is rare, but frequently fatal. It is not necessarily related to length of drug use or type of neuroleptic, but over 60% of patients are men.

☑ **Patient teaching**
• Warn patient to avoid activities that require alertness until CNS effects of drug are known.
• Warn patient to rise slowly, avoid hot showers, and use extra caution during first few days of therapy to avoid fainting.
• Advise patient to use caution in hot weather to prevent heatstroke.
• Tell patient to avoid alcohol.
• Tell patient to use sunblock and to wear protective clothing outdoors.
• Advise female patient to notify doctor if she is or plans to become pregnant during therapy.

thioridazine hydrochloride
Aldazine‡, Apo-Thioridazine†, Mellaril*, Mellaril Concentrate, Novo-Ridazine†, PMS-Thioridazine†

Pregnancy Risk Category: C

HOW SUPPLIED
Tablets: 10 mg, 15 mg, 25 mg, 50 mg, 100 mg, 150 mg, 200 mg
Oral suspension: 25 mg/5 ml, 100 mg/5 ml
Oral concentrate: 30 mg/ml, 100 mg/ml (3% to 4.2% alcohol)

ACTION
Unknown. A piperidine phenothiazine that probably blocks postsynaptic dopamine receptors in the brain.

Route	Onset	Peak	Duration
PO	Unknown	Unknown	Unknown

INDICATIONS & DOSAGE
Psychosis—
Adults: initially, 50 to 100 mg P.O. t.i.d., increased gradually to 800 mg daily in divided doses, if needed. Dosage varies.
Short-term treatment of moderate to marked depression with variable degrees of anxiety; treatment of multiple symptoms, such as agitation, anxiety, depressed mood, tension, sleep disturbances, and fears—
Adults: initially, 25 mg P.O. t.i.d. Maximum daily dosage is 200 mg.

Elderly: initially, 25 mg P.O. t.i.d. Maximum daily dosage is 200 mg.
Children 2 to 12 years: 0.5 to 3 mg/kg P.O. daily in divided doses.

ADVERSE REACTIONS
CNS: extrapyramidal reactions (low incidence), *tardive dyskinesia, sedation* (high incidence), EEG changes, dizziness.
CV: *orthostatic hypotension,* tachycardia, ECG changes.
EENT: *ocular changes, blurred vision,* retinitis pigmentosa.
GI: *dry mouth, constipation.*
GU: *urine retention,* dark urine, menstrual irregularities, gynecomastia, inhibited ejaculation.
Hematologic: *transient leukopenia, agranulocytosis,* hyperprolactinemia.
Hepatic: cholestatic jaundice.
Skin: *mild photosensitivity,* allergic reactions.
Other: weight gain; increased appetite; rarely, *neuroleptic malignant syndrome.*
After abrupt withdrawal of long-term therapy: gastritis, nausea, vomiting, dizziness, tremor, feeling of warmth or cold, diaphoresis, tachycardia, headache, insomnia.

INTERACTIONS
Drug-drug. *Antacids:* inhibited absorption of oral phenothiazines. Separate antacid and phenothiazine doses by at least 2 hours.
Barbiturates, lithium: may decrease phenothiazine effect. Observe patient.
Centrally acting antihypertensives: decreased antihypertensive effect. Monitor blood pressure.
Other CNS depressants: increased CNS depression. Use together cautiously.
Drug-lifestyle. *Alcohol use:* increased CNS depression. Avoid concomitant use.
Sun exposure: photosensitivity reactions may occur. Take precautions.

EFFECTS ON DIAGNOSTIC TESTS
Drug causes false-positive test results for urinary porphyrins, urobilinogen, amylase, and 5-hydroxyindoleacetic acid because of darkening of urine by metabolites; it also causes false-positive urine pregnancy results in tests using human chorionic gonadotropin as the indicator. Drug elevates test results for liver enzymes and protein-bound iodine and causes quinidine-like effects on the ECG.

CONTRAINDICATIONS
Contraindicated in patients with hypersensitivity to drug or in those experiencing coma, severe hypertensive or hypotensive cardiac disease, or CNS depression.

NURSING CONSIDERATIONS
• Use cautiously in elderly or debilitated patients and in patients with hepatic disease, CV disease, exposure to extreme heat or cold (including antipyretic therapy) or organophosphate insecticides, respiratory disorder, hypocalcemia, seizure disorder, or severe reactions to insulin or electroconvulsive therapy.
Alert: Remember that different liquid formulations have different concentrations. Check dosage carefully.
• Prevent contact dermatitis by keeping drug away from skin and clothes. Wear gloves when preparing liquid forms.
• Dilute liquid concentrate with water or fruit juice just before giving.
• Shake suspension well before using.
• Monitor patient for tardive dyskinesia, which may occur after prolonged use. It may not appear until months or years later and disappear spontaneously or persist for life, despite discontinuation of drug.
• Assess for neuroleptic malignant syndrome (extrapyramidal effects, hyperthermia, autonomic disturbance). It is rare, but frequently fatal. Not necessarily related to length of drug use or type of neuroleptic, but over 60% of patients are men.
• Monitor therapy with weekly bilirubin tests during 1st month, periodic blood tests (CBC and liver function), and ophthalmic tests (long-term use).
• Do not stop drug abruptly unless required by severe adverse reactions.
• Withhold dose and notify doctor if patient develops jaundice, blood dyscrasia (fever, sore throat, infection, cellulitis, weakness), or persistent extrapyramidal reactions, especially in pregnant patients or in children.

☑ Patient teaching

• Tell patient to shake suspension before use.

• Warn patient to avoid activities that require alertness until CNS effects of drug are known.

• Tell patient to watch for orthostatic hypotension, especially with parenteral administration. Advise patient to change positions slowly.

• Tell patient to avoid alcohol.

• Have patient report urine retention, constipation, or blurred vision.

• Tell patient that drug may discolor the urine.

• Advise patient to relieve dry mouth with sugarless gum or hard candy.

• Instruct patient to use sunblock and to wear protective clothing outdoors.

---

thiothixene
Navane

thiothixene hydrochloride
Navane*

Pregnancy Risk Category: C

HOW SUPPLIED
thiothixene
Capsules: 1 mg, 2 mg, 5 mg, 10 mg, 20 mg
thiothixene hydrochloride
Oral concentrate: 5 mg/ml (7% alcohol)
Injection: 2 mg/ml, 5 mg/ml

ACTION
Unknown. A thioxanthene that probably blocks postsynaptic dopamine receptors in the brain.

Route	Onset	Peak	Duration
PO, IM	Unknown	Unknown	Unknown

INDICATIONS & DOSAGE
Mild to moderate psychosis—
Adults: initially, 2 mg P.O. t.i.d. Increased gradually to 15 mg daily, p.r.n.
Severe psychosis—
Adults: initially, 5 mg P.O. b.i.d. Increased gradually to 20 to 30 mg daily, p.r.n. Maximum recommended dosage is 60 mg daily. Alternatively, 4 mg I.M. b.i.d. to q.i.d. Maximum dosage is 30 mg I.M. daily. Switch to oral form as soon as possible.

ADVERSE REACTIONS
CNS: *extrapyramidal reactions,* drowsiness, restlessness, agitation, insomnia, *tardive dyskinesia,* sedation, pseudoparkinsonism, EEG changes, dizziness.
CV: *hypotension,* tachycardia, ECG changes.
EENT: ocular changes, *blurred vision,* nasal congestion.
GI: *dry mouth, constipation.*
GU: *urine retention,* menstrual irregularities, gynecomastia, inhibited ejaculation.
Hematologic: *transient leukopenia,* leukocytosis, *agranulocytosis.*
Hepatic: jaundice.
Skin: *mild photosensitivity,* allergic reactions, pain at I.M. injection site, sterile abscess.
Other: weight gain, *neuroleptic malignant syndrome.*
After abrupt withdrawal of long-term therapy: gastritis, nausea, vomiting, dizziness, tremor, feeling of warmth or cold, diaphoresis, tachycardia, headache, insomnia.

INTERACTIONS
Drug-drug. *CNS depressants:* increased CNS depression. Avoid concomitant use.
Drug-herb. *Nutmeg:* may reduce effectiveness or interfere with drug therapy. Avoid concomitant use.
Drug-lifestyle. *Alcohol use:* increased CNS depression. Avoid concomitant use.
Sun exposure: photosensitivity reactions may occur. Take precautions.

EFFECTS ON DIAGNOSTIC TESTS
Drug causes false-positive test results for urinary porphyrins, urobilinogen, amylase, and 5-hydroxyindoleacetic acid because of darkening of urine by metabolites; it also causes false-positive urine pregnancy results in tests using human chorionic gonadotropin as the indicator. Thiothixene elevates test results for liver enzymes and protein-bound iodine and causes quinidine-like effects on the ECG.

CONTRAINDICATIONS
Contraindicated in patients with hypersensitivity to drug or in those experiencing circulatory collapse, coma, CNS depression, or blood dyscrasia.

NURSING CONSIDERATIONS
• Use with extreme caution in patients with history of seizure disorder or in a state of alcohol withdrawal.
• Use cautiously in elderly or debilitated patients and in those with CV disease (may cause sudden drop in blood pressure), hepatic disease, heat exposure, glaucoma, or prostatic hyperplasia.
• Prevent contact dermatitis by keeping drug off skin and clothes. Wear gloves when preparing liquid forms.
• Dilute liquid concentrate with fruit juice, milk, or semisolid food just before administering.
• Know that slight yellowing of injection or concentrate is common and does not affect potency. Discard markedly discolored solutions.
• Give I.M. only in upper outer quadrant of buttocks or midlateral thigh. Massage slowly afterward to prevent sterile abscess. Injection may sting.
• Monitor patient for tardive dyskinesia, which may occur after prolonged use; it may not appear until months or years later and disappear spontaneously or persist for life, despite discontinuation of drug.
• Assess for neuroleptic malignant syndrome (extrapyramidal effects, hyperthermia, autonomic disturbance). It is rare, but frequently fatal. Not necessarily related to length of drug use or type of neuroleptic, but over 60% of patients are men.
• Do not withdraw drug abruptly unless required by severe adverse reactions.
• Withhold dose and notify doctor if patient develops jaundice, blood dyscrasia (fever, sore throat, infection, cellulitis, weakness), or persistent extrapyramidal reactions, especially in pregnant patients.
• Monitor therapy with weekly bilirubin tests during 1st month, periodic blood tests (CBC and liver function), and ophthalmic tests (long-term use).
• Watch for orthostatic hypotension, especially with parenteral administration.

Keep the patient supine for 1 hour after drug administration and tell him to change positions slowly.

☑ **Patient teaching**
• Warn patient to avoid activities that require alertness until CNS effects of drug are known.
• Tell patient to watch for orthostatic hypotension. Advise him to change positions slowly.
• Instruct patient to dilute liquid appropriately.
• Tell patient to avoid alcohol.
• Have him report urine retention, constipation, or blurred vision.
• Instruct patient to use sunblock and to wear protective clothing outdoors.

---

trifluoperazine hydrochloride
Apo-Trifluoperazine†, Novo-Flurazine†, PMS-Trifluoperazine†, Solazine†, Stelazine, Stelazine Concentrate, Terfluzine†, Terfluzine Concentrate†

Pregnancy Risk Category: NR

HOW SUPPLIED
Tablets (regular and film-coated): 1 mg, 2 mg, 5 mg, 10 mg
Oral concentrate: 10 mg/ml
Injection: 2 mg/ml

ACTION
Unknown. A piperazine phenothiazine that probably blocks postsynaptic dopamine receptors in the brain.

Route	Onset	Peak	Duration
PO, IM	Unknown	Unknown	Unknown

INDICATIONS & DOSAGE
Anxiety states—
Adults: 1 to 2 mg P.O. b.i.d. Maximum dosage is 6 mg/day. Do not use drug for more than 12 weeks for this indication.
Schizophrenia and other psychotic disorders—
Adults: 2 to 5 mg P.O. b.i.d., gradually increased until therapeutic response. Or 1 to 2 mg deep I.M. q 4 to 6 hours, p.r.n. Most patients respond to 15 to 20 mg P.O. daily,

although some may require dosages of 40 mg/day or more. More than 6 mg I.M. in 24 hours is rarely required.

Children 6 to 12 years (hospitalized or under close supervision): 1 mg P.O. daily or b.i.d.; may increase gradually to 15 mg daily, if needed.

ADVERSE REACTIONS
CNS: *extrapyramidal reactions, tardive dyskinesia,* pseudoparkinsonism, dizziness, drowsiness, insomnia, fatigue, headache.
CV: *orthostatic hypotension,* tachycardia, ECG changes.
EENT: ocular changes, *blurred vision.*
GI: *dry mouth, constipation,* nausea.
GU: *urine retention.*
Hematologic: *transient leukopenia, agranulocytosis.*
Hepatic: cholestatic jaundice.
Skin: *photosensitivity,* allergic reactions, pain at I.M. injection site, sterile abscess, rash.
Other: weight gain; *neuroleptic malignant syndrome,* menstrual irregularities, gynecomastia, inhibited lactation.
After abrupt withdrawal of long-term therapy: gastritis, nausea, vomiting, dizziness, tremor, feeling of warmth or cold, diaphoresis, tachycardia, headache, insomnia, anorexia, muscle rigidity, altered mental status, evidence of autonomic instability.

INTERACTIONS
Drug-drug. *Antacids:* inhibited absorption of oral phenothiazines. Separate antacid and phenothiazine doses by at least 2 hours.
Barbiturates, lithium: may decrease phenothiazine effect. Monitor patient.
Centrally acting antihypertensives: decreased antihypertensive effect. Monitor blood pressure.
CNS depressants: increased CNS depression. Use together cautiously.
Propranolol: increased levels of both propranolol and trifluoperazine. Monitor closely.
Warfarin: decreased effect of oral anticoagulants. Monitor PT and INR.
Drug-lifestyle. *Alcohol use:* increased CNS depression. Avoid concomitant use.

Sun exposure: photosensitivity reactions may occur. Take precautions.

EFFECTS ON DIAGNOSTIC TESTS
Drug causes false-positive test results for urinary porphyrins, urobilinogen, amylase, and 5-hydroxyindoleacetic acid because of darkening of urine by metabolites; it also causes false-positive urine pregnancy results in tests using human chorionic gonadotropin as the indicator. Trifluoperazine elevates test results for liver enzymes and protein-bound iodine and causes quinidine-like effects on the ECG.

CONTRAINDICATIONS
Contraindicated in patients with hypersensitivity to phenothiazines or in those experiencing coma, CNS depression, bone marrow suppression, or liver damage.

NURSING CONSIDERATIONS
• Use cautiously in elderly or debilitated patients and in patients with CV disease (may cause drop in blood pressure), exposure to extreme heat, seizure disorder, glaucoma, or prostatic hyperplasia.
• Wear gloves when preparing liquid forms.
• Dilute liquid concentrate with 60 ml of tomato or fruit juice, carbonated beverages, coffee, tea, milk, water, or semisolid food just before giving.
• Protect drug from light. Slight yellowing of injection or concentrate is common and does not affect potency. Discard markedly discolored solutions.
• Give deeply I.M. only in upper outer quadrant of buttocks. Massage slowly afterward to prevent sterile abscess. Injection may sting.
• Watch for orthostatic hypotension, especially with parenteral administration. Keep patient supine for 1 hour after drug administration, and tell him to change positions slowly.
• Monitor patient for tardive dyskinesia, which may occur after prolonged use. It may not appear until months or years later and disappear spontaneously or persist for life, despite discontinuation of drug.
• Assess for neuroleptic malignant syn-

drome (extrapyramidal effects, hyperthermia, autonomic disturbance). It is rare, but frequently fatal. It is not necessarily related to length of drug use or type of neuroleptic, but over 60% of patients are men.

• Do not withdraw drug abruptly unless severe adverse reactions occur.

• Withhold dose and notify doctor if patient develops jaundice, symptoms of blood dyscrasia (fever, sore throat, infection, cellulitis, weakness), or persistent extrapyramidal reactions (longer than a few hours), especially in pregnant patients or in children.

• Monitor therapy with weekly bilirubin tests during 1st month, periodic blood tests (CBC and liver function), and ophthalmic tests (long-term use).

☑ Patient teaching

• Warn patient to avoid activities that require alertness until CNS effects of drug are known.

• Tell patient to avoid alcohol.

• Instruct patient to properly dilute liquid.

• Tell patient to report urine retention or constipation.

• Tell patient to use sunblock and to wear protective clothing outdoors.

• Advise patient to relieve dry mouth with sugarless gum or hard candy.

amphetamine sulfate
caffeine
dextroamphetamine sulfate
diethylpropion hydrochloride
doxapram hydrochloride
methamphetamine
  hydrochloride
methylphenidate hydrochloride
pemoline
phentermine hydrochloride

COMBINATION PRODUCTS

ADDERALL 5 MG: amphetamine aspartate 1.25 mg, amphetamine sulfate 1.25 mg, dextroamphetamine saccharate 1.25 mg, dextroamphetamine sulfate 1.25 mg, total amphetamine base equivalence 3.13 mg.
ADDERALL 10 MG: amphetamine aspartate 2.5 mg, amphetamine sulfate 2.5 mg, dextroamphetamine saccharate 2.5 mg, dextroamphetamine sulfate 2.5 mg, total amphetamine base equivalence 6.3 mg.
ADDERALL 20 MG: amphetamine aspartate 5 mg, amphetamine sulfate 5 mg, dextroamphetamine saccharate 5 mg, dextroamphetamine sulfate 5 mg, total amphetamine base equivalence 12.6 mg.
ADDERALL 30 MG: amphetamine aspartate 7.5 mg, amphetamine sulfate 7.5 mg, dextroamphetamine saccharate 7.5 mg, dextroamphetamine sulfate 7.5 mg, total amphetamine base equivalence 18.8 mg.

---

amphetamine sulfate

Controlled Substance Schedule II
Pregnancy Risk Category: C

HOW SUPPLIED
Tablets: 5 mg, 10 mg

ACTION
Unknown. Probably promotes nerve impulse transmission by releasing stored norepinephrine from nerve terminals in the brain. Main sites of activity appear to be the cerebral cortex and the reticular activating system.

Route	Onset	Peak	Duration
PO	Unknown	Unknown	Unknown

INDICATIONS & DOSAGE
Attention deficit disorder with hyperactivity—
Children 3 to 5 years: 2.5 mg P.O. daily, with dosage increases in 2.5-mg increments weekly, p.r.n.
Children 6 years and older: 5 mg P.O. daily to b.i.d., with dosage increases in 5-mg increments weekly, p.r.n. Give first dose on awakening; additional doses (one or two) at intervals of 4 to 6 hours. Dosage rarely exceeds 40 mg/day.
Narcolepsy—
Adults and children 12 years and older: 10 mg P.O. daily. Dosage increased in 10-mg increments weekly, p.r.n. Daily dosage may be divided with first dose given on awakening, additional doses at intervals of 4 to 6 hours.
Children 6 to 12 years: 5 mg P.O. daily. Dosage increased in 5-mg increments weekly, p.r.n. Daily dosage may be divided with first dose given on awakening, additional doses at intervals of 4 to 6 hours.
Short-term adjunct in exogenous obesity—
Adults: 5 to 30 mg P.O. daily in divided doses 30 to 60 minutes before meals.

ADVERSE REACTIONS
CNS: *restlessness,* tremor, *hyperactivity, talkativeness, insomnia,* irritability, dizziness, headache, chills, dysphoria, euphoria.
CV: *tachycardia, palpitations,* hypertension, *arrhythmias.*
GI: dry mouth, metallic taste, diarrhea, constipation, anorexia, weight loss.
GU: impotence.
Skin: urticaria.
Other: altered libido.

INTERACTIONS

Drug-drug. *Acetazolamide, antacids, sodium bicarbonate:* increased renal reabsorption. Monitor for enhanced effect.
Ammonium chloride, ascorbic acid: decreased serum levels and increased renal excretion of amphetamine. Monitor for decreased amphetamine effect.
Antihypertensives: reversal of antihypertensive action. Monitor blood pressure.
Haloperidol, phenothiazines, tricyclic antidepressants: altered CNS effect. Avoid concomitant use.
Insulin, oral antidiabetic agents: may decrease antidiabetic agent requirements. Monitor blood glucose level.
MAO inhibitors: may cause severe hypertension, possibly hypertensive crisis. Don't use together or within 14 days after an MAO inhibitor has been discontinued.
Drug-food. *Caffeine:* may increase amphetamine and related amine effects. Avoid concomitant use.

EFFECTS ON DIAGNOSTIC TESTS

Amphetamines may elevate plasma corticosteroid levels and also may interfere with urinary steroid determinations.

CONTRAINDICATIONS

Contraindicated in patients with symptomatic CV disease, hyperthyroidism, moderate to severe hypertension, glaucoma, advanced arteriosclerosis, history of drug abuse, or hypersensitivity or idiosyncrasy to sympathomimetic amines; within 14 days of MAO inhibitor therapy; and in agitated patients.

NURSING CONSIDERATIONS

• Use cautiously in elderly, debilitated, or hyperexcitable patients or those with psychopathic personalities or history of suicidal or homicidal tendencies.
• Know that drug is not recommended for first-line treatment of obesity or for treatment of obesity in children under 12 years. Use as an anorexigenic agent is prohibited in some states.
• Be aware that drug should not be used to combat fatigue.
• Make sure obese patient is on a weight-reduction program. Give drug 30 to 60 minutes before meals. Monitor dietary intake and count calories, if necessary.
• If tolerance to anorexigenic effect develops, know that drug should be discontinued. Notify doctor.

✓ **Patient teaching**
• To avoid sleep interference, tell patient to take drug at least 6 hours before bedtime.
• Warn patient to avoid activities that require alertness or good psychomotor coordination until CNS effects of the drug are known.
• Tell patient to report signs of excessive stimulation.
• Inform patient that fatigue may result as drug effects wear off.
• Advise patient to avoid caffeine while taking drug.
• Warn patient with seizure disorder that drug may decrease seizure threshold. Instruct him to notify doctor if seizure occurs.

---

caffeine
Caffedrine Caplets◇, Dexitac◇, NoDoz◇, Quick Pep◇, Tirend◇, Vivarin◇

Pregnancy Risk Category: C

HOW SUPPLIED
Tablets: 100 mg◇, 150 mg◇, 200 mg◇
Tablets (timed-release): 200 mg◇
Capsules (timed-release): 200 mg◇
Injection: caffeine (250 mg/ml) with sodium benzoate (250 mg/ml)

ACTION
Inhibits phosphodiesterase, the enzyme that degrades cAMP.

Route	Onset	Peak	Duration
PO	Unknown	50-75 min	Unknown
IM, IV	Unknown	Unknown	Unknown

INDICATIONS & DOSAGE
CNS stimulant—
Adults: 100 to 200 mg anhydrous caffeine P.O. q 3 to 4 hours, p.r.n. Alternatively, 500 mg to 1 g I.M. (or slow I.V.).

Total daily dosage should seldom exceed 2.5 g.

ADVERSE REACTIONS
CNS: *insomnia,* restlessness, nervousness, headache, excitement, agitation, muscle tremor, twitching.
CV: *tachycardia, palpitations,* extrasystoles.
GI: nausea, vomiting, diarrhea, stomach pain.
GU: *diuresis.*
Other: abrupt withdrawal symptoms (headache, irritability), tinnitus.

INTERACTIONS
Drug-drug. *Beta-adrenergic agonists, cimetidine, fluoroquinolones, oral contraceptives, phenylpropanolamine, theophylline:* excessive CNS stimulation. Avoid concomitant use.
Drug-food. *Caffeine-containing beverages:* excessive CNS stimulation. Use cautiously.

EFFECTS ON DIAGNOSTIC TESTS
Caffeine may increase blood glucose levels and cause false-positive urate levels; it may also cause false-positive test results for pheochromocytoma or neuroblastoma by increasing certain urinary catecholamines.

CONTRAINDICATIONS
Contraindicated in patients with hypersensitivity to drug.

NURSING CONSIDERATIONS
• Use cautiously in patients with history of peptic ulcer, symptomatic arrhythmias, or palpitations, and during the first several days to weeks after an acute MI.
• Know that caffeine does not reverse alcohol intoxication or CNS depressant effects of alcohol. Overly vigorous therapy with caffeine may aggravate depression in an already depressed patient.
Alert: Be aware single dose should not exceed 1 g.
• Be alert for signs of overdose such as GI pain, mild delirium, insomnia, diuresis, dehydration, and fever. Treat with short-acting barbiturates, gastric emesis, or lavage as ordered.

• Monitor patient for tolerance or psychological dependence.
• Be aware that sudden discontinuation of caffeine may cause headache and irritability.

☑ **Patient teaching**
• Stress importance of not exceeding recommended dosage.
• Instruct patient to stop taking caffeine if increased or abnormal heart rate, dizziness, or palpitations occur.
• Inform patient that caffeine is not intended for use as a substitute for sleep.
• Advise patient to minimize use of caffeine-containing beverages while taking drug.
• Tell patient to take drug at least 6 hours before bedtime to avoid sleep interference.
• Warn patient with seizure disorder that drug may decrease seizure threshold. Instruct him to notify doctor if seizure occurs.

---

dextroamphetamine sulfate
Dexedrine* **, Dexedrine Spansule, Ferndex

Controlled Substance Schedule II
Pregnancy Risk Category: C

HOW SUPPLIED
Tablets: 5 mg, 10 mg
Capsules (extended-release): 5 mg, 10 mg, 15 mg

ACTION
Unknown. Probably promotes nerve impulse transmission by releasing stored norepinephrine from nerve terminals in the brain. Main sites of activity appear to be the cerebral cortex and the reticular activating system. In children with hyperkinesis, dextroamphetamine has a paradoxical calming effect.

Route	Onset	Peak	Duration
PO	Unknown	2 hr	Unknown
PO (extended)	Unknown	8-10 hr	Unknown

INDICATIONS & DOSAGE
Narcolepsy—
Adults: 5 to 60 mg P.O. daily in divided doses.
Children 6 to 12 years: 5 mg P.O. daily. Dosage increased in 5-mg increments weekly, p.r.n.
Children 12 years and older: 10 mg P.O. daily. Dosage increased in 10-mg increments weekly, p.r.n. Give first dose on awakening; additional doses (one or two) at intervals of 4 to 6 hours.
Short-term adjunct in exogenous obesity—
Adults and children 12 years and older: 5 to 30 mg P.O. daily 30 to 60 minutes before meals in divided doses of 5 to 10 mg. Alternatively, one 10- or 15-mg extended-release capsule daily as a single dose in the morning.
Attention deficit disorder with hyperactivity—
Children 3 to 5 years: 2.5 mg P.O. daily. Dosage increased in 2.5-mg increments weekly, p.r.n.
Children 6 years and older: 5 mg P.O. once daily or b.i.d. Dosage increased in 5-mg increments weekly, p.r.n. Only in rare cases will it be necessary to exceed a total dosage of 40 mg/day.

ADVERSE REACTIONS
CNS: *restlessness,* tremor, *insomnia,* dizziness, headache, chills, overstimulation, dysphoria, euphoria.
CV: *tachycardia, palpitations,* hypertension, ***arrhythmias.***
GI: dry mouth, unpleasant taste, diarrhea, constipation, anorexia, weight loss, other GI disturbances.
GU: impotence.
Skin: urticaria.
Other: altered libido.

INTERACTIONS
Drug-drug. *Acetazolamide, alkalizing agents, antacids, sodium bicarbonate:* increased renal reabsorption. Monitor for enhanced amphetamine effects.
Acidifying agents, ammonium chloride, ascorbic acid: decreased blood levels and increased renal clearance of dextroamphetamine. Monitor for decreased amphetamine effects.

Adrenergic blockers: adrenergic blockers inhibited by amphetamines. Avoid concomitant use.
Chlorpromazine: inhibits the central stimulant effects of amphetamines. Can be used to treat amphetamine poisoning.
Haloperidol, phenothiazines, tricyclic antidepressants: increased CNS effects. Avoid concomitant use.
Insulin, oral antidiabetic agents: may decrease antidiabetic agent requirements. Monitor blood glucose levels.
Lithium carbonate: may inhibit antiobesity and stimulating effects of amphetamines. Monitor patient closely.
MAO inhibitors: may cause severe hypertension, possibly hypertensive crisis. Don't use together or within 14 days after MAO inhibitor has been discontinued.
Meperidine: amphetamines potentiate analgesic effect. Use together cautiously.
Methenamine: increased urinary excretion of amphetamines and efficacy reduced. Monitor effects.
Norepinephrine: amphetamines enhance the adrenergic effect of norepinephrine. Monitor patient.
Phenobarbital, phenytoin: amphetamines may delay absorption. Monitor patient closely.
Drug-food. *Caffeine:* may increase amphetamine and related amine effects. Use cautiously.

EFFECTS ON DIAGNOSTIC TESTS
Drug may elevate plasma corticosteroid levels and also interfere with urinary steroid determinations.

CONTRAINDICATIONS
Contraindicated in patients with hypersensitivity or idiosyncrasy to sympathomimetic amines; within 14 days of MAO inhibitor therapy; and in those with hyperthyroidism, moderate to severe hypertension, symptomatic CV disease, glaucoma, advanced arteriosclerosis, or history of drug abuse.

NURSING CONSIDERATIONS
• Use cautiously in patients with motor and phonic tics, with Tourette syndrome, and in agitated states.
• Be aware drug not recommended for

---

first-line treatment of obesity. Use as an anorexigenic agent is prohibited in some states.
• Be aware drug is not to be used to prevent fatigue.
• Make sure the obese patient is on a weight-reduction program.
• Know that drug may cause dependence.
• Be aware that overdose may cause seizures.
• If tolerance to anorexigenic effect develops, know that drug should be discontinued. Notify doctor.

☑ **Patient teaching**
• Tell patient to take drug 30 to 60 minutes before meals if used for weight reduction and at least 6 hours before bedtime to avoid sleep interference.
• Warn patient to avoid activities that require alertness or good psychomotor coordination until CNS effects of drug are known.
• Tell patient that fatigue may result as drug effects wear off.
• Ask patient to report signs of excessive stimulation.
• Advise patient to use caffeine-containing products cautiously.
• Warn patient with seizure disorder that drug may decrease seizure threshold. Instruct him to notify doctor if seizure occurs.

---

diethylpropion hydrochloride
Nobesine†, Tenuate, Tenuate Dospan, Tepanil Ten-Tab

Controlled Substance Schedule IV
Pregnancy Risk Category: B

HOW SUPPLIED
Tablets: 25 mg
Tablets (extended-release): 75 mg
Capsules (extended-release): 75 mg†

ACTION
Unknown. Probably promotes nerve impulse transmission by releasing stored norepinephrine from nerve terminals in the brain. Main sites of activity appear to be the cerebral cortex and the reticular activating system.

Route	Onset	Peak	Duration
PO	Unknown	Unknown	4-12 hr

INDICATIONS & DOSAGE
Short-term adjunct in exogenous obesity—
Adults: 25 mg P.O. before meals t.i.d.; or 75 mg extended-release tablet or capsule P.O. in midmorning.

ADVERSE REACTIONS
CNS: headache, *nervousness,* insomnia, fatigue, anxiety, drowsiness.
CV: *tachycardia, palpitations,* elevated blood pressure, **pulmonary hypertension,** ECG changes, **arrhythmias.**
EENT: blurred vision, mydriasis.
GI: dry mouth, nausea, abdominal cramps, diarrhea, constipation, unpleasant taste, vomiting.
GU: impotence.
Hematologic: decreased blood glucose levels.
Skin: urticaria, rash.
Other: altered libido, changes in menstruation.

INTERACTIONS
Drug-drug. *Guanethidine:* decrease antihypertensive effect. Monitor blood pressure.
Insulin, oral antidiabetic agents: may decrease antidiabetic agent requirements. Monitor blood glucose levels.
MAO inhibitors: may cause hypertension, possibly hypertensive crisis. Don't use together or within 14 days after MAO inhibitor has been discontinued.
Drug-food. *Caffeine:* may increase amphetamine and related amine effects. Avoid concomitant use.

EFFECTS ON DIAGNOSTIC TESTS
None reported.

CONTRAINDICATIONS
Contraindicated in patients with hypersensitivity or idiosyncrasy to sympathomimetic amines; within 14 days of MAO inhibitor therapy; in those with hyperthyroidism, severe hypertension, advanced

---

arteriosclerosis, glaucoma, or history of drug abuse; and in agitated patients.

NURSING CONSIDERATIONS
• Use cautiously in patients with mild to moderate hypertension, symptomatic CV disease (including arrhythmias), or seizure disorders.
• Be sure patient also is on a weight-reduction program.
• Monitor patient for habituation or psychic dependence.

☑**Patient teaching**
• Tell patient to take drug at least 6 hours before bedtime to avoid sleep interference, although it seldom causes insomnia.
• Instruct patient to notify doctor if tolerance to anorexigenic effect develops; drug may be discontinued.
• Tell patient to report signs of excessive stimulation.
• Inform patient that fatigue may result as drug effects wear off.
• Advise patient to avoid caffeine-containing beverages.
• Warn patient with seizure disorder that drug may decrease seizure threshold. Instruct him to notify doctor if seizure occurs.

---

doxapram hydrochloride
Dopram

Pregnancy Risk Category: B

HOW SUPPLIED
Injection: 20 mg/ml (benzyl alcohol 0.9%)

ACTION
Not clearly defined. Acts either directly on the central respiratory centers in the medulla or indirectly on chemoreceptors.

Route	Onset	Peak	Duration
IV	20-40 sec	1-2 min	5-12 min

INDICATIONS & DOSAGE
Postanesthesia respiratory stimulation—
Adults: 0.5 to 1 mg/kg as a single I.V. injection (not to exceed 1.5 mg/kg) or as multiple injections q 5 minutes, not to ex-

ceed 2 mg/kg total dosage. Alternatively, 250 mg in 250 ml of 0.9% NaCl solution or D$_5$W infused at an initial rate of 5 mg/minute I.V. until a satisfactory response is achieved. Maintain at 1 to 3 mg/minute. Recommended total dosage for infusion should not exceed 4 mg/kg.
Drug-induced CNS depression—
Adults: for injection, priming dose of 2 mg/kg I.V., repeated in 5 minutes and again q 1 to 2 hours until patient awakens (and if relapse occurs). Maximum daily dosage is 3 g.
   For infusion, priming dose of 2 mg/kg I.V., repeated in 5 minutes and again in 1 to 2 hours if needed. If response occurs, give I.V. infusion (1 mg/ml) at 1 to 3 mg/minute until patient awakens. Do not infuse for longer than 2 hours or administer more than 3 g/day. May resume I.V. infusion after a rest period of 30 minutes to 2 hours, if needed.
Chronic pulmonary disease associated with acute hypercapnia—
Adults: 1 to 2 mg/minute by I.V. infusion (using 2 mg/ml solution). Maximum dosage is 3 mg/minute for a maximum duration of 2 hours.

ADVERSE REACTIONS
CNS: *seizures, headache,* dizziness, apprehension, disorientation, hyperactivity, bilateral Babinski's signs, paresthesia.
CV: *chest pain and tightness, variations in heart rate, hypertension, arrhythmias.*
EENT: sneezing, *laryngospasm.*
GI: nausea, vomiting, diarrhea.
GU: urine retention, bladder stimulation with incontinence.
Respiratory: cough, *bronchospasm, dyspnea.*
Skin: pruritus.
Other: hiccups, rebound hypoventilation, muscle spasms, diaphoresis, flushing.

INTERACTIONS
Drug-drug. *MAO inhibitors, sympathomimetics:* potentiate adverse CV effects. Use together cautiously.

EFFECTS ON DIAGNOSTIC TESTS
Doxapram may cause T-wave depression on ECG, decreased erythrocyte and leukocyte counts, reduced hemoglobin

---

Reactions may be *common,* uncommon, *life-threatening,* or COMMON AND LIFE-THREATENING.

and hematocrit levels, increased BUN levels, and albuminuria.

CONTRAINDICATIONS
Contraindicated in patients with seizure disorders; head injury; CV disorders; frank, uncompensated heart failure; severe hypertension; CVA; respiratory failure or incompetence secondary to neuromuscular disorders, muscle paresis, flail chest, obstructed airway, pulmonary embolism, pneumothorax, restrictive respiratory disease, acute bronchial asthma, or extreme dyspnea; or hypoxia not associated with hypercapnia.

NURSING CONSIDERATIONS
• Use cautiously in patients with bronchial asthma, severe tachycardia or arrhythmias, cerebral edema or increased CSF pressure, hyperthyroidism, pheochromocytoma, or metabolic disorders.
• Be aware that drug is used only in surgical or emergency department situations.
Alert: Establish an adequate airway before administering drug. Prevent patients from aspirating vomitus by placing them on their side.
• Monitor blood pressure, heart rate, deep tendon reflexes, and arterial blood gases before giving drug and every 30 minutes afterward.
• Be alert for signs of overdosage: hypertension, tachycardia, arrhythmias, skeletal muscle hyperactivity, and dyspnea. Discontinue drug and notify doctor if patient shows signs of increased arterial carbon dioxide or oxygen tension, or if mechanical ventilation is necessary.

◖ I.V. administration
• Administer slowly; rapid infusion may cause hemolysis. Doxapram is physically incompatible with strongly alkaline drugs, such as thiopental sodium, aminophylline, and sodium bicarbonate. Drug is compatible with D_5W or $D_{10}W$ and 0.9% NaCl.
• Avoid extravasation, which may lead to thrombophlebitis and local skin irritation.

☑ Patient teaching
• Inform patient, if alert, and family of need for drug.

• Answer patient's questions and address his concerns.

methamphetamine hydrochloride
Desoxyn, Desoxyn Gradumet

Controlled Substance Schedule II
Pregnancy Risk Category: C

HOW SUPPLIED
Tablets: 5 mg
Tablets (long-acting): 5 mg, 10 mg, 15 mg**

ACTION
Unknown. Probably promotes nerve impulse transmission by releasing stored norepinephrine from nerve terminals in the brain. Main sites of activity appear to be the cerebral cortex and the reticular activating system. In children with hyperkinesis, methamphetamine has a paradoxical calming effect.

Route	Onset	Peak	Duration
PO	Unknown	Unknown	24 hr

INDICATIONS & DOSAGE
Attention deficit disorder with hyperactivity—
Children 6 years and older: 2.5 to 5 mg P.O. once daily or b.i.d., with 5-mg increments weekly, p.r.n. Usual effective dosage is 20 to 25 mg daily.
Short-term adjunct in exogenous obesity—
Adults: 2.5 to 5 mg P.O. b.i.d. or t.i.d., 30 minutes before meals; or 10- to 15-mg long-acting tablet daily before breakfast.

ADVERSE REACTIONS
CNS: *nervousness, insomnia,* irritability, *talkativeness,* dizziness, headache, hyperexcitability, tremor, euphoria.
CV: hypertension, *tachycardia,* palpitations, **arrhythmias.**
EENT: blurred vision, mydriasis.
GI: dry mouth, metallic taste, diarrhea, constipation, anorexia.
GU: impotence.
Skin: urticaria.
Other: altered libido.

INTERACTIONS

Drug-drug. *Acetazolamide, antacids, sodium bicarbonate:* increased renal reabsorption. Monitor for enhanced effects.
Ammonium chloride, ascorbic acid: decreased serum levels and increased renal excretion of methamphetamine. Monitor for decreased methamphetamine effects.
Haloperidol, phenothiazines, tricyclic antidepressants: altered CNS effects. Avoid concomitant use.
Insulin, oral antidiabetic agents: may decrease antidiabetic agent requirements. Monitor blood glucose levels.
MAO inhibitors: may cause severe hypertension, possibly hypertensive crisis. Don't use together or within 14 days after stopping MAO inhibitor.
Drug-herb. *Melatonin:* enhanced monoaminergic effects of methamphetamine; may exacerbate insomnia. Avoid concomitant use.
Drug-food. *Caffeine-containing beverages:* may increase amphetamine and related amine effects. Avoid concomitant use.

EFFECTS ON DIAGNOSTIC TESTS

Drug may elevate plasma corticosteroid levels and also interfere with urinary steroid determinations.

CONTRAINDICATIONS

Contraindicated in moderate to severe hypertension, hyperthyroidism, symptomatic CV disease, advanced arteriosclerosis, glaucoma, hypersensitivity or idiosyncrasy to sympathomimetic amines, or history of drug abuse; within 14 days of MAO inhibitor therapy; and in agitated patients.

NURSING CONSIDERATIONS

• Use cautiously in patients who are elderly, debilitated, asthenic, psychopathic, or who have a history of suicidal or homicidal tendencies.
• Be aware that drug is not recommended for first-line treatment of obesity. Use as an anorexigenic agent is prohibited in some states.
• When used for obesity, be sure patient is on a weight-reduction program.
• Monitor for tolerance or dependence.

☑ Patient teaching

• Tell patient to take drug at least 6 hours before bedtime to avoid sleep interference.
• Warn patient of high potential for abuse. Advise him that drug should not be used to prevent fatigue.
• If tolerance to anorexigenic effect develops, notify doctor because drug will need to be discontinued.
• Tell patient never to crush sustained-release tablets.
• Warn patient to avoid activities that require alertness or good psychomotor coordination until CNS effects of drug are known.
• Tell patient to avoid drinks containing caffeine, which increases the effects of amphetamines and related amines. Ask him to report signs of excessive stimulation.
• Warn patient with seizure disorder that drug may decrease seizure threshold. Instruct him to notify doctor if seizure occurs.

---

methylphenidate hydrochloride
PMS-Methylphenidate†, Ritalin, Ritalin-SR

Controlled Substance Schedule II
Pregnancy Risk Category: C

HOW SUPPLIED
Tablets: 5 mg, 10 mg, 20 mg
Tablets (sustained-release): 20 mg

ACTION
Unknown. Probably promotes nerve impulse transmission by releasing stored norepinephrine from nerve terminals in the brain. Main site of activity appears to be the cerebral cortex and the reticular activating system. In children with hyperkinesis, methylphenidate has a paradoxical calming effect.

Route	Onset	Peak	Duration
PO	Unknown	2-5 hr	Unknown

Reactions may be *common,* uncommon, *life-threatening*, or COMMON AND LIFE-THREATENING.

INDICATIONS & DOSAGE

Attention deficit disorder with hyperactivity—
Children 6 years and older: initial dose, 5 to 10 mg P.O. daily before breakfast and lunch, with 5- to 10-mg increments weekly p.r.n., up to 60 mg daily.
Narcolepsy—
Adults: 10 mg P.O. b.i.d. or t.i.d. 30 to 45 minutes before meals. Dosage varies with patient needs.

ADVERSE REACTIONS

CNS: *nervousness, insomnia,* Tourette syndrome, dizziness, headache, akathisia, dyskinesia, *seizures,* drowsiness.
CV: *palpitations,* angina, *tachycardia,* changes in blood pressure and pulse rate, *arrhythmias*.
GI: nausea, abdominal pain, anorexia, weight loss.
Hematologic: *thrombocytopenia,* thrombocytopenic purpura, *leukopenia,* anemia.
Skin: rash, urticaria, *exfoliative dermatitis, erythema multiforme*.

INTERACTIONS

Drug-drug. *Centrally acting antihypertensives:* decreased antihypertensive effect. Monitor blood pressure.
MAO inhibitors: may cause severe hypertension, possibly hypertensive crisis. Don't use together or within 14 days after an MAO inhibitor has been discontinued.
Tricyclic antidepressants: increased plasma levels of these drugs. Avoid concomitant use.
Drug-food. *Caffeine-containing beverages:* may increase amphetamine and related amine effects. Avoid concomitant use.

EFFECTS ON DIAGNOSTIC TESTS

None reported.

CONTRAINDICATIONS

Contraindicated in patients hypersensitive to drug and in those with glaucoma, motor tics, family history or diagnosis of Tourette syndrome, or history of marked anxiety, tension, or agitation.

NURSING CONSIDERATIONS

● Use cautiously in history of drug abuse, hypertension, history of seizures, or EEG abnormalities.
● Drug is not used to prevent fatigue.
● Drug may precipitate Tourette syndrome in children. Monitor patient, especially at start of therapy.
● Observe for signs of excessive stimulation. Monitor blood pressure.
● Monitor results of periodic CBC, differential, and platelet counts with long-term use.
● Monitor height and weight in children on long-term therapy. Drug may delay growth spurt, but children will attain normal height when drug is stopped.
● Monitor patient for tolerance or psychological dependence.

✓ Patient teaching

● Tell patient to take drug at least 6 hours before bedtime to prevent insomnia and after meals to reduce appetite-suppressant effects.
● Warn patient against chewing sustained-release tablets.
● Caution patient to avoid activities that require alertness or good psychomotor coordination until CNS effects of the drug are known.
● Warn patient with seizure disorder that drug may decrease seizure threshold. Instruct him to notify doctor if seizure occurs.
● Inform patient that he will need more rest as drug effects wear off.
● Advise patient to avoid caffeine-containing beverages while taking drug.

pemoline
Cylert, Cylert Chewable

Controlled Substance Schedule IV
Pregnancy Risk Category: B

HOW SUPPLIED

Tablets: 18.75 mg, 37.5 mg, 75 mg
Tablets (chewable): 37.5 mg

ACTION

Unknown. Probably promotes nerve impulse transmission by releasing stored

---

norepinephrine from nerve terminals in the brain. Main sites of activity appear to be the cerebral cortex and the reticular activating system.

Route	Onset	Peak	Duration
PO	Unknown	2-4 hr	Unknown

INDICATIONS & DOSAGE
Attention deficit disorder with hyperactivity—
Children 6 years and older: initially, 37.5 mg P.O. in the morning with daily dosage raised by 18.75 mg weekly, p.r.n. Usual effective dosage range is 56.25 to 75 mg daily; maximum dosage is 112.5 mg daily.

ADVERSE REACTIONS
CNS: *insomnia,* dyskinetic movements, irritability, fatigue, mild depression, dizziness, headache, drowsiness, hallucinations, **seizures,** *Tourette syndrome,* abnormal oculomotor function.
GI: anorexia, abdominal pain, nausea.
Hematologic: *aplastic anemia.*
Hepatic: acute hepatic failure, hepatitis, jaundice, *elevated liver enzymes.*
Skin: rash.

INTERACTIONS
Drug-drug. *Insulin, oral antidiabetic agents:* may decrease antidiabetic agent requirements. Monitor blood glucose levels.

EFFECTS ON DIAGNOSTIC TESTS
None reported.

CONTRAINDICATIONS
Contraindicated in patients with hepatic dysfunction and hypersensitivity or idiosyncrasy to drug.

NURSING CONSIDERATIONS
• Use cautiously in patients with impaired renal function.
• Be aware that liver function tests should be performed before starting, and periodically during, therapy. Liver function tests may not predict the onset of acute liver failure. Treatment should be initiated only in patients without liver disease and with normal baseline liver function tests.

• Closely monitor patients on long-term therapy for possible blood or hepatic function abnormalities and for growth suppression.
Alert: Be aware that drug should be discontinued if significant hepatic dysfunction is observed during its use.
• Be aware that drug is structurally dissimilar to amphetamines or methylphenidate; however, it may produce similar adverse reactions. Drug has greater potential for abuse and dependence than previously thought.
• Drug may precipitate Tourette syndrome in children. Monitor patient, especially at start of therapy.

☑**Patient teaching**
• Tell patient to take drug at least 6 hours before bedtime to avoid sleep interference.
• Tell patient to avoid activities that require alertness or good psychomotor coordination until CNS effects of drug are known.
• Warn patient with seizure disorder that drug may decrease seizure threshold. Instruct him to notify doctor if seizure occurs.

---

phentermine hydrochloride
Adipex-P, CD LONAMIN§, Duromine‡, Fastin, Obe-Nix, Obephen, OBY-CAP, Phentercot, Phentride, Phentrol, Phentrol 2, Phentrol 4, Phentrol 5, T-Diet

Controlled Substance Schedule IV
Pregnancy Risk Category: NR

HOW SUPPLIED
Tablets: 8 mg, 30 mg, 37.5 mg
Capsules: 15 mg, 18.75 mg, 30 mg, 37.5 mg
Capsules (resin complex, sustained-release): 15 mg, 30 mg

ACTION
Unknown. Probably promotes nerve impulse transmission by releasing stored norepinephrine from nerve terminals in the brain. Main sites of activity appear to

---

be the cerebral cortex and the reticular activating system.

Route	Onset	Peak	Duration
PO	Unknown	Unknown	12-14 hr

INDICATIONS & DOSAGE
Short-term adjunct in exogenous obesity—
Adults: 8 mg P.O. t.i.d. 30 minutes before meals. Alternatively, 15 to 30 mg (resin complex) or 15 to 37.5 mg (phentermine hydrochloride) P.O. daily as a single dose in the morning.

ADVERSE REACTIONS
CNS: overstimulation, headache, euphoria, dysphoria, dizziness, *insomnia.*
CV: *palpitations, tachycardia,* increased blood pressure.
GI: dry mouth, dysgeusia, constipation, diarrhea, other GI disturbances.
GU: impotence.
Skin: urticaria.
Other: altered libido.

INTERACTIONS
Drug-drug. *Acetazolamide, antacids, sodium bicarbonate:* increased renal reabsorption. Monitor for enhanced effects.
Ammonium chloride, ascorbic acid: decreased plasma levels and increased renal excretion of phentermine. Monitor for decreased phentermine effects.
Haloperidol, phenothiazines, tricyclic antidepressants: altered CNS effects. Avoid concomitant use.
Insulin, oral antidiabetic agents: may alter antidiabetic agent requirements. Monitor blood glucose levels.
MAO inhibitors: may cause severe hypertension, possibly hypertensive crisis. Don't use together or within 14 days after MAO inhibitor has been discontinued.
Drug-food. *Caffeine:* may increase CNS stimulation. Avoid concomitant use.

EFFECTS ON DIAGNOSTIC TESTS
None reported.

CONTRAINDICATIONS
Contraindicated in patients with hyperthyroidism, moderate to severe hypertension, advanced arteriosclerosis, symptomatic CV disease, glaucoma, or hypersensitivity or idiosyncrasy to sympathomimetic amines; within 14 days of MAO inhibitor therapy; and in agitated patients.

NURSING CONSIDERATIONS
• Use cautiously in patients with mild hypertension.
• Use drug in conjunction with a weight-reduction program.
• Monitor for tolerance or dependence.

✔Patient teaching
• Tell patient to take drug at least 6 hours before bedtime to avoid sleep interference.
• Advise patient to avoid drinks containing caffeine. Tell him to report signs of excessive stimulation.
• Warn patient that fatigue may result as drug effects wear off and that he will need more rest.

35

Antiparkinsonian drugs

amantadine hydrochloride
(See Chapter 17, ANTIVIRALS.)
benztropine mesylate
biperiden hydrochloride
biperiden lactate
bromocriptine mesylate
carbidopa-levodopa
levodopa
pergolide mesylate
pramipexole dihydrochloride
ropinirole hydrochloride
selegiline hydrochloride
tolcapone
trihexyphenidyl hydrochloride

COMBINATION PRODUCTS
MADOPAR‡: levodopa 200 mg and benser-azide 50 mg.
MADOPAR HBS‡: levodopa 100 mg and benserazide 25 mg.
MADOPAR Q‡: levodopa 50 mg and benserazide 12.5 mg.
SINEMET 10-100: carbidopa 10 mg and levodopa 100 mg.
SINEMET 25-100: carbidopa 25 mg and levodopa 100 mg.
SINEMET 25-250: carbidopa 25 mg and levodopa 250 mg.
SINEMET CR: carbidopa 50 mg and levo-dopa 200 mg, in extended-release tablets.

---

benztropine mesylate
Apo-Benztropine†, Bensylate†,
Cogentin, PMS-Benztropine†

Pregnancy Risk Category: NR

HOW SUPPLIED
Tablets: 0.5 mg, 1 mg, 2 mg
Injection: 1 mg/ml in 2-ml ampules

ACTION
Unknown. Thought to block central cholinergic receptors, helping to balance cholinergic activity in the basal ganglia.

Route	Onset	Peak	Duration
PO	1-2 hr	Unknown	24 hr
IV, IM	15 min	Unknown	24 hr

INDICATIONS & DOSAGE
Drug-induced extrapyramidal disorders (except tardive dyskinesia)—
Adults: 1 to 4 mg P.O. or I.M. once or twice daily.
Acute dystonic reaction—
Adults: 1 to 2 mg I.V. or I.M., followed by 1 to 2 mg P.O. b.i.d. to prevent recurrence.
Parkinsonism—
Adults: 0.5 to 6 mg P.O. or I.M. daily. Initial dose is 0.5 mg to 1 mg, increased by 0.5 mg q 5 to 6 days. Dosage adjusted to meet individual requirements. Maximum daily dosage 6 mg.

ADVERSE REACTIONS
CNS: disorientation, hallucinations, depression, toxic psychosis, confusion, memory impairment, nervousness.
CV: tachycardia.
EENT: dilated pupils, blurred vision.
GI: *dry mouth, constipation,* nausea, vomiting, paralytic ileus.
GU: urine retention, dysuria.
Other: decreased sweating.
   Some adverse reactions may result from atropine-like toxicity and are dose-related.

INTERACTIONS
Drug-drug. *Amantadine, phenothiazines, tricyclic antidepressants:* additive anticholinergic adverse reactions, such as confusion and hallucinations. Reduce dosage before administering.
Drug-herb. *Jimson weed:* may adversely effect CV function. Avoid concomitant use.

EFFECTS ON DIAGNOSTIC TESTS
None reported.

CONTRAINDICATIONS
Contraindicated in patients with narrow-angle glaucoma or hypersensitivity to drug or its components and in children under 3 years.

NURSING CONSIDERATIONS
• Use cautiously in hot weather, in patients with mental disorders, and in children 3 years and older. Also use cautiously in patients with prostatic hyperplasia, arrhythmias, and seizure disorders.
• Monitor vital signs carefully. Watch closely for adverse reactions, especially in elderly or debilitated patients. Call doctor promptly if they occur.
• Be aware that drug produces atropine-like adverse reactions and may aggravate tardive dyskinesia.
• Watch for intermittent constipation and abdominal distention and pain; may indicate onset of paralytic ileus.
Alert: Never discontinue drug abruptly. Reduce dosage gradually.

⚡ **I.V. administration**
• Route is seldom used because of small difference in onset when compared with I.M. route.

✅ **Patient teaching**
• Warn patient to avoid activities that require alertness until CNS effects of drug are known. If patient is to receive a single daily dose, tell him to take it at bedtime.
• Advise patient to report signs of urinary hesitancy or urine retention.
• Tell patient to relieve dry mouth with cool drinks, ice chips, sugarless gum, or hard candy.
• Advise patient to limit his activities during hot weather because drug-induced anhidrosis may cause hyperthermia.

---

biperiden hydrochloride
Akineton

biperiden lactate
Akineton Lactate

Pregnancy Risk Category: C

HOW SUPPLIED
biperiden hydrochloride
Tablets: 2 mg
biperiden lactate
Injection: 5 mg/ml in 1-ml ampules

ACTION
Unknown. Blocks central cholinergic receptors, helping to balance cholinergic activity in the basal ganglia.

Route	Onset	Peak	Duration
PO	1 hr	Unknown	6-12 hr
IV	< Few min	Unknown	1-8 hr
IM	10-30 min	Unknown	Unknown

INDICATIONS & DOSAGE
Drug-induced extrapyramidal disorders—
Adults: 2 mg P.O. once daily, b.i.d., or t.i.d., depending on severity. Usual dosage is 2 mg daily, or 2 mg I.M. or I.V. q 30 minutes, not to exceed four doses or 8 mg daily.
Parkinsonism—
Adults: 2 mg P.O. t.i.d. or q.i.d. Dosage is individualized and titrated to maximum of 16 mg in 24 hours.

ADVERSE REACTIONS
CNS: disorientation, euphoria, drowsiness, agitation.
CV: transient orthostatic hypotension (with parenteral use).
EENT: blurred vision.
GI: *dry mouth, constipation.*
GU: urine retention.
    Adverse reactions are dose-related and may resemble atropine toxicity.

INTERACTIONS
Drug-drug. *Amantadine, phenothiazines, tricyclic antidepressants:* excessive CNS anticholinergic effects. Avoid concomitant use.
Antacids: decreased biperiden absorption. Administer antacids at least 1 hour after biperiden.
Drug-lifestyle. *Alcohol use:* increased sedative effects. Avoid concomitant use.

EFFECTS ON DIAGNOSTIC TESTS
None reported.

CONTRAINDICATIONS

Contraindicated in patients with narrow-angle glaucoma, bowel obstruction, megacolon, or hypersensitivity to drug.

NURSING CONSIDERATIONS

• Use cautiously in patients with prostatic hyperplasia, arrhythmias, manifest glaucoma, and seizure disorder.
• To decrease adverse GI effects, give oral doses with or after meals.
• When giving parenterally, keep patient in supine position. Parenteral administration may cause transient orthostatic hypotension and coordination disturbances.
• Monitor vital signs carefully. Watch closely for adverse reactions, especially in elderly or debilitated patients. Call doctor promptly if they occur.
• Monitor patient for tolerance. If it develops, notify doctor because dosage will need to be increased.
• Know that in severe parkinsonism, tremors may increase as spasticity is relieved.

I.V. administration

• Administer drug very slowly.

Patient teaching

• Tell patient to take oral form of drug with or after meals to decrease adverse GI effects.
• Warn patient to avoid activities that require alertness until CNS effects of drug are known.
• Advise patient to report signs of urinary hesitancy or urine retention.
• Instruct patient to relieve dry mouth with cool drinks, ice chips, sugarless gum, or hard candy.
• Advise patient to avoid alcohol while taking drug.

---

bromocriptine mesylate
Parlodel

Pregnancy Risk Category: B

HOW SUPPLIED
Tablets: 2.5 mg
Capsules: 5 mg

ACTION

Inhibits secretion of prolactin and acts as a dopamine-receptor agonist by activating postsynaptic dopamine receptors.

Route	Onset	Peak	Duration
PO	2 hr	8 hr	24 hr

INDICATIONS & DOSAGE

Parkinson's disease—
Adults: 1.25 mg P.O. b.i.d. with meals. Dosage increased q 14 to 28 days, up to 100 mg daily.
Amenorrhea and galactorrhea associated with hyperprolactinemia; female infertility—
Adults: 1.25 to 2.5 mg P.O. daily, increased by 2.5 mg daily at 3- to 7-day intervals until desired effect is achieved. Therapeutic daily dosage is 2.5 to 15 mg. Safety and efficacy of doses exceeding 100 mg daily have not been established.
Acromegaly—
Adults: 1.25 to 2.5 mg P.O. with h.s. snack for 3 days. An additional 1.25 to 2.5 mg may be added q 3 to 7 days until patient receives therapeutic benefit. Maximum daily dosage is 100 mg.

ADVERSE REACTIONS

CNS: *dizziness, headache, fatigue,* mania, light-headedness, drowsiness, delusions, nervousness, insomnia, depression, *seizures.*
CV: *hypotension, stroke, acute MI.*
EENT: nasal congestion, blurred vision.
GI: *nausea,* vomiting, *abdominal cramps, constipation,* diarrhea, anorexia.
GU: urine retention, urinary frequency.
Skin: coolness and pallor of fingers and toes.

INTERACTIONS

Drug-drug. *Antihypertensives:* increased hypotensive effects. Adjust dosage of the antihypertensive.
Erythromycin: increased bromocriptine levels and potential adverse reactions. Use cautiously.
Haloperidol, loxapine, methyldopa, metoclopramide, MAO inhibitors, phenothiazines, reserpine: interferes with bromocriptine's effects. Bromocriptine dosage may need to be increased.

Reactions may be *common,* uncommon, *life-threatening,* or COMMON AND LIFE-THREATENING.

Levodopa: additive effects. Adjust dosage of levodopa.

Oral contraceptives, estrogens, progestins: interfere with effects of bromocriptine. Concurrent use not recommended.

Drug-lifestyle. *Alcohol use:* disulfiram-like reaction. Avoid concomitant use.

EFFECTS ON DIAGNOSTIC TESTS
Transient elevation of BUN, ALT, AST, CK, alkaline phosphatase, and uric acid levels may occur.

CONTRAINDICATIONS
Contraindicated in patients with uncontrolled hypertension, toxemia of pregnancy, severe ischemic heart disease, peripheral vascular disease, or hypersensitivity to ergot derivatives.

NURSING CONSIDERATIONS
• Use cautiously in patients with impaired renal or hepatic function and history of MI with residual arrhythmias.
• Know that for Parkinson's disease, bromocriptine usually is given in addition to either levodopa or carbidopa-levodopa. The carbidopa-levodopa dose may need to be reduced.
• Give drug with meals.
*Alert:*Monitor patient for adverse reactions. Incidence of adverse reactions is high (about 68%), particularly at beginning of therapy; however, most are mild to moderate, with nausea being the most common. Minimize adverse reactions by gradually titrating doses to effective levels as ordered. Adverse reactions are more frequent when drug is used for Parkinson's disease.
• Know that baseline and periodic evaluations of cardiac, hepatic, renal, and hematopoietic function are recommended during prolonged therapy.
• Drug may lead to early postpartum conception. Test for pregnancy every 4 weeks or whenever period is missed after menses resumes.

✓**Patient teaching**
• Instruct patient to take drug with meals.
• Advise patient to use contraceptive methods other than oral contraceptives or subdermal implants during treatment.

• Instruct patient to avoid dizziness and fainting by rising slowly to an upright position and avoiding sudden position changes.
• Inform patient that it may take 8 weeks or longer for menses to resume and galactorrhea to be suppressed.
• Advise patient to avoid alcohol while taking drug.

carbidopa-levodopa
Sinemet, Sinemet CR

Pregnancy Risk Category: C

HOW SUPPLIED
Tablets: carbidopa 10 mg with levodopa 100 mg (Sinemet 10-100), carbidopa 25 mg with levodopa 100 mg (Sinemet 25-100), carbidopa 25 mg with levodopa 250 mg (Sinemet 25-250)
Tablets (extended-release): carbidopa 50 mg with levodopa 200 mg (Sinemet CR)

ACTION
Decarboxylated to dopamine, countering the depletion of striatal dopamine in extrapyramidal centers. Carbidopa inhibits the peripheral decarboxylation of levodopa without affecting levodopa's metabolism within the CNS. Therefore, more levodopa is available to be decarboxylated to dopamine in the brain.

Route	Onset	Peak	Duration
PO	Unknown	40-150 min	Unknown

INDICATIONS & DOSAGE
Idiopathic Parkinson's disease, postencephalitic parkinsonism, and symptomatic parkinsonism resulting from carbon monoxide or manganese intoxication—
Adults: one tablet of 25 mg carbidopa/100 mg levodopa P.O. t.i.d. followed by an increase of one tablet daily or every other day, p.r.n., to maximum daily dosage of eight tablets. 25 mg carbidopa/250 mg levodopa or 10 mg carbidopa/100 mg levodopa tablets are substituted as required to obtain maximum response. Optimum daily dosage must be determined by careful titration for each patient.

Patients treated with conventional tablets may receive extended-release tablets; dosage is calculated on current levodopa intake. Initially, extended-release tablets given should amount to 10% more levodopa per day, increased, as needed and tolerated, to 30% more levodopa per day. Administered in divided doses at intervals of 4 to 8 hours.

ADVERSE REACTIONS
CNS: *choreiform, dystonic, dyskinetic movements; involuntary grimacing, head movements, myoclonic body jerks, ataxia,* tremor, muscle twitching; bradykinetic episodes; psychiatric disturbances, anxiety, disturbing dreams, euphoria, malaise, fatigue; severe depression, *suicidal tendencies,* dementia, delirium, hallucinations (may necessitate reduction or withdrawal of drug), confusion, insomnia, agitation.
CV: *orthostatic hypotension, cardiac irregularities.*
EENT: blepharospasm, blurred vision, diplopia, mydriasis or miosis, oculogyric crises, excessive salivation.
GI: dry mouth, bitter taste, *nausea, vomiting, anorexia,* weight loss (may occur at start of therapy); constipation; flatulence; diarrhea; abdominal pain.
GU: urinary frequency, urine retention, urinary incontinence, darkened urine, priapism.
Hematologic: *hemolytic anemia, thrombocytopenia, leukopenia, agranulocytosis.*
Hepatic: *hepatotoxicity.*
Other: dark perspiration, hyperventilation, hiccups, phlebitis.

INTERACTIONS
Drug-drug. *Antihypertensives:* additive hypotensive effects. Use together cautiously.
Iron salts: may reduce bioavailability of levodopa and carbidopa. Monitor closely.
MAO inhibitors: risk of severe hypertension. Avoid concomitant use.
Papaverine, phenytoin: antagonism of antiparkinsonian actions. Don't use together.
Phenothiazines, other antipsychotics: may antagonize antiparkinsonian actions. Use together cautiously.
Drug-herb. *Octacosanol:* may promote worsening of dyskinesias. Avoid concomitant use.
Drug-food. *Foods high in protein:* decreased absorption of levodopa. Don't give levodopa with high-protein foods.

EFFECTS ON DIAGNOSTIC TESTS
Drug elevates serum and urinary uric acid concentrations when colorimetric test methods are used; it may produce false-positive test results for urinary glucose when cupric sulfate reagent is used and false-negative results in tests using glucose oxidase. False-positive results may occur for urine ketone tests using sodium nitroprusside reagent. Levodopa interferes with urine screening tests for phenylketonuria, falsely elevates urinary catecholamine levels, and may falsely decrease urinary vanillylmandelic acid levels.

CONTRAINDICATIONS
Contraindicated in patients with narrow-angle glaucoma, melanoma, undiagnosed skin lesions, or hypersensitivity to drug and within 14 days of MAO inhibitor therapy.

NURSING CONSIDERATIONS
• Use cautiously in patients with severe CV, renal, hepatic, endocrine, or pulmonary disorders; history of peptic ulcer; psychiatric illness; MI with residual arrhythmias; bronchial asthma; emphysema; and well-controlled, chronic open-angle glaucoma.
• If patient is being treated with levodopa, discontinue drug at least 8 hours before starting carbidopa-levodopa.
• Know that carbidopa-levodopa typically decreases amount of levodopa needed by 75%, reducing the incidence of adverse reactions.
• Be aware that therapeutic and adverse reactions occur more rapidly with carbidopa-levodopa than with levodopa alone. Observe and monitor vital signs, especially while adjusting dosage. Report significant changes.
Alert: Muscle twitching and blepharospasm may be early signs of drug overdose; report immediately.
• Know that patients receiving long-term therapy should be tested regularly for dia-

betes and acromegaly and have periodic tests of liver, renal, and hematopoietic function as ordered.
• An accurate measure for urine glucose can be obtained if the paper strip is only partially immersed in the urine sample. Urine will migrate up the strip, as with an ascending chromatographic system. Read only the top of the strip.

☑ Patient teaching
• Tell patient to take drug with food to minimize GI upset. However, taking drug with high-protein meals can impair absorption and reduce effectiveness.
• Tell patient not to chew or crush extended-release formulation.
• Warn patient and caregivers not to increase dosage without doctor's orders.
• Caution patient of possible dizziness and orthostatic hypotension, especially at start of therapy. Tell him to change position slowly and dangle legs before getting out of bed. Elastic stockings may control this adverse reaction in some patients.
• Instruct patient to report adverse reactions and therapeutic effects.
• Inform patient that pyridoxine (vitamin B_6) does not reverse the beneficial effects of carbidopa-levodopa. Multivitamins can be taken without losing control of symptoms.

levodopa
Dopar, Larodopa

Pregnancy Risk Category: NR

HOW SUPPLIED
Tablets: 100 mg, 250 mg, 500 mg
Capsules: 100 mg, 250 mg, 500 mg

ACTION
Unknown. Thought to be decarboxylated to dopamine, countering the depletion of striatal dopamine in extrapyramidal centers, which is thought to produce parkinsonism.

Route	Onset	Peak	Duration
PO	Unknown	1-3 hr	5 hr

INDICATIONS & DOSAGE
Idiopathic parkinsonism, postencephalitic parkinsonism, and symptomatic parkinsonism after carbon monoxide or manganese intoxication or in association with cerebral arteriosclerosis—
Adults and children over 12 years: initially, 0.5 to 1 g P.O. daily, divided in two or more doses with food; increased by no more than 0.75 g daily q 3 to 7 days until maximum response is achieved. Do not exceed 8 g/day. Dosage adjusted to patient requirements, tolerance, and response. Higher dosage requires close supervision.

ADVERSE REACTIONS
CNS: *aggressive behavior; choreiform, dystonic, and dyskinetic movements; involuntary grimacing, head movements, myoclonic body jerks,* **seizures,** *ataxia, tremor, muscle twitching; bradykinetic episodes; psychiatric disturbances; mood changes, nervousness, anxiety, disturbing dreams, euphoria, malaise, fatigue; severe depression,* **suicidal tendencies,** *dementia, delirium, hallucinations* (may require reduction or withdrawal of drug).
CV: *orthostatic hypotension,* cardiac irregularities.
EENT: blepharospasm, blurred vision, diplopia, mydriasis or miosis, activation of latent Horner's syndrome, oculogyric crises, excessive salivation.
GI: dry mouth, bitter taste, *nausea, vomiting, anorexia,* weight loss (at start of therapy), constipation, flatulence, diarrhea, abdominal pain.
GU: urinary frequency, urine retention, incontinence, darkened urine, priapism.
Hematologic: **hemolytic anemia, leukopenia, agranulocytosis.**
Hepatic: **hepatotoxicity.**
Other: dark perspiration, hyperventilation, hiccups, phlebitis.

INTERACTIONS
Drug-drug. *Antacids:* increased absorption of levodopa. Administer antacids 1 hour after levodopa.
Inhalation anesthetics, sympathomimetic agents: increased risk of arrhythmias. Monitor closely.
MAO inhibitors, furazolidone, procar-

bazine: risk of severe hypertension. Avoid concomitant use.

Metoclopramide: accelerated gastric emptying of levodopa. Give metoclopramide 1 hour after levodopa.

Papaverine, phenothiazines, other antipsychotics, phenytoin, rauwolfia alkaloids: decreased levodopa effect. Avoid concomitant use, if possible.

Pyridoxine: reversal of antiparkinsonian effects. Check vitamin preparations and nutritional supplements for pyridoxine (vitamin B$_6$) content. Don't give together.

Drug-herb. *Jimson weed:* may adversely effect CV function. Avoid concomitant use.

Kava: increased Parkinsonian symptoms. Avoid concomitant use.

Drug-food. *Foods high in protein:* decreased absorption of levodopa. Don't give levodopa with high-protein foods.

Drug-lifestyle. *Cocaine use:* increased risk of arrhythmias. Monitor closely.

EFFECTS ON DIAGNOSTIC TESTS

Coombs' test occasionally becomes positive during extended therapy. Colorimetric test for uric acid has shown false elevations. Copper-reduction method has shown false-positive results for urine glucose; glucose oxidase method has shown false-negative results. Levodopa also may interfere with tests for urine ketones. Levodopa interferes with urine screening tests for phenylketonuria, falsely elevates urinary catecholamine levels, and may falsely decrease urinary vanillylmandelic acid levels. Alkaline phosphatase, AST, ALT, LD, bilirubin, BUN, and protein-bound iodine show transient elevations in patients receiving levodopa; WBC count, hemoglobin, and hematocrit show occasional reductions.

CONTRAINDICATIONS

Contraindicated in concurrent therapy with MAO inhibitors within 14 days and in patients with acute angle-closure glaucoma, melanoma, undiagnosed skin lesions, or hypersensitivity to drug.

NURSING CONSIDERATIONS

• Use cautiously in severe CV, renal, liver, and pulmonary disorders; peptic ulcer; psychiatric illness; MI with residual arrhythmias; bronchial asthma; emphysema; and endocrine disease.

• Know that patients who must undergo surgery should continue levodopa therapy as long as oral intake is permitted, generally 6 to 24 hours before surgery. Resume therapy as soon as patient is able to take drug orally.

• Be aware that carbidopa-levodopa typically decreases amount of levodopa needed by 75%, reducing the incidence of adverse reactions.

• Monitor vital signs, especially while adjusting dosage. Report changes.

• Watch for muscle twitching and blepharospasm, which may be early signs of drug overdose; report immediately.

• An accurate measure for urine glucose can be obtained if paper strip is only partially immersed in the urine sample. Urine will migrate up the strip, as with an ascending chromatographic system. Read only the top of the strip.

• Know that patients receiving long-term therapy should be tested regularly for diabetes and acromegaly; periodically monitor renal, liver, and hematopoietic function as ordered.

• A doctor-supervised period of drug discontinuance (called a drug holiday) may reestablish the effectiveness of a lower dosage regimen.

☑ Patient teaching

• Tell patient to take drug with food to minimize GI upset. However, taking drug with high-protein meals can impair absorption and reduce effectiveness.

• For patient who has difficulty swallowing pills, tell him and caregiver to crush tablets and mix with applesauce or baby food fruits.

• Warn patient and caregiver not to increase dosage unless ordered. Daily dosage should not exceed 8 g.

• Tell patient to protect drug from heat, light, and moisture. If preparation darkens, it has lost potency and should be discarded.

• Warn patient of possible dizziness and orthostatic hypotension, especially at start of therapy. Tell him to change position slowly and dangle legs before rising.

Elastic stockings may control this adverse reaction.

• Advise patient and caregivers that multivitamin preparations, fortified cereals, and certain OTC medications may contain pyridoxine (vitamin B_6), which can block the effects of levodopa by enhancing its peripheral metabolism.

pergolide mesylate
Celance§, Permax

Pregnancy Risk Category: B

HOW SUPPLIED
Tablets: 0.05 mg, 0.25 mg, 1 mg

ACTION
A dopamine agonist that directly stimulates dopamine receptors in the nigrostriatal system.

Route	Onset	Peak	Duration
PO	Unknown	Unknown	Unknown

INDICATIONS & DOSAGE
Adjunctive treatment with carbidopa-levodopa in the management of the symptoms in Parkinson's disease—
Adults: initially, 0.05 mg P.O. daily for first 2 days followed by increased dosage of 0.1 to 0.15 mg q third day over 12 days. Subsequent dosage increased by 0.25 mg q third day, if needed, until optimum response is seen. Drug usually is administered in divided doses t.i.d. Gradual reductions in carbidopa-levodopa dosage could be made during dosage titration.

ADVERSE REACTIONS
CNS: headache, asthenia, *dyskinesia, dizziness, hallucinations, dystonia, confusion, somnolence,* insomnia, anxiety, depression, tremor, abnormal dreams, personality disorder, psychosis, abnormal gait, akathisia, extrapyramidal syndrome, incoordination, akinesia, hypertonia, neuralgia, speech disorder, twitching.
CV: *orthostatic hypotension,* vasodilation, palpitations, hypotension, syncope, hypertension, ***arrhythmias, MI.***
EENT: *rhinitis,* epistaxis, abnormal vision, diplopia, eye disorder.

GI: dry mouth, taste perversion, abdominal pain, *nausea, constipation,* diarrhea, dyspepsia, anorexia, vomiting.
GU: urinary frequency, urinary tract infection, hematuria.
Skin: rash, diaphoresis, paresthesia.
Other: flulike syndrome; chest, neck, and back pain; chills; infection; facial, peripheral, or generalized edema; weight gain; arthralgia; bursitis; myalgia; dyspnea.
   Note: The preceding adverse reactions, although not always attributable to the drug, occurred in more than 1% of the study population.

INTERACTIONS
Drug-drug. *Butyrophenones, dopamine antagonists, metoclopramide, phenothiazines, thioxanthenes:* may antagonize effects of pergolide. Avoid concomitant use.

EFFECTS ON DIAGNOSTIC TESTS
None reported.

CONTRAINDICATIONS
Contraindicated in patients hypersensitive to drug or to ergot alkaloids.

NURSING CONSIDERATIONS
• Use cautiously in patients prone to arrhythmias.
Alert: Monitor blood pressure. Symptomatic orthostatic or sustained hypotension may occur especially at the start of therapy.

☑ **Patient teaching**
• Inform patient of potential adverse reactions, especially hallucinations and confusion (27% incidence).
• Warn patient to avoid activities that could result in injury from orthostatic hypotension and syncope.
• Advise patient to take drug with food.

pramipexole dihydrochloride
Mirapex

Pregnancy Risk Category: C

HOW SUPPLIED
Tablets: 0.125 mg, 0.25 mg, 1 mg, 1.5 mg

ACTION

Unknown, but thought to stimulate dopamine receptors in striatum.

Route	Onset	Peak	Duration
PO	Rapid	2 hr	8-12 hr

INDICATIONS & DOSAGE

Treatment of the signs and symptoms of idiopathic Parkinson's disease—
Adults: Initially, 0.375 mg P.O. daily given in three divided doses; do not increase more frequently than q 5 to 7 days. Maintenance range is 1.5 to 4.5 mg/day in three divided doses.
Adjust-a-dose: In patients with normal to mild renal impairment (creatinine clearance over 60 ml/minute), initial dose 0.125 mg P.O. t.i.d., up to 1.5 mg t.i.d.; in those with moderate impairment (creatinine clearance between 35 and 59 ml/minute), initial dose 1.25 mg P.O. b.i.d. up to 1.5 mg b.i.d.; and in those with severe impairment (creatinine clearance of 15 to 34 ml/minute), initial dose 0.125 mg P.O. daily, up to 1.5 mg daily.

ADVERSE REACTIONS

CNS: akathisia, amnesia, *asthenia, confusion,* delusions, *dizziness, dream abnormalities, dyskinesia,* dystonia, *extrapyramidal syndrome,* gait abnormalities, *hallucinations,* hypoesthesia, hypertonia, *insomnia,* myoclonus, paranoid reaction, *somnolence,* sleep disorders, thought abnormalities.
CV: chest pain, peripheral edema, *orthostatic hypotension.*
EENT: accommodation abnormalities, diplopia, dry mouth, rhinitis, vision abnormalities.
GI: anorexia, *constipation,* dysphagia, *nausea.*
GU: decreased libido, impotence, urinary frequency, urinary tract infection, urinary incontinence.
Respiratory: dyspnea, pneumonia.
Skin: skin disorders.
Other: *accidental injury,* arthritis, bursitis, fever, general edema, malaise, myasthenia, twitching, weight loss.

INTERACTIONS

Drug-drug. Butyrophenones, metoclo-

pramide, phenothiazines, thiothixenes: may diminish the effectiveness of pramipexole. Monitor closely.
Cimetidine, diltiazem, quinidine, quinine, ranitidine, triamterene, verapamil: decreased clearance of pramipexole. Adjust dose as needed.
Levodopa: increased adverse effects of levodopa. Adjust levodopa dose as needed.

EFFECTS ON DIAGNOSTIC TESTS

None reported.

CONTRAINDICATIONS

Contraindicated in patients with hypersensitivity to drug or its components.

NURSING CONSIDERATIONS

• Use with caution in patients with renal insufficiency. Dose may need to be decreased.
• Dosing may need to be adjusted in patients with renal impairment. It is not known if drug is excreted in breast milk. Use with caution.
• Withdraw drug over a 1-week period if drug needs to be discontinued.
• Know that drug may cause orthostatic hypotension, especially during dose escalation. Monitor patient carefully.
• Titrate dosage gradually. Increase dosage to achieve maximum therapeutic effect, balanced against the main adverse effects of dyskinesia, hallucinations, somnolence, and dry mouth.

☑ **Patient teaching**
• Instruct patient not to rise rapidly after sitting or lying down because of risk of orthostatic hypotension.
• Caution patient not to drive a car or operate complex machinery until response to drug is known.
• Tell patient to use caution before taking drug with other CNS depressants.
• Tell patient that hallucinations may occur, especially if he is elderly.
• Advise patient to take drug with food if nausea develops.
• Tell female patient to notify doctor if she is breast-feeding or intends to do so.
• Advise patient that it may take 4 weeks for effects of drug to be noticed due to slow titration schedule.

Reactions may be *common*, uncommon, ***life-threatening***, or COMMON AND LIFE-THREATENING.

ropinirole hydrochloride
Requip

Pregnancy Risk Category: C

HOW SUPPLIED
Tablets: 0.25 mg, 0.5 mg, 1 mg, 2 mg, 5 mg

ACTION
Unknown. A nonergoline dopamine agonist thought to stimulate postsynaptic dopamine D_2 receptors within the caudate-putamen in the brain.

Route	Onset	Peak	Duration
PO	Unknown	1-2 hr	6 hr

INDICATIONS & DOSAGE
Idiopathic Parkinson's disease—
Adults: initially, 0.25 mg t.i.d. Dosages can be titrated on a weekly basis. After week 4, dosage may be increased by 1.5 mg/day on a weekly basis up to a dose of 9 mg/day and then increased weekly by up to 3 mg/day to maximum of 24 mg/day.
Elderly: clearance is reduced in patients above 65 years, however, doses are individually titrated to clinical response.

ADVERSE REACTIONS
Early Parkinson's disease (without levodopa)—
CNS: hallucinations, *dizziness,* aggravated Parkinson's disease, *somnolence,* headache, confusion, hyperkinesia, hypoesthesia, vertigo, amnesia, impaired concentration.
CV: orthostatic hypotension, orthostatic symptoms, hypertension, *syncope,* edema, chest pain, extrasystoles, **atrial fibrillation,** palpitation, tachycardia.
EENT: pharyngitis, dry mouth, abnormal vision, eye abnormality, xerophthalmia, rhinitis, sinusitis.
GI: *nausea, vomiting, dyspepsia,* flatulence, abdominal pain, anorexia, constipation, abdominal pain.
GU: urinary tract infection, impotence (male).
Respiratory: bronchitis, dyspnea.
Skin: flushing.
Other: *fatigue,* malaise, *viral infection,* pain, increased sweating, asthenia, yawning, peripheral ischemia.
Advanced Parkinson's disease (with levodopa)—
CNS: *dizziness,* aggravated parkinsonism, *somnolence, headache,* insomnia, *hallucinations,* abnormal dreaming, confusion, tremor, anxiety, nervousness, amnesia, paresis, paresthesia.
CV: hypotension, syncope.
EENT: diplopia.
GI: *nausea,* abdominal pain, dry mouth, vomiting, constipation, diarrhea, dysphagia, flatulence.
GU: urinary tract infection, pyuria, urinary incontinence.
Hematologic: anemia.
Metabolic: weight decrease.
Musculoskeletal: arthralgia, arthritis.
Respiratory: upper respiratory infection, dyspnea.
Skin: increased sweating.
Other: *dyskinesia,* hypokinesia, injury, *falls,* viral infection, increased drug level, increased saliva, pain.

INTERACTIONS
Drug-drug. *Ciprofloxacin, inhibitors or substrates of cytochrome P-450:* altered clearance. Adjust ropinirole dose if drugs are started or stopped during treatment with ropinirole.
CNS depressants: increased CNS effects. Use cautiously.
Estrogens: reduced clearance of ropinirole. Adjust ropinirole dose if estrogens are started or stopped during treatment with ropinirole.
Drug-lifestyle. *Alcohol use:* increased sedative effects. Use cautiously.
Smoking: may increase clearance of ropinirole. Monitor closely.

EFFECTS ON DIAGNOSTIC TESTS
Drug suppresses serum prolactin, and may increase BUN and alkaline phosphatase.

CONTRAINDICATIONS
Contraindicated in patients with known hypersensitivity to drug.

NURSING CONSIDERATIONS
• Use cautiously in patients with severe hepatic or renal impairment.

Alert: Monitor patient carefully for orthostatic hypotension, especially during dose escalation.

• Drug can potentiate the dopaminergic adverse effects of levodopa and may cause or exacerbate existing dyskinesia. Dosage of drug may be decreased.

• Other adverse events reported with dopaminergic therapy could potentially occur with ropinirole (but have not been reported): withdrawal emergent hyperpyrexia and confusion; fibrotic complications.

• Syncope, with or without bradycardia, has been reported. Monitor carefully, especially after 4 weeks of initiation of therapy and with dose increases.

• Withdraw drug gradually over 7 days.

☑**Patient teaching**
• Advise patient to take drug with food if nausea is a problem.

• Advise patient that hallucinations can occur and the elderly are at greater risk than younger patients with Parkinson's disease.

• Instruct patient not to rise rapidly after sitting or lying down because of risk of orthostatic hypotension which may occur more frequently during initial therapy or with an increase in dose.

• Warn patient to use caution in driving or operating machinery until CNS effects are known.

• Advise patient to avoid alcohol.

• Tell female patient to notify doctor if pregnancy is suspected or is being planned; also tell her to inform doctor if she is breast-feeding.

• Advise patient not to double a dose if one is missed.

---

selegiline hydrochloride (L-deprenyl hydrochloride)
Eldepryl

Pregnancy Risk Category: C

HOW SUPPLIED
Tablets: 5 mg

ACTION
Unknown. May selectively inhibit MAO type B (found mostly in the brain). At higher-than-recommended doses, it is a nonselective inhibitor of MAO, including MAO type A (found in the GI tract). Also may directly increase dopaminergic activity by decreasing the reuptake of dopamine into nerve cells. Its active metabolites, amphetamine and methamphetamine, may contribute to this effect.

Route	Onset	Peak	Duration
PO	Unknown	0.5-2 hr	Unknown

INDICATIONS & DOSAGE
Adjunctive treatment with carbidopa-levodopa in the management of the symptoms in Parkinson's disease—
Adults: 10 mg P.O. daily, taken as 5 mg at breakfast and 5 mg at lunch. After 2 or 3 days, gradual decrease of carbidopa-levodopa dosage.

ADVERSE REACTIONS
CNS: *dizziness,* increased tremor, chorea, loss of balance, restlessness, increased bradykinesia, facial grimacing, stiff neck, dyskinesia, involuntary movements, twitching, increased apraxia, behavioral changes, fatigue, headache, confusion, hallucinations, vivid dreams, anxiety, insomnia, lethargy.
CV: orthostatic hypotension, hypertension, hypotension, *arrhythmias,* palpitations, new or increased anginal pain, tachycardia, peripheral edema, syncope.
EENT: blepharospasm.
GI: dry mouth, *nausea,* vomiting, constipation, weight loss, abdominal pain, anorexia or poor appetite, dysphagia, diarrhea, heartburn.
GU: slow urination, transient nocturia, prostatic hyperplasia, urinary hesitancy, urinary frequency, urine retention, sexual dysfunction.
Skin: rash, hair loss.
Other: malaise, diaphoresis.

INTERACTIONS
Drug-drug. *Adrenergic agents:* possible

Reactions may be *common,* uncommon, *life-threatening*, or COMMON AND LIFE-THREATENING.

increased pressor response, particularly in patients who have taken an overdose of selegiline. Use together cautiously.
Meperidine: may cause stupor, muscle rigidity, severe agitation, and elevated temperature. Avoid concomitant use.
Drug-herb. *Cacao tree:* potential vaso-pressor effects. Avoid concomitant use.
Ginseng: adverse reactions including headache, tremors, mania. Avoid concomitant use.
Drug-food. *Foods high in tyramine:* possible hypertensive crisis. Monitor blood pressure.

EFFECTS ON DIAGNOSTIC TESTS
None reported.

CONTRAINDICATIONS
Contraindicated in patients with hypersensitivity to drug and in those receiving meperidine.

NURSING CONSIDERATIONS
Alert: Some patients experience increased adverse reactions with levodopa and require a 10% to 30% reduction of carbidopa-levodopa dosage.

☑ **Patient teaching**
• Warn patient to move cautiously at the start of therapy because he may experience dizziness.
• Advise patient not to take more than 10 mg daily. A greater amount may increase adverse reactions.

▼ *NEW DRUG*

tolcapone
Tasmar

Pregnancy Risk Category: C

HOW SUPPLIED
Tablets: 100 mg, 200 mg

ACTION
Exact mechanism unknown. Thought to reversibly inhibit catechol-O-methyltransferase (COMT) when given in combination with carbidopa-levodopa, resulting in an increase in levodopa bioavailability.

Believed to result in a more constant dopaminergic stimulation in the brain.

Route	Onset	Peak	Duration
PO	Unknown	2 hr	Unknown

INDICATIONS & DOSAGE
Adjunct to levodopa and carbidopa for treatment of signs and symptoms of idiopathic Parkinson's disease—
Adults: initially, 100 mg P.O. t.i.d. (in combination with carbidopa-levodopa). Recommended daily dose is 100 mg P.O. t.i.d. although 200 mg P.O. t.i.d. can be given if the anticipated clinical benefit is justified. If treating with 200 mg t.i.d. and dyskinesia occurs, reduced dosage of levodopa may be necessary. Maximum daily dose is 600 mg. Discontinue drug if patient shows no benefit within 3 weeks.
Adjust-a-dose: Do not use doses over 100 mg t.i.d. in patients with severe renal dysfunction.

ADVERSE REACTIONS
CNS: *dyskinesia, sleep disorder, dystonia, excessive dreaming, somnolence,* dizziness, *confusion, headache, hallucinations,* hyperkinesia, hypertonia, fatigue, falling, syncope, balance loss, depression, tremor, speech disorder, paresthesia, agitation, irritability, mental deficiency, hyperactivity, hypokinesia.
CV: *orthostatic complaints,* chest pain, chest discomfort, palpitation, hypotension.
EENT: pharyngitis, tinnitus, sinus congestion.
GI: *nausea, anorexia, diarrhea,* flatulence, *vomiting,* constipation, abdominal pain, dyspepsia, dry mouth.
GU: urinary tract infection, urine discoloration, hematuria, micturition disorder, urinary incontinence, impotence.
Musculoskeletal: *muscle cramps,* stiffness, arthritis, neck pain.
Respiratory: bronchitis, dyspnea, upper respiratory infections.
Skin: increased sweating, rash.
Other: bleeding, burning, fever, influenza.

INTERACTIONS
Drug-drug. *Desipramine:* increased incidence of adverse effects. Use cautiously. *Nonselective MAO inhibitors (phenelzine, tranylcypromine):* possible hypertensive crisis. Avoid concomitant use.

EFFECTS ON DIAGNOSTIC TESTS
None reported.

CONTRAINDICATIONS
Contraindicated in patients with liver disease, elevated ALT or AST values, or hypersensitivity to drug or its components; in those who were withdrawn from tolcapone because of evidence of drug-induced hepatocellular injury; or in patients with history of nontraumatic rhabdomyolysis or hyperpyrexia and confusion possibly related to drug.

NURSING CONSIDERATIONS
• Use cautiously in patients with severe renal impairment and in breast-feeding women.
• Because of risk of liver toxicity, stop treatment if patient shows no benefit within 3 weeks.
• Use drug only in patients on levodopa and carbidopa who do not respond to or who are not appropriate candidates for other adjunctive therapies because of risk of potentially fatal liver failure.
• Know that patient should provide a written informed consent before drug is used.
• Monitor liver function test results before starting drug, then every 2 weeks for first year of therapy, then every 4 weeks for next 6 months, and then every 8 weeks thereafter. Stop drug if results are elevated or if patient appears jaundiced.
• Because of the highly protein-bound nature of tolcapone, drug is not expected to be removed significantly during dialysis.
• Monitor for orthostatic hypotension and syncope.
• Administer first dose of day with first daily dose of carbidopa-levodopa.
• Know that diarrhea commonly occurs, sometimes 2 to 12 weeks after therapy begins. Although it usually resolves with drug discontinuation, patient may require hospitalization in rare cases.

☑ **Patient teaching**
• Advise patient to take drug exactly as prescribed.
• Teach patient signs of liver injury (jaundice, fatigue, loss of appetite, persistent nausea, pruritus, dark urine, or right upper quadrant tenderness) and instruct him to report them immediately.
• Warn patient about risk of orthostatic hypotension; tell him to use caution when rising from a seated or recumbent position.
• Caution patient to avoid hazardous activities until CNS effects of drug are known.
• Tell patient that nausea may occur upon initiation of therapy.
• Advise patient about risk of increased dyskinesia or dystonia.
• Inform patient that hallucinations may occur.
• Tell patient to report if pregnancy is being planned or suspected during therapy.
• Tell patient to report adverse effects including diarrhea to doctor.
• Inform patient that drug may be taken without regard to meals.

trihexyphenidyl hydrochloride
Aparkanet†, Apo-Trihex†, Artane*, Artane Sequels, Novo-Hexidyl†, Trihexane, Trihexy-2, Trihexy-5

Pregnancy Risk Category: NR

HOW SUPPLIED
Tablets: 2 mg, 5 mg
Capsules (sustained-release): 5 mg
Elixir: 2 mg/5 ml

ACTION
Unknown. Blocks central cholinergic receptors, helping to balance cholinergic activity in the basal ganglia.

Route	Onset	Peak	Duration
PO	1 hr	Unknown	6-12 hr

INDICATIONS & DOSAGE
All forms of parkinsonism, drug-induced parkinsonism, and adjunctive treatment to levodopa in the management of parkinsonism—

Reactions may be *common,* uncommon, *life-threatening,* or COMMON AND LIFE-THREATENING.

Adults: 1 mg P.O. on day 1, 2 mg on day 2; then increased in 2-mg increments q 3 to 5 days until total of 6 to 10 mg is given daily. Usually given t.i.d. with meals, sometimes given q.i.d. (last dose h.s.) or switched to extended-release form b.i.d.

Postencephalitic parkinsonism may require total daily dosage of 12 to 15 mg.

ADVERSE REACTIONS
CNS: nervousness, dizziness, headache, hallucinations, drowsiness, weakness.
CV: tachycardia.
EENT: blurred vision, mydriasis, increased intraocular pressure.
GI: *dry mouth,* constipation, *nausea,* vomiting.
GU: urinary hesitancy, urine retention.

INTERACTIONS
Drug-drug. *Amantadine:* additive anticholinergic adverse reactions, such as confusion and hallucinations. Reduce dosage of trihexyphenidyl before administering.
Levodopa: decreased total bioavailability of levodopa. May require lower doses of both agents.
Drug-lifestyle. *Alcohol use:* increased sedative effects. Avoid concomitant use.

EFFECTS ON DIAGNOSTIC TESTS
None reported.

CONTRAINDICATIONS
Contraindicated in patients hypersensitive to drug.

NURSING CONSIDERATIONS
• Use cautiously in glaucoma; cardiac, hepatic, or renal disorders; obstructive disease of the GI and GU tracts; and prostatic hyperplasia.
• Be aware that dosage may need to be gradually increased in patients who develop a tolerance to drug.
• Monitor patient. Adverse reactions are dose-related and transient.
• Gonioscopic evaluation and monitoring of intraocular pressure are needed, especially in patients over 40 years.

☑ **Patient teaching**
• Advise patient that drug may cause nausea if given before meals.
• Tell patient to avoid activities that require alertness until CNS effects of drug are known.
• Advise patient to report signs of urinary hesitancy or urine retention.
• Tell patient to relieve dry mouth with cool drinks, ice chips, or sugarless gum or hard candy.
• Advise patient to avoid alcohol while taking drug.

bupropion hydrochloride
donepezil hydrochloride
droperidol
fluvoxamine maleate
lithium carbonate
lithium citrate
naratriptan hydrochloride
nicotine polacrilex
nicotine transdermal system
propofol
rizatriptan benzoate
sibutramine hydrochloride
   monohydrate
sumatriptan succinate
tacrine hydrochloride
zolmitriptan

COMBINATION PRODUCTS
None.

▼ NEW DRUG

bupropion hydrochloride
Zyban

Pregnancy Risk Category: B

HOW SUPPLIED
Tablets (sustained-release): 150 mg

ACTION
A relatively weak inhibitor of the neuronal uptake of norepinephrine, serotonin, and dopamine; drug does not inhibit MAO. Exact mechanism by which ability to abstain from smoking is enhanced is unknown.

Route	Onset	Peak	Duration
PO	Unknown	3 hr	Unknown

INDICATIONS & DOSAGE
Aid to smoking cessation treatment—
Adults: 150 mg P.O. daily for 3 days; increased to maximum of 300 mg P.O. daily given as two divided doses at least 8 hours apart.

ADVERSE REACTIONS
CNS: agitation, asthenia, depression, *dizziness,* headache, *insomnia,* irritability, somnolence, tremor, thinking or dream abnormalities, disturbed concentration, anxiety, nervousness.
CV: *complete AV block,* hypertension, hypotension, tachycardia, palpitations.
EENT: amblyopia, *dry mouth*, epistaxis, taste perversion, mouth ulcer, pharyngitis, sinusitis, tinnitus, *rhinitis.*
GI: anorexia, dyspepsia, increased appetite, abdominal pain, nausea, constipation, diarrhea, flatulence, vomiting.
GU: hot flashes, urinary frequency.
Musculoskeletal: arthralgia, leg cramps and twitching, myalgia.
Respiratory: bronchitis, increased cough, dyspnea.
Skin: dry skin, pruritus, rash, urticaria.
Other: allergic reactions, neck pain, injury, fever.

INTERACTIONS
Drug-drug. *Antipsychotics, antidepressants, theophylline, systemic steroids, treatment regimens (such as abrupt discontinuation of benzodiazepines):* may lower seizure threshold. Use cautiously.
Carbamazepine, phenobarbital, phenytoin: may induce metabolism of bupropion and decrease its effect. Monitor closely.
Cimetidine: may inhibit metabolism of bupropion and lead to increased levels. Monitor closely.
Levodopa: may lead to an increased incidence of adverse reactions when given concurrently with bupropion. If used concurrently, give small initial doses of bupropion and increase dose gradually.
MAO inhibitors (phenelzine): increased toxicity. Avoid concurrent use and allow at least 14 days to elapse between discontinuation of an MAO inhibitor and starting bupropion therapy.
Other medications containing bupropion (Wellbutrin, Wellbutrin SR): contain the same active ingredient as Zyban. Avoid concomitant use.

Drug-lifestyle. *Alcohol*: may increase risk of seizures. Avoid concomitant use.

EFFECTS ON DIAGNOSTIC TESTS
None reported.

CONTRAINDICATIONS
Contraindicated in patients with seizure disorders or with a current or prior diagnosis of bulimia or anorexia nervosa. Also contraindicated in patients known to be allergic to drug or its components and in those being treated with other medications containing bupropion (such as Wellbutrin, Wellbutrin SR) or MAO inhibitors. Allow at least 14 days to elapse between discontinuation of MAO inhibitors and initiation of drug treatment.

NURSING CONSIDERATIONS
• Use cautiously in patients with recent history of MI or unstable heart disease. Also use cautiously in patients with history of seizures, head trauma, and other predisposition to seizures, or in those being treated with agents that lower seizure threshold.
• Know that increased risk of seizures has been associated with excessive use of alcohol, abrupt withdrawal from alcohol or other sedatives, and addiction to cocaine, opiates, or stimulants. Seizure risk has also been associated with OTC stimulants and anorectics as well as diabetic patients being treated with oral antidiabetic agents or insulin.
• To reduce seizure risk, daily dose of 300 mg should not be exceeded. Divide dose (150 mg twice-daily) so that no single dose exceeds 150 mg.
• Be aware that therapy should be discontinued if patient has not made progress toward abstinence by week 7 of therapy.
• Know that dose does not require tapering before discontinuation of treatment.
Alert: Therapy should begin while patient is still smoking; approximately 1 week is needed to achieve steady-state plasma drug levels.

☑**Patient teaching**
• Stress importance of combining behavioral interventions, counseling, and support services with drug therapy.

• Advise patient to take doses at least 8 hours apart. If insomnia occurs, tell him not to take dose at bedtime.
• Tell patient not to chew, divide, or crush tablets.
• Advise patient that it may take 1 week for effects of drug to be evident. Also, tell him to set a target date for cessation of smoking during the second week of therapy.
• Tell patient that treatment usually lasts for 7 to 12 weeks.
• Inform patient that tablets may have a characteristic odor.
• Advise patient to avoid alcohol while taking drug.
• Advise patient to avoid activities that require mental alertness, such as driving or operating machinery, until drug's CNS effects are known.
• Warn patient not to use drug in combination with nicotine patches unless directed to do so under medical supervision. Doing so may lead to an increase in blood pressure.
• Inform patient that risk of seizures is increased if he has a seizure or eating disorder, exceeds the recommended dose, or takes other medications containing bupropion or those that lower seizure threshold.
• Advise patient to read accompanying patient information before starting drug.
• Advise patient to notify doctor if she is pregnant or plans to become pregnant while taking drug.

---

donepezil hydrochloride
Aricept

Pregnancy Risk Category: C

HOW SUPPLIED
Tablets: 5 mg, 10 mg

ACTION
Inhibits the enzyme acetylcholinesterase in the CNS, increasing the concentration of acetylcholine and may temporarily improve cognitive function in patients with Alzheimer's disease.

Route	Onset	Peak	Duration
PO	Unknown	3-4 hr	Unknown

INDICATIONS & DOSAGE
Mild to moderate dementia of the Alzheimer's type—
Adults: initially, 5 mg P.O. daily h.s. After 4 to 6 weeks, dosage may be increased to 10 mg daily.

ADVERSE REACTIONS
CNS: *headache, insomnia,* dizziness, depression, abnormal dreams, somnolence, *seizures,* tremor, irritability, paresthesia, aggression, vertigo, ataxia, restlessness, abnormal crying, nervousness, aphasia.
CV: syncope, chest pain, hypertension, vasodilation, *atrial fibrillation,* hot flashes, hypotension.
EENT: cataract, blurred vision, eye irritation.
GI: *nausea, diarrhea,* vomiting, anorexia, fecal incontinence, GI bleeding, bloating, epigastric pain.
GU: frequent urination.
Hematologic: ecchymosis.
Musculoskeletal: muscle cramps, arthritis, toothache, bone fracture.
Respiratory: dyspnea, sore throat, bronchitis.
Skin: pruritus, urticaria, diaphoresis.
Other: pain, fatigue, weight loss, influenza, dehydration, increased libido.

INTERACTIONS
Drug-drug. *Anticholinergics:* drug may interfere with anticholinergic activity. Monitor patient.
Bethanechol, succinylcholine: additive effects. Monitor patient closely.
Carbamazepine, dexamethasone, phenytoin, phenobarbital, rifampin: may increase rate of elimination of donepezil. Monitor patient.
Cholinomimetics, cholinesterase inhibitors: synergistic effect. Monitor patient closely.
Drug-herb. *Jaborandi tree:* may have additive effect when used concomitantly. Use cautiously to avoid risk of toxicity.
Pill-bearing spurge: additive effects may occur and risk of toxicity may be increased. Use together cautiously.

EFFECTS ON DIAGNOSTIC TESTS
None reported.

CONTRAINDICATIONS
Contraindicated in patients with known hypersensitivity to drug or piperidine derivatives.

NURSING CONSIDERATIONS
• Use cautiously in patients with CV disease, asthma or obstructive pulmonary disease, urinary outflow impairment, or history of ulcer disease, and in those patients presently taking NSAIDs.
• Know that drug should be used in pregnancy only if benefit justifies risk to fetus. Breast-feeding should be avoided.
• Monitor for symptoms of active or occult GI bleeding.

☑ **Patient teaching**
• Emphasize that drug does not alter underlying degenerative disease but can relieve symptoms. Effects of therapy depend on taking drug at regular intervals.
• Tell caregiver to give drug in the evening, just before bedtime.
• Advise patient and caregiver to immediately report significant adverse effects or changes in overall health status and to inform health care team if patient takes drug before he receives anesthesia.

droperidol
Droleptan§, Inapsine

Pregnancy Risk Category: C

HOW SUPPLIED
Injection: 2.5 mg/ml in 1-, 2- and 5-ml ampules, and 2-, 5-, and 10-ml vials

ACTION
Unknown. Produces marked tranquilization, sedation, and antiemetic effects while allowing for reflex alertness. Also causes mild alpha-adrenergic blockade.

Route	Onset	Peak	Duration
IV, IM	3-10 min	30 min	2-4 hr

INDICATIONS & DOSAGE
Premedication—
Adults and children over 12 years: 2.5 to 10 mg I.M. 30 to 60 minutes preoperatively.

Reactions may be *common,* uncommon, *life-threatening,* or COMMON AND LIFE-THREATENING.

Children 2 to 12 years: 1 to 1.5 mg per 9 to 11 kg (20 to 25 lb) of body weight I.M.
Elderly: reduce dose.
Adjust-a-dose: In debilitated patients and those who have received other depressant drugs, use reduced dose.
For induction as an adjunct to general anesthesia—
Adults and children over 12 years: 2.5 mg per 9 to 11 kg (20 to 25 lb) of body weight I.V. For maintenance, 1.25 to 2.5 mg, usually I.V.
Children 2 to 12 years: 1 to 1.5 mg per 9 to 11 kg (20 to 25 lb) of body weight I.V.
Use without a general anesthetic in diagnostic procedures—
Adults and children over 12 years: 2.5 to 10 mg I.M. 30 to 60 minutes before procedure. Additional doses of 1.25 to 2.5 mg, usually I.V., may be given.
Adjunct to regional anesthesia when additional sedation is required—
Adults: 2.5 to 5 mg I.M. or slow I.V.

ADVERSE REACTIONS
CNS: drowsiness, restlessness hyperactivity, anxiety, extrapyramidal symptoms, dizziness, hallucinations, *neuroleptic malignant syndrome.*
CV: hypotension, tachycardia.
Other: dysphoria, chills, shivering, *laryngospasm*, *bronchospasm.*

INTERACTIONS
Drug-drug. *CNS depressants:* additive CNS effects. Adjust dose as needed.
Fentanyl citrate: may cause hypertension, respiratory depression. Use together cautiously.

EFFECTS ON DIAGNOSTIC TESTS
Postoperative EEG returns to normal slowly.

CONTRAINDICATIONS
Contraindicated in patients with known hypersensitivity to drug.

NURSING CONSIDERATIONS
• Use cautiously in patients with hepatic or renal dysfunction and in breast-feeding patients.
• Use with caution in patients with suspected or diagnosed pheochromocytoma

because severe hypertension and tachycardia can occur.
• When used for induction of general anesthesia, use together with an analgesic.
• If used in procedures such as bronchoscopy, appropriate topical anesthesia is still necessary.
Alert: Have fluids and other measures to manage hypotension readily available.
• Monitor vital signs routinely.
• Monitor for symptoms of neuroleptic malignant syndrome (fever, altered consciousness, extrapyramidal symptoms, tachycardia).

◗ I.V. administration
• Administer I.V. doses slowly.

✓ Patient teaching
• Warn patient to rise slowly to prevent orthostatic hypotension.
• Advise patient to avoid alcohol for 24 hours after receiving droperidol.

---

fluvoxamine maleate
Faverin§, Luvox

Pregnancy Risk Category: C

HOW SUPPLIED
Tablets: 50 mg, 100 mg

ACTION
Unknown. Selectively inhibits the neuronal uptake of serotonin, which is thought to improve obsessive-compulsive disorders.

Route	Onset	Peak	Duration
PO	Unknown	3-8 hr	Unknown

INDICATIONS & DOSAGE
Obsessive-compulsive disorder—
Adults: initially, 50 mg P.O. daily h.s., increased in 50-mg increments q 4 to 7 days until maximum benefit achieved. Maximum daily dosage is 300 mg. Total daily doses of more than 100 mg should be given in two divided doses.

ADVERSE REACTIONS
CNS: *headache, asthenia, somnolence, insomnia, nervousness,* dizziness, tremor,

anxiety, hypertonia, *agitation*, depression, CNS stimulation, taste perversion.
CV: palpitations, vasodilation.
EENT: amblyopia.
GI: *nausea, diarrhea, constipation, dyspepsia*, anorexia, *vomiting*, flatulence, tooth disorder, dysphagia, *dry mouth*.
GU: abnormal ejaculation, urinary frequency, impotence, anorgasmia, urine retention.
Respiratory: upper respiratory tract infection, dyspnea, yawning.
Skin: sweating.
Other: flulike syndrome, chills, decreased libido.

INTERACTIONS
Drug-drug. *Astemizole:* may cause decreased metabolism, leading to increased levels of these antihistamines and cardiotoxicity. Avoid concomitant use.
Benzodiazepines, theophylline, warfarin: reduced clearance of these drugs by fluvoxamine. Use together cautiously (except for diazepam, which should not be administered with fluvoxamine). Dosage adjustments may be necessary.
Carbamazepine, clozapine, methadone, metopranolol, propranolol, tricyclic antidepressants: elevated serum levels of these drugs caused by fluvoxamine. Use together cautiously. Monitor patient closely for adverse reactions. Dosage adjustments may be necessary.
Diltiazem: bradycardia may occur. Monitor heart rate.
Lithium, tryptophan: may enhance effects of fluvoxamine. Use together cautiously.
MAO inhibitors: may cause severe excitation, hyperpyrexia, myoclonus, delirium, and coma. Avoid concomitant use.
Drug-lifestyle. *Smoking:* decreased effectiveness of drug. Encourage patient to stop smoking.

EFFECTS ON DIAGNOSTIC TESTS
None reported.

CONTRAINDICATIONS
Contraindicated in patients with hypersensitivity to drug or to other phenylpiperazine antidepressants and within 14 days of MAO inhibitor therapy.

NURSING CONSIDERATIONS
• Use cautiously in patients with hepatic dysfunction, concomitant conditions that may affect hemodynamic responses or metabolism, or history of mania or seizures.
Alert: Record mood changes. Monitor patient for suicidal tendencies, and allow only a minimum supply of drug.

☑ **Patient teaching**
• Warn patient not to engage in hazardous activity until drug's CNS effects are known.
• Instruct female patient who becomes pregnant or intends to become pregnant during therapy to notify doctor.
• Tell patient who develops a rash, hives, or a related allergic reaction to notify doctor.
• Inform patient that several weeks of therapy may be required to obtain the full antidepressant effect. Once improvement is seen, advise patient not to discontinue drug until directed by doctor.
• Advise patient to check with doctor before taking OTC medications; drug interactions can occur.

---

lithium carbonate
Camcolit§, Carbolith†, Duralith†, Eskalith, Eskalith CR, Lithane**, Lithicarb‡, Lithizine†, Lithobid, Lithonate, Lithotabs, Priadel§

lithium citrate
Cibalith-S*

Pregnancy Risk Category: D

HOW SUPPLIED
lithium carbonate
Tablets: 250 mg‡, 300 mg (300 mg equals 8.12 mEq lithium)
Tablets (controlled-release): 300 mg, 400 mg‡, 450 mg
Capsules: 150 mg, 300 mg, 600 mg
lithium citrate
Syrup (sugarless): 8 mEq (of lithium) per 5 ml
   Note: 5 ml of lithium citrate (liquid) contains 8 mEq lithium, equal to 300 mg of lithium carbonate.

Reactions may be *common*, uncommon, *life-threatening*, or COMMON AND LIFE-THREATENING.

ACTION
Unknown. Probably alters chemical transmitters in the CNS, possibly by interfering with ionic pump mechanisms in brain cells, and may compete with or replace sodium ions.

Route	Onset	Peak	Duration
PO	Unknown	0.5-3 hr	Unknown

INDICATIONS & DOSAGE
Prevention or control of mania—
Adults: 300 to 600 mg P.O. up to q.i.d. or 900 mg P.O. q 12 hours of controlled-release tablets; increase based on blood levels to achieve optimal dosage. Recommended therapeutic lithium blood levels are 1.5 mEq/L for acute mania, 0.6 to 1.2 mEq/L for maintenance therapy, and 2 mEq/L as maximum level.

ADVERSE REACTIONS
CNS: tremors, drowsiness, headache, confusion, restlessness, dizziness, psychomotor retardation, lethargy, *coma,* blackouts, *epileptiform seizures,* EEG changes, worsened organic mental syndrome, impaired speech, ataxia, muscle weakness, incoordination.
CV: reversible ECG changes, *arrhythmias,* hypotension, bradycardia, *peripheral vascular collapse* (rare).
EENT: tinnitus, blurred vision.
GI: dry mouth, metallic taste, nausea, vomiting, anorexia, diarrhea, *thirst,* abdominal pain, flatulence, indigestion.
GU: *polyuria,* glycosuria, decreased creatinine clearance, albuminuria; *renal toxicity* (with long-term use).
Hematologic: *leukocytosis with leukocyte count of 14,000 to 18,000/mm^3* (reversible).
Skin: pruritus, rash, diminished or absent sensation, drying and thinning of hair, psoriasis, acne, alopecia.
Other: transient hyperglycemia, goiter, hypothyroidism (lowered T_3, T_4, and protein-bound iodine, but elevated ^{131}I uptake), hyponatremia, ankle and wrist edema.

INTERACTIONS
Drug-drug. *Aminophylline, sodium bicarbonate, urine alkalinizers:* increased lithium excretion. Avoid excessive salt and monitor lithium levels.
Carbamazepine, fluoxetine, methyldopa, NSAIDs, probenecid: increased effect of lithium. Monitor for lithium toxicity.
Diuretics: increased reabsorption of lithium by kidneys, with possible toxic effect. Use with extreme caution and monitor lithium and electrolyte levels (especially sodium).
Neuroleptics: may cause encephalopathy. Watch for signs and symptoms (lethargy, tremor, extrapyramidal symptoms), and stop drug if it occurs.
Neuromuscular blockers: may cause prolonged paralysis or weakness. Monitor patient closely.
Thyroid hormones: may induce hypothyroidism. Monitor thyroid function.
Drug-herb. *Parsley:* may promote or produce serotonin syndrome. Avoid concomitant use.
Plantains: psyllium seed has been reported to inhibit GI absorption. Avoid concomitant use.

EFFECTS ON DIAGNOSTIC TESTS
Lithium causes false-positive test results on thyroid function tests; it also elevates neutrophil count.

CONTRAINDICATIONS
Contraindicated if therapy cannot be closely monitored.

NURSING CONSIDERATIONS
• Know that drug should not be administered during pregnancy.
• Use with extreme caution in patients receiving neuroleptics, neuromuscular blockers, and diuretics; in elderly or debilitated patients; and in patients with thyroid disease, seizure disorder, concomitant infection, renal or CV disease, severe debilitation or dehydration, and sodium depletion.
 *Alert:*Be aware that determination of lithium blood concentration is crucial to the safe use of drug. Do not use drug in patients who can't have regular lithium blood level checks. Monitor lithium blood levels 8 to 12 hours after first dose, usually before morning dose, two or three times weekly for the first month, then

weekly to monthly during maintenance therapy.

• Know that when blood levels of lithium are below 1.5 mEq/L, adverse reactions are usually mild.

• Monitor baseline ECG and thyroid and renal studies as well as electrolyte levels, as ordered.

• Check fluid intake and output, especially when surgery is scheduled.

• Weigh patient daily; check for signs of edema or sudden weight gain.

• Adjust fluid and salt ingestion to compensate if excessive loss occurs as a result of protracted diaphoresis or diarrhea. Under normal conditions, patients should have fluid intake of 2,500 to 3,000 ml daily and a balanced diet with adequate salt intake.

• Check urine specific gravity and report level below 1.005, which may indicate diabetes insipidus.

• Drug alters glucose tolerance in diabetics. Monitor blood glucose closely.

• Perform outpatient follow-up of thyroid and renal functions every 6 to 12 months. Palpate thyroid to check for enlargement.

☑ **Patient teaching**

• Tell patient to take drug with plenty of water and after meals to minimize GI upset.

• Explain that lithium has a narrow therapeutic margin of safety. A blood level that is even slightly high can be dangerous.

• Warn patient and caregivers to watch for evidence of toxicity (diarrhea, vomiting, tremor, drowsiness, muscle weakness, ataxia) and to expect transient nausea, polyuria, thirst, and discomfort during first few days.

• Instruct patient to withhold one dose and call the doctor if toxic symptoms appear, but not to stop drug abruptly.

• Warn ambulatory patient to avoid hazardous activities that require alertness and good psychomotor coordination until CNS effects of the drug are known.

• Tell patient not to switch brands of lithium or take other prescription or OTC drugs without doctor's guidance.

• Tell patient to carry medical identification at all times.

▼ *NEW DRUG*

naratriptan hydrochloride
Amerge

Pregnancy Risk Category: C

HOW SUPPLIED
Tablets: 1 mg, 2.5 mg

ACTION
Thought to activate receptors located in intracranial blood vessels leading to vasoconstriction and migraine headache relief. Another theory is that activation of receptors on sensory nerve endings in the trigeminal system results in the inhibition of proinflammatory neuropeptide release.

Route	Onset	Peak	Duration
PO	Unknown	2-3 hr	Unknown

INDICATIONS & DOSAGE
Treatment of acute migraine headache attacks with or without aura—
Adults: 1 or 2.5 mg P.O. as a single dose. If headache returns or if only partial response occurs, dose may be repeated after 4 hours, for maximum dose of 5 mg within 24 hours.
Adjust-a-dose: In patients with mild to moderate renal or hepatic impairment, a lower initial dose is recommended. Do not exceed maximum dose of 2.5 mg within a 24-hour period.

ADVERSE REACTIONS
CNS: paresthesias, dizziness, drowsiness, malaise, fatigue, vertigo, syncope.
CV: palpitation, increased blood pressure, ***tachyarrhythmias, abnormal ECG changes (PR, QTc prolongation, ST/T wave abnormalities, PVCs, atrial flutter or fibrillation), coronary vasospasm.***
EENT: ear, nose and throat infections, photophobia.
GI: nausea, hyposalivation, vomiting.
Other: warm or cold temperature sensations; pressure, tightness, heaviness sensations.

INTERACTIONS
Drug-drug. *Ergot-containing or ergot-type agents (methysergide, dihydroergota-*

---

mine), other 5HT₁ agonists: prolonged vasospastic reactions. Do not give within 24 hours of naratriptan.

Oral contraceptives: slightly higher concentrations of naratriptan. Monitor patient.

Selective serotonin reuptake inhibitors (fluoxetine, fluvoxamine, paroxetine, sertraline): may cause weakness, hyperreflexia, and incoordination. Monitor patient.

Drug-lifestyle. *Smoking:* increased clearance of naratriptan. Discourage concomitant use.

EFFECTS ON DIAGNOSTIC TESTS
None reported.

CONTRAINDICATIONS
Contraindicated in patients with hypersensitivity to drug or its components; history, symptoms, or signs of cardiac ischemia and cerebrovascular or peripheral vascular syndromes; or history of uncontrolled hypertension and in the elderly. Also contraindicated in patients with severe renal impairment (creatinine clearance below 15 ml/minute) or severe hepatic impairment [Child-Pugh grade C] and in those who have received ergot-containing, ergot-type, or other 5-HT₁ agonists within the past 24 hours.

NURSING CONSIDERATIONS
• Use cautiously in patients with risk factors for coronary artery disease, such as hypertension, hypercholesterolemia, obesity, diabetes, strong family history of coronary artery disease, women with surgical or physiologic menopause, men over 40 years, or smoking unless a CV evaluation has determined patient to be free from cardiac disease. For those with cardiac risk factors who have had a satisfactory CV evaluation, monitor closely after first dose.
• Use cautiously in patients with impaired renal or hepatic function.
• Assess cardiac status in patients who develop risk factors for coronary artery disease.

Alert: Know that drug can cause coronary artery vasospasm and increase risk of cerebrovascular events.

• Drug is not intended for prophylactic therapy of migraines or for use in managing hemiplegic or basilar migraine.
• Safety and effectiveness has not been established for cluster headaches or for treating more than four headaches in a 30-day period.
• Use drug after a definite diagnosis of migraine has been established.

☑ **Patient teaching**
• Instruct patient to take drug only as prescribed, and to read the accompanying patient instruction leaflet before using drug.
• Tell patient that drug is intended to relieve, not prevent migraine headaches.
• Instruct patient to take dose soon after headache starts. If no response occurs with first tablet, tell patient to seek medical approval before taking second tablet. Tell patient that if more relief is needed after first tablet (when a partial response occurs or if headache returns), and doctor has medically approved a second dose, he may take a second tablet but not sooner than 4 hours after first tablet. Inform him not to exceed two tablets within 24 hours.
• Instruct patient not to use drug during pregnancy or if it is suspected.
• Teach patient to alert doctor of risk factors for coronary artery disease or if bothersome adverse effects occur.

---

nicotine polacrilex (nicotine-polacrilin resin complex)
Nicorette ◇, Nicotinell§

Pregnancy Risk Category: X

HOW SUPPLIED
Chewing gum: 2 mg/square, 4 mg/square

ACTION
Provides nicotine, which stimulates nicotinic acetylcholine receptors in the CNS, neuromuscular junction, autonomic ganglia, and adrenal medulla.

Route	Onset	Peak	Duration
PO	Unknown	15-30 min	Unknown

INDICATIONS & DOSAGE
Relief of nicotine withdrawal symptoms in patients undergoing smoking cessation—
Adults: initially, one 2-mg square; highly dependent patients should start treatment with 4-mg squares. Patient should chew 1 piece of gum slowly and intermittently for 30 minutes whenever the urge to smoke occurs. Most patients require 9 to 12 pieces of gum daily during the first month. For patients using 4-mg squares, maximum dosage is 20 pieces daily. For patients using 2-mg squares, maximum dosage is 30 pieces daily.

ADVERSE REACTIONS
CNS: dizziness, light-headedness, irritability, insomnia, headache.
CV: *atrial fibrillation.*
EENT: *throat soreness, jaw muscle ache* (from chewing).
GI: nausea, vomiting, indigestion, eructation, anorexia, excessive salivation.
Other: *hiccups.*

INTERACTIONS
Drug-drug. *Beta blockers, methylxanthines, propoxyphene, propranolol:* decreased metabolism of these agents, increasing therapeutic effects. Dosage adjustments of these agents may be needed.
Drug-lifestyle. *Smoking:* reduced effectiveness of drug. Warn patient to avoid smoking while taking drug.

EFFECTS ON DIAGNOSTIC TESTS
None reported.

CONTRAINDICATIONS
Contraindicated in nonsmokers; in patients with recent MI, life-threatening arrhythmias, severe or worsening angina pectoris, or active temporomandibular joint disease; and during pregnancy.

NURSING CONSIDERATIONS
• Use cautiously in patients with hyperthyroidism, pheochromocytoma, insulin-dependent diabetes, peptic ulcer disease, history of esophagitis, oral or pharyngeal inflammation, or dental conditions that might be exacerbated by chewing gum.
• Know that smokers most likely to benefit from nicotine gum are those with high "physical" nicotine dependence—those who smoke more than 15 cigarettes daily, prefer brands of cigarettes with high nicotine levels, usually inhale the smoke, smoke the first cigarette within 30 minutes of rising, find the first morning cigarette the hardest to give up, smoke most frequently during the morning, find it difficult to refrain from smoking in places where it's forbidden, or smoke even when ill and confined to bed during the day.

✔ Patient teaching
• Instruct patient to chew gum slowly and intermittently (chew several times; then place between cheek and gum) for about 30 minutes to promote slow and even buccal absorption of nicotine. Gum must be chewed to release nicotine. Swallowing gum is ineffective. Fast chewing tends to produce more adverse reactions.
• Be sure that patient reads and understands the instruction sheet included in the package.
• Emphasize importance of withdrawing the gum gradually.
• Tell patient to gradually withdraw gum usage after 3 months. Use of the gum for longer than 6 months is not recommended. For gradual withdrawal, cut gum in halves or quarters and mix with other sugarless gum.

---

nicotine transdermal system
Habitrol, Nicoderm, Niconil§, Nicotrol, ProStep

Pregnancy Risk Category: D

HOW SUPPLIED
Transdermal system: designed to release nicotine at a fixed rate.
Habitrol—21 mg/day, 14 mg/day, 7 mg/day
Nicoderm—21 mg/day, 14 mg/day, 7 mg/day
Nicotrol—15 mg/16 hours, 10 mg/16 hours, 5 mg/16 hours
ProStep—22 mg/day, 11 mg/day

ACTION
Provides nicotine, which stimulates nicotinic acetylcholine receptors in the CNS,

neuromuscular junction, autonomic ganglia, and adrenal medulla.

Route	Onset	Peak	Duration
Trans-dermal	Unknown	3-9 hr	Unknown

INDICATIONS & DOSAGE

Relief of nicotine withdrawal symptoms in patients undergoing smoking cessation—
Adults: initially, one transdermal system, delivering the largest available dosage of nicotine in its dosage series, applied once daily to a nonhairy part of body. For Habitrol, Nicoderm, and ProStep, patch should be kept on for 24 hours, then removed and a new system applied to an alternate skin site. For Nicotrol, the patch should be applied upon awakening and removed h.s. After 4 to 12 weeks (depending on brand used), dosage tapered to next lowest available dosage of nicotine in its dosage series, followed in 2 to 4 weeks by lowest nicotine dosage system in series being used. Drug is then stopped in 2 to 4 weeks.

ADVERSE REACTIONS

CNS: somnolence, dizziness, *headache, insomnia,* paresthesia, abnormal dreams, nervousness.
EENT: pharyngitis, sinusitis.
GI: abdominal pain, constipation, dyspepsia, nausea, diarrhea, vomiting, dry mouth.
GU: dysmenorrhea.
Respiratory: increased cough, pharyngitis, sinusitis.
Skin: *local or systemic erythema, pruritus, burning at application site,* cutaneous hypersensitivity, rash.
Other: back pain, myalgia, diaphoresis, hypertension.

INTERACTIONS

Drug-drug. *Acetaminophen, imipramine, oxazepam, pentazocine, propranolol, theophylline:* may decrease induction of hepatic enzymes that help metabolize certain drugs. Dosage reductions may be necessary.
Adrenergic agonists (such as isoproterenol, phenylephrine): may decrease circulating catecholamines. Dosage increases may be necessary.
Adrenergic antagonists (such as labetalol, prazosin): may decrease circulating catecholamines. Dosage reductions may be necessary.
Insulin: may increase amount of S.C. insulin absorbed. Dosage reduction of insulin may be necessary.
Drug-herb. *Blue cohosh:* increased effects of nicotine. Avoid concomitant use.
Drug-food. *Caffeine:* may decrease induction of hepatic enzymes that help metabolize certain drugs. Dosage reductions may be necessary.

EFFECTS ON DIAGNOSTIC TESTS
None reported.

CONTRAINDICATIONS
Contraindicated in patients with hypersensitivity to nicotine or any component of transdermal system. Also contraindicated in nonsmokers; in patients with recent MI, life-threatening arrhythmias, and severe or worsening angina pectoris.

NURSING CONSIDERATIONS
• Use cautiously in patients with hyperthyroidism, pheochromocytoma, hypertension, insulin-dependent diabetes, or peptic ulcer disease.
• Know that health care workers' exposure to nicotine within transdermal systems is probably minimal; however, avoid unnecessary contact with the system. Wash hands with water alone because soap may enhance absorption.

☑ **Patient teaching**
• Inform patient that use of transdermal system for over 3 months is not recommended. Warn patient that chronic nicotine consumption by any route can be dangerous and habit-forming.
Alert: Warn patient not to smoke. If he continues to smoke while using the system, he may experience serious adverse effects because peak serum nicotine levels will be substantially higher than those achieved by smoking alone.
• Be sure that patient reads and understands the information that is dispensed with drug.

• Advise patient to apply patch promptly because nicotine can evaporate from the transdermal system once it's removed from its protective packaging. Patch should not be altered in any way (folded or cut) before application and not stored at temperatures above 86° F (30° C).

• Teach patient proper disposal of the transdermal system. After removal, fold the patch in half, bringing the adhesive sides together. If it comes in a protective pouch, place the used patch in the pouch that contained the system. Careful disposal is necessary to prevent accidental poisoning of children or pets.

• Tell patient who experiences persistent or severe local skin reactions or generalized rash to immediately discontinue use of the patch and notify doctor.

• Inform patient that those who cannot stop cigarette smoking during the initial 4 weeks of therapy probably will not benefit from the continued use of drug. Such patients may benefit from counseling to identify factors that led to treatment failure. Encourage patient to minimize or eliminate factors contributing to treatment failure and to try again, possibly after some time has passed.

propofol
Diprivan

Pregnancy Risk Category: B

HOW SUPPLIED
Injection: 10 mg/ml in 20 ml ampules; 50 ml prefilled syringes; 50-, 100-ml infusion vials.

ACTION
Unknown. Rapidly acting I.V. sedative-hypnotic agent.

Route	Onset	Peak	Duration
IV	< 40 sec	Unknown	10-15 min

INDICATIONS & DOSAGE
Induction of general anesthesia—
Adults under 55 years: 40 mg I.V. q 10 seconds until induction onset (2 to 2.5 mg/kg). In patients receiving cardiac anesthesia, 20 mg q 10 seconds (0.5 to 1.5 mg/kg) until induction onset. In neurosurgical patients, 20 mg q 10 seconds until induction onset (1 to 2 mg/kg).
Children 3 years or older: in healthy children, 2.5 to 3.5 mg/kg administered over 20 to 30 seconds.
Elderly: 20 mg q 10 seconds until induction onset (1 to 1.5 mg/kg).
Adjust-a-dose: In debilitated patients, or in patients classified as class III or IV by the American Society of Anesthesiologists (ASA), 20 mg q 10 seconds until induction onset (1 to 1.5 mg/kg).
Maintenance of general anesthesia: infusion—
Adults under 55 years: 100 to 200 mcg/kg/minute. In patients receiving cardiac anesthesia, 50 to 150 mcg/kg/minute. In neurosurgical patients, 100 to 200 mcg/kg/minute.
Children 3 years or older: in healthy children, 125 to 300 mcg/kg/minute.
Elderly: 50 to 100 mcg/kg/minute.
Adjust-a-dose: In debilitated or ASA class III or IV patients, 50 to 100 mcg/kg/minute.
Maintenance of general anesthesia—
Adults under 55 years: intermittent bolus in increments of 20 to 50 mg I.V. p.r.n.
Initiation of monitored anesthesia care (MAC) sedation—
Adults under 55 years: dosage individualized; 100 to 150 mcg/kg/minute infusion for 3 to 5 minutes, or slow injection over 3 to 5 minutes of 0.5 mg/kg followed immediately by I.V. infusion.
Maintenance of MAC sedation—
Adults under 55 years: 25 to 75 mcg/kg/minute infusion or incremental bolus doses of 10 to 20 mg I.V.
Elderly: 80% of healthy adult dose.
Adjust-a-dose: In debilitated, neurosurgical, or ASA class III or IV patients, 80% of healthy adult dose.
Initiation and maintenance of intensive care unit (ICU) sedation in intubated, mechanically ventilated patients—
Adults: dosage individualized. Initial infusion usually 5 mcg/kg/minute for 5 minutes. May increase rate at 5- to 10-minute intervals in increments of 5 to 10 mcg/kg/minute until desired level of sedation is achieved. Rates of 5 to

50 mcg/kg/minute or higher may be required.

ADVERSE REACTIONS
CNS: *movement.*
CV: bradycardia, *hypotension,* hypertension, decreased cardiac output.
Respiratory: APNEA, respiratory acidosis.
Skin: rash.
Other: *burning or stinging at injection site,* hyperlipemia.

INTERACTIONS
Drug-drug. *Inhaled anesthetics (such as enflurane, halothane, isoflurane), opioids (fentanyl, meperidine, morphine), sedatives (such as barbiturates, benzodiazepines, chloral hydrate, droperidol):* may increase anesthetic and sedative effects and may also result in a more pronounced decrease in blood pressure and cardiac output. Monitor closely.

EFFECTS ON DIAGNOSTIC TESTS
None reported.

CONTRAINDICATIONS
Contraindicated in patients hypersensitive to drug or its components (including egg lecithin, soybean oil, and glycerol) or when general anesthesia or sedation is contraindicated.

NURSING CONSIDERATIONS
● Use cautiously in patients with seizures. Because drug is excreted in breast milk, use is not recommended in breast-feeding patients.
● Always use strict aseptic technique during handling. Propofol can support the growth of microorganisms; do not use if contamination is suspected. Discard tubing and unused portions of drug after 12 hours.
● Do not use if there is evidence of separation of phases of emulsion.
● Allow an adequate time interval (3 to 5 minutes) between dose adjustments to assess effects.
● Titrate drug daily to achieve only minimum effective drug concentration.
● For general anesthesia or MAC sedation, drug should be administered by trained personnel not involved in the surgical or diagnostic procedure. For ICU sedation, drug should be administered by persons skilled in the management of critically ill patients and trained in cardiopulmonary resuscitation and airway management.
● Continuously monitor vital signs.
● Monitor patients at risk for hyperlipidemia for increases in serum triglycerides.
● Drug contains 0.1 g of fat (1.1 kcal)/ml. A reduction in concurrently administered lipids is necessary.
● Propofol contains ethylenediamine-tetraacetic acid (EDTA), a strong metal chelator. Consider supplemental zinc during prolonged therapy.
● When given in the ICU, assess patient's CNS function daily to determine minimum dose required.

◖ I.V. administration
● Protect drug from light. Shake well. Dilute only with D_5W. Do not dilute to a concentration below 2 g/ml. Do not infuse through a filter with a pore size smaller than 5 microns. Administer via larger veins of upper extremities to decrease injection site pain.
● Do not administer drug in the same I.V. line with blood or plasma.

☑ Patient teaching
● Advise patient that performance of activities requiring mental alertness, such as operating a motor vehicle or hazardous machinery, may be impaired for some time after drug use.

▼ *NEW DRUG*

rizatriptan benzoate
Maxalt, Maxalt-MLT

Pregnancy Risk Category: C

HOW SUPPLIED
Tablets: 5 mg, 10 mg
Tablets (orally disintegrating): 5 mg, 10 mg

ACTION
Believed to exert its effect by acting as an agonist at serotonin receptors on the ex-

tracerebral intracranial blood vessels, which results in vasoconstriction of the affected vessels, inhibition of neuropeptide release, and reduction of pain transmission in the trigeminal pathways.

Route	Onset	Peak	Duration
PO	Unknown	1-1.5 hr	Unknown

INDICATIONS & DOSAGE
Treatment of acute migraine headaches with or without aura—
Adults: initially, 5 or 10 mg P.O. If first dose is ineffective, another dose can be given at least 2 hours after first dose. Maximum dosage is 30 mg within a 24-hour period. For patients receiving propranolol, 5 mg P.O. up to maximum of three doses (15 mg) in 24 hours.

ADVERSE REACTIONS
CNS: dizziness, headache, somnolence, paresthesia, asthenia, fatigue, hypesthesia, decreased mental acuity, euphoria, tremor.
CV: chest pain, pressure or heaviness, palpitations.
EENT: neck, throat and jaw pain, pressure or heaviness.
GI: dry mouth, nausea, diarrhea, vomiting.
Respiratory: dyspnea.
Skin: flushing.
Other: pain, warm or cold sensations, hot flashes.

INTERACTIONS
Drug-drug. *Ergot-containing or ergot-type drugs (dihydroergotamine, methysergide), other 5-HT$_1$ agonists:* prolonged vasospastic reactions. Do not use within 24 hours of rizatriptan.
MAO inhibitors (moclobemide), nonselective MAO inhibitors (types A and B; isocarboxazid, pargyline, phenelzine, tranylcypromine): increased plasma concentrations of rizatriptan. Avoid concurrent use and allow at least 14 days to elapse between discontinuation of an MAO inhibitor and taking rizatriptan.
Propranolol: increased rizatriptan levels. Reduce rizatriptan dose to 5 mg.
Selective serotonin reuptake inhibitors (fluoxetine, fluvoxamine, paroxetine, ser-

traline): weakness, hyperreflexia, incoordination may occur. Monitor patient.

CONTRAINDICATIONS
Contraindicated in patients with ischemic heart disease (angina pectoris, history of MI, or documented silent ischemia) or in those with symptoms or findings consistent with ischemic heart disease, coronary artery vasospasm (Prinzmetal's variant angina), or other significant underlying CV disease. Also contraindicated in patients with uncontrolled hypertension or within 24 hours of treatment with another 5-HT$_1$ agonist, or an ergotamine-containing or ergot-type medication like dihydroergotamine or methysergide. Do not use within 2 weeks of discontinuation of MAO inhibitor. Also contraindicated in patients hypersensitive to drug or its inactive ingredients.

NURSING CONSIDERATIONS
• Use cautiously in patients with hepatic or renal impairment.
• Use with caution in patients with risk factors for coronary artery disease, (hypertension, hypercholesterolemia, smoking, obesity, diabetes, strong family history of coronary artery disease, women with surgical or physiological menopause, or men over 40 years), unless a cardiac evaluation provides evidence that patient is free from cardiac disease.
• For patients with risk factors that have a satisfactory cardiac evaluation, monitor closely after first dose.
• Assess CV status in patients who develop risk factors for coronary artery disease during treatment.
• Be aware that drug should be used only after a definite diagnosis of migraine is established.
• Do not use for prophylactic therapy of migraines or in patients with hemiplegic or basilar migraine or cluster headaches.
• Know that the safety of treating, on average, more than four headaches in a 30-day period has not been established.
• Safety and effectiveness have not been evaluated in children under 18 years.
• Know that the orally disintegrating tablets contain phenylalanine.

Reactions may be common, uncommon, ***life-threatening***, or COMMON AND LIFE-THREATENING.

☑ Patient teaching
- Inform patient that drug does not prevent migraine headache from occurring.
- For Maxalt-MLT, tell patient to remove blister pack from pouch, then remove drug from blister pack immediately before use. Tablet should not be popped out of blister pack, but pack should be carefully peeled away with dry hands, and tablet placed on tongue and allowed to dissolve. Tablet is then swallowed with the saliva. No water is necessary or recommended. Tell patient that orally dissolving tablet does not provide more rapid headache relief.
- Advise patient that if headache returns after initial dose, a second dose may be taken with medical approval at least 2 hours after the first dose. Do not take more than 30 mg in a 24-hour period.
- Inform patient that drug may cause somnolence and dizziness and warn him to avoid hazardous activities until effects are known.
- Tell patient that food may delay drug's onset of action.
- Advise patient to notify doctor if pregnancy occurs or is suspected.
- Instruct patient not to breast-feed because the effects on the infant are unknown.

---

sibutramine hydrochloride monohydrate
Meridia

Controlled Substance Schedule IV
Pregnancy Risk Category: C

HOW SUPPLIED
Capsules: 5 mg, 10 mg, 15 mg

ACTION
Produces its therapeutic effects by inhibiting the reuptake of norepinephrine, serotonin, and dopamine.

Route	Onset	Peak	Duration
PO	Unknown	3-4 hr	Unknown

INDICATIONS & DOSAGE
Management of obesity—
Adults: 10 mg P.O. administered once daily with or without food. May increase dose to 15 mg P.O. daily after 4 weeks if there is inadequate weight loss. Patients who do not tolerate the 10 mg dose may receive 5 mg P.O. daily. Doses above 15 mg daily are not recommended.

ADVERSE REACTIONS
CNS: *headache, insomnia,* dizziness, nervousness, anxiety, depression, paresthesia, somnolence, CNS stimulation, emotional lability, migraine.
CV: tachycardia, vasodilation, hypertension, palpitation, chest pain.
EENT: thirst, *dry mouth, rhinitis, pharyngitis,* sinusitis, taste perversion, ear disorder, ear pain.
GI: *anorexia, constipation,* increased appetite, nausea, dyspepsia, gastritis, vomiting, abdominal pain, rectal disorder.
GU: dysmenorrhea, urinary tract infection, vaginal monilia, metrorrhagia.
Musculoskeletal: arthralgia, myalgia, tenosynovitis, joint disorder, neck or back pain.
Respiratory: cough increase, laryngitis.
Skin: rash, sweating, herpes simplex, acne.
Other: back pain, flu syndrome, injury, accident, asthenia, neck pain, ***allergic reaction,*** generalized edema.

INTERACTIONS
Drug-drug. *CNS depressants:* may enhance CNS depression. Use with caution.
Dextromethorphan, dihydroergotamine, fentanyl, fluoxetine, fluvoxamine, lithium, MAO inhibitors, meperidine, paroxetine, pentazocine, sertraline, sumatriptan, tryptophan, venlafaxine: may cause hyperthermia, tachycardia, loss of consciousness. Avoid concomitant use.
Ephedrine, phenylpropanolamine, pseudoephedrine: may increase blood pressure or heart rate. Use with caution.
Drug-lifestyle. *Alcohol use:* enhanced CNS depression. Use with caution.

EFFECTS ON DIAGNOSTIC TESTS
Drug may cause elevated liver function tests.

CONTRAINDICATIONS
Contraindicated in patients taking MAO

inhibitors or other centrally acting appetite suppressant drugs, and in those with anorexia nervosa or hypersensitivity to drug or its active ingredients. Do not use drug in patients with severe renal or hepatic dysfunction, history of hypertension, coronary artery disease, heart failure, arrhythmias, or stroke

NURSING CONSIDERATIONS
• Use cautiously in patients with history of seizures or narrow angle-glaucoma.
• Know that drug is recommended for obese patients with an initial body mass index of 30 kg/m^2 or more or 27 kg/m^2 or more in the presence of other risk factors (such as hypertension, diabetes, or dyslipidemia).
• Rule out organic causes of obesity before starting therapy.
• Measure blood pressure and pulse before starting therapy, with dosage changes, and at regular intervals during therapy.
• Know that at least 2 weeks should elapse between stopping an MAO inhibitor and starting drug therapy, and vice versa.

☑ **Patient teaching**
• Advise patient to report rash, hives, or other allergic reactions immediately.
• Instruct patient to inform doctor before taking prescription or OTC drugs.
• Advise patient to have blood pressure and pulse monitored at regular intervals. Stress importance of regular follow-up visits with doctor.
• Advise patient to use drug with reduced-calorie diet.
• Tell patient that weight loss can precipitate gallstone formation. Teach patient signs and symptoms and to report them to doctor promptly.

---

sumatriptan succinate
Imigran§, Imitrex

Pregnancy Risk Category: C

HOW SUPPLIED
Tablets: 25 mg, 50 mg, 100 mg (base)†

Injection: 6 mg/0.5 ml (12 mg/ml) in 0.5-ml prefilled syringes and vials

ACTION
Unknown. Thought to selectively activate vascular serotonin (5-hydroxytryptamine, 5-HT) receptors. Stimulation of the specific receptor subtype 5-HT$_1$, present on cranial arteries and the dura mater, causes vasoconstriction of cerebral vessels but has minimal effects on systemic vessels, tissue perfusion, and blood pressure.

Route	Onset	Peak	Duration
PO	0.5 hr	1.5 hr	Unknown
SC	10-20 min	12 min	Unknown

INDICATIONS & DOSAGE
Acute migraine attacks (with or without aura)—
Adults: 6 mg S.C. Maximum recommended dosage is two 6-mg injections daily, with at least 1 hour allowed between injections. Alternatively, an initial dose of 25 to 100 mg P.O. and a second dose of up to 100 mg in 2 hours, if needed. Additional doses may be given q 2 hours, p.r.n., up to maximum P.O. dosage of 300 mg/day.

ADVERSE REACTIONS
CNS: *dizziness, vertigo,* drowsiness, headache, anxiety, malaise, fatigue, *burning sensation, tingling, warm or hot sensation,* feeling of strangeness, tight feeling in head, cold sensation; *heaviness, pressure, or tightness.*
CV: *atrial fibrillation, ventricular fibrillation, ventricular tachycardia, MI,* ECG changes such as ischemic ST-segment elevation (rare).
EENT: discomfort of throat, nasal cavity or sinus, mouth, jaw, or tongue; altered vision.
GI: abdominal discomfort, dysphagia.
Skin: flushing.
Other: pressure or tightness in chest; myalgia; muscle cramps; diaphoresis; neck pain; *injection site reaction.*

INTERACTIONS
Drug-drug. *Ergot and ergot derivatives:* prolonged vasospastic effects. Don't use

---

these drugs and sumatriptan within the same 24-hour period.
MAO inhibitors: increased effects of sumatriptan. Avoid concomitant use or within 2 weeks of discontinuing MAO inhibitor therapy.
Drug-herb. *Horehound:* may enhance serotonergic effects. Avoid concomitant use.

EFFECTS ON DIAGNOSTIC TESTS
None reported.

CONTRAINDICATIONS
Contraindicated in patients with uncontrolled hypertension or ischemic heart disease (such as angina pectoris, Prinzmetal's angina, history of MI, or documented silent ischemia), hemiplegic or basilar migraine, and hypersensitivity to drug. Also contraindicated in those taking ergotamine or within 14 days of MAO therapy.

NURSING CONSIDERATIONS
● Use cautiously in patients who are or intend to become pregnant.
● Also use cautiously in patients who may have unrecognized coronary artery disease, such as postmenopausal women; men over 40 years; or patients with risk factors such as hypertension, hypercholesterolemia, obesity, diabetes, smoking, or family history of coronary artery disease.
● When giving drug to patients at risk for unrecognized coronary artery disease, consider administering first dose in the doctor's office. Serious adverse cardiac effects can follow S.C. administration of drug, but such events are rare.
● After S.C. injection, most patients experience relief within 1 to 2 hours.
● Know that redness or pain at the injection site should subside within 1 hour after the injection.

☑ Patient teaching
● Inform patient that drug is intended only to treat migraine attacks, not to prevent or reduce their occurrence.
● Tell patient who is pregnant or intends to become pregnant not to use drug. Advise her to discuss with doctor the risks and benefits of using drug during pregnancy.
● Tell patient that drug may be given any time during a migraine attack, but should be given as soon as symptoms appear.
● Review information about drug's injectable form, which is available in a spring-loaded injector system that facilitates self-administration. Be sure patient understands how to load the injector, administer the injection, and dispose of the used syringes.
Alert: Tell patient to notify doctor immediately of persistent or severe chest pain. Warn him to stop using drug and call the doctor if he experiences pain or tightness in the throat, wheezing, heart throbbing, rash, lumps, hives, or swollen eyelids, face, or lips.

tacrine hydrochloride
Cognex

Pregnancy Risk Category: C

HOW SUPPLIED
Capsules: 10 mg, 20 mg, 30 mg, 40 mg

ACTION
Reversibly inhibits the enzyme cholinesterase in the CNS, preventing or blocking the breakdown of acetylcholine and thereby temporarily improving cognitive function in patients with Alzheimer's disease.

Route	Onset	Peak	Duration
PO	Unknown	0.5-3 hr	Unknown

INDICATIONS & DOSAGE
Mild to moderate dementia of the Alzheimer's type—
Adults: initially, 10 mg P.O. q.i.d. After 6 weeks and if the patient tolerates treatment and there are no transaminase elevations, dosage increased to 20 mg q.i.d. After 6 weeks, dosage titrated upward to 30 mg q.i.d. If still tolerated, dosage increased to 40 mg q.i.d. after another 6 weeks.

ADVERSE REACTIONS
CNS: agitation, ataxia, insomnia, abnor-

mal thinking, somnolence, depression, anxiety, *headache,* fatigue, *dizziness,* confusion.
GI: *nausea, vomiting, diarrhea,* dyspepsia, loose stools, changes in stool color, anorexia, abdominal pain, flatulence, constipation.
Respiratory: rhinitis, upper respiratory tract infection, cough.
Skin: rash, jaundice, facial flushing.
Other: myalgia, chest pain, weight loss.

INTERACTIONS
Drug-drug. *Anticholinergics:* may decrease effectiveness of anticholinergics. Monitor patient closely.
Cholinergics (such as bethanechol), cholinesterase inhibitors: additive effects. Monitor for toxicity.
Succinylcholine: enhanced neuromuscular blockade and prolonged duration of action. Monitor patient closely.
Theophylline: increased serum theophylline levels and prolonged theophylline half-life. Carefully monitor theophylline plasma levels and adjust dosage, as ordered.
Drug-food. *Any food:* delayed absorption of drug. Give drug 1 hour before meals.
Drug-lifestyle. *Smoking:* decreased plasma concentrations of drug. Monitor response.

EFFECTS ON DIAGNOSTIC TESTS
Drug may cause significant abnormalities in serum transaminase (ALT, AST), bilirubin, and GGT levels.

CONTRAINDICATIONS
Contraindicated in patients hypersensitive to drug or acridine derivatives. Also contraindicated in patients who have previously developed tacrine-related jaundice, which has been confirmed with an elevated total bilirubin level of more than 3 mg/dl.

NURSING CONSIDERATIONS
• Use cautiously in patients with sick sinus syndrome or bradycardia; in patients at risk for peptic ulceration (including patients taking NSAIDs or those with history of peptic ulcer); and in those with history of hepatic disease. Also use cautiously in patients with renal disease, asthma, prostatic hyperplasia, or other urinary outflow impairment.
• Monitor serum ALT levels weekly during the first 18 weeks of therapy as ordered. If ALT is modestly elevated after the first 18 weeks of monitoring (twice the upper limit of normal range), continue weekly monitoring. If no problems are detected, frequency of serum determinations is decreased to once every 3 months. On each occasion that dosage is increased, resume weekly monitoring for at least 6 weeks as ordered.
• Know that if drug is discontinued for 4 weeks or more, the full dosage titration and monitoring schedule must be restarted.

☑ **Patient teaching**
• Stress that drug does not alter the underlying degenerative disease, but can alleviate symptoms. Effect of therapy depends on drug administration at regular intervals.
Alert: Remind caregivers that dosage titration is an integral part of the safe use of drug. Abrupt discontinuation or a large reduction in daily dosage (80 mg/day or more) may precipitate behavioral disturbances and a decline in cognitive function.
• Tell caregiver to give patient drug between meals whenever possible. If GI upset becomes a problem, drug may be taken with meals, although doing so may reduce plasma levels by 30% to 40%.
• Advise patient and caregivers to immediately report significant adverse effects or changes in status.

zolmitriptan
Zomig

Pregnancy Risk Category: C

HOW SUPPLIED
Tablets (immediate-release): 2.5 mg, 5 mg

ACTION
A selective serotonin receptor agonist that can abort migraine headaches by causing

constriction of cranial blood vessels and inhibition of proinflammatory neuropeptide release.

Route	Onset	Peak	Duration
PO	Unknown	2 hr	3 hr

INDICATIONS & DOSAGE
Acute migraine headaches—
Adults: Initially, 2.5 mg or lower P.O. increased to 5 mg per dose p.r.n. If headache returns after initial dose, second dose may be administered after 2 hours. Maximum dosage is 10 mg in 24-hour period.
Adjust-a-dose: In patients with moderate to severe hepatic impairment, use a lower dose.

ADVERSE REACTIONS
CNS: somnolence, vertigo, *dizziness,* syncope.
CV: pain or heaviness in chest, *arrhythmias,* hypertension, *pain, tightness, or pressure in the neck, throat, or jaw.*
GI: dyspepsia, dysphagia, nausea.
Metabolic: hyperglycemia.
Other: hyperesthesias, paresthesias, warm or cold sensations, asthenia, myalgia.

INTERACTIONS
Drug-drug. *Cimetidine:* doubles half-life of zolmitriptan. Monitor patient.
Ergot-containing drugs: may cause additive vasospastic reactions. Avoid concomitant use.
Fluoxetine, fluvoxamine, paroxetine, sertraline: may cause weakness, hyperreflexia, and incoordination. Use cautiously.
MAO inhibitors: increased effects of drug. Avoid concomitant use.

EFFECTS ON DIAGNOSTIC TESTS
Hyperglycemia has been reported rarely.

CONTRAINDICATIONS
Contraindicated in patients with ischemic heart disease or other significant heart disease (including Wolff-Parkinson-White syndrome), uncontrolled hypertension, or hypersensitivity to drug. Do not give within 24 hours of ergot-containing medications or within 2 weeks of discontinuing MAO inhibitor therapy.

NURSING CONSIDERATIONS
• Use cautiously in patients with liver disease.
• Drug is not intended for prophylactic therapy of migraine headaches or for use in hemiplegic or basilar migraines.
• Safety has not been established for cluster headaches.
• Do not administer to patient who is or may be pregnant or one who is breast-feeding.

☑ Patient teaching
• Tell patient that drug is intended to relieve the symptoms of migraines and not to prevent them.
• Advise patient to take drug as prescribed. Do not take a second dose unless instructed by doctor. Tell patient that if a second dose is indicated and permitted, to only take it 2 hours after initial dose.
• Advise patient to report pain or tightness in the chest or throat, heart throbbing, rash, skin lumps, or swelling of the face, lips or eyelids immediately.
• Tell patient not to take drug if pregnancy is being planned or is suspected.

37

Cholinergics (parasympathomimetics)

bethanechol chloride
edrophonium chloride
neostigmine bromide
neostigmine methylsulfate
physostigmine salicylate
pyridostigmine bromide

COMBINATION PRODUCTS
None.

---

bethanechol chloride
Duvoid, Myotonachol, Myotonine§,
Urabeth, Urecholine, Urocarb
Liquid‡, Urocarb Tablets‡

Pregnancy Risk Category: C

HOW SUPPLIED
Tablets: 5 mg, 10 mg, 25 mg, 50 mg
Injection: 5 mg/ml

ACTION
Directly stimulates primarily muscarinic
cholinergic receptors, mimicking the action of acetylcholine, producing increased
tone and peristalsis in the GI tract and increasing contraction of the detrusor muscle of the urinary bladder.

Route	Onset	Peak	Duration
PO	30-90 min	1 hr	6 hr
SC	5-15 min	15-30 min	2 hr

INDICATIONS & DOSAGE
*Acute postoperative and postpartum non-
obstructive (functional) urine retention,
neurogenic atony of urinary bladder with
urine retention—*
Adults: 10 to 50 mg P.O. t.i.d. to q.i.d. Or,
2.5 to 5 mg S.C. Never give I.M. or I.V.
When used for urine retention, some patients may require 50 to 100 mg P.O. per
dose. Use such doses with extreme caution.
 Test dose is 2.5 mg S.C., repeated at
15- to 30-minute intervals to total of four
doses to determine the minimal effective
dose; then minimal effective dose used q

6 to 8 hours. All doses must be adjusted
individually.

ADVERSE REACTIONS
CNS: headache, malaise.
CV: bradycardia, *profound hypotension
with reflexive tachycardia.*
EENT: lacrimation, miosis.
GI: *abdominal cramps, diarrhea,* exces-
sive salivation, nausea, belching, borbo-
rygmus.
GU: urinary urgency.
Respiratory: *bronchoconstriction,* in-
creased bronchial secretions.
Skin: flushing, diaphoresis.

INTERACTIONS
Drug-drug. *Anticholinergic agents, atropine, procainamide, quinidine*: may reverse cholinergic effects. Observe for lack
of drug effect.
*Anticholinesterase agents, cholinergic ag-
onists*: may cause additive effects or increase toxicity. Avoid concomitant use.
Ganglionic blockers: may cause critical
fall in blood pressure usually preceded by
severe abdominal pain. Avoid concomitant use.

EFFECTS ON DIAGNOSTIC TESTS
Bethanechol increases serum levels of
amylase, lipase, bilirubin, and AST, and
increases sulfobromophthalein retention
time.

CONTRAINDICATIONS
Contraindicated for I.M. or I.V. use and in
patients with hypersensitivity to drug or
its components; in patients with uncertain
strength or integrity of bladder wall; when
increased muscular activity of the GI or
urinary tract is harmful; in patients with
mechanical obstructions of the GI or urinary tract; in patients with hyperthyroidism, peptic ulceration, latent or active
bronchial asthma, obstructive pulmonary
disease, pronounced bradycardia or hypotension, vasomotor instability, cardiac
or coronary artery disease, hypertension,

Reactions may be *common,* uncommon, *life-threatening,* or COMMON AND LIFE-THREATENING.

seizure disorder, Parkinson's disease, spastic GI disturbances, acute inflammatory lesions of the GI tract, peritonitis, or marked vagotonia.

NURSING CONSIDERATIONS

- Use cautiously in pregnant patients.
- Give drug on empty stomach; otherwise, may cause nausea and vomiting.
Alert: Never give I.M. or I.V.; could cause circulatory collapse, hypotension, severe abdominal cramping, bloody diarrhea, shock, or cardiac arrest.
- Monitor vital signs frequently, especially respirations. Always have atropine injection available and be prepared to give 0.6 mg S.C. or by slow I.V. push as ordered. Provide respiratory support if needed.
- Watch for toxicity, especially with S.C. administration. Edrophonium is not effective against muscle relaxation caused by bethanechol.
- Watch closely for adverse reactions that may indicate drug toxicity.
- Know that oral drug absorption is poor and variable, requiring larger oral doses. Oral and S.C. doses are not interchangeable.

☑ **Patient teaching**
- Instruct patient to take oral form on an empty stomach and at regular intervals.
- Inform patient that drug is usually effective within 30 to 90 minutes after oral administration and 5 to 15 minutes after S.C. administration.

---

edrophonium chloride
Enlon, Reversol, Tensilon

Pregnancy Risk Category: C

HOW SUPPLIED
Injection: 10 mg/ml in 1-ml ampules or in 10-ml or 15-ml vials

ACTION
Rapidly reversible inhibitor of acetylcholinesterase, thus blocking the destruction of acetylcholine released from the parasympathetic and somatic efferent nerves. Acetylcholine accumulates, promoting increased stimulation of the receptors.

Route	Onset	Peak	Duration
IV	< 1 min	Unknown	5-20 min
IM	2-10 min	Unknown	10-40 min

INDICATIONS & DOSAGE
As a curare antagonist (to reverse nondepolarizing neuromuscular blocking action)—
Adults: 10 mg I.V. given over 30 to 45 seconds. Dose may be repeated p.r.n. to 40 mg maximum dosage. Larger dosages may potentiate effect of curare.
Diagnostic aid in myasthenia gravis (Tensilon test)—
Adults: 1 to 2 mg I.V. over 15 to 30 seconds, then 8 mg if no response (increase in muscular strength and no cholinergic reaction) occurs. Alternatively, 10 mg I.M. If cholinergic reaction occurs, 2 mg I.M. 30 minutes later is given to rule out false-negative response.
Children weighing over 34 kg (75 lb): 2 mg I.V. If no response within 45 seconds, 1 mg q 45 seconds to maximum of 10 mg.
Children weighing up to 34 kg: 1 mg I.V. If no response within 45 seconds, 1 mg q 45 seconds to maximum of 5 mg.
  I.M. route may be used in children because of difficulty with I.V. route: for children under 34 kg, 2 mg I.M.; for children over 34 kg, 5 mg I.M. Expect same reactions as with I.V. test, but these appear after 2- to 10-minute delay.
To differentiate myasthenic crisis from cholinergic crisis—
Adults: 1 mg I.V. If no response in 1 minute, dose repeated once. Increased muscular strength confirms myasthenic crisis; no increase or exaggerated weakness confirms cholinergic crisis.

ADVERSE REACTIONS
CNS: *seizures,* weakness, dysarthria, dysphonia, dizziness, drowsiness, headache.
CV: hypotension, bradycardia, AV block, *cardiac arrest,* syncope.
EENT: excessive lacrimation, diplopia, miosis, conjunctival hyperemia.
GI: nausea, vomiting, *diarrhea, abdomi-*

---

nal cramps, excessive salivation, dysphagia.
GU: urinary frequency, incontinence.
Respiratory: *paralysis of respiratory muscles, central respiratory paralysis, bronchospasm, laryngospasm,* increased bronchial secretions, *respiratory depression, respiratory arrest,* dyspnea.
Skin: rash, flushing.
Other: muscle cramps, muscle fasciculation, diaphoresis.

INTERACTIONS
Drug-drug. *Aminoglycosides:* prolonged or enhanced muscle weakness. Monitor closely.
Cardiac glycosides: may increase the heart's sensitivity to edrophonium. Use together cautiously.
Cholinergics: increased effects. Stop all other cholinergics before giving drug, as ordered.
Corticosteroids, magnesium, procainamide, quinidine: may antagonize cholinergic effects. Observe for lack of drug effect.
Depolarizing muscle relaxants (decamethonium, succinylcholine): increased neuromuscular blocking effects, prolonged respiratory depression. Monitor closely.
Local and general anesthetics: may antagonize cholinergic effects. Observe for lack of drug effect.
Drug-herb. *Jaborandi tree, pill-bearing spurge:* may have an additive effect when used concomitantly. Use with caution to avoid risk of toxicity.

EFFECTS ON DIAGNOSTIC TESTS
None reported.

CONTRAINDICATIONS
Contraindicated in patients with mechanical obstruction of the intestine or urinary tract and hypersensitivity to anticholinesterase agents.

NURSING CONSIDERATIONS
• Use cautiously in patients with bronchial asthma or cardiac arrhythmias.
• Watch closely for adverse reactions; they may indicate toxicity.
• Keep in mind that drug is not effective

against neuromuscular block induced by decamethonium bromide and succinylcholine chloride.
• Be aware that this cholinergic has the most rapid onset but shortest duration; therefore, it is not used to treat myasthenia gravis.
• When giving drug to differentiate myasthenic crisis from cholinergic crisis, observe patient's muscle strength closely.

◖I.V. administration
• For easier parenteral administration, use tuberculin syringe with an I.V. needle.
• Monitor vital signs frequently, especially respirations. Always have atropine injection available and be prepared to give 0.5 to 1 mg S.C. or by slow I.V. push as ordered. Provide respiratory support as needed.
• If using as a test to distinguish myasthenic from cholinergic crisis, be sure to secure controlled ventilation if the patient is apneic before administering drug.

☑Patient teaching
• Teach patient to report adverse reactions promptly.
• Tell patient to alert nurse if discomfort occurs at I.V. site.

neostigmine bromide
Prostigmin

neostigmine methylsulfate
Prostigmin

Pregnancy Risk Category: C

HOW SUPPLIED
neostigmine bromide
Tablets: 15 mg
neostigmine methylsulfate
Injection: 0.25 mg/ml, 0.5 mg/ml, 1 mg/ml

ACTION
Competitive inhibitor of acetylcholinesterase, thus blocking the destruction of acetylcholine released from the parasympathetic and somatic efferent nerves. Acetylcholine accumulates, pro-

moting increased stimulation of the receptors.

Route	Onset	Peak	Duration
PO	45-75 min	1-2 hr	2-4 hr
IV	4-8 min	1-2 hr	2-4 hr
IM, SC	20-30 min	1-2 hr	2-4 hr

INDICATIONS & DOSAGE
Treatment of myasthenia gravis—
Adults: initially, 15 mg P.O. t.i.d., increase gradually p.r.n. Range 15 mg to 375 mg/day with intervals individualized. Average oral dose is 150 mg/day; or 0.5 to 2.0 mg S.C., I.M., or I.V. q 1 to 3 hours.
Children: 7.5 to 15 mg P.O. t.i.d. or q.i.d. or 0.01 to 0.04 mg/kg/dose I.M. or S.C. q 2 to 3 hours, p.r.n.

Dosage must be highly individualized, depending on response and tolerance of adverse effects. Therapy may be required day and night.
Diagnosis of myasthenia gravis—
Adults: 0.022 mg/kg I.M. 30 minutes after 0.011 mg/kg of atropine sulfate I.M.
Children: 0.025 to 0.04 mg/kg I.M. after 0.011 mg/kg atropine sulfate S.C.
Postoperative abdominal distention and bladder atony—
Adults: 0.5 to 1 mg I.M. or S.C. q 4 to 6 hours (treatment); 0.25 mg S.C. or I.M. q 4 to 6 hours for 2 to 3 days (prevention).
Antidote for nondepolarizing neuromuscular blocking agents—
Adults: 0.5 to 2.5 mg I.V. slowly. Repeat p.r.n. to a total of 5 mg. Before antidote dose, 0.6 to 1.2 mg atropine sulfate is given I.V.
Note: 1:1,000 solution of injectable solution contains 1 mg/ml; 1:2,000 solution contains 0.5 mg/ml.

ADVERSE REACTIONS
CNS: dizziness, headache, muscle weakness, loss of consciousness, drowsiness, *seizures.*
CV: bradycardia, hypotension, tachycardia, AV block, syncope, *cardiac arrest.*
EENT: blurred vision, lacrimation, miosis.
GI: *nausea, vomiting, diarrhea, abdominal cramps,* excessive salivation, flatulence, increased peristalsis.
GU: urinary frequency.

Respiratory: *bronchospasm,* dyspnea, *respiratory depression, respiratory arrest,* increased secretions, *laryngospasm, paralysis of respiratory muscles, central respiratory paralysis.*
Skin: rash, urticaria, diaphoresis, flushing.
Other: *muscle cramps,* muscle fasciculations, arthralgia, hypersensitivity reactions *(anaphylaxis).*

INTERACTIONS
Drug-drug. *Aminoglycosides, anticholinergic agents, atropine, corticosteroids, magnesium sulfate, procainamide, quinidine, local and general anesthetics:* may reverse cholinergic effects. Observe for lack of drug effect. Stop all other cholinergics before giving this drug, as ordered. *Succinylcholine:* may worsen blockade produced by succinylcholine when used to reverse the effects of nondepolarizing neuromuscular blockers in patients who have undergone surgery. Monitor patient.

EFFECTS ON DIAGNOSTIC TESTS
None reported.

CONTRAINDICATIONS
Contraindicated in patients with peritonitis, mechanical obstruction of the intestine or urinary tract, and hypersensitivity to cholinergics or bromides.

NURSING CONSIDERATIONS
• Use cautiously in patients with bronchial asthma, bradycardia, seizure disorders, recent coronary occlusion, vagotonia, hyperthyroidism, arrhythmias, and peptic ulcer.
• In myasthenia gravis, schedule doses before periods of fatigue. For example, if patient has dysphagia, schedule dose 30 minutes before each meal.
• Monitor vital signs frequently, especially respirations. Have atropine injection available and be prepared to give as ordered; provide respiratory support, as needed.
• Monitor and document patient's response after each dose. Optimum dosage is difficult to judge. Observe closely for improvement in strength, vision, and ptosis 45 to 60 minutes after each dose.

- I.M. neostigmine may be used instead of edrophonium to diagnose myasthenia gravis and may be preferable to edrophonium for lengthy procedures involving testing of limb strength.
- When drug is used to prevent abdominal distention and GI distress, be aware that doctor may order insertion of a rectal tube to help passage of gas.
- When drug is given for postoperative abdominal distention and bladder atony, mechanical obstruction should be ruled out before treatment doses are given. If there is no response within one hour after the first dose, the patient should be catheterized.
- Know that patient sometimes develops a resistance to neostigmine.
- If appropriate, obtain doctor's order for a hospitalized patient to have bedside supply of tablets. Many patients with long-standing disease insist on self-administration.

⬙ I.V. administration
- Give at a slow, controlled rate, not exceeding 1 mg/minute in adults.
- If patient's muscle weakness is severe, keep in mind that the doctor determines whether it is caused by drug-induced toxicity or exacerbation of myasthenia gravis. Test dose of edrophonium I.V. will aggravate drug-induced weakness but will temporarily relieve weakness caused by disease.

☑ Patient teaching
- Tell patient to take drug with food or milk to reduce adverse GI reactions.
- When using for myasthenia gravis, explain that drug will relieve ptosis, double vision, difficulty in chewing and swallowing, and trunk and limb weakness. Stress importance of taking drug exactly as ordered, including nighttime doses. Explain that drug may have to be taken for life.
- Show patient how to observe and record variations in muscle strength.
- Advise patient to wear medical identification bracelet indicating myasthenia gravis.

physostigmine salicylate (eserine salicylate)
Antilirium

Pregnancy Risk Category: C

HOW SUPPLIED
Injection: 1 mg/ml

ACTION
Reversible inhibitor of acetylcholinesterase, thus blocking the destruction of acetylcholine released from the parasympathetic and somatic efferent nerves. Acetylcholine accumulates, promoting increased stimulation of the receptor.

Route	Onset	Peak	Duration
IV	3-5 min	5 min	0.5-5 hr
IM	3-5 min	20-30 min	0.5-5 hr

INDICATIONS & DOSAGE
To reverse the CNS toxicity associated with clinical or toxic dosages of drugs capable of producing anticholinergic syndrome—
Adults: 0.5 to 2 mg I.M. or I.V. (1 mg/ minute I.V.) repeated q 20 minutes as necessary until response or adverse cholinergic effects occur. Additional doses of 1 to 4 mg I.M. or I.V. q 30 to 60 minutes may be given if life-threatening signs recur (coma, seizures, arrhythmias).
Children: reserved for life-threatening situations only. Requires dose of 0.02 mg/ kg I.M. or slow I.V., repeated q 5 to 10 minutes until response occurs. Maximum dosage is 2 mg.

ADVERSE REACTIONS
CNS: *seizures,* muscle weakness, *restlessness, excitability.*
CV: bradycardia, hypotension.
EENT: miosis.
GI: nausea, vomiting, epigastric pain, *diarrhea, excessive salivation.*
GU: urinary urgency.
Respiratory: *bronchospasm,* bronchial constriction, dyspnea, *respiratory paralysis.*
Other: diaphoresis.

INTERACTIONS
Drug-drug. *Anticholinergic agents, at-*

Reactions may be *common,* uncommon, *life-threatening,* or COMMON AND LIFE-THREATENING.

ropine, local and general anesthetics, procainamide, quinidine: may reverse cholinergic effects. Observe for lack of drug effect.
Ganglionic blockers: may decrease blood pressure. Avoid concomitant use.
Neuromuscular blockers (succinylcholine): increased neuromuscular blockade, respiratory depression. Use cautiously.
Drug-herb. *Jaborandi tree, pill-bearing spurge:* may have an additive effect when used concomitantly. Use with caution to avoid risk of toxicity.

EFFECTS ON DIAGNOSTIC TESTS
None reported.

CONTRAINDICATIONS
Contraindicated in patients with mechanical obstruction of the intestine or urogenital tract, asthma, gangrene, diabetes, CV disease, or vagotonia and in those receiving choline esters or depolarizing neuromuscular blockers.

NURSING CONSIDERATIONS
• Use cautiously in pregnant patients, in patients with epilepsy, Parkinsonian syndrome, or bradycardia.
• Use only clear solution. Darkening may indicate loss of potency.
• Watch closely for adverse reactions, particularly CNS disturbances. Raise side rails if patient becomes restless or hallucinates. Adverse reactions may indicate drug toxicity.
• Know that effectiveness is generally immediate and dramatic but that it may be transient and require repeated doses.

◖I.V. administration
• Give I.V. at controlled rate; use direct injection at no more than 1 mg/minute in adults or 0.5 mg/minute in children.
• Monitor vital signs frequently, especially respirations. Position patient to ease breathing. Have atropine injection available and be prepared to give 0.5 mg S.C. or by slow I.V. push as ordered. Provide respiratory support as needed. Best administered in presence of a doctor.

☑Patient teaching
• Inform patient of need for drug, explain

its use and adverse reactions, and answer any questions or concerns.
• Tell patient to report adverse reactions promptly.
• Instruct patient to alert nurse if discomfort occurs at I.V. site.

pyridostigmine bromide
Mestinon*, Mestinon-SR†,
Mestinon Timespans, Regonol

Pregnancy Risk Category: C

HOW SUPPLIED
Tablets: 60 mg
Tablets (extended-release): 180 mg
Syrup: 60 mg/5 ml
Injection: 5 mg/ml in 2-ml ampules or 5-ml vials

ACTION
Competitive inhibitor of acetylcholinesterase, thus blocking the destruction of acetylcholine released from the parasympathetic and somatic efferent nerves. Acetylcholine accumulates, promoting increased stimulation of the receptors.

Route	Onset	Peak	Duration
PO	20-30 min	1-2 hr	3-6 hr
PO (extended)	30-60 min	1-2 hr	6-12 hr
IV	2-5 min	Unknown	2-4 hr
IM	15 min	Unknown	2-4 hr

INDICATIONS & DOSAGE
Antidote for nondepolarizing neuromuscular blockers—
Adults: 10 to 20 mg I.V. preceded by atropine sulfate 0.6 to 1.2 mg I.V.
Myasthenia gravis—
Adults: 60 to 120 mg P.O. q 3 or 4 hours. Usual dosage is 600 mg daily but higher dosage may be needed (up to 1,500 mg daily). For I.M. or I.V. use, ⅓₀ of oral dosage is given. Dosage must be adjusted for each patient, based on patient's response and tolerance. Alternatively, 180 to 540 mg extended-release tablets (1 to 3 tablets) P.O. b.i.d., with at least 6 hours between doses.
Children: 7 mg/kg or 200 mg/m^2 daily in five or six divided doses.

Supportive treatment of neonates born to myasthenic mothers—
Neonates: 0.05 to 0.15 mg/kg I.M. q 4 to 6 hours. Dosage decreased daily until drug can be withdrawn.

ADVERSE REACTIONS
CNS: headache (with high doses), weakness, syncope.
CV: bradycardia, hypotension, *cardiac arrest.*
EENT: miosis.
GI: abdominal cramps, nausea, vomiting, diarrhea, excessive salivation, increased peristalsis.
Respiratory: *bronchospasm, bronchoconstriction,* increased bronchial secretions.
Skin: rash, diaphoresis.
Other: muscle cramps, muscle fasciculations, thrombophlebitis.

INTERACTIONS
Drug-drug. *Aminoglycosides:* prolonged or enhanced muscle weakness. Use together cautiously.
Anticholinergic agents, atropine, corticosteroids, general or local anesthetics, magnesium, procainamide, quinidine: may antagonize cholinergic effects. Observe for lack of drug effect.
Ganglionic blockers: increased risk of hypotension. Monitor closely.

EFFECTS ON DIAGNOSTIC TESTS
None reported.

CONTRAINDICATIONS
Contraindicated in patients with mechanical obstruction of the intestine or urinary tract and hypersensitivity to anticholinesterase agents or bromides.

NURSING CONSIDERATIONS
• Use cautiously in patients with bronchial asthma, bradycardia, arrhythmias, epilepsy, recent coronary occlusion, vagotonia, hyperthyroidism or peptic ulcer. Also use cautiously in pregnant women.
• Stop all other cholinergics before giving this drug, as ordered.
• Do not crush the extended-release tablets.

• When using sweet syrup for patients who have difficulty swallowing, give over ice chips if patient cannot tolerate flavor.
• Monitor and document patient's response after each dose. Optimum dosage is difficult to judge.
Alert: In the United States, be aware that Regonol contains benzyl ethanol preservative, which may cause toxicity in neonates if administered in high doses. The Canadian formulation of this drug does not contain benzyl ethanol.
• If appropriate, obtain a doctor's order for a hospitalized patient to have bedside supply of tablets. Many patients with long-standing disease insist on self-administration.

I.V. administration
• Administer I.V. injection no faster than 1 mg/minute. With rapid I.V. infusion, bradycardia and seizures may result. Monitor vital signs frequently, especially respirations. Position patient to ease breathing. Have atropine injection available and be prepared to give as ordered; provide respiratory support as needed.
• If patient's muscle weakness is severe, keep in mind that the doctor determines whether it is caused by drug-induced toxicity or exacerbation of myasthenia gravis. Test dose of edrophonium I.V. will aggravate drug-induced weakness, but will temporarily relieve weakness caused by disease.

Patient teaching
• When using for myasthenia gravis, stress importance of taking drug exactly as ordered, on time, in evenly spaced doses. If doctor has ordered extended-release tablets, explain that patient must take tablets at the same time each day, at least 6 hours apart.
• Advise patient not to crush or chew extended-release tablets.
• Explain that patient may have to take drug for life.
• Advise patient to wear a medical identification bracelet indicating he has myasthenia gravis.

Reactions may be *common*, uncommon, *life-threatening*, or COMMON AND LIFE-THREATENING.

atropine sulfate
(See Chapter 21, ANTIARRHYTHMICS.)
dicyclomine hydrochloride
glycopyrrolate
hyoscyamine
hyoscyamine sulfate
propantheline bromide
scopolamine
scopolamine butylbromide
scopolamine hydrobromide

COMBINATION PRODUCTS

BARBIDONNA NO. 2 TABLETS: atropine sulfate 0.025 mg, scopolamine hydrobromide 0.0074 mg, hyoscyamine hydrobromide or sulfate 0.1286 mg, and phenobarbital 32 mg.
BARBIDONNA TABLETS: atropine sulfate 0.025 mg, scopolamine hydrobromide 0.0074 mg, hyoscyamine hydrobromide or sulfate 0.1286 mg, and phenobarbital 16 mg.
DONNATAL ELIXIR*: atropine sulfate 0.0194 mg/5 ml, scopolamine hydrobromide 0.0065 mg/5 ml, ethanol 23%, hyoscyamine hydrobromide or sulfate 0.1037 mg/5 ml, and phenobarbital 16 mg/5 ml.
DONNATAL EXTENTABS: atropine sulfate 0.0582 mg, scopolamine hydrobromide 0.0195 mg, hyoscyamine sulfate 0.3111 mg, and phenobarbital 48.6 mg.
DONNATAL TABLETS AND CAPSULES: atropine sulfate 0.0194 mg, scopolamine hydrobromide 0.0065 mg, hyoscyamine hydrobromide or sulfate 0.1037 mg, and phenobarbital 16.2 mg.

---

dicyclomine hydrochloride
Antispas, A-Spas, Bemote, Bentyl, Bentylol†, Byclomine, Dibent, Di-Spaz, Formulex†, Lominet†, Merbentyl‡, Neoquess, Or-Tyl, Spasmoban†, Spasmoject

Pregnancy Risk Category: B

HOW SUPPLIED
Tablets: 10 mg‡, 20 mg
Capsules: 10 mg, 20 mg
Syrup: 5 mg/5 ml‡, 10 mg/5 ml
Injection: 10 mg/ml

ACTION
Inhibits action of acetylcholine on post-ganglionic, parasympathetic muscarinic receptors, decreasing GI motility. Also possesses local anesthetic properties that may be partly responsible for spasmolysis.

Route	Onset	Peak	Duration
PO, IM	Unknown	1-1.5 hr	Unknown

INDICATIONS & DOSAGE
Irritable bowel syndrome and other functional GI disorders—
Adults: initially, 20 mg P.O. q.i.d., increased to 40 mg q.i.d., or 20 mg I.M. q.i.d.

ADVERSE REACTIONS
CNS: *headache; dizziness;* insomnia; light-headedness; drowsiness; nervousness, confusion, excitement (in elderly patients).
CV: *palpitations,* tachycardia.
EENT: blurred vision, increased intraocular pressure, mydriasis, photophobia.
GI: nausea, vomiting, *constipation, dry mouth, thirst,* abdominal distention, heartburn, paralytic ileus.
GU: *urinary hesitancy, urine retention,* impotence.
Skin: urticaria, decreased sweating or possible anhidrosis, other dermal manifestations, local irritation.
Other: fever, allergic reactions. Dicyclomine is a synthetic tertiary derivative that may have atropine-like adverse reactions.
Note: Overdose may cause curare-like effects, such as respiratory paralysis.

INTERACTIONS
Drug-drug. *Amantadine, antihistamines,*

---

antiparkinsonian agents, disopyramide, glutethimide, meperidine, phenothiazines, procainamide, quinidine, tricyclic antidepressants: additive adverse effects. Avoid concomitant use.

Antacids: decreased absorption of oral anticholinergics. Separate administration times by 2 to 3 hours.

Ketoconazole: anticholinergics may interfere with ketoconazole absorption. Separate administration times by 2 to 3 hours.

Methotrimeprazine: anticholinergics may enhance risk of extrapyramidal reactions. Avoid concomitant use.

EFFECTS ON DIAGNOSTIC TESTS
None reported.

CONTRAINDICATIONS
Contraindicated in patients with obstructive uropathy, obstructive disease of the GI tract, reflux esophagitis, severe ulcerative colitis, toxic megacolon, myasthenia gravis, unstable CV status in acute hemorrhage, tachycardia secondary to cardiac insufficiency or thyrotoxicosis, glaucoma, or hypersensitivity to anticholinergics; in breast-feeding patients; and in children under 6 months.

NURSING CONSIDERATIONS
• Use cautiously in patients with autonomic neuropathy, hyperthyroidism, coronary artery disease, arrhythmias, heart failure, hypertension, hiatal hernia, hepatic or renal disease, prostatic hyperplasia, known or suspected GI infection and ulcerative colitis. Also use cautiously in patients in hot or humid environment. Drug-induced heat stroke can develop.
• Give drug 30 minutes to 1 hour before meals and h.s. Bedtime dose can be larger; give at least 2 hours after last meal of day.
Alert: Do not give S.C. or I.V.
• Be prepared to adjust dosage based on patient's needs and response, as ordered. Doses up to 40 mg P.O. q.i.d. have been used in adults, but safety and efficacy for more than 2 weeks have not been established.
• Monitor patient's vital signs and urine output carefully.

☑ Patient teaching
• Instruct patient when to take drug and stress importance of taking drug on time and in evenly spaced intervals.
• Advise patient to avoid driving and other hazardous activities if drowsiness, dizziness, or blurred vision occurs; to drink plenty of fluids to help prevent constipation; and to report rash or other skin eruption.

---

glycopyrrolate
Robinul, Robinul Forte

Pregnancy Risk Category: B

HOW SUPPLIED
Tablets: 1 mg, 2 mg
Injection: 0.2 mg/ml

ACTION
Inhibits cholinergic (muscarinic) actions of acetylcholine on autonomic effectors innervated by postganglionic cholinergic nerves.

Route	Onset	Peak	Duration
PO	Unknown	Unknown	8-12 hr
IV	1 min	Unknown	3-7 hr
IM, SC	15-30 min	30-45 min	3-7 hr

INDICATIONS & DOSAGE
Blockade of adverse cholinergic effects caused by anticholinesterase agents used to reverse neuromuscular blockade—
Adults and children: 0.2 mg I.V. for each 1 mg neostigmine or 5 mg of pyridostigmine. May be given I.V. without dilution or may be added to dextrose injection and given by infusion.
Preoperatively to diminish secretions and block cardiac vagal reflexes—
Adults and children 2 years and older: 0.0044 mg/kg of body weight I.M. 30 to 60 minutes before anesthesia.
Children under 2 years: 0.0088 mg/kg I.M. 30 to 60 minutes before anesthesia.
Adjunctive therapy in peptic ulcerations and other GI disorders—
Adults: 1 to 2 mg P.O. t.i.d. or 0.1 to 0.2 mg I.M. or I.V. t.i.d. or q.i.d. Dosage must be individualized. Maximum daily oral dosage is 8 mg.

Reactions may be *common*, uncommon, **life-threatening**, or COMMON AND LIFE-THREATENING.

ADVERSE REACTIONS

CNS: weakness, nervousness, insomnia, drowsiness, dizziness, headache, confusion or excitement (in elderly patients).
CV: palpitations, tachycardia.
EENT: *dilated pupils, blurred vision,* photophobia, increased intraocular pressure.
GI: *constipation, dry mouth,* nausea, loss of taste, abdominal distention, vomiting, epigastric distress.
GU: *urinary hesitancy, urine retention,* impotence.
Skin: urticaria, decreased sweating or anhidrosis, other dermal manifestations.
Other: allergic reactions *(anaphylaxis),* fever.

Note: Overdose may cause curare-like effects, such as respiratory paralysis.

INTERACTIONS

Drug-drug. *Amantadine, antihistamines, antiparkinsonian agents, disopyramide, glutethimide, meperidine, phenothiazines, procainamide, quinidine, tricyclic antidepressants:* additive adverse effects. Avoid concomitant use.
Antacids: decreased absorption of oral anticholinergics. Separate administration times by 2 to 3 hours.
Ketoconazole: anticholinergics may interfere with ketoconazole absorption. Separate administration times by 2 to 3 hours.
Methotrimeprazine: anticholinergics may enhance risk of extrapyramidal reactions. Avoid concomitant use.

EFFECTS ON DIAGNOSTIC TESTS

None reported.

CONTRAINDICATIONS

Contraindicated in patients with glaucoma, obstructive uropathy, obstructive disease of the GI tract, myasthenia gravis, paralytic ileus, intestinal atony, unstable CV status in acute hemorrhage, tachycardia secondary to cardiac insufficiency or thyrotoxicosis, severe ulcerative colitis, toxic megacolon, known or suspected GI infection, or hypersensitivity to drug.

NURSING CONSIDERATIONS

• Use cautiously in patients with autonomic neuropathy, hyperthyroidism, coronary artery disease, arrhythmias, heart failure, hypertension, hiatal hernia, hepatic or renal disease, ulcerative colitis and known or suspected GI infection. Also use cautiously in patients in hot or humid environment. Drug-induced heatstroke is possible.
• Administer oral form 30 minutes to 1 hour before meals.
Alert: Check all dosages carefully; slight overdose can lead to toxicity.
• Monitor vital signs carefully. Watch closely for adverse reactions, especially in elderly or debilitated patients. Call the doctor promptly if they occur.
• Be aware that elderly patients typically receive smaller dosages.

I.V. administration

• Administer by direct injection without dilution. Alternatively, inject into the tubing of a free-flowing I.V. solution.
• Do not mix with I.V. solution containing sodium bicarbonate or alkaline solutions with a pH higher than 6. Alkaline drugs, such as barbiturates, chloramphenicol, dexamethasone, dimenhydrinate, diazepam, methylprednisolone, and pentazocine are incompatible with glycopyrrolate.

Patient teaching

• Instruct patient to take oral drug 30 to 60 minutes before meals.
• Warn patient to avoid activities that require alertness until drug's CNS effects are known.
• Advise patient to report signs of urinary hesitancy or urine retention.

---

hyoscyamine
Cystospaz

hyoscyamine sulfate
Anaspaz, Cystospaz, Cystospaz-M, Gastrosed, Levbid, Levsin*, Levsin Drops*, Levsin/SL, Levsinex Timecaps, Neoquess

Pregnancy Risk Category: C

HOW SUPPLIED
hyoscyamine
Tablets: 0.15 mg
hyoscyamine sulfate
Tablets: 0.125 mg, 0.13 mg, 0.15 mg
Capsules (extended-release): 0.375 mg
Elixir: 0.125 mg/5 ml
Oral solution: 0.125 mg/ml
Injection: 0.5 mg/ml

ACTION
Competitively blocks the action of acetylcholine at muscarinic receptors, which decreases GI motility and inhibits gastric acid secretion.

Route	Onset	Peak	Duration
PO	20-30 min	0.5-1 hr	4-12 hr
PO (extended)	20-30 min	40-90 min	12 hr
IV	2 min	15-30 min	4 hr
IM, SC	Unknown	15-30 min	4-12 hr
SL	5-20 min	0.5-1 hr	4 hr

INDICATIONS & DOSAGE
GI tract disorders caused by spasm; to diminish secretions and block cardiac vagal reflexes preoperatively; adjunctive therapy for peptic ulcerations, cystitis, renal colic, as a "drying agent" in the relief of symptoms of allergic rhinitis—
Adults and children 12 years or older:
0.125 to 0.25 mg P.O. or S.L. t.i.d. or q.i.d. before meals and h.s.; 0.375 to 0.75 mg extended-release form P.O. q 8 to 12 hours; or 0.25 to 0.5 mg (1 or 2 ml) I.M., I.V., or S.C. b.i.d. to q.i.d. (Oral medication substituted when symptoms are controlled.) Maximum daily dosage is 1.5 mg.
Children under 12 years: dosage individualized according to weight.

ADVERSE REACTIONS
CNS: headache, insomnia, drowsiness, dizziness, *confusion or excitement* (in elderly patients), nervousness, weakness.
CV: *palpitations,* tachycardia.
EENT: *blurred vision,* mydriasis, increased intraocular pressure, cycloplegia, photophobia.
GI: *dry mouth,* dysphagia, *constipation,* heartburn, loss of taste, nausea, vomiting, *paralytic ileus.*

GU: *urinary hesitancy, urine retention,* impotence.
Skin: urticaria, decreased or lack of sweating, other skin conditions.
Other: fever, allergic reactions.
Note: Overdose may cause curare-like effects, such as respiratory paralysis.

INTERACTIONS
Drug-drug. *Amantadine, antihistamines, antiparkinsonian agents, disopyramide, glutethimide, meperidine, phenothiazines, procainamide, quinidine, tricyclic antidepressants:* additive adverse effects. Avoid concomitant use.
Antacids: decreased absorption of oral anticholinergics. Separate administration times by 2 to 3 hours.
Ketoconazole: anticholinergics may interfere with ketoconazole absorption. Separate administration times by 2 to 3 hours.
Methotrimeprazine: anticholinergics may enhance risk of extrapyramidal reactions. Avoid concomitant use.
Drug-herb. *Jimson weed:* may adversely affect CV function system. Avoid concomitant use.

EFFECTS ON DIAGNOSTIC TESTS
None reported.

CONTRAINDICATIONS
Contraindicated in patients with glaucoma, obstructive uropathy, obstructive disease of the GI tract, severe ulcerative colitis, myasthenia gravis, paralytic ileus, intestinal atony, unstable CV status in acute hemorrhage, tachycardia secondary to cardiac insufficiency of thyrotoxicosis, toxic megacolon, or hypersensitivity to anticholinergics.

NURSING CONSIDERATIONS
• Use cautiously in patients with autonomic neuropathy, hyperthyroidism, coronary artery disease, arrhythmias, heart failure, hypertension, hiatal hernia associated with reflux esophagitis, hepatic or renal disease, known or suspected GI infection, and ulcerative colitis. Also use cautiously in patients in hot or humid environment. Drug-induced heat stroke can develop.

Reactions may be *common*, uncommon, *life-threatening*, or COMMON AND LIFE-THREATENING.

• Give drug 30 minutes to 1 hour before meals and at bedtime. Bedtime dose can be larger; give at least 2 hours after last meal of day.
• Monitor patient's vital signs and urine output carefully.
• Be aware that injection contains sodium metabisulfite, which may cause allergic reaction in certain individuals.

☑**Patient teaching**
• Instruct patient to take drug as prescribed.
• Advise patient not to crush or chew extended-release tablets.
• Advise patient to avoid driving and other hazardous activities if drowsiness, dizziness, or blurred vision occurs; to drink plenty of fluids to help prevent constipation; and to report rash or other skin eruption.

---

propantheline bromide
Pro-Banthine, Propanthel†

Pregnancy Risk Category: C

HOW SUPPLIED
Tablets: 7.5 mg, 15 mg

ACTION
Competitively blocks the action of acetylcholine at muscarinic receptors, which decreases GI motility and inhibits gastric acid secretion.

Route	Onset	Peak	Duration
PO	1.5 hr	2-6 hr	6 hr

INDICATIONS & DOSAGE
Adjunctive treatment of peptic ulceration—
Adults: 15 mg P.O. t.i.d. before meals and 30 mg h.s.
Elderly: 7.5 mg P.O. t.i.d. before meals.

ADVERSE REACTIONS
CNS: headache, insomnia, drowsiness, dizziness, *confusion or excitement in elderly patients,* nervousness, weakness.
CV: *palpitations,* tachycardia.
EENT: *blurred vision,* mydriasis, increased intraocular pressure, cycloplegia, drying of salivary secretions.
GI: *dry mouth,* constipation, loss of taste, nausea, vomiting, paralytic ileus, bloated feeling.
GU: *urinary hesitancy, urine retention,* impotence.
Skin: urticaria, decreased sweating or possible anhidrosis, other dermal manifestations.
Other: allergic reactions *(anaphylaxis).*
Note: Overdose may cause curare-like effects, such as respiratory paralysis.

INTERACTIONS
Drug-drug. *Amantadine, antihistamines, antiparkinsonian agents, disopyramide, glutethimide, meperidine, phenothiazines, procainamide, quinidine, tricyclic antidepressants:* additive adverse effects. Avoid concomitant use.
Antacids: decreased absorption of oral anticholinergics. Separate administration times by 2 to 3 hours.
Digoxin: increased serum digoxin levels. Monitor closely for digitalis toxicity.
Ketoconazole: anticholinergics may interfere with ketoconazole absorption. Separate administration times by 2 to 3 hours.
Methotrimeprazine: anticholinergics may enhance risk of extrapyramidal reactions. Avoid concomitant use.

EFFECTS ON DIAGNOSTIC TESTS
None reported.

CONTRAINDICATIONS
Contraindicated in patients with angle-closure glaucoma, obstructive uropathy, obstructive disease of the GI tract, severe ulcerative colitis, myasthenia gravis, paralytic ileus, intestinal atony, unstable CV status in acute hemorrhage, tachycardia secondary to cardiac insufficiency or thyrotoxicosis, toxic megacolon, or hypersensitivity to anticholinergics

NURSING CONSIDERATIONS
• Use cautiously in patients with autonomic neuropathy, hyperthyroidism, coronary artery disease, arrhythmias, heart failure, hypertension, hiatal hernia associated with reflux esophagitis, hepatic or renal dis-

ease, known or suspected GI infection, and ulcerative colitis. Also use cautiously in patients in hot or humid environment. Drug-induced heat stroke can develop.
• Give drug 30 minutes to 1 hour before meals and h.s. Bedtime doses can be larger; give at least 2 hours after last meal of day.
• Monitor patient's vital signs and urine output carefully.
• Know that safety and efficacy have not been established in children.

☑ **Patient teaching**
• Instruct patient when to take drug.
• Advise patient to avoid driving and other hazardous activities if drowsiness, dizziness, or blurred vision occurs; to drink plenty of fluids to help prevent constipation; and to report rash or other skin eruption.

---

scopolamine (hyoscine)
Transderm-Scōp, Transderm-V†

scopolamine butylbromide (hyoscine butylbromide)
Buscopan†

scopolamine hydrobromide (hyoscine hydrobromide)
Scopolamine Hydrobromide Injection

Pregnancy Risk Category: C

HOW SUPPLIED
scopolamine
Transdermal patch: 1.5 mg/2.5 cm² (1 mg/72 hours)
scopolamine butylbromide
Capsules: 0.25 mg
Suppositories: 10 mg†
Tablets: 10 mg†
scopolamine hydrobromide
Injection: 0.3 mg, 0.4 mg, 0.5 mg, 0.6 mg, and 1 mg/ml in 1-ml vials and ampules; 0.86 mg/ml in 0.5-ml ampules

ACTION
Inhibits muscarinic actions of acetylcholine on autonomic effectors innervated by postganglionic cholinergic neurons.

Also may affect neural pathways originating in the labyrinth (inner ear) to inhibit nausea and vomiting.

Route	Onset	Peak	Duration
PO	1 hr	1-2 hr	4-6 hr
Transdermal	4 hr	Unknown	72 hr
Parenteral	0.5 hr	1 hr	4 hr
PR	Unknown	Unknown	Unknown

INDICATIONS & DOSAGE
Spastic states—
Adults: 10 to 20 mg P.O. t.i.d. or q.i.d. or 10 mg P.R. t.i.d. or q.i.d. Dosage adjusted p.r.n. Or 10 to 20 mg (butylbromide) S.C., I.M., or I.V. t.i.d. or q.i.d.
Delirium, preanesthetic sedation and obstetric amnesia in conjunction with analgesics—
Adults: 0.3 to 0.65 mg I.M., S.C., or I.V. Dilute solution with sterile water for injection before administering I.V.
Children: 0.006 mg/kg I.M., S.C., I.V.; maximum dose is 0.3 mg. Dilute solution with sterile water for injection before administering I.V.
Prevention of nausea and vomiting associated with motion sickness—
Adults: one Transderm-Scōp or Transderm-V patch (a circular flat unit) programmed to deliver 0.5 mg scopolamine daily over 3 days (72 hours), applied to the skin behind the ear at least 4 hours before the antiemetic is required. Or 300 to 600 mcg (hydrobromide) S.C., I.M., or I.V.
Children: 6 mcg/kg or 200 mcg/m² of body surface (hydrobromide) S.C., I.M., or I.V.

ADVERSE REACTIONS
CNS: disorientation, restlessness, irritability, dizziness, drowsiness, headache, confusion, hallucinations, delirium.
CV: palpitations, tachycardia, paradoxical bradycardia.
EENT: dilated pupils, blurred vision, photophobia, increased intraocular pressure, difficulty swallowing.
GI: *constipation, dry mouth, nausea, vomiting, epigastric distress.*
GU: urinary hesitancy, urine retention.

Reactions may be *common,* uncommon, ***life-threatening,*** or COMMON AND LIFE-THREATENING.

Respiratory: bronchial plugging, depressed respirations.
Skin: rash, flushing, dryness, contact dermatitis (with transdermal patch).
Other: fever.

Adverse reactions may be caused by pending atropine-like toxicity and are dose-related. Individual tolerance varies greatly.

Note: Overdose may cause curare-like effects, such as respiratory paralysis.

INTERACTIONS
Drug-drug. *Antacids:* decreased oral absorption of anticholinergics. Separate administration times by 2 to 3 hours.
Centrally acting anticholinergics (antihistamines, phenothiazines, tricyclic antidepressants, amantadine, antiparkinsonian agents, disopyramide, glutethimide, meperidine, procainamide, quinidine): increased incidence of adverse CNS reactions. Avoid concomitant use.
CNS depressants: increased incidence of CNS depression. Monitor patient closely.
Digoxin: increased digoxin levels. Monitor for digitalis toxicity.
Ketoconazole: anticholinergics may interfere with ketoconazole absorption. Separate administration times by 2 to 3 hours.
Methotrimeprazine: enhanced risk of extrapyramidal reactions. Avoid concomitant use.
Drug-herb. *Squaw vine:* tannic acid may decrease metabolic breakdown. Monitor patient.
Jaborandi tree: effects of these medications may be decreased with concomitant administration. Monitor closely.
Pill-bearing spurge: choline may decrease effect of scopolamine. Use cautiously.
Drug-lifestyle. *Alcohol use:* increased incidence of CNS depression. Monitor patient closely.

EFFECTS ON DIAGNOSTIC TESTS
None reported.

CONTRAINDICATIONS
Contraindicated in patients with angle-closure glaucoma, obstructive uropathy, obstructive disease of the GI tract, asthma, chronic pulmonary disease, myasthenia gravis, paralytic ileus, intestinal atony, unstable CV status in acute hemorrhage, tachycardia secondary to cardiac insufficiency, or toxic megacolon.

NURSING CONSIDERATIONS
• Use cautiously in patients with autonomic neuropathy, hyperthyroidism, coronary artery disease, arrhythmias, heart failure, hypertension, hiatal hernia associated with reflux esophagitis, hepatic or renal disease, known or suspected GI infection, ulcerative colitis and in children under 6 years. Also use cautiously in patients in hot or humid environment. Drug-induced heat stroke is possible.
• Raise the bed's side rails as a precaution because some patients become temporarily excited or disoriented or develop amnesia or drowsiness. Reorient patient as needed.
• Be aware that tolerance may develop when given over a long time.

⬛ I.V. administration
• Know that intermittent and continuous infusions are not recommended. For direct injection, dilute with sterile water and inject diluted drug at ordered rate through patent I.V. line.
• Protect I.V. solutions from freezing and light, and store at room temperature.

✅ Patient teaching
• Advise patient to apply patch the night before a planned trip. Transdermal method releases a controlled therapeutic amount of scopolamine. Transderm-Scōp is effective if applied 2 to 3 hours before experiencing motion, but more effective if applied 12 hours before.
• Instruct patient to wash and dry hands thoroughly before and after applying the transdermal patch on dry skin behind the ear and before touching the eye, as pupil may dilate. After removing the patch, discard it. Wash hands and application site thoroughly.
• Tell patient that if patch becomes displaced, he should remove it and apply another patch on a fresh skin site behind the ear.
• Alert patient to possible withdrawal

signs or symptoms (nausea, vomiting, headache, dizziness) when the transdermal system is used longer than 72 hours.

• Advise patient that eyes may be more sensitive to light as a result of wearing patch.

• Warn patient to avoid activities that require alertness until drug's CNS effects are known.

• Instruct patient to ask pharmacist for brochure that comes with the transdermal product.

• Advise patient to report signs of urinary hesitancy or urine retention.

Adrenergics (sympathomimetics)

dobutamine hydrochloride
dopamine hydrochloride
metaraminol bitartrate
norepinephrine bitartrate
phenylephrine hydrochloride
pseudoephedrine hydrochloride
pseudoephedrine sulfate

COMBINATION PRODUCTS
ENTEX: phenylephrine hydrochloride
5 mg, phenylpropanolamine hydrochloride 45 mg, and guaifenesin 200 mg.
ENTEX LIQUID*: phenylephrine hydrochloride 5 mg/5 ml, phenylpropanolamine hydrochloride 20 mg/5 ml, and guaifenesin 100 mg/5 ml (alcohol 5%).
ENTEX PSE: pseudoephedrine 120 mg and guaifenesin 600 mg.
SEMPREX-D: acrivastine 8 mg and pseudoephedrine hydrochloride 60 mg.

---

dobutamine hydrochloride
Dobutrex

Pregnancy Risk Category: B

HOW SUPPLIED
Injection: 12.5 mg/ml in 20-ml vials (parenteral)

ACTION
Directly stimulates beta$_1$ receptors of the heart to increase myocardial contractility and stroke volume. At therapeutic dosages, decreases peripheral vascular resistance (afterload), reduces ventricular filling pressure (preload), and may facilitate AV node conduction. Net result is increased cardiac output.

Route	Onset	Peak	Duration
IV	1-2 min	10 min	< 5 min after infusion ends

INDICATIONS & DOSAGE
Increase cardiac output in short-term treatment of cardiac decompensation caused by depressed contractility, such as during refractory heart failure; adjunct in cardiac surgery—
Adults: 2.5 to 15 mcg/kg/minute I.V. infusion. Infusion rates up to 40 mcg/kg/minute may be needed (rare).

ADVERSE REACTIONS
CNS: headache.
CV: *increased heart rate, hypertension, PVC,* angina, nonspecific chest pain, palpitations, hypotension.
GI: nausea, vomiting.
Respiratory: shortness of breath, *asthmatic episodes.*
Other: phlebitis, hypersensitivity reactions *(anaphylaxis).*

INTERACTIONS
Drug-drug. *Beta blockers:* may antagonize dobutamine effects. Don't use together.
Bretylium: may potentiate action of vasopressors on adrenergic receptors. Monitor closely for arrhythmias.
General anesthetics: greater incidence of ventricular arrhythmias. Monitor ECG closely.
Guanethidine, oxytocic drugs: may increase pressor response, possibly resulting in severe hypertension. Monitor closely.
Tricyclic antidepressants: may potentiate pressor response. Use with caution.
Drug-herb. *Rue:* increased inotropic potential. Use cautiously.

EFFECTS ON DIAGNOSTIC TESTS
None reported.

CONTRAINDICATIONS
Contraindicated in patients with idiopathic hypertrophic subaortic stenosis and hypersensitivity to drug or its ingredients.

NURSING CONSIDERATIONS
• Use cautiously in patients with history of hypertension. Drug may precipitate an exaggerated pressor response. Also use

---

*Liquid contains alcohol.   **May contain tartrazine.   †Canada   ‡Australia   §U.K.   ◇OTC

cautiously in patients with history of sulfite sensitivity.

• Before initiating therapy with dobutamine, correct hypovolemia with plasma volume expanders, as ordered.

• Administer a cardiac glycoside before dobutamine as ordered. Because drug increases AV node conduction, patients with atrial fibrillation may develop a rapid ventricular rate.

• Continuously monitor ECG, blood pressure, pulmonary artery wedge pressure, cardiac output, and urine output.

• Monitor serum electrolytes, as ordered. Drug may lower serum potassium levels.

◖I.V. administration
• Do not mix with sodium bicarbonate injection because drug is incompatible with alkaline solutions.

• Dilute concentrate for injection before administration. Compatible solutions include D₅W, 0.45% NaCl or 0.9% NaCl for injection and lactated Ringer's injection. The contents of one vial (250 mg) diluted with 1,000 ml of solution yields a concentration of 250 mcg/ml; diluted with 500 ml, a concentration of 500 mcg/ml; diluted with 250 ml, a concentration of 1,000 mcg/ml. Maximum concentration should not exceed 5 mg/ml.

• Be aware that oxidation of drug may slightly discolor admixtures containing dobutamine. This does not indicate a significant loss of potency provided drug is used within 24 hours of reconstitution.

• Administer through a central venous catheter or large peripheral vein. Titrate infusion according to doctor's orders and patient's condition. Use an infusion pump. Infusions for up to 72 hours produce no more adverse effects than shorter infusions.

• Avoid extravasation; may cause an inflammatory response. Change I.V. sites regularly to avoid phlebitis.

• Don't administer through the same I.V. line with other drugs. Drug is incompatible with heparin, hydrocortisone sodium succinate, cefazolin, cefamandole, neutral cephalothin, penicillin, and ethacrynate sodium.

• Keep in mind that I.V. solutions remain stable for 24 hours.

☑ Patient teaching
• Tell patient to report adverse reactions promptly, especially dyspnea and drug-induced headache.
• Instruct patient to report discomfort at I.V. insertion site.

---

dopamine hydrochloride
Intropin, Revimine†

Pregnancy Risk Category: C

HOW SUPPLIED
Injection: 40 mg/ml, 80 mg/ml, 160 mg/ml parenteral concentrate for injection for I.V. infusion; 0.8 mg/ml (200 or 400 mg) in dextrose 5%; 1.6 mg/ml (400 or 800 mg) in dextrose 5%, 3.2 mg/ml (800 mg) in dextrose 5% parenteral injection for I.V. infusion

ACTION
Dose related. Stimulates dopaminergic and alpha- and beta-adrenergic receptors of the sympathetic nervous system. High dose results in alpha stimulation.

Route	Onset	Peak	Duration
IV	5 min	Unknown	< 10 min after infusion ends

INDICATIONS & DOSAGE
To treat shock and correct hemodynamic imbalances; to improve perfusion to vital organs; to increase cardiac output; to correct hypotension—
Adults: initially, 1 to 5 mcg/kg/minute by I.V. infusion. Dosage titrated to desired hemodynamic or renal response; infusion may be increased by 1 to 4 mcg/kg/minute at 10- to 30-minute intervals.

ADVERSE REACTIONS
CNS: headache.
CV: ectopic beats, tachycardia, anginal pain, palpitations, *hypotension.* Less frequently, bradycardia, widening of QRS complex, conduction disturbances, vasoconstriction, hypertension.
GI: nausea, vomiting.
Other: necrosis and tissue sloughing with extravasation, piloerection, dyspnea, ***ana-***

---

phylactic reactions, asthmatic episodes, azotemia.

INTERACTIONS

Drug-drug. *Alpha blockers, beta blockers:* may antagonize dopamine's effects. Don't use together.

Ergot alkaloids: extreme elevations in blood pressure. Don't use together.

Inhalation anesthetics: increased risk of arrhythmias or hypertension. Monitor closely.

MAO inhibitors: may cause hypertensive crisis. Avoid if possible.

Oxytocic drugs: may cause severe, persistent hypertension. Use cautiously.

Phenytoin: may cause seizures, severe hypotension and bradycardia. Monitor carefully.

Tricyclics: decreased pressor response. Higher doses of dopamine may be needed.

EFFECTS ON DIAGNOSTIC TESTS

Dopamine may cause elevated urinary catecholamine levels. Drug may also cause increased serum glucose levels, though level usually doesn't rise above normal limits.

CONTRAINDICATIONS

Contraindicated in patients with uncorrected tachyarrhythmias, pheochromocytoma, or ventricular fibrillation.

NURSING CONSIDERATIONS

• Use cautiously in patients with occlusive vascular disease, cold injuries, diabetic endarteritis, and arterial embolism; in pregnant patients; in those with a history of sulfite sensitivity, and in those taking MAO inhibitors.

• Remember that drug is not a substitute for blood or fluid volume deficit. If deficit exists, replace fluid before administering vasopressors, as ordered.

• Discard after 24 hours (dopamine solutions deteriorate after 24 hours) or earlier if solution is discolored.

• During infusion, frequently monitor ECG, blood pressure, cardiac output, central venous pressure, pulmonary artery wedge pressure, pulse rate, urine output, and color and temperature of extremities.

• If a disproportionate rise in diastolic pressure (a marked decrease in pulse pressure) is observed in patients receiving dopamine, decrease infusion rate as ordered and observe carefully for further evidence of predominant vasoconstrictor activity, unless such an effect is desired.

• Observe patient closely for adverse effects; doctor may adjust dosage or discontinue drug.

• Check urine output often. If urine flow decreases without hypotension, notify doctor because dosage may need to be reduced.

Alert: After drug is stopped, watch closely for sudden drop in blood pressure. Taper dosage slowly to evaluate stability of blood pressure, as ordered.

• Be aware that acidosis decreases effectiveness of dopamine.

🔋 I.V. administration

• Use a central line or large vein, such as in the antecubital fossa, to minimize risk of extravasation. Watch infusion site carefully for signs of extravasation; if it occurs, stop infusion immediately and call doctor. Extravasation may require treatment by infiltration of the area with 5 to 10 mg phentolamine in 10 to 15 ml 0.9% NaCl solution.

• Don't mix with alkaline solutions, oxidizing agents, or iron salts. Use D_5W, 0.9% NaCl solution, or a combination of D_5W and 0.9% NaCl solution. Mix just before use.

• Use a continuous infusion pump to regulate flow rate. Know that patient response depends on dosage and pharmacologic effects. Dosages of 0.5 to 2 mcg/kg/minute predominantly stimulate dopamine receptors and produce vasodilation of the renal vasculature. Dosages of 2 to 10 mcg/kg/minute stimulate beta-adrenergic receptors for a positive inotropic effect. Higher dosages also stimulate alpha-adrenergic receptors, causing vasoconstriction and increased blood pressure. Know that most patients are satisfactorily maintained on dosages less than 20 mcg/kg/minute.

• Don't mix other drugs in I.V. container with dopamine. Don't give alkaline drugs through I.V. line containing dopamine.

☑ **Patient teaching**
• Tell patient to report adverse reactions promptly.
• Instruct patient to alert nurse if discomfort occurs at I.V. insertion site.

---

metaraminol bitartrate
Aramine

Pregnancy Risk Category: D

HOW SUPPLIED
Injection: 10 mg/ml

ACTION
Stimulates alpha- and beta$_1$-adrenergic receptors within the sympathetic nervous system, causing a rise in both systolic and diastolic blood pressure due to vasoconstriction.

Route	Onset	Peak	Duration
IV	1-2 min	Unknown	20 min
IM	10 min	Unknown	< 90 min
SC	5-20 min	Unknown	< 90 min

INDICATIONS & DOSAGE
Prevention of hypotension associated with spinal anesthesia—
Adults: 2 to 10 mg I.M. or S.C.
Treatment of hypotension associated with spinal anesthesia, hemorrhage, medication reaction, surgical complications, or shock associated with brain damage due to trauma or tumor—
Adults: 0.5 to 5 mg by direct I.V. injection, followed by I.V. infusion titrated to maintain blood pressure.
Children: 0.01 mg/kg as single I.V. injection; 1 mg/25 ml of D$_5$W as I.V. infusion. Rate adjusted to maintain blood pressure in normal range. Alternatively, 0.1 mg/kg I.M. as single dose, p.r.n. At least 10 minutes should elapse before dosage increased because maximum effect is not immediately apparent.

ADVERSE REACTIONS
CNS: apprehension, dizziness, headache, tremor.
CV: hypertension; hypotension; palpitations; *arrhythmias,* including sinus or *ventricular tachycardia, cardiac arrest.*

GI: nausea.
Skin: flushing, diaphoresis.
Other: abscess, necrosis, sloughing upon extravasation.

INTERACTIONS
Drug-drug. *Beta-adrenergic blockers:* mutual inhibition of drug effects, with possible hypertension, bradycardia, and heart block. Avoid concomitant use.
Cardiac glycosides, doxapram, ergot alkaloids, general anesthetics, levodopa, maprotiline, other sympathomimetics, thyroid hormones, tricyclic antidepressants: increased risk of adverse cardiac effects. Monitor closely.
Furazolidone, MAO inhibitors, procarbazine: may cause severe hypertension (hypertensive crisis) and increase action of metaraminol. Avoid this combination.
Guanadrel, guanethidine: metaraminol may decrease the hypotensive effect of these drugs; guanadrel and guanethidine may enhance the pressor effect of metaraminol. Avoid concomitant use.
Oxytocics: may cause severe, persistent hypertension. Use cautiously.
Drug-lifestyle. *Cocaine use:* increased risk of adverse cardiac effects. Monitor closely.

EFFECTS ON DIAGNOSTIC TESTS
None reported.

CONTRAINDICATIONS
Contraindicated in patients with hypersensitivity to drug and in those receiving anesthesia with cyclopropane and halogenated hydrocarbon anesthetics.

NURSING CONSIDERATIONS
• Use cautiously in patients with heart disease, hypertension, peripheral vascular disease, thyroid disease, diabetes, cirrhosis, history of malaria, or sulfite sensitivity and in patients receiving cardiac glycosides.
• Know that drug is not a substitute for blood or fluid volume deficit. If deficit exists, replace fluid before administering vasopressors, as ordered.
• Don't mix metaraminol with other drugs.
• During infusion, check blood pressure

Reactions may be common, *uncommon,* **life-threatening,** *or* **COMMON AND LIFE-THREATENING.**

every 5 minutes until stabilized; then check every 15 minutes. Frequently monitor ECG, blood pressure, cardiac output, central venous pressure, pulmonary artery wedge pressure, pulse rate, urine output, and color and temperature of extremities. Titrate infusion rate according to findings and the doctor's guidelines.

Alert: Keep in mind that blood pressure should be raised to slightly less than the patient's normal level. Be careful to avoid excessive blood pressure response. Headache may be a symptom of hypertension. Rapidly induced hypertensive response can cause acute pulmonary edema, arrhythmias, and cardiac arrest.

• Allow at least 10 minutes between doses. Drug effects are not always immediately apparent.

• Be aware that because of prolonged action, a cumulative effect is possible. With an excessive vasopressor response, elevated blood pressure may persist after drug is stopped.

• Observe patient closely for adverse effects; doctor may adjust dosage or discontinue drug.

• Keep emergency drugs on hand to reverse effects of metaraminol: atropine for reflex bradycardia; phentolamine to decrease vasopressor effects; and propranolol for arrhythmias.

• Report persistent decreased urine output. Urine output may decrease initially, then increase as blood pressure returns to normal level.

• Closely monitor patients with diabetes; insulin dosage may need to be adjusted.

• Keep solution in light-resistant container, away from heat. Use within 24 hours.

🌓 I.V. administration

• To prepare an I.V. infusion, mix 15 to 100 mg in 500 ml of 0.9% NaCl solution or D₅W. Aramine may be added to less than 500 ml of fluid if a smaller volume is desired. Adjust rate to maintain blood pressure.

• Use a central venous catheter or large vein, such as in the antecubital fossa, to minimize risk of extravasation. Use a continuous infusion pump to regulate infusion flow rate and a piggyback setup so I.V. line remains open if drug is stopped.

Watch infusion site carefully for signs of extravasation. If it occurs, stop infusion immediately and notify doctor.

• To treat extravasation, infiltrate site promptly with 10 to 15 ml of 0.9% NaCl for injection containing 5 to 10 mg phentolamine. Use a fine needle.

• When discontinuing drug, gradually slow infusion rate, as ordered. Continue monitoring vital signs, watching for possible severe drop in blood pressure. Keep equipment nearby to resume drug, if necessary. Do not reinstate vasopressor therapy until the systolic blood pressure falls below 70 to 80 mm Hg, as ordered.

✓ Patient teaching

• Tell patient to report adverse reactions promptly.

• Instruct patient to alert nurse if discomfort occurs at I.V. site.

---

norepinephrine bitartrate (levarterenol bitartrate, noradrenaline acid tartrate)
Levophed

Pregnancy Risk Category: C

HOW SUPPLIED
Injection: 1 mg/ml

ACTION
Stimulates alpha- and beta₁-adrenergic receptors within the sympathetic nervous system, primarily producing vasoconstriction and cardiac stimulation.

Route	Onset	Peak	Duration
IV	Immediate	Immediate	1-2 min after infusion ends

INDICATIONS & DOSAGE
To restore blood pressure in acute hypotensive states—
Adults: initially, 8 to 12 mcg/minute I.V. infusion, then adjusted to maintain normal blood pressure. Average maintenance dosage is 2 to 4 mcg/minute.
Children: 2 mcg/m²/minute I.V. infusion; dosage adjusted based on patient response.

Severe hypotension during cardiac arrest—
Children: initial I.V. infusion rate is 0.1 mcg/kg/minute. Rate adjusted based on patient response.

ADVERSE REACTIONS
CNS: *headache,* anxiety, weakness, dizziness, tremor, restlessness, insomnia.
CV: bradycardia, *severe hypertension, arrhythmias.*
Respiratory: respiratory difficulties, *asthmatic episodes.*
Other: *anaphylaxis,* irritation with extravasation, necrosis and gangrene secondary to extravasation.

INTERACTIONS
Drug-drug. *Alpha-adrenergic blockers:* may antagonize drug effects. Avoid concomitant use.
Antihistamines, ergot alkaloids, guanethidine, MAO inhibitors, methyldopa, oxytocics, tricyclic antidepressants: when given with sympathomimetics, may cause severe hypertension (hypertensive crisis). Don't give together.
Bretylium, inhalation anesthetics: increased risk of arrhythmias. Monitor closely.

EFFECTS ON DIAGNOSTIC TESTS
None reported.

CONTRAINDICATIONS
Contraindicated in patients with mesenteric or peripheral vascular thrombosis, profound hypoxia, hypercarbia, or hypotension resulting from blood volume deficit and during cyclopropane and halothane anesthesia.

NURSING CONSIDERATIONS
• Use with extreme caution in patients receiving MAO inhibitors or triptyline- or imipramine-type antidepressants. Use cautiously in patients with sulfite sensitivity.
• Know that drug is not a substitute for blood or fluid volume deficit. If deficit exists, replace fluid before administering vasopressors.
Alert: Never leave patient unattended during infusion. Also, check blood pressure

every 2 minutes until stabilized; then check every 5 minutes. In previously hypertensive patients, blood pressure should be raised no higher than 40 mm Hg below preexisting systolic pressure.
• Also during infusion, frequently monitor ECG, cardiac output, central venous pressure, pulmonary artery wedge pressure, pulse rate, urine output, and color and temperature of extremities. Titrate infusion rate according to findings and doctor's guidelines.
• Keep emergency drugs on hand to reverse effects of norepinephrine: atropine for reflex bradycardia; phentolamine for increased vasopressor effects; and propranolol for arrhythmias.
• Notify doctor of decreased urine output immediately.
• When discontinuing drug, gradually slow infusion rate, as ordered. Continue monitoring vital signs, watching for possible severe drop in blood pressure.

I.V. administration
• Avoid mixing with alkaline solutions, oxidizing agents, or iron salts.
• Use a central venous catheter or a large vein, such as in the antecubital fossa, to minimize risk of extravasation. Administer in dextrose 5% in 0.9% NaCl for injection; 0.9% NaCl for injection alone is not recommended. Use continuous infusion pump to regulate infusion flow rate and a piggyback setup so I.V. line remains open if norepinephrine is stopped.
• Check site frequently for signs of extravasation. If it occurs, stop infusion immediately and call doctor. He may counteract effect by infiltrating area with 5 to 10 mg phentolamine in 10 to 15 ml of 0.9% NaCl solution. Also check for blanching along course of infused vein; may progress to superficial sloughing.
• Protect drug from light. Discard discolored solutions or solutions that contain a precipitate. Norepinephrine solutions deteriorate after 24 hours.
• If prolonged I.V. therapy is necessary, change injection site frequently.

Patient teaching
• Tell patient to report adverse reactions promptly.

Reactions may be *common,* uncommon, *life-threatening,* or COMMON AND LIFE-THREATENING.

• Advise patient to alert nurse if discomfort occurs at I.V. insertion site.

---

phenylephrine hydrochloride
Neo-Synephrine

Pregnancy Risk Category: C

HOW SUPPLIED
Injection: 10 mg/ml

ACTION
Predominantly stimulates alpha-adrenergic receptors in the sympathetic nervous system causing vasoconstriction.

Route	Onset	Peak	Duration
IV	Immediate	Unknown	15-20 min
IM	10-15 min	Unknown	0.5-2 hr
SC	10-15 min	Unknown	50-60 min

INDICATIONS & DOSAGE
Hypotensive emergencies during spinal anesthesia—
Adults: initially, 0.2 mg I.V.; subsequent doses should not exceed the preceding dose by more than 0.2 mg. Maximum single dose should not exceed 0.5 mg.
Maintenance of blood pressure during spinal or inhalation anesthesia—
Adults: 2 to 3 mg S.C. or I.M. 3 to 4 minutes before anesthesia.
Children: 0.044 mg to 0.088 mg/kg S.C. or I.M.
Prolongation of spinal anesthesia—
Adults: 2 to 5 mg added to anesthetic solution.
Vasoconstrictor for regional anesthesia—
Adults: 1 mg phenylephrine added to 20 ml local anesthetic.
Mild to moderate hypotension—
Adults: 2 to 5 mg S.C. or I.M.; repeated in 1 to 2 hours as needed and tolerated. Initial dose should not exceed 5 mg. Alternatively, 0.1 to 0.5 mg slow I.V., not to be repeated more often than 10 to 15 minutes.
Children: 0.1 mg/kg I.M. or S.C.; repeated in 1 to 2 hours as needed and tolerated.
Severe hypotension and shock (including drug induced)—
Adults: 10 mg in 250 to 500 ml of D₅W or 0.9% NaCl for injection. I.V. infusion

started at 100 to 180 mcg/minute, then decreased to a maintenance infusion of 40 to 60 mcg/minute when blood pressure stabilizes.
Paroxysmal supraventricular tachycardia—
Adults: initially, 0.5 mg rapid I.V.; subsequent doses should not exceed the preceding dose by more than 0.1 to 0.2 mg and should not exceed 1 mg.
Note: Also used in eyedrops and OTC cold medications for decongestant effects.

ADVERSE REACTIONS
CNS: *headache,* excitability.
CV: bradycardia, *arrhythmias,* hypertension.
Other: tachyphylaxis (may occur with continued use), *anaphylaxis, asthmatic episodes,* decreased organ perfusion (with prolonged use), tissue sloughing (with extravasation).

INTERACTIONS
Drug-drug. *Alpha-adrenergic blockers, phenothiazines:* decreased vasopressor response. Monitor closely.
Beta-adrenergic blockers: blocked cardiostimulatory effects. Monitor closely.
Bretylium, halogenated hydrocarbon anesthetics, sympathomimetic agents: may cause serious arrhythmias. Use with extreme caution.
Guanethidine, oxytocics, tricyclic antidepressants: increased pressor response. Observe patient.
MAO inhibitors: may cause severe hypertension (hypertensive crisis). Don't use together.

EFFECTS ON DIAGNOSTIC TESTS
Drug may lower intraocular pressure in normal eyes or in open-angle glaucoma. It also may cause false-normal tonometry readings.

CONTRAINDICATIONS
Contraindicated in patients with severe hypertension, ventricular tachycardia, or hypersensitivity to drug.

NURSING CONSIDERATIONS
• Use with extreme caution in patients with heart disease, hyperthyroidism, se-

---

vere atherosclerosis, bradycardia, partial heart block, myocardial disease, or sulfite sensitivity and in elderly patients.
• Remember that drug causes little or no CNS stimulation.
• Keep in mind that drug is incompatible with butacaine sulfate, alkalis, ferric salts, and oxidizing agents.

🗋 I.V. administration
• For direct injection, dilute 10 mg (1 ml) with 9 ml sterile water for injection to provide a solution containing 1 mg/ml. I.V. infusions are usually prepared by adding 10 mg of drug to 500 ml of D_5W or 0.9% NaCl for injection. The initial infusion rate is usually 100 to 180 mcg/minute; the maintenance infusion rate is usually 40 to 60 mcg/minute.
• Use a central venous catheter or a large vein, as in the antecubital fossa, to minimize risk of extravasation. Use a continuous infusion pump to regulate infusion flow rate.
• To treat extravasation, infiltrate site promptly with 10 to 15 ml of 0.9% NaCl for injection containing 5 to 10 mg phentolamine, as ordered. Use a fine needle.
• With prolonged I.V. infusions, avoid abrupt withdrawal. During infusion, frequently monitor ECG, blood pressure, cardiac output, central venous pressure, pulmonary artery wedge pressure, pulse rate, urine output, and color and temperature of extremities. Titrate infusion rate according to findings and doctor's guidelines. Use a continuous infusion pump to regulate flow rate and avoid severe increase. Maintain blood pressure slightly below the patient's normal level, as ordered. In previously normotensive patients, maintain systolic blood pressure at 80 to 100 mm Hg; in previously hypertensive patients, maintain systolic blood pressure at 30 to 40 mm Hg below usual level.

✅ Patient teaching
• Tell patient to report adverse reactions promptly.
• Instruct patient to alert nurse if discomfort occurs at I.V. insertion site.

pseudoephedrine hydrochloride
Allermed◇, Cenafed◇, Children's Congestion Relief◇, Children's Sudafed Liquid◇, Congestac Caplets†◇, Congestion Relief◇, Decofed◇, Defed-60◇, Dorcol Children's Decongestant Liquid◇, Drixoral Non-Drowsy Formula◇, Efidac/24◇, Eltor 120†◇, Galpseud§, Genaphed◇, Halofed◇, Halofed Adult Strength◇, Maxenal†◇, Myfedrine◇, Novafed◇, Ornex◇, Pedia Care Infant's Decongestant◇, Pedia Care Infants' Oral Decongestant Drops◇, Pseudo◇, Pseudo-Gest◇, Seudotabs◇, Sinufed Timecelles◇, Sinustop Pro◇, Sudafed◇, Sudafed 12 Hour◇, Sufedrin◇

pseudoephedrine sulfate
Afrin◇, Drixoral†, Drixoral Non-Drowsy Formula◇

Pregnancy Risk Category: C

HOW SUPPLIED
pseudoephedrine hydrochloride
Tablets: 30 mg◇, 60 mg◇
Tablets (extended-release): 120 mg◇, 240 mg◇
Capsules: 60 mg
Capsules (extended-release): 120 mg
Oral solution: 7.5 mg/0.8 ml◇, 15 mg/5 ml◇, 30 mg/5 ml◇
Syrup: 30 mg/5 ml
pseudoephedrine sulfate
Tablets (extended-release): 120 mg (60 mg immediate-release, 60 mg delayed-release)◇

ACTION
Stimulates alpha-adrenergic receptors in the respiratory tract, producing vasoconstriction, causing shrinkage of swollen nasal mucous membranes, reduction of tissue hyperemia, edema, and nasal congestion, and an increase in airway patency.

Route	Onset	Peak	Duration
PO	0.5 hr	0.5-1 hr	4-12 hr

INDICATIONS & DOSAGE

Nasal and eustachian tube decongestion—
Adults: 60 mg P.O. q 4 hours. Maximum dosage is 240 mg daily. Or, 120 mg extended-release tablet P.O. q 12 hours or 240 mg extended-release (Efidac/24) once daily.
Children over 12 years: 60 mg P.O. q 4 to 6 hours. Maximum dosage is 240 mg daily. Or, 120 mg extended-release tablet P.O. q 12 hours or 240 mg extended-release (Efidac/24) once daily.
Children 6 to 12 years: 30 mg P.O. regular-release form q 4 to 6 hours. Maximum dosage is 120 mg daily.
Children 2 to 5 years: 15 mg P.O. regular-release form q 4 to 6 hours. Maximum dosage is 60 mg daily.
Children 1 to 2 years: 7 drops (0.2 ml)/ kg P.O. q 4 to q 6 hours up to four doses daily.
Children 3 to 12 months: 3 drops/kg P.O. q 4 to 6 hours up to four doses daily.

ADVERSE REACTIONS

CNS: *anxiety,* transient stimulation, tremor, dizziness, headache, insomnia, *nervousness.*
CV: *arrhythmias, palpitations,* tachycardia, *CV collapse.*
GI: anorexia, nausea, vomiting, dry mouth.
GU: difficulty urinating.
Respiratory: respiratory difficulties.
Skin: pallor.

INTERACTIONS

Drug-drug. *Antihypertensives:* may attenuate hypotensive effect. Monitor blood pressure closely.
MAO inhibitors: may cause severe hypertension (hypertensive crisis). Don't use together.
Methyldopa: may result in increased pressor response. Monitor closely.

EFFECTS ON DIAGNOSTIC TESTS

None reported.

CONTRAINDICATIONS

Contraindicated in patients with severe hypertension or severe coronary artery disease, in those receiving MAO inhibitors, and in breast-feeding patients. Extended-release preparations are contraindicated in children under 12 years.

NURSING CONSIDERATIONS

• Use cautiously in patients with hypertension, cardiac disease, diabetes, glaucoma, hyperthyroidism, and prostatic hyperplasia.
• Be aware that elderly patients are more sensitive to drug's effects. Extended-release tablets should not be administered to them until safety with short-acting preparations has been established.

☑**Patient teaching**
• Tell patient not to crush or break extended-release forms.
• Warn against using OTC products containing other sympathomimetics.
• Instruct patient not to take drug within 2 hours of bedtime because it can cause insomnia.
• Tell patient to stop drug if he becomes unusually restless and to notify doctor promptly.

**dihydroergotamine mesylate
ergotamine tartrate
methysergide maleate
propranolol hydrochloride**
(See Chapter 22, ANTIANGINALS.)

COMBINATION PRODUCTS
BELLERGAL-S**, BEL-PHEN-ERGOT-SR,
PHENERBEL-S: ergotamine tartrate 0.6 mg,
levorotatory belladonna alkaloids 0.2 mg,
and phenobarbital 40 mg.
CAFERGOT, ERCAF, WIGRAINE: ergotamine
tartrate 1 mg and caffeine 100 mg.
CAFERGOT SUPPOSITORIES, CAFETRATE
SUPPOSITORIES: ergotamine tartrate 2 mg
and caffeine 100 mg.
HYDERGINE: dihydroergocornine mesylate
0.167 mg, dihydroergocristine mesylate
0.167 mg, and dihydroergocryptine mesylate 0.167 mg.
WIGRAINE SUPPOSITORIES: ergotamine tartrate 2 mg and caffeine 100 mg.

---

dihydroergotamine mesylate
D.H.E. 45, Dihydergot‡,
Dihydroergotamine-Sandoz†

Pregnancy Risk Category: X

HOW SUPPLIED
Injection: 1 mg/ml

ACTION
Causes peripheral vasoconstriction primarily by stimulating alpha-adrenergic receptors; may abort vascular headaches by
direct vasoconstriction of dilated carotid
artery bed with a decline in amplitude of
pulsations. Also causes antagonistic effect
of serotonin $5HT_2$ receptors.

Route	Onset	Peak	Duration
IV	5 min	15 min	8 hr
IM	15-30 min	30 min	3-4 hr

INDICATIONS & DOSAGE
*To prevent or abort vascular or migraine
headache—*

Adults: 1 mg I.M. or I.V. repeated q 1 to
2 hours, p.r.n., up to total of 2 mg I.V. or
3 mg I.M. per attack. Maximum weekly
dosage is 6 mg.

ADVERSE REACTIONS
CV: transient tachycardia or bradycardia,
precordial distress and pain, increased arterial pressure.
GI: *nausea, vomiting.*
Skin: itching.
Other: weakness in legs, muscle pain in
extremities, localized edema, uterine contractions, numbness and tingling in fingers and toes.

INTERACTIONS
Drug-drug. *Erythromycin, other macrolides:* may cause symptoms of ergot toxicity (severe peripheral vasospasm with
possible ischemia, cyanosis and numbness).Vasodilators (nitroprusside, nifedipine, or prazosin) may be ordered to treat
such an attack. Monitor closely.
Propranolol, other beta blockers: blocked
natural pathway for vasodilation in patients receiving ergot alkaloids; may result in excessive vasoconstriction and
cold extremities. Watch closely if drugs
are used together.

EFFECTS ON DIAGNOSTIC TESTS
None reported.

CONTRAINDICATIONS
Contraindicated in patients with peripheral and occlusive vascular disease, coronary artery disease, uncontrolled hypertension, severe hepatic or renal dysfunction, malnutrition, severe pruritus, sepsis,
or hypersensitivity to drug and in pregnant or breast-feeding patients.

NURSING CONSIDERATIONS
• Know that drug is most effective when
used at first sign of migraine or soon after
onset.
• Avoid prolonged administration; don't
exceed recommended dosage, as ordered.

Reactions may be *common*, uncommon, **life-threatening**, or COMMON AND LIFE-THREATENING.

Adjust to most effective minimal dosage, as ordered, for best results.
• Be alert for ergotamine rebound, or an increase in frequency and duration of headache, which may occur when drug is stopped.

🔲 I.V. administration
• Directly inject solution into the vein over 3 minutes. Continuous and intermittent infusion are not recommended.
• Protect ampules from heat and light. Discard if solution is discolored.

✅ Patient teaching
• Instruct patient to lie down and relax in a quiet, low-light environment after administration of drug.
• Tell patient to report feeling of coldness in extremities or of tingling in fingers and toes. Severe vasoconstriction may result in tissue damage. Keep extremities warm and administer vasodilators as ordered.
• Help patient evaluate underlying causes of stress, which may precipitate attacks.
• Advise patient to notify doctor if pregnancy occurs or if planning to become pregnant.

---

ergotamine tartrate
Ergodryl Mono‡, Ergomar, Ergostat, Gynergen†, Lingraine§, Medihaler Ergotamine

Pregnancy Risk Category: X

HOW SUPPLIED
Capsules: 1 mg‡
Tablets: 1 mg†
Tablets (S.L.): 2 mg
Aerosol inhaler: 360 mcg/metered spray

ACTION
Stimulates alpha-adrenergic receptors, causing peripheral vasoconstriction. May abort vascular headaches by direct vasoconstriction of the dilated carotid artery bed with a concomitant decrease in the amplitude of pulsations. Also inhibits reuptake of norepinephrine, increasing vasoconstrictor activity. Also acts as an antagonist of serotonin receptors.

Route	Onset	Peak	Duration
PO	Variable	0.5-3 hr	Variable
SL, inhalation	Variable	Unknown	Variable

INDICATIONS & DOSAGE
To abort or prevent vascular or migraine headache—
Adults: initially, 2 mg P.O. or S.L., then 1 to 2 mg P.O. q hour or S.L. q 30 minutes, to maximum of 6 mg daily and 10 mg weekly. Alternatively, use aerosol inhaler: 1 spray (360 mcg) initially, repeated q 5 minutes p.r.n. to maximum of 6 sprays (2.16 mg) per 24 hours or 15 sprays (5.4 mg) per week.
Daily cluster headaches—
Adults: 1 to 2 mg P.O. h.s. for 10 to 14 days to help terminate a series of attacks.

ADVERSE REACTIONS
CV: transient tachycardia or bradycardia, precordial distress and pain, increased arterial pressure, angina pectoris, peripheral vasoconstriction.
GI: nausea, *vomiting*.
Skin: pruritus, localized edema.
Other: weakness in legs, muscle pain in extremities, uterine contractions, numbness and tingling in fingers and toes.

INTERACTIONS
Drug-drug. *Erythromycin, other macrolides:* may cause symptoms of ergot toxicity (severe peripheral vasospasm with possible ischemia, cyanosis, and numbness). Vasodilators (nifedipine, nitroprusside, or prazosin) may be ordered to treat such an attack. Monitor closely.
Propranolol, other beta blockers: blocked natural pathway for vasodilation in patients receiving ergot alkaloids; may result in excessive vasoconstriction. Watch closely if drugs are used together.

EFFECTS ON DIAGNOSTIC TESTS
None reported.

CONTRAINDICATIONS
Contraindicated in patients with peripheral and occlusive vascular diseases, coronary artery disease, hypertension, hepatic or renal dysfunction, malnutrition, severe

---

pruritus, sepsis, or hypersensitivity to ergot alkaloids and during pregnancy.

NURSING CONSIDERATIONS

• Obtain an accurate dietary history from the patient to determine if a relationship exists between certain foods and onset of headache.
• Be aware that drug is most effective when used during prodromal stage of headache or as soon as possible after onset.
• Avoid prolonged administration; don't exceed recommended dosage.
• Provide a quiet, low-light environment to help the patient relax.
• Be alert for ergotamine rebound, or an increase in frequency and duration of headache, which may occur if drug is suddenly discontinued.

✓ Patient teaching

• Advise patient to dissolve S.L. tablet under tongue, and not to chew or swallow it.
• Tell patient not to eat, drink, or smoke while the tablet is dissolving. S.L. tablet is preferred during early stage of attack because of its rapid absorption.
• Instruct patient to lie down and relax in a quiet, low-light environment after administration of drug.
• Warn patient not to increase dosage without first consulting doctor.
• Advise patient to avoid prolonged exposure to cold weather whenever possible. Cold may increase many of the adverse reactions to drug.
• Instruct patient on long-term therapy to check for and report feeling of coldness in extremities or of tingling in fingers and toes. Severe vasoconstriction may result in tissue damage. Keep extremities warm and administer vasodilators as ordered.
• Instruct patient how to use inhaler correctly.
• Help patient evaluate underlying causes of stress, which may precipitate attacks.
• Advise patient to notify doctor if pregnancy occurs or if planning to become pregnant.

methysergide maleate
Deseril‡, Sansert**

Pregnancy Risk Category: X

HOW SUPPLIED
Tablets: 1 mg‡, 2 mg

ACTION
Unknown. Specifically blocks serotonin (a neurotransmitter) in the peripheral nervous system. In CNS, drug may act as a serotonin agonist.

Route	Onset	Peak	Duration
PO	1-2 days after initiation	Unknown	1-2 days

INDICATIONS & DOSAGE
Prevention of frequent, severe, uncontrollable, or disabling migraine or other vascular headaches—
Adults: 4 to 8 mg P.O. daily with meals. There must be a drug-free interval of 3 to 4 weeks following each 6-month course of treatment.

ADVERSE REACTIONS
CNS: insomnia, drowsiness, *euphoria, vertigo,* ataxia, *light-headedness,* hyperesthesia, weakness, hallucinations or feelings of dissociation, rapid speech, lethargy.
CV: *fibrotic thickening of cardiac valves and aorta, inferior vena cava, and common iliac branches (retroperitoneal fibrosis);* vasoconstriction, causing chest pain, vascular insufficiency of lower limbs; cold, numb, painful extremities with or without paresthesia and diminished or absent pulses; orthostatic hypotension; tachycardia; peripheral edema; murmurs; bruits.
GI: abdominal pain, nausea, vomiting, diarrhea, constipation, heartburn.
Hematologic: *neutropenia,* eosinophilia.
Musculoskeletal: arthralgia, myalgia.
Respiratory: *pulmonary fibrosis* (causing dyspnea, tightness and pain in chest, pleural friction rubs, and effusion).
Skin: hair loss, flushing, rash.
Other: weight gain.

Reactions may be *common,* uncommon, *life-threatening,* or COMMON AND LIFE-THREATENING.

INTERACTIONS
Drug-drug. *Beta blockers:* may result in peripheral ischemia, cold extremities and possible gangrene. Monitor closely.

EFFECTS ON DIAGNOSTIC TESTS
None reported.

CONTRAINDICATIONS
Contraindicated in patients with severe hypertension or arteriosclerosis, peripheral vascular insufficiency, renal or hepatic disease, coronary artery disease, pulmonary disease, serious infections, phlebitis or cellulitis of lower limbs, collagen diseases, fibrotic processes, or valvular heart disease and in debilitated or pregnant patients.

NURSING CONSIDERATIONS
• Use cautiously in patients with peptic ulcerations or suspected coronary artery disease. ECG and cardiac status evaluation advisable before giving to patients over 40 years. Also use cautiously in patients sensitive to aspirin or tartrazine.
Alert: Know that drug is indicated only for patients who are unresponsive to other drugs and who can be kept under close medical supervision.
• Gradually introduce drug, as ordered, and administer with meals to prevent GI effects.
• Give drug, as ordered, for 3 weeks before evaluating effectiveness. If there is no response after 3 weeks, the drug is unlikely to be beneficial.
• Monitor laboratory studies of cardiac and renal function, CBC, and erythrocyte sedimentation rate before and during therapy.
• Know that drug should not be used for treatment of migraine or vascular headache or tension (muscle contraction) headaches.
• Be aware that drug may be withdrawn gradually every 6 months, then restarted after at least 3 weeks.

☑Patient teaching
• Instruct patient to take drug with meals.
• Instruct patient to keep daily weight record and report unusually rapid weight gain. Teach patient to check for peripheral edema. Explain and suggest low-sodium diet if necessary.
• Stress importance of keeping regular medical appointments as scheduled.
• Tell patient not to stop drug abruptly; may cause rebound headaches. Stop gradually over 2 to 3 weeks.
• Instruct patient to promptly notify doctor if the following symptoms occur: cold, numb, or painful hands and feet; leg cramps when walking; and pelvic, chest, or flank pain.
• Advise patient to notify doctor if pregnancy occurs or if planning to become pregnant.

41

Skeletal muscle relaxants

baclofen
carisoprodol
chlorzoxazone
cyclobenzaprine hydrochloride
dantrolene sodium
methocarbamol
tizanidine hydrochloride

COMBINATION PRODUCTS

NORGESIC: orphenadrine citrate 25 mg, aspirin 385 mg, and caffeine 30 mg.
NORGESIC FORTE: orphenadrine citrate 50 mg, aspirin 770 mg, and caffeine 60 mg.
ROBAXISAL: methocarbamol 400 mg and aspirin 325 mg.
SOMA COMPOUND: carisoprodol 200 mg and aspirin 325 mg.
SOMA COMPOUND WITH CODEINE: carisoprodol 200 mg, aspirin 325 mg, and codeine phosphate 16 mg.

---

baclofen
Clofen‡, Lioresal, Lioresal Intrathecal

Pregnancy Risk Category: C

HOW SUPPLIED
Tablets: 10 mg, 20 mg, 25 mg‡
Intrathecal injection: 500 mcg/ml, 2,000 mcg/ml

ACTION
Hyperpolarizes fibers to reduce impulse transmission. Appears to reduce transmission of impulses from the spinal cord to skeletal muscle, thus decreasing the frequency and amplitude of muscle spasms in patients with spinal cord lesions.

Route	Onset	Peak	Duration
PO	Hrs-wks	2-3 hr	Unknown
Intrathecal	0.5-1 hr	4 hr	4-8 hr

INDICATIONS & DOSAGE
Spasticity in multiple sclerosis, spinal cord injury—

Adults: initially, 5 mg P.O. t.i.d. for 3 days, then 10 mg t.i.d. for 3 days, 15 mg t.i.d. for 3 days, 20 mg t.i.d. for 3 days. Dosage increase based on response, up to maximum of 80 mg daily.
Management of severe spasticity in patients who do not respond to or cannot tolerate oral baclofen therapy—
Adults: *screening phase—*after test dose to check responsiveness, give drug by an implantable infusion pump. Administer test dose of 1 ml of 50-mcg/ml dilution into intrathecal space by barbotage over 1 minute or more. Significantly decreased severity or frequency of muscle spasm or reduced muscle tone should appear within 4 to 8 hours. If response is inadequate, give second test dose of 75 mcg/1.5 ml 24 hours after the first. If response is still inadequate, give final test dose of 100 mcg/2 ml after 24 hours. Patients unresponsive to the 100-mcg dose shouldn't be considered candidates for implantable pump.

*Maintenance therapy—*titrate initial dose based on screening dose that elicited an adequate response. Double this effective dose and administer over 24 hours. However, if screening dose efficacy was maintained for 12 hours or more, dose is not doubled. After the first 24 hours, increase dose slowly as needed and tolerated by 10% to 30% daily. During prolonged maintenance therapy, daily dose may be increased by 10% to 40% if needed; if patient experiences adverse effects, dosage may be decreased by 10% to 20%. Maintenance dosages have ranged from 12 mcg to 2,000 mcg daily; however, experience with dosages over 1,000 mcg daily is limited. Most patients need 300 to 800 mcg daily.
Adjust-a-dose: In patients with impaired renal function, oral and intrathecal dose decreased.

ADVERSE REACTIONS
CNS: *drowsiness, dizziness,* headache, *weakness, fatigue,* hypotonia, *confusion,*

---

insomnia, dysarthria, *seizures* (intrathecal).
CV: hypotension, hypertension.
EENT: blurred vision, nasal congestion, slurred speech.
GI: *nausea,* constipation, *vomiting.*
GU: urinary frequency.
Hepatic: increased AST and alkaline phosphatase levels.
Skin: rash, pruritus.
Other: excessive perspiration, hyperglycemia, weight gain, dyspnea.

INTERACTIONS
Drug-drug. *CNS depressants:* increased CNS depression. Avoid concomitant use.
Drug-lifestyle. *Alcohol use:* increased CNS depression. Avoid concomitant use.

EFFECTS ON DIAGNOSTIC TESTS
Drug therapy increases blood glucose, AST, and alkaline phosphatase levels.

CONTRAINDICATIONS
Contraindicated in patients with hypersensitivity to drug.

NURSING CONSIDERATIONS
• Use cautiously in patients with impaired renal function or seizure disorder or when spasticity is used to maintain motor function.
• Give oral form with meals or with milk to prevent GI distress.
• Know that orally administered drug should not be used to treat muscle spasm caused by rheumatic disorders, cerebral palsy, Parkinson's disease, or CVA because efficacy hasn't been established. Do not administer intrathecal injection by I.V., I.M., S.C., or epidural route.
• Watch for sensitivity reactions, such as fever, skin eruptions, and respiratory distress.
• Look for increased risk of seizures in patients with seizure disorder.
• Be aware that amount of relief determines whether dosage (and drowsiness) can be reduced.
• Do not withdraw drug abruptly after long-term use unless required by severe adverse reactions; may precipitate hallucinations or rebound spasticity.
• Know that experience with long-term

intrathecal use suggests that about 5% of patients may develop tolerance to drug. In some cases, this may be treated by hospitalizing patient and slowly withdrawing drug over a 2-week period.

✅Patient teaching
• Instruct patient to take oral form with meals or milk.
• Tell patient to avoid activities that require alertness until drug's CNS effects are known. Drowsiness usually is transient.
• Tell patient to avoid alcohol and OTC antihistamines while taking drug.
• Advise patient to follow doctor's orders regarding rest and physical therapy.

carisoprodol
Carisoma§, Soma, Vanadom

Pregnancy Risk Category: C

HOW SUPPLIED
Tablets: 350 mg

ACTION
Unknown. Drug appears to modify central perception of pain without modifying pain reflexes. Muscle relaxant effects may be related to its sedative properties.

Route	Onset	Peak	Duration
PO	0.5 hr	4 hr	4-6 hr

INDICATIONS & DOSAGE
As an adjunct in acute, painful musculoskeletal conditions—
Adults: 350 mg P.O. t.i.d. and h.s.

ADVERSE REACTIONS
CNS: *drowsiness, dizziness,* vertigo, ataxia, tremor, agitation, irritability, headache, depressive reactions, insomnia.
CV: *orthostatic hypotension,* tachycardia, facial flushing.
GI: nausea, vomiting, hiccups, epigastric distress.
Hematologic: eosinophilia.
Respiratory: asthmatic episodes.
Skin: rash, *erythema multiforme,* pruritus.
Other: fever, *angioedema, anaphylaxis.*

INTERACTIONS
Drug-drug. *CNS depressants:* increased CNS depression. Avoid concomitant use.
Drug-lifestyle. *Alcohol use:* increased CNS depression. Avoid concomitant use.

EFFECTS ON DIAGNOSTIC TESTS
None reported.

CONTRAINDICATIONS
Contraindicated in patients with intermittent porphyria or hypersensitivity to related compounds (such as meprobamate or tybamate).

NURSING CONSIDERATIONS
• Use cautiously in patients with impaired hepatic or renal function.
Alert: Watch for idiosyncratic reactions after first to fourth doses (weakness, ataxia, visual and speech difficulties, fever, skin eruptions, and mental changes) and for severe reactions, including bronchospasm, hypotension, and anaphylactic shock. Withhold dose and notify doctor immediately of unusual reactions.
• Record amount of relief to help doctor determine whether dosage can be reduced.
• Do not stop drug abruptly; mild withdrawal effects, such as insomnia, headache, nausea, and abdominal cramps, may result.
• Safety and efficacy in children under 12 years have not been established.

☑ **Patient teaching**
• Warn patient to avoid activities that require alertness until drug's CNS effects are known. Drowsiness is transient.
• Advise patient to avoid combining drug with alcohol or other CNS depressants.
• Tell patient to ask doctor before using OTC cold or hay fever remedies.
• Instruct patient to follow doctor's orders regarding rest and physical therapy.
• Advise patient to avoid sudden changes in posture if dizziness occurs.
• Tell patient to take drug with food or milk if GI upset occurs.

chlorzoxazone
Paraflex, Parafon Forte DSC, Remular-S

Pregnancy Risk Category: C

HOW SUPPLIED
Tablets: 250 mg, 500 mg
Caplets: 250 mg, 500 mg

ACTION
Unknown. Appears to modify central perception of pain without modifying pain reflexes. Inhibits reflex arcs in the spinal cord and subcortical areas of the brain to reduce muscle spasm, relieve pain, and increase mobility.

Route	Onset	Peak	Duration
PO	1 hr	1-2 hr	3-4 hr

INDICATIONS & DOSAGE
As an adjunct in acute, painful musculoskeletal conditions—
Adults: 250 to 750 mg P.O. t.i.d. or q.i.d.

ADVERSE REACTIONS
CNS: *drowsiness, dizziness, light-headedness,* malaise, headache, overstimulation, tremor.
GI: anorexia, nausea, vomiting, heartburn, abdominal distress, constipation, diarrhea.
GU: urine discoloration (orange or purplered).
Hepatic: hepatic dysfunction.
Skin: urticaria, redness, pruritus, petechiae, bruising.
Other: angioneurotic edema, *anaphylaxis.*

INTERACTIONS
Drug-drug. *CNS depressants:* increased CNS depression. Avoid concomitant use.
Drug-lifestyle. *Alcohol use:* increased CNS depression. Avoid concomitant use.

EFFECTS ON DIAGNOSTIC TESTS
None reported.

CONTRAINDICATIONS
Contraindicated in patients with impaired hepatic function or hypersensitivity to drug.

Reactions may be *common,* uncommon, *life-threatening,* or COMMON AND LIFE-THREATENING.

NURSING CONSIDERATIONS

• Use cautiously in patients with history of drug allergies.
• Know that the amount of relief determines if dosage (and drowsiness) can be reduced.
• Monitor patient's liver enzyme levels, as ordered. Watch for early signs of hepatic dysfunction or abnormal liver enzyme levels. If they occur, withhold dose and notify the doctor. Serious (including fatal) hepatocellular toxicity has been reported in patients receiving drug.

✓ **Patient teaching**
• Tell patient to take drug with meals or milk.
• Warn patient to avoid activities that require alertness until drug's CNS effects are known.
• Instruct patient to notify doctor immediately if fever, rash, anorexia, nausea, vomiting, fatigue, right upper quadrant pain, dark urine, or jaundice occurs because these may be signs or symptoms of hepatocellular toxicity, which warrants immediate discontinuation of drug.
• Warn patient to avoid alcohol and other CNS depressants; concomitant use with drug may increase risk of hepatocellular toxicity.
• Tell patient that drug may discolor urine orange or purple-red.
• Advise patient to follow doctor's orders regarding physical activity.

---

cyclobenzaprine hydrochloride
Flexeril

Pregnancy Risk Category: B

HOW SUPPLIED
Tablets: 10 mg

ACTION
Unknown. Relieves skeletal muscle spasm of local origin without interfering with muscle function.

Route	Onset	Peak	Duration
PO	1 hr	3-8 hr	12-24 hr

INDICATIONS & DOSAGE
Short-term treatment of muscle spasm—
Adults: 10 mg P.O. t.i.d. Maximum daily dosage 60 mg daily; maximum duration of treatment is 2 to 3 weeks.

ADVERSE REACTIONS
CNS: *drowsiness,* headache, insomnia, fatigue, asthenia, nervousness, confusion, paresthesia, *dizziness,* depression, *seizures,* dysarthria, ataxia.
CV: tachycardia, syncope, ***arrhythmias,*** palpitations, hypotension, vasodilation.
EENT: blurred vision, visual disturbances.
GI: dyspepsia, abnormal taste, constipation, *dry mouth,* nausea.
GU: urine retention, urinary frequency.
Skin: rash, urticaria, pruritus.
Other: with high doses, adverse reactions similar to those of other tricyclic antidepressants.

INTERACTIONS
Drug-drug. *Anticholinergics:* additive anticholinergic effects. Avoid concomitant use.
CNS depressants: increased CNS depression. Avoid concomitant use.
MAO inhibitors: Hyperpyretic crisis, seizures and death have occurred with concomitant administration of MAO inhibitors and tricyclics; the potential for this interaction with cyclobenzaprine also exists. Don't give within 14 days after discontinuing MAO inhibitors.
Drug-lifestyle. *Alcohol use:* increased CNS depression. Avoid concomitant use.

EFFECTS ON DIAGNOSTIC TESTS
None reported.

CONTRAINDICATIONS
Contraindicated in patients with hyperthyroidism, heart block, arrhythmias, conduction disturbances, heart failure, or hypersensitivity to drug and in those who have received MAO inhibitors within 14 days or who are in the acute recovery phase of MI.

NURSING CONSIDERATIONS
• Use cautiously in patients with history of urine retention, acute angle-closure

glaucoma, and increased intraocular pressure and in elderly or debilitated patients.
• Be alert for nausea, headache, and malaise, which may occur if drug is stopped abruptly after long-term use.
• Watch for symptoms of overdose, including possible cardiac toxicity. Notify doctor immediately.
• Safety and efficacy in children under 15 years have not been established.

☑ **Patient teaching**
• Advise patient to report urinary hesitancy or urine retention. If constipation is a problem, increase fluid intake and suggest a stool softener.
• Warn patient to avoid activities that require alertness until drug's CNS effects are known.
• Warn patient not to combine with alcohol or other CNS depressants, including OTC cold or allergy remedies.

---

dantrolene sodium
Dantrium, Dantrium Intravenous

Pregnancy Risk Category: C

HOW SUPPLIED
Capsules: 25 mg, 50 mg, 100 mg
Injection: 20 mg/vial

ACTION
Acts directly on skeletal muscle to decrease excitation and contraction coupling and reduce muscle strength by interfering with intracellular calcium movement.

Route	Onset	Peak	Duration
PO	Unknown	5 hr	Unknown
IV	Unknown	Unknown	3 hr after infusion ends

INDICATIONS & DOSAGE
Spasticity and sequelae secondary to severe chronic disorders (such as multiple sclerosis, cerebral palsy, spinal cord injury, CVA)—
Adults: 25 mg P.O. daily. Increased gradually in 25-mg increments, up to 100 mg b.i.d. to q.i.d., to maximum of 400 mg

daily. Maintain each dosage level for 4 to 7 days to determine response.
Children: initially, 0.5 mg/kg P.O. b.i.d.; increased to t.i.d. then q.i.d. Dosage increased p.r.n. by 0.5 mg/kg daily up to dose of 3 mg/kg b.i.d. to q.i.d. Maximum dosage is 100 mg q.i.d.
Management of malignant hyperthermia crisis—
Adults and children: 1 mg/kg I.V. push initially; dose repeated p.r.n. up to cumulative dosage of 10 mg/kg.
Prevention or attenuation of malignant hyperthermia crisis in susceptible patients who require surgery—
Adults: 4 to 8 mg/kg P.O. daily in three to four divided doses for 1 to 2 days before procedure. Final dose administered 3 to 4 hours before procedure.
Prevention of recurrence of malignant hyperthermia crisis—
Adults: 4 to 8 mg/kg/day P.O. in four divided doses for up to 3 days after hyperthermic crisis.

ADVERSE REACTIONS
CNS: *muscle weakness, drowsiness, dizziness,* light-headedness, *malaise, fatigue,* headache, confusion, nervousness, insomnia, *seizures.*
CV: tachycardia, blood pressure changes.
EENT: excessive lacrimation, speech disturbance, diplopia, visual disturbances.
GI: anorexia, constipation, cramping, dysphagia, metallic taste, severe diarrhea, GI bleeding.
GU: urinary frequency, hematuria, incontinence, nocturia, dysuria, crystalluria, difficult erection, urine retention.
Hepatic: *hepatitis.*
Musculoskeletal: myalgia, back pain.
Respiratory: pleural effusion with pericarditis, pulmonary edema.
Skin: eczematous eruption, pruritus, urticaria, abnormal hair growth, diaphoresis.
Other: chills, fever, phlebitis, thrombophlebitis.

INTERACTIONS
Drug-drug. *Clofibrate, warfarin:* may decrease plasma protein binding of dantrolene. Use together cautiously.

Reactions may be *common*, uncommon, *life-threatening*, or COMMON AND LIFE-THREATENING.

CNS depressants: increased CNS depression. Avoid concomitant use.
Estrogens: may increase risk of hepatotoxicity. Use together cautiously.
I.V. verapamil: may result in CV collapse. Stop verapamil before administering I.V. dantrolene.
Drug-lifestyle. *Alcohol use:* increased CNS depression. Avoid concomitant use.

EFFECTS ON DIAGNOSTIC TESTS
Drug therapy alters liver function test results (increased ALT, AST, alkaline phosphatase, and LD), BUN levels, and total serum bilirubin.

CONTRAINDICATIONS
Contraindicated in patients when spasticity is used to maintain motor function or for spasms in rheumatic disorders; in those with upper motor neuron disorders or active hepatic disease; and in breast-feeding patients.

NURSING CONSIDERATIONS
• Use cautiously in patients with severely impaired cardiac or pulmonary function or preexisting hepatic disease, in women, and in patients over 35 years.
• Because of risk of liver damage with long term use, therapy should be discontinued within 45 days if benefits are not seen.
• Obtain liver function tests at beginning of therapy.
• Prepare oral suspension for single dose by dissolving capsule contents in juice or other liquid. For multiple doses, use acid vehicle, and refrigerate. Use within several days.
• Watch for hepatitis (fever and jaundice), severe diarrhea, severe weakness, or sensitivity reactions (fever and skin eruptions). Withhold dose and notify doctor.
• Know that amount of relief in patient determines if dosage (and drowsiness) can be reduced.

🔲 I.V. administration
• Give as soon as malignant hyperthermia reaction is recognized, as ordered. Reconstitute each vial by adding 60 ml of sterile water for injection and shaking vial until clear. Don't use a diluent that contains a bacteriostatic agent. Protect contents from light, and use within 6 hours. Avoid extravasation.

✅ Patient teaching
• Instruct patient to take drug with meals or milk in four divided doses.
• Tell patient to use caution when eating to avoid choking. Some patients may experience difficulty swallowing during therapy.
• Warn patient to avoid driving and other hazardous activities until drug's CNS effects are known.
• Advise patient to avoid combining drug with alcohol and other CNS depressants.
• Advise patient to notify doctor if skin or eyes turn yellow, skin is itchy, or fever develops.
• Tell patient to avoid photosensitivity reactions by using sunblock and wearing protective clothing, to report abdominal discomfort or GI problems immediately, and to follow doctor's orders regarding rest and physical therapy.

---

methocarbamol
Carbacot, Robaxin, Robaxin-750, Skelex

Pregnancy Risk Category: C

HOW SUPPLIED
Tablets: 500 mg, 750 mg
Injection: 100 mg/ml

ACTION
Unknown. Probably modifies central perception of pain through sedative effects without modifying pain reflexes.

Route	Onset	Peak	Duration
PO	0.5 hr	2 hr	Unknown
IV	Immediate	Immediate	Unknown
IM	Unknown	Unknown	Unknown

INDICATIONS & DOSAGE
As an adjunct in acute, painful musculoskeletal conditions—
Adults: 1.5 g P.O. q.i.d. for 2 to 3 days, then 1 g P.O. q.i.d.; or not more than 500 mg (5 ml) I.M. into each gluteal region repeated q 8 hours p.r.n. Or 1 to 3 g

daily (10 to 30 ml) I.V. directly into vein at 3 ml/minute, or 10 ml may be added to no more than 250 ml of D_5W or 0.9% NaCl solution. Maximum I.V. or I.M. dosage is 3 g daily for not more than 3 days.

Supportive therapy in tetanus management—

Adults: 1 to 2 g by direct I.V. or 1 to 3 g as infusion q 6 hours until NG tube can be inserted; then give oral doses through NG tube. Maximum 24 g/day.

Children: 15 mg/kg I.V. q 6 hours.

ADVERSE REACTIONS

CNS: *drowsiness, dizziness, light-headedness*, headache, syncope, mild muscular incoordination (with I.M. or I.V. use), *seizures* (with I.V. use), vertigo.

CV: hypotension, bradycardia (with I.M. or I.V. use), thrombophlebitis.

EENT: blurred vision, conjunctivitis, nystagmus, diplopia.

GI: nausea, GI upset, metallic taste.

GU: hematuria (with I.V. use), discoloration of urine.

Skin: urticaria, pruritus, rash.

Other: extravasation (with I.V. use), fever, flushing, ***anaphylactic reactions*** (with I.M. or I.V. use).

INTERACTIONS

Drug-drug. *CNS depressants:* increased CNS depression. Avoid concomitant use.

Drug-lifestyle. *Alcohol use:* increased CNS depression. Avoid concomitant use.

EFFECTS ON DIAGNOSTIC TESTS

Drug therapy alters laboratory test results for urine 5-hydroxyindoleacetic acid using quantitative method of Udenfriend (false-positive) and urine vanillylmandelic acid (false-positive when Gitlow screening test used; no problem when quantitative method of Sunderman used).

CONTRAINDICATIONS

Contraindicated in patients with impaired renal function (injectable form), seizure disorder (injectable form), or hypersensitivity to drug.

NURSING CONSIDERATIONS

• For nasogastric tube administration, pre-

pare liquid by crushing tablets into water or NaCl solution.

• In tetanus management, be aware that methocarbamol is used with tetanus antitoxin, penicillin, tracheotomy, and aggressive supportive care. Long course of I.V. methocarbamol therapy is required.

• Give I.M. deeply, only into upper outer quadrant of buttocks, with maximum of 5 ml in each buttock.

• Do not give S.C.

• Watch for orthostatic hypotension, especially with parenteral administration. Keep the patient in a supine position for 15 minutes afterward, and supervise ambulation. Have patient get up slowly.

• Watch for sensitivity reactions, such as fever and skin eruptions.

• Have epinephrine, antihistamines, and corticosteroids available.

◖I.V. administration

• Dilute 10 ml of drug in not more than 250 ml of solution. Use D_5W or 0.9% NaCl for injection. Infuse slowly; maximum rate is 300 mg (3 ml)/minute.

• Know that drug irritates veins, may cause phlebitis, aggravate seizures, and cause fainting if injected rapidly. Make sure patient remains in a supine position during infusion. Drug is an irritant; avoid extravasation.

☑Patient teaching

• Instruct patient to take drug with food or milk at evenly spaced intervals, as ordered.

• Tell patient that a metallic taste may develop and urine may turn green, black, or brown.

• Advise patient to follow doctor's orders regarding physical activity.

• Warn patient to avoid activities that require alertness until drug's CNS effects are known.

• Advise patient to avoid combining drug with alcohol or other CNS depressants.

---

tizanidine hydrochloride
Zanaflex

Pregnancy Risk Category: C

HOW SUPPLIED
Tablets: 4 mg

ACTION
Unknown. Acts as an alpha$_2$-adrenergic agonist. Thought to reduce spasticity by increasing presynaptic inhibition of motor neurons at the level of the spinal cord.

Route	Onset	Peak	Duration
PO	Unknown	1-2 hr	3-6 hr

INDICATIONS & DOSAGE
Acute and intermittent management of increased muscle tone associated with spasticity—
Adults: initially, 4 mg P.O. q 6 to 8 hours p.r.n. to maximum of three doses in 24 hours. Dosage can be increased gradually in 2- to 4-mg increments. Maximum daily dose is 36 mg.
Adjust-a-dose: In patients with renal failure, reduce dosage. If higher dosages are needed, individual doses rather than frequency should be increased.

ADVERSE REACTIONS
CNS: *somnolence, sedation, asthenia, dizziness,* speech disorder, dyskinesia, nervousness, hallucinations.
CV: *hypotension, bradycardia.*
EENT: amblyopia, pharyngitis, rhinitis.
GI: *dry mouth,* constipation, vomiting.
GU: *urinary tract infection,* urinary frequency.
Hepatic: elevations of liver function tests, hepatic injury.
Other: infection, flulike syndrome.

INTERACTIONS
Drug-drug. *Antihypertensives, other alpha$_2$- adrenergic agonists:* may cause hypotension. Monitor patient closely. Do not use with other alpha$_2$-adrenergic agonists.
Baclofen, benzodiazepines, other CNS depressants: additive CNS depressant effects. Avoid concomitant use.
Oral contraceptives: decreased clearance of tizanidine. Dose of tizanidine may be reduced.
Drug-lifestyle. *Alcohol use:* increased CNS depression. Avoid concomitant use.

EFFECTS ON DIAGNOSTIC TESTS
Drug may increase liver function test results.

CONTRAINDICATIONS
Contraindicated in patients with known hypersensitivity to drug.

NURSING CONSIDERATIONS
• Use cautiously in patients who are currently taking antihypertensives, in those with renal and hepatic impairment, and in the elderly.
• Know that drug should be used in pregnancy only if the benefit justifies the risk to the fetus. Women taking drug should not breast-feed.
• Know that safety and effectiveness in children have not been established.
• Obtain baseline liver function test results as ordered before treatment; during treatment at 1, 3, and 6 months; and then periodically thereafter.

☑ **Patient teaching**
• Caution patient that drug may cause drowsiness and to avoid alcohol and activities such as driving and operating machinery that require alertness.
• Inform patient that orthostatic hypotension can be minimized by rising slowly and avoiding sudden position changes.

42

Neuromuscular blockers

atracurium besylate
cisatracurium besylate
doxacurium chloride
mivacurium chloride
pancuronium bromide
pipecuronium bromide
rocuronium bromide
succinylcholine chloride
tubocurarine chloride
vecuronium bromide

COMBINATION PRODUCTS
None.

atracurium besylate
Tracrium

Pregnancy Risk Category: C

HOW SUPPLIED
Injection: 10 mg/ml

ACTION
A nondepolarizing agent that prevents acetylcholine from binding to receptors on motor end plate, thus blocking neuromuscular transmission.

Route	Onset	Peak	Duration
IV	2 min	3-5 min	35-70 min

INDICATIONS & DOSAGE
Adjunct to general anesthesia to facilitate endotracheal intubation and to provide skeletal muscle relaxation during surgery or mechanical ventilation—
Dosage depends on anesthetic used, individual needs, and response. Dosages given here are representative only.
Adults and children over 2 years: 0.4 to 0.5 mg/kg by I.V. bolus. Maintenance dosage of 0.08 to 0.10 mg/kg within 20 to 45 minutes should be given during prolonged surgery. Maintenance dosages may be given q 12 to 25 minutes in patients receiving balanced anesthesia. For prolonged procedures, a constant infusion of 5 to 9 mcg/kg/minute may be used.

Children 1 month to 2 years: initial dose, 0.3 to 0.4 mg/kg. Frequent maintenance doses may be needed.

ADVERSE REACTIONS
CV: bradycardia, hypotension, tachycardia.
Respiratory: *prolonged, dose-related apnea;* wheezing; increased bronchial secretions; dyspnea; *bronchospasm; laryngospasm.*
Skin: *skin flushing,* erythema, pruritus, urticaria, rash.
Other: *anaphylaxis.*

INTERACTIONS
Drug-drug. *Aminoglycoside antibiotics (amikacin, gentamicin, kanamycin, neomycin, streptomycin); clindamycin; general anesthetics (enflurane, halothane, isoflurane); polymyxin antibiotics (colistin, polymyxin B sulfate); quinidine, verapamil, procainamide, trimethaphan, thiazide diuretics:* potentiated neuromuscular blockade, leading to increased skeletal muscle relaxation and prolonged effect. Use cautiously during and after surgery.
Corticosteroids: prolonged weakness may occur. Monitor closely.
Edrophonium, neostigmine, pyridostigmine: inhibition of drug and reversed neuromuscular block. Monitor closely.
Lithium, magnesium salts, opioid analgesics: potentiated neuromuscular blockade, leading to increased skeletal muscle relaxation and possible respiratory paralysis. Reduce dose of atracurium.
Phenytoin, theophylline: resistance to or reversal of neuromuscular blockade. Monitor closely.
Succinylcholine: quickens onset and may increase depth of neuromuscular blockade. Monitor patient.

EFFECTS ON DIAGNOSTIC TESTS
None reported.

CONTRAINDICATIONS
Contraindicated in patients with hypersensitivity to drug.

NURSING CONSIDERATIONS
• Use cautiously in those with CV disease; severe electrolyte disorder; bronchogenic carcinoma; hepatic, renal, or pulmonary impairment; neuromuscular disease; or myasthenia gravis and in elderly or debilitated patients.
• Administer analgesics, as ordered, for pain. Remember that patient may have pain but not be able to express it.
• Do not give by I.M. injection.
• Once spontaneous recovery starts, be prepared to reverse atracurium-induced neuromuscular blockade with an anticholinesterase agent (such as neostigmine or edrophonium), as ordered. Usually given together with an anticholinergic (such as atropine). Complete reversal of neuromuscular blockade is generally achieved within 8-10 minutes after administration of a cholinesterase inhibitor.
• Monitor respirations closely until patient has fully recovered from neuromuscular blockade, as evidenced by tests of muscle strength (hand grip, head lift, and ability to cough).
• A nerve stimulator and train-of-four monitoring are recommended to confirm antagonism of neuromuscular blockade and recovery of muscle strength. Evidence of spontaneous recovery should be seen before attempting reversal with neostigmine.
• Know that prior administration of succinylcholine doesn't prolong duration of action but quickens onset and may deepen neuromuscular blockade.

I.V. administration
• Use drug only under direct medical supervision by personnel skilled in the use of neuromuscular blockers and techniques for maintaining a patent airway. Have emergency respiratory support equipment (endotracheal equipment, ventilator, oxygen, atropine, edrophonium, neostigmine, and epinephrine) available.
• Administer sedatives or general anesthetics before neuromuscular blockers,

which don't obtund consciousness or alter pain threshold.
• Drug usually is administered by rapid I.V. bolus injection but may be given by intermittent infusion or continuous infusion. At concentrations of 0.2 mg/ml to 0.5 mg/ml, atracurium is compatible for 24 hours in D_5W, 0.9% NaCl for injection, or dextrose 5% in 0.9% NaCl for injection.
• Do not use lactated Ringer's solution. In lactated Ringer's injection, atracurium is stable for 8 hours at a concentration of 0.5 mg/ml. However, because of increased degradation in this solution, it is not recommended.
• Do not mix with alkaline solutions (such as barbiturates) because precipitates may form.

✔ Patient teaching
• Explain all events and procedures to patient because he can still hear.

cisatracurium besylate
Nimbex

Pregnancy Risk Category: B

HOW SUPPLIED
Injection: 2 mg/ml, 10 mg/ml

ACTION
A nondepolarizing agent that binds to cholinergic receptors on the motor end plate, antagonizing acetylcholine and blocking neuromuscular transmission.

Route	Onset	Peak	Duration
IV	1-3.3 min	2-5 min	25-44 min

INDICATIONS & DOSAGE
Dosage requirements vary widely among patients.
Adjunct to general anesthesia, to facilitate tracheal intubation, and to provide skeletal muscle relaxation during surgery—
Adults: initial dose of 0.15 mg/kg I.V., followed by maintenance doses of 0.03 mg/kg I.V. q 40 to 50 minutes p.r.n. (or initial dose of 0.20 mg/kg I.V., followed by maintenance doses of 0.03 mg/

kg I.V. q 50 to 60 minutes p.r.n.). Alternatively, after initial dose, a maintenance infusion may be given at 3 mcg/kg/minute, reduced to 1 to 2 mcg/kg/minute p.r.n.
Children 2 to 12 years: 0.1 mg/kg I.V. over 5 to 10 seconds. After initial dose, a maintenance infusion may be given at 3 mcg/kg/minute, reduced to 1 to 2 mcg/kg/minute p.r.n.
Maintenance of neuromuscular blockade during mechanical ventilation in intensive care unit—
Adults: after initial dose, 3 mcg/kg/minute (range, 0.5 to 10.2 mcg/kg/minute) I.V. infusion.

ADVERSE REACTIONS
CV: bradycardia, hypotension.
Respiratory: *bronchospasm; prolonged, dose-related apnea*.
Skin: flushing, rash.

INTERACTIONS
Drug-drug. *Aminoglycosides, bacitracin, clindamycin, colistin, lincomycin, lithium, local anesthetics, magnesium salts, polymyxins, procainamide, quinidine, sodium colistimethate, tetracyclines:* may enhance neuromuscular blocking action of cisatracurium. Use together cautiously.
Carbamazepine, phenytoin: may cause slightly shorter duration of neuromuscular block, requiring higher infusion rate. Monitor closely.
Enflurane or isoflurane administered with nitrous oxide/oxygen: may prolong duration of action of cisatracurium. Be aware that patient may require less frequent maintenance dosing, lower maintenance doses, or reduced infusion rate of cisatracurium.
Succinylcholine: shorter time to onset of maximum neuromuscular block. Monitor patient.

EFFECTS ON DIAGNOSTIC TESTS
None reported.

CONTRAINDICATIONS
Contraindicated in patients with hypersensitivity to drug, other bis-benzylisoquinolinium agents, or benzyl alcohol (found in 10-ml vial).

NURSING CONSIDERATIONS
• Drug is not recommended for rapid-sequence endotracheal intubation because of its intermediate onset.
• Use cautiously in pregnant or breast-feeding women.
• Monitor neuromuscular function with nerve stimulator during administration. If stimulation does not elicit a response, stop infusion until response returns.
• To avoid inaccurate dosing, perform neuromuscular monitoring on a nonparetic limb in patients with hemiparesis or paraparesis.
• In patients with neuromuscular disease (myasthenia gravis and myasthenic syndrome [Eaton-Lambert syndrome]), prolonged neuromuscular block is possible. Use of a peripheral nerve stimulator and a dose of not more than 0.02 mg/kg is recommended to assess the level of neuromuscular block and to monitor dosage requirements.
• Because patients with burns have been shown to develop resistance to nondepolarizing neuromuscular blocking agents, they may require increased dosing. Monitor closely.
• Monitor acid-base balance and electrolyte levels, as ordered. Abnormalities may potentiate or antagonize the action of cisatracurium.
• Monitor patient for malignant hyperthermia.
• Administer analgesics, if appropriate. Patient can feel pain but cannot indicate its presence.

⬛ I.V. administration
• Use only under direct medical supervision by personnel skilled in the use of neuromuscular blockers and techniques for maintaining airway patency. Do not use unless facilities and equipment for artificial respiration, mechanical ventilation and oxygen therapy are within reach.
• Drug has no known effect on consciousness, pain threshold, or cerebration. To avoid patient distress, do not induce neuromuscular block before unconsciousness.
• Know that 20-ml vial is intended for use in intensive care unit only. Drug is not compatible with propofol injection or ke-

torolac injection for Y-site administration. Drug is acidic and may not be compatible with an alkaline solution having a pH greater than 8.5 (such as barbiturate solutions for Y-site administration). Drug should not be diluted in lactated Ringer's injection because of chemical instability.

• Drug is colorless to slightly yellow or green-yellow. Inspect vials for particulate and discoloration before administration. Unclear solutions or those with visible particulate should not be used.

☑**Patient teaching**
• Explain drug's purpose.
• Assure patient that monitoring will be continuous.
• Explain all procedures and events; drug does not interfere with patient's ability to hear.

---

doxacurium chloride
Nuromax

Pregnancy Risk Category: C

HOW SUPPLIED
Injection: 1 mg/ml

ACTION
A nondepolarizing neuromuscular blocking agent that competes with acetylcholine for receptor sites at the motor end plate; because this action may be antagonized by cholinesterase inhibitors, doxacurium is considered a competitive antagonist.

Route	Onset	Peak	Duration
IV	Variable	Variable	Variable

INDICATIONS & DOSAGE
To provide skeletal muscle relaxation during surgery as an adjunct to general anesthesia—
Dosage is highly individualized. All times of onset and duration are averages; considerable individual variation is normal.
Adults: 0.05 mg/kg rapid I.V. produces adequate conditions for endotracheal intubation in 5 minutes in about 90% of patients when used as part of a thiopental-narcotic induction technique. Lower doses

may require longer delay before intubation is possible. Neuromuscular blockade at this dose lasts for an average of 100 minutes.
Children over 2 years: an initial dose of 0.03 mg/kg I.V. given during halothane anesthesia produces effective blockade in 7 minutes with duration of 30 minutes. Under the same conditions, 0.05 mg/kg produces blockade in 4 minutes with duration of 45 minutes.
Maintenance of neuromuscular blockade during long procedures—
Adults: after initial dose of 0.05 mg/kg I.V., maintenance doses of 0.005 to 0.01 mg/kg will prolong neuromuscular blockade for an average of 30 to 45 minutes.

ADVERSE REACTIONS
Respiratory: dyspnea, *respiratory depression, respiratory insufficiency or apnea.*
Other: prolonged muscle weakness.

INTERACTIONS
Drug-drug. *Alkaline solutions:* physically incompatible; precipitate may form. Do not administer through same I.V. line.
Aminoglycosides (gentamicin, kanamycin, neomycin, and streptomycin), bacitracin, clindamycin, colistimethate, colistin, lincomycin, polymyxin B, tetracyclines: potentiated neuromuscular blockade leading to increased skeletal muscle relaxation and prolonged effect. Use together cautiously.
Carbamazepine, phenytoin: may prolong the time to maximal block or shorten the duration of block with neuromuscular blockers. Monitor patient.
Inhalation anesthetics: may enhance or prolong action of nondepolarizing neuromuscular blockers. Monitor patient.
Lithium, local anesthetics, magnesium salts, procainamide, quinidine: may enhance neuromuscular blockade. Monitor for excessive weakness.

EFFECTS ON DIAGNOSTIC TESTS
None reported.

CONTRAINDICATIONS
Contraindicated in patients with hyper-

sensitivity to drug and in neonates. Drug contains benzyl alcohol, which has been associated with fatalities in newborns.

NURSING CONSIDERATIONS
• Use cautiously, possibly at reduced dosage, in elderly or debilitated patients; in patients with metastatic cancer, severe electrolyte disturbances, renal or hepatic impairment, or neuromuscular diseases; and in those in whom potentiation or difficulty in reversal of neuromuscular blockade is anticipated. Patients with myasthenia gravis or myasthenic syndrome (Eaton-Lambert syndrome) are particularly sensitive to the effects of nondepolarizing relaxants. Shorter-acting agents are recommended for use in such patients.
• Because of lack of data supporting drug's safety, be aware that it is not recommended for use in patients requiring prolonged mechanical ventilation in the intensive care unit, before or after administration of nondepolarizing neuromuscular blocking agents, or during cesarean section.
• Drug is not metabolized; it is excreted in urine and bile. Patients with renal or hepatic insufficiency may require dosage adjustment.
• Keep in mind that dosage should be adjusted to ideal body weight in obese patients (patients 30% or more above their ideal weight) to avoid prolonged neuromuscular blockade.
• Know that higher initial doses may be required in patients with severe burns and in some patients with severe liver disease. Higher doses (0.8 mg/kg) will produce intubating conditions more rapidly (4 minutes), with neuromuscular blockade for 160 minutes or more. Consequently, these higher doses should be reserved for long procedures. Administration during steady-state anesthesia with enflurane, halothane, or isoflurane may allow 33% reduction of dose.
• Be aware that a nerve stimulator and train-of-four monitoring are recommended to document antagonism of neuromuscular blockade and recovery of muscle strength. Before attempting pharmacologic reversal with neostigmine, some evidence of spontaneous recovery should be present.
• Because drug has minimal vagolytic action, monitor for bradycardia, which may occur during anesthesia.
• Monitor respirations until patient is fully recovered from neuromuscular blockade, as evidenced by tests of muscle strength (hand grip, head lift, and ability to cough).
• Know that experimental evidence suggests that acid-base and electrolyte balance may influence the actions of nondepolarizing neuromuscular blockers. Alkalosis may counteract paralysis; acidosis may enhance it.

◖ I.V. administration
• Use drug only under direct medical supervision by personnel skilled in the use of neuromuscular blockers and techniques for maintaining a patent airway. Do not use unless facilities and equipment for mechanical ventilation, oxygen therapy, and intubation and an antagonist are within reach.
• To avoid patient distress, do not give drug until patient's consciousness is obtunded by general anesthetic. Drug has no effect on consciousness or pain threshold.
• Prepare drug for I.V. use with D_5W, 0.9% NaCl for injection, dextrose 5% in 0.9% NaCl for injection, lactated Ringer's injection, and dextrose 5% in lactated Ringer's injection.
• Administer product immediately after reconstitution. Diluted solutions are stable for 24 hours at room temperature; however, because reconstitution dilutes the preservative, risk of contamination increases. Discard unused solutions after 8 hours.
• When diluted as directed, remember that drug is compatible with alfentanil, fentanyl, and sufentanil.

☑ Patient teaching
• Inform patient of need for drug.
• Reassure patient and family that he will be monitored at all times.

---

mivacurium chloride
Mivacron

Pregnancy Risk Category: C

HOW SUPPLIED
Injection: 2 mg/ml in 5-ml and 10-ml vials
Infusion: 0.5 mg/ml in 50 ml of D_5W

ACTION
A nondepolarizing agent that competes with acetylcholine for receptor sites at the motor end plate, blocking neuromuscular transmission. Because this action may be antagonized by cholinesterase inhibitors, mivacurium is considered a competitive antagonist. Drug is a mixture of three stereoisomers, each possessing neuromuscular blocking activity.

Route	Onset	Peak	Duration
IV	1-2 min	2-5 min	20-35 min

INDICATIONS & DOSAGE
Adjunct to general anesthesia, to facilitate endotracheal intubation, and to relax skeletal muscles during surgery or mechanical ventilation—
Adults: dosage is highly individualized. Usually, 0.15 mg/kg I.V. push over 5 to 15 seconds provides adequate muscle relaxation within 2½ minutes for endotracheal intubation. Supplemental doses of 0.1 mg/kg I.V. q 15 minutes are usually sufficient to maintain muscle relaxation.

Alternatively, maintain neuromuscular blockade with a continuous infusion of 4 mcg/kg/minute begun simultaneously with the initial dose, or 9 to 10 mcg/kg/minute started after spontaneous recovery caused by the initial dose is evident. When used with isoflurane or enflurane anesthesia, dosage usually is reduced up to 40%.
Children 2 to 12 years: 0.2 mg/kg I.V. push administered over 5 to 15 seconds. Neuromuscular blockade is usually evident in less than 2 minutes. Maintenance doses are generally required more frequently in children.

Alternatively, neuromuscular blockade can be maintained with a continuous I.V. infusion titrated to effect. Most children respond to 5 to 31 mcg/kg/minute (average, 14 mcg/kg/minute).

ADVERSE REACTIONS
CNS: dizziness.
CV: *flushing,* tachycardia, bradycardia, *arrhythmias,* hypotension.
Respiratory: *bronchospasm,* wheezing, *respiratory insufficiency or apnea.*
Skin: rash, urticaria, erythema.
Other: prolonged muscle weakness, phlebitis, muscle spasms.

INTERACTIONS
Drug-drug. *Alkaline solutions (such as barbiturate solutions):* physically incompatible; precipitate may form. Do not administer through same I.V. line.
Aminoglycosides (gentamicin, kanamycin, neomycin, streptomycin), bacitracin, clindamycin, colistimethate, colistin, lincomycin, polymyxin B sulfate, tetracyclines: potentiated neuromuscular blockade, leading to increased skeletal muscle relaxation and prolonged effect. Use together cautiously.
Carbamazepine, phenytoin: may prolong time to maximal blockade or shorten duration of blockade with neuromuscular blockers. Monitor patient.
Inhalation anesthetics (especially enflurane, isoflurane): may enhance or prolong action of nondepolarizing neuromuscular blockers. Monitor for excessive weakness.
Lithium, local anesthetics, magnesium salts, procainamide, quinidine: may enhance neuromuscular blockade. Monitor for excessive weakness.

EFFECTS ON DIAGNOSTIC TESTS
None reported.

CONTRAINDICATIONS
Contraindicated in patients with hypersensitivity to drug, other bis-benzylisoquinolinium agents, or benzyl alcohol.

NURSING CONSIDERATIONS
• Use cautiously in patients with significant CV disease and in those who may be adversely affected by release of histamine (such as asthmatic patients). To avoid hypotension, use lower initial dose of drug

or give drug over longer period (60 seconds).

• Also use cautiously, possibly at reduced dosage, in debilitated patients; in those with metastatic cancer, severe electrolyte disturbances, or neuromuscular diseases; and in those in whom potentiation or difficulty in reversal of neuromuscular blockade is anticipated. Patients with myasthenia gravis or myasthenic syndrome (Eaton-Lambert syndrome) are particularly sensitive to effects of nondepolarizing relaxants. Test dose of 0.015 to 0.02 mg/kg may be used to assess the patient's sensitivity to drug.

Alert: Use very cautiously, if at all, in patients who are homozygous for the atypical plasma pseudocholinesterase gene. Drug is metabolized to inactive compound by plasma pseudocholinesterase.

• Administer a test dose to assess patient's sensitivity to drug. Patients with severe burns are known to develop resistance to nondepolarizing neuromuscular blockers; however, they also may have reduced plasma pseudocholinesterase activity.

• Keep in mind that dosage should be adjusted to ideal body weight in obese patients (patients 30% or more above their ideal weight) to avoid prolonged neuromuscular blockade.

• Be aware that like other neuromuscular blockers, dosage requirements for children are higher on a milligram per kilogram basis than those for adults. Onset and recovery of neuromuscular blockade occur more rapidly in children.

• A nerve stimulator and train-of-four monitoring are recommended to document antagonism of neuromuscular blockade and recovery of muscle strength. Before attempting pharmacologic reversal with neostigmine or edrophonium, some signs of spontaneous recovery should be evident.

• Monitor respirations closely until patient is fully recovered from neuromuscular blockade, as evidenced by tests of muscle strength (hand grip, head lift, and ability to cough).

• Know that experimental evidence suggests that acid-base and electrolyte balances may influence the actions of nondepolarizing neuromuscular blockers. Alkalosis may counteract the paralysis; acidosis may enhance it.

• Know that duration of drug effect is increased about 150% in patients with end-stage renal disease and 300% in patients with hepatic dysfunction.

I.V. administration

• Use only under direct medical supervision by personnel skilled in the use of neuromuscular blockers and techniques for maintaining a patent airway. Do not use unless facilities and equipment for artificial respiration, mechanical ventilation, oxygen therapy, and intubation and an antagonist are within reach.

• To avoid patient distress, do not administer until patient's consciousness is obtunded by general anesthetic because drug has no effect on consciousness or pain threshold.

• Prepare drug for I.V. use with D_5W, 0.9% NaCl for injection, dextrose 5% in 0.9% NaCl for injection, lactated Ringer's injection, and dextrose 5% in lactated Ringer's injection. Diluted solutions are stable for 24 hours at room temperature.

• For drug available as premixed infusion in D_5W, remove the protective outer wrap, then check container for minor leaks by squeezing the bag before administering. Do not add other drugs to the container, and do not use the container in series connections.

• Remember that when diluted as directed, mivacurium is compatible with alfentanil, fentanyl, sufentanil, droperidol, and midazolam.

Patient teaching

• Explain drug's purpose.
• Reassure patient and family that he will be monitored at all times.

---

pancuronium bromide
Pavulon

Pregnancy Risk Category: C

HOW SUPPLIED
Injection: 1 mg/ml, 2 mg/ml

ACTION
A nondepolarizing agent that prevents acetylcholine from binding to receptors on the motor end plate, thus blocking neuromuscular transmission.

Route	Onset	Peak	Duration
IV	30-45 sec	3-4.5 min	35-65 min

INDICATIONS & DOSAGE
Adjunct to anesthesia to induce skeletal muscle relaxation; to facilitate intubation; to assist with mechanical ventilation—
Dosage depends on anesthetic used, individual needs, and response. Dosages are representative only.
Adults and children 1 month and over: initially, 0.04 to 0.1 mg/kg I.V.; then 0.01 mg/kg q 30 to 60 minutes.
Neonates: individualized.

ADVERSE REACTIONS
CV: tachycardia, increased blood pressure.
Respiratory: *prolonged, dose-related respiratory insufficiency or apnea.*
Skin: transient rashes.
Other: excessive salivation, residual muscle weakness, allergic or idiosyncratic hypersensitivity reactions.

INTERACTIONS
Drug-drug. *Aminoglycoside antibiotics (including amikacin, gentamicin, kanamycin, neomycin, streptomycin); clindamycin; general anesthetics (such as enflurane, halothane, isoflurane); lincomycin; magnesium sulfate, polymyxin antibiotics (colistin, polymyxin B sulfate); quinidine:* potentiated neuromuscular blockade, leading to increased skeletal muscle relaxation and prolonged effect. Use cautiously during surgical and postoperative periods.
Azathioprine: may reverse neuromuscular blockade induced by pancuronium. Monitor patient.
Lithium, opioid analgesics: potentiated neuromuscular blockade, leading to increased skeletal muscle relaxation and possible respiratory paralysis. Use with extreme caution, and reduce dose of pancuronium.

Succinylcholine: increased intensity and duration of neuromuscular blockade. Allow effects of succinylcholine to subside before administering pancuronium.

EFFECTS ON DIAGNOSTIC TESTS
None reported.

CONTRAINDICATIONS
Contraindicated in patients with preexisting tachycardia or hypersensitivity to bromides and in those for whom even a minor increase in heart rate is undesirable.

NURSING CONSIDERATIONS
• Use cautiously in elderly or debilitated patients; in patients with renal, hepatic, or pulmonary impairment; and in those with respiratory depression, myasthenia gravis, myasthenic syndrome (Eaton-Lambert syndrome) of lung cancer or bronchogenic carcinoma, dehydration, thyroid disorders, CV disease, collagen diseases, porphyria, electrolyte disturbances, hyperthermia, and toxemic states. Also use large doses cautiously in patients undergoing cesarean section.
• Know that drug should be used only by personnel skilled in airway management.
• Allow succinylcholine effects to subside before giving pancuronium.
• Monitor baseline electrolyte determinations (electrolyte imbalance can potentiate neuromuscular effects) and vital signs, especially respirations and heart rate.
• Measure fluid intake and output; renal dysfunction may prolong duration of action because 25% of the drug is excreted unchanged in the urine.
• Keep in mind that a nerve stimulator and train-of-four monitoring are recommended to confirm antagonism of neuromuscular blockade and recovery of muscle strength. Before attempting pharmacologic reversal with neostigmine, some evidence of spontaneous recovery should be seen.
• Monitor respirations closely until patient has fully recovered from neuromuscular blockade, as evidenced by tests of muscle strength (hand grip, head lift, and ability to cough).
• Once spontaneous recovery starts, pancuronium-induced neuromuscular block-

ade may be reversed with an anti-cholinesterase agent (such as neostigmine or edrophonium), which is usually administered with an anticholinergic (such as atropine).
• Know that drug does not cause histamine release or hypotension but may raise heart rate and blood pressure.
• Give analgesics, as ordered, for pain.

◖ I.V. administration
• Administer sedatives or general anesthetics before neuromuscular blockers, as ordered. Neuromuscular blockers do not obtund consciousness or alter the pain threshold.
• Have emergency respiratory support equipment (endotracheal equipment, ventilator, oxygen, atropine, edrophonium, epinephrine, and neostigmine) immediately available.
• Do not mix with alkaline solutions, such as barbiturate solutions, because precipitate will form; use only fresh solutions.
• Store in refrigerator. Do not store in plastic containers or syringes, although plastic syringes may be used for administration.

☑ Patient teaching
• Explain all events and procedures to patient because he can still hear.

pipecuronium bromide
Arduan

Pregnancy Risk Category: C

HOW SUPPLIED
Powder for injection: 10-mg vial

ACTION
A nondepolarizing neuromuscular blocking agent that competes with acetylcholine for receptor sites at the motor end plate. Because this action may be antagonized by cholinesterase inhibitors, pipecuronium is considered a competitive antagonist.

Route	Onset	Peak	Duration
IV	1-2 min	5 min	24 min

INDICATIONS & DOSAGE
To provide skeletal muscle relaxation during surgery as adjunct to general anesthesia for procedures expected to last 90 minutes or more—
Dosage is highly individualized. The following doses may serve as a guide for use in nonobese patients with normal renal function.
Adults and children: initially, 70 to 85 mcg/kg I.V. provides conditions considered ideal for endotracheal intubation and maintains paralysis for 1 to 2 hours. If succinylcholine is used for endotracheal intubation, initial dose of 50 mcg/kg I.V. provides good relaxation for 45 minutes or more. Maintenance dose of 10 to 15 mcg/kg provides relaxation for about 50 minutes.
Adjust-a-dose: In renally impaired patients, dosage adjustment is required.

ADVERSE REACTIONS
CV: *hypotension,* bradycardia, hypertension, myocardial ischemia, *CVA,* thrombosis, atrial fibrillation, *ventricular extrasystole.*
GU: anuria.
Respiratory: dyspnea, *respiratory depression, respiratory insufficiency or apnea.*
Skin: rash, urticaria.
Other: prolonged muscle weakness, increased creatinine levels.

INTERACTIONS
Drug-drug. *Aminoglycosides (gentamicin, kanamycin, neomycin, streptomycin), bacitracin, colistimethate, colistin, polymyxin B sulfate, tetracyclines:* potentiated neuromuscular blockade, leading to increased skeletal muscle relaxation and prolonged effect. Use together cautiously.
Inhalation anesthetics, quinidine: enhances or prolongs action of nondepolarizing neuromuscular blockers. Monitor patient.
Magnesium salts: may enhance neuromuscular blockade. Monitor for excessive weakness.

EFFECTS ON DIAGNOSTIC TESTS
None reported.

CONTRAINDICATIONS
Contraindicated in patients with hypersensitivity to drug.

NURSING CONSIDERATIONS
• Use cautiously and with dosage adjustments in patients with renal failure because drug is excreted by the kidneys. No information is available regarding use of drug in patients with hepatic disease.
• Because of lack of data supporting drug's safety, know that it is not recommended for use in patients requiring prolonged mechanical ventilation in the intensive care unit, before or after administration of other nondepolarizing neuromuscular blockers, or during cesarean section.
• Be aware that patients with myasthenia gravis or myasthenic syndrome (Eaton-Lambert syndrome) are particularly sensitive to the effects of nondepolarizing relaxants. Shorter-acting agents are recommended.
• Keep in mind that drug is not recommended for use in neonates and infants under 3 months. Limited evidence suggests that infants and children (1 to 14 years) under balanced anesthesia or halothane anesthesia may be less sensitive than adults.
• Know that dosage should be adjusted to ideal body weight in obese patients (30% or more over their ideal weight) to avoid prolonged neuromuscular blockade.
Alert: Because of its prolonged duration of action, keep in mind that pipecuronium is recommended only for procedures that take 90 minutes or longer.
• Monitor respirations closely until patient is fully recovered from neuromuscular blockade, as evidenced by tests of muscle strength (hand grip, head lift, and ability to cough).
• Monitor for bradycardia during anesthesia.
• Know that a nerve stimulator and train-of-four monitoring are recommended to document antagonism of neuromuscular blockade and recovery of muscle strength. Before attempting pharmacologic reversal with neostigmine, some evidence of spontaneous recovery should be present.
• Be aware that experimental evidence suggests that acid-base and electrolyte balances may influence the actions of nondepolarizing neuromuscular blockers. Alkalosis may counteract the paralysis, and acidosis may enhance it.

◖I.V. administration
• Use drug under direct medical supervision by personnel skilled in use of neuromuscular blockers and techniques for maintaining a patent airway. Do not use drug unless facilities and equipment for artificial respiration, mechanical ventilation, oxygen therapy, and intubation and an antagonist are within reach.
• Give patient sedatives or general anesthetics before neuromuscular blockers are administered, as ordered. Neuromuscular blockers do not obtund consciousness or alter pain threshold.
• Reconstitute with 10 ml solution before use to yield a solution of 1 mg/ml. Using a large volume of diluent or adding drug to a hanging I.V. solution is not recommended.
• After reconstitution with sterile water for injection or other compatible I.V. solutions (such as 0.9% NaCl for injection, D_5W, lactated Ringer's injection, dextrose 5% in 0.9% NaCl for injection), drug is stable for 24 hours if refrigerated.
• Know that after reconstitution with bacteriostatic water for injection, drug is stable for 5 days at room temperature or in the refrigerator. Bacteriostatic water contains benzyl alcohol and is not intended for use in neonates.
• After reconstitution with solutions other than bacteriostatic water for injection, discard unused drug.
• Administer pipecuronium after succinylcholine when the latter is used to facilitate intubation.
• Store powder at room temperature or in refrigerator (36° to 86° F [2° to 30° C]).

✅Patient teaching
• Explain drug's purpose.
• Reassure patient and family that he will be monitored at all times.

rocuronium bromide
Zemuron

Pregnancy Risk Category: B

HOW SUPPLIED
Injection: 10 mg/ml

ACTION
A nondepolarizing agent that prevents acetylcholine from binding to receptors on the motor end plate, thus blocking neuromuscular transmission.

Route	Onset	Peak	Duration
IV	1 min	2 min	22-67 min

INDICATIONS & DOSAGE
Adjunct to general anesthesia to facilitate endotracheal intubation and to provide skeletal muscle relaxation during surgery or mechanical ventilation—
Dosage depends on anesthetic used, individual needs, and response. Dosages are representative and must be adjusted.
Adults: initially, 0.6 mg/kg I.V. bolus. In most patients, tracheal intubation may be performed within 2 minutes; muscle paralysis should last about 31 minutes. A maintenance dosage of 0.1 mg/kg should provide an additional 12 minutes of muscle relaxation; 0.15 mg/kg will add 17 minutes; or 0.2 mg/kg will add 24 minutes to the duration of effect.

ADVERSE REACTIONS
CV: tachycardia, abnormal ECG, *arrhythmias* (rare), transient hypotension, hypertension.
GI: nausea, vomiting.
Respiratory: asthma, *respiratory insufficiency, apnea.*
Skin: rash, edema, pruritus.
Other: hiccups.

INTERACTIONS
Drug-drug. *Aminoglycoside antibiotics (including amikacin, gentamicin, kanamycin, neomycin, streptomycin); anticonvulsants; clindamycin; general anesthetics (such as enflurane, halothane, isoflurane); magnesium salts; opiate analgesics; polymyxin antibiotics (colistin, polymyxin B sulfate); quinidine; succinylcholine; tetracyclines:* potentiated neuromuscular blockade, leading to increased skeletal muscle relaxation and potentiated effect. Use cautiously during surgical and postoperative periods.

EFFECTS ON DIAGNOSTIC TESTS
None reported.

CONTRAINDICATIONS
Contraindicated in patients with hypersensitivity to drug or bromides.

NURSING CONSIDERATIONS
• Use cautiously in patients with altered circulation time caused by CV disease, old age, and edematous states; hepatic disease; severe obesity; bronchogenic carcinoma; electrolyte disturbances; and neuromuscular disease.
• Drug is not recommended for use during rapid sequence induction for cesarean section.
• Know that drug should be used only by personnel skilled in airway management.
• Be alert that rocuronium provides conditions for intubation within 3 minutes.
• Know that a nerve stimulator and train-of-four monitoring are recommended to confirm antagonism of neuromuscular blockade and recovery of muscle strength. Before attempting pharmacologic reversal with neostigmine, some evidence of spontaneous recovery should be present.
• Keep in mind that prior administration of succinylcholine may enhance neuromuscular blocking effect and duration of action.
• Monitor patients with liver disease because they may require higher doses of drug to achieve adequate muscle relaxation. However, such patients exhibit prolonged effects from drug.
• Monitor respirations closely until patient is fully recovered from neuromuscular blockade, as evidenced by tests of muscle strength (hand grip, head lift, and ability to cough).
• Know that rocuronium is well tolerated in patients with renal failure.
• Give analgesics, as ordered, for pain.

Reactions may be *common*, uncommon, *life-threatening*, or COMMON AND LIFE-THREATENING.

◖ I.V. administration
● Administer sedatives or general anesthetics before neuromuscular blockers, as ordered. Neuromuscular blockers do not obtund consciousness or alter the pain threshold.
● Administer by rapid I.V. injection. Alternatively, give by continuous I.V. infusion. Infusion rates are highly individualized. Compatible solutions include D_5W, 0.9% NaCl for injection, dextrose 5% in 0.9% NaCl for injection, sterile water for injection, and lactated Ringer's injection.
● Keep airway clear. Have emergency respiratory support equipment (endotracheal equipment, ventilator, oxygen, atropine, edrophonium, epinephrine, and neostigmine) available.
● Know that vials can be stored at room temperature for up to 30 days. Diluted infusion solutions should be used within 24 hours.

☑ Patient teaching
● Explain all events and procedures to patient because he can still hear.

---

succinylcholine chloride
(suxamethonium chloride)
Anectine, Anectine Flo-Pack, Quelicin, Scoline‡, Sucostrin

Pregnancy Risk Category: C

HOW SUPPLIED
Injection: 20 mg/ml, 50 mg/ml, 100 mg/ml; 100-mg vial, 500-mg vial, 1-g vial

ACTION
Binds with a high affinity to cholinergic receptors, prolonging depolarization of the motor end plate and ultimately producing muscle paralysis.

Route	Onset	Peak	Duration
IV	0.5-1 sec	1-2 min	4-10 min
IM	2-3 min	Unknown	10-30 min

INDICATIONS & DOSAGE
Adjunct to anesthesia to induce skeletal muscle relaxation for surgery and orthopedic manipulations; to facilitate intuba-
tion and assist with mechanical ventilation; to lessen muscle contractions in pharmacologically or electrically induced seizures—
Dosage depends on anesthetic used, individual needs, and response. Dosages are representative only.
Adults: 0.6 mg/kg I.V. given over 10 to 30 seconds. For longer response, administer continuous infusion at rate of 0.5 to 10 mg/minute or 0.04 to 0.07 mg/kg intermittently p.r.n. to maintain relaxation.
Children: 1 to 2 mg/kg I.V. or 3 to 4 mg/kg I.M. Maximum I.M. dosage is 150 mg. (Children may be less sensitive to succinylcholine than adults.)

ADVERSE REACTIONS
CV: bradycardia, tachycardia, hypertension, hypotension, *arrhythmias,* flushing, *cardiac arrest.*
EENT: increased intraocular pressure.
Respiratory: *prolonged respiratory depression, apnea, bronchoconstriction.*
Other: *malignant hyperthermia,* muscle fasciculation, *postoperative muscle pain,* myoglobinemia, *rhabdomyolysis (with possible myoglobinuric acute renal failure,* excessive salivation, hyperkalemia, rash), allergic or idiosyncratic hypersensitivity reactions *(anaphylaxis).*

INTERACTIONS
Drug-drug. *Aminoglycoside antibiotics (including amikacin, gentamicin, kanamycin, neomycin, streptomycin); cholinesterase inhibitors (such as echothiophate, edrophonium, neostigmine, physostigmine, pyridostigmine); general anesthetics (such as enflurane, halothane, isoflurane); polymyxin antibiotics (colistin, polymyxin B sulfate):* potentiated neuromuscular blockade, leading to increased skeletal muscle relaxation and potentiated effect. Use cautiously during and after surgery.
Cardiac glycosides: may cause arrhythmias. Use together cautiously.
Cyclophosphamide, lithium, MAO inhibitors: prolonged apnea. Use with caution.
Methotrimeprazine, opioid analgesics: potentiated neuromuscular blockade, leading to increased skeletal muscle re-

laxation and possible respiratory paralysis. Use with extreme caution.
Parenteral magnesium sulfate: potentiated neuromuscular blockade, increased skeletal muscle relaxation, and possible respiratory paralysis. Use with caution, preferably with reduced doses.
Drug-herb. *Melatonin:* potentiates blocking properties of succinylcholine. Avoid concomitant use.

EFFECTS ON DIAGNOSTIC TESTS
Use of succinylcholine may increase serum potassium concentrations.

CONTRAINDICATIONS
Contraindicated in patients with abnormally low plasma pseudocholinesterase, angle-closure glaucoma, personal or family history of malignant hyperthermia, myopathies associated with elevated CK, penetrating eye injuries, or hypersensitivity to drug.

NURSING CONSIDERATIONS
• Use cautiously in elderly or debilitated patients; in patients receiving quinidine or cardiac glycoside therapy; in patients with hepatic, renal, or pulmonary impairment; in those with respiratory depression, severe burns or trauma, electrolyte imbalances, hyperkalemia, paraplegia, spinal neuraxis injury, CVA, degenerative or dystrophic neuromuscular disease, myasthenia gravis, myasthenic syndrome (Eaton-Lambert syndrome) of lung cancer or bronchogenic carcinoma, dehydration, thyroid disorders, collagen diseases, porphyria, fractures, muscle spasms, eye surgery, and pheochromocytoma. Also use large doses cautiously in patients undergoing cesarean section.
• Know that succinylcholine is the drug of choice for short procedures (less than 3 minutes) and for orthopedic manipulations; use caution in fractures or dislocations.
• Be aware that succinylcholine should be used only by personnel skilled in airway management.
• When giving drug I.M., inject deeply, preferably high into deltoid muscle.
• Store injectable form in refrigerator. Store powder form at room temperature in tightly closed container. Use immediately after reconstitution. Do not mix with alkaline solutions (thiopental sodium, sodium bicarbonate, or barbiturates).
• Monitor baseline electrolyte determinations and vital signs (check respirations every 5 to 10 minutes during infusion).
• Monitor respirations closely until patient is fully recovered from neuromuscular blockade, as evidenced by tests of muscle strength (hand grip, head lift, and ability to cough).
Alert: Don't use reversing agents. Unlike nondepolarizing agents, neostigmine or edrophonium may worsen neuromuscular blockade.
• Know that repeated or continuous infusions of succinylcholine are not advisable; they may cause reduced response or prolonged muscle relaxation and apnea.
• Give analgesics, as ordered, for pain.
• Keep airway clear. Have emergency respiratory support equipment (endotracheal equipment, ventilator, oxygen, atropine, and epinephrine) immediately available.

I.V. administration
• Administer sedatives or general anesthetics before neuromuscular blockers, which do not obtund consciousness or alter the pain threshold.
• Give test dose (5 to 10 mg I.V.) after patient has been anesthetized. Normal response (no respiratory depression or transient depression for up to 5 minutes) indicates drug may be given. Do not give if patient develops respiratory paralysis sufficient to permit endotracheal intubation. (Recovery within 30 to 60 minutes.)

Patient teaching
• Explain all events and procedures to patient because he can still hear.
• Reassure patient that postoperative stiffness is normal and will soon subside.

---

tubocurarine chloride
Tubarine†

Pregnancy Risk Category: C

HOW SUPPLIED
Injection: 3 mg (20 units)/ml

ACTION
A nondepolarizing neuromuscular blocking agent that prevents acetylcholine from binding to receptors on the motor end plate, thus blocking neuromuscular transmission.

Route	Onset	Peak	Duration
IV	1 min	2-5 min	25-90 min

INDICATIONS & DOSAGE
Adjunct to anesthesia to induce skeletal muscle relaxation; to facilitate intubation, orthopedic manipulations as an adjunct during pharmacologically or electrically induced convulsive therapy—
Dosage depends on anesthetic used, individual needs, and response. Dosages listed are representative and must be adjusted.
Adults: 1.1 unit/kg or 0.165 mg/kg I.V. slowly over 60 to 90 seconds. Average dose is initially 40 to 60 units I.V. May give 20 to 30 units in 3 to 5 minutes. For longer procedures, give 20 units p.r.n.
To assist with mechanical ventilation—
Adults and children: initially, 0.0165 mg/kg I.V. (average: 1 mg or 7 units); then adjust subsequent doses to patient response.
To lessen muscle contractions in pharmacologically or electrically induced seizures—
Adults and children: 1.1 unit/kg or 0.165 mg/kg over 60 to 90 seconds. As a precaution, initial dose should be 20 units (3 mg) less than calculated dose.
Diagnosis of myasthenia gravis—
Adults: 4 to 33 mcg/kg as a single I.V. dose.

ADVERSE REACTIONS
CV: hypotension, ***arrhythmias, cardiac arrest,*** bradycardia.
Respiratory: ***respiratory depression or apnea, bronchospasm.***
Other: profound and prolonged muscle relaxation, ***hypersensitivity reactions,*** idiosyncrasy, residual muscle weakness, increased salivation.

INTERACTIONS
Drug-drug. *Aminoglycoside antibiotics (including amikacin, gentamicin, kanamycin, neomycin, streptomycin); clin-*damycin, general anesthetics (such as enflurane, halothane, isoflurane); lincomycin, magnesium salts, polymyxin antibiotics (colistin, polymyxin B sulfate):* potentiated neuromuscular blockade, leading to increased skeletal muscle relaxation and potentiated effect. Use cautiously during and after surgery.
Amphotericin B, ethacrynic acid, furosemide, methotrimeprazine, opioid analgesics, propranolol, thiazide diuretics, verapamil: potentiated neuromuscular blockade, leading to increased skeletal muscle relaxation and possible respiratory paralysis. Use with extreme caution during surgical and postoperative periods.
Quinidine: prolonged neuromuscular blockade. Use together with caution. Monitor closely.

EFFECTS ON DIAGNOSTIC TESTS
Large doses result in production of a factor that interferes with the detection of urinary catecholamines by fluorometric measures in patients with tetanus.

CONTRAINDICATIONS
Contraindicated in patients with hypersensitivity to drug and in those for whom histamine release is a hazard (asthmatic patients).

NURSING CONSIDERATIONS
• Use cautiously in elderly or debilitated patients and in those with hepatic or pulmonary impairment, hypothermia, respiratory depression, myasthenia gravis, myasthenic syndrome (Eaton-Lambert syndrome) of lung cancer or bronchogenic carcinoma, in those with sulfite sensitivity, dehydration, thyroid disorders, collagen diseases, porphyria, electrolyte disturbances, fractures, and muscle spasms. Also use large doses cautiously in patients undergoing cesarean section.
• Know that only personnel skilled in airway management should administer tubocurarine.
• Assess baseline electrolyte determinations (electrolyte imbalance can potentiate neuromuscular blocking effects).
• Check vital signs every 15 minutes. Notify doctor at once of changes.

• Measure fluid intake and output; renal dysfunction prolongs duration of action because much of drug is excreted unchanged in urine.

• Know that a nerve stimulator and train-of-four monitoring are recommended to confirm antagonism of neuromuscular blockade and recovery of muscle strength. Before attempting pharmacologic reversal with neostigmine, some evidence of spontaneous recovery should be present.

• Monitor respirations closely until patient is fully recovered from neuromuscular blockade, as evidenced by tests of muscle strength (hand grip, head lift, and ability to cough).

• Give analgesics, as ordered, for pain.

• Premedication with an antihistamine will decrease the release of histamine-associated hypotension.

☐I.V. administration
• Administer sedatives or general anesthetics before neuromuscular blockers, which do not obtund consciousness or alter the pain threshold.

• Keep airway clear. Have emergency respiratory support equipment (endotracheal equipment, ventilator, oxygen, atropine, edrophonium, epinephrine, and neostigmine) available.

• Allow succinylcholine effects to subside before giving tubocurarine.

• Give I.V. over 60 to 90 seconds.

• Do not mix with barbiturates or other alkaline solutions because a precipitate will form. Use only fresh solutions and discard if discolored.

☑Patient teaching
• Explain all events and procedures to patient because he still can hear.

---

vecuronium bromide
Norcuron

Pregnancy Risk Category: C

HOW SUPPLIED
Injection: 10-mg, 20-mg vials

ACTION
A nondepolarizing agent that prevents acetylcholine from binding to receptors on the motor end plate, thus blocking neuromuscular transmission.

Route	Onset	Peak	Duration
IV	1 min	3-5 min	15-25 min

INDICATIONS & DOSAGE
Adjunct to general anesthesia to facilitate endotracheal intubation and to provide skeletal muscle relaxation during surgery or mechanical ventilation—
Dosage depends on anesthetic used, individual needs, and response. Dosages are representative and must be adjusted.
Adults and children over 9 years: initially, 0.08 to 0.1 mg/kg I.V. bolus. Maintenance doses of 0.01 to 0.015 mg/kg within 25 to 40 minutes of initial dose should be administered during prolonged surgical procedures. Maintenance doses may be given q 12 to 15 minutes in patients receiving balanced anesthesia.
Children 1 to 9 years: may require a slightly higher initial dose and also may require supplementation slightly more often than adults. Alternatively, drug may be given by continuous I.V. infusion of 1 mcg/kg/minute initially, then 0.8 to 1.2 mcg/kg/minute.
Children 7 weeks to 1 year: doses comparable to those used in adults are appropriate, but less frequent administration of maintenance doses may be required.

ADVERSE REACTIONS
Respiratory: *prolonged, dose-related respiratory insufficiency or apnea.*
Other: skeletal muscle weakness.

INTERACTIONS
Drug-drug. *Aminoglycoside antibiotics (including amikacin, gentamicin, kanamycin, neomycin, streptomycin); bacitracin; clindamycin; general anesthetics (such as enflurane, halothane, isoflurane); magnesium salts, other skeletal muscle relaxants; polymyxin antibiotics (colistin, polymyxin B sulfate); quinidine; succinylcholine, tetracyclines:* potentiated neuromuscular blockade, leading to increased skeletal muscle relaxation and potentiated effect. Use cautiously during and after surgery.

Opioid analgesics: potentiated neuromuscular blockade, leading to increased skeletal muscle relaxation and possible respiratory paralysis. Use with extreme caution, and reduce dose of vecuronium.

EFFECTS ON DIAGNOSTIC TESTS
None reported.

CONTRAINDICATIONS
Contraindicated in patients with hypersensitivity to drug or bromides.

NURSING CONSIDERATIONS
• Use cautiously in elderly patients; in patients with altered circulation caused by CV disease and edematous states; and in those with hepatic disease, severe obesity, bronchogenic carcinoma, electrolyte disturbances, and neuromuscular disease.
• Know that drug should be used only by personnel skilled in airway management.
• Know that a nerve stimulator and train-of-four monitoring are recommended to confirm antagonism of neuromuscular blockade and recovery of muscle strength. Before attempting pharmacologic reversal with neostigmine, some evidence of spontaneous recovery should be seen.
• Monitor respirations closely until patient has fully recovered from neuromuscular blockade as evidenced by tests of muscle strength (hand grip, head lift, and ability to cough).
• Keep in mind that prior administration of succinylcholine may enhance the neuromuscular blocking effect and duration of action.
• Know that vecuronium is well tolerated in patients with renal failure.
• Give analgesics, as ordered, for pain.

I.V. administration
• Administer sedatives or general anesthetics before neuromuscular blockers, which do not obtund consciousness or alter the pain threshold.
• Keep airway clear. Have emergency respiratory support equipment (endotracheal equipment, ventilator, oxygen, atropine, edrophonium, epinephrine, and neostigmine) available.
• Administer by rapid I.V. injection. Alternatively, 10 to 20 mg may be added to 100 ml of a compatible solution and given by I.V. infusion. Compatible solutions include D_5W, 0.9% NaCl for injection, dextrose 5% in 0.9% NaCl for injection, and lactated Ringer's injection.
• Do not mix with alkaline solutions such as barbiturates.
• Store reconstituted solution in refrigerator. Discard after 24 hours.

☑ Patient teaching
• Explain all events and procedures to patient because he can still hear.

43

Antihistamines

astemizole
brompheniramine maleate
cetirizine hydrochloride
chlorpheniramine maleate
clemastine fumarate
cyproheptadine hydrochloride
diphenhydramine hydrochloride
fexofenadine hydrochloride
loratadine
promethazine hydrochloride
promethazine theoclate
triprolidine hydrochloride

COMBINATION PRODUCTS

ALLEREST MAXIMUM STRENGTH
TABLETS ◊ : pseudoephedrine hydrochloride 30 mg and chlorpheniramine maleate 2 mg.
CHLOR-TRIMETON ALLERGY 4-HOUR DECONGESTANT ◊ : chlorpheniramine maleate 4 mg and pseudoephedrine sulfate 60 mg.
CHLOR-TRIMETON 12 HOUR RELIEF TABLETS ◊ : chlorpheniramine maleate 8 mg and pseudoephedrine sulfate 120 mg.
CLARITIN-D: loratadine 5 mg and pseudoephedrine sulfate 120 mg.
CONTAC 12-HOUR ◊ : phenylpropanolamine 75 mg and chlorpheniramine maleate 8 mg.
CONTAC MAXIMUM STRENGTH 12-HOUR CAPLETS ◊ : phenylpropanolamine 75 mg and chlorpheniramine maleate 12 mg.
CORICIDIN "D" DECONGESTANT TABLETS ◊ : chlorpheniramine maleate 2 mg, acetaminophen 325 mg, and phenylpropanolamine hydrochloride 12.5 mg.
DECONAMINE: pseudoephedrine hydrochloride 60 mg and chlorpheniramine maleate 4 mg.
DIMETAPP EXTENTABS: brompheniramine maleate 12 mg and phenylpropanolamine hydrochloride 75 mg.
DRIZE: phenylpropanolamine hydrochloride 75 mg and chlorpheniramine maleate 12 mg.

FEDAHIST: pseudoephedrine hydrochloride 60 mg and chlorpheniramine maleate 4 mg.
NALDECON: phenylephrine hydrochloride 10 mg, phenylpropanolamine hydrochloride 40 mg, phenyltoloxamine citrate 15 mg, and chlorpheniramine maleate 5 mg.
NOLAMINE: chlorpheniramine maleate 4 mg, phenindamine tartrate 24 mg, and phenylpropanolamine hydrochloride 50 mg.
NOVAFED A: pseudoephedrine hydrochloride 120 mg and chlorpheniramine maleate 8 mg.
NOVAHISTINE ELIXIR ◊*: phenylephrine 5 mg, chlorpheniramine maleate 2 mg, and alcohol 5% per 5 ml.
ORNADE SPANSULES: phenylpropanolamine hydrochloride 75 mg and chlorpheniramine maleate 12 mg.
P-V-TUSSIN SYRUP*: chlorpheniramine maleate 2 mg/5 ml, phenindamine tartrate 5 mg/5 ml, phenylephrine hydrochloride 5 mg/5 ml, and pyrilamine maleate 6 mg/5 ml.
SUDAFED PLUS ◊ : pseudoephedrine hydrochloride 60 mg and chlorpheniramine maleate 4 mg.
TAVIST-D ◊ : clemastine fumarate 1.34 mg and phenylpropanolamine 75 mg.
TRIAMINIC-12: phenylpropanolamine hydrochloride 75 mg and chlorpheniramine maleate 12 mg.
TRINALIN REPETABS: azatadine maleate 1 mg and pseudoephedrine sulfate 120 mg.

astemizole
Hismanal

Pregnancy Risk Category: C

HOW SUPPLIED
Tablets: 10 mg
Oral suspension: 2 mg/ml*‡

Reactions may be *common*, uncommon, *life-threatening*, or COMMON AND LIFE-THREATENING.

ACTION
Blocks effects of histamine at H_1 receptors. Astemizole is a nonsedating antihistamine; its chemical structure prevents entry into the CNS.

Route	Onset	Peak	Duration
PO	Unknown	1 hr	24 hr (slow)

INDICATIONS & DOSAGE
Relief of symptoms associated with chronic idiopathic urticaria and seasonal allergic rhinitis—
Adults and children over 12 years: 10 mg P.O. daily.
Children 6 to 12 years: 5 mg P.O. daily.
Children under 6 years: 0.2 mg/kg P.O. once daily.

ADVERSE REACTIONS
CNS: headache, nervousness, dizziness, drowsiness.
CV: *arrhythmias* (with high plasma levels).
EENT: dry mouth, pharyngitis, conjunctivitis.
GI: abdominal pain, increased appetite, nausea, diarrhea.
Other: arthralgia, weight gain, cholestatic jaundice.

INTERACTIONS
Drug-drug. *Itraconazole, ketoconazole, macrolide antibiotics (such as clarithromycin, erythromycin), quinine:* risk of serious adverse cardiac reactions. Don't use together.
Protease inhibitors (indinavir, nelfinavir, ritonavir, saquinavir), zileuton: may increase astemizole plasma levels, leading to potential for serious CV events. Avoid concomitant administration.
Serotonin reuptake inhibitors (fluoxetine, fluvoxamine, nefazodone, paroxetine, sertraline): may increase astemizole's plasma levels, leading to potential for serious CV events. Avoid concomitant use.
Drug-food. *Grapefruit juice:* can inhibit hepatic metabolism of astemizole. Avoid use together.
Drug-lifestyle. *Alcohol use:* increased CNS depression. Use cautiously.

EFFECTS ON DIAGNOSTIC TESTS
Discontinue drug 4 days before performing diagnostic skin tests; it can prevent, reduce, or mask positive skin test response.

CONTRAINDICATIONS
Contraindicated in patients with hepatic failure or hypersensitivity to astemizole and in those taking the antifungal agents itraconazole or ketoconazole or macrolide antibiotics, including erythromycin, and quinine.

NURSING CONSIDERATIONS
• Avoid use in patients with hepatic disease. Use cautiously in patients with renal disease. Also use cautiously in patients with lower respiratory tract diseases (including asthma); drying effects can increase the risk of bronchial mucus plug formation.
• See package insert for events causing serious CV adverse effects.

☑ Patient teaching
• Instruct patient to take drug only once daily. Warn patient not to increase dosage without consulting doctor. High doses may increase risk of arrhythmias.
• Instruct patient to take drug on an empty stomach at least 2 hours after a meal and to avoid eating for at least 1 hour after dosing.
• Tell patient to stop drug 4 to 6 weeks before allergy skin tests to preserve accuracy of tests.
• Warn patient to avoid alcohol and driving or other activities that require alertness until drug's CNS effects are known.
• Tell patient to avoid consumption of grapefruit juice within 2 hours of taking dose.
• Instruct patient to report symptoms of palpitations to doctor immediately.

---

brompheniramine maleate
Bromphen*◇, Chlorphed◇,
Codimal-A, Conjec-B◇,
Cophene-B, Dehist, Diamine T.D.,
Dimetane*◇, Dimetane
Extentabs◇, Dimotane§, Histaject
Modified, Nasahist B, ND-Stat
Revised, Oraminic II

Pregnancy Risk Category: C

HOW SUPPLIED
Tablets: 4 mg◇, 8 mg, 12 mg
Tablets (extended-release): 8 mg◇,
12 mg◇
Elixir: 2 mg/5 ml*◇
Injection: 10 mg/ml

ACTION
Competes with histamine for H₁-receptor sites on effector cells. Prevents, but does not reverse, histamine-mediated responses.

Route	Onset	Peak	Duration
PO	15-60 min	2-5 hr	3-24 hr
IV, IM, SC	Unknown	Unknown	Unknown

INDICATIONS & DOSAGE
Rhinitis, allergy symptoms—
Adults: 4 to 8 mg P.O. t.i.d. or q.i.d.; or 8 to 12 mg extended-release P.O. b.i.d. or t.i.d. Maximum oral dosage is 24 mg daily. Or, 5 to 20 mg q 6 to 12 hours I.M., I.V., or S.C. Maximum parenteral dosage is 40 mg daily.
Children 6 to 12 years: 2 to 4 mg P.O. t.i.d. or q.i.d.; or 8 to 12 mg extended-release P.O. q 12 hours; or 0.5 mg/kg I.M., I.V., or S.C. daily in divided doses t.i.d. or q.i.d.
Children under 6 years: 0.5 mg/kg P.O., I.M., I.V., or S.C. daily in divided doses t.i.d. or q.i.d.
   Note: Children under 12 years should use only as directed by doctor.

ADVERSE REACTIONS
CNS: dizziness, tremors, irritability, insomnia, syncope, *drowsiness, stimulation.*
CV: hypotension, palpitations.
GI: anorexia, nausea, vomiting, *dry mouth and throat.*
GU: urine retention.

Hematologic: *thrombocytopenia, agranulocytosis.*
Skin: urticaria, rash.
Other: (after parenteral administration) local stinging, diaphoresis.

INTERACTIONS
Drug-drug. *CNS depressants:* increased sedation. Use together cautiously.
MAO inhibitors: increased anticholinergic effects. Don't use together.
Drug-lifestyle. *Alcohol use:* increased CNS depression. Use cautiously.

EFFECTS ON DIAGNOSTIC TESTS
Discontinue drug 4 days before performing diagnostic skin tests; it can prevent, reduce, or mask positive skin test response.

CONTRAINDICATIONS
Contraindicated in patients hypersensitive to drug's ingredients; in those with acute asthma, severe hypertension, coronary artery disease, angle-closure glaucoma, urine retention, symptomatic prostatic hypertrophy, pyloroduodenal obstruction, or peptic ulcer; and within 14 days of MAO inhibitor therapy.

NURSING CONSIDERATIONS
• Use cautiously in elderly patients and in those with increased intraocular pressure, diabetes, ischemic heart disease, hyperthyroidism, hypertension, bronchial asthma, and prostatic hyperplasia.
• Monitor blood count during long-term therapy, as ordered; observe for signs of blood dyscrasias.

⬛I.V. administration
• Injectable form containing 10 mg/ml can be given diluted or undiluted very slowly I.V.

✅Patient teaching
• Instruct patient to reduce GI distress by taking drug with food or milk.
• Warn patient to avoid alcohol and activities that require alertness until drug's CNS effects are known.
• Advise patient to notify doctor if unusual bleeding or bruising occurs.
• Tell patient that coffee or tea may reduce drowsiness and to use cautiously if

---

Reactions may be *common*, uncommon, *life-threatening*, or COMMON AND LIFE-THREATENING.

palpitations develop. Causes less drowsiness than some other antihistamines.
- Inform patient that sugarless gum, sugarless sour hard candy, or ice chips may relieve dry mouth.
- Tell patient to notify doctor if tolerance develops because a different antihistamine may need to be prescribed.

cetirizine hydrochloride
Zyrtec

Pregnancy Risk Category: B

HOW SUPPLIED
Tablets: 5 mg, 10 mg
Oral solution: 5 mg/5 ml

ACTION
A nonsedating antihistamine that selectively inhibits peripheral H_1 receptors.

Route	Onset	Peak	Duration
PO	20-60 min	0.5-1.5 hr	24 hr

INDICATIONS & DOSAGE
Seasonal allergic rhinitis, perennial allergic rhinitis, chronic urticaria—
Adults and children 12 years and older: 5 or 10 mg P.O. daily depending on symptom severity.
Children 6 to 11 years: 5 or 10 mg (1 or 2 tsp) P.O. once daily depending on symptom severity.
Adjust-a-dose: In renally impaired patients with creatinine clearance of 11 to 31 ml/minute, those on dialysis (creatinine clearance less than 7 ml/minute) or those with hepatic impairment, 5 mg P.O. daily.

ADVERSE REACTIONS
CNS: *somnolence,* fatigue, dizziness, headache.
EENT: pharyngitis.
GI: dry mouth, nausea, vomiting, abdominal distress.

INTERACTIONS
Drug-drug. *CNS depressants:* possible additive effect. Avoid concomitant use.
Theophylline: may cause decreased clearance of cetirizine. Monitor patient closely.

Drug-lifestyle. *Alcohol use:* possible additive effect. Avoid concomitant use.

EFFECTS ON DIAGNOSTIC TESTS
Discontinue drug 4 days before performing diagnostic skin tests; it can prevent, reduce, or mask positive skin test response.

CONTRAINDICATIONS
Contraindicated in patients with hypersensitivity to drug or hydroxyzine.

NURSING CONSIDERATIONS
- Use cautiously in patients with renal impairment or liver impairment.
- Drug is not recommended for use in breast-feeding women.
- Safety of drug has not been established in children under 6 years.

☑ **Patient teaching**
- Warn patient not to drive or perform hazardous activities if he experiences somnolence, a common adverse reaction.
- Advise patient not to use alcohol or other CNS depressants while taking drug.
- Warn patient to avoid driving or other activities that require alertness until drug's CNS effects are known.
- Tell patient that coffee or tea may reduce drowsiness. Suggest sugarless gum, sugarless sour hard candy, or ice chips to relieve dry mouth.

chlorpheniramine maleate
Aller-Chlor* ◇, Chlo-Amine ◇, Chlor-100 ◇, Chlorate ◇, Chlor-Niramine ◇, Chlor-Pro, Chlor-Pro 10, Chlorspan-12, Chlortab-4, Chlortab-8, Chlor-Trimeton* ◇, Chlor-Trimeton 12 Hour Relief ◇, Chlor-Tripolon† ◇, GenAllerate ◇, Novo-Pheniram† ◇, Pfeiffer's Allergy ◇, Phenetron*, Piriton§, Telachlor, Teldrin ◇, Trymegen ◇

Pregnancy Risk Category: B

HOW SUPPLIED
Tablets: 4 mg ◇, 8 mg ◇, 12 mg ◇
Tablets (chewable): 2 mg ◇
Tablets (timed-release): 8 mg ◇, 12 mg ◇

Capsules (timed-release): 6 mg◇,
8 mg◇, 12 mg◇
Syrup: 2 mg/5 ml*◇
Injection: 10 mg/ml, 100 mg/ml

ACTION
Competes with histamine for H_1-receptor sites on effector cells. Prevents, but does not reverse, histamine-mediated responses.

Route	Onset	Peak	Duration
PO	15-60 min	2-6 hr	24 hr
IV	15-60 min	Immediate	24 hr
IM, SC	15-60 min	Unknown	24 hr

INDICATIONS & DOSAGE
Rhinitis, allergy symptoms—
Adults: 4 mg P.O. q 4 to 6 hours, not to exceed 24 mg/day; or 8 to 12 mg timed-release P.O. q 8 to 12 hours, not to exceed 24 mg daily. Alternatively, 5 to 20 mg I.M., I.V., or S.C. as a single dose. Maximum recommended parenteral dosage is 40 mg per 24 hours.
Children 6 to 12 years: 2 mg P.O. q 4 to 6 hours, not to exceed 12 mg daily. Alternatively, may give 8 mg timed-release P.O. h.s.
Children 2 to 6 years: 1 mg P.O. q 4 to 6 hours, not to exceed 4 mg daily.
Children under 2 years: 0.35 mg/kg/day in divided doses q 4 to 6 hours.

ADVERSE REACTIONS
CNS: *stimulation,* sedation, *drowsiness,* excitability (in children).
CV: hypotension, palpitations, weak pulse.
GI: epigastric distress, *dry mouth.*
GU: urine retention.
Respiratory: thick bronchial secretions.
Skin: rash, urticaria.
Other: local stinging, burning sensation (after parenteral administration), pallor.

INTERACTIONS
Drug-drug. *CNS depressants:* increased sedation. Use together cautiously.
MAO inhibitors: increased anticholinergic effects. Don't use together.
Drug-lifestyle. *Alcohol use:* increased CNS depression. Use cautiously.

EFFECTS ON DIAGNOSTIC TESTS
Discontinue drug 4 days before diagnostic skin tests; antihistamines can prevent, reduce, or mask positive skin test response.

CONTRAINDICATIONS
Contraindicated in patients having acute asthmatic attacks, in those with narrow-angle glaucoma, symptomatic prostatic hypertrophy, pyloroduodenal obstruction, or bladder neck obstruction, and in patients taking MAO inhibitors. Antihistamines are not recommended for breast-feeding patients because small amounts of drug are excreted in breast milk.

NURSING CONSIDERATIONS
• Use cautiously in elderly patients and in those with increased intraocular pressure, hyperthyroidism, CV or renal disease, hypertension, bronchial asthma, urine retention, prostatic hyperplasia, and stenosing peptic ulcerations.
• Injectable form contains benzyl alcohol. Avoid use in infants.
• If symptoms occur during or after parenteral dose, discontinue drug and notify doctor.

⬛ I.V. administration
• Drug is available in 10 mg/ml ampules for I.V. use. It is compatible with most I.V. solutions. Check with pharmacist before mixing with I.V. solutions to verify specific compatibilities. Give injection over 1 minute.
Alert: Do not give the 100 mg/ml strength I.V.

✅ Patient teaching
• Warn patient to avoid alcohol and other CNS depressants and driving and other activities that require alertness until drug's CNS effects are known.
• Tell patient that coffee or tea may reduce drowsiness. Suggest sugarless gum, sugarless sour hard candy, or ice chips to relieve dry mouth.
• Instruct patient to notify doctor if tolerance develops because a different antihistamine may need to be prescribed.
• Tell parent that drug, including extended-release products, should not be used in

---

children under 12 years unless directed by doctor.

clemastine fumarate
Tavist, Tavist-1 ◊, Antihist-1

Pregnancy Risk Category: B

HOW SUPPLIED
Tablets: 1.34 mg ◊, 2.68 mg
Syrup*: 0.67 mg/5 ml

ACTION
Competes with histamine for H_1-receptor sites on effector cells. Prevents, but does not reverse, histamine-mediated responses.

Route	Onset	Peak	Duration
PO	15-60 min	5-7 hr	12 hr

INDICATIONS & DOSAGE
Rhinitis, allergy symptoms—
Adults and children 12 years and over: 1.34 mg P.O. q 12 hours, or 2.68 mg P.O. once to three times daily, p.r.n. Do not exceed daily dosage of 8.04 mg.
Children 6 to 12 years: 0.67 to 1.34 mg P.O. b.i.d. Do not exceed daily dosage of 4.02 mg.

ADVERSE REACTIONS
CNS: *sedation, drowsiness, seizures,* nervousness, tremor, confusion, restlessness, vertigo, headache, *sleepiness, dizziness, incoordination,* fatigue.
CV: hypotension, palpitations, tachycardia.
GI: *epigastric distress,* anorexia, diarrhea, nausea, vomiting, constipation, *dry mouth.*
GU: urine retention, urinary frequency.
Hematologic: hemolytic anemia, ***thrombocytopenia, agranulocytosis.***
Respiratory: *thick bronchial secretions.*
Skin: rash, urticaria, photosensitivity, diaphoresis.
Other: *anaphylactic shock.*

INTERACTIONS
Drug-drug. *CNS depressants:* increased sedation. Use together cautiously.
MAO inhibitors: increased anticholinergic effects. Don't use together.

Drug-lifestyle. *Alcohol use:* increased CNS depression. Use cautiously.
Sun exposure: photosensitivity reactions may occur. Avoid prolonged or unprotected sun exposure.

EFFECTS ON DIAGNOSTIC TESTS
Discontinue drug 4 days before diagnostic skin tests; antihistamines can prevent, reduce, or mask positive skin test response.

CONTRAINDICATIONS
Contraindicated in patients with acute asthma, narrow-angle glaucoma, stenosing peptic ulcer, symptomatic prostatic hypertrophy, bladder neck obstruction, pyloroduodenal obstruction, or hypersensitivity to drug or other antihistamines of similar chemical structure. Also contraindicated in neonates, premature infants, or breast-feeding women. Avoid use in those taking MAO inhibitors.

NURSING CONSIDERATIONS
• Use cautiously in elderly patients and in those with increased intraocular pressure, hyperthyroidism, CV disease, hypertension, bronchial asthma, and prostatic hyperplasia.
• Know that children under 12 years should use only as directed by a doctor.
• Monitor blood counts during long-term therapy, as ordered; observe for signs of blood dyscrasias.

✅ Patient teaching
• Warn patient to avoid alcohol and driving or other activities that require alertness until drug's CNS effects are known.
• Tell patient that coffee or tea may reduce drowsiness and to use cautiously if palpitations develop. Suggest sugarless gum, sugarless sour hard candy, or ice chips to relieve dry mouth.
• Warn patient of possible photosensitivity reactions. Advise use of a sunblock.
• Tell patient to notify doctor if tolerance develops because a different antihistamine may need to be prescribed.

cyproheptadine hydrochloride
Periactin

Pregnancy Risk Category: B

HOW SUPPLIED
Tablets: 4 mg
Syrup: 2 mg/5 ml

ACTION
Competes with histamine for H_1-receptor sites on effector cells. Prevents, but does not reverse, histamine-mediated responses; also has antiserotonergic activity.

Route	Onset	Peak	Duration
PO	15-60 min	6-9 hr	Unknown

INDICATIONS & DOSAGE
Allergy symptoms, pruritus—
Adults: 4 to 20 mg P.O. daily in divided doses. Maximum dosage is 0.5 mg/kg daily.
Children 7 to 14 years: 4 mg P.O. b.i.d. or t.i.d. Maximum dosage is 16 mg/day.
Children 2 to 6 years: 2 mg P.O. b.i.d. or t.i.d. Maximum dosage is 12 mg daily.
Children under 2 years: 0.25 mg/kg/day in two or three divided doses.

ADVERSE REACTIONS
CNS: *drowsiness,* dizziness, headache, fatigue, sedation, sleepiness, incoordination, confusion, restlessness, insomnia, nervousness, tremor, *seizures.*
CV: hypotension, palpitations, tachycardia.
GI: nausea, vomiting, epigastric distress, *dry mouth,* diarrhea, constipation.
GU: urine retention, urinary frequency.
Hematologic: hemolytic anemia, *leukopenia, agranulocytosis, thrombocytopenia.*
Skin: rash, urticaria, photosensitivity.
Other: weight gain, *anaphylactic shock.*

INTERACTIONS
Drug-drug. *CNS depressants:* increased sedation. Use together cautiously.
MAO inhibitors: increased anticholinergic effects. Don't use together.
Drug-lifestyle. *Alcohol use:* increased CNS depression. Use cautiously.

Sun exposure: photosensitivity reactions may occur. Avoid prolonged or unprotected sun exposure.

EFFECTS ON DIAGNOSTIC TESTS
Discontinue drug 4 days before diagnostic skin tests; antihistamines can prevent, reduce, or mask positive skin test response.

CONTRAINDICATIONS
Contraindicated in patients with acute asthma, angle-closure glaucoma, stenosing peptic ulcer, symptomatic prostatic hyperplasia, bladder-neck obstruction, pyloroduodenal obstruction, and hypersensitivity to drug or other drugs of similar chemical structure; in those who are in concurrent therapy with MAO inhibitors; in neonates or premature infants; in elderly or debilitated patients; and in breast-feeding women.

NURSING CONSIDERATIONS
• Use cautiously in patients with increased intraocular pressure, hyperthyroidism, CV disease, hypertension, or bronchial asthma.
• Know that children under 14 years should use only as directed by a doctor.

☑ **Patient teaching**
• Tell patient that GI distress can be reduced by taking drug with food or milk.
• Warn patient to avoid alcohol and driving or other activities that require alertness until drug's CNS effects are known.
• Tell patient that coffee or tea may reduce drowsiness and to use cautiously if palpitations develop. Suggest sugarless gum, sugarless sour hard candy, or ice chips to relieve dry mouth.
• Warn patient of possible photosensitivity reactions. Advise use of a sunblock.
• Instruct patient to notify doctor if tolerance develops because a different antihistamine may need to be prescribed.

Reactions may be *common,* uncommon, *life-threatening,* or COMMON AND LIFE-THREATENING.

diphenhydramine hydrochloride

Allerdryl†◇, AllerMax Allergy and Cough Formula, AllerMax Caplets◇, Allermed◇, Banophen◇, Banophen Caplets◇, Beldin◇, Belix◇, Bena-D 10, Bena-D 50, Benadryl◇, Benadryl Allergy, Benadryl 25◇, Benadryl Kapseals◇, Benahist 10, Benahist 50, Ben-Allergin-50, Benoject-10, Benoject-50, Benylin Cough◇, Bydramine Cough◇, Compoz◇, Diphenacen-50, Diphenadryl◇, Diphen Cough◇, Diphenhist◇, Diphenhist Captabs◇, Dormarex 2◇, Fynex◇, Genahist◇, Gen-D-phen◇, Hydramine◇, Hydramine Cough◇, Hydramyn◇, Hydril◇, Hyrexin-50, Insomnal†◇, Nervine Nighttime Sleep-Aid◇, Nidryl◇, Noradryl◇, Nordryl◇, Nordryl Cough◇, Nytol Maximum Strength◇, Nytol with DPH◇, Phendry◇, Phendry Children's Allergy Medicine◇, Sleep-Eze 3◇, Sominex Formula 2◇, Tusstat◇, Twilite Caplets◇, Uni-Bent Cough◇, Wehdryl-10, Wehdryl-50

Pregnancy Risk Category: B

HOW SUPPLIED
Tablets: 25 mg◇, 50 mg◇
Capsules: 25 mg◇, 50 mg◇
Elixir*: 12.5 mg/5 ml (14% alcohol)◇
Liquid: 6.25 mg/5 ml
Syrup*: 12.5 mg/5 ml◇
Injection: 10 mg/ml, 50 mg/ml

ACTION
Competes with histamine for H_1-receptor sites on effector cells. Prevents, but does not reverse, histamine-mediated responses, particularly histamine's effects on the smooth muscle of the bronchial tubes, GI tract, uterus, and blood vessels. Structurally related to local anesthetics, diphenhydramine provides local anesthesia by preventing initiation and transmission of nerve impulses. Also suppresses cough reflex by a direct effect in the medulla of the brain.

Route	Onset	Peak	Duration
PO	15 min	1-4 hr	6-8 hr
IV	Immediate	1-4 hr	6-8 hr
IM	Unknown	1-4 hr	6-8 hr

INDICATIONS & DOSAGE
Rhinitis, allergy symptoms, motion sickness, Parkinson's disease—
Adults and children 12 years and over: 25 to 50 mg P.O. t.i.d. or q.i.d.; or 10 to 50 mg deep I.M. or I.V. Maximum I.M. or I.V. dosage is 400 mg daily.
Children under 12 years: 5 mg/kg/day P.O., deep I.M., or I.V. in divided doses q.i.d. Maximum dosage is 300 mg daily.
Sedation—
Adults: 25 to 50 mg P.O., or deep I.M., p.r.n.
Nighttime sleep aid—
Adults: 25 to 50 mg P.O. h.s.
Nonproductive cough—
Adults: 25 mg P.O. q 4 to 6 hours (not to exceed 150 mg daily).
Children 6 to 12 years: 12.5 mg P.O. q 4 to 6 hours (not to exceed 75 mg daily).
Children 2 to 6 years: 6.25 mg P.O. q 4 to 6 hours (not to exceed 25 mg daily).

ADVERSE REACTIONS
CNS: *drowsiness,* confusion, insomnia, headache, vertigo, *sedation, sleepiness, dizziness, incoordination,* fatigue, restlessness, tremor, nervousness, **seizures.**
CV: palpitations, hypotension, tachycardia.
EENT: diplopia, blurred vision, nasal congestion, tinnitus.
GI: *nausea,* vomiting, diarrhea, *dry mouth,* constipation, *epigastric distress,* anorexia.
GU: dysuria, urine retention, urinary frequency.
Hematologic: hemolytic anemia, **thrombocytopenia, agranulocytosis.**
Respiratory: *thickening of bronchial secretions.*
Skin: urticaria, photosensitivity, rash.
Other: *anaphylactic shock.*

INTERACTIONS
Drug-drug. *CNS depressants:* increased sedation. Use together cautiously.
MAO inhibitors: increased anticholinergic effects. Don't use together.
Drug-lifestyle. *Alcohol use:* increased CNS depression. Use cautiously.
Sun exposure: photosensitivity reactions may occur. Avoid prolonged or unprotected sun exposure.

EFFECTS ON DIAGNOSTIC TESTS
Discontinue drug 4 days before diagnostic skin tests; antihistamines can prevent, reduce, or mask positive skin test response.

CONTRAINDICATIONS
Contraindicated in patients with narrow-angle glaucoma, stenosing peptic ulcer, symptomatic prostatic hypertrophy, bladder neck obstruction, pyloroduodenal obstruction, or hypersensitivity to drug; during acute asthmatic attacks; and in newborns, premature neonates, or breast-feeding women. Avoid use in patients taking MAO inhibitors.

NURSING CONSIDERATIONS
• Use with extreme caution in patients with prostatic hyperplasia, asthma or COPD, increased intraocular pressure, hyperthyroidism, CV disease and hypertension.
• Know that children under 12 years should use only as directed by a doctor.
• Alternate injection sites to prevent irritation. Administer I.M. injection deeply into large muscle.

◘ I.V. administration
• Be sure the I.V. site is patent. Drug given perivascularly causes tissue irritation.

☑ Patient teaching
• Instruct patient to take 30 minutes before travel to prevent motion sickness.
• Tell patient to take diphenhydramine with food or milk to reduce GI distress.
• Warn patient to avoid alcohol and driving or other hazardous activities that require alertness until drug's effect on the CNS is known.
• Tell patient that coffee or tea may reduce drowsiness and to use cautiously if palpitations develop. Suggest sugarless gum, sugarless sour hard candy, or ice chips to relieve dry mouth.
• Tell patient to notify doctor if tolerance develops because a different antihistamine may need to be prescribed.
• Warn patient of possible photosensitivity reactions. Advise use of a sunblock.

---

fexofenadine hydrochloride
Allegra, Telfast‡

Pregnancy Risk Category: C

HOW SUPPLIED
Capsules: 60 mg

ACTION
A nonsedating antihistamine in which the principal effects are mediated through a selective inhibition of peripheral H_1 receptors.

Route	Onset	Peak	Duration
PO	Unknown	3 hr	14 hr

INDICATIONS & DOSAGE
Seasonal allergic rhinitis—
Adults and children age 12 and over: 60 mg P.O. b.i.d.
Adjust-a-dose: For patients with impaired renal function or currently on dialysis, 60 mg daily.

ADVERSE REACTIONS
CNS: fatigue, drowsiness.
GI: nausea, dyspepsia.
Other: viral infection, dysmenorrhea.

INTERACTIONS
Drug-lifestyle. *Alcohol use:* increased CNS depression. Use cautiously.

EFFECTS ON DIAGNOSTIC TESTS
Discontinue drug 4 days before performing diagnostic skin tests; it can prevent, reduce, or mask positive skin test response.

CONTRAINDICATIONS
Contraindicated in patients with hypersensitivity to drug or its components.

NURSING CONSIDERATIONS
• Use cautiously in patients with impaired renal function.
• Safety and effectiveness in children under 12 years have not been established.
• It is not known whether drug is excreted in breast milk; caution is recommended when administering drug to breast-feeding women. Advise women taking drug to avoid breast-feeding.

☑**Patient teaching**
• Caution patient not to perform hazardous activities if drowsiness occurs as a result of drug use.
• Instruct patient not to exceed prescribed dosage and to take drug only when needed.
• Warn patient to avoid alcohol and driving or other activities that require alertness until drug's CNS effects are known.
• Tell patient that coffee or tea may reduce drowsiness. Suggest sugarless gum, sugarless sour hard candy, or ice chips to relieve dry mouth.

---

loratadine
Claratyne‡, Clarinase‡, Claritin, Claritin Reditabs, Claritin Syrup

Pregnancy Risk Category: B

HOW SUPPLIED
Tablets: 10 mg
Tablets (rapidly disintegrating): 10 mg
Syrup: 1 mg/ml

ACTION
Blocks effects of histamine at H_1-receptor sites. Loratadine is a nonsedating antihistamine; its chemical structure prevents entry into the CNS.

Route	Onset	Peak	Duration
PO	1-3 hr	8-10 hr	24 hr

INDICATIONS & DOSAGE
Symptomatic treatment of seasonal allergic rhinitis, chronic urticaria—
Adults and children 6 years and over: 10 mg P.O. daily.
*Adjust-a-dose:*In renally impaired patients with glomerular filtration rate below 30 ml/minute and in those with hepatic failure, initial dose is 10 mg every other day.

ADVERSE REACTIONS
CNS: headache, somnolence (with high doses), fatigue.
GI: dry mouth.
Skin: photosensitivity reactions.

INTERACTIONS
Drug-drug. *Cimetidine, macrolide antibiotics (clarithromycin, erythromycin, troleandomycin):* increased loratadine plasma concentrations. Monitor patient closely.
Drug-herb. *Licorice:* may prolong the QT interval and be potentially additive. Use together cautiously.
Drug-lifestyle. *Alcohol use:* increased CNS depression. Use cautiously.
Sun exposure: photosensitivity reactions may occur. Avoid prolonged or unprotected sun exposure.

EFFECTS ON DIAGNOSTIC TESTS
Discontinue drug 4 days before performing diagnostic skin tests; it can prevent, reduce, or mask positive skin test response.

CONTRAINDICATIONS
Contraindicated in patients with hypersensitivity to drug.

NURSING CONSIDERATIONS
• Use cautiously in patients with liver impairment and in breast-feeding patients.
• Be aware that administration of loratadine can affect the results of allergy skin tests.

☑**Patient teaching**
• Make sure that patient understands that drug should only be taken once daily. If symptoms persist or worsen, tell him to contact the doctor.
• Advise patients taking Claritin Reditabs to place tablet on the tongue, where it disintegrates within a few seconds. It can be swallowed with or without water.
• Warn patient to avoid alcohol and driving or other activities that require alertness until drug's CNS effects are known.
• Warn patient of possible photosensitivity reactions. Advise use of a sunblock.

• Tell patient that dry mouth can be relieved with sugarless gum, sugarless sour hard candy, or ice chips.

---

promethazine hydrochloride
Anergan 25, Anergan 50, Histantil†, Pentazine, Phencen-50, Phenergan*, Phenergan Fortis*, Phenergan Plain*, Phenoject-50, PMS-Promethazine†, Pro-50, Promethegan, Prorex-25, Prorex-50, Prothazine*, Prothazine Plain, V-Gan-25, V-Gan-50

promethazine theoclate
Avomine‡

Pregnancy Risk Category: C

HOW SUPPLIED
promethazine hydrochloride
Tablets: 12.5 mg, 25 mg, 50 mg
Syrup: 5 mg/5 ml‡*, 6.25 mg/5 ml*, 10 mg/5 ml†*, 25 mg/5 ml*
Injection: 25 mg/ml, 50 mg/ml
Suppositories: 12.5 mg, 25 mg, 50 mg
promethazine theoclate
Tablets: 25 mg‡

ACTION
A phenothiazine derivative that competes with histamine for H_1-receptor sites on effector cells. Prevents, but does not reverse, histamine-mediated responses. At high doses, promethazine also exhibits local anesthetic effects.

Route	Onset	Peak	Duration
PO	15-60 min	Unknown	< 12 hr
IV	3-5 min	Unknown	< 12 hr
IM, PR	20 min	Unknown	< 12 hr

INDICATIONS & DOSAGE
Motion sickness—
Adults: 25 mg P.O. b.i.d.
Children: 12.5 to 25 mg P.O. or P.R. b.i.d. Or 0.5 mg/kg 30 minutes to 1 hour before departure.
Nausea—
Adults: 12.5 to 25 mg P.O., I.M., or P.R. q 4 to 6 hours, p.r.n.
Children: 12.5 to 25 mg P.O. or P.R. q 4

to 6 hours, p.r.n. Or 0.25 to 1 mg/kg q 4 to 6 hours, p.r.n. Or 6.25 to 12.5 mg I.M. q 4 to 6 hours, p.r.n.
Rhinitis, allergy symptoms—
Adults: 12.5 mg P.O. q.i.d.; or 25 mg P.O. h.s.
Children: 6.25 to 12.5 mg P.O. t.i.d. or 25 mg P.O. or P.R. h.s. Or, 0.1 mg/kg q 6 hours during the day and 0.5 mg/kg h.s.
Sedation—
Adults: 25 to 50 mg P.O. or I.M. h.s. or p.r.n.
Children: 12.5 to 25 mg P.O., I.M., or P.R. h.s. Or 0.5 to 1 mg/kg q 6 hours, p.r.n.
Routine preoperative or postoperative sedation or adjunct to analgesics—
Adults: 25 to 50 mg I.M., I.V., or P.O.
Children: 12.5 to 25 mg I.M., I.V., or P.O.

ADVERSE REACTIONS
CNS: *sedation,* confusion, sleepiness, dizziness, disorientation, extrapyramidal symptoms, *drowsiness.*
CV: hypotension, hypertension.
EENT: blurred vision.
GI: nausea, vomiting, *dry mouth.*
GU: urine retention.
Hematologic: *leukopenia, agranulocytosis, thrombocytopenia.*
Other: photosensitivity, rash.

INTERACTIONS
Drug-drug. *Anticholinergics, phenothiazines, tricyclic antidepressants:* increased effects. Don't give together.
CNS depressants: increased sedation. Use together cautiously.
Epinephrine: promethazine may block or reverse the effects of epinephrine. Use other pressor agents instead.
Levodopa: promethazine may decrease levodopa's antiparkinsonian action. Avoid concomitant use.
Lithium: promethazine may reduce GI absorption or enhance renal elimination of lithium. Avoid concomitant use.
MAO inhibitors: increased extrapyramidal effects. Don't use together.
Drug-lifestyle. *Alcohol use:* increased sedation. Use together cautiously.
Sun exposure: photosensitivity reactions

---

may occur. Encourage patient to use sun-block and other protection.

EFFECTS ON DIAGNOSTIC TESTS
Discontinue drug 4 days before diagnostic skin tests; antihistamines can prevent, re-duce, or mask positive skin test response. Drug may cause hyperglycemia and either false-positive or false-negative pregnancy test results. It may also interfere with blood grouping in the ABO system.

CONTRAINDICATIONS
Contraindicated in patients with intestinal obstruction, prostatic hyperplasia, bladder-neck obstruction, narrow-angle glaucoma, seizure disorders, coma, CNS depression, stenosing peptic ulcerations, or hypersensitivity to drug; in newborns, premature neonates, and breast-feeding patients; and in acutely ill or dehydrated children.

NURSING CONSIDERATIONS
• Use cautiously in patients with pul-monary, hepatic, CV disease, or asthma.
• Know that pronounced sedative effect limits use in many ambulatory patients.
• Know that promethazine is used as an adjunct to analgesics (usually to increase sedation) and that it has no analgesic ac-tivity.
• Reduce GI distress by giving drug with food or milk.
• Inject deep I.M. into large muscle mass. Rotate injection sites.
Alert: Don't administer via S.C. route.
• Be aware that drug may be mixed with meperidine in same syringe.
• In patients scheduled for a myelogram, discontinue drug 48 hours before proce-dure and do not resume drug until 24 hours after procedure, as ordered, because of the risk of seizures.

◖I.V. administration
• Don't give in a concentration greater than 25 mg/ml or at a rate exceeding 25 mg/minute. Shield I.V. infusion from direct light.

✔Patient teaching
• Tell patient to take oral form with food or milk.

• When treating motion sickness, tell pa-tient to take first dose 30 to 60 minutes before travel. On succeeding days of trav-el, patient should take dose upon rising and with evening meal.
• Warn patient to avoid alcohol and dri-ving or other activities that require alert-ness until drug's CNS effects are known.
• Tell patient that coffee or tea may re-duce drowsiness. Suggest sugarless gum, sugarless sour hard candy, or ice chips to relieve dry mouth.
• Warn patient about possible photosensi-tivity reactions and precautions to take.

---

triprolidine hydrochloride
Actidil ◇ , Myidyl

Pregnancy Risk Category: C

HOW SUPPLIED
Tablets: 2.5 mg ◇
Syrup*: 1.25 mg/5 ml ◇

ACTION
Competes with histamine for H_1-receptor sites on effector cells. Prevents, but does not reverse, histamine-mediated respons-es.

Route	Onset	Peak	Duration
PO	15-60 min	2-3 hr	4-8 hr

INDICATIONS & DOSAGE
Colds and seasonal allergy symptoms, chronic urticaria—
Adults and children 12 years and over: 2.5 mg P.O. q 4 to 6 hours. Maximum dai-ly dosage is 10 mg.
Children 6 to 12 years: 1.25 mg P.O. q 4 to 6 hours. Maximum daily dosage is 5 mg.
Children 4 to 6 years: 0.938 mg P.O. q 4 to 6 hours. Maximum daily dosage is 3.744 mg.
Children 2 to 4 years: 0.625 mg P.O. q 4 to 6 hours. Maximum daily dosage is 2.5 mg.
Children 4 months to 2 years: 0.313 mg P.O. q 4 to 6 hours. Maximum daily dosage is 1.252 mg.

ADVERSE REACTIONS

CNS: *drowsiness, dizziness,* confusion, restlessness, insomnia, headache, *sedation, sleepiness, incoordination,* fatigue, anxiety, nervousness, tremor, **seizures, stimulation.**

CV: hypotension, palpitations, tachycardia.

EENT: *dry nose and throat.*

GI: anorexia, diarrhea, constipation, nausea, vomiting, *dry mouth,* epigastric distress.

GU: urinary frequency, urine retention.

Hematologic: hemolytic anemia, **thrombocytopenia, agranulocytosis.**

Skin: urticaria, rash, photosensitivity, diaphoresis.

Other: **anaphylactic shock,** chills, thickening of bronchial secretions.

INTERACTIONS

Drug-drug. *CNS depressants:* increased sedation. Use together cautiously.
MAO inhibitors: increased anticholinergic effects. Don't use together.
Drug-lifestyle. *Alcohol use:* increased CNS depression. Use cautiously.
Sun exposure: photosensitivity reactions may occur. Avoid prolonged or unprotected sun exposure.

EFFECTS ON DIAGNOSTIC TESTS

Discontinue drug 4 days before diagnostic skin tests; antihistamines can prevent, reduce, or mask positive skin test response.

CONTRAINDICATIONS

Contraindicated in patients with acute asthma, narrow-angle glaucoma, stenosing peptic ulcer, symptomatic prostatic hypertrophy, bladder neck obstruction, pyloroduodenal obstruction, or hypersensitivity to drug and in neonates, premature infants, or breast-feeding patients. Avoid use in patients taking MAO inhibitors.

NURSING CONSIDERATIONS

• Use with extreme caution in patients with increased intraocular pressure, hyperthyroidism, CV disease, hypertension, bronchial asthma, and prostatic hyperplasia.
• Know that children under 12 years should use only as directed by a doctor.

☑Patient teaching

• Tell patient to take drug with food or milk to reduce GI distress.
• Warn patient to avoid alcohol and driving or other activities that require alertness until drug's CNS effects are known.
• Tell patient that coffee or tea may reduce drowsiness. Suggest sugarless gum, sugarless sour hard candy, or ice chips to relieve dry mouth.
• Warn patient of possible photosensitivity reactions. Advise use of a sunblock.

Reactions may be *common,* uncommon, **life-threatening,** or COMMON AND LIFE-THREATENING.

44

Bronchodilators

albuterol
albuterol sulfate
aminophylline
atropine sulfate
(See Chapter 21, ANTIARRHYTHMICS.)
ephedrine sulfate
epinephrine
epinephrine bitartrate
epinephrine hydrochloride
ipratropium bromide
isoproterenol
isoproterenol hydrochloride
isoproterenol sulfate
metaproterenol sulfate
oxtriphylline
pirbuterol
salmeterol xinafoate
terbutaline sulfate
theophylline

COMBINATION PRODUCTS

Inhalants

DUO-MEDIHALER: isoproterenol hydrochloride 0.16 mg and phenylephrine bitartrate 0.24 mg per dose.

Oral bronchodilators

ASBRON G INLAY-TABS: theophylline 150 mg and guaifenesin 100 mg.
BRONCHIAL CAPSULES: theophylline 150 mg and guaifenesin 90 mg.
DILOR-G TABLETS: dyphylline 200 mg and guaifenesin 200 mg.
DYFLEX-G TABLETS: dyphylline 200 mg and guaifenesin 200 mg.
DYLINE-GG TABLETS: dyphylline 200 mg and guaifenesin 200 mg.
GLYCERYL-T CAPSULES: theophylline 150 mg and guaifenesin 90 mg.
MARAX*: theophylline 130 mg, ephedrine sulfate 25 mg, and hydroxyzine hydrochloride 10 mg.
MUDRANE GG-2 TABLETS: theophylline 111 mg and guaifenesin 100 mg.
NEOTHYLLINE-GG: dyphylline 200 mg and guaifenesin 200 mg.
QUIBRON CAPSULES: theophylline 150 mg and guaifenesin 90 mg.
QUIBRON-300 CAPSULES: theophylline 300 mg and guaifenesin 180 mg.
SLO-PHYLLIN GG SYRUP: theophylline 150 mg and guaifenesin 90 mg.
SYNOPHYLATE-GG SYRUP*: guaifenesin 33.3 mg/5 ml and theophylline sodium glycinate 100 mg/5 ml.

Decongestants

ACTIFED ◊ : pseudoephedrine hydrochloride 60 mg and triprolidine hydrochloride 2.5 mg.
DRISTAN COLD MULTI-SYMPTOM ◊ : phenylephrine hydrochloride 5 mg, chlorpheniramine maleate 2 mg, and acetaminophen 325 mg.
ELIXOPHYLLIN-KI ELIXIR: theophylline 80 mg, potassium iodide 130 mg.
MARAX-DF SYRUP: theophylline 97.5 mg, ephedrine sulfate 18.75 mg, hydroxyzine hydrochloride 7.5 mg.
NALDECON SYRUP: 10 ml contains phenylpropanolamine hydrochloride 40 mg, phenylephrine hydrochloride 10 mg, chlorpheniramine maleate 5 mg, and phenyltoloxamine citrate 15 mg.
SEMPREX-D CAPSULES: acrivastine 8 mg and pseudoephedrine hydrochloride 60 mg.

albuterol (salbutamol)

Asmol‡, Proventil, Ventolin

albuterol sulfate (salbutamol sulfate)

Aerolin Autoinhaler Airomir§, Proventil, Proventil Repetabs, Respolin Autohaler‡, Respolin Inhaler‡, Respolin Respirator Solution‡, Steri-Neb Salamol§, Ventolin, Ventolin Obstetric Injection‡, Ventolin Rotacaps, Volmax

Pregnancy Risk Category: C

HOW SUPPLIED

albuterol

Aerosol inhaler: 90 mcg/metered spray, 100 mcg/metered spray‡

*Liquid contains alcohol. **May contain tartrazine. †Canada ‡Australia §U.K. ◊ OTC

albuterol sulfate
Capsules for inhalation: 200 mcg
Tablets: 2 mg, 4 mg
Tablets (extended-release): 4 mg, 8 mg
Syrup: 2 mg/5 ml
Solution for inhalation: 0.083%, 0.5%
Injection: 1 mg/ml‡

ACTION
Relaxes bronchial, uterine, and vascular smooth muscle by stimulating beta$_2$-adrenergic receptors.

Route	Onset	Peak	Duration
PO	15-30 min	2-3 hr	6-12 hr
IV	Variable	Unknown	4-6 hr
Inhalation	5-15 min	0.5-2 hr	2-6 hr

INDICATIONS & DOSAGE
To prevent or treat bronchospasm in patients with reversible obstructive airway disease and the prevention of bronchospasm due to exercise—
Adults and children 12 years and older: dosage and frequency vary with dosage form.
*Aerosol inhalation—*1 to 2 inhalations q 4 to 6 hours. More frequent administration or a greater number of inhalations is not recommended.
*Solution for inhalation—*2.5 mg t.i.d. or q.i.d. by nebulizer. To prepare solution, use 0.5 ml of the 0.5% solution diluted with 2.5 ml of 0.9% NaCl. Alternatively, use 3 ml of the 0.083% solution.
*Capsules for inhalation—*200 mcg inhaled q 4 to 6 hours using a Rotahaler inhalation device. Some patients may need 400 mcg q 4 to 6 hours.
*Oral tablets—*2 to 4 mg P.O. t.i.d. or q.i.d. Maximum dosage is 8 mg q.i.d.
*Extended-release tablets—*4 to 8 mg P.O. q 12 hours. Maximum dosage is 16 mg b.i.d.
Children 6 to 14 years: 2 mg (1 tsp) P.O. t.i.d. or q.i.d.
Children 2 to 6 years: 0.1 mg/kg P.O. t.i.d., not to exceed 2 mg (1 tsp) t.i.d.
Adults over 65 years: 2 mg P.O. t.i.d. or q.i.d.
To prevent exercise-induced asthma—
Adults: 2 inhalations 15 minutes before exercise.
Prevention of premature labor‡—

Adults: initially, 10 mcg/minute by continuous I.V. infusion (via an infusion pump). Dosage should be increased at 10-minute intervals until desired response is achieved.

ADVERSE REACTIONS
CNS: *tremor, nervousness,* dizziness, insomnia, *headache, hyperactivity,* weakness, CNS stimulation, malaise.
CV: *tachycardia, palpitations,* hypertension.
EENT: dry and irritated nose and throat (with inhaled form), nasal congestion, epistaxis, hoarseness.
GI: heartburn, *nausea, vomiting,* anorexia, bad taste in mouth, increased appetite.
Respiratory: *bronchospasm,* cough, wheezing, dyspnea, bronchitis, increased sputum.
Other: muscle cramps, hypokalemia (with high doses), hypersensitivity reactions.

INTERACTIONS
Drug-drug. *CNS stimulants:* increased CNS stimulation. Avoid concomitant use.
Digoxin: digoxin serum levels may be decreased. Monitor closely.
MAO inhibitors, tricyclic antidepressants: increased adverse CV effects. Monitor patient closely.
Propranolol, other beta blockers: mutual antagonism. Monitor patient carefully.

EFFECTS ON DIAGNOSTIC TESTS
Albuterol may decrease sensitivity of spirometry used for diagnosis of asthma.

CONTRAINDICATIONS
Contraindicated in patients with hypersensitivity to drug or its ingredients.

NURSING CONSIDERATIONS
• Use cautiously in patients with CV disorders (including coronary insufficiency and hypertension), hyperthyroidism, or diabetes mellitus and in those who are unusually responsive to adrenergics.
• Use extended-release tablets cautiously in patients with preexisting GI narrowing.
• Know that when switching from regular release to extended release tablets, a regular release 2 mg tablet every 6 hours is

---

equivalent to an extended release 4 mg tablet every 12 hours.
• Know that pleasant-tasting syrup may be taken by children as young as 2 years; it contains no alcohol or sugar.
• Know that aerosol form may be used 15 minutes before exercise to prevent exercise-induced bronchospasm.
• Know that patient may use tablets and aerosol concomitantly. Monitor closely for toxicity.
• When used to prevent premature labor, monitor maternal heart rate closely. It should not exceed 140 beats/minute.

I.V. administration
• Where available, I.V. form may be used to prepare infusion using NaCl for injection, dextrose for injection, or NaCl and dextrose for injection. Do not administer drug without dilution. Do not mix with other medications. Discard unused diluted solution after 24 hours.
• After uterine contractions have ceased, drip rate of drug should be maintained for 1 hour, then gradually tapered at 50% increments in six hourly intervals. Do not continue infusions for more than 48 hours. If therapy needs to continue over 48 hours, doctor may prescribe 4 to 8 mg P.O. q.i.d.

☑ Patient teaching
• Warn patient about possibility of paradoxical bronchospasm. If this occurs, discontinue drug immediately.
• Teach patient to perform oral inhalation correctly. Give the following instructions for using metered-dose inhaler:
–Shake the inhaler.
–Clear nasal passages and throat.
–Breathe out, expelling as much air from lungs as possible.
–Place mouthpiece well into mouth as dose from inhaler is released, and inhale deeply.
–Hold breath for several seconds, remove mouthpiece, and exhale slowly.
    Alternatively, inhaler may be held approximately 1″ (two finger widths) from open mouth; inhale while dose is released.
• If more than 1 inhalation is ordered, advise patient to wait at least 2 minutes before repeating procedure.
• Tell patient that use with an aerochamber may improve drug delivery to the lungs.
• If patient is also using a steroid inhaler, instruct him to use the bronchodilator first and then wait about 5 minutes before using the steroid. This allows the bronchodilator to open the air passages for maximum effectiveness.
• Tell patient to remove canister and wash inhaler with warm, soapy water at least once a week.

aminophylline (theophylline ethylenediamine)
Aminophyllin, Pecram§, Phyllocontin, Phyllocontin Continus§, Phyllocontin-350, Truphylline

Pregnancy Risk Category: C

HOW SUPPLIED
Tablets: 100 mg, 200 mg
Tablets (extended-release): 225 mg, 350 mg†
Oral liquid: 105 mg/5 ml
Injection: 250 mg/10 ml, 500 mg/20 ml, 100 mg/100 ml in 0.45% NaCl, 200 mg/100 ml in 0.45% NaCl
Rectal suppositories: 250 mg, 500 mg

ACTION
Inhibits phosphodiesterase, the enzyme that degrades cAMP. Results in relaxation of smooth muscle of the bronchial airways and pulmonary blood vessels.

Route	Onset	Peak	Duration
PO (solution)	15-60 min	1-7 hr	Variable
IV	15 min	Immediate	Variable
PR	Unknown	Unknown	Unknown

INDICATIONS & DOSAGE
Symptomatic relief of bronchospasm—
Patients not currently receiving theophylline products who require rapid relief of symptoms: loading dose is 6 mg/kg (equivalent to 4.7 mg/kg anhydrous the-

ophylline) I.V. (25 mg/minute or less); then maintenance infusion.

Adults (nonsmokers): 0.7 mg/kg/hour I.V. for 12 hours; then 0.5 mg/kg/hour.

Children 9 to 16 years: 1 mg/kg/hour I.V. for 12 hours; then 0.8 mg/kg/hour.

Children 6 months to 9 years: 1.2 mg/kg/hour for 12 hours; then 1 mg/kg/hour.

Elderly: 0.6 mg/kg/hour I.V. for 12 hours; then 0.3 mg/kg/hour.

Adjust-a-dose: In otherwise healthy adult smokers, 1 mg/kg/hour I.V. for 12 hours; then 0.8 mg/kg/hour.

In adults with cor pulmonale, 0.6 mg/kg/hour I.V. for 12 hours; then 0.3 mg/kg/hour.

In adults with heart failure or liver disease, 0.5 mg/kg/hour I.V. for 12 hours; then 0.1 to 0.2 mg/kg/hour.

Patients currently receiving theophylline products: first determine time, amount, route of administration, and dosage form of patient's last theophylline dose. Aminophylline infusions of 0.63 mg/kg (0.5 mg/kg anhydrous theophylline) will increase plasma levels of theophylline by 1 mcg/ml. Some doctors recommend a dose of 3.1 mg/kg (2.5 mg/kg anhydrous theophylline) if no obvious signs of theophylline toxicity are present. *Chronic bronchial asthma—* Dosage is highly individualized.

Adults and children: usual initial oral dose is 16 mg/kg or 400 mg (whichever is less) P.O. daily in three or four divided doses q 6 to 8 hours if using rapidly absorbed dosage forms. Dosage may be increased, if tolerated, in increments of 25% q 2 to 3 days. Alternatively, if using extended-release preparations, 12 mg/kg or 400 mg (whichever is less) P.O. daily in two to three divided doses q 8 to 12 hours. Dosage may be increased, if tolerated, by 2 to 3 mg/kg daily q 3 days.

Regardless of dosage form, the following are recommended maximum dosages. For adults and children 16 years and older, 13 mg/kg daily or 900 mg/day, whichever is less; children 12 to 16 years, 18 mg/kg daily; children 9 to 12 years, 20 mg/kg daily; and children 1 to 9 years, 24 mg/kg daily.

When recommended maximum dosage is reached, dosage adjustment is based on measurement of peak serum theophylline concentrations. Target theophylline concentrations are generally between 10 and 20 mcg/ml.

Note: P.R. dosage is same as that recommended for P.O. dosage.

ADVERSE REACTIONS

CNS: *nervousness, restlessness,* headache, *insomnia, **seizures,*** muscle twitching, irritability, *dizziness.*

CV: *palpitations, sinus tachycardia,* extrasystoles, flushing, marked hypotension, ***arrhythmias.***

GI: *nausea, vomiting,* diarrhea, epigastric pain, hematemesis.

Respiratory: tachypnea, ***respiratory arrest.***

Skin: urticaria.

Other: irritation (with rectal suppositories), hyperglycemia, fever, hypersensitivity reactions.

INTERACTIONS

Drug-drug. *Adenosine:* decreased antiarrhythmic effectiveness. Higher doses of adenosine may be necessary.

Alkali-sensitive drugs: reduced activity. Do not add to I.V. fluids containing aminophylline.

Barbiturates, nicotine, phenytoin, rifampin: enhanced metabolism and decreased theophylline blood levels. Monitor for decreased aminophylline effect.

Beta-adrenergic blockers: antagonism. *Propranolol* and *nadolol,* especially, may cause bronchospasm in sensitive patients. Use together cautiously.

Calcium channel blockers, cimetidine, disulfiram, influenza virus vaccine, interferon, macrolide antibiotics (such as erythromycin), methotrexate, oral contraceptives, quinolone antibiotics (such as ciprofloxacin): decreased hepatic clearance of theophylline; elevated theophylline levels. Monitor for signs of toxicity.

Carbamazepine, isoniazid, loop diuretics: may increase or decrease theophylline levels. Monitor closely.

Ephedrine, other sympathomimetics: theophylline may exhibit synergistic toxicity with these agents, predisposing patients to arrhythmias. Monitor patient closely.

Lithium: theophylline may increase excre-

tion of lithium. Monitor patient closely.
Drug-lifestyle. *Smoking:* increased elimination of theophylline, increasing dosing requirements. Monitor theophylline response and serum concentrations.

EFFECTS ON DIAGNOSTIC TESTS
Aminophylline may alter the assay for uric acid, depending on method used, and increases plasma levels of free fatty acids and urinary catecholamines. Theophylline levels are falsely elevated in the presence of furosemide, phenylbutazone, probenecid, theobromine, caffeine, tea, chocolate, cola beverages, and acetaminophen, depending on type of assay used.

CONTRAINDICATIONS
Contraindicated in patients with hypersensitivity to xanthine compounds (caffeine, theobromine) and ethylenediamine and in those with active peptic ulcer disease and seizure disorders (unless adequate anticonvulsant therapy is given). Rectal suppositories are also contraindicated in patients who have an irritation or infection of the rectum or lower colon.

NURSING CONSIDERATIONS
• Use cautiously in neonates and infants under 1 year, young children, and elderly patients; also use cautiously in patients with heart failure or other cardiac or circulatory impairment, COPD, cor pulmonale, renal or hepatic disease, hyperthyroidism, diabetes mellitus, glaucoma, peptic ulcer, severe hypoxemia, and hypertension.
• Relieve GI symptoms by giving oral drug with full glass of water at meals, although food in stomach delays absorption. No evidence exists that antacids reduce adverse GI reactions. Know that enteric-coated tablets also may delay and impair absorption.
Alert: Before giving loading dose, ensure that patient has not had recent theophylline therapy.
• Suppositories are slowly and erratically absorbed. Administer rectal suppository if patients cannot take drug orally, as ordered. Schedule after evacuation, if possible; may be retained better if given before

meal. Have patients remain recumbent 15 to 20 minutes after insertion.
• Monitor vital signs; measure and record fluid intake and output. Expected clinical effects include improved quality of pulse and respirations.
• Aminophylline is a soluble salt of theophylline. Know that dosage is adjusted by monitoring response, tolerance, pulmonary function, and serum theophylline levels. Monitor serum theophylline levels as ordered. Theophylline concentrations should range from 10 to 20 mcg/ml; toxicity has been reported with levels above 20 mcg/ml.
• Know that signs of toxicity include tachycardia, anorexia, nausea, vomiting, diarrhea, restlessness, irritability and headache. The presence of any of these signs in patients taking theophylline warrants checking theophylline levels and dose adjustment as indicated.
• Be aware that patients who experience urticaria may still tolerate other theophylline preparations. Urticaria may be caused by the ethylenediamine salt.

🔵 I.V. administration
• I.V. drug administration can cause burning; dilute with compatible I.V. solution, and inject at a rate no faster than 25 mg/minute. Drug is compatible with most I.V. solutions except invert sugar, fructose, and fat emulsions.

✅ Patient teaching
• Supply instructions for home care administration of form prescribed and dosage schedule. Some patients may require an around-the-clock dosage schedule.
• Warn elderly patient that dizziness, a common adverse reaction at start of therapy, may occur.
• Warn patient to check with the doctor or pharmacist before combining aminophylline with other drugs. Prescription or OTC remedies may contain ephedrine in combination with theophylline salts; excessive CNS stimulation may result.
• Advise patient to avoid switching brand without first checking with doctor.
• Tell patient who is a smoker to notify doctor if he has quit smoking.

ephedrine sulfate
Vicks Vatronol

Pregnancy Risk Category: C

HOW SUPPLIED
Capsules: 25 mg, 50 mg
Injection: 25 mg/ml, 30 mg/ml‡,
50 mg/ml

ACTION
Stimulates alpha- and beta-adrenergic receptors; a direct- and indirect-acting sympathomimetic. Relaxes bronchial smooth
muscle by beta-2 adrenergic receptor
stimulation.

Route	Onset	Peak	Duration
PO	15-60 min	Unknown	3-5 hr
IV	5 min	Unknown	1 hr
IM, SC	10-20 min	Unknown	0.5-1 hr

INDICATIONS & DOSAGE
To correct hypotension—
Adults: 25 mg one to four times daily
P.O., 25 to 50 mg I.M. or S.C., or 10 to
25 mg I.V. p.r.n. to maximum of
150 mg/24 hours.
Children: 3 mg/kg or 25 to 100 mg/m^2
S.C. or I.V. daily, in four to six divided
doses.
Bronchodilation or nasal decongestion—
Adults and children over 12 years: 12.5
to 25 mg P.O. b.i.d., t.i.d., or q.i.d. Maximum dosage is 150 mg daily in four to six
divided doses.
Children 6 to 12 years: 6.25 to 12.5 mg q
4 hours, not to exceed 75 mg in 24 hours.
Children over 2 years: 2 to 3 mg/kg or
100 mg/m^2 P.O. daily in four to six divided doses.

ADVERSE REACTIONS
CNS: *insomnia, nervousness,* dizziness,
headache, muscle weakness, euphoria,
confusion, delirium, tremor, ***cerebral hemorrhage.***
CV: *palpitations,* tachycardia, hypertension, precordial pain, ***arrhythmias.***
EENT: dry nose and throat.
GI: nausea, vomiting, anorexia.
GU: urine retention, painful urination due
to visceral sphincter spasm.

Other: diaphoresis.

INTERACTIONS
Drug-drug. *Acetazolamide:* increased
serum ephedrine levels. Monitor for toxicity.
Alpha-adrenergic blockers: unopposed
beta-adrenergic effects, resulting in hypotension. Avoid concomitant use.
Antihypertensives: decreased effects.
Monitor blood pressure.
Beta-adrenergic blockers: unopposed
alpha-adrenergic effects, resulting in hypertension. Monitor blood pressure.
*Cardiac glycosides, general anesthetics
(halogenated hydrocarbons):* increased
risk of ventricular arrhythmias. Monitor
ECG closely.
Ergot alkaloids: decreased vasoconstrictor activity. Monitor patient closely.
Guanadrel, guanethidine: decreased pressor effects of ephedrine. Monitor patient
closely.
Levodopa: enhanced risk of ventricular
arrhythmias. Monitor ECG closely.
MAO inhibitors, tricyclic antidepressants:
when given with sympathomimetics, may
cause severe hypertension (hypertensive
crisis). Monitor patient and blood pressure closely.
Methyldopa, reserpine: may inhibit
ephedrine effects. Use cautiously.

EFFECTS ON DIAGNOSTIC TESTS
None reported.

CONTRAINDICATIONS
Contraindicated in patients with porphyria, severe coronary artery disease, arrhythmias, angle-closure glaucoma, psychoneurosis, angina pectoris, substantial
organic heart disease, CV disease, or hypersensitivity to ephedrine and other sympathomimetics and in those receiving
MAO inhibitors or general anesthesia
with cyclopropane or halothane.

NURSING CONSIDERATIONS
• Use with extreme caution in the elderly
and in those with hypertension, hyperthyroidism, nervous or excitable states, diabetes, and prostatic hyperplasia.
Alert: Know that hypoxia, hypercapnia,
and acidosis, which may reduce effective-

ness or increase the incidence of adverse reactions, must be identified and corrected before or during ephedrine therapy.
• Drug is not a substitute for blood or fluid volume replenishment. Know that volume deficit must be corrected before administering vasopressors.
• To prevent insomnia, avoid giving within 2 hours of bedtime.
• Effectiveness decreases after 2 to 3 weeks, as tolerance develops. Doctor may need to increase dosage. Drug is not addictive.
• Ephedrine should be used in children under 12 years of age only under the direction of a doctor.
• Rebound congestion and tachyphylaxis may occur with topical decongestant formulations.

◖ I.V. administration
• Give 10 to 25 mg by I.V. injection slowly; repeat in 5 to 10 minutes if necessary. Compatible with most common I.V. solutions.

✅ Patient teaching
• Tell patient taking oral form of drug at home to take last dose of day at least 2 hours before bedtime.
• Warn patient not to take OTC drugs or herbal agents that contain ephedrine without informing doctor.

epinephrine (adrenaline)
Bronkaid Mist ◇ , Bronkaid Mistometer† , Primatene Mist ◇

epinephrine bitartrate
AsthmaHaler Mist ◇ , Bronitin Mist ◇ , Bronkaid Mist ◇ , Primatene Mist* , Primatene Mist Suspension ◇

epinephrine hydrochloride
Adrenalin Chloride, AsthmaNefrin ◇ , Epi-Pen, Epi-Pen Jr., microNefrin ◇ , Nephron ◇ , Sus-Phrine, Vaponefrin

Pregnancy Risk Category: C

HOW SUPPLIED
Aerosol inhaler: 160 mcg ◇ , 200 mcg ◇ , 220 mcg ◇ , 250 mcg/metered spray ◇
Nebulizer inhaler: 1% (1:100)† ◇ , 1.25%† ◇ , 2.25%† ◇
Injection: 0.01 mg/ml (1:100,000), 0.1 mg/ml (1:10,000), 0.5 mg/ml (1:2,000), 1 mg/ml (1:1,000) parenteral; 5 mg/ml (1:200) parenteral suspension

ACTION
Stimulates alpha- and beta-adrenergic receptors within the sympathetic nervous system. Relaxes bronchial smooth muscle by beta-2 adrenergic receptor stimulation.

Route	Onset	Peak	Duration
IV	Immediate	5 min	Short
IM	Variable	Unknown	1-4 hr
SC	5-15 min	0.5 hr	1-4 hr
Inhalation	1-5 min	Unknown	1-3 hr

INDICATIONS & DOSAGE
Bronchospasm, hypersensitivity reactions, anaphylaxis—
Adults: 0.1 to 0.5 ml of 1:1,000 S.C. or I.M. Repeated q 10 to 15 minutes, p.r.n. Or 0.1 to 0.25 ml of 1:1,000 (1 to 2.5 ml of a commercially available 1:10,000 injection or of a 1:10,000 dilution prepared by diluting 1 ml of a commercially available 1:1,000 injection with 10 ml of water for injection or 0.9% NaCl for injection) I.V. slowly over 5 to 10 minutes.
Children: 0.01 ml/kg (10 mcg) of 1:1,000 solution S.C.; repeated q 20 minutes to 4 hours p.r.n. Maximum single dose should not exceed 0.5 mg. Or, 0.004 to 0.005 ml/kg of 1:200 (Sus-Phrine) S.C.; repeated q 8 to 12 hours p.r.n. Maximum single dose should not exceed 0.75 mg.
Hemostasis—
Adults: 1:50,000 to 1:1,000, sprayed or applied topically.
Acute asthmatic attacks—
Adults and children 4 years and over: 160 to 250 mcg (metered aerosol) which is equivalent to 1 inhalation, repeated once if necessary after at least 1 minute; subsequent doses should not be administered for at least 3 hours. Alternatively, 1% (1:100) solution of epinephrine or 2.25% solution of racepinephrine admin-

istered with a hand-bulb nebulizer as 1 to 3 deep inhalations, repeated q 3 hours, p.r.n.

To prolong local anesthetic effect—
Adults and children: in conjunction with local anesthetics, may be used in concentrations of 1:500,000 to 1:50,000. The most commonly used concentration is 1:200,000.

To restore cardiac rhythm in cardiac arrest—
Adults: usual adult dose is 0.5 to 1 mg I.V. Doses may be repeated q 3 to 5 minutes if needed. Higher dose epinephrine may be used if 1-mg doses fail: 3 to 5 mg (approximately 0.1 mg/kg) doses of epinephrine repeated q 3 to 5 minutes.

Children: usual dose is 0.01 mg/kg (0.1 ml/kg of 1:10,000 injection) I.V. Usual initial dose through an endotracheal tube is 0.1 mg/kg (0.1 ml/kg of a 1:1,000 injection) diluted in 1 to 2 ml of 0.45% or 0.9% NaCl solution. Subsequent I.V. or intratracheal doses range from 0.1 to 0.2 mg/kg (0.1 to 0.2 ml/kg of a 1:1,000 injection). I.V. or intratracheal doses may be repeated q 3 to 5 minutes if needed.

Note: 1 mg equals 1 ml of 1:1,000 or 10 ml of 1:10,000.

ADVERSE REACTIONS
CNS: *nervousness, tremor,* vertigo, *headache,* disorientation, agitation, *drowsiness,* fear, pallor, dizziness, weakness, ***cerebral hemorrhage, CVA.***
CV: *palpitations;* widened pulse pressure; hypertension; tachycardia; ***ventricular fibrillation; shock;*** anginal pain; ECG changes, including a decreased T-wave amplitude.
GI: *nausea, vomiting.*
Respiratory: dyspnea.
Skin: urticaria, pain, hemorrhage at injection site.
Other: tissue necrosis.

INTERACTIONS
Drug-drug. *Alpha-adrenergic blockers:* hypotension due to unopposed beta-adrenergic effects. Avoid concomitant use.
Antihistamines, thyroid hormones, tricyclic antidepressants: when given with sympathomimetics, may cause severe

adverse cardiac effects. Avoid giving together.
Beta blockers (such as propranolol): may cause vasoconstriction and reflex bradycardia. Monitor patient carefully.
Cardiac glycosides, general anesthetics (halogenated hydrocarbons): increased risk of ventricular arrhythmias. Monitor ECG closely.
Doxapram, mazindol, methylphenidate: enhanced CNS stimulation or pressor effects. Monitor patient closely.
Ergot alkaloids: decreased vasoconstrictor activity. Monitor patient closely.
Guanadrel, guanethidine: enhanced pressor effects of epinephrine. Monitor patient closely.
Levodopa: enhanced risk of arrhythmias. Monitor ECG closely.
MAO inhibitors: increased risk of hypertensive crisis. Monitor blood pressure closely.

EFFECTS ON DIAGNOSTIC TESTS
Epinephrine therapy alters blood glucose and serum lactic acid levels (both may be increased), increases BUN levels, and interferes with tests for urinary catecholamines.

CONTRAINDICATIONS
Contraindicated in patients with angle-closure glaucoma, shock (other than anaphylactic shock), organic brain damage, cardiac dilation, arrhythmias, coronary insufficiency, or cerebral arteriosclerosis. Also contraindicated in patients during general anesthesia with halogenated hydrocarbons or cyclopropane and in patients in labor (may delay second stage).

Some commercial products contain sulfites: contraindicated in patients with sulfite allergies except when epinephrine is being used for treatment of serious allergic reactions or other emergency situations.

In conjunction with local anesthetics, epinephrine is contraindicated for use in fingers, toes, ears, nose, or genitalia.

NURSING CONSIDERATIONS
• Use with extreme caution in patients with long-standing bronchial asthma and emphysema who have developed degener-

ative heart disease. Also use cautiously in elderly patients and in those with hyperthyroidism, CV disease, hypertension, psychoneurosis, and diabetes.

• In patients with Parkinson's disease, drug increases rigidity and tremor.

• Be aware that epinephrine is drug of choice in emergency treatment of acute anaphylactic reactions.

• Discard epinephrine solutions after 24 hours or if solution is discolored or contains precipitate. Keep solution in light-resistant container, and don't remove before use.

Alert: Avoid I.M. administration of parenteral suspension into buttocks. Gas gangrene may occur because epinephrine reduces oxygen tension of the tissues, encouraging the growth of contaminating organisms.

• Massage site after I.M. injection to counteract possible vasoconstriction. Repeated local injection can cause necrosis resulting from vasoconstriction at injection site.

• Observe patient closely for adverse reactions. Notify doctor if adverse reactions develop; dose adjustment or drug discontinuance may be warranted.

• Know that if a sharp blood pressure rise occurs, rapid-acting vasodilators, such as nitrates or alpha-adrenergic blockers, can be given to counteract the marked pressor effect of large doses of epinephrine.

• Know that epinephrine is rapidly destroyed by oxidizing agents, such as iodine, chromates, nitrites, oxygen, and salts of easily reducible metals (such as iron).

■ **I.V. administration**

• Don't mix with alkaline solutions. Use D_5W, 0.9% NaCl for injection, lactated Ringer's injection, or combinations of dextrose in NaCl. Mix just before use.

• When administering I.V., monitor blood pressure, heart rate, and ECG when therapy is initiated and frequently thereafter.

☑ **Patient teaching**

• Teach patient to perform oral inhalation correctly. Give the following instructions for using a metered-dose inhaler:
–Clear nasal passages and throat.

–Breathe out, expelling as much air from lungs as possible.
–Place mouthpiece well into mouth as dose from inhaler is released, and inhale deeply.
–Hold breath for several seconds, remove mouthpiece, and exhale slowly.

Alternatively, inhaler may be held approximately 1″ (two finger widths) from open mouth; inhale while dose is released.

• If more than 1 inhalation is ordered, advise patient to wait at least 2 minutes before repeating procedure.

• Tell patient that use with an aerochamber may improve drug delivery to the lungs.

• If patient is also using a steroid inhaler, instruct him to use the bronchodilator first and then wait about 5 minutes before using the steroid. This allows the bronchodilator to open the air passages for maximum effectiveness.

• Instruct patient to wash inhaler with warm, soapy water at least once weekly. Remove canister before washing.

• If patient has acute hypersensitivity reactions, such as to bee stings, it may be necessary to instruct him to self-inject epinephrine at home.

---

ipratropium bromide
Atrovent

Pregnancy Risk Category: B

HOW SUPPLIED
Inhaler: each metered dose supplies 18 mcg
Solution (for inhalation): 0.02% (500 mcg/vial)
Solution (for nebulizer): 0.025% (250 mcg/ml)‡
Nasal spray: 0.03% (each metered dose supplies 21 mcg), 0.06% (each metered dose supplies 42 mcg)

ACTION
Inhibits vagally mediated reflexes by antagonizing acetylcholine at muscarinic receptors on bronchial smooth muscle.

Route	Onset	Peak	Duration
Inhalation	5-15 min	1-2 hr	3-6 hr

INDICATIONS & DOSAGE
Bronchospasm associated with COPD—
Adults and children over 12 years: 1 to 2 inhalations q.i.d. Additional inhalations may be needed. However, total inhalations should not exceed 12 in 24 hours. Alternatively, use inhalation solution. Give 500 mcg dissolved in 0.9% NaCl and administer by nebulizer q 6 to 8 hours.
Children 5 to 12 years: give 125 to 250 mcg nebulizer solution dissolved in 0.9% NaCl and administer by nebulizer q 4 to 6 hours.
Perennial rhinitis—
Adults and children over 12 years: usual dosage of 0.03% nasal spray is 2 sprays (42 mcg) per nostril b.i.d. or t.i.d.
Common cold-induced rhinorrhea—
Adults and children over 12 years: usual dosage of 0.06% nasal spray is 2 sprays (84 mcg) per nostril t.i.d. or q.i.d.
Infants and children: nebulization 25 mcg/kg t.i.d.
❊ *NEW INDICATION: Symptomatic relief of rhinorrhea associated with allergic and nonallergic perennial rhinitis—*
Adults and children 6 years and older: 2 sprays (42 mcg) of 0.03% nasal spray per nostril b.i.d. or t.i.d. (total dose 168 to 252 mcg/day)

ADVERSE REACTIONS
CNS: dizziness, headache, nervousness.
CV: palpitations, hypertension.
EENT: cough, blurred vision, rhinitis, pharyngitis, sinusitis, epistaxis.
GI: nausea, GI distress, dry mouth.
Respiratory: *upper respiratory tract infection, bronchitis,* cough, dyspnea, ***bronchospasm,*** increased sputum.
Skin: rash.
Other: pain, back pain, chest pain, flulike symptoms, hypersensitivity reactions.

INTERACTIONS
Drug-drug. *Anticholinergics:* increased anticholinergic effects. Avoid concomitant use.
Drug-herb. *Jaborandi tree:* effects of ipratropium may be decreased with concurrent administration. Monitor closely.
Pill-bearing spurge: choline may decrease effect of ipratropium. Use together cautiously.

EFFECTS ON DIAGNOSTIC TESTS
None reported.

CONTRAINDICATIONS
Contraindicated in patients with hypersensitivity to drug, atropine, or its derivatives and in those with history of hypersensitivity to soy lecithin or related food products, such as soybeans and peanuts.

NURSING CONSIDERATIONS
• Use cautiously in patients with angle-closure glaucoma, prostatic hyperplasia, and bladder-neck obstruction.
• If using a face mask for a nebulizer, take care to avoid leakage around the mask; temporary blurring of vision or eye pain may occur.
• Safety and efficacy of use beyond 4 days in patients with the common cold have not been established.

☑ **Patient teaching**
• Warn patient that drug is not effective for treating acute episodes of bronchospasm where rapid response is required.
• Teach patient to perform oral inhalation correctly. Give the following instructions for using a metered-dose inhaler:
–Clear nasal passages and throat.
–Breathe out, expelling as much air from lungs as possible.
–Place mouthpiece well into mouth as dose from inhaler is released, and inhale deeply.
–Hold breath for several seconds, remove mouthpiece, and exhale slowly.
• Inform patient that use of aerochamber with metered-dose inhaler may improve drug delivery to lungs.
• Warn patient to avoid accidentally spraying into eyes. Temporary blurring of vision may result.
• If more than 1 inhalation is ordered, tell patient to wait at least 2 minutes before repeating procedure.
• Instruct patient to wash inhaler in warm, soapy water at least once weekly. Remove canister before washing.
• Tell patient who is also using a steroid inhaler to use ipratropium first, then wait about 5 minutes before using the steroid. This allows the bronchodilator to open air passages for maximum effectiveness.

Reactions may be *common,* uncommon, ***life-threatening,*** or COMMON AND LIFE-THREATENING.

• Inform patient to take missed dose as soon as remembered unless it's almost time for the next dose. In that case, he should skip the missed dose and never double dose.

---

isoproterenol (isoprenaline)
Isuprel, Medihaler-Iso

isoproterenol hydrochloride
Isuprel, Isuprel Mistometer

isoproterenol sulfate
Medihaler-Iso

Pregnancy Risk Category: C

HOW SUPPLIED
isoproterenol
Nebulizer inhaler: 0.25%, 0.5%, 1%
isoproterenol hydrochloride
Tablets (S.L.): 10 mg, 15 mg
Aerosol inhaler: 131 mcg/metered spray
Injection: 20 mcg/ml, 200 mcg/ml
isoproterenol sulfate
Aerosol inhaler: 80 mcg/metered spray

ACTION
Relaxes bronchial smooth muscle by stimulating beta$_2$-adrenergic receptors. As a cardiac stimulant, acts on beta$_1$-adrenergic receptors in the heart.

Route	Onset	Peak	Duration
IV	Immediate	Unknown	< 1 hr
SL	15-30 min	Unknown	1-2 hr
Inhalation	2-5 min	Unknown	0.5-2 hr

INDICATIONS & DOSAGE
Bronchial asthma and reversible bronchospasm—
Adults: 10 to 20 mg hydrochloride S.L. t.i.d. or q.i.d. Do not exceed daily S.L. dosage of 60 mg.
Children: 5 to 10 mg hydrochloride S.L. t.i.d. Do not exceed daily S.L. dosage of 30 mg.
Bronchospasm—
Adults and children: acute dyspneic episodes: 1 inhalation of sulfate form initially. Repeated if needed after 2 to 5 minutes. No more than 6 inhalations should

be taken during any single hour in a 24-hour period.
Maintenance dosage is 1 to 2 inhalations four to six times daily.
Bronchospasm in COPD—
Administered via IPPB or for nebulization by compressed air or oxygen.
Adults: 2 ml of 0.125% or 2.5 ml of 0.1% solution (prepared by diluting 0.5 ml of 0.5% solution to 2 or 2.5 ml, respectively, or by diluting 0.25 ml of 1% solution to 2 or 2.5 ml, respectively, with water or 0.45% or 0.9% NaCl solution) up to five times daily.
Children: 2 ml of a 0.0625% solution or 2.5 ml of 0.05% solution (prepared by diluting 0.25 ml of 0.5% solution to 2 or 2.5 ml, respectively, with water or 0.45% or 0.9% NaCl solution) up to five times daily.
Heart block and ventricular arrhythmias—
Adults: (hydrochloride) initially, 0.02 to 0.06 mg I.V. Subsequent doses 0.01 to 0.2 mg I.V. or 5 mcg/minute I.V.; or 0.2 mg I.M. initially, then 0.02 to 1 mg, p.r.n.
Children: (hydrochloride) I.V. infusion of 2.5 mcg/minute or 0.1 mcg/kg/minute. Dosage is adjusted based on patient's response.
Shock—
Adults and children: (hydrochloride) 0.5 to 5 mcg/minute by continuous I.V. infusion. Usual concentration is 1 mg (5 ml) in 500 ml D$_5$W. Rate adjusted according to heart rate, CVP, blood pressure, and urine flow.

ADVERSE REACTIONS
CNS: *headache, mild tremor,* weakness, dizziness, *nervousness,* insomnia, ***Adams-Stokes seizures.***
CV: *palpitations, tachycardia, anginal pain,* **arrhythmias, cardiac arrest,** *rapid rise and fall in blood pressure.*
GI: *nausea, vomiting, heartburn.*
Respiratory: ***bronchospasm,*** bronchitis, sputum increase, pharyngitis, pulmonary edema.
Other: diaphoresis, hyperglycemia; swelling of parotid glands with prolonged use, pharyngitis.

INTERACTIONS
Drug-drug. *Epinephrine, other sympath-omimetics:* increased risk of arrhythmias. Use together cautiously.
Halogenated general anesthetics or cyclopropane: increased risk of arrhythmias. Avoid concomitant use.
Propranolol, other beta blockers: blocked bronchodilating effect of isoproterenol. Monitor patient carefully if used together.

EFFECTS ON DIAGNOSTIC TESTS
Drug may reduce sensitivity of spirometry in the diagnosis of asthma.

CONTRAINDICATIONS
Contraindicated in patients with tachycardia or AV block caused by digitalis intoxication, preexisting arrhythmias (other than those that may respond to treatment with isoproterenol), angina pectoris, or narrow-angle glaucoma and with concurrent use of general anesthetics with halogenated agents or cyclopropane.

NURSING CONSIDERATIONS
• Use cautiously in the elderly and in patients with renal or CV disease, coronary insufficiency, diabetes, hyperthyroidism, or history of sensitivity to sympathomimetic amines.
• Know that drug is not a substitute for blood or fluid volume deficit. Volume deficit should be corrected before administering vasopressors.
• Do not use injection or inhalation solution if it's discolored or contains precipitate.
Alert: If heart rate exceeds 110 beats/minute with I.V. infusion, notify doctor. Doses sufficient to increase the heart rate to more than 130 beats/minute may induce ventricular arrhythmias.
• Do not administer S.L. doses more frequently than every 3 to 4 hours or more than three times daily.
• If drug is administered via inhalation with oxygen, be sure oxygen concentration will not suppress respiratory drive.
• Follow same instructions for metered powder nebulizer, although deep inhalation is not necessary.
• Be aware that drug may aggravate ventilation-perfusion abnormalities; even while ease of breathing is improved, arterial oxygen tension may fall paradoxically.
• Be aware that isoproterenol may cause a slight rise in systolic blood pressure and a slight to marked drop in diastolic blood pressure.
• Monitor patient for adverse reactions.

◖ I.V. administration
• Give by direct injection or I.V. infusion. For infusion, drug may be diluted with most common I.V. solutions. However, do not use with sodium bicarbonate injection; drug decomposes rapidly in alkaline solutions.
• When administering I.V. isoproterenol to treat shock, closely monitor blood pressure, CVP, ECG, arterial blood gas measurements, and urine output. Carefully adjust infusion rate according to these measurements, as ordered. Use a continuous infusion pump to regulate flow rate.

✓ Patient teaching
• Teach patient to perform oral inhalation correctly. Give the following instructions for using a metered-dose inhaler:
–Clear nasal passages and throat.
–Breathe out, expelling as much air from lungs as possible.
–Place mouthpiece well into mouth as dose from inhaler is released, and inhale deeply.
–Hold breath for several seconds, remove mouthpiece, and exhale slowly.
• If more than 1 inhalation is ordered, tell patient to wait at least 2 minutes before repeating procedure.
• Alternatively, inhaler may be held approximately 1″ (two finger widths) from open mouth; inhale as dose is released.
• Use of aerochamber may improve drug delivery to the lungs.
• If patient is also using a steroid inhaler, instruct him to use the bronchodilator first and then wait about 5 minutes before using the steroid. This allows the bronchodilator to open the air passages for maximum effectiveness.
• Instruct patient to wash inhaler with warm, soapy water at least once weekly. Remove canister before washing.

Reactions may be *common*, uncommon, *life-threatening*, or COMMON AND LIFE-THREATENING.

- Warn patient using oral inhalant that drug may turn sputum and saliva pink.
- Teach patient to take S.L. tablet properly. Instruct patient to hold tablet under tongue and not to swallow saliva until tablet dissolves and is absorbed. Instruct him to rinse mouth with water between doses to help prevent oropharyngeal dryness.
- Caution patient that prolonged use of S.L. tablets can cause tooth decay.
- Tell patient not to use drug at bedtime, if possible; it interrupts sleep patterns.
- Inform patient to discontinue drug immediately and notify doctor if drug causes precordial distress or anginal pain or if an increase in chest tightness or dyspnea occurs.
- Warn patient against overuse; tolerance may develop.

---

metaproterenol sulfate
Alupent, Arm-A-Med
Metaproterenol, Dey-Lute
Metaproterenol, Metaprel

Pregnancy Risk Category: C

HOW SUPPLIED
Tablets: 10 mg, 20 mg
Syrup: 10 mg/5 ml
Aerosol inhaler: 0.65 mg/metered spray
Nebulizer inhaler: 0.4%, 0.6%, 5% solution

ACTION
Relaxes bronchial smooth muscle by stimulating beta$_2$-adrenergic receptors.

Route	Onset	Peak	Duration
PO	15 min	1 hr	1-4 hr
Inhalation	1 min	1 hr	1-2.5 hr
Nebulizer	5-30 min	1 hr	1-2.5 hr

INDICATIONS & DOSAGE
Acute episodes of bronchial asthma—
Adults and children 12 years and over: 2 to 3 inhalations. Do not repeat inhalations more often than q 3 to 4 hours. Do not exceed 12 inhalations daily.
Bronchial asthma and reversible bronchospasm—
Adults: 20 mg P.O. q 6 to 8 hours.

Children over 9 years or weighing over 27 kg (60 lb): 20 mg P.O. q 6 to 8 hours.
Children 6 to 9 years or weighing less than 27 kg: 10 mg P.O. q 6 to 8 hours.
Children under 6 years: 1.3 to 2.6 mg/kg/day in divided doses of syrup. Alternatively, via IPPB or nebulizer:
Adults and children 12 years and over: 0.2 to 0.3 ml of 5% solution diluted in approximately 2.5 ml of 0.45% or 0.9% NaCl or 2.5 ml of a commercially available 0.4% or 0.6% solution q 4 hours, p.r.n.
Children 6 to 12 years: 0.1 to 0.2 ml of a 5% solution diluted in 0.9% NaCl to final volume of 3 ml q 4 hours, p.r.n.

ADVERSE REACTIONS
CNS: *nervousness,* weakness, drowsiness, *tremor,* vertigo, headache.
CV: *tachycardia,* hypertension, palpitations, *cardiac arrest* (with excessive use).
GI: *vomiting, nausea,* heartburn, dry mouth.
Respiratory: paradoxical bronchiolar constriction (with excessive use), cough, dry and irritated throat.
Skin: rash, hypersensitivity reactions.

INTERACTIONS
Drug-drug. *Epinephrine, other sympathomimetics:* increased risk of arrhythmias. Use together cautiously.
Levodopa: risk of arrhythmias. Avoid concomitant use.
Propranolol, other beta blockers: blocked bronchodilating effect of metaproterenol. Monitor patient carefully if used together.

EFFECTS ON DIAGNOSTIC TESTS
Drug may reduce the sensitivity of spirometry in the diagnosis of asthma.

CONTRAINDICATIONS
Contraindicated in patients with hypersensitivity to drug or its ingredients and in use during anesthesia with cyclopropane or halogenated hydrocarbon general anesthetics and in those with tachycardia or arrhythmias associated with tachycardia, peripheral or mesenteric vascular thrombosis, profound hypoxia or hypercapnia.

NURSING CONSIDERATIONS
• Use cautiously in patients with hypertension, hyperthyroidism, heart disease, diabetes, or cirrhosis and in those who are receiving cardiac glycosides.
• Be aware that patients may use tablets and aerosol concomitantly. Monitor closely for toxicity.
• Know that inhalant solution can be administered by IPPB with drug diluted in 0.9% NaCl solution or with a hand nebulizer at full strength.

☑ **Patient teaching**
• Teach patient to perform oral inhalation correctly. Give the following instructions for using a metered-dose inhaler:
–Shake canister.
–Clear nasal passages and throat.
–Breathe out, expelling as much air from lungs as possible.
–Place mouthpiece well into mouth as dose from inhaler is released, and inhale deeply.
–Hold breath for several seconds, remove mouthpiece, and exhale slowly. Allow two minutes between inhalations.
  Alternatively, inhaler may be held approximately 1″ (2 finger widths) from open mouth; inhale while dose is released.
• Inform patient that use of aerochamber with metered-dose inhalers may improve drug delivery to lungs.
• Advise patient to store drug in light-resistant container.
• Tell patient who is also using a steroid inhaler to use bronchodilator first, then wait about 5 minutes before using the steroid. This allows bronchodilator to open air passages for maximum effectiveness.
• Tell patient to wash inhaler in warm, soapy water at least once weekly; remove canister before washing.
• Warn patient to discontinue immediately if paradoxical bronchospasm occurs and to notify doctor.
• Warn patient to notify doctor if no response is derived from dosage or to request dosage adjustment.

oxtriphylline (choline salt of theophyllinate)
Choledyl SA

Pregnancy Risk Category: C

HOW SUPPLIED
Tablets: 100 mg, 200 mg
Tablets (extended-release): 400 mg, 600 mg
Syrup: 50 mg/5 ml
Elixir*: 100 mg/5 ml

ACTION
Inhibits phosphodiesterase, the enzyme that degrades cAMP. Results in relaxation of smooth muscle of the bronchial airways and pulmonary blood vessels. Oxtriphylline is equivalent to 64% anhydrous theophylline.

Route	Onset	Peak	Duration
PO	Unknown	2 hr	Unknown

INDICATIONS & DOSAGE
Acute bronchial asthma and reversible bronchospasm associated with chronic bronchitis and emphysema—
Adults (nonsmokers): 4.7 mg/kg P.O. q 8 hours.
Adults (smokers) and children 9 to 16 years: 4.7 mg/kg q 6 hours.
Children 1 to 9 years: 6.2 mg/kg P.O. q 6 hours.
  Note: If total daily maintenance dosage is established at approximately 800 to 1,200 mg, one sustained-action tablet q 12 hours may be substituted.

ADVERSE REACTIONS
CNS: *restlessness, dizziness,* headache, *insomnia,* irritability, **seizures,** muscle twitching.
CV: *palpitations, sinus tachycardia,* extrasystoles, flushing, marked hypotension, **arrhythmias.**
GI: *nausea, vomiting,* epigastric pain, diarrhea.
Respiratory: tachypnea, ***respiratory arrest.***

INTERACTIONS
Drug-drug. *Adenosine:* decreased antiar-

---

rhythmic effectiveness. Higher doses of adenosine may be necessary.

Allopurinol (high-dose): increased serum theophylline levels. Monitor for toxicity.

Barbiturates, nicotine, phenytoin, rifampin: enhanced metabolism and decreased theophylline blood levels. Monitor for decreased effect.

Beta-adrenergic blockers: antagonism. Propranolol and nadolol, especially, may cause bronchospasm in sensitive patients. Use together cautiously.

Calcium channel blockers, cimetidine, influenza virus vaccine, macrolide antibiotics (such as erythromycin), oral contraceptives, quinolone antibiotics (such as ciprofloxacin): decreased hepatic clearance of theophylline; elevated theophylline levels. Monitor for signs of toxicity.

Carbamazepine, isoniazid, loop diuretics: may increase or decrease theophylline levels. Monitor closely.

Lithium: increased renal excretion of lithium. Monitor for decreased effect.

EFFECTS ON DIAGNOSTIC TESTS
Drug may falsely elevate serum uric acid levels measured by colorimetric methods. Theophylline levels may be falsely elevated in patients using furosemide, phenylbutazone, probenecid, some cephalosporins, sulfa medications, theobromine, caffeine, tea, chocolate, cola beverages, and acetaminophen, depending on assay method used.

CONTRAINDICATIONS
Contraindicated in patients with preexisting arrhythmias, especially tachyarrhythmias, active peptic ulcer disease, poorly controlled seizure disorders, or hypersensitivity to xanthines (caffeine, theobromine).

NURSING CONSIDERATIONS
• Use cautiously in young children, in elderly patients, and in those with peptic ulceration, COPD, heart failure, cor pulmonale, renal or hepatic impairment, glaucoma, severe hypoxemia, hypertension, compromised cardiac or circulatory function, angina, acute MI, sulfite sensitivity, hyperthyroidism, and diabetes.

• Do not combine with products containing ephedrine; excessive CNS stimulation (nervousness, tremor, akathisia) may result.

• Administer drug after meals and at bedtime.

• Know that oxtriphylline is a soluble salt of theophylline. Dosage is adjusted by monitoring response, tolerance, pulmonary function, and serum theophylline levels. Ensure that theophylline concentrations range from 10 to 20 mcg/ml; toxicity has been reported with levels above 20 mcg/ml.

• Know that signs of toxicity include tachycardia, anorexia, nausea, vomiting, diarrhea, restlessness, irritability, and headache. The presence of any of these signs in patients taking theophylline warrants checking theophylline levels and adjusting dose as indicated.

• Monitor therapy carefully. Individuals metabolize theophyllines at different rates. Dosage adjustments are necessary in elderly patients; in those with heart failure, cor pulmonale, and hepatic disease; and in smokers.

• Store at 59° to 86° F (15° to 30° C). Protect elixir from light and tablets from moisture.

☑ **Patient teaching**
• Tell patient to report GI distress, palpitations, irritability, restlessness, nervousness, or insomnia; may indicate excessive CNS stimulation.

• Inform patient that tablets should not be chewed, crushed, or dissolved. Instruct him when to take drug.

• Inform elderly patients that dizziness, a common adverse reaction at the start of therapy, may occur.

pirbuterol
Maxair, Maxair Autohaler

Pregnancy Risk Category: C

HOW SUPPLIED
Inhaler: 0.2 mg/metered dose

ACTION

Relaxes bronchial smooth muscle by stimulating beta₂-adrenergic receptors.

Route	Onset	Peak	Duration
Inhalation	5 min	0.5-1 hr	5 hr

INDICATIONS & DOSAGE

Prevention and reversal of bronchospasm, asthma—

Adults and children 12 years and over: 1 or 2 inhalations (0.2 to 0.4 mg) repeated q 4 to 6 hours. Do not to exceed 12 inhalations daily.

ADVERSE REACTIONS

CNS: tremor, nervousness, dizziness, insomnia, headache, vertigo.
CV: tachycardia, palpitations, chest tightness.
EENT: dry or irritated throat, dry mouth, cough.
GI: nausea, vomiting, diarrhea.

INTERACTIONS

Drug-drug. *Beta-adrenergic blockers, propranolol:* decreased bronchodilating effects. Avoid concomitant use.
MAO inhibitors, tricyclic antidepressants: may potentiate action of beta-adrenergic agonist on vascular system. Use together cautiously.

EFFECTS ON DIAGNOSTIC TESTS

None reported.

CONTRAINDICATIONS

Contraindicated in patients with hypersensitivity to drug.

NURSING CONSIDERATIONS

• Use cautiously in patients with CV disorders, hyperthyroidism, diabetes, and seizure disorders or in those who are unusually responsive to sympathomimetic amines.

☑**Patient teaching**
• Teach patient to perform oral inhalation correctly. Give the following instructions for using a metered-dose inhaler:
–Clear nasal passages and throat.
–Breathe out, expelling as much air from lungs as possible.

–Place mouthpiece well into mouth as dose from inhaler is released, and inhale deeply.
–Hold breath for several seconds, remove mouthpiece, and exhale slowly.
• If more than 1 inhalation is ordered, tell patient to wait at least 2 minutes before repeating procedure.
• Give the following instructions for using an autohaler:
–Remove mouthpiece cover by pulling down lip on back cover. Inspect mouthpiece for foreign objects. Locate "Up" arrows and air vents.
–Hold autohaler upright so that arrows point up while raising lever until it snaps into place.
–Hold autohaler around the middle, and shake gently several times.
–Continue to hold upright and not block air vents at bottom. Exhale normally before use.
–Seal lips around mouthpiece. Inhale deeply through mouthpiece with steady, moderate force. A click will be heard and a soft puff will be felt when inhaling triggers the release of medication. Continue to take a full, deep breath.
–Take autohaler away from mouth when done inhaling. Hold breath for 10 seconds; then exhale slowly.
–Continue to hold autohaler upright while lowering lever. Lower lever after each puff. If additional puffs are ordered, wait 1 minute between each puff and repeat process.
• Tell patient who is also using a steroid inhaler to use bronchodilator first, then wait about 5 minutes before using the steroid. This allows the bronchodilator to open air passages for maximum effectiveness.
• Instruct patient who experiences increased bronchospasm after using drug to call doctor.
• Advise patient to seek medical attention if a previously effective dosage does not control symptoms; this may signify worsening of disease.

Reactions may be *common*, uncommon, ***life-threatening***, or **COMMON AND LIFE-THREATENING**.

salmeterol xinafoate
Serevent, Serevent Diskus

Pregnancy Risk Category: C

HOW SUPPLIED
Inhalation aerosol: 21 mcg/metered spray
Inhalation powder: 50 mcg/blister

ACTION
Not clearly defined. Selectively activates
beta$_2$-adrenergic receptors, which results
in bronchodilation. Also blocks the release of allergic mediators from mast cells
lining the respiratory tract.

Route	Onset	Peak	Duration
Inhalation	10-20 min	3 hr	12 hr

INDICATIONS & DOSAGE
*Long-term maintenance treatment of asth-
ma; prevention of bronchospasm in patients with nocturnal asthma or reversible
obstructive airway disease who require
regular treatment with short-acting beta
agonists—*
For inhalation aerosol—
Adults and children over 12 years: 2 inhalations q 12 hours, in the morning and
evening.
For inhalation powder—
Adults and children over 4 years: 1 inhalation q 12 hours, in the morning and
evening.
*Prevention of exercise-induced broncho-
spasm—*
For inhalation aerosol—
Adults and children 12 years and over:
2 inhalations at least 30 to 60 minutes before exercise.
For inhalation powder—
Adults and children 4 years and older:
1 inhalation at least 30 minutes before exercise.
✳ *NEW INDICATION: Maintenance treatment of bronchospasm associated with
COPD (including emphysema and chronic bronchitis)—*
Adults: 2 inhalations (42 mcg; inhalation
aerosol) q 12 hours, in the morning and
evening.

ADVERSE REACTIONS
CNS: headache, sinus headache, tremor,
nervousness, giddiness, dizziness.
CV: tachycardia, palpitations, *ventricular
arrhythmias.*
EENT: *upper respiratory infection, nasopharyngitis,* nasal cavity or sinus disorder.
GI: nausea, vomiting, diarrhea, heartburn.
Respiratory: cough, lower respiratory infection, *bronchospasm,* pharyngitis.
Other: hypersensitivity reactions (rash,
urticaria), joint and back pain, myalgia.

INTERACTIONS
Drug-drug. *Beta-adrenergic agonists,
other methylxanthines, theophylline:* possible adverse cardiac effects with excessive use. Monitor closely.
MAO inhibitors: risk of severe adverse
CV effects. Avoid use within 14 days of
MAO therapy.
Tricyclic antidepressants: risk of moderate to severe adverse CV effects. Use with
extreme caution.

EFFECTS ON DIAGNOSTIC TESTS
None reported.

CONTRAINDICATIONS
Contraindicated in patients with hypersensitivity to drug or its ingredients.

NURSING CONSIDERATIONS
• Use cautiously in patients with coronary
insufficiency, arrhythmias, hypertension,
other CV disorders, thyrotoxicosis, or
seizure disorders and in those who are unusually responsive to sympathomimetics.

☑ **Patient teaching**
• Remind patient to take drug at approximately 12-hour intervals for optimum effect and to take the drug even when feeling better.
• If patient is taking drug to prevent exercise-induced bronchospasm, tell him he
should take it 30 to 60 minutes before exercise.
Alert: Tell patient that although drug is a
beta agonist, it should not be used to treat
acute bronchospasm. He must be provid-

ed with a short-acting beta agonist (such as albuterol) to treat such exacerbations.
• Tell patient to contact doctor if the short-acting agonist no longer provides sufficient relief or if more than 4 inhalations are needed daily. This may be a sign that the asthma symptoms are worsening. Tell him not to increase the dosage of salmeterol.
• If patient is taking an inhaled corticosteroid, he should continue to use it on a regular basis. Warn patient not to take other medications without doctor's consent.
• If taking the inhalation powder (diskus device), instruct patient not to exhale into the device. The device should only be activated and used in a level, horizontal position.
• Tell patient not to use diskus device with a spacer.
• Instruct patient never to wash the mouthpiece or any part of the diskus device; it must be kept dry.

terbutaline sulfate
Brethaire, Brethine, Bricanyl

Pregnancy Risk Category: B

HOW SUPPLIED
Tablets: 2.5 mg, 5 mg
Aerosol inhaler: 200 mcg/metered spray
Injection: 1 mg/ml

ACTION
Relaxes bronchial smooth muscle by stimulating beta$_2$-adrenergic receptors. Also relaxes uterine smooth muscle.

Route	Onset	Peak	Duration
PO	30 min	2-3 hr	4-8 hr
SC	15 min	30 min	1.5-4 hr
Inhalation	5-30 min	1-2 hr	3-6 hr

INDICATIONS & DOSAGE
Bronchospasm in patients with reversible obstructive airway disease—
Adults and children 12 years and older: dosage varies with dosage form.
*Aerosol inhaler—*2 inhalations separated by 60-second interval, repeated q 4 to 6 hours.

*Injection—*0.25 mg S.C. May be repeated in 15 to 30 minutes p.r.n. Dosage should not exceed 0.5 mg in 4 hours.
*Tablets in adults—*2.5 to 5 mg P.O. q 6 hours t.i.d. during waking hours. Maximum dosage is 15 mg/day.
Tablets in children 12 to 15 years— 2.5 mg P.O. q 6 hours t.i.d. during waking hours. Maximum dosage is 7.5 mg/day.
Note: Drug is not recommended for children under 12 years.

ADVERSE REACTIONS
CNS: *nervousness, tremor, drowsiness, dizziness, headache,* weakness.
CV: *palpitations,* tachycardia, **arrhythmias,** flushing.
EENT: dry and irritated nose and throat (with inhaled form).
GI: *vomiting, nausea,* heartburn.
Respiratory: *paradoxical bronchospasm with prolonged usage,* dyspnea.
Other: hypokalemia (with high doses), diaphoresis.

INTERACTIONS
Drug-drug. *Cardiac glycosides, cyclopropane, halogenated inhalation anesthetics, levodopa:* increased risk of arrhythmias. Monitor closely, and avoid concomitant use with levodopa.
CNS stimulants: increased CNS stimulation. Avoid concomitant use.
MAO inhibitors: when given with sympathomimetics, may cause severe hypertension (hypertensive crisis). Avoid concomitant use.
Propranolol, other beta blockers: blocked bronchodilating effects of terbutaline. Avoid concomitant use.

EFFECTS ON DIAGNOSTIC TESTS
Terbutaline may reduce the sensitivity of spirometry for the diagnosis of bronchospasm.

CONTRAINDICATIONS
Contraindicated in patients with hypersensitivity to drug or sympathomimetic amines.

NURSING CONSIDERATIONS
• Use cautiously in patient with CV disor-

Reactions may be *common,* uncommon, *life-threatening,* or COMMON AND LIFE-THREATENING.

ders, hyperthyroidism, diabetes, or seizure disorders.
- Give S.C. injections in lateral deltoid area.
- Protect injection from light. Do not use if discolored.
- Know that patient may use tablets and aerosol concomitantly. Monitor closely for toxicity.

☑ **Patient teaching**
- Ensure that patient and caregivers understand why drug is necessary.
- Teach patient to perform oral inhalation correctly. Give the following instructions for using a metered-dose inhaler:
–Clear nasal passages and throat.
–Breathe out, expelling as much air from lungs as possible.
–Place mouthpiece well into mouth as dose from inhaler is released, and inhale deeply.
–Hold breath for several seconds, remove mouthpiece, and exhale slowly. Alternatively, inhaler may be held on 1″ (two finger widths) from open mouth; inhale while drug is released.
- If more than 1 inhalation is ordered, tell patient to wait at least 2 minutes before repeating procedure.
- Tell patient that use of an aerochamber may improve drug delivery to the lungs.
- Tell patient who is also using a steroid inhaler to use bronchodilator first, then wait about 5 minutes before using steroid. This allows bronchodilator to open air passages for maximum effectiveness.
- Instruct patient to wash inhaler with warm, soapy water at least once a week; remove canister before washing.
- Warn patient to discontinue drug immediately and notify doctor if paradoxical bronchospasm occurs.
- Warn patient that tolerance may develop with prolonged use.

theophylline

Immediate-release liquids: Accurbron*, Aerolate, Aquaphyllin, Asmalix*, Bronkodyl*, Elixomin*, Elixophyllin*, Lanophyllin*, Slo-Phyllin, Theoclear-80, Theolair Liquid, Theostat 80*

Immediate-release tablets and capsules: Bronkodyl, Elixophyllin, Nuelin‡, Quibron-T Dividose, Slo-Phyllin

Timed-release tablets: Constant-T, Lasma§, Quibron-T/SR, Respbid, Sustaire, Theochron, Theo-Dur, Theolair-SR, Theo-Sav, Theo-Time, T-phyl, Uniphyl, Uniphyllin Continus§

Timed-release capsules: Aerolate, Elixophyllin SR, Nuelin-SR‡, Slo-bid Gyrocaps, Slo-Phyllin, Theo-24, Theobid Duracaps, Theobid Jr. Duracaps, Theochron, Theoclear L.A., Theo-Dur Sprinkle, Theospan-SR, Theovent Long-Acting

Pregnancy Risk Category: C

HOW SUPPLIED
Tablets: 100 mg, 125 mg, 200 mg, 250 mg, 300 mg
Tablets (chewable): 100 mg
Tablets (extended-release): 100 mg, 200 mg, 250 mg, 300 mg, 400 mg, 450 mg, 500 mg
Capsules: 100 mg, 200 mg
Capsules (extended-release): 50 mg, 60 mg, 65 mg, 75 mg, 100 mg, 125 mg, 130 mg, 200 mg, 250 mg, 260 mg, 300 mg
Elixir: 27 mg/5 ml*, 50 mg/5 ml*
Oral solution: 27 mg/5 ml, 50 mg/5 ml
Syrup: 27 mg/5 ml, 50 mg/5 ml
Dextrose 5% injection: 200 mg in 50 ml or 100 ml; 400 mg in 100 ml, 250 ml, 500 ml, or 1,000 ml; 800 mg in 500 ml or 1,000 ml

ACTION
Inhibits phosphodiesterase, the enzyme that degrades cAMP. Results in relaxation

of smooth muscle of the bronchial airways and pulmonary blood vessels.

Route	Onset	Peak	Duration
PO	15-60 min	1-2 hr	Unknown
PO (extended)	15-60 min	4-7 hr	Unknown
IV	15 min	15-30 min	Unknown

INDICATIONS & DOSAGE

Extended-release preparations should not be used for the treatment of acute bronchospasm.

Oral theophylline for acute bronchospasm in patients not currently receiving theophylline—

Adults (nonsmokers): 5 mg/kg P.O., followed by 3 mg/kg q 6 hours for two doses. Maintenance dosage is 3 mg/kg q 8 hours.

Children 9 to 16 years: 5 mg/kg P.O., followed by 3 mg/kg q 4 hours for three doses. Maintenance dosage is 3 mg/kg q 6 hours.

Children 6 months to 9 years: 5 mg/kg P.O., followed by 4 mg/kg q 4 hours for three doses. Maintenance dosage is 4 mg/kg q 6 hours.

Adjust-a-dose: In otherwise healthy adult smokers, 5 mg/kg P.O., followed by 3 mg/kg q 4 hours for three doses. Maintenance dosage is 3 mg/kg q 6 hours.

In older adults and patients with cor pulmonale, 5 mg/kg P.O., followed by 2 mg/kg q 6 hours for two doses. Maintenance dosage is 2 mg/kg q 8 hours.

In adults with heart failure or liver disease, 5 mg/kg P.O., followed by 2 mg/kg q 8 hours for two doses. Maintenance dosage is 1 to 2 mg/kg q 12 hours.

Parenteral theophylline for patients not currently receiving theophylline—

Loading dose: 4.7 mg/kg I.V. slowly; then maintenance infusion.

Adults (nonsmokers): 0.55 mg/kg/hour I.V. for 12 hours, then 0.39 mg/kg/hour.

Children 9 to 16 years: 0.79 mg/kg/hour I.V. for 12 hours; then 0.63 mg/kg/hour.

Children 6 months to 9 years: 0.95 mg/kg/hour I.V. for 12 hours; then 0.79 mg/kg/hour.

Adjust-a-dose: In otherwise healthy adult smokers, 0.79 mg/kg/hour I.V. for 12 hours; then 0.63 mg/kg/hour.

In older adults and patients with cor pulmonale, 0.47 mg/kg/hour I.V. for 12 hours; then 0.24 mg/kg/hour.

In adults with heart failure or liver disease, 0.39 mg/kg/hour I.V. for 12 hours; then 0.08 to 0.16 mg/kg/hour.

Oral and parenteral theophylline for acute bronchospasm in patients currently receiving theophylline—

Adults and children: each 0.5 mg/kg I.V. or P.O. (loading dose) will increase plasma levels by 1 mcg/ml. Ideally, dose is based on current theophylline level. In emergency situations, some clinicians recommend a 2.5 mg/kg P.O. dose of rapidly absorbed form if no obvious signs of theophylline toxicity are present.

Chronic bronchospasm—

Adults and children: initial dosage is 16 mg/kg or 400 mg P.O. daily (whichever is less) given in three or four divided doses at 6- to 8-hour intervals. Alternatively, 12 mg/kg or 400 mg P.O. daily (whichever is less) in an extended-release preparation given in two or three divided doses at 8- or 12-hour intervals. Dosage may be increased as tolerated at 2- to 3-day intervals to maximum dosage as follows:

Adults and children 16 years and over: 13 mg/kg or 900 mg P.O. daily (whichever is less).

Children 12 to 16 years: 18 mg/kg P.O. daily.

Children 9 to 12 years: 20 mg/kg P.O. daily.

Children under 9 years: 24 mg/kg P.O. daily.

ADVERSE REACTIONS

CNS: *restlessness, dizziness,* headache, *insomnia,* irritability, **seizures,** muscle twitching.

CV: *palpitations, sinus tachycardia,* extrasystoles, flushing, marked hypotension, **arrhythmias.**

GI: *nausea, vomiting,* diarrhea, epigastric pain.

Respiratory: tachypnea, *respiratory arrest.*

Reactions may be *common*, uncommon, *life-threatening*, or COMMON AND LIFE-THREATENING.

INTERACTIONS

Drug-drug. *Adenosine:* decreased antiarrhythmic effectiveness. Higher doses of adenosine may be necessary.

Allopurinol, calcium channel blockers, cimetidine, disulfiram, influenza virus vaccine, interferon, macrolide antibiotics (such as erythromycin), methotrexate, oral contraceptives, quinolone antibiotics (such as ciprofloxacin): decreased hepatic clearance of theophylline; elevated theophylline levels. Monitor for signs of toxicity.

Barbiturates, nicotine, phenytoin, rifampin: enhanced metabolism and decreased theophylline blood levels. Monitor for decreased effect.

Beta-adrenergic blockers: antagonism. Propranolol and nadolol, especially, may cause bronchospasm in sensitive patients. Use together cautiously.

Carbamazepine, isoniazid, loop diuretics: may increase or decrease theophylline levels. Monitor closely.

Ephedrine, other sympathomimetics: theophylline may exhibit synergistic toxicity with these agents, predisposing patients to arrhythmias. Monitor patient closely.

Lithium: theophylline may increase lithium excretion. Monitor patient closely.

Drug-herb. *Cacao tree:* possible inhibition of theophylline metabolism. Avoid concomitant ingestion of large amounts of cocoa.

Guarana: may cause additive CNS and CV effects. Avoid concomitant use of guarana and other sources of caffeine.

Drug-food. *Any food:* accelerated release of theophylline from SR products. Tell patient to take Theo-24 on an empty stomach.

Caffeine: decreased hepatic clearance of theophylline; elevated theophylline levels. Monitor for signs of toxicity.

Drug-lifestyle. *Smoking:* increased elimination of theophylline, increasing dosage requirements. Monitor theophylline response and serum concentrations.

EFFECTS ON DIAGNOSTIC TESTS

Theophylline increases plasma levels of free fatty acids and urinary catecholamines. Depending on assay used, theophylline levels may be falsely elevated in the presence of furosemide, phenylbutazone, probenecid, theobromine, caffeine, tea, chocolate, cola beverages, and acetaminophen.

CONTRAINDICATIONS

Contraindicated in patients with active peptic ulcer, poorly controlled seizure disorders, or hypersensitivity to xanthine compounds (caffeine, theobromine).

NURSING CONSIDERATIONS

● Use cautiously in young children, infants under 1 year, and neonates; in elderly patients; and in those with COPD, cardiac failure, cor pulmonale, renal or hepatic disease, peptic ulceration, hyperthyroidism, diabetes mellitus, glaucoma, severe hypoxemia, hypertension, compromised cardiac or circulatory function, angina, acute MI, or sulfite sensitivity.

● Be careful not to confuse extended-release dosage forms with regular-release dosage forms.

● Know that drug dosage may need to be increased in cigarette smokers and in habitual marijuana smokers because smoking causes the drug to be metabolized faster.

● Give drug around-the-clock, using extended-release product at bedtime, as ordered.

● Monitor vital signs; measure and record fluid intake and output. Expected clinical effects include improved quality of pulse and respirations.

● Know that individuals metabolize xanthines at different rates; dosage is determined by monitoring response, tolerance, pulmonary function, and serum theophylline levels. Serum theophylline concentrations should range from 10 to 20 mcg/ml; toxicity has been reported with levels above 20 mcg/ml.

● Know that signs of toxicity include tachycardia, anorexia, nausea, vomiting, diarrhea, restlessness, irritability, and headache. The presence of any of these signs in patients taking theophylline warrants checking theophylline levels and adjusting dose as indicated.

---

*Liquid contains alcohol.   **May contain tartrazine.   †Canada   ‡Australia   §U.K.   ◇OTC

I.V. administration
• Use commercially available infusion solution, or mix in D_5W. Use infusion pump for continuous infusion.

✓ Patient teaching
• Supply instructions for home care and dosage schedule.
• Warn patient not to dissolve, crush, or chew extended-release products. Small children unable to swallow these can ingest (without chewing) the contents of capsules sprinkled over soft food.
• Tell patient to relieve GI symptoms by taking oral drug with full glass of water after meals, although food in stomach delays absorption.
• Warn patient to take drug regularly, as directed. Patients tend to want to take extra "breathing pills."
• Inform elderly patient that dizziness, a common adverse reaction at start of therapy, may occur.
• Warn patient to check with doctor or pharmacist about *any* other drugs used. OTC remedies may contain ephedrine in combination with theophylline salts; excessive CNS stimulation may result.

45

Expectorants and antitussives

benzonatate
codeine phosphate
(See Chapter 28, NARCOTIC AND OPIOID ANALGESICS.)
codeine sulfate
(See Chapter 28, NARCOTIC AND OPIOID ANALGESICS.)
dextromethorphan hydrobromide
diphenhydramine hydrochloride
(See Chapter 43, ANTIHISTAMINES.)
guaifenesin
hydromorphone hydrochloride
(See Chapter 28, NARCOTIC AND OPIOID ANALGESICS.)

COMBINATION PRODUCTS
Preparations are available in the following combinations:
● expectorants with decongestants or antihistamines, or both
● antitussives with decongestants or antihistamines, or both
● expectorants and antitussives
● expectorants and antitussives with decongestants or antihistamines, or both.

---

benzonatate
Tessalon

Pregnancy Risk Category: C

HOW SUPPLIED
Capsules: 100 mg

ACTION
Suppresses the cough reflex by direct action on the cough center in the medulla and through an anesthetic action on stretch receptors of vagal afferent fibers in the respiratory passages, lungs and pleura.

Route	Onset	Peak	Duration
PO	15-20 min	Unknown	3-8 hr

INDICATIONS & DOSAGE
Symptomatic relief of cough—
Adults and children over 10 years:
100 mg P.O. t.i.d.; up to 600 mg daily may be needed.
Children 10 years and younger: 8 mg/kg daily in three to six divided doses.

ADVERSE REACTIONS
CNS: dizziness, headache, sedation.
EENT: nasal congestion, burning sensation in eyes.
GI: nausea, constipation, GI upset.
Skin: hypersensitivity reactions (rash).
Other: chills.

INTERACTIONS
None significant.

EFFECTS ON DIAGNOSTIC TESTS
None reported.

CONTRAINDICATIONS
Contraindicated in patients hypersensitive to drug or related compounds.

NURSING CONSIDERATIONS
● Use cautiously in patients hypersensitive to PABA anesthetics (procaine, tetracaine) because cross-sensitivity reactions may occur.
● Do not use benzonatate when cough is a valuable diagnostic sign or is beneficial (as after thoracic surgery).
● Monitor cough type and frequency.
● Use with percussion and chest vibration.

☑ **Patient teaching**
● Warn patient not to chew capsules or dissolve in mouth. Produces either local anesthesia that may result in aspiration or CNS stimulation that may cause restlessness, tremor, and seizures.
● Instruct patient to report adverse reactions.
Alert: Ensure that patient understands that persistent cough may indicate a serious condition and that he should contact a doctor if cough lasts longer than 1 week, recurs frequently, or is associated with high fever, rash, or severe headache.

---

dextromethorphan hydrobromide

Balminil D.M. ◇, Benylin DM ◇, Broncho-Grippol-DM†, Buckley's Mixture, Children's Hold ◇, Delsym, DM Syrup ◇, Hold ◇, Koffex†, Mediquell ◇, Neo-DM†, Ornex-DM 15 ◇, Ornex-DM 30 ◇, Pertussin Cough Suppressant ◇, Pertussin CS ◇, Pertussin ES ◇, Robidex†, Robitussin Pediatric ◇, Sedatuss†, St. Joseph Cough Suppressant for Children ◇, Sucrets Cough Control Formula ◇, Trocal ◇, Vicks Formula 44 Pediatric Formula ◇

More commonly available in combination products, such as:
Anti-Tuss DM Expectorant ◇, Benylin Expectorant ◇, Cheracol D Cough ◇, Extra Action Cough ◇, Glycotuss dM ◇, Guiamid D.M. Liquid ◇, Guiatuss-DM ◇, Halotussin-DM Expectorant ◇, Kolephrin GG/DM ◇, Mytussin DM ◇, Naldecon Senior DX ◇, Pertussin CS ◇, Rhinosyn-DMX Expectorant ◇, Robitussin-DM ◇, Scot-Tussin DM Cough Chasers ◇, Silexin Cough ◇, Tolu-Sed DM ◇, Tuss-DM ◇, Unproco ◇, Vicks Pediatric Formula 44e ◇

Pregnancy Risk Category: C

HOW SUPPLIED
Liquid (extended-release): 30 mg/5 ml ◇
Lozenges: 5 mg ◇, 7.5 mg ◇
Solution: 3.5 mg/5 ml, 5 mg/5 ml* ◇, 7.5 mg/5 ml ◇, 10 mg/5 ml* ◇, 15 mg/5 ml* ◇, 15 mg/15 ml* ◇, 12.5 mg/5 ml

ACTION
An antitussive that suppresses the cough reflex by direct action on the cough center in the medulla.

Route	Onset	Peak	Duration
PO	< 0.5 hr	Unknown	3-6 hr

INDICATIONS & DOSAGE
Nonproductive cough—
Adults and children 12 years and over: 10 to 20 mg P.O. q 4 hours, or 30 mg q 6 to 8 hours. Or, 60 mg extended-release liquid b.i.d. Maximum dosage is 120 mg daily.
Children 6 to 12 years: 5 to 10 mg P.O. q 4 hours, or 15 mg q 6 to 8 hours. Or, 30 mg extended-release liquid b.i.d. Maximum dosage is 60 mg daily.
Children 2 to 6 years: 2.5 to 5 mg P.O. q 4 hours, or 7.5 mg q 6 to 8 hours. Or, 15 mg extended-release liquid b.i.d. Maximum dosage is 30 mg daily.
Children under 2 years: dosages must be individualized.

ADVERSE REACTIONS
CNS: drowsiness, dizziness.
GI: nausea, vomiting, stomach pain.

INTERACTIONS
Drug-drug. *MAO inhibitors:* risk of hypotension, coma, hyperpyrexia, and death. Avoid concomitant use.
Selegiline: risk of confusion, coma, hyperpyrexia. Avoid concurrent use.
Drug-herb. *Parsley:* may promote or produce serotonin syndrome. Avoid concomitant use.

EFFECTS ON DIAGNOSTIC TESTS
None reported.

CONTRAINDICATIONS
Contraindicated in patients currently taking MAO inhibitors or within 2 weeks of discontinuing MAO inhibitors.

NURSING CONSIDERATIONS
• Use with caution in atopic children, sedated or debilitated patients, and patients confined to the supine position. Also use cautiously in patients with sensitivity to aspirin or tartrazine dyes.
• Do not use dextromethorphan when cough is a valuable diagnostic sign or is beneficial (as after thoracic surgery).
• Know that dextromethorphan 15 to 30 mg is equivalent to 8 to 15 mg codeine as an antitussive.
• Be aware that drug produces no analge-

sia or addiction and little or no CNS depression.
• Use drug with chest percussion and vibration.
• Monitor cough type and frequency.

✓ Patient teaching
• Instruct patient to take exactly as prescribed.
• Tell patient to report adverse reactions.
Alert: Ensure that patient understands that persistent cough may indicate a serious condition and that he should contact a doctor if cough lasts longer than 1 week, recurs frequently, or is associated with high fever, rash, or severe headache.

guaifenesin (glyceryl guaiacolate)
Anti-Tuss* ◊, Balminil Expectorant†, Breonesin ◊, Fenesin, Gee-Gee ◊, GG-CEN* ◊, Glyate* ◊, Glycotuss ◊, Glytuss ◊, Guiatuss* ◊, Halotussin, Humibid L.A., Humibid Sprinkle, Hytuss* ◊, Hytuss-2X ◊, Naldecon Senior EX ◊, Resyl† ◊, Robitussin* ◊, Scot-Tussin Expectorant ◊, Uni-tussin* ◊

Pregnancy Risk Category: C

HOW SUPPLIED
Tablets: 100 mg ◊, 200 mg ◊
Tablets (extended-release): 600 mg
Capsules: 200 mg ◊
Capsules (extended-release): 300 mg
Solution: 100 mg/5 ml* ◊, 200 mg/5 ml ◊

ACTION
Increases production of respiratory tract fluids to help liquefy and reduce the viscosity of tenacious secretions.

Route	Onset	Peak	Duration
PO	Unknown	Unknown	Unknown

INDICATIONS & DOSAGE
Expectorant—
Adults and children 12 years and over: 200 to 400 mg P.O. q 4 hours, or 600 to 1,200 mg extended-release capsules or tablets q 12 hours. Maximum dosage is 2,400 mg daily.
Children 6 to 12 years: 100 to 200 mg P.O. q 4 hours. Maximum dosage is 1,200 mg daily.
Children 2 to 6 years: 50 to 100 mg P.O. q 4 hours. Maximum dosage is 600 mg daily.

ADVERSE REACTIONS
CNS: dizziness, headache.
GI: vomiting, nausea (with large doses).
Skin: rash.

INTERACTIONS
None significant.

EFFECTS ON DIAGNOSTIC TESTS
Drug may cause color interference with tests for 5-hydroxyindoleacetic acid and vanillylmandelic acid.

CONTRAINDICATIONS
Contraindicated in patients hypersensitive to drug.

NURSING CONSIDERATIONS
• Be aware that drug is used to liquefy thick, tenacious sputum. There is evidence that guaifenesin is effective as an expectorant but no evidence to support its role as an antitussive.
• Monitor cough type and frequency.

✓ Patient teaching
Alert: Ensure that patient understands that persistent cough may indicate a serious condition and that he should contact a doctor if cough lasts longer than 1 week, recurs frequently, or is associated with high fever, rash, or severe headache.
• Inform patient that drug should not be used for chronic or persistent cough such as that occurring with smoking, asthma, chronic bronchitis, or emphysema.
• Advise patient to take each dose with one glass of water; increasing fluid intake may prove beneficial.
• Encourage deep-breathing exercises.

46

Miscellaneous respiratory drugs

acetylcysteine
beclomethasone dipropionate
beractant
budesonide
calfactant
cromolyn sodium
dexamethasone sodium
   phosphate inhalation
dornase alfa
epoprostenol sodium
flunisolide
fluticasone propionate
montelukast sodium
nedocromil sodium
palivizumab
triamcinolone acetonide
zafirlukast
zileuton

COMBINATION PRODUCTS
None.

---

acetylcysteine
Mucomyst, Mucomyst-10, Mucosil-10, Mucosil-20, Parvolex†‡

Pregnancy Risk Category: B

HOW SUPPLIED
Solution: 10%, 20%
Injection: 200 mg/ml‡

ACTION
A mucolytic that reduces the viscosity of pulmonary secretions by splitting disulfide linkages between mucoprotein molecular complexes. Also restores liver stores of glutathione to treat acetaminophen toxicity.

Route	Onset	Peak	Duration
PO, IV, inhalation	Unknown	Unknown	Unknown

INDICATIONS & DOSAGE
Adjuvant therapy for abnormal viscid or inspissated mucus secretions in patients with pneumonia, bronchitis, bronchiectasis, primary amyloidosis of the lung, tu-

berculosis, cystic fibrosis, emphysema, atelectasis (adjunct), pulmonary complications of thoracic surgery, and CV surgery—
Adults and children: 1 to 2 ml 10% or 20% solution by direct instillation into trachea as often as q hour; or 1 to 10 ml of 20% solution or 2 to 20 ml of 10% solution by nebulization q 2 to 6 hours p.r.n.
Acetaminophen toxicity—
P.O.—
Adults and children: initially, 140 mg/kg P.O., followed by 70 mg/kg P.O. q 4 hours for 17 doses.
I.V.‡—
Adults: dilute initial dose (150 mg/kg) in 200 ml of D_5W and infuse over 15 minutes. Dilute second dose of 50 mg/kg in 500 ml of D_5W and give over 4 hours. Dilute final dose of 100 mg/kg in 1,000 ml of D_5W and infuse over 16 hours.

ADVERSE REACTIONS
CV: tachycardia, hypotension, hypertension.
EENT: *rhinorrhea.*
GI: *stomatitis, nausea, vomiting.*
Respiratory: ***bronchospasm*** (especially in asthmatic patients).
Skin: rash.
Other: fever, clamminess, chest tightness, ***angioedema.***

INTERACTIONS
Drug-drug. *Activated charcoal:* limits acetylcysteine's effectiveness. Avoid concomitant use in treating acetaminophen toxicity or lavage before administering acetylcysteine.

EFFECTS ON DIAGNOSTIC TESTS
None reported.

CONTRAINDICATIONS
Contraindicated in patients hypersensitive to drug.

NURSING CONSIDERATIONS
• Use cautiously in elderly or debilitated

---

patients with severe respiratory insufficiency.
• Use plastic, glass, stainless steel, or another nonreactive metal when administering by nebulization. Hand-bulb nebulizers are not recommended because output is too small and particle size too large.
• Drug is physically or chemically incompatible with tetracyclines, erythromycin lactobionate, amphotericin B, and ampicillin sodium. If administered by aerosol inhalation, these drugs should be nebulized separately. Iodized oil, trypsin, and hydrogen peroxide are physically incompatible with acetylcysteine; don't add to nebulizer.
• Monitor cough type and frequency.
• After opening, store in refrigerator; use within 96 hours.
Alert: Acetylcysteine is administered to treat acetaminophen overdose within 24 hours after ingestion. Start treatment immediately as prescribed; do not wait for results of acetaminophen blood levels.
• When used orally to treat acetaminophen overdose, dilute oral doses with cola, fruit juice, or water before administering. Dilute the 20% solution to a concentration of 5% (add 3 ml of diluent to each ml of acetylcysteine). If patient vomits within 1 hour of receiving loading or maintenance dose, repeat dose.

◐ I.V. administration‡
• To prepare I.V. infusion, dilute calculated dose in D_5W.

☑ Patient teaching
• Warn patient that drug may have a foul taste or smell that some patients find distressing.
• For maximum effect, instruct patient to clear his airway by coughing before aerosol administration.

---

beclomethasone dipropionate
Beclodisk†, Becloforte Inhaler‡, Beclovent, Beclovent Rotacaps†, Vanceril

Pregnancy Risk Category: C

HOW SUPPLIED
Oral inhalation aerosol: 42 mcg/metered spray, 50 mcg/metered spray‡

ACTION
Unknown. May decrease inflammation by decreasing the number and activity of inflammatory cells, inhibiting bronchoconstrictor mechanisms producing direct smooth muscle relaxation, and decreasing airway hyperresponsiveness.

Route	Onset	Peak	Duration
Inhalation	1-4 wk	Unknown	Unknown

INDICATIONS & DOSAGE
Chronic asthma—
Adults and children 12 years and over: 2 inhalations t.i.d. or q.i.d. or 4 inhalations b.i.d. Maximum dosage is 20 inhalations daily (840 mcg).
Children 6 to 12 years: 1 to 2 inhalations t.i.d. or q.i.d. or 2 to 4 inhalations b.i.d. Maximum dosage is 10 inhalations daily (420 mcg).

ADVERSE REACTIONS
EENT: *hoarseness,* fungal infection of throat, *throat irritation.*
GI: dry mouth, *fungal infection of mouth.*
Respiratory: *bronchospasm,* wheezing, cough.
Skin: hypersensitivity reactions (urticaria, rash).
Other: *angioedema,* suppression of hypothalamic-pituitary-adrenal function, *adrenal insufficiency,* facial edema.

INTERACTIONS
None significant.

EFFECTS ON DIAGNOSTIC TESTS
None reported.

CONTRAINDICATIONS
Contraindicated in patients with status asthmaticus or hypersensitivity to drug or its ingredients (fluorocarbons, oleic acid).

NURSING CONSIDERATIONS
• Use with extreme caution, if at all, in patients with tuberculosis, fungal or bacterial infections, ocular herpes simplex, or systemic viral infections.

• Do not use drug in patients with asthma controlled by bronchodilators or other noncorticosteroids alone or for those with nonasthmatic bronchial diseases.

• Use with caution in patients receiving systemic corticosteroid therapy.

• Be aware a spacer device may help ensure delivery of the proper dose and decrease local (oral) adverse effects.

• Check mucous membranes frequently for signs of fungal infection.

• Keep in mind that during times of stress (trauma, surgery, or infection) systemic corticosteroids may be needed to prevent adrenal insufficiency in previously steroid-dependent patients.

• Know that periodic measurement of growth and development may be necessary during high-dose or prolonged therapy in children.

Alert: Taper oral glucocorticoid therapy slowly as ordered. Acute adrenal insufficiency and death have occurred in asthmatics who changed abruptly from oral corticosteroids to beclomethasone.

☑ **Patient teaching**

• Inform patient that drug doesn't provide relief for acute asthma attacks.

• Tell patient requiring a bronchodilator to use it several minutes before beclomethasone.

• Instruct patient to carry a medical identification card indicating his need for supplemental systemic glucocorticoids during stress.

• If using a metered-dose inhaler, instruct patient to shake canister well before use.

• Advise patient to allow 1 minute to elapse before taking subsequent puffs of medication and to hold his breath for a few seconds to enhance action of drug.

• Instruct patient to contact his doctor if response to therapy decreases or if symptoms don't improve within 3 weeks; dosage may need to be adjusted. Tell him not to exceed recommended dosage on his own.

• Tell patient to keep inhaler clean and unobstructed. He should wash it with warm water and dry it thoroughly.

• Advise patient to prevent oral fungal infections by gargling or rinsing mouth with

water after each use, but not to swallow the water.

• Tell patient to report symptoms associated with corticosteroid withdrawal, including fatigue, weakness, arthralgia, orthostatic hypotension, and dyspnea.

• Instruct patient to store medication between 59° and 86° F (15° and 30° C). Advise patient to ensure delivery of proper dose by gently warming canister to room temperature before using.

---

beractant (natural lung surfactant)
Survanta

Pregnancy Risk Category: NR

HOW SUPPLIED
Suspension for intratracheal instillation: 25 mg/ml

ACTION
Lowers the surface tension on alveolar surfaces during respiration and stabilizes the alveoli against collapse. An extract of bovine lung containing neutral lipids, fatty acids, surfactant-associated proteins, and phospholipids, which mimics naturally occurring surfactant; palmitic acid, tripalmitin, and colfosceril palmitate are added to standardize the solution's composition.

Route	Onset	Peak	Duration
Intratra-cheal	0.5-2 hr	Unknown	2-3 days

INDICATIONS & DOSAGE
Prevention of respiratory distress syndrome (RDS), also known as hyaline membrane disease, in premature neonates weighing 1,250 g (2 lb, 12 oz) or less at birth or having symptoms consistent with surfactant deficiency—
Neonates: 4 ml/kg intratracheally. Divide each dose into four quarter-doses and administer each quarter-dose with infant in a different position to ensure homogenous distribution of drug; between quarter-doses, use a handheld resuscitation bag at a rate of 60 breaths/minute and sufficient oxygen to prevent cyanosis. Give drug as

soon as possible, preferably within 15 minutes of birth. Repeat in 6 hours if respiratory distress continues. Give no more than four doses in 48 hours.

Rescue treatment of RDS in premature infants—

Neonates: 4 ml/kg intratracheally; before administering, increase ventilator rate to 60 breaths/minute with an inspiratory time of 0.5 second and a fraction of inspired oxygen of 1. Divide each dose into four quarter-doses and administer each quarter-dose with infant in a different position to ensure homogenous distribution of drug; between quarter-doses, continue mechanical ventilation for at least 30 seconds or until stable. Give dose as soon as RDS is confirmed by X-ray, preferably within 8 hours of birth. Repeat in 6 hours if respiratory distress continues. Give no more than four doses in 48 hours.

ADVERSE REACTIONS
CV: *transient bradycardia,* vasoconstriction, hypotension.
Hematologic: decreased oxygen saturation, hypocapnia, hypercapnia.
Other: endotracheal tube reflux or blockage, pallor, *apnea.*

INTERACTIONS
None significant.

EFFECTS ON DIAGNOSTIC TESTS
None reported.

CONTRAINDICATIONS
No known contraindications.

NURSING CONSIDERATIONS
• Beractant should be administered only by personnel experienced in the care of clinically unstable premature neonates. Such personnel should have knowledge of neonatal intubation and airway management.
• Accurate determination of weight is essential to proper measurement of dosage.
• Continuously monitor neonate before, during, and after beractant administration. The endotracheal tube may be suctioned before giving drug; allow neonate to stabilize before proceeding with administration.

• Refrigerate at 36° to 46° F (2° to 8° C). Warm before administration by allowing drug to stand at room temperature for at least 20 minutes or by holding in hand for at least 8 minutes. Do not use artificial warming methods. Unopened vials that have been warmed to room temperature may be returned to the refrigerator within 8 hours; however, warm and return drug to the refrigerator only once. Vials are for single use only—discard unused drug.
• Beractant does not require sonication or reconstitution before use. Inspect contents before giving; ensure that the color is off-white to light brown and the contents are uniform. If settling occurs, swirl vial gently; do not shake. Some foaming is normal.
• Use a large-bore needle (20G or larger) to draw up drug; do not use a filter. Administer drug using a #5 French end-hole catheter. Premeasure and shorten catheter before use. Fill catheter with beractant and discard excess drug so that only total dose to be given remains in the syringe. Insert catheter into neonate's endotracheal tube; make sure catheter tip protrudes just beyond end of tube above neonate's carina. Do not instill drug into a mainstem bronchus.
• Homogeneous distribution of drug is important. In clinical trials, each dose of drug was given in four quarter-doses, with patient positioned differently after each administration. Each quarter-dose was given over 2 to 3 seconds; the catheter was removed and patient ventilated between quarter-doses. With the head and body inclined slightly downward, the first quarter-dose was given with the head turned to the right; the second quarter-dose, with the head turned to the left. Then the head and body were inclined slightly upward; the third quarter-dose was given with the head turned to the right; the fourth quarter-dose, with the head turned to the left.
• Immediately after administration, moist breath sounds and crackles can occur. *Do not* suction the neonate for 1 hour unless other signs of airway obstruction are evident.
• Continuous monitoring of ECG and transcutaneous oxygen saturation are es-

sential; frequent arterial blood pressure monitoring and frequent arterial blood gas sampling are highly desirable.

• Transient bradycardia and oxygen desaturation are common after dosing.

Alert: Know that beractant can rapidly affect oxygenation and lung compliance. Peak ventilator inspiratory pressures may need to be adjusted if chest expansion improves substantially after drug administration. Notify doctor and adjust immediately as directed because lung overdistention and fatal pulmonary air leakage may result.

• Know that audiovisual materials that describe dosage and administration procedures are available from the manufacturer.

☑**Patient teaching**
• Inform parents of need for drug and explain drug action and administration.
• Encourage parents to ask questions and address any concerns raised by them.

---

budesonide
Pulmicort Turbuhaler

Pregnancy Risk Category: C

HOW SUPPLIED
Dry powder inhaler: 200 mcg/dose

ACTION
Anti-inflammatory corticosteroid that exhibits potent glucocorticoid activity and weak mineralocorticoid activity. The exact mechanism of the corticosteroids is not known, but they have been shown to have a wide range of inhibitory activities against cell types such as mast cells and macrophages and mediators such as leukotrienes involved in allergic and nonallergic inflammation.

Route	Onset	Peak	Duration
Inhalation	24 hr	1-2 wk	Unknown

INDICATIONS & DOSAGE
Prophylactic therapy in the maintenance treatment of asthma—
In all patients, use lowest effective dose after stabilization of asthma has occurred.
Adults previously on bronchodilators

alone: initially, inhaled dose of 200 to 400 mcg b.i.d. to maximum of 400 mcg b.i.d.
Adults previously on inhaled corticosteroids: initially, inhaled dose of 200 to 400 mcg b.i.d. to maximum of 800 mcg b.i.d.
Adults previously on oral corticosteroids: initially, inhaled dose of 400 to 800 mcg b.i.d. to maximum of 800 mcg b.i.d.
Children over 6 years previously on bronchodilators alone or inhaled corticosteroids: initially, inhaled dose of 200 mcg b.i.d. to maximum of 400 mcg b.i.d.
Children over 6 years previously on oral corticosteroids: highest recommended dose is 400 mcg b.i.d.

ADVERSE REACTIONS
CNS: *headache,* asthenia, insomnia, syncope, hypertonia.
EENT: *sinusitis, pharyngitis,* rhinitis, voice alteration.
GI: oral candidiasis, dyspepsia, gastroenteritis, nausea, dry mouth, taste perversion, vomiting, abdominal pain.
Musculoskeletal: pain, back pain, fractures, myalgias.
Respiratory: *respiratory infections,* increased cough, **bronchospasm.**
Other: weight gain, ecchymosis, flulike symptoms, fever, **hypersensitivity reactions.**

INTERACTIONS
Drug-drug. *Ketoconazole:* may inhibit metabolism of budesonide and increase plasma levels. Monitor patient.

EFFECTS ON DIAGNOSTIC TESTS
None reported.

CONTRAINDICATIONS
Contraindicated in patients with hypersensitivity to drug or in the treatment of status asthmaticus or other acute episodes of asthma.

NURSING CONSIDERATIONS
• Use cautiously, if at all, in patients with active or quiescent tuberculosis of the respiratory tract; untreated systemic fungal,

bacterial, viral, or parasitic infections; or ocular herpes simplex.

• When transferring from systemic steroid to budesonide, use caution and gradually decrease steroid dose to prevent adrenal insufficiency.

• Drug does not replace the need for systemic corticosteroid therapy in some situations.

• If bronchospasm occurs after using the budesonide, stop therapy and treat with a bronchodilator.

Note: Improved lung function has been observed within 24 hours of initiating treatment with budesonide, although the maximum benefit may not be achieved for 1 to 2 weeks or longer.

• Watch for *Candida* infections of the mouth or pharynx.

• Corticosteroid use may increase the risk of developing serious or fatal infections in individuals exposed to viral illnesses such as chickenpox or measles.

• In rare cases, inhaled steroids have been associated with increased intraocular pressure and cataract development. If local irritation occurs with use, the product should be discontinued.

☑ **Patient teaching**

• Tell patient that the budesonide inhaler is not a bronchodilator and is not intended to treat acute episodes of asthma.

• Instruct patient to use the inhaler at regular intervals as follows because effectiveness depends on twice-daily administration on a regular basis:

–Pulmicort Turbuhaler must be in the upright position (mouthpiece on top) during the loading in order to provide the correct dose.

–Turbuhaler must be primed when the unit is used for the very first time. To prime, hold the unit in an upright position and turn the brown grip fully to the right, then fully to the left until it clicks. Repeat.

–To load the first dose, turn grip to the right and fully to the left until it clicks.

–On subsequent doses, load in the upright position, turn the brown grip fully to the right and then the left until it clicks.

–During inhalation, Turbuhaler must be in the upright or horizontal position.

–Do not shake inhaler.

–Place mouthpiece between lips and inhale forcefully and deeply.

–Tell patient that he may not taste the medication but this does not mean it is not effective.

–Tell patient not to exhale through the Turbuhaler.

–Due to the small volume of powder, patient may not taste or sense the presence of medication entering the lungs.

–Rinse the mouth with water without swallowing after each dose to decrease the risk of developing oral candidiasis.

–When there are 20 doses remaining in the Turbuhaler, a red mark appears in the indicator window.

–Do not use with a spacer device.

–Do not chew or bite the mouthpiece.

–Replace mouthpiece cover after use and keep it clean and dry at all times.

• Know that improvement in asthma control may be seen within 24 hours, although the maximum benefit may not be evident for 1 to 2 weeks. If symptoms worsen during this time, patient should contact doctor.

• Advise patient to avoid exposure to chickenpox or measles and contact doctor if there is exposure.

• Instruct patient to carry medical identification indicating need for supplementary steroids during periods of stress or an asthma attack.

• Tell patient to read and follow the patient information leaflet contained in the package.

▼ *NEW DRUG*

calfactant
Infasurf

Pregnancy Risk Category: NR

HOW SUPPLIED
Intratracheal suspension: 35 mg phospholipids and 0.65 mg proteins/ml; 6-ml vial

ACTION
A nonpyrogenic lung surfactant that mod-

ifies alveolar surface tension, thereby stabilizing the alveoli.

Route	Onset	Peak	Duration
Intratracheal	24-48 hr	Unknown	Unknown

INDICATIONS & DOSAGE

Prevention of respiratory distress syndrome (RDS) in premature infants under 29 weeks gestational age at high risk for RDS; treatment of infants under 72 hours of age who develop RDS (confirmed by clinical and radiologic findings) and require endotracheal intubation—
Newborns: 3 ml/kg body weight at birth intratracheally, administered in two aliquots of 1.5 ml/kg each, q 12 hours for total of three doses.

ADVERSE REACTIONS
CV: BRADYCARDIA.
Respiratory: AIRWAY OBSTRUCTION, APNEA, *hypoventilation.*
Other: *cyanosis, reflux of drug into endotracheal tube,* dislodgement of endotracheal tube.

INTERACTIONS
None reported.

EFFECTS ON DIAGNOSTIC TESTS
None reported.

CONTRAINDICATIONS
None known.

NURSING CONSIDERATIONS
• Know that drug should be administered under supervision of doctors experienced in the acute care of newborn infants with respiratory failure who require intubation.
• Store drug at 36° to 46° F (2° to 8° C). It is not necessary to warm drug before use.
• Be aware that unopened, unused vials that have warmed to room temperature can be returned to refrigerated storage within 24 hours for future use. Avoid repeated warming to room temperature.
• Know that suspension settles during storage. Gentle swirling or agitation of the vial is often necessary for redispersion. *Do not shake.* Visible flecks in the suspension and foaming at the surface are normal.
• Drug is intended for intratracheal use only; administer to infants for prophylaxis of RDS as soon as possible after birth, preferably within 30 minutes.
• Withdraw dose into a syringe from single-use vial using a 20G or larger needle; avoid excessive foaming.
• Administer through a side-port adapter into the endotracheal tube. Two medical personnel should be present during dosing. Administer dose in two aliquots of 1.5 ml/kg each. After each aliquot is instilled, infant should be positioned on either side. Administration is made while ventilation is continued over 20 to 30 breaths for each aliquot, with small bursts timed only during the inspiratory cycles. Evaluate respiratory status and reposition infant between each aliquot.
• Monitor for reflux of drug into endotracheal tube, cyanosis, bradycardia, or airway obstruction during the dosing procedure. If these occur, stop drug and take appropriate measures to stabilize infant. After infant is stable, resume dosing with appropriate monitoring.
• After giving drug, carefully monitor infant so that oxygen therapy and ventilatory support can be modified in response to improvements in oxygenation and lung compliance.
• Know that each single-use vial should be entered only once; discard unused material after use.

☑ **Patient teaching**
• Explain to parents reason for use of medication for the prevention and treatment of RDS.
• Notify parents that although infant may improve rapidly after treatment, he may continue to require intubation and mechanical ventilation.
• Notify parents of the potential adverse effects of drug, including bradycardia, reflux into endotracheal tube, airway obstruction, cyanosis, dislodgment of endotracheal tube, and hypoventilation.
• Reassure parents that infant will be carefully monitored.

---

cromolyn sodium (sodium cromoglycate)
Crolom, Gastrocrom, Intal, Intal Nebulizer Solution, Intal Spray Aerosol, Nasalcrom, Rynacrom†

Pregnancy Risk Category: B

HOW SUPPLIED
Capsules (for oral solution): 100 mg
Aerosol: 800 mcg/metered spray
Nasal solution: 5.2 mg/metered spray (40 mg/ml)
Solution (for nebulization): 20 mg/2 ml
Ophthalmic solution: 4%

ACTION
Inhibits the degranulation of sensitized mast cells that occurs after a patient's exposure to specific antigens. Also inhibits release of histamine and slow-reacting substance of anaphylaxis.

Route	Onset	Peak	Duration
PO, inhalation, intranasal, ophthalmic	Unknown	Unknown	Unknown

INDICATIONS & DOSAGE
Mild to moderate persistent asthma—
Adults and children 5 years and over: 2 metered sprays using inhaler q.i.d. at regular intervals. Alternatively, 20 mg via nebulization q.i.d. at regular intervals.
Prevention and treatment of seasonal and perennial allergic rhinitis—
Adults and children over 6 years: 1 spray in each nostril t.i.d. or q.i.d. Maximal administration is six times daily.
Prevention of exercise-induced bronchospasm—
Adults and children 5 years or over: 2 metered sprays inhaled no more than 1 hour before anticipated exercise.
Conjunctivitis—
Adults and children 4 years and older: 1 to 2 drops in each eye four to six times daily at regular intervals.
Systemic mastocytosis—
Adults and children over 12 years: 200 mg P.O. q.i.d. before meals and h.s.
Children 2 to 12 years: 100 mg P.O. q.i.d. 30 minutes before meals or h.s.

ADVERSE REACTIONS
CNS: dizziness, headache.
EENT: *irritated throat and trachea,* lacrimation, nasal congestion, pharyngeal irritation, *sneezing,* nasal burning and irritation, epistaxis.
GI: nausea, esophagitis, abdominal pain, *bad taste in mouth.*
GU: dysuria, urinary frequency.
Respiratory: *bronchospasm* (after inhalation of dry powder), *cough,* wheezing, eosinophilic pneumonia.
Skin: rash, urticaria.
Other: joint swelling and pain, swollen parotid gland, *angioedema.*

INTERACTIONS
None significant.

EFFECTS ON DIAGNOSTIC TESTS
None reported.

CONTRAINDICATIONS
Contraindicated in patients experiencing acute asthma attacks and status asthmaticus and in those hypersensitive to drug.

NURSING CONSIDERATIONS
• Administer with caution in children. Use of cromolyn oral inhalation solution is *not* recommended in children under 2 years; cromolyn powder or aerosol for oral inhalation, not recommended in children under 5 years; cromolyn ophthalmic solution, not recommended in children under 4 years; and cromolyn nasal solution, not recommended in children under 6 years.
• Use inhalation form cautiously in patients with coronary artery disease or a history of arrhythmias.
• Know that drug (except for ophthalmic solution) should be used only when acute episode of asthma has been controlled, airway is cleared, and the patient can breathe independently.
• Be aware that oral cromolyn sodium should be used in full-term neonates and infants *only* for a severe, incapacitating disease when benefits clearly outweigh the risks.
• Dissolve powder in capsules for oral dose in hot water, and further dilute with

cold water before ingestion. Do not mix with fruit juice, milk, or food.
• Discontinue drug if eosinophilic pneumonia (indicated by eosinophilia and infiltrates on chest X-ray) develops.
• Watch for recurrence of asthmatic symptoms when dosage is decreased, especially when corticosteroids are also used.

☑ **Patient teaching**
• Instruct patient how to administer form of drug prescribed.
• Instruct patient that full effects of drug may not be noted for 4 weeks.
• Tell patient that esophagitis may be relieved by antacids or a glass of milk.
• Warn patient using nasal solution that stinging or sneezing may occur.

---

dexamethasone sodium phosphate inhalation
Dexacort Phosphate Respihaler

Pregnancy Risk Category: C

HOW SUPPLIED
Inhalation aerosol: 100 mcg dexamethasone/metered spray

ACTION
Unknown. May decrease inflammation through inhibitory activities against cell types such as mast cells and macrophages and mediators such as leukotrienes.

Route	Onset	Peak	Duration
Inhalation	1-4 wk	Unknown	Unknown

INDICATIONS & DOSAGE
Persistent asthma—
Adults: initially, 3 inhalations t.i.d. or q.i.d. Decreased as needed and tolerated; most patients respond to 2 inhalations b.i.d. Maximum dosage is 12 inhalations daily. No more than 3 inhalations should be given per dose.
Children: 2 inhalations t.i.d. or q.i.d. Decreased as needed and tolerated; most patients respond to 2 inhalations b.i.d. Maximum dosage is 8 inhalations daily or 2 inhalations per dose.

ADVERSE REACTIONS
EENT: *hoarseness,* fungal infection of throat, *throat irritation.*
GI: dry mouth, *fungal infection of mouth.*
Other: rash, wheezing, facial edema.

INTERACTIONS
None significant.

EFFECTS ON DIAGNOSTIC TESTS
None reported.

CONTRAINDICATIONS
Contraindicated in patients with status asthmaticus, persistent positive sputum cultures for *Candida albicans,* systemic fungal infections, or hypersensitivity to drug or its ingredients (fluorocarbons, ethanol).

NURSING CONSIDERATIONS
• Do not use drug in patients with asthma controlled by bronchodilators or other noncorticosteroids alone or for those with nonasthmatic bronchial diseases.
• Use cautiously in patients with ocular herpes simplex, nonspecific ulcerative colitis, diverticulitis, fresh intestinal anastomoses, peptic ulcer, renal insufficiency, hypertension, osteoporosis, and myasthenia gravis.
• Know that spacer device may help ensure delivery of proper dose and decrease local (oral) adverse effects.
• Check mucous membranes frequently for signs of fungal infection.
• Monitor patient for adverse effects. With prolonged use of high doses, systemic effects are likely because up to 50% of a dose is absorbed.
• Conduct periodic measurements of growth and development during high-dose or prolonged therapy in children.
• Know that during times of stress (trauma, surgery, or infection), systemic corticosteroids may be needed to prevent adrenal insufficiency in previously steroid-dependent patients.
Alert: Taper oral glucocorticoid therapy slowly as ordered. Acute adrenal insufficiency and death have occurred in asthmatics who switched abruptly from oral corticosteroids to inhaled steroids. Be sure patients report symptoms associated

---

with corticosteroid withdrawal, including fatigue, weakness, arthralgia, orthostatic hypotension, and dyspnea.

☑**Patient teaching**
• Inform patient that drug doesn't provide relief for acute asthma attacks.
• Instruct patient to store medication between 59° and 86° F (15° and 30° C). Tell him to use it at room temperature. If canister is cold, proper dose may not be delivered.
• Advise patient to ensure delivery of the proper dose by gently warming the canister to room temperature before using. Some patients carry the canister in a pocket to keep it warm.
• Advise patient requiring bronchodilator to use it several minutes before dexamethasone.
• Tell patient to allow 1 minute to elapse before taking subsequent puffs of medication and to hold his breath for a few seconds to enhance action of drug.
• Instruct patient to contact doctor if response to therapy decreases or if symptoms don't improve within 3 weeks of initiating therapy; doctor may need to adjust the dosage. Tell patient not to exceed recommended dosage on his own.
• Advise patient to prevent oral fungal infection by gargling or rinsing mouth with water after each use, but not to swallow water.
• Teach patient to keep inhaler clean and unobstructed. He should wash it with warm water and dry it thoroughly.
• Instruct patient to carry a card indicating need for supplemental systemic glucocorticoids during stress.

---

dornase alfa
Pulmozyme

Pregnancy Risk Category: B

HOW SUPPLIED
Inhalation solution: 2.5-mg ampule (1 mg/ml)

ACTION
Hydrolyzes DNA in sputum of cystic fi-

brosis patients, causing decreased viscosity and elasticity of pulmonary secretions.

Route	Onset	Peak	Duration
Inhalation	3-7 days	9 days	Unknown

INDICATIONS & DOSAGE
To improve pulmonary function and decrease the frequency of moderate to severe respiratory infections in patients with cystic fibrosis—
Adults and children 5 years and over: 1 ampule (2.5 mg) inhaled once daily. Treatment usually takes 10 to 15 minutes. Use drug only with an approved nebulizer.

ADVERSE REACTIONS
EENT: *pharyngitis, voice alteration,* laryngitis, conjunctivitis.
Skin: *rash,* urticaria.
Other: *chest pain.*

INTERACTIONS
None significant.

EFFECTS ON DIAGNOSTIC TESTS
None reported.

CONTRAINDICATIONS
Contraindicated in patients hypersensitive to drug or products derived from the Chinese hamster ovary cell.

NURSING CONSIDERATIONS
• Know that drug is used in conjunction with other standard therapies for cystic fibrosis.
• Some patients (those over 21 years or those with forced vital capacity exceeding 85%) may benefit from twice-daily administration.
• Be aware that safety and efficacy in children under 5 years or with forced vital capacity of less than 40% of normal value, or use for more than 12 months have not been established.
• Administer only with the following nebulizers and compressors: the Hudson T Up-draft II disposable jet nebulizer and the Marquest Acorn II disposable jet nebulizer along with the Pulmo-Aide compressor or the PARI LC Jet+ reusable nebulizer along with the PARI PRONEB compressor.

• Discard cloudy or discolored solution.
• Do not mix with other drugs in the nebulizer. Doing so could lead to a physical or chemical reaction that may inactivate dornase alfa.
• Refrigerate drug in its protective foil pouch to protect it from strong light.
• Once opened, the entire ampule must be used or discarded.

☑ **Patient teaching**
• Instruct patient how to administer drug at home.
• Remind patient to breathe only through his mouth when using the nebulizer. If this is difficult, suggest use of a nose clip.
• Tell patient that if he begins coughing during treatment to turn off nebulizer without spilling drug. To resume, he should turn on nebulizer and continue breathing through the mouthpiece until the nebulizer cup is empty or mist is no longer produced.

---

epoprostenol sodium
Flolan

Pregnancy Risk Category: B

HOW SUPPLIED
Injection: 0.5 mg (500,000 ng)/17 ml, 1.5 mg (1,500,000 ng)/17 ml

ACTION
Causes direct vasodilation of pulmonary and systemic arterial vascular beds and inhibits platelet aggregation.

Route	Onset	Peak	Duration
IV	Unknown	Unknown	Unknown

INDICATIONS & DOSAGE
Long-term I.V. treatment of primary pulmonary hypertension in New York Heart Association classes III and IV patients—
Adults: initially, 2 ng/kg/minute as I.V. infusion, increased in increments of 2 ng/kg/minute q 15 minutes or longer until dose-limiting pharmacologic effects are elicited. Maintenance dosing is begun with 4 ng/kg/minute less than the maximum tolerated rate determined during initial dosing. If the maximum rate is less than 5 ng/kg/minute, the maintenance infusion is started at 50% the maximum rate. Subsequent adjustments are made based on persistence, recurrence, or worsening of symptoms; such increases should be made gradually in 1- to 2-ng/kg/minute increments q 15 minutes or longer. Occurrence of adverse events from excessive doses may necessitate a gradual decrease in dosage in 2-ng/kg/minute increments q 15 minutes or longer.

ADVERSE REACTIONS
After initial dosing—
CNS: *headache, anxiety, nervousness, agitation,* dizziness, hypoesthesia, paresthesia.
CV: *hypotension, chest pain,* bradycardia, tachycardia.
GI: *nausea, vomiting,* abdominal pain, dyspepsia.
Musculoskeletal: musculoskeletal pain, back pain.
Respiratory: dyspnea.
Skin: *flushing,* sweating.
During maintenance dosing—
CNS: *headache, anxiety, nervousness,* dizziness, hypoesthesia, hyperesthesia, paresthesia, tremor.
CV: *tachycardia.*
GI: *nausea, vomiting, diarrhea.*
Hematologic: *thrombocytopenia.*
Musculoskeletal: *jaw pain, myalgia, nonspecific musculoskeletal pain.*
Skin: *flushing.*
Other: *flulike symptoms, chills, fever, sepsis.*

INTERACTIONS
Drug-drug. *Anticoagulants, antiplatelet agents:* may increase risk of bleeding. Monitor closely for bleeding.
Antihypertensive agents, diuretics, other vasodilators: additional reductions in blood pressure may occur. Monitor blood pressure closely.

EFFECTS ON DIAGNOSTIC TESTS
None reported.

CONTRAINDICATIONS
Contraindicated in patients with hypersensitivity to drug or structurally related compounds. Chronic use is contraindicat-

ed in patients with heart failure due to severe left ventricular systolic dysfunction and in patients who develop pulmonary edema during initial dosing.

NURSING CONSIDERATIONS
● Use cautiously in elderly patients and in pregnant or breast-feeding women.
● Safety and efficacy in children have not been established.
● Drug should be used only by clinicians experienced in diagnosis and treatment of primary pulmonary hypertension. The appropriate dose must be determined in a setting with adequate personnel and equipment for physiologic monitoring and emergency care.
● Reconstituted solutions must be protected from light and refrigerated at 36° to 46° F (2° to 8° C) if not used immediately. Do not freeze reconstituted solutions. Discard frozen solution or solution that has been refrigerated for more than 48 hours.
● To facilitate extended use at ambient temperatures above 77° F (25° C), a cold pouch with frozen gel packs can be used. The pouch must be able to maintain the drug at a temperature of 36° to 46° F for 12 hours. When such a pouch is used, reconstituted solution may be administered up to 24 hours with use of two pouches.
● Administer anticoagulant therapy during maintenance infusion, unless contraindicated. Monitor PT closely.
● To reduce risk of infection, aseptic technique must be used when reconstituting and administering the drug and when performing routine catheter care.
● All orders for epoprostenol are distributed only by Quantum Healthcare, Inc. To order the drug or request reimbursement assistance, call 1-800-622-1820.

◨ I.V. administration
● Reconstitute drug only as directed, using sterile diluent for Flolan. Do not reconstitute or mix drug with other parenteral medications or solutions before or during administration.
● Follow manufacturer guidelines for reconstituting drug. The prescribed concentration should be compatible with the infusion pump's minimum and maximum flow rates and reservoir capacity and with other criteria recommended by manufacturer. When used for maintenance infusion, drug should be prepared in a drug delivery reservoir appropriate for the infusion pump, with a total reservoir volume of at least 100 ml. Drug should be prepared using two vials of sterile diluent for use during 24 hours.
● Maintenance dosing should be given by continuous I.V. infusion via a permanent indwelling central venous catheter using an ambulatory infusion pump. During establishment of dosing range, drug may be administered peripherally.
● After establishment of a maintenance infusion rate, observe patient closely and monitor standing and supine blood pressure and heart rate for several hours to ensure tolerance.
● Avoid abrupt withdrawal of drug or sudden, large reductions in infusion rate. Ensure that a backup infusion pump and I.V. infusion set are available to avoid potential interruptions in drug delivery. A multilumen catheter should be considered if other I.V. therapies are routinely administered.
● Adjust infusion rates only under doctor's direction, except in life-threatening situations.

☑ Patient teaching
● Discuss patient's long-term need for drug. Ensure that patient or family member can care for a permanent I.V. catheter and infusion pump.
● Show patient and family how to reconstitute, administer, and store drug; how to use the infusion pump; and how to switch to a new pump in the event of pump failure. Stress importance of maintaining continuous drug therapy.
● Urge patient to report adverse reactions immediately; dosage adjustments may be necessary.
● Provide patient with the telephone number of an organization that offers 24-hour support.

flunisolide
AeroBid, AeroBid-M, Bronalide†

Pregnancy Risk Category: C

HOW SUPPLIED
Oral inhalant: 250 mcg/metered spray (at least 100 metered inhalations/container)

ACTION
Unknown. May decrease inflammation through inhibitory activities against cell types such as mast cells and macrophages and mediators such as leukotrienes.

Route	Onset	Peak	Duration
Inhalation	1-4 wk	Unknown	Unknown

INDICATIONS & DOSAGE
Chronic asthma—
Adults: 2 inhalations (500 mcg) b.i.d. Maximum total daily dose is 2,000 mcg (8 inhalations daily).
Children 6 to 15 years: 2 inhalations (500 mcg) b.i.d. Higher dosages have not been studied. Maximum total daily dose is 1,000 mcg.

ADVERSE REACTIONS
CNS: dizziness, irritability, nervousness.
CV: palpitations, chest pain.
EENT: throat irritation, hoarseness, nasopharyngeal fungal infections, *sore throat, nasal congestion.*
GI: *nausea, vomiting,* dry mouth, *unpleasant taste, diarrhea, upset stomach,* abdominal pain, decreased appetite.
Respiratory: *upper respiratory tract infection, cold symptoms.*
Skin: rash, pruritus.
Other: *flu,* edema, fever.

INTERACTIONS
None significant.

EFFECTS ON DIAGNOSTIC TESTS
None reported.

CONTRAINDICATIONS
Contraindicated in patients with status asthmaticus, respiratory infections, or hypersensitivity to drug.

NURSING CONSIDERATIONS
• Drug is not recommended in patients with asthma controlled by bronchodilators or other noncorticosteroids alone or for those with nonasthmatic bronchial diseases.
• Know that a spacer device may help to ensure proper dosage administration and decrease local (oral) adverse effects.
• Store medication between 59° and 86° F (15° and 30° C).
• Withdraw drug slowly as ordered in patients who have received long-term oral corticosteroid therapy.
• Be aware that after withdrawal of systemic corticosteroids, patient may still need supplementation of systemic steroids if patient show signs and symptoms of adrenal insufficiency when exposed to trauma, surgery, or infections.

☑ Patient teaching
• Warn patient that flunisolide doesn't relieve emergency asthma attacks.
• Advise patient to ensure delivery of proper dose by gently warming the canister to room temperature before using. Some patients carry the canister in a pocket to keep it warm.
• Tell patient who also is using a bronchodilator to use it several minutes before he uses flunisolide.
• Instruct patient to allow 1 minute to elapse before repeating inhalations and to hold his breath for a few seconds to enhance drug action.
• Teach patient to keep inhaler clean and unobstructed. He should wash it with warm water and dry it thoroughly after use.
• Teach patient to check mucous membranes frequently for signs of fungal infection.
• Advise patient to prevent oral fungal infections by gargling or rinsing mouth with water after each inhaler use. Caution him not to swallow the water.
• Advise parents of children receiving long-term therapy that the child should have periodic growth measurements and be checked for evidence of hypothalamic-pituitary-adrenal axis suppression.

fluticasone propionate
Flixotide§, Flovent Inhalation
Aerosol, Flovent Rotadisk

Pregnancy Risk Category: C

HOW SUPPLIED
Oral inhalation aerosol: 44 mcg,
110 mcg, 220 mcg
Oral inhalation powder: 50 mcg,
100 mcg, 250 mcg

ACTION
Synthetic glucocorticoid with potent anti-inflammatory activity. Inflammation is an important component in the pathogenesis of asthma. Glucocorticoids inhibit many cell types and mediator production or secretion involved in the asthmatic response. These anti-inflammatory actions of fluticasone may contribute to its efficacy in asthma.

Route	Onset	Peak	Duration
Inhalation	24 hr	1-2 wk	Several days

INDICATIONS & DOSAGE
Maintenance treatment of asthma as prophylactic therapy and for patients requiring oral corticosteroid treatment for chronic asthma—
Flovent Inhalation Aerosol
Adults and children 12 years and over: in those previously taking bronchodilators alone, initially, inhaled dose of 88 mcg b.i.d. to maximum of 440 mcg b.i.d.
Patients previously taking inhaled corticosteroids: initially, inhaled dose of 88 to 220 mcg b.i.d. to maximum of 440 mcg b.i.d.
Patients previously taking oral corticosteroids: inhaled dose of 880 mcg b.i.d.
Flovent Rotadisk
Adults and adolescents: in patients previously taking bronchodilators alone, initially, inhaled dose of 100 mcg b.i.d. to maximum of 500 mcg b.i.d.
Patients previously taking inhaled corticosteroids: initially, inhaled dose of 100 to 250 mcg b.i.d. to maximum of 500 mcg b.i.d.
Patients previously taking oral corticosteroids: inhaled dose of 1,000 mcg b.i.d.

Children 4 to 11 years: For patients previously on bronchodilators alone or on inhaled corticosteroids, initially, inhaled dose of 50 mcg b.i.d. to maximum of 100 mcg b.i.d.

ADVERSE REACTIONS
CNS: *headache,* dizziness, migraine, nervousness.
EENT: *pharyngitis,* acute nasopharyngitis, nasal congestion, sinusitis, dysphonia, rhinitis, otitis media, tonsillitis, nasal discharge, earache, laryngitis, epistaxis, sneezing, hoarseness, conjunctivitis, irritation of the eye, dental problems.
GI: mouth irritation, *oral candidiasis,* diarrhea, abdominal pain, viral gastroenteritis, colitis, abdominal discomfort, nausea, vomiting.
GU: dysmenorrhea, candidiasis of vagina, pelvic inflammatory disease, vaginitis, vulvovaginitis, irregular menstrual cycle.
Metabolic: cushingoid features, growth retardation in children, weight gain.
Musculoskeletal: pain in joint, aches and pains, disorder or symptoms of neck sprain or strain, muscular soreness.
Respiratory: *upper respiratory infection,* influenza, bronchitis, chest congestion, dyspnea, irritation due to inhalant.
Skin: dermatitis, urticaria.
Other: fever.

INTERACTIONS
Drug-drug. *Ketoconazole:* increased mean fluticasone concentrations. Use care when coadministering fluticasone with long-term ketoconazole and other known cytochrome P-450 3A4 inhibitors.

EFFECTS ON DIAGNOSTIC TESTS
Some patients on high doses of fluticasone may have an abnormal response to the 6-hour cosyntropin stimulation test.

CONTRAINDICATIONS
Contraindicated in primary treatment of patients with status asthmaticus or other acute episodes of asthma in which intensive measures are required. Contraindicated in patients with hypersensitivity to ingredients in these preparations.

NURSING CONSIDERATIONS

• Use cautiously in breast-feeding patients.
• Because of risk of systemic absorption of inhaled corticosteroids, observe patient carefully for evidence of systemic corticosteroid effects.
• Monitor patient especially postoperatively or during periods of stress for evidence of inadequate adrenal response.
• During withdrawal from oral corticosteroids, some patients may experience symptoms of systemically active corticosteroid withdrawal, such as joint or muscular pain, lassitude, and depression, despite maintenance or even improvement of respiratory function.
• For patients starting therapy who are currently receiving oral corticosteroid therapy, reduce dose of prednisone to no more than 2.5 mg/day on a weekly basis, beginning after at least 1 week of therapy with fluticasone.
• As with other inhaled asthma medications, bronchospasm may occur with an immediate increase in wheezing after dosing. If bronchospasm occurs following dosing with fluticasone inhalation aerosol, it should be treated immediately with a fast-acting inhaled bronchodilator.

☑ Patient teaching
• Tell patient that drug is not indicated for the relief of acute bronchospasm.
• For proper use of drug and to attain maximum improvement, tell patient to follow carefully the accompanying patient instructions.
• Advise patient to use drug at regular intervals as directed.
• Instruct patient not to increase dosage but to contact doctor if symptoms do not improve or if condition worsens.
• Instruct patient to contact doctor immediately when episodes of asthma that are not responsive to bronchodilators occur during course of treatment with fluticasone. During such episodes, patients may require therapy with oral corticosteroids.
• Warn patient to avoid exposure to chickenpox or measles and, if exposed, to consult doctor immediately.
• Tell patient to carry medical identification indicating he may need supplementary corticosteroids during stress or a severe asthma attack.
• During periods of stress or a severe asthma attack, instruct patient who has been withdrawn from systemic corticosteroids to resume oral corticosteroids (in large doses) immediately and to contact doctor for further instruction. Instruct him to rinse his mouth after inhalation.
• Advise patient to avoid spraying inhalation aerosol into eyes.
• Instruct patient to shake canister well before using inhalation aerosol.
• Advise patient to store fluticasone powder in a dry place.

▼ *NEW DRUG*

montelukast sodium
Singulair

Pregnancy Risk Category: B

HOW SUPPLIED
Tablets (film-coated): 10 mg
Tablets (chewable): 5 mg

ACTION
Drug causes inhibition of airway cysteinyl leukotriene ($CysLT_1$) receptors. It binds with high affinity and selectivity to the $CysLT_1$ receptor and inhibits physiologic action of the cysteinyl leukotriene LTD_4. This receptor inhibition reduces early- and late-phase bronchoconstriction due to antigen challenge.

Route	Onset	Peak	Duration
PO (film-coated)	Unknown	3-4 hr	Unknown
PO (chewable)	Unknown	2-2.5 hr	Unknown

INDICATIONS & DOSAGE
For prophylaxis and chronic treatment of asthma—
Adults and children 15 years and older: 10 mg (film-coated tablet) P.O. once daily in evening.
Children 6 to 14 years: 5 mg (chewable tablet) P.O. once daily in evening.

ADVERSE REACTIONS
CNS: *headache,* dizziness, fatigue, asthenia.
EENT: nasal congestion, dental pain.
GI: dyspepsia, infectious gastroenteritis, abdominal pain.
GU: pyuria.
Hepatic: increased ALT and AST.
Respiratory: cough.
Skin: rash.
Other: fever, trauma, influenza.

INTERACTIONS
Drug-drug. *Phenobarbital, rifampin:* may decrease bioavailability of montelukast due to induction of hepatic metabolism. Monitor closely.

EFFECTS ON DIAGNOSTIC TESTS
None reported.

CONTRAINDICATIONS
Contraindicated in patients with hypersensitivity to drug or its ingredients.

NURSING CONSIDERATIONS
• Use cautiously and with appropriate monitoring in patients when dosages of their systemic corticosteroid medications are reduced.
• Assess patient's underlying condition and monitor for effectiveness.
• Safety and efficacy for patients under 6 years have not been established.
• Although dose of inhaled corticosteroids may be reduced gradually, do not abruptly substitute drug for inhaled or oral corticosteroids.
• Be aware that drug is not indicated for use in patients with acute asthmatic attacks, status asthmaticus, or as monotherapy for management of exercise-induced bronchospasm. Appropriate rescue medication should be continued for acute exacerbations.

☑ **Patient teaching**
• Advise patient to take drug daily, even if asymptomatic, and to contact doctor if asthma is not well controlled.
• Warn patient not to reduce or stop taking other prescribed antiasthma medications without doctor's approval.
• Advise patient to seek medical attention if short-acting inhaled bronchodilators are needed more often than usual during drug therapy.
• Warn patient that drug is not beneficial in acute asthma attacks or in exercise-induced bronchospasm, and advise him to keep appropriate rescue medications available.
• Advise patient with known aspirin sensitivity to continue to avoid using aspirin and NSAIDs during drug therapy.
• Advise patient with phenylketonuria that chewable tablet contains phenylalanine.

---

nedocromil sodium
Tilade

Pregnancy Risk Category: B

HOW SUPPLIED
Inhalation aerosol: 1.75 mg/activation

ACTION
Reduces inflammatory changes in the airway by blocking the release of inflammation mediators (such as leukotrienes, histamine, and prostaglandins) from mast cells, eosinophils, monocytes, neutrophils, macrophages, and other immune cells.

Route	Onset	Peak	Duration
Inhalation	Unknown	30 min	3.5 hr

INDICATIONS & DOSAGE
Maintenance in mild to moderate bronchial asthma—
Adults and children 12 years and older: 2 inhalations q.i.d. at regular intervals.

ADVERSE REACTIONS
CNS: headache, dysphonia, fatigue.
EENT: pharyngitis, rhinitis.
GI: nausea, vomiting, dyspepsia, abdominal pain, *unpleasant taste,* dry mouth.
Respiratory: upper respiratory tract infection, cough, increased sputum, bronchitis, dyspnea, *bronchospasm.*
Other: chest pain, viral infection.

INTERACTIONS
None significant.

EFFECTS ON DIAGNOSTIC TESTS
None reported.

CONTRAINDICATIONS
Contraindicated in patients hypersensitive to the formulation or in those experiencing an acute asthmatic attack or acute bronchospasm.

NURSING CONSIDERATIONS
• Know that drug should not be used during acute bronchospasm because drug action has a slow onset and is not therapeutic in aborting an acute attack.

☑Patient teaching
• Warn patient that drug has no direct bronchodilating action and cannot replace bronchodilators during an acute asthmatic attack.
• Tell patient that drug is an adjunct to the regular bronchodilator regimen and may reduce the need for corticosteroids or bronchodilators.
• Emphasize that regular use of drug will help him feel better. Most patients report benefits after 1 week of use; some require longer treatment before improvement occurs.
• Teach patient how to use inhaler. Instruct him to shake canister before use and to invert it just before actuation.
• Advise patient that the use of an aerochamber may improve drug delivery to the lungs.
• Advise patient to clean inhaler at least twice weekly and to remove canister before rinsing inhaler in hot running water. Then let inhaler air-dry overnight.

▼ NEW DRUG

palivizumab
Synagis

Pregnancy Risk Category: C

HOW SUPPLIED
Injection: 100 mg vial

ACTION
Exhibits neutralizing and fusion-inhibitory activity against respiratory syncytial virus (RSV) which inhibits RSV replication.

Route	Onset	Peak	Duration
IM	Unknown	Unknown	Unknown

INDICATIONS & DOSAGE
Prevention of serious lower respiratory tract disease caused by RSV in children at high risk—
Children: 15 mg/kg I.M. monthly throughout RSV season. Administer first dose before beginning of RSV season.

ADVERSE REACTIONS
CNS: nervousness.
EENT: *otitis media, rhinitis,* pharyngitis, sinusitis, conjunctivitis, oral candidiasis.
GI: diarrhea, vomiting, gastroenteritis.
Hematologic: anemia.
Hepatic: liver function abnormality (increased ALT, AST).
Respiratory: *upper respiratory infection,* cough, wheeze, bronchiolitis, *apnea,* pneumonia, bronchitis, asthma, croup, dyspnea.
Skin: *rash,* fungal dermatitis, eczema, seborrhea.
Other: pain, hernia, failure to thrive, injection site reaction, viral infection, flu syndrome.

INTERACTIONS
None reported.

EFFECTS ON DIAGNOSTIC TESTS
None reported.

CONTRAINDICATIONS
Contraindicated in children with history of a severe prior reaction to drug or its components.

NURSING CONSIDERATIONS
• Use cautiously in patients with thrombocytopenia or other coagulation disorders.
• Be aware that patients should receive monthly doses throughout RSV season, even if patient develops RSV infection. In the northern hemisphere, RSV season typically lasts from November to April.
• To reconstitute, slowly add 1 ml of sterile water for injection into a 100-mg vial.

Reactions may be *common,* uncommon, *life-threatening,* or COMMON AND LIFE-THREATENING.

Gently swirl the vial for 30 seconds to avoid foaming. Do not shake vial. Let reconstituted solution stand at room temperature for 20 minutes. Administer within 6 hours of reconstitution.
• Administer drug in anterolateral aspect of thigh. Do not use gluteal muscle routinely as an injection site because of risk of damage to sciatic nerve. Injection volumes over 1 ml should be given as a divided dose.
Alert: Anaphylactoid reactions following administration of drug have not been observed, but can occur following the administration of proteins. If anaphylaxis or severe allergic reaction occurs, administer epinephrine (1:1,000) and provide supportive care as required.

☑ **Patient teaching**
• Explain to parent or caregiver that drug is used to prevent RSV and not to treat it.
• Advise parent that monthly injections are recommended throughout RSV season (November to April in the northern hemisphere).
• Advise parent to report adverse reactions immediately.

---

triamcinolone acetonide
Azmacort

Pregnancy Risk Category: C

HOW SUPPLIED
Inhalation aerosol: 100 mcg/metered spray

ACTION
Unknown. May decrease inflammation through inhibitory activities against cell types such as mast cells and macrophages and mediators such as leukotrienes.

Route	Onset	Peak	Duration
Inhalation	1-4 wk	Unknown	Unknown

INDICATIONS & DOSAGE
Persistent asthma—
Adults: 2 inhalations t.i.d. to q.i.d. Maximum dosage is 16 inhalations daily. In some patients, maintenance can be accomplished when total daily dosage is given b.i.d.
Children 6 to 12 years: 1 to 2 inhalations t.i.d. to q.i.d. Maximum dosage is 12 inhalations daily.

ADVERSE REACTIONS
Most adverse reactions to corticosteroids are dose- or duration-dependent.
EENT: dry or irritated nose or throat, hoarseness, *pharyngitis,* oral candidiasis, dry or irritated tongue or mouth.
Metabolic: hypothalamic-pituitary-adrenal function suppression, adrenal insufficiency.
Respiratory: cough, wheezing.
Other: facial edema.

INTERACTIONS
None significant.

EFFECTS ON DIAGNOSTIC TESTS
None reported.

CONTRAINDICATIONS
Contraindicated in patients with status asthmaticus or hypersensitivity to drug or its ingredients.

NURSING CONSIDERATIONS
• It is not known if drug is excreted in breast milk. Because of risk of severe adverse effects, breast-feeding is not recommended during therapy.
• Use with extreme caution, if at all, in patients with tuberculosis of the respiratory tract; untreated fungal, bacterial, or systemic viral infections; or ocular herpes simplex.
• Unlike other available corticosteroids, drug has a spacer built into the drug-delivery device.
• Use cautiously in patients receiving systemic corticosteroids.
• Know that patients who have recently been switched from systemic administration of steroids to oral inhaled steroids may need to resume systemic steroid therapy during periods of stress or severe asthma attacks.
• Taper oral therapy slowly as ordered.
• Store medication between 59° and 86° F (15° and 30° C).

☑ **Patient teaching**

• Inform patient that inhaled corticosteroids don't provide relief for emergency asthma attacks.

• Advise patient to warm canister to room temperature before using. Some patients carry canister in a pocket to keep it warm.

• Tell patient requiring a bronchodilator to use it several minutes before triamcinolone. Tell patient to allow 1 minute to elapse before repeat inhalations and to hold breath for a few seconds to enhance drug action.

• Teach patient to check mucous membranes frequently for signs of fungal infection.

• Tell patient to prevent oral fungal infections by gargling or rinsing mouth with water after each use of the inhaler, but not to swallow the water.

• Tell patient to keep inhaler clean and unobstructed and to wash it with warm water and dry it thoroughly after use.

• Instruct patient to contact doctor if response to therapy decreases; dosage may require adjustment. Tell him not to exceed recommended dosage on his own.

• Instruct patient to carry a card indicating his need for supplemental systemic glucocorticoids during periods of stress.

---

zafirlukast
Accolate

Pregnancy Risk Category: B

HOW SUPPLIED
Tablets: 20 mg

ACTION
Selectively competes for leukotriene receptor sites, blocking inflammatory action.

Route	Onset	Peak	Duration
PO	Rapid	3 hr	Unknown

INDICATIONS & DOSAGE
Prophylaxis and chronic treatment of asthma—

Adults and children 12 years and older: 20 mg P.O. b.i.d. taken 1 hour before or 2 hours after meals.

ADVERSE REACTIONS
CNS: *headache,* asthenia, dizziness.
GI: nausea, diarrhea, abdominal pain, vomiting, dyspepsia.
Musculoskeletal: pain, myalgia, back pain.
Other: infection, accidental injury, fever, ALT elevation.

INTERACTIONS
Drug-drug. *Aspirin:* increased plasma levels of zafirlukast. Monitor patient.
Erythromycin, theophylline: decreased plasma levels of zafirlukast. Monitor patient.
Warfarin: increased PT. Monitor PT and INR levels, and adjust dosage of anticoagulant, as ordered.

EFFECTS ON DIAGNOSTIC TESTS
Drug may elevate liver enzyme levels.

CONTRAINDICATIONS
Contraindicated in patients with known hypersensitivity to drug.

NURSING CONSIDERATIONS
• Know that drug is not indicated for use in the reversal of bronchospasm in acute asthma attacks.

• Administer with caution in patients with hepatic impairment and in the elderly.

• Use drug in pregnant patients only if clearly needed. Do not use in breast-feeding women.

• Reduction of oral steroid dose in patients on drug therapy has been followed in rare cases by eosinophilia, vasculitic rash, worsening pulmonary symptoms, cardiac complications, or neuropathy, sometimes presenting as Churg-Strauss syndrome.

• Safety and effectiveness in patients under 12 years have not been established.

☑ **Patient teaching**

• Tell patient that drug is used for chronic treatment of asthma and to keep taking drug even if symptoms disappear.

• Advise patient to continue taking other antiasthma drugs as ordered.

• Instruct patient not to take drug with food. Drug should be taken 1 hour before or 2 hours after meals.

---

zileuton
Zyflo

Pregnancy Risk Category: C

HOW SUPPLIED
Tablets: 600 mg

ACTION
Inhibits enzyme responsible for the formation of leukotrienes, thus reducing inflammatory response.

Route	Onset	Peak	Duration
PO	Rapid	2 hr	Unknown

INDICATIONS & DOSAGE
Prophylaxis and chronic treatment of asthma—
Adults and children 12 years and older: 600 mg P.O. q.i.d.

ADVERSE REACTIONS
CNS: *headache,* asthenia, dizziness, insomnia, nervousness, somnolence, malaise.
CV: chest pain.
EENT: conjunctivitis.
GI: dyspepsia, nausea, abdominal pain, constipation, flatulence, vomiting.
GU: urinary tract infection, vaginitis.
Hematologic: *leukopenia.*
Musculoskeletal: myalgia, arthralgia, hypertonia, neck pain, rigidity.
Skin: pruritus.
Other: pain, accidental injury, fever, lymphadenopathy, ALT elevation.

INTERACTIONS
Drug-drug. *Propranolol, other beta blockers:* increased beta-blocker effect. Monitor patient and reduce dosage of beta blocker as needed.
Theophylline: decreased theophylline clearance (on average, serum theophylline concentrations double). Reduce theophylline dose, as ordered, and monitor serum levels.
Warfarin: increased PT. Monitor PT and INR and adjust dosage of anticoagulant, as ordered.

EFFECTS ON DIAGNOSTIC TESTS
Drug may elevate liver enzyme levels and temporarily lower WBC count.

CONTRAINDICATIONS
Contraindicated in patients with active liver disease, transaminase elevations at least three times the upper limit of normal, or known hypersensitivity to drug.

NURSING CONSIDERATIONS
• Know that drug is not indicated for use in the reversal of bronchospasm in acute asthma attacks.
• Administer with caution in patients with hepatic impairment or history of heavy alcohol use.
• Drug should be used in pregnancy only if the benefit of use outweighs the potential risk to the fetus. Breast-feeding women should not take drug.
• Safety and effectiveness in patients under 12 years have not been established.
• Obtain baseline and periodic liver enzyme levels, as ordered.

☑**Patient teaching**
• Tell patient that drug is used for chronic treatment of asthma and to keep taking drug even if symptoms disappear.
• Caution patient that drug is not a bronchodilator and should not be used to treat an acute asthma attack.
• Advise patient to continue taking other antiasthma drugs, as ordered.
• Instruct patient to notify doctor if his short-acting bronchodilator doesn't relieve symptoms.
• Inform patient that he must undergo periodic testing of liver enzyme levels.
• Tell patient to notify doctor immediately if he develops signs and symptoms of liver dysfunction (right upper quadrant pain, nausea, fatigue, pruritus, jaundice, malaise).
• Tell patient to avoid alcohol and to consult his doctor first before taking OTC or new prescription drugs.

47

Antacids, adsorbents, and antiflatulents

aluminum carbonate
aluminum hydroxide
calcium carbonate
magaldrate
magnesium hydroxide
  (See Chapter 50, LAXATIVES.)
magnesium oxide
simethicone
sodium bicarbonate
  (See Chapter 64, ACIDIFIERS AND
  ALKALINIZERS.)

COMBINATION PRODUCTS
ALKA-SELTZER GOLD ◊ : sodium bicarbonate 958 mg, citric acid 832 mg, and potassium bicarbonate 312 mg.
ALKA-SELTZER ORIGINAL ◊ : aspirin 325 mg, citric acid 1,000 mg and phenylalanine 9 mg.
ALUDROX ◊ : aluminum hydroxide 307 mg and magnesium hydroxide 103 mg.
DI-GEL ADVANCED FORMULA ◊ : magnesium hydroxide 128 mg, and calcium carbonate 280 mg.
EXTRA STRENGTH ALKA-SELTZER ◊ : aspirin 500 mg and citric acid 1,000 mg.
GAVISCON TABLETS ◊ : aluminum hydroxide 80 mg and magnesium trisilicate 20 mg.
GELUSIL ◊ : aluminum hydroxide 200 mg, magnesium hydroxide 200 mg, and simethicone 25 mg.
MAALOX TABLETS ◊ : aluminum hydroxide 200 mg, magnesium hydroxide 200 mg, and simethicone 25 mg.
MAALOX EXTRA STRENGTH TABLETS ◊ : aluminum hydroxide 350 mg, magnesium hydroxide 350 mg and simethicone 30 mg.
MAALOX PLUS ◊ : aluminum hydroxide 200 mg, magnesium hydroxide 200 mg, and simethicone 25 mg.
MAALOX THERAPEUTIC CONCENTRATE SUSPENSION: aluminum hydroxide 600 mg and magnesium hydroxide 300 mg/5 ml.
MYLANTA LIQUID: aluminum hydroxide 200 mg, magnesium hydroxide 200 mg, and simethicone 20 mg/5 ml.

MYLANTA TABLETS ◊ : aluminum hydroxide 200 mg, magnesium hydroxide 200 mg, and simethicone 20 mg.
RIOPAN PLUS CHEWABLE TABLETS ◊ : magaldrate 480 mg and simethicone 20 mg.
RIOPAN PLUS DOUBLE STRENGTH CHEWABLE TABLETS: magaldrate 1,080 mg and simethicone 20 mg.
RIOPAN PLUS DOUBLE STRENGTH SUSPENSION: magaldrate 1,080 mg and simethicone 40 mg/5 ml.
RIOPAN PLUS SUSPENSION ◊ : magaldrate 540 mg and simethicone 40 mg/5 ml.
TITRALAC PLUS ◊ : calcium carbonate 420 mg and simethicone 21 mg.
UNIVOL† ◊ : aluminum hydroxide and magnesium carbonate co-dried gel 300 mg and magnesium hydroxide 100 mg.

---

aluminum carbonate
Basaljel ◊

Pregnancy Risk Category: NR

HOW SUPPLIED
Tablets or capsules: equivalent to aluminum hydroxide 500 mg ◊
Oral suspension: equivalent to aluminum hydroxide 400 mg/5 ml ◊

ACTION
An antacid that reduces total acid load in the GI tract, elevates gastric pH to reduce pepsin activity, strengthens the gastric mucosal barrier, and increases esophageal sphincter tone.

Route	Onset	Peak	Duration
PO	20 min	Unknown	20-180 min

INDICATIONS & DOSAGE
Antacid—
Adults: 5 to 10 ml of suspension P.O. q 2 hours p.r.n.; or 1 to 2 tablets or capsules P.O. q 2 hours p.r.n. Maximum dosage is 24 capsules, tablets, or teaspoonfuls per 24 hours.

To prevent formation of urinary phosphate stones (in conjunction with low-phosphate diet)—
Adults: 15 to 30 ml of suspension in water or juice P.O. 1 hour after meals and h.s.; or 2 to 6 tablets or capsules 1 hour after meals and h.s.

ADVERSE REACTIONS
CNS: encephalopathy.
GI: *constipation,* intestinal obstruction.
Other: hypophosphatemia, osteomalacia.

INTERACTIONS
Drug-drug. *Allopurinol, antibiotics (including quinolones, tetracyclines), corticosteroids, diflunisal, digoxin, ethambutol, H_2 antagonists, iron salts, isoniazid, penicillamine, phenothiazines, thyroid hormones, ticlopidine:* decreased pharmacologic effect because of possible impaired absorption. Separate administration times by 1 to 2 hours.
Enteric-coated drugs: may be released prematurely in stomach. Separate doses by at least 1 hour.

EFFECTS ON DIAGNOSTIC TESTS
Aluminum carbonate may interfere with imaging techniques using sodium pertechnetate Tc99m and thus impair evaluation of Meckel's diverticulum. It may also interfere with reticuloendothelial imaging of liver, spleen, or bone marrow using technetium Tc99m sulfur colloid. It may antagonize pentagastrin's effect during gastric acid secretion tests. Drug may increase serum gastrin levels and decrease serum phosphate levels.

CONTRAINDICATIONS
No known contraindications.

NURSING CONSIDERATIONS
• Use cautiously in patients with chronic renal disease.
• When administering through nasogastric tube, make sure tube is placed correctly and is patent; after instilling, flush tube with water to ensure passage to stomach and to clear tube.
• Monitor long-term, high-dose use in patients on restricted sodium intake. Each tablet, capsule, or 5 ml of suspension contains about 3 mg of sodium.
• Record stool amount and consistency. Manage constipation with laxatives or stool softeners as ordered. Alternate with magnesium-containing antacids (unless patient has renal disease).
• Monitor serum phosphate levels.
• Watch for symptoms of hypophosphatemia (anorexia, malaise, muscle weakness) with prolonged use; can also lead to resorption of calcium and bone demineralization.
• Because drug contains aluminum, keep in mind that it is used in patients with renal failure to help control hyperphosphatemia by binding with phosphate in the GI tract.
• Know that Basaljel liquid contains no sugar.

☑**Patient teaching**
• Warn patient not to take aluminum carbonate indiscriminately or to switch antacids without doctor's advice.
• Tell patient to shake suspension well and to take with small amount of water or fruit juice to facilitate passage.
• Instruct patient to notify doctor of signs of bleeding, tarry stools, or coffee-ground vomitus.
• Instruct pregnant patients to seek medical advice before taking drug.

aluminum hydroxide
AlternaGEL◇, Alu-Cap◇§, Aluminum Hydroxide Gel◇, Aluminum Hydroxide Gel Concentrated◇, Alu-Tab◇, Amphojel◇, Dialume◇

Pregnancy Risk Category: NR

HOW SUPPLIED
Tablets: 300 mg◇, 500 mg◇, 600 mg◇
Capsules: 400 mg◇, 500 mg◇
Oral suspension: 320 mg/5 ml◇, 450 mg/5 ml◇, 600 mg/5 ml◇, 675 mg/5 ml◇

ACTION
An antacid that reduces total acid load in the GI tract, elevates gastric pH to reduce

pepsin activity, strengthens the gastric mucosal barrier, and increases esophageal sphincter tone.

Route	Onset	Peak	Duration
PO	Variable	Unknown	20-180 min

INDICATIONS & DOSAGE
Antacid—
Adults: 500 to 1,500 mg P.O. (5 to 30 ml of most suspension products) 1 hour after meals and h.s.; alternatively, 300-mg tablet or 600-mg tablet (chewed before swallowing) taken with milk or water five to six times daily after meals and h.s.

ADVERSE REACTIONS
CNS: encephalopathy.
GI: *constipation,* intestinal obstruction.
Other: hypophosphatemia, osteomalacia.

INTERACTIONS
Drug-drug. *Allopurinol, antibiotics (including quinolones, tetracyclines), corticosteroids, diflunisal, digoxin, ethambutol, H_2 antagonists, iron salts, isoniazid, penicillamine, phenothiazines, thyroid hormones, ticlopidine:* decreased pharmacologic effect because of possible impaired absorption. Separate administration times.
Enteric-coated drugs: may be released prematurely in stomach. Separate doses by at least 1 hour.

EFFECTS ON DIAGNOSTIC TESTS
Aluminum hydroxide therapy may interfere with imaging techniques using sodium pertechnetate Tc99m and thus impair evaluation of Meckel's diverticulum. It may also interfere with reticuloendothelial imaging of liver, spleen, or bone marrow using technetium Tc99m sulfur colloid. It may antagonize pentagastrin's effect during gastric acid secretion tests. Drug may increase serum gastrin levels and decrease serum phosphate levels.

CONTRAINDICATIONS
No known contraindications.

NURSING CONSIDERATIONS
• Use cautiously in patients with chronic renal disease.

• When administering through nasogastric tube, make sure tube is placed correctly and is patent; after instilling, flush tube with water to ensure passage to stomach and to clear tube.
• Monitor long-term, high-dose use in patient on restricted sodium intake. Each tablet, capsule, or 5 ml of suspension contains 2 to 3 mg of sodium.
• Record amount and consistency of stools. Manage constipation with laxatives or stool softeners as ordered; alternate with magnesium-containing antacids (if patient does not have renal disease).
• Monitor serum phosphate levels.
• Watch for symptoms of hypophosphatemia (anorexia, malaise, and muscle weakness) with prolonged use; can also lead to resorption of calcium and bone demineralization.
• Because drug contains aluminum, keep in mind that it is used in patients with renal failure to help control hyperphosphatemia by binding with phosphate in the GI tract.

☑**Patient teaching**
• Instruct patient to shake suspension well and to follow with small amount of milk or water to facilitate passage.
• Advise patient not to take aluminum hydroxide indiscriminately or to switch antacids without doctor's advice.
• Instruct patient to notify doctor of signs of bleeding, tarry stools, or coffee-ground vomitus.
• Instruct pregnant patients to seek medical advice before taking drug.

calcium carbonate
Alka-Mints ◇, Amitone ◇, Cal-Sup‡, Chooz ◇, Dicarbosil ◇, Maalox Antacid Caplets ◇, Rolaids Calcium Rich ◇, Tums ◇, Tums E-X ◇, Tums Ultra ◇

Pregnancy Risk Category: NR

HOW SUPPLIED
Calcium carbonate contains 40% calcium; 20 mEq calcium per gram.
Tablets (chewable): 350 mg ◇, 420 mg ◇,

500 mg ◊, 750 mg, 850 mg, 1,000 mg, 1,250 mg‡
Tablets: 500 mg ◊, 600 mg ◊, 650 mg ◊, 1,000 mg ◊, 1,250 mg ◊
Chewing gum: 500 mg/piece
Oral suspension: 1,250 mg/5 ml
Lozenges: 600 mg ◊

ACTION
An antacid that reduces total acid load in the GI tract, elevates gastric pH to reduce pepsin activity, strengthens the gastric mucosal barrier, and increases esophageal sphincter tone.

Route	Onset	Peak	Duration
PO	20 min	Unknown	20-180 min

INDICATIONS & DOSAGE
Antacid, calcium supplement—
Adults: 350 mg to 1.5 g P.O. or 2 pieces of chewing gum 1 hour after meals and h.s. p.r.n.

ADVERSE REACTIONS
CNS: headache, irritability, weakness.
GI: rebound hyperacidity, *nausea.*

INTERACTIONS
Drug-drug. *Antibiotics (including quinolones, tetracyclines), hydantoins, iron salts, isoniazid, salicylates:* decreased pharmacologic effect because of possible impaired absorption. Separate administration times.
Enteric-coated drugs: may be released prematurely in stomach. Separate doses by at least 1 hour.
Drug-food. *Milk, other foods high in vitamin D:* possible milk-alkali syndrome (headache, confusion, distaste for food, nausea, vomiting, hypercalcemia, hypercalciuria). Avoid concomitant use.

EFFECTS ON DIAGNOSTIC TESTS
Drug may alter serum phosphate levels.

CONTRAINDICATIONS
Contraindicated in patients with ventricular fibrillation or hypercalcemia.

NURSING CONSIDERATIONS
• Use cautiously, if at all, in patients with sarcoidosis or renal or cardiac disease,

and in patients receiving cardiac glycosides.
• Record amount and consistency of stools. Manage constipation with laxatives or stool softeners as ordered.
• Monitor serum calcium levels, especially in patients with mild renal impairment.
• Watch for signs and symptoms of hypercalcemia (nausea, vomiting, headache, confusion, and anorexia).

☑ Patient teaching
• Advise patient not to take calcium carbonate indiscriminately or to switch antacids without doctor's advice.
• Tell patient taking chewable tablets to chew thoroughly before swallowing and follow with a glass of water.
• Tell patient using suspension form to shake well and take with a small amount of water to facilitate passage.
• Instruct patient to notify doctor of signs of bleeding, tarry stools, or coffee-ground vomitus.

magaldrate (aluminum-magnesium complex)
Lowsium ◊, Riopan ◊

Pregnancy Risk Category: NR

HOW SUPPLIED
Oral suspension: 540 mg/5 ml ◊

ACTION
An antacid that reduces total acid load in the GI tract, elevates gastric pH to reduce pepsin activity, strengthens the gastric mucosal barrier, and increases esophageal sphincter tone.

Route	Onset	Peak	Duration
PO	20 min	Unknown	20-180 min

INDICATIONS & DOSAGE
Antacid—
Adults: 540 to 1,080 mg (5 to 10 ml) of suspension P.O. with water between meals and h.s.

ADVERSE REACTIONS
GI: mild constipation, diarrhea.

INTERACTIONS
Drug-drug. *Allopurinol, antibiotics (including quinolones, tetracyclines), diflunisal, digoxin, iron salts, isoniazid, salicylates, penicillamine, phenothiazines, quinidine, ticlopidine:* decreased pharmacologic effect because of possible impaired absorption. Separate administration times by 1 to 2 hours.
Enteric-coated drugs: may be released prematurely in stomach. Separate doses by at least 1 hour.

EFFECTS ON DIAGNOSTIC TESTS
Drug may antagonize pentagastrin's effect during gastric acid secretion tests; it may decrease serum potassium levels and increase serum gastrin and urine pH levels.

CONTRAINDICATIONS
Contraindicated in patients with severe renal disease.

NURSING CONSIDERATIONS
• Use cautiously in patients with mild kidney impairment.
• When giving through nasogastric tube, make sure tube is placed properly and is patent. After instilling, flush tube with water to ensure passage to stomach and to clear tube.
• Monitor serum magnesium level in patients with mild kidney impairment. Symptomatic hypermagnesemia usually occurs only in severe renal failure.
Alert: Keep in mind that drug is not typically used in patients with renal failure to help control hypophosphatemia because it contains magnesium, which may accumulate.
• Be aware that drug has a low sodium content and is good for patients on restricted sodium intake.

☑ Patient teaching
• Instruct patient to shake suspension well and to follow with water.
• Tell patient taking chewable tablets to chew thoroughly and to follow with a glass of water.
• Advise patient not to take magaldrate indiscriminately or to switch antacids without doctor's advice.
• Instruct patient to notify doctor of signs of bleeding, tarry stools, or coffee-ground vomitus.

magnesium oxide
Mag-Ox 400 ◊ , Maox ◊ ,
Uro-Mag ◊

Pregnancy Risk Category: NR

HOW SUPPLIED
Tablets: 400 mg ◊ , 420 mg ◊ , 500 mg
Capsules: 140 mg ◊

ACTION
Reduces total acid load in the GI tract, elevates gastric pH, strengthens the gastric mucosal barrier, and increases esophageal sphincter tone.

Route	Onset	Peak	Duration
PO	20 min	Unknown	20-180 min

INDICATIONS & DOSAGE
Antacid—
Adults: 140 mg P.O. with water or milk after meals and h.s.
Laxative—
Adults: 4 g P.O. with water or milk, usually h.s.
Oral replacement therapy in mild hypomagnesemia—
Adults: 400 to 840 mg P.O. daily. Monitor serum magnesium level.

ADVERSE REACTIONS
GI: *diarrhea,* nausea, abdominal pain.
Other: hypermagnesemia.

INTERACTIONS
Drug-drug. *Allopurinol, antibiotics, digoxin, iron salts, penicillamine, phenothiazines:* decreased effect because of possible impaired absorption. Separate administration times by 1 to 2 hours.
Enteric-coated drugs: may be released prematurely in stomach. Separate doses by at least 1 hour.

EFFECTS ON DIAGNOSTIC TESTS
None reported.

Reactions may be *common*, uncommon, **life-threatening**, or COMMON AND LIFE-THREATENING.

CONTRAINDICATIONS
Contraindicated in patients with severe renal disease.

NURSING CONSIDERATIONS
• Use cautiously in patients with mild renal impairment.
• When used as laxative, do not give within 1 to 2 hours of other oral drugs.
• Monitor serum magnesium levels. With prolonged use and renal impairment, watch for signs and symptoms of hypermagnesemia (hypotension, nausea, vomiting, depressed reflexes, respiratory depression, and coma).
• If diarrhea occurs, be prepared to suggest alternative preparation.

✅ **Patient teaching**
• Advise patient not to take magnesium oxide indiscriminately or to switch antacids without doctor's advice.
• Instruct patient to report bleeding, tarry stools, or coffee-ground vomitus.

---

simethicone
Flatulex ◇, Gas Relief ◇, Gas-X ◇, Gas-X Extra Strength ◇, Mylanta Gas ◇, Mylanta Gas Maximum Strength ◇, Mylicon ◇, Ovol†, Ovol-40†, Ovol-80†, Phazyme ◇, Phazyme 95 ◇, Phazyme 125 Maximum Strength ◇

Pregnancy Risk Category: NR

HOW SUPPLIED
Tablets: 40 mg ◇, 55 mg† ◇, 60 mg ◇, 80 mg ◇, 95 mg ◇, 125 mg ◇
Capsules: 125 mg
Drops: 40 mg/0.6 ml ◇

ACTION
By its defoaming action, disperses or prevents formation of mucus-surrounded gas pockets in the GI tract.

Route	Onset	Peak	Duration
PO	Immediate	Immediate	Unknown

INDICATIONS & DOSAGE
Flatulence, functional gastric bloating—
Adults and children over 12 years: 40 to 125 mg P.O. after each meal and h.s., up to 500 mg daily. For drops, 40 to 80 mg P.O. after each meal and h.s., up to 500 mg daily.

ADVERSE REACTIONS
GI: expulsion of excessive liberated gas as belching, rectal flatus.

INTERACTIONS
None significant.

EFFECTS ON DIAGNOSTIC TESTS
None reported.

CONTRAINDICATIONS
Contraindicated in patients hypersensitive to drug.

NURSING CONSIDERATIONS
• Know that drug is not recommended in treating infant colic because of limited information on safety in children.
• Be aware that medication does not prevent formation of gas.

✅ **Patient teaching**
• Tell patient to chew tablet before swallowing.
• Advise patient to change positions often and ambulate to aid flatus passage.

48

Digestive enzymes and gallstone solubilizers

pancreatin
pancrelipase
ursodiol

COMBINATION PRODUCTS
DONNAZYME TABLETS: pancreatin
300 mg, pepsin 150 mg, bile salts
150 mg, hyoscyamine sulfate 0.0518 mg,
atropine sulfate 0.0097 mg, scopolamine
hydrobromide 0.0033 mg, and phenobarbital 8.1 mg.
PANCREASE CAPSULES: lipase 4,000 units,
protease 25,000 units, and amylase
20,000 units in enteric-coated microspheres.

---

pancreatin
Creon, Donnazyme, Entozyme,
Hi-Vegi-Lip Tablets ◇ , 4X
Pancreatin 600 mg ◇ , 8X
Pancreatin 900 mg ◇ ,
Pancrezyme 4X Tablets ◇

Pregnancy Risk Category: C

HOW SUPPLIED
Creon
Microspheres (enteric-coated): 300 mg
pancreatin, 8,000 units lipase,
13,000 units protease, 30,000 units amylase
Donnazyme
Tablets: 500 mg pancreatin, 1,000 units lipase, 12,500 units protease, and
12,500 units amylase
Entozyme
Tablets: 300 mg pancreatin, 600 units lipase, 7,500 units protease, 7,500 units
amylase
Hi-Vegi-Lip Tablets
Tablets (enteric-coated): 2,400 mg pancreatin, 4,800 units lipase, 60,000 units
protease, and 60,000 units amylase ◇
4X Pancreatin 600 mg
Tablets (enteric-coated): 2,400 mg pancreatin, 12,000 units lipase, 60,000 units
protease, and 60,000 units amylase ◇

8X Pancreatin 900 mg
Tablets (enteric-coated): 7,200 mg pancreatin, 22,500 units lipase, 180,000 units
protease, and 180,000 units amylase ◇
Pancrezyme 4X Tablets
Tablets (enteric-coated): 2,400 mg pancreatin, 12,000 units lipase, 60,000 units
protease, and 60,000 units amylase ◇

ACTION
Replaces endogenous exocrine pancreatic
enzymes and aids digestion of starches,
fats, and proteins.

Route	Onset	Peak	Duration
PO	Unknown	Unknown	1-2 hr

INDICATIONS & DOSAGE
*Exocrine pancreatic secretion insufficien-
cy; digestive aid in diseases associated
with deficiency of pancreatic enzymes,
such as cystic fibrosis—*
Adults and children: dosage varies with
condition being treated. Usual initial
dosage is 8,000 to 24,000 units of lipase
activity P.O. before or with each meal or
snack. Total daily dose may also be given
in divided doses at 1- to 2-hour intervals
throughout day.

ADVERSE REACTIONS
GI: nausea, diarrhea (with high doses).
Other: allergic reactions, perianal irrita-
tion.

INTERACTIONS
Drug-drug. *Antacids:* may negate pancreatin's beneficial effect. Avoid concomitant
use.
Oral iron: may decrease serum iron response. Monitor for decreased effectiveness.

EFFECTS ON DIAGNOSTIC TESTS
Pancreatin, particularly in large doses, increases serum uric acid concentrations.

Reactions may be *common*, uncommon, *life-threatening*, or COMMON AND LIFE-THREATENING.

CONTRAINDICATIONS

Contraindicated in patients acute pancreatitis, acute exacerbations of chronic pancreatitis, or hypersensitivity to drug or pork protein or enzymes.

NURSING CONSIDERATIONS

• Use with caution in pregnant or breast-feeding patients.
• Be aware that minimal USP standards dictate that each milligram of bovine or porcine pancreatin contains lipase 2 units, protease 25 units, and amylase 25 units.
• To avoid indigestion, monitor patient's dietary intake to ensure a proper balance of fat, protein, and starch intake. Dosage varies according to degree of maldigestion and malabsorption, amount of fat in diet, and enzyme activity of individual preparations.
• Keep in mind that fewer bowel movements and improved stool consistency indicate effective therapy.
• Know that drug is not effective in GI disorders unrelated to pancreatic enzyme deficiency.
• Know that enteric coating on some products may reduce available enzyme in upper portion of jejunum.

☑ **Patient teaching**
• Instruct patient to take before or with meals and snacks.
• Tell patient not to crush or chew enteric-coated forms. Capsules containing enteric-coated microspheres may be opened and sprinkled on a small quantity of cooled, soft food. Stress importance of swallowing immediately without chewing and following with glass of water or juice.
• Warn patient not to inhale powder form or powder from capsules; may irritate skin or mucous membranes.
• Tell patient to store in airtight containers at room temperature.
• Instruct patient not to change brands without consulting doctor.

pancrelipase

Cotazym Capsules, Cotazym-S Capsules, Creon 5 Capsules, Creon 10 Capsules, Creon 20 Capsules, Ilozyme Tablets, Ku-Zyme HP Capsules, Pancrease Capsules, Pancrease MT4, Pancrease MT10, Pancrease MT16, Pancrease MT20, Pancrelipase Capsules, Protilase Capsules, Ultrase MT12, Ultrase MT18, Ultrase MT20, Ultrase MT24, Viokase Powder, Viokase Tablets, Zymase Capsules

Pregnancy Risk Category: C

HOW SUPPLIED
Cotazym
Capsules: 8,000 units lipase, 30,000 units protease, 30,000 units amylase, and 25 mg calcium carbonate
Cotazym-S
Capsules (enteric-coated spheres): 5,000 units lipase, 20,000 units protease, and 20,000 units amylase
Creon 5
Capsules (delayed-release): 5,000 units lipase, 18,750 units protease, and 16,600 units amylase
Creon 10
Capsules (delayed-release): 10,000 units lipase, 37,500 units protease, and 33,200 units amylase
Creon 20
Capsules (delayed-release): 20,000 units lipase, 75,000 units protease, and 66,400 units amylase
Ilozyme
Tablets: 11,000 units lipase, 30,000 units protease, and 30,000 units amylase
Ku-Zyme HP
Capsules: 8,000 units lipase, 30,000 units protease, and 30,000 units amylase
Pancrease
Capsules (enteric-coated microspheres): 4,000 units lipase, 25,000 units protease, and 20,000 units amylase
Pancrease MT4
Capsules (enteric-coated microtablets): 4,500 units lipase, 12,000 units protease, and 12,000 units amylase

Pancrease MT10
Capsules (enteric-coated microtablets):
10,000 units lipase, 30,000 units protease,
and 30,000 units amylase
Pancrease MT16
Capsules (enteric-coated microtablets):
16,000 units lipase, 48,000 units protease,
and 48,000 units amylase
Pancrease MT20
Capsules (enteric-coated microtablets):
20,000 units lipase, 44,000 units protease,
and 56,000 units amylase
Pancrelipase
Capsules (enteric-coated pellets):
4,000 units lipase, 25,000 units protease,
and 20,000 units amylase
Protilase
Capsules (enteric-coated spheres):
4,000 units lipase, 25,000 units protease,
and 20,000 units amylase
Ultrase MT12
Capsules (delayed-release): 12,000 units
lipase, 39,000 units protease, and
39,000 units amylase
Ultrase MT18
Capsules (delayed-release): 18,000 units
lipase, 58,500 units protease, and
58,000 units amylase
Ultrase MT20
Capsules (delayed-release): 20,000 units
lipase, 65,000 units protease, and
65,000 units amylase
Ultrase MT24
Capsules (delayed-release): 24,000 units
lipase, 78,000 units protease, and
78,000 units amylase
Viokase
Powder: 16,800 units lipase, 70,000 units
protease, and 70,000 units amylase per
0.7 g powder
Tablets: 8,000 units lipase, 30,000 units
protease, and 30,000 units amylase
Zymase
Capsules (enteric-coated spheres):
12,000 units lipase, 24,000 units protease,
and 24,000 units amylase

ACTION
Replaces endogenous exocrine pancreatic
enzymes and aids digestion of starches,
fats, and proteins.

Route	Onset	Peak	Duration
PO	Variable	Variable	Variable

INDICATIONS & DOSAGE
*Exocrine pancreatic secretion insufficien-
cy, cystic fibrosis in adults and children,
steatorrhea and other disorders of fat metabolism secondary to insufficient pancreatic enzymes—*
Adults and children 12 years and older:
dosage titrated to patient's response. Usual initial dosage 4,000 to 48,000 units of
lipase with each meal.
Children 7 to 12 years: 4,000 to
12,000 units (more, if needed) of lipase
activity with each meal or snack.
Children 1 to 6 years: 4,000 to
8,000 units of lipase with each meal and
4,000 units of lipase with each snack.
Children 6 months to 1 year:
2,000 units of lipase with each meal.
Children under 6 months: dosage not
established.

ADVERSE REACTIONS
GI: *nausea,* cramping, diarrhea (high
doses).

INTERACTIONS
Drug-drug. *Antacids:* may destroy enteric coating and result in enhanced
degradation of pancrelipase. Avoid concomitant use.
Oral iron: may decrease serum iron response. Monitor for decreased effectiveness.

EFFECTS ON DIAGNOSTIC TESTS
Pancrelipase, particularly in large doses,
increases serum uric acid concentrations.

CONTRAINDICATIONS
Contraindicated in patients with acute
pancreatitis, acute exacerbations of chronic pancreatic diseases, or severe hypersensitivity to pork.

NURSING CONSIDERATIONS
• Know that drug should be used only for
confirmed exocrine pancreatic insufficiency. It's not effective in GI disorders
unrelated to enzyme deficiency.
• Know that lipase activity is greater than
with other pancreatic enzymes.
• For infants, mix powder with applesauce
and give with meals. Avoid contact with
or inhalation of powder because it may be

very irritating. Older children may take capsules with food.
- Monitor patient's stools. Adequate replacement decreases number of bowel movements and improves stool consistency.
- Know that minimal USP standards dictate that each milligram of pancrelipase contains 24 units lipase, 100 units protease, and 100 units amylase.
- Be aware that dosage varies with degree of maldigestion and malabsorption, amount of fat in diet, and enzyme activity of individual preparations.
- Know that enteric coating on some products may reduce available enzyme in upper portion of jejunum.

☑ **Patient teaching**
- Instruct patient to take before or with meals and snacks.
- Advise patient not to crush or chew enteric-coated forms. Capsules containing enteric-coated microspheres may be opened and sprinkled on a small quantity of cooled, soft food. Stress importance of swallowing immediately without chewing and following with glass of water or juice.
- Warn patient not to inhale powder form or powder from capsules; it may irritate skin or mucous membranes.
- Tell patient to store in airtight containers at room temperature.
- Instruct patient not to change brands without consulting doctor.

ursodiol
Actigall

Pregnancy Risk Category: B

HOW SUPPLIED
Capsules: 300 mg

ACTION
Unknown. A naturally occurring bile acid that probably suppresses hepatic synthesis and secretion of cholesterol as well as intestinal cholesterol absorption. After long-term use, ursodiol can solubilize cholesterol from gallstones.

Route	Onset	Peak	Duration
PO	Unknown	1-3 hr	Unknown

INDICATIONS & DOSAGE
Dissolution of gallstones less than 20 mm in diameter when surgery precluded—
Adults: 8 to 10 mg/kg P.O. daily in two or three divided doses.
Prevention of gallstone formation in obese patients with rapid weight loss—
Adults: 300 mg P.O. b.i.d.

ADVERSE REACTIONS
CNS: *headache*, fatigue, anxiety, depression, *dizziness*, sleep disorders.
EENT: rhinitis.
GI: *nausea, vomiting, dyspepsia*, metallic taste, *abdominal pain*, biliary pain, cholecystitis, *diarrhea, constipation*, stomatitis, flatulence.
Musculoskeletal: arthralgia, myalgia, *back pain.*
Respiratory: cough.
Skin: pruritus, rash, dry skin, urticaria, hair thinning, diaphoresis.
Other: *urinary tract infection.*

INTERACTIONS
Drug-drug. *Aluminum-containing antacids, cholestyramine, colestipol:* bind ursodiol and prevent its absorption. Avoid concomitant use.
Clofibrate, estrogens, oral contraceptives: increased hepatic cholesterol secretion; may counteract the effects of ursodiol. Avoid concomitant use.

EFFECTS ON DIAGNOSTIC TESTS
None reported.

CONTRAINDICATIONS
Contraindicated in patients with chronic hepatic disease, unremitting acute cholecystitis, cholangitis, biliary obstruction, gallstone-induced pancreatitis, biliary fistula, and hypersensitivity to ursodiol or other bile acids.

NURSING CONSIDERATIONS
- Know that drug won't dissolve calcified cholesterol stones, radiolucent bile pigment stones, or radiopaque stones.
Alert: Monitor liver function test results, including AST and ALT, at the start of therapy and after 1 month, 3 months, and then every 6 months during therapy, as ordered. Abnormal tests may indicate a

worsening of the disease. A theoretical risk exists that a hepatotoxic metabolite of ursodiol may form in some patients.

• Know that therapy usually is long-term, with ultrasound images of the gallbladder taken every 6 months. If partial stone dissolution does not occur within 12 months, eventual success is unlikely. Safety of use for longer than 24 months has not been established.

✔Patient teaching

• Advise patient about alternative therapies, including "watchful waiting" (no intervention) and cholecystectomy because the relapse rate may be as high as 50% after 5 years.

• Tell patient to report adverse effects.

49

Antidiarrheals

attapulgite
bismuth subsalicylate
calcium polycarbophil
  (See Chapter 50, LAXATIVES.)
diphenoxylate hydrochloride and
  atropine sulfate
loperamide
octreotide acetate
opium tincture
opium tincture, camphorated

COMBINATION PRODUCTS
KAODENE NON-NARCOTIC ◊: 3.9 g kaolin
and 194.4 mg pectin in 30-ml bismuth
subsalicylate liquid.
KAPECTOLIN: 90 g kaolin and 2 g pectin in
30-ml suspension.
K-C ◊: 5.2 g kaolin, 260 mg pectin,
260 mg bismuth subsalicylate in 30-ml
suspension.

---

attapulgite
Children's Kaopectate, Diasorb,
Donnagel, Fowler's†, Kaopectate
Advanced Formula, Kaopectate
Maximum Strength, K-Pek,
Parepectolin, Rheaban Maximum
Strength

Pregnancy Risk Category: NR

HOW SUPPLIED
Tablets: 300 mg, 600 mg†, 630 mg†,
750 mg
Tablets (chewable): 300 mg, 600 mg
Oral suspension: 600 mg/15 ml, 750 mg/
5 ml, 750 mg/15 ml†, 900 mg/15 ml†
Caplets: 750 mg

ACTION
A hydrated magnesium aluminum silicate
that is thought to adsorb large numbers of
bacteria and toxins and reduce water loss.

Route	Onset	Peak	Duration
PO	Unknown	Unknown	Unknown

INDICATIONS & DOSAGE
Acute, nonspecific diarrhea—
**Adults and children older than 12
years:** 1.2 to 1.5 g (up to 3 g if using Diasorb) P.O. after each loose bowel movement, not to exceed 9 g in 24 hours.
Children 6 to 12 years: 600 mg (suspension) or 750 mg (tablet) P.O. after each
loose bowel movement, not to exceed
4.2 g (suspension) or 4.5 g (tablet) in 24
hours.
Children 3 to 6 years: 300 mg P.O. after
each loose bowel movement, not to exceed 2.1 g in 24 hours.

ADVERSE REACTIONS
GI: constipation.

INTERACTIONS
Drug-drug. *Oral medications:* potential
for impaired absorption of oral medications when administered concurrently
with attapulgite. Administer attapulgite
not less than 2 hours before or 3 hours after these medications, and monitor for decreased effectiveness.

EFFECTS ON DIAGNOSTIC TESTS
None reported.

CONTRAINDICATIONS
Contraindicated in patients with dysen-
tery or suspected bowel obstruction.

NURSING CONSIDERATIONS
• Use cautiously in patients with dehydration. Promote adequate fluid intake to
compensate for fluid loss from diarrhea.
• Be aware that drug should not be used if
diarrhea is accompanied by fever or by
blood or mucus in the stool. If these signs
occur during treatment, withhold drug
and notify doctor.

☑ **Patient teaching**
• Tell patient to take drug after each loose
bowel movement until diarrhea is controlled.
• Instruct patient to notify doctor if diar-

---

*Liquid contains alcohol.   **May contain tartrazine.   †Canada   ‡Australia   §U.K.   ◊OTC

rhea is not controlled within 48 hours or if fever develops.

bismuth subsalicylate
Bismatrol ◇, Bismatrol Extra Strength ◇, Pepto-Bismol ◇, Pepto-Bismol Maximum Strength Liquid ◇, Pink Bismuth ◇

Pregnancy Risk Category: NR

HOW SUPPLIED
Tablets (chewable): 262 mg ◇
Oral suspension: 262 mg/15 ml ◇, 524 mg/15 ml ◇

ACTION
Unknown. Has a mild water-binding capacity; also may adsorb toxins and provide protective coating for mucosa.

Route	Onset	Peak	Duration
PO	1 hr	Unknown	Unknown

INDICATIONS & DOSAGE
Mild, nonspecific diarrhea—
Adults: 30 ml or 2 tablets P.O. q 30 minutes to 1 hour, up to maximum of eight doses and for no longer than 2 days.
Children 3 to 6 years: 5 ml or ⅓ tablet P.O.
Children 6 to 9 years: 10 ml or ⅔ tablet P.O.
Children 9 to 12 years: 15 ml or 1 tablet P.O.

ADVERSE REACTIONS
GI: temporary darkening of tongue and stools.
Other: salicylism (with high doses).

INTERACTIONS
Drug-drug. *Aspirin, other salicylates:* risk of salicylate toxicity. Monitor closely.
Oral anticoagulants, oral antidiabetic agents: theoretical risk of increased effects of these agents after high doses of bismuth subsalicylate. Monitor patient closely.
Tetracycline: decreased tetracycline absorption. Separate administration times by at least 2 hours.

EFFECTS ON DIAGNOSTIC TESTS
Because bismuth is radiopaque, it may interfere with radiologic examination of the GI tract.

CONTRAINDICATIONS
Contraindicated in patients hypersensitive to salicylates.

NURSING CONSIDERATIONS
• Use cautiously in patients taking aspirin. Discontinue if tinnitus occurs.
• Be aware salicylate absorption may occur from bismuth subsalicylate. Use cautiously in patients with bleeding disorders or salicylate sensitivity and in children.
• Avoid use before GI radiologic procedures because bismuth is radiopaque and may interfere with X-rays.

☑**Patient teaching**
• Advise patient that bismuth subsalicylate contains salicylate (each tablet has 102 mg salicylate; the regular-strength liquid has 130 mg/15 ml, and the extra-strength liquid has 230 mg/15 ml).
• Instruct patient to chew tablets well before swallowing or to shake liquid before measuring dose.
• Tell patient to call doctor if diarrhea persists for more than 2 days or is accompanied by high fever.
• Tell patient to consult with doctor before giving bismuth subsalicylate to children or teenagers during or after recovery from the flu or chickenpox.
• Inform patient that all forms of Pepto-Bismol are effective against traveler's diarrhea. Tablets and caplets may be more convenient to carry.

diphenoxylate hydrochloride and atropine sulfate
Logen, Lomanate, Lomotil*, Lonox

Controlled Substance Schedule V
Pregnancy Risk Category: C

HOW SUPPLIED
Tablets: 2.5 mg (with atropine sulfate 0.025 mg)
Liquid: 2.5 mg/5 ml (with atropine sulfate 0.025 mg/5 ml)*

ACTION
Unknown. Probably increases smooth muscle tone in the GI tract, inhibits motility and propulsion, and diminishes secretions.

Route	Onset	Peak	Duration
PO	45-60 min	3 hr	3-4 hr

INDICATIONS & DOSAGE
Acute, nonspecific diarrhea—
Adults: initially, 5 mg P.O. q.i.d.; then adjusted p.r.n.
Children 2 to 12 years: 0.3 to 0.4 mg/kg liquid form P.O. daily in four divided doses. For maintenance, initial dosage reduced p.r.n., up to 75%.

ADVERSE REACTIONS
CNS: *sedation, dizziness,* headache, drowsiness, lethargy, restlessness, depression, euphoria, malaise, confusion, numbness in extremities.
CV: tachycardia.
EENT: mydriasis.
GI: *dry mouth,* nausea, vomiting, abdominal discomfort or distention, *paralytic ileus,* anorexia, fluid retention in bowel or megacolon (may mask depletion of extracellular fluid and electrolytes, especially in young children treated for acute gastroenteritis), pancreatitis, swollen gums, possible physical dependence with long-term use.
GU: urine retention.
Respiratory: *respiratory depression.*
Skin: pruritus, rash, dry skin.
Other: *angioedema, anaphylaxis.*

INTERACTIONS
Drug-drug. *Barbiturates, CNS depressants, narcotic agents, tranquilizers:* enhanced CNS depression. Closely monitor patient.
MAO inhibitors: possible hypertensive crisis. Avoid concomitant use.
Drug-lifestyle. *Alcohol use:* enhanced CNS depression. Closely monitor patient.

EFFECTS ON DIAGNOSTIC TESTS
None reported.

CONTRAINDICATIONS
Contraindicated in patients with jaundice or hypersensitivity to diphenoxylate or atropine and in children under 2 years. Also contraindicated in those with acute diarrhea resulting from poison (until toxic material is eliminated from GI tract), from organisms that penetrate intestinal mucosa, or from antibiotic-induced pseudomembranous enterocolitis.

NURSING CONSIDERATIONS
• Use cautiously in children 2 years and over; in patients with hepatic disease, narcotic dependence, or acute ulcerative colitis; and in pregnant patients. Stop therapy immediately if abdominal distention or other signs of toxic megacolon develop and notify doctor.
• Monitor fluid and electrolyte balance. Correct fluid and electrolyte disturbances before starting drug. Dehydration, especially in young children, may increase risk of delayed toxicity.
• Know that drug is not indicated for treating antibiotic-induced diarrhea.
• Be aware that drug is unlikely to be effective if no response occurs within 48 hours.
• Know that risk of physical dependence increases with high dosage and long-term use. Atropine sulfate helps discourage abuse.

☑ **Patient teaching**
• Tell patient not to exceed recommended dosage.
• Warn patient not to use drug to treat acute diarrhea for longer than 2 days and to seek medical attention if diarrhea continues.
• Advise patient to avoid hazardous activities, such as driving, until CNS effects of drug are known.

loperamide
Imodium, Imodium A-D ◊,
Kaopectate II Caplets ◊, Maalox
Anti-Diarrheal Caplets ◊, Pepto
Diarrhea Control ◊

Pregnancy Risk Category: B

HOW SUPPLIED
Caplets: 2 mg ◊

---

*Liquid contains alcohol.   **May contain tartrazine.   †Canada   ‡Australia   §U.K.   ◊OTC

Capsules: 2 mg
Oral liquid: 1 mg/5 ml ◇

ACTION
Inhibits peristaltic activity, prolonging transit of intestinal contents.

Route	Onset	Peak	Duration
PO	Unknown	2.5-5 hr	24 hr

INDICATIONS & DOSAGE
Acute, nonspecific diarrhea—
Adults: initially, 4 mg P.O.; then 2 mg after each unformed stool. Maximum dosage is 16 mg daily.
Children 2 to 5 years: 5 ml P.O. t.i.d. on first day. If diarrhea persists, contact doctor.
Children 6 to 8 years: 10 ml (2 mg) P.O. b.i.d. on first day. If diarrhea persists, contact doctor. Do not exceed 4 mg daily.
Children 8 to 12 years: 10 ml (2 mg) t.i.d. P.O. on first day. (Subsequent doses of 5 ml [1 mg]/10 kg of body weight may be administered after each unformed stool.) Maximum dosage is 6 mg daily.
Chronic diarrhea—
Adults: initially, 4 mg P.O., then 2 mg after each unformed stool until diarrhea subsides. Dosage adjusted to individual response.

ADVERSE REACTIONS
CNS: drowsiness, fatigue, dizziness.
GI: dry mouth; abdominal pain, distention, or discomfort; *constipation;* nausea; vomiting.
Skin: rash, *hypersensitivity reactions.*

INTERACTIONS
None significant.

EFFECTS ON DIAGNOSTIC TESTS
None reported.

CONTRAINDICATIONS
Contraindicated in patients with hypersensitivity and when constipation must be avoided. Also contraindicated in children under 2 years.

NURSING CONSIDERATIONS
• Use cautiously in patients with hepatic disease.

• Be aware that the drug produces antidiarrheal action similar to diphenoxylate but without as many adverse CNS effects.
Alert: Monitor children closely for CNS effects; they may be more sensitive to CNS effects of drug than adults.

✅ Patient teaching
• Advise patient not to exceed recommended dosage.
• Tell patient with acute diarrhea to discontinue drug and seek medical attention if no improvement occurs within 48 hours; in chronic diarrhea, tell him to notify doctor and discontinue drug if no improvement occurs after taking 16 mg daily for at least 10 days.
• Advise patient with acute colitis to stop drug immediately if abdominal distention or other symptoms develop and notify doctor.
• Warn patient to avoid activities that require mental alertness until CNS effects of drug are known.
• Tell patient to report nausea, abdominal pain, or abdominal discomfort.
• Advise patient to relieve dry mouth with ice chips or sugarless gum.

octreotide acetate
Sandostatin

Pregnancy Risk Category: B

HOW SUPPLIED
Injection ampules: 0.05 mg, 0.1 mg, 0.5 mg
Injection-multidose vials: 0.2 mg/ml, 1 mg/ml

ACTION
Mimics the action of naturally occurring somatostatin.

Route	Onset	Peak	Duration
SC	0.5 hr	0.5 hr	< 12 hr

INDICATIONS & DOSAGE
Flushing and diarrhea associated with carcinoid tumors—
Adults: 0.1 to 0.6 mg daily S.C. in two to four divided doses for first 2 weeks of therapy (usual daily dosage is 0.3 mg).

Reactions may be *common,* uncommon, *life-threatening,* or COMMON AND LIFE-THREATENING.

Subsequent dosage based on individual response.

Watery diarrhea associated with vasoactive intestinal polypeptide secreting tumors (VIPomas)—
Adults: 0.2 to 0.3 mg daily S.C. in two to four divided doses for first 2 weeks of therapy. Subsequent dosage based on individual response; typically, don't exceed 0.45 mg daily.

Acromegaly—
Adults: initially, 50 mcg S.C. t.i.d., then adjusted based on somatomedin C levels q 2 weeks.

ADVERSE REACTIONS
CNS: dizziness, light-headedness, fatigue, headache.
CV: sinus bradycardia, conduction abnormalities, *arrhythmias.*
EENT: blurred vision.
GI: *nausea, diarrhea, abdominal pain or discomfort, loose stools,* vomiting, fat malabsorption, gallbladder abnormalities, flatulence, constipation.
GU: pollakiuria, urinary tract infection.
Metabolic: hyperglycemia, hypoglycemia, hypothyroidism.
Musculoskeletal: backache, joint pain.
Skin: flushing, edema, wheal, erythema or pain at injection site, alopecia.
Other: pain or burning at the S.C. injection site, cold symptoms, flulike symptoms.

INTERACTIONS
Drug-drug. *Cyclosporine:* may decrease plasma levels of cyclosporine. Monitor patient closely.

EFFECTS ON DIAGNOSTIC TESTS
Octreotide suppresses secretion of growth hormone and of the gastroenterohepatic peptides gastrin, vasoactive intestinal polypeptide, insulin, glucagon, secretin, motilin, and pancreatic polypeptide.

CONTRAINDICATIONS
Contraindicated in patients hypersensitive to drug or its components.

NURSING CONSIDERATIONS
• Monitor baseline thyroid function tests as ordered.

• Monitor somatomedin C levels every 2 weeks as ordered. Know that dosage adjustments are based on this level.
• Monitor laboratory tests periodically, such as thyroid function tests, blood glucose, urine 5-hydroxyindoleacetic acid, plasma serotonin, and plasma substance P (for carcinoid tumors).
• Monitor patient regularly for gallbladder disease. Octreotide therapy may be associated with development of cholelithiasis because of its effect on gallbladder motility or fat absorption.
• Monitor closely for symptoms of glucose imbalance. Be alert that insulin-dependent diabetic patients and patients receiving oral antidiabetic agents or oral diazoxide may require dosage adjustments during therapy. Monitor blood glucose levels.
• Keep in mind that octreotide therapy may alter fluid and electrolyte balance and may require adjustment of other drugs used to control symptoms of the disease, such as beta blockers.
• Be aware that half-life may be altered in patients in end-stage renal failure who are receiving dialysis.

☑ **Patient teaching**
• Instruct patient to report signs of abdominal discomfort immediately.
• Stress importance of need for periodic laboratory testing during octreotide therapy.

opium tincture*

Controlled Substance Schedule II

opium tincture, camphorated* (paregoric)

Controlled Substance Schedule III
Pregnancy Risk Category: NR

HOW SUPPLIED
opium tincture
Oral solution: equivalent to morphine 10 mg/ml*
opium tincture, camphorated
Oral solution: each 5 ml contains morphine, 2 mg; anise oil, 0.2 ml; benzoic

---

acid, 20 mg; camphor, 20 mg; glycerin, 0.2 ml; and ethanol to make 5 ml*

ACTION
Increases smooth muscle tone in the GI tract, inhibits motility and propulsion, and diminishes secretions.

Route	Onset	Peak	Duration
PO	Unknown	Unknown	Unknown

INDICATIONS & DOSAGE
Acute, nonspecific diarrhea—
Note: Do not confuse opium tincture with camphorated opium tincture.
opium tincture
Adults: 0.6 ml (range 0.3 to 1 ml) P.O. q.i.d. Maximum dosage is 6 ml daily.
opium tincture, camphorated
Adults: 5 to 10 ml P.O. once daily, b.i.d., t.i.d., or q.i.d. until diarrhea subsides.
Children: 0.25 to 0.5 ml/kg P.O. once daily, b.i.d., t.i.d., or q.i.d. until diarrhea subsides.

ADVERSE REACTIONS
CNS: dizziness, light-headedness.
GI: nausea, vomiting, physical dependence after long-term use.

INTERACTIONS
None significant.

EFFECTS ON DIAGNOSTIC TESTS
Opium tincture and camphorated opium tincture may prevent delivery of Tc99m disofenin to small intestine during hepatobiliary imaging tests; delay test until 24 hours after last dose. They also may raise serum amylase and lipase levels by inducing contractions of sphincter of Oddi and raising biliary tract pressure.

CONTRAINDICATIONS
Contraindicated in patients with acute diarrhea caused by poisoning until toxic material is removed from GI tract or in those with diarrhea caused by organisms that penetrate intestinal mucosa.

NURSING CONSIDERATIONS
• Use cautiously in patients with asthma, prostatic hyperplasia, hepatic disease, and history of opioid dependence.

Alert: Be aware that opium tincture has 25 times more opium content than camphorated opium tincture. Camphorated opium tincture is more dilute, and teaspoon doses are easier to measure than dropper quantities of opium tincture.
Alert: For overdose, use the narcotic antagonist naloxone, as ordered, to reverse respiratory depression.
• Mix with sufficient water to ensure passage to stomach.
• Know that a milky fluid forms when camphorated opium tincture is added to water.
• Store in tightly capped, light-resistant container.

✔Patient teaching
• Advise patient against using drug for more than 2 days; risk of physical dependence increases with long-term use.
• Instruct patient to measure dosage carefully to avoid overdose.
• Tell patient to notify doctor if diarrhea persists.

bisacodyl
calcium polycarbophil
cascara sagrada
cascara sagrada aromatic
    fluidextract
cascara sagrada fluidextract
castor oil
docusate calcium
docusate sodium
glycerin
lactulose
magnesium citrate
magnesium hydroxide
magnesium sulfate
methylcellulose
mineral oil
polyethylene glycol and
    electrolyte solution
psyllium
senna
sodium phosphates

COMBINATION PRODUCTS

Note: The U.S. FDA proposed a ban on the use of phenolphthalein due to long-term safety concerns.

AGORAL ◊: mineral oil 4.2 g and white phenolphthalein 0.2 g per 15 ml, with tragacanth, agar, egg albumin, acacia, glycerin and saccharin.

DIALOSE PLUS ◊: docusate sodium 100 mg and casanthranol 30 mg.

DOXIDAN ◊: docusate calcium 60 mg and phenolphthalein 65 mg.

D-S-S PLUS ◊: docusate sodium 100 mg and casanthranol 30 mg.

HALEY'S M-O ◊: mineral oil 3.75 ml and magnesium hydroxide 900 mg per 15 ml.

KONDREMUL WITH PHENOLPHTHALEIN ◊: heavy mineral oil 55%, white phenolphthalein 150 mg/15 ml, and Irish moss as emulsifier.

MODANE PLUS ◊: docusate sodium 100 mg and white phenolphthalein 65 mg.

PERI-COLACE CAPSULES ◊: docusate sodium 100 mg and casanthranol 30 mg.

PERI-COLACE SYRUP ◊: docusate sodium 60 mg and casanthranol 30 mg/15 ml.

SENOKOT-S ◊: docusate sodium 50 mg and standardized senna concentrate 187 mg.

UNILAX CAPSULE: docusate sodium 230 mg and yellow phenolphthalein 130 mg.

---

bisacodyl

Bisacolax† ◊, Bisalax‡, Bisco-Lax** ◊, Dulcagen ◊, Dulcolax ◊, Durolax‡, Fleet Bisacodyl ◊, Fleet Bisacodyl Prep ◊, Fleet Laxative ◊, Laxit† ◊

Pregnancy Risk Category: NR

HOW SUPPLIED
Tablets (enteric-coated): 5 mg ◊
Enema: 0.33 mg/ml ◊, 10 mg/5 ml (microenema)‡
Powder for rectal solution (bisacodyl tannex): 1.5 mg bisacodyl and 2.5 g tannic acid
Suppositories: 5 mg ◊, 10 mg ◊

ACTION
Unknown. A stimulant laxative that increases peristalsis probably by direct effect on the smooth muscle of the intestine. Thought to either irritate the musculature or stimulate the colonic intramural plexus. Also promotes fluid accumulation in the colon and small intestine.

Route	Onset	Peak	Duration
PO	6-12 hr	Variable	Variable
PR	15-60 min	Variable	Variable

INDICATIONS & DOSAGE
Chronic constipation; preparation for delivery, surgery, or rectal or bowel examination—
Adults and children 12 years and over: 10 to 15 mg P.O. in evening or before breakfast. Up to 30 mg P.O. as needed and ordered, or 10 mg P.R. for evacuation before examination or surgery.
Children 6 to 12 years: 5 mg P.O. or P.R. h.s. or before breakfast. Oral dose is not

recommended if child cannot swallow tablet whole.

ADVERSE REACTIONS
CNS: muscle weakness (with excessive use), dizziness, faintness.
GI: *nausea, vomiting, abdominal cramps,* diarrhea (with high doses), *burning sensation in rectum* (with suppositories), laxative dependence (with long-term or excessive use).
Other: alkalosis, hypokalemia, tetany, fluid and electrolyte imbalance; protein-losing enteropathy (with excessive use).

INTERACTIONS
Drug-drug. *Antacids:* gastric irritation or dyspepsia from premature dissolution of enteric coating. Do not administer together.
Drug-food. *Milk:* gastric irritation or dyspepsia from premature dissolution of enteric coating. Do not administer together.

EFFECTS ON DIAGNOSTIC TESTS
None reported.

CONTRAINDICATIONS
Contraindicated in patients with rectal bleeding, gastroenteritis, intestinal obstruction, abdominal pain, nausea, vomiting, other symptoms of appendicitis or acute surgical abdomen, or hypersensitivity to drug or its components.

NURSING CONSIDERATIONS
• Time administration of drug so as not to interfere with scheduled activities or sleep. Soft, formed stools are usually produced 15 to 60 minutes after rectal administration.
• Before giving for constipation, determine if the patient has adequate fluid intake, exercise, and diet.
• Know that tablets and suppositories are used together to clean the colon before and after surgery and before barium enema.
• Insert suppository as high as possible into the rectum, and try to position the suppository against the rectal wall. Avoid embedding within fecal material because this may delay the onset of action.

✅ **Patient teaching**
• Advise patient to swallow enteric-coated tablet whole to avoid GI irritation. Don't give within 1 hour of milk or antacid intake.
• Tell patient drug is for short-term (1 week) treatment only (stimulant laxatives are frequently abused). Discourage excessive use.
• Advise patient to report adverse effects to doctor.
• Teach patient about dietary sources of bulk, which include bran and other cereals, fresh fruit, and vegetables.
• Tell patient to take drug with a full glass of water or juice.

---

calcium polycarbophil
Equalactin◇, Fiberall◇,
FiberCon◇, Fiber-Lax◇,
Mitrolan◇

Pregnancy Risk Category: NR

HOW SUPPLIED
Tablets: 500 mg◇, 625 mg◇
Tablets (chewable): 500 mg◇, 1,250 mg◇

ACTION
A bulk-forming laxative that absorbs water and expands to increase bulk and moisture content of stools. The increased bulk encourages peristalsis and bowel movement. As an antidiarrheal, absorbs free fecal water, thereby producing formed stools.

Route	Onset	Peak	Duration
PO	12-24 hr	3 days	Variable

INDICATIONS & DOSAGE
Constipation—
Adults: 1 g P.O. q.i.d., p.r.n. Maximum dosage is 6 g in 24-hour period.
Children 3 to 6 years: use must be directed by doctor. 500 mg P.O. b.i.d., p.r.n. Maximum dosage is 1.5 g in 24-hour period.
Children 6 to 12 years: 500 mg P.O. one to three times daily, p.r.n. Maximum dosage is 3 g in 24-hour period.
Diarrhea associated with irritable bowel

---

syndrome, as well as acute nonspecific diarrhea—
Adults: 1 g P.O. q.i.d., p.r.n. Maximum dosage is 6 g in 24-hour period.
Children 2 to 6 years: use must be directed by doctor. 500 mg P.O. b.i.d., p.r.n. Maximum dosage is 1.5 g in 24-hour period.
Children 6 to 12 years: 500 mg P.O. t.i.d., p.r.n. Maximum dosage is 3 g in 24-hour period.

ADVERSE REACTIONS
GI: abdominal fullness and increased flatus, intestinal obstruction.
Other: laxative dependence (with long-term or excessive use).

INTERACTIONS
Drug-drug. *Tetracyclines:* impaired absorption of tetracyclines. Avoid use together.

EFFECTS ON DIAGNOSTIC TESTS
None reported.

CONTRAINDICATIONS
Contraindicated in patients with signs of GI obstruction.

NURSING CONSIDERATIONS
• Before giving for constipation, determine if patient has adequate fluid intake, exercise, and diet.
Alert: Be aware that rectal bleeding or failure to respond to therapy may indicate need for surgery.

☑ **Patient teaching**
• Advise patient to chew Equalactin or Mitrolan tablets thoroughly before swallowing and to drink a full glass of water with each dose. When used as an antidiarrheal, tell patient not to drink a glass of water.
• Teach patient about dietary sources of bulk, which include bran and other cereals, fresh fruit, and vegetables.
• For severe diarrhea, advise patient to repeat dose every 30 minutes, but not to exceed maximum daily dosage.

cascara sagrada ◇
cascara sagrada aromatic fluidextract* ◇
cascara sagrada fluidextract* ◇
Pregnancy Risk Category: C

HOW SUPPLIED
Tablets: 325 mg ◇
Aromatic fluidextract: 1 g/ml* ◇
Fluidextract: 1 g/ml* ◇

ACTION
Unknown. A stimulant laxative that increases peristalsis probably by direct effect on the smooth muscle of the intestine. Thought to either irritate the musculature or stimulate the colonic intramural plexus. Also promotes fluid accumulation in the colon and small intestine.

Route	Onset	Peak	Duration
PO	6-10 hr	Variable	Variable

INDICATIONS & DOSAGE
Acute constipation; preparation for bowel or rectal examination—
Adults and children 12 years and over: one 325 mg tablet of cascara sagrada P.O. once daily h.s.; 0.5 to 1.5 ml of cascara sagrada fluidextract P.O. once daily, or 2 to 6 ml of aromatic cascara fluidextract P.O. once daily.
Children 2 to 12 years: ½ adult dosage.
Children under 2 years: ¼ adult dosage.

ADVERSE REACTIONS
GI: *nausea;* vomiting; diarrhea; loss of normal bowel function with excessive use; *abdominal cramps,* especially in severe constipation; malabsorption of nutrients; "cathartic colon" (syndrome resembling ulcerative colitis radiologically and pathologically; with chronic misuse); discoloration of rectal mucosa (after long-term use).
Other: hypokalemia, protein enteropathy, electrolyte imbalance (with excessive use), laxative dependence (with long-term or excessive use).

---

*Liquid contains alcohol.   **May contain tartrazine.   †Canada   ‡Australia   §U.K.   ◇OTC

INTERACTIONS
None significant.

EFFECTS ON DIAGNOSTIC TESTS
Drug turns alkaline urine pink to red, red to violet, or red to brown and turns acidic urine yellow to brown in the phenolsulfonphthalein excretion test.

CONTRAINDICATIONS
Contraindicated in patients with abdominal pain, nausea, vomiting, or other symptoms of appendicitis or acute surgical abdomen; acute surgical delirium; fecal impaction; and intestinal obstruction or perforation.

NURSING CONSIDERATIONS
• Use cautiously when rectal bleeding is present.
• Before giving for constipation, determine if patient has adequate fluid intake, exercise, and diet.
• Monitor serum electrolytes during prolonged use.
• Be aware that cascara sagrada aromatic fluidextract is less active and less bitter than the nonaromatic fluidextract.
• Know that liquid preparations are more reliable than solid dosage forms.

☑ **Patient teaching**
• Warn patient that drug may turn alkaline urine red-pink and acidic urine yellow-brown.
• Teach patient about dietary sources of bulk, which include bran and other cereals, fresh fruit, and vegetables.
• Tell patient to take with a full glass of water.

---

castor oil
Castor Oil Capsules, Emulsoil ◇,
Fleet Flavored Castor Oil ◇

Pregnancy Risk Category: X

HOW SUPPLIED
Capsules: 0.62 ml
Oral liquid: 67% (Fleet ◇), 95% (Emulsoil ◇, Purge ◇)

ACTION
Unknown. A stimulant laxative that increases peristalsis probably by direct effect on the smooth muscle of the intestine. Thought to either irritate the musculature or stimulate the colonic intramural plexus. Also promotes fluid accumulation in the colon and small intestine.

Route	Onset	Peak	Duration
PO	2-6 hr	Variable	Variable

INDICATIONS & DOSAGE
Preparation for rectal or bowel examination or for surgery—
Adults and children 12 years and older: 15 to 60 ml P.O.
Children 2 to 12 years: 5 to 15 ml P.O.
Children under 2 years: 2.5 to 7.5 ml P.O. Increased dose produces no greater effect.
   For all patients, administered as a single dose about 16 hours before surgery or procedure.

ADVERSE REACTIONS
GI: *nausea;* vomiting; diarrhea; loss of normal bowel function with excessive use; *abdominal cramps,* especially in severe constipation; malabsorption of nutrients; "cathartic colon" (syndrome resembling ulcerative colitis radiologically and pathologically) with chronic misuse; laxative dependence with long-term or excessive use. May cause constipation after catharsis.
Other: hypokalemia, protein-losing enteropathy, other electrolyte imbalances (with excessive use).

INTERACTIONS
None significant.

EFFECTS ON DIAGNOSTIC TESTS
None reported.

CONTRAINDICATIONS
Contraindicated in patients with ulcerative bowel lesions; abdominal pain, nausea, vomiting, or other symptoms of appendicitis or acute surgical abdomen; anal or rectal fissures, fecal impaction, or intestinal obstruction or perforation; and during menstruation or pregnancy.

Reactions may be *common*, uncommon, *life-threatening*, or COMMON AND LIFE-THREATENING.

NURSING CONSIDERATIONS
• Use cautiously in patients with rectal bleeding.
• Give castor oil with juice or carbonated beverage to mask oily taste. Have patient stir mixture and drink it promptly. Ice held in the mouth before taking drug will help prevent tasting it.
• Shake emulsion well before measuring dose. Emulsion is better tolerated but is more expensive. Store below 40° F (4.4° C). Don't freeze.
• Give on empty stomach for best results.
• Time drug administration so that it doesn't interfere with scheduled activities or sleep.
• Know that increased intestinal motility lessens absorption of concomitantly administered oral drugs. Separate administration times.
Alert: Be aware that failure to respond to drug may indicate acute condition requiring surgery.

☑**Patient teaching**
• Tell patient not to expect another bowel movement for 1 to 2 days after castor oil has emptied bowel.
• Warn patient about potential adverse reactions.

---

docusate calcium (dioctyl calcium sulfosuccinate)
DC Softgels ◇, Pro-Cal-Sof ◇, Sulfalax Calcium ◇, Surfak ◇

docusate sodium (dioctyl sodium sulfosuccinate)
Colace ◇, Coloxyl‡, Coloxyl Enema Concentrate‡, Diocto ◇, Dioctyl§, Dioeze ◇, Diosuccin ◇, Disonate ◇, Di-Sosul ◇, DOS ◇, Doxinate ◇, D-S-S ◇, Duosol ◇, Fletcher's Enemette§, Modane Soft ◇, Norgalax Micro-enema§, Pro-Sof ◇, Regulax SS ◇, Regulex† ◇, Regutol ◇

Pregnancy Risk Category: C

HOW SUPPLIED
docusate calcium
Capsules: 50 mg ◇, 240 mg ◇

docusate sodium
Tablets: 100 mg ◇, 50 mg ◇
Capsules: 50 mg ◇, 100 mg ◇, 240 mg ◇, 250 mg ◇
Oral liquid: 150 mg/15 ml ◇
Oral solution: 50 mg/ml ◇, 10 mg/ml ◇
Syrup: 20 mg/5 ml, 50 mg/15 ml ◇, 60 mg/15 ml ◇
Enema concentrate: 18 g/100 ml (must be diluted)‡

ACTION
A stool softener that reduces surface tension of interfacing liquid contents of the bowel. This detergent activity promotes incorporation of additional liquid into stools, thus forming a softer mass.

Route	Onset	Peak	Duration
PO, PR	24-72 hr	24-72 hr	24-72 hr

INDICATIONS & DOSAGE
Stool softener—
Adults and children older than 12 years: 50 to 500 mg P.O. daily until bowel movements are normal. Alternatively, give enema (where available). Dilute 1:24 with sterile water before administration, and give 100 to 150 ml (retention enema), 300 to 500 ml (evacuation enema), or 0.5 to 1.5 L (flushing enema) P.R.
Children 6 to 12 years: 40 to 120 mg docusate sodium P.O. daily.
Children 3 to 6 years: 20 to 60 mg docusate sodium P.O. daily.
Children under 3 years: 10 to 40 mg docusate sodium P.O. daily.
  Higher dosages used for initial therapy. Dosage adjusted to individual response. Usual dosage in children and adults with minimal needs is 50 to 150 mg (calcium) P.O. daily.

ADVERSE REACTIONS
GI: bitter taste, mild abdominal cramping, diarrhea, laxative dependence (with long-term or excessive use).

INTERACTIONS
Drug-drug. *Mineral oil:* may increase mineral oil absorption and cause toxicity and lipoid pneumonia. Separate administration times.

EFFECTS ON DIAGNOSTIC TESTS
None reported.

CONTRAINDICATIONS
Contraindicated in patients with intestinal obstruction, undiagnosed abdominal pain, vomiting or other signs of appendicitis, fecal impaction, acute surgical abdomen, or hypersensitivity to drug.

NURSING CONSIDERATIONS
• Give liquid in milk, fruit juice, or infant formula to mask bitter taste.
• Before giving for constipation, determine if patient has adequate fluid intake, exercise, and diet.
• Know that drug is not for use in treating existing constipation but prevents constipation from developing.
• Be aware that drug is laxative of choice for patients who should not strain during defecation, including patients recovering from MI or rectal surgery; for those with rectal or anal disease that makes passage of firm stools difficult; and for those with postpartum constipation.
• Store drug at 59° to 86° F (15° to 30° C), and protect liquid from light.

☑ **Patient teaching**
• Teach patient about dietary sources of bulk, which include bran and other cereals, fresh fruit, and vegetables.
• Instruct patient to use only occasionally and not for more than 1 week without the doctor's knowledge.
• Tell patient to discontinue if severe cramping occurs and to notify doctor.
• Notify patient that it may take from 1 to 3 days to soften stools.

---

glycerin
Fleet Babylax ◊ , Sani-Supp ◊

Pregnancy Risk Category: NR

HOW SUPPLIED
Enema (pediatric): 4 ml/applicator ◊
Suppositories: adult, children, and infant sizes ◊

ACTION
A hyperosmolar laxative that draws water from the tissues into the feces and thus stimulates evacuation.

Route	Onset	Peak	Duration
PR	15-60 min	15-60 min	15-60 min

INDICATIONS & DOSAGE
Constipation—
Adults and children 6 years and over: 2 to 3 g as a rectal suppository or 5 to 15 ml as an enema.
Children 2 to 6 years: 1 to 1.7 g as a rectal suppository; or 2 to 5 ml as an enema.

ADVERSE REACTIONS
GI: *cramping pain,* rectal discomfort, hyperemia of rectal mucosa.

INTERACTIONS
None significant.

EFFECTS ON DIAGNOSTIC TESTS
None reported.

CONTRAINDICATIONS
Contraindicated in patients with intestinal obstruction, undiagnosed abdominal pain, vomiting or other signs of appendicitis, fecal impaction, acute surgical abdomen, or hypersensitivity to drug.

NURSING CONSIDERATIONS
• Know that drug is used mainly to reestablish proper toilet habits in laxative-dependent patients.

☑ **Patient teaching**
• Tell patient that drug must be retained for at least 15 minutes and that it usually acts within 1 hour. Entire suppository need not melt to be effective.
• Warn patient about adverse GI reactions.

---

lactulose
Cephulac, Cholac, Chronulac, Constilac, Constulose, Duphalac, Enulose, Evalose, Heptalac, Lactulax†

Pregnancy Risk Category: B

HOW SUPPLIED
Syrup: 10 g/15 ml

ACTION
Produces an osmotic effect in the colon; resulting distention promotes peristalsis. Also decreases blood ammonia, probably as a result of bacterial degradation, which decreases the pH of colon contents.

Route	Onset	Peak	Duration
PO	24-48 hr	Variable	Variable
PR	Unknown	Unknown	Unknown

INDICATIONS & DOSAGE
Constipation—
Adults: 10 to 20 g (15 to 30 ml) P.O. daily, increased to 60 ml/day, if needed.
To prevent and treat hepatic encephalopathy, including hepatic precoma and coma in patients with severe hepatic disease—
Adults: initially, 20 to 30 g (30 to 45 ml) P.O. t.i.d. or q.i.d., until two or three soft stools are produced daily. Usual dosage is 60 to 100 g daily in divided doses. Alternatively, 200 g (300 ml) diluted with 700 ml of water or 0.9% NaCl solution and given as a retention enema P.R. q 4 to 6 hours p.r.n.

ADVERSE REACTIONS
GI: *abdominal cramps, belching, diarrhea, gaseous distention, flatulence,* nausea, vomiting.

INTERACTIONS
Drug-drug. *Antacids, antibiotics, orally administered neomycin:* decreased effectiveness of lactulose. Avoid concomitant use.

EFFECTS ON DIAGNOSTIC TESTS
None reported.

CONTRAINDICATIONS
Contraindicated in patients on a low-galactose diet.

NURSING CONSIDERATIONS
• Use cautiously in patients with diabetes mellitus.
• To minimize sweet taste, dilute with water or fruit juice or give with food.
• Prepare enema (not commercially available) by adding 200 g (300 ml) to 700 ml of water or 0.9% NaCl solution. The diluted solution is administered as a retention enema for 30 to 60 minutes. Use a rectal balloon.
• If enema is not retained for at least 30 minutes, be prepared to repeat dose.
• Monitor serum sodium level for possible hypernatremia, especially when giving in higher doses to treat hepatic encephalopathy.
• Monitor mental status when given to patients with hepatic encephalopathy.
• Be prepared to replace fluid loss.

☑**Patient teaching**
• Instruct home care patient how to mix and then administer drug.
• Inform patient about adverse reactions and tell him to notify doctor if they become bothersome or if diarrhea occurs.
• Instruct patient not to take other laxatives while on lactulose therapy.

magnesium citrate
(citrate of magnesia)
Citroma ◇, Citro-Mag†, Citro-Nesia ◇

magnesium hydroxide
(milk of magnesia)
Milk of Magnesia ◇, Milk of Magnesia Concentrated ◇, Phillips' Milk of Magnesia ◇

magnesium sulfate
(epsom salts) ◇

Pregnancy Risk Category: NR

HOW SUPPLIED
magnesium citrate
Oral solution: approximately 168 mEq magnesium/240 ml ◇
magnesium hydroxide
Oral suspension: 7% to 8.5% (approximately 80 mEq magnesium/30 ml) ◇
magnesium sulfate
Granules: approximately 40 mEq magnesium/5 g ◇

ACTION
A saline laxative that produces an osmotic

effect in the small intestine by drawing water into the intestinal lumen.

Route	Onset	Peak	Duration
PO	0.5-3 hr	Variable	Variable

INDICATIONS & DOSAGE

Constipation; to evacuate bowel before surgery—
Adults and children 12 years and older: 11 to 25 g magnesium citrate P.O. daily as a single dose or divided; 2.4 to 4.8 g (30 to 60 ml) magnesium hydroxide P.O. daily as a single dose or divided; 10 to 30 g magnesium sulfate P.O. daily as a single dose or divided.
Children 6 to 12 years: 5.5 to 12.5 g magnesium citrate P.O. daily as a single dose or divided; 1.2 to 2.4 g (15 to 30 ml) magnesium hydroxide P.O. daily as a single dose or divided; 5 to 10 g magnesium sulfate P.O. daily as a single dose or divided.
Children 2 to 6 years: 2.7 to 6.25 g magnesium citrate P.O. daily as a single dose or divided; 0.4 to 1.2 g (5 to 15 ml) magnesium hydroxide P.O. daily as a single dose or divided; 2.5 to 5 g magnesium sulfate P.O. daily as a single dose or divided.
Antacid—
Adults: 5 to 15 ml milk of magnesia P.O. t.i.d. or q.i.d.

ADVERSE REACTIONS

GI: *abdominal cramping, nausea, diarrhea,* laxative dependence (with long-term or excessive use).
Other: fluid and electrolyte disturbances (with daily use).

INTERACTIONS

Drug-drug. *Orally administered drugs:* impaired absorption. Separate administration times.

EFFECTS ON DIAGNOSTIC TESTS

None reported.

CONTRAINDICATIONS

Contraindicated in patients with abdominal pain, nausea, vomiting, or other symptoms of appendicitis or acute surgical abdomen; in those with myocardial damage, heart block, fecal impaction, rectal fis-

sures, intestinal obstruction or perforation, or renal disease; and in pregnant patients about to deliver.

NURSING CONSIDERATIONS

• Use cautiously in patients with rectal bleeding.
• Time drug administration so that it doesn't interfere with scheduled activities or sleep. Drug produces watery stools in 3 to 6 hours.
• Before giving for constipation, determine if the patient has adequate fluid intake, exercise, and diet.
• Chill magnesium citrate before use to make it more palatable.
• Shake suspension well; give with large amount of water when used as laxative. When administering through nasogastric tube, make sure tube is placed properly and is patent. After instilling, flush tube with water to ensure passage to stomach and maintain tube patency.
Alert: Monitor serum electrolytes as ordered during prolonged use. Magnesium may accumulate in patients with renal insufficiency.
• Keep in mind that drug is for short-term therapy only.
• Know that magnesium sulfate is more potent than other saline laxatives.

☑ **Patient teaching**
• Instruct patient on drug administration.
• Teach patient about dietary sources of bulk, which include bran and other cereals, fresh fruit, and vegetables.
• Warn patient that frequent or prolonged use as a laxative may cause dependence.

---

methylcellulose
Citrucel ◊, Citrucel Orange Flavor ◊, Citrucel Sugar-Free Orange Flavor ◊

Pregnancy Risk Category: NR

HOW SUPPLIED
Powder: 2 g/tbs (heaping) ◊

ACTION
A bulk-forming laxative that absorbs water and expands to increase bulk and

---

moisture content of stools. The increased bulk encourages peristalsis and bowel movement.

Route	Onset	Peak	Duration
PO	12-24 hr	< 3 days	Variable

INDICATIONS & DOSAGE
Chronic constipation—
Adults: 1 to 3 tbs (heaping) in 8 oz (240 ml) of cold water daily to t.i.d. Usual dose up to 6 g daily (3 tbs).
Children 6 to 12 years: 1 to 1½ level tbs in 4 oz (120 ml) of cold water daily to t.i.d. Usual dose up to 3 g daily (1½ tbs).

ADVERSE REACTIONS
GI: *nausea,* vomiting, diarrhea (with excessive use); esophageal, gastric, small intestinal, or colonic strictures when drug is chewed or taken in dry form; *abdominal cramps,* especially in severe constipation; laxative dependence (with long-term or excessive use).

INTERACTIONS
None significant.

EFFECTS ON DIAGNOSTIC TESTS
None reported.

CONTRAINDICATIONS
Contraindicated in patients with abdominal pain, nausea, vomiting, or other symptoms of appendicitis or acute surgical abdomen and in those with intestinal obstruction or ulceration, disabling adhesions, or difficulty swallowing.

NURSING CONSIDERATIONS
• Before giving for constipation, determine if patient has adequate fluid intake, exercise, and diet.
• Be aware that drug is especially useful in debilitated patients and in those with postpartum constipation, irritable bowel syndrome, diverticulitis, and colostomies. It's also used to treat laxative abuse and to empty colon before barium enema examinations.
• Know that drug is not absorbed systemically and is nontoxic.

☑ **Patient teaching**
• Tell patient to take drug with at least 8 oz (240 ml) of liquid to mask grittiness.
• Teach patient about food sources of bulk: bran, cereals, fruits, vegetables.
• Tell patient to increase fluid intake.

mineral oil (liquid petrolatum)
Fleet Mineral Oil Enema◊,
Kondremul◊, Kondremul Plain◊,
Lansoÿl†, Liqui-Doss◊,
Milkinol◊, Neo-Cultol◊,
Petrogalar Plain◊

Pregnancy Risk Category: C

HOW SUPPLIED
Emulsion: 2.75 ml/5 ml◊, 4.75 ml/5 ml◊
Oral liquid: in pints, quarts, gallons◊
Enema: 120 ml◊, 133 ml◊

ACTION
A lubricant laxative that increases water retention in stools by creating a barrier between colon wall and feces that prevents colonic reabsorption of fecal water.

Route	Onset	Peak	Duration
PO	6-8 hr	Variable	Variable
PR	2-15 min	Unknown	Unknown

INDICATIONS & DOSAGE
Constipation; preparation for bowel studies or surgery—
Adults and children 12 years and older: 15 to 45 ml P.O. h.s.; or 120 ml P.R. (as enema).
Children 6 to 12 years: 5 to 20 ml P.O. h.s.; or 30 to 60 ml P.R. (as enema).
Children 2 to 6 years: 30 to 60 ml P.R. (as enema).

ADVERSE REACTIONS
GI: *nausea;* vomiting; diarrhea (with excessive use); *abdominal cramps,* especially in severe constipation; decreased absorption of nutrients and fat-soluble vitamins, resulting in deficiency; slowed healing after hemorrhoidectomy.
Other: laxative dependence (with long-term or excessive use), anal pruritus, anal

irritation, hemorrhoids, perianal discomfort, *lipid pneumonia.*

INTERACTIONS
Drug-drug. *Docusate salts:* may increase mineral oil absorption and cause lipid pneumonia. Separate administration times.
Fat-soluble vitamins (A, D, E, K): possible decreased absorption after prolonged administration. Monitor for vitamin deficiency.

EFFECTS ON DIAGNOSTIC TESTS
None reported.

CONTRAINDICATIONS
Contraindicated in patients with abdominal pain, nausea, vomiting, or other symptoms of appendicitis or acute surgical abdomen and in those with fecal impaction or intestinal obstruction or perforation.

NURSING CONSIDERATIONS
• Use cautiously in young children; in elderly or debilitated patients because of susceptibility to lipid pneumonia through aspiration, absorption, and transport from intestinal mucosa; and in patients with rectal bleeding.
• Before giving for constipation, determine if the patient has adequate fluid intake, exercise, and diet.
• Give drug on an empty stomach because it delays passage of food from stomach; drug is more active on an empty stomach.
• Give with fruit juice or carbonated drink to disguise taste.
• Keep in mind that drug may be used when patient needs to ease the strain of evacuation.

☑Patient teaching
• Advise patient to take drug only at bedtime on an empty stomach and not to take it for more than 1 week. Tell him to take drug with fruit juice or carbonated drink to disguise taste.
• To avoid soiling clothing, advise patient of possible rectal leakage from excessive dosages.
• Teach patient about dietary sources of bulk, which include bran and other cereals, fresh fruit, and vegetables.

polyethylene glycol and electrolyte solution
Co-Lav, Colovage, CoLyte, Glycoprep‡, Go-Evac, GoLYTELY, NuLYTELY, OCL

Pregnancy Risk Category: C

HOW SUPPLIED
Powder for oral solution: polyethylene glycol (PEG) 3350 (6 g), anhydrous sodium sulfate (568 mg), NaCl (146 mg), potassium chloride (74.5 mg)/100 ml (Colovage); PEG 3350 (120 g), sodium sulfate (3.36 g), NaCl (2.92 g), potassium chloride (1.49 g)/2 L (CoLyte); PEG 3350 (60 g), NaCl (1.46 g), potassium chloride (0.745 g), sodium bicarbonate (1.68 g), sodium sulfate (5.68 g)/L (Co-Lav); PEG 3350 (60 g), NaCl (1.46 g), potassium chloride (745 mg), sodium bicarbonate (1.68 g), sodium sulfate (5.68 g)/L (Glycoprep‡); PEG 3350 (236 g), sodium sulfate (22.74 g), sodium bicarbonate (6.74 g), NaCl (5.86 g), potassium chloride (2.97 g)/4.8 L (GoLYTELY); PEG 3350 (59 g), sodium sulfate (5.685 g), sodium bicarbonate (1.685 g), NaCl (1.465 g), potassium chloride (0.743 g)/L (Go-Evac); PEG 3350 (420 g), sodium bicarbonate (5.72 g), NaCl (11.2 g), potassium chloride (1.48 g)/4 L (NuLYTELY); PEG 3350 (6 g), sodium sulfate decahydrate (1.29 g), NaCl (146 mg), potassium chloride (75 mg), polysorbate-80 (30 mg)/100 ml (OCL)

ACTION
PEG 3350, a nonabsorbable solution, acts as an osmotic agent. Sodium sulfate greatly reduces sodium absorption. The electrolyte concentration causes virtually no net absorption or secretion of ions.

Route	Onset	Peak	Duration
PO	1 hr	Variable	Variable

INDICATIONS & DOSAGE
Bowel preparation before GI examination—
Adults: 240 ml P.O. q 10 minutes until 4 L are consumed or until the watery stool is clear. Typically, administer 4

hours before examination, allowing 3 hours for drinking and 1 hour for bowel evacuation.

ADVERSE REACTIONS
GI: *nausea, bloating, cramps, vomiting, abdominal fullness.*
Skin: urticaria, dermatitis, allergic reaction.
Other: anal irritation, rhinorrhea.

INTERACTIONS
Drug-drug. *Orally administered drugs:* decreased absorption if administered within 1 hour of starting therapy. Administer at least 2 to 3 hours before starting therapy.

EFFECTS ON DIAGNOSTIC TESTS
Patient preparation for barium enema may be less satisfactory with this solution as it may interfere with the barium coating of the colonic mucosa using the double-contrast technique.

CONTRAINDICATIONS
Contraindicated in patients with GI obstruction or perforation, gastric retention, toxic colitis, or megacolon.

NURSING CONSIDERATIONS
• Use tap water to reconstitute powder. Shake vigorously to ensure that all powder is dissolved. Refrigerate reconstituted solution but use within 48 hours.
Alert: Do not add flavoring or additional ingredients to the solution or administer chilled solution. Hypothermia has been reported after ingestion of large amounts of chilled solution.
• Administer solution early in the morning if patient is scheduled for a midmorning examination. Orally administered solution induces diarrhea (onset 30 to 60 minutes) that rapidly cleans the bowel, usually within 4 hours.
• When used as preparation for barium enema, administer solution the evening before the examination to avoid interfering with barium coating of the colonic mucosa.
• If administered to semiconscious patients or to patients with impaired gag reflex, take care to prevent aspiration.

• Be aware that no major shifts in fluid or electrolyte balance have been reported.

☑ **Patient teaching**
• Tell patient to fast for 3 to 4 hours before taking the solution and thereafter ingest only clear fluids until the examination is complete.
• Warn patient about adverse reactions.

---

psyllium
Effer-Syllium Instant Mix◊, Fiberall◊, Fibrepur†◊, Genfiber◊, Hydrocil Instant◊, Karacil†◊, Konsyl◊, Konsyl-D◊, Maalox Daily Fiber Therapy◊, Metamucil◊, Metamucil Effervescent Sugar Free◊, Metamucil Sugar-Free◊, Modane Bulk◊, Muci-Lax◊, Mylanta Natural Fiber Supplement◊, Perdiem Fiber◊, Prodiem Plain†◊, Reguloid Natural◊, Restore◊, Serutan◊, Siblin◊, Syllact◊, Unilax◊, V-Lax◊

Pregnancy Risk Category: NR

HOW SUPPLIED
Chewable pieces: 1.7 g/piece◊, 3.4 g/piece◊
Effervescent powder: 3.4 g/packet◊, 3.7 g/packet◊
Granules: 2.5 g/tsp◊, 4.03 g/tsp◊
Powder: 3.3 g/tsp◊, 3.4 g/tsp◊, 3.5 g/tsp◊, 4.94 g/tsp◊
Wafers: 3.4 g/wafer◊

ACTION
A bulk-forming laxative that absorbs water and expands to increase bulk and moisture content of the stool, thus encouraging peristalsis and bowel movement.

Route	Onset	Peak	Duration
PO	12-24 hr	3 days	Variable

INDICATIONS & DOSAGE
Constipation; bowel management—
Adults: 1 to 2 tsp (rounded) P.O. in full glass of liquid once daily, b.i.d., or t.i.d., followed by second glass of liquid; or 1

packet dissolved in water once daily, b.i.d., or t.i.d.
Children over 6 years: 1 tsp (level) P.O. in half a glass of liquid h.s.

ADVERSE REACTIONS
GI: nausea, vomiting, diarrhea (with excessive use); esophageal, gastric, small intestinal, and rectal obstruction when drug is taken in dry form; abdominal cramps, especially in severe constipation.

INTERACTIONS
None significant.

EFFECTS ON DIAGNOSTIC TESTS
None reported.

CONTRAINDICATIONS
Contraindicated in patients with abdominal pain, nausea, vomiting, or other symptoms of appendicitis; intestinal obstruction or ulceration; disabling adhesions; difficulty swallowing; or hypersensitivity to drug.

NURSING CONSIDERATIONS
• Before giving for constipation, determine if the patient has adequate fluid intake, exercise, and diet.
• Mix with at least 8 oz (240 ml) of cold, pleasant-tasting liquid, such as orange juice, to mask grittiness, and stir only a few seconds. Have patient drink mixture immediately so it does not congeal. Follow with additional glass of liquid.
• For dosages in children under 6 years, consult doctor.
• Know that drug may reduce appetite if taken before meals.
• Be aware that drug is not absorbed systemically and is nontoxic. It is especially useful in debilitated patients and those with postpartum constipation, irritable bowel syndrome, and diverticular disease. It's also used to treat chronic laxative abuse and in combination with other laxatives to empty colon before barium enema examinations.

☑**Patient teaching**
• Teach patient how to properly mix medication. Tell him to take drug with plenty

of water. Advise patient that inhaling powder may cause allergic reactions.
• Tell patient that laxative effect usually occurs in 12 to 24 hours but may be delayed 3 days.
• Advise diabetic patient to check the label and use a brand of psyllium that does not contain sugar.
• Teach patient about dietary sources of bulk, which include bran and other cereals, fresh fruit, and vegetables.

senna
Black-Draught◊, Fletcher's Castoria◊, Senexon◊, Senna-Gen◊, Senokot◊, Senokotxtra◊, X-Prep Liquid*◊

Pregnancy Risk Category: C

HOW SUPPLIED
Tablets: 187 mg◊, 217 mg◊, 600 mg◊
Granules: 326 mg/tsp◊, 1.65 g/½ tsp◊
Suppositories: 652 mg◊
Syrup: 218 mg/5 ml◊

ACTION
Unknown. A stimulant laxative that increases peristalsis probably by direct effect on the smooth muscle of the intestine. Thought to either irritate the musculature or stimulate the colonic intramural plexus. Also promotes fluid accumulation in the colon and small intestine.

Route	Onset	Peak	Duration
PO	6-10 hr	Variable	Variable
PR	0.5-2 hr	Unknown	Unknown

INDICATIONS & DOSAGE
Acute constipation; preparation for bowel or rectal examination—
Adults: dosage range for Senokot is 1 to 8 tablets P.O.; ½ to 4 tsp of granules added to liquid P.O.; 1 to 2 suppositories P.R. h.s.; or 1 to 4 tsp syrup P.O. h.s. Dosage for Black-Draught is 2 tablets or ¼ to ½ tsp (level) of granules mixed with water.
   X-Prep Liquid used solely as single dose for preradiographic bowel evacuation. Give 20 g powder dissolved in juice or 75 ml liquid P.O. between 2 p.m. and 4

p.m. on day before X-ray procedure. Use in divided doses, if needed, for elderly or debilitated patients.
Children weighing over 27 kg (60 lb): one-half adult dose of tablets, granules, or syrup (except Black-Draught tablets and granules—not recommended for children).
Children 1 month to 1 year: 1.25 to 2.5 ml Senokot syrup P.O. h.s.

ADVERSE REACTIONS
GI: *nausea;* vomiting; diarrhea; loss of normal bowel function with excessive use; *abdominal cramps,* especially in severe constipation; malabsorption of nutrients; "cathartic colon" (syndrome resembling ulcerative colitis radiologically) with chronic misuse; possible constipation after catharsis; yellow or yellow-green cast to feces; diarrhea in breast-feeding infants of mothers receiving senna; darkened pigmentation of rectal mucosa with long-term use (usually reversible within 4 to 12 months after stopping drug); laxative dependence with excessive use.
GU: red-pink discoloration in alkaline urine; yellow-brown color to acidic urine.
Other: protein-losing enteropathy, electrolyte imbalance (such as hypokalemia).

INTERACTIONS
None significant.

EFFECTS ON DIAGNOSTIC TESTS
In the phenolsulfonphthalein excretion test, senna may turn urine pink to red, red to violet, or red to brown.

CONTRAINDICATIONS
Contraindicated in patients with ulcerative bowel lesions; nausea, vomiting, abdominal pain, or other symptoms of appendicitis or acute surgical abdomen; fecal impaction; or intestinal obstruction or perforation.

NURSING CONSIDERATIONS
• Before giving for constipation, determine if patient has adequate fluid intake, exercise, and diet.
• Limit diet to clear liquids after X-Prep Liquid is taken.

• Avoid exposing product to excessive heat or light.
• Know that drug is used for short-term therapy.
• Know that senna is one of the most effective laxatives for counteracting constipation caused by narcotic analgesics.

☑ Patient teaching
• Teach patient about dietary sources of bulk, including bran and other cereals, fresh fruit, and vegetables.
• Tell patient to report persistent or severe reactions.

sodium phosphates
Fleet Phospho-Soda ◊

Pregnancy Risk Category: NR

HOW SUPPLIED
Liquid: 2.4 g/5 ml sodium phosphate and 900 mg sodium biphosphate/5 ml ◊
Enema: 160 mg/ml sodium phosphate and 60 mg/ml sodium biphosphate ◊

ACTION
A saline laxative that produces an osmotic effect in the small intestine by drawing water into the intestinal lumen.

Route	Onset	Peak	Duration
PO	0.5-3 hr	Variable	Variable
PR	5-10 min	With effect	With effect

INDICATIONS & DOSAGE
Constipation—
Adults: 20 to 30 ml solution mixed with 120 ml cold water P.O.; or 60 to 135 ml P.R. (as enema).
Children: 5 to 15 ml solution mixed with 120 ml of cold water P.O.; or 67.5 ml P.R. (as enema).

ADVERSE REACTIONS
GI: *abdominal cramping.*
Other: fluid and electrolyte disturbances (hypernatremia, hyperphosphatemia) with daily use; laxative dependence with long-term or excessive use.

INTERACTIONS
None significant.

EFFECTS ON DIAGNOSTIC TESTS
None reported.

CONTRAINDICATIONS
Contraindicated in patients with abdominal pain, nausea, vomiting, or other symptoms of appendicitis or acute surgical abdomen; intestinal obstruction or perforation; edema; heart failure; megacolon; or impaired renal function and in patients on sodium-restricted diets.

NURSING CONSIDERATIONS
• Use cautiously in patients with large hemorrhoids or anal excoriations.
• Before giving for constipation, determine if patient has adequate fluid intake, exercise, and diet.
Alert: Be aware that up to 10% of sodium content of drug may be absorbed.

☑ **Patient teaching**
• Teach patient about dietary sources of bulk, which include bran and other cereals, fresh fruit, and vegetables.
• Warn patient about adverse reactions and stress importance of using only for short-term therapy.

chlorpromazine hydrochloride
(See Chapter 33, ANTIPSYCHOTICS.)
dimenhydrinate
dolasetron mesylate
dronabinol
granisetron hydrochloride
meclizine hydrochloride
metoclopramide hydrochloride
ondansetron hydrochloride
perphenazine
(See Chapter 33, ANTIPSYCHOTICS.)
prochlorperazine
prochlorperazine edisylate
prochlorperazine maleate
promethazine hydrochloride
(See Chapter 43, ANTIHISTAMINES.)
scopolamine
(See Chapter 38, ANTICHOLINERGICS.)
thiethylperazine maleate
trimethobenzamide hydrochloride

COMBINATION PRODUCTS
None.

dimenhydrinate
Andrumin‡, Apo-Dimenhydri-
nate†, Calm-X ◇, Children's
Dramamine ◇, Dimetabs, Dinate,
Dramamine ◇*, Dramamine
Chewable ◇**, Dramamine
Liquid ◇*, Dramanate, Dymenate,
Gravol†, Gravol L/A†, Hydrate,
Nausetrol†, Novo-Dimenate†,
PMS-Dimenhydrinate†,
Travamine†, Triptone Caplets ◇

Pregnancy Risk Category: B

HOW SUPPLIED
Tablets: 50 mg ◇
Tablets (chewable): 50 mg ◇
Elixir: 15 mg/5 ml†
Syrup: 12.5 mg/4 ml* ◇, 15.62 mg/5 ml
Injection: 50 mg/ml

ACTION
Unknown. An antihistamine that may affect neural pathways originating in the
labyrinth to inhibit nausea and vomiting.

Route	Onset	Peak	Duration
PO	15-30 min	Unknown	3-6 hr
IV	Immediate	Unknown	3-6 hr
IM	20-30 min	Unknown	3-6 hr

INDICATIONS & DOSAGE
*Prevention and treatment of motion sick-
ness—*
Adults and children 12 years and over:
50 to 100 mg P.O. q 4 to 6 hours; 50 mg
I.M., p.r.n.; or 50 mg I.V. diluted in 10 ml
0.9% NaCl for injection, injected over 2
minutes. Maximum dosage is 400 mg daily. For prevention take 30 minutes prior to
motion exposure.
Children 6 to 12 years: 25 to 50 mg P.O.
q 6 to 8 hours, not to exceed 150 mg in 24
hours. Alternatively, 1.25 mg/kg or
37.5 mg/m^2 I.M. q.i.d. Maximum dosage
is 300 mg daily.
Children 2 to 6 years: 12.5 to 25 mg P.O.
q 6 to 8 hours, not to exceed 75 mg in 24
hours. Alternatively, 1.25 mg/kg or
37.5 mg/m^2 I.M. q.i.d. Maximum dosage
is 300 mg daily.

ADVERSE REACTIONS
CNS: *drowsiness,* headache, dizziness,
confusion, nervousness, insomnia (especially in children), vertigo, tingling and
weakness of hands, lassitude, excitation.
CV: palpitations, hypotension, tachycardia.
EENT: blurred vision, dry respiratory
passages, diplopia, nasal congestion.
GI: dry mouth, nausea, vomiting, diarrhea, epigastric distress, constipation,
anorexia.
Respiratory: wheezing, thickened
bronchial secretions.
Skin: photosensitivity, urticaria, rash.
Other: *anaphylaxis,* tightness of chest.

INTERACTIONS
Drug-drug. *CNS depressants:* additive
CNS depression. Avoid concomitant use.

---

*Liquid contains alcohol.   **May contain tartrazine.   †Canada   ‡Australia   §U.K.   ◇OTC

Drug-lifestyle. *Alcohol use:* additive CNS depression. Avoid concomitant use.

EFFECTS ON DIAGNOSTIC TESTS

Drug may alter or confuse test results for xanthines (caffeine, aminophylline) because of its 8-chlorotheophylline content; discontinue drug 4 days before diagnostic skin tests to avoid preventing, reducing, or masking test response.

CONTRAINDICATIONS

Contraindicated in patients hypersensitive to drug or its components.

NURSING CONSIDERATIONS

• Use cautiously in patients with seizures, acute angle-closure glaucoma, or enlarged prostate gland, or in patients receiving ototoxic drugs.
• Know that undiluted solution irritates veins and may cause sclerosis.
• Because incompatibilities are common, avoid mixing parenteral preparation with other drugs.
• Like other antiemetics, know that drug may mask symptoms of ototoxicity, brain tumor, or intestinal obstruction.

▮I.V. administration

• Before administration, dilute each ml of drug with 10 ml of sterile water for injection, D_5W, or 0.9% NaCl for injection. Give by direct injection over not less than 2 minutes.
Alert: Be aware that most I.V. products contain benzyl alcohol, which has been associated with a fatal "gasping syndrome" in premature infants and low birth weight infants.

☑Patient teaching

• Advise patient to avoid activities that require alertness until CNS effects of the drug are known.
• Instruct patient to report adverse reactions promptly.

---

dolasetron mesylate
Anzemet

Pregnancy Risk Category: B

HOW SUPPLIED

Tablets: 50 mg, 100 mg
Injection: 20 mg/ml as 12.5 mg/0.625 ml ampule or 100 mg/5 ml vials

ACTION

A selective serotonin 5-HT_3 receptor antagonist that blocks the action of serotonin. Blocking the activity of the serotonin receptors prevents serotonin from stimulating the vomiting reflex.

Route	Onset	Peak	Duration
PO	Rapid	1 hr	8 hr
IV	Rapid	36 min	7 hr

INDICATIONS & DOSAGE

Prevention of nausea and vomiting associated with cancer chemotherapy—
Adults: 100 mg P.O. given as a single dose 1 hour before chemotherapy; or 1.8 mg/kg (or a fixed dose of 100 mg) as a single I.V. dose given 30 minutes before chemotherapy.
Children 2 to 16 years: 1.8 mg/kg P.O. given 1 hour before chemotherapy, or 1.8 mg/kg as a single I.V. dose given 30 minutes before chemotherapy. Injectable formulation can be mixed with apple juice and administered P.O. Maximum dose of 100 mg.
Prevention of postoperative nausea and vomiting—
Adults: 100 mg P.O. within 2 hours before surgery; 12.5 mg as a single I.V. dose approximately 15 minutes before cessation of anesthesia.
Children 2 to 16 years: 1.2 mg/kg P.O. given within 2 hours before surgery, up to a maximum of 100 mg; or 0.35 mg/kg (up to 12.5 mg) given as a single I.V. dose approximately 15 minutes before the cessation of anesthesia. Injectable formulation can be mixed with apple juice and administered P.O.
Treatment of postoperative nausea and vomiting—
Adults: 12.5 mg as a single I.V. dose as soon as nausea or vomiting presents.
Children 2 to 16 years: 0.35 mg/kg, up to a maximum dose of 12.5 mg, given as a single I.V. dose as soon as nausea or vomiting presents.

Reactions may be *common,* uncommon, *life-threatening*, or COMMON AND LIFE-THREATENING.

ADVERSE REACTIONS
CNS: *headache*, dizziness, drowsiness, fatigue.
CV: *arrhythmias*, ECG changes, hypotension, hypertension, tachycardia.
GI: *diarrhea*, dyspepsia, abdominal pain, constipation, anorexia.
GU: oliguria, urinary retention.
Skin: pruritus, rash.
Other: fever, elevation of liver function tests, chills, pain at injection site.

INTERACTIONS
Drug-drug. *Drugs that prolong ECG intervals (such as antiarrhythmia drugs):* increased risk of arrhythmia. Monitor patient closely.
Drugs that inhibit the P-450 enzymes (such as cimetidine): increased hydrodolasetron levels. Monitor patient for adverse effects.
Drugs that induce the P-450 enzymes (such as rifampin): decreased hydrodolasetron levels. Monitor patient for decreased efficacy of antiemetic.

EFFECTS ON DIAGNOSTIC TESTS
None reported.

CONTRAINDICATIONS
Contraindicated in patients hypersensitive to drug.

NURSING CONSIDERATIONS
Alert: Administer with caution in patients who have or may develop prolonged cardiac conduction intervals, such as those with electrolyte abnormalities, history of arrhythmia, and cumulative high-dose anthracycline therapy.
• Drug is not recommended for use in children under 2 years. Use cautiously in breast-feeding women.
• Injection for oral administration is stable in apple or in apple-grape juice for 2 hours at room temperature.

◖I.V. administration
• Injection can be infused as rapidly as 100 mg/30 seconds or diluted in 50 ml compatible solution and infused over 15 minutes.

☑Patient teaching
• Tell patient about potential adverse effects.
• Instruct patient not to mix injection in juice for oral administration until just before dosing.
• Tell patient to report nausea or vomiting.

dronabinol (delta-9-tetrahydrocannabinol)
Marinol

Controlled Substance Schedule II
Pregnancy Risk Category: B

HOW SUPPLIED
Capsules: 2.5 mg, 5 mg, 10 mg

ACTION
Unknown. A derivative of marijuana.

Route	Onset	Peak	Duration
P.O.	Unknown	2-4 hr	4-6 hr

INDICATIONS & DOSAGE
Nausea and vomiting associated with cancer chemotherapy—
Adults: 5 mg/m² P.O. 1 to 3 hours before administration of chemotherapy. Then same dose q 2 to 4 hours after chemotherapy for total of four to six doses daily. If needed, dosage increased in 2.5-mg/m² increments to maximum of 15 mg/m² per dose.
Anorexia and weight loss in patients with AIDS—
Adults: 2.5 mg P.O. b.i.d. before lunch and dinner. If unable to tolerate, decrease dose to 2.5 mg P.O. given as a single dose daily in evening or h.s. May gradually increase dosage to maximum of 20 mg/day.

ADVERSE REACTIONS
CNS: *dizziness, drowsiness, euphoria, ataxia,* depersonalization, hallucinations, somnolence, headache, muddled thinking, asthenia, amnesia, confusion, *paranoia*.
CV: tachycardia, orthostatic hypotension, palpitations, vasodilation.
EENT: visual disturbances.
GI: *dry mouth, nausea, vomiting, abdominal pain,* diarrhea.

---

*Liquid contains alcohol.   **May contain tartrazine.   †Canada   ‡Australia   §U.K.   ◇OTC

INTERACTIONS
Drug-drug. *CNS depressants, psychotomimetic substances, sedatives:* additive CNS depression. Avoid concomitant use.
Drug-lifestyle. *Alcohol use:* additive CNS depression. Avoid concomitant use.

EFFECTS ON DIAGNOSTIC TESTS
None reported.

CONTRAINDICATIONS
Contraindicated in patients hypersensitive to sesame oil or cannabinoids.

NURSING CONSIDERATIONS
• Use cautiously in elderly, pregnant, or breast-feeding patients and in those with heart disease, psychiatric illness, and history of drug abuse.
• Expect drug to be prescribed only for patients who have not responded satisfactorily to other antiemetics.
• Know that dronabinol is principal active substance in *Cannabis sativa* (marijuana). This substance can produce both physical and psychological dependence and has a high potential for abuse.
• Keep in mind that CNS effects are intensified at higher drug dosages.
• Be aware that drug's effects may persist for days after treatment ends.

☑ **Patient teaching**
• Tell patient drug may induce unusual changes in mood or other adverse behavioral effects.
• Advise patient against activities that require alertness until CNS effects of drug are known.
• Warn caregivers to supervise patient during and immediately after treatment.
• Advise patient to take drug 1 to 3 hours before chemotherapy administration.

---

granisetron hydrochloride
Kytril

Pregnancy Risk Category: B

HOW SUPPLIED
Tablets: 1 mg
Injection: 1 mg/ml

ACTION
A selective antagonist of a specific type of serotonin receptor ($5\text{-}HT_3$) located in the CNS in the chemoreceptor trigger zone and in the peripheral nervous system on nerve terminals of the vagus nerve. Drug's blocking action may occur at both sites.

Route	Onset	Peak	Duration
PO, IV	Unknown	Unknown	Unknown

INDICATIONS & DOSAGE
Prevention of nausea and vomiting associated with emetogenic cancer chemotherapy—
Adults and children 2 to 16 years: 10 mcg/kg I.V. infused over 5 minutes. Begin infusion within 30 minutes before administration of chemotherapy. Alternatively, 1 mg P.O. up to 1 hour before chemotherapy and dosage repeated 12 hours later; or 2 mg P.O. daily given up to 1 hour before chemotherapy.

ADVERSE REACTIONS
CNS: *headache, asthenia,* somnolence, dizziness, anxiety.
CV: hypertension.
GI: diarrhea, *constipation,* abdominal pain, *nausea,* vomiting, decreased appetite.
Hematologic: *leukopenia,* anemia, ***thrombocytopenia.***
Other: fever, alopecia, elevated liver function tests.

INTERACTIONS
Drug-herb. *Horehound:* may enhance serotoninergic effects. Avoid concomitant use.

EFFECTS ON DIAGNOSTIC TESTS
None reported.

CONTRAINDICATIONS
Contraindicated in patients hypersensitive to drug.

NURSING CONSIDERATIONS
• Know that drug regimen is given only on days when chemotherapy is given. Treatment at other times has not been found to be useful.

Reactions may be *common,* uncommon, ***life-threatening,*** or COMMON AND LIFE-THREATENING.

• Do not mix with other drugs; data regarding compatibility are limited.

◖ I.V. administration
• Dilute drug with 0.9% NaCl for injection or D₅W to a volume of 20 to 50 ml. Infuse over 5 minutes, beginning within 30 minutes before initiating chemotherapy, and only on the days chemotherapy is given. Diluted solutions are stable for 24 hours at room temperature.

✅ Patient teaching
• Stress importance of taking second dose of oral drug 12 hours later for maximum effectiveness.
• Instruct patient to report adverse reactions immediately.

---

meclizine hydrochloride (meclozine hydrochloride)
Antivert, Antivert/25 ◇, Antivert/50, Bonamine†, Bonine ◇, Dizmiss ◇, Meni-D, Ru-Vert-M, Vergon ◇

Pregnancy Risk Category: B

HOW SUPPLIED
Tablets: 12.5 mg, 25 mg ◇, 50 mg
Tablets (chewable): 25 mg ◇
Capsules: 25 mg

ACTION
Unknown. An antihistamine that may affect neural pathways originating in the labyrinth to inhibit nausea and vomiting.

Route	Onset	Peak	Duration
PO	1 hr	Unknown	8-24 hr

INDICATIONS & DOSAGE
Vertigo—
Adults: 25 to 100 mg P.O. daily in divided doses. Dosage varies with response.
Motion sickness—
Adults: 25 to 50 mg P.O. 1 hour before travel, then daily for duration of trip.

ADVERSE REACTIONS
CNS: *drowsiness,* restlessness, excitation, nervousness, auditory and visual hallucinations.

CV: hypotension, palpitations, tachycardia.
EENT: blurred vision, diplopia, tinnitus, dry nose and throat.
GI: dry mouth, constipation, anorexia, nausea, vomiting, diarrhea.
GU: urine retention, urinary frequency.
Skin: urticaria, rash.

INTERACTIONS
Drug-drug. *CNS depressants:* increased drowsiness. Use together cautiously.

EFFECTS ON DIAGNOSTIC TESTS
Discontinue drug 4 days before diagnostic skin tests to avoid interference with test response.

CONTRAINDICATIONS
Contraindicated in patients hypersensitive to drug.

NURSING CONSIDERATIONS
• Use cautiously in patients with asthma, glaucoma, or prostatic hyperplasia.
• Like other antiemetics, be alert that drug may mask symptoms of ototoxicity, brain tumor, or intestinal obstruction.

✅ Patient teaching
• Advise patient to avoid hazardous activities that require alertness until CNS effects of drug are known.
• Instruct patient to report persistent or serious adverse reactions promptly.

---

metoclopramide hydrochloride
Apo-Metoclop†, Clopra, Emext†, Maxeran†, Maxolon‡, Octamide PFS, Pramin‡, Reclomide, Reglan

Pregnancy Risk Category: B

HOW SUPPLIED
Tablets: 5 mg, 10 mg
Syrup: 5 mg/5 ml
Injection: 5 mg/ml

ACTION
Stimulates motility of the upper GI tract, also increases lower esophageal sphincter

---

tone and blocks dopamine receptors at the chemoreceptor trigger zone.

Route	Onset	Peak	Duration
PO	0.5-1 hr	1-2 hr	1-2 hr
IV	1-3 min	Unknown	1-2 hr
IM	10-15 min	Unknown	1-2 hr

INDICATIONS & DOSAGE

Prevention or reduction of nausea and vomiting associated with emetogenic cancer chemotherapy—
Adults: 1 to 2 mg/kg I.V. 30 minutes before cancer chemotherapy, then repeated q 2 hours for two doses, then q 3 hours for three doses.

Prevention or reduction of postoperative nausea and vomiting—
Adults: 10 to 20 mg I.M. near end of surgical procedure, repeated q 4 to 6 hours, p.r.n.

To facilitate small-bowel intubation and to aid in radiologic examinations—
Adults and children over 14 years: 10 mg (2 ml) I.V. as a single dose over 1 to 2 minutes.
Children under 6 years: 0.1 mg/kg I.V.
Children 6 to 14 years: 2.5 to 5 mg I.V. (0.5 to 1 ml).

Delayed gastric emptying secondary to diabetic gastroparesis—
Adults: 10 mg P.O. for mild symptoms, slow I.V. (1 to 2 minutes) for severe symptoms 30 minutes before meals and h.s. I.V. dose may be necessary for up to 10 days, then P.O. dose may be started to continue for rest of 2 to 8 weeks.

Gastroesophageal reflux disease—
Adults: 10 to 15 mg P.O. q.i.d., p.r.n., 30 minutes before meals and h.s.

Adjust-a-dose: In renally impaired patients with creatinine clearance below 40 ml/minute, decrease initial dosage by half the recommended dose.

ADVERSE REACTIONS

CNS: *restlessness, anxiety, drowsiness, fatigue, lassitude,* depression, akathisia, insomnia, confusion, **suicide ideation, seizures,** hallucinations, headache, dizziness, extrapyramidal symptoms, tardive dyskinesia, *dystonic reactions.*
CV: transient hypertension, hypotension.
GI: nausea, bowel disorders, diarrhea.

Hematologic: *neutropenia, agranulocytosis.*
Skin: rash, urticaria.
Other: fever, prolactin secretion, loss of libido, urinary frequency, incontinence.

INTERACTIONS

Drug-drug. *Anticholinergics, opioid analgesics:* antagonized GI motility effects of metoclopramide. Use together cautiously.
CNS depressants: additive CNS effects. Avoid concomitant use.
Phenothiazines: increased risk of extrapyramidal effects. Monitor closely.
Drug-lifestyle. *Alcohol use*: additive CNS effects. Avoid concomitant use.

EFFECTS ON DIAGNOSTIC TESTS

Drug may increase serum aldosterone and prolactin levels.

CONTRAINDICATIONS

Contraindicated in patients in whom stimulation of GI motility might be dangerous (for example, those with hemorrhage, obstruction, or perforation) and in those with pheochromocytoma, seizure disorders, or hypersensitivity to drug.

NURSING CONSIDERATIONS

• Use cautiously in patients with history of depression, Parkinson's disease, and hypertension.
• Monitor bowel sounds.
• Know that drug is compatible with D_5W, 0.9% NaCl for injection, and dextrose 5% in NaCl 0.45%, NaCl 0.9% (preferred), Ringer's injection, and lactated Ringer's injection.
• Know that safety and effectiveness have not been established for therapy that continues longer than 12 weeks.

🔲 I.V. administration

• Give lower doses (10 mg or less) by direct injection over 1 to 2 minutes. Dilute doses larger than 10 mg in 50 ml of a compatible diluent, and infuse over at least 15 minutes. Protection from light is unnecessary if infusion mixture is administered within 24 hours. If infusion mixture is protected from light and refrigerated, stability is 48 hours.

Reactions may be *common,* uncommon, *life-threatening*, or COMMON AND LIFE-THREATENING.

• Closely monitor blood pressure in patients receiving I.V. form of drug.
Alert: Use diphenhydramine 25 mg I.V. as ordered to counteract the extrapyramidal adverse effects associated with high metoclopramide doses.

☑**Patient teaching**
• Tell patient to avoid activities requiring alertness for 2 hours after doses.
• Instruct patient to report persistent or serious adverse reactions promptly.
• Advise patient to avoid alcohol ingestion.

ondansetron hydrochloride
Zofran

Pregnancy Risk Category: B

HOW SUPPLIED
Tablets: 4 mg, 8 mg
Injection: 2 mg/ml
Premixed injection: 32 mg/50 ml

ACTION
A selective antagonist of a specific type of serotonin receptor ($5\text{-}HT_3$) located in the CNS at the area postrema (chemoreceptor trigger zone) and in the peripheral nervous system on nerve terminals of the vagus nerve. Drug's blocking action may occur at both sites.

Route	Onset	Peak	Duration
PO, IV	Unknown	Unknown	Unknown

INDICATIONS & DOSAGE
Prevention of nausea and vomiting associated with emetogenic chemotherapy—
Adults and children 12 years and over: 8 mg P.O. 30 minutes before start of chemotherapy. Then 8 mg P.O. 8 hours after first dose. Then 8 mg q 12 hours for 1 to 2 days. Or, administer a single dose of 32 mg by I.V. infusion over 15 minutes beginning 30 minutes before chemotherapy; or three divided doses of 0.15 mg/kg I.V. (first dose 30 minutes before chemotherapy; subsequent doses given 4 and 8 hours after first dose). Infuse drug over 15 minutes.
Children 4 to 12 years: 4 mg P.O. 30

minutes before start of chemotherapy. Then 4 mg P.O. 4 and 8 hours after first dose. Follow with 4 mg q 8 hours for 1 to 2 days. Alternatively, three doses of 0.15 mg/kg I.V. Give first dose 30 minutes before chemotherapy; administer subsequent doses 4 and 8 hours after first dose. Infuse drug over 15 minutes.
Prevention of postoperative nausea and vomiting—
Adults: 4 mg I.V. (undiluted) over 2 to 5 minutes. Alternatively, 16 mg P.O. 1 hour before induction of anesthesia.
Prevention of nausea and vomiting associated with radiotherapy in patients receiving total body irradiation, single high-dose fraction to abdomen, or daily fractions to abdomen—
Adults: 8 mg P.O. t.i.d.
Adjust-a-dose: In patients with severe liver failure, total daily dose should not exceed 8 mg.

ADVERSE REACTIONS
CNS: *headache, malaise, fatigue, dizziness, sedation.*
GI: *diarrhea, constipation,* abdominal pain, xerostomia.
Hepatic: transient elevations in AST and ALT levels.
Skin: rash.
Other: *musculoskeletal pain,* chills, urine retention, chest pain, injection-site reaction, fever, hypoxia, gynecologic disorders.

INTERACTIONS
Drug-drug. *Drugs that alter hepatic drug metabolizing enzymes (such as cimetidine, phenobarbital):* may alter pharmacokinetics of ondansetron. No dosage adjustment appears necessary.
Drug-herb. *Horehound:* may enhance serotoninergic effects. Avoid concomitant use.

EFFECTS ON DIAGNOSTIC TESTS
Drug may increase ALT and AST levels.

CONTRAINDICATIONS
Contraindicated in patients with known hypersensitivity to drug.

NURSING CONSIDERATIONS
• Use cautiously in patients with liver failure. Monitor liver function tests. Dose should not exceed 8 mg in this population.

🔋 I.V. administration
• Dilute drug in 50 ml of D_5W injection or 0.9% NaCl for injection before administration.
• Know that drug is also stable for up to 48 hours after dilution in 5% dextrose in 0.9% NaCl for injection, 5% dextrose in 0.45% NaCl for injection, and 3% NaCl for injection.
Alert: Administer as I.V. infusion over 15 minutes.

☑ Patient teaching
• Instruct patient to alert nurse immediately if difficulty in breathing occurs after drug administration.
• Tell patient receiving drug I.V. to report discomfort at insertion site.

---

prochlorperazine
Compazine, PMS Prochlorperazine†, Prorazin†, Stemetil†

prochlorperazine edisylate
Compazine, Compazine Syrup

prochlorperazine maleate
Compazine, Compazine Spansule, PMS Prochlorperazine†, Prorazin†, Stemetil†

Pregnancy Risk Category: C

HOW SUPPLIED
prochlorperazine
Tablets: 5 mg, 10 mg
Injection: 5 mg/ml
Suppositories: 2.5 mg, 5 mg, 25 mg
prochlorperazine edisylate
Syrup: 5 mg/5 ml
Injection: 5 mg/ml
prochlorperazine maleate
Tablets: 5 mg, 10 mg, 25 mg
Capsules (sustained-release): 10 mg, 15 mg, 30 mg

ACTION
Acts on the chemoreceptor trigger zone to inhibit nausea and vomiting; in larger doses, partially depresses vomiting center.

Route	Onset	Peak	Duration
PO	30-40 min	Unknown	3-12 hr
IV	Unknown	Unknown	Unknown
IM	10-20 min	Unknown	3-4 hr
PR	1 hr	Unknown	3-4 hr

INDICATIONS & DOSAGE
Preoperative nausea control—
Adults: 5 to 10 mg I.M. 1 to 2 hours before induction of anesthesia; repeat once in 30 minutes, if necessary. Or, 5 to 10 mg I.V. 15 to 30 minutes before induction of anesthesia; repeat once if necessary.
Severe nausea and vomiting—
Adults: 5 to 10 mg P.O., t.i.d. or q.i.d.; 15 mg sustained-release form P.O. on rising; 10 mg sustained-release form P.O. q 12 hours; 25 mg P.R., b.i.d.; or 5 to 10 mg I.M. repeated q 3 to 4 hours, p.r.n. Maximum I.M. dosage is 40 mg daily. Alternatively, 2.5 to 10 mg I.V. at a rate not to exceed 5 mg/minute.
Children weighing 18 to 39 kg (40 to 86 lb): 2.5 mg P.O. or P.R., t.i.d.; or 5 mg P.O. or P.R., b.i.d. Maximum dosage is 15 mg daily. Or, give 0.132 mg/kg by deep I.M. injection. Control usually is obtained with one dose.
Children weighing 14 to 17 kg (30 to 38 lb): 2.5 mg P.O. or P.R., b.i.d. or t.i.d. Maximum dosage is 10 mg daily. Or give 0.132 mg/kg by deep I.M. injection. Control usually is obtained with one dose.
Children weighing 9 to 13 kg (20 to 29 lb): 2.5 mg P.O. or P.R. once daily or b.i.d. Maximum dosage is 7.5 mg daily. Or give 0.132 mg/kg by deep I.M. injection. Control usually is obtained with one dose.
To manage symptoms of psychotic disorders—
Adults: 5 to 10 mg P.O., t.i.d. or q.i.d.
Children 2 to 12 years: 2.5 mg P.O. or P.R., b.i.d. or t.i.d. Do not exceed 10 mg on day 1. Increase dosage gradually to recommended maximum (if necessary). In children 2 to 5 years, maximum daily

---

dosage is 25 mg. In children 6 to 10 years, maximum daily dosage is 25 mg.
To manage symptoms of severe psychosis—
Adults: 10 to 20 mg I.M. repeated in 1 to 4 hours, if needed. Rarely, patients may receive 10 to 20 mg q 4 to 6 hours. Institute oral therapy after symptoms are controlled.
Children 2 to 12 years: 0.13 mg/kg I.M.
Nonpsychotic anxiety—
Adults: 5 to 10 mg by deep I.M. injection q 3 to 4 hours, not to exceed 20 mg daily or for longer than 12 weeks; or 5 to 10 mg P.O., t.i.d. or q.i.d. Alternatively, give 15 mg extended-release capsule once daily or 10 mg extended-release capsule q 12 hours.

ADVERSE REACTIONS
CNS: *extrapyramidal reactions,* sedation, pseudoparkinsonism, EEG changes, dizziness.
CV: *orthostatic hypotension,* tachycardia, ECG changes.
EENT: *ocular changes, blurred vision.*
GI: *dry mouth, constipation.*
GU: *urine retention,* dark urine, menstrual irregularities, inhibited ejaculation.
Hematologic: *transient leukopenia, agranulocytosis.*
Hepatic: cholestatic jaundice.
Skin: *mild photosensitivity,* allergic reactions, *exfoliative dermatitis.*
Other: hyperprolactinemia, gynecomastia, weight gain, increased appetite.

INTERACTIONS
Drug-drug. *Antacids:* inhibited absorption of oral phenothiazines. Separate antacid and phenothiazine doses by at least 2 hours.
Anticholinergics, including antidepressants and antiparkinsonian agents: increased anticholinergic activity and aggravated parkinsonian symptoms. Use together cautiously.
Barbiturates: may decrease phenothiazine effect. Monitor patient for decreased antiemetic effect.

EFFECTS ON DIAGNOSTIC TESTS
Drug causes false-positive results for urinary porphyrins, urobilinogen, amylase,

and 5-hydroxyindoleacetic acid; it causes false-positive urine pregnancy results in tests using human chorionic gonadotropin. Drug elevates liver enzymes and protein-bound iodine levels and causes quinidine-like ECG effects.

CONTRAINDICATIONS
Contraindicated in patients hypersensitive to phenothiazines and in those with CNS depression including coma; during pediatric surgery; when using spinal or epidural anesthetic, adrenergic blockers, or ethanol; and in children under 2 years.

NURSING CONSIDERATIONS
• Use cautiously in patients with impaired CV function, glaucoma, seizure disorders; in those who have been exposed to extreme heat; and in children with acute illness.
• Dilute oral solution with tomato or fruit juice, milk, coffee, carbonated beverage, tea, water, or soup or mix with pudding.
• For I.M. use, inject deeply into upper outer quadrant of gluteal region.
• Do not give S.C. or mix in syringe with another drug.
• To prevent contact dermatitis, avoid getting concentrate or injection solution on hands or clothing.
• Monitor CBC and liver function studies during long-term therapy as ordered.
Alert: Know that drug is used only when vomiting can't be controlled by other measures or when only a few doses are required. If more than four doses are needed in 24 hours, notify doctor.
• Store in light-resistant container. Slight yellowing does not affect potency; discard extremely discolored solutions.

◪I.V. administration
• 15 to 30 minutes before induction, add 20 mg of prochlorperazine per liter of D_5W and 0.9% NaCl solution. Infusion rate should not exceed 5 mg/minute. Maximum parenteral dosage is 40 mg daily. Infuse slowly, never as a bolus.
• Watch for orthostatic hypotension, especially when giving drug I.V.

---

*Liquid contains alcohol.   **May contain tartrazine.   †Canada   ‡Australia   §U.K.   ◇OTC

☑ **Patient teaching**
• Teach patient what to use to dilute oral solution.
• Advise patient to wear protective clothing when exposed to sunlight.
• Tell patient to call doctor if more than four doses are needed within 24 hours.

---

thiethylperazine maleate
Norzine, Torecan**

Pregnancy Risk Category: X

HOW SUPPLIED
Tablets: 10 mg
Injection: 5 mg/ml

ACTION
Unknown. Probably acts on the chemoreceptor trigger zone to inhibit nausea and vomiting.

Route	Onset	Peak	Duration
PO, IM	0.5 hr	Unknown	4 hr

INDICATIONS & DOSAGE
Nausea and vomiting—
Adults: 10 mg P.O., or I.M., once daily, b.i.d. or t.i.d.

ADVERSE REACTIONS
CNS: *extrapyramidal reactions* (high incidence), sedation (low incidence), pseudoparkinsonism, EEG changes, dizziness, confusion (especially in elderly patients).
CV: *orthostatic hypotension,* tachycardia, ECG changes.
EENT: *ocular changes, blurred vision.*
GI: *dry mouth, constipation.*
GU: *urine retention,* dark urine, menstrual irregularities, inhibited ejaculation, gynecomastia.
Hematologic: *transient leukopenia, agranulocytosis.*
Hepatic: *cholestatic jaundice.*
Skin: *mild photosensitivity,* allergic reactions.
Other: hyperprolactinemia, weight gain, increased appetite.

INTERACTIONS
Drug-drug. *Antacids:* inhibited absorption of oral phenothiazines. Separate antacid and phenothiazine doses by at least 2 hours.
Anticholinergics, including antidepressants and antiparkinsonian agents: increased anticholinergic activity and increased risk of parkinsonian-like symptoms. Use together cautiously.
Barbiturates: may decrease phenothiazine effect. Monitor patient for decreased antiemetic effect.

EFFECTS ON DIAGNOSTIC TESTS
Drug may alter immunologic urine pregnancy test results.

CONTRAINDICATIONS
Contraindicated in patients with severe CNS depression, hepatic disease, or hypersensitivity to phenothiazines; in patients experiencing coma; and during pregnancy.

NURSING CONSIDERATIONS
• Use cautiously in patients with aspirin or tartrazine hypersensitivity.
Alert: Don't give I.V. May cause severe hypotension.
• For nausea and vomiting associated with anesthesia and surgery, give deep I.M. injection shortly before or when terminating anesthesia.
• If drug gets on skin, wash off at once to prevent contact dermatitis.
• Use only when vomiting can't be controlled by other measures or when only a few doses are required.

☑ **Patient teaching**
• Warn patient about hypotension; suggest that he stay in bed for 1 hour after receiving drug.
• Instruct patient to report decreased urine output, visual changes, and CNS effects immediately.

Photoguide to tablets and capsules

This photoguide provides full-color photographs of some of the most commonly prescribed tablets and capsules in the United States. Shown in actual size, the drugs are organized alphabetically by trade or generic name for quick reference.

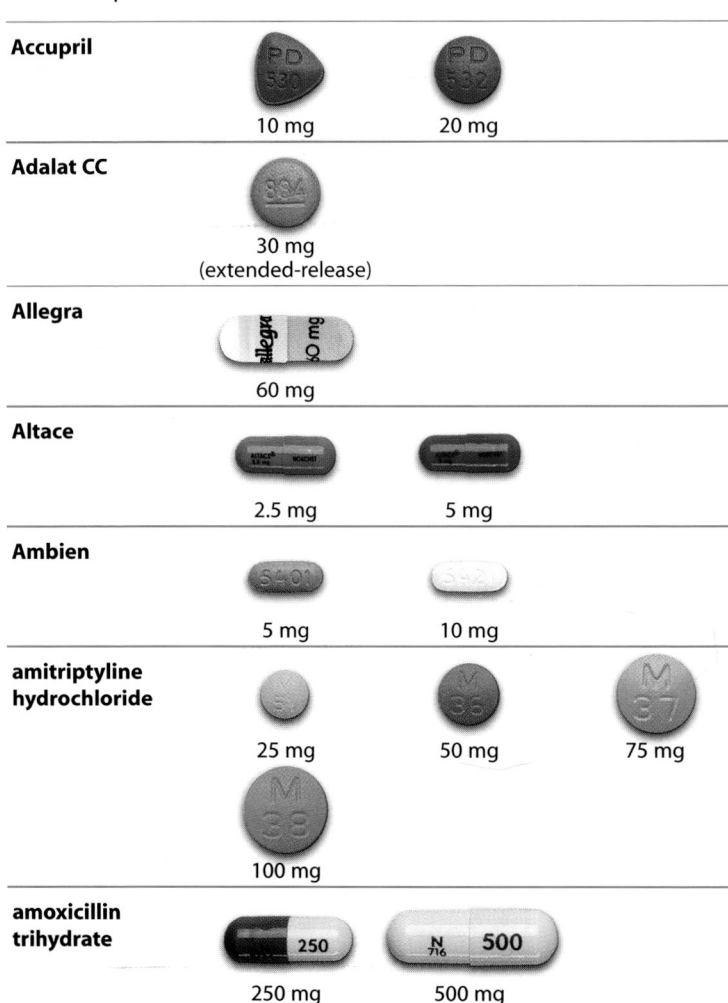

Accupril

10 mg   20 mg

Adalat CC

30 mg
(extended-release)

Allegra

60 mg

Altace

2.5 mg   5 mg

Ambien

5 mg   10 mg

amitriptyline hydrochloride

25 mg   50 mg   75 mg

100 mg

amoxicillin trihydrate

250 mg   500 mg

C2 PHOTOGUIDE TO TABLETS AND CAPSULES

Amoxil

125 mg
(chewable)

250 mg
(chewable)

250 mg

500 mg

atenolol

25 mg

Ativan

0.5 mg

1 mg

Augmentin

250 mg/125 mg

500 mg/125 mg

125 mg/31.25 mg
(chewable)

250 mg/62.5 mg
(chewable)

Axid

150 mg

300 mg

Biaxin

250 mg

500 mg

Bumex

0.5 mg

1 mg

2 mg

BuSpar

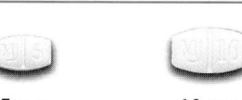
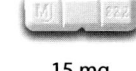

5 mg

10 mg

15 mg

Calan

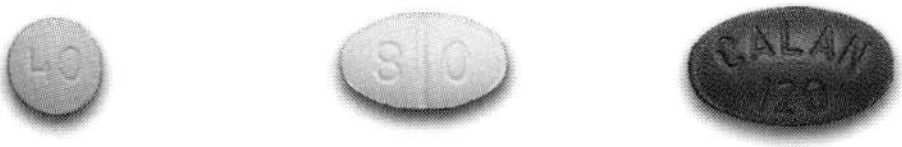

40 mg   80 mg   120 mg

Capoten

12.5 mg   25 mg

Carafate

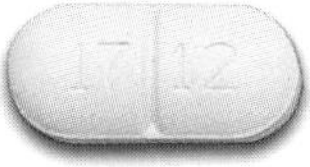

1 g

Cardizem

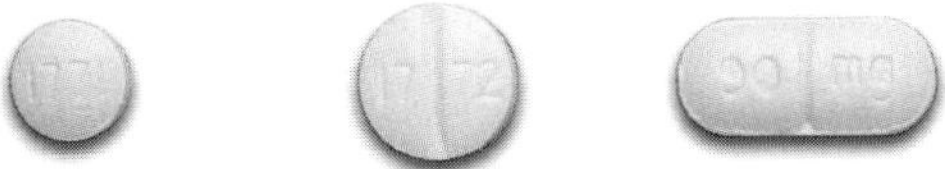

30 mg   60 mg   90 mg

Cardizem CD
(extended-release)

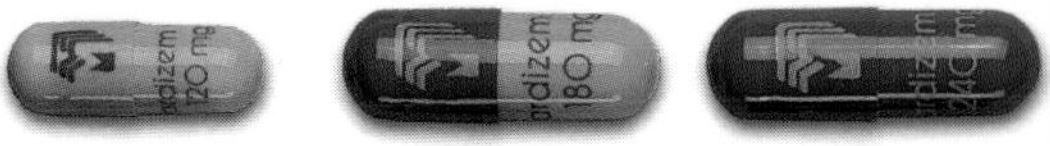

120 mg   180 mg   240 mg

Cardura

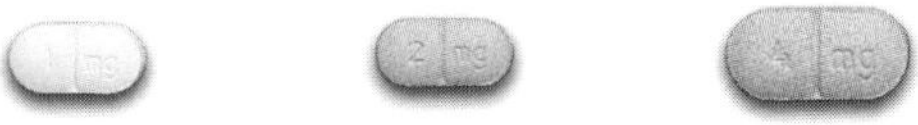

1 mg   2 mg   4 mg

Ceclor

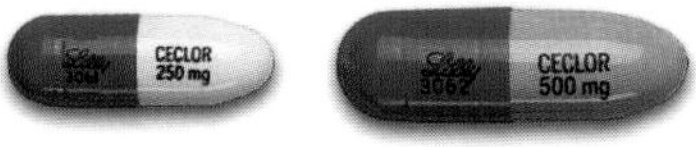

250 mg   500 mg

Ceftin

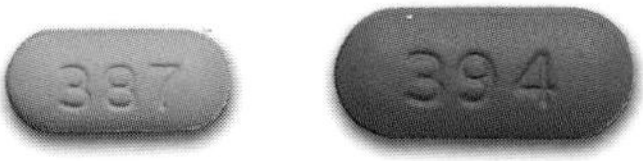

250 mg   500 mg

Cefzil

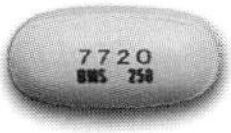

250 mg

cephalexin

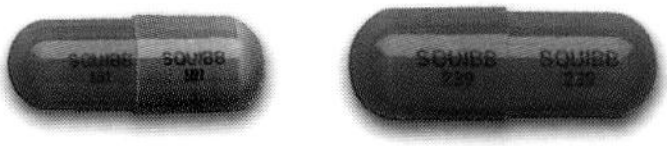

250 mg   500 mg

cimetidine

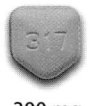 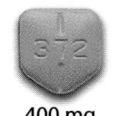

300 mg   400 mg

C4 PHOTOGUIDE TO TABLETS AND CAPSULES

Cipro			
250 mg	500 mg	750 mg	

Claritin
10 mg

Compazine
SKF C66 — 5 mg
SKF C67 — 10 mg

Cordarone
200 mg

Coreg
3.125 mg | 6.25 mg | 12.5 mg
25 mg

Coumadin
1 mg | 2 mg | 2.5 mg
5 mg | 7.5 mg | 10 mg

Cozaar
25 mg | 50 mg

cyclobenzaprine hydrochloride
10 mg

Darvocet-N 100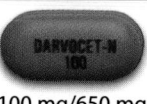
DARVOCET-N 100
100 mg/650 mg

Daypro

600 mg

Deltasone

2.5 mg

5 mg

10 mg

20 mg

Depakote
(delayed-release)

125 mg

250 mg

500 mg

Depakote Sprinkle

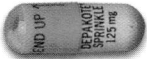

125 mg

DiaBeta

1.25 mg

2.5 mg

5 mg

Diflucan

100 mg

150 mg

200 mg

Dilacor XR

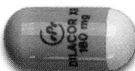

180 mg

240 mg

Dilantin Infatabs

50 mg

Dilantin Kapseals

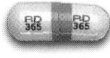

30 mg

100 mg

**doxepin
hydrochloride**

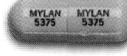

75 mg

C6 PHOTOGUIDE TO TABLETS AND CAPSULES

Duricef

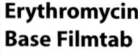

500 mg

Dyazide

25 mg/37.5 mg

E.E.S.

400 mg

Effexor

25 mg   37.5 mg   50 mg

75 mg   100 mg

E-Mycin
(delayed-release)

250 mg   333 mg

Ery-Tab
(delayed-release)

250 mg   333 mg

**Erythrocin
Stearate Filmtab**

250 mg

**Erythromycin
Base Filmtab**

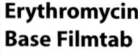

250 mg   500 mg

Estrace

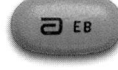   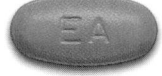

1 mg   2 mg

**Fiorinal with
Codeine**

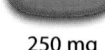

325 mg aspirin, 50 mg butalbital, 40 mg caffeine, 30 mg codeine phosphate

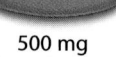

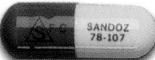

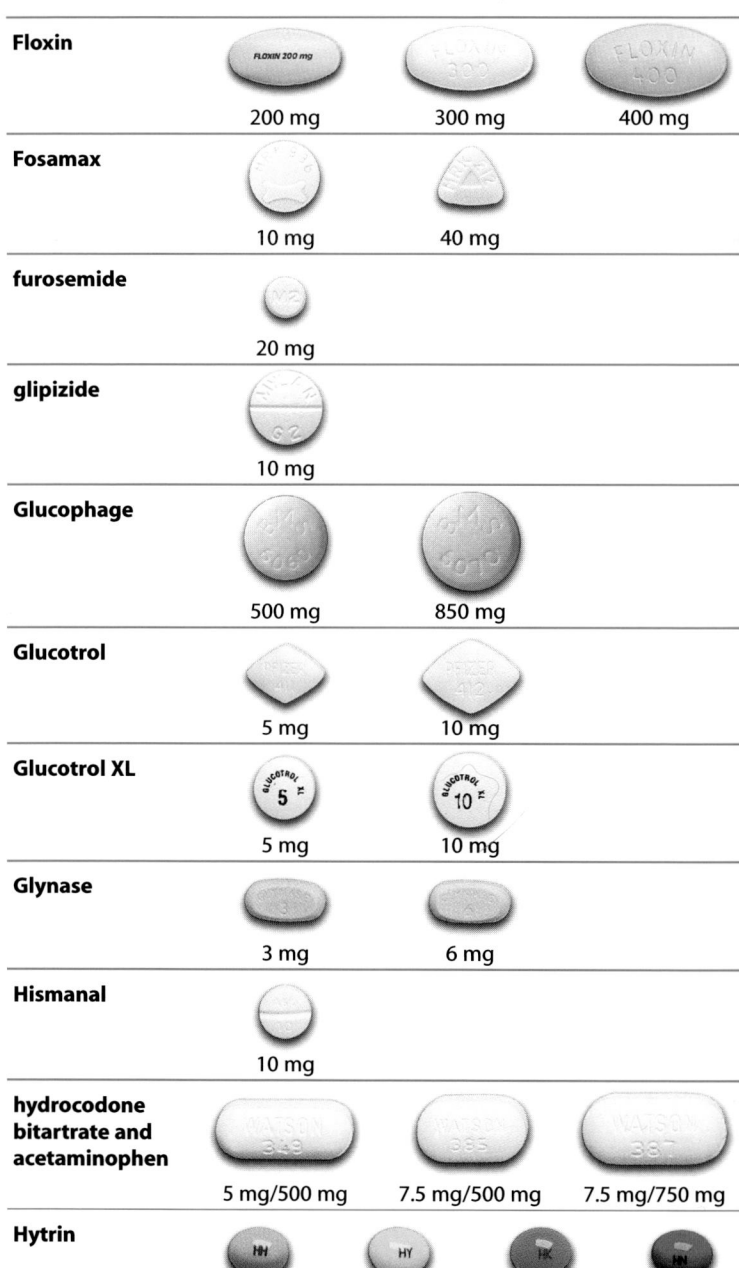

Floxin

200 mg   300 mg   400 mg

Fosamax

10 mg   40 mg

furosemide

20 mg

glipizide

10 mg

Glucophage

500 mg   850 mg

Glucotrol

5 mg   10 mg

Glucotrol XL

5 mg   10 mg

Glynase

3 mg   6 mg

Hismanal

10 mg

hydrocodone bitartrate and acetaminophen

5 mg/500 mg   7.5 mg/500 mg   7.5 mg/750 mg

Hytrin

1 mg   2 mg   5 mg   10 mg

ibuprofen

IBU 400	IBU 600	IBU 800
400 mg	600 mg	800 mg

Inderal

10 mg	20 mg	40 mg

60 mg

K-Dur

10 mEq	20 mEq

Klonopin

0.5 mg	1 mg	2 mg

Lanoxin

0.125 mg	0.25 mg

Lasix

20 mg	40 mg

Levoxyl

0.025 mg	0.05 mg	0.075 mg
0.088 mg	0.1 mg	0.112 mg
0.125 mg	0.137 mg	0.15 mg
0.175 mg	0.2 mg	0.3 mg

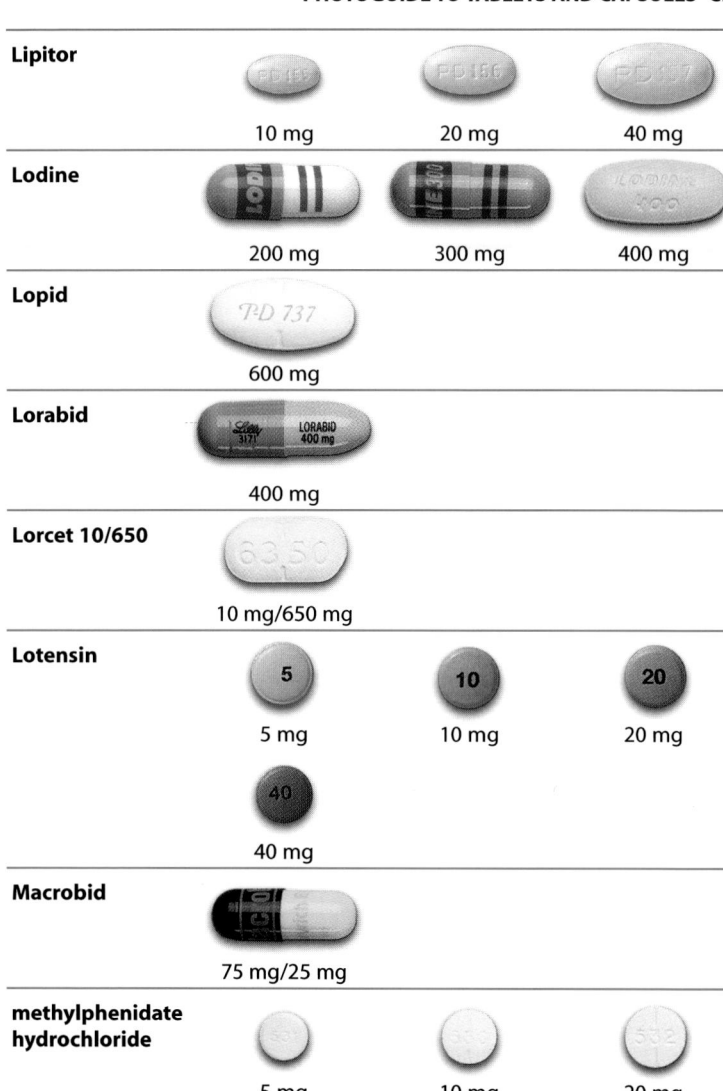

Lipitor

10 mg 20 mg 40 mg

Lodine

200 mg 300 mg 400 mg

Lopid

600 mg

Lorabid

400 mg

Lorcet 10/650

10 mg/650 mg

Lotensin

5 mg 10 mg 20 mg

40 mg

Macrobid

75 mg/25 mg

methylphenidate hydrochloride

5 mg 10 mg 20 mg

20 mg
(extended-release)

C10 PHOTOGUIDE TO TABLETS AND CAPSULES

Mevacor	10 mg	20 mg	40 mg

Micro-K Extencaps (controlled-release)	10 mEq (750 mg)

Micronase	2.5 mg	5 mg

Motrin	400 mg	600 mg	800 mg

Naprosyn	250 mg	375 mg	500 mg

naproxen	375 mg	500 mg

Nitrostat	0.3 mg	0.4 mg	0.6 mg

Nolvadex	10 mg

nortriptyline hydrochloride	10 mg	25 mg	50 mg

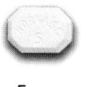
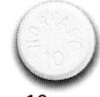

Norvasc	5 mg	10 mg

Oruvail	100 mg	150 mg	200 mg

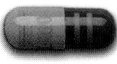
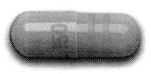
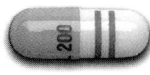

Pamelor

10 mg 25 mg 50 mg

75 mg

Paxil

20 mg 30 mg

PCE

333 mg 500 mg

Pepcid

20 mg 40 mg

Percocet

5 mg/325 mg

potassium chloride

10 mEq
(extended-release)

Pravachol

  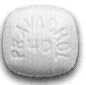

10 mg 20 mg 40 mg

Premarin

 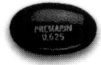 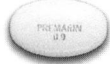

0.3 mg 0.625 mg 0.9 mg

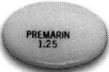 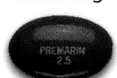

1.25 mg 2.5 mg

Prevacid

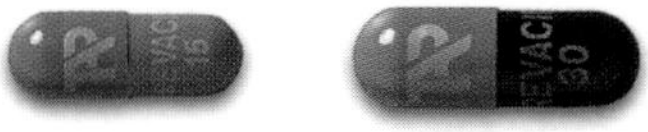

15 mg   30 mg

Prilosec

10 mg   20 mg

Prinivil

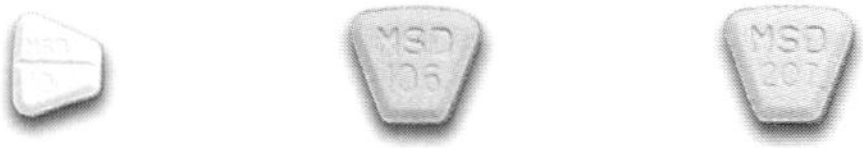

5 mg   10 mg   20 mg

Procardia XL
(extended-release)

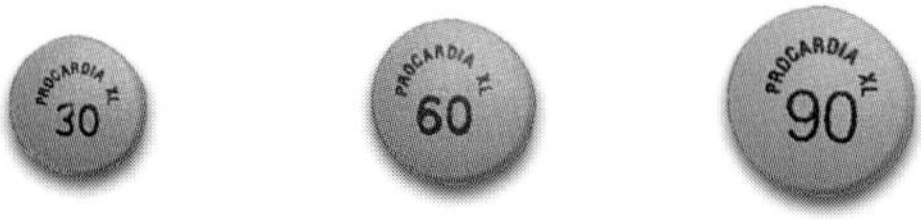

30 mg   60 mg   90 mg

propoxyphene napsylate with acetaminophen

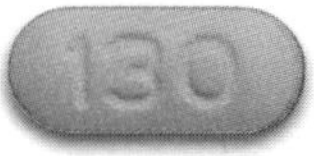

100 mg/650 mg

Propulsid

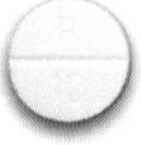

10 mg

Provera

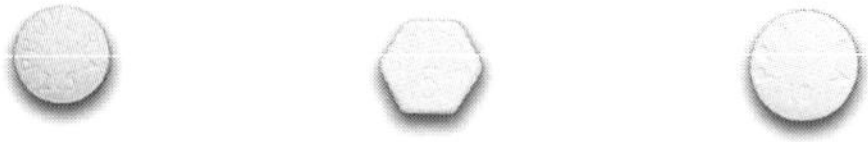

2.5 mg   5 mg   10 mg

Prozac

10 mg   20 mg

Relafen

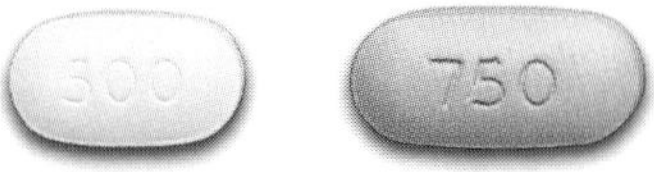

500 mg   750 mg

Risperdal

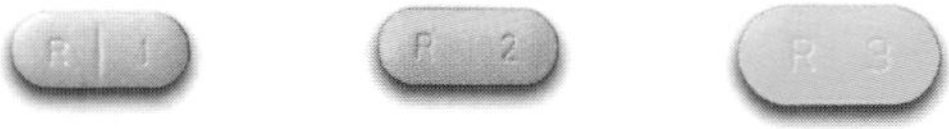

1 mg   2 mg   3 mg

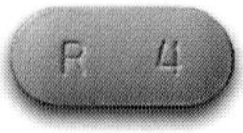

4 mg

Roxicet

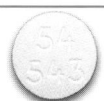

5 mg/325 mg

Sinemet

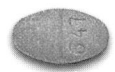 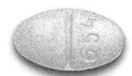

10 mg/100 mg · 25 mg/250 mg

Sinemet CR

25 mg/100 mg
(extended-release)

Slo-bid Gyrocaps
(extended-release)

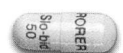 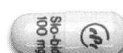

50 mg · 75 mg · 100 mg

200 mg · 300 mg

Sumycin

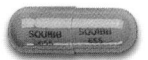

250 mg

Synthroid

25 mcg · 50 mcg · 75 mcg

88 mcg · 100 mcg · 112 mcg

125 mcg · 150 mcg · 175 mcg

200 mcg · 300 mcg

Tagamet

200 mg · 300 mg

C14 PHOTOGUIDE TO TABLETS AND CAPSULES

Tenormin
25 mg   50 mg   100 mg

Theo-Dur
(extended-release)
100 mg   200 mg   300 mg

450 mg

Ticlid
250 mg

Toprol XL
50 mg   100 mg   200 mg

Toradol
10 mg

Trental
400 mg

Trimox
250 mg   500 mg

Tylenol with Codeine No. 3
300 mg/30 mg

Ultram
50 mg

Valium
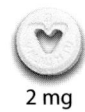 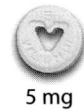 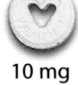
2 mg   5 mg   10 mg

Vasotec

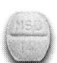

2.5 mg   5 mg   10 mg

20 mg

Veetids

250 mg   500 mg

verapamil hydrochloride

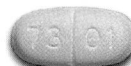

180 mg
(sustained-release)

Verelan
(sustained-release)

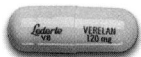   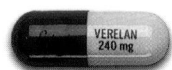

120 mg   240 mg

Vicodin

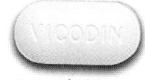

5 mg/500 mg

Vicodin ES

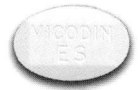

7.5 mg/750 mg

Xanax

0.25 mg   0.5 mg   1 mg

Zantac

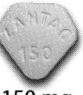   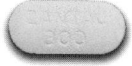

150 mg   300 mg

Zantac EFFERdose

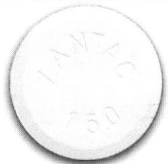

150 mg

Zestril

5 mg

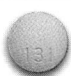

10 mg

20 mg

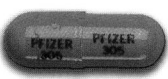

40 mg

Zithromax

250 mg

Zocor

5 mg

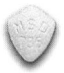

10 mg

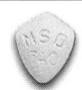

20 mg

Zoloft

50 mg

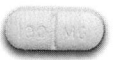

100 mg

Zovirax

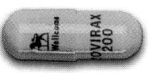

200 mg

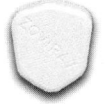

400 mg

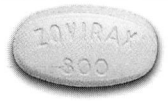

800 mg

Zyrtec

5 mg

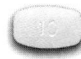

10 mg

trimethobenzamide hydrochloride
Arrestin, Tebamide, Tegamide, T-Gen, Ticon, Tigan, Triban, Trimazide

Pregnancy Risk Category: C

HOW SUPPLIED
Capsules: 100 mg, 250 mg
Injection: 100 mg/ml
Suppositories: 100 mg, 200 mg

ACTION
Unknown. Probably acts on the chemoreceptor trigger zone to inhibit nausea and vomiting.

Route	Onset	Peak	Duration
PO	10-20 min	Unknown	3-4 hr
IM	15-35 min	Unknown	2-3 hr
PR	Unknown	Unknown	Unknown

INDICATIONS & DOSAGE
Nausea and vomiting—
Adults: 250 mg P.O., t.i.d. or q.i.d.; or 200 mg I.M. or P.R., t.i.d. or q.i.d.
Children weighing under 13 kg (29 lb): 100 mg P.R. t.i.d. or q.i.d.
Children weighing 13 to 40 kg (29 to 88 lb): 100 to 200 mg P.O. or P.R., t.i.d. or q.i.d.

ADVERSE REACTIONS
CNS: *drowsiness,* dizziness (in large doses), headache, disorientation, depression, parkinsonian-like symptoms, ***coma, seizures.***
CV: hypotension.
GI: diarrhea.
Hepatic: jaundice.
Other: hypersensitivity reactions (pain, stinging, burning, redness, swelling at I.M. injection site); blurred vision; muscle cramps.

INTERACTIONS
Drug-drug. *CNS depressants:* additive CNS depression. Avoid concomitant use.
Drug-lifestyle. *Alcohol use:* additive CNS depression. Avoid concomitant use.

EFFECTS ON DIAGNOSTIC TESTS
None reported.

CONTRAINDICATIONS
Contraindicated in patients with hypersensitivity to drug. Suppositories contraindicated in patients hypersensitive to benzocaine hydrochloride or similar local anesthetic.

NURSING CONSIDERATIONS
• Use cautiously in children; drug may be associated with Reye's syndrome.
• For I.M. administration, inject deeply into upper outer quadrant of gluteal region to reduce pain and local irritation.
• Drug may mask evidence of overdose of toxic agents or of intestinal obstruction, brain tumor, or other conditions.
• Withhold drug if skin hypersensitivity reaction occurs.

☑ **Patient teaching**
• Instruct patient to refrigerate suppositories.
• Advise patient of possible drowsiness and dizziness; caution against driving or other activities requiring alertness until CNS effects of drug are known.

---

*Liquid contains alcohol. **May contain tartrazine. †Canada ‡Australia §U.K. ◇OTC

cimetidine
famotidine
lansoprazole
misoprostol
nizatidine
omeprazole
ranitidine bismuth citrate
ranitidine hydrochloride
sucralfate

COMBINATION PRODUCTS
None.

---

cimetidine
Tagamet, Tagamet HBL,
Tagamet HCl, Tagamet Tiltab

Pregnancy Risk Category: B

HOW SUPPLIED
Tablets: 100 mg ◊, 200 mg, 300 mg,
400 mg, 800 mg
Tablets (effervescent): 800 mg‡
Oral liquid: 300 mg/5 ml
Injection: 100 mg/ml‡, 300 mg/2 ml;
300 mg in 50 ml 0.9% NaCl solution

ACTION
Competitively inhibits the action of H_2 at
receptor sites of the parietal cells, decreasing gastric acid secretion.

Route	Onset	Peak	Duration
PO	Unknown	45-90 min	4-5 hr
IV	Unknown	Immediate	Unknown
IM	Unknown	Unknown	Unknown

INDICATIONS & DOSAGE
Duodenal ulcer (short-term treatment and maintenance)—
Adults and children 16 years and over:
800 mg P.O. h.s. Alternatively, 400 mg
P.O. b.i.d. or 300 mg q.i.d. (with meals
and h.s.). Treatment continued for 4 to 6
weeks unless endoscopy shows healing.
For maintenance therapy, 400 mg h.s. For
parenteral therapy, 300 mg diluted to
20 ml with 0.9% NaCl solution or other
compatible I.V. solution by I.V. push over
at least 5 minutes q 6 hours; or 300 mg
diluted in 50 ml D_5W or other compatible
I.V. solution by I.V. infusion over 15 to 20
minutes q 6 hours; or 300 mg I.M. q 6
hours (no dilution necessary). Parenteral
dosage increased by giving 300-mg doses
more frequently to maximum daily dosage of 2,400 mg p.r.n. Alternatively,
900 mg/day (37.5 mg/hour) I.V. diluted in
100 to 1,000 ml of compatible solution by
continuous I.V. infusion.
Active benign gastric ulceration—
Adults: 800 mg P.O. h.s., or 300 mg P.O.
q.i.d. (with meals and h.s.) for up to 6
weeks.
*Pathologic hypersecretory conditions
(such as Zollinger-Ellison syndrome, systemic mastocytosis, and multiple endocrine adenomas)—*
Adults and children 16 years and over:
300 mg P.O. q.i.d. with meals and h.s.; adjusted to patient needs. Maximum oral
daily dosage is 2,400 mg.
   For parenteral therapy, 300 mg diluted
to 20 ml with 0.9% NaCl solution or other
compatible I.V. solution by I.V. push over
at least 5 minutes q 6 hours; or 300 mg
diluted in 50 ml D_5W or other compatible
I.V. solution by I.V. infusion over 15 to 20
minutes q 6 hours. Parenteral dosage increased by giving 300-mg doses more frequently to maximum daily dosage of
2,400 mg, p.r.n.
Gastroesophageal reflux disease—
Adults: 800 mg P.O. b.i.d. or 400 mg
q.i.d. before meals and h.s. for up to 12
weeks.
*Prevention of upper GI bleeding in criti-
cally ill patients—*
Adults: 50 mg/hour by continuous I.V. infusion for up to 7 days; 25 mg/hour to patients with creatinine clearance below
30 ml/minute.
Heartburn—
Adults: 200 mg (Tagamet HB only) P.O.
with water as symptoms occur, or as directed, up to b.i.d. Maximum dosage is

---

400 mg daily. Drug shouldn't be taken daily for longer than 2 weeks.

ADVERSE REACTIONS
CNS: confusion, dizziness, headache, peripheral neuropathy, somnolence, hallucinations.
GI: *mild and transient diarrhea.*
GU: transient elevations in serum creatinine levels, impotence, mild gynecomastia if used longer than 1 month.
Hematologic: *agranulocytosis* (rare), *neutropenia, thrombocytopenia* (rare), *aplastic anemia* (rare).
Hepatic: jaundice (rare).
Other: hypersensitivity reactions, muscle pain, arthralgia.

INTERACTIONS
Drug-drug. *Antacids:* interference with cimetidine absorption. Separate administration by at least 1 hour if possible.
Lidocaine, phenytoin, propranolol, some benzodiazepines, theophylline, warfarin: inhibited hepatic microsomal enzyme metabolism of these drugs. Monitor serum levels.
Drug-herb. *Guarana:* may increase caffeine serum levels or prolong serum caffeine half-life. Monitor patient.
Pennyroyal: may change the rate of formation of toxic metabolites of pennyroyal. Monitor patient.
Yerba maté: may decrease clearance of yerba maté methylxanthines and cause toxicity. Use together cautiously.

EFFECTS ON DIAGNOSTIC TESTS
Drug may antagonize pentagastrin's effect during gastric acid secretion tests; it may cause false-negative results in skin tests using allergen extracts. Drug therapy increases prolactin levels and serum alkaline phosphatase and creatinine levels.

FD and C blue dye #2 used in Tagamet tablets may impair interpretation of Hemoccult and Gastroccult tests on gastric content aspirate. Wait at least 15 minutes after tablet administration before drawing the sample and follow test manufacturer's instructions closely.

CONTRAINDICATIONS
Contraindicated in patients hypersensitive to drug.

NURSING CONSIDERATIONS
● Use cautiously in elderly or debilitated patients because they may be more susceptible to cimetidine-induced confusion.
● Assess for abdominal pain. Note any blood in emesis, stool, or gastric aspirate.
● Identify tablet strength when obtaining a drug history.
● Schedule cimetidine dose at end of hemodialysis treatment. Hemodialysis reduces blood levels of cimetidine. Adjust dosage as ordered in patients with renal failure.
● Keep in mind that effectiveness for treatment of gastric ulcer is not as great as for duodenal ulcer.
● Know that up to 10 g overdose can occur without adverse reactions.

🔲 **I.V. administration**
● Dilute I.V. solutions with 0.9% NaCl solution, D_5W, and $D_{10}W$ (and combinations of these), lactated Ringer's solution, or 5% sodium bicarbonate injection. Do not dilute with sterile water for injection. Cimetidine is also frequently added to total parenteral nutrition solutions with or without fat emulsion.
Alert: Drug must be diluted before direct injection and given over 5 minutes. A rapid I.V. injection may result in arrhythmias and hypotension. Some authorities recommend infusing drug over at least 30 minutes to minimize risk of adverse cardiac effects. Sometimes given as continuous I.V. infusion. Use infusion pump if given in a total volume of 250 ml over 24 hours or less.

✅ **Patient teaching**
● Remind patient taking cimetidine once daily to take it at bedtime. If drug is being taken more than once a day, instruct him to take it with meals.
● Instruct patient taking Tagamet HB not to exceed recommended dosage and not to take daily for longer than 14 days.
● Warn patient receiving drug I.M. that injection may be painful.
● Urge patient to avoid cigarette smoking

because it may increase gastric acid secretion and worsen disease.
- Advise patient to report abdominal pain and blood in stools or emesis.

---

famotidine
Pepcid, Pepcid AC ◇, Pepcidine‡

Pregnancy Risk Category: B

HOW SUPPLIED
Tablets: 10 mg, 20 mg, 40 mg
Powder for oral suspension: 40 mg/5 ml after reconstitution
Injection: 10 mg/ml
Premixed injection: 20 mg/50 ml in 0.9% NaCl

ACTION
Competitively inhibits the action of H_2 at receptor sites of the parietal cells, decreasing gastric acid secretion.

Route	Onset	Peak	Duration
PO	1 hr	1-3 hr	12 hr
IV	Unknown	30 min	12 hr

INDICATIONS & DOSAGE
Duodenal ulcer (short-term treatment)—
Adults: For acute therapy, 40 mg P.O. once daily h.s. or 20 mg P.O. b.i.d. For maintenance therapy, give 20 mg P.O. once daily h.s.
Benign gastric ulcer (short-term treatment)—
Adults: 40 mg P.O. daily h.s. for 8 weeks.
Pathologic hypersecretory conditions (such as Zollinger-Ellison syndrome)—
Adults: 20 mg P.O. q 6 hours up to 160 mg q 6 hours.
Hospitalized patients with intractable ulcerations or hypersecretory conditions or patients who cannot take oral medication—
Adults: 20 mg I.V. q 12 hours.
Gastroesophageal reflux disease (GERD)—
Adults: 20 mg P.O. b.i.d. for up to 6 weeks. For esophagitis caused by GERD, 20 to 40 mg b.i.d. for up to 12 weeks.
Prevention or treatment of heartburn—
Adults: 10 mg (Pepcid AC only) P.O. 1 hour before meals (prevention) or 10 mg (Pepcid AC only) P.O. with water when symptoms occur. Maximum dosage is 20 mg daily. Drug should not be taken daily for longer than 2 weeks.
Adjust-a-dose: In patients with severe renal insufficiency and creatinine clearance of below 10 ml/minute, 20 mg I.V. or P.O. h.s. or prolong dosing interval to q 36 to 48 hours.

ADVERSE REACTIONS
CNS: *headache,* dizziness, vertigo, malaise, paresthesia.
EENT: tinnitus, orbital edema.
GI: diarrhea, constipation, anorexia, taste disorder, dry mouth.
GU: increased BUN and creatinine levels.
Skin: acne, dry skin, flushing.
Other: transient irritation (at I.V. site), musculoskeletal pain, palpitations, fever.

INTERACTIONS
None significant.

EFFECTS ON DIAGNOSTIC TESTS
Drug may antagonize pentagastrin during gastric acid secretion tests. It may also elevate hepatic enzyme levels. In skin tests using allergen extracts, drug may cause false-negative results.

CONTRAINDICATIONS
Contraindicated in patients hypersensitive to drug.

NURSING CONSIDERATIONS
- Assess for abdominal pain. Note any blood in emesis, stool, or gastric aspirate.
- Store reconstituted suspension below 86° F (30° C). Discard after 30 days.

🔔 I.V. administration
- To prepare I.V. injection, dilute 2 ml (20 mg) famotidine with compatible I.V. solution to a total volume of either 5 or 10 ml, and inject over at least 2 minutes. Compatible solutions include sterile water for injection, 0.9% NaCl for injection, D_5W or $D_{10}W$ injection, 5% sodium bicarbonate injection, and lactated Ringer's injection. Famotidine can also be added to total parenteral nutrition solutions.
- Alternatively, give famotidine by intermittent I.V. infusion. Dilute 20 mg (2 ml)

Reactions may be *common,* uncommon, ***life-threatening,*** or COMMON AND LIFE-THREATENING.

famotidine in 100 ml of compatible solution, and infuse over 15 to 30 minutes. Solution is stable for 48 hours at room temperature after dilution.
• Store I.V. injection in refrigerator at 36° to 46° F (2° to 8° C).

☑ **Patient teaching**
• Instruct patient on proper use of OTC product (Pepcid AC), if appropriate.
• Tell patient to take prescription drug with a snack if desired.
• Remind patient that prescription drug is most effective if taken at bedtime. Tell patient taking 20 mg b.i.d. to take at least one dose at bedtime.
• Advise patient not to take prescription drug for more than 8 weeks, unless ordered by doctor, and to limit use of OTC drug to no more than 2 weeks.
• With doctor's knowledge, allow patient to take antacids concomitantly, especially at the beginning of therapy when pain is severe.
• Urge patient to avoid cigarette smoking because it may increase gastric acid secretion and worsen disease.
• Advise patient to report abdominal pain and blood in stools or emesis.

lansoprazole
Prevacid, Zoton§

Pregnancy Risk Category: B

HOW SUPPLIED
Capsules (delayed-release): 15 mg, 30 mg

ACTION
Inhibits the activity of the proton pump and binds to hydrogen-potassium adenosine triphosphatase, located at the secretory surface of the gastric parietal cells, to block the formation of gastric acid.

Route	Onset	Peak	Duration
PO	Unknown	1.7 hr	Unknown

INDICATIONS & DOSAGE
Short-term treatment of active duodenal ulcer—
Adults: 15 mg P.O. daily before eating for 4 weeks.

Short-term treatment of active benign gastric ulcer—
Adults: 30 mg P.O. once daily for up to 8 weeks.
Short-term treatment of erosive esophagitis—
Adults: 30 mg P.O. daily before eating for up to 8 weeks. If healing doesn't occur, 8 more weeks of therapy may be given. Maintenance dose for healing is 15 mg P.O. daily.
Long-term treatment of pathologic hypersecretory conditions, including Zollinger-Ellison syndrome—
Adults: initially, 60 mg P.O. once daily. Dosage increased p.r.n. Daily dosages of more than 120 mg should be given in divided doses.
Maintenance of healed duodenal ulcers—
Adults: 15 mg P.O. daily.
Helicobacter pylori *eradication to reduce risk of duodenal ulcer recurrence—*
Adults: in patients receiving dual therapy, 30 mg P.O. lansoprazole with 1 g P.O. amoxicillin, each given q 8 hours for 14 days. In patients receiving triple therapy, 30 mg P.O. lansoprazole with 1 g P.O. amoxicillin and 500 mg P.O. clarithromycin, all given q 12 hours for 14 days.
✳ *NEW INDICATION: Short-term treatment of symptomatic gastroesophageal reflux disease—*
Adults: 15 mg P.O. once daily for up to 8 weeks.

ADVERSE REACTIONS
GI: diarrhea, nausea, abdominal pain.

INTERACTIONS
Drug-drug. *Ampicillin esters, digoxin, iron salts, ketoconazole:* lansoprazole may inhibit absorption. Monitor patient closely.
Sucralfate: delayed lansoprazole absorption. Give lansoprazole at least 30 minutes prior to sucralfate.
Theophylline: may cause mild increase in theophylline clearance. Use together cautiously. Dosage adjustment of theophylline may be needed when lansoprazole is started or stopped.
Drug-herb. *Male fern:* male fern is inactivated in alkaline environments. Do not give concurrently.

---

*Liquid contains alcohol.   **May contain tartrazine.   †Canada   ‡Australia   §U.K.   ◇OTC

EFFECTS ON DIAGNOSTIC TESTS
None reported.

CONTRAINDICATIONS
Contraindicated in patients hypersensitive to drug.

NURSING CONSIDERATIONS
• Know that no dosage adjustment is necessary in patients with renal insufficiency or in elderly patients. For patients with severe liver disease, dosage adjustment may be necessary.
• Be aware that lansoprazole should not be used as maintenance therapy for treatment of patients with duodenal ulcer or erosive esophagitis.
• Know that safety and efficacy have not been established in children.
• For patients who have a nasogastric tube in place, capsules can be opened, the intact granules mixed in 40 ml of apple juice, and administered through the tube into the stomach. After administering the granules, the nasogastric tube should be flushed with additional apple juice to clear the tube.
• Because it is not known if lansoprazole is excreted in breast milk, be aware that a decision to discontinue breast-feeding or drug should be made when drug is prescribed for breast-feeding women.

☑ **Patient teaching**
• Instruct patient to take drug before eating.
• Tell patient who has trouble swallowing capsules to open and sprinkle contents over applesauce.

---

misoprostol
Cytotec

Pregnancy Risk Category: X

HOW SUPPLIED
Tablets: 100 mcg, 200 mcg

ACTION
A synthetic prostaglandin E_1 analogue that replaces gastric prostaglandins depleted by NSAID therapy. Misoprostol also decreases basal and stimulated gastric acid secretion and may increase gastric mucus and bicarbonate production.

Route	Onset	Peak	Duration
PO	30 min	10-15 min	3 hr

INDICATIONS & DOSAGE
Prevention of NSAID-induced gastric ulcer in elderly or debilitated patients at high risk for complications from gastric ulcer and in patients with history of NSAID-induced ulcer—
Adults: 200 mcg P.O. q.i.d. with food; if not tolerated, may be decreased to 100 mcg P.O. q.i.d. Dosage should be given for duration of NSAID therapy. Last dose should be given h.s.

ADVERSE REACTIONS
CNS: headache.
GI: *diarrhea, abdominal pain,* nausea, flatulence, dyspepsia, vomiting, constipation.
GU: hypermenorrhea, dysmenorrhea, spotting, cramps, menstrual disorders.

INTERACTIONS
Drug-drug. *Antacids:* reduced plasma levels when administered concomitantly. Not considered significant.

EFFECTS ON DIAGNOSTIC TESTS
Drug causes a modest decrease in basal pepsin secretion.

CONTRAINDICATIONS
Contraindicated in pregnant or breast-feeding patients.

NURSING CONSIDERATIONS
• Know that drug should not be routinely given to women of childbearing age unless they are at high risk for developing ulcers or complications from NSAID-induced ulcers.
Alert: Take special precautions to prevent use of drug during pregnancy. Make sure patient understands the dangers of drug to a fetus and that she receives both oral and written warnings about these dangers. Also ensure that she can comply with effective contraception and that she has a

---

negative serum pregnancy test within 2 weeks of initiating therapy.

☑**Patient teaching**
• Instruct patient not to share misoprostol. Remind pregnant patient that drug may cause miscarriage, often with potentially life-threatening bleeding.
• Advise female patient not to begin misoprostol therapy until the second or third day of the next normal menstrual period.
• Advise patient to take drug as prescribed for duration of NSAID therapy.

---

nizatidine
Axid, Tazac‡

Pregnancy Risk Category: C

HOW SUPPLIED
Capsules: 150 mg, 300 mg

ACTION
Competitively inhibits the action of H_2 at receptor sites of the parietal cells, decreasing gastric acid secretion.

Route	Onset	Peak	Duration
PO	0.5 hr	0.5-3 hr	12 hr

INDICATIONS & DOSAGE
Active duodenal ulcer—
Adults: 300 mg P.O. daily h.s. Alternatively, 150 mg P.O. b.i.d.
Maintenance therapy for duodenal ulcer—
Adults: 150 mg P.O. daily h.s.
Benign gastric ulcer—
Adults: 150 mg P.O. b.i.d. or 300 mg h.s. for 8 weeks.
Gastroesophageal reflux disease (GERD)—
Adults: 150 mg P.O. b.i.d.
Adjust-a-dose: In renally impaired patients with creatinine clearance of 20 to 50 ml/minute, 150 mg P.O. daily for treatment of active duodenal ulcer, benign gastric ulcer, or GERD; or 150 mg every other day for maintenance therapy. If creatinine clearance is below 20 ml/minute, 150 mg P.O. every other day for treat-

ment, or 150 mg every third day for maintenance.

ADVERSE REACTIONS
CNS: *somnolence.*
CV: *arrhythmias.*
Hematologic: eosinophilia.
Skin: *diaphoresis,* rash, urticaria.
Other: hyperuricemia, fever, hepatocellular injury, elevated liver function tests.

INTERACTIONS
Drug-drug. *Aspirin:* possibly elevated serum salicylate levels (with high doses).
Drug-food. *Tomato-based mixed-vegetable juices:* may decrease potency of drug when used concomitantly. Don't use together.

EFFECTS ON DIAGNOSTIC TESTS
False-positive test results for urobilinogen may occur during drug therapy.

CONTRAINDICATIONS
Contraindicated in patients hypersensitive to H_2-receptor antagonists.

NURSING CONSIDERATIONS
• Use cautiously and in reduced dosages in patients with renal impairment.
• If necessary, open capsules and mix contents with apple juice. However, be aware that drug loses some potency when combined with tomato-based mixed-vegetable juices. Ask pharmacist about compatibility.
• Assess patient for abdominal pain. Note presence of blood in emesis, stool, or gastric aspirate.

☑**Patient teaching**
• Tell patient who has difficulty swallowing capsules that contents may be mixed with apple juice but not with tomato-based mixed-vegetable juices.
• Urge patient to avoid cigarette smoking because it may increase gastric acid secretion and worsen disease.
• Advise patient to report abdominal pain and blood in stools or emesis.

---

omeprazole
Losec†‡, Prilosec

Pregnancy Risk Category: C

HOW SUPPLIED
Capsules (delayed-release): 10 mg, 20 mg, 40 mg

ACTION
Inhibits the activity of the acid (proton) pump, and binds to hydrogen-potassium adenosine triphosphatase, located at the secretory surface of the gastric parietal cells to block the formation of gastric acid.

Route	Onset	Peak	Duration
PO	1 hr	2 hr	< 3 days

INDICATIONS & DOSAGE
Symptomatic gastroesophageal reflux disease (GERD) without esophageal lesions—
Adults: 20 mg P.O. daily for 4 to 8 weeks for patients poorly responsive to customary medical treatment usually including an adequate course of H_2 receptor antagonists.
Erosive esophagitis and accompanying symptoms due to GERD—
Adults: 20 mg P.O. daily for 4 to 8 weeks.
Maintenance of healing erosive esophagitis—
Adults: 20 mg P.O. daily.
Pathologic hypersecretory conditions (such as Zollinger-Ellison syndrome)—
Adults: initially, 60 mg P.O. daily; dosage titrated based on patient response. If daily dosage exceeds 80 mg, administer in divided doses. Dosages up to 120 mg t.i.d. have been given. Continue therapy as long as clinically indicated.
Duodenal ulcer (short-term treatment)—
Adults: 20 mg P.O. daily for 4 to 8 weeks.
Treatment of Helicobacter pylori *infection and duodenal ulcer disease to eradicate* H. pylori *in combination with clarithromycin (dual therapy)—*
Adults: 40 mg P.O. every morning in conjunction with clarithromycin 500 mg P.O. t.i.d for days 1 to 14. For patients with an ulcer present at initiation of therapy, an

additional 14 days of omeprazole 20 mg P.O. once daily is recommended.
Short-term treatment of active benign gastric ulcer—
Adults: 40 mg P.O. once daily for 4 to 8 weeks.
✳ *NEW INDICATION: Treatment of* H. pylori *infection and duodenal ulcer disease to eradicate* H. pylori *in combination with clarithromycin and amoxicillin (triple therapy)—*
Adults: 20 mg P.O. in conjunction with clarithromycin 500 mg P.O. and amoxicillin 1,000 mg P.O., each given b.i.d. for 10 days. For patients with an ulcer present at initiation of therapy, an additional 18 days of omeprazole 20 mg P.O. once daily is recommended.

ADVERSE REACTIONS
CNS: headache, dizziness, asthenia.
GI: diarrhea, abdominal pain, nausea, vomiting, constipation, flatulence.
Respiratory: cough, upper respiratory infection.
Skin: rash.
Other: back pain.

INTERACTIONS
Drug-drug. *Ampicillin esters, iron derivatives, ketoconazole:* may exhibit poor bioavailability in patients taking omeprazole because optimal absorption of these drugs requires a low gastric pH. Avoid concomitant use.
Diazepam, phenytoin, warfarin: decreased hepatic clearance, possibly leading to increased serum levels. Monitor closely.
Drug-herb. *Male fern:* male fern is inactivated in alkaline environments. Separate administration.
Pennyroyal: may change the rate of formation of toxic metabolites of pennyroyal. Avoid concurrent use.

EFFECTS ON DIAGNOSTIC TESTS
Serum gastrin levels rise in most patients during the first 2 weeks of therapy.

CONTRAINDICATIONS
Contraindicated in patients hypersensitive to drug or its formulation.

NURSING CONSIDERATIONS
• Know that dosage adjustments are not needed for patients with renal or hepatic impairment.
• Know that omeprazole increases its own bioavailability with repeated dosages. Drug is labile in gastric acid; less drug is lost to hydrolysis because the drug increases gastric pH.

☑ **Patient teaching**
• Tell patient to swallow capsules whole and not to open, crush, or chew them.
• Instruct patient to take drug before meals.
• Caution patient not to perform hazardous activities if dizziness occurs.

---

ranitidine bismuth citrate
Tritec

Pregnancy Risk Category: C

HOW SUPPLIED
Tablets: 400 mg

ACTION
Reduces gastric acid secretion by competitively inhibiting histamine at the H_2 receptor of the gastric parietal cells. Bismuth is a topical agent that disrupts the integrity of bacterial cell walls and prevents adhesion of *Helicobacter pylori* to gastric epithelium.

Route	Onset	Peak	Duration
PO	Unknown	Variable	Variable

INDICATIONS & DOSAGE
In combination with clarithromycin for treatment of active duodenal ulcer associated with H. pylori *infection—*
Adults: 400 mg P.O. b.i.d for 28 days in conjunction with clarithromycin 500 mg P.O. t.i.d for first 14 days.

ADVERSE REACTIONS
CNS: headache.
GI: constipation, darkening of tongue and stool, diarrhea.

INTERACTIONS
Drug-drug. *Delavirdine, enoxacin, itra-conazole, ketoconazole:* ranitidine will decrease absorption of delavirdine, enoxacin, itraconazole, and ketoconazole by increasing gastric pH. Avoid concomitant use.
Glipizide: possible increased hypoglycemic effect. Monitor glucose levels.
Warfarin: concomitant use may increase warfarin's hypoprothrombinemic effects. Monitor PT and INR and adjust dose if needed.

EFFECTS ON DIAGNOSTIC TESTS
Drug may cause false-positive results in urine protein tests using Multistix; test with sulfosalicylic acid if necessary.

CONTRAINDICATIONS
Contraindicated in patients with known hypersensitivity to drug or its components.

NURSING CONSIDERATIONS
• Use caution when administering drug to breast-feeding patients because it is not known if drug is excreted in breast milk.
• Do not use drug in combination with clarithromycin in patients with history of acute porphyria.
• Drug is not recommended in patients with creatinine clearance below 25 ml/minute.
• Drug should not be prescribed alone for treatment of active duodenal ulcers.
• Patients not eradicated of *H. pylori* infection following drug therapy in combination with clarithromycin should be considered to have clarithromycin-resistant *H. pylori* and should not be retreated with a regimen containing clarithromycin.
• Drug may cause a temporary and harmless darkening of the tongue or stool. Do not confuse with blood in the stool.

☑ **Patient teaching**
• Inform patient that drug may be administered without regard to food.
• Instruct patient to take drug as directed, even after pain has subsided.
• Tell patient that it is important to take clarithromycin with drug for specified length of time.
• Inform patient that a temporary and

---

harmless darkening of the tongue or stool may occur with drug use.

ranitidine hydrochloride
Apo-Ranitidine†, Zantac*, Zantac-C†, Zantac 75 ◇, Zantac 150, Zantac 150 EFFERdose, Zantac 150 GELdose, Zantac 300, Zantac 300 GELdose

Pregnancy Risk Category: B

HOW SUPPLIED
Tablets: 75 mg ◇, 150 mg, 300 mg
Tablets (dispersible): 150 mg‡
Tablets (effervescent): 150 mg
Granules (effervescent): 150 mg
Syrup: 15 mg/ml*
Injection: 25 mg/ml
Infusion: 0.5 mg/ml in 100-ml containers

ACTION
Competitively inhibits the action of H_2 at receptor sites of the parietal cells, decreasing gastric acid secretion.

Route	Onset	Peak	Duration
PO	1 hr	1-3 hr	13 hr
IV	Unknown	Unknown	Unknown

INDICATIONS & DOSAGE
Duodenal and gastric ulcer (short-term treatment); pathologic hypersecretory conditions, such as Zollinger-Ellison syndrome—
Adults: 150 mg P.O. b.i.d. or 300 mg daily h.s. Alternatively, 50 mg I.V. or I.M. q 6 to 8 hours. Patients with Zollinger-Ellison syndrome may require dosages up to 6 g P.O. daily.
Maintenance therapy for duodenal or gastric ulcer—
Adults: 150 mg P.O. h.s.
Gastroesophageal reflux disease—
Adults: 150 mg P.O. b.i.d.
Erosive esophagitis—
Adults: 150 mg P.O. q.i.d. Maintenance therapy is 150 mg P.O. b.i.d.
Treatment for heartburn—
Adults: 75 mg (Zantac 75 only) P.O. as symptoms occur, not to exceed 150 mg daily.

Adjust-a-dose: In renally impaired patients with creatinine clearance below 50 ml/minute, 150 mg P.O. q 24 hours or 50 mg I.V. q 18 to 24 hours.

ADVERSE REACTIONS
CNS: vertigo, malaise.
EENT: blurred vision.
Hematologic: reversible leukopenia, pancytopenia.
Hepatic: elevated liver enzymes, jaundice.
Other: burning and itching at injection site, *anaphylaxis,* angioneurotic edema.

INTERACTIONS
Drug-drug. *Antacids:* may interfere with ranitidine absorption. Stagger doses if possible.
Diazepam: decreased absorption of diazepam. Monitor closely.
Glipizide: possible increased hypoglycemic effect. Adjust glipizide dosage as necessary.
Procainamide: possible decreased renal clearance of procainamide. Monitor patient closely for toxicity.
Warfarin: possible interference with warfarin clearance. Monitor closely.

EFFECTS ON DIAGNOSTIC TESTS
Drug may cause false-positive results in urine protein tests using Multistix. It may increase serum creatinine, lactate dehydrogenase, alkaline phosphatase, AST, ALT, and total bilirubin levels. Drug may also decrease WBC, RBC, and platelet counts.

CONTRAINDICATIONS
Contraindicated in patients hypersensitive to drug.

NURSING CONSIDERATIONS
• Use cautiously in patients with hepatic dysfunction. Adjust dosage in patients with impaired renal function as ordered.
• Assess patient for abdominal pain. Note presence of blood in emesis, stool, or gastric aspirate.
• Ranitidine may be added to total parenteral nutrition solutions.

Reactions may be *common,* uncommon, *life-threatening*, or COMMON AND LIFE-THREATENING.

⬛ I.V. administration

• When administering by I.V. push, dilute to a total volume of 20 ml, and inject over a period of 5 minutes. No dilution is necessary when administering I.M.

• When giving by intermittent I.V. infusion, dilute 50 mg (2 ml) ranitidine in 100 ml of compatible solution, and infuse over 15 to 20 minutes. Compatible solutions include 0.9% NaCl for injection, D_5W or $D_{10}W$ injection, 5% sodium bicarbonate injection, or lactated Ringer's injection. Or, give by continuous I.V. infusion: 150 mg in 250 ml of compatible solution. Administer at 6.25 mg/hour using an infusion pump.

• When administering premixed I.V. infusion, give by slow I.V. drip (over 15 to 20 minutes). Don't add other drugs to the solution. If used with a primary I.V. fluid system, discontinue the primary solution during the infusion.

☑ Patient teaching

• Instruct patient on proper use of OTC preparation, as indicated.

• Remind patient taking prescription drug once daily to take it at bedtime for best results.

• Instruct patient to take without regard to meals because absorption is not affected by food.

• Tell patient taking EFFERdose to dissolve drug in 6 to 8 ounces of water before taking.

• Urge patient to avoid cigarette smoking because it may increase gastric acid secretion and worsen disease.

• Advise patient to report abdominal pain and blood in stool or emesis.

---

sucralfate
Antepsin§, Carafate

Pregnancy Risk Category: B

HOW SUPPLIED
Tablets: 1 g
Suspension: 1 g/10 ml

ACTION
Unknown. Probably adheres to and protects the ulcer's surface by forming a barrier.

Route	Onset	Peak	Duration
PO	Unknown	Unknown	6 hr

INDICATIONS & DOSAGE
Short-term (up to 8 weeks) treatment of duodenal ulcer—
Adults: 1 g P.O. q.i.d. 1 hour before meals and h.s.
Maintenance therapy for duodenal ulcer—
Adults: 1 g P.O. b.i.d.

ADVERSE REACTIONS
CNS: dizziness, sleepiness, headache, vertigo.
GI: *constipation,* nausea, gastric discomfort, diarrhea, bezoar formation, vomiting, flatulence, dry mouth, indigestion.
Skin: rash, pruritus.
Other: back pain.

INTERACTIONS
Drug-drug. *Antacids:* may decrease binding of drug to gastroduodenal mucosa, impairing effectiveness. Don't administer within 30 minutes of each other.
Cimetidine, ciprofloxacin, digoxin, ketoconazole, norfloxacin, phenytoin, quinidine, ranitidine, tetracycline, theophylline: decreased absorption. Separate administration times by at least 2 hours.

EFFECTS ON DIAGNOSTIC TESTS
None reported.

CONTRAINDICATIONS
No known contraindications.

NURSING CONSIDERATIONS
• Use cautiously in patients with chronic renal failure.

• Reconstitute drug before instillation through nasogastric tube. Flush tube with water to ensure passage into stomach.

• Know that drug is minimally absorbed and has a low incidence of adverse reactions.

• Monitor for severe, persistent constipation.

• Be aware that studies suggest that sucralfate is as effective as cimetidine in healing duodenal ulcer.

• Know that drug contains aluminum but isn't classified as an antacid.

☑ Patient teaching

• Tell patient to take sucralfate on an empty stomach (1 hour before each meal and at bedtime).
• Instruct patient to continue prescribed regimen to ensure complete healing. Pain and ulcerative symptoms may subside within first few weeks of therapy.
• Urge patient to avoid cigarette smoking because it may increase gastric acid secretion and worsen disease.

53
Corticosteroids

betamethasone
betamethasone acetate and
  betamethasone sodium
  phosphate
betamethasone sodium
  phosphate
cortisone acetate
dexamethasone
dexamethasone acetate
dexamethasone sodium
  phosphate
fludrocortisone acetate
hydrocortisone
hydrocortisone acetate
hydrocortisone cypionate
hydrocortisone sodium
  phosphate
hydrocortisone sodium
  succinate
methylprednisolone
methylprednisolone acetate
methylprednisolone sodium
  succinate
prednisolone
prednisolone sodium
  phosphate
prednisolone tebutate
prednisone
triamcinolone
triamcinolone acetonide

COMBINATION PRODUCTS
DECADRON PHOSPHATE WITH XYLOCAINE:
dexamethasone phosphate 4 mg and lidocaine hydrochloride 10 mg per ml.
PREDNISOLONE ACETATE AND PRED-
NISOLONE SODIUM PHOSPHATE: prednisolone acetate 80 mg/ml and prednisolone sodium phosphate 20 mg/ml.

betamethasone
Betnelan†, Celestone*

betamethasone acetate and betamethasone sodium phosphate
Celestone Chronodose‡,
Celestone Soluspan

betamethasone sodium phosphate
Betnesol§, Celestone Phosphate,
Selestoject

Pregnancy Risk Category: C

HOW SUPPLIED
betamethasone
Tablets: 600 mcg, 500 mcg
Tablets (effervescent): 500 mcg†
Syrup: 600 mcg/5 ml
**betamethasone acetate and betametha-
sone sodium phosphate**
Injection (suspension): betamethasone acetate 3 mg and betamethasone sodium
phosphate (equivalent to 3-mg base)
per ml
betamethasone sodium phosphate
Injection: 4 mg (equivalent to 3-mg
base)/ml in 5-ml vials

ACTION
Not completely defined. Decreases inflammation, mainly by stabilizing leukocyte lysosomal membranes; suppresses
the immune response; stimulates bone
marrow; and influences protein, fat, and
carbohydrate metabolism.

Route	Onset	Peak	Duration
PO	Prompt	Unknown	3-25 days
IM	Unknown	Unknown	7-14 days

INDICATIONS & DOSAGE
Betamethasone sodium phosphate and betamethasone acetate suspension combination product should *not* be used for I.V.
administration.

---

*Liquid contains alcohol. **May contain tartrazine. †Canada ‡Australia §U.K. ◊OTC

Conditions with severe inflammation; conditions requiring immunosuppression—
Adults: 0.6 to 7.2 mg P.O. daily; or 0.5 to 9 mg I.M., or into joint or soft tissue daily. Betamethasone sodium phosphate-acetate suspension 1.5 to 12 mg injected into large joints or 1.5 to 6 mg injected into smaller joints. Both injections may be given q 1 to 2 weeks, p.r.n.
Children: not recommended for chronic use; especially likely to inhibit growth. 17.5 mcg/kg or 500 mcg/m² of body surface area; given in three divided doses q 3 days. *Or,* 5.8 to 8.75 mcg/kg or 166 to 250 mcg/m² of body surface area once daily.

ADVERSE REACTIONS

Most adverse reactions to corticosteroids are dose- or duration-dependent.
CNS: *euphoria, insomnia,* psychotic behavior, pseudotumor cerebri, vertigo, headache, paresthesia, **seizures.**
CV: **heart failure,** hypertension, edema, **arrhythmias,** thrombophlebitis, **thromboembolism.**
EENT: cataracts, glaucoma.
Endocrine: menstrual irregularities, cushingoid state (moonface, buffalo hump, central obesity).
GI: *peptic ulceration,* GI irritation, increased appetite, pancreatitis, nausea, vomiting.
Skin: delayed wound healing, acne, various skin eruptions.
Other: muscle weakness, osteoporosis, hirsutism, susceptibility to infections; hypokalemia, hyperglycemia, and carbohydrate intolerance; growth suppression in children; *acute adrenal insufficiency may follow increased stress (infection, surgery, or trauma) or abrupt withdrawal after long-term therapy.*
After abrupt withdrawal: rebound inflammation, fatigue, weakness, arthralgia, fever, dizziness, lethargy, depression, fainting, orthostatic hypotension, dyspnea, anorexia, hypoglycemia. *After prolonged use, sudden withdrawal may be fatal.*

INTERACTIONS

Drug-drug. *Antidiabetic agents, including insulin:* decreased response. May need dose adjustment.
Aspirin, indomethacin, other NSAIDs: increased risk of GI distress and bleeding. Give together cautiously.
Barbiturates, phenytoin, rifampin: decreased corticosteroid effect. Corticosteroid dosage may need to be increased.
Cardiac glycosides: increased arrhythmia possibility due to hypokalemia. May need dosage adjustment.
Oral anticoagulants: altered dosage requirements. Monitor PT and INR closely.
Potassium-depleting drugs (such as thiazide diuretics): enhanced potassium-wasting effects of betamethasone. Monitor serum potassium levels.
Salicylates: reduced serum salicylate levels with corticosteroids. Monitor for lack of salicylate effectiveness.
Skin-test antigens: decreased response. Defer skin testing until therapy is completed.
Toxoids, vaccines: decreased antibody response and increased risk of neurologic complications. Avoid concomitant use.
Drug-lifestyle. *Alcohol use:* increased risk of gastric irritation and GI ulceration. Advise patient to avoid alcohol use.

EFFECTS ON DIAGNOSTIC TESTS

Adrenocorticoid therapy suppresses reactions to skin tests, causes false-negative results in the nitroblue tetrazolium tests for systemic bacterial infections, and decreases ¹³¹I uptake and protein-bound iodine concentrations in thyroid function tests. It may increase serum glucose and cholesterol levels; decrease serum potassium, calcium, T₄, and T₃ levels; and increase urine glucose and calcium levels.

CONTRAINDICATIONS

Contraindicated in patients with viral or bacterial infections (except in life-threatening situations), systemic fungal infections, or hypersensitivity to drug.

NURSING CONSIDERATIONS

• Use with extreme caution in a patient with recent MI or active peptic ulcer (used only in life-threatening situations).
• Use cautiously in patients with renal disease, hypertension, osteoporosis, dia-

betes mellitus, hypothyroidism, cirrhosis, diverticulitis, nonspecific ulcerative colitis, recent intestinal anastomoses, thromboembolic disorders, seizures, myasthenia gravis, heart failure, tuberculosis, ocular herpes simplex, emotional instability, and psychotic tendencies. Because some formulations contain sulfite preservatives, also use cautiously in patients with hypersensitivity to sulfites.

• Check for sensitivity to other corticosteroid medications.

Alert: Know that drug should not be used for alternate-day therapy.

• Obtain baseline weight before starting therapy, and weigh patients daily; report any sudden weight gain to the doctor.

• For better results and less toxicity, give a once-daily dose in the morning.

• To reduce GI irritation, give with milk or food.

• To prevent muscle atrophy, give I.M. injection deeply. Rotate injection sites.

• Be aware that drug should always be titrated to lowest effective dose.

• Monitor blood glucose and serum potassium levels regularly, as ordered. Diabetic patients may require adjustments in insulin dosage.

• Monitor for depression or mood changes, especially in patients receiving long-term therapy.

• A calorie- or sodium-restricted diet with protein supplementation may be necessary for patients receiving long-term therapy.

• Know that elderly patients may be more susceptible to osteoporosis with long-term use.

• Be aware that adrenal suppression may last up to 1 year after drug is stopped.

• Gradually reduce drug dosage after long-term therapy, as ordered.

• Observe for signs of infection, especially after steroid withdrawal.

☑ **Patient teaching**

• Tell patient not to stop drug abruptly or without doctor's consent.

• Instruct patient to take drug with food or milk; tell patient using effervescent tablets to dissolve them in water immediately before ingestion.

• Teach patient about drug's effects. Warn patient on long-term therapy about cush-

ingoid symptoms and to notify doctor of sudden weight gain or swelling.

• Instruct patient to report symptoms associated with corticosteroid withdrawal, including fatigue, weakness, arthralgia, orthostatic hypotension, and dyspnea.

• Tell patient to contact doctor if symptoms worsen or the medication is no longer effective. Tell patient not to increase dosage without doctor's consent.

• Advise elderly patient receiving long-term therapy to consider exercise or physical therapy. Tell him to ask his doctor about vitamin D or calcium supplement.

• Advise patients receiving prolonged therapy to have periodic ophthalmic examinations.

• Tell patient to report slow healing of wounds.

• Instruct patient to carry a card indicating his need for supplemental glucocorticoids during stress. This card should contain doctor's name, medication, and dose being taken.

• Advise patient to avoid exposure to infections (such as chickenpox or measles) and to notify doctor if exposure occurs.

---

cortisone acetate
Cortate‡, Cortisyl§, Cortone Acetate

Pregnancy Risk Category: C

HOW SUPPLIED
Tablets: 5 mg, 10 mg, 25 mg
Injection (suspension): 50 mg/ml

ACTION
Not completely defined. Decreases inflammation, mainly by stabilizing leukocyte lysosomal membranes; suppresses the immune response; stimulates bone marrow; and influences protein, fat, and carbohydrate metabolism.

Route	Onset	Peak	Duration
PO, IM	Variable	Variable	Variable

INDICATIONS & DOSAGE
Adrenal insufficiency, allergy, inflammation—
Adults: 25 to 300 mg P.O. or 20 to

300 mg I.M. daily. Dosages are highly individualized, depending on severity of disease.

ADVERSE REACTIONS

Most adverse reactions to corticosteroids are dose- or duration-dependent.

CNS: *euphoria, insomnia,* psychotic behavior, pseudotumor cerebri, vertigo, headache, paresthesia, *seizures.*

CV: *heart failure,* hypertension, edema, *arrhythmias,* thrombophlebitis, *thromboembolism.*

EENT: cataracts, glaucoma.

Endocrine: menstrual irregularities, cushingoid state (moonface, buffalo hump, central obesity).

GI: *peptic ulceration,* GI irritation, increased appetite, pancreatitis, nausea, vomiting.

Skin: delayed wound healing, acne, various skin eruptions; atrophy (at I.M. injection site).

Other: muscle weakness, osteoporosis, hirsutism, susceptibility to infections; possible hypokalemia, hyperglycemia, and carbohydrate intolerance; growth suppression in children; *acute adrenal insufficiency may follow increased stress (infection, surgery, or trauma) or abrupt withdrawal after long-term therapy.*

After abrupt withdrawal: rebound inflammation, fatigue, weakness, arthralgia, fever, dizziness, lethargy, depression, fainting, orthostatic hypotension, dyspnea, anorexia, hypoglycemia. *After prolonged use, sudden withdrawal may be fatal.*

INTERACTIONS

Drug-drug. *Antidiabetic agents, including insulin:* decreased response. May need dose adjustment.

Aspirin, indomethacin, other NSAIDs: increased risk of GI distress and bleeding. Give together cautiously.

Barbiturates, phenytoin, rifampin: decreased corticosteroid effect. Increase corticosteroid dosage, as ordered.

Live attenuated virus vaccines, other toxoids and vaccines: decreased antibody response and increased risk of neurologic complications. Avoid concomitant use.

Oral anticoagulants: altered dosage requirements. Monitor PT and INR closely.

Potassium-depleting drugs (such as thiazide diuretics): enhanced potassium-wasting effects of cortisone. Monitor serum potassium levels.

Salicylates: decreased serum salicylate levels with corticosteroids. Monitor for lack of salicylate effectiveness.

Skin-test antigens: decreased response. Defer skin testing until therapy is completed.

Drug-lifestyle. *Alcohol use:* increased risk of gastric irritation and GI ulceration. Advise patient to avoid alcohol use.

EFFECTS ON DIAGNOSTIC TESTS

Cortisone therapy suppresses reactions to skin tests, causes false-negative results in the nitroblue tetrazolium test for systemic bacterial infections, and decreases ^{131}I uptake and protein-bound iodine concentrations in thyroid function tests. It may increase serum glucose and cholesterol levels; decrease serum potassium, calcium, T_4, and T_3 levels; and increase urine glucose and calcium levels.

CONTRAINDICATIONS

Contraindicated in patients with systemic fungal infections and hypersensitivity to drug or its ingredients.

NURSING CONSIDERATIONS

• Use with extreme caution in a patient with recent MI.

• Use cautiously in patients with GI ulcer, renal disease, hypertension, osteoporosis, diabetes mellitus, hypothyroidism, cirrhosis, diverticulitis, nonspecific ulcerative colitis, recent intestinal anastomoses, thromboembolic disorders, seizures, myasthenia gravis, heart failure, tuberculosis, ocular herpes simplex, emotional instability, and psychotic tendencies.

• Check for sensitivity to any other corticosteroid medications.

• To reduce GI irritation, give with milk or food. Patient may require medication to prevent GI irritation.

• For better results and less toxicity, give a once-daily dose in the morning.

• I.M. route causes slow onset of action. Should not be used in acute conditions

---

where a rapid effect is required. May be used on a twice-daily schedule matching diurnal variation. Rotate injection sites to prevent muscle atrophy.

• Mixing or diluting parenteral suspension may alter absorption rate and decrease drug's effectiveness.

Alert: Know that drug is not for I.V. use.

• Know that drug should always be titrated to lowest effective dose.

• Monitor serum electrolyte and blood glucose levels, as ordered. Diabetic patients may require adjustment in insulin dose.

• Monitor patient for fluid and electrolyte imbalances. Patients may need low-sodium diet and potassium supplements.

• Know that elderly patients may be more susceptible to osteoporosis with long-term administration.

• Gradually reduce drug dosage after long-term therapy, as ordered.

• Observe for signs of infection, especially after steroid withdrawal.

☑ **Patient teaching**

• Tell patient not to discontinue drug abruptly or without doctor's consent.

• Instruct patient to take drug with milk or food.

• Advise patient receiving long-term therapy to consider exercise or physical therapy. Also tell him to ask his doctor about vitamin D or calcium supplement.

• Tell patient to report slow healing of wounds.

• Warn patient on long-term therapy about cushingoid symptoms and to notify doctor of sudden weight gain or swelling.

• Instruct patient to carry a card indicating his need for supplemental glucocorticoids during stress. This card should contain doctor's name, medication, and dose taken.

• Instruct patient to avoid exposure to infections (such as measles and chickenpox) and to notify doctor if such exposure occurs.

dexamethasone
Decadron*, Deronil†, Dexasone†, Dexone 0.5, Dexone 0.75, Dexone 1.5, Dexone 4, Hexadrol*, Mymethasone*

dexamethasone acetate
Dalalone D.P., Dalalone L.A., Decadron-LA, Decaject-L.A., Dexacen LA-8, Dexasone-LA, Dexone LA, Solurex-LA

dexamethasone sodium phosphate
Dalalone, Decadron Phosphate, Decaject, Dexacen-4, Dexone, Hexadrol Phosphate, Solurex

Pregnancy Risk Category: C

HOW SUPPLIED
dexamethasone
Tablets: 0.25 mg, 0.5 mg, 0.75 mg, 1 mg, 1.5 mg, 2 mg, 4 mg, 6 mg
Oral solution: 0.5 mg/5 ml, 1 mg/ml
Elixir: 0.5 mg/5 ml*
dexamethasone acetate
Injection: 8 mg/ml, 16 mg/ml suspension
dexamethasone sodium phosphate
Injection: 4 mg/ml, 10 mg/ml, 20 mg/ml, 24 mg/ml

ACTION
Not clearly defined. Decreases inflammation, mainly by stabilizing leukocyte lysosomal membranes; suppresses the immune response; stimulates bone marrow; and influences protein, fat, and carbohydrate metabolism.

Route	Onset	Peak	Duration
PO	1-2 hr	1-2 hr	2.5 days
IV	1 hr	1 hr	Variable
IM	1 hr	1 hr	6 days
IM (acetate)	1 hr	8 hr	Unknown

INDICATIONS & DOSAGE
Cerebral edema—
Adults: initially, 10 mg (phosphate) I.V.; then 4 to 6 mg I.M. q 6 hours until symptoms subside (usually 2 to 4 days); then tapered over 5 to 7 days.

Inflammatory conditions, allergic reactions, neoplasias—
Adults: 0.75 to 9 mg/day P.O. or 0.5 to 9 mg/day (phosphate) I.M.; or 4 to 16 mg (acetate) I.M. into joint or soft tissue q 1 to 3 weeks; or 0.8 to 1.6 mg (acetate) into lesions q 1 to 3 weeks.
Shock—
Adults: 20 mg (phosphate) as a single initial dose, then 3 mg/kg per 24 hours via continuous I.V. infusion *or* 1 to 6 mg/kg (phosphate) I.V. as a single dose; or 40 mg I.V. q 2 to 6 hours, p.r.n.; continued only until patient is stabilized (usually not longer than 48 to 72 hours).
Dexamethasone suppression test for Cushing's syndrome—
Adults: after determining baseline 24-hour levels of 17-hydroxycorticosteroids, 0.5 mg P.O. q 6 hours for 48 hours; *or* 1 mg as a single dose at 11:00 pm; 24-hour urine collection made for determination of 17-hydroxycorticosteroid excretion again during second 24 hours of dexamethasone administration.
Adrenocortical insufficiency—
Children: 23.3 mcg/kg daily in three divided doses.

ADVERSE REACTIONS
Most adverse reactions to corticosteroids are dose- or duration-dependent.
CNS: *euphoria, insomnia,* psychotic behavior, pseudotumor cerebri, vertigo, headache, paresthesia, *seizures.*
CV: *heart failure,* hypertension, edema, *arrhythmias,* thrombophlebitis, *thromboembolism.*
EENT: cataracts, glaucoma.
Endocrine: menstrual irregularities, cushingoid state (moonface, buffalo hump, central obesity).
GI: *peptic ulceration,* GI irritation, increased appetite, pancreatitis, nausea, vomiting.
Skin: delayed wound healing, acne, various skin eruptions; atrophy (at I.M. injection site).
Other: muscle weakness, osteoporosis, hirsutism, susceptibility to infections; hypokalemia, hyperglycemia, and carbohydrate intolerance; growth suppression in children; *acute adrenal insufficiency may follow increased stress (infection,*

surgery, or trauma) or abrupt withdrawal after long-term therapy.
After abrupt withdrawal: rebound inflammation, fatigue, weakness, arthralgia, fever, dizziness, lethargy, depression, fainting, orthostatic hypotension, dyspnea, anorexia, hypoglycemia. *After prolonged use, sudden withdrawal may be fatal.*

INTERACTIONS
Drug-drug. *Antidiabetic agents, including insulin:* decreased response. May need dose adjustment
Aspirin, indomethacin, other NSAIDs: increased risk of GI distress and bleeding. Give together cautiously.
Barbiturates, phenytoin, rifampin: decreased corticosteroid effect. Increase corticosteroid dosage, as ordered.
Cardiac glycosides: increased arrhythmia possibility due to hypokalemia. May warrant dosage adjustment.
Oral anticoagulants: altered dosage requirements. Monitor PT and INR closely.
Potassium-depleting drugs (such as thiazide diuretics): enhanced potassium-wasting effects of dexamethasone. Monitor serum potassium levels.
Salicylates: decreased serum salicylate levels. Monitor for lack of salicylate effectiveness.
Skin-test antigens: decreased response. Defer skin testing until therapy is completed.
Toxoids, vaccines: decreased antibody response and increased risk of neurologic complications. Avoid concomitant use.
Drug-lifestyle. *Alcohol use:* increased risk of gastric irritation and GI ulceration. Advise patient to avoid alcohol use.

EFFECTS ON DIAGNOSTIC TESTS
Drug suppresses reactions to skin tests, causes false-negative results in the nitroblue tetrazolium test for systemic bacterial infections, and decreases ^{131}I uptake and protein-bound iodine concentrations in thyroid function tests. It may increase serum glucose and cholesterol levels; decrease serum potassium, calcium, T_4, and T_3 levels; and increase urine glucose and calcium levels.

Reactions may be *common*, uncommon, *life-threatening*, or COMMON AND LIFE-THREATENING.

CONTRAINDICATIONS
Contraindicated in patients with systemic fungal infections and hypersensitivity to drug or its ingredients.

NURSING CONSIDERATIONS
• Use with extreme caution in patient with recent MI.
• Use cautiously in patients with GI ulcer, renal disease, hypertension, osteoporosis, diabetes mellitus, hypothyroidism, cirrhosis, diverticulitis, nonspecific ulcerative colitis, recent intestinal anastomoses, thromboembolic disorders, seizures, myasthenia gravis, heart failure, tuberculosis, ocular herpes simplex, emotional instability, and psychotic tendencies. Because some formulations contain sulfite preservatives, also use cautiously in patients sensitive to sulfites.
• Determine if patient is sensitive to other corticosteroid medications.
• For better results and less toxicity, give once-daily dose in the morning.
• Give oral dose with food when possible. Patient may require medication to prevent GI irritation.
• Give I.M. injection deeply into gluteal muscle. Rotate injection sites to prevent muscle atrophy. Avoid S.C. injection because atrophy and sterile abscesses may occur.
• Always titrate to lowest effective dose, as ordered.
• Monitor patient's weight, blood pressure, and serum electrolyte levels.
• Watch for depression or psychotic episodes, especially in high-dose therapy.
• Keep in mind that diabetic patients may need increased insulin. Monitor blood glucose levels.
• Know that drug may mask or exacerbate infections, including latent amebiasis.
• Know that elderly patients may be more susceptible to osteoporosis with long-term use.
• Inspect patient's skin for petechiae.
• Gradually reduce drug dosage after long-term therapy, as ordered.

I.V. administration
• When administering as direct injection, inject undiluted over at least 1 minute. When administering as an intermittent or continuous infusion, dilute solution according to the manufacturer's instructions and give over the prescribed duration. If used for continuous infusion, change solution every 24 hours.

☑ Patient teaching
• Tell patient not to discontinue drug abruptly or without doctor's consent.
• Instruct patient to take drug with food or milk.
• Teach patient the signs of early adrenal insufficiency: fatigue, muscular weakness, joint pain, fever, anorexia, nausea, dyspnea, dizziness, and fainting.
• Instruct patient to carry a card indicating his need for supplemental systemic glucocorticoids during stress, especially when dosage is decreased. This card should contain doctor's name, medication, and dose taken.
• Warn patient on long-term therapy about cushingoid symptoms and to notify doctor of sudden weight gain or swelling.
• Warn patient about easy bruising.
• Advise patient receiving long-term therapy to consider exercise or physical therapy. Give vitamin D or calcium supplement, as ordered.
• Instruct patient receiving long-term therapy to have periodic ophthalmic examinations.
• Advise patient to avoid exposure to infections (such as measles and chickenpox) and to notify doctor if such exposure occurs.

---

fludrocortisone acetate
Florinef

Pregnancy Risk Category: C

HOW SUPPLIED
Tablets: 0.1 mg

ACTION
Increases sodium reabsorption and potassium and hydrogen secretion at the nephrons' distal convoluted tubules.

Route	Onset	Peak	Duration
PO	Variable	2 hr	1-2 days

INDICATIONS & DOSAGE
Salt-losing adrenogenital syndrome—
Adults: 0.1 mg P.O. daily. Decrease dosage to 0.05 mg daily if transient hypertension develops as a result of drug therapy.

ADVERSE REACTIONS
CV: *sodium and water retention,* hypertension, cardiac hypertrophy, edema, *heart failure.*
Skin: bruising, diaphoresis, urticaria, allergic rash.
Other: hypokalemia.

INTERACTIONS
Drug-drug. *Barbiturates, phenytoin, rifampin:* increased clearance of fludrocortisone acetate. Monitor for possible diminished effect of steroid. Steroid dose may need to be increased.
Potassium-depleting drugs (such as thiazide diuretics): enhanced potassium-wasting effects of fludrocortisone. Monitor serum potassium levels.
Drug-food. *Sodium-containing medications or foods:* may increase blood pressure. Sodium intake may need to be adjusted.

EFFECTS ON DIAGNOSTIC TESTS
Drug therapy increases serum sodium levels and decreases serum potassium levels. Glucose tolerance tests should be performed only if necessary, because addisonian patients tend to develop severe hypoglycemia within 3 hours of the test.

CONTRAINDICATIONS
Contraindicated in patients with systemic fungal infections and hypersensitivity to drug.

NURSING CONSIDERATIONS
• Use cautiously in patients with hypothyroidism, cirrhosis, ocular herpes simplex, emotional instability, and psychotic tendencies, nonspecific ulcerative colitis, diverticulitis, fresh intestinal anastomoses, active or latent peptic ulcer, renal insufficiency, hypertension, osteoporosis, and myasthenia gravis.
• Be aware that drug is used with cortisone or hydrocortisone in adrenal insufficiency.
Alert: Monitor patient's blood pressure and serum electrolyte levels. If hypertension occurs, notify doctor and expect dosage to be decreased by 50%.
• Weigh patient daily; notify doctor of sudden weight gain.
• Unless contraindicated, give low-sodium diet that's high in potassium and protein. Be aware that potassium supplements may be needed.

☑ **Patient teaching**
• Tell patient to notify doctor if symptoms, such as hypotension, weakness, cramping, and palpitations, worsen.
• Warn patient that mild peripheral edema is common.

---

hydrocortisone
Cortef, Cortenema, Hydrocortone

hydrocortisone acetate
Cortifoam, Hydrocortone Acetate

hydrocortisone cypionate
Cortef

hydrocortisone sodium phosphate
Hydrocortone Phosphate

hydrocortisone sodium succinate
A-hydroCort, Solu-Cortef

Pregnancy Risk Category: C

HOW SUPPLIED
hydrocortisone
Tablets: 5 mg, 10 mg, 20 mg
Enema: 100 mg/60 ml
hydrocortisone acetate
Injection: 25 mg/ml*, 50 mg/ml* suspension
Enema: 10% aerosol foam (provides 90 mg/application)
hydrocortisone cypionate
Oral suspension: 2 mg/ml
hydrocortisone sodium phosphate
Injection: 50 mg/ml solution

---

hydrocortisone sodium succinate
Injection: 100-mg vial*, 250-mg vial*,
500-mg vial*, 1,000-mg vial*

ACTION

Not clearly defined. Decreases inflammation, mainly by stabilizing leukocyte lysosomal membranes; suppresses the immune response; stimulates bone marrow; and influences protein, fat, and carbohydrate metabolism.

Route	Onset	Peak	Duration
PO, IV, IM, PR	Variable	Variable	Variable

INDICATIONS & DOSAGE

Severe inflammation, adrenal insufficiency—
Adults: 5 to 30 mg P.O. b.i.d., t.i.d., or q.i.d. (as much as 80 mg q.i.d. may be given in acute situations); or initially, 100 to 500 mg succinate I.M. or I.V., and then 50 to 100 mg I.M., as indicated; or 15 to 240 mg phosphate I.M. or I.V. daily in divided doses q 12 hours; or 5 to 75 mg acetate into joints or soft tissue repeated at 2- to 3-week intervals. Dosage varies with size of joint. Local anesthetics often are injected with dose.
Shock—
Adults: initially, 50 mg/kg succinate I.V., repeated in 4 hours. Repeat dosage q 24 hours p.r.n. Alternatively, 100 to 500 mg to 2 g q 2 to 6 hours; continued until patient is stabilized (usually not longer than 48 to 72 hours).
Children: phosphate (I.M.) or succinate (I.M. or I.V.) 0.186 to 0.28 mg/kg or 10 to 12 (base) mg/m² daily in three divided doses.
Adjunct for ulcerative colitis and proctitis—
Adults: 1 enema (100 mg) P.R. nightly for 21 days. Alternatively, 1 applicator (90-mg foam) P.R. daily or b.i.d. for 14 to 21 days.

ADVERSE REACTIONS

Most adverse reactions to corticosteroids are dose- or duration-dependent.
CNS: *euphoria, insomnia,* psychotic behavior, pseudotumor cerebri, vertigo, headache, paresthesia, *seizures.*

CV: *heart failure,* hypertension, edema, *arrhythmias,* thrombophlebitis, *thromboembolism.*
EENT: cataracts, glaucoma.
Endocrine: menstrual irregularities, cushingoid state (moonface, buffalo hump, central obesity).
GI: *peptic ulceration,* GI irritation, increased appetite, pancreatitis, nausea, vomiting.
Skin: delayed wound healing, acne, various skin eruptions, easy bruising.
Other: muscle weakness, osteoporosis, hirsutism, susceptibility to infections; possible hypokalemia, hyperglycemia, and carbohydrate intolerance; growth suppression in children; *acute adrenal insufficiency may occur with increased stress (infection, surgery, or trauma) or abrupt withdrawal after long-term therapy.*
After abrupt withdrawal: rebound inflammation, fatigue, weakness, arthralgia, fever, dizziness, lethargy, depression, fainting, orthostatic hypotension, dyspnea, anorexia, hypoglycemia. *After prolonged use, sudden withdrawal may be fatal.*

INTERACTIONS

Drug-drug. *Aspirin, indomethacin, other NSAIDs:* increased risk of GI distress and bleeding. Give together cautiously.
Barbiturates, phenytoin, rifampin: decreased corticosteroid effect. Increase corticosteroid dosage, as ordered.
Live attenuated virus vaccines, other toxoids and vaccines: decreased antibody response and increased risk of neurologic complications. Avoid concomitant use.
Oral anticoagulants: altered dosage requirements. Monitor PT and INR closely.
Potassium-depleting drugs (such as thiazide diuretics): enhanced potassium-wasting effects of hydrocortisone. Monitor serum potassium levels.
Skin-test antigens: decreased response. Defer skin testing until after therapy.

EFFECTS ON DIAGNOSTIC TESTS

Drug suppresses reactions to skin tests, causes false-negative results in the nitroblue tetrazolium test for systemic bacterial infections, and decreases ¹³¹I uptake and protein-bound iodine concentrations in

---

*Liquid contains alcohol.   **May contain tartrazine.   †Canada   ‡Australia   §U.K.   ◊OTC

thyroid function tests. It may increase serum glucose and cholesterol levels; decrease serum potassium, calcium, T_4, and T_3 levels; and increase urine glucose and calcium levels.

CONTRAINDICATIONS

Contraindicated in patients with systemic fungal infections or hypersensitivity to drug or its ingredients and in premature infants (succinate).

NURSING CONSIDERATIONS

• Use with extreme caution in patient with recent MI.
• Use cautiously in patients with GI ulcer, renal disease, hypertension, osteoporosis, diabetes mellitus, hypothyroidism, cirrhosis, diverticulitis, nonspecific ulcerative colitis, recent intestinal anastomoses, thromboembolic disorders, seizures, myasthenia gravis, heart failure, tuberculosis, ocular herpes simplex, emotional instability, and psychotic tendencies.
• Determine if patient is sensitive to other corticosteroid medications.
• For better results and less toxicity, give a once-daily dose in the morning.
• Give oral dose with food when possible. Patient may require medication to prevent GI irritation.
• Give I.M. injection deeply into gluteal muscle. Rotate injection sites to prevent muscle atrophy. Avoid S.C. injection because atrophy and sterile abscesses may occur.
Alert: Do not confuse Solu-Cortef with Solu-Medrol (methylprednisolone sodium succinate).
• Know that injectable forms are not used for alternate-day therapy.
• Enema may produce same systemic effects as other forms of hydrocortisone. If enema therapy must exceed 21 days, discontinue gradually by reducing administration to every other night for 2 or 3 weeks, as ordered.
• Be aware that high-dose therapy is usually not continued beyond 48 hours.
• Always titrate to lowest effective dose, as ordered.
• Monitor patient's weight, blood pressure, and serum electrolyte levels.
• Unless contraindicated, give low-sodium diet that's high in potassium and protein. Administer potassium supplements, as ordered.
• Know that drug may mask or exacerbate infections, including latent amebiasis.
• Know that stress (fever, trauma, surgery, and emotional problems) may increase adrenal insufficiency. Increase dosage, as ordered.
• Watch for depression or psychotic episodes, especially during high-dose therapy.
• Inspect patient's skin for petechiae.
• Keep in mind that diabetic patients may need increased insulin. Monitor blood glucose levels.
• Know that periodic measurement of growth and development may be necessary during high-dose or prolonged therapy in children.
• Know that elderly patients may be more susceptible to osteoporosis with prolonged use.
• Gradually reduce drug dosage after long-term therapy, as ordered. May affect patient's sleep.

◘ I.V. administration

• Do not use the acetate or suspension form for I.V. use. When administering as direct injection, inject directly into vein or an I.V. line containing a free-flowing compatible solution over 30 seconds to several minutes. When administering as an intermittent or continuous infusion, dilute solution according to manufacturer's instructions, and give over the prescribed duration. If used for continuous infusion, change solution every 24 hours.
• Hydrocortisone sodium phosphate may be added directly to D_5W or 0.9% NaCl for I.V. administration.
• Reconstitute hydrocortisone sodium succinate with bacteriostatic water or bacteriostatic NaCl solution before adding to I.V. solutions. When giving by direct I.V. injection, inject over a period of 30 seconds to 10 minutes. For infusion, dilute with D_5W, 0.9% NaCl, or dextrose 5% in 0.9% NaCl to a concentration of 1 mg/ml or less.

Reactions may be *common*, uncommon, *life-threatening*, or COMMON AND LIFE-THREATENING.

☑Patient teaching
• Tell patient not to discontinue drug abruptly or without doctor's consent.
• Instruct patient to take oral form of drug with milk or food.
• Warn patient on long-term therapy about cushingoid symptoms and to notify doctor of sudden weight gain or swelling.
• Teach patient the signs of early adrenal insufficiency: fatigue, muscular weakness, joint pain, fever, anorexia, nausea, dyspnea, dizziness, and fainting.
• Instruct patient to carry a card identifying his need for supplemental systemic glucocorticoids during stress. This card should contain doctor's name, medication and dose taken.
• Warn patient about easy bruising.
• Advise patient receiving long-term therapy to consider exercise or physical therapy. Also tell him to ask his doctor about vitamin D or calcium supplement.
• Advise patient receiving long-term therapy to have periodic ophthalmic examinations.
• Advise patient to avoid exposure to infections (such as chicken pox or measles) and to notify doctor if such exposure occurs.

methylprednisolone
Medrol**, Medrone§

methylprednisolone acetate
depMedalone 40, depMedalone 80, Depoject-40, Depoject-80, Depo-Medrol, Depo-Medrone§, Depopred-40, Depopred-80, Depo-Predate 40, Depo-Predate 80, Duralone-40, Duralone-80, Medralone-40, Medralone-80, Rep-Pred 40, Rep-Pred 80

methylprednisolone sodium succinate
A-methaPred, Solu-Medrol

Pregnancy Risk Category: C

HOW SUPPLIED
methylprednisolone
Tablets: 2 mg, 4 mg, 8 mg, 16 mg, 24 mg, 32 mg

methylprednisolone acetate
Injection (suspension): 20 mg/ml, 40 mg/ml, 80 mg/ml
methylprednisolone sodium succinate
Injection: 40-mg vial, 125-mg vial, 500-mg vial, 1,000-mg vial, 2,000-mg vial

ACTION
Not clearly defined. Decreases inflammation, mainly by stabilizing leukocyte lysosomal membranes; suppresses the immune response; stimulates bone marrow; and influences protein, fat, and carbohydrate metabolism.

Route	Onset	Peak	Duration
PO	Rapid	2-3 hr	30-36 hr
IV	Rapid	Immediate	7 days
IM	6-48 hr	4-8 days	1-4 wk
Intra-articular	Rapid	7 days	1-5 wk

INDICATIONS & DOSAGE
Severe inflammation or immunosuppression—
Adults: 4 to 48 mg as a single dose or in divided doses; 10 to 80 mg acetate I.M. daily, or 10 to 250 mg succinate I.M., 10 to 40 mg (base) repeated as necessary or I.V. up to q 4 hours; or 4 to 40 mg acetate into smaller joints or 20 to 80 mg acetate into larger joints. Intralesional administration is usually 20 to 60 mg acetate. Intralesional and intra-articular injections may be repeated q 1 to 5 weeks.
Children: 0.03 to 0.2 mg/kg succinate or 1 to 6.25 mg/m² I.M. once daily or b.i.d.
Shock—
Adults: 100 to 250 mg succinate I.V. at 2- to 6-hour intervals; or 30 mg/kg I.V. initially, repeated q 4 to 6 hours p.r.n. Continue therapy for 2 to 3 days or until patient is stable.

ADVERSE REACTIONS
Most adverse reactions to corticosteroids are dose- or duration-dependent.
CNS: *euphoria, insomnia,* psychotic behavior, pseudotumor cerebri, vertigo, headache, paresthesia, *seizures.*
CV: *heart failure,* hypertension, edema, *arrhythmias,* thrombophlebitis, *thromboembolism, fatal arrest, or circulatory*

collapse (following rapid administration of large I.V. doses).

EENT: cataracts, glaucoma.

Endocrine: menstrual irregularities, cushingoid state (moonface, buffalo hump, central obesity).

GI: *peptic ulceration,* GI irritation, increased appetite, pancreatitis, nausea, vomiting.

Skin: delayed wound healing, acne, various skin eruptions.

Other: muscle weakness, osteoporosis, hirsutism, susceptibility to infections; hypokalemia, hyperglycemia, and carbohydrate intolerance; growth suppression in children; *acute adrenal insufficiency may occur with increased stress (infection, surgery, or trauma) or abrupt withdrawal after long-term therapy.*

After abrupt withdrawal: rebound inflammation, fatigue, weakness, arthralgia, fever, dizziness, lethargy, depression, fainting, orthostatic hypotension, dyspnea, anorexia, hypoglycemia. *After prolonged use, sudden withdrawal may be fatal.*

INTERACTIONS

Drug-drug. *Aspirin, indomethacin, other NSAIDs:* increased risk of GI distress and bleeding. Give together cautiously.

Barbiturates, phenytoin, rifampin: decreased corticosteroid effect. Increase corticosteroid dosage, as ordered.

Oral anticoagulants: altered dosage requirements. Monitor PT and INR closely.

Potassium-depleting drugs (such as thiazide diuretics): enhanced potassium-wasting effects of methylprednisolone. Monitor serum potassium levels.

Salicylates: decreased serum salicylate levels. Monitor for lack of salicylate effectiveness.

Skin-test antigens: decreased response. Defer skin testing until after therapy.

Toxoids, vaccines: decreased antibody response and increased risk of neurologic complications. Avoid concomitant use.

EFFECTS ON DIAGNOSTIC TESTS

Methylprednisolone suppresses reactions to skin tests, causes false-negative results in the nitroblue tetrazolium test for systemic bacterial infections, and decreases ^{131}I uptake and protein-bound iodine concentrations in thyroid function tests. It may increase serum glucose and cholesterol levels; may decrease serum potassium, calcium, T_4, and T_3 levels; and may increase urine glucose and calcium levels.

CONTRAINDICATIONS

Contraindicated in patients with systemic fungal infections or hypersensitivity to drug or its ingredients and in premature infants (acetate and succinate).

NURSING CONSIDERATIONS

• Use cautiously in patients with GI ulceration or renal disease, hypertension, osteoporosis, diabetes mellitus, hypothyroidism, cirrhosis, diverticulitis, nonspecific ulcerative colitis, recent intestinal anastomoses, thromboembolic disorders, seizures, myasthenia gravis, heart failure, tuberculosis, ocular herpes simplex, emotional instability, and psychotic tendencies.

• Determine if patient is sensitive to other corticosteroid medications.

• Know that drug may be used for alternate-day therapy.

• For better results and less toxicity, give a once-daily dose in the morning.

• Give oral dose with food when possible. Know that critically ill patients may require concomitant antacid or H_2-receptor antagonist therapy.

• Do not confuse Solu-Medrol with Solu-Cortef (hydrocortisone sodium succinate).

Alert: The manufacturers state that Solu-Medrol should not be given intrathecally because severe adverse reactions have been reported.

• Give I.M. injection deeply into gluteal muscle. Avoid S.C. injection because atrophy and sterile abscesses may occur.

• Dermal atrophy may occur with large doses of acetate salt. Use multiple small injections rather than a single large dose and rotate injection sites.

• Don't use acetate salt when immediate onset of action is needed.

• Discard reconstituted solutions after 48 hours.

• Always titrate to lowest effective dose, as ordered.

• Monitor patient's weight, blood pres-

sure, serum electrolyte levels, and sleep patterns. Euphoria may initially interfere with sleep, but patients generally adjust to the medication after 1 to 3 weeks.
• Know that drug may mask or exacerbate infections, including latent amebiasis.
• Watch for depression or psychotic episodes, especially in high-dose therapy.
• Keep in mind that diabetic patients may need increased insulin. Monitor blood glucose levels.
• Watch for an enhanced response to drug in patients with hypothyroidism or cirrhosis.
• Watch for allergic reaction to the dye tartrazine in patients with sensitivity to aspirin.
• Unless contraindicated, give low-sodium diet that's high in potassium and protein. Administer potassium supplements as needed.
• Know that elderly patients may be more susceptible to osteoporosis with prolonged use.
• Gradually reduce drug dosage after long-term therapy, as ordered.

◖ I.V. administration
• Use only methylprednisolone sodium succinate; never use acetate form for I.V. use. Reconstitute according to the manufacturer's directions using the supplied diluent, or use bacteriostatic water for injection with benzyl alcohol.
• When administering as direct injection, inject diluted drug into a vein or free-flowing compatible I.V. solution over at least 1 minute. For treatment of shock, give massive doses over at least 10 minutes to prevent arrhythmias and circulatory collapse. When administering as an intermittent or continuous infusion, dilute solution according to manufacturer's instructions, and give over the prescribed duration. If used for continuous infusion, change solution every 24 hours.
• Compatible solutions include D_5W, 0.9% NaCl, and dextrose 5% in 0.9% NaCl.

☑ Patient teaching
• Tell patient not to discontinue drug abruptly or without doctor's consent.

• Instruct patient to take oral form of drug with milk or food.
• Teach patient the signs of early adrenal insufficiency: fatigue, muscular weakness, joint pain, fever, anorexia, nausea, dyspnea, dizziness, and fainting.
• Instruct patient to carry a card identifying his need for supplemental systemic glucocorticoids during stress. This card should contain doctor's name, medication, and dose taken.
• Warn patient on long-term therapy about cushingoid symptoms and to notify doctor of sudden weight gain or swelling.
• Advise patient receiving long-term therapy to consider exercise or physical therapy. Also tell patient to ask doctor about vitamin D or calcium supplement.
• Instruct patient to avoid exposure to infections (such as chickenpox or measles) and to contact doctor if such exposure occurs.

---

prednisolone
Delta-Cortef, Panafcortelone‡, Precortisyl Forte§, Predenema§, Prelone, Solone‡

prednisolone sodium phosphate
Hydeltrasol, Key-Pred-SP, Pediapred, Predate S, Predicort-RP, Predsol Retention Enema‡, Predsol Suppositories‡

prednisolone tebutate
Hydeltra-T.B.A., Nor-Pred T.B.A., Predalone T.B.A., Predate TBA, Predcor-TBA

Pregnancy Risk Category: C

HOW SUPPLIED
prednisolone
Tablets: 1 mg‡, 5 mg, 25 mg‡
Syrup: 15 mg/5 ml
prednisolone sodium phosphate
Oral solution: 5 mg/5 ml
Injection: 20 mg/ml
Retention enema: 20 mg/100 ml‡
Suppositories: 5 mg‡
prednisolone tebutate
Injection (suspension): 20 mg/ml

ACTION

Not clearly defined. Decreases inflammation, mainly by stabilizing leukocyte lysosomal membranes; suppresses the immune response; stimulates bone marrow; and influences protein, fat, and carbohydrate metabolism.

Route	Peak	Onset	Duration
PO	Rapid	1-2 hr	3-36 hr
IV	Rapid	1 hr	Unknown
IM	Rapid	1 hr	4 wk
Intra-articular	1-2 days	Unknown	< 4 wk
PR	Unknown	Unknown	Unknown

INDICATIONS & DOSAGE

Severe inflammation or immunosuppression—
Adults: 2.5 to 15 mg P.O. b.i.d., t.i.d., or q.i.d.; 2 to 30 mg I.M. (phosphate) or I.V. (phosphate) q 12 hours; or 2 to 30 mg (phosphate) into joints (depending on joint size), lesions, or soft tissue; or 4 to 40 mg (tebutate) into joints (depending on joint size) and lesions, p.r.n.
Adrenocortical insufficiency—
Children: 0.14 mg/kg or 4 mg/m² of body surface area daily in three divided doses.
Proctitis‡—
Adults: 1 suppository b.i.d., preferably in the morning and h.s.
Ulcerative colitis‡—
Adults: 1 retention enema h.s. nightly for 2 to 4 weeks. The contents of the enema should be retained overnight.
Acute exacerbations of multiple sclerosis—
Adults: 200 mg/day as a single or divided dose for 7 days, followed by 80 mg every other day for 1 month.

ADVERSE REACTIONS

Most adverse reactions to corticosteroids are dose- or duration-dependent.
CNS: *euphoria, insomnia,* psychotic behavior, pseudotumor cerebri, vertigo, headache, paresthesia, *seizures.*
CV: *heart failure,* hypertension, edema, *arrhythmias,* thrombophlebitis, *thromboembolism.*
EENT: cataracts, glaucoma.
Endocrine: menstrual irregularities, cushingoid state (moonface, buffalo hump, central obesity).
GI: *peptic ulceration,* GI irritation, increased appetite, pancreatitis, nausea, vomiting.
Skin: delayed wound healing, acne, various skin eruptions.
Other: muscle weakness, osteoporosis, hirsutism, susceptibility to infections; hypokalemia, hyperglycemia, and carbohydrate intolerance; growth suppression in children; *acute adrenal insufficiency may occur with increased stress (infection, surgery, or trauma) or abrupt withdrawal after long-term therapy.*
After abrupt withdrawal: rebound inflammation, fatigue, weakness, arthralgia, fever, dizziness, lethargy, depression, fainting, orthostatic hypotension, dyspnea, anorexia, hypoglycemia. *After prolonged use, sudden withdrawal may be fatal.*

INTERACTIONS

Drug-drug. *Aspirin, indomethacin, other NSAIDs:* increased risk of GI distress and bleeding. Give together cautiously.
Barbiturates, phenytoin, rifampin: decreased corticosteroid effect. Increase corticosteroid dosage, as ordered.
Oral anticoagulants: altered dosage requirements. Monitor PT and INR closely.
Potassium-depleting drugs (such as thiazide diuretics): enhanced potassium-wasting effects of prednisolone. Monitor serum potassium levels.
Salicylates: decreased serum salicylate levels. Monitor for lack of salicylate effectiveness.
Skin-test antigens: decreased response. Defer skin testing until therapy is completed.
Toxoids, vaccines: decreased antibody response and increased risk of neurologic complications. Avoid concomitant use.

EFFECTS ON DIAGNOSTIC TESTS

Drug suppresses reactions to skin tests, causes false-negative results in the nitroblue tetrazolium test for systemic bacterial infections, and decreases ^{131}I uptake and protein-bound iodine concentrations in thyroid function tests. It may increase serum glucose and cholesterol levels; may decrease serum potassium, calcium, T₄, and T₃ levels; and may increase urine glucose and calcium levels.

CONTRAINDICATIONS

Contraindicated in patients with systemic fungal infections and hypersensitivity to drug or its ingredients.

NURSING CONSIDERATIONS

• Use with extreme caution in a patient with recent MI.
• Use cautiously in patients with GI ulcer, renal disease, hypertension, osteoporosis, diabetes mellitus, hypothyroidism, cirrhosis, diverticulitis, nonspecific ulcerative colitis, recent intestinal anastomoses, thromboembolic disorders, seizures, myasthenia gravis, heart failure, tuberculosis, ocular herpes simplex, emotional instability, and psychotic tendencies.
• Determine if patient is sensitive to other corticosteroid medications.
Alert: Don't confuse with prednisone.
• Always titrate to lowest effective dose, as ordered.
• Be aware that prednisolone salts (sodium phosphate and tebutate) are used parenterally less often than other corticosteroids that have more potent anti-inflammatory action.
• Know that drug may be used for alternate-day therapy.
• Give oral dose with food when possible to reduce GI irritation. Patient may require medication to prevent GI irritation.
• Give I.M. injection deeply into gluteal muscle. Rotate injection sites to prevent muscle atrophy. Avoid S.C. injection because atrophy and sterile abscesses may occur.
• Monitor patient's weight, blood pressure, and serum electrolyte levels.
• Watch for depression or psychotic episodes, especially in high-dose therapy.
• Keep in mind that diabetic patients may need increased insulin. Monitor blood glucose levels.
• Unless contraindicated, give low-sodium diet that's high in potassium and protein. Administer potassium supplements as needed.
• Know that drug may mask or exacerbate infections, including latent amebiasis.
• Know that elderly patients may be more susceptible to osteoporosis with long-term use.
• Gradually reduce drug dosage after long-term therapy as ordered.

◻ I.V. administration

• Use only prednisolone sodium phosphate. When administering as direct injection, inject undiluted over at least 1 minute. When administering as an intermittent or continuous infusion, dilute solution according to manufacturer's instructions, and give over the prescribed duration. D₅W or 0.9% NaCl is recommended as diluent for I.V. infusion.

☑ Patient teaching

• Tell patient not to discontinue drug abruptly or without doctor's consent.
• Instruct patient to take oral form of drug with food or milk.
• Teach patient the signs of early adrenal insufficiency: fatigue, muscular weakness, joint pain, fever, anorexia, nausea, dyspnea, dizziness, and fainting.
• Instruct patient to carry a card identifying his need for supplemental systemic glucocorticoids during stress. This card should contain doctor's name, medication, and dose taken.
• Warn patient on long-term therapy about cushingoid symptoms and to notify doctor of sudden weight gain or swelling.
• Tell patient to report slow healing.
• Advise patient receiving long-term therapy to consider exercise or physical therapy. Also tell him to ask doctor about vitamin D or calcium supplement.
• Instruct patient to avoid exposure to infections and to notify doctor if exposure occurs.
• Tell patient to avoid immunizations while taking drug.

prednisone
Apo-Prednisone†, Deltasone, Liquid Pred*, Meticorten, Novo-Prednisone†, Orasone, Panafcort‡, Prednicen-M, Prednisone Intensol*, Sone‡, Sterapred, Winpred†

Pregnancy Risk Category: C

HOW SUPPLIED
Tablets: 1 mg, 2.5 mg, 5 mg, 10 mg, 20 mg, 50 mg
Oral solution: 5 mg/5 ml*, 5 mg/ml (concentrate)*
Syrup: 5 mg/5 ml*

ACTION
Not clearly defined. Decreases inflammation, mainly by stabilizing leukocyte lysosomal membranes; suppresses the immune response; stimulates bone marrow; and influences protein, fat, and carbohydrate metabolism.

Route	Onset	Peak	Duration
PO	Variable	Variable	Variable

INDICATIONS & DOSAGE
Severe inflammation or immunosuppression—
Adults: 5 to 60 mg P.O. daily in a single dose or as two to four divided doses. Maintenance dosage given once daily or every other day. Dosage must be individualized.
Children: 0.14 to 2 mg/kg or 4 to 60 mg/ m^2 daily P.O. in four divided doses.
Acute exacerbations of multiple sclerosis—
Adults: 200 mg P.O. daily for 7 days, then 80 mg P.O. every other day for 1 month.

ADVERSE REACTIONS
Most adverse reactions to corticosteroids are dose- or duration-dependent.
CNS: *euphoria, insomnia,* psychotic behavior, pseudotumor cerebri, vertigo, headache, paresthesia, *seizures.*
CV: *heart failure,* hypertension, edema, *arrhythmias,* thrombophlebitis, *thromboembolism.*
EENT: cataracts, glaucoma.
Endocrine: menstrual irregularities, cushingoid state (moonface, buffalo hump, central obesity).
GI: *peptic ulceration,* GI irritation, increased appetite, pancreatitis, nausea, vomiting.
Skin: delayed wound healing, acne, various skin eruptions.
Other: muscle weakness, osteoporosis, hirsutism, susceptibility to infections; hypokalemia, hyperglycemia, and carbohydrate intolerance; growth suppression in children; *acute adrenal insufficiency may occur with increased stress (infection, surgery, or trauma) or abrupt withdrawal after long-term therapy.*
After abrupt withdrawal: rebound inflammation, fatigue, weakness, arthralgia, fever, dizziness, lethargy, depression, fainting, orthostatic hypotension, dyspnea, anorexia, hypoglycemia. *After prolonged use, sudden withdrawal may be fatal.*

INTERACTIONS
Drug-drug. *Aspirin, indomethacin, other NSAIDs:* increased risk of GI distress and bleeding. Give together cautiously.
Barbiturates, phenytoin, rifampin: decreased corticosteroid effect. Increase corticosteroid dosage, as ordered.
Oral anticoagulants: altered dosage requirements. Monitor PT and INR closely.
Potassium-depleting drug (such as thiazide diuretics): enhanced potassium-wasting effects of prednisone. Monitor serum potassium levels.
Salicylates: decreased serum salicylate levels. Monitor for lack of salicylate effectiveness.
Skin-test antigens: decreased response. Defer skin testing until therapy is completed.
Toxoids, vaccines: decreased antibody response and increased risk of neurologic complications. Avoid concomitant use.

EFFECTS ON DIAGNOSTIC TESTS
Drug suppresses reactions to skin tests, causes false-negative results in the nitro-blue tetrazolium test for systemic bacterial infections, and decreases ^{131}I uptake and protein-bound iodine concentrations in thyroid function tests. It may increase serum glucose and cholesterol levels; may decrease serum potassium, calcium, T_4, and T_3 levels; and may increase urine glucose and calcium levels.

CONTRAINDICATIONS
Contraindicated in patients with systemic fungal infections and hypersensitivity to drug.

Reactions may be *common,* uncommon, *life-threatening,* or COMMON AND LIFE-THREATENING.

NURSING CONSIDERATIONS

• Use cautiously in patients with GI ulcer, renal disease, hypertension, osteoporosis, diabetes mellitus, hypothyroidism, cirrhosis, diverticulitis, nonspecific ulcerative colitis, recent intestinal anastomoses, thromboembolic disorders, seizures, myasthenia gravis, heart failure, tuberculosis, ocular herpes simplex, emotional instability, and psychotic tendencies.

• Determine if patient is sensitive to other corticosteroid medications.

Alert: Don't confuse with prednisolone.

• Know that drug may be used for alternate-day therapy.

• Always titrate to lowest effective dose as ordered.

• For better results and less toxicity, give a once-daily dose in the morning.

• Unless contraindicated, give oral dose with food when possible to reduce GI irritation. Patient may require medication to prevent GI irritation.

• Monitor patient's blood pressure, sleep patterns, and serum potassium levels.

• Weigh patient daily; report sudden weight gain to doctor.

• Watch for depression or psychotic episodes, especially in high-dose therapy.

• Diabetic patients may need increased insulin; monitor blood glucose levels.

• Know that elderly patients may be more susceptible to osteoporosis with long-term use.

• Know that drug may mask or exacerbate infections, including latent amebiasis.

• Unless contraindicated, give low-sodium diet that's high in potassium and protein. Administer potassium supplements as needed.

• Gradually reduce drug dosage after long-term therapy, as ordered.

☑ Patient teaching

• Tell patient not to discontinue drug abruptly or without doctor's consent.

• Instruct patient to take drug with food or milk.

• Teach patient signs of early adrenal insufficiency: fatigue, muscular weakness, joint pain, fever, anorexia, nausea, dyspnea, dizziness, and fainting.

• Instruct patient to carry a card identifying his need for supplemental systemic glucocorticoids during stress. This card should contain doctor's name, medication, and dose taken.

• Warn patient on long-term therapy about cushingoid symptoms and to notify doctor of sudden weight gain or swelling.

• Advise patient receiving long-term therapy to consider exercise or physical therapy. Also tell patient to ask doctor about vitamin D or calcium supplement.

• Tell patient to report slow healing.

• Advise patient receiving long-term therapy to have periodic ophthalmic examinations.

• Instruct patient to avoid exposure to infections and to contact doctor if exposure occurs.

---

triamcinolone
Adcortyl Intra-articular/
Intradermal§, Aristocort, Atolone,
Kenacort**

triamcinolone acetonide
Cenocort A-40, Cinonide 40,
Kenaject-40, Kenalog-10,
Kenalog-40, Tac-3, Triam-A,
Triamonide 40, Tri-Kort, Trilog

Pregnancy Risk Category: C

HOW SUPPLIED
triamcinolone
Tablets: 1 mg, 2 mg, 4 mg, 8 mg
triamcinolone acetonide
Injection (suspension): 3 mg/ml, 10 mg/ml, 40 mg/ml

ACTION
Not clearly defined. Decreases inflammation, mainly by stabilizing leukocyte lysosomal membranes; suppresses the immune response; stimulates bone marrow; and influences protein, fat, and carbohydrate metabolism.

Route	Onset	Peak	Duration
PO, IM, intralesion, intra-articular	Variable	Variable	Variable

INDICATIONS & DOSAGE
Severe inflammation or immunosuppression—
Adults: 4 to 48 mg P.O. daily in a single dose or divided doses; 40 to 80 mg I.M. (acetonide) at 4-week intervals; 1 mg (acetonide) into lesions; 2.5 to 15 mg (acetonide) into joints (depending on joint size) or soft tissue. A local anesthetic often is injected along with triamcinolone into the joint.
Adrenocortical insufficiency—
Children: 0.117 mg/kg/day or 3.3 mg/m^2/day P.O. as one dose or in divided doses.

ADVERSE REACTIONS
Most adverse reactions to corticosteroids are dose- or duration-dependent.
CNS: *euphoria, insomnia,* psychotic behavior, pseudotumor cerebri, vertigo, headache, paresthesia, **seizures.**
CV: *heart failure,* hypertension, edema, **arrhythmias,** thrombophlebitis, **thromboembolism.**
EENT: cataracts, glaucoma.
Endocrine: menstrual irregularities, cushingoid state (moonface, buffalo hump, central obesity).
GI: *peptic ulceration,* GI irritation, increased appetite, pancreatitis, nausea, vomiting.
Skin: delayed wound healing, acne, various skin eruptions.
Other: muscle weakness, osteoporosis, hirsutism, susceptibility to infections; hypokalemia, hyperglycemia, and carbohydrate intolerance; growth suppression in children; *acute adrenal insufficiency may occur with increased stress (infection, surgery, or trauma) or abrupt withdrawal after long-term therapy.*
After abrupt withdrawal: rebound inflammation, fatigue, weakness, arthralgia, fever, dizziness, lethargy, depression, fainting, orthostatic hypotension, dyspnea, anorexia, hypoglycemia. *After prolonged use, sudden withdrawal may be fatal.*

INTERACTIONS
Drug-drug. *Aspirin, indomethacin, other NSAIDs:* increased risk of GI distress and bleeding. Give together cautiously.
Barbiturates, phenytoin, rifampin: de-creased corticosteroid effect. Increase corticosteroid dosage, as ordered.
Oral anticoagulants: altered dosage requirements. Monitor PT and INR closely.
Potassium-depleting drugs (such as thiazide diuretics): enhanced potassium-wasting effects of triamcinolone. Monitor serum potassium levels.
Salicylates: decreased serum salicylate levels. Monitor for lack of salicylate effectiveness.
Skin-test antigens: decreased response. Defer skin testing until after therapy.
Toxoids, vaccines: decreased antibody response and increased risk of neurologic complications. Avoid concomitant use.

EFFECTS ON DIAGNOSTIC TESTS
Triamcinolone suppresses reactions to skin tests, causes false-negative results in the nitroblue tetrazolium test for systemic bacterial infections, and decreases ^{131}I uptake and protein-bound iodine concentrations in thyroid function tests. It may increase serum glucose and cholesterol levels; may decrease serum potassium, calcium, T_4, and T_3 levels; and may increase urine glucose and calcium levels.

CONTRAINDICATIONS
Contraindicated in patients with systemic fungal infections and hypersensitivity to drug or its ingredients.

NURSING CONSIDERATIONS
● Use cautiously in patients with GI ulcer, renal disease, hypertension, osteoporosis, diabetes mellitus, hypothyroidism, cirrhosis, diverticulitis, nonspecific ulcerative colitis, recent intestinal anastomoses, thromboembolic disorders, seizures, myasthenia gravis, heart failure, tuberculosis, ocular herpes simplex, emotional instability, and psychotic tendencies.
● Determine if patient is sensitive to other corticosteroid medications.
● Know that drug is not used for alternate-day therapy.
● Always titrate to lowest effective dose, as ordered.
● For better results and less toxicity, give a once-daily oral dose in the morning with food.

• Know that parenteral form is *not* for I.V. use.
• Don't use the 40 mg/ml strength for intradermal or intralesion administration.
• Don't use the 10 mg/ml strength for I.M. administration.
• Don't use diluents that contain preservatives; flocculation may occur.
• Give I.M. injection deeply into gluteal muscle. Rotate injection sites to prevent muscle atrophy.
• Monitor patient's weight, blood pressure, and serum electrolyte levels.
• Watch for allergic reaction to the dye tartrazine in patients with sensitivity to aspirin.
• Watch for depression or psychotic episodes, especially in high-dose therapy.
• Keep in mind that diabetic patients may need increased insulin. Monitor blood glucose levels.
• Know that drug may mask or exacerbate infections, including latent amebiasis.
• Know that elderly patients may be more susceptible to osteoporosis with long-term use.
• Unless contraindicated, give low-sodium diet that's high in potassium and protein. Administer potassium supplements as needed.
• Gradually reduce drug dosage after long-term therapy, as ordered. Drug may affect patient's sleep.

☑ **Patient teaching**
• Tell patient not to discontinue drug abruptly or without doctor's consent.
• Instruct patient to take drug with food or milk.
• Teach patient signs of early adrenal insufficiency: fatigue, muscular weakness, joint pain, fever, anorexia, nausea, dyspnea, dizziness, and fainting.
• Instruct patient to carry a card identifying his need for supplemental systemic glucocorticoids during stress. This card should contain doctor's name, medication, and dose taken.
• Warn patient on long-term therapy about cushingoid symptoms and to notify doctor of sudden weight gain and swelling.
• Tell patient to report slow healing.
• Advise patient receiving long-term therapy to consider exercise or physical therapy. Also tell patient to ask doctor about vitamin D or calcium supplement.
• Instruct patient to avoid exposure to infections and to notify doctor if exposure occurs.

54

Androgens and anabolic steroids

danazol
fluoxymesterone
methyltestosterone
nandrolone decanoate
nandrolone phenpropionate
testosterone
testosterone cypionate
testosterone enanthate
testosterone propionate
testosterone transdermal system

COMBINATION PRODUCTS

ANDROGYN L.A., DELADUMONE, VALERTEST
NO. 1: testosterone enanthate 90 mg/ml and
estradiol valerate 4 mg/ml in sesame oil.
DEPANDROGYN, DEPO-TESTADIOL, DEPO-
TESTOGEN, DUO-CYP, DURATESTRIN, TEST-
ESTRO CYPIONATE (oil): testosterone cypionate 50 mg and estradiol cypionate 2 mg.
ESTRATEST: esterified estrogens 1.25 mg
and methyltestosterone 2.5 mg.
ESTRATEST H.S.: esterified estrogens
0.625 mg and methyltestosterone 1.25 mg.
HALODRIN: fluoxymesterone 1 mg with
ethinyl estradiol 0.02 mg.
PREMARIN WITH METHYLTESTOSTERONE:
conjugated estrogens 0.625 mg and methyltestosterone 5 mg; or conjugated estrogens
1.25 mg and methyltestosterone 10 mg.

---

danazol
Cycloment†, Danocrine, Danol§

Pregnancy Risk Category: X

HOW SUPPLIED
Capsules: 50 mg, 100 mg, 200 mg

ACTION
Danazol binds to receptor sites of gonadal
steroids at target organs. It thus suppresses the pituitary-ovarian axis and depresses the output of follicle-stimulating hormone
(FSH) and luteinizing hormone.

Route	Onset	Peak	Duration
PO	1 mo	6-8 wk	Variable

INDICATIONS & DOSAGE
Mild endometriosis—
Women: initially, 100 to 200 mg P.O.
b.i.d. uninterrupted for 3 to 6 months;
may be continued for 9 months. Subsequent dosage based on patient response.
Moderate to severe endometriosis—
Women: 400 mg P.O. b.i.d. uninterrupted
for 3 to 6 months; may be continued for 9
months.
Fibrocystic breast disease—
Women: 100 to 400 mg P.O. daily in two
divided doses uninterrupted for 2 to 6
months.
Prevention of hereditary angioedema—
Adults: 200 mg P.O. b.i.d. to t.i.d., continued until favorable response is achieved.
Then dosage decreased by 50% at 1- to 3-
month intervals.

ADVERSE REACTIONS
CNS: dizziness, headache, sleep disorders, fatigue, tremor, irritability, excitation, lethargy, mental depression, paresthesia.
CV: elevated blood pressure.
EENT: visual disturbances.
GI: gastric irritation, nausea, vomiting,
diarrhea, constipation, change in appetite.
GU: hematuria, hypoestrogenic effects
(flushing, diaphoresis, vaginitis [includ-
ing itching, dryness, burning], vaginal
bleeding, nervousness, emotional lability,
menstrual irregularities), decreased testicular size.
Hepatic: reversible jaundice, elevated liver enzyme levels, hepatic dysfunction.
Other: muscle cramps or spasms; androgenic effects in women *(weight gain, hirsutism,* hoarseness, clitoral enlargement,
decreased breast size, acne, edema,
changes in libido, *oily skin or hair,* voice
deepening), chills; *allergic reactions.*

INTERACTIONS
Drug-drug. *Carbamazepine:* may increase
carbamazepine levels. Monitor closely.
Cyclosporine: can increase cyclosporine

Reactions may be *common,* uncommon, *life-threatening,* or COMMON AND LIFE-THREATENING.

levels and increase chance of nephrotoxicity. Monitor patient closely.

Warfarin: may prolong PT in patients stabilized on warfarin. Monitor PT and INR.

EFFECTS ON DIAGNOSTIC TESTS
Plasma proteins, lipids, CK, lipoproteins and glucose tolerance test results may be abnormal. Total serum T_4 may be decreased; T_3 may be increased. PT (especially in patients on anticoagulant therapy) may be prolonged.

CONTRAINDICATIONS
Contraindicated in patients with undiagnosed abnormal genital bleeding, porphyria, or impaired renal, cardiac, or hepatic function. Also contraindicated in pregnant and breast-feeding women.

NURSING CONSIDERATIONS
• Know that therapy should begin during menstruation.
• Use cautiously in patients with seizure disorders or migraine headache.
Alert: Avoid use in women of childbearing age until pregnancy is ruled out.
• Unless contraindicated, use with diet high in calories and protein.
• Monitor closely for signs of virilization. Some androgenic effects, such as deepening of voice, may not be reversible upon discontinuation of drug.
• Periodically evaluate hepatic function as ordered. Semen evaluation is routinely performed every 3 to 4 months, especially in adolescent boys.
• Know that periodic dosage decreases or gradual drug withdrawal is best.
• After withdrawal of treatment, ovulation and cyclic menstrual bleeding usually return in 2 to 3 months; fibrocystic disease symptoms return within 1 year for 50% of patients.
• Keep in mind that diabetic patient may require increased dosages of insulin.

☑ **Patient teaching**
• Advise patient taking danazol for fibrocystic breast disease to examine breasts regularly and to call doctor immediately if breast nodules enlarge.
• Make sure patient understands impor-

tance of using an effective nonhormonal contraceptive during therapy.
• Instruct patient to report adverse reactions, especially signs of virilization, promptly.
• Advise female patient to wash after intercourse to decrease risk of vaginitis. Instruct her to wear only cotton underwear.

---

fluoxymesterone
Android-F, Halotestin**

Controlled Substance Schedule III
Pregnancy Risk Category: X

HOW SUPPLIED
Tablets: 2 mg, 5 mg, 10 mg

ACTION
Stimulates target tissues to develop normally in androgen-deficient men.

Route	Onset	Peak	Duration
PO	Unknown	Unknown	9 hr

INDICATIONS & DOSAGE
Hypogonadism caused by testicular deficiency—
Adults: 5 to 20 mg P.O. daily.
Delayed puberty—
Adolescent: highly individualized; usually 2.5 to 10 mg daily, duration of therapy 4 to 6 months.
Palliation of breast cancer in women—
Adults: 10 to 40 mg P.O. daily in divided doses. All dosages are individualized and reduced to minimum when effect is noted.

ADVERSE REACTIONS
CNS: headache, anxiety, depression, paresthesia, sleep apnea syndrome.
CV: edema.
GI: nausea.
GU: *hypoestrogenic effects in women (flushing; diaphoresis; vaginitis, including itching, dryness, and burning; vaginal bleeding; nervousness; emotional lability; menstrual irregularities);* excessive hormonal effects in men (prepubertal—*premature epiphyseal closure, acne, priapism, growth of body and facial hair,* phallic enlargement; postpubertal—testicular atrophy, oligospermia, decreased

ejaculatory volume, impotence, gynecomastia, epididymitis).
Hematologic: polycythemia, elevated serum lipid levels, suppression of clotting factors.
Hepatic: reversible jaundice, peliosis hepatis, elevated liver enzyme levels, *liver cell tumors.*
Other: hypercalcemia; hypersensitivity skin manifestations; androgenic effects in women (acne, edema, *weight gain, hirsutism,* hoarseness, clitoral enlargement, deepening voice, *decreased breast size,* changes in libido, male-pattern baldness, *oily skin or hair).*

INTERACTIONS
Drug-drug. *Hepatotoxic medications:* increased risk of hepatotoxicity. Monitor closely.
Insulin, oral antidiabetic agents: altered dosage requirements. Monitor blood glucose levels in diabetic patients.
Oral anticoagulants: increased sensitivity to oral anticoagulants; altered dosage requirements. Monitor INR.

EFFECTS ON DIAGNOSTIC TESTS
Drug may cause abnormal results of the glucose tolerance test. Thyroid function test results (protein-bound iodine, radioactive iodine uptake, thyroid-binding capacity) may decrease. PT may be prolonged. Abnormal liver function tests may occur. Because of drug anabolic activity, serum sodium, potassium, calcium, phosphate, and cholesterol levels may all rise.

CONTRAINDICATIONS
Contraindicated in patients with hypersensitivity to drug; in males with breast cancer or known or suspected prostate cancer; in those with cardiac, hepatic, or renal decompensation; during pregnancy; and in breast-feeding patients.

NURSING CONSIDERATIONS
● Use cautiously in prepubertal males or patients with benign prostatic hyperplasia or aspirin sensitivity.
Alert: Avoid use in women of childbearing age until pregnancy is ruled out.
● Monitor INR in patients on oral antico-

agulant therapy because dosage may need adjustment.
● Unless contraindicated, use with diet high in calories and protein. Give small, frequent feedings.
● Watch for symptoms of jaundice and periodically evaluate hepatic function, as ordered. Dosage adjustment may reverse condition. If liver function test results are abnormal, notify doctor because therapy should be stopped.
● Know that edema can be controlled with sodium restriction or diuretics. Monitor weight routinely.
● Monitor male patients for signs of excessive sexual stimulation or priapism.
● Be aware that semen evaluation is routinely performed every 3 to 4 months, especially in adolescent boys.
Alert: Know that hypercalcemia symptoms may be difficult to distinguish from symptoms associated with condition being treated, unless anticipated and thought of as a symptom cluster. Hypercalcemia is particularly likely to occur in immobilized patients or patients with metastatic breast cancer and may indicate bone metastases.
Alert: Know that drug should not be used for enhancement of athletic performance or physique.
● Watch for symptoms of hypoglycemia in diabetic patients. Check blood glucose levels. Dosage of antidiabetic drug may need adjustment.
● When used in breast cancer, subjective effects may not occur for about 1 month; objective effects on clinical symptoms may take 3 months.

☑**Patient teaching**
● If GI upset occurs, tell patient to take drug with food or meals.
● Make sure patient understands importance of using an effective nonhormonal contraceptive during therapy.
● Advise female patient to wash after intercourse to decrease the risk of vaginitis. Instruct her to wear only cotton underwear.
● Tell women to report menstrual irregularities and to discontinue therapy pending etiologic determination.
● Explain to patient taking drug for palliation of breast cancer that virilization usu-

---

ally occurs. Give emotional support. Tell patient to report androgenic effects immediately. Stopping drug will prevent further androgenic changes but will probably not reverse existing effects.

• Warn diabetic patients to be alert for signs and symptoms of hypoglycemia; report them to doctor.

• Alert patient to report sudden weight gain.

---

methyltestosterone
Android, Metandren†**,
Oreton Methyl, Testred, Virilon

Controlled Substance Schedule III
Pregnancy Risk Category: X

HOW SUPPLIED
Tablets: 10 mg, 25 mg
Tablets (buccal): 10 mg
Capsules: 10 mg

ACTION
Stimulates target tissues to develop normally in androgen-deficient men.

Route	Onset	Peak	Duration
PO	Unknown	2 hr	Unknown
Buccal	Unknown	1 hr	Unknown

INDICATIONS & DOSAGE
Breast cancer in women 1 to 5 years postmenopausal—
Adults: 50 to 200 mg P.O. daily; or 25 to 100 mg buccally daily.
Male hypogonadism—
Adults: 10 to 50 mg P.O. daily; or 5 to 25 mg buccally daily.
Postpubertal cryptorchidism—
Adults: 30 mg P.O. daily; or 15 mg buccally daily.

ADVERSE REACTIONS
CNS: headache, anxiety, depression, paresthesia.
CV: edema.
GI: irritation of oral mucosa (with buccal administration), nausea.
GU: *hypoestrogenic effects in women (flushing; diaphoresis; vaginitis, including itching, dryness, and burning; vaginal bleeding; nervousness; emotional lability;*

menstrual irregularities); excessive hormonal effects in men (prepubertal—*premature epiphyseal closure, acne,* priapism, *growth of body and facial hair,* phallic enlargement; postpubertal—testicular atrophy, oligospermia, decreased ejaculatory volume, impotence, gynecomastia, epididymitis).
Hepatic: reversible jaundice, cholestatic hepatitis, abnormal liver enzyme levels.
Other: hypercalcemia; polycythemia; hypersensitivity skin manifestations; suppression of clotting factors; muscle cramps or spasms; androgenic effects in women (acne, edema, *weight gain, hirsutism,* hoarseness, clitoral enlargement, *decreased breast size,* deepening voice, changes in libido, male-pattern baldness, *oily skin or hair*).

INTERACTIONS
Drug-drug. *Hepatotoxic medications:* increased risk of hepatotoxicity. Monitor closely.
Insulin, oral antidiabetic agents: decreased serum glucose may alter dosage requirements. Monitor blood glucose levels in diabetic patients.
Oral anticoagulants: increased sensitivity to oral anticoagulants may alter dosage requirements. Monitor PT and INR.

EFFECTS ON DIAGNOSTIC TESTS
Drug may cause abnormal results of the glucose tolerance test. Thyroid function test results (protein-bound iodine, radioactive iodine uptake, thyroid-binding capacity) may decrease. PT (especially in patients on anticoagulant therapy) may be prolonged. Abnormal liver function tests may occur. Because of this agent's anabolic activity, serum sodium, potassium, calcium, phosphate, and cholesterol levels all may rise.

CONTRAINDICATIONS
Contraindicated in pregnant or breast-feeding patients and in males with breast cancer or known or suspected prostate cancer.

NURSING CONSIDERATIONS
• Use cautiously in elderly patients; patients with cardiac, renal, or hepatic dis-

---

ease; or healthy males with delayed puberty.

• Avoid use in women of childbearing age until pregnancy is ruled out.

• In children, X-rays of the wrist bones should be taken before therapy begins to establish the level of bone maturation. During treatment, bone maturation may proceed more rapidly than linear growth; ensure intermittent dosage and periodically review X-ray results to monitor bone maturation.

• Know that drug is typically used only for intermittent therapy. Because of potential hepatotoxicity, watch closely for jaundice.

• Promptly report signs of virilization in women.

• Unless contraindicated, use with diet high in calories and protein. Give small, frequent feedings.

• Periodically check hemoglobin and hematocrit values, serum cholesterol and calcium levels, and cardiac and liver function test results, as ordered.

• Check weight regularly. Edema can be controlled with sodium restriction or diuretics.

Alert: Therapeutic response in breast cancer is usually apparent within 3 months. Know therapy should be stopped if signs of disease progression appear.

• Report signs of hypercalcemia. In metastatic breast cancer, hypercalcemia may indicate progression of bone metastases.

• Know that semen evaluation is routinely performed every 3 to 4 months, especially in adolescent boys.

Alert: Know that drug should not be used for enhancement of athletic performance or physique.

☑ **Patient teaching**
• Make sure patient understands importance of using an effective nonhormonal contraceptive during therapy.

• Buccal tablets are twice as potent as oral tablets. Tell patient to avoid eating, drinking, chewing, or smoking while buccal tablet is in place and not to swallow tablet. Place in upper or lower buccal pouch between cheek and gum; tablet requires 30 to 60 minutes to dissolve. In

struct patient to change tablet absorption site with each dose to minimize risk of buccal irritation.

• Review signs and symptoms of virilization with female patient and instruct her to notify doctor immediately if any occur.

• Teach patient the signs of hypoglycemia and method for checking blood glucose level; drug enhances hypoglycemia. Instruct patient to report hypoglycemia immediately.

• Advise female patient to wash after intercourse to decrease risk of vaginitis. Instruct her to wear only cotton underwear.

nandrolone decanoate
Androlone-D, Deca-Durabolin, Hybolin Decanoate, Kabolin, Neo-Durabolic

nandrolone phenpropionate
Durabolin, Hybolin Improved, Nandrobolic

Controlled Substance Schedule III
Pregnancy Risk Category: X

HOW SUPPLIED
nandrolone decanoate
Injection (in oil): 50 mg/ml, 100 mg/ml, 200 mg/ml
nandrolone phenpropionate
Injection (in oil): 25 mg/ml, 50 mg/ml

ACTION
Anabolic steroid that promotes tissue-building processes, reverses catabolism, and stimulates erythropoiesis.

Route	Onset	Peak	Duration
IM (deca-noate)	Unknown	3-6 days	Unknown
IM (phen-propionate)	Unknown	1-2 days	Unknown

INDICATIONS & DOSAGE
Severe debility or disease states, refractory anemias—
Adults: 50 to 100 mg decanoate I.M. at 1- to 4-week intervals for females; 50 to 200 mg decanoate I.M. at 1- to 4-week intervals for males. Therapy should be in

termittent and discontinued if no improvement in 6 months.

Children 2 to 13 years: 25 to 50 mg decanoate I.M. q 3 to 4 weeks.

Control of metastatic breast cancer—
Adults: 25 to 100 mg phenpropionate I.M. weekly.

ADVERSE REACTIONS

CNS: excitation, insomnia, habituation, depression.
CV: edema.
GI: nausea, vomiting, diarrhea.
GU: bladder irritability, *hypoestrogenic effects in women (flushing; diaphoresis; vaginitis, including itching, dryness, and burning; vaginal bleeding; nervousness; emotional lability; menstrual irregularities);* excessive hormonal effects in men (prepubertal—*premature epiphyseal closure, acne,* priapism, *growth of body and facial hair,* phallic enlargement; postpubertal—testicular atrophy, oligospermia, decreased ejaculatory volume, impotence, gynecomastia, epididymitis).
Hematologic: elevated serum lipid levels, suppression of clotting factors.
Hepatic: reversible jaundice, peliosis hepatis, elevated liver enzyme levels, *liver cell tumors.*
Skin: pain, induration (at injection site).
Other: androgenic effects in women (acne, edema, *weight gain, hirsutism,* hoarseness, clitoral enlargement, *decreased breast size,* changes in libido, male-pattern baldness, *oily skin or hair*).

INTERACTIONS

Drug-drug. *Hepatotoxic medications:* increased risk of hepatotoxicity. Monitor closely.
Insulin, oral antidiabetic agents: altered dosage requirements. Monitor blood glucose levels in diabetic patients.
Oral anticoagulants: altered dosage requirements. Monitor PT and INR.

EFFECTS ON DIAGNOSTIC TESTS

Drug may cause abnormal results of fasting plasma glucose, glucose tolerance, and metyrapone tests. Thyroid function test results (protein-bound iodine, radioactive iodine uptake, thyroid-binding capacity) and 17-ketosteroid levels may de-

crease. Liver function test results, PT (especially in patients receiving anticoagulant therapy), and serum-creatinine levels may be elevated. Because of this agent's anabolic activity, serum sodium, potassium, calcium, phosphate, and cholesterol levels may all rise.

CONTRAINDICATIONS

Contraindicated in patients with hypersensitivity to anabolic steroids, in those with nephrosis or experiencing the nephrotic phase of nephritis, in males with breast cancer or known or suspected prostate cancer, in women with breast cancer and hypercalcemia, and in pregnant or breast-feeding patients.

NURSING CONSIDERATIONS

● Use cautiously in patients with diabetes; cardiac, renal, or hepatic disease; epilepsy; or migraine or other conditions that may be aggravated by fluid retention.
● Avoid use in women of childbearing age until pregnancy is ruled out.
● In children, X-rays of the wrist bones should be taken before surgery to establish the level of bone maturation. During treatment, bone maturation may proceed more rapidly than linear growth; ensure intermittent dosage and periodically review X-ray results to monitor bone maturation.
● Inject I.M. drug deeply, preferably into upper outer quadrant of gluteal muscle in adults. Rotate injection sites to prevent muscle atrophy.
● Unless contraindicated, use with diet high in calories and protein. Give small, frequent feedings.
● Watch for signs of virilization, which may be irreversible despite prompt discontinuation of therapy.
● Closely observe boys under 7 years for precocious development of male sexual characteristics.
● Know that semen evaluation is routinely performed every 3 to 4 months, especially in adolescent boys.
Alert: Periodically evaluate hepatic function, as ordered. Watch for jaundice; dosage adjustment may reverse condition. If liver function test results are abnormal, therapy should be stopped.

• Check weight regularly. Edema generally can be controlled with sodium restrictions or diuretics.

• Watch for symptoms of hypoglycemia in diabetic patients. Check blood glucose levels. Adjust dosage of antidiabetic agent, as ordered.

• Check quantitative urine and serum calcium levels. Hypercalcemia is most likely to occur in patients with breast cancer.

• When used to promote erythropoiesis in refractory anemias, make sure patients have adequate daily iron intake.

• Be aware that anabolic steroids may alter results of laboratory studies performed during therapy and for 2 to 3 weeks after therapy ends.

☑ **Patient teaching**
• Make sure patient understands importance of using an effective nonhormonal contraceptive during therapy.

• Review signs and symptoms of virilization with female patient, and instruct her to notify doctor immediately if they occur.

• Advise patient to wash after intercourse to decrease risk of vaginitis. Instruct her to wear only cotton underwear.

• Warn diabetic patients also to be alert for signs and symptoms of hypoglycemia; report them to doctor.

• Alert patient to report sudden weight gain to doctor.

• Tell female patient to report menstrual irregularities and to discontinue therapy pending etiologic determination.

---

testosterone
Andro 100, Histerone-50, Histerone 100, Testamone 100, Testaqua, Testoject-50

testosterone cypionate
Andro-Cyp 100, Andro-Cyp 200, Andronate 100, Andronate 200, depAndro 100, depAndro 200, Depotest, Depo-Testosterone, Duratest-100, Duratest-200, T-Cypionate, Testa-C, Testoject-LA, Testred Cypionate 200, Virilon IM

testosterone enanthate
Delatest, Delatestryl

testosterone propionate
Malogen†, Testex, Virormone§

Controlled Substance Schedule III
Pregnancy Risk Category: X

HOW SUPPLIED
testosterone
Injection (aqueous suspension): 25 mg/ml, 50 mg/ml, 100 mg/ml
testosterone cypionate
Injection (in oil): 100 mg/ml, 200 mg/ml
testosterone enanthate
Injection (in oil): 100 mg/ml, 200 mg/ml
testosterone propionate
Injection (in oil): 50 mg/ml; 100 mg/ml

ACTION
Stimulates target tissues to develop normally in androgen-deficient men. Testosterone may have some antiestrogen properties, making it useful to treat certain estrogen-dependent breast cancers. Its action in postpartum breast engorgement is not known because testosterone does not suppress lactation.

Route	Onset	Peak	Duration
IM	Unknown	10-100 min	Unknown

INDICATIONS & DOSAGE
Male hypogonadism—
Adults: 10 to 25 mg (testosterone) I.M. two to three times weekly, or 50 to 400 mg (cypionate or enanthate) I.M. q 2 to 4 weeks.
Metastatic breast cancer in women 1 to 5 years postmenopausal—
Adults: 50 to 100 mg I.M. three times weekly; or 200 to 400 mg (enanthate) I.M. q 2 to 4 weeks.
Postpartum breast pain and engorgement—
Adults: 25 to 50 mg I.M. of testosterone or testosterone propionate daily for 3 to 4 days.

ADVERSE REACTIONS
CNS: headache, anxiety, depression, paresthesia, sleep apnea syndrome.
GU: hypoestrogenic effects in women

(flushing; diaphoresis; vaginitis, including itching, drying, and burning; vaginal bleeding; menstrual irregularities); excessive hormonal effects in men (prepubertal—premature epiphyseal closure, *acne,* priapism, *growth of body and facial hair,* phallic enlargement; postpubertal—testicular atrophy, oligospermia, decreased ejaculatory volume, impotence, gynecomastia, epididymitis).
Hepatic: reversible jaundice, cholestatic hepatitis, abnormal liver enzyme levels.
Skin: pain, induration (at injection site); local edema.
Other: edema, nausea, hypercalcemia; polycythemia; hypersensitivity skin manifestations; suppression of clotting factors; androgenic effects in women.

INTERACTIONS
Drug-drug. *Hepatotoxic medications:* increased risk of hepatotoxicity. Monitor closely.
Insulin, oral antidiabetic agents: decreased serum glucose; altered dosage requirements. Monitor blood glucose levels in diabetic patients.
Oral anticoagulants: increased sensitivity; altered dosage requirements. Monitor PT and INR.

EFFECTS ON DIAGNOSTIC TESTS
Testosterone may cause abnormal results of glucose tolerance tests. Thyroid function test results and serum 17-ketosteroid levels may decrease. Liver function test results, PT, INR, and serum creatinine levels may be elevated. Increased serum sodium, potassium, calcium, phosphate, and cholesterol levels may occur.

CONTRAINDICATIONS
Contraindicated in male patients with breast or known or suspected prostate cancer; in patients with hypercalcemia; in those with cardiac, hepatic, or renal decompensation; and in pregnant or breast-feeding patients.

NURSING CONSIDERATIONS
• Use cautiously in elderly patients.
• Avoid use in women of childbearing age until pregnancy is ruled out.
• Store I.M. preparations at room temper-

ature. If crystals appear, warm and shake the bottle to disperse them.
• Inject deep into upper outer quadrant of gluteal muscle. Rotate injection sites. Report soreness at site.
• Unless contraindicated, administer with diet high in calories and protein. Provide small, frequent feedings to help avoid nausea.
• Monitor patient's liver function test results.
• Be aware that in patients with metastatic breast cancer, hypercalcemia usually indicates progression of bone metastases. Report signs and symptoms of hypercalcemia.
• Report signs of virilization in women.
• Monitor patient's weight and blood pressure routinely.
• Monitor prepubertal boys by X-ray for rate of bone maturation.
Alert: Therapeutic response in breast cancer is usually apparent within 3 months. Know that therapy should be stopped if disease progresses.
• Know that androgens may alter results of laboratory studies during therapy and for 2 to 3 weeks after therapy ends.

☑ Patient teaching
• Make sure patient understands importance of using an effective nonhormonal contraceptive during therapy.
• Review signs and symptoms of virilization with female patient and instruct her to notify doctor if they occur.
• Advise female patient to wash after intercourse to decrease risk of vaginitis. Instruct her to wear cotton underwear.
• Instruct male patient to report priapism, reduced ejaculatory volume, and gynecomastia. Notify doctor if these occur.
• Teach patient how to recognize signs and symptoms of hypoglycemia. Instruct him to report these immediately if they occur.
• Warn diabetic patients to be alert for signs and symptoms of hypoglycemia; report them to the doctor.
• Alert patient to report sudden weight gain.

testosterone transdermal system
Androderm, Testoderm

Controlled Substance Schedule III
Pregnancy Risk Category: X

HOW SUPPLIED
Transdermal system: 2.5 mg/day, 4 mg/day, 5 mg/day, 6 mg/day

ACTION
Releases testosterone, which stimulates target tissues to develop normally in androgen-deficient men.

Route	Onset	Peak	Duration
Transdermal	Unknown	2-4 hr	2 hr

INDICATIONS & DOSAGE
Primary or hypogonadotropic hypogonadism in men—
Adults: *Testoderm*—one 6-mg/day patch applied to scrotal area daily. If scrotal area is too small for 6-mg/day patch, therapy started with 4 mg/day patch. Patch worn for 22 to 24 hours daily.
Androderm—two systems applied h.s. for a total dose of 5 mg/day. Apply to clean, dry skin on back, abdomen, upper arms, or thigh.

ADVERSE REACTIONS
CNS: *CVA,* headache, depression.
GU: gynecomastia, prostatitis, prostate abnormalities, urinary tract infection, breast tenderness.
Skin: acne irritation, *blister under system,* allergic contact dermatitis; burning, induration (at injection site).
Other: *pruritus,* GI bleeding.

INTERACTIONS
Drug-drug. *Insulin:* altered insulin dosage requirements. Monitor blood glucose levels.
Oral anticoagulants: altered anticoagulant dosage requirements. Monitor PT and INR.
Oxyphenbutazone: may increase oxyphenbutazone levels. Monitor patient.

EFFECTS ON DIAGNOSTIC TESTS
Androgens may decrease levels of thyroxine-binding globulin, resulting in decreased total T_4 serum levels and increased resin uptake of T_3 and T_4.

CONTRAINDICATIONS
Contraindicated in patients hypersensitive to drug, in women, and in men with known or suspected breast or known or suspected prostate cancer.

NURSING CONSIDERATIONS
• Use cautiously in elderly men. Use cautiously in patients with preexisting renal, hepatic, or cardiac disease.
• Periodically assess liver function tests, serum lipid profiles, hemoglobin and hematocrit (with chronic use), prostatic acid phosphatase and prostate-specific antigen levels, as ordered.

☑ **Patient teaching**
• Teach patient how to apply transdermal system. Warn him that adequate serum levels will *not* be attained if the Testoderm patch is not applied to genital skin. Tell patient using Androderm that patch is *not* to be applied to scrotum. Application site should be rotated with an interval of 7 days between applications to the same site. Avoid bony prominences.
• Warn diabetic patient that testosterone may decrease serum glucose levels and that he should be alert for signs and symptoms of hypoglycemia.
• Tell male patient that topical testosterone has caused virilization in female partners, who should report acne or changes in body hair distribution.
• Advise patient to report persistent erections, nausea, vomiting, changes in skin color, ankle edema, or sudden weight gain to the doctor.
• Tell patient that Androderm does not have to be removed during sexual intercourse or while showering.

Reactions may be *common,* uncommon, *life-threatening,* or COMMON AND LIFE-THREATENING.

55

Estrogens and progestins

chlorotrianisene
diethylstilbestrol
diethylstilbestrol diphosphate
esterified estrogens
estradiol
estradiol cypionate
estradiol/norethindrone acetate
   transdermal system
estradiol valerate
estrogens, conjugated
estropipate
ethinyl estradiol
ethinyl estradiol and desogestrel
ethinyl estradiol and ethynodiol
   diacetate
ethinyl estradiol and
   levonorgestrel
ethinyl estradiol and
   norethindrone
ethinyl estradiol and
   norethindrone acetate
ethinyl estradiol and norgestimate
ethinyl estradiol and norgestrel
ethinyl estradiol, norethindrone
   acetate, and ferrous fumarate
levonorgestrel
medroxyprogesterone acetate
mestranol and norethindrone
norethindrone
norethindrone acetate
norgestrel
progesterone

COMBINATION PRODUCTS

ESTRATEST: esterified estrogens 125 mg and methyltestosterone 1.25 mg.
PMB 200: conjugated estrogens 0.45 mg and meprobamate 200 mg.
PMB 400: conjugated estrogens 0.45 mg and meprobamate 400 mg.
PREMPHASE: conjugated estrogens 0.625 mg and conjugated estrogens 0.625 mg/medroxyprogesterone acetate 5 mg.
PREMPRO 0.625 mg/2.5 mg: conjugated estrogens 0.625 mg/medroxyprogesterone acetate 2.5 mg.
PREMPRO 0.625 mg/5 mg: conjugated estrogens 0.625 mg/medroxyprogesterone acetate 5 mg.

chlorotrianisene
Tace**

Pregnancy Risk Category: X

HOW SUPPLIED
Capsules: 12 mg, 25 mg

ACTION
Increases the synthesis of DNA, RNA, and protein in responsive tissues and reduces release of follicle-stimulating hormone and luteinizing hormone from the pituitary gland.

Route	Onset	Peak	Duration
PO	Unknown	Unknown	24 hr

INDICATIONS & DOSAGE
Prostate cancer—
Adults: 12 to 25 mg P.O. daily.
Female hypogonadism—
Adults: 12 to 25 mg P.O. for 21 days, followed by one dose of progesterone 100 mg I.M. or 5 days of oral progestin concurrently with last 5 days of chlorotrianisene (for example, medroxyprogesterone 5 to 10 mg).
Vasomotor symptoms associated with menopausal symptoms, atrophic vaginitis, kraurosis vulvae—
Adults: 12 to 25 mg P.O. daily for 30 days or cyclic (3 weeks on, 1 week off).

ADVERSE REACTIONS
CNS: headache, dizziness, chorea, migraine, depression, *seizures.*
CV: thrombophlebitis; *thromboembolism;* hypertension; edema; *increased risk of CVA, pulmonary embolism, MI.*
EENT: worsening of myopia or astigmatism, intolerance of contact lenses.
GI: *nausea,* vomiting, abdominal cramps, bloating, colitis, acute pancreatitis, anorexia, increased appetite, excessive thirst, weight changes.
GU: breakthrough bleeding, altered menstrual flow, dysmenorrhea, *increased risk*

of endometrial cancer, possibility of increased risk of breast cancer, amenorrhea, cervical erosion or abnormal secretions, enlargement of uterine fibromas, vaginal candidiasis (in women); *gynecomastia, testicular atrophy, impotence* (in men).
Hepatic: cholestatic jaundice, *hepatic adenoma.*
Skin: melasma, urticaria, hirsutism or hair loss, erythema nodosum, dermatitis.
Other: breast changes (tenderness, enlargement, secretion), hypercalcemia.

INTERACTIONS
Drug-drug. *Carbamazepine, phenobarbital, rifampin:* decreased effectiveness of estrogen therapy. Monitor closely.
Corticosteroids: possible enhanced effects of corticosteroids. Monitor closely.
Cyclosporine: increased risk of toxicity. Use together with caution and frequently monitor cyclosporine levels.
Dantrolene, other hepatotoxic medications: increased risk of hepatotoxicity. Monitor closely.
Oral anticoagulants: effect of anticoagulant may be decreased. Dosage adjustments may be necessary. Monitor PT and INR, as ordered.
Tamoxifen: estrogens may interfere with effectiveness of tamoxifen. Avoid concomitant use.
Drug-food. *Caffeine:* may increase serum caffeine concentrations. Monitor effects.
Drug-lifestyle. *Smoking:* increased risk of adverse CV effects. If smoking continues, may need alternative therapy.

EFFECTS ON DIAGNOSTIC TESTS
In patients with diabetes, drug may increase blood glucose levels, necessitating dosage adjustment of insulin or oral hypoglycemic drugs. Drug has the potential to decrease the effects of warfarin-type anticoagulants.

CONTRAINDICATIONS
Contraindicated in patients with thrombophlebitis or thromboembolic disorders; breast, reproductive organ, or genital cancer; undiagnosed abnormal genital bleeding; and during pregnancy.

NURSING CONSIDERATIONS
● Use cautiously in patients with cerebrovascular or coronary artery disease; asthma; bone disease; migraine; seizures; cardiac, hepatic, or renal dysfunction; hypercalcemia from metastatic breast disease; and family history (mother, grandmother, sister) of breast or genital tract cancer, or who have breast nodules, fibrocystic breasts, or abnormal mammographic findings.
● Ensure that patient has a thorough physical examination before initiating estrogen therapy. Periodically monitor blood pressure, hepatic function, and serum lipid levels.
● Monitor weight regularly and recommend sodium restriction, as needed. May cause fluid retention and edema.
● Notify pathologist about patient receiving estrogen therapy when specimens are obtained and sent to pathology for evaluation.
● Because of risk of thromboembolism, know that therapy should be stopped at least 1 month before procedures associated with prolonged immobilization or thromboembolism, such as knee or hip surgery.

☑ **Patient teaching**
● Tell patient that package insert describing estrogen's adverse effects is available; also explain effects.
Alert: Warn patient to report immediately suspected pregnancy; abdominal pain; pain, numbness, or stiffness in legs or buttocks; pressure or pain in chest; shortness of breath; severe headaches; visual disturbances, such as blind spots, flashing lights, or blurriness; vaginal bleeding or discharge; breast lumps; swelling of hands or feet; yellow skin and sclera; dark urine; and light-colored stools.
● Explain to patient on cyclic therapy for postmenopausal symptoms that, although withdrawal bleeding may occur during week off drug, fertility is not restored. Pregnancy cannot occur because patient does not ovulate.
● Teach female patient how to perform routine breast self-examination.
● Tell diabetic patient to report elevated

blood glucose test results so that antidiabetic medication dosage can be adjusted.
• Emphasize importance of regular physical examinations. Studies suggest that postmenopausal women who use estrogen replacement for more than 5 years to treat menopausal symptoms may be at increased risk for endometrial cancer. This risk is reduced by using cyclic rather than continuous therapy and the lowest possible dosages of estrogen. Adding progestins to the regimen decreases the incidence of endometrial hyperplasia; however, it isn't known if progestins affect the incidence of endometrial cancer. Most studies show no increased risk of breast cancer.
• Teach patient how to reduce risk of thromboembolism.

---

diethylstilbestrol (stilboestrol)
DES

diethylstilbestrol diphosphate
DES, Honvol†, Stilphostrol

Pregnancy Risk Category: X

HOW SUPPLIED
diethylstilbestrol
Tablets: 1 mg, 5 mg
diethylstilbestrol diphosphate
Tablets: 50 mg, 83 mg†
Injection: 50 mg/ml

ACTION
Increases the synthesis of DNA, RNA, and protein in responsive tissues. Also reduces release of follicle-stimulating hormone and luteinizing hormone from the pituitary gland.

Route	Onset	Peak	Duration
PO, IV	Unknown	Unknown	Unknown

INDICATIONS & DOSAGE
Prostate cancer—
Men: initially, 1 to 3 mg P.O. daily; may be reduced to 1 mg daily, or 50 mg P.O. diphosphate t.i.d. Then increased up to 200 mg or more p.r.n. t.i.d. or 0.5 g I.V., followed by 1 g daily for 5 or more days

p.r.n. Maintenance dosage is 0.25 to 0.5 g I.V. once or twice weekly.
Metastatic, advanced breast cancer—
Men and postmenopausal women:
15 mg P.O. daily.

ADVERSE REACTIONS
CNS: headache, dizziness, chorea, depression, *seizures.*
CV: thrombophlebitis, *thromboembolism,* hypertension, *edema, increased risk of CVA, pulmonary embolism, MI.*
EENT: worsening of myopia or astigmatism, intolerance of contact lenses.
GI: *nausea,* vomiting, abdominal cramps, bloating, anorexia, increased appetite, excessive thirst, weight changes, pancreatitis.
GU: breakthrough bleeding, altered menstrual flow, dysmenorrhea, amenorrhea, cervical erosion, *increased risk of endometrial cancer, possibility of increased risk of breast cancer,* altered cervical secretions, enlargement of uterine fibromas, vaginal candidiasis, loss of libido (in women); gynecomastia, testicular atrophy, impotence (in men).
Hepatic: cholestatic jaundice, *hepatic adenoma.*
Skin: melasma, urticaria, hirsutism or hair loss, erythema nodosum, dermatitis.
Other: *breast tenderness or enlargement,* hypercalcemia, gallbladder disease.

INTERACTIONS
Drug-drug. *Carbamazepine, phenobarbital, rifampin:* decreased effectiveness of estrogen therapy. Monitor closely.
Corticosteroids: possible enhanced effects of corticosteroids. Monitor closely.
Cyclosporine: increased risk of toxicity. Use together with caution and frequently monitor cyclosporine levels.
Dantrolene, other hepatotoxic medications: increased risk of hepatotoxicity. Monitor closely.
Oral anticoagulants: effect of anticoagulant may be decreased. Dosage adjustments may be necessary. Monitor PT and INR, as ordered.
Tamoxifen: estrogens may interfere with effectiveness of tamoxifen. Avoid concomitant use.

---

*Liquid contains alcohol.   **May contain tartrazine.   †Canada   ‡Australia   §U.K.   ◇OTC

Drug-food. *Caffeine:* may increase serum caffeine concentrations. Monitor effects.
Drug-lifestyle. *Smoking:* increased risk of adverse CV effects. If smoking continues, may need alternative therapy.

EFFECTS ON DIAGNOSTIC TESTS

Drug may cause increases in blood glucose levels, necessitating dosage adjustment of insulin or oral hypoglycemic drugs. It increases sulfobromophthalein retention, prothrombin and clotting factors VII to X, and norepinephrine-induced platelet aggregation. Increases in thyroid-binding globulin concentrations may occur, resulting in increased total thyroid concentrations (measured by protein-bound iodine or total T_4) and decreased uptake of free T_3 resin. Antithrombin III concentrations decrease; serum folate and pyridoxine concentrations and pregnanediol excretion may decrease; triglyceride, glucose, and phospholipid levels may increase. Glucose tolerance may be impaired. Reduced response to metyrapone test.

CONTRAINDICATIONS

Contraindicated in patients with known or suspected breast cancer, except in selected patients being treated for metastatic disease; in patients with active thrombophlebitis or thromboembolic disorders, estrogen-dependent neoplasia, undiagnosed abnormal genital bleeding, during pregnancy, and history of thrombophlebitis, thrombosis, or thromboembolic disorders associated with estrogen use.

NURSING CONSIDERATIONS

• Use cautiously in patients with hypertension, mental depression, bone disease, migraine, seizures, diabetes mellitus, cardiac, hepatic, or renal dysfunction, and cerebrovascular or coronary artery disease.
• Know that diabetic patients may require increased dose of insulin. Monitor carefully.
• Ensure that patient has a physical examination before initiating therapy. Patients receiving long-term therapy should be examined annually. Monitor weight, blood pressure, hepatic function, and serum lipid levels.

Alert: Know that a high incidence of gross nonmalignant genital changes may occur in offspring of women taking drug during pregnancy. Female offspring have a higher than normal risk of developing cervical and vaginal adenocarcinoma. Male offspring may have a higher than normal risk of developing testicular tumors, epididymal cysts, and impaired fertility.
• If patient experiences GI upset, give drug with or immediately after meals.
• Notify pathologist about patient receiving estrogen therapy when specimens are obtained and sent to pathology for evaluation.
• Know that increased number of CV deaths reported in men taking diethylstilbestrol tablet (5 mg daily) for prostate cancer for a long time. This effect is not associated with 1-mg daily dose.
• Because of risk of thromboembolism, know that therapy should be discontinued at least 1 month before procedures associated with prolonged immobilization or thromboembolism, such as knee or hip surgery.

⬛ I.V. administration

• Mix ordered dose in 250 to 500 ml of D_5W or 0.9% NaCl. Infuse at 1 to 2 ml/minute for first 15 minutes; if no adverse reactions occur, increase infusion rate to administer entire dose within 1 hour.

☑ Patient teaching

• Tell patient that package insert describing estrogen's adverse effects is available; however, also give patient verbal explanation.
• Teach patient methods of decreasing risk of thromboembolism.
• Tell patient not to crush, break, or chew enteric-coated tablets. Instruct patient to take with food if stomach upset occurs.
Alert: Warn patient to immediately report abdominal pain; pain, numbness, or stiffness in legs or buttocks; pressure or pain in chest; shortness of breath; severe headache; visual disturbances, such as blind spots, flashing lights, or blurriness; vaginal bleeding or discharge; breast lumps; sudden weight gain; swelling of

hands or feet; yellow sclera or skin; dark urine; and light-colored stools.
• Teach female patient how to perform routine breast self-examination.
• Tell diabetic patient to report elevated blood glucose test results so that antidiabetic medication dosage can be adjusted.
• Advise patient of childbearing age of risks of using DES during pregnancy.

esterified estrogens
Estratab, Menest, Neo-Estrone†

Pregnancy Risk Category: X

HOW SUPPLIED
Tablets: 0.3 mg, 0.625 mg, 1.25 mg, 2.5 mg
Tablets (film-coated): 0.3 mg, 0.625 mg, 1.25 mg, 2.5 mg

ACTION
Increases the synthesis of DNA, RNA, and protein in responsive tissues. Also reduces release of follicle-stimulating hormone and luteinizing hormone from the pituitary gland.

Route	Onset	Peak	Duration
PO	Unknown	Unknown	Unknown

INDICATIONS & DOSAGE
Inoperable prostate cancer—
Men: 1.25 to 2.5 mg P.O. t.i.d.
Breast cancer—
Men and postmenopausal women: 10 mg P.O. t.i.d. for 3 or more months.
Female hypogonadism—
Women: 2.5 to 7.5 mg daily in divided doses in cycles of 20 days on, 10 days off.
Castration, primary ovarian failure—
Women: 1.25 mg daily in cycles of 3 weeks on, 1 week off. Adjust for symptoms. Can be given continuously.
Vasomotor menopausal symptoms—
Women: average dosage is 1.25 mg P.O. daily in cycles of 3 weeks on, 1 week off.
Atrophic vaginitis and atrophic urethritis—
Women: 0.3 to 1.25 mg or more P.O. daily in cycles of 3 weeks on, 1 week off.

✷ *NEW INDICATION: Prevention of osteoporosis (Estratab, Neo-Estrone†)—*
Adults: initially, 0.3 mg P.O. daily; may be increased to maximum daily dose of 1.25 mg.

ADVERSE REACTIONS
CNS: headache, dizziness, chorea, depression, *seizures.*
CV: thrombophlebitis; *thromboembolism;* hypertension; *edema; increased risk of CVA, pulmonary embolism, MI.*
EENT: worsening of myopia or astigmatism, intolerance of contact lenses.
GI: *nausea,* vomiting, abdominal cramps, bloating, anorexia, increased appetite, weight changes, pancreatitis, increased risk of gallbladder disease.
GU: breakthrough bleeding, altered menstrual flow, dysmenorrhea, amenorrhea, *increased risk of endometrial cancer, possibility of increased risk of breast cancer,* cervical erosion, altered cervical secretions, enlargement of uterine fibromas, vaginal candidiasis (in women); gynecomastia, testicular atrophy, impotence (in men).
Hepatic: cholestatic jaundice, *hepatic adenoma.*
Skin: melasma, rash, hirsutism or hair loss, erythema nodosum, dermatitis.
Other: *breast changes (tenderness, enlargement, secretion),* gallbladder disease, hypercalcemia.

INTERACTIONS
Drug-drug. *Carbamazepine, phenobarbital, rifampin:* decreased effectiveness of estrogen therapy. Monitor closely.
Corticosteroids: possible enhanced effects. Monitor closely.
Cyclosporine: increased risk of toxicity. Use together with caution and frequently monitor cyclosporine levels.
Dantrolene, other hepatotoxic medications: increased risk of hepatotoxicity. Monitor closely.
Oral anticoagulants: effect of anticoagulant may be decreased. Dosage adjustments may be necessary. Monitor PT and INR, as ordered.
Tamoxifen: estrogens may interfere with effectiveness of tamoxifen. Avoid concomitant use.

---

*Liquid contains alcohol. **May contain tartrazine. †Canada ‡Australia §U.K. ◇OTC

Drug-food. *Caffeine:* may increase serum caffeine concentrations. Monitor effects.
Drug-lifestyle. *Smoking:* increased risk of adverse CV effects. If smoking continues, may need alternative therapy.

EFFECTS ON DIAGNOSTIC TESTS
Drug therapy increases sulfobromophthalein retention, PT and clotting factors VII to X, and norepinephrine-induced platelet aggregation. Increases in the thyroid-binding globulin concentration may occur, resulting in increased total thyroid concentrations (measured by protein-bound iodine or total T_4) and decreased uptake of free T_3 resin. Serum folate, pyridoxine, and antithrombin III concentrations may decrease; triglyceride, glucose, and phospholipid levels may increase. Glucose tolerance may be impaired. Pregnanediol excretion may decrease. Reduced response to metyrapone test.

CONTRAINDICATIONS
Contraindicated in patients with breast cancer (except metastatic disease), estrogen-dependent neoplasia, active thrombophlebitis or thromboembolic disorders, undiagnosed abnormal genital bleeding, hypersensitivity to drug, history of thromboembolic disease, or during pregnancy.

NURSING CONSIDERATIONS
• Use cautiously in patients with history of hypertension, mental depression, cardiac or renal dysfunction, liver impairment, or bone diseases, migraine, seizures, or diabetes mellitus.
• When used for vasomotor symptoms in menstruating women, cyclic administration is started on day 5 of bleeding.
• Ensure that patient has a thorough physical examination before initiating estrogen therapy. Patients receiving long-term therapy should have repeat examinations yearly. Periodically monitor body weight, blood pressure, serum lipid levels, and hepatic function.
• Notify pathologist of patient receiving estrogen therapy when specimens are obtained and sent to pathology for evaluation.
• Because of risk of thromboembolism, know that therapy should be discontinued at least 1 month before procedures associated with prolonged immobilization or thromboembolism, such as knee or hip surgery.

☑ **Patient teaching**
• Tell patient that package insert describing estrogen's adverse effects is available; however, also give patient verbal explanation.
• Emphasize importance of regular physical examinations. Studies suggest that postmenopausal women who use estrogen replacement for over 5 years to treat menopausal symptoms may be at increased risk for endometrial cancer. This risk is reduced by using cyclic rather than continuous therapy and the lowest possible dosages of estrogen. Adding progestins to the regimen decreases the incidence of endometrial hyperplasia; however, it isn't known if progestins affect the incidence of endometrial cancer. Most studies show no increased risk of breast cancer.
Alert: Warn patient to immediately report abdominal pain; pain, numbness, or stiffness in legs or buttocks; pressure or pain in chest; shortness of breath; severe headaches; visual disturbances, such as blind spots, flashing lights, or blurriness; vaginal bleeding or discharge; breast lumps; swelling of hands or feet; yellow skin or sclera; dark urine; and light-colored stools.
• Tell diabetic patient to report elevated blood glucose test results so that antidiabetic medication dosage can be adjusted.
• Explain to patient on cyclic therapy for postmenopausal symptoms that, although she may experience withdrawal bleeding during week off drug, fertility is not restored. Pregnancy cannot occur because patient does not ovulate.
• Teach female patient to perform routine breast self-examination.
• Advise patient of childbearing age to consult doctor before taking this drug, and to advise doctor immediately if pregnancy occurs.
• Teach patient methods to decrease risk of thromboembolism.

Reactions may be *common*, uncommon, *life-threatening*, or COMMON AND LIFE-THREATENING.

estradiol (oestradiol)
Climara, Estrace**, Estrace
Vaginal Cream, Estraderm,
FemSeven§, Menorest§,
Ovestin§, Vivelle, Zumenon§

estradiol cypionate
depGynogen, Depo-Estradiol,
Depogen, Dura-Estrin,
E-Cypionate, Estragyn LA 5,
Estro-Cyp, Estrofem, Estroject-LA

estradiol valerate
(oestradiol valerate)
Clinagen LA 40, Deladiol 40,
Delestrogen, Dioval 40, Dioval XX,
Duragen-20, Duragen-40,
Estra-L 40, Estro-Span, Femogex,
Gynogen L.A., Menaval, Primogyn
Depot‡, Progynova§, Valergen-10,
Valergen-20, Valergen-40

Pregnancy Risk Category: X

HOW SUPPLIED
estradiol
Tablets (micronized): 0.5 mg, 1 mg, 2 mg
Transdermal: 0.0375 mg/24 hours,
0.05 mg/24 hours; 0.075 mg/24 hours;
0.1 mg/24 hours; 4 mg/10 cm² (delivers
0.05 mg/24 hours); 8 mg/20 cm² (delivers
0.1 mg/24 hours)
Vaginal cream (in nonliquefying base):
0.1 mg/g
estradiol cypionate
Injection (in oil): 1 mg/ml, 5 mg/ml
estradiol valerate
Injection (in oil): 10 mg/ml, 20 mg/ml,
40 mg/ml

ACTION
Increases the synthesis of DNA, RNA,
and protein in responsive tissues. Also reduces release of follicle-stimulating hormone and luteinizing hormone from the
pituitary gland.

Route	Onset	Peak	Duration
PO, IM, transdermal, intravaginal	Unknown	Unknown	Unknown

INDICATIONS & DOSAGE
*Vasomotor menopausal symptoms, female
hypogonadism, female castration, primary
ovarian failure—*
Adults: 0.5 to 2 mg P.O. (estradiol) daily
in cycles of 21 days on and 7 days off; or
cycles of 5 days on and 2 days off; or one
transdermal system (Estraderm) delivering 0.05 mg/24 hours applied twice weekly; or as a system (Vivelle) delivering either 0.05 mg/24 hours or 0.0375 mg/24
hours applied twice weekly; or as a system (Climara) delivering either 0.05 mg
24 hours or 0.1 mg/24 hours and applied
once weekly, in cycles of 3 weeks on and
1 week off.
  Note: Transdermal systems are sometimes used on a continuous basis (not
cyclic). Alternatively, 1 to 5 mg (cypionate) I.M. q 3 to 4 weeks or 10 to 20 mg
(valerate) I.M. q 4 weeks, p.r.n.
Atrophic vaginitis, kraurosis vulvae—
Adults: 0.05 mg/24 hours (Estraderm)
applied twice weekly in a cyclic regimen;
or 0.05 mg/24 hours (Climara) applied
weekly in a cyclic regimen; or 2 to 4 g intravaginal applications of cream daily for
1 to 2 weeks. When vaginal mucosa is restored, maintenance dosage is 1 g one to
three times weekly in a cyclic regimen.
Alternatively, 10 to 20 mg (valerate) I.M.
q 4 weeks, p.r.n.
*Palliative treatment of advanced, inopera-
ble breast cancer—*
Men and postmenopausal women:
10 mg P.O. (estradiol) t.i.d. for 3 months.
*Palliative treatment of advanced inopera-
ble prostate cancer—*
Men: 30 mg (valerate) I.M. q 1 to 2
weeks, or 1 to 2 mg P.O. (estradiol) t.i.d.

ADVERSE REACTIONS
CNS: headache, dizziness, chorea, depression, *seizures.*
CV: thrombophlebitis, *thromboembolism,* hypertension, *edema, increased
risk of CVA, pulmonary embolism and
MI.*
EENT: worsening of myopia or astigmatism, intolerance of contact lenses.
GI: *nausea,* vomiting, abdominal cramps,
bloating, increased appetite, weight
changes, pancreatitis, anorexia.
GU: breakthrough bleeding, altered men-

---

strual flow, dysmenorrhea, amenorrhea, *increased risk of endometrial cancer, possibility of increased risk of breast cancer,* cervical erosion, altered cervical secretions, enlargement of uterine fibromas, vaginal candidiasis (in women); gynecomastia, testicular atrophy, impotence (in men).
Hepatic: cholestatic jaundice, *hepatic adenoma.*
Skin: melasma, urticaria, erythema nodosum, dermatitis, hair loss.
Other: *breast changes (tenderness, enlargement, secretion),* gallbladder disease, hypercalcemia.

INTERACTIONS
Drug-drug. *Carbamazepine, phenobarbital, rifampin:* decreased effectiveness of estrogen therapy. Monitor closely.
Corticosteroids: possible enhanced effects of corticosteroids. Monitor closely.
Cyclosporine: increased risk of toxicity. Use together with caution and monitor cyclosporine levels frequently.
Dantrolene, other hepatotoxic medications: increased risk of hepatotoxicity. Monitor closely.
Oral anticoagulants: effect of anticoagulant may be decreased. Dosage adjustments may be necessary. Monitor PT and INR, as ordered.
Tamoxifen: estrogens may interfere with effectiveness of tamoxifen. Avoid concomitant use.
Drug-food. *Caffeine:* may increase serum caffeine concentrations. Monitor effects.
Drug-lifestyle. *Smoking:* increased risk of adverse CV effects. If smoking continues, may need alternative therapy.

EFFECTS ON DIAGNOSTIC TESTS
Estradiol increases sulfobromophthalein retention, PT and clotting factors VII to X, and norepinephrine-induced platelet aggregation. Increases in thyroid-binding globulin concentrations may occur, resulting in increased total thyroid concentrations (measured by protein-bound iodine or total T_4) and decreased uptake of free T_3 resin. Serum folate, pyridoxine, and antithrombin III concentrations may decrease; triglyceride, glucose, and phospholipid levels may increase. Glucose tol-

erance may be impaired. Pregnanediol excretion may decrease. Reduced response to metyrapone test.

CONTRAINDICATIONS
Contraindicated in patients with thrombophlebitis or thromboembolic disorders, estrogen-dependent neoplasia, breast or reproductive organ cancer (except for palliative treatment), or undiagnosed abnormal genital bleeding and during pregnancy. Also contraindicated in patients with history of thrombophlebitis or thromboembolic disorders associated with previous estrogen use (except for palliative treatment of breast and prostate cancer).

NURSING CONSIDERATIONS
• Use cautiously in patients with cerebrovascular or coronary artery disease; asthma; bone diseases; migraine; seizures; cardiac, hepatic, or renal dysfunction; or in women with a strong family history of breast cancer or who have breast nodules, fibrocystic breasts, or abnormal mammographic findings.
• Ensure that patient has a physical examination before initiating therapy. Patients receiving long-term therapy should be examined yearly. Monitor serum lipid levels, blood pressure, body weight, and hepatic function as ordered.
• Ask patient about allergies, especially to foods or plants. Estradiol is available as an aqueous solution or as a solution in peanut oil; estradiol cypionate, as a solution in cottonseed oil; estradiol valerate, as a solution in castor oil or sesame oil.
• To administer as an I.M. injection, make sure drug is well dispersed in solution by rolling vial between palms. Inject deep I.M. into large muscle. Rotate injection sites to prevent muscle atrophy. Never give drug I.V.
• Apply transdermal patch to clean, dry, hairless, intact skin on abdomen or buttocks. Do not apply it to breasts, waistline, or other areas where clothing can loosen the patch. When applying, ensure good contact with the skin, especially around the edges, and hold in place with the palm for about 10 seconds. Rotate application sites.
• Know that in women who are currently

taking oral estrogen, treatment with the Estraderm transdermal patch can begin 1 week after withdrawal of oral therapy or sooner if menopausal symptoms appear before the end of the week.

• Because of risk of thromboembolism, know that therapy should be discontinued at least 1 month before procedures associated with prolonged immobilization or thromboembolism, such as knee or hip surgery.

• Notify pathologist of patient receiving estrogen therapy when specimens are obtained and sent to pathology for evaluation.

☑ **Patient teaching**
• Tell patient that package insert describing estrogen's adverse effects is available; however, also give patient verbal explanation.

• Emphasize importance of regular physical examinations. Postmenopausal women who use estrogen replacement for over 5 years may be at increased risk for endometrial cancer. This risk is reduced by using cyclic rather than continuous therapy and the lowest possible dosages of estrogen. Adding progestins to the regimen decreases the incidence of endometrial hyperplasia; however, it isn't known if progestins affect the incidence of endometrial cancer. Most studies show no increased risk of breast cancer.

• Tell patient how to use cream. Patient should wash vaginal area with soap and water before applying and take drug at bedtime or lie flat for 30 minutes after instillation to minimize drug loss.

• Tell patient how to use transdermal. Rotate sites and do not apply to breasts or waist area.

Alert: Warn patient to immediately report abdominal pain; pain, numbness, or stiffness in legs or buttocks; pressure or pain in chest; shortness of breath; severe headaches; visual disturbances; vaginal bleeding or discharge; breast lumps; swelling of hands or feet; yellow skin or sclera; dark urine; and light-colored stools.

• Explain to patient on cyclic therapy that, although postmenopausal symptoms may occur during week off drug, fertility is not restored.

Pregnancy cannot occur because patient does not ovulate.

• Tell diabetic patient to report elevated blood glucose test results so that antidiabetic medication dosage can be adjusted.

• Teach female patient how to perform routine breast self-examination.

• Teach patient methods to decrease risk of thromboembolism.

• Advise patient not to become pregnant while on estrogen therapy.

▼ *NEW DRUG*

estradiol/norethindrone acetate transdermal system
CombiPatch

Pregnancy Risk Category: X

HOW SUPPLIED
Transdermal: 9 cm^2 system releasing 0.05 mg estradiol and 0.14 mg norethindrone acetate per day; 16 cm^2 system releasing 0.05 mg estradiol and 0.25 mg norethindrone acetate per day

ACTION
A matrix transdermal system, in which the estradiol and norethindrone are released continuously. Estrogen replacement therapy can reduce the frequency of menopausal symptoms and the release of follicle-stimulating hormone and luteinizing hormone from the pituitary gland in postmenopausal women.

Route	Onset	Peak	Duration
Transdermal	12-24 hr	Unknown	3-4 days

INDICATIONS & DOSAGE
Moderate-to-severe vasomotor symptoms associated with menopause, vulvar and vaginal atrophy, and hypoestrogenemia due to hypogonadism, castration, or primary ovarian failure in women with an intact uterus—
Adults: *Continuous combined regimen—* 9 cm^2 patch worn continuously on the lower abdomen. Old system should be removed and new system applied twice weekly during a 28-day cycle. May increase to 16 cm^2 patch.
*Continuous sequential regimen—*patch

can be applied as a sequential regimen in combination with an estradiol transdermal system (such as Alora, Esclim, Estraderm, Vivelle). A 0.05-mg estradiol transdermal patch is worn for first 14 days of a 28-day cycle; replace system twice weekly. For rest of 28-day cycle, the 9 cm^2 patch system should be worn on the lower abdomen. May increase to 16 cm^2 patch, p.r.n.

Women not currently receiving continuous estrogen or estrogen/progestin therapy may start therapy at any time.

Women currently receiving continuous hormone replacement therapy should complete the current cycle of therapy before initiating therapy. Women often experience withdrawal bleeding at the completion of the cycle; first day of withdrawal bleeding would be an appropriate time to initiate therapy.

ADVERSE REACTIONS
CNS: *asthenia*, depression, insomnia, nervousness, dizziness, *headache.*
EENT: tooth disorder, pharyngitis, *rhinitis, sinusitis.*
GI: *abdominal pain, diarrhea*, dyspepsia, flatulence, *nausea*, constipation.
GU: *dysmenorrhea, leukorrhea, menstrual disorder*, suspicious Papanicolaou smears, *vaginitis*, menorrhagia, vaginal hemorrhage.
Musculoskeletal: arthralgia, *back pain.*
Respiratory: *respiratory disorder*, bronchitis.
Skin: application site reactions, acne.
Other: *accidental injury, flu syndrome, pain, breast pain*, peripheral edema, breast enlargement, infection.

INTERACTIONS
None reported.

EFFECTS ON DIAGNOSTIC TESTS
Drug may cause a reduced response to the metyrapone test as well as reduced serum folate concentrations.

CONTRAINDICATIONS
Contraindicated in women who may be pregnant, have known or suspected breast cancer, known or suspected estrogen-dependent neoplasia, undiagnosed abnormal genital bleeding, active thrombophlebitis, thromboembolic disorders or stroke, or known hypersensitivity to estrogen, progestin, or any component of the patch.

NURSING CONSIDERATIONS
● Use cautiously in patients with impaired liver function, asthma, epilepsy, migraine, and cardiac or renal dysfunction. Also use cautiously in breast-feeding patients.
● Store norethindrone patches in refrigerator before dispensing. Patient may then store patches at room temperature for up to 3 months.
● Advise patient not to store patches where extreme temperatures can occur.
● Reevaluate therapy at 3- to 6-month intervals. Combination estrogen/progestin regimens are indicated for women with an intact uterus.
● Be aware that progestins taken with estrogen drugs significantly reduce, but do not eliminate, the risk of endometrial cancer associated with the use of estrogen.
● Know that blood pressure increases have been associated with estrogen use. Monitor patient's blood pressure regularly.
● Be aware that treatment of post-menopausal symptoms is usually initiated during menopausal stage when vasomotor symptoms occur.
● Apply patch system to a smooth (fold-free), clean, dry, nonirritated area of skin on the lower abdomen, avoiding the waistline. Application sites should be rotated, with an interval of at least 1 week between applications to the same site.
● Do not apply patch on or near the breasts.
● Avoid application to areas that may get prolonged sun exposure.
● Reapply system, if necessary, to another area of the lower abdomen. If the system fails to adhere, replace with a new one.
● Know that INR, activated partial thromboplastin time, and platelet aggregation times may be altered; platelet count and fibrinogen activity may increase. Increased thyroid-binding globulin may lead to increased T_4 and T_3 levels and decreased T_3 resin uptake. A decrease in serum total cholesterol, high-density lipoprotein cholesterol, low-density

---

Reactions may be *common*, uncommon, ***life-threatening***, or COMMON AND LIFE-THREATENING.

lipoprotein cholesterol, and triglyceride concentrations may also occur.

☑ **Patient teaching**
• Teach patient how to apply system properly. Only one system should be worn at any time during the dosing intervals.
• Tell patient an oil-based cream or lotion may help remove the adhesive from the skin once a system has been removed and the area allowed to dry for 15 minutes.
• Advise patient not to use patch if pregnancy occurs or is being planned.
• Instruct patient that, for the continuous combined regimen, irregular bleeding may occur, particularly in the first 6 months, but generally decreases with time, often to an amenorrheic state.
• Tell patient that, for the continuous sequential regimen, monthly withdrawal bleeding often occurs.
• Advise patient to alert doctor and discontinue patch at first sign of thrombotic disorders (thrombophlebitis, cerebrovascular disorders, and pulmonary embolism).
• Instruct patient to discontinue patch and call doctor if a partial or complete loss of vision, sudden onset of proptosis (a downward displacement of the eyeball), double vision, or migraine occurs.

---

estrogens, conjugated (estrogenic substances, conjugated; oestrogens, conjugated)
C.E.S.†, Premarin, Premarin Intravenous

Pregnancy Risk Category: X

HOW SUPPLIED
Tablets: 0.3 mg, 0.625 mg, 0.9 mg, 1.25 mg, 2.5 mg
Injection: 25 mg/5 ml
Vaginal cream: 0.625 mg/g

ACTION
Increases the synthesis of DNA, RNA, and protein in responsive tissues. Also reduces release of follicle-stimulating hor-

mone and luteinizing hormone from the pituitary gland.

Route	Onset	Peak	Duration
PO, IV, IM, intravaginal	Unknown	Unknown	Unknown

INDICATIONS & DOSAGE
Abnormal uterine bleeding (hormonal imbalance)—
Women: 25 mg I.V. or I.M., repeated in 6 to 12 hours p.r.n.
Palliative treatment of breast cancer (at least 5 years after menopause)—
Men and postmenopausal women: 10 mg P.O. t.i.d. for 3 months or more.
Female castration, primary ovarian failure—
Women: 1.25 mg P.O. daily in cycles of 3 weeks on and 1 week off. Can be given continuously.
Osteoporosis—
Postmenopausal women: 0.625 mg P.O. daily in cyclic regimen (3 weeks on, 1 week off). Can be given continuously.
Hypogonadism—
Women: 2.5 to 7.5 mg daily in divided doses for 20 days followed by 10 days off.
Vasomotor menopausal symptoms—
Women: 0.3 to 1.25 mg P.O. daily in cycles of 3 weeks on and 1 week off. Can be given continuously.
Atrophic vaginitis, kraurosis vulvae—
Women: 0.5 to 2 g intravaginally once daily on a cyclical basis (3 weeks on and 1 week off).
Palliative treatment of inoperable prostate cancer—
Men: 1.25 to 2.5 mg P.O. t.i.d.

ADVERSE REACTIONS
CNS: headache, dizziness, chorea, depression, *seizures.*
CV: thrombophlebitis; *thromboembolism;* hypertension; *edema; increased risk of CVA, pulmonary embolism, MI.*
EENT: worsening of myopia or astigmatism, intolerance of contact lenses.
GI: *nausea,* vomiting, abdominal cramps, bloating, anorexia, increased appetite, weight changes, pancreatitis.
GU: breakthrough bleeding, altered menstrual flow, dysmenorrhea, amenorrhea,

increased risk of endometrial cancer, possibility of increased risk of breast cancer, cervical erosion, altered cervical secretions, enlargement of uterine fibromas, vaginal candidiasis (in women); gynecomastia, testicular atrophy, impotence (in men).
Hepatic: cholestatic jaundice, *hepatic adenoma.*
Skin: melasma, urticaria, flushing (with rapid I.V. administration), hirsutism or hair loss, erythema nodosum, dermatitis.
Other: *breast changes (tenderness, enlargement, secretion),* hypercalcemia, gallbladder disease.

INTERACTIONS
Drug-drug. *Carbamazepine, phenobarbital, rifampin:* decreased effectiveness of estrogen therapy. Monitor closely.
Corticosteroids: possible enhanced effects of corticosteroids. Monitor closely.
Cyclosporine: increased risk of toxicity. Use together with caution and frequently monitor cyclosporine levels.
Dantrolene, other hepatotoxic medications: increased risk of hepatotoxicity. Monitor closely.
Oral anticoagulants: effect of anticoagulant may be decreased. Dosage adjustments may be necessary. Monitor PT and INR, as ordered.
Tamoxifen: estrogens may interfere with effectiveness of tamoxifen. Avoid concomitant use.
Drug-food. *Caffeine:* may increase serum caffeine concentrations. Monitor effects.
Drug-lifestyle. *Smoking:* increased risk of adverse CV effects. If smoking continues, may need alternative therapy.

EFFECTS ON DIAGNOSTIC TESTS
Therapy with estrogens increases sulfobromophthalein retention, PT and clotting factors VII to X, and norepinephrine-induced platelet aggregation. Increases in thyroid-binding globulin concentration may occur, resulting in increased total thyroid concentration (measured by protein-bound iodine or total T_4) and decreased uptake of free T_3 resin. Reduced response to metyrapone test. Serum folate, pyridoxine, and antithrombin III concentrations may decrease; triglyceride,

glucose, and phospholipid levels may increase. Glucose tolerance may be impaired. Pregnanediol excretion may decrease.

CONTRAINDICATIONS
Contraindicated in patients with thrombophlebitis or thromboembolic disorders, estrogen-dependent neoplasia, breast or reproductive cancer (except for palliative treatment), undiagnosed abnormal genital bleeding, and during pregnancy.

NURSING CONSIDERATIONS
• Use cautiously in patients with cerebrovascular or coronary artery disease; asthma; bone disease; migraine; seizures; cardiac, hepatic, or renal dysfunction; or in women with family history (mother, grandmother, sister) of breast or genital tract cancer or who have breast nodules, fibrocystic breasts, or abnormal mammographic findings.
• Ensure that patient has a thorough physical examination before initiating estrogen therapy. Patients receiving long-term therapy should have annual examinations. Periodically monitor serum lipid levels, blood pressure, body weight, and hepatic function, as ordered.
• Know that I.M. or I.V. use is preferred for rapid treatment of dysfunctional uterine bleeding or reduction of surgical bleeding.
• When administering by I.M. injection, inject deeply into large muscle. Rotate injection sites to prevent muscle atrophy.
• Notify pathologist of patient receiving estrogen therapy when specimens are obtained and sent to pathology for evaluation.
• Because of risk of thromboembolism, know that therapy should be discontinued at least 1 month before procedures associated with prolonged immobilization or thromboembolism, such as knee or hip surgery.

🔲 I.V. administration
• When giving by direct I.V. injection, administer slowly to avoid flushing reaction. I.V. solution is *not* compatible with protein hydrolysate, ascorbic acid or solutions with an acid pH. Mix only with nor-

mal saline, dextrose, or invert sugar solutions.
• Refrigerate before reconstituting. Agitate gently after adding diluent.

☑ **Patient teaching**
• Tell patient that package insert describing estrogen's adverse effects is available; also explain effects.
• Emphasize importance of regular physical examinations. Studies suggest that postmenopausal women who use estrogen replacement for over 5 years to treat menopausal symptoms may be at increased risk for endometrial cancer. This risk is reduced by using cyclic rather than continuous therapy and the lowest possible dosages of estrogen. Adding progestins to the regimen decreases the incidence of endometrial hyperplasia; however, it isn't known if progestins affect the incidence of endometrial cancer. Most studies show no increased risk of breast cancer.
• Teach patient how to use vaginal cream. Patient should wash the vaginal area with soap and water before applying. Tell her to use drug at bedtime or to lie flat for 30 minutes after instillation to minimize drug loss.
• Explain to patient on cyclic therapy for postmenopausal symptoms that, although withdrawal bleeding may occur during week off drug, fertility is not restored. Pregnancy cannot occur because patient does not ovulate.
Alert: Warn patient to immediately report abdominal pain; pain, numbness, or stiffness in legs or buttocks; pressure or pain in chest; shortness of breath; severe headaches; visual disturbances, such as blind spots, flashing lights, or blurriness; vaginal bleeding or discharge; breast lumps; swelling of hands or feet; yellow skin or sclera; dark urine; and light-colored stools.
• Tell diabetic patient to report elevated blood glucose test results so that antidiabetic medication dosage can be adjusted.
• Teach female patient how to perform routine breast self-examination.
• Tell patient not to become pregnant while on estrogen therapy.

estropipate (piperazine estrone sulfate)
Harmogen§, Ogen, Ortho-Est

Pregnancy Risk Category: X

HOW SUPPLIED
Tablets: 0.75 mg, 1.5 mg, 3 mg, 6 mg
Vaginal cream: 1.5 mg/g

ACTION
Increases the synthesis of DNA, RNA, and proteins in responsive tissues. Also reduces release of follicle-stimulating hormone and luteinizing hormone from the pituitary gland.

Route	Onset	Peak	Duration
PO, intra-vaginal	Unknown	Unknown	Unknown

INDICATIONS & DOSAGE
Vulval and vaginal atrophy—
Women: 0.75 to 6 mg P.O. daily 3 weeks on, 1 week off, or 2 to 4 g of vaginal cream daily. Typically, dosage given on a cyclical, short-term basis. Can be given continuously.
Primary ovarian failure, female castration, female hypogonadism—
Women: administered on a cyclical basis—1.5 to 9 mg P.O. daily for the first 3 weeks, followed by a rest period of 8 to 10 days. If bleeding does not occur by the end of the rest period, cycle repeated. Can be given continuously.
Vasomotor menopausal symptoms—
Women: 0.75 mg to 6 mg P.O. daily in cyclic method of 3 weeks on, 1 week off. Can be given continuously.
Prevention of osteoporosis—
Women: 0.625 mg (0.75 mg estropipate) tablet P.O. daily for 25 days of a 31-day cycle.

ADVERSE REACTIONS
CNS: depression, headache, dizziness, migraine, *seizures.*
CV: *edema;* thrombophlebitis; *increased risk of CVA, pulmonary embolism, MI; thromboembolism.*
GI: nausea, vomiting, abdominal cramps, bloating, weight changes.

GU: increased size of uterine fibromas, *increased risk of endometrial cancer, possibility of increased risk of breast cancer,* vaginal candidiasis, cystitis-like syndrome, dysmenorrhea, amenorrhea, breakthrough bleeding, condition resembling premenstrual syndrome.

Hepatic: cholestatic jaundice, *hepatic adenoma.*

Skin: hemorrhagic eruption, erythema nodosum, *erythema multiforme,* hirsutism, melasma, hair loss.

Other: breast engorgement or enlargement, hypercalcemia, gallbladder disease, aggravation of porphyria, libido changes.

INTERACTIONS

Drug-drug. *Carbamazepine, phenobarbital, rifampin:* decreased effectiveness of estrogen therapy. Monitor closely.
Corticosteroids: possible enhanced effects of corticosteroids. Monitor closely.
Cyclosporine: increased risk of toxicity. Use together with caution and frequently monitor serum cyclosporine concentrations.
Dantrolene, other hepatotoxic medications: increased risk of hepatotoxicity. Monitor closely.
Oral anticoagulants: effect of anticoagulant may be decreased. Dosage adjustments may be necessary. Monitor PT and INR, as ordered.
Tamoxifen: estrogens may interfere with effectiveness of tamoxifen. Avoid concomitant use.

Drug-food. *Caffeine:* may increase serum caffeine concentrations. Monitor effects.

Drug-lifestyle. *Smoking:* increased risk of adverse CV effects. If smoking continues, may need alternative therapy.

EFFECTS ON DIAGNOSTIC TESTS

Therapy with estrogens increases sulfobromophthalein retention, PT and clotting factors VII to X, and norepinephrine-induced platelet aggregation. Increases in thyroid-binding globulin concentration may occur, resulting in increased total thyroid concentration (measured by protein-bound iodine or total T_4) and decreased uptake of free T_3 resin. Reduced response to metyrapone test. Serum folate, pyridoxine, and antithrombin III concentrations may decrease; triglyceride, glucose, and phospholipid levels may increase. Glucose tolerance may be impaired. Pregnanediol excretion may decrease.

CONTRAINDICATIONS

Contraindicated in patients with active thrombophlebitis or thromboembolic disorders; estrogen-dependent neoplasia; breast, reproductive organ, or genital cancer; or in those with undiagnosed genital bleeding; and during pregnancy.

NURSING CONSIDERATIONS

• Use cautiously in patients with cerebrovascular or coronary artery disease; asthma; mental depression; bone disease; migraine; seizures; cardiac, hepatic, or renal dysfunction; and in women with a family history (mother, grandmother, sister) of breast or genital tract cancer or who have breast nodules, fibrocystic breasts, or abnormal mammographic findings.

• Ensure that patient has a thorough physical examination before initiating estrogen therapy. Patients receiving long-term therapy should have examinations yearly. Periodically monitor serum lipid levels, blood pressure, body weight, and hepatic function as ordered.

• Know that when used to treat hypogonadism, the duration of therapy necessary to produce withdrawal bleeding depends on the patient's endometrial response to the drug. If satisfactory withdrawal bleeding does not occur, an oral progestin is added to the regimen, as ordered. Explain to the patient that, despite the return of withdrawal bleeding, pregnancy cannot occur because she does not ovulate.

• Be aware of the following estropipate/estrone equivalents:

0.75 mg estropipate = 0.625 mg estrone
1.5 mg estropipate = 1.25 mg estrone
3 mg estropipate = 2.5 mg estrone
6 mg estropipate = 5 mg estrone

• Because of risk of thromboembolism, know that therapy should be discontinued at least 1 month before procedures associated with prolonged immobilization or thromboembolism, such as knee or hip surgery.

Reactions may be *common*, uncommon, *life-threatening*, or COMMON AND LIFE-THREATENING.

☑ Patient teaching

• Tell patient that package insert describing estrogen's adverse effects is available; also explain effects.

• Tell diabetic patient to notify doctor of elevated glucose levels.

• Stress importance of regular physical examinations. Postmenopausal women who use estrogen replacement for over 5 years may have increased risk for endometrial cancer. Using cyclic therapy and lowest possible estrogen dosage reduces risk. Adding progestins to regimen decreases incidence of endometrial hyperplasia; however, it isn't known if progestins affect incidence of endometrial cancer. Most studies show no increased risk of breast cancer.

Alert: Warn patient to immediately report abdominal pain; pain, stiffness, or numbness in the legs or buttocks; pressure or pain in the chest; shortness of breath; severe headaches; visual disturbances, such as blind spots or flashing lights; vaginal bleeding or discharge; breast lumps; swelling of the hands or feet; yellow skin or sclera; dark urine; and light-colored stools.

• Teach female patient how to perform routine breast self-examination.

• Advise patient not to become pregnant while on estrogen therapy.

---

ethinyl estradiol
(ethinyloestradiol)
Estinyl**

Pregnancy Risk Category: X

HOW SUPPLIED
Tablets: 0.02 mg, 0.05 mg, 0.5 mg

ACTION
Increases the synthesis of DNA, RNA, and protein in responsive tissues. Also reduces release of follicle-stimulating hormone and luteinizing hormone from the pituitary gland.

Route	Onset	Peak	Duration
PO	Unknown	Unknown	Unknown

INDICATIONS & DOSAGE
Palliative treatment of metastatic breast cancer (at least 5 years after menopause)—
Women: 1 mg P.O. t.i.d. for at least 3 months.
Female hypogonadism—
Women: 0.05 mg P.O. once daily to t.i.d. 2 weeks per month, followed by 2 weeks of progesterone therapy; continued for 3 to 6 monthly dosing cycles, followed by 2 months off. Can be given continuously.
Vasomotor menopausal symptoms—
Women: 0.02 to 0.05 mg P.O. daily for cycles of 3 weeks on and 1 week off. Can be given continuously.
Palliative treatment of metastatic inoperable prostate cancer—
Men: 0.15 to 2 mg P.O. daily.

ADVERSE REACTIONS
CNS: headache, dizziness, chorea, depression, *seizures.*
CV: thrombophlebitis; *thromboembolism; hypertension; edema, increased risk of CVA, pulmonary embolism, MI.*
EENT: worsening of myopia or astigmatism, intolerance to contact lenses.
GI: *nausea,* vomiting, abdominal cramps, bloating, anorexia, increased appetite, weight changes.
GU: breakthrough bleeding, altered menstrual flow, dysmenorrhea, amenorrhea, cervical erosion, *increased risk of endometrial cancer, possibility of increased risk of breast cancer,* altered cervical secretions, enlargement of uterine fibromas, vaginal candidiasis (in women); gynecomastia, testicular atrophy, impotence (in men).
Hepatic: cholestatic jaundice, *hepatic adenoma.*
Skin: melasma, urticaria, acne, seborrhea, oily skin, hirsutism or hair loss, erythema nodosum, dermatitis.
Other: *breast changes (tenderness, enlargement, secretion),* hypercalcemia, gallbladder disease.

INTERACTIONS
Drug-drug. *Carbamazepine, phenobarbital, rifampin:* decreased effectiveness of estrogen therapy. Monitor closely.

Corticosteroids: possible enhanced effects of corticosteroids. Monitor closely.

Cyclosporine: increased risk of toxicity. Use together with caution and frequently monitor cyclosporine levels.

Dantrolene other hepatotoxic medications: increased risk of hepatotoxicity. Monitor closely.

Oral anticoagulants: effect of anticoagulant may be decreased. Dosage adjustments may be necessary. Monitor PT and INR, as ordered.

Tamoxifen: estrogens may interfere with effectiveness of tamoxifen. Avoid concomitant use.

Drug-food. *Caffeine:* may increase serum caffeine concentrations. Monitor effects.

Drug-lifestyle. *Smoking:* increased risk of adverse CV effects. If smoking continues, may need alternative therapy.

EFFECTS ON DIAGNOSTIC TESTS

Drug therapy increases sulfobromophthalein retention, PT and clotting factors VII to X, and norepinephrine-induced platelet aggregation. Increases in thyroid-binding globulin concentration may occur, resulting in increased total thyroid concentration (measured by protein-bound iodine or total T_4) and decreased uptake of free T_3 resin. Serum folate, pyridoxine, and antithrombin III concentrations may decrease; triglyceride, glucose, and phospholipid levels may increase. Glucose tolerance may be impaired. Pregnanediol excretion may decrease. Reduced response to metyrapone test.

CONTRAINDICATIONS

Contraindicated in patients with thrombophlebitis, thromboembolic disorders, estrogen-dependent neoplasia, breast or reproductive organ cancer (except for palliative treatment), or undiagnosed abnormal genital bleeding and during pregnancy.

NURSING CONSIDERATIONS

• Use cautiously in patients with cerebrovascular or coronary artery disease; asthma; mental depression; bone disease; cardiac, hepatic, or renal dysfunction; or in women with a family history (mother, grandmother, sister) of breast or genital tract cancer, or who have breast nodules, fibrocystic breasts, or abnormal mammographic findings.

• Ensure that patient has a thorough physical examination before initiating estrogen therapy. Patients receiving long-term therapy should have examinations yearly. Periodically monitor serum lipid levels, blood pressure, body weight, and hepatic function as ordered.

• Because of risk of thromboembolism, know that therapy should be discontinued at least 1 month before procedures associated with prolonged immobilization or thromboembolism, such as knee or hip surgery.

• Notify pathologist of patient receiving estrogen therapy when specimens are obtained and sent to pathology for evaluation.

☑ Patient teaching

• Tell patient that package insert describing estrogen's adverse effects is available; however, also give patient verbal explanation.

• Emphasize importance of regular physical examinations. Studies suggest that postmenopausal women who use estrogen replacement for over 5 years to treat menopausal symptoms may be at increased risk for endometrial cancer. This risk is reduced by using cyclic rather than continuous therapy and the lowest possible dosages of estrogen. Adding progestins to the regimen decreases the incidence of endometrial hyperplasia; however, it isn't known if progestins affect the incidence of endometrial cancer. Most studies show no increased risk of breast cancer.

• Explain to patient on cyclic therapy for postmenopausal symptoms that, although withdrawal bleeding may occur during week off drug, fertility is not restored. Pregnancy cannot occur because patient does not ovulate.

Alert: Warn patient to immediately report abdominal pain; pain, numbness, or stiffness in legs or buttocks; pressure or pain in chest; shortness of breath; severe headaches; visual disturbances such as blind spots, flashing lights, or blurriness;

vaginal bleeding or discharge; breast lumps; swelling of hands or feet; yellow skin or sclera; dark urine; or light-colored stools.

• Tell diabetic patient to report elevated blood glucose test results; antidiabetic medication dosage may be adjusted.

• Teach female patient how to perform routine breast self-examination.

• Teach patient methods to decrease risk of thromboembolism.

---

ethinyl estradiol and desogestrel
monophasic: Desogen, Marvelon§, Ortho-Cept

ethinyl estradiol and ethynodiol diacetate
monophasic: Demulen 1/35, Demulen 1/50

ethinyl estradiol and levonorgestrel
monophasic: Alesse-21, Alesse-28, Levlen, Levora-21, Levora-28, Nordette-21, Nordette-28

triphasic: Microgynon-30§, Ovran-30§, Ovranette§, Tri-Levlen, Triphasil

ethinyl estradiol and norethindrone
monophasic: Brevicon, Genora 0.5/35, Genora 1/35, ModiCon, N.E.E. 1/35, Nelova 0.5/35E, Nelova 1/35E, Norethin 1/35E, Norinyl 1 + 35, Ortho-Novum 1/35, Ovcon-35, Ovcon-50

biphasic: Jenest, Nelova 10/11, Ortho-Novum 10/11

triphasic: Ortho-Novum 7/7/7, Tri-Norinyl

ethinyl estradiol and norethindrone acetate
monophasic: Loestrin 1/20, Loestrin 1.5/30

ethinyl estradiol and norgestimate
monophasic: Ortho-Cyclen

triphasic: Ortho Tri-Cyclen

ethinyl estradiol and norgestrel
monophasic: Lo/Ovral, Ovral

ethinyl estradiol, norethindrone acetate, and ferrous fumarate
monophasic: Loestrin Fe 1/20, Loestrin Fe 1.5/30

mestranol and norethindrone
monophasic: Genora 1/50, Nelova 1/50M, Norethin 1/50M, Norinyl 1/50, Ortho-Novum 1/50

Pregnancy Risk Category: X

HOW SUPPLIED
Monophasic oral contraceptives
ethinyl estradiol and desogestrel
Tablets: ethinyl estradiol 30 mcg and desogestrel 0.15 mg (Desogen, Ortho-Cept)
ethinyl estradiol and ethynodiol diacetate
Tablets: ethinyl estradiol 35 mcg and ethynodiol diacetate 1 mg (Demulen 1/35); ethinyl estradiol 50 mcg and ethynodiol diacetate 1 mg (Demulen 1/50)
ethinyl estradiol and levonorgestrel
Tablets: ethinyl estradiol 30 mcg and levonorgestrel 0.15 mg (Levlen, Levora, Micregynon 30, Ovran 30, Ovranette, Nordette-21, Nordette-28); ethinylestradiol 20 mg and levonorgestrel 0.1 mg (Alesse-21, Alesse-28)
ethinyl estradiol and norethindrone
Tablets: ethinyl estradiol 35 mcg and norethindrone 0.4 mg (Ovcon-35); ethinyl estradiol 35 mcg and norethindrone 0.5 mg (Brevicon, Genora 0.5/35, ModiCon, Nelova 0.5/35 E); ethinyl estradiol 35 mcg and norethindrone 1 mg (Genora 1/35, N.E.E. 1/35, Nelova 1/35 E, Norethin 1/35 E, Norinyl 1/35, Ortho-Novum 1/35); ethinyl estradiol 50 mcg and norethindrone 1 mg (Ovcon-50)

---

ethinyl estradiol and norethindrone acetate
Tablets: ethinyl estradiol 20 mcg and norethindrone acetate 1 mg (Loestrin 1/20); ethinyl estradiol 30 mcg and norethindrone acetate 1.5 mg (Loestrin 1.5/30)

ethinyl estradiol and norgestimate
Tablets: ethinyl estradiol 35 mcg and norgestimate 0.25 mg (Ortho-Cyclen)

ethinyl estradiol and norgestrel
Tablets: ethinyl estradiol 30 mcg and norgestrel 0.3 mg (Lo/Ovral); ethinyl estradiol 50 mcg and norgestrel 0.5 mg (Ovral)

ethinyl estradiol, norethindrone acetate, and ferrous fumarate
Tablets: ethinyl estradiol 20 mcg, norethindrone acetate 1 mg, and ferrous fumarate 75 mg (Loestrin Fe 1/20); ethinyl estradiol 30 mcg, norethindrone acetate 1.5 mg, and ferrous fumarate 75 mg (Loestrin Fe 1.5/30)

mestranol and norethindrone
Tablets: mestranol 50 mcg and norethindrone 1 mg (Genora 1/50, Nelova 1/50 M, Norethin 1/50 M, Norinyl 1/50, Ortho-Novum 1/50)

Biphasic oral contraceptives
ethinyl estradiol and norethindrone
Tablets: ethinyl estradiol 35 mcg and norethindrone 0.5 mg during phase 1 (10 days); ethinyl estradiol 35 mcg and norethindrone 1 mg during phase 2 (11 days) (Jenest 7/14, Nelova 10/11, Ortho-Novum 10/11)

Triphasic oral contraceptives
ethinyl estradiol and levonorgestrel
Tablets: (Tri-Levlen, Triphasil) ethinyl estradiol 30 mcg and levonorgestrel 0.05 mg during phase 1 (6 days); ethinyl estradiol 40 mcg and levonorgestrel 0.075 mg during phase 2 (5 days); ethinyl estradiol 30 mcg and levonorgestrel 0.125 mg during phase 3 (10 days); ethinyl estradiol 30 mcg and levonorgestrel 0.15 mg (Microgynon 30§, Ovran 30§, Ovranette§)

ethinyl estradiol and norethindrone
Tablets: (Tri-Norinyl) ethinyl estradiol 35 mcg and norethindrone 0.5 mg during phase 1 (7 days); ethinyl estradiol 35 mcg and norethindrone 1 mg during phase 2 (9 days); ethinyl estradiol 35 mcg and norethindrone 0.5 mg during phase 3 (5 days); (Ortho-Novum 7/7/7) ethinyl estradiol 35 mcg and norethindrone 0.5 mg during phase 1 (7 days); ethinyl estradiol 35 mcg and norethindrone 0.75 mg during phase 2 (7 days); ethinyl estradiol 35 mcg and norethindrone 1 mg during phase 3 (7 days)

ethinyl estradiol and norgestimate
Tablets: (Ortho Tri-Cyclen) ethinyl estradiol 35 mcg and norgestimate 0.18 mg during phase 1 (7 days); ethinyl estradiol 35 mcg and norgestimate 0.215 mg during phase 2 (7 days); ethinyl estradiol 35 mcg and norgestimate 0.25 mg during phase 3 (7 days)

ACTION

Oral contraceptives inhibit ovulation through a negative feedback mechanism directed at the hypothalamus. They also may prevent transport of the ovum through the fallopian tubes.

Estrogen suppresses secretion of follicle-stimulating hormone, blocking follicular development and ovulation.

Progestin suppresses secretion of luteinizing hormone so ovulation cannot occur even if the follicle develops. Progestin thickens cervical mucus, which interferes with sperm migration, and also causes endometrial changes that prevent implantation of the fertilized ovum.

Route	Onset	Peak	Duration
PO	Unknown	0.5-4 hr	Unknown

INDICATIONS & DOSAGE

Contraception—
Adults: *Monophasic oral contraceptives:* 1 tablet P.O. daily, beginning on day 5 of menstrual cycle (first day of menstrual flow is day 1). With 20- and 21-tablet packages, new dosing cycle begins 7 days after last tablet taken. With 28-tablet packages, dosage is 1 tablet daily without interruption; extra tablets are placebos or contain iron.
Biphasic oral contraceptives: 1 color tablet P.O. daily for 10 days; then next color tablet for 11 days. With 21-tablet packages, new dosing cycle begins 7 days after last tablet taken. With 28-tablet

packages, dosage is 1 tablet daily without interruption.

Triphasic oral contraceptives: 1 tablet P.O. daily in the sequence specified by the brand. With 21-tablet packages, new dosing cycle begins 7 days after last tablet taken. With 28-tablet packages, dosage is 1 tablet daily without interruption.

ADVERSE REACTIONS
CNS: *headache, dizziness,* depression, lethargy, migraine.
CV: *thromboembolism,* hypertension, edema, *pulmonary embolism, CVA.*
EENT: worsening of myopia or astigmatism, intolerance of contact lenses, exophthalmos, diplopia.
GI: *nausea,* vomiting, abdominal cramps, bloating, anorexia, changes in appetite, weight gain, pancreatitis.
GU: *breakthrough bleeding, spotting,* granulomatous colitis, dysmenorrhea, amenorrhea, cervical erosion or abnormal secretions, enlargement of uterine fibromas, vaginal candidiasis.
Hepatic: gallbladder disease, cholestatic jaundice, *liver tumors.*
Skin: rash, acne, *erythema multiforme.*
Other: breast changes (*tenderness,* enlargement, secretion); hypercalcemia.

INTERACTIONS
Drug-drug. *Carbamazepine, phenobarbital, phenytoin, rifampin:* decreased effectiveness of estrogen therapy. Monitor closely.
Corticosteroids: possible enhanced effects of corticosteroids. Monitor closely.
Griseofulvin, penicillins, sulfonamides, tetracyclines: may decrease effectiveness of oral contraceptives. Avoid concomitant use, if possible.
Insulin, sulfonylureas: glucose intolerance may decrease effects of antidiabetic agents. Monitor effects.
Oral anticoagulants: effect of anticoagulant may be decreased. Dosage adjustments may be necessary. Monitor PT and INR, as ordered.
Tamoxifen: estrogens may interfere with effectiveness of tamoxifen. Avoid concomitant use.
Drug-food. *Caffeine:* may increase serum caffeine concentrations. Monitor effects.

Drug-lifestyle. *Smoking:* increased risk of adverse CV effects. If smoking continues, may need alternative therapy.

EFFECTS ON DIAGNOSTIC TESTS
Therapy with ethinyl estradiol increases sulfobromophthalein retention, PT and clotting factors VII to X, and norepinephrine-induced platelet aggregation. Increases in thyroid-binding globulin concentration may occur, resulting in increased total thyroid concentration (measured by protein-bound iodine or total T_4) and decreased uptake of free T_3 resin. Serum folate, pyridoxine, and antithrombin III concentrations may decrease; triglyceride, glucose, and phospholipid levels may increase. Glucose tolerance may be impaired. Pregnanediol excretion may decrease.

CONTRAINDICATIONS
Contraindicated in patients with thromboembolic disorders, cerebrovascular or coronary artery disease, diplopia or any ocular lesion arising from ophthalmic vascular disease, classical migraine, MI, known or suspected breast cancer, known or suspected estrogen-dependent neoplasia, benign or malignant liver tumors, active liver disease or history of cholestatic jaundice with pregnancy or prior use of oral contraceptives, and undiagnosed abnormal vaginal bleeding; in known or suspected pregnancy; and in breast-feeding patients.

NURSING CONSIDERATIONS
● Use cautiously in patients with cardiac, renal, or hepatic insufficiency; hyperlipidemia; hypertension; migraine; seizure disorders; or asthma.
● Be aware that triphasic oral contraceptives may cause fewer adverse reactions, such as breakthrough bleeding and spotting.
● Know that the Centers for Disease Control and Prevention reports that the use of oral contraceptives *may decrease* the incidence of ovarian and endometrial cancers. Also, oral contraceptives do not appear to increase a woman's risk of breast cancer. However, the FDA reports that oral con-

---

traceptives may be linked to an increased risk of cervical cancer.

• Monitor serum lipid levels, blood pressure, body weight, and hepatic function, as ordered.

• Know that many laboratory tests are affected by oral contraceptives.

• Estrogens and progestins may alter glucose tolerance, thus changing dosage requirements for antidiabetic drugs. Monitor blood glucose levels.

• Discontinue if patient develops granulomatous colitis while on oral contraceptives and notify doctor.

• Know that drug should be discontinued at least 1 week before surgery to decrease risk of thromboembolism. Tell patient to use an alternative method of birth control.

☑ Patient teaching

• Tell patient to take tablets at same time each day; nighttime dosing may reduce nausea and headaches.

• Advise patient to use an additional method of birth control, such as condoms or a diaphragm with spermicide, for the first week of administration in the initial cycle.

• Tell patient missed doses in midcycle greatly increase likelihood of pregnancy.

• If one tablet is missed, tell patient to take it as soon as she remembers or to take two tablets the next day and continue regular schedule. If patient misses 2 consecutive days, instruct her to take two tablets daily for 2 days and then resume normal schedule. Also advise her to use an additional method of birth control for 7 days after two missed doses. If three or more doses are missed, tell patient to discard remaining tablets in monthly package and to substitute another contraceptive method. If next menstrual period doesn't begin on schedule, warn patient to rule out pregnancy before starting new dosing cycle. If menstrual period begins, have patient start new dosing cycle 7 days after last tablet was taken.

• Warn patient that headache, nausea, dizziness, breast tenderness, spotting, and breakthrough bleeding are common at first. These effects should diminish after three to six dosing cycles (months).

• Instruct patient to weigh herself at least twice a week and to report any sudden weight gain or edema to doctor.

• Warn patient to avoid exposure to ultraviolet light or prolonged exposure to sunlight.

Alert: Warn patient to immediately report abdominal pain; numbness, stiffness, or pain in legs or buttocks; pressure or pain in chest; shortness of breath; severe headache; visual disturbances such as blind spots, blurriness, or flashing lights; undiagnosed vaginal bleeding or discharge; two consecutive missed menstrual periods; lumps in the breast; swelling of hands or feet; or severe pain in the abdomen (tumor rupture in the liver).

• Advise patient of increased risks associated with simultaneous use of cigarettes and oral contraceptives.

• If one menstrual period is missed and tablets have been taken on schedule, tell patient to continue taking them. If two consecutive menstrual periods are missed, tell patient to stop drug and have pregnancy test. Progestins may cause birth defects if taken early in pregnancy.

• Advise patient not to take same drug for longer than 12 months without consulting the doctor. Stress importance of Papanicolaou tests and annual gynecologic examinations.

• Advise patient to check with doctor about how soon pregnancy may be attempted after hormonal therapy is stopped. Many doctors recommend that women not become pregnant within 2 months after stopping drug.

• Warn patient of possible delay in achieving pregnancy when drug is discontinued.

• Tell patient many doctors advise women on long-term therapy (5 years or longer) to stop drug and use other birth control methods. Periodically reassess patient while off hormone therapy.

• Teach patient how to perform routine breast self-examination.

• Teach patient methods to decrease risk of thromboembolism.

• Advise patient to use additional form of birth control with oral contraceptives during concurrent treatment with certain antibiotics.

Reactions may be *common*, uncommon, *life-threatening*, or COMMON AND LIFE-THREATENING.

levonorgestrel
Norplant System

Pregnancy Risk Category: X

HOW SUPPLIED
Implants: 36 mg per capsule; each kit contains six capsules

ACTION
Slowly releases the synthetic progestin levonorgestrel into the bloodstream. How progestins provide contraception is not fully understood, but they alter the mucus covering the cervix, prevent implantation of the egg, and, in some patients, prevent ovulation.

Route	Onset	Peak	Duration
Subdermal	24 hr	24 hr	Unknown

INDICATIONS & DOSAGE
Prevention of pregnancy—
Women: six capsules implanted subdermally in the midportion of the upper arm, about 8 cm above the elbow crease, during first 7 days of onset of menses. Capsules are placed in fanlike position, 15 degrees apart (total of 75 degrees). Contraceptive efficacy lasts for 5 years.

ADVERSE REACTIONS
CNS: headache, nervousness, dizziness.
GI: nausea, *abdominal discomfort,* appetite change.
GU: *amenorrhea, many days of bleeding or prolonged bleeding, spotting,* irregular onset of bleeding, frequent onset of bleeding, scanty bleeding, cervicitis, vaginitis, leukorrhea.
Skin: dermatitis, acne, hirsutism, hypertrichosis, alopecia, infection at implant site, transient pain or itching at implant site.
Other: adnexal enlargement, mastalgia, weight gain, musculoskeletal pain, *removal difficulty,* breast discharge.

INTERACTIONS
Drug-drug. *Carbamazepine, phenytoin, rifampin:* may reduce the contraceptive efficacy of levonorgestrel implants. Monitor closely.

Drug-food. *Caffeine:* may increase serum caffeine concentrations. Monitor effects.
Drug-lifestyle. *Smoking:* increased risk of adverse CV effects. If smoking continues, may need alternative therapy.

EFFECTS ON DIAGNOSTIC TESTS
Decreased sex hormone-binding globulin and T_4 concentrations and increased T_3 uptake have been reported.

CONTRAINDICATIONS
Contraindicated in patients with active thrombophlebitis or thromboembolic disorders, undiagnosed abnormal genital bleeding, acute liver disease, malignant or benign liver tumors, known or suspected breast cancer, and in known or suspected pregnancy.

NURSING CONSIDERATIONS
• Use cautiously in patients with history of depression or hyperlipidemia and in diabetic or prediabetic patients.
• Drug can be used 5 days postpartum after lactation has been established.
• Know that most patients develop variations in menstrual bleeding patterns, including irregular bleeding, prolonged bleeding, spotting, and amenorrhea. In most patients, these irregularities diminish over time.
• Be aware that irregular bleeding may mask symptoms of cervical or endometrial cancer.
• Closely monitor patient with condition that may be aggravated by fluid retention because steroid hormones may cause fluid retention.
• Be aware laboratory tests for sex hormone-binding globulin and T_4 concentrations may show decreased values; for T_3 uptake, increased values.
• Know that implants do not contain estrogen. Levonorgestrel is a totally synthetic progestin.
• Expect implants to be removed if patient develops active thrombophlebitis or thromboembolic disease or will be immobilized for a significant length of time because of illness or some other factor.
• If jaundice develops, expect implants to be removed because steroid hormone me-

---

tabolism is impaired in patients with liver failure.

• Although retinal thrombosis after use of oral contraceptives has been reported, no similar incidents have been documented after use of the implant system. However, patients with sudden unexplained vision problems, including users of contact lenses who develop vision changes or changes in lens tolerance, should be immediately evaluated by an ophthalmologist.

☑ **Patient teaching**
Alert: Tell patient to notify doctor immediately if one of the implanted capsules falls out (before the skin heals over the implant). Contraceptive efficacy may be impaired.

• Warn patient that missed menstrual periods are not an accurate indicator of early pregnancy because drug may induce amenorrhea. Advise patient that 6 weeks or more of amenorrhea (after a pattern of regular menstrual periods) could indicate pregnancy. If pregnancy is confirmed, implants must be removed.

• Teach patient how to perform breast self-examination.

• Encourage regular (at least annual) physical examinations.

• Teach patient methods to decrease risk of thromboembolism.

---

medroxyprogesterone acetate
Amen, Cycrin, Depo-Provera, Provera

Pregnancy Risk Category: X

HOW SUPPLIED
Tablets: 2.5, 5 mg, 10 mg
Injection (suspension): 150 mg/ml, 400 mg/ml

ACTION
Suppresses ovulation, possibly by inhibiting pituitary gonadotropin secretion, thus preventing follicular maturation and causing endometrial thinning.

Route	Onset	Peak	Duration
PO, IM	Unknown	Unknown	Unknown

INDICATIONS & DOSAGE
Abnormal uterine bleeding caused by hormonal imbalance—
Adults: 5 to 10 mg P.O. daily for 5 to 10 days beginning on day 16 of menstrual cycle. If patient also has received estrogen—10 mg P.O. daily for 10 days beginning on day 16 or 21 of cycle.
Secondary amenorrhea—
Adults: 5 to 10 mg P.O. daily for 5 to 10 days. Start at any time during the menstrual cycle (usually during latter half of cycle).
Endometrial or renal cancer—
Adults: 400 to 1,000 mg I.M. weekly. (Dose may be decreased to 400 mg/month when disease has stabilized).
Contraception in women—
Adults: 150 mg I.M. once q 3 months.

ADVERSE REACTIONS
CNS: depression.
CV: thrombophlebitis, *pulmonary embolism,* edema, *thromboembolism, CVA.*
EENT: exophthalmos, diplopia.
GU: *breakthrough bleeding,* dysmenorrhea, *amenorrhea,* cervical erosion, abnormal secretions, *bloating, abdominal pain.*
Hepatic: cholestatic jaundice.
Skin: rash, pain, induration, sterile abscesses, acne, pruritus, melasma, alopecia, hirsutism.
Other: breast tenderness, enlargement, or secretion; changes in weight.

INTERACTIONS
Drug-drug. *Aminoglutethimide, carbamazepine, phenobarbital, phenytoin, rifampin:* decreased progestin effects. Monitor for diminished therapeutic response. Tell patient to use a nonhormonal contraceptive during therapy with these drugs.
Drug-food. *Caffeine:* may increase serum caffeine concentrations. Monitor effects.
Drug-lifestyle. *Smoking:* increased risk of adverse CV effects. If smoking continues, may need alternative therapy.

EFFECTS ON DIAGNOSTIC TESTS
Pregnanediol excretion may decrease; serum alkaline phosphatase and amino acid levels may increase. Glucose tolerance has been shown to decrease in a

---

small percentage of patients receiving this drug. Reduced response to metyrapone test. Increased liver function tests. Increased thyroid-binding globulin; decreased T₃ uptake.

CONTRAINDICATIONS
Contraindicated in patients with hypersensitivity to drug, active thromboembolic disorders, or past history of thromboembolic disorders or of cerebral vascular disease or apoplexy, breast cancer, undiagnosed abnormal vaginal bleeding, missed abortion, or hepatic dysfunction and during pregnancy. Tablets are also contraindicated in patients with liver dysfunction or known or suspected malignant disease of the genital organs.

NURSING CONSIDERATIONS
• Use cautiously in patients with diabetes mellitus, seizures, migraine, cardiac or renal disease, asthma, and mental depression.
• Know that drug should not be used as test for pregnancy; it may cause birth defects and masculinization of female fetus.
• I.M. injection may be painful. Monitor sites for evidence of sterile abscess. Rotate injection sites to prevent muscle atrophy.

☑Patient teaching
• Know that FDA regulations require that, before receiving first dose, patient reads package insert explaining possible adverse effects of progestins. Also, give patient verbal explanation.
 Alert:Tell patient to report unusual symptoms immediately and to stop drug and call doctor if visual disturbances or migraine occur.
• Teach patient how to perform routine monthly breast self-examination.
• Advise patient that injection must be administered every 3 months to maintain adequate contraceptive effects.

norethindrone
Micronor, Nor-QD

norethindrone acetate
Aygestin

Pregnancy Risk Category: X

HOW SUPPLIED
norethindrone
Tablets: 0.35 mg
norethindrone acetate
Tablets: 5 mg

ACTION
Suppresses ovulation, possibly by inhibiting pituitary gonadotropin secretion, and forms thick cervical mucus.

Route	Onset	Peak	Duration
PO	Unknown	Unknown	Unknown

INDICATIONS & DOSAGE
Amenorrhea, abnormal uterine bleeding—
Adults: 2.5 to 10 mg norethindrone acetate P.O. daily on days 5 to 25 of menstrual cycle.
Endometriosis—
Adults: 5 mg norethindrone acetate P.O. daily for 14 days; then increased by 2.5 mg daily q 2 weeks, up to 15 mg daily.
Contraception in women—
Adults: initially, 0.35 mg norethindrone P.O. on first day of menstruation; then 0.35 mg daily.

ADVERSE REACTIONS
CNS: depression.
CV: thrombophlebitis, *pulmonary embolism,* edema, *thromboembolism, CVA.*
EENT: exophthalmos, diplopia.
GI: *bloating, abdominal pain or cramping.*
GU: *breakthrough bleeding,* dysmenorrhea, *amenorrhea,* cervical erosion, abnormal secretions.
Hepatic: cholestatic jaundice.
Skin: melasma, rash, acne, pruritus.
Other: breast tenderness, enlargement, or secretion; changes in weight.

INTERACTIONS
Drug-drug. *Barbiturates, carbamazepine, phenytoin, rifampin:* decreased progestin effects. Monitor for diminished therapeutic response.
Drug-food. *Caffeine:* may increase serum caffeine concentrations. Monitor effects.
Drug-lifestyle. *Smoking:* increased risk of adverse CV effects. If smoking continues, may need alternative therapy.

EFFECTS ON DIAGNOSTIC TESTS
Pregnanediol excretion may decrease; serum alkaline phosphatase and amino acid levels may increase. Glucose tolerance has been shown to decrease in a small percentage of patients receiving drug. Increased liver function tests. Increased thyroid-binding globulin, decreased T_3 uptake. Reduced response to metyrapone test.

CONTRAINDICATIONS
Contraindicated in patients with thromboembolic disorders, cerebral apoplexy, or history of these conditions; hypersensitivity to drug; breast cancer, undiagnosed abnormal vaginal bleeding, severe hepatic disease, or missed abortion and during pregnancy.

NURSING CONSIDERATIONS
• Use cautiously in patients with diabetes mellitus, seizures, migraine, cardiac or renal disease, asthma, and mental depression.
• Norethindrone acetate is twice as potent as norethindrone. Know that norethindrone acetate should not be used for contraception.
• Know that use as test for pregnancy is not appropriate; drug may cause birth defects and masculinization of female fetus.
• Know that preliminary estrogen treatment is usually needed in menstrual disorders.
• Watch patient carefully for signs of edema.
• Monitor blood pressure.

☑ **Patient teaching**
• Know that FDA regulations require that, before receiving first dose, patient reads package insert explaining possible adverse effects of progestin. Also give patient verbal explanation.
• Tell patient that drug needs to be taken at same time every day of the year when used as a contraceptive.
Alert: Tell patient to report unusual symptoms immediately and to stop drug and call doctor if visual disturbances or migraine occurs.
• Teach patient how to perform routine monthly breast self-examination.
• Inform patient what to do if dose is missed.

---

norgestrel
Ovrette**

Pregnancy Risk Category: X

HOW SUPPLIED
Tablets: 0.075 mg

ACTION
Unknown. Probably suppresses ovulation, possibly by inhibiting pituitary gonadotropin secretion, and forms thick cervical mucus.

Route	Onset	Peak	Duration
PO	Unknown	Unknown	Unknown

INDICATIONS & DOSAGE
Contraception in women—
Adults: 0.075 mg P.O. daily starting on first day of menstruation.

ADVERSE REACTIONS
CNS: cerebral thrombosis or hemorrhage, migraine, depression.
CV: thrombophlebitis, *pulmonary embolism*, *edema*, *thromboembolism, CVA*, hypertension.
EENT: exophthalmos, diplopia.
GI: *bloating, abdominal pain/cramping.*
GU: *breakthrough bleeding, change in menstrual flow,* dysmenorrhea, spotting, *amenorrhea,* cervical erosion.
Hepatic: cholestatic jaundice, benign hepatic adenomas.
Skin: melasma, rash, acne, pruritus.
Other: breast tenderness, enlargement, or secretion; changes in weight.

Reactions may be *common*, uncommon, *life-threatening*, or COMMON AND LIFE-THREATENING.

INTERACTIONS

Drug-drug. *Ampicillin, barbiturates, carbamazepine, griseofulvin, phenylbutazone, phenytoin, rifampin, tetracycline:* decreased progestin effects. Monitor for diminished therapeutic response.

Drug-food. *Caffeine:* may increase serum caffeine concentrations. Monitor effects.

Drug-lifestyle. *Smoking:* increased risk of adverse CV effects. If smoking continues, may need alternative therapy.

EFFECTS ON DIAGNOSTIC TESTS

Pregnanediol excretion may decrease; serum alkaline phosphatase and amino acid levels may increase. Glucose tolerance has been shown to decrease in a small percentage of patients receiving drug. Increased liver function tests. Increased thyroid-binding globulin; decreased T_3 uptake. Reduced response to metyrapone test.

CONTRAINDICATIONS

Contraindicated in patients with thromboembolic disorders, cerebral apoplexy, or history of these conditions; hypersensitivity to drug; breast cancer, undiagnosed abnormal vaginal bleeding, severe hepatic disease, or missed abortion and during pregnancy.

NURSING CONSIDERATIONS

• Use cautiously in patients with diabetes mellitus, seizures, migraine, cardiac or renal disease, asthma, and mental depression.
• Be aware that norgestrel is a progestin-only oral contraceptive known as the "minipill."

☑ **Patient teaching**
• Know that FDA regulations require that, before receiving first dose, patient reads package insert explaining possible adverse effects of progestins. Also provide verbal explanation.
• Tell patient to take pill every day, at the same time, even if menstruating.
• Be aware that risk of pregnancy increases with each tablet missed. Tell patient who misses one tablet to take it as soon as she remembers and then to take the next tablet at the regular time. Advise patient

who misses two tablets to take one as soon as she remembers. She must then take the next regular dose at the usual time and use a nonhormonal method of contraception in addition to norgestrel until 14 tablets have been taken. Instruct patient who misses three or more tablets to discontinue drug and use a nonhormonal method of contraception until after menses. If menstrual period does not occur within 45 days, pregnancy testing is necessary.
• Advise patient using oral contraceptives of the increased risk of serious adverse CV reactions associated with heavy cigarette smoking (15 or more cigarettes per day). These risks are quite marked in women over age 35.
• Instruct patient to immediately report excessive bleeding or bleeding between menstrual cycles, breast pain or tenderness, vaginal discharge, or swelling of the hands or feet.
Alert: Tell patient to report unusual symptoms immediately and to stop drug and call doctor if visual disturbances, migraine, or numbness or tingling in limbs occur.
• Teach patient how to perform routine breast self-examination.

progesterone
Gesterol 50, Gestone§

Pregnancy Risk Category: X

HOW SUPPLIED
Injection (in oil): 50 mg/ml

ACTION
Suppresses ovulation, possibly by inhibiting pituitary gonadotropin secretion, and forms thick cervical mucus.

Route	Onset	Peak	Duration
IM	Unknown	Unknown	Unknown

INDICATIONS & DOSAGE
Amenorrhea—
Adults: 5 to 10 mg I.M. daily for 6 to 10 days, usually beginning 8 to 10 days before the anticipated start of menstruation. Or as a single 100- to 150-mg I.M. dose.

Dysfunctional uterine bleeding—
Adults: 5 to 10 mg I.M. daily for six doses.

ADVERSE REACTIONS
CNS: depression.
CV: thrombophlebitis, ***thromboembolism, CVA, pulmonary embolism,*** *edema,* hypertension.
GU: *breakthrough bleeding,* dysmenorrhea, *amenorrhea,* cervical erosion, abnormal secretions.
Hepatic: cholestatic jaundice.
Skin: melasma, rash, acne, pruritus, *pain at injection site.*
Other: breast tenderness, enlargement, or secretion.

INTERACTIONS
Drug-drug. *Barbiturates, carbamazepine, phenytoin, rifampin:* decreased progestin effects. Monitor for diminished therapeutic response.

EFFECTS ON DIAGNOSTIC TESTS
Pregnanediol excretion may decrease; serum alkaline phosphatase and amino acid levels may increase. Glucose tolerance has been shown to decrease in some patients receiving drug. Increase in prothrombin factors VII, VIII, IX, and X. Abnormal thyroid function tests are reflected by increase in protein-binding iodine and butanol extractable iodine and a decrease in T_3 uptake values. Altered liver function test results and a reduced response to metyrapone test may occur.

CONTRAINDICATIONS
Contraindicated in patients with thromboembolic disorders, cerebral apoplexy, or history of these conditions; hypersensitivity to drug; breast cancer, undiagnosed abnormal vaginal bleeding, severe hepatic disease, missed abortion and during pregnancy. Be aware that due to possible allergic reaction, this drug should not be administered to patients allergic to peanuts or sesame.

NURSING CONSIDERATIONS
• Use cautiously in patients with diabetes mellitus, seizures, migraine, cardiac or renal disease, asthma, and mental depression.
• Know preliminary estrogen treatment is usually needed in menstrual disorders.
• Give oil solutions (peanut oil or sesame oil) via deep I.M. injection. Check sites frequently for irritation. Rotate injection sites.

✓**Patient teaching**
• Know that FDA regulations require that, before receiving first dose, patient reads package insert explaining possible adverse effects of progestins. Also give patient verbal explanation.
Alert: Tell patient to report unusual symptoms immediately and to stop drug and call doctor if visual disturbances or migraine occur.
Alert: Tell patient to report increased depression immediately; drug may need to be discontinued.
• Teach patient how to perform routine breast self-examination.

56
Gonadotropins

gonadorelin acetate
histrelin acetate
menotropins

COMBINATION PRODUCTS
None.

gonadorelin acetate
Lutrepulse

Pregnancy Risk Category: B

HOW SUPPLIED
Injection: 0.8 mg/10 ml, 3.2 mg/10-ml vials; supplied as kit with I.V. supplies with or without ambulatory infusion pump

ACTION
Mimics action of gonadotropin-releasing hormone, resulting in the synthesis and release of luteinizing hormone (LH) from anterior pituitary gland. LH then acts upon reproductive organs to regulate hormone synthesis.

Route	Onset	Peak	Duration
IV	Unknown	Unknown	10-40 min

INDICATIONS & DOSAGE
Induction of ovulation in women with primary hypothalamic amenorrhea—
Adults: 5 mcg I.V. q 90 minutes for 21 days. If no response follows three treatment intervals, increase dosage as ordered.

ADVERSE REACTIONS
Skin: hematoma, local infection, inflammation, mild phlebitis, urticaria, pruritus.
Other: multiple pregnancy, ovarian hyperstimulation including ascites, pleural effusion, hemoconcentration, and fluid and electrolyte imbalance.

INTERACTIONS
Drug-drug. *Other ovulation stimulators:* additive effects. Avoid concomitant use.

EFFECTS ON DIAGNOSTIC TESTS
None reported.

CONTRAINDICATIONS
Contraindicated in patients hypersensitive to drug; in those with ovarian cysts or conditions that could be complicated by pregnancy (such as prolactinoma); and in patients who are anovulatory from causes other than a hypothalamic disorder. Also contraindicated in conditions that may be worsened by reproductive hormones, such as estrogen dependent tumors.

NURSING CONSIDERATIONS
• Know that patient usually needs pelvic ultrasound on days 7 and 14 after a baseline scan. Some doctors prefer shorter intervals between scans.

⚡ I.V. administration
• To mimic the naturally occurring hormone, administer gonadorelin in a pulsatile fashion with the available ambulatory infusion pump. Set the pulse period at 1 minute (infuse drug over 1 minute) and the pulse interval at 90 minutes.
• To give 2.5 mcg/pulse, reconstitute the 0.8-mg vial with 8 ml of supplied diluent, and set the pump to deliver 25 microliters/pulse. To administer 5 mcg/pulse, use same dosage strength and dilution, but set the pump to deliver 50 microliters/pulse.
• Some patients may need higher I.V. doses. To give 10 mcg/pulse, reconstitute the 3.2-mg vial with 8 ml of supplied diluent, and set pump to deliver 25 microliters/pulse. To give 20 mcg/pulse, use same dosage strength and dilution, but set pump to deliver 50 microliters/pulse.
• Inspect I.V. site at each visit.

☑ Patient teaching
• Ensure that patient understands that multiple pregnancy is possible (incidence is about 12%). Monitoring of dosage and ovarian ultrasonography to monitor drug response are needed.
• Instruct patient about proper aseptic

technique and care of I.V. site. Cannula and I.V. site should be changed every 48 hours. Written instructions are available for patient.
• Know that anaphylaxis has been reported with similar drugs. Teach patient symptoms of hypersensitivity reactions (rash, hives, wheezing, difficulty breathing, rapid heartbeat), and encourage her to report these at once.
• Tell patient to report signs of infection, hematoma, inflammation, or phlebitis at injection site. She also should report severe abdominal pain, bloating, swelling of the hands or feet, nausea, vomiting, diarrhea, substantial weight gain, or shortness of breath.
• Encourage patient to adhere to close monitoring schedule required by therapy. Regular pelvic examinations, midluteal-phase serum progesterone determinations, and multiple ovarian ultrasound scans are necessary.

---

histrelin acetate
Supprelin

Pregnancy Risk Category: X

HOW SUPPLIED
Injection: 120 mcg/0.6 ml, 300 mcg/0.6 ml, 600 mcg/0.6 ml

ACTION
An agonist that mimics the effects of gonadotropin-releasing hormone (GnRH; also called luteinizing hormone-releasing hormone) but is more potent. Chronic administration desensitizes responsiveness of the pituitary gonadotropin, decreasing sex hormone production by the testes or ovaries.

Route	Onset	Peak	Duration
SC	Unknown	Unknown	Unknown

INDICATIONS & DOSAGE
Centrally mediated (idiopathic or neurogenic) precocious puberty—
Children (girls 2 to 8 years; boys 2 to 9½ years): 10 mcg/kg S.C. daily.

ADVERSE REACTIONS
CNS: *mood changes, nervousness, dizziness, depression, headache, libido changes, insomnia, anxiety,* paresthesia, cognitive changes, syncope, somnolence, lethargy, impaired consciousness, tremor, hyperkinesia, *seizures,* hot flashes, conduct disorder, fatigue.
CV: *vasodilation,* edema, palpitations, pallor, tachycardia, hypertension.
EENT: epistaxis, ear congestion, abnormal pupillary function, otalgia, visual disturbances, hearing loss, polyopia, photophobia, rhinorrhea, sinusitis, nasal infections.
GI: *abdominal pain, nausea, vomiting, diarrhea, flatulence, decreased appetite, dyspepsia,* cramps, constipation, thirst, gastritis, GI distress.
GU: *menstrual changes, vaginal dryness, leukorrhea, hypermenorrhea, vaginal bleeding, vaginitis, dysmenorrhea,* polyuria, incontinence, dysuria, hematuria, nocturia, tenderness of female genitalia, glycosuria.
Hematologic: hyperlipidemia, anemia.
Respiratory: *upper respiratory infection, respiratory congestion, cough,* asthma, breathing disorder, bronchitis, hyperventilation.
Skin: *redness, swelling, acne, rash, diaphoresis,* urticaria, pruritus, alopecia.
Other: *fever, arthralgia, muscle stiffness, muscle cramps, breast pain or edema,* breast discharge, decreased breast size, *weight gain, body pains,* chills, malaise, purpura, acute hypersensitivity reactions *(anaphylaxis, angioedema).*

INTERACTIONS
None significant.

EFFECTS ON DIAGNOSTIC TESTS
None reported.

CONTRAINDICATIONS
Contraindicated in patients hypersensitive to drug or its ingredients and in pregnant or breast-feeding patients.

NURSING CONSIDERATIONS
• Be aware drug is indicated only for patients who will comply with the daily schedule. Noncompliance or inadequate

---

Reactions may be *common,* uncommon, *life-threatening,* or COMMON AND LIFE-THREATENING.

dosing may result in inadequate control of the pubertal process, which can result in recurrence of symptoms, including onset of menses, breast development, or testicular growth; long-term consequences may involve decreased adult height.

• Know that a complete physical and endocrinologic evaluation should be performed before initiating drug therapy; several indices should be reexamined at 3 months, then every 6 to 12 months thereafter. Such evaluations should include determinations of height and weight, hand and wrist X-rays for bone-age determination, sex steroid (estradiol or testosterone) levels, and GnRH stimulation test. Monitor these tests periodically to determine effectiveness of therapy.

• Be aware that further tests to rule out other causes of precocious puberty include beta human chorionic gonadotropin levels (to detect chorionic gonadotropin-secreting tumor); pelvic/adrenal/testicular ultrasound (to detect steroid-secreting tumor); and computed tomography scan of the head (to detect previously undiagnosed intracranial tumors). Workup also sets baseline of gonad size for serial monitoring.

• Refrigerate drug (36° to 46° F [2° to 8° C]) and protect from light in its original container. Use vials only once because drug does not contain preservatives. Allow drug to reach room temperature before use.

• Give S.C. and rotate injection sites to minimize local reactions.

• Know that decreases in follicle-stimulating hormone, luteinizing hormone, and sex steroid levels occur within 3 months.

• Reevaluate patient if prepubertal levels of sex steroids or GnRH test responses are not achieved within 3 months of therapy.

• Know that safety and efficacy have not been established in children under 2 years.

☑ **Patient teaching**
• Before therapy, make sure patient and caregiver understands importance of adhering to daily schedules. Tell parents to give drug at same time each day to aid compliance and ensure adequate dosing.

• Drug is dispensed as a 30-day kit that contains a patient information leaflet. Ensure that caregiver reads and understands the leaflet.

• Inform patient that because drug is a peptide, it is destroyed in the GI tract and so must be given parenterally.

• Explain importance of rotating injection sites daily. Sites should include upper arms, thighs, and abdomen.

• Warn patient of the potential risks of therapy and potential adverse effects. During the first month of treatment, girls commonly experience a slight menstrual flow, which probably is related to decreasing estrogen levels brought on by treatment. As estrogen levels drop, menses begins because estrogens support the endometrium.

• Advise patient to seek medical attention immediately if signs of hypersensitivity reactions occur—sudden development of rash, difficulty breathing or swallowing, or rapid heartbeat. Also tell her to notify doctor if severe or persistent swelling, redness, or irritation occurs at the injection site.

---

menotropins
Humegon, Menogen§, Pergonal, Repronex

Pregnancy Risk Category: X

HOW SUPPLIED
Injection: 75 IU of luteinizing hormone (LH) and 75 IU of follicle-stimulating hormone (FSH) activity per ampule; 150 IU of LH and 150 IU of FSH activity per ampule

ACTION
When given to women who have not had primary ovarian failure, mimics FSH in inducing follicular growth and LH in aiding follicular maturation; induces spermatogenesis in men.

Route	Onset	Peak	Duration
IM	9-12 days	Unknown	Unknown

INDICATIONS & DOSAGE

Anovulation—
Women: 75 IU each of FSH and LH I.M. daily for 7 to 12 days, followed by 5,000 to 10,000 units of human chorionic gonadotropin (HCG) I.M. 1 day after last dose of menotropins. Repeated for one to three menstrual cycles until ovulation occurs.

Infertility with ovulation—
Women: 75 IU each of FSH and LH I.M. daily for 7 to 12 days, then 5,000 to 10,000 units HCG I.M. 1 day after last dose of menotropins. Repeated for two menstrual cycles, then 150 IU each of FSH and LH daily for 7 to 12 days, followed by 5,000 to 10,000 units HCG I.M. 1 day after last dose of menotropins. Repeated for two menstrual cycles.

Infertility in men—
Men: prior treatment with HCG of 5,000 units three times a week for 4 to 6 months; then 75 IU each of FSH and LH I.M. three times weekly (given with 2,000 units of HCG twice weekly) for at least 4 months. If increased spermatogenesis does not occur, increase to 150 IU each of FSH and LH three times weekly (dosage of HCG remains unchanged).

ADVERSE REACTIONS

CNS: headache, malaise, dizziness, *CVA.*
CV: tachycardia, venous thrombophlebitis.
GI: nausea, vomiting, diarrhea, abdominal cramps, bloating.
GU: *ovarian enlargement with pain and abdominal distention,* multiple births, ovarian hyperstimulation syndrome, ovarian cysts, ectopic pregnancy.
Respiratory: *atelectasis, acute respiratory distress syndrome, pulmonary embolism, pulmonary infarction, arterial occlusion,* dyspnea, tachypnea.
Other: fever, *gynecomastia, hypersensitivity and anaphylactic reactions,* chills, musculoskeletal aches, joint pains, rash.

INTERACTIONS

None significant.

EFFECTS ON DIAGNOSTIC TESTS

None reported.

CONTRAINDICATIONS

Contraindicated in patients with primary ovarian failure, uncontrolled thyroid or adrenal dysfunction, pituitary tumor, abnormal uterine bleeding, uterine fibromas, ovarian cysts or enlargement, or hypersensitivity to drug; during pregnancy; and in men with normal pituitary function, primary testicular failure, or infertility disorders other than hypogonadotropic hypogonadism.

NURSING CONSIDERATIONS

• Monitor closely to ensure adequate ovarian stimulation without hyperstimulation.
• Watch for ovarian hyperstimulation syndrome. This may progress rapidly to become a serious medical event characterized by dramatic increase in vascular permeability resulting in rapid accumulation of fluid in the peritoneal cavity, thorax, and pericardium. Clinical signs and symptoms include hypovolemia, hemoconcentration, electrolyte imbalance, ascites, hemoperitoneum, pleural effusion, hydrothorax, and thromboembolitic events. Cases are more common and severe if pregnancy occurs.
• Reconstitute with 1 to 2 ml of sterile 0.9% NaCl for injection. Use immediately.
• Rotate injection sites.

☑ **Patient teaching**
• Tell patient about possibility of multiple births.
• In infertility, encourage daily intercourse from day before HCG is given until ovulation occurs.
• Tell patient that pregnancy usually occurs 4 to 6 weeks after therapy.
• Instruct patient to immediately report severe abdominal pain, bloating, swelling of the hands or feet, nausea, vomiting, diarrhea, substantial weight gain, or shortness of breath.

Reactions may be *common,* uncommon, *life-threatening,* or **COMMON AND LIFE-THREATENING.**

57

Antidiabetic drugs and glucagon

acarbose
chlorpropamide
glimepiride
glipizide
glucagon
glyburide
insulins
metformin hydrochloride
repaglinide
troglitazone

COMBINATION PRODUCTS
HUMULIN 50/50 ◊ : isophane insulin suspension (human) 50% and insulin injection (human) 50%, 100 units/ml.
HUMULIN 70/30 ◊, NOVOLIN 70/30 ◊ : isophane insulin suspension (human) 70% and insulin injection (human) 30%, 100 units/ml.

acarbose
Glucobay§, Prandase†, Precose

Pregnancy Risk Category: B

HOW SUPPLIED
Tablets: 50 mg, 100 mg

ACTION
An alpha-glucosidase inhibitor that delays digestion of carbohydrates, resulting in a smaller rise in blood glucose concentration.

Route	Onset	Peak	Duration
PO	Unknown	1 hr	2-4 hr

INDICATIONS & DOSAGE
Adjunct to diet to lower blood glucose in patients with type 2 (non-insulin-dependent) diabetes mellitus whose hyperglycemia cannot be managed by diet alone or by diet and a sulfonylurea—
Adults: individualized. Initially, 25 mg P.O. t.i.d. at start of each main meal. Subsequent dosage adjustment made q 4 to 8 weeks, based on 1-hour postprandial glucose level and tolerance. Maintenance dosage is 50 mg to 100 mg P.O. t.i.d.
Adjust-a-dose: In patients weighing below 60 kg (132 lb), do not exceed 50 mg P.O. t.i.d. In patients weighing above 60 kg, do not exceed 100 mg P.O. t.i.d.

ADVERSE REACTIONS
GI: *abdominal pain, diarrhea, flatulence.*
Other: elevated serum transaminase level.

INTERACTIONS
Drug-drug. *Calcium channel blockers, corticosteroids, estrogens, isoniazid, nicotinic acid, oral contraceptives, phenothiazine, phenytoin, sympathomimetics, thiazides and other diuretics, thyroid products:* may cause hyperglycemia during concomitant use or hypoglycemia when withdrawn. Monitor blood glucose level.
Digestive enzyme preparations containing carbohydrate-splitting enzymes (such as amylase, pancreatin), intestinal adsorbents (such as activated charcoal): may reduce effect of acarbose. Do not administer concomitantly.

EFFECTS ON DIAGNOSTIC TESTS
Acarbose therapy, particularly in doses exceeding 50 mg t.i.d., may cause elevations of serum transaminase and, in rare cases, bilirubin levels. Also associated with low serum calcium and plasma vitamin B_6 levels.

CONTRAINDICATIONS
Contraindicated in patients with diabetic ketoacidosis, cirrhosis, inflammatory bowel disease, colonic ulceration, partial intestinal obstruction, predisposition to intestinal obstruction, chronic intestinal disease associated with marked disorder of digestion or absorption, conditions that may deteriorate because of increased intestinal gas formation, or hypersensitivity to drug.

NURSING CONSIDERATIONS
• Drug is not recommended for use in pa-

tients with serum creatinine levels over 2 mg/dl, in pregnant or breast-feeding women, or in patients with cirrhosis.

• Use cautiously in patients receiving a sulfonylurea or insulin. Drug is not recommended for renally impaired patients. Acarbose may increase hypoglycemic potential of the sulfonylurea. Monitor patient receiving both drugs closely. If hypoglycemia occurs, treat patient with oral glucose (dextrose). Severe hypoglycemia may require I.V. glucose infusion or glucagon administration. Because dosage adjustments may be needed to prevent further hypoglycemia, report hypoglycemia and treatment required to doctor. Insulin therapy may be needed during increased stress (infection, fever, surgery, or trauma). Monitor patient closely for hyperglycemia.

• Know that safety and efficacy of drug have not been established in children.

• Monitor patient's 1-hour postprandial plasma glucose level to determine therapeutic effectiveness of acarbose and to identify appropriate dose. Report hyperglycemia to doctor. Thereafter, glycosylated hemoglobin should be measured every 3 months.

• Monitor serum transaminase level every 3 months in first year of therapy and periodically thereafter in patients receiving doses in excess of 50 mg t.i.d. Report abnormalities; dosage adjustment or drug withdrawal may be needed.

✅ Patient teaching

• Tell patient to take drug daily with first bite of each of three main meals.

• Explain that therapy relieves symptoms but does not cure the disease.

• Stress importance of adhering to specific diet, weight reduction, exercise, and hygiene programs. Show patient how to monitor blood glucose level and to recognize and treat hyperglycemia.

• Teach patient taking a sulfonylurea how to recognize hypoglycemia, and to treat symptoms with a form of dextrose rather than with a product containing table sugar.

• Urge patient to carry medical identification at all times.

• Instruct patient about nature of disease, importance of following therapeutic regimen, adhering to specific diet, and weight reduction.

chlorpropamide
Apo-Chlorpropamide†, Diabinese, Novo-Propamide†

Pregnancy Risk Category: C

HOW SUPPLIED
Tablets: 100 mg, 250 mg

ACTION
Unknown. A sulfonylurea that probably stimulates insulin release from the pancreatic beta cells and reduces glucose output by the liver. An extrapancreatic effect increases peripheral sensitivity to insulin. Also exerts an antidiuretic effect in patients with diabetes insipidus.

Route	Onset	Peak	Duration
PO	1 hr	2-4 hr	24 hr

INDICATIONS & DOSAGE
Adjunct to diet to lower blood glucose level in patients with type 2 (non-insulin-dependent) diabetes mellitus—
Adults: 250 mg P.O. daily with breakfast. Initial dosage increased after 5 to 7 days because of extended duration of action; then increased q 3 to 5 days by 50 to 125 mg, if needed, to maximum of 750 mg daily. Some patients with mild diabetes respond well to dosages of 100 mg or less daily.
Elderly: in patients over 65 years, initially 100 to 125 mg P.O. daily, then increase as with adult dose.
Adjust-a-dose: In patients with renal insufficiency, increase dosage as tolerated.
To change from insulin to oral therapy—
Adults: if insulin dosage is less than 40 units daily, insulin is stopped and oral therapy started as above. If insulin dosage is 40 units or more daily, oral therapy started as above with insulin reduced 50%. Insulin dosage reduced further according to response.

ADVERSE REACTIONS
CNS: paresthesia, fatigue, dizziness, vertigo, malaise, headache.

EENT: tinnitus.
GI: nausea, heartburn, epigastric distress.
GU: tea-colored urine.
Hematologic: leukopenia, *thrombocytopenia, aplastic anemia, agranulocytosis,* hemolytic anemia.
Skin: rash, pruritus, erythema, urticaria.
Other: *hypersensitivity reactions, prolonged hypoglycemia, dilutional hyponatremia.*

INTERACTIONS

Drug-drug. *Anabolic steroids, chloramphenicol, clofibrate, guanethidine, MAO inhibitors, salicylates, sulfonamides:* increased hypoglycemic activity. Monitor blood glucose level.
Beta blockers: prolonged hypoglycemic effect and masked symptoms of hypoglycemia. Use together cautiously.
Corticosteroids, glucagon, rifampin, thiazide diuretics: decreased hypoglycemic response. Monitor blood glucose level.
Hydantoins: increased blood levels of hydantoins. Monitor blood levels.
Oral anticoagulants: increased hypoglycemic activity or enhanced anticoagulant effect. Monitor blood glucose level and PT.
Drug-lifestyle. *Alcohol use:* altered glycemic control, most commonly hypoglycemia. May also cause a disulfiram-like reaction. Discourage concomitant use.

EFFECTS ON DIAGNOSTIC TESTS

Drug alters cholesterol, alkaline phosphatase, bilirubin, urine phenylketone, porphyrias, protein levels, and cephalin flocculation (thymol turbidity). May elevate AST, LD, BUN, and creatinine levels.

CONTRAINDICATIONS

Contraindicated for treating type 1 diabetes (insulin-dependent) or diabetes that can be adequately controlled by diet. Also contraindicated in patients with type 2 diabetes complicated by ketosis, acidosis, diabetic coma, major surgery, severe infections, or severe trauma; during pregnancy or breast-feeding; and in those hypersensitive to drug.

NURSING CONSIDERATIONS

• Use cautiously in patients with porphyria or impaired hepatic or renal function, or in debilitated, malnourished, or elderly patients.
• Know that elderly patients may be more sensitive to adverse effects.
• Know that drug may accumulate in patients with renal insufficiency. Watch for and report signs of impending renal insufficiency, such as dysuria, anuria, and hematuria.
Alert: Know that adverse effects of drug, especially hypoglycemia, may be more frequent or severe than with some other sulfonylureas because of the drug's long duration of action. If hypoglycemia occurs, monitor patient closely for a minimum of 3 to 5 days.
• Know that patients transferring from another oral antidiabetic agent usually need no transition period.
• Be aware that patients may require hospitalization during transition from insulin therapy to an oral antidiabetic agent. Monitor patient's blood glucose levels at least three times daily before meals.

☑ Patient teaching

• Instruct patient about nature of disease, importance of following therapeutic regimen, adhering to specific diet, weight reduction, exercise, and personal hygiene programs, and about avoiding infection. Explain how and when to perform self-monitoring of blood glucose level, and teach recognition of and intervention for hypoglycemia and hyperglycemia.
• Make sure patient understands that therapy only relieves symptoms.
• Tell patient not to change drug dosage without doctor's consent and to report abnormal blood or urine glucose test results.
• Teach patient to carry candy or other simple sugars to treat mild hypoglycemic episodes. Severe episodes may require hospital treatment.
• Advise patient not to take other drugs, including OTC drugs, without checking with doctor.
• Advise patient to avoid intake of alcohol. Chlorpropamide-alcohol flush is characterized by facial flushing, light-headedness, headache, and occasional

---

*Liquid contains alcohol.   **May contain tartrazine.   †Canada   ‡Australia   §U.K.   ◇OTC

breathlessness. Even very small amounts of alcohol can produce this reaction.
• Advise patient to carry medical identification at all times.
Alert: Tell patient to report rash, skin eruptions, and other signs and symptoms of hypersensitivity to doctor immediately.

---

glimepiride
Amaryl

Pregnancy Risk Category: C

HOW SUPPLIED
Tablets: 1 mg, 2 mg, 4 mg

ACTION
Exact mechanism of drug's ability to lower blood glucose may depend on stimulating the release of insulin from functioning pancreatic beta cells. Drug can also lead to increased sensitivity of peripheral tissues to insulin.

Route	Onset	Peak	Duration
PO	Unknown	2-3 hr	> 24 hr

INDICATIONS & DOSAGE
Adjunct to diet and exercise to lower blood glucose in patients with type 2 (non-insulin-dependent) diabetes mellitus whose hyperglycemia cannot be managed by diet and exercise alone—
Adults: initially, 1 to 2 mg P.O. once daily with first main meal of day; usual maintenance dosage is 1 to 4 mg P.O. once daily. After reaching dosage of 2 mg, dosage is increased in increments not exceeding 2 mg q 1 to 2 weeks, based on patient's blood glucose response. Maximum dose is 8 mg/day.
Adjunct to insulin therapy in patients with type 2 diabetes mellitus whose hyperglycemia cannot be managed by diet and exercise in conjunction with oral hypoglycemic agents—
Adults: 8 mg P.O. once daily with first main meal of day; used in combination with low-dose insulin. Insulin adjusted upward weekly p.r.n., based on patient's blood glucose response.
Adjust-a-dose: In renally impaired patients, initial dose 1 mg P.O. once daily with first main meal of day, followed by appropriate dose titrated, p.r.n.

ADVERSE REACTIONS
CNS: dizziness, asthenia, headache.
EENT: changes in accommodation.
GI: nausea.
Hematologic: leukopenia, hemolytic anemia, agranulocytosis, ***thrombocytopenia, aplastic anemia, pancytopenia.***
Hepatic: cholestatic jaundice.
Skin: allergic skin reactions (pruritus, erythema, urticaria, and morbilliform or maculopapular eruptions).
Other: hypoglycemia, dilutional hyponatremia.

INTERACTIONS
Drug-drug. *Beta-adrenergic blocking agents:* may mask symptoms of hypoglycemia.
Drugs that tend to produce hyperglycemia (such as corticosteroids, estrogens, isoniazid, nicotinic acid, oral contraceptives, other diuretics, phenothiazines, phenytoin, sympathomimetic thiazides, thyroid products): may lead to loss of glucose control. Adjust dosage as ordered.
Insulin: may increase potential for hypoglycemia. Avoid concomitant use.
NSAIDs, other drugs that are highly protein-bound (such as beta-adrenergic blocking agents, chloramphenicol, coumarins, MAO inhibitors, probenecid, salicylates, sulfonamides): may potentiate hypoglycemic action of sulfonylureas such as glimepiride. Monitor blood glucose levels carefully.
Drug-lifestyle. *Alcohol use:* altered glycemic control, most commonly hypoglycemia. May also cause disulfiram-like reaction. Discourage concomitant use.

EFFECTS ON DIAGNOSTIC TESTS
Drug may elevate transaminase levels, LD, alkaline phosphatase, BUN, and creatinine.

CONTRAINDICATIONS
Contraindicated in patients hypersensitive to drug or in those with diabetic ketoacidosis, which should be treated with insulin.

NURSING CONSIDERATIONS
• Use cautiously in debilitated or malnourished patients and in those with adrenal, pituitary, hepatic, or renal insufficiency; these patients are more susceptible to the hypoglycemic action of glucose-lowering drugs. Its use is not recommended in elderly patients.
• Glimepiride and insulin may be used concurrently in secondary failure patients (those who lose glucose control after initially responding to therapy).
• Monitor fasting blood glucose periodically to determine therapeutic response. Also monitor glycosylated hemoglobin, usually every 3 to 6 months to precisely assess long-term glycemic control.
• Know that oral hypoglycemic agents have been associated with an increased risk of CV mortality compared with diet alone or with diet and insulin therapy.
• Know that safety and effectiveness in children have not been established.
• It is not known whether drug is excreted in breast milk. Do not administer drug to breast-feeding women due to potential for hypoglycemia in breast-fed infants.
• Know that no transition period is needed when changing patients from other hypoglycemic agents (sulfonylureas) to glimepiride.

☑**Patient teaching**
• Tell patient to take drug with first meal of the day.
• Make sure patient understands that therapy relieves symptoms but does not cure the disease. He should also understand potential risks and advantages of taking drug and other treatment methods.
• Stress importance of adhering to diet, weight reduction, exercise, and personal hygiene programs. Explain to patient and family how and when to perform self-monitoring of blood glucose levels, and teach recognition of and intervention for signs and symptoms of hyperglycemia and hypoglycemia.
• Advise patient to carry medical identification about his condition at all times.
• Advise female patient who is planning a pregnancy to consult doctor before becoming pregnant. Insulin may be required during pregnancy and breast-feeding.

• Teach patient to carry candy or other simple sugars to treat mild hypoglycemic episodes. Severe episodes may require hospital treatment.
• Inform the patient that alcohol lowers blood sugar, and therefore intake should be limited.

glipizide
Glibenese§, Glucotrol,
Glucotrol XL, Minidiab‡

Pregnancy Risk Category: C

HOW SUPPLIED
Tablets: 5 mg, 10 mg
Tablets (extended-release): 5 mg, 10 mg

ACTION
Unknown. A sulfonylurea that probably stimulates insulin release from the pancreatic beta cells and reduces glucose output by the liver. An extrapancreatic effect increases peripheral sensitivity to insulin.

Route	Onset	Peak	Duration
PO	15-30 min	1-3 hr	4 hr
PO (extended)	2-3 hr	6-12 hr	24 hr

INDICATIONS & DOSAGE
Adjunct to diet to lower blood glucose level in patients with type 2 (non-insulin-dependent) diabetes mellitus—
Adults: initially, 5 mg P.O. daily 30 minutes before breakfast. Maximum once-daily dose is 15 mg. Doses above 15 mg should be divided; maximum total daily dosage is 40 mg for immediate-release tablets.
Elderly: in patients over 65 years, initial dose is 2.5 mg P.O. daily.
Adjust-a-dose: In patients with liver disease, initial dose is 2.5 mg P.O. daily.
Extended-release tablets: initially, 5 mg P.O. daily. Titrate in 5-mg increments q 3 months depending on level of glycemic control. Maximum daily dosage is 20 mg.
To replace insulin therapy—
Adults: if insulin dosage is more than 20 units daily, patient is started at usual dosage in addition to 50% of insulin. If insulin dosage is less than 20 units, in-

sulin may be discontinued on initiation of glipizide.

ADVERSE REACTIONS
CNS: dizziness, drowsiness, headache.
GI: nausea, constipation, diarrhea.
Hematologic: leukopenia, hemolytic anemia, *agranulocytosis, thrombocytopenia, aplastic anemia.*
Hepatic: cholestatic jaundice.
Skin: rash, pruritus.
Other: *hypoglycemia.*

INTERACTIONS
Drug-drug. *Anabolic steroids, chloramphenicol, clofibrate, guanethidine, MAO inhibitors, probenecid, salicylates, sulfonamides:* increased hypoglycemic activity. Monitor blood glucose level.
Beta blockers: prolonged hypoglycemic effect and masked symptoms of hypoglycemia. Use together cautiously.
Corticosteroids, glucagon, rifampin, thiazide diuretics: decreased hypoglycemic response. Monitor blood glucose level.
Hydantoins: increased blood levels of hydantoins. Monitor blood levels.
Oral anticoagulants: increased hypoglycemic activity or enhanced anticoagulant effect. Monitor blood glucose levels and PT.
Drug-lifestyle. *Alcohol use:* altered glycemic control, most commonly hypoglycemia. May also cause disulfiram-like reaction. Discourage concomitant use.

EFFECTS ON DIAGNOSTIC TESTS
Drug therapy alters cholesterol, alkaline phosphatase, AST, LD, BUN, and creatinine levels.

CONTRAINDICATIONS
Contraindicated in patients hypersensitive to drug or in those with diabetic ketoacidosis with or without coma, and in pregnant or breast-feeding women.

NURSING CONSIDERATIONS
• Use cautiously in patients with renal and hepatic disease and in debilitated, malnourished, or elderly patients.
• Give drug about 30 minutes before meals.
• Know that some patients may attain ef-

fective control on a once-daily regimen, whereas others respond better with divided dosing.
• Be aware that glipizide is a second-generation sulfonylurea. The frequency of adverse reactions appears to be lower than with first-generation drugs, such as chlorpropamide.
• During periods of increased stress, patient may require insulin therapy. Monitor patient closely for hyperglycemia in these situations.
• Know that patient transferring from insulin therapy to an oral antidiabetic agent requires blood glucose monitoring at least three times daily before meals. Patient may require hospitalization during transition.

☑ **Patient teaching**
• Instruct patient about disease, importance of following therapeutic regimen, adhering to diet, weight reduction, exercise, personal hygiene programs, and avoiding infection. Explain how and when to perform self-monitoring of blood glucose level, and teach recognition of hypoglycemia and hyperglycemia.
• Tell patient to carry candy or other simple sugars to treat mild hypoglycemic episodes. Severe episodes may require hospital treatment.
• Instruct patient not to change drug dosage without doctor's consent and to report abnormal blood or urine glucose test results.
• Tell patient not to take other medications, including OTC drugs, without checking with doctor.
• Advise patient to carry medical identification at all times.
• Inform patient that alcohol lowers blood sugar, and therefore should be avoided.

glucagon

Pregnancy Risk Category: B

HOW SUPPLIED
Powder for injection: 1-mg (1 unit) vial, 10-mg (10 units) vial

ACTION
Raises blood glucose level by promoting catalytic depolymerization of hepatic glycogen to glucose.

Route	Onset	Peak	Duration
IV	Immediate	0.5 hr	Unknown
IM, SC	Unknown	Unknown	Unknown

INDICATIONS & DOSAGE
Hypoglycemia—
Adults and children weighing over 20 kg (44 lb): 1 mg S.C., I.M., or I.V.
Children weighing 20 kg or less: 0.025 USP units or 25 mcg/kg S.C., I.M., or I.V.; maximum dose 1 mg.
Note: May repeat in 20 minutes, if necessary. I.V. glucose must be given if patient fails to respond. When patient responds, supplemental carbohydrate needs to be given immediately.
Diagnostic aid for radiologic examination—
Adults: 0.25 to 2 mg I.V. or I.M. before radiologic procedure.

ADVERSE REACTIONS
CV: hypotension.
GI: nausea, vomiting.
Respiratory: respiratory distress.
Other: hypersensitivity reactions (***bronchospasm,*** rash, dizziness, light-headedness).

INTERACTIONS
Drug-drug. *Phenytoin:* inhibited glucagon-induced insulin release. Use cautiously.

EFFECTS ON DIAGNOSTIC TESTS
Glucagon lowers serum potassium levels.

CONTRAINDICATIONS
Contraindicated in patients with pheochromocytoma or hypersensitivity to drug.

NURSING CONSIDERATIONS
• Use cautiously in those with history of insulinoma or pheochromocytoma.
Alert: Arouse patient from coma as quickly as possible and give additional carbohydrates orally to prevent secondary hypoglycemic reactions.

I.V. administration
• Reconstitute 1-unit vial with 1 ml of diluent; reconstitute 10-unit vial with 10 ml of diluent. Use only the diluent supplied by the manufacturer when preparing doses of 2 mg or less. For larger doses, dilute with sterile water for injection.
• For I.V. drip infusion, use dextrose solution, which is compatible with glucagon (drug forms a precipitate in chloride solutions). Inject directly into vein or into I.V. tubing of a free-flowing compatible solution over 2 to 5 minutes. Interrupt primary infusion during glucagon injection if using the same I.V. line.
• Unstable hypoglycemic diabetic patients may not respond to glucagon; give dextrose I.V. instead, as ordered.

Patient teaching
• Instruct patient and caregivers in proper glucagon administration and recognition of hypoglycemia.
• Explain importance of calling doctor at once in emergencies.

---

glyburide (glibenclamide)
Daonil§, DiaBeta**, Euglucon†, Glynase PresTab, Micronase, Semi-Daonil§

Pregnancy Risk Category: B

HOW SUPPLIED
Tablets: 1.25 mg, 2.5 mg, 5 mg
Tablets (micronized): 1.5 mg, 3 mg, 6 mg

ACTION
Unknown. A sulfonylurea that probably stimulates insulin release from the pancreatic beta cells and reduces glucose output by the liver. An extrapancreatic effect increases peripheral sensitivity to insulin and causes a mild diuretic effect.

Route	Onset	Peak	Duration
PO	1-4 hr	4 hr	24 hr

INDICATIONS & DOSAGE
Adjunct to diet to lower blood glucose level in patients with type 2 (non-insulin-dependent) diabetes mellitus—
Adults: initially, 2.5 to 5 mg regular

tablets P.O. once daily with breakfast or first main meal. Usual maintenance dosage is 1.25 to 20 mg daily as a single dose or in divided doses.

Alternatively, micronized formulation may be used. Initial dosage is 1.5 to 3 mg daily. Usual maintenance dosage of the micronized formulation is 0.75 to 12 mg/day. Patients receiving above 6 mg/day may have a better response with b.i.d. dosing.

Adjust-a-dose: In patients who are more sensitive to antidiabetic agents, initially 1.25 mg daily. Patients with adrenal or pituitary insufficiency should start with 1.25 mg daily. When using micronized tablets, patients who are more sensitive to antidiabetic agents should be started at 0.75 mg daily.

To replace insulin therapy—
Adults: if insulin dosage is below 40 units/day, patient may be switched directly to glyburide when insulin is discontinued. If insulin dosage is 40 or more units/day, initially 5-mg regular tablets or 3-mg micronized formulation P.O. once daily in addition to 50% of insulin dosage.

ADVERSE REACTIONS
EENT: changes in accommodation or blurred vision.
GI: nausea, epigastric fullness, heartburn.
Hematologic: leukopenia, hemolytic anemia, *agranulocytosis, thrombocytopenia, aplastic anemia.*
Hepatic: cholestatic jaundice, hepatitis, abnormal liver function.
Skin: rash, pruritus, other allergic reactions.
Other: *hypoglycemia,* arthralgia, myalgia, angioedema.

INTERACTIONS
Drug-drug. *Anabolic steroids, chloramphenicol, clofibrate, guanethidine, MAO inhibitors, salicylates, sulfonamides:* increased hypoglycemic activity. Monitor blood glucose level.
Beta blockers: prolonged hypoglycemic effect and masked symptoms of hypoglycemia. Use together cautiously.
Corticosteroids, glucagon, rifampin, thi-

azide diuretics: decreased hypoglycemic response. Monitor blood glucose level.
Hydantoins: increased blood levels of hydantoins. Monitor blood levels.
Oral anticoagulants: increased hypoglycemic activity or enhanced anticoagulant effect. Monitor blood glucose level and PT.
Drug-lifestyle. *Alcohol use:* altered glycemic control, most commonly hypoglycemia. May also cause disulfiram-like reaction. Discourage concomitant use.

EFFECTS ON DIAGNOSTIC TESTS
Glyburide therapy alters cholesterol, alkaline phosphatase, and BUN levels.

CONTRAINDICATIONS
Contraindicated in patients hypersensitive to drug or in those with diabetic ketoacidosis with or without coma, and during pregnant or breast-feeding women.

NURSING CONSIDERATIONS
• Use cautiously in patients with hepatic or renal impairment, or in debilitated, malnourished, or elderly patients.
• Know that elderly patients may be more sensitive to adverse effects.
Alert: Know that micronized glyburide (Glynase PresTab) contains drug in a smaller particle size and is not bioequivalent to regular glyburide tablets. Patients who have been taking Micronase or DiaBeta need to be retitrated.
• Know that although most patients may take glyburide once daily, those taking more than 10 mg daily may achieve better results with twice-daily dosage.
• Know that glyburide is a second-generation sulfonylurea. The frequency of adverse effects appears to be lower than with first-generation drugs, such as chlorpropamide.
• During periods of increased stress, such as infection, fever, surgery, or trauma, patients may require insulin therapy. Monitor patient closely for hyperglycemia in these situations.
• Know that patient transferring from insulin to an oral antidiabetic agent requires blood glucose monitoring at least three times daily before meals. Patient may require hospitalization during transition.

☑Patient teaching
• Instruct patient about nature of disease, importance of following therapeutic regimen, adhering to specific diet, weight reduction, exercise, and personal hygiene programs, and about avoiding infection. Explain how and when to perform self-monitoring of blood glucose levels, and teach recognition of and intervention for hypoglycemia and hyperglycemia.
• Tell patient not to change drug dosage without doctor's consent and to report abnormal blood or urine glucose test results.
• Teach patient to carry candy or other simple sugars to treat mild hypoglycemic episodes. Severe episodes may require hospital treatment.
• Advise patient not to take other medications, including OTC drugs, without first checking with doctor.
• Advise patient to carry medical identification at all times.
Alert: Instruct patient to report episodes of hypoglycemia to doctor immediately; severe hypoglycemia is sometimes fatal in patients receiving as little as 2.5 to 5 mg glyburide daily.
• Inform patient that alcohol may lower blood glucose levels and should be avoided.

---

insulins
insulin injection (regular insulin, crystalline zinc insulin)
Actrapid‡, Actrapid Penfill‡, Humulin-R◇, Hypurin Neutral‡, Insulin 2 Neutral‡, Novolin R◇, Novolin R PenFill◇, Pork Regular Iletin II◇, Regular (Concentrated) Iletin II, Regular Iletin I◇, Regular Purified Pork Insulin◇, Velosulin Human BR†

insulin (lispro)
Humalog

insulin zinc suspension, prompt (semilente)
Human Monotard§, Hypurin Lente§, Lentard MC§

isophane insulin suspension (neutral protamine Hagedorn insulin, NPH)
Humulin N◇, Humulin NPH‡, Hypurin Isophane‡, Isotard MC‡, Novolin N◇, Novolin N Penfill◇, NPH insulin◇, NPH Purified Pork◇, Purified Pork NPH Iletin II◇, Protaphane‡, Protaphane Penfill‡

isophane insulin suspension with insulin injection
Humulin 50/50◇, Humulin 70/30◇, Novolin 70/30, Novolin 70/30 PenFill◇

insulin zinc suspension (lente)
Humulin L◇, Lente Iletin II◇, Lente Insulin◇, Lente MC‡, Lente Purified Pork Insulin◇, Novolin L◇

protamine zinc suspension (PZI)
Hypurin Bovine Protamine Zinc§

insulin zinc suspension, extended (ultralente)
Humulin-U◇, Ultralente Insulin◇

Pregnancy Risk Category: NR

HOW SUPPLIED
insulin injection
Injection (human): 100 units/ml (Humulin-R◇, Novolin R◇, Velosulin Human BR‡); 100 units/ml in 1.5-ml cartridge system◇ (Novolin R PenFill◇)
Injection (from pork): 100 units/ml◇
Injection (purified beef): 100 units/ml (Hypurin Neutral‡, Insulin 2 Neutral‡)
Injection (purified pork): 100 units/ml (Actrapid‡, Pork Regular Iletin II◇, Regular Purified Pork Insulin◇); 100 units/ml in 1.5-ml cartridge system‡ (Actrapid Penfill‡); 100 units/ml in 2-ml cartridge system‡; 500 units/ml (Regular [Concentrated] Iletin II)
insulin lispro injection
Injection (human): 100 units/ml (Humalog)

---

insulin zinc suspension, prompt
Injection (purified pork): 100 units/ml ◇
isophane insulin suspension
Injection (from beef): 100 units/ml ◇
(NPH Insulin ◇)
Injection (human, recombinant):
100 units/ml (Humulin N ◇, Humulin
NPH‡, Novolin N ◇); 100 units/ml in
1.5-ml cartridge system (Novolin N
PenFill ◇, Protaphane HM PenFill‡)
Injection (purified beef): 100 units/ml
(Hypurin Isophane‡, Isotard MC‡)
Injection (purified pork): 100 units/ml
(NPH Purified Pork ◇, Pork NPH Iletin
II, Protaphane‡)
**isophane insulin suspension 50% with
insulin injection 50%**
Injection (human): 100 units/ml
(Humulin 50/50 ◇)
**isophane insulin suspension 70% with
insulin injection 30%**
Injection (human): 100 units/ml
(Humulin 70/30 ◇, Novolin 70/30 ◇);
100 units/ml in 1.5-ml cartridge system
(Novolin 70/30 PenFill ◇)
insulin zinc suspension
Injection (from beef): 100 units/ml (Lente
Insulin ◇, Lente MC‡)
Injection (purified beef): 100 units/ml
(Lente MC‡)
Injection (purified pork): 100 units/ml
(Lente Iletin II, Lente Purified Pork
Insulin ◇)
Injection (human): 100 units/ml ◇
(Humulin L ◇, Novolin I ◇)
protamine zinc suspension
Injection (purified beef): 100 units/ml
(Protamine Zinc Insulin§)
insulin zinc suspension, extended
Injection (from beef): 100 units/ml ◇
(Ultralente Insulin ◇)
Injection (human): 100 units/ml
(Humulin U ◇)

ACTION
Increases glucose transport across muscle
and fat cell membranes to reduce blood
glucose level. Promotes conversion of
glucose to its storage form, glycogen;
triggers amino acid uptake and conversion
to protein in muscle cells and inhibits protein degradation; stimulates triglyceride
formation and inhibits release of free fatty
acids from adipose tissue; and stimulates
lipoprotein lipase activity, which converts
circulating lipoproteins to fatty acids.

Route	Onset	Peak	Duration
IV (rapid)	10-30 min	15-30 min	0.5-1 hr
SC (rapid)	0.5-1.5 hr	2-3 hr	5-7 hr
SC (inter-mediate)	1-2.5 hr	4-15 hr	12-24 hr
SC (long-acting)	4-8 hr	10-30 hr	36 hr

INDICATIONS & DOSAGE
*Diabetic ketoacidosis (use regular insulin
only)—*
Adults: 0.33 units/kg as an I.V. bolus, followed by 0.1 units/kg/hour by continuous
infusion. Continue infusion until blood
glucose level drops to 250 mg/dl; then
S.C. insulin is begun with dosage, and
dosage interval is adjusted according to
patient's blood glucose concentration.
    Alternatively, 50 to 100 units I.V. and
50 to 100 units S.C. immediately; then
additional doses q 2 to 6 hours based on
blood glucose levels.
    To prepare infusion, add 100 units of
regular insulin and 1 g of albumin to
100 ml of 0.9% NaCl solution. Insulin
concentration will be 1 unit/ml. (The albumin will adhere to plastic, preventing
insulin from adhering to plastic.)
Children: 0.1 unit/kg as an I.V. bolus,
then 0.1 unit/kg hourly by continuous infusion until blood glucose level drops to
250 mg/dl; then S.C. insulin started. Alternatively, 1 to 2 units/kg in two divided
doses, one I.V. and the other S.C., followed by 0.5 to 1 unit/kg I.V. q 1 to 2
hours based on blood glucose levels.
*Type 1 (insulin-dependent) diabetes, ad-
junct to type 2 (non-insulin-dependent)
diabetes inadequately controlled by diet
and oral antidiabetic agents—*
Adults and children: therapeutic regimen is prescribed by doctor and adjusted
based on patient's blood glucose concentrations.

ADVERSE REACTIONS
Skin: urticaria, pruritus, swelling, redness, stinging, warmth at injection site.
Other: *lipoatrophy, lipohypertrophy,* hypersensitivity reactions (***anaphylaxis,***

Reactions may be *common*, uncommon, *life-threatening*, or COMMON AND LIFE-THREATENING.

rash), *hypoglycemia,* hyperglycemia (rebound, or Somogyi effect).

INTERACTIONS
Drug-drug. *Anabolic steroids, beta blockers, clofibrate, fenfluramine, guanethidine, MAO inhibitors, salicylates, tetracycline:* prolonged hypoglycemic effect. Monitor blood glucose level carefully.
Corticosteroids, dextrothyroxine, epinephrine, thiazide diuretics, thyroid hormone: diminished insulin response. Monitor for hyperglycemia.
Diazoxide, phenytoin (high doses): may inhibit endogenous insulin secretion and cause hypoglycemia in diabetic patients. Carefully adjust insulin dosage when using with these drugs.
Oral contraceptives: may decrease glucose tolerance in diabetic patients. Monitor blood glucose levels and adjust insulin dosage carefully.
Drug-herb. *Basil, bay, bee pollen, burdock, sage:* may affect glycemic control. Monitor blood sugar closely.
Garlic dust, ginseng: may decrease blood glucose concentrations. Monitor for effects.
Drug-lifestyle. *Alcohol use:* hypoglycemic effect. Discourage concomitant use.
Marijuana use: may increase serum glucose concentrations. Patients should take action to reduce this risk.
Smoking: may increase glucose concentrations and decrease response to insulin administration. Monitor glucose levels.

EFFECTS ON DIAGNOSTIC TESTS
Physiologic effects of insulin may decrease serum magnesium, potassium, or inorganic phosphate concentrations.

CONTRAINDICATIONS
Contraindicated in patients with history of systemic allergic reaction to pork.

NURSING CONSIDERATIONS
● Know that insulin is drug of choice to treat diabetes during pregnancy. Insulin requirements increase in pregnant diabetic patients and then decline immediately postpartum. Monitor patient closely.
● Dosage is always expressed in USP units.

Remember to use only the syringes calibrated for the particular concentration of insulin administered. U-500 insulin must be administered with a U-100 syringe because no syringes are made for this strength.
● Be aware that some patients may develop insulin resistance and require large insulin doses to control symptoms of diabetes. U-500 insulin is available as Regular (Concentrated) Iletin II for such patients. Although not every pharmacy may stock it, it is available. Be sure to give the hospital pharmacy sufficient notice before requesting refill of in-house prescription. Never store U-500 insulin in same area with other insulin preparations because of danger of severe overdose if given accidentally to other patients.
● To mix insulin suspension, swirl vial gently or rotate between palms or between palm and thigh. Do not shake vigorously—this causes bubbling and air in syringe.
● Know that lente, semilente, and ultralente insulins may be mixed in any proportion. Regular insulin may be mixed with NPH or lente insulins in any proportion. When mixing regular insulin with intermediate or long-acting insulin, always draw up regular insulin into syringe first.
● Note that switching from separate injections to a prepared mixture may alter patient response. Whenever NPH or lente is mixed with regular insulin in the same syringe, give it immediately to avoid loss of potency.
● Lispro insulin may be mixed with Humulin N or Humulin U and should be given within 15 minutes before a meal to prevent a hypoglycemic reaction.
● Do not use insulin that changes color or becomes clumped or granular in appearance.
● Check expiration date on vial before using contents.
● Know that usual administration route is S.C. For proper S.C. administration, remember to pinch a fold of skin with the fingers at least 3" (7.6 cm) apart, and insert needle at a 45- to 90-degree angle.
● Press but do not rub site after injection. Rotate injection sites and chart to avoid

overuse of one area. Know that diabetic patients may achieve better control if injection site is rotated within same anatomic region.

• Store insulin in cool area. Refrigeration is desirable but not essential, except with regular insulin (concentrated).

I.V. administration
• Administer only regular insulin I.V. Inject directly into vein at ordered rate through an intermittent infusion device or into a port close to I.V. access site. Intermittent infusion is not recommended. If given by continuous infusion, infuse drug diluted in 0.9% NaCl at the prescribed rate.

Alert: Know that regular insulin is used in patients with circulatory collapse, diabetic ketoacidosis, or hyperkalemia. Do not use regular insulin (concentrated), 500 units/ml, I.V. Do not use intermediate- or long-acting insulins for coma or other emergency requiring rapid drug action. Also know that ketosis-prone type 1, severely ill, and newly diagnosed diabetic patients with very high blood glucose levels may require hospitalization and I.V. treatment with regular fast-acting insulin.

✔Patient teaching
• Make sure patient knows that therapy only relieves symptoms.

• Instruct patient about nature of disease, importance of following the therapeutic regimen, adhering to specific diet, weight reduction, exercise, and personal hygiene program, and about avoiding infection. Emphasize the importance of the timing of injections and eating, and that meals must not be omitted.

• Stress that accuracy of measurement is important, especially with concentrated regular insulin. Aids, such as magnifying sleeve or dose magnifier, may improve accuracy. Instruct patient and caregivers how to measure and administer insulin.

• Advise patient not to alter the order of mixing insulins or change the model or brand of insulin, syringe, or needle.

• Teach patient that self-monitoring of blood glucose levels and urine ketone tests are essential guides to dosage and success of therapy. It is important for pa-

tient to recognize hyperglycemic and hypoglycemic symptoms. Insulin-induced hypoglycemia is hazardous and may cause brain damage if prolonged; most adverse effects are self-limiting and temporary. Instruct patient in insulin peak times and their importance.

• Instruct patient on proper use of equipment for performing self-monitoring of blood glucose levels.

• Advise patient not to smoke within 30 minutes after insulin injection. Cigarette smoking decreases the amount of absorption of insulin administered S.C.

• Tell patient that marijuana use may increase insulin requirements.

• Advise patient to wear a medical identification bracelet at all times, to carry ample insulin and syringes on trips, to have carbohydrates (lump of sugar or candy) on hand for emergencies, and to note time zone changes for dosage schedule when traveling.

---

metformin hydrochloride
Glucophage

Pregnancy Risk Category: B

HOW SUPPLIED
Tablets: 500 mg, 850 mg

ACTION
Decreases hepatic glucose production and intestinal absorption of glucose and improves insulin sensitivity (increases peripheral glucose uptake and utilization).

Route	Onset	Peak	Duration
PO	Unknown	Unknown	Unknown

INDICATIONS & DOSAGE
Adjunct to diet to lower blood glucose level in patients with type 2 (non-insulin-dependent) diabetes mellitus—
Adults: initially, 500 mg P.O. b.i.d. given with morning and evening meals, or 850 mg P.O. once daily given with morning meal. When 500-mg dose form used, dosage increased 500 mg weekly to maximum dosage of 2,500 mg P.O. daily in divided doses p.r.n. When 850-mg dose form used, dosage increased 850 mg

---

every other week to maximum dosage of 2,550 mg P.O. daily in divided doses, p.r.n.
Elderly: in patients over 65 years, dosing should be conservative because of potential decrease in renal function.
Adjust-a-dose: In debilitated patients, dosing should be conservative because of potential decrease in renal function.

ADVERSE REACTIONS
GI: diarrhea, nausea, vomiting, abdominal bloating, flatulence, anorexia, unpleasant or metallic taste.
Hematologic: megaloblastic anemia.
Other: *lactic acidosis.*

INTERACTIONS
Drug-drug. *Calcium channel blockers, corticosteroids, estrogens, isoniazid, nicotinic acid, oral contraceptives, phenothiazines, phenytoin, sympathomimetics, thiazide and other diuretics, thyroid agents:* may produce hyperglycemia. Monitor patient's glycemic control. Metformin dosage may need to be increased.
Cationic drugs (such as amiloride, cimetidine, digoxin, morphine, procainamide, quinidine, quinine, ranitidine, triamterene, trimethoprim, vancomycin): have the potential to compete for common renal tubular transport systems, which may increase metformin plasma levels. Monitor patient's blood glucose level.
Nifedipine: increased metformin plasma levels. Monitor patient closely. Metformin dosage may need to be decreased.
Radiologic contrast dye: can result in acute renal failure. Withhold metformin for 24 hours before procedure.
Drug-lifestyle. *Alcohol use:* potentiated drug's effects. Avoid concurrent use.

EFFECTS ON DIAGNOSTIC TESTS
None reported.

CONTRAINDICATIONS
Contraindicated in patients with renal disease, metabolic acidosis, or hypersensitivity to drug. Drug should be temporarily withheld in patients undergoing radiologic studies involving parenteral administration of iodinated contrast materials because use of such products may result in acute renal dysfunction. Drug should also be promptly discontinued if patient enters a hypoxic state. Avoid use in patients with hepatic disease.

NURSING CONSIDERATIONS
● Use caution when giving drug to elderly, debilitated, or malnourished patients and to those with adrenal or pituitary insufficiency because of increased risk of hypoglycemia.
● Know that before therapy begins, and at least annually thereafter, patient's renal function should be assessed. If renal impairment is detected, expect doctor to switch patient to a different antidiabetic agent. This is particularly important in elderly patients.
● Administer with meals; once-daily dosage should be given with breakfast and twice-daily dosage with breakfast and dinner.
● Know that when transferring patients from standard oral hypoglycemic agents (except chlorpropamide) to metformin, no transition period generally is necessary. When switching patients from chlorpropamide to metformin, care should be exercised during the first 2 weeks of metformin therapy because the prolonged retention of chlorpropamide increases risk of hypoglycemia during this time.
● Monitor patient's blood glucose levels regularly to evaluate effectiveness of therapy. Notify doctor if blood glucose levels become elevated despite therapy.
● Be aware that if patient has not responded to 4 weeks of therapy using the maximum dosage, doctor may add an oral sulfonylurea while continuing metformin at the maximum dosage. If patient still does not respond after several months of concomitant therapy at maximum dosages, doctor may discontinue both agents and institute insulin therapy.
● Monitor patient closely during times of increased stress, such as infection, fever, surgery, or trauma. Insulin therapy may be needed in these situations.
● Be aware that incidence of drug-induced lactic acidosis is very low. Reported cases have occurred primarily in diabetic patients with significant renal insufficiency; with multiple, concomitant medical or surgical problems; and with multiple,

concomitant drug regimens. The risk increases with the degree of renal impairment and patient's age.

Alert: Know that drug should be discontinued immediately and doctor notified if patient develops a condition associated with hypoxemia or dehydration because of risk of lactic acidosis associated with these conditions.

• Expect drug therapy to be temporarily suspended for any surgical procedure (except minor procedures not associated with restricted intake of food and fluids), and for patients undergoing radiologic studies involving the use of contrast media containing iodine. Therapy should not be restarted until the patient's oral intake has resumed and renal function has been evaluated as normal, as instructed by doctor.

• Monitor patient's hematologic status for evidence of megaloblastic anemia. Patients with inadequate vitamin B_{12} or calcium intake or absorption appear to be predisposed to developing subnormal vitamin B_{12} levels. These patients should have routine serum vitamin B_{12} level determinations every 2 to 3 years.

☑**Patient teaching**

Alert: Instruct patient about nature of diabetes, importance of following therapeutic regimen, adhering to specific diet, weight reduction, exercise, personal hygiene programs, and avoiding infection. Explain how and when to perform self-monitoring of blood glucose level, and teach signs of hypoglycemia and hyperglycemia and emergency measures.

• Instruct patient to discontinue drug and notify doctor immediately if unexplained hyperventilation, myalgia, malaise, unusual somnolence, or other nonspecific symptoms of early lactic acidosis occur.

• Warn patient not to consume excessive alcohol while taking drug.

• Tell patient not to change drug dosage without doctor's consent. Encourage patient to report abnormal blood glucose results.

• Advise patient not to take other medications, including OTC drugs, without checking with doctor.

• Instruct patient to carry medical identification at all times.

▼ *NEW DRUG*

repaglinide
Prandin

Pregnancy Risk Category: C

HOW SUPPLIED
Tablets: 0.5 mg, 1 mg, 2 mg

ACTION
Stimulates the release of insulin from the beta cells in the pancreas by closing ATP-dependent potassium channels in the beta cell membrane, which causes opening of the calcium channels. The increased calcium influx induces insulin secretion; the overall effect is to lower the blood glucose level.

Route	Onset	Peak	Duration
PO	Unknown	1 hr	Unknown

INDICATIONS & DOSAGE
Adjunct to diet and exercise in lowering blood glucose in patient with type 2 (non-insulin-dependent) diabetes mellitus whose hyperglycemia cannot be controlled by diet and exercise alone; in combination with metformin to lower blood glucose in patients whose hyperglycemia cannot be controlled by exercise, diet, and either repaglinide or metformin alone—
Adults: for patients not previously treated or whose glycosylated hemoglobin (HbA_{1c}) is below 8%, initially 0.5 mg P.O. taken immediately to 30 minutes before each meal; for those previously treated with glucose-lowering drugs and whose HbA_{1c} is 8% or more, initially 1 to 2 mg P.O. taken immediately to 30 minutes before each meal. Recommended dosage range is 0.5 to 4 mg with meals divided b.i.d., t.i.d., or q.i.d. Maximum daily dosage is 16 mg.

ADVERSE REACTIONS
CNS: *headache,* paresthesia.
CV: angina, chest pain.
EENT: rhinitis, sinusitis, tooth disorder.
GI: constipation, diarrhea, dyspepsia, nausea, vomiting.
GU: urinary tract infection.

Reactions may be *common,* uncommon, *life-threatening,* or COMMON AND LIFE-THREATENING.

Metabolic: HYPOGLYCEMIA, hyperglycemia.
Musculoskeletal: arthralgia, back pain.
Respiratory: bronchitis, *upper respiratory infection.*

INTERACTIONS
Drug-drug. *Barbiturates, carbamazepine, rifampin, troglitazone:* may increase metabolism of repaglinide. Monitor glucose level.
Beta-adrenergic blocking agents, chloramphenicol, coumarins, MAO inhibitors, NSAIDs, others drugs that are highly protein-bound, probenecid, salicylates, sulfonamides: may potentiate hypoglycemic action of repaglinide. Monitor glucose level.
Calcium channel blocking drugs, corticosteroids, estrogens, isoniazid, nicotinic acid, oral contraceptives, phenothiazines, phenytoin, sympathomimetics, thiazides and other diuretics, thyroid products: may produce hyperglycemia resulting in a loss of glycemic control. Monitor glucose level.
Erythromycin, inhibitors of P-450 cytochrome system 3A4, ketoconazole, miconazole: may inhibit the metabolism of repaglinide. Monitor glucose levels.

EFFECTS ON DIAGNOSTIC TESTS
None reported.

CONTRAINDICATIONS
Contraindicated in patients with type 1 (insulin-dependent) diabetes mellitus, diabetic ketoacidosis, or hypersensitivity to drug or its inactive ingredients.

NURSING CONSIDERATIONS
• Use cautiously in patients with hepatic insufficiency in whom reduced metabolism could cause elevated blood levels of repaglinide and hypoglycemia.
• Use cautiously in elderly, debilitated, or malnourished patients and those with adrenal or pituitary insufficiency because they are more susceptible to the hypoglycemic effect of glucose-lowering drugs.
• Make increases in drug dosage carefully in patients with impaired renal function or renal failure requiring dialysis.
• Adjust dosage by blood glucose response. May double dosage up to 4 mg

with each meal until satisfactory blood glucose response is achieved. At least 1 week should elapse between dosage adjustments to assess response to each dose.
• Know that metformin may be added if repaglinide monotherapy is inadequate.
• Know that administration of oral antidiabetic drugs has been reported to be associated with increased CV mortality compared with diet alone or diet plus insulin treatment. Although drug was not included in original study, this warning may also apply to repaglinide.
• Be aware that loss of glycemic control can occur during stress, such as fever, trauma, infection, or surgery. Discontinue drug as ordered and administer insulin.
• Know that hypoglycemia may be difficult to recognize in the elderly and in patients taking beta-adrenergic blocking agents.

☑ Patient teaching
• Instruct patient on importance of diet and exercise in combination with drug therapy.
• Discuss symptoms of hypoglycemia with patient and family.
• Advise patient to monitor blood glucose periodically to determine minimum effective dose.
• Encourage patient to keep regular appointments and have his HbA_{1c} levels checked every 3 months to determine long-term glucose control.
• Tell patient to administer drug before meals, usually 15 minutes before start of meal; however, time can vary from immediately preceding meal to up to 30 minutes before meal.
• Tell patient that if a meal is skipped or an extra meal added, he should skip the dose or add an extra dose of drug for that meal.
• Instruct patient to monitor blood glucose carefully along with what to do when he is ill, undergoing surgery, or under added stress.

---

troglitazone
Rezulin

Pregnancy Risk Category: B

HOW SUPPLIED
Tablets: 200 mg, 400 mg

ACTION
Inhibits hepatic glucose production and enhances effects of circulating insulin.

Route	Onset	Peak	Duration
PO	Rapid	2-3 hr	Unknown

INDICATIONS & DOSAGE
Adjunct to diet and insulin therapy in patients with type 2 (non-insulin-dependent) diabetes mellitus whose hyperglycemia is inadequately controlled with insulin therapy of over 30 units/day given as multiple injections—
Adults: initially, continue with current insulin and begin concomitant therapy with 200 mg P.O. once daily, taken with a meal. May increase dosage after 2 to 4 weeks if needed. Usual daily dose is 400 mg; maximum daily dose is 600 mg. Insulin dose may be decreased by 10% to 25% when fasting glucose levels are below 120 mg/dl in patients receiving both troglitazone and insulin.
In combination with sulfonylureas in patients with type 2 diabetes mellitus—
Adults: initially, 200 mg P.O. daily; continue current sulfonylurea dose. Increase dosage after 2 to 4 weeks p.r.n. to maximum dose of 600 mg/day. Sulfonylurea dose may have to be lowered.
As monotherapy for patients with type 2 diabetes mellitus not controlled with diet alone—
Adults: initially, 400 mg P.O. once daily. Dosage may be increased to 600 mg after 1 month if needed. For patients not responding to 600 mg after 1 month, discontinue drug and consider alternative therapeutic options.

ADVERSE REACTIONS
CNS: *headache,* asthenia, dizziness.
CV: peripheral edema.
EENT: rhinitis, pharyngitis.
GI: nausea, diarrhea.
GU: urinary tract infection.
Hepatic: *hepatotoxicity*.
Musculoskeletal: back pain.
Other: *infection, pain,* accidental injury.

INTERACTIONS
Drug-drug. *Cholestyramine:* reduced absorption of troglitazone. Avoid concomitant use.
Oral contraceptives: may reduce plasma concentrations of hormones, resulting in loss of contraceptive properties. Additional form of contraception is recommended.
Drug-food. *Any food:* increased absorption. Take drug with food.

EFFECTS ON DIAGNOSTIC TESTS
Drug may cause transient elevations in AST and ALT levels, small increases in serum lipid levels, and small decreases in hemoglobin, hematocrit, and neutrophil counts.

CONTRAINDICATIONS
Contraindicated in patients with active liver disease or known hypersensitivity to drug. Rare cases of severe idiosyncratic hepatocellular injury have been reported. The injury is usually reversible, but very rare cases of hepatic failure, including death, have been reported. Injury has occurred after both short- and long-term treatment. Drug should not be initiated in patients with ALT levels over 1.5 times the upper limit of normal.

NURSING CONSIDERATIONS
• Use cautiously in heart failure patients with New York Heart Association class III and IV status.
Alert: Be aware that liver enzyme levels should be measured at start of therapy, every month for first 8 months of treatment, then every 2 months for rest of year, and periodically thereafter. In addition, liver function tests should be performed on patient receiving drug who develops symptoms of liver dysfunction, such as nausea, vomiting, fatigue, loss of appetite, jaundice, or dark urine. Discontinue drug if patient has jaundice or if results of liver function tests suggest liver injury.

Reactions may be *common*, uncommon, ***life-threatening***, or COMMON AND LIFE-THREATENING.

• Know that drug should be used in pregnancy only if the benefit justifies the potential risk to the fetus. The preferred antidiabetic agent to be used during pregnancy is insulin. Breast-feeding women should not take troglitazone.

• Safety and effectiveness in children have not been established.

• Be aware that drug does not stimulate insulin secretion; it should not be used to treat patients with type 1 diabetes or ketoacidosis.

• When used concomitantly with insulin, monitor patient for hypoglycemia. Know that dose of insulin may need to be reduced.

• Before starting drug therapy, investigate and address secondary causes of poor glycemic control (including infection and poor injection technique).

• Monitor glucose levels, especially during times of increased stress, such as infection, fever, surgery, and trauma.

✓ Patient teaching

• Instruct patient about nature of diabetes, importance of following treatment, avoiding infection, and adhering to specific diet, weight reduction, exercise, and personal hygiene programs. Explain how and when to perform self-monitoring of blood glucose level; teach patient and family members signs of hypoglycemia and hyperglycemia and explain what to do if those conditions occur.

• Tell patient that drug should be taken with a meal; if a dose is missed, it may be taken with the next meal, but do not take two doses the next day.

• Instruct patient to notify doctor immediately if signs of liver injury develop, like fatigue, nausea, vomiting, yellow skin or eyes, or dark urine.

• Inform patient that drug may cause resumption of ovulation in premenopausal, anovulatory women, increasing the risk for pregnancy.

• Instruct patient to carry medical identification at all times.

58

Thyroid hormones

levothyroxine sodium
liothyronine sodium
liotrix
thyroid

COMBINATION PRODUCTS
None.

---

levothyroxine sodium (T₄, L-thyroxine sodium)

Eltroxin†, Levo-T, Levothroid, Levoxine, Levoxyl, Oroxine‡, Synthroid**

Pregnancy Risk Category: A

HOW SUPPLIED
Tablets: 25 mcg, 50 mcg, 75 mcg, 88 mcg, 100 mcg, 112 mcg, 125 mcg, 137 mcg, 150 mcg, 175 mcg, 200 mcg, 300 mcg
Injection: 200-mcg vial, 500-mcg vial

ACTION
Not completely defined. Stimulates metabolism of all body tissues by accelerating rate of cellular oxidation.

Route	Onset	Peak	Duration
PO	24 hr	Unknown	Unknown
IV	Unknown	Unknown	Unknown

INDICATIONS & DOSAGE
Cretinism—
Children up to 6 months: 25 to 50 mcg or 5 to 6 mcg/kg P.O. daily.
Children 6 to 12 months: 50 to 75 mcg or 5 to 6 mcg/kg P.O. daily.
Children 1 to 5 years: 75 to 100 mcg or 3 to 5 mcg/kg P.O. daily.
Children 6 to 12 years: 100 to 150 mcg or 4 to 5 mcg/kg P.O. daily.
Children over 12 years: over 150 mcg or 2 to 3 mcg/kg P.O. daily.
Myxedema coma—
Adults: 200 to 500 mcg I.V.; then 100 to 300 mcg given on second day, followed by parenteral maintenance dosage of 50 to 200 mcg I.V. daily. Switch patient to oral maintenance as soon as possible.
Thyroid hormone replacement—
Adults: initially, 25 to 50 mcg P.O. daily, increased by 25 mcg P.O. q 2 to 4 weeks until desired response occurs. Maintenance dosage is 75 to 200 mcg P.O. daily. May administer I.V. or I.M. when P.O. ingestion is precluded for long periods. However, dosage adjustment is necessary.
Elderly: in patients over 65 years, 12.5 to 50 mcg P.O. daily. Increased by 12.5 to 25 mcg at 3- to 8-week intervals, depending on response.
Children: in children under 1 year, initial dose is 25 to 50 mcg P.O. daily; in children 1 year and older, 3 to 5 mcg/kg P.O. daily. Gradually increased by 25 to 50 mcg q 2 to 4 weeks until desired response occurs.

ADVERSE REACTIONS
CNS: *nervousness, insomnia, tremor,* headache.
CV: *tachycardia, palpitations,* **arrhythmias,** *angina pectoris,* **cardiac arrest.**
GI: diarrhea, vomiting.
Other: weight loss, diaphoresis, heat intolerance, fever, menstrual irregularities, allergic skin reactions.

INTERACTIONS
Drug-drug. *Cholestyramine, colestipol:* impaired levothyroxine absorption. Separate doses by 4 to 5 hours.
Estrogens: decreased free levothyroxines. Monitor for decreased effectiveness of thyroid hormone.
Insulin, oral antidiabetic agents: altered serum glucose levels. Monitor blood glucose levels. Dosage adjustments may be necessary.
I.V. phenytoin: free thyroid released. Monitor for tachycardia.
Oral anticoagulants: altered PT. Monitor PT and INR; dosage adjustments may be necessary.
Sympathomimetics (such as epinephrine):

Reactions may be *common,* uncommon, ***life-threatening,*** or **COMMON AND LIFE-THREATENING.**

increased risk of coronary insufficiency. Monitor closely.

EFFECTS ON DIAGNOSTIC TESTS
Drug therapy alters radioactive iodine (^{131}I) thyroid uptake, protein-bound iodine levels, and liothyronine uptake.

CONTRAINDICATIONS
Contraindicated in patients with acute MI uncomplicated by hypothyroidism, untreated thyrotoxicosis, uncorrected adrenal insufficiency, or hypersensitivity to drug.

NURSING CONSIDERATIONS
● Use with extreme caution in elderly patients and those with angina pectoris, hypertension, other CV disorders, renal insufficiency, or ischemia.
● Use cautiously in those with diabetes mellitus, insipidus, or myxedema. Patients with diabetes mellitus may require increased doses of antidiabetic medication when beginning thyroid hormone replacement.
● Rapid replacement in patients with arteriosclerosis may precipitate angina, coronary occlusion, or CVA. Use cautiously in these patients. Also, in patients with coronary artery disease who must receive thyroid hormone, observe carefully for possible coronary insufficiency.
● Know that thyroid hormone replacement requirements are about 25% lower in patients over 60 years than in young adults.
● Also know that patients with adult hypothyroidism are unusually sensitive to thyroid hormone. Patient should be started at lowest dosage and titrated to higher dosages according to patient's symptoms and laboratory data until euthyroid state is reached.
● When changing from levothyroxine to liothyronine (T_3), levothyroxine should be stopped and liothyronine begun. Dosage should be increased in small increments after residual effects of levothyroxine have disappeared. When changing from liothyronine to levothyroxine, levothyroxine is started several days before withdrawing liothyronine to avoid relapse.
● Know that thyroid hormones alter thyroid function test results.

● Be aware that patients taking levothyroxine who need to have ^{131}I uptake studies performed must discontinue drug 4 weeks before test.
● Know that patients on anticoagulant therapy may need their dose modified; also careful monitoring of coagulation status is necessary.

◖ I.V. administration
● Prepare I.V. dose immediately before injection. Do not mix with other solutions. Inject into vein over 1 to 2 minutes.
● Monitor blood pressure and heart rate closely. High initial I.V. dosage is usually well tolerated by patients in myxedema coma. Normal serum levels of T_4 should occur within 24 hours, followed by a threefold increase in serum T_3 in 3 days.

✓ Patient teaching
● Make sure patient understands importance of compliance. Tell him to take thyroid hormones at same time each day, preferably before breakfast, to maintain constant hormone levels. Suggest morning dosage to prevent insomnia.
● Make sure patient understands that replacement therapy is for a lifetime.
● Warn patient (especially elderly patient) to notify doctor at once if chest pain, palpitations, sweating, nervousness, shortness of breath, or other signs of overdose or aggravated CV disease occur.
● Advise patient who has achieved stable response not to change brands.
● Tell patient to report unusual bleeding and bruising.

---

liothyronine sodium (T_3)
Cytomel, Tertroxin‡, Triostat

Pregnancy Risk Category: A

HOW SUPPLIED
Tablets: 5 mcg, 25 mcg, 50 mcg
Injection: 10 mcg/ml

ACTION
Not clearly defined. Enhances oxygen consumption by most tissues of the body; increases the basal metabolic rate and the

metabolism of carbohydrates, lipids, and proteins.

Route	Onset	Peak	Duration
PO	Unknown	2-3 days	3 days
IV	Unknown	Unknown	Unknown

INDICATIONS & DOSAGE

Congenital hypothyroidism—
Children: 5 mcg P.O. daily with a 5-mcg increase q 3 to 4 days until desired response achieved.
Myxedema—
Adults: initially, 2.5 to 5 mcg P.O. daily, increased by 5 to 10 mcg q 1 or 2 weeks until daily dosage reaches 25 mcg. Then, increased by 12.5 to 25 mcg daily q 1 to 2 weeks. Maintenance dosage is 50 to 100 mcg daily.
Myxedema coma, premyxedema coma—
Adults: initially, 10 to 20 mcg I.V. for patients with known or suspected CV disease; 25 to 50 mcg I.V. for patients not known to have CV disease. Subsequent dosage adjustments made as indicated by patient's condition and response. Switch patient to oral therapy as soon as possible.
Nontoxic goiter—
Adults: initially, 5 mcg P.O. daily; may increase by 5 to 10 mcg daily q 1 to 2 weeks, until daily dosage reaches 25 mcg. Then, increase by 12.5 to 25 mcg daily q 1 to 2 weeks. Usual maintenance dosage is 75 mcg daily.
Thyroid hormone replacement—
Adults: initially, 25 mcg P.O. daily, increased by 12.5 to 25 mcg q 1 to 2 weeks until satisfactory response occurs. Usual maintenance dosage is 25 to 50 mcg daily.
Elderly: in patients over 65 years, 5 mcg daily, increased in 5-mcg daily increments.
T_3 suppression test to differentiate hyperthyroidism from euthyroidism—
Adults: 75 to 100 mcg P.O. daily for 7 days.

ADVERSE REACTIONS

CNS: *nervousness, insomnia, tremor,* headache.
CV: *tachycardia,* **arrhythmias,** angina pectoris, **cardiac decompensation and collapse.**
GI: diarrhea, vomiting.
Other: weight loss, heat intolerance, diaphoresis, accelerated bone maturation in infants and children, menstrual irregularities, skin reactions.

INTERACTIONS

Drug-drug. *Cholestyramine, colestipol:* impaired liothyronine absorption. Separate doses by 4 to 5 hours.
Insulin, oral antidiabetic agents: initial thyroid replacement therapy may cause increases in insulin or oral hypoglycemic requirements. Monitor blood glucose levels. Dosage adjustments may be necessary.
Oral anticoagulants: altered PT. Monitor PT; dosage adjustments may be necessary.
Sympathomimetics (such as epinephrine): increased risk of coronary insufficiency. Monitor closely.

EFFECTS ON DIAGNOSTIC TESTS

Drug therapy alters radioactive iodine (^{131}I) uptake, protein-bound iodine levels, and liothyronine uptake.

CONTRAINDICATIONS

Contraindicated in patients with acute MI uncomplicated by hypothyroidism, untreated thyrotoxicosis, uncorrected adrenal insufficiency, or hypersensitivity to drug.

NURSING CONSIDERATIONS

• Use with extreme caution in elderly patients and those with angina pectoris, hypertension, other CV disorders, renal insufficiency, or ischemia.
• Use cautiously in patients with diabetes mellitus, insipidus, or myxedema.
• Rapid replacement in patients with arteriosclerosis may precipitate angina, coronary occlusion, or CVA. Use cautiously in these patients. In patients with coronary artery disease who must receive thyroid hormones, observe carefully for possible coronary insufficiency.
Alert: Know that levothyroxine is usually the preferred agent for thyroid hormone replacement therapy. Liothyronine may be used when a rapid onset or a rapidly reversible agent is desirable, or in patients with impaired peripheral conversion of levothyroxine to liothyronine.
• Be aware that regulation of liothyronine dosage is difficult.

Reactions may be *common,* uncommon, *life-threatening,* or COMMON AND LIFE-THREATENING.

• Know that thyroid hormone replacement requirements are about 25% lower in patients over 60 years than in young adults.
• Monitor pulse and blood pressure.
• Know that thyroid hormones alter thyroid function tests. Monitor PT; patients taking these hormones usually require decreased anticoagulant dosage.
• When changing from levothyroxine to liothyronine, levothyroxine should be stopped and liothyronine begun at a low dosage. Dosage should be increased in small increments after residual effects of levothyroxine have disappeared. When changing from liothyronine to levothyroxine, levothyroxine is started several days before withdrawing liothyronine to avoid relapse.
• Know that patients taking liothyronine who need ^{131}I uptake studies done must discontinue drug 7 to 10 days before test.

◖I.V. administration
• Repeat dosages should be administered longer than 4 hours but less than 12 hours apart. Do not administer injection I.M. or S.C.

☑Patient teaching
• Make sure patient understands importance of compliance. Tell him to take thyroid hormones at same time each day, preferably before breakfast, to maintain constant hormone levels. Suggest morning dosage to prevent insomnia.
• Make sure patient understands that replacement therapy is for a lifetime.
• Advise patient who has achieved a stable response not to change brands.
• Warn patient (especially elderly patient) to notify doctor at once if chest pain, palpitations, sweating, nervousness, or other signs of overdose or aggravated CV disease occur.
• Tell patient to report unusual bleeding and bruising.

liotrix
Euthroid**, Thyrolar

Pregnancy Risk Category: A

HOW SUPPLIED
Tablets: levothyroxine sodium (T$_4$) 30 mcg and liothyronine sodium (T$_3$) 7.5 mcg (Euthroid-½); levothyroxine sodium 60 mcg and liothyronine sodium 15 mcg (Euthroid-1); levothyroxine sodium 120 mcg and liothyronine sodium 30 mcg (Euthroid-2); levothyroxine sodium 180 mcg and liothyronine sodium 45 mcg (Euthroid-3); levothyroxine sodium 12.5 mcg and liothyronine sodium 3.1 mcg (Thyrolar-¼); levothyroxine sodium 25 mcg and liothyronine sodium 6.25 mcg (Thyrolar-½); levothyroxine sodium 50 mcg and liothyronine sodium 12.5 mcg (Thyrolar-1); levothyroxine sodium 100 mcg and liothyronine sodium 25 mcg (Thyrolar-2); levothyroxine sodium 150 mcg and liothyronine sodium 37.5 mcg (Thyrolar-3)

ACTION
Not clearly defined. Stimulates metabolism of all body tissues by accelerating the rate of cellular oxidation and provides both T$_3$ and T$_4$ to the tissues.

Route	Onset	Peak	Duration
PO	Unknown	Unknown	Unknown

INDICATIONS & DOSAGE
Hypothyroidism—
Dosages are expressed in thyroid equivalents and must be individualized to approximate the deficit in the patient's thyroid secretion.
Adults: initially, a single dose of Thyrolar-¼, Thyrolar-½, or Euthroid-½. Dosage is adjusted at 2-week intervals.

ADVERSE REACTIONS
CNS: *nervousness, insomnia, tremor,* headache.
CV: *tachycardia,* **arrhythmias,** angina pectoris, **cardiac decompensation and collapse.**
GI: diarrhea, vomiting.
Other: weight loss, heat intolerance, diaphoresis, accelerated rate of bone maturation in infants and children, menstrual irregularities, allergic skin reactions.

INTERACTIONS
Drug-drug. *Cholestyramine, colestipol:*

---

impaired liotrix absorption. Separate doses by 4 to 5 hours.

Insulin, oral antidiabetic agents: altered serum glucose levels. Monitor blood glucose levels. Dosage adjustments may be necessary.

I.V. phenytoin: free thyroid released. Monitor for tachycardia.

Oral anticoagulants: altered PT. Monitor PT and INR. Dosage adjustments may be necessary.

Sympathomimetics (such as epinephrine): increased risk of coronary insufficiency. Monitor closely.

EFFECTS ON DIAGNOSTIC TESTS
Drug therapy alters radioactive iodine (^{131}I) thyroid uptake, protein-bound iodine levels, and T_3 uptake.

CONTRAINDICATIONS
Contraindicated in patients acute MI uncomplicated by hypothyroidism, untreated thyrotoxicosis, uncorrected adrenal insufficiency, or hypersensitivity to drug.

NURSING CONSIDERATIONS
• Use with extreme caution in elderly patients and those with angina pectoris, hypertension, other CV disorders, renal insufficiency, or ischemia.

• Use cautiously in patients with myxedema, diabetes mellitus, or insipidus.

• Rapid replacement in patients with arteriosclerosis may precipitate angina, coronary occlusion, or CVA. Use cautiously in these patients.

• In patients with coronary artery disease who must receive thyroid hormones, observe carefully for possible coronary insufficiency. Also observe carefully during surgery because arrhythmias can be precipitated.

• Know that thyroid hormone replacement requirements are about 25% lower in patients over 60 years than in young adults.

• Monitor pulse and blood pressure.

• Know that thyroid hormones alter thyroid function test results.

• Know that patients taking liotrix who need ^{131}I uptake studies done must discontinue drug 7 to 10 days before test.

✓ Patient teaching
• Make sure patient understands importance of compliance. He should take thyroid hormones at same time each day, preferably before breakfast, to maintain constant hormone levels. Morning dosage may prevent insomnia.

• Warn patient (especially elderly patient) to notify doctor at once if chest pain, palpitations, sweating, nervousness, or other signs of overdose or aggravated CV disease occur.

• The two commercially prepared liotrix drugs contain different amounts of each ingredient; tell patient not to switch brands.

• Tell patient to report unusual bleeding and bruising.

thyroid
Armour Thyroid, S-P-T, Thyrar, Thyroid Strong, Westhroid

Pregnancy Risk Category: A

HOW SUPPLIED
Tablets: 15 mg, 30 mg, 60 mg, 65 mg, 90 mg, 120 mg, 130 mg, 180 mg, 240 mg, 300 mg
Tablets (Thyrar; bovine origin): 30 mg, 60 mg, 120 mg
Tablets (S-P-T; pork origin): 15 mg, 30 mg, 60 mg, 120 mg, 200 mg, 250 mg, 300 mg
Tablets (enteric-coated): 60 mg, 120 mg
Strong tablets (50% stronger than thyroid USP, and containing 0.3% iodine): 32.5 mg, 65 mg, 130 mg, 200 mg
Capsules (pork origin): 60 mg, 120 mg, 180 mg, 300 mg

ACTION
Not clearly defined. Stimulates metabolism of all body tissues by accelerating the rate of cellular oxidation.

Route	Onset	Peak	Duration
PO	Unknown	Unknown	Unknown

INDICATIONS & DOSAGE
Mild hypothyroidism—
Adults: initially, 60 mg P.O. daily, increased by 60 mg q 30 days until desired

response occurs. Usual maintenance dosage is 60 to 120 mg daily as a single dose.

Severe hypothyroidism—
Adults: initially, 15 mg P.O. daily, increased by 30 mg daily after 2 weeks, and 2 weeks later increased to 60 mg daily. After 2 months, increased to 120 mg daily, p.r.n., for 2 months; then to 120 mg daily, p.r.n.

Congenital or severe hypothyroidism in children—
Children: same as adults with severe hypothyroidism.
Elderly: in patients over 65 years, 7.5 to 15 mg daily. This may be doubled q 6 to 8 weeks until desired result is obtained.

ADVERSE REACTIONS
CNS: *nervousness, insomnia,* tremor, headache.
CV: *tachycardia,* **arrhythmias,** angina pectoris, **cardiac decompensation and collapse.**
GI: diarrhea, vomiting.
Other: weight loss, heat intolerance, diaphoresis, accelerated rate of bone maturation in infants and children, menstrual irregularities, allergic skin reactions.

INTERACTIONS
Drug-drug. *Cholestyramine:* impaired thyroid absorption. Separate doses by 4 to 5 hours.
Insulin, oral antidiabetic agents: altered serum glucose levels. Monitor glucose levels, and adjust dosage as needed.
Oral anticoagulants: altered PT. Monitor PT and INR. Adjust dosage as needed.
Sympathomimetics (such as epinephrine): increased risk of coronary insufficiency. Monitor closely.

EFFECTS ON DIAGNOSTIC TESTS
Thyroid USP therapy alters radioactive iodine (^{131}I) thyroid uptake, protein-bound iodine levels, and liothyronine uptake.

CONTRAINDICATIONS
Contraindicated in patients with acute MI uncomplicated by hypothyroidism, untreated thyrotoxicosis, uncorrected adrenal insufficiency, or hypersensitivity to drug.

NURSING CONSIDERATIONS
• Use with extreme caution in elderly patients and those with angina pectoris, hypertension, other CV disorders, renal insufficiency, or ischemia.
• Use cautiously in patients with myxedema or diabetes mellitus or insipidus.
• In patients with coronary artery disease, check for coronary insufficiency.
• Know that thyroid hormone replacement requirements are about 25% lower in patients over 60 years.
• Monitor pulse and blood pressure.
• Be aware that in children, sleeping pulse rate and basal morning temperature guide treatment.
• Know that thyroid hormones alter thyroid function test results.
• Realize that patient must discontinue thyroid 7 to 10 days before undergoing ^{131}I studies.

☑**Patient teaching**
• Tell patient to take thyroid hormones at same time each day, preferably before breakfast, to maintain constant hormone levels. Advise patient that taking dose in the morning may prevent insomnia.
• Advise patient who has achieved stable response not to change brands.
• Warn patient (especially elderly patient) to notify doctor at once if chest pain, palpitations, or other signs of overdose or aggravated CV disease occur.
• Tell patient to report unusual bleeding and bruising.

---

*Liquid contains alcohol.   **May contain tartrazine.   †Canada   ‡Australia   §U.K.   ◇OTC

59

Thyroid hormone antagonists

methimazole
potassium iodide
potassium iodide, saturated
    solution
strong iodine solution
propylthiouracil
radioactive iodine (sodium
    iodide) [131]I

COMBINATION PRODUCTS
None.

---

methimazole
Tapazole

Pregnancy Risk Category: D

HOW SUPPLIED
Tablets: 5 mg, 10 mg

ACTION
Inhibits oxidation of iodine in thyroid
gland, blocking iodine's ability to combine with tyrosine to form T_4. Also may
prevent coupling of monoiodotyrosine
and diiodotyrosine to form T_4 and T_3.

Route	Onset	Peak	Duration
PO	< 5 days	0.5-1 hr	Unknown

INDICATIONS & DOSAGE
Hyperthyroidism—
Adults: if mild, 15 mg P.O. daily; if moderately severe, 30 to 40 mg daily; if severe, 60 mg daily. Dose once daily or in
two divided doses. Maintenance dosage is
5 to 15 mg daily.
Children: 0.4 mg/kg P.O. once or in divided doses daily. Maintenance dosage is
0.2 mg/kg once or in divided doses daily.

ADVERSE REACTIONS
CNS: headache, drowsiness, vertigo,
paresthesia, neuritis, neuropathies, CNS
stimulation, depression.
GI: diarrhea, nausea, vomiting (may be
dose-related), salivary gland enlargement,
loss of taste, epigastric distress.

GU: nephritis.
Hematologic: *agranulocytosis, leukopenia, thrombocytopenia, aplastic anemia.*
Hepatic: jaundice, hepatic dysfunction,
hepatitis.
Skin: rash, urticaria, discoloration, pruritus, erythema nodosum, exfoliative dermatitis, lupus-like syndrome.
Other: arthralgia, myalgia, fever, lymphadenopathy, hypothyroidism (mental
depression; cold intolerance; hard, nonpitting edema; hypoprothrombinemia; and
bleeding).

INTERACTIONS
Drug-drug. *Aminophylline, oxtriphylline,
theophylline:* decreased clearance. May
need dosage adjustment.
Anticoagulants: may alter dose requirements. Monitor PT, PTT, and INR.
Cardiac glycosides: increase serum levels. May need to decrease digitalis dose.
Potassium iodide: may decrease response
to drug. May need to increase dosage of
methimazole.

EFFECTS ON DIAGNOSTIC TESTS
Drug therapy alters selenomethionine
(^{75}Se) uptake by the pancreas and ^{123}I or
^{131}I uptake by the thyroid. Hepatotoxicity
may be evident by elevations of PT, ALT,
and AST, bilirubin, alkaline phosphatase,
and LD levels.

CONTRAINDICATIONS
Contraindicated in patients with hypersensitivity to drug and in breast-feeding
patients.

NURSING CONSIDERATIONS
• Use with extreme caution during pregnancy. Pregnant women may require less
drug as pregnancy progresses. Monitor
thyroid function studies closely. Thyroid
may be added to regimen. Drug may be
stopped during last few weeks of pregnancy.
• Monitor CBC periodically as ordered to
detect impending leukopenia, thrombocy-

Reactions may be *common*, uncommon, *life-threatening*, or COMMON AND LIFE-THREATENING.

topenia, and agranulocytosis. Also monitor hepatic function.

*Alert:*Dosages over 30 mg/day increase the risk of agranulocytosis.

*Alert:*Patients over 40 years may have an increased risk of developing drug-induced agranulocytosis.

• Watch for signs of hypothyroidism (mental depression; cold intolerance; hard, nonpitting edema); notify doctor because dosage may need to be adjusted as necessary.

• Discontinue drug and notify doctor if severe rash or enlarged cervical lymph nodes develop.

☑**Patient teaching**

• Tell patient to take drug with meals to reduce adverse GI reactions.

• Warn patient to report fever, sore throat, mouth sores, skin eruptions, anorexia, pruritus, right upper quadrant pain, yellow skin or sclera.

• Tell patient to ask doctor about using iodized salt and eating shellfish. The iodine in these may make the medication less effective.

• Warn patient against OTC cough medicines; many contain iodine.

• Instruct patient to store drug in light-resistant container.

• Teach patient to watch for signs and symptoms of hypothyroidism (unexplained weight gain, fatigue, cold intolerance) and to notify doctor if they occur.

potassium iodide
losat, Pima, Thyro-Block

potassium iodide, saturated solution (SSKI)

strong iodine solution (Lugol's solution)

Pregnancy Risk Category: D

HOW SUPPLIED
potassium iodide
Tablets: 130 mg
Oral solution: 500 mg/15 ml
Syrup: 325 mg/5 ml

potassium iodide, saturated solution
Oral solution: 1 g/ml
strong iodine solution
Oral solution: iodine 50 mg/ml and potassium iodide 100 mg/ml

ACTION
Inhibits thyroid hormone formation, limits iodide transport into the thyroid gland, and blocks thyroid hormone release.

Route	Onset	Peak	Duration
PO	< 24 hr	10-15 days	Unknown

INDICATIONS & DOSAGE
Preparation for thyroidectomy—
Adults and children: strong iodine solution (USP), 0.1 to 0.3 ml P.O. t.i.d., or potassium iodide, saturated solution (SSKI), 1 to 5 drops in water P.O. t.i.d. after meals for 10 to 14 days before surgery.
Thyrotoxic crisis—
Adults and children: 500 mg P.O. q 4 hours (about 10 drops of SSKI) or 1 ml of strong iodine solution t.i.d.
Radiation protectant for thyroid gland—
Adults and children 1 year and over: 130 mg P.O. daily for 7 to 14 days after radiation exposure.
Children up to 1 year: 65 mg P.O. daily for 7 to 14 days after exposure.

ADVERSE REACTIONS
EENT: periorbital edema.
GI: diarrhea, inflammation of salivary glands, burning mouth and throat, sore teeth and gums, *metallic taste.*
Skin: acneiform rash.
Other: fever; *hypersensitivity reactions, potassium toxicity* (confusion, irregular heartbeat, numbness, tingling, pain or weakness of hands or feet, tiredness).

INTERACTIONS
Drug-drug. *ACE inhibitors, potassium-sparing diuretics:* risk of hyperkalemia. Avoid concomitant use.
Antithyroid medications: potassium iodide may potentiate hypothyroid or goitrogenic effects. Monitor closely.
Lithium carbonate: hypothyroidism may occur. Use with caution.

EFFECTS ON DIAGNOSTIC TESTS
Potassium iodide may alter the results of thyroid function tests.

CONTRAINDICATIONS
Contraindicated in patients with tuberculosis, acute bronchitis, iodide hypersensitivity, or hyperkalemia. Some formulations contain sulfites, which may precipitate allergic reactions in hypersensitive patients.

NURSING CONSIDERATIONS
• Use cautiously in patients with hypocomplementemic vasculitis, goiter, or autoimmune thyroid disease.
• Know that drug is usually given with other antithyroid drugs.
• Know that doctor may avoid prescribing enteric-coated tablets, which have been associated with small-bowel lesions and can lead to serious complications, including perforation, hemorrhage, or obstruction.
• Dilute oral solutions in water, milk, or fruit juice, and give after meals to prevent gastric irritation, to hydrate the patient, and to mask salty taste.
• Give iodides through straw to avoid tooth discoloration.
Alert: Know that earliest signs of delayed hypersensitivity reactions caused by iodides are irritation and swollen eyelids.
• Store in light-resistant container.

☑ Patient teaching
• Instruct patient how to mask salty taste of oral solution. Tell him to take all forms of the drug after meals.
• Warn patient that sudden withdrawal may precipitate thyroid crisis.
• Tell patient to ask doctor about using iodized salt and eating shellfish. These foods contain iodine and may alter drug's effectiveness.

---

propylthiouracil (PTU)
Propyl-Thyracil†

Pregnancy Risk Category: D

HOW SUPPLIED
Tablets: 50 mg, 100 mg

ACTION
Inhibits oxidation of iodine in thyroid gland, blocking iodine's ability to combine with tyrosine to form T_4, and may prevent coupling of monoiodotyrosine and diiodotyrosine to form T_4 and T_3.

Route	Onset	Peak	Duration
PO	Unknown	1-1.5 hr	Unknown

INDICATIONS & DOSAGE
Hyperthyroidism—
Adults: 300 to 900 mg P.O. daily in one to four divided doses; up to 1,200 mg daily have been used in severe cases. Maintenance dose is variable but generally ranges from 100 to 150 mg daily.
Children over 10 years: 150 to 300 mg P.O. daily in divided doses t.i.d. Maintenance dosage determined by patient response.
Children 6 to 10 years: 50 to 150 mg P.O. daily in divided doses t.i.d or q.i.d. Maintenance dosage determined by patient's response.
Thyrotoxic crisis—
Adults and children: 200 mg P.O. q 4 to 6 hours on first day; once full control of symptoms is achieved, dosage is gradually reduced to usual maintenance levels.

ADVERSE REACTIONS
CNS: headache, drowsiness, vertigo, paresthesia, neuritis, neuropathies, CNS stimulation, depression.
CV: vasculitis.
EENT: visual disturbances.
GI: diarrhea, *nausea, vomiting* (may be dose-related), epigastric distress, salivary gland enlargement, loss of taste.
GU: nephritis.
Hematologic: *agranulocytosis, leukopenia, thrombocytopenia, aplastic anemia.*
Hepatic: jaundice, *hepatotoxicity.*
Skin: rash, urticaria, skin discoloration, pruritus, erythema nodosum, exfoliative dermatitis, lupus-like syndrome.
Other: arthralgia, myalgia, fever, lymphadenopathy; dose-related hypothyroidism (mental depression; hypoprothrombinemia and bleeding; cold intolerance; hard, nonpitting edema).

Reactions may be *common,* uncommon, *life-threatening,* or COMMON AND LIFE-THREATENING.

INTERACTIONS

Drug-drug. *Aminophylline, oxtriphylline, theophylline*: decreased clearance. Dosage may need to be altered.

Anticoagulants: anticoagulant effects may be increased. Monitor PT and INR.

Cardiac glycosides: increased serum levels of glycosides. May need dosage reduction.

Potassium iodide: may decrease response to drug. May need to increase dosage of antithyroid drug.

EFFECTS ON DIAGNOSTIC TESTS

PTU therapy alters selenomethionine (^{75}Se) levels and PT; it also alters AST, ALT, and LD levels as well as liothyronine uptake.

CONTRAINDICATIONS

Contraindicated in patients with hypersensitivity to drug and in breast-feeding patients.

NURSING CONSIDERATIONS

• Use cautiously in pregnant patients. Pregnant women may require less drug as pregnancy progresses. Monitor thyroid function studies closely. Thyroid may be added to regimen. Drug may be stopped during last few weeks of pregnancy.

Alert: Patients older than 40 years may have an increased risk of developing propylthiouracil-induced agranulocytosis.

• Give drug with meals to reduce adverse GI reactions.

• Watch for signs of hypothyroidism (mental depression; cold intolerance; hard, nonpitting edema); adjust dosage as ordered.

• Monitor CBC periodically to detect impending leukopenia, thrombocytopenia, and agranulocytosis.

Alert: Discontinue drug and notify doctor if severe rash or enlarged cervical lymph nodes develop.

• Store drug in light-resistant container.

✅ Patient teaching

• Instruct patient to take drug with meals.

• Warn patient to report fever, sore throat, mouth sores, and skin eruptions.

• Tell patient to ask doctor about using iodized salt and eating shellfish. These foods contain iodine and may alter the effectiveness of the medication.

• Warn patient against taking OTC cough medicines; many contain iodine.

• Teach patient to watch for signs and symptoms of hypothyroidism (unexplained weight gain, fatigue, cold intolerance) and to notify their doctor if such occur.

---

radioactive iodine (sodium iodide) ^{131}I

Iodotope, Sodium Iodide ^{131}I Therapeutic

Pregnancy Risk Category: X

HOW SUPPLIED

All radioactivity concentrations are determined at time of calibration.

iodotope therapeutic

Capsules: radioactivity range is 1 to 50 millicuries (mCi)/capsule at time of calibration

Oral solution: radioactivity concentration is 7.05 mCi/ml at time of calibration; in vials containing approximately 7, 14, 28, 70, or 106 mCi at time of calibration

sodium iodide ^{131}I therapeutic

Capsules: radioactivity range is 0.8 to 100 mCi/capsule at time of calibration

Oral solution: radioactivity range is 3.5 to 150 mCi/vial at time of calibration

ACTION

Limits thyroid hormone secretion by destroying thyroid tissue. The affinity of thyroid tissue for radioactive iodine facilitates uptake of drug by cancerous thyroid tissue that has metastasized to other sites in the body.

Route	Onset	Peak	Duration
PO	Unknown	1-1.5 hr	Unknown

INDICATIONS & DOSAGE

Hyperthyroidism—

Adults: usual dosage is 4 to 10 mCi P.O. Dosage is based on estimated weight of thyroid gland and thyroid uptake. Treatment repeated after 6 weeks, based on serum T_4 level.

Thyroid cancer—
Adults: initially, 30 to 100 mCi P.O. with subsequent doses of 100 to 200 mCi. Dosage is based on estimated malignant thyroid tissue and metastatic tissue as determined by total body scan. Treatment repeated according to clinical status.

ADVERSE REACTIONS

CV: chest pain, tachycardia.
EENT: *fullness in neck,* pain on swallowing, sore throat, cough.
Hematologic: anemia; blood dyscrasia; leukopenia; *thrombocytopenia;* possible increased risk of *leukemia* later (after sufficient ^{131}I dose for thyroid ablation following cancer surgery).
Skin: rash, pruritus, urticaria.
Other: hypothyroidism; radiation-induced thyroiditis; radiation sickness (nausea, vomiting); *death;* temporary thinning of hair; allergic-type reactions; possible increased risk of birth defects in offspring after sufficient ^{131}I dose for thyroid ablation after cancer surgery.

INTERACTIONS

Drug-drug. *Lithium carbonate:* hypothyroidism may occur. Use with caution.

The following drugs can interfere with the action of ^{131}I and should be withheld for the specified time before administering the ^{131}I dose:
Adrenocorticoids: 1 week.
Benzodiazepines: 1 month.
Cholecystographic agents: 6 to 9 months.
Contrast media containing iodine: 1 to 2 months.
Iodine-containing products, including antitussives, expectorants, topical agents, and vitamins: 2 weeks.
Salicylates: 1 to 2 weeks.

EFFECTS ON DIAGNOSTIC TESTS

^{131}I therapy alters ^{131}I thyroid uptake and protein-bound iodine levels.

CONTRAINDICATIONS

Contraindicated during pregnancy (except to treat thyroid cancer) and in breast-feeding patients.

NURSING CONSIDERATIONS

• Know that all antithyroid medications and thyroid preparations must be stopped 1 week before ^{131}I dose. If this is not possible, patient may receive thyroid-stimulating hormone for 3 days before ^{131}I dose. When treating female of childbearing age, give dose during menstruation or within 7 days afterward.
• Know that after therapy for hyperthyroidism, patient should not resume antithyroid drugs but should continue propranolol or other drugs used to treat symptoms of hyperthyroidism until onset of full ^{131}I effect occurs (usually 6 weeks).
• Monitor thyroid function via serum T_4 levels, as ordered.
• Institute full radiation precautions. Have patient use proper disposal methods when coughing and expectorating. After dose for hyperthyroidism, patient's urine and saliva are slightly radioactive for 24 hours; vomitus is highly radioactive for 6 to 8 hours.
• Be aware that after dose for thyroid cancer, patient's urine, saliva, and perspiration are radioactive for 3 days. Isolate patient and observe these precautions: Do not allow pregnant personnel to care for patient; provide disposable eating utensils and linens; instruct patient to save urine in lead container for 24 to 48 hours; limit contact with patient to 30 minutes per shift per person on day 1, and increase time, as necessary, to 1 hour on day 2 and longer on day 3.

☑ Patient teaching

• Tell patient to fast overnight before administration and to drink as much fluid as possible for 48 hours afterwards.
• Instruct patient about appropriate radiation exposure precautions to use after drug administration.
• Warn patient who is discharged less than 7 days after ^{131}I dose for thyroid cancer to avoid close contact with small children and not to sleep in same room with spouse for 7 days after treatment.
• Teach patient the signs and symptoms of hypothyroidism (unexplained weight gain, fatigue, cold intolerance) and instruct them to notify doctor if these occur.

Reactions may be *common,* uncommon, *life-threatening,* or COMMON AND LIFE-THREATENING.

60

Pituitary hormones

corticotropin
cosyntropin
desmopressin acetate
leuprolide acetate
(See Chapter 72, ANTINEOPLASTICS
THAT ALTER HORMONE BALANCE.)
repository corticotropin
somatrem
somatropin
vasopressin

COMBINATION PRODUCTS
None.

corticotropin (adrenocorticotropic hormone, ACTH)
ACTH, Acthar

repository corticotropin
Acthar Gel (H.P.)†, H.P. Acthar Gel

Pregnancy Risk Category: C

HOW SUPPLIED
Aqueous injection: 25-unit vial, 40 units/vial
Repository injection: 40 units/ml, 80 units/ml

ACTION
By replacing the body's own tropic hormone, stimulates the adrenal cortex to secrete its entire spectrum of hormones.

Route	Onset	Peak	Duration
IV, IM	Rapid	1 hr	2-4 hr
IM (repository)	Unknown	Unknown	3 days
SC	Unknown	Unknown	Unknown

INDICATIONS & DOSAGE
Diagnostic test of adrenocortical function—
Adults: 40 units I.M. (repository) q 12 hours for 1 to 2 days; or 10 to 25 units aqueous form in 500 ml of D_5W I.V. over 8 hours, between blood samplings.

Individual dosages vary with adrenal glands' sensitivity to stimulation as well as with specific disease. Infants and younger children require larger doses per kilogram than do older children and adults.
For therapeutic use—
Adults: 40 units aqueous form S.C. or I.M. in four divided doses; or 40 to 80 units q 24 to 72 hours (repository form).

ADVERSE REACTIONS
CNS: *seizures, dizziness,* vertigo, *increased intracranial pressure with papilledema,* pseudotumor cerebri.
CV: hypertension, heart failure, necrotizing angiitis, *shock.*
EENT: cataracts, glaucoma.
GI: peptic ulceration with perforation and hemorrhage, pancreatitis, abdominal distention, ulcerative esophagitis, nausea, vomiting.
Musculoskeletal: muscle weakness, steroid myopathy, loss of muscle mass, osteoporosis, vertebral compression fractures.
Skin: impaired wound healing, thin fragile skin, petechiae, ecchymoses, facial erythema, diaphoresis, acne, hyperpigmentation, allergic reactions, hirsutism.
Other: pneumonia, abscess and septic infection, cushingoid symptoms, suppression of growth in children, activation of latent diabetes mellitus, progressive increase in antibodies, loss of corticotropin stimulatory effect, hypersensitivity reactions (rash, *bronchospasm*), *sodium and fluid retention,* calcium and potassium loss, hypokalemic alkalosis, negative nitrogen balance, menstrual irregularities.

INTERACTIONS
Drug-drug. *Amphotericin B, potassium-wasting diuretics:* increased risk of hypokalemia. Monitor serum potassium levels.
Anticonvulsants, barbiturates, rifampin: increased metabolism of corticotropin and decreased effectiveness. Monitor for lack of effect.

Antidiabetic agents: may increase requirements of antidiabetic agents due to intrinsic hyperglycemic activity of corticotropin. Monitor blood glucose levels closely.
Estrogens: may potentiate the effects of cortisol. Dosage adjustments may be necessary.
NSAIDs, salicylates: increased risk of GI bleeding. Avoid concomitant use.
Oral anticoagulants: altered PT. Monitor PT and INR. Dosage adjustments may be necessary.
Vaccines: risk of neurologic complications and lack of antibody response. Smallpox vaccine should not be used and other immunizations should be considered with extreme caution.

EFFECTS ON DIAGNOSTIC TESTS
Drug therapy alters blood and urinary glucose levels; sodium and potassium levels; protein-bound iodine levels; radioactive iodine (^{131}I) uptake and T_3 uptake; total protein values; serum amylase, urine amino acid, serotonin, uric acid, calcium and 17-ketosteroid levels; and leukocyte counts.

High plasma cortisol concentrations may be reported erroneously in patients receiving spironolactone, cortisone, or hydrocortisone when fluorometric analysis is used. This does not occur with the radioimmunoassay or competitive protein-binding method. However, therapy can be maintained with prednisone, dexamethasone, or betamethasone because they are not detectable by the fluorometric method.

CONTRAINDICATIONS
Contraindicated in patients with peptic ulcer, scleroderma, osteoporosis, systemic fungal infections, ocular herpes simplex, peptic ulceration, heart failure, hypertension, adrenocortical hyperfunction or primary insufficiency, Cushing's syndrome, or sensitivity to pork and pork products. Also contraindicated after recent surgery.

NURSING CONSIDERATIONS
• Use cautiously during pregnancy and in women of childbearing age. Also use cautiously in patients being immunized and those with latent tuberculosis or tuberculin reactivity, hypothyroidism, cirrhosis, acute gouty arthritis, psychotic tendencies, renal insufficiency, diverticulitis, nonspecific ulcerative colitis, thromboembolic disorders, seizures, uncontrolled hypertension, or myasthenia gravis.
• Know that corticotropin treatment should be preceded by verification of adrenal responsiveness and testing for hypersensitivity and allergic reactions.
• If administering gel, warm it to room temperature, draw into large needle, and give slowly as deep I.M. injection with 21G or 22G needle.
• Know that corticotropin may mask signs of chronic disease and decrease host resistance and ability to localize infection.
• Note and record weight changes, fluid exchange, and resting blood pressures until minimal effective dosage is achieved.
• Watch neonates of corticotropin-treated mothers for signs of hypoadrenalism.
• Unusual stress may require additional use of rapidly acting corticosteroids. When possible, gradually reduce corticotropin dosage to smallest effective dose as ordered to minimize induced adrenocortical insufficiency. Know that therapy can be reinstituted if stressful situation (trauma, surgery, severe illness) occurs shortly after stopping drug.

◐ I.V. administration
• Use only the aqueous form for I.V. administration. Dilute in 500 ml of D_5W and infuse over 8 hours.
• Refrigerate reconstituted solution and use within 24 hours.

☑ Patient teaching
• Warn patient that injection is painful.
• Stress importance of informing all members of health care team about therapeutic use of drug because unusual stress may require additional use of rapidly acting corticosteroids.
• Instruct patient how to handle troublesome adverse reactions, such as limiting sodium intake to reduce severity of edema and increasing protein intake to combat nitrogen loss.
• Advise patient about need for close follow-up care.

• Instruct patient to avoid individuals with known or suspected varicella infections.

---

cosyntropin
Cortrosyn

Pregnancy Risk Category: C

HOW SUPPLIED
Injection: 0.25-mg vial

ACTION
By replacing the body's own tropic hormone, stimulates the adrenal cortex to secrete its entire spectrum of hormones.

Route	Onset	Peak	Duration
IV	Rapid	45-60 min	Unknown
IM, SC	Unknown	45-60 min	Unknown

INDICATIONS & DOSAGE
Diagnostic test of adrenocortical function—
Adults and children 2 years and over: 0.25 mg I.M. or I.V over 2 minutes or 40 mcg/hour over 6 hours (unless label prohibits I.V. administration) between blood samplings.
Children under 2 years: 0.125 mg I.M. or I.V.

ADVERSE REACTIONS
CNS: *seizures,* dizziness, vertigo, *increased intracranial pressure with papilledema,* pseudotumor cerebri.
EENT: cataracts, glaucoma.
GI: peptic ulceration, pancreatitis, abdominal distension, ulcerative esophagitis, nausea, vomiting.
Skin: pruritus; impaired wound healing; thin, fragile skin; petechiae; ecchymoses; facial erythema; diaphoresis; acne; hyperpigmentation; hirsutism.
Other: flushing, *hypersensitivity reactions,* muscle weakness, steroid myopathy, loss of muscle mass, osteoporosis, vertebral compression, fractures, cushingoid symptoms, menstrual irregularities.

INTERACTIONS
Drug-drug. *Blood, plasma products:* inactivates cosyntropin. Avoid concomitant administration.

Cortisone, hydrocortisone: may interfere with test results of cortisol levels if administered on test day. Avoid concomitant use.
Spironolactone: may interfere with fluorometric analysis of cortisol levels. Avoid concomitant use.

EFFECTS ON DIAGNOSTIC TESTS
Drug therapy alters blood glucose levels.

CONTRAINDICATIONS
Contraindicated in patients with hypersensitivity to drug.

NURSING CONSIDERATIONS
• Use cautiously in patients hypersensitive to natural corticotropin.
• Know that drug is synthetic duplication of the biologically active part of the corticotropin molecule. It is less likely to produce sensitivity than natural corticotropin derived from animal sources.
• Monitor patient for allergic reactions, rash, dyspnea, wheezing, or evidence of anaphylaxis.

🔲 I.V. administration
• Reconstitute with 1 ml of supplied diluent. For direct injection, administer over at least 2 minutes. May be further diluted with D_5W or 0.9% NaCl and infused over 6 hours. Solution is stable for 12 hours at room temperature.

☑ Patient teaching
• Explain test procedure to patient.
• Tell patient to report adverse reactions immediately.

---

desmopressin acetate
DDAVP, Desmospray§, Minirin‡, Stimate

Pregnancy Risk Category: B

HOW SUPPLIED
Tablets: 0.1 mg, 0.2 mg
Nasal solution: 0.1 mg/ml, 1.5 mg/ml
Injection: 4 mcg/ml

ACTION
Increases the permeability of the renal tubular epithelium to adenosine mono-

phosphate and water; the epithelium promotes reabsorption of water and produces a concentrated urine. Desmopressin also increases factor VIII activity by releasing endogenous factor VIII from plasma storage sites.

Route	Onset	Peak	Duration
PO	1 hr	1-1.5 hr	8-12 hr
IV	15-30 min	Unknown	4-12 hr
Nasal	1 hr	1-5 hr	8-12 hr

INDICATIONS & DOSAGE

Nonnephrogenic diabetes insipidus, temporary polyuria and polydipsia associated with pituitary trauma—
Adults: 0.1 to 0.4 ml intranasally daily in one to three doses. Morning and evening doses adjusted separately for adequate diurnal rhythm of water turnover. Most adults require 0.2 ml daily in divided doses. Alternatively, injectable form administered in dosage of 0.5 to 1 ml I.V. or S.C. daily, usually in two divided doses.
Children 3 months to 12 years: 0.05 to 0.3 ml intranasally daily in one or two doses.
Hemophilia A and von Willebrand's disease—
Adults and children: 0.3 mcg/kg diluted in 0.9% NaCl and infused I.V. over 15 to 30 minutes. Dose repeated if necessary as indicated by laboratory response and patient's clinical condition.
Primary nocturnal enuresis—
Children 6 years and older: initially, 20 mcg (0.2 ml) intranasally h.s. (10 mcg each nostril). Dosage adjusted based on response. Maximum recommended dosage is 40 mcg daily.
✱ *NEW INDICATION: Management of primary nocturnal enuresis (with oral therapy)—*
Children 6 years and older: initially, 0.2 mg P.O. h.s. May be titrated up to 0.6 mg to achieve desired response. For patients previously on intranasal DDAVP therapy, start tablet the night following (24 hours after) last intranasal dose.

ADVERSE REACTIONS
CNS: headache.
CV: slight rise in blood pressure at high dosage.

EENT: rhinitis, epistaxis, sore throat, cough.
GI: nausea, abdominal cramps.
GU: vulval pain.
Other: flushing, local erythema, swelling or burning after injection.

INTERACTIONS
Drug-drug. *Carbamazepine, chlorpropamide:* potentiate ADH, may potentiate effects of desmopressin. Avoid concomitant use.
Clofibrate: enhanced and prolonged effects of desmopressin. Monitor carefully.
Demeclocycline, epinephrine, heparin, lithium: increased risk of adverse effects. Monitor closely.
Drug-lifestyle. *Alcohol use:* increased risk of adverse effects. Avoid concomitant use.

EFFECTS ON DIAGNOSTIC TESTS
None reported.

CONTRAINDICATIONS
Contraindicated in patients with type IIB von Willebrand's disease or hypersensitivity to drug.

NURSING CONSIDERATIONS
• Use cautiously in breast-feeding women; it is not known whether drug occurs in breast milk.
• Use cautiously in patients with coronary artery insufficiency or hypertensive CV disease or in patients with conditions associated with fluid and electrolyte imbalances such as cystic fibrosis because these patients are prone to hyponatremia.
• Know that desmopressin injection should not be used to treat hemophilia A with factor VIII levels of up to 5% or severe cases of von Willebrand's disease.
• Be aware that intranasal use can cause changes in the nasal mucosa resulting in erratic, unreliable absorption. Report a worsening condition to doctor, who may prescribe injectable DDAVP.
• Adjust fluid intake to reduce risk of water intoxication and sodium depletion, especially in children or elderly patients.
Alert: Overdose may cause oxytocic or vasopressor activity. Withhold drug and notify doctor. Use furosemide if fluid retention is excessive, as ordered.

Reactions may be *common*, uncommon, *life-threatening*, or COMMON AND LIFE-THREATENING.

◖ I.V. administration
• For adults and children weighing over 10 kg (22 lb), dilute with 50 ml sterile physiologic saline. For children weighing under 10 kg, 10 ml of diluent is recommended.
• Monitor blood pressure and pulse during infusion.
• Inspect for particulate matter and discoloration before infusing drug.

☑ Patient teaching
• Instruct patient to clear nasal passages before administering drug.
• Some patients may have difficulty measuring and inhaling drug into nostrils. Teach patient and caregivers correct method of administration.
• Advise patient to report nasal congestion, allergic rhinitis, or upper respiratory infections to doctor; a dosage adjustment may be needed.
• Teach patient using S.C. desmopressin to rotate injection sites to prevent tissue damage.
• Warn patient to drink only enough water to satisfy thirst.
• Inform patient that, when treating hemophilia A and von Willebrand's disease, taking desmopressin may avoid the hazards of using blood products.
• Advise patient to wear medical identification indicating use of drug.

---

somatrem
Protropin

Pregnancy Risk Category: C

HOW SUPPLIED
Injectable lyophilized powder: 5-mg (about 15-IU) vial, 10-mg (about 30-IU) vial

ACTION
Purified growth hormone (GH) of recombinant DNA origin that stimulates linear, skeletal muscle, and organ growth.

Route	Onset	Peak	Duration
IM, SC	Unknown	3-5 hr	Unknown

INDICATIONS & DOSAGE
Long-term treatment of children who have growth failure because of lack of adequate endogenous GH secretion—
Children (prepuberty): highly individualized; up to 0.3 mg/kg/week S.C. (preferred) or I.M, divided into appropriate daily dose for injection (six or seven times weekly).

ADVERSE REACTIONS
Metabolic: hypothyroidism, hyperglycemia.
Other: *antibodies to GH.*

INTERACTIONS
Drug-drug. *Glucocorticoids:* may inhibit growth-promoting action of somatrem. Adjust glucocorticoid dosage as necessary.

EFFECTS ON DIAGNOSTIC TESTS
Drug therapy alters glucose tolerance test (reduced with high doses) and total protein and thyroid function tests (T_4-binding capacity and radioactive uptake may be decreased).

CONTRAINDICATIONS
Contraindicated in patients with epiphyseal closure, active neoplasia, or hypersensitivity to benzyl alcohol.

NURSING CONSIDERATIONS
• Use cautiously in patients with hypothyroidism and in those whose GH deficiency is caused by an intracranial lesion.
• Be sure to check product's expiration date.
• To prepare solution, inject supplied bacteriostatic water for injection into vial containing drug. Then swirl vial with a gentle rotary motion until contents are completely dissolved. Do not shake vial.
• After reconstitution, vial solution should be clear. Do not inject solution if it is cloudy or contains particles.
• If prepared for other than neonatal use, store reconstituted vial in refrigerator; use within 14 days.
Alert: Know that toxicity in neonates has occurred from exposure to benzyl alcohol used in drug as a preservative. If drug is administered to neonates, reconstitute im-

---

mediately before use with sterile water for injection (without bacteriostat). Use vial once, then discard.

• Know that regular checkups, including monitoring of height and of blood and radiologic studies, are necessary.

• Observe patient for signs of glucose intolerance and hyperglycemia.

• Monitor for slipped capital femoral epiphysis or progression of scoliosis in patients with rapid growth.

• Monitor periodic thyroid function tests for hypothyroidism as ordered, which may require treatment with a thyroid hormone.

• Funduscopic examination of patient for intracranial hypertension should be done at the onset of therapy and periodically thereafter.

☑**Patient teaching**

• Reassure patient and caregivers that somatrem is *pure* and *safe*. Drug replaces pituitary-derived human GH, which was removed from the market in 1985 because of its association with a rare but fatal viral infection (Creutzfeldt-Jakob disease).

• Review the signs and symptoms of hypothyroidism and hyperglycemia. Instruct patient and parents to report such signs or symptoms promptly.

---

somatropin
Genotropin§, Humatrope, Norditropin, Nutropin, Nutropin AQ, Saizen, Serostim, Zomacton§

Pregnancy Risk Category: C

HOW SUPPLIED
Injection: 2-mg (about 6-IU [Humatrope]) vial†, 5-mg (about 15-IU [Humatrope]) vial, 10-mg (about 30-IU [Nutropin]) vial
Genotropin injection: 1.5 mg (about 4 IU/ml), 5.8 mg (about 15 IU/ml)
Norditropin injection: 4 mg (about 12 IU/ml), 8 mg (about 24 IU/ml)
Serostim injection: 5 mg (about 15 IU/vial), 6 mg (about 18 IU/ml)
Saizen injection: 5 mg (about 15 IU/vial)
Nutropin injection: 5 mg (about 15 IU/vial), 10 mg (about 30 IU/vial)

Nutropin AQ injection: 10 mg (about 30 IU/vial)

ACTION
Purified growth hormone (GH) of recombinant DNA origin that stimulates skeletal, linear, muscle, and organ growth.

Route	Onset	Peak	Duration
IM, SC	Unknown	3-5 hr	12-48 hr

INDICATIONS & DOSAGE
Long-term treatment of growth failure in children with inadequate secretion of endogenous GH—
Children: 0.18 mg/kg body weight S.C. or I.M. weekly divided equally and given on 3 alternate days, six times weekly or daily using Humatrope; or 0.30 mg/kg body weight S.C. weekly in daily divided doses using Nutropin; or 0.06 mg/kg I.M. or S.C. three times weekly using Saizen; or 0.024 to 0.034 mg/kg S.C., six to seven times weekly using Norditropin.
Growth failure in children associated with chronic renal insufficiency up to time of renal transplantation (Nutropin only)—
Children: 0.35 mg/kg body weight S.C. weekly in daily divided doses.
Long-term treatment of short stature associated with Turner's syndrome—
Children: up to 0.375 mg/kg/week (approximately 1.125 IU/kg/week) S.C. divided into equal doses given three to seven times weekly.
❊ *NEW INDICATION: Replacement of endogenous GH in adult patients with GH deficiency—*
Adults: initially, not more than 0.006 mg/kg SC daily. May be increased to maximum of 0.025 mg/kg daily in patients under 35 years or 0.0125 mg/kg daily in patients over 35 years.

ADVERSE REACTIONS
CNS: headache, weakness.
CV: mild, transient edema.
Hematologic: *leukemia.*
Metabolic: mild hyperglycemia, hypothyroidism.
Other: injection site pain, localized muscle pain, antibodies to GH.

INTERACTIONS
Drug-drug. *Corticosteroids, corticotropin:* long-term use inhibits growth response to growth hormone. Monitor for lack of effect.

EFFECTS ON DIAGNOSTIC TESTS
Serum levels of inorganic phosphorus, alkaline phosphatase, and parathyroid hormone may increase with somatropin therapy. Laboratory measurements of thyroid hormone may also change.

CONTRAINDICATIONS
Contraindicated in patients with closed epiphyses or an active underlying intracranial lesion. Humatrope should not be reconstituted with supplied diluent for patients with known sensitivity to either *m*-cresol or glycerin.

NURSING CONSIDERATIONS
• Use cautiously in children with hypothyroidism and in those whose GH deficiency is caused by an intracranial lesion. Be aware that these children should be examined frequently for progression or recurrence of the underlying disease.
• To prepare solution, inject supplied diluent into vial containing drug by aiming stream of liquid against glass wall of vial. Then swirl vial with a gentle rotary motion until contents are completely dissolved. Do *not* shake vial.
• After reconstitution, vial solution should be clear. Do not inject solution if it is cloudy or contains particles.
• Know that patients on dialysis require changes in drug administration schedule as follows:
–Hemodialysis: administer before bedtime or 3 to 4 hours after dialysis.
–Chronic cycling peritoneal dialysis: administer in the morning after completion of dialysis.
–Chronic ambulatory peritoneal dialysis: administer in the evening at the time of the overnight exchange.
• Store reconstituted vial in refrigerator; use within 14 days.
• If sensitivity to diluent should occur, vials may be reconstituted with sterile water for injection. When drug is reconstituted in this manner, use only 1 reconstituted

dose per vial; refrigerate solution if it is not used immediately after reconstitution; use reconstituted dose within 24 hours; and discard unused portion.
• Monitor child's height regularly. Know that regular checkups, including monitoring of blood and radiologic studies, also are necessary.
• Monitor patient's blood glucose levels regularly because GH may induce a state of insulin resistance.
• Know that excessive glucocorticoid therapy will inhibit the growth-promoting effect of somatropin. Patients with a coexisting corticotropin deficiency should have their glucocorticoid replacement dosage carefully adjusted to avoid an inhibitory effect on growth.
• Monitor for slipped capital femoral epiphysis or progression of scoliosis in patients with rapid growth.
• Monitor periodic thyroid function tests, as ordered, for hypothyroidism, which may require treatment with a thyroid hormone.
• Funduscopic examination of patient for intracranial hypertension should be done at the onset of, and periodically during, therapy.

☑ **Patient teaching**
• Inform parents that child with endocrine disorders (including GH deficiency) may develop slipped capital epiphyses more frequently. Tell them that if they notice their child is limping, they should notify the doctor.
• Stress importance of close follow-up care.

---

vasopressin (ADH)
Pitressin

Pregnancy Risk Category: C

HOW SUPPLIED
Injection: 0.5-ml and 1-ml ampules, 20 units/ml

ACTION
Increases the permeability of the renal tubular epithelium to adenosine monophosphate and water; the epithelium pro-

motes reabsorption of water and produces a concentrated urine.

Route	Onset	Peak	Duration
IM, SC, nasal	2-8 hr	Unknown	Unknown

INDICATIONS & DOSAGE
Nonnephrogenic, nonpsychogenic diabetes insipidus—
Adults: 5 to 10 units I.M. or S.C. b.i.d. to q.i.d., p.r.n.; or intranasally (aqueous solution used as spray or applied to cotton balls) in individualized dosages, based on response.
Children: 2.5 to 10 units I.M. or S.C. b.i.d. to q.i.d., p.r.n.; or intranasally (aqueous solution used as spray or applied to cotton balls) in individualized doses.

ADVERSE REACTIONS
CNS: tremor, headache, vertigo.
CV: angina in patients with vascular disease; vasoconstriction, *arrhythmias, cardiac arrest*, myocardial ischemia, circumoral pallor, decreased cardiac output.
GI: abdominal cramps, nausea, vomiting, flatulence.
Other: water intoxication (drowsiness, listlessness, headache, confusion, weight gain, *seizures, coma*), hypersensitivity reactions (urticaria, angioedema, *bronchoconstriction, anaphylaxis*), diaphoresis, cutaneous gangrene.

INTERACTIONS
Drug-drug. *Carbamazepine, chlorpropamide, clofibrate, fludrocortisone, tricyclic antidepressants:* increased antidiuretic response. Use together cautiously.
Demeclocycline, heparin, lithium, norepinephrine: reduced antidiuretic activity. Use together cautiously.
Drug-lifestyle. *Alcohol use:* reduced antidiuretic activity. Avoid use.

EFFECTS ON DIAGNOSTIC TESTS
None reported.

CONTRAINDICATIONS
Contraindicated in patients with chronic nephritis accompanied by nitrogen retention.

NURSING CONSIDERATIONS
• Use cautiously in children, elderly patients, pregnant patients, preoperative and postoperative polyuric patients, and in those with seizure disorders, migraine headache, asthma, CV disease, heart failure, renal disease, goiter with cardiac complications, arteriosclerosis, or fluid overload.
• Know that synthetic desmopressin is sometimes preferred because of its longer duration of action and less frequent adverse reactions. Desmopressin also is available commercially as a nasal solution.
• Drug may be used for transient polyuria resulting from ADH deficiency related to neurosurgery or head injury.
• Know that minimum effective dosage should be used to reduce adverse reactions.
• Give with 1 to 2 glasses of water to reduce adverse reactions and to improve therapeutic response.
• Monitor specific gravity of urine and fluid intake and output to aid evaluation of drug effectiveness.
• To prevent possible seizures, coma, and death, observe patient closely for early signs of water intoxication.
• Monitor blood pressure of patient taking vasopressin twice daily. Watch for excessively elevated blood pressure or lack of response to drug, which may be indicated by hypotension. Also monitor daily weight.

☑ Patient teaching
• Instruct patient to rotate injection sites to prevent tissue damage.
• Tell patient to report adverse reactions promptly.

Reactions may be *common*, uncommon, *life-threatening*, or COMMON AND LIFE-THREATENING.

61
Parathyroid-like drugs

calcifediol
calcitonin (human)
calcitonin (salmon)
calcitriol
dihydrotachysterol
etidronate disodium

COMBINATION PRODUCTS
None.

---

calcifediol
Calderol

Pregnancy Risk Category: C

HOW SUPPLIED
Capsules: 20 mcg, 50 mcg

ACTION
A vitamin D analogue that stimulates calcium absorption from the GI tract and promotes secretion of calcium from bone to blood.

Route	Onset	Peak	Duration
PO	Unknown	4 hr	15-20 days

INDICATIONS & DOSAGE
Metabolic bone disease and hypocalcemia associated with chronic renal failure—
Adults: initially, 300 to 350 mcg P.O. weekly. Dosage increased at 4-week intervals if necessary.

ADVERSE REACTIONS
Vitamin D intoxication associated with hypercalcemia:
CNS: headache, somnolence, weakness, irritability, psychosis (rare).
CV: hypertension, *arrhythmias.*
EENT: conjunctivitis, rhinorrhea.
GI: constipation, nausea, vomiting, polydipsia, pancreatitis, metallic taste, dry mouth, anorexia, diarrhea.
GU: polyuria, nocturia.
Skin: pruritus, photosensitivity reactions.
Other: bone and muscle pain, weight

loss, hyperthermia, nephrocalcinosis, decreased libido.

INTERACTIONS
Drug-drug. *Cardiac glycosides:* increased risk of arrhythmias. Avoid concomitant use.
Cholestyramine, colestipol: decreased absorption of orally administered vitamin D analogues. Avoid concomitant use.
Corticosteroids: counteract vitamin D analogue effects. Do not use together.
Magnesium-containing antacids: possible hypermagnesemia, especially in patients with chronic renal failure. Avoid concomitant use.
Other vitamin D analogues: increased toxicity. Avoid concomitant use.
Phenytoin: may increase metabolism of vitamin to inactive metabolites. Avoid concomitant use.
Products containing calcium, thiazide diuretics: increased risk of hypercalcemia. Use with caution.

EFFECTS ON DIAGNOSTIC TESTS
Drug may falsely elevate cholesterol determinations made using the Zlatkis-Zak reaction. Alters concentrations of serum alkaline phosphatase concentrations and may alter electrolytes, such as magnesium, phosphate, and calcium, in the serum and urine.

CONTRAINDICATIONS
Contraindicated in patients with hypercalcemia or vitamin D toxicity.

NURSING CONSIDERATIONS
• Monitor serum calcium level as ordered; serum calcium level multiplied by serum phosphate level should not exceed 70. During titration, serum calcium level should be determined at least weekly.
• If hypercalcemia occurs, discontinue calcifediol and notify doctor. Drug may be resumed after serum calcium level returns to normal.

☑ **Patient teaching**
• Teach patient to report signs and symptoms of hypercalcemia.
• Instruct patient about importance of getting an adequate daily intake of calcium. Inform patient about foods high in calcium and how much to consume daily to meet RDA.

---

calcitonin (human)
Cibacalcin

calcitonin (salmon)
Calcimar, Calsynar§, Miacalcin, Miacalcin Nasal Spray, Osteocalcin, Salmonine

Pregnancy Risk Category: C

HOW SUPPLIED
calcitonin human
Injection: 0.5 mg/vial
calcitonin salmon
Injection: 100 IU/ml, 1-ml ampules; 200 IU/ml, 2-ml ampules
Nasal spray: 200 IU/activation in 2-ml bottle

ACTION
Decreases osteoclastic activity by inhibiting osteocytic osteolysis and decreases mineral release and matrix or collagen breakdown in bone.

Route	Onset	Peak	Duration
IM, SC	15 min	4 hr	8-24 hr
Intranasal	Rapid	0.5 hr	1 hr

INDICATIONS & DOSAGE
Paget's disease of bone (osteitis deformans)—
Adults: initially, 100 IU of calcitonin (salmon) daily S.C. or I.M.; maintenance dosage is 50 to 100 IU daily S.C. or I.M., every other day, or three times weekly. Alternatively, calcitonin (human) 0.5 mg daily, reduced to 0.25 mg daily. Some patients may need up to 0.5 mg b.i.d.
Hypercalcemia—
Adults: 4 IU/kg of calcitonin (salmon) q 12 hours I.M. If response inadequate after 1 or 2 days, dose increased to 8 IU/kg I.M. q 12 hours. If response remains unsatisfactory after 2 more days, dosage increased to maximum of 8 IU/kg I.M. q 6 hours.
Postmenopausal osteoporosis—
Adults: 100 IU of calcitonin (salmon) daily I.M. or S.C. Alternatively, 200 IU (one activation) of calcitonin (salmon) daily intranasally, alternating nostrils daily. Patients should receive adequate vitamin D and calcium supplements (1.5 g of calcium carbonate daily and 400 units of vitamin D daily).

ADVERSE REACTIONS
CNS: headache, weakness, dizziness, paresthesia.
EENT: eye pain, nasal congestion.
GI: *transient nausea,* unusual taste, diarrhea, anorexia, *vomiting,* epigastric discomfort, abdominal pain.
GU: *increased urinary frequency,* nocturia.
Skin: *facial flushing,* rash, pruritus of ear lobes, *inflammation at injection site.*
Other: hypersensitivity reactions *(anaphylaxis),* edema of feet, chills, chest pressure, shortness of breath, tender palms and soles.

INTERACTIONS
None significant.

EFFECTS ON DIAGNOSTIC TESTS
In Paget's disease, maximum reductions of serum alkaline phosphatase and urinary hydroxyproline excretion may take 6 to 24 months of continuous treatment.

CONTRAINDICATIONS
Contraindicated in patients hypersensitive to salmon calcitonin. Human calcitonin has no contraindications.

NURSING CONSIDERATIONS
• Be aware that skin test is usually done before therapy.
• Systemic allergic reactions possible because hormone is protein. Keep epinephrine nearby.
• Know that calcitonin (human) is especially indicated in patients who have developed resistance to calcitonin (salmon). Calcitonin (human) is associated with risk of diminishing efficacy caused by antibody formation or hypersensitivity reactions.

Reactions may be *common,* uncommon, *life-threatening,* or COMMON AND LIFE-THREATENING.

• Administer at bedtime when possible to minimize nausea and vomiting.
• I.M. route is preferred if volume of dose to be administered exceeds 2 ml.
• Use freshly reconstituted solution within 2 hours.
• Observe patient for signs of hypocalcemic tetany during therapy (muscle twitching, tetanic spasms, and seizures when hypocalcemia is severe).
• Monitor serum calcium level closely. Watch for signs of hypercalcemia relapse: bone pain, renal calculi, polyuria, anorexia, nausea, vomiting, thirst, constipation, lethargy, bradycardia, muscle hypotonicity, pathologic fracture, psychosis, and coma.
• Know that periodic examinations of urine sediment are advisable.
• Monitor periodic serum alkaline phosphatase and 24-hour urine hydroxyproline levels to evaluate drug effect, as ordered.
• In patients with good initial clinical response to calcitonin who suffer relapse, expect to evaluate for antibody response to the hormone protein.
• If symptoms have been relieved after 6 months, know that treatment may be discontinued until symptoms or radiologic signs recur.
• Store calcitonin (human) at room temperature (77° F [25° C]) and protect from light; refrigerate calcitonin (salmon) at 36° to 46° F (2° to 8° C).

✓ **Patient teaching**
• When administered for postmenopausal osteoporosis, remind the patient to take adequate calcium and vitamin D supplements.
• Instruct home care patient or family member on how to administer drug. Tell them to administer drug at bedtime if only one dose is required daily. If nasal spray is prescribed, tell patient to alternate nostrils daily.
• Inform patient that facial flushing and warmth occur in 20% to 30% of all patients within minutes of injection and usually last about 1 hour. Reassure patient that this is a transient effect.
• Tell patient to report signs and symptoms of hypercalcemia promptly. Inform patient that if calcitonin loses its hypocal-

cemic activity, other drugs or increased dosages will not help.
• Advise patient to notify doctor immediately if signs of an allergic response occur.

---

calcitriol (1,25-dihydroxy-cholecalciferol)
Calcijex, Rocaltrol

Pregnancy Risk Category: C

HOW SUPPLIED
Capsules: 0.25 mcg, 0.5 mcg
Injection: 1 mcg/ml, 2 mcg/ml

ACTION
A vitamin D analogue that stimulates calcium absorption from the GI tract and promotes secretion of calcium from bone to blood.

Route	Onset	Peak	Duration
PO	2-6 hr	3-6 hr	3-5 days
IV	Immediate	Unknown	3-5 days

INDICATIONS & DOSAGE
Hypocalcemia in patients undergoing chronic dialysis—
Adults: initially, 0.25 mcg P.O. daily. Dosage may be increased by 0.25 mcg daily at 4 to 8 week intervals. Maintenance dosage is 0.5 to 3 mcg daily.
  Or, 0.5 mcg I.V. three times weekly approximately every other day. If response is inadequate to initial dose, may increase by 0.25 to 0.5 mcg at 2- to 4-week intervals. Maintenance dose is 0.5 to 3 mcg I.V. three times weekly.
Hypoparathyroidism and pseudohypoparathyroidism—
Adults and children 6 years and over: initially, 0.25 mcg P.O. daily. Dosage may be increased at 2- to 4-week intervals. Maintenance dose is 0.25 to 2.7 mcg P.O. daily.
Hypoparathyroidism—
Children 1 to 6 years: 0.04 to 0.08 mcg/ kg P.O. daily.

ADVERSE REACTIONS
Vitamin D intoxication associated with hypercalcemia:

CNS: headache, somnolence, weakness, irritability, psychosis (rare).
CV: hypertension, *arrhythmias.*
EENT: conjunctivitis, photophobia, rhinorrhea.
GI: nausea, vomiting, constipation, polydipsia, pancreatitis, metallic taste, dry mouth, anorexia.
GU: polyuria, nocturia.
Skin: pruritus.
Other: bone and muscle pain, weight loss, hyperthermia, nephrocalcinosis, decreased libido.

INTERACTIONS
Drug-drug. *Cardiac glycosides:* increased risk of arrhythmias. Avoid concomitant use.
Cholestyramine, colestipol, excessive use of mineral oil: decreased absorption of orally administered vitamin D analogues. Avoid concomitant use.
Corticosteroids: counteract vitamin D analogue effects. Do not use together.
Magnesium-containing antacids: may induce hypermagnesemia, especially in patients with chronic renal failure. Avoid concomitant use.

EFFECTS ON DIAGNOSTIC TESTS
Drug therapy may falsely elevate cholesterol determinations made using the Zlatkis-Zak reaction. It also alters serum alkaline phosphatase concentrations and may alter electrolytes, such as magnesium, phosphate, and calcium in serum and urine.

CONTRAINDICATIONS
Contraindicated in patients with hypercalcemia or vitamin D toxicity. Withhold all preparations containing vitamin D.

NURSING CONSIDERATIONS
• Use cautiously in patients receiving cardiac glycosides and in those with sarcoidosis or hyperparathyroidism.
• Monitor serum calcium level; serum calcium level multiplied by the serum phosphate level should not exceed 70. During titration, determine serum calcium level twice weekly. Discontinue if hypercalcemia occurs and notify doctor, but resume after serum calcium level returns to

normal. Patient should receive adequate daily intake of calcium. Observe for hypocalcemia, bone pain, and weakness prior to and throughout therapy.
• Protect drug from heat and light.

◖ I.V. administration
• For hypocalcemic patients with chronic renal failure undergoing hemodialysis, may give drug by rapid I.V. injection through the catheter at end of hemodialysis session.

☑ Patient teaching
• Tell patient to report immediately early symptoms of vitamin D intoxication: weakness, nausea, vomiting, dry mouth, constipation, muscle or bone pain, or metallic taste.
• Instruct patient to adhere to diet and calcium supplementation and to avoid unapproved OTC drugs and magnesium-containing antacids.
Alert: Tell patient that drug must not be taken by anyone for whom it was not prescribed. It is the most potent form of vitamin D available.

---

dihydrotachysterol
AT-10‡, DHT Intensol*, Hytakerol

Pregnancy Risk Category: C

HOW SUPPLIED
Tablets: 0.125 mg, 0.2 mg, 0.4 mg
Capsules: 0.125 mg
Oral solution: 0.2 mg/5 ml, 0.2 mg/ml* (DHT Intensol*), 0.25 mg/ml (in sesame oil)
   Note: 1 mg of dihydrotachysterol is equal to 120,000 units ergocalciferol (vitamin D_2).

ACTION
A vitamin D analogue that stimulates calcium absorption from the GI tract and promotes secretion of calcium from bone to blood.

Route	Onset	Peak	Duration
PO	Several hr	1-2 wk	9 wk

INDICATIONS & DOSAGE

Hypocalcemia associated with hypopara-thyroidism and pseudohypoparathy-roidism—
Adults: initially, 0.75 to 2.5 mg P.O. daily for 3 days. Maintenance dosage is 0.2 to 1.0 mg daily.
Children: initially, 1 to 5 mg P.O. for 4 days. Maintenance dosage is 0.5 to 1.5 mg daily.
Prophylaxis of hypocalcemic tetany following thyroid surgery—
Adults: initially, 0.75 to 2.5 mg P.O. daily for 3 days. Maintenance dose is 0.25 mg weekly to 1 mg daily, p.r.n. (with calcium supplements).

ADVERSE REACTIONS

Vitamin D intoxication associated with hypercalcemia:
CNS: headache, somnolence, irritability, psychosis (rare).
CV: hypertension, *arrhythmias.*
EENT: conjunctivitis, photophobia, rhinorrhea.
GI: nausea, vomiting, constipation, polydipsia, pancreatitis, metallic taste, dry mouth, anorexia, diarrhea.
GU: polyuria, nocturia.
Other: weakness, bone and muscle pain, weight loss, hyperthermia, decreased libido, nephrocalcinosis.

INTERACTIONS

Drug-drug. *Cardiac glycosides:* increased risk of arrhythmias. Avoid concomitant use.
Cholestyramine, colestipol, excessive use of mineral oil: decreased absorption of orally administered vitamin D analogues. Avoid concomitant use.
Corticosteroids: counteract vitamin D analogue effects. Do not use together.
Magnesium-containing antacids: possible hypermagnesemia, especially in patients with chronic renal failure. Avoid concomitant use.
Other vitamin D analogues: increased toxicity. Avoid concomitant use.
Thiazide diuretics: may cause hypercalcemia. Use together cautiously.

EFFECTS ON DIAGNOSTIC TESTS

Drug alters serum alkaline phosphatase concentrations and cholesterol levels and may alter electrolyte levels, such as magnesium, phosphate, and calcium, in serum and urine.

CONTRAINDICATIONS

Contraindicated in patients with hypercalcemia or vitamin D toxicity.

NURSING CONSIDERATIONS

● Monitor serum calcium level as ordered; serum calcium level multiplied by serum phosphate level should not exceed 70. During titration, determine serum calcium level twice weekly. Discontinue if hypercalcemia occurs and notify doctor. Know that drug can be resumed after serum calcium level returns to normal. Adequate daily intake of calcium is 1,000 mg.
● Monitor urine calcium level.
● Store in tightly closed, light-resistant container. Do not refrigerate.

☑ Patient teaching

● Tell patient to report early signs of hypercalcemia: thirst, headache, vertigo, tinnitus, or anorexia promptly.
● Instruct patient to adhere to diet and calcium supplementation and to avoid OTC drugs and magnesium-containing antacids unless approved by doctor.

etidronate disodium
Didronel

Pregnancy Risk Category: C

HOW SUPPLIED

Tablets: 200 mg, 400 mg
Injection: 50 mg/ml

ACTION

Decreases osteoclastic activity by inhibiting osteocytic osteolysis and decreases mineral release and matrix or collagen breakdown in bone.

Route	Onset	Peak	Duration
PO	1 mo (in Paget's)	Unknown	Unknown
IV	24 hr	After 3rd infusion	Unknown

INDICATIONS & DOSAGE

Symptomatic Paget's disease of bone (osteitis deformans)—
Adults: 5 to 10 mg/kg P.O. daily (not to exceed 6 months of therapy) or 11 to 20 mg/kg P.O. daily (not to exceed 3 months of therapy) in single dose 2 hours before a meal with water or juice. Treatment is initiated only after an etidronate-free period of at least 90 days, and when there is specific evidence of active disease process.

Heterotopic ossification in spinal cord injuries—
Adults: 20 mg/kg P.O. daily for 2 weeks, then 10 mg/kg daily for 10 weeks. Total treatment period is 12 weeks.

Heterotopic ossification after total hip replacement—
Adults: 20 mg/kg P.O. daily for 1 month before total hip replacement and for 3 months afterward.

Malignancy-associated hypercalcemia—
Adults: 7.5 mg/kg I.V. daily for 3 consecutive days; a period of at least 7 days should elapse between courses of I.V. therapy. Maintenance dosage is 20 mg/kg P.O. daily for 30 days, initiated day after last I.V. dosage. May be used for a maximum of 90 days.

ADVERSE REACTIONS

GI: diarrhea, increased frequency of bowel movements, nausea, constipation, stomatitis (with dosage of 20 mg/kg daily).
Other: increased or recurrent bone pain, pain at previously asymptomatic sites, increased risk of fracture, *elevated serum phosphate level,* fever, fluid overload, dyspnea, **seizures,** abnormal hepatic function, hypersensitivity reactions.

INTERACTIONS

Drug-drug. *Antacids containing calcium, magnesium, or aluminum; mineral supplements containing calcium, iron, magnesium, or aluminum:* can inhibit absorption. Avoid use within 2 hours of dose.
Drug-food. *Foods containing large amounts of calcium (such as milk and dairy products):* can prevent oral absorption. Avoid use within 2 hours of dose.

EFFECTS ON DIAGNOSTIC TESTS

Drug may elevate serum phosphate levels.

CONTRAINDICATIONS

Contraindicated in patients with clinically overt osteomalacia or known hypersensitivity to drug. Also, I.V. etidronate disodium is contraindicated in patients with serum creatinine concentrations of 5 mg/dl or more.

NURSING CONSIDERATIONS

• Use cautiously in patients with impaired renal function.
• Monitor renal function before and during therapy, as ordered.
• Do not give drug with food, milk, or antacids; may reduce absorption.
• To monitor drug effects, review serum alkaline phosphatase and urinary hydroxyproline excretion.
• Be aware that elevated serum phosphate level may occur, especially in patients receiving higher doses. Phosphate level usually returns to normal 2 to 4 weeks after drug is discontinued.

⬗ I.V. administration

• Dilute daily dose in at least 250 ml of 0.9% NaCl solution or D_5W, and infuse over at least 2 hours. Diluted solution may be stored at room temperature for up to 48 hours.
• Know that some patients may receive I.V. drug for up to 7 days. Risk of hypokalemia increases after 3 days.

☑ Patient teaching

• Stress importance of a diet high in calcium and vitamin D.
• Tell patient not to eat for 2 hours after daily dose.
• Tell patient that improvement may not occur for up to 3 months and may continue for months after drug is stopped.

Reactions may be *common*, uncommon, *life-threatening*, or COMMON AND LIFE-THREATENING.

acetazolamide
acetazolamide sodium
amiloride hydrochloride
bumetanide
chlorthalidone
ethacrynate sodium
ethacrynic acid
furosemide
hydrochlorothiazide
indapamide
mannitol
methazolamide
metolazone
spironolactone
torsemide
triamterene
urea

COMBINATION PRODUCTS
ALDACTAZIDE 25/25: spironolactone
25 mg and hydrochlorothiazide 25 mg.
ALDACTAZIDE 50/50: spironolactone
50 mg and hydrochlorothiazide 50 mg.
DYAZIDE: triamterene 37.5 mg and
hydrochlorothiazide 25 mg.
MAXZIDE: triamterene 75 mg and hydrochlorothiazide 50 mg.
MAXZIDE-25MG: triamterene 37.5 mg
and hydrochlorothiazide 25 mg.
MODURETIC: amiloride hydrochloride
5 mg and hydrochlorothiazide 50 mg.
ZIAC 2.5: bisoprolol fumarate 2.5 mg and
hydrochlorothiazide 6.25 mg.
ZIAC 5: bisoprolol fumarate 5 mg and
hydrochlorothiazide 6.25 mg.
ZIAC 10: bisoprolol fumarate 10 mg and
hydrochlorothiazide 6.25 mg.

---

acetazolamide
Acetazolam†, Apo-Acetazolamide†,
Dazamide, Diamox, Diamox
Sequels

acetazolamide sodium
Diamox

Pregnancy Risk Category: C

HOW SUPPLIED
acetazolamide
Tablets: 125 mg, 250 mg
Capsules (extended-release): 500 mg
acetazolamide sodium
Injection: 500-mg vial

ACTION
Blocks the action of carbonic anhydrase,
promoting renal excretion of sodium,
potassium, bicarbonate, water, and decreases secretion of aqueous humor in the
eye, thereby lowering intraocular pressure. As an anticonvulsant, may inhibit
carbonic anhydrase in the CNS and decrease abnormal paroxysmal or excessive
neuronal discharge. In acute mountain
sickness, carbonic anhydrase inhibitors
produce a respiratory and metabolic acidosis that may stimulate ventilation, increase cerebral blood flow, promote the
release of oxygen from hemoglobin, and
increase ventilation.

Route	Onset	Peak	Duration
PO	1-1.5 hr	2-4 hr	8-12 hr
PO (extended)	2 hr	3-6 hr	18-24 hr
IV	2 min	15 min	1-5 hr

INDICATIONS & DOSAGE
*Secondary glaucoma and preoperative
treatment of acute angle-closure glaucoma*—
Adults: 250 mg P.O. q 4 hours; or 250 mg
P.O. b.i.d. for short-term therapy. To rapidly lower intraocular pressure, initially,
500 mg I.V., then 125 to 250 mg I.V. q 4
hours.
Children: 8 to 30 mg/kg P.O. daily in divided doses. For acute angle-closure glaucoma, 5 to 10 mcg/kg I.V. q 6 hours.
Chronic open-angle glaucoma—
Adults: 250 mg to 1 g P.O. daily in divided doses q.i.d., or 500 mg (extended-
release) P.O. b.i.d.
*Prevention or amelioration of acute
mountain sickness*—
Adults: 500 mg to 1 g P.O. daily in divid-

---

ed doses q 8 to 12 hours, or 500 mg (extended release) P.O. b.i.d. Treatment started 24 to 48 hours before ascent, and continued for 48 hours while at high altitude.
Adjunctive treatment of myoclonic, refractory, generalized tonic-clonic, absence, or mixed seizures—
Adults and children: 4 to 30 mg/kg P.O. daily in divided doses. For adults, the optimum dosage range is 375 mg to 1 g daily. Usually given with other anticonvulsants.

ADVERSE REACTIONS
CNS: drowsiness, paresthesia, confusion, depression, *seizures,* weakness.
EENT: transient myopia, hearing dysfunction, tinnitus.
GI: nausea, vomiting, anorexia, altered (metallic) taste, diarrhea, black tarry stools.
GU: polyuria, hematuria, crystalluria, glycosuria, renal calculus.
Hematologic: *aplastic anemia,* hemolytic anemia, leukopenia.
Skin: rash.
Other: *pain* (at injection site), sterile abscesses, hyperchloremic acidosis, hypokalemia, asymptomatic hyperuricemia.

INTERACTIONS
Drug-drug. *Amphetamines, anticholinergics, mecamylamine, procainamide, quinidine:* decreased renal clearance of these agents, increasing toxicity. Monitor closely.
Cyclosporine: increased cyclosporine levels, which may cause nephrotoxicity and neurotoxicity. Monitor closely.
Diflunisal: increased incidence of side effects of acetazolamide; significant decrease in intracranial pressure if used concurrently. Use with caution.
Lithium: increased excretion of lithium resulting in decreased effectiveness. Monitor closely.
Methenamine: reduced effectiveness of acetazolamide. Avoid concomitant use.
Primidone: serum and urine concentrations of primidone may be decreased. Monitor patient closely.
Salicylates: possible accumulation and toxicity of acetazolamide, including CNS depression and metabolic acidosis. Monitor closely.

EFFECTS ON DIAGNOSTIC TESTS
Because it alkalinizes urine, acetazolamide may cause false-positive proteinuria in Albustix or Albutest. Acetazolamide may also decrease thyroid iodine uptake.

CONTRAINDICATIONS
Contraindicated in patients receiving long-term treatment for chronic noncongestive angle-closure glaucoma and in those with hyponatremia or hypokalemia, renal or hepatic disease or dysfunction, renal calculi, adrenal gland failure, hyperchloremic acidosis, or hypersensitivity to drug.

NURSING CONSIDERATIONS
• Use cautiously in patients with respiratory acidosis, emphysema, or chronic pulmonary disease and in those receiving other diuretics.
• Know that cross-sensitivity between antibacterial sulfonamides and sulfonamide derivative diuretics such as acetazolamide has been reported.
• If patient is unable to swallow oral forms, check with the pharmacist. He may make a suspension using crushed acetazolamide tablets in a highly flavored syrup, such as cherry, raspberry, or chocolate. Although concentrations up to 500 mg/5 ml are feasible, concentrations of 250 mg/5 ml are more palatable. Refrigeration improves palatability but does not improve stability. Suspensions are stable for 1 week.
• Monitor fluid intake and output, glucose, and electrolytes, especially serum potassium, bicarbonate, and chloride. When used in diuretic therapy, consult doctor and dietitian about providing a high-potassium diet.
• Monitor elderly patients closely because they are especially susceptible to excessive diuresis.
• Weigh patient daily. Rapid or excessive fluid loss causes weight loss and hypotension.
• Keep in mind that diuretic effect decreases when acidosis occurs but can be reestablished by withdrawing drug, as or-

---

Reactions may be *common,* uncommon, *life-threatening,* or COMMON AND LIFE-THREATENING.

dered, for several days and then restarting, or by using intermittent administration schedules.

• Because bicarbonate ion excretion makes patient's urine alkaline, be aware that drug may cause false-positive urine protein tests.

• Know that drug may increase blood glucose and cause glycosuria.

▶ I.V. administration

• Inject 100 to 500 mg/minute into a large vein using a 21G or 23G needle. Intermittent or continuous infusion is not recommended.

• Reconstitute 500-mg vial with at least 5 ml of sterile water for injection. Use within 24 hours of reconstitution.

☑ Patient teaching

• Tell patient to take oral form with food if GI upset occurs.

• Caution patient not to perform hazardous activities if adverse CNS reactions occur.

• Tell patient to monitor blood glucose and urine for sugar.

---

amiloride hydrochloride
Kaluril‡, Midamor

Pregnancy Risk Category: B

HOW SUPPLIED
Tablets: 5 mg

ACTION
A potassium-sparing diuretic that inhibits sodium reabsorption and potassium excretion in the distal tubules.

Route	Onset	Peak	Duration
PO	2 hr	6-10 hr	24 hr

INDICATIONS & DOSAGE
Hypertension; hypokalemia; edema associated with heart failure, usually in patients also taking thiazide or other potassium-wasting diuretics—
Adults: usual dosage is 5 mg P.O. daily. Increased to 10 mg daily, if necessary, then 15 mg. Maximum dosage is 20 mg daily.

ADVERSE REACTIONS
CNS: *headache,* weakness, dizziness, encephalopathy.
CV: orthostatic hypotension.
GI: *nausea, anorexia, diarrhea, vomiting,* abdominal pain, constipation, appetite changes.
GU: impotence.
Hematologic: *aplastic anemia,* neutropenia.
Other: hyperkalemia, fatigue, muscle cramps, dyspnea, hyponatremia.

INTERACTIONS
Drug-drug. *ACE inhibitors, potassium-sparing diuretics, potassium supplements:* possible hyperkalemia. Avoid concomitant use.
Lithium: decreased lithium clearance, increasing risk of lithium toxicity. Monitor lithium level.
NSAIDs: decreased diuretic effectiveness. Avoid concomitant use.
Drug-food. *Foods high in potassium (such as bananas, oranges), potassium-containing salt substitutes:* possible hyperkalemia. Choose diet with caution. Use low-potassium salt substitutes.

EFFECTS ON DIAGNOSTIC TESTS
Transient abnormal renal and hepatic function tests have been noted. Amiloride therapy causes severe hyperkalemia in diabetic patients after glucose tolerance testing; discontinue amiloride at least 3 days before testing.

CONTRAINDICATIONS
Contraindicated in patients with elevated serum potassium level (greater than 5.5 mEq/L). Do not administer to patients receiving other potassium-sparing diuretics, such as spironolactone and triamterene. Also contraindicated in patients with anuria, acute or chronic renal insufficiency, diabetic nephropathy, and hypersensitivity to drug.

NURSING CONSIDERATIONS
• Use cautiously in patients with diabetes mellitus, cardiopulmonary disease, and severe, existing hepatic insufficiency and in elderly or debilitated patients.

• To prevent nausea, administer drug with meals.
• If drug is not taken concurrently with a potassium-wasting drug, monitor potassium level because of increased risk of hyperkalemia. Alert doctor immediately if potassium level exceeds 6.5 mEq/L, and expect drug to be discontinued.

☑ **Patient teaching**
• Advise patient to avoid sudden postural changes and to rise slowly to avoid orthostatic hypotension.
• Caution patient not to perform hazardous activities if adverse CNS reactions occur.
• To prevent serious hyperkalemia, warn patient to avoid excessive ingestion of potassium-rich foods, potassium-containing salt substitutes, and potassium supplements.
• Advise patient to report signs of hyperkalemia: paresthesia, muscular weakness, fatigue, paralysis of extremities.
• Instruct patient to check with doctor or pharmacist before taking new prescription or OTC medications.

---

bumetanide
Bumex, Burinex‡§

Pregnancy Risk Category: C

HOW SUPPLIED
Tablets: 0.5 mg, 1 mg, 2 mg
Injection: 0.25 mg/ml

ACTION
A potent loop diuretic that inhibits sodium and chloride reabsorption at the ascending portion of the loop of Henle.

Route	Onset	Peak	Duration
PO	0.5-1 hr	1-2 hr	4-6 hr
IV	Within minutes	15-30 min	0.5-1 hr
IM	40 min	Unknown	5-6 hr

INDICATIONS & DOSAGE
Edema in heart failure, or hepatic or renal disease—
Adults: 0.5 to 2 mg P.O. once daily. If diuretic response is not adequate, a second or third dose may be given at 4- to 5-hour

intervals. Maximum dosage is 10 mg/day. May be administered parenterally if P.O. not feasible. Usual initial dose is 0.5 to 1 mg given I.V. or I.M. If response is not adequate, a second or third dose may be given at 2- to 3-hour intervals. Maximum dosage is 10 mg/day.

ADVERSE REACTIONS
CNS: dizziness, headache, vertigo.
CV: volume depletion and dehydration, orthostatic hypotension, ECG changes, chest pain, increased cholesterol levels.
EENT: transient deafness, tinnitus.
GI: nausea, vomiting, upset stomach, dry mouth, diarrhea, pain.
GU: *renal failure,* premature ejaculation, difficulty maintaining erection, oliguria.
Hematologic: azotemia, *thrombocytopenia.*
Skin: rash, pruritus, diaphoresis.
Other: hypokalemia; hypochloremic alkalosis; hypomagnesemia, asymptomatic hyperuricemia; weakness; arthritic pain; fluid and electrolyte imbalances, including dilutional hyponatremia, hypocalcemia, hyperglycemia, and glucose intolerance impairment; muscle pain and tenderness.

INTERACTIONS
Drug-drug. *Aminoglycoside antibiotics:* potentiated ototoxicity. Use together cautiously.
Antihypertensives: increased risk of hypotension. Use together cautiously.
Cardiac glycosides: increased risk of digitalis toxicity from bumetanide-induced hypokalemia. Monitor potassium and digitalis levels.
Indomethacin, NSAIDs, probenecid: inhibited diuretic response. Use together cautiously.
Lithium: decreased lithium clearance, increasing risk of lithium toxicity. Monitor lithium level.
Metolazone: profound diuresis and potential electrolyte loss. Monitor the patient for fluid and electrolyte disorders.
Other potassium-wasting drugs (such as amphotericin B, corticosteroids): increased risk of hypokalemia. Use together cautiously.

Reactions may be *common,* uncommon, *life-threatening,* or **COMMON AND LIFE-THREATENING.**

EFFECTS ON DIAGNOSTIC TESTS
Drug therapy alters electrolyte balance and liver and renal function tests.

CONTRAINDICATIONS
Contraindicated in patients with anuria, hepatic coma, or hypersensitivity to drug or sulfonamides (possible cross-sensitivity) and in those in states of severe electrolyte depletion.

NURSING CONSIDERATIONS
• Use cautiously in patients with hepatic cirrhosis and ascites, in the elderly, and in those with depressed renal function.
• To prevent nocturia, give in the morning. If second dose is necessary, give in early afternoon.
• Be aware that safest and most effective dosage schedule for control of edema is intermittent dosage given on alternate days, or for 3 to 4 days with 1 or 2 days of rest periods.
• Monitor fluid intake and output, weight, and serum electrolyte, BUN, creatinine, and carbon dioxide levels frequently.
• Watch for evidence of hypokalemia, such as muscle weakness and cramps. Instruct patient to report these symptoms.
• Consult doctor and dietitian about a high-potassium diet. Foods rich in potassium include citrus fruits, tomatoes, bananas, dates, and apricots.
• Monitor blood glucose levels in diabetic patients.
• Monitor blood uric acid levels, especially in patients with history of gout.
• Monitor blood pressure and pulse rate during rapid diuresis. Bumetanide can lead to profound water and electrolyte depletion.
• If oliguria or azotemia develops or increases, know that doctor may stop drug.
• Keep in mind that bumetanide can be safely used in patients allergic to furosemide; 1 mg of bumetanide equals 40 mg of furosemide.

◘ I.V. administration
• Give I.V. doses directly, using a 21G or 23G needle over 1 to 2 minutes. For intermittent infusion, give diluted drug through an intermittent infusion device or piggyback into an I.V. line containing a free-flowing, compatible solution. Infuse at ordered rate. Continuous infusion not recommended.

☑ Patient teaching
• Tell patient to take drug in morning to prevent nocturia, and if second dose is prescribed to take it in early afternoon. Also instruct patient to take drug with food or milk if adverse GI reactions occur.
• Advise patient to stand up slowly to prevent dizziness, and to limit alcohol intake and strenuous exercise in hot weather to avoid exacerbating orthostatic hypotension.
• Instruct patient to weigh himself daily to monitor fluid status.

chlorthalidone
Apo-Chlorthalidone†, Hygroton, Novo-Thalidone†, Thalitone, Uridon†

Pregnancy Risk Category: B

HOW SUPPLIED
Tablets: 15 mg, 25 mg, 50 mg, 100 mg

ACTION
Although not a thiazide, chlorthalidone acts similarly, increasing sodium and water excretion by inhibiting sodium and chloride reabsorption in the nephron's distal segment.

Route	Onset	Peak	Duration
PO	2-3 hr	2-6 hr	2-3 days

INDICATIONS & DOSAGE
Edema, hypertension—
Adults: initially, 25 to 100 mg P.O. daily, or up to 200 mg P.O. on alternate days.
Children: 2 mg/kg or 60 mg/m² P.O. three times weekly.

ADVERSE REACTIONS
CNS: dizziness, vertigo, headache, paresthesia, weakness, restlessness.
CV: volume depletion and dehydration, orthostatic hypotension, vasculitis, increased cholesterol and triglyceride levels.
GI: anorexia, nausea, pancreatitis, vomit-

ing, abdominal pain, diarrhea, constipation.

GU: impotence.

Hematologic: *aplastic anemia, agranulocytosis,* leukopenia, thrombocytopenia.

Hepatic: jaundice.

Skin: dermatitis, photosensitivity, rash, purpura, urticaria.

Other: hypersensitivity reactions; *hypokalemia;* asymptomatic hyperuricemia; hyperglycemia and impairment of glucose tolerance; fluid and electrolyte imbalances, including dilutional hyponatremia and hypochloremia, metabolic alkalosis, hypercalcemia; gout.

INTERACTIONS

Drug-drug. *Amphotericin B:* increased risk of hypokalemia. Monitor closely.

Antidiabetic agents: decreased effectiveness; dosage adjustments may be necessary. Monitor blood glucose levels.

Barbiturates, opiates: increased orthostatic hypotensive effect. Monitor closely.

Cardiac glycosides: increased risk of digitalis toxicity from chlorthalidone-induced hypokalemia. Monitor potassium and digitalis levels.

Cholestyramine, colestipol: decreased intestinal absorption of thiazides. Separate doses.

Corticosteroids: increased risk of hypokalemia. Monitor closely.

Diazoxide: increased antihypertensive, hyperglycemic, and hyperuricemic effects. Use together cautiously.

Lithium: decreased lithium clearance, increasing risk of lithium toxicity. Monitor lithium level.

NSAIDs: increased risk of NSAID-induced renal failure. Monitor closely.

Drug-lifestyle. *Alcohol use:* increased orthostatic hypotensive effect. Monitor closely.

Sun exposure: photosensitivity reactions may occur. Take precautions.

EFFECTS ON DIAGNOSTIC TESTS

Drug therapy may alter serum electrolyte levels and may increase serum uric acid, glucose, cholesterol, and triglyceride levels. It may interfere with tests for parathyroid functions and should be discontinued before such tests.

CONTRAINDICATIONS

Contraindicated in patients with anuria and hypersensitivity to thiazides or other sulfonamide-derived drugs.

NURSING CONSIDERATIONS

● Use cautiously in patients with severe renal disease and impaired hepatic function.

● To prevent nocturia, give drug in the morning.

● Monitor fluid intake and output, weight, blood pressure, and serum electrolyte levels.

● Watch for signs of hypokalemia, such as muscle weakness, and cramps. Know that drug may be used with potassium-sparing diuretic to prevent potassium loss.

● Consult doctor and dietitian about a high-potassium diet. Foods rich in potassium include citrus fruits, tomatoes, bananas, apricots, and dates.

● Monitor serum creatinine and BUN levels regularly. Cumulative effects of drug may occur with impaired renal function.

● Monitor blood uric acid levels, especially in patients with history of gout.

● Monitor blood glucose levels, and check insulin requirements in diabetic patients.

● Monitor elderly patients, who are especially susceptible to excessive diuresis.

Alert: Do not use Hygroton and Thalitone interchangeably; they have different bioavailabilities.

● As ordered, discontinue thiazides and thiazide-like diuretics before parathyroid function tests.

● In patients with hypertension, be aware that therapeutic response may be delayed several weeks.

Alert: Do not confuse Uridon tablets (available in Canada only) with the urinary anti-infective Uridon Modified (available in the United States).

☑ **Patient teaching**

● Instruct patient to take in morning to prevent nocturia.

● Tell patient to avoid sudden posture changes and to rise slowly to avoid orthostatic hypotension.

● Advise patient to use a sunblock to prevent photosensitivity reactions.

Reactions may be *common,* uncommon, *life-threatening,* or COMMON AND LIFE-THREATENING.

ethacrynate sodium
Edecrin Sodium

ethacrynic acid
Edecril‡, Edecrin

Pregnancy Risk Category: B

HOW SUPPLIED
ethacrynic acid
Tablets: 25 mg, 50 mg
ethacrynate sodium
Injection: 50 mg (with 62.5 mg of mannitol and 0.1 mg of thimerosal)

ACTION
A potent loop diuretic that inhibits sodium and chloride reabsorption at the proximal and distal tubules and the ascending loop of Henle.

Route	Onset	Peak	Duration
PO	30 min	2 hr	6-8 hr
IV	5 min	15-30 min	2 hr

INDICATIONS & DOSAGE
Acute pulmonary edema—
Adults: 50 mg or 0.5 to 1 mg/kg I.V. Usually only one dose is necessary, although a second dose may be required.
Edema—
Adults: 50 to 200 mg P.O. daily. Refractory cases may require up to 200 mg b.i.d.
Children: initial dose is 25 mg P.O., increased cautiously in 25-mg increments daily until desired effect is achieved.

ADVERSE REACTIONS
CNS: confusion, fatigue, vertigo, headache, nervousness.
CV: volume depletion and dehydration, orthostatic hypotension.
EENT: transient or permanent deafness (with too-rapid I.V. injection), blurred vision, tinnitus, hearing loss.
GI: cramping, diarrhea, anorexia, nausea, vomiting, *GI bleeding, pancreatitis.*
GU: oliguria, hematuria, nocturia, polyuria, frequent urination.
Hematologic: *agranulocytosis,* neutropenia, *thrombocytopenia,* azotemia.
Other: hypokalemia; hypochloremic alkalosis; asymptomatic hyperuricemia; rash; fever; chills; malaise; fluid and electrolyte imbalances, including dilutional hyponatremia, hypocalcemia, hypomagnesemia; hyperglycemia and impaired glucose tolerance.

INTERACTIONS
Drug-drug. *Aminoglycoside antibiotics:* potentiated ototoxic adverse reactions of both drugs. Use together cautiously.
Antihypertensives: increased risk of hypotension. Use together cautiously.
Cardiac glycosides: increased risk of digitalis toxicity from ethacrynate-induced hypokalemia. Monitor potassium and digitalis levels.
Cisplatin: increased risk of ototoxicity. Avoid concomitant use.
Lithium: decreased lithium clearance, increasing risk of lithium toxicity. Monitor lithium level.
Metolazone: profound diuresis and enhanced electrolyte loss. Use together cautiously.
NSAIDs: decreased diuretic effectiveness. Use together cautiously.
Warfarin: potentiated anticoagulant effect. Use together cautiously.

EFFECTS ON DIAGNOSTIC TESTS
Drug therapy alters electrolyte balance and liver and renal function tests.

CONTRAINDICATIONS
Contraindicated in infants and in patients with anuria or hypersensitivity to drug.

NURSING CONSIDERATIONS
• Use cautiously in patients with electrolyte abnormalities or hepatic impairment.
• Give oral doses in the morning to prevent nocturia.
• Do not give S.C. or I.M. because of local pain and irritation.
• Monitor fluid intake and output, weight, blood pressure, and serum electrolyte levels.
• Watch for signs of hypokalemia, such as muscle weakness and cramps.
• Consult doctor and dietitian about providing a high-potassium diet. Foods rich in potassium include citrus fruits, tomatoes, bananas, dates, and apricots. Know

---

that potassium chloride and sodium supplements may be needed.
• Monitor elderly patients, who are especially susceptible to excessive diuresis.
• Monitor blood uric acid levels, especially in patients with a history of gout.
Alert: Be aware that severe diarrhea will necessitate discontinuing drug. Know that patient should not receive drug again after diarrhea has resolved.

I.V. administration
• Add to vial 50 ml of D_5W or 0.9% NaCl solution. Give slowly through tubing of running infusion over several minutes. Discard unused solution after 24 hours. Do not use cloudy or opalescent solutions.
• If more than one I.V. dose is necessary, use a new injection site to avoid thrombophlebitis.
• Do not mix with whole blood or its derivatives.

Patient teaching
• Instruct patient to take oral form of drug in morning to prevent nocturia and if second dose is required, to take it in early afternoon. Also tell patient to take drug with food or milk if adverse GI reactions occur.
• Advise patient to avoid sudden posture changes and to rise slowly to avoid orthostatic hypotension.
• Caution patient not to perform hazardous activities if drowsiness occurs.
• Advise diabetic patient to closely monitor blood glucose levels.

---

furosemide (frusemide†‡)
Apo-Furosemide†, Furoside†, Lasix*, Novo-Semide†, Urex‡, Urex-M‡, Uritol†

Pregnancy Risk Category: C

HOW SUPPLIED
Tablets: 20 mg, 40 mg, 80 mg, 500 mg†‡
Oral solution: 10 mg/ml, 40 mg/5 ml
Injection: 10 mg/ml

ACTION
A potent loop diuretic that inhibits sodium and chloride reabsorption at the proximal and distal tubules and the ascending loop of Henle.

Route	Onset	Peak	Duration
PO	20-60 min	1-2 hr	6-8 hr
IV	5 min	30 min	2 hr

INDICATIONS & DOSAGE
Acute pulmonary edema—
Adults: 40 mg I.V. injected slowly over 1 to 2 minutes; then 80 mg I.V. in 1 to 1½ hours if needed.
Edema—
Adults: 20 to 80 mg P.O. daily in the morning, second dose in 6 to 8 hours; carefully titrated up to 600 mg daily if needed. Or, 20 to 40 mg I.M. or I.V., increased by 20 mg q 2 hours until desired response is achieved. Give I.V. dose slowly over 1 to 2 minutes.
Infants and children: 2 mg/kg P.O. daily, increased by 1 to 2 mg/kg in 6 to 8 hours if needed; carefully titrated up to 6 mg/kg daily if needed.
Hypertension—
Adults: 40 mg P.O. b.i.d. Dosage adjusted based on response. May be used as adjunct to other antihypertensive agents if necessary.

ADVERSE REACTIONS
CNS: vertigo, headache, dizziness, paresthesia, restlessness.
CV: volume depletion and dehydration, orthostatic hypotension, increased cholesterol levels.
EENT: transient deafness (with too-rapid I.V. injection), blurred or yellowed vision.
GI: abdominal discomfort and pain, diarrhea, anorexia, nausea, vomiting, constipation, pancreatitis.
GU: nocturia, polyuria, frequent urination, oliguria.
Hematologic: *agranulocytosis, leukopenia, thrombocytopenia,* azotemia, anemia, *aplastic anemia.*
Skin: dermatitis, purpura, photosensitivity.
Other: hepatic dysfunction; hypokalemia; hypochloremic alkalosis; asymptomatic hyperuricemia; gout; fever; muscle spasm; weakness; fluid and electrolyte imbalances, including dilutional hyponatremia, hypocalcemia, hypomagnesemia;

hyperglycemia and impaired glucose tolerance; transient pain at injection site (with I.M. administration); thrombophlebitis (with I.V. administration).

INTERACTIONS
Drug-drug. *Aminoglycoside antibiotics, cisplatin:* potentiated ototoxicity. Use together cautiously.
Amphotericin B, corticosteroids, corticotropin, metolazone: increased risk of hypokalemia. Monitor potassium levels closely.
Antidiabetic agents: decreased hypoglycemic effects. Monitor blood glucose levels.
Antihypertensives: increased risk of hypotension. Use together cautiously.
Cardiac glycosides, neuromuscular blockers: increased toxicity of these agents from furosemide-induced hypokalemia. Monitor potassium levels.
Ethacrynic acid: may increase risk of ototoxicity. Do not use concomitantly.
Lithium: decreased lithium excretion, resulting in lithium toxicity. Monitor lithium level.
NSAIDs: inhibited diuretic response. Use together cautiously.
Salicylates: may cause salicylate toxicity. Use together cautiously.
Sucralfate: may reduce diuretic and antihypertensive effect. Separate administration time by 2 hours.
Drug-herb. *Aloe:* possible increased drug effects. Use together cautiously.
Drug-lifestyle. *Sun exposure:* photosensitivity reactions may occur. Take precautions.

EFFECTS ON DIAGNOSTIC TESTS
Drug therapy alters electrolyte balance and liver and renal function tests.

CONTRAINDICATIONS
Contraindicated in patients with anuria or history of hypersensitivity to drug.

NURSING CONSIDERATIONS
● Use cautiously in patients with hepatic cirrhosis. Know that furosemide should be used during pregnancy only if potential benefits clearly outweigh possible risks to fetus.

● To prevent nocturia, give P.O. and I.M. preparations in the morning. Give second doses in early afternoon.
Alert: Monitor weight, blood pressure, and pulse rate routinely with chronic use and during rapid diuresis. Furosemide can lead to profound water and electrolyte depletion.
● Be aware that if oliguria or azotemia develops or increases, it may require stopping drug.
● Monitor fluid intake and output and serum electrolyte, BUN, and carbon dioxide levels frequently.
● Watch for signs of hypokalemia, such as muscle weakness and cramps.
● Consult doctor and dietitian about a high-potassium diet. Foods rich in potassium include citrus fruits, tomatoes, bananas, and dates.
● Monitor blood glucose levels in diabetic patients.
● Know that furosemide may not be well absorbed orally in severe heart failure. Drug may need to be given I.V. even if patient is taking other oral medications.
● Monitor blood uric acid, especially in patients with a history of gout.
● Monitor elderly patients, who are especially susceptible to excessive diuresis, with potential for circulatory collapse and thromboembolic complications.
● Store tablets in light-resistant container to prevent discoloration (does not affect potency). Do not use discolored (yellow) injectable preparation. Refrigerate oral furosemide solution to ensure drug stability.

I.V. administration
● Given by direct injection over 1 to 2 minutes. Alternatively, dilute with D_5W, 0.9% NaCl solution, or lactated Ringer's solution, and infuse no faster than 4 mg/minute to avoid ototoxicity. Use prepared infusion solution within 24 hours.

Patient teaching
● Advise patient to take drug with food to prevent GI upset. Also tell him to take drug in morning to prevent nocturia; if second dose is required, tell patient to take the second dose in early afternoon, 6 to 8 hours after morning dose.

• Inform patient of possible need for potassium or magnesium supplements.

• Instruct patient to stand slowly to prevent dizziness and to limit alcohol intake and strenuous exercise in hot weather to avoid exacerbating orthostatic hypotension.

• Advise patient to immediately report ringing in ears, severe abdominal pain, or sore throat and fever; may indicate furosemide toxicity.

• Discourage patient taking furosemide at home from storing different types of medication in the same container, increasing the risk of drug errors. The most popular strengths of furosemide and digoxin are white tablets approximately equal in size.

• Tell patient to check with doctor or pharmacist before taking OTC medications.

• Teach patient to avoid direct sunlight and use protective clothing and a sunblock; there is a risk of photosensitivity.

---

hydrochlorothiazide
Apo-Hydro†, Dichlotride‡, Diuchlor H†, Esidrix, Ezide, HydroDIURIL, Hydro-Par, HydroSaluric§, Neo-Codema†, Novo-Hydrazide†, Oretic, Urozide†

Pregnancy Risk Category: B

HOW SUPPLIED
Tablets: 25 mg, 50 mg, 100 mg
Oral solution: 50 mg/5 ml, 100 mg/ml

ACTION
A thiazide diuretic that increases sodium and water excretion by inhibiting sodium and chloride reabsorption in the nephron's distal segment.

Route	Onset	Peak	Duration
PO	2 hr	4-6 hr	6-12 hr

INDICATIONS & DOSAGE
Edema—
Adults: 25 to 100 mg P.O. daily or intermittently. May go to 200 mg initially for several days until dry weight is attained.
Children 2 to 12 years: 1 to 2 mg/kg

once or twice daily not to exceed 37.5 to 100 mg daily.
Children 6 months to 2 years: 1 to 2 mg/kg once or twice daily within a range of 12.5 to 37.5 mg daily.
Infants under 6 months: up to 3 mg/kg P.O. daily in two divided doses. Total daily dosage may range from 12.5 to 37.5 mg.
Hypertension—
Adults: 25 to 50 mg P.O. daily as a single dose or divided b.i.d. Daily dosage increased or decreased according to blood pressure.

Doses exceeding 50 mg/day are not required when combined with other antihypertensives.

ADVERSE REACTIONS
CNS: dizziness, vertigo, headache, paresthesia, weakness, restlessness.
CV: volume depletion and dehydration, orthostatic hypotension, allergic myocarditis, vasculitis.
GI: anorexia, nausea, pancreatitis, epigastric distress, vomiting, abdominal pain, diarrhea, constipation.
GU: polyuria, frequent urination, *renal failure,* interstitial nephritis.
Hematologic: *aplastic anemia, agranulocytosis,* leukopenia, *thrombocytopenia,* hemolytic anemia.
Hepatic: jaundice.
Respiratory: respiratory distress, pneumonitis.
Skin: dermatitis, photosensitivity, rash, purpura, alopecia.
Other: hypersensitivity reactions; hypokalemia; asymptomatic hyperuricemia; hyperglycemia and impaired glucose tolerance; fluid and electrolyte imbalances, including dilutional hyponatremia and hypochloremia, metabolic alkalosis, hypercalcemia; gout; muscle cramps; *anaphylactic reactions.*

INTERACTIONS
Drug-drug. *Amphotericin B, corticosteroids:* increased risk of hypokalemia. Monitor closely.
Antidiabetic agents: decreased effectiveness of hypoglycemic agents; dosage adjustments may be necessary. Monitor blood glucose levels.

Reactions may be *common,* uncommon, *life-threatening,* or COMMON AND LIFE-THREATENING.

Antihypertensives: additive antihypertensive effect. Use together cautiously.

Barbiturates, opiates: increased orthostatic hypotensive effect. Monitor closely.

Cardiac glycosides: increased risk of digitalis toxicity from hydrochlorothiazide-induced hypokalemia. Monitor potassium and digitalis levels.

Cholestyramine, colestipol: decreased intestinal absorption of thiazides. Separate doses.

Diazoxide: increased antihypertensive, hyperglycemic, and hyperuricemic effects. Use together cautiously.

Lithium: decreased lithium excretion, increasing risk of lithium toxicity. Monitor lithium level.

NSAIDs: increased risk of NSAID-induced renal failure. Monitor closely.

Drug-lifestyle. *Alcohol use:* increased orthostatic hypotensive effect. Monitor closely.

EFFECTS ON DIAGNOSTIC TESTS
Drug therapy may alter serum electrolyte levels and may increase serum uric acid, glucose, cholesterol, and triglyceride levels. It also may interfere with tests for parathyroid function and should be discontinued before such tests.

CONTRAINDICATIONS
Contraindicated in patients with anuria and hypersensitivity to other thiazides or other sulfonamide derivatives.

NURSING CONSIDERATIONS
• Use cautiously in children and in patients with severe renal disease, impaired hepatic function, and progressive hepatic disease.
• To prevent nocturia, give in the morning.
• Monitor fluid intake and output, weight, blood pressure, and serum electrolyte levels.
• Watch for signs of hypokalemia, such as muscle weakness and cramps. Drug may be used with potassium-sparing diuretic to prevent potassium loss.
• Consult doctor and dietitian about a high-potassium diet. Foods rich in potassium include citrus fruits, tomatoes, bananas, apricots, and dates.

• Monitor serum creatinine and BUN levels regularly. Cumulative effects of the drug may occur with impaired renal function.
• Monitor blood uric acid levels, especially in patients with history of gout.
• Monitor blood glucose levels, especially in diabetic patients.
• Monitor elderly patients, who are especially susceptible to excessive diuresis.
• As ordered, discontinue thiazides and thiazide-like diuretics before parathyroid function tests.
• In patients with hypertension, know that therapeutic response may be delayed several weeks.

☑ **Patient teaching**
• Instruct patient to take drug with food to minimize GI upset. Also tell him to take drug in morning to avoid nocturia; if second dose is needed, have him take it in early afternoon.
• Advise patient to avoid sudden posture changes and to rise slowly to avoid orthostatic hypotension.
• Encourage patient to use a sunblock to prevent photosensitivity reactions.
• Tell patient to check with doctor or pharmacist before taking OTC medications or alcohol.

indapamide
Lozide†, Lozol, Natrilix‡

Pregnancy Risk Category: B

HOW SUPPLIED
Tablets: 1.25 mg, 2.5 mg

ACTION
Unknown. A thiazide-like diuretic that probably inhibits sodium reabsorption in the nephron's distal segment. Also has a direct vasodilating effect that may be a result of calcium channel-blocking action.

Route	Onset	Peak	Duration
PO	Unknown	2-5 hr	18 hr

INDICATIONS & DOSAGE
Edema—
Adults: initially, 2.5 mg P.O. daily in the

morning. Increased to 5 mg daily after 1 week, if needed.

Hypertension—

Adults: initially, 1.25 mg P.O. daily in morning. Increased to 2.5 mg daily after 4 weeks, if needed. Increased to 5 mg daily after 4 more weeks, if needed.

ADVERSE REACTIONS

CNS: headache, nervousness, dizziness, light-headedness, weakness, vertigo, restlessness, drowsiness, fatigue, anxiety, depression, numbness of extremities, irritability, agitation.

CV: volume depletion and dehydration, orthostatic hypotension, palpitations, PVC, irregular heartbeat, vasculitis.

GI: anorexia, nausea, epigastric distress, vomiting, abdominal pain, diarrhea, constipation.

GU: nocturia, polyuria, frequent urination, impotence.

Skin: rash, pruritus, urticaria, flushing.

Other: muscle cramps and spasms; asymptomatic hyperuricemia; fluid and electrolyte imbalances, including dilutional hyponatremia and hypochloremia, metabolic alkalosis, hypokalemia; gout; rhinorrhea; weight loss.

INTERACTIONS

Drug-drug. *Amphotericin B:* increased risk of hypokalemia. Monitor closely.
Cardiac glycosides: increased risk of digitalis toxicity from indapamide-induced hypokalemia. Monitor potassium and digitalis levels.
Corticosteroids: increased risk of hypokalemia. Monitor closely.
Diazoxide: increased antihypertensive, hyperglycemic, and hyperuricemic effects. Use together cautiously.
Lithium: decreased lithium clearance that may increase lithium toxicity. Avoid concomitant use.
NSAIDs: increased risk of NSAID-induced renal failure. Monitor patient for signs of renal failure.

EFFECTS ON DIAGNOSTIC TESTS

Drug therapy may alter serum electrolyte levels and may increase serum uric acid, glucose, cholesterol, and triglyceride levels. It also may interfere with tests for parathyroid function and should be discontinued before such tests.

CONTRAINDICATIONS

Contraindicated in patients with anuria or hypersensitivity to other sulfonamide-derived drugs.

NURSING CONSIDERATIONS

• Use cautiously in patients with severe renal disease, impaired hepatic function, and progressive hepatic disease.

• To prevent nocturia, give drug in the morning.

• Monitor fluid intake and output, weight, blood pressure, and serum electrolyte levels.

• Watch for signs of hypokalemia, such as muscle weakness and cramps. Know that drug may be used with potassium-sparing diuretic to prevent potassium loss.

• Consult doctor and dietitian about a high-potassium diet. Foods rich in potassium include citrus fruits, tomatoes, bananas, apricots, and dates.

• Monitor serum creatinine and BUN levels regularly. Cumulative effects of drug may occur with impaired renal function.

• Monitor blood uric acid levels, especially in patients with a history of gout.

• Monitor blood glucose levels, especially in diabetic patients.

• Monitor elderly patients, who are especially susceptible to excessive diuresis.

• Discontinue thiazides and thiazide-like diuretics before parathyroid function tests, as ordered.

• Be aware that therapeutic response may be delayed several weeks in patients with hypertension. Also, if dose needs to be increased to 5 mg, concomitant therapy may be considered.

☑ **Patient teaching**
• Instruct patient to take drug in morning to prevent nocturia and with food if GI upset occurs.

• Advise patient to avoid sudden posture changes and to rise slowly to avoid orthostatic hypotension.

Reactions may be *common,* uncommon, *life-threatening,* or COMMON AND LIFE-THREATENING.

mannitol
Osmitrol

Pregnancy Risk Category: C

HOW SUPPLIED
Injection: 5%, 10%, 15%, 20%, 25%

ACTION
An osmotic diuretic that increases the osmotic pressure of glomerular filtrate, inhibiting tubular reabsorption of water and electrolytes, and that elevates blood plasma osmolality, resulting in enhanced water flow into extracellular fluid.

Route	Onset	Peak	Duration
IV	1-3 hr	0.5-1 hr	3-8 hr

INDICATIONS & DOSAGE
Test dose for marked oliguria or suspected inadequate renal function—
Adults and children over 12 years:
200 mg/kg or 12.5 g as a 15% to 20% I.V. solution over 3 to 5 minutes. Response is adequate if 30 to 50 ml urine/hour is excreted over 2 to 3 hours; if response is inadequate, a second test dose is given. If still no response after the second dose, mannitol should not be continued.
Oliguria—
Adults and children over 12 years: 50 to 100 g I.V. as a 15% to 25% solution over 1½ to several hours.
Prevention of oliguria or acute renal failure—
Adults and children over 12 years: 50 to 100 g I.V. of a concentrated solution, followed by a 5% to 10% solution. Exact concentration determined by fluid requirements.
Reduction of intraocular or intracranial pressure—
Adults and children over 12 years: 1.5 to 2 g/kg as a 15% to 20% I.V. solution over 30 to 60 minutes.
Diuresis in drug intoxication—
Adults and children over 12 years: 5% to 10% solution continuously up to 200 g I.V., while maintaining 100 to 500 ml urine output/hour and a positive fluid balance.

Irrigating solution during transurethral resection of the prostate gland—
Adults: 2.5% to 5% solution, p.r.n.

ADVERSE REACTIONS
CNS: *seizures,* dizziness, headache.
CV: edema, thrombophlebitis, hypotension, hypertension, *heart failure,* tachycardia, angina-like chest pain, vascular overload.
EENT: blurred vision, rhinitis.
GI: thirst, dry mouth, nausea, vomiting, *diarrhea.*
GU: urine retention.
Other: fluid and electrolyte imbalance, dehydration, local pain, fever, chills, urticaria.

INTERACTIONS
Drug-drug. *Lithium:* increased urinary excretion of lithium. Monitor closely.

EFFECTS ON DIAGNOSTIC TESTS
Drug therapy alters electrolyte balance. It also may interfere with tests for inorganic phosphorus concentration or blood ethylene glycol.

CONTRAINDICATIONS
Contraindicated in patients with anuria, severe pulmonary congestion, frank pulmonary edema, severe heart failure, severe dehydration, metabolic edema, progressive renal disease or dysfunction, active intracranial bleeding except during craniotomy, and hypersensitivity to drug.

NURSING CONSIDERATIONS
● To redissolve crystallized solution (occurs at low temperatures or in concentrations greater than 15%), warm bottle in hot water bath and shake vigorously. *Cool to body temperature before giving.* Do not use solution with undissolved crystals.
● For maximum intraocular pressure reduction before surgery, give 1 to 1½ hours preoperatively, as ordered.
● Monitor vital signs, including central venous pressure, and fluid intake and output hourly. Report increasing oliguria. Check weight, renal function, fluid balance, and serum and urine sodium and potassium levels daily.
● Insert urethral catheter in comatose or

incontinent patients because therapy is based on strict evaluation of fluid intake and output. In patients with urethral catheters, use an hourly urometer collection bag to facilitate accurate evaluation of output.

• Be aware that drug can be used to measure glomerular filtration rate.

• To relieve thirst, give frequent mouth care or fluids as permitted.

• When used as an irrigating solution for prostate surgery, keep in mind that concentrations of 3.5% or greater are needed to avoid hemolysis.

• Know that drug is commonly used in chemotherapy regimens to enhance diuresis of renally-toxic agents.

⬛ I.V. administration

• Administer as intermittent or continuous infusion at prescribed rate, using an in-line filter and an infusion pump. Direct injection is not recommended. Check I.V. line patency at infusion site before and during administration.

• Avoid infiltration; if it occurs, observe for inflammation, edema, and necrosis.

☑ Patient teaching

• Tell patient that he may feel thirsty or experience mouth dryness, and emphasize importance of drinking only the amount of fluids ordered.

• Instruct patient to report adverse reactions promptly and to alert nurse if discomfort occurs at I.V. site.

---

methazolamide
Neptazane

Pregnancy Risk Category: C

HOW SUPPLIED
Tablets: 25 mg, 50 mg

ACTION
A carbonic anhydrase inhibitor that decreases secretion of aqueous humor, lowering intraocular pressure.

Route	Onset	Peak	Duration
PO	2-4 hr	6-8 hr	10-18 hr

INDICATIONS & DOSAGE
Glaucoma (chronic open-angle or secondary, or preoperatively in obstructive or acute angle-closure)—
Adults: 50 to 100 mg P.O. b.i.d. or t.i.d.

ADVERSE REACTIONS
CNS: drowsiness, paresthesia, fatigue, malaise, confusion.
EENT: transient myopia, hearing dysfunction, tinnitus.
GI: nausea, vomiting, anorexia, taste alteration, diarrhea.
GU: crystalluria, renal calculi.
Skin: urticaria.
Other: metabolic acidosis, electrolyte imbalance.

INTERACTIONS
Drug-drug. *Amphetamines, anticholinergics, mecamylamine, procainamide, quinidine:* decreased renal clearance of these agents, increasing risk of toxicity. Avoid concomitant use.
Methenamine compounds: reduced methenamine effectiveness. Avoid concomitant use.
Salicylates: accumulation and toxicity of methazolamide may occur. Monitor closely.

EFFECTS ON DIAGNOSTIC TESTS
Because methazolamide alkalizes urine, it may cause false-positive proteinuria when Albustix or Albutest test is performed. Methazolamide also may decrease iodine uptake by the thyroid.

CONTRAINDICATIONS
Contraindicated for long-term use in patients with angle-closure glaucoma, depressed serum sodium or potassium levels, renal or hepatic disease or dysfunction, adrenal gland dysfunction, or hyperchloremic acidosis.

NURSING CONSIDERATIONS
• Use cautiously in patients with emphysema and pulmonary obstruction.
• Monitor fluid intake and output, weight, and serum electrolyte levels.
• Monitor elderly patients, who are especially susceptible to excessive diuresis.
• Know that drug may cause false-

---

positive urine protein tests by alkalinizing urine.

• Evaluate patient for eye pain to ensure drug is effective in decreasing intraocular pressure.

☑ **Patient teaching**
• Caution patient to comply with prescribed dosage to lessen risk of metabolic acidosis. Effects may decrease in acidosis.
• Warn patient not to perform hazardous activities if adverse CNS reactions occur.

metolazone
Metenix-5§, Mykrox, Zaroxolyn**

Pregnancy Risk Category: B

HOW SUPPLIED
Tablets (extended-release): 2.5 mg, 5 mg, 10 mg (Zaroxolyn)
Tablets (prompt-release): 0.5 mg (Mykrox)

ACTION
Increases sodium and water excretion by inhibiting sodium reabsorption in the cortical diluting site of the ascending loop of Henle.

Route	Onset	Peak	Duration
PO	1 hr	2-8 hr	12-24 hr

INDICATIONS & DOSAGE
Edema in heart failure or renal disease—
Adults: 5 to 20 mg (extended-release) P.O. daily.
Hypertension—
Adults: 2.5 to 5 mg (extended-release) P.O. daily. Maintenance dosage based on patient's blood pressure. Or 0.5 mg (prompt-release) P.O. once daily in morning, increased to 1 mg P.O. daily, p.r.n. If response is inadequate, another antihypertensive is added.

ADVERSE REACTIONS
CNS: *dizziness,* headache, fatigue, vertigo, paresthesia, weakness, restlessness, drowsiness, anxiety, depression, nervousness, blurred vision.
CV: volume depletion and dehydration,

orthostatic hypotension, palpitations, vasculitis, increased cholesterol levels.
GI: anorexia, nausea, pancreatitis, epigastric distress, vomiting, abdominal pain, diarrhea, constipation, dry mouth.
GU: nocturia, polyuria, frequent urination, impotence.
Hematologic: *aplastic anemia, agranulocytosis,* leukopenia.
Hepatic: jaundice, hepatitis.
Skin: dermatitis, photosensitivity, rash, purpura, pruritus, urticaria.
Other: hyperglycemia and glucose tolerance impairment; fluid and electrolyte imbalances, including hypokalemia, hypomagnesemia, dilutional hyponatremia and hypochloremia, metabolic alkalosis, hypercalcemia; muscle cramps.

INTERACTIONS
Drug-drug. *Amphotericin B:* increased risk of hypokalemia. Monitor closely.
Anticoagulants: may affect hypoprothrombinemic response. Monitor PT and INR.
Antidiabetic agents: may alter blood glucose level requiring dosage adjustment of antidiabetic agents. Monitor blood glucose levels.
Barbiturates, opiates: increased orthostatic hypotensive effect. Monitor closely.
Cardiac glycosides: increased risk of digitalis toxicity from metolazone-induced hypokalemia. Monitor potassium and digitalis levels.
Cholestyramine, colestipol: decreased intestinal absorption of thiazides. Separate doses.
Corticosteroids: increased risk of hypokalemia. Monitor closely.
Diazoxide: increased antihypertensive, hyperglycemic, and hyperuricemic effects. Use together cautiously.
Lithium: decreased lithium clearance, increasing risk of lithium toxicity. Monitor lithium level.
NSAIDs: increased risk of NSAID-induced renal failure. Monitor patient for signs of renal failure.
Other antihypertensives: may have additive effects. Use together cautiously.
Drug-lifestyle. *Alcohol use:* increased orthostatic hypotensive effect. Monitor closely.

Sun exposure: photosensitivity reactions may occur. Take precautions.

EFFECTS ON DIAGNOSTIC TESTS
Drug therapy may alter serum electrolyte levels and may increase serum uric acid, glucose, cholesterol, and triglyceride levels. It also may interfere with tests for parathyroid function and should be discontinued before such tests.

CONTRAINDICATIONS
Contraindicated in patients with anuria, hepatic coma or precoma, or hypersensitivity to thiazides or other sulfonamide-derived drugs.

NURSING CONSIDERATIONS
• Use cautiously in patients with impaired renal or hepatic function.
• To prevent nocturia, give in the morning.
• Keep in mind that Mykrox (prompt-release) tablets are more rapidly and completely absorbed than other brands, mimicking an oral solution. Do not interchange Mykrox with Zaroxolyn (extended-release) tablets.
• Monitor fluid intake and output, weight, blood pressure, and serum electrolyte levels.
• Watch for signs and symptoms of hypokalemia, such as muscle weakness and cramps. Know that drug may be used with potassium-sparing diuretic to prevent potassium loss.
• Consult doctor and dietitian about a high-potassium diet. Foods rich in potassium include citrus fruits, tomatoes, bananas, dates, and apricots.
• Monitor blood glucose levels, especially in diabetic patients.
• Monitor blood uric acid levels, especially in patients with a history of gout.
• Monitor elderly patients, who are especially susceptible to excessive diuresis.
• In patients with hypertension, know that therapeutic response may be delayed several weeks.
• Keep in mind that unlike thiazide diuretics, metolazone is effective in patients with decreased renal function.
• Be aware that drug is used as an adjunct in furosemide-resistant edema.

• As ordered, discontinue thiazides and thiazide-like diuretics before parathyroid function tests.

☑ **Patient teaching**
• Tell patient to take drug in morning to prevent nocturia.
• Advise patient to avoid sudden posture changes and to rise slowly to avoid orthostatic hypotension.
• Instruct patient to use a sunblock to prevent photosensitivity reactions.

spironolactone
Aldactone, Novospiroton†, Spiractin‡, Spiroctan§

Pregnancy Risk Category: D

HOW SUPPLIED
Tablets: 25 mg, 50 mg, 100 mg

ACTION
A potassium-sparing diuretic that antagonizes aldosterone in the distal tubules, increasing sodium and water excretion.

Route	Onset	Peak	Duration
PO	1-2 days	2-3 days	2-3 days

INDICATIONS & DOSAGE
Edema—
Adults: 25 to 200 mg P.O. daily or in two to four divided doses.
Children: 3.3 mg/kg P.O. daily or in divided doses.
Hypertension—
Adults: 50 to 100 mg P.O. daily or in divided doses.
Diuretic-induced hypokalemia—
Adults: 25 to 100 mg P.O. daily.
Detection of primary hyperaldosteronism—
Adults: 400 mg P.O. daily for 4 days (short test) or 3 to 4 weeks (long test). If hypokalemia and hypertension are corrected, a presumptive diagnosis of primary hyperaldosteronism is made.
Management of primary hyperaldosteronism—
Adults: 100 to 400 mg P.O. daily. Use lowest effective dose.

ADVERSE REACTIONS

CNS: headache, drowsiness, lethargy, confusion, ataxia.
GI: diarrhea, gastric bleeding, ulceration, cramping, gastritis, vomiting.
Skin: urticaria, hirsutism, maculopapular eruptions.
Other: *hyperkalemia,* dehydration, hyponatremia, transient elevation in BUN, mild acidosis, inability to maintain erection, gynecomastia, breast soreness and menstrual disturbances in women, drug fever, *agranulocytosis, anaphylaxis.*

INTERACTIONS

Drug-drug. *ACE inhibitors, indomethacin, other potassium-sparing diuretics, potassium supplements:* increased risk of hyperkalemia. Use together cautiously, especially in patients with renal impairment.
Aspirin: possible blocked diuretic effect of spironolactone. Watch for diminished spironolactone response.
Digoxin: may alter digoxin clearance, increasing risk of digoxin toxicity. Monitor digoxin levels.
Drug-herb. *Licorice:* may block ulcer healing and aldosterone-like effects of licorice. Avoid concomitant use.
Drug-food. *Potassium-containing salt substitutes, potassium-rich foods (such as citrus fruits, tomatoes):* increased risk of hyperkalemia. Use low-potassium salt substitutes. Ingest high-potassium foods cautiously.

EFFECTS ON DIAGNOSTIC TESTS

Drug therapy alters fluorometric determinations of plasma and urinary 17-hydroxycorticosteroid levels and may cause false elevations on radioimmunoassay of serum digoxin.

CONTRAINDICATIONS

Contraindicated in patients with anuria, acute or progressive renal insufficiency, hyperkalemia, or known hypersensitivity to drug.

NURSING CONSIDERATIONS

● Use cautiously in patients with fluid or electrolyte imbalances, impaired renal function, and hepatic disease.
● Drug or its metabolites may cross the placental barrier. Use with extreme caution in pregnancy.
● To enhance absorption, give drug with meals.
● Protect drug from light.
● Monitor serum electrolytes, fluid intake and output, weight, and blood pressure.
● Monitor elderly patients, who are more susceptible to excessive diuresis.
● Inform laboratory that patient is taking spironolactone, because it may interfere with some laboratory tests that measure digoxin levels.
● Be aware that drug is less potent than thiazide and loop diuretics; useful as an adjunct to other diuretic therapy. Diuretic effect delayed 2 to 3 days when used alone.
● Keep in mind that maximum antihypertensive response may be delayed for up to 2 weeks.
● Watch for hyperchloremic metabolic acidosis, which may occur during therapy, because of danger in patients with hepatic cirrhosis.
● Know that breast cancer has been reported in some patients taking spironolactone.

☑ Patient teaching

● Instruct patient to take drug in morning to prevent nocturia; if second dose is needed, tell him to take it in early afternoon. Also tell patient to take it with food.
Alert: Warn patient to avoid excessive ingestion of potassium-rich foods (such as citrus fruits, tomatoes, bananas, dates, and apricots), potassium-containing salt substitutes, and potassium supplements to prevent serious hyperkalemia.
● Caution patient not to perform hazardous activities if adverse CNS reactions occur.
● Advise male patient about potential adverse effects of breast tenderness or gynecomastia.

---

*Liquid contains alcohol.   **May contain tartrazine.   †Canada   ‡Australia   §U.K.   ◇OTC

torsemide
Demadex, Torem§

Pregnancy Risk Category: B

HOW SUPPLIED
Tablets: 5 mg, 10 mg, 20 mg, 100 mg
Injection: 10 mg/ml

ACTION
A loop diuretic that enhances excretion of sodium, chloride, and water by acting on the ascending portion of the loop of Henle.

Route	Onset	Peak	Duration
PO	1 hr	1-2 hr	6-8 hr
IV	10 min	1 hr	6-8 hr

INDICATIONS & DOSAGE
Diuresis in patients with heart failure—
Adults: initially, 10 to 20 mg P.O. or I.V. once daily. If response is inadequate, dose is doubled until a response is obtained. Maximum dosage is 200 mg daily.
Diuresis in patients with chronic renal failure—
Adults: initially, 20 mg P.O. or I.V. once daily. If response is inadequate, dose is doubled until a response is obtained. Maximum dosage is 200 mg daily.
Diuresis in patients with hepatic cirrhosis—
Adults: initially, 5 to 10 mg P.O. or I.V. once daily with an aldosterone antagonist or a potassium-sparing diuretic. If response is inadequate, dose is doubled until a response is obtained. Maximum dosage is 40 mg daily.
Hypertension—
Adults: initially, 5 mg P.O. daily. Increased to 10 mg if needed and tolerated. If response is still inadequate, another antihypertensive should be added.

ADVERSE REACTIONS
CNS: dizziness, headache, nervousness, insomnia, syncope.
CV: ECG abnormalities, chest pain, edema, increased cholesterol level, *dehydration,* orthostatic hypotension.
EENT: rhinitis, cough, sore throat.
GI: diarrhea, constipation, nausea, dyspepsia, *hemorrhage.*
GU: *excessive urination*, impotence.
Other: asthenia, arthralgia, myalgia, rash, *electrolyte imbalances including hypokalemia and hypomagnesemia,* increased uric acid, *excessive thirst*, hypochloremic alkalosis.

INTERACTIONS
Drug-drug. *Cholestyramine:* decreased absorption of torsemide. Separate administration times by at least 3 hours.
Digoxin: decreased torsemide clearance. No dosage adjustments are necessary.
Indomethacin: decreased diuretic effectiveness in sodium-restricted patients. Avoid concomitant use.
Lithium, ototoxic drugs (such as aminoglycosides, ethacrynic acid): possible increased toxicity of these agents. Avoid concomitant use.
NSAIDs: may potentiate nephrotoxicity of NSAIDs. Use together cautiously.
Probenecid: decreased diuretic effectiveness. Avoid concomitant use.
Salicylates: decreased excretion, possibly leading to salicylate toxicity. Avoid concomitant use.
Spironolactone: decreased renal clearance of spironolactone. No dosage adjustments are necessary.

EFFECTS ON DIAGNOSTIC TESTS
Drug therapy alters electrolyte balance and renal function tests. It also may mildly affect glucose, serum lipid, and alkaline phosphatase levels, CBC, and platelet count.

CONTRAINDICATIONS
Contraindicated in patients with anuria and hypersensitivity to drug or other sulfonylurea derivatives.

NURSING CONSIDERATIONS
• Use cautiously in patients with hepatic disease and associated cirrhosis and ascites; sudden changes in fluid and electrolyte balance may precipitate hepatic coma in these patients.
• To prevent nocturia, give drug in the morning.
• Monitor fluid intake and output, serum electrolyte levels, blood pressure, weight, and pulse rate during rapid diuresis and

---

Reactions may be *common,* uncommon, *life-threatening,* or COMMON AND LIFE-THREATENING.

routinely with chronic use. Drug can cause profound diuresis and water and electrolyte depletion.
• Watch for signs of hypokalemia, such as muscle weakness and cramps.
• Consult doctor and dietitian about providing a high-potassium diet. Foods rich in potassium include citrus fruits, tomatoes, bananas, dates, and apricots.
• Monitor elderly patients, who are especially susceptible to excessive diuresis with potential for circulatory collapse and thromboembolic complications.

I.V. administration
• Inspect ampules for precipitate or discoloration before use.
• Drug may be given by direct injection over at least 2 minutes. Rapid injection may cause ototoxicity. Do not give more than 200 mg at a time.

Patient teaching
• Tell patient to take drug in morning to prevent nocturia.
• Advise patient to change positions slowly to prevent dizziness, and to limit alcohol intake and strenuous exercise in hot weather to prevent orthostatic hypotension.
• Advise patient to immediately report ringing in ears. May indicate toxicity.
• Tell patient to check with doctor or pharmacist before taking OTC medications.

triamterene
Dyrenium, Dytac§

Pregnancy Risk Category: B

HOW SUPPLIED
Capsules: 50 mg, 100 mg

ACTION
A potassium-sparing diuretic that inhibits sodium reabsorption and potassium and hydrogen excretion by direct action on the distal tubules.

Route	Onset	Peak	Duration
PO	2-4 hr	2-4 hr	7-9 hr

INDICATIONS & DOSAGE
Edema—
Adults: initially, 100 mg P.O. b.i.d. after meals. Total dosage should not exceed 300 mg daily.

ADVERSE REACTIONS
CNS: dizziness, weakness, fatigue, headache.
CV: hypotension.
GI: dry mouth, nausea, vomiting, diarrhea.
GU: interstitial nephritis, nephrolithiasis.
Hematologic: megaloblastic anemia related to low folic acid levels, ***thrombocytopenia, agranulocytosis.***
Skin: photosensitivity, rash.
Other: ***anaphylaxis, hyperkalemia,*** muscle cramps, transient elevation in BUN or creatinine levels, acidosis, hypokalemia, hyponatremia, hyperglycemia, azotemia, jaundice, increased liver enzyme abnormalities.

INTERACTIONS
Drug-drug. *ACE inhibitors, potassium supplements:* increased risk of hyperkalemia. Use together as long as serum potassium is monitored.
Amantadine: increased risk of amantadine toxicity. Do not use together.
Folic acid: may antagonize folate. Use leucovorin calcium.
Lithium: decreased lithium clearance, increasing risk of lithium toxicity. Monitor lithium level.
NSAIDs: may enhance risk of nephrotoxicity. Use together cautiously.
Quinidine: may interfere with some laboratory tests that measure quinidine levels. Inform laboratory that patient is taking triamterene.
Drug-food. *Potassium-containing salt substitutes, potassium-rich foods:* increased risk of hyperkalemia. Use cautiously and monitor serum potassium levels.
Drug-lifestyle. *Sun exposure:* photosensitivity reactions may occur. Take precautions.

EFFECTS ON DIAGNOSTIC TESTS
Drug therapy may interfere with enzyme assays that use fluorometry, such as serum quinidine determinations.

CONTRAINDICATIONS
Contraindicated in patients with anuria, severe or progressive renal disease or dysfunction, severe hepatic disease, hyperkalemia, or hypersensitivity to drug.

NURSING CONSIDERATIONS
• Use cautiously in patients with impaired hepatic function or diabetes mellitus and in elderly or debilitated patients.
• To minimize nausea, give drug after meals.
• Monitor blood pressure, blood uric acid, CBC, blood glucose, BUN, and serum electrolyte levels.
• Watch for blood dyscrasia.
• To minimize excessive rebound potassium excretion, withdraw drug gradually, as ordered.
• Know that drug is less potent than thiazides and loop diuretics and is useful as an adjunct to other diuretic therapy. Usually used with potassium-wasting diuretics. Full effect is delayed 2 to 3 days when used alone.

☑**Patient teaching**
• Tell patient to take drug after meals to minimize nausea.
• If a single daily dose is prescribed, instruct the patient to take it in the morning to prevent nocturia.
Alert: Warn patient to avoid excessive ingestion of potassium-rich foods (such as citrus fruits, tomatoes, bananas, dates, and apricots), potassium-containing salt substitutes, and potassium supplements to prevent serious hyperkalemia.
• Teach patient to avoid direct sunlight, wear protective clothing, and use a sunblock to prevent photosensitivity reactions.
• Tell patient urine may turn blue.

---

urea (carbamide)
Ureaphil

Pregnancy Risk Category: C

HOW SUPPLIED
Injection: 40 g/150 ml

ACTION
An osmotic diuretic that increases the osmotic pressure of glomerular filtrate, inhibiting tubular reabsorption of water and electrolytes. Also elevates blood plasma osmolality, resulting in enhanced water flow into extracellular fluid.

Route	Onset	Peak	Duration
IV	30-45 min	1-2 hr	3-10 hr

INDICATIONS & DOSAGE
Elevated intracranial or intraocular pressure—
Adults: 1 to 1.5 g/kg as a 30% solution by slow I.V. infusion over 1 to 2½ hours. Rate should not exceed 4 ml/minute. Maximum dosage is 120 g daily.
Children: 0.1 to 1.5 g/kg by slow I.V. infusion (rate not to exceed 4 ml/minute) or 35 g/m^2 in 24 hours. Children under 2 years may receive as little as 0.1 g/kg by slow I.V. infusion.

ADVERSE REACTIONS
CNS: *headache,* syncope, disorientation.
CV: hypotension, tachycardia, dizziness, ECG changes.
GI: *nausea, vomiting.*
Other: irritation or necrotic sloughing with extravasation, hemolysis (with rapid administration), fluid overload, *hyponatremia,* hypokalemia.

INTERACTIONS
Drug-drug. *Lithium:* increased lithium clearance and decreased lithium effectiveness. Monitor lithium level.

EFFECTS ON DIAGNOSTIC TESTS
Urea therapy alters electrolyte balance.

CONTRAINDICATIONS
Contraindicated in patients with severely impaired renal function, marked dehydration, frank hepatic failure, active intracranial bleeding, and sickle-cell disease with CNS involvement.

NURSING CONSIDERATIONS
• Use cautiously in patients with cardiac disease or hepatic or renal impairment and in pregnant or breast-feeding women.

Reactions may be *common,* uncommon, *life-threatening,* or COMMON AND LIFE-THREATENING.

• Assess breath sounds for crackles, indicating pulmonary edema.
• Watch for signs and symptoms of hyponatremia (nausea, vomiting, tachycardia) or hypokalemia (muscle weakness, lethargy); these may indicate electrolyte depletion before serum levels are reduced.
• Maintain adequate hydration; monitor blood pressure, fluid intake and output, and serum electrolyte levels.
• Monitor BUN level in patients with renal disease.
• To ensure bladder emptying in comatose patients, use an indwelling urinary catheter, and use an hourly urometer collection bag for accurate evaluation of diuresis.
• If satisfactory diuresis does not occur in 6 to 12 hours, be aware that urea should be discontinued and renal function reevaluated.

⚠ I.V. administration
• Avoid rapid I.V. infusion; may cause hemolysis or increased capillary bleeding. Maximum infusion rate is 4 ml/minute.
Alert: Avoid extravasation; may cause reactions ranging from mild irritation to necrosis.
• To prepare 135 ml of 30% solution, mix contents of 40-g vial of urea with 105 ml of D_5W or dextrose 10% in water or 10% invert sugar in water. Each ml of 30% solution provides 300 mg urea.
• Use freshly reconstituted urea only for I.V. infusion; solution becomes ammonia upon standing. Use within minutes of reconstitution and discard within 24 hours.

☑ Patient teaching
• Instruct patient to report adverse reactions promptly.
• Tell patient to alert nurse if discomfort occurs at I.V. insertion site.

CHAPTER 283

63

Electrolytes and replacement solutions

calcium acetate
calcium carbonate
calcium chloride
calcium citrate
calcium glubionate
calcium gluceptate
calcium gluconate
calcium lactate
calcium phosphate, dibasic
calcium phosphate, tribasic
dextran, high-molecular-weight
dextran, low-molecular-weight
hetastarch
magnesium chloride
magnesium sulfate
potassium acetate
potassium bicarbonate
potassium chloride
potassium gluconate
Ringer's injection
Ringer's injection, lactated
sodium chloride

COMBINATION PRODUCTS
CITRACAL +D: calcium 316.5 mg with
200 units cholecalciferol.
DICAL-D; DIOSTATE D: calcium 116.7 mg
(as phosphate tribasic) with 133 mg
choiecalciferol.
DICAL-D WAFERS: calcium 232 mg (as
phosphate tribasic) with cholecalciferol
200 units.
KLORVESS*: potassium and chloride
20 mEq each (from potassium chloride,
potassium bicarbonate, and l-lysine
monohydrochloride).
K-LYTE-CL: potassium 25 mEq, chloride
25 mEq (from potassium chloride, potassium bicarbonate, and lysine hydrochloride).
KOLYUM: potassium 20 mEq, chloride
3.4 mEq per 15 ml (from potassium gluconate and potassium chloride).
NEUTRA-PHOS: phosphorus 250 mg, sodium 164 mg, potassium 278 mg (from
dibasic and monobasic sodium and potassium phosphate).
POSTURE-D: calcium 600 mg (as phosphate
tribasic) with cholecalciferol 125 units.

TWIN-K: 15 ml supplies 20 mEq of potassium ions as a combination of potassium
gluconate and potassium citrate.
TWIN-K: 20 mEq/15 ml potassium from
potassium acetate, potassium bicarbonate,
potassium citrate.

---

calcium acetate
Phos-Lo

calcium carbonate
Apo-Cal† ◇, Cal Carb-HD ◇,
Calci-Chew ◇, Calciday 667 ◇,
Calci-Mix ◇, Calcite 500† ◇,
Calcium 600 ◇, Calglycine ◇,
Cal-Plus ◇, Calsant† ◇, Caltrate
600 ◇, Chooz ◇, Dicarbosil ◇,
Gencalc 600 ◇, Mallamint ◇,
Nephro-Calci ◇, Nu-Cal† ◇,
Os-Cal† ◇, Os-Cal 500 ◇, Os-Cal
Chewable† ◇, Oysco ◇, Oysco
500 Chewable ◇, Oyst-Cal 500 ◇,
Oystercal 500 ◇, Oyster Shell
Calcium-500 ◇, Rolaids Calcium
Rich ◇, Super Calcium '1200' ◇,
Titralac ◇, Tums ◇, Tums E-X ◇

calcium chloride ◇
Calciject†

calcium citrate ◇
Citracal ◇, Citracal Liquitab† ◇

calcium glubionate
Calcium-Sandoz†, Neo-Calglucon

calcium gluceptate ◇

calcium gluconate

calcium lactate ◇

calcium phosphate, dibasic ◇

calcium phosphate, tribasic
Posture ◇

Pregnancy Risk Category: C

Reactions may be *common*, uncommon, *life-threatening*, or COMMON AND LIFE-THREATENING.

HOW SUPPLIED
calcium acetate
Contains 253 mg or 12.7 mEq of elemental calcium/g
Tablets: 250 mg ◊, 500 mg ◊, 667 mg, 668 mg ◊, 1,000 mg ◊
Injection: 0.5 mEq Ca^{++} per ml
calcium carbonate
Contains 400 mg or 20 mEq of elemental calcium/g
Tablets: 650 mg ◊, 1.25 g ◊, 1.5 g ◊
Tablets (chewable): 350 mg ◊, 420 mg ◊, 500 mg ◊, 550 mg ◊, 625 mg ◊†, 750 mg ◊, 835 mg ◊, 850 mg ◊, 1 g ◊, 1.25 g ◊
Capsules: 600 mg ◊, 1.25 g ◊
Oral suspension: 1 g/5 ml ◊, 1.25 g/5 ml ◊
Powder packets: 6.5 g (2,400 mg calcium) per packet ◊
calcium chloride
Contains 270 mg or 13.5 mEq of elemental calcium/g
Injection: 10% solution in 10-ml ampules, vials, and syringes
calcium citrate
Contains 211 mg or 10.6 mEq of elemental calcium/g
Tablets: 950 mg ◊, 1.04 g
Tablets (effervescent): 2.376 g ◊
calcium glubionate
Contains 64 mg or 3.2 mEq elemental calcium/g
Syrup: 1.8 g/5 ml
calcium gluceptate
Contains 82 mg or 4.1 mEq elemental calcium/g
Injection: 1.1 g/5 ml in 5-ml ampules or 10-ml vials
calcium gluconate
Contains 90 mg or 4.5 mEq of elemental calcium/g
Tablets: 500 mg ◊, 650 mg ◊, 1 g ◊
Injection: 10% solution in 10-ml ampules and vials, 10-ml or 50-ml vials
calcium lactate
Contains 130 mg or 6.5 mEq of elemental calcium/g
Tablets: 325 mg, 650 mg
calcium phosphate, dibasic
Contains 230 mg or 11.5 mEq of elemental calcium/g
Tablets: 500 mg ◊
calcium phosphate, tribasic

Contains 400 mg or 20 mEq of elemental calcium/g
Tablets: 300 mg ◊, 600 mg ◊

ACTION
Replaces and maintains calcium.

Route	Onset	Peak	Duration
PO	Unknown	Unknown	Unknown
IV	Immediate	Immediate	0.5-2 hr

INDICATIONS & DOSAGE
Hypocalcemic emergency—
Adults: 7 to 14 mEq calcium I.V. May be given as a 10% calcium gluconate solution, 2% to 10% calcium chloride solution, or a 22% calcium glucceptate solution.
Children: 1 to 7 mEq calcium I.V.
Infants: up to 1 mEq calcium I.V.
Hypocalcemic tetany—
Adults: 4.5 to 16 mEq calcium I.V. Repeated until tetany is controlled.
Children: 0.5 to 0.7 mEq/kg calcium I.V. three to four times a day until tetany is controlled.
Neonates: 2.4 mEq/kg I.V. daily in divided doses.
Adjunctive treatment of cardiac arrest—
Adults: 0.027 to 0.054 mEq/kg calcium chloride I.V., 4.5 to 6.3 mEq calcium glucceptate I.V., or 2.3 to 3.7 mEq calcium gluconate I.V.
Children: 0.27 mEq/kg calcium chloride I.V. Repeated in 10 minutes if necessary; determine serum calcium levels before administering further doses.
Adjunctive treatment of magnesium intoxication—
Adults: initially, 7 mEq I.V. Subsequent doses must be based on patient's response.
During exchange transfusions—
Adults: 1.35 mEq I.V. concurrently with each 100 ml citrated blood.
Neonates: 0.45 mEq I.V. after each 100 ml citrated blood.
Hyperphosphatemia—
Adults: 1,334 to 2,000 mg P.O. calcium acetate or 2 to 5.2 g calcium ion t.i.d. with meals. Most dialysis patients will require three to four tablets with each meal.
Dietary supplement—
Adults: 500 mg to 2 g P.O. daily.

ADVERSE REACTIONS

CNS: tingling sensations, sense of oppression or heat waves (with I.V. use); syncope (with rapid I.V. injection).

CV: mild fall in blood pressure; vasodilation, bradycardia, *arrhythmias, cardiac arrest (*with rapid I.V. injection).

GI: irritation, *constipation* (with oral use); chalky taste (with I.V. use); *hemorrhage,* nausea, vomiting, thirst, abdominal pain (with oral calcium chloride).

GU: hypercalcemia, polyuria, renal calculi.

Skin: local reactions including burning, necrosis, tissue sloughing, cellulitis, soft tissue calcification (with I.M. use).

Other: pain, irritation (with S.C. injection); *vein irritation* (with I.V. use).

INTERACTIONS

Drug-drug. *Atenolol, fluoroquinolones, tetracyclines:* decreased bioavailability of these agents and calcium when oral preparations are taken together. Separate administration times.

Calcium channel blockers: decreased calcium effectiveness. Avoid concomitant use.

Cardiac glycosides: increased digitalis toxicity. Give calcium cautiously (if at all) to digitalized patients.

Phenytoin: concomitant use decreases absorption of both drugs. Avoid concomitant use or monitor levels carefully.

Sodium polystyrene sulfonate: risk of metabolic acidosis in patients with renal disease. Avoid concomitant use.

Thiazide diuretics: risk of hypercalcemia. Avoid concomitant use.

Drug-food. *Foods containing oxalic acid (rhubarb, spinach), phytic acid (bran, whole cereals), and phosphorus (milk, dairy products):* may interfere with calcium absorption. Avoid concomitant use.

EFFECTS ON DIAGNOSTIC TESTS

I.V. calcium may produce transient elevation of plasma 11-hydroxycorticosteroid concentrations (Glenn-Nelson technique) and false-negative values for serum and urine magnesium as measured by the Titan yellow method.

CONTRAINDICATIONS

Contraindicated in patients with ventricular fibrillation, hypercalcemia, hypophosphatemia, or renal calculi and in cancer patients with bone metastases.

NURSING CONSIDERATIONS

● Use all calcium products with extreme caution in patients with sarcoidosis and renal or cardiac disease, and in digitalized patients. Use calcium chloride cautiously in patients with cor pulmonale, respiratory acidosis, and respiratory failure.

● Give I.M. injection in the gluteal region in adults, lateral thigh in infants. Use I.M. route only in emergencies when no I.V. route is available due to irritability of calcium salts to tissue.

● Ensure that doctor specifies the form of calcium to be given; crash carts usually contain both calcium gluconate and calcium chloride.

● Monitor blood calcium levels frequently. Hypercalcemia may result after large doses in chronic renal failure. Report abnormalities.

◖ I.V. administration

● Give calcium chloride I.V. only. When adding to parenteral solutions that contain other additives (especially phosphorus or phosphate), watch for precipitate. Use an in-line filter.

● Give calcium gluconate I.V. only.

● Monitor ECG when giving calcium I.V. Stop if patient complains of discomfort and notify doctor. After I.V. injection, patient should remain recumbent for 15 minutes.

Alert: Be aware that severe necrosis and tissue sloughing can occur after extravasation. Calcium gluconate is less irritating to veins and tissues than calcium chloride.

Direct injection

● Warm solutions to body temperature before administration.

● Administer slowly through a small needle into a large vein or through an I.V. line containing a free-flowing, compatible solution at a rate not exceeding 1 ml/minute (1.5 mEq/minute) for calcium chloride, 1.5 to 5 ml/minute for calcium gluconate, and 2 ml/minute for calcium gluceptate. Do not use scalp veins in children.

Reactions may be *common,* uncommon, *life-threatening,* or COMMON AND LIFE-THREATENING.

Intermittent infusion

• Infuse diluted solution through an I.V. line containing a compatible solution. Maximum rate of 200 mg/minute suggested for calcium gluceptate and calcium gluconate.

• Know that drug will precipitate if administered I.V. with sodium bicarbonate or other alkaline drugs.

☑ Patient teaching

• Tell patient to take oral calcium 1 to 1½ hours after meals if GI upset occurs.

• Warn patient to avoid oxalic acid (found in rhubarb and spinach), phytic acid (in bran and whole cereals), and phosphorus (in dairy products) in the meal preceding calcium consumption; these substances may interfere with calcium absorption.

---

dextran, low-molecular-weight (dextran 40)

Dextran 40, Gentran 40, LMD 10%, Rheomacrodex

Pregnancy Risk Category: C

HOW SUPPLIED

Injection: 10% dextran 40 in D_5W or 0.9% NaCl solution

ACTION

Expands plasma volume via colloidal osmotic effect, drawing fluid from interstitial to intravascular space, providing fluid replacement.

Route	Onset	Peak	Duration
IV	Immediate	Immediate	3 hr

INDICATIONS & DOSAGE

Plasma volume expansion—
Adults: dosage by I.V. infusion depends on amount of fluid loss. First 10 ml/kg of dextran infused rapidly with central venous pressure monitoring; the remaining dose slowly. Total dosage not to exceed 20 ml/kg body weight daily. If therapy continues longer than 24 hours, do not exceed 10 ml/kg daily, continued for no longer than 5 days.
Prophylaxis of venous thrombosis—
Adults: 10 ml/kg (500 to 1,000 ml) I.V.

on day of procedure; 500 ml on days 2 and 3.
Hemodiluent in extracorporeal circulation—
Adults: 10 to 20 ml/kg added to the perfusion circuit, not to exceed total dosage of 20 ml/kg.

ADVERSE REACTIONS

GI: nausea, vomiting.
GU: tubular stasis and blocking, increased urine viscosity.
Hematologic: *decreased hemoglobin and hematocrit levels;* increased bleeding time (with higher doses).
Hepatic: increased AST and ALT levels.
Skin: *hypersensitivity reactions,* urticaria.
Other: *anaphylaxis,* thrombophlebitis.

INTERACTIONS

None significant.

EFFECTS ON DIAGNOSTIC TESTS

Falsely elevated blood glucose levels may occur in patients receiving dextran 40 or 70 if the test uses high concentrations of acid. Dextran may cause turbidity, which interferes with bilirubin assays that use alcohol, total protein levels using biuret reagent, and blood glucose levels using the orthotoluidine method. Blood typing and cross-matching using enzyme techniques may give unreliable readings if the samples are taken after the dextran infusion.

Dextran 40 administration has been associated with abnormal renal and hepatic function test results.

CONTRAINDICATIONS

Contraindicated in patients with marked hemostatic defects, marked cardiac decompensation, renal disease with severe oliguria or anuria, and hypersensitivity to drug.

NURSING CONSIDERATIONS

• Use cautiously in patients with active hemorrhage, thrombocytopenia, or diabetes mellitus.

• Assess hydration before starting therapy; otherwise, use urine or serum osmolality because urine specific gravity is affected by urine dextran concentration.

---

*Liquid contains alcohol.   **May contain tartrazine.   †Canada   ‡Australia   §U.K.   ◊OTC

• Watch for circulatory overload and a rise in central venous pressure. Provides plasma expansion slightly greater than volume infused.

• Monitor urine flow rate during administration. If oliguria or anuria occurs or is not relieved, stop dextran and give loop diuretic as ordered.

• Check hemoglobin and hematocrit levels; if values fall below 30% by volume, notify doctor.

• Be aware that drug may interfere with analyses of blood grouping, cross-matching, bilirubin, blood glucose, and protein.

• Monitor blood glucose levels before and during infusion. Know that drug metabolizes to glucose.

🔲 I.V. administration
• Observe patient closely during early phase of infusion when most anaphylactic reactions occur.

• Use D_5W solution instead of 0.9% NaCl solution for patients with heart failure, as ordered.

• Know that doctor may order dextran 1 to protect against dextran-induced anaphylaxis. Administer 20 ml of dextran 1 (containing 150 mg/ml) I.V. over 60 seconds, 1 to 2 minutes before I.V. infusion of dextran.

• Store drug at constant 77° F (25° C). May precipitate in storage but can be heated to dissolve if necessary.

• Discard partially used containers.

☑ Patient teaching
• Explain use and administration of dextran to patient and family.

• Tell patient to report adverse effects.

---

dextran, high-molecular-weight (dextran 70, dextran 75)
Dextran 75, Gendex 75, Gentran 70, Macrodex

Pregnancy Risk Category: C

HOW SUPPLIED
Injection: 6% dextran 70 in 0.9% NaCl solution or dextrose 5%; 6% dextran 75 in 0.9% NaCl solution or dextrose 5%

ACTION
Expands plasma volume via colloidal osmotic effect, drawing fluid from interstitial to intravascular space, providing fluid replacement.

Route	Onset	Peak	Duration
IV	Immediate	Immediate	Unknown

INDICATIONS & DOSAGE
Plasma expander—
Adults: 30 g (500 ml of 6% solution) I.V. In emergencies, may be given at 1.2 to 2.4 g (20 to 40 ml)/minute. In normovolemic or nearly normovolemic patients, rate of infusion should not exceed 240 mg (4 ml)/minute.

Total dosage during first 24 hours not to exceed 1.2 g/kg; actual dosage depends on amount of fluid loss and resultant hemoconcentration and must be determined for each patient.

ADVERSE REACTIONS
GI: nausea, vomiting.
GU: increased specific gravity and viscosity of urine, tubular stasis and blocking, oliguria, anuria.
Hematologic: decreased hemoglobin and hematocrit levels; with doses of 15 ml/kg body weight, prolonged bleeding time and significant suppression of platelet function.
Hepatic: increased AST and ALT levels.
Skin: *hypersensitivity reactions,* urticaria.
Other: fever, arthralgia, nasal congestion, fluid overload, *anaphylaxis,* thrombophlebitis.

INTERACTIONS
Drug-drug. *Abciximab, aspirin, heparin, thrombolytics, warfarin:* increased bleeding if given in combination. Use together with extreme caution.

EFFECTS ON DIAGNOSTIC TESTS
Falsely elevated blood glucose levels may occur in patients receiving dextran 40 or 70 if the test uses high concentrations of acid. Dextran may cause turbidity, which interferes with bilirubin assays that use alcohol, total protein levels using biuret reagent, and blood glucose levels using

---

the orthotoluidine method. Blood typing and cross-matching using enzyme techniques may give unreliable readings if the samples are taken after the dextran infusion.

Dextran 40 administration has been associated with abnormal renal and hepatic function test results.

CONTRAINDICATIONS
Contraindicated in patients with marked hemostatic defects, marked cardiac decompensation, renal disease with severe oliguria or anuria, hypervolemic conditions, severe bleeding disorders, and hypersensitivity to dextran.

NURSING CONSIDERATIONS
• Use cautiously in patients with active hemorrhage, thrombocytopenia, impaired renal clearance, chronic liver disease, and abdominal conditions or in patients undergoing bowel surgery.
• Assess hydration before starting therapy; otherwise, use urine or serum osmolality because urine specific gravity is affected by the urine dextran concentration.
• Have blood samples drawn before starting infusion.
• Monitor urine flow rate during administration. If oliguria or anuria occurs or is not relieved by infusion, stop dextran and give loop diuretic.
• Watch for circulatory overload. Provides plasma expansion slightly greater than volume infused.
• Monitor hemoglobin and hematocrit levels; if values fall below 30% by volume, notify doctor.
• Be aware that drug may interfere with analyses of blood grouping, cross-matching, bilirubin, blood glucose, and protein.
• Know that drug may precipitate in storage but can be heated to dissolve if necessary.
• Monitor blood glucose levels before and during infusion. Know that drug metabolizes to glucose.

◖ I.V. administration
Alert: Observe patient closely during early phase of infusion when most anaphylactic reactions occur.
• Be aware that doctor may order dextran 1 to protect against dextran-induced anaphylaxis. Give 20 ml of dextran 1 (containing 150 mg/ml) I.V. over 60 seconds, 1 to 2 minutes before I.V. infusion of dextran 70.
• As ordered, use D₅W solution instead of 0.9% NaCl solution for patients with heart failure.

☑ Patient teaching
• Explain use and administration of dextran to patient and family.
• Tell patient to report adverse effects.

hetastarch
Hespan

Pregnancy Risk Category: C

HOW SUPPLIED
Injection: 500 ml (6 g/100 ml in 0.9% NaCl solution)

ACTION
Expands plasma volume and provides fluid replacement.

Route	Onset	Peak	Duration
IV	Immediate	Immediate	Unknown

INDICATIONS & DOSAGE
Plasma expander—
Adults: 500 to 1,000 ml I.V., depending on amount of blood lost and resultant hemoconcentration. Total daily dosage should not exceed 1,500 ml.

ADVERSE REACTIONS
CNS: headache.
CV: peripheral edema of lower extremities.
EENT: periorbital edema.
GI: nausea, vomiting.
Respiratory: wheezing.
Skin: rash, urticaria.
Other: mild fever, chills, muscle pain, fluid overload, *hypersensitivity reaction,* dilution of clotting factors.

INTERACTIONS
None significant.

EFFECTS ON DIAGNOSTIC TESTS
When added to whole blood, hetastarch increases the erythrocyte sedimentation rate.

CONTRAINDICATIONS
Contraindicated in patients with severe bleeding disorders, severe heart failure, or renal failure with oliguria and anuria, or known hypersensitivity to drug.

NURSING CONSIDERATIONS
• Use cautiously in patients with liver disease.
• Know that hetastarch is not a substitute for blood or plasma.
• To avoid circulatory overload, monitor patients with impaired renal function carefully.
• When used in continuous-flow centrifugation, know that leukapheresis ratio is usually one part hetastarch to eight parts venous whole blood.
• Discontinue if allergic or sensitivity reactions occur and notify doctor. If necessary, administer an antihistamine as ordered.

🔲 **I.V. administration**
• Up to 20 ml/kg hourly may be used in hemorrhagic shock. Slower rates of administration are generally used in patients with burns or septic shock.
• Discard partially used bottles.

✅ **Patient teaching**
• Explain use and administration of drug to patient and family.
• Tell patient to report adverse reactions promptly.

magnesium chloride
Slow-Mag ◇

magnesium sulfate

Pregnancy Risk Category: D

HOW SUPPLIED
magnesium chloride
Tablets (delayed-release): 64 mg
magnesium sulfate
Injectable solutions: 10%, 12.5%, 50% in 2-ml, 5-ml, 10-ml, 20-ml, and 30-ml ampules, vials, and prefilled syringes

ACTION
Replaces and maintains magnesium levels; as an anticonvulsant, reduces muscle contractions by interfering with release of acetylcholine at myoneural junction.

Route	Onset	Peak	Duration
PO	Unknown	4 hr	4-6 hr
IV	Immediate	Unknown	30 min
IM	1 hr	Unknown	3-4 hr

INDICATIONS & DOSAGE
Mild hypomagnesemia—
Adults: 1 g I.V. by piggyback or I.M. q 6 hours for four doses, depending on serum magnesium level. Alternatively, 3 g P.O. q 6 hours for four doses.
Severe hypomagnesemia (serum magnesium 0.8 mEq/L or less, with symptoms)—
Adults: 2 to 5 g I.V. in 1 L of solution over 3 hours. Subsequent doses depend on serum magnesium levels.
Magnesium supplementation—
Adults: 64 mg (one tablet) P.O. t.i.d.
Magnesium supplementation in total parenteral nutrition (TPN)—
Adults: 4 to 24 mEq I.V. daily added to TPN solution.
Infants: 2 to 10 mEq I.V. daily added to TPN solution. Each 2 ml of 50% solution contains 1 g, or 8.12 mEq, magnesium sulfate.

ADVERSE REACTIONS
CNS: toxicity, *weak or absent deep tendon reflexes,* flaccid paralysis, hypothermia, drowsiness, stupor.
CV: slow, weak pulse; *arrhythmias* (caused by hypocalcemia); *hypotension; circulatory collapse* (with toxicity).
GI: diarrhea.
Respiratory: *respiratory paralysis.*
Skin: flushing, diaphoresis.
Other: hypocalcemia.

INTERACTIONS
Drug-drug. *Alendronate, nitrofurantoin, penicillamine, quinolones, sodium polystyrene sulfonate, tetracyclines:* decreased bioavailability with oral magnesium sup-

plements. Separate administration by 2 to 3 hours.

Cardiac glycosides: possible serious cardiac conduction changes. Administer with extreme caution.

CNS depressants: may have additive effect. Use cautiously.

Neuromuscular blockers: possible increased neuromuscular blockage. Use cautiously.

EFFECTS ON DIAGNOSTIC TESTS
None reported.

CONTRAINDICATIONS
Contraindicated in patients with myocardial damage or heart block and in actively progressing labor.

NURSING CONSIDERATIONS
• Use parenteral magnesium with extreme caution in patients with impaired renal function.
• Be aware that undiluted 50% solutions may be given by deep I.M. injection to adults. Dilute solutions to 20% or less for use in children.
• Keep I.V. calcium available to reverse magnesium intoxication.
• Test knee-jerk and patellar reflexes before each additional dose. If absent, notify doctor and give no more magnesium until reflexes return; otherwise, patient may develop temporary respiratory failure and need cardiopulmonary resuscitation or I.V. administration of calcium.
• Check magnesium level after repeated doses.
• Monitor fluid intake and output. Output should be 100 ml or more during 4-hour period before dose.
• After giving to toxemic patient within 24 hours before delivery, watch neonate for signs of magnesium toxicity, including neuromuscular and respiratory depression.

I.V. administration
• Inject I.V. bolus dose slowly, using infusion pump for continuous infusion, if available, to avoid respiratory or cardiac arrest. Maximum infusion rate is 150 mg/minute. Rapid drip causes feeling of heat.
Alert: When giving I.V. for severe hypo-

magnesemia, watch for respiratory depression and signs of heart block. Respirations should be over 16 breaths/minute before dose is given.
• Know that drug is incompatible with alkalis, including carbonates and bicarbonates. Precipitate may form if mixed with solutions containing ethanol, arsenates, barium, calcium, clindamycin, heavy metals, hydrocortisone sodium succinate, phosphates, polymyxin B sulfate, procaine, salicylates, or tartrates.

☑ **Patient teaching**
• Explain use and administration of drug to patient and family.
• Tell patient to report adverse effects.

potassium acetate

Pregnancy Risk Category: C

HOW SUPPLIED
Injection: 2 mEq/ml in 20-ml, 30-ml vials; 4 mEq/ml in 50-ml vials

ACTION
Replaces and maintains potassium level.

Route	Onset	Peak	Duration
IV	Immediate	Immediate	Unknown

INDICATIONS & DOSAGE
Treatment of hypokalemia—
Adults: no more than 20 mEq hourly in concentration of 40 mEq/L or less. Total 24-hour dosage should not exceed 150 mEq (3 mEq/kg in children). Potassium replacement should be done with ECG monitoring and frequent serum potassium determinations. I.V. route should be used only for life-threatening hypokalemia or when oral replacement is not feasible.
Prevention of hypokalemia—
Adults: dosage is individualized to patient's needs, not to exceed 150 mEq/day. Administered as an additive to I.V. infusions. Usual dose is 20 mEq/L infused at a rate not to exceed 20 mEq/hour.
Children: individualized dosage not to exceed 3 mEq/kg/day. Administered as an additive to I.V. infusions.

ADVERSE REACTIONS
Signs and symptoms of hyperkalemia—
CNS: paresthesia of the extremities, listlessness, mental confusion, weakness or heaviness of legs, flaccid paralysis.
CV: hypotension, *arrhythmias, heart block,* ECG changes, *cardiac arrest.*
GI: nausea, vomiting, abdominal pain, diarrhea.
Respiratory: *respiratory paralysis.*
Other: pain and redness at infusion site, fever, hyperkalemia.

INTERACTIONS
Drug-drug. *ACE inhibitors, potassium-sparing diuretics:* increased risk of hyperkalemia. Use with extreme caution.

EFFECTS ON DIAGNOSTIC TESTS
None reported.

CONTRAINDICATIONS
Contraindicated in patients with severe renal impairment with oliguria, anuria, or azotemia; untreated Addison's disease; and acute dehydration, heat cramps, hyperkalemia, hyperkalemic form of familial periodic paralysis, or conditions associated with extensive tissue breakdown.

NURSING CONSIDERATIONS
• Use cautiously in patients with cardiac disease or renal impairment.
• During therapy, monitor ECG, renal function, fluid intake and output, and serum potassium, serum creatinine, and BUN levels. Never give potassium postoperatively until urine flow is established.

I.V. administration
• Give by I.V. infusion only, never I.V. push or I.M. Watch for pain and redness at infusion site. Large-bore needle reduces local irritation.
Alert: Give slowly as diluted solution; potentially fatal hyperkalemia may result from too-rapid infusion.

✓ Patient teaching
• Explain use and administration to patient and family.
• Tell patient to report adverse effects, especially pain at insertion site.

potassium bicarbonate
K+Care ET, Klor-Con/EF, K-Lyte, K-Vescent

Pregnancy Risk Category: C

HOW SUPPLIED
Tablets (effervescent): 25 mEq

ACTION
Replaces and maintains potassium.

Route	Onset	Peak	Duration
PO	Unknown	4 hr	Unknown

INDICATIONS & DOSAGE
Hypokalemia—
Adults: 25 to 50 mEq dissolved in 4 to 8 oz (120 to 240 ml) of water once daily to q.i.d.

ADVERSE REACTIONS
CNS: paresthesia of the extremities, listlessness, mental confusion, weakness or heaviness of legs, flaccid paralysis.
CV: *arrhythmias,* ECG changes, hypotension, *heart block, cardiac arrest.*
GI: *nausea, vomiting, abdominal pain,* diarrhea.

INTERACTIONS
Drug-drug. *ACE inhibitors, potassium-sparing diuretics:* risk of hyperkalemia. Use with extreme caution.

EFFECTS ON DIAGNOSTIC TESTS
None reported.

CONTRAINDICATIONS
Contraindicated in patients with severe renal impairment with oliguria, anuria, or azotemia; untreated Addison's disease; and acute dehydration, heat cramps, hyperkalemia, hyperkalemic form of familial periodic paralysis, or other conditions associated with extensive tissue breakdown.

NURSING CONSIDERATIONS
• Use cautiously in patients with cardiac disease or renal impairment.
• Dissolve potassium bicarbonate tablets

Reactions may be *common*, uncommon, *life-threatening*, or COMMON AND LIFE-THREATENING.

completely in 4 to 8 oz (120 to 240 ml) of cold water.
• Ask patient's flavor preference. Available in lime fruit punch, citrus and orange flavors.
• Do not administer potassium supplements postoperatively until urine flow has been established.
• Never switch potassium products without doctor's order. Potassium chloride cannot be given instead of potassium bicarbonate.
• Monitor BUN, serum potassium, and creatinine levels and fluid intake and output.

☑ **Patient teaching**
• Tell patient to take drug with meals and sip slowly over 5 to 10 minutes.
• Tell patient to report adverse effects.
• Warn patient not to use salt substitutes concurrently, except with doctor's permission.

potassium chloride
Cena-K, K + 10, Kaochlor 10%*, Kaochlor S-F 10%*, Kaon-Cl, Kaon-Cl 20%*, Kay-Cee-L§, Kay Ciel*, K + Care, K-Dur, K-Lease, K-Lor, Klor-Con, Klor-Con/25, Klorvess, Klotrix, K-Lyte/Cl, K-Norm, K-Tab, Micro-K Extencaps, Rum-K, Slow-K, Ten-K

Pregnancy Risk Category: C

HOW SUPPLIED
Tablets (controlled-release): 6.7 mEq (500 mg), 8 mEq (600 mg), 10 mEq (750 mg), 20 mEq (1,500 mg)
Tablets (film-coated): 2.5 mEq (200 mg), 8 mEq (600 mg), 10 mEq (750 mg)
Capsules (controlled-release): 8 mEq (600 mg), 10 mEq (750 mg)
Oral liquid: 10% (20 mEq/15 ml), 15% (30 mEq/15 ml), 20% (40 mEq/15 ml)
Powder for oral use: 15-mEq packet, 20-mEq packet, 25-mEq packet, 25-mEq dose
Injection: 20-mEq, 40-mEq ampules; additive syringes containing 30-mEq or 40-mEq; 10-mEq, 20-mEq, 30-mEq,
40-mEq, 60-mEq, 100-mEq, 200-mEq, 400-mEq, or 1,000-mEq vials

ACTION
Replaces and maintains potassium level.

Route	Onset	Peak	Duration
PO	Unknown	Unknown	Unknown
IV	Immediate	Immediate	Unknown

INDICATIONS & DOSAGE
Hypokalemia—
Adults: 40 to 100 mEq P.O. daily in three or four divided doses for treatment; 10 to 20 mEq for prevention. Further dosage based on serum potassium level.
Children: 3 mEq/kg daily. Total daily dosage not to exceed 40 mEq/m².

Use I.V. route only when oral replacement is not feasible or when hypokalemia is life-threatening. If serum potassium level is below 2 mEq/ml, maximum infusion rate is 40 mEq/hour; maximum infusion concentration is 80 mEq/L; and maximum 24-hour dose is 400 mEq. If serum potassium level is greater than 2 mEq/ml, maximum infusion rate is 10 mEq/hour; maximum infusion concentration is 40 mEq/L; and maximum 24-hour dose is 200 mEq. For routine supplementation, the usual dose is 10 to 20 mEq hourly in concentration of 40 mEq/L or less.

ADVERSE REACTIONS
Signs and symptoms of hyperkalemia—
CNS: paresthesia of the extremities, listlessness, mental confusion, weakness or heaviness of limbs, flaccid paralysis.
CV: *arrhythmias, heart block, possible cardiac arrest,* ECG changes, hypotension.
GI: nausea, vomiting, abdominal pain, diarrhea.
Respiratory: *respiratory paralysis.*
Other: *postinfusion phlebitis,* hyperkalemia.

INTERACTIONS
Drug-drug. *ACE inhibitors, potassium-sparing diuretics:* risk of hyperkalemia. Use with extreme caution.

EFFECTS ON DIAGNOSTIC TESTS
None reported.

CONTRAINDICATIONS

Contraindicated in patients with severe renal impairment with oliguria, anuria, or azotemia; with untreated Addison's disease; and acute dehydration, heat cramps, hyperkalemia, hyperkalemic form of familial periodic paralysis, or other conditions associated with extensive tissue breakdown.

NURSING CONSIDERATIONS

• Give oral potassium supplements with extreme caution because different forms deliver varying amounts of potassium. Never switch products without doctor's order.

• Make sure powders are completely dissolved before administering.

• Realize that enteric-coated tablets are not recommended because of increased potential for GI bleeding and small-bowel ulcerations.

• Know that tablets in wax matrix sometimes lodge in esophagus and cause ulceration in cardiac patients who have esophageal compression from enlarged left atrium. Use liquid form in such patients and in those with esophageal stasis or obstruction.

• Know that drug is often used orally with potassium-wasting diuretics to maintain potassium levels.

• Be aware that sugar-free liquid is available (Kaochlor S-F 10%); use if tablet or capsule passage is likely to be delayed, such as in GI obstruction. Have patients sip slowly to minimize GI irritation.

• Do not crush sustained-release potassium products.

• Monitor ECG and serum electrolyte levels during therapy.

• Monitor renal function. Potassium should not be given during immediate postoperative period until urine flow is established.

• Use cautiously in patients with cardiac disease or renal impairment.

☐ I.V. administration

Alert: Give by infusion only, never I.V. push or I.M. Give slowly as dilute solution; potentially fatal hyperkalemia may result from too-rapid infusion.

☑ Patient teaching

• Instruct patient how to prepare (powders) and administer drug form prescribed. Tell patient to take with or after meals with full glass of water or fruit juice to lessen GI distress.

• Teach patient the signs and symptoms of hyperkalemia, and tell patient to notify doctor if they occur.

• Tell patient to alert nurse if discomfort occurs at I.V. insertion site.

• Warn patient not to use salt substitutes concurrently, except with doctor's permission.

---

potassium gluconate
Glu-K, Kaon, Kaylixir*, K-G Elixir*

Pregnancy Risk Category: C

HOW SUPPLIED
Tablets: 500 mg (2 mEq K$^+$)
Elixir: 4.68 g (20 mEq K$^+$)/15 ml*

ACTION
Replaces and maintains intracellular and extracellular potassium.

Route	Onset	Peak	Duration
PO	Unknown	Unknown	4 hr

INDICATIONS & DOSAGE
Hypokalemia—
Adults: 40 to 100 mEq P.O. daily in three or four divided doses for treatment; 10 to 20 mEq daily for prevention. Further dosage adjustments are based on serum potassium determinations.

ADVERSE REACTIONS
CNS: paresthesia of the extremities, listlessness, mental confusion, weakness or heaviness of legs, flaccid paralysis.
CV: *arrhythmias*, ECG changes.
GI: *nausea, vomiting, abdominal pain*, diarrhea.

INTERACTIONS
Drug-drug. *ACE inhibitors, potassium-sparing diuretics:* risk of hyperkalemia. Use with extreme caution.

Reactions may be *common*, uncommon, *life-threatening*, or COMMON AND LIFE-THREATENING.

EFFECTS ON DIAGNOSTIC TESTS
None reported.

CONTRAINDICATIONS
Contraindicated in patients with severe renal impairment with oliguria, anuria, or azotemia; untreated Addison's disease; and in those with acute dehydration, heat cramps, hyperkalemia, hyperkalemic form of familial periodic paralysis, or other conditions associated with extensive tissue breakdown.

NURSING CONSIDERATIONS
• Give oral potassium supplements with extreme caution because different forms deliver varying amounts of potassium. Never switch products without doctor's order.
• Use cautiously in patients with cardiac disease and in those with renal impairment.
• Do not administer potassium supplements postoperatively until urine flow has been established.
• Monitor ECG, serum potassium, and creatinine levels, BUN, and fluid intake and output.

☑ **Patient teaching**
• Advise patient to sip liquid potassium slowly to minimize GI irritation. Also tell him to take drug with or after meals with a full glass of water or fruit juice.
• Warn patient not to use salt substitutes concurrently, except with doctor's permission.

Ringer's injection

Pregnancy Risk Category: NR

HOW SUPPLIED
Injection: 250 ml, 500 ml, 1,000 ml

ACTION
Replaces fluids and electrolytes.

Route	Onset	Peak	Duration
IV	Immediate	Immediate	Unknown

INDICATIONS & DOSAGE
Fluid and electrolyte replacement—
Adults and children: dosage highly indi-

vidualized, but usually 1.5 to 3 L (2% to 6% body weight), infused I.V. over 18 to 24 hours.

ADVERSE REACTIONS
CV: fluid overload.
Other: electrolyte imbalance.

INTERACTIONS
None significant.

EFFECTS ON DIAGNOSTIC TESTS
None reported.

CONTRAINDICATIONS
Contraindicated in patients with renal failure, except as emergency volume expander.

NURSING CONSIDERATIONS
• Use cautiously in patients with heart failure, circulatory insufficiency, renal dysfunction, hypoproteinemia, and pulmonary edema.
• Be aware that Ringer's injection contains sodium, 147 mEq/L; potassium, 4 mEq/L; calcium, 4.5 mEq/L; and chloride, 155.5 mEq/L.
• Know that electrolyte content is insufficient for treating severe electrolyte deficiencies but does provide electrolytes in levels approximately equal to those of the blood.

◖ **I.V. administration**
• Administer at ordered rate via an infusion device.

☑ **Patient teaching**
• Explain use and administration of drug to patient and family.
• Tell patient to report unusual signs or symptoms promptly.

Ringer's injection, lactated (Ringer's lactate solution)

Pregnancy Risk Category: NR

HOW SUPPLIED
Injection: 150 ml, 250 ml, 500 ml, 1,000 ml

ACTION
Replaces fluids and electrolytes.

Route	Onset	Peak	Duration
IV	Immediate	Immediate	Unknown

INDICATIONS & DOSAGE
Fluid and electrolyte replacement—
Adults and children: dosage highly individualized, but usually 1.5 to 3 L (2% to 6% body weight) infused I.V. over 18 to 24 hours.

ADVERSE REACTIONS
CV: fluid overload.
Other: electrolyte imbalance.

INTERACTIONS
None significant.

EFFECTS ON DIAGNOSTIC TESTS
None reported.

CONTRAINDICATIONS
Contraindicated in patients with renal failure, except as emergency volume expander.

NURSING CONSIDERATIONS
• Use cautiously in patients with heart failure, circulatory insufficiency, renal dysfunction, hypoproteinemia, and pulmonary edema.
• Know that lactated Ringer's injection contains sodium, 130 mEq/L; potassium, 4 mEq/L; calcium, 3 mEq/L; chloride, 109.7 mEq/L; and lactate, 28 mEq/L.
• Be aware that lactated Ringer's injection more closely approximates the electrolyte concentration in blood plasma.

🔲 **I.V. administration**
• Administer at ordered rate via an infusion device.

☑ **Patient teaching**
• Explain use and administration of drug to patient and family.
• Tell patient to report unusual signs or symptoms promptly.

sodium chloride
Slow-Sodium§

Pregnancy Risk Category: C

HOW SUPPLIED
Tablets: 650 mg
Tablets (slow-release): 600 mg, 1 g, 2.25 g
Injection: 0.45% NaCl solution 25 ml, 50 ml, 150 ml, 250 ml, 500 ml, 1,000 ml; 0.9% NaCl solution 2 ml, 3 ml, 5 ml, 10 ml, 20 ml, 25 ml, 30 ml, 50 ml, 100 ml, 150 ml, 250 ml, 500 ml, 1,000 ml; 3% NaCl solution 500 ml; 5% NaCl solution 500 ml; 14.6% NaCl solution 20 ml, 40 ml, 200 ml; 23.4% NaCl solution 30 ml, 50 ml, 100 ml, and 200 ml

ACTION
Replaces and maintains sodium and chloride levels.

Route	Onset	Peak	Duration
PO	Unknown	Unknown	Unknown
IV	Immediate	Immediate	Unknown

INDICATIONS & DOSAGE
Fluid and electrolyte replacement in hyponatremia caused by electrolyte loss or in severe salt depletion—
Adults: dosage is individualized. 3% or 5% solution used only with frequent electrolyte determination and given only slow I.V. With 0.45% solution: 3% to 8% of body weight, according to deficiencies, over 18 to 24 hours; with 0.9% solution: 2% to 6% of body weight, according to deficiencies, over 18 to 24 hours.
Management of heat cramp caused by excessive perspiration—
Adults: 1 g P.O. with each glass of water.

ADVERSE REACTIONS
CV: aggravation of heart failure; edema (when given too rapidly or in excess).
Respiratory: *pulmonary edema* (when given too rapidly or in excess).
Other: hypernatremia, aggravation of existing metabolic acidosis (with excessive infusion); serious electrolyte disturbances, loss of potassium; local tenderness, abscess, tissue necrosis (at injection site); thrombophlebitis.

INTERACTIONS
None significant.

EFFECTS ON DIAGNOSTIC TESTS
None reported.

CONTRAINDICATIONS
Contraindicated in patients with conditions in which sodium and chloride administration is detrimental. Sodium chloride 3% and 5% injections are contraindicated in patients with increased, normal, or only slightly decreased serum electrolyte concentrations.

NURSING CONSIDERATIONS
• Use cautiously in patients with heart failure, circulatory insufficiency, renal dysfunction, and hypoproteinemia and in elderly or postoperative patients.
• Monitor serum electrolyte levels.

I.V. administration
• Do not confuse concentrates (14.6%, 23.4%) available to add to parenteral nutrient solutions with 0.9% NaCl injection, and never give without diluting. Read labels carefully.
Alert: Infuse 3% and 5% solutions slowly and cautiously to avoid pulmonary edema. Use only for critical situations, and observe the patient continually.
• Never use bacteriostatic NaCl injection with newborns.

Patient teaching
• Explain use and administration of drug to patient and family.
• Tell patient to report adverse reactions promptly.

64

Acidifiers and alkalinizers

sodium bicarbonate
sodium lactate
tromethamine

COMBINATION PRODUCTS
None.

---

sodium bicarbonate ◇
Arm and Hammer Pure Baking
Soda, Bell/ans, Citrocarbonate,
Soda Mint

Pregnancy Risk Category: C

HOW SUPPLIED
Tablets ◇ : 325 mg, 650 mg
Injection: 4% (2.4 mEq/5 ml), 4.2%
(5 mEq/10 ml), 5% (297.5 mEq/500 ml),
7.5% (8.92 mEq/10 ml and 44.6 mEq/
50 ml), 8.4% (10 mEq/10 ml and 50 mEq/
50 ml)

ACTION
Restores buffering capacity of the body
and neutralizes excess acid.

Route	Onset	Peak	Duration
PO	Unknown	Unknown	Unknown
IV	Immediate	Immediate	Unknown

INDICATIONS & DOSAGE
Cardiac arrest—
Adults and children: 1 mEq/kg I.V. of
7.5% or 8.4% solution, followed by
0.5 mEq/kg I.V. q 10 minutes, depending
on arterial blood gases (ABG). Further
dosages based on results of ABG analysis.
If ABG results are unavailable, use
0.5 mEq/kg I.V. q 10 minutes until spontaneous circulation returns.
Infants up to 2 years: not to exceed
8 mEq/kg I.V. daily of 4.2% solution.
Metabolic acidosis—
Adults and children: dosage depends on
blood carbon dioxide content, pH, and patient's clinical condition. Generally, 2 to
5 mEq/kg I.V. infused over 4- to 8-hour
period.

Systemic or urinary alkalinization—
Adults: initially, 4 g P.O., followed by 1
to 2 g q 4 hours.
Children: 84 to 840 mg/kg P.O. daily.
Antacid—
Adults: 300 mg to 2 g P.O. up to q.i.d.
taken with glass of water.

ADVERSE REACTIONS
GI: gastric distention, belching, flatulence.
Other: hypokalemia, *metabolic alkalosis*,
hypernatremia, hyperosmolarity (with
overdose); pain, irritation (at injection site).

INTERACTIONS
Drug-drug. *Anorexiants, flecainide,
mecamylamine, methenamine, quinidine,
sympathomimetics:* urine alkalinization
causes decreased renal clearance of these
drugs and increased risk of toxicity. Monitor closely.
*Chlorpropamide, lithium, methotrexate,
salicylates, tetracycline:* increased urine
alkalinization causes increased renal
clearance of these drugs and reduced effectiveness. Monitor closely.
Enteric-coated drugs: may be released
prematurely in stomach. Avoid concomitant use.
Ketoconazole: concurrent use may decrease absorption. Use with caution.

EFFECTS ON DIAGNOSTIC TESTS
Sodium bicarbonate therapy may alter
serum electrolyte levels and may increase
serum lactate levels.

CONTRAINDICATIONS
Contraindicated in patients with metabolic
or respiratory alkalosis; in patients who
are losing chlorides by vomiting or from
continuous GI suction; in those receiving
diuretics known to produce hypochloremic
alkalosis; and in those with hypocalcemia
in which alkalosis may produce tetany, hypertension, seizures, or heart failure. Orally administered sodium bicarbonate is
contraindicated in patients with acute ingestion of strong mineral acids.

NURSING CONSIDERATIONS
• Use with extreme caution in patients with heart failure or other edematous or sodium-retaining conditions or renal insufficiency.
• To avoid risk of alkalosis, obtain blood pH, partial pressure of arterial oxygen, partial pressure of arterial carbon dioxide, and serum electrolytes. Keep the doctor informed of serum laboratory results.

◖ **I.V. administration**
• Drug may be added to other I.V. fluids. Sodium bicarbonate inactivates such catecholamines as norepinephrine and dopamine, and forms precipitate with calcium. Do not mix sodium bicarbonate with I.V. solutions of these agents, and flush I.V. line adequately.
Alert: Be aware that sodium bicarbonate is not routinely recommended for use in cardiac arrest because it may produce a paradoxical acidosis from carbon dioxide production. It should not be routinely administered during the early stages of resuscitation unless preexisting acidosis is clearly present.
• Know that 4% sodium bicarbonate is usually used for neutralizing certain I.V. medications (such as erythromycin). Consult a pharmacist prior to use.

☑ **Patient teaching**
• Tell patient not to take drug with milk. Drug may cause hypercalcemia, alkalosis, and possibly renal calculi.

sodium lactate

Pregnancy Risk Category: NR

HOW SUPPLIED
Injection: 1/6 M solution (167 mEq/L)
Injection: 5 mEq/ml

ACTION
Metabolized to sodium bicarbonate, producing buffering effect.

Route	Onset	Peak	Duration
IV	Immediate	1-2 hr	Unknown

INDICATIONS & DOSAGE
Alkalinize urine—
Adults: 30 ml of 1/6 M solution/kg of body weight I.V., given in divided doses over 24 hours.
Metabolic acidosis—
Adults: 1/6 M injection (167 mEq lactate/L I.V.); dosage depends on degree of bicarbonate deficit.

ADVERSE REACTIONS
Other: fever, infection, thrombophlebitis (at injection site); *metabolic alkalosis*, hypernatremia, hyperosmolarity (with overdose).

INTERACTIONS
None significant.

EFFECTS ON DIAGNOSTIC TESTS
None reported.

CONTRAINDICATIONS
Contraindicated in patients with hypernatremia, lactic acidosis, or conditions in which sodium administration is detrimental, such as heart failure or corticosteroid administration.

NURSING CONSIDERATIONS
• Use with extreme caution in patients with metabolic or respiratory alkalosis, severe hepatic or renal disease, heart failure, shock, hypoxia, or beriberi.
• Monitor serum electrolyte levels to avoid alkalosis.

◖ **I.V. administration**
• Add sodium lactate to other I.V. solutions, or give as an isotonic 1/6 M solution. Drug is compatible with most common I.V. solutions.
• Do not mix with sodium bicarbonate; drugs are incompatible.

☑ **Patient teaching**
• Explain use and administration of drug to patient and family.
• Tell patient to report unusual signs and symptoms.

tromethamine
Tham

Pregnancy Risk Category: C

HOW SUPPLIED
Injection: 18 g/500 ml

ACTION
Combines with hydrogen ions and associated acid anions; resulting salts are excreted. Also has osmotic diuretic effect.

Route	Onset	Peak	Duration
IV	Immediate	Immediate	Unknown

INDICATIONS & DOSAGE
Metabolic acidosis associated with cardiac bypass surgery or with cardiac arrest—
Adults: dosage depends on bicarbonate deficit. Calculate as follows: each ml of 0.3 M tromethamine solution required equals weight in kg multiplied by bicarbonate deficit (mEq/L). Additional therapy based on serial determinations of existing bicarbonate deficit. Administer over at least 1 hour; individual doses should not exceed 500 mg/kg.
Acidosis during bypass surgery: Average dose of 9 ml/kg (2.7 mEq/kg or 0.32 g/kg); total single dose of 500 ml (150 mEq or 18 g) is adequate for most adults; not to exceed 500 mg/kg over a period of less than 1 hour.
Cardiac arrest: 3.6 to 10.8 g (111 to 333 ml) injected into large peripheral vein.

ADVERSE REACTIONS
Respiratory: *respiratory depression.*
Other: hypoglycemia, *hyperkalemia* (with decreased urine output), venospasm; I.V. thrombosis; inflammation, necrosis, sloughing (if extravasation occurs); hemorrhagic hepatic necrosis; fever.

INTERACTIONS
None significant.

EFFECTS ON DIAGNOSTIC TESTS
Drug alters serum electrolyte levels. Transient decreases in blood glucose concentrations may occur.

CONTRAINDICATIONS
Contraindicated in patients with anuria, uremia, or chronic respiratory acidosis, or during pregnancy (except in acute, life-threatening situations).

NURSING CONSIDERATIONS
• Use cautiously in patients with renal disease and poor urine output. Monitor ECG and serum potassium levels.
• Make these determinations before, during, and after therapy: blood pH; carbon dioxide tension; bicarbonate, glucose, and electrolyte levels.
• Have mechanical ventilation available for patients with associated respiratory acidosis.
• To prevent blood pH from rising above normal, be prepared to adjust dosage carefully, as ordered.

🔲 I.V. administration
• Give slowly through 18G to 20G needle into largest antecubital vein, or by indwelling I.V. catheter.
• If extravasation occurs, infiltrate area with 1% procaine and 150 units hyaluronidase, as ordered.

☑ Patient teaching
• Explain use of drug to patient and family.
• Tell patient to report adverse reactions.

65
Hematinics

ferrous fumarate
ferrous gluconate
ferrous sulfate
ferrous sulfate, dried
iron dextran
iron sorbitol
polysaccharide-iron complex

COMBINATION PRODUCTS
FERRO-DOSS, FERROUS DS, FERRO-DSS: ferrous fumarate 150 mg and docusate sodium 100 mg.
FERRO-SEQUELS ◇: ferrous fumarate 150 mg and docusate sodium 100 mg.

---

ferrous fumarate
Femiron ◇, Feostat ◇, Feostat Drops ◇, Fersamal§, Hemocyte ◇, Ircon ◇, Nephro-Fer ◇, Novofumar†, Palafer†, Palafer Pediatric Drops†, Span-FF ◇

Pregnancy Risk Category: A

HOW SUPPLIED
Each 100 mg of ferrous fumarate provides 33 mg of elemental iron
Tablets ◇: 63 mg, 200 mg, 324 mg, 325 mg, 350 mg
Tablets (chewable): 100 mg ◇
Oral suspension: 100 mg/5 ml ◇
Drops: 45 mg/0.6 ml ◇

ACTION
Provides elemental iron, an essential component in the formation of hemoglobin.

Route	Onset	Peak	Duration
PO	4 days	7-10 days	2-4 mo

INDICATIONS & DOSAGE
Iron deficiency—
Adults: 50 to 100 mg of elemental iron t.i.d.
Children: 4 to 6 mg/kg/day of elemental iron in three divided doses.

ADVERSE REACTIONS
GI: *nausea, epigastric pain, vomiting, constipation, diarrhea, black stools, anorexia.*
Other: suspension and drops may temporarily stain teeth.

INTERACTIONS
Drug-drug. *Antacids, cholestyramine resin, cimetidine, vitamin E:* decreased iron absorption. Separate doses by at least 2 hours.
Chloramphenicol: delayed response to iron therapy. Monitor patient.
Fluoroquinolones, penicillamine, tetracyclines: decreased GI absorption, possibly resulting in decreased serum levels or efficacy. Separate doses by 2 to 4 hours.
Levodopa, methyldopa: decreased absorption and efficacy of levodopa and methyldopa. Monitor for decreased effect of these agents.
L-thyroxine: decreased L-thyroxine absorption. Separate doses by at least 2 hours. Monitor thyroid function.
Vitamin C: may increase iron absorption. Give together.
Drug-herb. *Oregano:* may reduce iron absorption. Separate administration of oregano by at least 2 hours when given with iron supplements or iron-containing foods.
Drug-food. *Cereals, cheese, coffee, eggs, milk, tea, whole-grain breads, yogurt:* may impair oral iron absorption. Do not administer together.

EFFECTS ON DIAGNOSTIC TESTS
Ferrous fumarate blackens feces and may interfere with tests for occult blood in the stool; the guaiac test and orthotoluidine test may yield false-positive results, but benzidine test is usually not affected. Iron overload may decrease uptake of Tc99m and thus interfere with skeletal imaging.

CONTRAINDICATIONS
Contraindicated in patients with primary hemochromatosis or hemosiderosis, he-

---

molytic anemia unless iron deficiency anemia is also present, peptic ulcer disease, regional enteritis, or ulcerative colitis and in those receiving repeated blood transfusions.

NURSING CONSIDERATIONS
• Use cautiously on long-term basis.
• Keep in mind that GI upset may be related to dose. Between-meal doses are preferable, but can be given with some foods, although absorption may be decreased. Enteric-coated products reduce GI upset but also reduce amount of iron absorbed.
• Check for constipation; record color and amount of stools.
• Be aware that oral iron may turn stools black. Although this unabsorbed iron is harmless, it could mask the presence of melena.
• Monitor hemoglobin and hematocrit levels and reticulocyte count during therapy, as ordered.
• Know that combination products, such as Ferro-Sequels and Ferocyl, contain stool softeners, which help prevent constipation, a common adverse reaction.

☑ **Patient teaching**
• Tell patient to take tablets with juice (preferably orange juice) or water, but not with milk or antacids.
• To avoid staining teeth, tell patient to take suspension with straw and place drops at back of throat.
• Caution patient not to crush tablets or to chew extended-release iron preparations.
• Advise patient not to substitute one iron salt for another; the amount of elemental iron may vary.
• Inform parents that as little as three or four tablets can cause serious poisoning in children.

---

ferrous gluconate
Fergon*◊, Fertinic†, Novoferrogluc†

Pregnancy Risk Category: A

HOW SUPPLIED
Each 100 mg of ferrous gluconate provides 11.6 mg of elemental iron.
Tablets: 240 mg◊, 325 mg◊

ACTION
Provides elemental iron, an essential component in the formation of hemoglobin.

Route	Onset	Peak	Duration
PO	4 days	7-10 days	2-4 mo

INDICATIONS & DOSAGE
Iron deficiency—
Adults: 100 to 200 mg of elemental iron t.i.d.
Children: 4 to 6 mg/kg/day of elemental iron in three divided doses.

ADVERSE REACTIONS
GI: *nausea,* epigastric pain, vomiting, *constipation,* diarrhea, *black stools,* anorexia.

INTERACTIONS
Drug-drug. *Antacids, cholestyramine resin, cimetidine, vitamin E:* decreased iron absorption. Separate doses by at least 2 hours.
Chloramphenicol: delayed response to iron therapy. Monitor patient.
Fluoroquinolones, penicillamine, tetracyclines: decreased GI absorption, possibly resulting in decreased serum levels or efficacy. Separate doses by 2 to 4 hours.
Levodopa, methyldopa: decreased absorption and efficacy of levodopa and methyldopa. Monitor for decreased effect of these agents.
L-thyroxine: decreased L-thyroxine absorption. Separate doses by at least 2 hours. Monitor thyroid function.
Vitamin C: may increase iron absorption. Give together.
Drug-herb. *Oregano:* may reduce iron absorption. Separate administration of oregano by at least 2 hours when given with iron supplements or iron-containing foods.
Drug-food. *Cereals, cheese, coffee, eggs, milk, tea, whole-grain breads, yogurt:* may impair oral iron absorption. Do not administer together.

EFFECTS ON DIAGNOSTIC TESTS
Ferrous gluconate blackens feces and may interfere with test for occult blood in the stools; the guaiac test and orthotoluidine test may yield false-positive results, but benzidine test is usually not affected. Iron overload may decrease uptake of Tc99m and thus interfere with skeletal imaging.

CONTRAINDICATIONS
Contraindicated in patients with peptic ulceration, regional enteritis, ulcerative colitis, hemosiderosis, primary hemochromatosis, or hemolytic anemia (unless an iron deficiency anemia is also present) and in those receiving repeated blood transfusions.

NURSING CONSIDERATIONS
• Use cautiously on long-term basis.
• Keep in mind that GI upset may be related to dose. Between-meal doses are preferable, but can be given with some foods, although absorption may be decreased. Enteric-coated products reduce GI upset but also reduce amount of iron absorbed.
• Check for constipation; record color and amount of stools.
• Be aware that oral iron may turn stools black. This unabsorbed iron is harmless; however, it could mask melena.
• Monitor hemoglobin and hematocrit levels and reticulocyte count during therapy.

☑ **Patient teaching**
• To promote absorption, tell patient to take tablets with orange juice.
• Inform parents that as few as three or four tablets can cause serious iron poisoning in children.
• Caution patient not to substitute one iron salt for another as the amounts of elemental iron vary.

ferrous sulfate
Apo-Ferrous Sulfate†, Feosol*◊, Fer-gen-sol, Fer-In-Sol Drops*◊, Fer-In-Sol Syrup*◊, Fer-Iron Drops◊, Fero-Grad, Mol-Iron*◊

ferrous sulfate, dried
Fe⁵⁰, Feosol◊, Feospan§, Feratab, Novoferrosulfa†, PMS-Ferrous Sulfate†, Slow Fe◊

Pregnancy Risk Category: A

HOW SUPPLIED
Ferrous sulfate is 20% elemental iron; dried and powdered, about 32% elemental iron.
Tablets: 324 mg, 325 mg◊; 200 mg (dried)
Tablets (extended-release): 160 mg (dried)◊, 525 mg
Caplets (extended-release): 160 mg (dried)
Capsules: 250 mg◊
Elixir: 220 mg/5 ml*◊
Syrup: 90 mg/5 ml◊
Drops: 125 mg/ml

ACTION
Provides elemental iron, an essential component in the formation of hemoglobin.

Route	Onset	Peak	Duration
PO	4 days	7-10 days	2-4 mo

INDICATIONS & DOSAGE
Iron deficiency—
Adults: 100 to 200 mg of elemental iron t.i.d.
Children: 4 to 6 mg/kg/day of elemental iron in three divided doses.

ADVERSE REACTIONS
GI: *nausea,* epigastric pain, vomiting, *constipation, black stools,* diarrhea, anorexia.
Other: liquid forms may temporarily stain teeth.

INTERACTIONS
Drug-drug. *Antacids, cholestyramine resin, cimetidine, vitamin E:* decreased iron absorption. Separate doses if possible.

Chloramphenicol: delayed response to iron therapy. Monitor patient.

Fluoroquinolones, penicillamine, tetracyclines: decreased GI absorption, possibly resulting in decreased serum levels or efficacy. Separate doses by 2 to 4 hours.

Levodopa, methyldopa: decreased absorption and efficacy of levodopa and methyldopa. Monitor for decreased effect of these agents.

L-thyroxine: decreased L-thyroxine absorption. Separate doses by at least 2 hours. Monitor thyroid function.

Vitamin C: may increase iron absorption. Give together.

Drug-herb. *Oregano:* may reduce iron absorption. Separate administration of oregano by at least 2 hours when given with iron supplements or iron-containing foods.

Drug-food. *Cereals, cheese, coffee, eggs, milk, tea, whole-grain breads, yogurt:* may impair oral iron absorption. Do not administer together.

EFFECTS ON DIAGNOSTIC TESTS

Ferrous sulfate blackens feces and may interfere with tests for occult blood in the stool; the guaiac test and orthotoluidine test may yield false-positive results, but benzidine test is usually not affected. Iron overload may decrease uptake of Tc99m and thus interfere with skeletal imaging.

CONTRAINDICATIONS

Contraindicated in patients with hemosiderosis, primary hemochromatosis, hemolytic anemia (unless iron deficiency anemia is also present), peptic ulceration, ulcerative colitis, or regional enteritis and in those receiving repeated blood transfusions.

NURSING CONSIDERATIONS

• Use cautiously on long-term basis.
• Keep in mind that GI upset may be related to dose. Between-meal doses are preferable, but can be given with some foods, although absorption may be decreased. Enteric-coated products reduce GI upset but also reduce amount of iron absorbed.
• Be aware that oral iron may turn stools black. Although this unabsorbed iron is harmless, it could mask melena.

• Monitor hemoglobin and hematocrit levels and reticulocyte count during therapy, as ordered.

☑ Patient teaching
• Tell patient to take with juice.
• Instruct patient not to crush or chew extended-release preparations.
• Inform parents that as little as three to four tablets can cause serious iron poisoning in children.
• Caution patient not to substitute one iron salt for another as the amounts of elemental iron vary.
• Advise patient to report constipation and change in stool color or consistency.

---

iron dextran
DexFerrum, InFeD

iron sorbitol

Pregnancy Risk Category: C

HOW SUPPLIED
1 ml iron dextran provides 50 mg elemental iron
Injection: 50 mg elemental iron/ml

ACTION
Provides elemental iron, an essential component in the formation of hemoglobin.

Route	Onset	Peak	Duration
IM	72 hr	Unknown	3-4 wk

INDICATIONS & DOSAGE
Iron deficiency anemia—
Adults and children: I.M. or I.V. test dose required before administration.

I.M. (by Z-track method): 0.5-ml test dose injected. If no reactions occur in 1 hour, remainder of dose is given. Daily dosage should ordinarily not exceed 0.5 ml (25 mg) for infants under 5 kg (11 lb); 1 ml (50 mg) for children under 10 kg (22 lb); 2 ml (100 mg) for heavier children and adults.

I.V.: 0.5-ml test dose injected over 30 seconds. If no reactions occur in 1 hour, remainder of therapeutic I.V. dose is given. Therapeutic dose repeated I.V. daily.

Reactions may be *common*, uncommon, *life-threatening*, or COMMON AND LIFE-THREATENING.

Single dose should not exceed 100 mg. Give slowly (1 ml/minute).

ADVERSE REACTIONS
CNS: headache, transitory paresthesia, arthralgia, myalgia, dizziness, malaise.
CV: *hypotensive reaction, peripheral vascular flushing* (with overly rapid I.V. administration).
GI: nausea, anorexia.
Respiratory: *bronchospasm,* dyspnea.
Skin: rash, urticaria.
Other: *soreness, inflammation, brown skin discoloration* (at I.M. injection site); *local phlebitis* (at I.V. injection site); sterile abscess, necrosis, atrophy, fibrosis, *anaphylaxis,* delayed sensitivity reactions, fever, chills.

INTERACTIONS
None reported.

EFFECTS ON DIAGNOSTIC TESTS
Large doses (over 250 mg iron) may color the serum brown. Iron dextran may cause false elevations of serum bilirubin level and false reductions in serum calcium level. Iron dextran prevents meaningful measurement of serum iron concentration and total iron binding capacity for up to 3 weeks; I.M. injection may cause dense areas of activity for 1 to 6 days on bone scans using Tc99m diphosphonate.

CONTRAINDICATIONS
Contraindicated in patients with hypersensitivity to drug, acute infectious renal disease, and all anemias except iron-deficiency anemia.

NURSING CONSIDERATIONS
• Do not administer iron dextran concomitantly with oral iron preparations.
• Use with extreme caution in patients with serious hepatic impairment, rheumatoid arthritis, and other inflammatory diseases because these patients may be at higher risk for certain delays and reactions.
• Use cautiously in patients with history of significant allergies or asthma.
• Keep in mind that I.M. or I.V. injections of iron are advisable only for patients in whom oral administration is impossible or ineffective.

• For I.M. route, inject deeply into upper outer quadrant of buttock—never into arm or other exposed area—with a 2″ to 3″ 19G or 20G needle. Use Z-track method to avoid leakage into S.C. tissue and staining of skin. After drawing up medication, use a new sterile needle to administer injection.
• Monitor hemoglobin and hematocrit levels and reticulocyte count, as ordered.

◖ I.V. administration
• Check hospital policy before administering I.V. Do not mix with other parenteral medication or nutritional solutions containing liquid emulsions.
• Upon completion of I.V. dose, flush the vein with 10 ml of 0.9% NaCl solution. Patient should rest 15 to 30 minutes after I.V. administration.
• Know that drug can also be given as an I.V. infusion over 1 to 6 hours. This is a nonlabeled use.

☑ Patient teaching
• Teach patient symptoms of hypersensitivity or iron toxicity and tell him to report them.

polysaccharide-iron complex
Hytinic, Niferex, Niferex-150, Nu-Iron, Nu-Iron 150

Pregnancy Risk Category: NR

HOW SUPPLIED
Tablets (film-coated): 50 mg
Capsules: 150 mg
Solution: 100 mg/5 ml

ACTION
Provides elemental iron, an essential component in the formation of hemoglobin.

Route	Onset	Peak	Duration
PO	Few days	2-10 days	2 mo

INDICATIONS & DOSAGE
Treatment of uncomplicated iron deficiency anemia—
Adults: 100 to 200 mg of elemental iron t.i.d.

Children: 4 to 6 mg/kg/day of elemental iron in three divided doses.

ADVERSE REACTIONS
Although nausea, constipation, black stools, and epigastric pain are common adverse reactions associated with iron therapy, few, if any, occur with polysaccharide iron complex.

INTERACTIONS
Drug-drug. *Antacids, cholestyramine resin, cimetidine, vitamin E:* decreased iron absorption. Separate doses by 2 to 4 hours.
Chloramphenicol: delayed response to iron therapy. Monitor patient.
Fluoroquinolones, penicillamine, tetracyclines: decreased GI absorption, possibly resulting in decreased serum levels or efficacy. Separate doses if possible.
Levodopa, methyldopa: decreased absorption and efficacy of levodopa and methyldopa. Monitor for decreased effect of these agents.
Vitamin C: may increase iron absorption. Give together.
Drug-herb. *Oregano:* may reduce iron absorption. Separate administration of oregano by at least 2 hours when given with iron supplements or iron-containing foods.
Drug-food. *Cereals, cheese, coffee, eggs, milk, tea, whole-grain breads, yogurt:* may impair oral iron absorption. Do not administer together.

EFFECTS ON DIAGNOSTIC TESTS
Polysaccharide iron complex may blacken feces and may interfere with test for occult blood in stool; guaiac and orthotoluidine tests may yield false-positive results. Benzidine test is usually not affected. Iron overload may decrease uptake of Tc99m and, thus, interfere with skeletal imaging.

CONTRAINDICATIONS
Contraindicated in patients with hemochromatosis, hemosiderosis, and hypersensitivity to drug or its ingredients.

NURSING CONSIDERATIONS
• Know that oral iron may turn stools black. This unabsorbed iron is harmless; however, it may mask melena.
• Monitor hemoglobin and hematocrit values and reticulocyte count during therapy.

☑ **Patient teaching**
• Tell patient to take with juice.
• Inform parents that as few as three tablets can cause serious iron poisoning in children.
• Caution patient not to substitute one iron salt for another because the amounts of elemental iron vary.

---

ardeparin sodium
dalteparin sodium
danaparoid sodium
enoxaparin sodium
heparin calcium
heparin sodium
warfarin sodium

COMBINATION PRODUCTS
None.

---

ardeparin sodium
Normiflo Injection

Pregnancy Risk Category: C

HOW SUPPLIED
Injection: 5,000 antifactor Xa units/
0.5 ml, 10,000 antifactor Xa units/0.5 ml

ACTION
Low-molecular-weight heparin that binds
to and accelerates the activity of antithrombin III. This results in an inactivation of factor Xa and thrombin, which
prevents the formation of clots.

Route	Onset	Peak	Duration
SC	Unknown	3 hr	Unknown

INDICATIONS & DOSAGE
*Prevention of deep venous thrombosis
that may lead to pulmonary embolism following knee replacement surgery—*
Adults: 50 anti-Xa units/kg S.C. q 12
hours for 14 days or until patient is ambulatory, whichever is shorter. Give initial
dose in evening of day of surgery or following morning.

ADVERSE REACTIONS
CNS: dizziness, headache, *CVA,* insom-
nia.
CV: chest pain, peripheral edema.
GI: nausea, vomiting.
Hematologic: anemia, ecchymosis, *hem-
orrhage,* injection site hematoma, *throm-
bocytopenia.*

Skin: pruritus, rash, local reaction, urticaria.
Other: arthralgia, dyspnea, fever, pain.

INTERACTIONS
Drug-drug. *Anticoagulants, antiplatelet
agents, including aspirin, NSAIDs:* concomitant use may increase risk of bleeding. Avoid use together. Monitor patient,
PT, PTT, and INR.

EFFECTS ON DIAGNOSTIC TESTS
None reported.

CONTRAINDICATIONS
Contraindicated in patients with active
major bleeding, thrombocytopenia associated with antiplatelet antibodies in presence of drug, and known hypersensitivity
to drug or pork products.

NURSING CONSIDERATIONS
• Use with extreme caution in patients
with history of heparin-induced thrombocytopenia and known hypersensitivity to
parabens or sulfites.
• Use cautiously in patients at increased
risk for hemorrhage such as those with
bacterial endocarditis, congenital or acquired bleeding disorders, active ulcerative disease, angiodysplastic GI disease,
hemorrhagic stroke, or severe uncontrolled hypertension; in those receiving
concomitant antiplatelet agents; and
shortly after brain, spinal, or ophthalmic
surgery. Monitor vital signs.
• It is not known if drug is excreted in
breast milk. Use cautiously when administering to breast-feeding patients.
• Use cautiously in patients with severe
renal failure.
Alert: Be aware that bleeding is the principal sign of drug overdose. To stop most
bleeding, discontinue drug, apply pressure
to the site, and replace hemostatic blood
elements, if necessary. Protamine sulfate
can also be administered. Dose of protamine should be equal to dose of drug administered (1 mg of protamine neutralizes

---

100 anti-Xa units of ardeparin). If bleeding persists after 2 hours, blood should be drawn and residual anti-Xa levels determined. Administer additional protamine if clinically important bleeding persists or anti-Xa levels remain high.
• Base ardeparin dose on actual body weight.
Alert: Be aware that ardeparin cannot be used interchangeably (unit for unit) with heparin sodium or other low-molecular-weight heparins.
• Routinely monitor CBC, platelet counts, urinalysis, and occult blood in stools throughout therapy. Routine monitoring of coagulation parameters is not required.
• Do not mix with other injections or infusions.
• Administer drug with deep S.C. injection. Injection sites include the abdomen (avoiding the navel), outer aspect of upper arm, or anterior thigh with patient sitting or lying down. Extrude air and excess medication before administration. Introduce the full length of the needle into the skin fold held between the thumb and forefinger. Hold skin fold throughout the injection. Do not rub injection site.
• Rotate injection site.
• Do not give drug I.M. to avoid possible hematoma at injection site.
• Monitor patient closely for bleeding if drug is given during or immediately following spinal or epidural puncture.

☑ **Patient teaching**
• Instruct patient to report abnormal bruising, bleeding, or dark stools.
• Instruct patient to observe for hematoma at injection site.
• Tell patient to avoid use of OTC medications such as aspirin or NSAIDs.

dalteparin sodium
Fragmin

Pregnancy Risk Category: B

HOW SUPPLIED
Syringe: 2,500 antifactor Xa IU/0.2 ml, 5,000 antifactor Xa IU/0.2 ml

ACTION
Low-molecular-weight heparin derivative that enhances the inhibition of factor Xa and thrombin by antithrombin.

Route	Onset	Peak	Duration
SC	Unknown	4 hr	Unknown

INDICATIONS & DOSAGE
Prophylaxis against deep vein thrombosis (DVT) in patients undergoing abdominal surgery who are at risk for thromboembolic complications—
Adults: 2,500 IU S.C. daily, starting 1 to 2 hours before surgery and repeated once daily for 5 to 10 days postoperatively.

ADVERSE REACTIONS
Hematologic: *thrombocytopenia.*
Skin: pruritus, rash; *hematoma* (at injection site); pain, skin necrosis (rare) (at injection site).
Other: *hemorrhage,* ecchymoses, bleeding complications, fever, *anaphylactoid reactions* (rare).

INTERACTIONS
Drug-drug. *Antiplatelet agents, oral anticoagulants:* may increase risk of bleeding. Use together cautiously.

EFFECTS ON DIAGNOSTIC TESTS
Drug may falsely elevate transaminase levels (AST, ALT).

CONTRAINDICATIONS
Contraindicated in patients with active major bleeding, thrombocytopenia associated with positive in vitro tests for antiplatelet antibody in the presence of drug, and hypersensitivity to drug, heparin, or pork products.

NURSING CONSIDERATIONS
• Use with extreme caution in patients with history of heparin-induced thrombocytopenia; in those at increased risk for hemorrhage, such as those with severe uncontrolled hypertension, bacterial endocarditis, congenital or acquired bleeding disorders, active ulceration or angiodysplastic GI disease or hemorrhagic stroke; and shortly after brain, spinal, or ophthalmic surgery. Monitor vital signs.

• Use with caution in patients with bleeding diathesis, thrombocytopenia, platelet defects, severe hepatic or renal insufficiency, hypertensive or diabetic retinopathy, and recent GI bleeding.

• Know that patients who are candidates for therapy are at risk for DVT, including patients who are over 40 years, obese, undergoing surgery under general anesthesia lasting longer than 30 minutes, or have additional risk factors (such as malignancy or history of deep vein thrombosis or pulmonary embolism).

• Have patient assume a sitting or supine position when administering drug. Give S.C. injection deeply. Injection sites include a U-shaped area around the navel, upper outer side of thigh, and upper outer quadrangle of buttock. Rotate sites daily. When the area around the navel or the thigh is used, use thumb and forefinger to lift up a fold of skin while giving the injection. The entire length of the needle should be inserted at a 45- to 90-degree angle.

• Never administer drug I.M.

• Do not mix with other injections or infusions unless specific compatibility data support such mixing.

Alert: Be aware that drug is not interchangeable (unit for unit) with unfractionated heparin or other low-molecular-weight heparin.

• Know that periodic, routine CBC and fecal occult blood tests are recommended during the course of treatment. Patients do not require regular monitoring of PT or activated PTT.

• Monitor patient closely for thrombocytopenia.

• Be aware that drug should be discontinued if a thromboembolic event occurs despite dalteparin prophylaxis.

☑ **Patient teaching**
• Instruct patient and family to watch for and report signs of bleeding.
• Tell patient to avoid OTC drugs containing aspirin or other salicylates.

danaparoid sodium
Orgaran

Pregnancy Risk Category: B

HOW SUPPLIED
Ampule: 750 anti-Xa units/0.6 ml
Syringe: 750 anti-Xa units/0.6 ml

ACTION
Prevents fibrin formation by inhibiting generation of thrombin by factor Xa and factor IIa.

Route	Onset	Peak	Duration
SC	Unknown	2-5 hr	Unknown

INDICATIONS & DOSAGE
Prophylaxis against postoperative deep vein thrombosis (DVT) in patients undergoing elective hip replacement surgery—
Adults: 750 anti-Xa units S.C. b.i.d. starting 1 to 4 hours preoperatively, and then not sooner than 2 hours after surgery. Treatment continued for 7 to 10 days postoperatively or until risk of DVT has diminished.

ADVERSE REACTIONS
CNS: insomnia, headache, asthenia, dizziness.
CV: peripheral edema, *hemorrhage.*
GI: *nausea, constipation,* vomiting.
GU: urinary tract infection, urine retention.
Hematologic: anemia.
Musculoskeletal: joint disorder.
Skin: rash, pruritus.
Other: *fever, injection site pain,* infection.

INTERACTIONS
Drug-drug. *Oral anticoagulants, platelet inhibitors:* may increase risk of bleeding. Use together cautiously. Monitor PT and INR.

EFFECTS ON DIAGNOSTIC TESTS
Drug may cause unreliable PT and Thrombotest results within 5 hours after administration.

CONTRAINDICATIONS
Contraindicated in patients with severe hemorrhagic diathesis (such as hemophilia or idiopathic thrombocytopenic purpura), active major bleeding, thrombocytopenia associated with positive in vitro tests for antiplatelet antibody in presence of drug, and hypersensitivity to drug or pork products.

NURSING CONSIDERATIONS
• Use with extreme caution in patients at increased risk of hemorrhage, such as in severe uncontrolled hypertension, acute bacterial endocarditis, congenital or acquired bleeding disorders, active ulcerative and angiodysplastic GI disease, nonhemorrhagic stroke, postoperative use of indwelling epidural catheter, or shortly after brain, spinal, or ophthalmic surgery. Monitor vital signs.
• Know that drug contains sodium sulfite, which can cause allergic reactions in some people, especially asthmatics.
• Use with caution in patients with impaired renal function.
• Know that drug should be used in pregnancy only if clearly needed. Use cautiously in breast-feeding women.
• Know that the safety and effectiveness of drug in pediatric patients have not been established.
• Danaparoid should never be given I.M. To administer drug, have patient lie down. Give S.C. injection deeply, using a 25G to 26G needle. Injection sites should be alternated between the left and right anterolateral and posterolateral abdominal wall. Gently pull up a skin fold with thumb and forefinger and insert entire length of the needle into tissue. Don't rub afterward.
Alert: Be aware that drug is not interchangeable (unit for unit) with heparin or low-molecular-weight heparin.
• Know that periodic, routine CBC (including platelet count) and fecal occult blood tests are recommended during therapy. Patients don't require regular monitoring of PT and PTT.
• Know that drug has little effect on PT, PTT, fibrinolytic activity, and bleeding time.
Alert: Monitor patient's hematocrit and blood pressure closely; a decrease in either may signal hemorrhage.
• If serious bleeding occurs, drug should be stopped and blood products transfused as ordered.
• Store ampules at room temperature; syringes should be refrigerated at 36° to 46° F (2° to 8° C). Protect drug from light.

✓ **Patient teaching**
• Instruct patient and family to watch for and report signs of bleeding.
• Tell patient to avoid OTC drugs containing aspirin or other salicylates.

---

enoxaparin sodium
Lovenox

Pregnancy Risk Category: B

HOW SUPPLIED
Injection: 30 mg/0.3 ml, 40 mg/0.4 ml, 60 mg/0.6 ml, 80 mg/0.8 ml, 100 mg/1 ml

ACTION
Low-molecular-weight heparin derivative that accelerates formation of antithrombin III-thrombin complex and deactivates thrombin, preventing conversion of fibrinogen to fibrin. Enoxaparin has a higher antifactor Xa- to antifactor IIa-activity ratio.

Route	Onset	Peak	Duration
SC	Unknown	3-5 hr	24 hr

INDICATIONS & DOSAGE
To prevent pulmonary embolism and deep vein thrombosis (DVT) after hip or knee replacement surgery—
Adults: 30 mg S.C. q 12 hours for 7 to 10 days. Initial dose given between 12 and 24 hours postoperatively provided hemostasis has been established. Treatment should continue throughout the postoperative period until risk of DVT has diminished. Hip replacement patients may receive a dose of 40 mg S.C. given 12 hours preoperatively. After the initial phase of therapy, hip replacement patients should continue with 40 mg S.C. daily for 3 weeks.

To prevent pulmonary embolism and DVT after abdominal surgery—
Adults: 40 mg S.C. daily with initial dose 2 hours before surgery. Subsequent dose, provided hemostasis has been established, is given 24 hours after the initial preoperative dose and continued once daily for 7 to 10 days. Treatment should continue during postoperative period until risk of DVT has diminished.

✳*NEW INDICATION: Prevention of ischemic complications of unstable angina and non-Q-wave MI in conjunction with oral aspirin therapy—*
Adults: 1 mg/kg S.C. q 12 hours until clinical stabilization (minimum, 2 days) in conjunction with aspirin 100 to 325 mg P.O. once daily.

ADVERSE REACTIONS
CNS: confusion, *neurologic injury* when used with spinal or epidural puncture.
CV: edema, peripheral edema, *CV toxicity* (chest pain, dizziness, irregular heartbeat).
GI: nausea.
Hematologic: hypochromic anemia, *thrombocytopenia.*
Other: irritation, pain, hematoma, erythema (at injection site); fever; pain; *hemorrhage;* ecchymoses; bleeding complications, *angioedema,* rash, hives.

INTERACTIONS
Drug-drug. *Anticoagulants, antiplatelet agents, NSAIDs:* increased risk of bleeding. May also lead to spinal or epidural hematomas in patients with spinal punctures or epidural or spinal anesthesia. Don't use together.
Plicamycin, valproic acid: may cause hypoprothrombinemia and inhibit platelet aggregation. Monitor closely.

EFFECTS ON DIAGNOSTIC TESTS
Drug may decrease platelet count and may increase transaminase levels (AST and ALT).

CONTRAINDICATIONS
Contraindicated in patients with active major bleeding, thrombocytopenia, or hypersensitivity to drug, heparin, or pork products and in those who demonstrate antiplatelet antibodies in presence of drug.

NURSING CONSIDERATIONS
• Use with extreme caution in patients with history of heparin-induced thrombocytopenia, aneurysms, cerebrovascular hemorrhage, uncontrolled hypertension, or threatened abortion.
• Be aware that the vascular access sheath for instrumentation should remain in place for 6 to 8 hours following a dose and the next dose given no sooner than 6 to 8 hours after sheath removal. Monitor vital signs.
• Use cautiously in the elderly and in patients with conditions that place them at increased risk for hemorrhage, such as bacterial endocarditis; congenital or acquired bleeding disorders; ulcer disease; angiodysplastic GI disease; hemorrhagic stroke; or recent spinal, eye, or brain surgery. Also use cautiously in patients with regional or lumbar block anesthesia, blood dyscrasias, recent childbirth, pericarditis or pericardial effusion, renal insufficiency, or severe CNS trauma.
Alert: Patients receiving low-molecular-weight heparins or heparinoids who have epidural or spinal anesthesia, or spinal puncture, are at risk for developing epidural or spinal hematoma that can result in long-term paralysis. Risk is increased with the use of epidural catheters, use of drugs affecting hemostasis, or traumatic or repeated epidural or spinal punctures. Monitor these patients frequently for signs of neurologic impairment. Urgent treatment is necessary.
• Draw blood to establish baseline coagulation parameters before therapy.
• Never administer drug I.M.
• Don't massage after S.C. injection. Watch for signs of bleeding at site. Rotate sites and keep record.
• Avoid excessive I.M. injections of other drugs to prevent or minimize hematomas. If possible, don't give I.M. injections at all.
• Monitor platelet counts regularly. Patients with normal coagulation won't require close monitoring of PT or PTT.
• Regularly inspect patient for bleeding gums, bruises on arms or legs, petechiae,

nosebleeds, melena, tarry stools, hematuria, hematemesis.
• To treat severe overdose, give protamine sulfate (a heparin antagonist) by slow I.V. infusion at a concentration of 1% to equal the dosage of drug injected, as ordered.

☑ **Patient teaching**
• Instruct patient and family to watch for signs of bleeding and to notify doctor immediately.
• Tell patient to avoid OTC drugs containing aspirin or other salicylates.

---

heparin calcium
Calcilean†, Caprin‡, Uniparin-Ca‡

heparin sodium
Hepalean†, Heparin Leo†, Heparin Lock Flush Solution (with Tubex), Heparin Sodium Injection, Hep-Lock, Monoparin§, Multiparin§, Pump-Hep§, Unihep§, Uniparin‡

Pregnancy Risk Category: C

HOW SUPPLIED
Products are derived from beef lung or pork intestinal mucosa.
heparin calcium
Ampule: 12,500 units/0.5 ml; 20,000 units/0.8 ml
Syringe: 5,000 units/0.2 ml
heparin sodium
Carpuject: 5,000 units/ml
Disposable syringes: 1,000 units/ml, 2,500 units/ml, 5,000 units/ml, 7,500 units/ml, 10,000 units/ml, 15,000 units/ml, 20,000 units/ml, 40,000 units/ml
Premixed I.V. solutions: 1,000 units in 500 ml of 0.9% NaCl solution; 2,000 units in 1,000 ml of 0.9% NaCl solution; 12,500 units in 250 ml of 0.45% NaCl solution; 25,000 units in 250 ml of 0.45% NaCl solution; 25,000 units in 500 ml of 0.45% NaCl solution; 10,000 units in 100 ml of D_5W; 12,500 units in 250 ml of D_5W; 25,000 units in 250 ml D_5W; 25,000 units in 500 ml D_5W; 20,000 units in 500 ml of D_5W

Unit-dose vials: 1,000 units/ml, 5,000 units/ml, 10,000 units/ml, 20,000 units/ml, 40,000 units/ml
Vials: 1,000 units/ml, 2,000 units/ml, 2,500 units/ml, 5,000 units/ml, 7,500 units/ml, 10,000 units/ml, 20,000 units/ml, 40,000 units/ml
heparin sodium flush
Disposable syringes: 10 units/ml, 100 units/ml
Vials: 10 units/ml, 100 units/ml

ACTION
Accelerates formation of antithrombin III-thrombin complex and deactivates thrombin, preventing conversion of fibrinogen to fibrin.

Route	Onset	Peak	Duration
IV	Immediate	Unknown	Variable
SC	20-60 min	2-4 hr	Variable

INDICATIONS & DOSAGE
Dosage is highly individualized, depending upon disease state, age, and renal and hepatic status.
Full-dose continuous I.V. infusion therapy for deep vein thrombosis (DVT), MI, pulmonary embolism—
Adults: initially, 5,000 units by I.V. bolus, followed by 750 to 1,500 units/hour by I.V. infusion with pump. Hourly rate adjusted 8 hours after bolus dose and based on PTT results.
Children: initially, 50 units/kg I.V. followed by 25 units/kg/hour or 20,000 units/m^2 daily by I.V. infusion pump. Dosage adjusted based on PTT.
Full-dose S.C. therapy for DVT, MI, pulmonary embolism—
Adults: initially, 5,000 units I.V. bolus and 10,000 to 20,000 units in a concentrated solution S.C., followed by 8,000 to 10,000 units S.C. q 8 hours or 15,000 to 20,000 units in a concentrated solution q 12 hours.
Full-dose intermittent I.V. therapy for DVT, MI, pulmonary embolism—
Adults: initially, 10,000 units by I.V. bolus and then adjusted according to PTT, and 5,000 to 10,000 units I.V. q 4 to 6 hours.
Children: initially, 100 units/kg by I.V. bolus followed by 50 to 100 units/kg q 4 hours.

Reactions may be *common*, uncommon, *life-threatening*, or COMMON AND LIFE-THREATENING.

Fixed low-dose therapy for venous thrombosis, pulmonary embolism, atrial fibrillation with embolism, postoperative DVT, and prevention of embolism—
Adults: 5,000 units S.C. q 12 hours. In surgical patients, first dose given 2 hours before procedure, followed by 5,000 units S.C. q 8 to 12 hours for 5 to 7 days or until patient can walk.
Consumptive coagulopathy (such as disseminated intravascular coagulation)—
Adults: 50 to 100 units/kg by I.V. bolus or continuous I.V. infusion q 4 hours.
Children: 25 to 50 units/kg by I.V. bolus or continuous I.V. infusion q 4 hours. If no improvement within 4 to 8 hours, discontinue heparin.
Open-heart surgery—
Adults: (total body perfusion) 150 to 300 units/kg by continuous I.V infusion.
Patency maintenance of I.V. indwelling catheters—
Adults: 10 to 100 units I.V. flush. Use sufficient volume to fill the device. Not intended for therapeutic use.

ADVERSE REACTIONS
Hematologic: *hemorrhage* (with excessive dosage), *overly prolonged clotting time,* **thrombocytopenia.**
Other: irritation; mild pain; hematoma; ulceration; cutaneous or subcutaneous necrosis; *"white clot" syndrome; hypersensitivity reactions,* including chills, fever, pruritus, rhinitis, urticaria, *anaphylactoid reactions.*

INTERACTIONS
Drug-drug. *Oral anticoagulants:* increased additive anticoagulation. Monitor PT, INR, and PTT.
Salicylates, other antiplatelet agents: increased anticoagulant effect. Don't use together.
Thrombolytics: increased risk of hemorrhage. Monitor closely.
Drug-herb. *Motherwort, red clover:* risk of increased bleeding. Avoid concomitant use.

EFFECTS ON DIAGNOSTIC TESTS
Heparin therapy prolongs PT, may falsely elevate AST and serum ALT levels, and may cause false elevations in some tests for serum thyroxine levels.

CONTRAINDICATIONS
Contraindicated in patients hypersensitive to drug. Conditionally contraindicated in patients with active bleeding, blood dyscrasia, or bleeding tendencies, such as hemophilia, thrombocytopenia, or hepatic disease with hypoprothrombinemia; suspected intracranial hemorrhage; suppurative thrombophlebitis; inaccessible ulcerative lesions (especially of GI tract) and open ulcerative wounds; extensive denudation of skin; ascorbic acid deficiency and other conditions that cause increased capillary permeability; during or after brain, eye, or spinal cord surgery; during spinal tap or spinal anesthesia; during continuous tube drainage of stomach or small intestine; in subacute bacterial endocarditis; shock; advanced renal disease; threatened abortion; severe hypertension.
   Although heparin use is clearly hazardous in these conditions, its risks and its benefits must be evaluated.

NURSING CONSIDERATIONS
● Use cautiously during menses; in patients with mild hepatic or renal disease, alcoholism, occupations with high risk of physical injury; immediately postpartum; and in patients with history of allergies, asthma, or GI ulcerations.
● Draw blood to establish baseline coagulation parameters before therapy.
● Know that when patient requires anticoagulation during pregnancy, most clinicians use heparin.
● Keep in mind that drug requirements are higher in early phases of thrombogenic diseases and febrile states; lower when the patient's condition stabilizes.
● Be aware that elderly patients should usually start at lower doses.
● Check order and vial carefully. Heparin comes in various concentrations.
● Give low-dose injections sequentially between iliac crests in lower abdomen deep into S.C. fat. Inject drug S.C. slowly into fat pad. Leave needle in place for 10 seconds after injection; then withdraw needle. Don't massage after S.C. injection, and watch for signs of bleeding at in-

---

*Liquid contains alcohol.   **May contain tartrazine.   †Canada   ‡Australia   §U.K.   ◊OTC

jection site. Alternate sites every 12 hours—right for morning, left for evening.
• For S.C. injections, PTT should be drawn 4 to 6 hours after dose administered.
• Avoid excessive I.M. injections of other drugs to prevent or minimize hematomas. If possible, don't give I.M. injections at all.
• Measure PTT carefully and regularly. Anticoagulation is present when PTT values are one and one-half to two times the control values.
• Monitor platelet count regularly. Thrombocytopenia caused by heparin may be associated with a type of arterial thrombosis known as "white clot" syndrome.
• Regularly inspect patient for bleeding gums, bruises on arms or legs, petechiae, nosebleeds, melena, tarry stools, hematuria, hematemesis.
• Monitor vital signs.
Alert: To treat severe heparin calcium or sodium overdose, use protamine sulfate, a heparin antagonist, as ordered. Dosage is based on the dose of heparin, its route of administration, and the time elapsed since it was given. Generally, 1 to 1.5 mg of protamine/100 units of heparin is given if only a few minutes have elapsed; 0.5 to 0.75 mg protamine/100 units heparin if 30 to 60 minutes have elapsed, 0.25 to 0.375 mg protamine/100 units heparin if 2 hours or more have elapsed. Do not give more than 50 mg protamine in a 10-minute period.
• Know that abrupt withdrawal may cause increased coagulability, and heparin therapy is usually followed by oral anticoagulants for prophylaxis.

I.V. administration
• Administer I.V. using infusion pump to provide maximum safety because of long-term effect and irregular absorption when given S.C. Check constant I.V. infusions regularly, even when pumps are in good working order, to prevent overdosage or underdosage. Place notice above patient's bed to inform I.V. team or laboratory personnel to apply pressure dressings after taking blood.
• During intermittent I.V. therapy, always draw blood 30 minutes before next scheduled dose to avoid falsely elevated PTT. Blood for PTT may be drawn any time after 8 hours of initiation of continuous I.V. heparin therapy. Blood for PTT should never be drawn from the I.V. tubing of the heparin infusion or from the infused vein. Falsely elevated PTT will result. Always draw blood from the opposite arm.
• Don't skip a dose or "catch up" with an I.V. containing heparin. If I.V. runs out, restart it as soon as possible, and reschedule bolus dose immediately.
• Know that concentrated heparin solutions (greater than 100 units/ml) can irritate blood vessels.
• Never piggyback other drugs into an infusion line while the heparin infusion is running. Never mix another drug and heparin in the same syringe when giving a bolus.

☑ Patient teaching
• Instruct patient and family to watch for signs of bleeding and notify doctor immediately.
• Tell patient to avoid OTC medications containing aspirin, other salicylates, or drugs that may interact with heparin.

warfarin sodium
Coumadin, Warfilone†

Pregnancy Risk Category: X

HOW SUPPLIED
Tablets: 1 mg, 2 mg, 2.5 mg, 3 mg, 4 mg, 5 mg, 6 mg, 7.5 mg, 10 mg
Injection: 2 mg/ml (powder)

ACTION
Inhibits vitamin K-dependent activation of clotting factors II, VII, IX, and X, formed in the liver.

Route	Onset	Peak	Duration
PO	0.5-3 days	Unknown	2-5 days
IV	Unknown	Unknown	Unknown

INDICATIONS & DOSAGE
Pulmonary embolism associated with deep vein thrombosis, MI, rheumatic heart disease with heart valve damage,

prosthetic heart valves, chronic atrial fibrillation—
Adults: 2 to 5 mg P.O. daily for 2 to 4 days, then dosage based on daily PT and INR. Usual maintenance dosage is 2 to 10 mg P.O. daily; I.V. dosage would be same as that used P.O.

ADVERSE REACTIONS

GI: anorexia, nausea, vomiting, cramps, *diarrhea,* mouth ulcerations, sore mouth, melena.
GU: hematuria, excessive menstrual bleeding.
Hematologic: *hemorrhage* (with excessive dosage).
Hepatic: hepatitis, elevated liver function tests, jaundice.
Skin: dermatitis, urticaria, necrosis, gangrene, alopecia, *rash.*
Other: *fever,* headache.

INTERACTIONS

Drug-drug. *Acetaminophen:* may increase bleeding with long-term (longer than 2 weeks) therapy with high doses (more than 2 g/day) of acetaminophen. Monitor very carefully.
Allopurinol, amiodarone, anabolic steroids, cephalosporins, chloramphenicol, cimetidine, ciprofloxacin, clofibrate, danazol, diazoxide, diflunisal, disulfiram, erythromycin, ethacrynic acid, fenoprofen calcium, fluconazole, fluoroquinolones, glucagon, heparin, ibuprofen, influenza virus vaccine, isoniazid, itraconazole, ketoprofen, lovastatin, meclofenamate, methimazole, methylthiouracil, metronidazole, miconazole, nalidixic acid, neomycin (oral), norfloxacin, ofloxacin, omeprazole, pentoxifylline, propafenone, propoxyphene, propylthiouracil, quinidine, simvastatin, streptokinase, sulfinpyrazone, sulfonamides, sulindac, tamoxifen, tetracyclines, thiazides, thyroid drugs, tricyclic antidepressants, urokinase, vitamin E: increased PT. Monitor patient carefully for bleeding. Consider anticoagulant dosage reduction.
Anticonvulsants: increased serum levels of phenytoin and phenobarbital. Monitor closely.
Barbiturates, carbamazepine, corticosteroids, corticotropin, dicloxacillin, *ethchlorvynol, griseofulvin, haloperidol, meprobamate, mercaptopurine, methaqualone, nafcillin, oral contraceptives containing estrogen, rifampin, spironolactone, sucralfate, trazodone:* decreased PT with reduced anticoagulant effect. Monitor patient carefully.
Chloral hydrate, glutethimide, propylthiouracil, sulfinpyrazone: increased or decreased PT. Avoid use if possible, and monitor patient carefully.
Cholestyramine: decreased response when administered too closely together. Administer 6 hours after oral anticoagulants.
NSAIDs, salicylates: increased PT; ulcerogenic effects. Don't use together.
Sulfonylureas (oral antidiabetic agents): increased hypoglycemic response. Monitor blood glucose levels.
Drug-food. *Foods or enteral products containing vitamin K:* may impair anticoagulation. Patient should maintain consistent daily intake of leafy green vegetables.
Drug-herb. *Angelica:* significantly prolonged prothrombin time when *Angelica sinensis* is administered with warfarin. Avoid concomitant use.
Motherwort, red clover: risk for increased bleeding. Avoid concomitant use.
Drug-lifestyle. *Alcohol use*: enhanced anticoagulant effects may occur. Tell patient to avoid large amounts of alcohol.

EFFECTS ON DIAGNOSTIC TESTS

Warfarin prolongs PT, INR, and PTT; it may enhance uric acid excretion, elevate serum transaminase levels, increase lactate dehydrogenase activity, and cause false-negative serum theophylline levels.

CONTRAINDICATIONS

Contraindicated in patients with known hypersensitivity to drug; during pregnancy, threatened abortion, eclampsia, or preeclampsia; in those with blood dyscrasias or hemorrhagic tendencies; recent surgery involving large open areas, eye, brain, or spinal cord; recent prostatectomy; major regional lumbar block anesthesia, spinal puncture, diagnostic or therapeutic invasive procedures; bleeding from the GI, GU, or respiratory tracts; aneurysm; cerebrovascular hemorrhage; severe or malignant hypertension; severe renal or hepatic disease; subacute bacterial endocarditis, pericarditis, or pericardial effusion; history of warfarin-induced necrosis; unsupervised patients with senility, alcoholism, or psychosis; or situations where there are inadequate laboratory facilities for coagulation testing.

NURSING CONSIDERATIONS

• Use cautiously in patients with diverticulitis, colitis, mild or moderate hypertension, and mild or moderate hepatic or renal disease; with drainage tubes in any orifice; with regional or lumbar block anesthesia; or in any condition that increases risk of hemorrhage and in breast-feeding patients.
• Draw blood to establish baseline coagulation parameters before therapy.
• Know that PT and INR determinations are essential for proper control. Doctors typically try to maintain PT at one and one-half to two times normal; high incidence of bleeding when PT exceeds two and one-half times the control values.
• Give warfarin at the same time daily. INR range for chronic atrial fibrillation is 2 to 3.
• Be aware that I.M. administration is not recommended.
• Regularly inspect the patient for bleeding gums, bruises on arms or legs, petechiae, nosebleeds, melena, tarry stools, hematuria, and hematemesis.
• Observe breast-fed infants of patients on drug for unexpected bleeding.
Alert: Withhold drug and call doctor at once if fever or rash (signal severe adverse reactions) occurs.
• Be aware that half-life of warfarin's anticoagulant effect is 36 to 44 hours. Effect can be neutralized by vitamin K injections.
• Know that drug is the best oral anticoagulant for patient taking antacids or phenytoin.
• Know that elderly patients and patients with renal or hepatic failure are especially sensitive to warfarin effect.

I.V. administration

• I.V. form may be ordered in the rare instances that oral therapy cannot be given.

Reconstitute powder with 2.7 ml sterile water, or as instructed in manufacturer guidelines. Give I.V. as a slow bolus injection over 1 to 2 minutes into a peripheral vein.
• Because onset of action is delayed, keep in mind that heparin sodium is often given during first few days of treatment. When heparin is being given simultaneously, blood for PT and INR should not be drawn within 5 hours of intermittent I.V. heparin administration. However, blood for PT and INR may be drawn at any time during continuous heparin infusion.

✓ Patient teaching

• Stress importance of complying with prescribed dosage and follow-up appointments. Tell patient to carry a card that identifies him as a potential bleeder.
• Tell patient and family to watch for signs of bleeding and to call doctor at once if they occur.
• Warn patient to avoid OTC products containing aspirin, other salicylates, or drugs that may interact with warfarin.
• Instruct female patient to notify doctor if menses is heavier than usual; may require dosage adjustment.
• Tell patient to use electric razor when shaving to avoid scratching skin and to use a soft toothbrush.
• Warn patient to read food labels. Food and enteral feedings that contain vitamin K may impair anticoagulation.
• Tell patient to eat a daily, consistent amount of leafy green vegetables, which contain vitamin K. Eating different amounts daily may alter anticoagulant effects.

Reactions may be *common*, uncommon, *life-threatening*, or COMMON AND LIFE-THREATENING.

67

Blood derivatives

albumin 5%
albumin 25%
antihemophilic factor
anti-inhibitor coagulant complex
antithrombin III, human
factor IX (human)
factor IX complex
plasma protein fractions

COMBINATION PRODUCTS
None.

albumin 5%
Albuminar-5, Albutein 5%,
Buminate 5%, Plasbumin-5

albumin 25%
Albuminar-25, Albutein 25%,
Buminate 25%, Plasbumin-25

Pregnancy Risk Category: C

HOW SUPPLIED
albumin 5%
Injection: 50-ml, 250-ml, 500-ml,
1,000-ml vials
albumin 25%
Injection: 20-ml, 50-ml, 100-ml vials

ACTION
Albumin 5% supplies colloid to the blood
and expands plasma volume. Albumin
25% provides intravascular oncotic pressure in a 5:1 ratio, causing a fluid shift
from interstitial spaces to the circulation
and slightly increasing plasma protein
concentration.

Route	Onset	Peak	Duration
IV	< 15 min	< 15 min	Several hr

INDICATIONS & DOSAGE
Hypovolemic shock—
Adults: initially, 500 to 750 ml 5% solu-
tion by I.V. infusion, repeated q 30 min-
utes, p.r.n. Alternatively, 100 to 200 ml
I.V. of 25% solution, repeated after 10 to

30 minutes, if needed. Dosage varies with
patient's condition and response.
Children: 12 to 20 ml 5% solution/kg by
I.V. infusion, repeated in 15 to 30 minutes
if response is not adequate. Alternatively,
2.5 to 5 ml I.V. of 25% solution/kg, repeated after 10 to 30 minutes if needed.
Hypoproteinemia—
Adults: 200 to 300 ml of 25% albumin.
Dosage varies with patient's condition and
response.
Hyperbilirubinemia—
Infants: 1 g albumin (4 ml 25%)/kg during or 1 to 2 hours before exchange transfusion.

ADVERSE REACTIONS
CNS: headache.
CV: *vascular overload after rapid infu-
sion,* hypotension, tachycardia.
GI: increased salivation, nausea, vomiting.
Respiratory: altered respiration, dys-
pnea, *pulmonary edema.*
Skin: urticaria, rash.
Other: chills, fever, back pain.

INTERACTIONS
None significant.

EFFECTS ON DIAGNOSTIC TESTS
Preparations of albumin derived from placental tissue may increase serum alkaline
phosphatase level; all products may
slightly increase plasma albumin levels.

CONTRAINDICATIONS
Contraindicated in patients with severe
anemia, cardiac failure, or hypersensitivity to drug.

NURSING CONSIDERATIONS
• Use with extreme caution in patients
with hypertension, low cardiac reserve,
hypervolemia, pulmonary edema, or hypoalbuminemia with peripheral edema.
• Watch for hemorrhage or shock after
surgery or injury. Rapid rise in blood
pressure may cause bleeding from sites
that are not apparent at lower pressures.

---

*Liquid contains alcohol.   **May contain tartrazine.   †Canada   ‡Australia   §U.K.   ◇OTC

• Monitor vital signs carefully.
• Watch for signs of vascular overload (heart failure or pulmonary edema).
• Monitor fluid intake and output and hemoglobin, hematocrit, serum protein, and electrolyte levels during therapy.
• Follow storage instructions on bottle. Freezing may cause bottle to break.

🖐 I.V. administration
• Make sure patient is properly hydrated before infusion.
• Take care when preparing and administering drug to minimize waste. This product is expensive, and random supply shortages occur often.
• Avoid rapid I.V. infusion. Specific rate is individualized according to patient's age, condition, and diagnosis. Know that 5% albumin is infused undiluted; 25% albumin may be infused undiluted or diluted with sterile water for injection, 0.9% NaCl solution, or D_5W injection. Use solution promptly. Discard unused solution. Don't use cloudy solutions or those containing sediment. Solution should be clear amber color.
Alert: Do not give more than 250 g in 48 hours.

☑ Patient teaching
• Explain use and administration of albumin to patient and family.
• Tell patient to report adverse reactions promptly.

---

antihemophilic factor (AHF)
Alphanate, Helixate, Hemofil M, Humate-P, Koate-HP, Kogenate, Monoclate-P, Recombinate

Pregnancy Risk Category: C

HOW SUPPLIED
Injection: vials, with diluent. Units specified on label

ACTION
Directly replaces deficient clotting factor.

Route	Onset	Peak	Duration
IV	Immediate	1-2 hr	Unknown

INDICATIONS & DOSAGE
Spontaneous hemorrhage in patients with hemophilia A (factor VIII deficiency)—
Adults and children: calculate dosage using this formula:

$$\text{AHF required (IU)} = \text{body weight (kg)} \times \text{desired factor VIII increase (\% of normal)} \times 0.5$$

To prevent spontaneous hemorrhage, the desired level of factor VIII is 5% of normal; for mild hemorrhage, 30% of normal; for moderate hemorrhage and minor surgery, 30% to 50% of normal; for severe hemorrhage, 80% to 100% of normal.

Treatment of bleeding in patients with hemophilia A (factor VIII deficiency)—
Adults and children: for minor hemorrhage into muscle and joints, 8 to 10 IU/kg I.V. (or calculated dose to raise plasma factor VIII levels to 20% to 40% of normal) q 8 to 12 hours for 1 to 3 days as needed. For overt bleeding, an initial dose of 15 to 25 IU/kg I.V., followed by 8 to 15 IU/kg q 8 to 12 hours for 3 to 4 days. To treat massive bleeding or hemorrhage involving major organs, an initial dose of 40 to 50 IU/kg I.V., followed by 20 to 25 IU/kg I.V. q 8 to 12 hours.

Prevention of bleeding in hemophilic patients requiring surgery—
Adults: 25 to 30 IU/kg I.V. 1 hour before surgery, followed by 50% of initial dosage 5 hours later. Dosage adjusted to achieve a level of AHF 80% to 100% of normal during surgery and maintained at 30% to 60% of normal for at least 10 to 14 days postoperatively.

ADVERSE REACTIONS
CV: tightness in chest.
GI: nausea.
Respiratory: wheezing.
Skin: *urticaria.*
Other: chills, *fever, **thrombosis, hemolytic anemia, thrombocytopenia,** hypersensitivity reactions, (stinging at injection site, fever, **anaphylaxis**), risk of hepatitis B and HIV.*

INTERACTIONS
None significant.

Reactions may be *common,* uncommon, *life-threatening,* or COMMON AND LIFE-THREATENING.

EFFECTS ON DIAGNOSTIC TESTS
None reported.

CONTRAINDICATIONS
Monoclonal prepared AHF is contraindicated in patients with hypersensitivity to drug or murine (mouse) protein.

NURSING CONSIDERATIONS
• Use cautiously in neonates, infants, and patients with hepatic disease because of their susceptibility to hepatitis, which may be transmitted in antihemophilic factor.
• Monitor coagulation studies before therapy.
• Monitor patients with blood types A, B, and AB for possible hemolysis.
• Know that change in urine color to an orange or red hue can signify a hemolytic reaction.
• As ordered, administer hepatitis B vaccine before administering antihemophilic factor.
• Do not use S.C. or I.M.
• Monitor vital signs regularly.
• Monitor coagulation studies frequently during therapy.
• Monitor patient for allergic reactions.
• Be aware that some patients develop inhibitors to factor VIII, resulting in decreased response to drug.
• Keep in mind that risk of hepatitis must be weighed against risk of patient not receiving drug.
• Because of manufacturing process, be aware that the risk of HIV transmission is extremely low.

🖰 **I.V. administration**
• Refrigerate concentrate until ready to use. Warm concentrate and diluent bottles to room temperature before reconstituting. To mix drug, gently roll vial between hands.
• Use reconstituted solution within 3 hours. Store away from heat and do not refrigerate. Refrigeration after reconstitution may cause the active ingredient to precipitate. Don't shake or mix with other I.V. solutions. Solution should be filtered before administration.
• Take baseline pulse rate before I.V. administration. Use plastic syringe; drug

may interact with glass syringe and bind to its surface. If pulse rate increases significantly, flow rate should be reduced or administration stopped.

☑ **Patient teaching**
• Explain use and administration of AHF to patient and family.
• Advise patient to report adverse reactions promptly.
• Advise patient to wear medical identification tag.
• Tell patient to notify doctor if medication seems less effective; a change may signify the development of antibodies.

anti-inhibitor coagulant complex
Autoplex T, Feiba VH Immuno

Pregnancy Risk Category: C

HOW SUPPLIED
Injection: number of units of factor VIII correctional activity indicated on label of vial

ACTION
Unknown. It has been suggested that efficacy may be related in part to the presence of the activated factors, which leads to more complete factor X activation in conjunction with tissue factor, phospholipid, and ionic calcium and allows the coagulation process to proceed beyond those stages where factor VIII is needed.

Route	Onset	Peak	Duration
IV	10-30 min	Unknown	Unknown

INDICATIONS & DOSAGE
Prevention and control of hemorrhagic episodes in patients with hemophilia A who have developed inhibitor antibodies to antihemophilic factor; management of bleeding in patients with acquired hemophilia who have spontaneously acquired inhibitors to factor VIII—
Adults and children: highly individualized and varies among manufacturers. For Autoplex T, 25 to 100 units/kg I.V., depending on the severity of hemorrhage. If

no hemostatic improvement occurs within 6 hours after initial administration, dosage repeated. For Feiba VH Immuno, 50 to 100 units/kg I.V. q 6 or 12 hours until clear signs of improvement. Maximum daily dosage is 200 units/kg.

ADVERSE REACTIONS
CNS: headache.
CV: changes in blood pressure, *acute MI*, *thromboembolic events.*
GI: nausea, vomiting.
Hematologic: *disseminated intravascular coagulation (DIC).*
Skin: flushing, rash, urticaria.
Other: fever, chills, hypersensitivity reactions, *anaphylaxis*, lethargy, *risk of hepatitis B and HIV.*

INTERACTIONS
Drug-drug. *Antifibrinolytic agents:* may alter effects of anti-inhibitor coagulant complex. Do not use together.

EFFECTS ON DIAGNOSTIC TESTS
None reported.

CONTRAINDICATIONS
Contraindicated in patients with DIC or a normal coagulation mechanism and in those showing signs of fibrinolysis.

NURSING CONSIDERATIONS
• Use with caution in patients with liver disease.
• As ordered, administer hepatitis B vaccine before administering drug.
• Keep epinephrine available to treat anaphylaxis.
• Know that Feiba VH Immuno should not be used with newborns, but Autoplex T can be used with caution.
• Monitor patient closely for hypersensitivity reactions.
• Monitor vital signs regularly, and report significant changes to the doctor.
• Reassure patient that because of the manufacturing process, the risk of HIV transmission is extremely low.

I.V. administration
• Warm drug and diluent to room temperature before reconstitution. Reconstitute according to manufacturer's directions.

Use the filter needle provided by manufacturer to withdraw reconstituted solution from vial into syringe; filter needle should then be replaced with a sterile injection needle for administration. Administer as soon as possible. If drug is given as an I.V. infusion, the administration set must contain a filter. Autoplex T infusions should be completed within 1 hour after reconstitution; Feiba VH Immuno infusions, within 3 hours.
• Individualize rate of administration based on patient's response. Autoplex T infusions may begin at a rate of 2 ml/minute; if well tolerated, the infusion rate may be increased gradually to 10 ml/minute. Feiba VH Immuno infusion rate should not exceed 2 units/kg/minute.
Alert: If flushing, lethargy, headache, transient chest discomfort, or changes in blood pressure or pulse rate develop because of a rapid rate of infusion, stop drug and notify doctor. Know that these symptoms usually disappear with cessation of the infusion. The infusion may then be resumed at a slower rate, as ordered.

☑ Patient teaching
• Explain use and administration of anti-inhibitor coagulant complex to patient and family.
• Tell patient to report adverse reactions promptly.

---

antithrombin III, human (AT-III, heparin cofactor I)
ATnativ, Thrombate III

Pregnancy Risk Category: C

HOW SUPPLIED
Injection: 500 IU

ACTION
Replaces deficient AT-III in patients with hereditary AT-III deficiency, normalizing coagulation inhibition and inhibiting thromboembolism formation. Also deactivates plasmin (to lesser extent than the clotting factor).

Route	Onset	Peak	Duration
IV	Immediate	Unknown	4 days

Reactions may be *common*, uncommon, *life-threatening*, or COMMON AND LIFE-THREATENING.

INDICATIONS & DOSAGE

Thromboembolism associated with hereditary AT-III deficiency—

Adults and children: initial dose is individualized to quantity required to increase AT-III activity to 120% of normal activity as determined 30 minutes after administration. Usual dose is 50 to 100 IU/minute I.V., not to exceed 100 IU/minute. Dose is calculated based on anticipated 1% increase in plasma AT-III activity produced by 1 IU/kg of body weight using the formula:

$$\text{Dose required (IU)} = \frac{(\text{desired activity [\%]} - \text{baseline activity [\%]}) \times \text{weight (kg)}}{1.4}$$

Maintenance dosage is individualized to quantity required to increase AT-III activity to 80% of normal activity and is administered at 24-hour intervals.

To calculate subsequent dosages, multiply desired AT-III activity (as percentage of normal) minus baseline AT-III activity (as percentage of normal) by body weight (in kg). Divide by actual increase in AT-III activity (as percentage) produced by 1 IU/kg as determined 30 minutes after initial dose is given.

Treatment is usually continued for 2 to 8 days but may be prolonged in pregnancy or when used with surgery or immobilization.

ADVERSE REACTIONS

CNS: dizziness.
CV: vasodilation, lowered blood pressure.
GI: nausea, foul taste.
GU: diuresis.
Other: chills.

INTERACTIONS

Drug-drug. *Heparin:* increased anticoagulant effect of both drugs. Heparin dosage reduction may be necessary.

EFFECTS ON DIAGNOSTIC TESTS

Plasma levels of AT-III may be measured with clotting assays or amidolytic assays using synthetic chromogenic substrates. Immunoassays may not detect all congenital AT-III deficiencies.

CONTRAINDICATIONS

No known contraindications.

NURSING CONSIDERATIONS

● Use with extreme caution in children and neonates because safety and efficacy have not been established.
● Use drug cautiously. Prepared from pooled plasma from human donors, it carries minimal risk of transmission of viruses, including hepatitis and HIV.
Alert: Because of risk of neonatal thromboembolism (sometimes fatal) in children of parents with hereditary AT-III deficiency, anticipate obtaining AT-III levels immediately after birth.
● Bring solution to room temperature prior to administration. Use solution within 3 hours of preparation.
● Obtain AT-III activity levels twice daily until dosage requirement has stabilized, then daily immediately before dose. Functional assays are preferred because quantitative immunologic test results may be normal despite decreased AT-III activity.
● Monitor for dyspnea and increased blood pressure, which may occur if administration rate is too rapid.
● Keep in mind that 1 IU is equivalent to the quantity of endogenous AT-III present in 1 ml of normal human plasma.
● Know that heparin binds to AT-III lysine binding sites, increasing heparin efficacy.
● Know that drug is not recommended for long-term prophylaxis of thrombotic episodes.
● Store drug at 36° to 46° F (2° to 8° C).

◖ I.V. administration
● Reconstitute using 10 ml of sterile water (provided), 0.9% NaCl solution, or D₅W. Do not shake vial. Dilute further in same diluent solution if desired.

☑ Patient teaching
● Explain use and administration of AT-III, human to patient and parents.
● Instruct patient to report adverse reactions promptly.

---

factor IX (human)
AlphaNine SD, Mononine

factor IX complex
Konyne 80, Profilnine SD, Proplex T

Pregnancy Risk Category: C

HOW SUPPLIED
Injection: vials, with diluent. Units specified on label

ACTION
Directly replaces deficient clotting factor.

Route	Onset	Peak	Duration
IV	Immediate	10-30 min	Unknown

INDICATIONS & DOSAGE
Factor IX deficiency (hemophilia B or Christmas disease), anticoagulant overdosage—
Adults and children: approximate units required factor IX = For human product: use 1 unit/kg; (for recombinant product: use 1.2 units/kg; for Proplex T: use 0.5 units/kg) × body weight in kilograms × percentage of desired increase of factor IX level. Infusion rates vary with product and patient comfort. Dosage is highly individualized, depending on degree of deficiency, level of factor IX desired, patient weight, and severity of bleeding.

ADVERSE REACTIONS
CNS: headache.
CV: *thromboembolic reactions, MI, disseminated intravascular coagulation, pulmonary embolism,* changes in blood pressure.
GI: nausea, vomiting.
Skin: urticaria.
Other: *transient fever, chills, flushing, tingling.*

INTERACTIONS
Drug-drug. *Aminocaproic acid:* increased risk of thrombosis. Avoid concomitant use.

EFFECTS ON DIAGNOSTIC TESTS
None reported.

CONTRAINDICATIONS
Contraindicated in patients with hepatic disease in whom intravascular coagulation or fibrinolysis is suspected. Mononine is contraindicated in patients with hypersensitivity to murine (mouse) protein.

NURSING CONSIDERATIONS
• Use cautiously in neonates and infants because of susceptibility to hepatitis, which may be transmitted with factor IX complex.
• Administer hepatitis B vaccine before giving factor IX complex, as ordered.
• Observe patient for allergic reactions, and monitor vital signs regularly.
• Know that risk of hepatitis must be weighed against risk of not receiving drug.
• Be aware that risk of HIV transmission is extremely low due to manufacturing process.

I.V. administration
• Avoid rapid infusion. If tingling sensation, fever, chills, or headache develops, decrease flow rate and notify doctor.
• Reconstitute with 20 ml of sterile water for injection for each vial of lyophilized drug. Keep refrigerated until ready to use; warm to room temperature before reconstituting. Use within 3 hours. Unstable in solution. Don't shake, refrigerate, or mix with other I.V. solutions. Store away from heat.

Patient teaching
• Explain use and administration of factor IX to patient and family.
• Tell patient to report adverse reactions promptly and discontinue drug.
• Advise patient to report chest tightness, wheezing, or hypotension.

plasma protein fractions
Plasmanate, Plasma-Plex, Plasmatein, Protenate

Pregnancy Risk Category: C

HOW SUPPLIED
Injection: 5% solution in 50-ml, 250-ml, 500-ml vials

ACTION
Supplies colloid to the blood and expands plasma volume.

Route	Onset	Peak	Duration
IV	Immediate	Immediate	Unknown

INDICATIONS & DOSAGE
Shock—
Adults: varies with patient's condition and response, but usual dose is 250 to 500 ml I.V. (12.5 to 25 g protein), usually no faster than 10 ml/minute.
Children: 6.6 to 33 ml/kg (0.33 to 1.65 g/kg of protein) I.V., 5 to 10 ml/minute.
Hypoproteinemia—
Adults: 1,000 to 1,500 ml I.V. daily. Maximum infusion rate is 8 ml/minute.

ADVERSE REACTIONS
CNS: headache.
CV: hypotension (after rapid infusion or intra-arterial administration); *vascular overload* (after rapid infusion); tachycardia.
GI: nausea, vomiting, hypersalivation.
Respiratory: dyspnea, *pulmonary edema.*
Skin: rash.
Other: flushing, chills, fever, back pain.

INTERACTIONS
None significant.

EFFECTS ON DIAGNOSTIC TESTS
Plasma protein fraction slightly increases plasma protein levels.

CONTRAINDICATIONS
Contraindicated in patients with severe anemia or heart failure and in those undergoing cardiac bypass.

NURSING CONSIDERATIONS
• Use cautiously in patients with hepatic or renal failure, low cardiac reserve, and restricted sodium intake.
• Be aware that hypotension risk is greater when infusion rates exceed 10 ml/minute.
• Monitor blood pressure. Be prepared to slow or stop infusion if hypotension suddenly occurs. Vital signs should return to normal gradually; monitor hourly.

• Watch for signs of vascular overload (heart failure or pulmonary edema).
• Watch for hemorrhage or shock after surgery or injury. A rapid rise in blood pressure may cause bleeding from sites that are not apparent at lower pressures.
• Report decreased urine output.
• Keep in mind that drug contains 130 to 160 mEq sodium/L.

I.V. administration
• Check expiration date before using. Don't use solutions that are cloudy, contain sediment, or have been frozen. Discard solutions in containers opened for more than 4 hours because solution contains no preservatives.
• Don't infuse solutions containing amino acids or alcohol through same I.V. line; proteins may precipitate.
• If patient is dehydrated, give additional fluids either P.O. or I.V., as ordered.
• Do not give more than 250 g or 5,000 ml in 48 hours.

✓ Patient teaching
• Explain use and administration of drug to patient and family.
• Tell patient to report adverse reactions promptly.

alteplase
anistreplase
reteplase, recombinant
streptokinase
urokinase

COMBINATION PRODUCTS
None.

---

alteplase (tissue plasminogen activator, recombinant; t-PA)
Actilyse‡, Activase

Pregnancy Risk Category: C

HOW SUPPLIED
Injection: 20-mg (11.6 million–IU),
50-mg (29 million–IU), 100 mg
(58 million–IU) vials

ACTION
Binds to fibrin in a thrombus, and locally
converts plasminogen to plasmin, which
initiates local fibrinolysis.

Route	Onset	Peak	Duration
IV	Immediate	45 min	4 hr

INDICATIONS & DOSAGE
Lysis of thrombi obstructing coronary arteries in acute MI—
Adults: 100 mg I.V. infusion over 3 hours
as follows: 60 mg in first hour, of which 6
to 10 mg is given as a bolus over first 1 to
2 minutes. Then 20 mg/hour infusion for
2 hours. Smaller adults (under 143 lb
[65 kg]) should receive 1.25 mg/kg in a
similar fashion (60% in first hour, 10% as
a bolus; then 20% of total dose per hour
for 2 hours).
*Management of acute massive pulmonary
embolism—*
Adults: 100 mg I.V. infusion over 2
hours. Heparin begun at end of the infusion when PTT or thrombin time returns
to twice normal or less. Do not exceed
100-mg dose. Higher doses may increase
risk of intracranial bleeding.

Acute ischemic stroke—
Adults: 0.9 mg/kg I.V. infusion over 1
hour with 10% of total dose administered
as an initial I.V. bolus over 1 minute.
Maximum total dosage is 90 mg.
   Note: Administer within 3 hours after
symptoms occur and only when intracranial bleeding has been ruled out.

ADVERSE REACTIONS
CNS: *cerebral hemorrhage,* fever.
CV: hypotension, *arrhythmias,* edema.
GI: nausea, vomiting.
Hematologic: *severe, spontaneous bleeding* (cerebral, retroperitoneal, GU, GI).
Other: bleeding (at puncture sites), *cholesterol embolization, hypersensitivity reactions (anaphylaxis).*

INTERACTIONS
Drug-drug. *Aspirin, coumadin anticoagulants, dipyridamole, heparin:* increased
risk of bleeding. Monitor patient carefully.

EFFECTS ON DIAGNOSTIC TESTS
Altered results may be expected in coagulation and fibrinolytic tests. Use of aprotinin (150 to 200 units/ml) in blood sample may attenuate this interference.

CONTRAINDICATIONS
Contraindicated in patients with active internal bleeding, intracranial neoplasm,
arteriovenous malformation, aneurysm,
and severe uncontrolled hypertension.
Also contraindicated in patients with history of CVA, recent (within 2 months) intraspinal or intracranial trauma or surgery,
or known bleeding diathesis. Also contraindicated in patients with history or current evidence of intracranial hemorrhage,
suspicion of subarachnoid hemorrhage, or
seizure at onset of stroke when used for
acute ischemic stroke.

NURSING CONSIDERATIONS
• Use cautiously in patients with recent
(within 10 days) major surgery when
bleeding is difficult to control because of

Reactions may be *common,* uncommon, *life-threatening,* or COMMON AND LIFE-THREATENING.

its location; in pregnancy and first 10 days postpartum; organ biopsy; trauma (including cardiopulmonary resuscitation); GI or GU bleeding; cerebrovascular disease; hypertension (systolic pressure of 180 mm Hg or higher or diastolic pressure of 110 mm Hg or higher); mitral stenosis, atrial fibrillation, or other condition that may lead to left heart thrombus; acute pericarditis or subacute bacterial endocarditis; hemostatic defects due to hepatic or renal impairment; septic thrombophlebitis; diabetic hemorrhagic retinopathy; in patients receiving anticoagulants; and in patients 75 years and older.

• Know that recanalization of occluded coronary arteries and improvement of heart function require initiation of treatment with alteplase as soon as possible after the onset of symptoms.

• Be aware that anticoagulant and antiplatelet therapy is frequently initiated during or after treatment with alteplase to decrease the risk of rethrombosis.

• Monitor vital signs and neurologic status carefully. Patient should be kept on strict bed rest.

• Have antiarrhythmics readily available, and carefully monitor ECG. Coronary thrombolysis is associated with arrhythmias induced by reperfusion of ischemic myocardium. Such arrhythmias do not differ from those commonly associated with MI.

• Avoid invasive procedures during thrombolytic therapy. Carefully monitor the patient for signs of internal bleeding, and frequently check all puncture sites. Bleeding is the most common adverse effect and may occur internally and at external puncture sites.

• If uncontrollable bleeding occurs, stop infusion (and concomitant heparin) and notify doctor.

▌ I.V. administration
• Administer alteplase I.V. only, using a controlled infusion device.

• Reconstitute drug with sterile water for injection (without preservatives) only. (Check manufacturer's labeling for specific information.) Do not use vial if the vacuum is not present in 50-mg vials, but know that 100-mg vials don't have a vac-

uum. Reconstitute with a large-bore (18G) needle, directing the stream of sterile water at the lyophilized cake. Do not shake. Slight foaming is common (allow foaming to settle before use), and solution should be clear or pale yellow.

• Keep in mind that drug may be administered as reconstituted (1 mg/ml) or diluted with an equal volume of 0.9% NaCl solution or D_5W to make a 0.5 mg/ml solution. Adding other drugs to the infusion is not recommended.

• Reconstitute alteplase solution immediately before use, and administer it within 8 hours.

✓ Patient teaching
• Explain use and administration of alteplase to patient and family.

• Tell patient to report adverse reactions promptly.

anistreplase (anisoylated plasminogen-streptokinase activator complex; APSAC)
Eminase

Pregnancy Risk Category: C

HOW SUPPLIED
Injection: 30 units-vial

ACTION
Anistreplase, derived from Lys-plasminogen and streptokinase, is formulated into a fibrinolytic enzyme plus activator complex with the activator temporarily blocked by an anisoyl group. Drug is activated in vivo by a nonenzymatic process that removes the anisoyl group. Active drug converts plasminogen to plasmin, resulting in thrombolysis.

Route	Onset	Peak	Duration
IV	Immediate	45 min	6 hr-2 days

INDICATIONS & DOSAGE
Lysis of coronary artery thrombi following acute MI—
Adults: 30 units I.V. over 2 to 5 minutes by direct injection.

ADVERSE REACTIONS
CNS: *intracranial hemorrhage.*
CV: ARRHYTHMIAS, *conduction disorders, hypotension.*
EENT: hemoptysis, gum or mouth hemorrhage.
GI: *hemorrhage.*
GU: hematuria.
Hematologic: *bleeding tendency,* eosinophilia.
Skin: hematoma, urticaria, pruritus, flushing, delayed (2 weeks after therapy) purpuric rash.
Other: bleeding (at puncture sites), *anaphylaxis or anaphylactoid reactions* (rare), arthralgia.

INTERACTIONS
Drug-drug. *Drugs that alter platelet function (including aspirin and dipyridamole), heparin, oral anticoagulants:* may increase risk of bleeding. Use together cautiously.

EFFECTS ON DIAGNOSTIC TESTS
Drug prolongs activated PTT, PT, and thrombin time; it remains active in vivo and can cause degeneration of fibrinogen in blood samples drawn for analysis. Decreases in alpha$_2$-antiplasmin, factor V, factor VIII, fibrinogen, and plasminogen activities have been reported, as well as moderate reductions in hematocrit and hemoglobin. Concentrations of fibrinogen- and fibrin-degeneration products are increased.

CONTRAINDICATIONS
Contraindicated in patients with history of severe allergic reaction to anistreplase or streptokinase; active internal bleeding, CVA, recent (within past 2 months) intraspinal or intracranial surgery or trauma, aneurysm, arteriovenous malformation, intracranial neoplasm, uncontrolled hypertension, or known bleeding diathesis.

NURSING CONSIDERATIONS
• Use cautiously in patients with recent (within 10 days) major surgery (when bleeding is difficult to control because of its location); trauma (including cardiopulmonary resuscitation); GI or GU bleeding; cerebrovascular disease; hypertension (systolic pressure of 180 mm Hg or higher or diastolic pressure of 110 mm Hg or higher); mitral stenosis, atrial fibrillation, or other conditions that may lead to left heart thrombus; acute pericarditis or subacute bacterial endocarditis; hemostatic defects due to hepatic or renal impairment; septic thrombophlebitis; diabetic hemorrhagic retinopathy; in pregnancy and first 10 days postpartum; in patients receiving anticoagulants; and in those 75 years and older.
• Carefully monitor ECG during treatment. Be prepared to treat bradycardia or ventricular irritability. Thrombolytic therapy is associated with reperfusion arrhythmias that may signify successful thrombolysis. These arrhythmias are similar to those seen in the course of an acute MI and may include sinus bradycardia, accelerated idioventricular rhythm, ventricular tachycardia, or premature ventricular depolarizations.
• Carefully monitor patient; avoid I.M. injections and nonessential handling or moving of patient. Bleeding is the most common adverse reaction and may occur internally and at external puncture sites.
• Be aware that anticoagulant or antiplatelet therapy may be used with drug treatment to decrease the risk of rethrombosis.
• Be aware that anistreplase is derived from human plasma. No cases of hepatitis or HIV infection have been reported to date. The manufacturing process is designed to purify the plasma used in preparation of drug.
Alert: Keep in mind that drug efficacy may be limited if antistreptokinase antibodies are present. Antibody levels may be elevated if more than 5 days have elapsed since previous treatment with anistreplase or streptokinase, or if patient has had a recent streptococcal infection.
• Be aware that in vitro coagulation tests will be affected by the presence of anistreplase. This can be attenuated if blood samples are collected in the presence of aprotinin (150 to 200 units/ml).

I.V. administration
• Unlike other thrombolytics that must be infused, administer anistreplase by direct

injection into an I.V. line over 2 to 5 minutes.
• Reconstitute drug by slowly adding 5 ml of sterile water for injection. Direct the stream against the side of vial, not at drug itself. Gently roll vial to mix dry powder and water. To avoid excessive foaming, don't shake vial. Reconstituted solution should be colorless to pale yellow. Inspect for precipitate. If drug is not administered within 30 minutes of reconstituting, discard vial.
• Do not mix drug with other medications; do not dilute solution after reconstitution.

☑**Patient teaching**
• Explain use and administration of anistreplase to patient and family.
• Tell patient to report adverse reactions promptly.

reteplase, recombinant
Rapilysin§, Retavase

Pregnancy Risk Category: C

HOW SUPPLIED
Injection: 10.8 units (18.8 mg)/vial. Supplied in a kit with components for reconstitution for two single-use vials.

ACTION
Enhances the cleavage of plasminogen to generate plasmin, which leads to fibrinolysis.

Route	Onset	Peak	Duration
IV	Unknown	Unknown	Unknown

INDICATIONS & DOSAGE
Management of acute MI—
Adults: double-bolus injection of 10 + 10 units. Give each bolus I.V. over 2 minutes. If complications, such as serious bleeding or an anaphylactoid reaction do not occur after first bolus, give second bolus 30 minutes after start of first bolus.

ADVERSE REACTIONS
CNS: *intracranial hemorrhage.*
CV: *arrhythmias, cholesterol embolization, hemorrhage.*
GI: *hemorrhage.*
GU: hematuria.
Hematologic: *bleeding tendency,* anemia.
Other: bleeding (at puncture sites).

INTERACTIONS
Drug-drug. *Heparin, oral anticoagulants, platelet inhibitors (abciximab, aspirin, dipyridamole):* may increase risk of bleeding. Use together cautiously.

EFFECTS ON DIAGNOSTIC TESTS
Reteplase may alter coagulation studies; drug remains active in vitro and can lead to degradation of fibrinogen in sample. Collect blood samples in the presence of PPACK (chloromethylketone) at 2-micromolar concentrations.

CONTRAINDICATIONS
Contraindicated in patients with active internal bleeding, known bleeding diathesis, history of cerebrovascular accident, recent intracranial or intraspinal surgery or trauma, severe uncontrolled hypertension, intracranial neoplasm, arteriovenous malformation, or aneurysm.

NURSING CONSIDERATIONS
• Use cautiously in patients with recent (within 10 days) major surgery, obstetric delivery, organ biopsy, or trauma; previous puncture of noncompressible vessels; cerebrovascular disease; recent GI or GU bleeding; hypertension (systolic pressure of 180 mm Hg or more or diastolic pressure of 110 mm Hg or more); conditions that may lead to left heart thrombus including mitral stenosis; acute pericarditis or subacute bacterial endocarditis; hemostatic defects; diabetic hemorrhagic retinopathy; septic thrombophlebitis; other conditions in which bleeding would be difficult to manage; and in patients 75 years or older. Use cautiously in breast-feeding women.
• Carefully monitor ECG during treatment. Coronary thrombolysis may result in arrhythmias associated with reperfusion. Be prepared to treat bradycardia or ventricular irritability.
• Carefully monitor patient for bleeding. Avoid I.M. injections, invasive proce-

dures, and nonessential handling of patient. Bleeding is the most common adverse reaction and may occur internally or at external puncture sites. Should local measures not control serious bleeding, discontinue concomitant anticoagulation therapy and notify doctor. Withhold second bolus of reteplase.

• Know that drug should be used in pregnancy only if the benefit justifies the potential risk to the fetus.

• Know that safety and effectiveness in children have not been established.

• Be aware that potency is expressed in terms of units specific for reteplase and not comparable to other thrombolytic agents.

• Use of noncompressible pressure sites should be avoided during therapy. If an arterial puncture is needed, an upper extremity vessel that can be compressed manually should be used. Apply pressure for at least 30 minutes; then apply a pressure dressing. Check site frequently.

I.V. administration

• Know that reteplase is administered I.V. as a double-bolus injection. If bleeding or anaphylactoid reactions occur after the first bolus, notify doctor; second bolus may be withheld.

• Reconstitute drug according to manufacturer's instructions using items provided in the kit. Reconstitute with sterile water for injection, USP (without preservatives). Reconstituted solution should be colorless; the resulting concentration will be 1 U/ml. If foaming occurs, allow vial to stand for several minutes. Inspect for precipitation. Use within 4 hours of reconstitution; discard unused portions.

• Do not administer drug with other I.V. medications through same I.V. line. Note that heparin and reteplase are incompatible in solution.

✅ Patient teaching

• Explain use and administration of reteplase to patient and family.

• Tell patient to report adverse reactions immediately.

streptokinase
Kabikinase, Streptase

Pregnancy Risk Category: C

HOW SUPPLIED
Injection: 250,000 IU, 750,000 IU, 1,500,000 IU in vials for reconstitution

ACTION
Activates plasminogen in two steps: Plasminogen and streptokinase form a complex that exposes the plasminogen-activating site; plasminogen is then converted to plasmin by cleavage of the peptide bond, which leads to fibrinolysis.

Route	Onset	Peak	Duration
IV	Immediate	20 min-2 hr	4 hr

INDICATIONS & DOSAGE
Arteriovenous cannula occlusion—
Adults: 250,000 IU in 2 ml I.V. solution by I.V. pump infusion into each occluded limb of the cannula over 25 to 35 minutes. Clamp off cannula for 2 hours. Then aspirate contents of cannula; flush with NaCl solution, and reconnect.
Venous thrombosis, pulmonary embolism, and arterial thrombosis and embolism—
Adults: loading dose is 250,000 IU by I.V. infusion over 30 minutes. Sustaining dose is 100,000 IU/hour I.V. infusion for 72 hours for deep vein thrombosis and 100,000 IU/hour over 24 to 72 hours by I.V. infusion pump for pulmonary embolism and arterial thrombosis or embolism.
Lysis of coronary artery thrombi following acute MI—
Adults: loading dose is 20,000 IU bolus via coronary catheter, followed by infusion of a maintenance dose of 2,000 IU/minute over 60 minutes. Alternatively, may be administered as an I.V. infusion. Usual adult dose is 1.5 million IU infused I.V. over 60 minutes.

ADVERSE REACTIONS
CNS: polyradiculoneuropathy, headache.
CV: *reperfusion arrhythmias,* hypotension, vasculitis.
EENT: periorbital edema.

Reactions may be *common,* uncommon, *life-threatening,* or COMMON AND LIFE-THREATENING.

GI: nausea.
Hematologic: *bleeding.*
Respiratory: minor breathing difficulty, *bronchospasm, pulmonary edema.*
Skin: urticaria, pruritus, flushing.
Other: phlebitis (at injection site), hypersensitivity reactions *(anaphylaxis), delayed hypersensitivity reactions* (interstitial nephritis, serum sickness–like reactions), musculoskeletal pain, *angioedema, fever.*

INTERACTIONS

Drug-drug. *Anticoagulants:* increased risk of bleeding. Monitor patient closely.
Antifibrinolytic agents: streptokinase activity is inhibited and reversed by antifibrinolytic agents such as aminocaproic acid. Avoid concurrent use.
Aspirin, dipyridamole, drugs affecting platelet activity, indomethacin, phenylbutazone: increased risk of bleeding. Monitor patient closely.

EFFECTS ON DIAGNOSTIC TESTS

Drug increases thrombin time, activated PPT, and PT; it moderately decreases hematocrit.

CONTRAINDICATIONS

Contraindicated in patients with ulcerative wounds, active internal bleeding, and recent CVA; recent trauma with possible internal injuries; visceral or intracranial malignant neoplasms; ulcerative colitis; diverticulitis; severe hypertension; acute or chronic hepatic or renal insufficiency; uncontrolled hypocoagulation; chronic pulmonary disease with cavitation; subacute bacterial endocarditis or rheumatic valvular disease; recent cerebral embolism, thrombosis, hemorrhage; or severe allergic reaction to streptokinase.

Also contraindicated within 10 days after intra-arterial diagnostic procedure or any surgery, including liver or kidney biopsy, lumbar puncture, thoracentesis, paracentesis, or extensive or multiple cutdowns.

I.M. injections and other invasive procedures are contraindicated during streptokinase therapy.

NURSING CONSIDERATIONS

● Use cautiously when treating arterial embolism that originates from left side of heart because of danger of cerebral infarction.
● Know that only doctors with wide experience in thrombotic disease management, where clinical and laboratory monitoring can be performed, should use streptokinase.
● Before using streptokinase to clear an occluded arteriovenous cannula, try flushing with heparinized NaCl solution, as ordered.
● Keep aminocaproic acid available to treat bleeding, and corticosteroids to treat allergic reactions.
● Before initiating therapy, draw blood for coagulation studies, hematocrit, platelet count, and type and crossmatching. Rate of I.V. infusion depends on thrombin time and streptokinase resistance.
● To check for hypersensitivity reactions, give 100 IU intradermally as ordered; a wheal and flare response within 20 minutes means patient is probably allergic. Monitor vital signs frequently.
● Be aware that if patient has had either a recent streptococcal infection or recent treatment with streptokinase, a higher loading dose may be necessary.
● Know that combined therapy with low-dose aspirin (162.5 mg) or dipyridamole has improved acute and long-term results.
● Monitor patient for excessive bleeding every 15 minutes for first hour, every 30 minutes for second through eighth hours, then every 4 hours. If bleeding is evident, stop therapy and notify doctor. Know that pretreatment with heparin or drugs that affect platelets causes high risk of bleeding, but may improve long-term results. Monitor closely.
● Monitor pulses, color, and sensation of extremities every hour.
● Maintain the involved extremity in straight alignment to prevent bleeding from the infusion site.
● Avoid unnecessary handling of patient; pad side rails. Bruising is more likely during therapy.
● Keep a laboratory flow sheet on patient's chart to monitor PTT, PT, thrombin time, and hemoglobin and hematocrit lev-

---

els. Monitor vital signs and neurologic status.

• Avoid I.M. injection. Keep venipuncture sites to a minimum; use pressure dressing on puncture sites for at least 15 minutes.
Alert: Watch for signs of hypersensitivity. Notify doctor immediately. Antihistamines or corticosteroids may be used to treat mild allergic reactions. If a severe reaction occurs, stop infusion immediately and notify doctor.

• Keep in mind that thrombolytic therapy in patients with acute MI may decrease infarct size, improve ventricular function, and decrease incidence of heart failure. Streptokinase must be administered within 6 hours of the onset of symptoms for optimal effect.

◗ I.V. administration
• Reconstitute each vial with 5 ml of 0.9% NaCl solution for injection or D_5W solution. Further dilute to 45 ml (if necessary, total volume may be increased to 500 ml in a glass or 50 ml in a plastic container). Don't shake; roll gently to mix. Some flocculation may be present after reconstituting; discard if large amounts are present. Filter solution with 0.8-micron or larger filter. Use within 8 hours. Store powder at room temperature and refrigerate after reconstitution.
• Do not mix with other medications or give other drugs through the same I.V. line.
• Be aware that heparin by continuous infusion is usually started within 1 to 4 hours after stopping streptokinase. Use infusion pump to administer heparin.

☑ Patient teaching
• Explain use and administration of streptokinase to patient and family.
• Tell patient to report adverse reactions promptly.

---

urokinase
Abbokinase, Abbokinase
Open-Cath, Ukidan‡

Pregnancy Risk Category: B

HOW SUPPLIED
Injection: 5,000 units (IU) per unit-dose vial; 9,000 units (IU) per unit-dose vial; 250,000-IU vial

ACTION
Activates plasminogen to plasmin by directly cleaving peptide bonds at two different sites, causing fibrinolysis.

Route	Onset	Peak	Duration
IV	Immediate	20 min-4 hr	4 hr

INDICATIONS & DOSAGE
Lysis of acute massive pulmonary embolism and lysis of pulmonary embolism accompanied by unstable hemodynamics—
Adults: for I.V. infusion *only* by constant infusion pump.
Priming dose: 4,400 IU/kg of urokinase—0.9% NaCl or D_5W solution admixture, given over 10 minutes. Followed with 4,400 IU/kg/hour for 12 hours. Therapy followed with continuous I.V. infusion of heparin, then oral anticoagulants.
Coronary artery thrombosis—
Adults: after a bolus dose of heparin ranging from 2,500 to 10,000 units, 6,000 IU/minute of urokinase is infused into the occluded artery for up to 2 hours. Average total dosage is 500,000 IU. Urokinase therapy should be initiated within 6 hours of onset of symptoms.
Venous catheter occlusion—
Adults: solution containing 5,000 IU/ml is instilled into occluded line and, after 5 minutes, is aspirated. Aspiration attempts repeated q 5 minutes for 30 minutes. If not patent after 30 minutes, the line is capped and urokinase left to work for 30 to 60 minutes before aspirating again. May require second instillation. Flush with 10 ml 0.9% NaCl after patency restored.

ADVERSE REACTIONS
CV: *reperfusion arrhythmias*, hypotension.
Hematologic: *bleeding.*
Respiratory: *bronchospasm*, minor breathing difficulties.
Other: phlebitis (at injection site), fever, chills, nausea, vomiting, *hypersensitivity reaction.*

Reactions may be *common*, uncommon, *life-threatening*, or COMMON AND LIFE-THREATENING.

INTERACTIONS
Drug-drug. *Anticoagulants:* increased risk of bleeding. Monitor patient closely. *Aspirin, dipyridamole, indomethacin, phenylbutazone, other drugs affecting platelet activity:* increased risk of bleeding. Monitor patient.

EFFECTS ON DIAGNOSTIC TESTS
Drug increases thrombin time, PT, and activated PPT; it sometimes moderately decreases hematocrit.

CONTRAINDICATIONS
Contraindicated in patients with active internal bleeding, history of CVA, aneurysm, arteriovenous malformation, known bleeding diathesis, recent trauma with possible internal injuries, visceral or intracranial malignancy, pregnancy and first 10 days postpartum, ulcerative colitis, diverticulitis, severe hypertension, hemostatic defects including those secondary to severe hepatic or renal insufficiency, uncontrolled hypocoagulation, chronic pulmonary disease with cavitation, subacute bacterial endocarditis or rheumatic valvular disease, and recent cerebral embolism, thrombosis, or hemorrhage.

Also contraindicated within 10 days after intra-arterial diagnostic procedure or any surgery (liver or kidney biopsy, lumbar puncture, thoracentesis, paracentesis, or extensive or multiple cutdowns) or within 2 months after intracranial or intraspinal surgery.

I.M. injections and other invasive procedures are contraindicated during urokinase therapy.

NURSING CONSIDERATIONS
• Have typed and crossmatched RBCs, whole blood, plasma expanders (other than dextran), and aminocaproic acid available to treat bleeding, and corticosteroids, epinephrine, and antihistamines to treat allergic reactions.

• Know that only doctors with extensive experience in thrombotic disease management should use urokinase in institutions where clinical and laboratory monitoring can be performed.

• Monitor patient for excessive bleeding every 15 minutes for first hour; every 30 minutes for second through eighth hours; then once every 4 hours. Pretreatment with drugs affecting platelets places patient at high risk of bleeding.

• Monitor pulse, color, and sensation of extremities every hour.

• Although the incidence of hypersensitivity reactions is low, watch for signs of this reaction.

• Keep a laboratory flow sheet on patient's chart to monitor PTT, PT, thrombin time, and hemoglobin and hematocrit levels.

• Monitor vital signs and neurologic status. Don't take blood pressure in lower extremities because this could dislodge a clot.

• Keep venipuncture sites to a minimum; use pressure dressing on puncture sites for at least 15 minutes.

• Maintain involved extremity in straight alignment to prevent bleeding from the infusion site.

• Avoid unnecessary handling of patient; pad side rails. Bruising is more likely during therapy.

I.V. administration
• Reconstitute according to manufacturer's directions. Gently roll vial; do not shake. Don't use bacteriostatic water for injection to reconstitute; it contains preservatives. Dilute further with 0.9% NaCl solution or D_5W solution before infusion. Urokinase solutions may be filtered through a 0.45-micron or smaller cellulose-membrane filter before administration. Discard unused solution.

• Do not mix with other medications. Administer through separate I.V. line.

• Be aware that heparin by continuous infusion is usually started within 3 to 4 hours after urokinase has been stopped to prevent recurrent thrombosis.

Patient teaching
• Explain use and administration of urokinase to patient and family.

• Instruct patient to report adverse reactions promptly.

---

*Liquid contains alcohol.   **May contain tartrazine.   †Canada   ‡Australia   §U.K.   ◊OTC

Alkylating drugs

busulfan
carboplatin
carmustine
chlorambucil
cisplatin
cyclophosphamide
ifosfamide
lomustine
mechlorethamine hydrochloride
melphalan
streptozocin
thiotepa

COMBINATION PRODUCTS
None.

---

busulfan
Mylevan

Pregnancy Risk Category: D

HOW SUPPLIED
Tablets: 2 mg

ACTION
Unknown. Thought to cross-link strands of cellular DNA and interferes with RNA transcription, causing an imbalance of growth that leads to cell death. Cell cycle–nonspecific.

Route	Onset	Peak	Duration
PO	1-2 wk	Unknown	Unknown

INDICATIONS & DOSAGE
Chronic myelocytic (granulocytic) leukemia—
Adults: 4 to 8 mg P.O. daily, until WBC count falls to 15,000/mm^3; drug stopped until WBC count rises to 50,000/mm^3, and then resumed as before; or 4 to 8 mg P.O. daily until WBC count falls to 10,000 to 20,000/mm^3; then daily dosage reduced p.r.n. to maintain WBC count at this level. Dosage highly variable; range, 2 mg/week to 4 mg/day.
Children: 0.06 to 0.12 mg/kg/day or 1.8 to 4.6 mg/m^2/day P.O.; dosage adjusted to maintain WBC count at 20,000/mm^3, but never less than 10,000/mm^3.

ADVERSE REACTIONS
CNS: unusual tiredness or weakness, fatigue.
EENT: cataracts.
GI: cheilosis, dry mouth, anorexia.
Hematologic: *leukopenia* (WBC count falling after about 10 days and continuing to fall for 2 weeks after stopping drug), *thrombocytopenia, anemia, severe pancytopenia.*
Respiratory: *irreversible pulmonary fibrosis (commonly called "busulfan lung").*
Skin: alopecia, *transient hyperpigmentation,* rash, urticaria, anhidrosis.
Other: gynecomastia, Addison-like wasting syndrome, profound hyperuricemia caused by increased cell lysis, jaundice.

INTERACTIONS
Drug-drug. *Anticoagulants, aspirin:* increased risk of bleeding. Avoid concomitant use.
Cyclophosphamide: may increase risk of cardiac tamponade in patients with thalassemia. Monitor patient.
Myelosuppressive agents: concomitant use can cause additive myelosuppression. Monitor patient.
Thioguanine: may cause hepatotoxicity, esophageal varices, or portal hypertension. Use together cautiously.

EFFECTS ON DIAGNOSTIC TESTS
Drug-induced cellular dysplasia may interfere with interpretation of cytologic studies. Busulfan therapy may increase blood and urine levels of uric acid as a result of increased purine catabolism that accompanies cell destruction.

CONTRAINDICATIONS
Contraindicated in patients with chronic myelogenous leukemia that has demonstrated prior resistance to drug. Not useful with chronic lymphocytic leukemia or

---

Reactions may be *common*, uncommon, ***life-threatening***, or COMMON AND LIFE-THREATENING.

acute leukemia or in the blastic crisis of chronic myelogenous leukemia.

NURSING CONSIDERATIONS
• Use cautiously in patients recently given other myelosuppressants or radiation treatment and in those with depressed neutrophil or platelet count. Because high-dose therapy has been associated with seizures, use such therapy cautiously in patients with a history of head trauma or seizures or in patients receiving other drugs that lower the seizure threshold.
• Follow institutional policy regarding preparation and handling of drug. Label as a hazardous drug.
• Know that therapeutic effects are often accompanied by toxicity.
• To prevent bleeding, avoid all I.M. injections when platelet count is below 100,000/mm^3.
• Monitor patient response (increased appetite and sense of well-being, decreased total WBC count, reduced size of spleen), which usually begins within 1 to 2 weeks.
• Monitor serum uric acid. To prevent hyperuricemia with resulting uric acid nephropathy, know that allopurinol may be ordered in addition to keeping patient adequately hydrated.
• Anticipate possible blood transfusion during treatment because of cumulative anemia. Be aware that patients may receive injections of RBC colony stimulating factors to promote RBC production and decrease the need for blood transfusions.
Alert: Be aware that pulmonary fibrosis may occur as late as 8 months to 10 years after treatment with busulfan. (Average duration of therapy is 4 years.)

☑ **Patient teaching**
• Advise patient to watch for signs of infection (fever, sore throat, fatigue) and bleeding (easy bruising, nosebleeds, bleeding gums, melena). Tell patient to take temperature daily.
• Instruct patient to report symptoms of toxicity so dosage adjustments can be made. Persistent cough and progressive dyspnea with alveolar exudate, suggestive of pneumonia, may be the result of drug toxicity.

• Instruct patient to avoid OTC products containing aspirin.
• Inform patient that drug may cause darkening of skin.
• Advise women of childbearing age to avoid becoming pregnant during therapy. Recommend patient consult with doctor before becoming pregnant.
• Warn breast-feeding patient to discontinue breast-feeding because of risk of infant toxicity.
• Instruct patient to take drug on an empty stomach to decrease nausea and vomiting.
• Because of incidence of impotence and male sterility, advise men of childbearing potential about sperm banking.

carboplatin
Paraplatin, Paraplatin-AQ†

Pregnancy Risk Category: D

HOW SUPPLIED
Injection: 50-mg, 150-mg, 450-mg vials

ACTION
Unknown. An alkylating agent that probably produces cross-linking of DNA strands. Cell cycle–nonspecific.

Route	Onset	Peak	Duration
IV	Unknown	Unknown	Unknown

INDICATIONS & DOSAGE
Palliative treatment of ovarian cancer—
Adults: 360 mg/m^2 I.V. on day 1 q 4 weeks or 300 mg/m^2 when used in combination with other chemotherapy agents; doses should not be repeated until platelet count exceeds 100,000/mm^3 and neutrophil count exceeds 2,000/mm^3. Subsequent doses are based on blood counts.
Adjust-a-dose: In renally impaired patients with creatinine clearance of 41 to 59 ml/minute, initial dose is 250 mg/m^2; if it is between 16 and 40 ml/minute, initial dose is 200 mg/m^2. Drug is not recommended for patients with creatinine clearance of 15 ml/minute or less.

ADVERSE REACTIONS
CNS: dizziness, confusion, peripheral

neuropathy, ototoxicity, central neurotoxicity, paresthesia, *CVA.*
CV: *cardiac failure, embolism.*
EENT: visual disturbances.
GI: constipation, diarrhea, *nausea, vomiting,* mucositis, change in taste, stomatitis.
Hematologic: THROMBOCYTOPENIA, *leukopenia,* **neutropenia,** anemia, BONE MARROW SUPPRESSION.
Other: alopecia; *hypersensitivity reactions; increased BUN, creatinine, AST, or alkaline phosphatase levels; pain; asthenia;* **anaphylaxis;** *decreased serum electrolyte levels.*

INTERACTIONS
Drug-drug. *Aspirin:* increased risk of bleeding. Avoid concomitant use.
Bone marrow suppressants, including radiation therapy: increased hematologic toxicity. Monitor closely.
Myelosuppressive agents: concomitant use can cause additive myelosuppression. Monitor patient.
Nephrotoxic agents, especially aminoglycosides: enhanced nephrotoxicity of carboplatin. Use cautiously.

EFFECTS ON DIAGNOSTIC TESTS
High doses may cause elevated bilirubin, alkaline phosphatase, AST, serum creatinine, and BUN levels.

CONTRAINDICATIONS
Contraindicated in patients with severe bone marrow suppression, bleeding, and history of hypersensitivity to cisplatin, platinum-containing compounds, or mannitol.

NURSING CONSIDERATIONS
• Determine serum electrolyte, creatinine, and BUN levels; CBC; and creatinine clearance before the first infusion and before each course of treatment.
• Keep in mind that bone marrow suppression may be more severe in patients with creatinine clearance below 60 ml/minute; dosage adjustments are recommended for such patients.
• Follow institutional policy to reduce risks because preparation and administration of parenteral form of this drug is as-

sociated with mutagenic, teratogenic, and carcinogenic risks for personnel.
• Check ordered dose against laboratory test results carefully. Only one increase in dosage is recommended. Subsequent doses should not exceed 125% of starting dose.
• Know that therapeutic effects are often accompanied by toxicity.
• To prevent bleeding, avoid all I.M. injections when platelet count is below $100,000/mm^3$.
• Monitor vital signs during infusion.
• Monitor CBC and platelet count frequently during therapy and, when indicated, until recovery. WBC and platelet count nadirs usually occur by day 21. Levels usually return to baseline by day 28. Know that dose should not be repeated unless platelet count exceeds $100,000/mm^3$. Administer WBC colony stimulating factors as ordered to promote cell line growth.
• Administer antiemetic therapy, as ordered. Carboplatin can produce severe vomiting.
• Anticipate possible blood transfusions during treatment because of cumulative anemia. Patient may receive injections of RBC colony stimulating factors to promote cell production.
• Know that hydration or diuresis before or after treatment is not necessary.
• Be aware that patients over 65 years are at greater risk for neurotoxicity.

☐ I.V. administration
Alert: Have epinephrine, corticosteroids, and antihistamines available when administering carboplatin because anaphylactoid reactions may occur within minutes of administration.
• Reconstitute with D_5W, 0.9% NaCl solution, or sterile water for injection to make a concentration of 10 mg/ml. Add 5 ml of diluent to 50-mg vial, 15 ml of diluent to 150-mg vial, or 45 ml of diluent to 450-mg vial. It can then be further diluted for infusion with 0.9% NaCl solution or D_5W. A concentration as low as 0.5 mg/ml can be prepared. Give drug by continuous or intermittent infusion over at least 15 minutes.
• Do not use needles or I.V. administra-

tion sets containing aluminum to administer carboplatin; precipitation and loss of drug's potency may occur.
• Store unopened vials at room temperature. Once reconstituted and diluted as directed, drug is stable at room temperature for 8 hours. Because the drug does not contain antibacterial preservatives, discard unused drug after 8 hours.

☑ **Patient teaching**
• Advise patient of most common adverse reactions: nausea, vomiting, bone marrow suppression, anemia, thrombocytopenia.
• Advise patient to watch for signs of infection (fever, sore throat, fatigue) and bleeding (easy bruising, nosebleeds, bleeding gums, melena). Tell patient to take temperature daily.
• Instruct patient to avoid OTC products containing aspirin.
• Because of incidence of impotence, sterility, and amenorrhea, advise patients (male and female) of childbearing age before initiating therapy. Also recommend that women patients consult with the doctor before becoming pregnant.
• Because of risk of infant toxicity, advise breast-feeding patient taking carboplatin to discontinue breast-feeding.

---

carmustine (BCNU)
BiCNU, Gliadel

Pregnancy Risk Category: D

HOW SUPPLIED
Injection: 100-mg vial (lyophilized), with a 3-ml vial of absolute alcohol supplied as a diluent
Wafer: 7.7 mg, for intracavitary use

ACTION
Inhibits enzymatic reactions involved with DNA synthesis, cross-links strands of cellular DNA, and interferes with RNA transcription, causing an imbalance of growth that leads to cell death. Cell cycle–nonspecific.

Route	Onset	Peak	Duration
IV, intra-cavitary	Unknown	Unknown	Unknown

INDICATIONS & DOSAGE
Brain tumors, Hodgkin's disease, malignant lymphoma, and multiple myeloma—
Adults: 75 to 100 mg/m^2 I.V. by slow infusion daily for 2 days; repeated q 6 weeks if platelet count is above 100,000/mm^3 and WBC count is above 4,000/mm^3.
Adjust-a-dose: Dosage is reduced by 50% when WBC count is 3,000 to 3,999/mm^3. Dosage is reduced by 75% when WBC count is 2,000 to 2,999/mm^3 and platelet count is 25,000 to 75,000/mm^3. Dosage is held when WBC count is less than 2,000/mm^3 and platelet count is less than 25,000/mm^3.
Adjunct to surgery to prolong survival in patients with recurrent glioblastoma multiforme for whom surgical resection is indicated—
Adults: *(for wafer)* recommendation—8 wafers be placed in the resection cavity if the size and shape of cavity allows. If 8 wafers cannot be accommodated, maximum number of wafers as allowed should be used.
Alternatively, 150 to 200 mg/m^2 I.V. by slow infusion as a single dose, repeated q 6 to 8 weeks.

ADVERSE REACTIONS
CNS: ataxia, drowsiness.
EENT: ocular toxicities.
GI: *nausea* beginning in 2 to 6 hours (can be severe), *vomiting, stomatitis.*
GU: *nephrotoxicity,* azotemia, *renal failure.*
Hematologic: *cumulative bone marrow suppression,* delayed 4 to 6 weeks, lasting 1 to 2 weeks; *leukopenia; thrombocytopenia; acute leukemia or bone marrow dysplasia* (may occur after long-term use); anemia.
Hepatic: *hepatotoxicity.*
Respiratory: *pulmonary fibrosis.*
Skin: facial flushing, hyperpigmentation.
Other: *intense pain at infusion site from venous spasm;* possible hyperuricemia in lymphoma patients when rapid cell lysis occurs.

INTERACTIONS
Drug-drug. *Anticoagulants, aspirin:* in-

creased risk of bleeding. Avoid concomitant use.

Cimetidine: may increase carmustine's bone marrow toxicity. Avoid combination if possible.

Myelosuppressive agents: concomitant use can cause additive myelosuppression. Monitor patient.

EFFECTS ON DIAGNOSTIC TESTS
Drug may increase BUN, serum alkaline phosphatase, AST, and bilirubin levels.

CONTRAINDICATIONS
Contraindicated in patients with hypersensitivity to drug.

NURSING CONSIDERATIONS
• Be aware that pulmonary toxicity appears to be dose related and may occur 9 days to 15 years after treatment. Obtain pulmonary function tests as ordered before and during therapy.
• To reduce nausea, give antiemetic before administering drug, as ordered.
• Avoid contact with skin because carmustine will cause a brown stain. If drug comes into contact with skin, wash off thoroughly.
• Perform liver, renal function, and pulmonary function tests periodically, as ordered.
• Monitor CBC, as ordered.
• Monitor serum uric acid level, as ordered. To prevent hyperuricemia with resulting uric acid nephropathy, know that allopurinol may be used with adequate hydration.
• Be aware that therapeutic effects are often accompanied by toxicity.
• To prevent bleeding, avoid all I.M. injections when platelet count is below 100,000/mm³.
• Anticipate possible blood transfusions during treatment because of cumulative anemia. Patient may receive injections of RBC colony stimulating factors to promote cell production.
• Unopened foil pouches of wafer may be kept at ambient room temperature for a maximum of 6 hours at a time.
• Be aware that wafers broken in half may be used; however discard wafers broken in more than two pieces.

⬛ I.V. administration
• Follow institutional policy to reduce risks because preparation and administration of parenteral form of this drug is associated with carcinogenic, mutagenic, and teratogenic risks for personnel. Manufacturer recommends wearing gloves when handling either form.
• To reconstitute, dissolve 100 mg of carmustine in the 3 ml of absolute alcohol provided by the manufacturer. Dilute solution with 27 ml of sterile water for injection. Resultant solution contains 3.3 mg of carmustine/ml in 10% alcohol. Dilute in 0.9% NaCl solution or D_5W for I.V. infusion. Give at least 250 ml over 1 to 2 hours. To reduce pain on infusion, dilute further or slow infusion rate.
• Discard drug if powder liquefies or appears oily (decomposition has occurred).
• Administer only in glass containers. Solution is unstable in plastic I.V. bags.
• Don't mix with other drugs during administration.
• Store reconstituted solution in refrigerator for 24 hours or at room temperature for 8 hours. May decompose at temperatures above 80° F (27° C).

☑ Patient teaching
• Advise patient about common adverse reactions to drug.
• Tell patient to watch for signs and symptoms of infection (fever, sore throat, fatigue) and bleeding (easy bruising, nosebleeds, bleeding gums, melena). Tell him to take temperature daily.
• Instruct patient to avoid OTC products containing aspirin.
• Advise breast-feeding patient to discontinue breast-feeding during therapy because of possible infant toxicity.
• Caution women of childbearing age to avoid becoming pregnant during therapy. Recommend patient consult with doctor before becoming pregnant.

---

chlorambucil
Leukeran

Pregnancy Risk Category: D

HOW SUPPLIED
Tablets: 2 mg

ACTION
Cross-links strands of cellular DNA and interferes with RNA transcription, causing an imbalance of growth that leads to cell death. Cell cycle–nonspecific.

Route	Onset	Peak	Duration
PO	3-4 wk	1 hr	Unknown

INDICATIONS & DOSAGE
Chronic lymphocytic leukemia; malignant lymphomas including lymphosarcoma, giant follicular lymphoma, and Hodgkin's disease—
Adults: 0.1 to 0.2 mg/kg P.O. daily for 3 to 6 weeks; then adjusted for maintenance (usually 4 to 10 mg daily).

ADVERSE REACTIONS
CNS: *seizures,* peripheral neuropathy, tremor, muscle twitching, confusion, agitation, ataxia, flaccid paresis.
GI: *nausea, vomiting,* stomatitis, diarrhea.
GU: *azoospermia, infertility,* sterile cystitis.
Hematologic: *neutropenia,* delayed up to 3 weeks, lasting up to 10 days after last dose; *bone marrow suppression; thrombocytopenia; anemia; myelosuppression* (usually moderate, gradual, and rapidly reversible).
Hepatic: *hepatotoxicity.*
Respiratory: interstitial pneumonitis, *pulmonary fibrosis* (rare).
Skin: rash, including erythema multiforme, epidermal necrolysis, and *Stevens-Johnson syndrome; hypersensitivity.*
Other: allergic febrile reaction.

INTERACTIONS
Drug-drug. *Anticoagulants, aspirin:* increased risk of bleeding. Avoid concomitant use.
Myelosuppressive agents: concomitant use can cause additive myelosuppression. Monitor patient.

EFFECTS ON DIAGNOSTIC TESTS
Drug may increase concentrations of serum alkaline phosphatase, AST, and blood and urine uric acid.

CONTRAINDICATIONS
Contraindicated in patients with hypersensitivity or resistance to previous therapy. Patients hypersensitive to other alkylating agents may also be hypersensitive to chlorambucil.

NURSING CONSIDERATIONS
• Use cautiously in patients with history of head trauma or seizures or in patients receiving other drugs that lower the seizure threshold. Also use cautiously within 4 weeks of a full course of radiation or chemotherapy.
• Monitor CBC, as ordered.
• Monitor serum uric acid level, as ordered. To prevent hyperuricemia with resulting uric acid nephropathy, know that allopurinol may be used with adequate hydration.
• If WBC count falls below 2,000/mm³ or granulocyte count falls below 1,000/mm³, follow institutional policy for infection control in immunocompromised patients. Patients may receive injections of WBC colony stimulating factors to decrease risk for infection. Severe neutropenia is reversible up to cumulative dosage of 6.5 mg/kg in a single course.
• Be aware that therapeutic effects are often accompanied by toxicity.
• To prevent bleeding, avoid all I.M. injections when platelet count is below 100,000/mm³.
• Anticipate possible blood transfusions during treatment because of cumulative anemia. Patient may receive injections of RBC colony stimulating factors to promote RBC production and decrease need for blood transfusions.

☑ Patient teaching
• Advise patient to watch for signs of infection (fever, sore throat, fatigue) and bleeding (easy bruising, nosebleeds, bleeding gums, melena). Tell patient to take temperature daily.
• Instruct patient to avoid OTC products containing aspirin.
• Tell breast-feeding patient to discontin-

---

ue breast-feeding during therapy because of possible infant toxicity.
• Advise women of childbearing age to avoid becoming pregnant during therapy and to notify doctor immediately if pregnancy is suspected.

---

cisplatin (cis-platinum, CDDP)
Platinol AQ

Pregnancy Risk Category: D

HOW SUPPLIED
Injection: 0.5 mg/ml†, 1 mg/ml

ACTION
Unknown. Probably cross-links strands of cellular DNA and interferes with RNA transcription, causing an imbalance of growth that leads to cell death. Cell cycle–nonspecific.

Route	Onset	Peak	Duration
IV	Unknown	Unknown	Several days

INDICATIONS & DOSAGE
Adjunctive therapy in metastatic testicular cancer—
Adults: 20 mg/m² I.V. daily for 5 days. Repeated q 3 weeks for three cycles or longer.
Adjunctive therapy in metastatic ovarian cancer—
Adults: 100 mg/m² I.V.; repeated q 4 weeks. Or 75 to 100 mg/m² I.V. once q 4 weeks in combination with cyclophosphamide.
Advanced bladder cancer—
Adults: 50 to 70 mg/m² I.V. q 3 to 4 weeks. Patients who have received other antineoplastic agents or radiation therapy should receive 50 mg/m² q 4 weeks.

ADVERSE REACTIONS
CNS: *peripheral neuritis, **seizures.***
EENT: *tinnitus, hearing loss, ototoxicity,* vestibular toxicity, optic neuritis, papilledema, cerebral blindness, blurred vision.
GI: loss of taste, *nausea, vomiting* (beginning 1 to 4 hours after dose and lasting 24 hours).
GU: more prolonged and SEVERE RENAL TOXICITY with repeated courses of therapy.

Hematologic: MYELOSUPPRESSION; *leukopenia, thrombocytopenia, anemia;* nadirs in circulating platelet and WBC counts on days 18 to 23, with recovery by day 39.
Other: *anaphylactoid reaction, hypomagnesemia,* hypokalemia, hypocalcemia, hyponatremia, hypophosphatemia, hyperuricemia.

INTERACTIONS
Drug-drug. *Aminoglycoside antibiotics:* additive nephrotoxicity. Monitor renal function studies very carefully.
Aspirin: increased risk of bleeding. Avoid concurrent use.
Bumetanide, ethacrynic acid, furosemide: additive ototoxicity. Avoid concomitant use.
Myelosuppressive agents: concomitant use can cause additive myelosuppression. Monitor patient.
Phenytoin: decreased serum phenytoin levels. Monitor serum levels.

EFFECTS ON DIAGNOSTIC TESTS
Drug may increase BUN, serum creatinine, and serum uric acid levels. It may decrease creatinine clearance, serum calcium, magnesium, phosphate, and potassium levels, indicating nephrotoxicity.

CONTRAINDICATIONS
Contraindicated in patients with severe renal disease, hearing impairment, myelosuppression, and hypersensitivity to drug or other platinum-containing compounds.

NURSING CONSIDERATIONS
• Use cautiously in patients previously treated with radiation or cytotoxic agents, in those with preexisting peripheral neuropathies, and with other ototoxic and nephrotoxic drugs.
• Monitor CBC, electrolyte levels (especially potassium and magnesium), platelet count, and renal function studies before initial and subsequent dosages, as ordered.
• To detect hearing loss, perform audiometry before initial dosage and subsequent courses, as ordered.
• Be aware that prehydration and manni-

tol diuresis may reduce renal toxicity and ototoxicity significantly.
• Know that therapeutic effects are often accompanied by toxicity.
• Check current protocol. Some clinicians use I.V. sodium thiosulfate to minimize toxicity.
• Administer antiemetics, as ordered. Nausea and vomiting may be severe and protracted; however incidence and severity have been significantly reduced with the use of ondansetron and granisetron. Monitor intake and output. Continue I.V. hydration until patient can tolerate adequate oral intake.
• Some clinicians combine metoclopramide with dexamethasone and antihistamines, or ondansetron or granisetron with dexamethasone.
• Be aware that delayed-onset vomiting (3 to 5 days after treatment) has been reported. Patients may need prolonged antiemetic treatment.
• Know that renal toxicity is cumulative. Renal function must return to normal before next dose can be given.
• Know that dosage should not be repeated unless platelet count is over 100,000/mm³, WBC count is over 4,000/mm³, creatinine level is under 1.5 mg/dl, or BUN level is under 25 mg/dl.
• To prevent bleeding, avoid all I.M. injections when platelet counts are below 100,000/mm³.
• Anticipate blood transfusions during treatment because of cumulative anemia.
Alert: Immediately administer epinephrine, corticosteroids, or antihistamines for anaphylactoid reactions, as ordered.
• Know that pediatric dosages have not been safely established.

I.V. administration
• As ordered, administer mannitol or furosemide boluses or infusions before and concurrent with cisplatin infusion to maintain diuresis of 100 to 400 ml/hour during and for 24 hours after therapy.
• Hydrate patient with 0.9% NaCl solution before giving drug, as ordered. Maintain urine output of at least 100 ml/hour for 4 consecutive hours before therapy and for 24 hours after therapy.
• Follow institutional policy to reduce

risks because preparation and administration of parenteral form of this drug is associated with carcinogenic, mutagenic, and teratogenic risks for personnel.
• Reconstitute powder using sterile water for injection. Add 10 ml to the 10-mg vial or 50 ml to the 50-mg vial to make a solution containing 1 mg/ml. If necessary, further dilute with dextrose 5% in 0.3% NaCl injection or dextrose 5% in 0.45% NaCl injection. Solutions are stable for 20 hours at room temperature. Don't refrigerate.
• Keep in mind that infusions are most stable in chloride-containing solutions (such as 0.9% NaCl, 0.45% NaCl, and 0.22% NaCl).
• Be aware that the manufacturer recommends administering drug as an I.V. infusion in 2 L of dextrose 5% in 0.45% NaCl or dextrose 5% in 0.22% NaCl solution with 37.5 g of mannitol over 6 to 8 hours.
• Do not use needles or I.V. administration sets that contain aluminum because it will displace the platinum, causing a loss of potency and formation of a black precipitate.
• To prevent hypokalemia, know that potassium chloride (10 to 20 mEq/L) is frequently added to I.V. fluids before and after cisplatin therapy.

✓ Patient teaching
• Advise patient to watch for signs of infection (fever, sore throat, fatigue) and bleeding (easy bruising, nosebleeds, bleeding gums, melena). Tell patient to take temperature daily.
• Tell patient to report tinnitus or numbness in hands or feet immediately.
• Instruct patient to avoid OTC products containing aspirin.
• Advise breast-feeding patient taking drug to discontinue breast-feeding because of the possibility of infant toxicity.
• Caution women of childbearing age to avoid becoming pregnant during therapy. Also recommend consulting with doctor before becoming pregnant.

---

*Liquid contains alcohol.   **May contain tartrazine.   †Canada   ‡Australia   §U.K.   ◊OTC

cyclophosphamide
Cycloblastin‡, Cytoxan**, Cytoxan
Lyophilized, Endoxan-Asta‡,
Neosar, Procytox†

Pregnancy Risk Category: D

HOW SUPPLIED
Tablets: 25 mg, 50 mg
Injection: 100-mg, 200-mg, 500-mg, 1-g,
2-g vials

ACTION
Cross-links strands of cellular DNA and
interferes with RNA transcription, causing an imbalance of growth that leads to
cell death. Cell cycle–nonspecific.

Route	Onset	Peak	Duration
PO, IV	Unknown	Unknown	Unknown

INDICATIONS & DOSAGE
*Breast and ovarian cancers, Hodgkin's
disease, chronic lymphocytic leukemia,
chronic myelocytic leukemia, acute lymphoblastic leukemia, acute myelocytic
and monocytic leukemia, neuroblastoma,
retinoblastoma, malignant lymphoma,
multiple myeloma, mycosis fungoides,
sarcoma—*
Adults and children: initially, 40 to
50 mg/kg I.V. in divided doses over 2 to 5
days. Alternatively, 10 to 15 mg/kg I.V. q
7 to 10 days, 3 to 5 mg/kg I.V. twice
weekly, or 1 to 5 mg/kg P.O. daily, depending on patient tolerance. Subsequent
dosages adjusted according to evidence of
antitumor activity or leukopenia.
*"Minimal change" nephrotic syndrome in
children—*
Children: 2.5 to 3 mg/kg P.O. daily for
60 to 90 days.

ADVERSE REACTIONS
CV: *cardiotoxicity* (with very high doses
and in combination with doxorubicin).
GI: anorexia, *nausea and vomiting* (beginning within 6 hours), abdominal pain,
stomatitis, mucositis.
GU: HEMORRHAGIC CYSTITIS, impaired
fertility.
Hematologic: *leukopenia,* nadir between

days 8 to 15, recovery in 17 to 28 days;
thrombocytopenia; anemia.
Respiratory: *pulmonary fibrosis* (with
high doses).
Skin: *reversible alopecia,* rash, pigmentation, nail changes, flushing, itching.
Other: *secondary malignant disease,
anaphylaxis, hypersensitivity reactions,
hepatotoxicity.*

INTERACTIONS
Drug-drug. *Allopurinol:* increased myelosuppression. Monitor toxicity.
Aspirin: increased risk of bleeding. Avoid
concurrent use.
Barbiturates: increased pharmacologic effect and enhanced cyclophosphamide toxicity due to induction of hepatic enzymes.
Monitor patient closely.
Cardiotoxic drugs: additive adverse cardiac effects. Monitor for toxicity.
Chloramphenicol, corticosteroids: reduced activity of cyclophosphamide. Use
cautiously.
Digoxin: may decrease serum digoxin
levels. Monitor levels closely.
Myelosuppressive agents: concomitant
use can cause additive myelosuppression.
Monitor patient.
Succinylcholine: prolonged neuromuscular blockade. Don't use together.

EFFECTS ON DIAGNOSTIC TESTS
Drug may suppress positive reaction to
Candida, mumps, Trichophyton, and tuberculin TB skin test. A false-positive result for the Papanicolaou test may occur.
Drug therapy may also increase serum
uric acid levels and decrease serum pseudocholinesterase levels.

CONTRAINDICATIONS
Contraindicated in patients with severe
bone marrow suppression or hypersensitivity to drug.

NURSING CONSIDERATIONS
• Use cautiously in patients with leukopenia, thrombocytopenia, malignant cell infiltration of bone marrow, or hepatic or
renal disease and in those who have recently undergone radiation therapy or
chemotherapy.
• Don't give drug at bedtime; infrequent

Reactions may be *common*, uncommon, *life-threatening*, or COMMON AND LIFE-THREATENING.

urination during the night may increase the possibility of cystitis. If cystitis occurs, discontinue drug and notify doctor. Cystitis can occur months after therapy ceases. Mesna may be given to lower the incidence and severity of bladder toxicity.

• Monitor CBC and renal and liver function tests, as ordered.

• Monitor serum uric acid level, as ordered. To prevent hyperuricemia with resulting uric acid nephropathy, know that allopurinol may be used with adequate hydration.

Alert: Monitor for cyclophosphamide toxicity if patient's corticosteroid therapy is discontinued.

• To prevent bleeding, avoid all I.M. injections when platelet count is below 100,000/mm^3.

• Anticipate possible blood transfusions because of cumulative anemia. Patients may receive injections of RBC colony stimulating factors to promote RBC production and decrease need for blood transfusions.

• Know that therapeutic effects are often accompanied by toxicity.

⬤ I.V. administration

• Follow institutional policy to reduce risks. Preparation and administration of parenteral form of this drug is associated with carcinogenic, mutagenic, and teratogenic risks for personnel.

• Reconstitute powder using sterile water for injection or bacteriostatic water for injection containing only parabens. For the nonlyophilized product, add 5 ml to 100-mg vial, 10 ml to 200-mg vial, 25 ml to 500-mg vial, 50 ml to 1-g vial, or 100 ml to 2-g vial to produce a solution containing 20 mg/ml. Shake to dissolve; this may take up to 6 minutes, and it may be difficult to completely dissolve drug. Lyophilized preparation is much easier to reconstitute; check package insert for quantity of diluent needed to reconstitute drug.

• After reconstitution, administer as ordered by direct I.V. injection or infusion. For I.V. infusion, further dilute with D$_5$W, dextrose 5% in 0.9% NaCl injection, dextrose 5% in Ringer's injection, lactated

Ringer's injection, sodium lactate injection, or 0.45% NaCl injection.

• Check reconstituted solution for small particles. Filter solution if necessary.

• Know that reconstituted solution is stable for 6 days refrigerated or 24 hours at room temperature. However, use stored solutions cautiously because drug contains no preservatives.

✅ Patient teaching

• Warn patient that alopecia is likely to occur but that it is reversible.

• Advise patient to watch for signs of infection (fever, sore throat, fatigue) and bleeding (easy bruising, nosebleeds, bleeding gums, melena). Tell patient to take temperature daily.

• Instruct patient to avoid OTC products containing aspirin.

• To minimize the risk of hemorrhagic cystitis, encourage patient to void every 1 to 2 hours while awake and to drink at least 3 L of fluid daily. If patient is taking oral form of drug, instruct him to avoid taking it at bedtime because infrequent urination increases risk of cystitis.

• Advise male and female patients to practice contraception while taking drug and for 4 months after; drug is potentially teratogenic.

• Advise breast-feeding patient taking drug to discontinue breast-feeding because of the possibility of infant toxicity.

• Drug can cause irreversible sterility in both male and female patients. Counsel patients of childbearing potential before initiating therapy. Also recommend female patient consults with doctor before becoming pregnant.

---

ifosfamide
Ifex, Mitoxana§

Pregnancy Risk Category: D

HOW SUPPLIED
Injection: 1 g, 2 g†, 3 g

ACTION
Cross-links strands of cellular DNA and interferes with RNA transcription, caus-

ing an imbalance of growth that leads to cell death. Cell cycle–nonspecific.

Route	Onset	Peak	Duration
IV	Unknown	Unknown	Unknown

INDICATIONS & DOSAGE
Testicular cancer—
Adults: 1.2 g/m^2/day I.V. for 5 consecutive days. Treatment is repeated q 3 weeks or after patient recovers from hematologic toxicity.

ADVERSE REACTIONS
CNS: *somnolence, confusion,* **coma,** **seizures,** ataxia, hallucinations, depressive psychosis, dizziness, disorientation, cranial nerve dysfunction.
GI: *nausea, vomiting.*
GU: *hemorrhagic cystitis, hematuria,* **nephrotoxicity.**
Hematologic: *leukopenia, thrombocytopenia, myelosuppression.*
Hepatic: elevated liver enzyme levels, liver dysfunction.
Other: *alopecia, metabolic acidosis,* infection, phlebitis.

INTERACTIONS
Drug-drug. *Allopurinol:* may produce excessive ifosfamide effect by prolonging half-life. Monitor for enhanced toxicity.
Anticoagulants, aspirin: increased risk of bleeding. Avoid concomitant use.
Barbiturates, chloral hydrate, phenytoin: may increase ifosfamide toxicity by inducing hepatic enzymes that hasten the formation of toxic metabolites. Monitor patient closely.
Corticosteroids: may inhibit hepatic enzymes, reducing ifosfamide's effect. Monitor for enhanced ifosfamide toxicity if concurrent steroid dosage is suddenly reduced or discontinued.
Cyclophosphamides: may increase risk of cardiac tamponade in patients with thalassemia. Monitor concomitant use.
Myelosuppressants: enhanced hematologic toxicity. Dosage adjustment may be necessary.

EFFECTS ON DIAGNOSTIC TESTS
Drug therapy may increase serum levels of AST, ALT, BUN, LD, bilirubin, creatinine, and alkaline phosphatase.

CONTRAINDICATIONS
Contraindicated in patients with severe bone marrow suppression or hypersensitivity to drug.

NURSING CONSIDERATIONS
• Use cautiously in patients with renal impairment or compromised bone marrow reserve as indicated by leukopenia, granulocytopenia, extensive bone marrow metastases, prior radiation therapy, or prior therapy with cytotoxic agents.
• Administer antiemetics, as ordered, before giving ifosfamide to help decrease nausea.
• Don't give drug at bedtime; infrequent voiding during the night may increase the possibility of cystitis. If cystitis develops, discontinue drug and notify doctor.
• Be aware that bladder irrigation with 0.9% NaCl solution may decrease the possibility of cystitis.
• Monitor CBC and renal and liver function tests, as ordered.
• To prevent bleeding, avoid all I.M. injections when platelet count is below 100,000/mm^3.
• Anticipate possible blood transfusions because of cumulative anemia. Patients may receive injections of RBC colony stimulating factors to promote RBC production and decrease need for blood transfusions.
• Assess patient for mental status changes; dosage may have to be decreased.

◖I.V. administration
• Follow institutional policy to reduce risks. Preparation and administration of parenteral form of this drug is associated with carcinogenic, mutagenic, and teratogenic risks for personnel.
• Reconstitute each gram of drug with 20 ml of diluent to yield a solution of 50 mg/ml. Use sterile water for injection or bacteriostatic water for injection. Solutions may then be further diluted with sterile water, dextrose 2.5% or 5% in water, 0.45% or 0.9% NaCl for injection, 5%

dextrose and 0.9% NaCl for injection, or lactated Ringer's injection.
• Infuse each dose over at least 30 minutes.
• As ordered, administer ifosfamide with a protecting agent (mesna) to prevent hemorrhagic cystitis. Obtain urinalysis before each dose. If microscopic hematuria is present, mesna must be given concomitantly with or before ifosfamide to prevent cystitis. (Dosage adjustments of mesna given concomitantly may be necessary.) Adequate fluid intake (2 L/day, either P.O. or I.V.) is essential before and 72 hours after therapy.
• Know that ifosfamide and mesna are physically compatible and may be mixed in the same I.V. solution.
• Keep in mind that reconstituted solution is stable for 1 week at room temperature or 6 weeks if refrigerated. However, use solution within 6 hours if drug was reconstituted with sterile water without a preservative (such as benzyl alcohol or parabens).

☑ **Patient teaching**
• Remind patient to void frequently to minimize contact of drug and its metabolites with the bladder mucosa.
• Advise patient to watch for signs of infection (fever, sore throat, fatigue) and bleeding (easy bruising, nosebleeds, bleeding gums, melena). Tell patient to take temperature daily.
• Instruct patient to avoid OTC products containing aspirin.
• Advise breast-feeding patient to discontinue breast-feeding during therapy because of possible infant toxicity.
• Caution women of childbearing age to avoid becoming pregnant during therapy. Also recommend consulting with doctor before becoming pregnant.

---

lomustine (CCNU)
CeeNu

Pregnancy Risk Category: D

HOW SUPPLIED
Capsules: 10 mg, 40 mg, 100 mg, dose pack (two 10-mg, two 40-mg, two 100-mg capsules)

ACTION
Cross-links strands of cellular DNA and interferes with RNA transcription, causing an imbalance of growth that leads to cell death. Cell cycle–nonspecific.

Route	Onset	Peak	Duration
PO	Unknown	Unknown	Unknown

INDICATIONS & DOSAGE
Brain tumor, Hodgkin's disease—
Adults and children: 100 to 130 mg/m^2 P.O. as a single dose q 6 weeks. Repeat doses should not be given until WBC count is more than 4,000/mm^3 and platelet count is more than 100,000/mm^3.
Adjust-a-dose: Dosage reduced according to degree of bone marrow suppression or when used with other myelosuppressive drugs. Dosage should be reduced by 25% for WBC count 3,000 to 3,999/mm^3; by 50% for WBC count 2,000 to 2,999/mm^3; drug dosage should be held for WBC count less than 2,000/mm^3.

ADVERSE REACTIONS
CNS: disorientation, lethargy, ataxia.
GI: *nausea, vomiting,* stomatitis.
GU: *nephrotoxicity,* progressive azotemia, *renal failure.*
Hematologic: *anemia, leukopenia,* delayed up to 6 weeks, lasting 1 to 2 weeks; *thrombocytopenia,* delayed up to 4 weeks, lasting 1 to 2 weeks; *bone marrow suppression,* delayed up to 4 to 6 weeks.
Other: *hepatotoxicity, secondary malignant disease, pulmonary fibrosis,* alopecia.

INTERACTIONS
Drug-drug. *Anticoagulants, aspirin:* increased risk of bleeding. Avoid concomitant use.
Myelosuppressive agents: concomitant use can cause additive myelosuppression. Monitor patient

EFFECTS ON DIAGNOSTIC TESTS
Drug therapy may cause transient increases in liver function tests.

CONTRAINDICATIONS
Contraindicated in patients with hypersensitivity to drug.

NURSING CONSIDERATIONS
• Use cautiously in patients with decreased platelet, WBC, or RBC counts and in those receiving other myelosuppressants.
• To avoid nausea, give antiemetic before administering, as ordered.
• Give 2 to 4 hours after meals; drug will be more completely absorbed if taken when the stomach is empty.
• Monitor CBC weekly, as ordered. Usually not administered more often than every 6 weeks; bone marrow toxicity is cumulative and delayed, usually occurring in 4 to 6 weeks after drug administration.
• Periodically monitor liver function tests, as ordered.
• To prevent bleeding, avoid all I.M. injections when platelet count is below 100,000/mm³.
• Anticipate possible blood transfusions because of cumulative anemia. Patients may receive RBC colony stimulating factors to promote RBC production and decrease need for blood transfusions.
• Know that therapeutic effects are often accompanied by toxicity.
• Store capsules at room temperature. Avoid exposure to moisture and protect from temperatures above 104° F (40° C).

☑ **Patient teaching**
• Advise patient to watch for signs of infection (fever, sore throat, fatigue) and bleeding (easy bruising, nosebleeds, bleeding gums, melena). Tell patient to take temperature daily.
• Instruct patient to avoid OTC products containing aspirin.
• Advise breast-feeding patients to discontinue breast-feeding during therapy because of possible infant toxicity.
• Caution women of childbearing age to avoid becoming pregnant during therapy. Also recommend consulting with doctor before becoming pregnant.

mechlorethamine hydrochloride (nitrogen mustard)
Mustargen

Pregnancy Risk Category: D

HOW SUPPLIED
Injection: 10-mg vials

ACTION
Cross-links strands of cellular DNA and interferes with RNA transcription, causing an imbalance of growth that leads to cell death. Cell cycle–nonspecific.

Route	Onset	Peak	Duration
IV, intra-cavitary	Few seconds-few minutes	Unknown	Unknown

INDICATIONS & DOSAGE
Polycythemia vera, chronic lymphocytic leukemia, chronic myelocytic leukemia, malignant effusions (pericardial, peritoneal, pleural), mycosis fungoides, Hodgkin's disease, lymphosarcoma, bronchogenic cancer—
Adults: 0.4 mg/kg I.V. as a single dose or in divided doses of 0.1 to 0.2 mg/kg/day. Given through running I.V. infusion. Subsequent courses of therapy given when patient has recovered hematologically from previous course (usually 3 to 6 weeks).
Malignant effusions—
Adults: 0.4 mg/kg intracavitarily, although 0.2 mg/kg has been used intraperi-cardially.

ADVERSE REACTIONS
CNS: weakness, vertigo, neurotoxicity.
EENT: tinnitus; deafness (with high doses).
GI: *nausea, vomiting,* and *anorexia* beginning within minutes, lasting 8 to 24 hours; diarrhea; metallic taste.
Hematologic: *thrombocytopenia,* lymphocytopenia, *agranulocytosis,* nadir of myelosuppression occurring by days 4 to 10 and lasting 10 to 21 days; mild anemia begins in 2 to 3 weeks.
Skin: *alopecia,* rash, sloughing; severe ir-

ritation (if drug extravasates or touches skin).

Other: precipitation of herpes zoster, **anaphylaxis, secondary malignant disease,** hyperuricemia, *thrombophlebitis,* amyloidosis, jaundice, menstrual irregularities, impaired spermatogenesis.

INTERACTIONS
Drug-drug. *Anticoagulants, aspirin:* increased risk of bleeding. Avoid concomitant use.
Myelosuppressive agents: concomitant use can cause additive myelosuppression. Monitor patient.

EFFECTS ON DIAGNOSTIC TESTS
Drug therapy increases blood and urine uric acid levels. Renal, hepatic, and bone marrow function abnormalities have been reported.

CONTRAINDICATIONS
Contraindicated in patients with known infectious diseases or hypersensitivity to drug.

NURSING CONSIDERATIONS
● Use cautiously in patients with severe anemia, depressed neutrophil or platelet count, or in those who have recently undergone radiation therapy or chemotherapy. Monitor CBC.
● When given intracavitarily for sclerosing effect, dilute using up to 100 ml of 0.9% NaCl for injection. Turn patient from side to side every 5 to 10 minutes for 1 hour to distribute drug.
● Monitor serum uric acid level, as ordered. To prevent hyperuricemia with resulting uric acid nephropathy, know that mechlorethamine may be used with adequate hydration.
● Know that therapeutic effects are often accompanied by toxicity.
● Be aware that neurotoxicity increases with dose and patient age.
● To prevent bleeding, avoid all I.M. injections when platelet count is below 100,000/mm³.
● Anticipate possible blood transfusions because of cumulative anemia. Patients may receive RBC colony stimulating fac-

tors to promote RBC cell production and decrease the need for blood transfusions.

◖ I.V. administration
● Follow institutional policy to reduce risks. Preparation and administration of parenteral form of this drug is associated with carcinogenic, mutagenic, and teratogenic risks for personnel.
● Reconstitute drug using 10 ml of sterile water for injection or 0.9% NaCl injection. Resulting solution contains 1 mg/ml of mechlorethamine. Give by direct injection into a vein or into the tubing of a free-flowing I.V. solution.
● Prepare immediately before infusion. Very unstable solution. Visually inspect before using; use within 15 minutes, and discard unused solution.
● Dispose of equipment used in the preparation and administration of mechlorethamine properly and according to institutional policy. Neutralize unused solution with an equal volume of 5% sodium bicarbonate and 5% sodium thiosulfate for 45 minutes.
Alert: Make sure I.V. solution doesn't infiltrate. Mechlorethamine is a potent vesicant. If drug extravasates, apply cold compresses for 6 to 12 hours, and infiltrate the area with isotonic sodium thiosulfate, as ordered.

☑ Patient teaching
● Advise patient to watch for signs of infection (fever, sore throat, fatigue) and bleeding (easy bruising, nosebleeds, bleeding gums, melena). Tell patient to take temperature daily.
● Instruct patient to avoid OTC products containing aspirin.
● Advise women of childbearing age to avoid becoming pregnant during therapy. Suggest consulting with doctor before becoming pregnant.
● Caution breast-feeding patient taking drug to discontinue breast-feeding because of the possibility of infant toxicity.

melphalan
(L-phenylalanine mustard)
Alkeran

Pregnancy Risk Category: D

HOW SUPPLIED
Tablets (scored): 2 mg
Injection: 50 mg

ACTION
Cross-links strands of cellular DNA and interferes with RNA transcription, causing an imbalance of growth that leads to cell death. Cell cycle–nonspecific.

Route	Onset	Peak	Duration
PO, IV	Unknown	Unknown	Unknown

INDICATIONS & DOSAGE
Multiple myeloma—
Adults: initially, 6 mg P.O. daily for 2 to 3 weeks; then drug is stopped for up to 4 weeks or until WBC and platelet counts stop dropping and begin to rise again; maintenance dosage of 2 mg daily then given. Alternative therapy: 0.15 mg/kg P.O. daily for 7 days, or 0.25 mg/kg for 4 days; repeated q 4 to 6 weeks.

Alternatively, administered I.V. to patients who can't tolerate oral therapy. 16 mg/m^2 given by infusion over 15 to 20 minutes at 2-week intervals for four doses. After patient has recovered from toxicity, drug given at 4-week intervals.
Adjust-a-dose: In patients with renal insufficiency, dosage is reduced up to 50%.
Nonresectable advanced ovarian cancer—
Adults: 0.2 mg/kg P.O. daily for 5 days. Repeated q 4 to 6 weeks, depending on bone marrow recovery.

ADVERSE REACTIONS
CV: hypotension, tachycardia, edema.
GI: nausea, vomiting, diarrhea, oral ulceration, stomatitis.
Hematologic: *thrombocytopenia, leukopenia, bone marrow suppression,* hemolytic anemia.
Respiratory: *pneumonitis, pulmonary fibrosis,* dyspnea, bronchospasm.

Skin: pruritus, alopecia, urticaria; ulceration (at injection site).
Other: *anaphylaxis, hypersensitivity, hepatotoxicity,* hyperuricemia.

INTERACTIONS
Drug-drug. *Anticoagulants, aspirin:* increased risk of bleeding. Avoid concomitant use.
Antigout agents: decreased effectiveness. Dosage adjustments may be necessary.
Bone marrow suppressants: additive toxicity. Monitor closely.
Cyclosporine: severe renal failure may occur. Monitor closely.
Myelosuppressive agents: concomitant use can cause additive myelosuppression. Monitor patient
Vaccines: decreased effectiveness of killed-virus vaccines and increased risk of toxicity from live-virus vaccines. Postpone routine immunization for at least 3 months after last dose of melphalan.
Drug-food. *Any food:* decreased oral drug absorption. Give oral drug on an empty stomach.

EFFECTS ON DIAGNOSTIC TESTS
Drug therapy may increase blood and urine levels of uric acid.

CONTRAINDICATIONS
Contraindicated in patients with hypersensitivity to drug and in those whose disease is known to be resistant to drug. Patients hypersensitive to chlorambucil may have cross-sensitivity to melphalan.

NURSING CONSIDERATIONS
● Be aware that drug is not recommended in patients with severe leukopenia, thrombocytopenia, or anemia or in those with chronic lymphocytic leukemia. Use cautiously in patients receiving concurrent radiation and chemotherapy.
● Keep in mind that dosage may need to be reduced in patients with renal impairment.
● Know that melphalan is drug of choice in combination with prednisone in patients with multiple myeloma.
● Give oral form on empty stomach. Food decreases drug absorption.

Reactions may be *common,* uncommon, *life-threatening*, or COMMON AND LIFE-THREATENING.

• Monitor serum uric acid level and CBC, as ordered.
• To prevent bleeding, avoid all I.M. injections when platelet count is below 100,000/mm^3.
• Anticipate possible blood transfusions because of cumulative anemia. Patients may receive RBC colony stimulating factors to promote RBC production and decrease the need for blood transfusions.

◖ **I.V. administration**
• Follow institutional policy to reduce risks. Preparation and administration of parenteral form of drug are associated with carcinogenic, mutagenic, and teratogenic risks for personnel.
• Because drug isn't stable in solution, reconstitute immediately before administering with the 10 ml of sterile diluent supplied by the manufacturer. Shake vigorously until a solution is clear. The resultant solution will contain 5 mg/ml of melphalan. Immediately dilute required dose in 0.9% NaCl for injection. Final concentration shouldn't exceed 0.45 mg/ml. Give infusion over 15 to 20 minutes.
• Promptly dilute and administer; reconstituted product begins to degrade within 30 minutes. After final dilution, nearly 1% of drug degrades every 10 minutes. Don't refrigerate reconstituted product because a precipitate will form. Administration of drug must be completed within 60 minutes of reconstitution.

☑ **Patient teaching**
• Advise patient to watch for signs of infection (fever, sore throat, fatigue) and bleeding (easy bruising, nosebleeds, bleeding gums, melena). Tell patient to take temperature daily.
• Instruct patient to avoid OTC products containing aspirin.
• Advise women of childbearing age to avoid becoming pregnant during therapy. Suggest consulting with doctor before becoming pregnant.
• Caution breast-feeding patient taking drug to discontinue breast-feeding because of risk of infant toxicity.

streptozocin
Zanosar

Pregnancy Risk Category: C

HOW SUPPLIED
Injection: 1-g vials

ACTION
Unknown. Probably cross-links strands of cellular DNA and interferes with RNA transcription, causing an imbalance of growth that leads to cell death. Cell cycle–nonspecific.

Route	Onset	Peak	Duration
IV	Unknown	Unknown	Unknown

INDICATIONS & DOSAGE
Metastatic islet cell carcinoma of the pancreas—
Adults and children: 500 mg/m^2 I.V. for 5 consecutive days q 6 weeks until maximum benefit or toxicity is observed. Alternatively, 1,000 mg/m^2 at weekly intervals for the first 2 weeks. Not to exceed a single dose of 1,500 mg/m^2.

ADVERSE REACTIONS
CNS: confusion, lethargy, depression.
GI: *nausea, vomiting,* diarrhea.
GU: *renal toxicity* (evidenced by azotemia, glycosuria, and renal tubular acidosis), mild proteinuria.
Hematologic: *anemia, leukopenia, thrombocytopenia.*
Hepatic: elevated liver enzyme levels, jaundice, *liver dysfunction.*
Other: hyperglycemia, hypoglycemia, diabetes mellitus.

INTERACTIONS
Drug-drug. *Doxorubicin:* prolonged elimination half-life of doxorubicin. Dose of doxorubicin should be reduced.
Other potentially nephrotoxic drugs (such as aminoglycosides): increased risk of renal toxicity. Use cautiously.
Phenytoin: may decrease effectiveness of streptozocin in patients with pancreatic cancer. Monitor carefully.
Myelosuppressive agents: concomitant

use can cause additive myelosuppression. Monitor patient.

EFFECTS ON DIAGNOSTIC TESTS

Drug therapy may decrease serum albumin and increase liver function test values; these increases are a sign of hepatotoxicity. BUN and serum creatinine levels may be increased, indicating nephrotoxicity. Drug may decrease blood glucose levels because of a sudden release of insulin.

CONTRAINDICATIONS

No known contraindications.

NURSING CONSIDERATIONS

• Use cautiously in patients with renal disease.
• Obtain renal function tests before therapy, as ordered.
• Monitor renal function tests after each course of therapy, as ordered. Renal toxicity resulting from streptozocin therapy is dose-related and cumulative. Urinalysis, BUN, creatinine, serum electrolyte levels, and creatinine clearance should be obtained at least weekly during drug therapy. Weekly monitoring should continue for 4 weeks after each course.
• Test urine for protein and glucose levels each nursing shift. Mild proteinuria is one of the first signs of renal toxicity; notify doctor, who may reduce the dosage.
• Monitor CBC and liver function studies at least weekly, as ordered.
• Make sure patients are being treated with an antiemetic. Nausea and vomiting occur in most patients.
• Know that therapeutic effects are often accompanied by toxicity.

⬛I.V. administration

• Follow institutional policy to reduce risks. Preparation and administration of parenteral form of this drug is associated with carcinogenic, mutagenic, and teratogenic risks for personnel.
• Reconstitute streptozocin powder with 9.5 ml of D_5W or 0.9% NaCl for injection. This will produce a pale gold solution. May be further diluted with D_5W or 0.9% NaCl for injection. Infuse over at least 15 minutes to minimize the risk of phlebitis.

• Refrigerate unopened vials.
Alert: If extravasation occurs, stop infusion at once and notify doctor.
• Use within 12 hours of reconstitution. The product contains no preservatives and is not intended as a multiple-dose vial.

☑Patient teaching

• Advise patient to watch for signs of infection (fever, sore throat, fatigue) and bleeding (easy bruising, nosebleeds, bleeding gums, melena). Tell patient to take temperature daily.
• Caution breast-feeding patient taking drug to discontinue breast-feeding due to risk of infant toxicity.

---

thiotepa (TESPA, triethylenethiophosphoramide, TSPA)
Thioplex

Pregnancy Risk Category: D

HOW SUPPLIED

Injection: 15-mg vials

ACTION

Cross-links strands of cellular DNA and interferes with RNA transcription, causing an imbalance of growth that leads to cell death. Cell cycle–nonspecific.

Route	Onset	Peak	Duration
IV, intra-cavitary	Unknown	Unknown	Unknown

INDICATIONS & DOSAGE

Breast and ovarian cancers, lymphoma, Hodgkin's disease—
Adults and children over 12 years: 0.3 to 0.4 mg/kg I.V. q 1 to 4 weeks or 0.2 mg/kg for 4 to 5 days at intervals of 2 to 4 weeks.
Bladder tumor—
Adults and children over 12 years: 30 to 60 mg in 30 to 60 ml of NaCl instilled in bladder for 2 hours once weekly for 4 weeks.
Neoplastic effusions—
Adults and children over 12 years: 0.6 to 0.8 mg/kg intracavitarily q 1 to 4 weeks.

ADVERSE REACTIONS

CNS: headache, dizziness, fatigue, weakness.

EENT: blurred vision, laryngeal edema, conjunctivitis.

GI: *nausea, vomiting,* abdominal pain, anorexia, stomatitis.

GU: amenorrhea, decreased spermatogenesis, dysuria, urine retention, hemorrhagic cystitis.

Hematologic: *leukopenia* begins within 5 to 10 days; *thrombocytopenia; neutropenia; anemia.*

Respiratory: asthma.

Skin: hives, rash, dermatitis, alopecia; pain (at injection site).

Other: fever, *hypersensitivity, anaphylactic shock.*

INTERACTIONS

Drug-drug. *Anticoagulants, aspirin:* increased risk of bleeding. Avoid concomitant use.

Myelosuppressive agents: concomitant use can cause additive myelosuppression. Monitor patient.

Neuromuscular blocking agents: may prolong muscular paralysis. Monitor closely.

Other alkylating agents, irradiation therapy: may intensify toxicity rather than enhance therapeutic response. Avoid concurrent use.

Succinylcholine: increased apnea with concomitant use. Avoid concurrent use.

EFFECTS ON DIAGNOSTIC TESTS

Drug therapy may increase blood and urine levels of uric acid and decrease plasma pseudocholinesterase concentrations.

CONTRAINDICATIONS

Contraindicated in patients with severe bone marrow, hepatic, or renal dysfunction and hypersensitivity to drug.

NURSING CONSIDERATIONS

● Know that use in pregnancy is not recommended except in situations where the benefits outweigh the risk of teratogenicity involved.

● Use cautiously in patients with mild bone marrow suppression and renal or hepatic dysfunction.

● For bladder instillation: Dehydrate patient 8 to 10 hours before therapy. Instill drug into bladder by catheter; ask patient to retain solution for 2 hours. Know that volume may be reduced to 30 ml if discomfort is too great with 60 ml. Reposition patient every 15 minutes for maximum area contact.

● Monitor CBC weekly for at least 3 weeks after last dose, as ordered.

● Be aware that drug should be discontinued if patient's WBC count drops below 3,000/mm³ or if platelet count falls below 150,000/mm³. If that occurs, notify doctor. If WBC count falls below 2,000/mm³ or granulocyte count falls below 1,000/mm³, follow institutional policy for infection control in immunocompromised patients.

● Monitor serum uric acid levels, as ordered. To prevent hyperuricemia with resulting uric acid nephropathy, know that allopurinol may be used with adequate hydration.

● Know that therapeutic effects are often accompanied by toxicity.

● To prevent bleeding, avoid all I.M. injections when platelet count is below 100,000/mm³.

● Anticipate blood transfusions because of cumulative anemia. Patient may require injections of RBC colony stimulating factors to promote RBC production and decrease need for blood transfusions.

● Refrigerate and protect dry powder from direct sunlight to avoid possible drug breakdown.

◖I.V. administration

● Follow institutional policy to minimize risks. Preparation and administration of parenteral form of this drug is linked with mutagenic, teratogenic, and carcinogenic risks to personnel.

● Reconstitute with 1.5 ml of sterile water for injection. Do not reconstitute with any other solution. Further dilute with 0.9% NaCl for injection, D_5W, dextrose 5% in 0.9% NaCl for injection, Ringer's injection, or lactated Ringer's injection. Solutions should be used in 8 hours.

● If pain occurs at insertion site, dilute drug further or use a local anesthetic, as

---

ordered, to reduce pain. Make sure drug does not infiltrate.

• Discard if solution appears grossly opaque or has a precipitate. Solutions should be clear to slightly opaque. To eliminate haze, filter solutions through a 0.22-micron filter before administration.

☑ Patient teaching

• Advise patient to watch for signs of infection (fever, sore throat, fatigue) and bleeding (easy bruising, nosebleeds, bleeding gums, melena). Tell patient to take temperature daily. Tell patient to report even mild infections.

• Instruct patient to avoid OTC products containing aspirin.

• Advise breast-feeding patient to stop breast-feeding during therapy because of possible infant toxicity.

• Caution women of childbearing age to avoid becoming pregnant during therapy. Suggest consulting with doctor before becoming pregnant.

capecitabine
cladribine
cytarabine
floxuridine
fludarabine phosphate
fluorouracil
hydroxyurea
mercaptopurine
methotrexate
methotrexate sodium
thioguanine

COMBINATION PRODUCTS
None.

▼ *NEW DRUG*

capecitabine
Xeloda

Pregnancy Risk Category: D

HOW SUPPLIED
Tablets: 150 mg, 500 mg

ACTION
Capecitabine is converted to the active drug 5-fluorouracil (5-FU). 5-FU is metabolized by both normal and tumor cells to metabolites that cause cellular injury via two different mechanisms: interference with DNA synthesis to inhibit cell division and interference with RNA processing and protein synthesis.

Route	Onset	Peak	Duration
PO	Unknown	1.5-2 hr	Unknown

INDICATIONS & DOSAGE
Treatment of patients with metastatic breast cancer resistant to both paclitaxel and an anthracycline-containing chemotherapy regimen or resistant to paclitaxel and for whom further anthracycline therapy is not indicated—
Adults: 2,500 mg/m^2 P.O. daily in two divided doses (approximately 12 hours apart) at end of a meal for 2 weeks, followed by a 1-week rest period given as 3-week cycles.

Adjust-a-dose: National Cancer Institute of Canada (NCIC) Common Toxicity Criteria: NCIC grade 2: first appearance, interrupt treatment until resolved to grade 0 to 1, then restart at 100% of starting dose for next cycle; second appearance, interrupt treatment until resolved to grade 0 to 1 and use 75% of starting dose for next cycle; third appearance, interrupt treatment until resolved to grade 0 to 1 and use 50% of starting dose for next cycle; fourth appearance, discontinue treatment permanently.

NCIC grade 3: first appearance, interrupt treatment until resolved to grade 0 to 1 and use 75% of starting dose for next cycle; second appearance, interrupt treatment until resolved to grade 0 to 1 and use 50% of starting dose for next cycle; third appearance, discontinue treatment permanently.

NCIC grade 4: first appearance, discontinue treatment permanently or interrupt treatment until resolved to grade 0 to 1 and use 50% of starting dose for next cycle.

Note: Toxicity criteria relate to degrees of severity of diarrhea, nausea, vomiting, stomatitis, and hand/foot syndrome. Refer to capecitabine package insert for specific toxicity definitions.

ADVERSE REACTIONS
CNS: dizziness, *fatigue,* headache, insomnia, *paresthesia.*
CV: edema.
EENT: eye irritation.
GI: *diarrhea, nausea, vomiting, stomatitis, abdominal pain, constipation, anorexia,* anemia, *dyspepsia.*
Hematologic: NEUTROPENIA, THROMBOCYTOPENIA, *anemia, lymphopenia.*
Hepatic: *hyperbilirubinemia.*
Musculoskeletal: myalgia, pain in limb.
Skin: *hand-and-foot syndrome, dermatitis,* nail disorder.
Other: *pyrexia,* dehydration.

INTERACTIONS
Drug-drug. *Leucovorin*: increased concentration of 5-FU with enhanced toxicity. Monitor patient carefully.

EFFECTS ON DIAGNOSTIC TESTS
None reported.

CONTRAINDICATIONS
Contraindicated in patients with known hypersensitivity to 5-FU.

NURSING CONSIDERATIONS
• Use cautiously in patients with history of coronary artery disease, mild-to-moderate hepatic dysfunction due to liver metastases, hyperbilirubinemia, renal insufficiency, and in the elderly. Safety and effectiveness have not been established in patients 18 years or younger.
• Know that patients older than 80 years may experience a greater incidence of GI adverse effects.
• Monitor for and notify doctor if severe diarrhea occurs. Give fluid and electrolyte replacement as ordered if patient becomes dehydrated. Drug may need to be immediately interrupted until diarrhea resolves or decreases in intensity.
• Monitor for hand-and-foot syndrome (characterized by numbness, paresthesia, tingling, painless or painful swelling, erythema, desquamation, blistering and severe pain of hands or feet), hyperbilirubinemia, and severe nausea. Drug therapy will need to be immediately adjusted.
• Know that hyperbilirubinemia may require stopping drug.
Alert: Monitor patient carefully for toxicity. Toxicity may be managed by symptomatic treatment, dose interruptions, and dosage adjustments.

☑ Patient teaching
• Inform patient and caregiver of expected adverse effects of drug, especially nausea, vomiting, diarrhea, and hand-and-foot syndrome (pain, swelling or redness of hands or feet). Tell them that patient-specific dose adaptations during therapy are expected and necessary.
Alert: Instruct patient to stop taking drug and contact doctor immediately if the following adverse effects occur: diarrhea (over four bowel movements daily or diarrhea at night), vomiting (two to five episodes in a 24-hour period), nausea, appetite loss or decrease in amount of food taken each day, stomatitis (pain, redness, swelling or sores in mouth), hand-and-foot syndrome, fever of 100.5° F (38° C) or greater or other evidence of infection.
• Tell patient that most adverse effects improve within 2 to 3 days after stopping drug. If these don't improve, tell him to contact doctor.
• Tell patient how to take the medication. Drug is usually taken for 14 days followed by a 7-day rest period (no drug) given as a 21-day cycle. The doctor determines the number of treatment cycles.
• Instruct patient to take drug with water within 30 minutes after end of a meal (breakfast and dinner).
• If a combination of tablets is prescribed, teach patient importance of correctly identifying the tablets to avoid possible misdosing.
• For missed doses, instruct patient not to take the missed dose and not to double the next one. Instead, he should continue with regular dosing schedule and check with the doctor.
• Instruct patient to inform doctor if he is taking the vitamin folic acid.
• Advise women of childbearing age to avoid becoming pregnant while receiving treatment.
• Advise breast-feeding patient to discontinue breast-feeding while on drug therapy.

cladribine (CdA, 2-chlorodeoxyadenosine)
Leustat§, Leustatin

Pregnancy Risk Category: D

HOW SUPPLIED
Injection: 1 mg/ml, 10-mg vial, preservative-free

ACTION
Unknown. A purine nucleoside analogue that enters tumor cells, is phosphorylated by deoxycytidine kinase, and is subsequently converted into an active triphosphate deoxynucleotide. This metabolite

probably impairs synthesis of new DNA, inhibits repair of existing DNA, and disrupts cellular metabolism.

Route	Onset	Peak	Duration
IV	4 mo	Unknown	> 8 mo

INDICATIONS & DOSAGE
Active hairy cell leukemia—
Adults: 0.09 mg/kg daily by continuous I.V. infusion for 7 days.

ADVERSE REACTIONS
CNS: *headache, fatigue,* dizziness, insomnia, asthenia.
CV: tachycardia, edema.
EENT: epistaxis.
GI: *nausea, decreased appetite, vomiting, diarrhea,* constipation, abdominal pain.
Hematologic: NEUTROPENIA, *anemia, thrombocytopenia.*
Respiratory: *abnormal breath or chest sounds, cough,* shortness of breath.
Skin: *rash, pruritus, erythema, purpura,* petechiae.
Other: *fever,* INFECTION, *chills, diaphoresis, malaise, trunk pain, myalgia, arthralgia,* hyperuricemia, insomnia; *local reaction* (at injection site).

INTERACTIONS
None significant.

EFFECTS ON DIAGNOSTIC TESTS
Drug frequently alters hematologic studies because of its suppressive effect on bone marrow. It may increase blood and urine concentrations of uric acid.

CONTRAINDICATIONS
Contraindicated in patients hypersensitive to drug.

NURSING CONSIDERATIONS
• Use cautiously in patients with renal or hepatic impairment.
• Because of risk of hyperuricemia from tumor lysis, administer allopurinol, as ordered, during therapy.
• Monitor hematologic function closely, as ordered, especially during the first 4 to 8 weeks of therapy. Cladribine is a toxic drug, and some toxicity is expected during treatment. Severe bone marrow suppression, including neutropenia, anemia, and thrombocytopenia, has commonly been observed in patients treated with drug; many patients also have preexisting hematologic impairment from their disease.
• Keep in mind that fever is common during the first month of therapy. In clinical trials, virtually all patients received parenteral antibiotics.
• To prevent bleeding, avoid all I.M. injections when platelet count is below 100,000/mm³.
• If WBC count falls below 2,000/mm³ or granulocyte count falls below 1,000/mm³, follow institutional policy for infection control in immunocompromised patients.
• Anticipate possible blood transfusions because of cumulative anemia. Patient may receive injections of RBC colony stimulating factors to promote RBC production and decrease need for blood transfusions.

◘I.V. administration
• For a 24-hour infusion, add the calculated dose to a 500-ml infusion bag of 0.9% NaCl for injection. Once diluted, administer promptly or store in refrigerator for no more than 8 hours. Don't use solutions that contain dextrose because studies have shown increased degradation of drug. Repeat preparation daily for 7 consecutive days.
Alert: Because drug product doesn't contain bacteriostatic agents, use strict aseptic technique to prepare the daily admixture.
• Alternatively, prepare a 7-day infusion solution, using bacteriostatic NaCl for injection, which contains 0.9% benzyl alcohol. Studies have shown acceptable physical and chemical stability using Pharmacia Deltec medication cassettes. First, pass the calculated amount of drug through a disposable 0.22-micron hydrophilic syringe filter into a sterile infusion reservoir. Next, add sufficient bacteriostatic NaCl injection to bring the total volume to 100 ml. Clamp off the line; then disconnect and discard the filter. If necessary, aseptically aspirate air bubbles from the reservoir using a new filter or a sterile vent filter assembly.

• Be aware that because the calculated dose dilutes the benzyl alcohol preservative, 7-day infusion solutions prepared for patients weighing over 85 kg (187 lb) may have reduced preservative effectiveness.

• Refrigerate unopened vials at 36° to 46° F (2° to 8° C) and protect from light. Although freezing doesn't adversely affect drug, a precipitate may form; this will disappear if drug is allowed to warm to room temperature gradually and vial is vigorously shaken. Don't heat or microwave; don't refreeze.

☑ **Patient teaching**

• Instruct patient to watch for signs of infection and bleeding (easy bruising, nosebleeds, bleeding gums, melena). Tell patient to take temperature daily.

• Caution women of childbearing age to avoid becoming pregnant because of risk of fetal malformations.

• Advise breast-feeding patient to discontinue breast-feeding during therapy because of possible infant toxicity.

---

cytarabine (ara-C, cytosine arabinoside)
Cytosar†, Cytosar-U

Pregnancy Risk Category: D

HOW SUPPLIED
Injection: 100-mg, 500-mg, 1-g, 2-g vials

ACTION
Inhibits DNA synthesis.

Route	Onset	Peak	Duration
IV, intrathecal	Unknown	Unknown	Unknown
SC	Unknown	20-60 min	Unknown

INDICATIONS & DOSAGE
Acute nonlymphocytic leukemia, acute lymphocytic leukemia, blast phase of chronic myelocytic leukemia—
Adults and children: 100 mg/m² daily by continuous I.V. infusion or 100 mg/m² I.V. q 12 hours. Given for 7 days and repeated q 2 weeks. For maintenance, 1 mg/kg S.C. once or twice weekly.

Meningeal leukemia—
Adults and children: highly variable from 5 to 75 mg/m² intrathecally. Frequency also varies from once daily for 4 days to once q 4 days. The most frequently used dosage is 30 mg/m², q 4 days until CSF fluid is normal, followed by one additional dose.

ADVERSE REACTIONS
CNS: neurotoxicity, malaise, dizziness, headache.
EENT: conjunctivitis.
GI: *nausea, vomiting, diarrhea, anorexia, anal ulceration,* abdominal pain; oral ulcers in 5 to 10 days; projectile vomiting, bowel necrosis (high dose given rapid I.V.).
GU: urine retention, renal dysfunction.
Hematologic: *leukopenia,* with initial WBC count nadir 7 to 9 days after drug is stopped and a second (more severe) nadir 15 to 24 days after drug is stopped; anemia; reticulocytopenia; *thrombocytopenia,* with platelet count nadir occurring on day 12 to 15; *megaloblastosis.*
Hepatic: *hepatotoxicity* (usually mild and reversible), jaundice.
Skin: *rash,* pruritus, alopecia, freckling.
Other: flulike syndrome, hyperuricemia, infection, *fever, thrombophlebitis,* myalgia, bone pain, **anaphylaxis,** edema.

INTERACTIONS
Drug-drug. *Digoxin:* may decrease digoxin absorption. Monitor closely. Digoxin oral liquid and liquid-filled capsules may not be affected.
Flucytosine: decreased flucytosine activity. Avoid concomitant use.
Gentamicin: decreased activity against *Klebsiella pneumoniae.* Avoid concomitant use.

EFFECTS ON DIAGNOSTIC TESTS
Drug therapy may increase blood and urine levels of uric acid. It may also increase serum alkaline phosphatase, AST, and bilirubin concentrations, which indicate drug-induced hepatotoxicity.

CONTRAINDICATIONS
Contraindicated in patients hypersensitive to drug.

Reactions may be *common,* uncommon, ***life-threatening***, or COMMON AND LIFE-THREATENING.

NURSING CONSIDERATIONS

• Use cautiously in patients with hepatic or renal compromise, gout, or myelosuppression.

• For intrathecal administration, use preservative-free 0.9% NaCl. Add 5 ml to the 100-mg vial or 10 ml to 500-mg vial. Use immediately after reconstitution. Discard unused drug.

• Monitor fluid intake and output carefully. Maintain high fluid intake and give allopurinol, if ordered, to avoid urate nephropathy in leukemia-induction therapy. Monitor serum uric acid level, as ordered.

• Monitor hepatic and renal function studies and CBC, as ordered.

• Know that therapy may be modified or stopped if granulocyte count is below 1,000/mm³ or if platelet count is below 50,000/mm³.

• Know that corticosteroid eyedrops are prescribed to prevent drug-induced keratitis.

• Provide diligent mouth care to help prevent stomatitis.

Alert: Assess patient receiving high doses for neurotoxicity, which may first appear as nystagmus, but can progress to ataxia and cerebellar dysfunction.

• To prevent bleeding, avoid all I.M. injections when platelet count is below 100,000/mm³.

• Anticipate possible blood transfusions because of cumulative anemia. Patient may receive RBC colony stimulating factors to promote RBC production and decrease need for blood transfusions.

• Know that therapeutic effects are often accompanied by toxicity.

⬛ I.V. administration
• To reduce nausea, give antiemetic before administering, as ordered. Nausea and vomiting are more frequent when large doses are administered rapidly by I.V. push. These reactions are less frequent when given by infusion.

• Follow institutional policy to reduce risks. Preparation and administration of parenteral form of drug is associated with carcinogenic, mutagenic, and teratogenic risks for personnel.

• Reconstitute drug using the provided diluent, which is bacteriostatic water for injection containing benzyl alcohol. Avoid this diluent when preparing drug for neonates or for intrathecal use. Reconstitute 100-mg vial with 5 ml of diluent or 500-mg vial with 10 ml of diluent. Reconstituted solution is stable for 48 hours. Discard cloudy reconstituted solution.

• For I.V. infusion, further dilute using 0.9% NaCl for injection or D_5W.

☑ Patient teaching
• Instruct patient to watch for signs of infection (fever, sore throat, fatigue) and bleeding (easy bruising, nosebleeds, bleeding gums, melena). Tell patients to take temperature daily.

• Advise breast-feeding patient to discontinue breast-feeding during therapy because of possible infant toxicity.

• Caution women of childbearing age to avoid becoming pregnant during therapy. Also recommend consulting with doctor before becoming pregnant. Drug may harm the fetus.

---

floxuridine
(fluorodeoxyuridine)
FUDR

Pregnancy Risk Category: D

HOW SUPPLIED
Powder for injection: 500 mg for reconstitution (5-ml, 10-ml vials)
Preservative-free injection: 100 mg/ml (5-ml vials)

ACTION
Inhibits DNA synthesis.

Route	Onset	Peak	Duration
Intra-arterial	Unknown	Unknown	Unknown

INDICATIONS & DOSAGE
GI adenocarcinoma metastatic to the liver—
Adults: 0.1 to 0.6 mg/kg daily by intra-arterial infusion for 14 to 21 days or until toxicity occurs; or 0.4 to 0.6 mg/kg daily into hepatic artery.

ADVERSE REACTIONS
CNS: malaise, weakness, headache, lethargy, disorientation, confusion, euphoria.
CV: *myocardial ischemia,* angina.
EENT: blurred vision, nystagmus, photophobia, epistaxis.
GI: *anorexia, stomatitis, nausea, vomiting, diarrhea, bleeding, abdominal pain, enteritis,* GI ulceration, intra- and extrahepatic biliary sclerosis, acalculous cholecystitis.
Hematologic: *leukopenia, anemia, thrombocytopenia, agranulocytosis.*
Skin: *erythema,* dermatitis, pruritus, rash, alopecia, photosensitivity.
Other: thrombophlebitis, *anaphylaxis,* fever.

INTERACTIONS
Drug-lifestyle. *Sun exposure:* may increase skin reaction. Take precautions.

EFFECTS ON DIAGNOSTIC TESTS
Drug therapy may increase serum concentrations of ALT, AST, alkaline phosphatase, bilirubin, and LD; these increases indicate drug-induced hepatotoxicity.

CONTRAINDICATIONS
Contraindicated in patients with poor nutritional state, bone marrow suppression, or serious infection.

NURSING CONSIDERATIONS
• Use cautiously following high-dose pelvic radiation therapy or use of alkylating agents and in patients with impaired hepatic or renal function.
• Check line for bleeding, blockage, displacement, or leakage.
• Monitor fluid intake and output, CBC, and renal and hepatic function, as ordered.
• Know that use of antacid eases but won't prevent GI distress. An H_2 antihistamine is recommended to prevent peptic ulcer disease during drug therapy.
• Provide diligent mouth care to help prevent stomatitis.
• Be aware that severe skin and adverse GI reactions require stopping drug.
• Know that drug should be discontinued if patient's WBC count drops below 3,500/mm³ or if his platelet count falls

below 100,000/mm³. If either occurs, notify doctor. If WBC count falls below 2,000/mm³ or granulocyte count falls below 1,000/mm³, follow institutional policy for infection control in immunocompromised patients.
• To prevent bleeding, avoid all I.M. injections when platelet count is below 100,000/mm³.
• Anticipate possible blood transfusions because of cumulative anemia. Patients may receive injections of RBC colony-stimulating factors to promote RBC production and decrease need for blood transfusions.

🔆 I.V. administration
• Follow institutional policy to reduce risks. Preparation and administration of parenteral form of drug are associated with carcinogenic, mutagenic, and teratogenic risks for personnel.
• Reconstitute with sterile water for injection. To prepare infusion, dilute in D_5W or 0.9% NaCl solution.
• Refrigerated solution is stable for no more than 2 weeks.
• Use an infusion pump with intra-arterial infusions.

✅ Patient teaching
• Inform patient that therapeutic effect may be delayed 1 to 6 weeks.
• Inform patient receiving medication at home to monitor placement of needle into catheter site and to call his infusion provider immediately if the needle becomes dislodged.
• Advise patient to watch for signs of infection (fever, sore throat, fatigue) and bleeding (easy bruising, nosebleeds, bleeding gums, melena). Tell patient to take temperature daily.
• Tell patient that exposure to sun may initiate or intensify skin reaction.
• Advise breast-feeding patient to discontinue breast-feeding during therapy because of possible infant toxicity.
• Caution women of childbearing age to avoid becoming pregnant during therapy. Also recommend consulting with doctor before becoming pregnant.

---

fludarabine phosphate
Fludara

Pregnancy Risk Category: D

HOW SUPPLIED
Powder for injection: 50 mg

ACTION
Unknown. An antineoplastic antimetabolite that may have multifaceted actions. After conversion to its active metabolite, fludarabine interferes with DNA synthesis by inhibiting DNA polymerase alpha, ribonucleotide reductase, and DNA primase.

Route	Onset	Peak	Duration
IV	7-21 wk	Unknown	Unknown

INDICATIONS & DOSAGE
B-cell chronic lymphocytic leukemia in patients who have either not responded or responded inadequately to at least one standard alkylating agent regimen—
Adults: 25 mg/m² I.V. over 30 minutes for 5 consecutive days. Cycle repeated q 28 days.

ADVERSE REACTIONS
CNS: *fatigue, malaise, weakness, paresthesia,* peripheral neuropathy, headache, sleep disorder, depression, cerebellar syndrome, ***CVA,*** transient ischemic attack, agitation, *confusion;* ***coma, death*** (with very high doses).
CV: *edema,* angina, phlebitis, ***arrhythmias, heart failure, MI,*** supraventricular tachycardia, deep venous thrombosis, ***aneurysm, hemorrhage.***
EENT: *visual disturbances,* hearing loss, delayed blindness (with high doses), sinusitis, pharyngitis, sinusitis, epistaxis.
GI: *nausea, vomiting, diarrhea,* constipation, *anorexia,* stomatitis, *GI bleeding,* esophagitis, mucositis.
GU: dysuria, *urinary infection* or hesitancy, proteinuria, hematuria, ***renal failure.***
Hematologic: ***hemolytic anemia,*** MYELO-SUPPRESSION.
Hepatic: ***liver failure,*** cholelithiasis.
Respiratory: *cough, pneumonia, dyspnea, upper respiratory tract infection,* allergic pneumonitis, hemoptysis, hypoxia, bronchitis.
Skin: *rash,* pruritus, alopecia, seborrhea.
Other: *fever, chills, pain, myalgia,* tumor lysis syndrome, INFECTION, ***anaphylaxis,*** diaphoresis, hypocalcemia, hyperkalemia, hyperglycemia, dehydration, hyperuricemia, hyperphosphatemia.

INTERACTIONS
Drug-drug. *Other myelosuppressants:* increased toxicity. Avoid concomitant use.
Pentostatin: increases risk of pulmonary toxicity, which can be fatal. Avoid concomitant administration.

EFFECTS ON DIAGNOSTIC TESTS
Drug may increase alkaline phosphatase, AST, and uric acid levels.

CONTRAINDICATIONS
Contraindicated in patients hypersensitive to drug or its components.

NURSING CONSIDERATIONS
• Use cautiously in patients with renal insufficiency.
Alert: Monitor patient closely and expect modified dosage based on toxicity. Most toxic effects are dose-dependent. Advanced age, renal insufficiency, and bone marrow impairment may predispose patients to increased or excessive toxicity.
• Know that careful hematologic monitoring is required, especially of neutrophil and platelet counts. Bone marrow suppression can be severe.
• To prevent bleeding, avoid all I.M. injections when platelet count is below 100,000/mm³.
• Anticipate possible blood transfusions because of cumulative anemia. Patients may receive RBC colony-stimulating factors to promote RBC production and decrease need for blood transfusions.
• Know that optimal duration of therapy is not yet determined. Current recommendations suggest three additional cycles after achieving maximal response before discontinuing therapy.
• Take preventive measures before starting drug treatment. Hyperuricemia, hypocalcemia, hyperkalemia, and renal

failure may result from rapid lysis of tumor cells.
• Store drug in refrigerator at 36° to 46° F (2° to 8° C).

I.V. administration
• Follow institutional policy to reduce risks. Preparation and administration of parenteral form of drug are associated with mutagenic, teratogenic, and carcinogenic risks for personnel.
• To prepare solution, add 2 ml of sterile water for injection to the solid cake of fludarabine. Dissolution should occur within 15 seconds; each milliliter will contain 25 mg of drug. Dilute further in 100 or 125 ml of D_5W or 0.9% NaCl for injection. Use within 8 hours of reconstitution.

Patient teaching
• Instruct patient to watch for signs of infection (fever, sore throat, fatigue) and bleeding (easy bruising, nosebleeds, bleeding gums, melena). Tell patient to take temperature daily.
• Advise women of childbearing age to avoid becoming pregnant during therapy. Also recommend consulting with doctor before becoming pregnant.
• Caution breast-feeding patient to discontinue breast-feeding during therapy because of possible infant toxicity.

---

fluorouracil
(5-fluorouracil, 5-FU)
Adrucil, Efudex, Fluoroplex

Pregnancy Risk Category: D (injection), X (topical form)

HOW SUPPLIED
Injection: 50 mg/ml
Cream: 1%, 5%
Topical solution: 1%, 2%, 5%

ACTION
Thought to inhibit DNA and RNA synthesis.

Route	Onset	Peak	Duration
IV, topical	Unknown	Unknown	Unknown

INDICATIONS & DOSAGE
Colon, rectal, breast, stomach, and pancreatic cancers—
Adults: initially, 12 mg/kg I.V. daily for 4 days; if no toxicity, 6 mg/kg given on days 6, 8, 10, and 12; then a single weekly maintenance dose of 10 to 15 mg/kg I.V. begun after toxicity (if any) from initial course has subsided. (Dosages recommended based on actual body weight unless patient is obese or retaining fluid.) Maximum single recommended dose is 800 mg/day.
Palliative treatment of advanced colorectal cancer—
Adults: 425 mg/m² I.V. daily for 5 consecutive days. Given with 20 mg/m² of leucovorin I.V. Repeated at 4-week intervals for two additional courses; then repeated at intervals of 4 to 5 weeks if tolerated.
Multiple actinic (solar) keratoses; superficial basal cell carcinoma—
Adults: apply cream or topical solution once or twice daily. Usual duration of treatment is 2 to 6 weeks.

ADVERSE REACTIONS
CNS: acute cerebellar syndrome, confusion, disorientation, euphoria, ataxia, headache, nystagmus, *weakness, malaise.*
CV: *myocardial ischemia,* angina.
EENT: epistaxis, photophobia, lacrimation, lacrimal duct stenosis, visual changes.
GI: *stomatitis, GI ulcer* (may precede leukopenia), *nausea, vomiting, diarrhea, anorexia,* GI bleeding.
Hematologic: *leukopenia, thrombocytopenia, agranulocytosis,* anemia; WBC count nadir 9 to 14 days after first dose; platelet count nadir in 7 to 14 days.
Hepatic: May increase alkaline phosphatase, serum transaminases, bilirubin, and LD.
Skin: *dermatitis; erythema; scaling; pruritus;* nail changes; pigmented palmar creases; erythematous, contact dermatitis, desquamative rash of hands and feet ("hand-and-foot syndrome" with long-term use); photosensitivity, *reversible alopecia.*
Other: *pain, burning,* soreness, suppura-

---

tion, swelling (with topical use), *anaphylaxis,* thrombophlebitis.

INTERACTIONS
Drug-drug. *Leucovorin calcium, prior treatment with alkylating agents:* increased toxicity of fluorouracil. Use with extreme caution.
Drug-lifestyle. *Sun exposure:* photosensitivity reactions may occur. Take precautions.

EFFECTS ON DIAGNOSTIC TESTS
Drug may decrease plasma albumin concentrations because of drug-induced protein malabsorption. Drug may also increase 5-hydroxyintole acetic acid in urine.

CONTRAINDICATIONS
Contraindicated in patients hypersensitive to drug; in those who are in a poor nutritional state; in patients with bone marrow suppression (WBC counts of $5,000/mm^3$ or less or platelet counts of $100,000/mm^3$ or less), or potentially serious infections; and in those who have had major surgery within the previous month.

NURSING CONSIDERATIONS
• Use cautiously after high-dose pelvic radiation therapy or use of alkylating agents, or in patients with impaired hepatic or renal function or widespread neoplastic infiltration of bone marrow.
• Apply topical form with caution near eyes, nose, and mouth.
• Avoid occlusive dressings with topical dressings because they increase the risk of inflammatory reactions in adjacent normal skin.
• Wash hands immediately after handling topical form of medication. Apply topical form with a nonmetal applicator or suitable gloves.
• Expect to use 1% topical concentration on the face. Higher concentrations are used for thicker-skinned areas or resistant lesions.
• Expect to use 5% topical strength for superficial basal cell carcinoma confirmed by biopsy.
• Be aware that ingestion and systemic absorption of topical form may cause

leukopenia, thrombocytopenia, stomatitis, diarrhea, or GI ulceration, bleeding, and hemorrhage. Application to large ulcerated areas may cause systemic toxicity.
• Watch for stomatitis or diarrhea (signs of toxicity). May use topical oral anesthetic to soothe lesions, as ordered. Discontinue drug if diarrhea occurs and notify doctor.
• Encourage diligent oral hygiene to prevent superinfection of denuded mucosa.
• Monitor WBC and platelet counts daily, as ordered. Watch for ecchymoses, petechiae, easy bruising, and anemia.
• Monitor fluid intake and output, CBC, and renal and hepatic function tests, as ordered.
• Be aware that dermatologic adverse effects are reversible when drug is stopped.
• To prevent bleeding, avoid all I.M. injections when platelet count is below $100,000/mm^3$.
• Anticipate possible blood transfusions because of cumulative anemia. Patient may receive injections of RBC colony-stimulating factors to promote RBC production and decrease need for blood transfusions.
Alert: Be alert that fluorouracil toxicity may be delayed for 1 to 3 weeks.
• Know that drug is sometimes ordered as 5-fluorouracil or 5-FU. The numeral 5 is part of drug name and should not be confused with dosage units.

█ I.V. administration
• Follow institutional policy to reduce risks. Preparation and administration of parenteral form of drug are associated with carcinogenic, mutagenic, and teratogenic risks for personnel.
• Give antiemetic, as ordered, before administering drug to reduce nausea.
• Know that drug may be administered by direct injection without dilution. For I.V. infusion, drug may be diluted with D_5W, sterile water for injection, or 0.9% NaCl for injection. Discard unused portion of vial after 1 hour.
• Don't use cloudy solution. If crystals form, redissolve by warming.
• Use plastic I.V. containers for administering continuous infusions. Solution is

---

more stable in plastic I.V. bags than in glass bottles.
• Don't refrigerate fluorouracil. Protect drug from sunlight.

☑ **Patient teaching**
• Warn patient that alopecia may occur, but that it's reversible.
• Caution patient to avoid prolonged exposure to sunlight or ultraviolet light when topical form is used.
• Tell patient to use highly protective sunblock to avoid inflammatory erythematous dermatitis. Long-term use of drug is associated with erythematous, desquamative rash of the hands and feet. May be treated with pyridoxine (50 to 150 mg P.O. daily) for 5 to 7 days.
• Warn patient that topically treated area may be unsightly during therapy and for several weeks after therapy. Complete healing may take 1 or 2 months.
• Caution women of childbearing age to avoid becoming pregnant during therapy. Also recommend consulting with doctor before becoming pregnant.
• Advise breast-feeding patient to discontinue breast-feeding during therapy because of possible infant toxicity.

---

hydroxyurea
Droxia, Hydrea**

Pregnancy Risk Category: D

HOW SUPPLIED
Capsules: 200, 300, 400, 500 mg

ACTION
Unknown. Thought to inhibit DNA synthesis.

Route	Onset	Peak	Duration
PO	Unknown	2 hr	24 hr

INDICATIONS & DOSAGE
Melanoma; resistant chronic myelocytic leukemia; recurrent, metastatic, or inoperable ovarian cancer; head and neck cancers—
Adults: 80 mg/kg P.O. as single dose q 3 days; or 20 to 30 mg/kg P.O. as a single daily dose.

✳ *NEW INDICATION: Reduce frequency of painful crises and need for blood transfusions in adult patients with sickle cell anemia with recurrent moderate-to-severe painful crises—*
Adults: 15 mg/kg P.O. once daily. If blood counts are in acceptable range, dose may be increased by 5 mg/kg/day q 12 weeks until maximum tolerated dose or 35 mg/kg/day has been reached. If blood counts are considered toxic, withhold drug until hematologic recovery occurs. Resume treatment after reducing dose by 2.5 mg/kg/day. Every 12 weeks, drug may then be titrated up or down in 2.5 mg/kg/day increments until patient is at stable, nontoxic dose for 24 weeks.

ADVERSE REACTIONS
CNS: hallucinations, headache, dizziness, disorientation, *seizures,* malaise.
GI: *anorexia, nausea, vomiting, diarrhea,* stomatitis, constipation.
GU: increased BUN and serum creatinine levels.
Hematologic: *leukopenia, thrombocytopenia,* anemia, megaloblastosis; *dose-limiting and dose-related bone marrow suppression,* with rapid recovery.
Skin: alopecia (rare), rash, itching.
Other: fever, chills.

INTERACTIONS
Drug-drug. *Cytotoxic drugs, radiation therapy:* enhanced toxicity of hydroxyurea. Use together cautiously.

EFFECTS ON DIAGNOSTIC TESTS
Drug therapy elevates BUN, serum creatinine, and serum uric acid levels.

CONTRAINDICATIONS
Contraindicated in patients hypersensitive to drug and in those with marked bone marrow depression (leukopenia [less than 2,500/mm³ WBCs], thrombocytopenia [less than 100,000/mm³ platelets], or severe anemia).

NURSING CONSIDERATIONS
• Use cautiously in patients with renal dysfunction.
• Routinely measure BUN, uric acid, and serum creatinine levels. Be aware that

---

blood counts must be monitored every 2 weeks.

• Know that acceptable blood counts during dose titration are for neutrophils, 2,500 cells/mm^3 or more; platelets, 95,000/mm^3 or more; hemoglobin over 5.3 g/dl; and reticulocytes (if Hg is below 9 g/dl) over 95,000/mm^3. Toxic levels are considered when neutrophil count is below 2,000 cells/mm^3, platelets are below 80,000/mm^3, hemoglobin is under 4.5 g/dl, and reticulocytes (if Hg is below 9 g/dl) are below 80,000/mm^3.

• Monitor fluid intake and output; keep patient hydrated.

• To prevent bleeding, avoid all I.M. injections when platelet count is below 100,000/mm^3.

• Anticipate possible blood transfusions because of cumulative anemia. Patient may receive injections of RBC colony-stimulating factors to promote RBC production and decrease need for blood transfusions.

• Be aware that dosage modification may be required after chemotherapy or radiation therapy.

• Be aware that auditory and visual hallucinations and hematologic toxicity increase when decreased renal function exists.

• Know that drug crosses blood-brain barrier.

• Realize that concomitant radiation therapy may increase incidence or severity of GI distress or stomatitis.

☑ **Patient teaching**

• Tell patient who can't swallow capsules that he may empty contents into water and take immediately. Patient should rinse mouth with water after taking drug this way. Inform patient that some inert material may not dissolve.

• Advise patient to watch for signs of infection (fever, sore throat, fatigue) and bleeding (easy bruising, nosebleeds, bleeding gums, melena). He should also take his temperature daily.

• Caution female patient of childbearing age to avoid becoming pregnant during therapy. Also recommend consulting with doctor before becoming pregnant.

mercaptopurine
(6-mercaptopurine, 6-MP)
Purinethol

Pregnancy Risk Category: D

HOW SUPPLIED
Tablets (scored): 50 mg

ACTION
Inhibits RNA and DNA synthesis.

Route	Onset	Peak	Duration
PO	Unknown	Unknown	Unknown

INDICATIONS & DOSAGE
Acute myeloblastic leukemia, chronic myelocytic leukemia—
Adults: 80 to 100 mg/m^2 (rounded to nearest 25 mg) P.O. daily as a single dose, up to 5 mg/kg/day.
Children: 75 mg/m^2 (rounded to nearest 25 mg) P.O. daily.
Acute lymphoblastic leukemia—
Children: 75 mg/m^2 (rounded to nearest 25 mg) P.O. daily.
   Usual maintenance for adults and children: 1.5 to 2.5 mg/kg/day.

ADVERSE REACTIONS
GI: nausea, vomiting, anorexia, painful oral ulcers, diarrhea, pancreatitis, GI ulceration.
Hematologic: *leukopenia, thrombocytopenia, anemia*—all may persist for several days after drug is stopped.
Hepatic: *jaundice, hepatotoxicity.*
Skin: rash, hyperpigmentation.
Other: hyperuricemia.

INTERACTIONS
Drug-drug. *Allopurinol:* slowed inactivation of mercaptopurine. Decrease mercaptopurine to 25% or 33% of normal dose.
Hepatotoxic drugs: may enhance hepatotoxicity of mercaptopurine. Monitor for hepatotoxicity.
Nondepolarizing neuromuscular blockers: antagonized muscle relaxant effect. Notify anesthesiologist that patient is receiving mercaptopurine.
Trimethoprim/sulfamethoxazole: en-

hanced bone marrow suppression has occurred; monitor carefully.
Warfarin: antagonized or potentiated anticoagulant effect. Monitor PT and INR.

EFFECTS ON DIAGNOSTIC TESTS
Drug therapy may cause falsely elevated serum glucose and uric acid values when sequential multiple analyzer is used.

CONTRAINDICATIONS
Contraindicated in patients whose disease has shown resistance to drug.

NURSING CONSIDERATIONS
• Be aware that dosage modifications may be required after chemotherapy or radiation therapy in patients with depressed neutrophil or platelet counts and in those with impaired hepatic or renal function.
• Know that drug is sometimes ordered as 6-mercaptopurine or 6-MP. The numeral 6 is part of drug name and does not signify number of dosage units.
• Monitor blood counts and serum transaminase, alkaline phosphatase, and bilirubin levels weekly during induction and monthly during maintenance, as ordered.
• Observe for signs of bleeding and infection.
• Monitor fluid intake and output. Encourage adequate fluid intake (3 L daily).
Alert: Watch for jaundice, clay-colored stools, and frothy, dark urine. Hepatic dysfunction is reversible when drug is stopped. If hepatic tenderness occurs, drug should be stopped and doctor notified.
• Monitor serum uric acid level, as ordered. If allopurinol is ordered, use cautiously.
• To prevent bleeding, avoid all I.M. injections when platelet count is below 100,000/mm^3.
• Anticipate possible blood transfusions because of cumulative anemia. Patient may receive injections of RBC colony-stimulating factors to promote RBC production and decrease need for blood transfusions.
• Be alert that GI adverse reactions are less common in children than in adults.

☑ **Patient teaching**
• Instruct patient to watch for signs of infection (fever, sore throat, fatigue) and

bleeding (easy bruising, nosebleeds, bleeding gums, melena). Tell patient to take temperature daily.
• Caution women of childbearing age to avoid becoming pregnant during therapy. Also recommend consulting with doctor before becoming pregnant.
• Advise breast-feeding patient to discontinue breast-feeding during therapy because of possible infant toxicity.

---

methotrexate (amethopterin, MTX)

methotrexate sodium
Folex, Folex PFS, Rheumatrex

Pregnancy Risk Category: X

HOW SUPPLIED
Tablets (scored): 2.5 mg
Injection: 20-mg, 25-mg, 50-mg, 100-mg, 250-mg vials, lyophilized powder, preservative free; 25-mg/ml vials, preservative-free solution; 2.5-mg/ml, 25-mg/ml vials, lyophilized powder, preserved

ACTION
Prevents reduction of folic acid to tetrahydrofolate by binding to dihydrofolate reductase.

Route	Onset	Peak	Duration
PO	Unknown	1-2 hr	Unknown
IV	Unknown	Immediate	Unknown
IM	Unknown	0.5-1 hr	Unknown
Intrathecal	Unknown	Unknown	Unknown

INDICATIONS & DOSAGE
Trophoblastic tumors (choriocarcinoma, hydatidiform mole)—
Adults: 15 to 30 mg P.O. or I.M. daily for 5 days. Repeated after 1 or more weeks, according to response or toxicity. Maximum number of courses is 3 to 5.
Acute lymphocytic leukemia—
Adults and children: 3.3 mg/m^2/day P.O., I.M., or I.V. for 4 to 6 weeks or until remission occurs; then 20 to 30 mg/m^2 P.O. or I.M. weekly in two divided doses or 2.5 mg/kg I.V. q 14 days.
Meningeal leukemia—
Adults and children: 12 mg/m^2 or less

(maximum 15 mg) intrathecally q 2 to 5 days until CSF is normal, then one additional dose.

Burkitt's lymphoma (stage I, II, or III)—
Adults: 10 to 25 mg P.O. daily for 4 to 8 days with 1-week rest intervals.

Lymphosarcoma (stage III)—
Adults: 0.625 to 2.5 mg/kg daily P.O., I.M., or I.V.

Osteosarcoma—
Adults: initially, 12 g/m² I.V. as 4-hour infusion. Subsequent doses 12 to 15 g/m² I.V. as 4-hour I.V. infusion given at 4th, 5th, 6th, 7th, 11th, 12th, 15th, 16th, 29th, 30th, 44th, 45th weeks after surgery. Given with leucovorin, 15 mg P.O., I.M., or I.V. q 6 hours for 10 doses, beginning 24 hours after start of methotrexate infusion.

Mycosis fungoides—
Adults: 2.5 to 10 mg P.O. daily, or 50 mg I.M. weekly, or 25 mg I.M. twice weekly.

Psoriasis—
Adults: 10 to 25 mg P.O., I.M., or I.V. as single weekly dose; or 2.5 mg P.O. every 12 hours for three doses. Dosage should not exceed 30 mg/week.

Rheumatoid arthritis—
Adults: initially, 7.5 mg P.O. weekly, either in a single dose or divided as 2.5 mg P.O. q 12 hours for three doses once a week. Dosage may be gradually increased to a maximum of 20 mg weekly.

ADVERSE REACTIONS

CNS: *arachnoiditis* within hours of intrathecal use; subacute neurotoxicity, which may begin a few weeks later; *leukoencephalopathy;* demyelination; malaise; fatigue; dizziness; headache; aphasia; hemiparesis; drowsiness; *seizures.*
EENT: pharyngitis, blurred vision.
GI: gingivitis, *stomatitis, diarrhea,* abdominal distress, anorexia, GI ulceration and bleeding, enteritis, *nausea, vomiting.*
GU: nephropathy, *tubular necrosis, renal failure,* hematuria, menstrual dysfunction, defective spermatogenesis, infertility, abortion, cystitis.
Hematologic: WBC and platelet count nadirs occurring on day 7; *anemia, leukopenia, thrombocytopenia* (all dose-related).
Hepatic: *acute toxicity* (elevated

transaminase level), *chronic toxicity* (cirrhosis, *hepatic fibrosis*).
Respiratory: *pulmonary fibrosis; pulmonary interstitial infiltrates;* pneumonitis; dry, nonproductive cough.
Skin: *urticaria,* pruritus, hyperpigmentation, erythematous rashes, ecchymoses; psoriatic lesions (aggravated by exposure to sun), rash, photosensitivity, alopecia, acne.
Other: osteoporosis (in children, with long-term use), fever, chills, reduced resistance to infection, septicemia, hyperuricemia, arthralgia, myalgia, diabetes, *sudden death.*

INTERACTIONS

Drug-drug. *Acyclovir:* concurrent use with intrathecal MTX may cause neurologic abnormalities. Monitor closely.
Digoxin: may decrease serum digoxin levels. Monitor closely.
Folic acid derivatives: antagonized methotrexate effect. Avoid concomitant use, except for leucovorin rescue with high-dose methotrexate therapy.
Hepatotoxic drugs: may increase risk of hepatotoxicity. Monitor closely.
NSAIDs, phenylbutazone, probenecid, salicylates, sulfonamides: increased methotrexate toxicity. Avoid use together.
Oral antibiotics: may decrease absorption of methotrexate. Monitor closely.
Phenytoin: may decrease serum phenytoin levels. Monitor closely.
Theophylline: may increase level of theophylline. Monitor closely.
Vaccines: immunizations may be ineffective; risk of disseminated infection with live-virus vaccines. Defer immunization, if possible.
Drug-food. *Any food:* may delay the absorption and reduce peak concentration of methotrexate. Avoid concomitant use.
Drug-lifestyle. *Alcohol use:* may increase hepatotoxicity. Discourage concomitant use.
Sun exposure: photosensitivity reactions may occur. Take precautions.

EFFECTS ON DIAGNOSTIC TESTS

Drug therapy may increase blood and urine levels of uric acid and serum AST. It may alter results of laboratory assay for folate, thus interfering with the detection of folic acid deficiency.

CONTRAINDICATIONS

Contraindicated in patients hypersensitive to drug; in those with psoriasis or rheumatoid arthritis who also have alcoholism, alcoholic liver, chronic liver disease, immunodeficiency syndromes, or preexisting blood dyscrasias; and in pregnant or breast-feeding patients.

NURSING CONSIDERATIONS

• Use cautiously and at modified dosage in patients with impaired hepatic or renal function, bone marrow suppression, aplasia, leukopenia, thrombocytopenia, or anemia. Also use cautiously in patients with infection, peptic ulceration, and ulcerative colitis and in very young, elderly, or debilitated patients.
• Monitor pulmonary function tests periodically, as ordered, and fluid intake and output daily. Encourage fluid intake of 2 to 3 L daily.
• Monitor serum uric acid level, as ordered.
Alert: Alkalinize urine as ordered by giving sodium bicarbonate tablets to prevent precipitation of drug, especially with high doses. Maintain urine pH at more than 6.5. Reduce dosage, as ordered, if BUN level is 20 to 30 mg/dl or creatinine level is 1.2 to 2 mg/dl. Stop drug if BUN level exceeds 30 mg/dl or creatinine level is over 2 mg/dl and notify doctor.
• Use preservative-free formulation for intrathecal administration.
• Watch for increases in AST, ALT, and alkaline phosphatase levels, which may signal hepatic dysfunction.
• Watch for signs of bleeding (especially GI) and infection.
• To prevent bleeding, avoid all I.M. injections when platelet count is below 100,000/mm^3.
• Anticipate blood transfusions because of cumulative anemia. Patient may receive injections of RBC colony-stimulating factors to promote RBC production and decrease need for blood transfusions.
• Know that rash, redness, or ulcerations in mouth or adverse pulmonary reactions may signal serious complications.

• Know that leucovorin rescue is necessary with high-dose (over 100 mg) protocols and is started 24 hours after beginning methotrexate therapy.
• Monitor methotrexate levels and adjust leucovorin dose, as ordered.

I.V. administration
• Follow institutional policy to reduce risks. Preparation and administration of parenteral form of drug are associated with carcinogenic, mutagenic, and teratogenic risks for personnel.
• Know that dilution of drug depends on product and that infusion guidelines vary, depending on dose.
• Reconstitute solutions without preservatives immediately before use, and discard unused drug.

Patient teaching
• Advise patient to watch for signs of infection (fever, sore throat, fatigue) and bleeding (easy bruising, nosebleeds, bleeding gums, melena). Tell patient to take temperature daily.
• Teach and encourage diligent mouth care to reduce the risk of superinfection in the mouth.
• Tell patient to use highly protective sunblock when exposed to sunlight.
• Warn patient to avoid conception during and immediately after therapy because of possible abortion or congenital anomalies.
• Advise breast-feeding patient to discontinue breast-feeding during therapy because of possible infant toxicity.

---

thioguanine
(6-TG, 6-thioguanine)
Lanvist†

Pregnancy Risk Category: D

HOW SUPPLIED
Tablets (scored): 40 mg

ACTION
Inhibits DNA and (to a lesser degree) RNA synthesis.

Route	Onset	Peak	Duration
PO	Unknown	Unknown	Unknown

Reactions may be *common,* uncommon, *life-threatening,* or COMMON AND LIFE-THREATENING.

INDICATIONS & DOSAGE

Acute nonlymphocytic leukemia, chronic myelogenous leukemia—
Adults and children: initially, 2 mg/kg P.O. daily (usually calculated to nearest 20 mg). If after 4 weeks at 2 mg/kg there is no clinical improvement, dosage may be cautiously increased to 3 mg/kg/day if not contraindicated.

ADVERSE REACTIONS

GI: nausea, vomiting, stomatitis, diarrhea, anorexia.
Hematologic: *leukopenia, anemia, thrombocytopenia* (occurs slowly over 2 to 4 weeks).
Hepatic: *hepatotoxicity,* jaundice, hepatic fibrosis, toxic hepatitis.
Other: hyperuricemia.

INTERACTIONS

Drug-drug. *Myelosuppressants:* increased risk of toxicity, especially myelosuppression, bleeding, and hepatotoxicity. Use together cautiously.

EFFECTS ON DIAGNOSTIC TESTS

Drug therapy may increase blood and urine levels of uric acid.

CONTRAINDICATIONS

Contraindicated in patients whose disease has shown resistance to drug. There is usually complete cross-resistance between mercaptopurine and thioguanine.

NURSING CONSIDERATIONS

● Use cautiously and with dosage modification in patients with renal or hepatic dysfunction.
● Monitor CBC daily during induction and then weekly during maintenance therapy, as ordered. Be aware that leukocyte and/or platelet count depression is a contraindication to increasing medication dosage.
● Monitor serum uric acid level, as ordered. Hyperuricemia can be minimized by increased urine alkalization and the administration of allopurinol.
● Watch for jaundice; may be reversible if drug is stopped promptly.
● To prevent bleeding, avoid all I.M. in-

jections when platelet count is below 100,000/mm^3.
● Anticipate possible blood transfusions because of cumulative anemia. Patient may receive injections of RBC colony-stimulating factors to promote RBC production and decrease need for blood transfusions.
● Know that drug is sometimes ordered as 6-thioguanine. The numeral 6 is part of drug name and does not signify dosage units.

☑ Patient teaching

● Instruct patient to watch for signs of infection (fever, sore throat, fatigue) and bleeding (easy bruising, nosebleeds, bleeding gums, melena). Tell patient to take temperature daily.
● Caution women of childbearing age to avoid becoming pregnant during therapy. Also recommend consulting with doctor before becoming pregnant.
● Advise breast-feeding patient to discontinue breast-feeding during therapy because of possible infant toxicity.

bleomycin sulfate
dactinomycin
daunorubicin hydrochloride
doxorubicin hydrochloride
idarubicin hydrochloride
mitomycin
pentostatin
plicamycin

COMBINATION PRODUCTS
None.

---

bleomycin sulfate
Blenoxane

Pregnancy Risk Category: D

HOW SUPPLIED
Injection: 15-unit vials, 30-unit vials

ACTION
Unknown. Thought to inhibit DNA synthesis and cause scission of single- and double-stranded DNA.

Route	Onset	Peak	Duration
IV, SC	Unknown	Unknown	Unknown
IM	Unknown	30-60 min	Unknown

INDICATIONS & DOSAGE
Dosage and indications may vary. Check treatment protocol with doctor.
Squamous cell carcinoma (head and neck, skin, penis, cervix, and vulva), lymphosarcoma, reticulum cell carcinoma, testicular carcinoma—
Adults: 10 to 20 units/m² I.V., I.M., or S.C. once or two times weekly to total of 300 to 400 units.
Hodgkin's disease—
Adults: 10 to 20 units/m² I.V., I.M., or S.C. one or two times weekly. After 50% response, maintenance dosage is 1 unit I.M. or I.V. daily or 5 units I.M. or I.V. weekly.
Treatment of malignant pleural effusion; prevention of recurrent pleural effusions—

Adults: 60 units administered as a single-dose bolus intrapleural injection.

ADVERSE REACTIONS
GI: *stomatitis, anorexia, nausea, vomiting,* diarrhea.
Respiratory: pulmonary toxicity such as PNEUMONITIS, *pulmonary fibrosis.*
Skin: *erythema, hyperpigmentation, acne, rash, striae, skin tenderness, pruritus, reversible alopecia,* hyperkeratosis, nail changes.
Other: *chills,* weight loss, fever, *anaphylactoid reactions.*

INTERACTIONS
Drug-drug. *Anesthesia:* may increase oxygen requirements. Monitor closely.
Cardiac glycosides: decreased serum digoxin levels. Monitor closely.
Phenytoin: decreased serum phenytoin levels. Monitor closely.

EFFECTS ON DIAGNOSTIC TESTS
Drug therapy may increase blood and urine concentrations of uric acid.

CONTRAINDICATIONS
Contraindicated in patients hypersensitive to drug.

NURSING CONSIDERATIONS
• Use cautiously in patients with renal or pulmonary impairment.
• Obtain pulmonary function tests as ordered. Drug should be stopped if tests show a marked decline.
• For I.M. use, dilute drug in 1 to 5 ml of sterile water for injection, bacteriostatic water for injection, or 0.9% NaCl for injection.
• For intrapleural use, dissolve drug in 50 to 100 ml 0.9% NaCl injection and administer through a thoracotomy tube after drainage of excess pleural fluid and confirmation of complete lung expansion.
• Monitor injection site for irritation.
Alert: Adverse pulmonary reactions are more common in patients over 70 years.

Reactions may be *common,* uncommon, *life-threatening,* or COMMON AND LIFE-THREATENING.

Pulmonary fibrosis is fatal in 1% of patients, especially when cumulative dosage exceeds 400 units. Also, pulmonary toxic adverse effects may be increased in patients receiving radiation therapy.

• Monitor chest X-ray, as ordered, and listen to lungs regularly.

• If patient's condition requires sclerosis, drug may be instilled when chest tube drainage is 100 to 300 ml/24 hours before therapy; ideally, drainage should be under 100 ml. Following instillation, thoracotomy tube is clamped and patient is moved alternately from the supine to left and right lateral positions for the next 4 hours. The clamp is then removed and suction reestablished. The amount of time the chest tube is left in place after sclerosis depends on patient's condition.

• Monitor for fever, which may be treated with antipyretics. This reaction usually occurs within 3 to 6 hours of administration.

• Watch for hypersensitivity reactions, which may be delayed for several hours, especially in patients with lymphoma. (Test dose of 1 to 2 units should be given before first two doses in these patients. If no reaction occurs, regular dosage is followed.)

• Don't use adhesive dressings on skin.

🔲 I.V. administration

• Follow institutional policy to reduce risks. Preparation and administration of parenteral form of drug is associated with carcinogenic, mutagenic, and teratogenic risks for personnel.

• Reconstitute drug with 5 ml or more of 0.9% NaCl for injection. For I.V. infusion, dilute with 50 to 100 ml 0.9% NaCl for injection. Administer over 10 minutes.

• Refrigerate unopened vials containing dry powder. Refrigerated, reconstituted solution is stable for 4 weeks; at room temperature, for 2 weeks. Bleomycin may adsorb to plastic I.V. bags. For prolonged stability, use glass containers.

✅ Patient teaching

• Warn patient that alopecia may occur, but that it's usually reversible.

• Tell patient to report adverse reactions promptly and to take infection-control and bleeding precautions.

• Instruct patient that if he is to ever receive anesthesia, he must inform the anesthesiologist of prior treatment with bleomycin. The pulmonary toxicity of drug may be enhanced by high inspired oxygen concentrations during surgery.

dactinomycin (actinomycin D)
Cosmegen

Pregnancy Risk Category: C

HOW SUPPLIED
Injection: 500 mcg-vial

ACTION
Unknown. May interfere with DNA-dependent RNA synthesis by intercalation.

Route	Onset	Peak	Duration
IV	Unknown	Unknown	Unknown

INDICATIONS & DOSAGE
Dosage and indications vary. Check treatment protocol with doctor.
Sarcoma, trophoblastic tumors in women, testicular cancer—
Adults: 500 mcg (0.5 mg) I.V. daily for 5 days. Maximum dosage is 15 mcg/kg or 400 to 600 mcg/m^2/day for 5 days. After bone marrow recovery, and at least 3 weeks, course may be repeated.
Wilms' tumor, rhabdomyosarcoma, Ewing's sarcoma—
Children: 10 to 15 mcg/kg or 400 to 500 mcg/m^2/day I.V. for 5 days. Maximum dosage is 500 mcg/day. Or 2.5 mg/m^2 I.V. in equally divided daily doses over 7 days. After bone marrow recovery, course may be repeated. Not recommended for infants under 6 months.

ADVERSE REACTIONS
GI: *anorexia, nausea, vomiting,* abdominal pain, diarrhea, *stomatitis,* ulceration, proctitis.
Hematologic: *anemia, leukopenia, thrombocytopenia, pancytopenia, aplastic anemia, agranulocytosis.*
Hepatic: *hepatotoxicity.*
Skin: *erythema;* desquamation; reversible alopecia; *hyperpigmentation of skin, especially in previously irradiated areas;*

acne-like eruptions (reversible); "radiation recall effect."
Other: phlebitis and severe damage to soft tissue at injection site, malaise, fatigue, lethargy, fever, myalgia, hypocalcemia, ***anaphylactoid reaction, death.***

INTERACTIONS
Drug-drug. *Bone marrow suppressants:* additive toxicity. Monitor closely.
Vitamin K derivatives: decreased effectiveness. Monitor closely.

EFFECTS ON DIAGNOSTIC TESTS
Drug therapy may increase blood and urine concentrations of uric acid, as well as serum liver enzymes; it may also interfere with determination of antibiotic drug levels (peak and trough).

CONTRAINDICATIONS
Contraindicated in patients with chickenpox or herpes zoster.

NURSING CONSIDERATIONS
• If skin contact occurs, irrigate with water for at least 15 minutes.
Alert: Be aware that dosage must be reduced in patients who have recently been treated with, or who will receive concomitant treatment with, radiation therapy or other chemotherapy drugs.
• In the event of a spill, use a solution of trisodium phosphate 5% to inactivate drug.
• Monitor CBC and platelet counts and renal and hepatic functions, as ordered.
• If WBC count falls below 2,000/mm³ or granulocyte count falls below 1,000/mm³, follow institutional policy for infection control in immunocompromised patients.
• Monitor for stomatitis, diarrhea, leukopenia, or thrombocytopenia.
• To reduce nausea, give antiemetic before drug, as ordered.

🔲 I.V. administration
• Follow institutional policy to reduce risks. Preparation and administration of parenteral form of drug are associated with carcinogenic, mutagenic, and teratogenic risks for personnel.
• Use only sterile water (without preservatives) as diluent for reconstitution. Add

1.1 ml to vial to yield gold-colored solution containing 0.5 mg/ml. Give by direct injection into a vein or through tubing of a free-flowing I.V. solution of 0.9% NaCl for injection or D₅W. Be aware that an in-line cellulose ester membrane filter should not be used during dactinomycin administration.
• For I.V. infusion, dilute with up to 50 ml of D₅W or 0.9% NaCl for injection; infuse over 15 minutes.
• Administer through a running I.V. line with good blood return. Drug is a vesicant; if extravasation occurs, severe tissue necrosis may result. If infiltration occurs, apply cold compresses to area and notify doctor.
• Discard unused solutions.

☑ Patient teaching
• Advise patient to watch for signs of infection (fever, sore throat, fatigue) and bleeding (easy bruising, nosebleeds, bleeding gums, melena), and to take temperature daily.
• Tell patient that alopecia may occur, but that it's usually reversible.
• Inform patient who received a course of radiation therapy that he may experience "radiation recall effect".

---

daunorubicin hydrochloride
Cerubidine

Pregnancy Risk Category: D

HOW SUPPLIED
Injection: 20 mg-vial

ACTION
May interfere with DNA-dependent RNA synthesis by intercalation.

Route	Onset	Peak	Duration
IV	Unknown	Unknown	Unknown

INDICATIONS & DOSAGE
Dosage and indications vary. Check treatment protocol with doctor.
Remission induction in acute nonlymphocytic (myelogenous, monocytic, erythroid) leukemia—
Adults: in combination, 30 to 45 mg/m²/

---

day I.V. on days 1, 2, and 3 of first course and on days 1 and 2 of subsequent courses with cytarabine infusions.
Remission induction in acute lymphocytic leukemia—
Adults: in combination 45 mg/m²/day I.V. on days 1, 2, and 3 of first course.
Children 2 years and older: 25 mg/m² I.V. on day 1 q week, for up to 6 weeks, if needed.
Children under 2 years or body surface area under 0.5 m²: dose based on body weight (1 mg/kg), not surface area.

ADVERSE REACTIONS
CV: IRREVERSIBLE CARDIOMYOPATHY (dose-related), ECG changes.
GI: *nausea, vomiting,* diarrhea.
GU: red urine (transient).
Hematologic: *bone marrow suppression* (lowest blood counts 10 to 14 days after administration).
Hepatic: *hepatotoxicity.*
Skin: rash, *reversible alopecia,* darkening or redness of previously irradiated areas.
Other: *severe cellulitis, tissue sloughing* (if drug extravasates); *anaphylactoid reaction,* fever, chills, hyperuricemia.

INTERACTIONS
Drug-drug. *Dexamethasone, heparin:* may form a precipitate. Don't mix together.
Doxorubicin: additive cardiotoxicity. Monitor closely.
Hepatotoxic drugs: increased risk of additive hepatotoxicity. Monitor closely.

EFFECTS ON DIAGNOSTIC TESTS
Drug therapy may increase blood and urine concentration of uric acid; it may also cause an increase in serum alkaline phosphatase, AST, and bilirubin levels, indicating drug-induced hepatotoxicity.

CONTRAINDICATIONS
No known contraindications.

NURSING CONSIDERATIONS
● Use cautiously in patients with myelosuppression or impaired cardiac, renal, or hepatic function.
● Take preventive measures (including adequate hydration) before starting treatment. Hyperuricemia may result from rapid lysis of leukemic cells. Allopurinol may be ordered.
● Know that cardiac function studies (including ECG) should be performed before treatment and then periodically throughout therapy.
● Never give drug I.M. or S.C.
● Be aware that cumulative adult dosage is limited to 400-550 mg/m² (450 mg/m² when patients are also receiving or have received cyclophosphamide or radiation therapy to cardiac area).
● Know that therapeutic effects are often accompanied by toxicity.
● Monitor CBC and hepatic function tests, as ordered; monitor ECG every month during therapy.
● Monitor pulse rate closely. Light resting pulse rate is a sign of cardiac adverse reactions. Notify doctor if this occurs.
Alert: Stop drug immediately and notify doctor if signs of heart failure or cardiomyopathy develop.
● Monitor for nausea and vomiting, which may last 24 to 48 hours.
● Anticipate the need for blood transfusions to combat anemia. Patient may receive injections of RBC colony-stimulating factors to promote red blood cell production and decrease need for blood transfusions.
● Know that reddish color is similar to that of doxorubicin. Take care to avoid confusing the two drugs.
● Optimally, use within 8 hours of preparation. Reconstituted solution is stable for 24 hours at room temperature or 48 hours if refrigerated.

⬛ I.V. administration
● Follow institutional policy to reduce risks. Preparation and administration of parenteral form of drug are associated with carcinogenic, mutagenic, and teratogenic risks for personnel.
● Reconstitute drug using 4 ml of sterile water for injection to produce a 5 mg/ml solution.
● Withdraw the desired dose into a syringe containing 10 to 15 ml of 0.9% NaCl for injection. Inject into the tubing of a free-flowing I.V. solution of D₅W or 0.9% NaCl for injection over 2 to 3 min-

utes. Alternatively, dilute in 50 ml of 0.9% NaCl for injection and infuse over 10 to 15 minutes, or dilute in 100 ml and infuse over 30 to 45 minutes.

• If extravasation occurs, discontinue I.V. infusion immediately, apply ice to area for 24 to 48 hours, and notify doctor. Drug is a vesicant; if extravasation occurs, severe tissue necrosis may result.

☑ **Patient teaching**
• Advise patient to watch for signs of infection (fever, sore throat, fatigue) and bleeding (easy bruising, nosebleeds, bleeding gums, melena) and to take temperature daily.
• Inform patient that red urine for 1 to 2 days is normal and does not indicate the presence of blood in urine.
• Advise patient that alopecia may occur, but that it's usually reversible.
• Caution women of childbearing age to avoid becoming pregnant during therapy and to consult with doctor before becoming pregnant.

---

doxorubicin hydrochloride
Adriamycin‡, Adriamycin PFS, Adriamycin RDF, Rubex

Pregnancy Risk Category: D

HOW SUPPLIED
Injection (preservative-free): 2 mg/ml
Powder for injection: 10-mg, 20-mg, 50-mg, 100-mg, 150-mg vials

ACTION
Unknown. May interfere with DNA-dependent RNA synthesis by intercalation.

Route	Onset	Peak	Duration
IV	Unknown	Unknown	Unknown

INDICATIONS & DOSAGE
Dosage and indications vary. Check treatment protocol with doctor.
Bladder, breast, lung, ovarian, stomach, and thyroid cancers; Hodgkin's disease; acute lymphoblastic and myeloblastic leukemia; Wilms' tumor; neuroblastoma; lymphoma; sarcoma—
Adults: 60 to 75 mg/m^2 I.V. as single

dose q 3 weeks; or 30 mg/m^2 I.V. in single daily dose, days 1 to 3 of 4-week cycle. Alternatively, 20 mg/m^2 I.V. once weekly. Maximum cumulative dosage is 550 mg/m^2.
Elderly: may require reduced dosage.
Adjust-a-dose: In patients with myelosuppression or impaired cardiac or liver function, dosage may be reduced. Be prepared to decrease dosage if serum bilirubin level rises: 50% of the dosage should be given when bilirubin is 1.2 to 3 mg/100 ml; 25% when it is over 3 mg/100 ml.

ADVERSE REACTIONS
CV: cardiac depression, seen in such ECG changes as sinus tachycardia, T-wave flattening, ST-segment depression, voltage reduction; *arrhythmias; acute left ventricular failure; irreversible cardiomyopathy.*
EENT: conjunctivitis.
GI: *nausea, vomiting,* diarrhea, *stomatitis,* esophagitis, anorexia.
GU: red urine (transient).
Hematologic: *leukopenia* during days 10 to 15 with recovery by day 21; *thrombocytopenia;* MYELOSUPPRESSION.
Skin: urticaria, facial flushing, *complete alopecia within 3 to 4 weeks* (hair may regrow 2 to 5 months after drug is stopped), hyperpigmentation of nail beds and dermal creases, "radiation recall effect."
Other: *severe cellulitis, tissue sloughing* (if drug extravasates); hyperuricemia; fever; chills; *anaphylaxis.*

INTERACTIONS
Drug-drug. *Aminophylline, cephalothin, dexamethasone, fluorouracil, heparin, hydrocortisone:* may form a precipitate. Don't mix together.
Calcium channel blockers: may potentiate cardiotoxic effects. Monitor closely.
Digoxin: may decrease serum digoxin levels. Monitor closely.
Phenytoin: decreased serum levels of phenytoin. Check levels.
Streptozocin: increased and prolonged blood levels. Dosage may have to be adjusted.
Drug-herb. *Green tea:* may enhance the antitumor activity of doxorubicin. Monitor patient.

Reactions may be *common,* uncommon, *life-threatening,* or COMMON AND LIFE-THREATENING.

EFFECTS ON DIAGNOSTIC TESTS
Drug therapy may increase blood and urine concentrations of uric acid.

CONTRAINDICATIONS
Contraindicated in patients with marked myelosuppression induced by previous treatment with other antitumor agents or by radiotherapy and in patients who have received lifetime cumulative dosage of 550 mg/m^2 of doxorubicin or daunorubicin.

NURSING CONSIDERATIONS
• Know that cardiac function studies (including ECG) should be performed before treatment and then periodically throughout therapy. Be aware that dexrazoxane may be administered concomitantly with doxorubicin if the accumulated dose of doxorubicin has reached 300 mg/m^2.

• Take preventive measures (including adequate hydration) before starting treatment. Hyperuricemia may result from rapid lysis of leukemic cells. Allopurinol may be ordered.

• Premedicate with antiemetic, as ordered, to reduce nausea.

• If skin or mucosal contact occurs, immediately wash with soap and water.

• In the event of a leak or spill, inactivate drug with 5% sodium hypochlorite solution (household bleach).

• Never give drug I.M. or S.C.

• Know that dosage modification may be required in patients with myelosuppression, in those with impaired cardiac or hepatic function, and in elderly patients.

• Monitor CBC and hepatic function tests, as ordered; monitor ECG monthly during therapy. If WBC count falls below 2,000/mm^3 or granulocyte count falls below 1,000/mm^3, follow institutional policy for infection control in immunocompromised patients.

• Be prepared to stop drug or slow rate of infusion if tachycardia develops and notify doctor.

Alert: If signs of heart failure develop, stop drug and notify doctor. Heart failure can often be prevented by limiting cumulative dosage to 550 mg/m^2 (400 mg/m^2 when patient is also receiving or has received cyclophosphamide or radiation therapy to cardiac area).

• Know that reddish color is similar to that of daunorubicin. Take care to avoid confusing the two drugs.

• Keep in mind that esophagitis is very common in patients who have also received radiation therapy.

I.V. administration
• Follow institutional policy to reduce risks. Preparation and administration of parenteral form of drug are associated with carcinogenic, mutagenic, and teratogenic risks for personnel.

• Reconstitute using preservative-free 0.9% NaCl for injection. Add 5 ml to 10-mg vial, 10 ml to 20-mg vial, or 25 ml to 50-mg vial. Shake vial and allow drug to dissolve; final concentration will be 2 mg/ml. Give by direct injection into the tubing of a free-flowing I.V. solution containing D$_5$W or 0.9% NaCl for injection. Administration rate should not be less than 3 minutes. Drug is a severe vesicant; if extravasation occurs, tissue necrosis may result.

• Don't place I.V. line over joints or in extremities with poor venous or lymphatic drainage. If extravasation occurs, discontinue I.V. infusion immediately, apply ice to area for 24 to 48 hours, and notify doctor. Monitor area closely because extravasation may be progressive. Early consultation with a plastic surgeon may be advisable.

• If vein streaking occurs, slow administration rate. However, if welts occur, stop administration and notify doctor.

• Know that refrigerated, reconstituted solution is stable for 48 hours; at room temperature, it's stable for 24 hours.

Patient teaching
• Advise patient to watch for signs of infection (fever, sore throat, fatigue) and bleeding (easy bruising, nosebleeds, bleeding gums, melena) and to take temperature daily.

• Advise patient that orange to red urine for 1 to 2 days is normal and does not indicate presence of blood.

• Inform patient that alopecia may occur, but that it's usually reversible.

idarubicin hydrochloride
Idamycin, Zavedos§

Pregnancy Risk Category: D

HOW SUPPLIED
Powder for injection: 5 mg, 10 mg, 20 mg

ACTION
Unknown. Probably inhibits nucleic acid synthesis by intercalation and interacts with the enzyme topoisomerase II. It is highly lipophilic, which results in an increased rate of cellular uptake.

Route	Onset	Peak	Duration
IV	Unknown	Few min	Unknown

INDICATIONS & DOSAGE
Dosage and indications vary. Check treatment protocol with doctor.
Acute myeloid leukemia, including FAB (French-American-British) classifications M1 through M7, in combination with other approved antileukemic agents—
Adults: 12 mg/m^2/day for 3 days by slow I.V. injection (over 10 to 15 minutes) in combination with 100 mg/m^2/day of cytarabine for 7 days by continuous I.V. infusion; or as a 25 mg/m^2 bolus (cytarabine), followed by 200 mg/m^2/day (cytarabine) for 5 days by continuous infusion. A second course may be administered if needed.
Adjust-a-dose: If patient experiences severe mucositis, administration is delayed until recovery is complete and dosage reduced by 25%. Dosage should also be reduced in patients with hepatic or renal impairment. Idarubicin should not be given if bilirubin level is above 5 mg/dl.

ADVERSE REACTIONS
CNS: *headache, changed mental status,* peripheral neuropathy, *seizures.*
CV: *heart failure,* atrial fibrillation, chest pain, *MI,* asymptomatic decline in left ventricular ejection fraction, *myocardial insufficiency, arrhythmias,* HEMORRHAGE, *myocardial toxicity.*
GI: *nausea, vomiting, cramps, diarrhea, mucositis, severe enterocolitis with perforation* (rare).

GU: decreased renal function, red urine.
Hematologic: *myelosuppression.*
Hepatic: changes in hepatic function.
Skin: *alopecia, rash, urticaria, bullous erythrodermatous rash on palms and soles,* hives at injection site, erythema at previously irradiated sites, tissue necrosis at injection site (if extravasation occurs).
Other: INFECTION, *fever,* hyperuricemia, *hypersensitivity reactions.*

INTERACTIONS
Drug-drug. *Alkaline solutions, heparin:* incompatibility. Do not mix idarubicin with other drugs unless specific compatibility data are available.

EFFECTS ON DIAGNOSTIC TESTS
None reported.

CONTRAINDICATIONS
No known contraindications.

NURSING CONSIDERATIONS
• Use with extreme caution in patients with bone marrow suppression induced by previous drug therapy or radiotherapy, impaired hepatic or renal function, prior treatment with anthracyclines or cardiotoxic agents, or a preexisting cardiac condition.
• Cardiotoxicity is the dose-limiting toxicity of drug.
• Take preventive measures (including adequate hydration) before starting treatment. Hyperuricemia may result from rapid lysis of leukemic cells. Allopurinol may be ordered.
• Assess patient for systemic infection and ensure that it's controlled before therapy begins.
• Give antiemetics, as ordered, to prevent or treat nausea and vomiting.
• Know that drug must never be given I.M. or S.C.
• Monitor hepatic and renal function tests and CBC frequently, as ordered.
• To prevent bleeding, avoid all I.M. injections when platelet count is below 100,000/mm^3.
• Anticipate need for blood transfusions to combat anemia. Patient may receive injections of RBC colony-stimulating fac-

---

Reactions may be *common,* uncommon, *life-threatening,* or COMMON AND LIFE-THREATENING.

tors to promote RBC production and decrease need for blood transfusions.
• Notify doctor if signs or symptoms of heart failure occur.

🅘 I.V. administration
• Follow institutional policy to reduce risks. Preparation and administration of parenteral form of drug are associated with carcinogenic, mutagenic, and teratogenic risks for personnel.
• Reconstitute to a final concentration of 1 mg/ml using 0.9% NaCl for injection without preservatives. Add 5 ml to 5-mg vial, 10 ml to 10-mg vial, or 20 ml to 20-mg vial. Do *not* use bacteriostatic NaCl. Vial is under negative pressure.
• Administer over 10 to 15 minutes into a free-flowing I.V. infusion of 0.9% NaCl or D$_5$W solution running into a large vein.
• Drug is a vesicant; tissue necrosis may result. If extravasation occurs, discontinue infusion immediately and notify doctor. Treat with intermittent ice packs—for ½ hour immediately, and then for ½ hour four times daily for 4 days.
• Know that reconstituted solutions are stable for 3 days (72 hours) at room temperature (59° to 86° F [15° to 30° C]); 7 days if refrigerated. Label any unused solutions with CHEMOTHERAPY HAZARD label.

☑ Patient teaching
• Instruct patient to recognize signs and symptoms of extravasation and to call the doctor or nurse if these occur.
• Warn patient to watch for signs of infection (fever, sore throat, fatigue) and bleeding (easy bruising, nosebleeds, bleeding gums, melena).
• Advise patient that red urine for several days is normal and does not indicate presence of blood.
• Caution women of childbearing age to avoid becoming pregnant during therapy and to consult with doctor before becoming pregnant.

---

mitomycin (mitomycin-C)
Mutamycin

Pregnancy Risk Category: NR

HOW SUPPLIED
Injection: 5-mg, 20-mg, 40-mg vials

ACTION
Acts like an alkylating agent, cross-linking strands of DNA. This causes an imbalance of cell growth, leading to cell death.

Route	Onset	Peak	Duration
IV	Unknown	Unknown	Unknown

INDICATIONS & DOSAGE
Dosage and indications vary. Check treatment protocol with doctor.
Disseminated adenocarcinoma of stomach or pancreas—
Adults: 10 to 20 mg/m^2 as an I.V. single dose. Cycle repeated after 6 to 8 weeks when WBC and platelet counts have returned to normal.

ADVERSE REACTIONS
CNS: headache, neurologic abnormalities, confusion, drowsiness, fatigue.
GI: *nausea, vomiting, anorexia, diarrhea.*
Hematologic: THROMBOCYTOPENIA, LEUKOPENIA (may be delayed up to 8 weeks and may be cumulative with successive doses).
Respiratory: *interstitial pneumonitis,* pulmonary edema, dyspnea, nonproductive cough, adult respiratory distress syndrome.
Skin: *reversible alopecia,* purple bands on nails, rash.
Other: induration, desquamation, pruritus, *pain at injection site; septicemia;* cellulitis, ulceration, sloughing with extravasation; *fever; microangiopathic hemolytic anemia (characterized by thrombocytopenia, renal failure, and hypertension);* blurred vision, pain.

INTERACTIONS
Drug-drug. *Vinca alkaloids:* may cause acute respiratory distress when administered concomitantly. Monitor closely.

EFFECTS ON DIAGNOSTIC TESTS
Drug therapy, through drug-induced renal toxicity, may increase serum creatinine and BUN concentrations. Drug may also

decrease hemoglobin, hematocrit, leukocyte, and platelet counts.

CONTRAINDICATIONS
Contraindicated in patients hypersensitive to drug and in those with thrombocytopenia, coagulation disorders, or an increase in bleeding tendency due to other causes.

NURSING CONSIDERATIONS
• Never give drug I.M. or S.C.
• Continue CBC and blood studies, as ordered, at least 8 weeks after therapy is stopped. Leukopenia and thrombocytopenia are cumulative. If WBC count falls below 2,000/mm³ or granulocyte count falls below 1,000/mm³, follow institutional policy for infection control in immunocompromised patients.
• To prevent bleeding, avoid all I.M. injections when platelet count is below 100,000/mm³.
• Anticipate need for blood transfusions to combat anemia. Patients may receive injections of RBC colony-stimulating factors to promote red blood cell production and decrease need for blood transfusions.
• Monitor patient for dyspnea with nonproductive cough; chest X-ray may show infiltrates.
• Monitor renal function tests, as ordered.

◖ I.V. administration
• Follow institutional policy to reduce risks. Preparation and administration of parenteral form of drug is associated with mutagenic, teratogenic, and carcinogenic risks to personnel.
• Using sterile water for injection, reconstitute the 5-mg vials with 10 ml, the 20-mg vials with 40 ml, and the 40-mg vials with 80 ml. Know that when reconstituted with sterile water, the solution is stable for 14 days under refrigeration and 7 days at room temperature.
• For infusion, dilute with 0.9% NaCl for injection, D₅W, or sodium lactate for injection. After dilution, drug is stable for 3 hours in D₅W, 12 hours in 0.9% NaCl for injection, and 24 hours in sodium lactate for injection at room temperature.
• Avoid extravasation. Stop infusion immediately if extravasation occurs because of the potential for severe ulceration and necrosis, and notify doctor.

☑ Patient teaching
• Warn patient to watch for signs of infection (fever, sore throat, fatigue) and bleeding (easy bruising, nosebleeds, bleeding gums, melena). Tell patient to take temperature daily.
• Inform patient that alopecia may occur, but that it's usually reversible.

pentostatin (2′-deoxycoformycin)
Nipent

Pregnancy Risk Category: D

HOW SUPPLIED
Powder for injection: 10 mg-vial

ACTION
Inhibits the enzyme adenosine deaminase (ADA), causing an increase in intracellular levels of deoxyadenosine triphosphate. This leads to cell damage and death. Because the greatest activity of ADA is in cells of the lymphoid system (especially malignant T cells), pentostatin is useful in treating leukemias.

Route	Onset	Peak	Duration
IV	Unknown	Unknown	Unknown

INDICATIONS & DOSAGE
Alpha-interferon–refractory hairy-cell leukemia—
Adults: 4 mg/m² I.V. every other week.

ADVERSE REACTIONS
CNS: *headache, neurologic symptoms,* anxiety, confusion, depression, dizziness, insomnia, nervousness, paresthesia, somnolence, abnormal thinking, *fatigue.*
CV: *arrhythmias,* abnormal ECG, *MI,* angina, *heart failure,* thrombophlebitis, peripheral edema, *hemorrhage.*
EENT: abnormal vision, conjunctivitis, ear pain, eye pain, *epistaxis, pharyngitis, rhinitis,* sinusitis.
GI: *abdominal pain, nausea, vomiting, anorexia, diarrhea,* constipation, flatulence, *stomatitis.*

Reactions may be *common,* uncommon, *life-threatening*, or **COMMON AND LIFE-THREATENING**.

GU: hematuria, dysuria, increased BUN and creatinine levels.
Hematologic: *myelosuppression,* LEUKOPENIA, *anemia,* THROMBOCYTOPENIA, lymphadenopathy.
Hepatic: *elevated liver enzyme levels.*
Respiratory: *cough, bronchitis, dyspnea, pulmonary edema,* pneumonia, *upper respiratory infection.*
Skin: *ecchymosis, petechiae, rash,* eczema, dry skin, herpes simplex or zoster, maculopapular rash, vesiculobullous rash, *pruritus, seborrhea, discoloration, diaphoresis.*
Other: *fever,* INFECTION, *pain,* HYPERSENSITIVITY REACTIONS, *chills, sepsis, death, neoplasm,* chest pain, back pain, flulike syndrome, *asthenia,* malaise, *myalgia,* arthralgia, weight loss.

INTERACTIONS
Drug-drug. *Cytarabine, vidarabine:* increased incidence or severity of adverse effects associated with either drug. Avoid concomitant use.
Fludarabine: risk of severe or fatal pulmonary toxicity. Don't use together.

EFFECTS ON DIAGNOSTIC TESTS
Drug may increase serum alkaline phosphatase, ALT, AST, LD, creatinine, and uric acid levels.

CONTRAINDICATIONS
Contraindicated in patients hypersensitive to drug.

NURSING CONSIDERATIONS
● Use cautiously and only under the supervision of a doctor qualified and experienced in the use of chemotherapeutic agents. Adverse reactions after pentostatin therapy are common.
● Know that use in patients with renal damage (creatinine clearance of 60 ml/minute or less) should be avoided.
● Treat all spills and waste products with 5% sodium hypochlorite (household bleach).
● Know that optimal duration of therapy is unknown. Current recommendations suggest two additional courses of therapy after a complete response. If a partial response is not evident after 6 months of

therapy, drug will be discontinued. If a partial response is evident, drug will be continued for another 6 months.
Alert: Withhold or discontinue drug in patients with evidence of CNS toxicity, a severe rash, or an active infection, and notify doctor. Drug may be resumed when the infection clears.
● Temporarily withhold drug if absolute neutrophil count falls below 200/mm^3 and the pretreatment level was over 500/mm^3, and notify doctor. No recommendations exist regarding dosage adjustments in patients with anemia, neutropenia, or thrombocytopenia.
● If WBC count falls below 2,000/mm^3 or granulocyte falls below 1,000/mm^3, follow institutional policy for infection control in immunocompromised patients.
● Anticipate possible blood transfusion during treatment because of cumulative anemia. Patient may receive injections of RBC colony-stimulating factors to promote RBC production and decrease need for blood transfusions.
● Be aware that drug should be used only in patients who have hairy-cell leukemia refractory to alpha-interferon. This is defined as disease that progresses after a minimum of 3 months of treatment with alpha-interferon or disease that does not exhibit a response after 6 months of therapy.
● Monitor renal function.

🩸 I.V. administration
● Make sure patient is adequately hydrated before therapy. Administer 500 to 1,000 ml of D$_5$W in 0.45% NaCl solution, as ordered, for hydration. Ensure at least 2 L of urine output daily while on therapy.
● Follow institutional policy to reduce risks. Preparation and administration of parenteral form of drug are associated with mutagenic, teratogenic, and carcinogenic risks to personnel.
● Add 5 ml of sterile water for injection to vial containing pentostatin powder for injection. Mix thoroughly to make a solution of 2 mg/ml. Drug may be administered by I.V. bolus injection or diluted further in 25 or 50 ml of D$_5$W or 0.9% NaCl for injection and infused over 20 to 30 minutes.

• Use reconstituted solution within 8 hours; it contains no preservatives.
• Give an additional 500 ml of D₅W, as ordered, for hydration after drug is administered.

☑ **Patient teaching**
• Advise patient to watch for signs of infection (fever, sore throat, fatigue) and bleeding (easy bruising, nosebleeds, bleeding gums, melena), and to take temperature daily.
• Caution women of childbearing age to avoid becoming pregnant during therapy and to consult with doctor before becoming pregnant.

---

plicamycin (mithramycin)
Mithracin

Pregnancy Risk Category: X

HOW SUPPLIED
Injection: 2.5-mg vials (contains mannitol 100 mg)

ACTION
Unknown. Thought to form a complex with DNA, thus inhibiting RNA synthesis. Also inhibits osteocytic activity, blocking calcium and phosphorus resorption from bone.

Route	Onset	Peak	Duration
IV	1-2 days	3 days	7-10 days

INDICATIONS & DOSAGE
Dosage and indications vary. Check treatment protocol with doctor.
Hypercalcemia and hypercalciuria associated with advanced malignant disease—
Adults: 15 to 25 mcg/kg/day I.V. over 4 to 6 hours for 3 to 4 days. Dosage repeated at weekly intervals until desired response is obtained.
Testicular cancer—
Adults: 25 to 30 mcg/kg/day I.V. for 8 to 10 days or until toxicity occurs. Do not use more than 10 daily doses, or 30 mcg/kg individual daily doses.

ADVERSE REACTIONS
CNS: drowsiness, weakness, lethargy, depression, headache, malaise.
GI: *nausea, vomiting,* anorexia, diarrhea, stomatitis.
GU: increased BUN and serum creatinine levels.
Hematologic: *leukopenia, thrombocytopenia; bleeding syndrome* (from epistaxis to generalized hemorrhage).
Hepatic: *elevated liver enzyme levels, hepatotoxicity.*
Skin: facial flushing, rash; pain, redness, swelling (at injection site).
Other: *decreased serum calcium,* potassium, and phosphorus levels; *death,* fever, cellulitis with extravasation, phlebitis.

INTERACTIONS
None significant.

EFFECTS ON DIAGNOSTIC TESTS
Because of drug-induced toxicity, drug therapy may increase serum concentrations of alkaline phosphatase, AST, ALT, LD, and bilirubin; it may also increase serum creatinine and BUN levels through nephrotoxicity.

CONTRAINDICATIONS
Contraindicated in patients with thrombocytopenia, bone marrow suppression, or coagulation and bleeding disorders and in women who are or who may become pregnant.

NURSING CONSIDERATIONS
• Use with extreme caution in patients with significant renal or hepatic impairment.
• Obtain baseline platelet count and PT before therapy, as ordered.
• To reduce nausea, give antiemetic before administering, as ordered.
• Use ideal body weight to calculate dose if patient has edema or fluid retention.
• Avoid contact with skin or mucous membranes.
• Monitor platelet count and PT during therapy, as ordered. Discontinue drug and notify doctor if patient's WBC count falls below 4,000/mm³, if his platelet count falls below 150,000/mm³, or if his PT is

---

prolonged more than 4 seconds longer than control.

Alert: Know that facial flushing is an early indicator of bleeding. The first evidence of a bleeding syndrome may manifest in epistaxis (nosebleed).

• To prevent bleeding, avoid all I.M. injections when platelet count is below 100,000/mm³.

• Anticipate need for blood transfusions to combat anemia. Patient may receive injections of RBC colony-stimulating factors to promote RBC production and decrease need for blood transfusions.

• Monitor LD, AST, ALT, alkaline phosphatase, BUN, creatinine, potassium, calcium, and phosphorus levels, as ordered.

• Monitor patient for tetany, carpopedal spasm, Chvostek's sign, and muscle cramps; check serum calcium level. Precipitous drop in calcium level is possible.

• Be aware that patients receiving drug for treatment of testicular cancer may require calcium supplementation.

I.V. administration

• Follow institutional policy to reduce risks. Preparation and administration of parenteral form of drug are associated with carcinogenic, mutagenic, and teratogenic risks for personnel.

• To prepare solution, add 4.9 ml of sterile water for injection to vial and shake to dissolve. Then dilute for I.V infusion in 1,000 ml of D₅W or 0.9% NaCl. Administer by infusion over 4 to 6 hours. Discard unused drug.

• Be aware that slow infusion reduces nausea that develops with I.V. push.

• Avoid extravasation. Plicamycin is a vesicant and tissue necrosis may result. If I.V. solution infiltrates, stop immediately, notify doctor, and use ice packs. Restart I.V. line.

• Store lyophilized powder in refrigerator and protect from light.

✓ Patient teaching

• Advise patient to watch for signs of infection (fever, sore throat, fatigue) and bleeding (easy bruising, nosebleeds, bleeding gums, melena), and to take temperature daily.

• Caution women of childbearing age to avoid becoming pregnant during therapy and to consult with doctor before becoming pregnant.

72

Antineoplastics that alter hormone balance

anastrozole
bicalutamide
diethylstilbestrol
(See Chapter 55, ESTROGENS AND PROGESTINS.)
estramustine phosphate sodium
flutamide
goserelin acetate
letrozole
leuprolide acetate
megestrol acetate
nilutamide
tamoxifen citrate
testolactone
toremifene citrate

COMBINATION PRODUCTS
None.

anastrozole
Arimidex

Pregnancy Risk Category: D

HOW SUPPLIED
Tablets: 1 mg

ACTION
Selective nonsteroidal aromatase inhibitor that significantly lowers serum estradiol concentrations, thereby inhibiting stimulation of breast cancer cell growth in postmenopausal women.

Route	Onset	Peak	Duration
PO	< 24 hr	Unknown	< 6 days

INDICATIONS & DOSAGE
Treatment of advanced breast cancer in postmenopausal women with disease progression after tamoxifen therapy—
Adults: 1 mg P.O. daily.

ADVERSE REACTIONS
CNS: *headache,* dizziness, depression, paresthesia.
CV: chest pain, edema.
GI: *nausea,* vomiting, diarrhea, constipation, abdominal pain, anorexia, dry mouth.
GU: vaginal hemorrhage, vaginal dryness.
Respiratory: dyspnea, increased cough, pharyngitis.
Skin: *hot flushes, alopecia,* rash, sweating.
Other: *asthenia, pain, back pain,* bone pain, peripheral edema, pelvic pain, thromboembolic disease, weight gain.

INTERACTIONS
None reported.

EFFECTS ON DIAGNOSTIC TESTS
Drug may elevate alkaline phosphatase, ALT, AST, GGT, low-density lipoprotein, and total cholesterol levels.

CONTRAINDICATIONS
No known contraindications.

NURSING CONSIDERATIONS
- Use cautiously in breast-feeding patients.
- Know that pregnancy must be ruled out before treatment.
- Be aware that drug should be administered under supervision of a qualified doctor experienced in the use of anticancer drugs.

☑ **Patient teaching**
- Instruct patient to report adverse reactions.
- Stress need for follow-up care.
- Counsel patient of childbearing age about potential risks to pregnancy during therapy.

bicalutamide
Casodex

Pregnancy Risk Category: X

HOW SUPPLIED
Tablets: 50 mg

ACTION

A nonsteroidal antiandrogen that binds to cytosol androgen receptors in target tissue.

Route	Onset	Peak	Duration
PO	Unknown	Unknown	Unknown

INDICATIONS & DOSAGE

Adjunct therapy in combination with a luteinizing hormone-releasing hormone (LHRH) analogue for treatment of advanced prostate cancer—
Adults: 50 mg P.O. once daily in morning or evening, at same time each day.

ADVERSE REACTIONS

CNS: anxiety, depression, headache, dizziness, paresthesia, insomnia.
CV: *hot flashes,* hypertension, chest pain, peripheral edema.
GI: *constipation, nausea, diarrhea,* abdominal pain, flatulence, vomiting.
GU: nocturia, hematuria, urinary tract infection, impotence, urinary incontinence.
Hepatic: increased liver enzymes.
Hematologic: hypochromic anemia, iron deficiency anemia.
Respiratory: dyspnea.
Skin: rash, sweating, dry skin, pruritus.
Other: *general pain, back pain, gynecomastia, breast pain, pelvic pain, asthenia, infection,* flulike syndrome, hyperglycemia, bone pain, weight loss.

INTERACTIONS

Drug-drug. *Coumadin anticoagulants:* displacement of these drugs from their protein-binding sites. Monitor PT closely, and know that anticoagulant dose may need adjustment.

EFFECTS ON DIAGNOSTIC TESTS

Drug may elevate bilirubin, BUN, and creatinine levels and decrease hemoglobin and WBC counts.

CONTRAINDICATIONS

Contraindicated in patients with hypersensitivity to drug or its components and during pregnancy.

NURSING CONSIDERATIONS

• Use cautiously in patients with moder-ate-to-severe hepatic impairment (drug is extensively metabolized by the liver).
• Bicalutamide is used in combination with an LHRH analogue. Treatment should be started at same time for both drugs.
• Give drug at same time each day.
• Regularly monitor serum prostate specific antigen (PSA) levels, as ordered. PSA levels help in assessing response to therapy. Report elevated levels to doctor, who should evaluate patient to determine disease progression.
• Monitor liver function studies, as ordered. When patient develops jaundice or exhibits laboratory evidence of liver injury in the absence of liver metastases, drug should be discontinued. Abnormalities are usually reversible on discontinuation.

☑ **Patient teaching**
• Tell patient to take drug at same time each day, without regard to meals.
• Urge patient not to stop drug therapy without consulting doctor.

---

estramustine phosphate sodium
Emcyt, Estracyt‡ , Estracyt§

Pregnancy Risk Category: NR

HOW SUPPLIED

Capsules: 140 mg

ACTION

Unknown. A combination of estrogen and an alkylating agent; probably acts by its ability to bind selectively to a protein present in the prostate gland.

Route	Onset	Peak	Duration
PO	Unknown	Unknown	Unknown

INDICATIONS & DOSAGE

Palliative treatment of metastatic or progressive prostate cancer—
Adults: 10 to 16 mg/kg/day P.O. in three or four divided doses. Usual dosage is 14 mg/kg daily. Therapy continued for up to 3 months and, if successful, maintained as long as patient responds.

ADVERSE REACTIONS

CNS: lethargy, insomnia, headache, anxiety.

CV: *MI,* sodium and fluid retention, chest pain, thrombophlebitis, *heart failure, stroke.*

GI: *nausea, vomiting,* diarrhea, anorexia, flatulence, GI bleeding, thirst.

Hematologic: *leukopenia, thrombocytopenia.*

Respiratory: *pulmonary embolism,* dyspnea.

Skin: rash, pruritus, dry skin, thinning of hair, flushing.

Other: *edema, painful gynecomastia and breast tenderness,* leg cramps, decreased libido.

INTERACTIONS

Drug-drug. *Calcium-containing drugs (such as antacids):* impaired absorption of estramustine. Do not administer at same time.

Drug-food. *Calcium-rich foods (dairy products, milk):* impaired absorption of estramustine. Do not administer concurrently.

EFFECTS ON DIAGNOSTIC TESTS

Drug therapy may increase norepinephrine-induced platelet aggregation and may reduce response to the metyrapone test. Glucose tolerance may be decreased. May increase AST, ALT, LD, ceruloplasmin, cortisol, phospholipids, prolactin PT, sodium, and triglycerides. May decrease serum folate, pregnanediol and pyridoxine levels, and phosphate.

CONTRAINDICATIONS

Contraindicated in patients hypersensitive to estradiol and nitrogen mustard. Also contraindicated in those with active thrombophlebitis or thromboembolic disorders, except when the actual tumor mass is the cause of the thromboembolic phenomenon.

NURSING CONSIDERATIONS

● Use cautiously in patients with history of thrombophlebitis or thromboembolic disorders and cerebrovascular or coronary artery disease. Monitor weight regularly in these patients. Estramustine may exag-

gerate preexisting peripheral edema or heart failure.

● Also use cautiously in patients with impaired liver function. Monitor liver function periodically throughout therapy.

● Be aware that each 140-mg capsule contains 12.5 mg of sodium.

● Monitor blood pressure and blood glucose periodically throughout therapy. Drug may increase blood pressure and decrease blood glucose.

● Keep in mind that estramustine is a combination of estrogen estradiol and a nitrogen mustard, shown to be effective in patients refractory to estrogen therapy alone.

● Be aware that patient may continue therapy as long as response is favorable. Some patients have taken drug for more than 3 years.

● Store capsules in refrigerator.

✅ Patient teaching

● Tell patient to take drug on an empty stomach (1 hour before or 2 hours after meals) and to avoid taking with milk or dairy products.

● Because of risk of mutagenic effects, advise patient and partner to use contraception if woman is of childbearing age.

---

flutamide
Drogenil§, Euflex†, Eulexin

Pregnancy Risk Category: D

HOW SUPPLIED
Capsules: 125 mg, 250 mg†

ACTION
Inhibits androgen uptake or prevents binding of androgens in nucleus of cells within target tissues.

Route	Onset	Peak	Duration
PO	Unknown	2 hr	Unknown

INDICATIONS & DOSAGE
Metastatic prostate cancer (stage B$_2$, C, D$_2$) in combination with luteinizing hormone-releasing hormone analogues such as leuprolide acetate—
Adults: 250 mg P.O. q 8 hours.

ADVERSE REACTIONS
CNS: drowsiness, confusion, depression, anxiety, nervousness.
CV: peripheral edema, hypertension.
GI: *diarrhea, nausea, vomiting,* anorexia.
GU: *impotence, loss of libido.*
Hematologic: anemia, *leukopenia, thrombocytopenia,* hemolytic anemia.
Hepatic: elevated liver enzyme levels, hepatitis, encephalopathy.
Skin: rash, photosensitivity.
Other: *hot flashes,* gynecomastia, paresthesia.

INTERACTIONS
Drug-drug. *Warfarin:* may increase PT. Monitor PT and INR.
Drug-lifestyle. *Sun exposure:* may cause sensitivity reactions. Warn patient to take appropriate precautions.

EFFECTS ON DIAGNOSTIC TESTS
Elevation of plasma testosterone and estradiol levels has been reported. Serum ALT, AST, bilirubin, and creatinine levels may be increased.

CONTRAINDICATIONS
Contraindicated in patients hypersensitive to drug.

NURSING CONSIDERATIONS
• Monitor liver function tests and CBC periodically, as ordered.
• Know that flutamide must be taken continuously with agent used for medical castration (such as leuprolide acetate) to allow the full benefit of therapy. Leuprolide suppresses testosterone production while flutamide inhibits testosterone action at the cellular level. Together, they can impair the growth of androgen-responsive tumors.

☑ Patient teaching
• Advise patient not to discontinue drug therapy without consulting doctor.
• Instruct patient to report adverse reactions promptly.

goserelin acetate
Zoladex

Pregnancy Risk Category: X (endometriosis and endometrial thinning); D (breast cancer)

HOW SUPPLIED
Implants: 3.6 mg, 10.8 mg

ACTION
A luteinizing hormone-releasing hormone (LHRH) analogue that acts on the pituitary to decrease the release of follicle-stimulating hormone and luteinizing hormone, resulting in dramatically lowered serum levels of sex hormones.

Route	Onset	Peak	Duration
SC	2-4 wk	12-15 days	Throughout therapy

INDICATIONS & DOSAGE
Endometriosis, palliative treatment of advanced prostate cancer—
Adults: 3.6 mg S.C. q 28 days into upper abdominal wall. For endometriosis, maximum duration of therapy is 6 months. For prostate cancer, 10.8 mg S.C. into upper abdominal wall q 12 weeks.
Palliative treatment of advanced breast cancer in pre- and perimenopausal women—
Adults: 3.6 mg S.C. q 28 days into upper abdominal wall.
Endometrial thinning agent for use before endometrial ablation—
Adults: 3.6 mg S.C. into upper abdominal wall. One or two depots are recommended (each given 4 weeks apart).

ADVERSE REACTIONS
CNS: lethargy, pain (worsened in the first 30 days), dizziness, *insomnia,* anxiety, *depression, headache,* chills, *emotional lability.*
CV: edema, *heart failure, arrhythmias, peripheral edema, CVA,* hypertension, *MI,* peripheral vascular disorder, chest pain.
GI: nausea, vomiting, diarrhea, constipation, ulcer, anorexia, abdominal pain.
GU: *impotence, sexual dysfunction, lower*

urinary tract symptoms, renal insufficiency, urinary obstruction, *vaginitis,* urinary tract infection, amenorrhea.

Hematologic: anemia.

Respiratory: COPD, upper respiratory infection.

Skin: rash, *diaphoresis, acne, seborrhea,* hirsutism.

Other: *hot flashes,* gout, hyperglycemia, weight increase, breast swelling and tenderness, *changes in breast size,* breast pain, *changes in libido, asthenia, infection,* breast pain, back pain, hypercalcemia.

INTERACTIONS
None significant.

EFFECTS ON DIAGNOSTIC TESTS
Serum testosterone levels increase during first week of therapy and then decrease. Serum acid phosphatase may increase initially and will decrease by week 4. Serum lipid levels may be increased.

CONTRAINDICATIONS
Contraindicated in patients with hypersensitivity to LHRH, LHRH agonist analogues, or to goserelin acetate. Also contraindicated during pregnancy or breastfeeding and in patients with obstructive uropathy or vertebral metastases. The 10.8-mg implant is contraindicated in women because data are insufficient to support reliable suppression of serum estradiol.

NURSING CONSIDERATIONS
• Because use of drug is associated with a loss of bone mineral density in women, use cautiously in patients with other risk factors for osteoporosis, such as family history of osteoporosis, chronic alcohol or tobacco abuse, or the use of drugs such as corticosteroids or anticonvulsants that affect bone density.

• Before administering to female patient, rule out pregnancy.

• Never administer by I.V. injection.

• Administer drug into upper abdominal wall using aseptic technique. After cleaning area with an alcohol swab (and injecting a local anesthetic), stretch patient's skin with one hand while grasping the barrel of the syringe with the other. Insert needle into the subcutaneous fat; then change direction of needle so that it parallels the abdominal wall. Then push needle in until hub touches patient's skin; withdraw about 1 cm (this creates a gap for drug to be injected) before depressing plunger completely.

• To avoid need for a new syringe and injection site, do not aspirate after inserting needle. If needle penetrates a blood vessel, blood will be seen in the syringe chamber. Withdraw needle, and inject with a new syringe elsewhere.

Alert: Know that the implant comes in a preloaded syringe. If package is damaged, do not use the syringe. Make sure that drug is visible in the translucent chamber of the syringe.

• When used for prostate cancer, be aware that LHRH analogues such as goserelin may initially cause a worsening of prostatic cancer symptoms because drug initially increases testosterone serum levels. Some patients may experience increased bone pain. Rarely, disease exacerbation (either spinal cord compression or ureteral obstruction) has occurred.

• When used for endometrial thinning, surgery should be performed at 4 weeks if one depot is administered. When two depots are given, surgery should be performed within 2 to 4 weeks after administration of second depot.

☑ Patient teaching
• Advise patient to report every 28 days for a new implant. A delay of a couple of days is permissible.

• Tell female patient to use a nonhormonal form of contraception during treatment. Caution patient about significant risks to fetus should pregnancy occur.

• Tell patient to call doctor if menstruation persists or if breakthrough bleeding occurs. Menstruation should stop during treatment.

• Inform patient that she may experience a delayed return of menses after therapy ends. Persistent amenorrhea is rare.

Reactions may be *common,* uncommon, *life-threatening,* or COMMON AND LIFE-THREATENING.

letrozole
Femara

Pregnancy Risk Category: D

HOW SUPPLIED
Tablets: 2.5 mg

ACTION
A nonsteroidal competitive inhibitor of the aromatase enzyme system, which results in the inhibition of the conversion of androgens to estrogens. Decreased estrogens lead to decreased tumor mass or delayed progression of tumor growth in some women.

Route	Onset	Peak	Duration
PO	Unknown	2 days	Unknown

INDICATIONS & DOSAGE
Metastatic breast cancer in postmenopausal women with disease progression following antiestrogen therapy—
Adults: 2.5 mg P.O. as a single daily dose.

ADVERSE REACTIONS
CNS: headache, somnolence, dizziness.
CV: hypertension, *thromboembolism,* chest pain.
GI: *nausea,* vomiting, constipation, diarrhea, abdominal pain, anorexia.
Musculoskeletal: *bone pain, extremities pain, back pain,* arthralgias.
Respiratory: dyspnea, coughing.
Skin: hot flashes, rash, pruritus.
Other: fatigue, edema, weight gain, hypercholesterolemia, viral infections, mood changes.

INTERACTIONS
None reported.

EFFECTS ON DIAGNOSTIC TESTS
None reported.

CONTRAINDICATIONS
Contraindicated in patients with known hypersensitivity to drug or its components.

NURSING CONSIDERATIONS
• Know that no dose adjustment is needed in renally impaired patients with creatinine clearance of 10 ml/minute or more.
• Use cautiously in patients with severe liver impairment. No dosage adjustment is needed for mild to moderate liver dysfunction.
• Know that food does not affect drug absorption.

☑ **Patient teaching**
• Instruct patient to take drug exactly as prescribed.
• Tell patient that drug can be taken with or without food.
• Inform patient about potential adverse reactions.

leuprolide acetate
Lucrin‡, Lupron, Lupron Depot, Lupron Depot-Ped, Lupron Depot-3 Month, Lupron Depot-4 Month, Lupron for Pediatric Use

Pregnancy Risk Category: X

HOW SUPPLIED
Injection: 1 mg/0.2 ml (5 mg/ml) in 2.8-ml multiple-dose vials
Depot injection: 3.75 mg, 7.5 mg, 11.25 mg, 15 mg, 22.5 mg, 30 mg

ACTION
Initially stimulates but then inhibits the release of follicle-stimulating hormone and luteinizing hormone, resulting in testosterone suppression.

Route	Onset	Peak	Duration
IM, SC	< 2-4 wk	1-2 mo	60-90 days

INDICATIONS & DOSAGE
Advanced prostate cancer—
Adults: 1 mg S.C. daily. Alternatively, 7.5 mg I.M. (depot injection) monthly or 22.5 mg I.M. q 3 months (depot injection) or 30 mg I.M. q 4 months (depot injection).
Endometriosis—
Adults: 3.75 mg I.M (depot injection only) as single injection once monthly for up to 6 months or 11.25 mg I.M. q 3 months for up to 6 months.

Central precocious puberty—
Children: initially, 0.3 mg/kg (minimum 7.5 mg) I.M. (depot injection only) as single injection q 4 weeks. Dosage may be increased in increments of 3.75 mg q 4 weeks, if needed. Therapy should be discontinued before female child reaches 11 years and before male child reaches 12 years.

ADVERSE REACTIONS
CNS: *dizziness, depression, headache, pain,* insomnia.
CV: ***arrhythmias,*** angina, ***MI,*** *peripheral edema, ECG changes,* hypotension, hypertension, murmur.
GI: *nausea, vomiting,* anorexia, constipation.
GU: *impotence, vaginitis,* urinary frequency, hematuria, urinary tract infection, gynecomastia, amenorrhea.
Hepatic: elevated liver enzyme levels.
Respiratory: dyspnea, sinus congestion, pulmonary fibrosis.
Other: transient bone pain during first week of treatment, *hot flashes,* skin reactions at injection site, androgen-like effects, joint disorder, myalgia, neuromuscular disorder, paresthesias, *weight gain or loss,* anemia, dermatitis, *asthenia.*

INTERACTIONS
None significant.

EFFECTS ON DIAGNOSTIC TESTS
Serum acid phosphatase and testosterone levels initially increase, then decrease with continued therapy.

CONTRAINDICATIONS
Contraindicated in patients hypersensitive to drug or other gonadotropin-releasing hormone analogues, in women with undiagnosed vaginal bleeding, and in pregnant or breast-feeding patients. The 30-mg depot injection is contraindicated in women.

NURSING CONSIDERATIONS
• Use cautiously in patients hypersensitive to benzyl alcohol.
• Never administer by I.V. injection.
• Know that depot injections should be administered under medical supervision. Use supplied diluent to reconstitute drug

(extra diluent is provided and remainder should be discarded). Draw 1 ml into a syringe with a 22G needle. (When preparing Lupron Depot-3 Month 22.5 mg, use a 23G or larger needle.) Withdraw 1.5 ml from ampule for the 3-month formulation. Inject into vial; then shake well. Suspension will appear milky. Although the suspension is stable for 24 hours after reconstitution, it contains no bacteriostatic agent. Use immediately.
• When using prefilled dual-chamber syringes: Prepare for injection by screwing white plunger into end stopper until stopper begins to turn. Remove and discard tab around base of needle. Hold syringe upright and release diluent by slowly pushing plunger until first stopper is at blue line in middle of barrel. Gently shake syringe to form a uniform milky suspension. If particles adhere to stopper, tap syringe against your finger. Remove needle guard and advance plunger to expel air from syringe. Inject entire contents I.M. as you would for a normal injection.
• Know that a fractional dose of drug formulated to give q 3 months is not equivalent to same dose of once-a-month formulation.
• Be aware that response to the treatment of central precocious puberty should be monitored q 1 to 2 months after the start of therapy with a gonadotropin-releasing hormone stimulation test and sex steroid levels. Measurement of bone age for advancement should be done q 6 to 12 months.
• Know that drug use may cause an increase in the signs and symptoms being treated during first few weeks of therapy.

☑ Patient teaching
• Prior to starting a child on treatment of central precocious puberty, ensure that parents understand the importance of continuous therapy.
• Carefully instruct patient who will self-administer S.C. injection about proper administration techniques and advise them to use only the syringes provided by manufacturer.
• Advise patient that if another syringe must be substituted, a low-dose insulin syringe (U-100, 0.5 ml) may be an appropri-

ate choice but that needle gauge should not be smaller than 22G (except when using Lupron Depot-3 Month 22.5 mg).
• Instruct patient to store drug at room temperature, protected from heat and light.
• Inform patient with history of undesirable effects from other endocrine therapies that drug is easier to tolerate.
• Reassure patient that effects disappear after about 1 week. Worsening of prostate cancer symptoms or central precocious puberty symptoms may occur initially.
• Advise female patient of childbearing age to use a nonhormonal form of contraception during treatment.

megestrol acetate
Megace, Megostat‡

Pregnancy Risk Category: D

HOW SUPPLIED
Tablets: 20 mg, 40 mg
Oral suspension: 40 mg/ml

ACTION
A progestin that changes the tumor's hormonal environment and alters the neoplastic process. Mechanism responsible for appetite stimulation is unknown.

Route	Onset	Peak	Duration
PO	Unknown	Unknown	Unknown

INDICATIONS & DOSAGE
Breast cancer—
Adults: 40 mg P.O. q.i.d.
Endometrial cancer—
Adults: 40 to 320 mg P.O. daily in divided doses.
Treatment of anorexia, cachexia, or unexplained significant weight loss in patients with AIDS—
Adults: 800 mg P.O. (oral suspension) daily.

ADVERSE REACTIONS
CV: thrombophlebitis, *heart failure,* hypertension.
GI: nausea, vomiting, diarrhea, flatulence, constipation, dry mouth.
GU: breakthrough menstrual bleeding, impotence, vaginal bleeding or discharge, urinary tract infection.
Respiratory: *pulmonary embolism,* dyspnea.
Skin: alopecia, rash.
Other: weight gain, increased appetite, carpal tunnel syndrome, hyperglycemia, tumor flare, gynecomastia.

INTERACTIONS
None significant.

EFFECTS ON DIAGNOSTIC TESTS
Pregnanediol excretion may decrease; serum alkaline phosphatase and amino acid concentrations may increase. Glucose tolerance has been shown to decrease in a small percentage of patients.

CONTRAINDICATIONS
Contraindicated in patients hypersensitive to drug or as a diagnostic test for pregnancy.

NURSING CONSIDERATIONS
• Use cautiously in patients with history of thrombophlebitis.
• Know that blood glucose levels may increase in diabetic patients.
• Know that megestrol is a relatively nontoxic drug with a low incidence of adverse effects.
• Be aware that 2 months is an adequate trial when treating patients with cancer.

☑ **Patient teaching**
• Inform patient that therapeutic response isn't immediate.
• Advise breast-feeding patient to discontinue breast-feeding during therapy because of possible infant toxicity.
• Advise women of childbearing age to use an effective form of contraception while receiving drug.

nilutamide
Nilandron

Pregnancy Risk Category: C

HOW SUPPLIED
Tablets: 50 mg

ACTION

This nonsteroidal antiandrogen interacts with the androgen receptor and prevents normal androgenic response.

Route	Onset	Peak	Duration
PO	Unknown	Unknown	Unknown

INDICATIONS & DOSAGE

Adjunct therapy with surgical castration for the treatment of metastatic prostate cancer—
Adults: 6 tablets (50 mg each) P.O. once daily for total of 300 mg/day for 30 days; then 3 tablets once daily for total of 150 mg/day thereafter.

ADVERSE REACTIONS

CNS: dizziness.
CV: hypertension.
EENT: *impaired adaptation to darkness*, photophobia, abnormal vision.
GI: nausea, constipation, diarrhea.
GU: urinary tract infection, impotence.
Hepatic: elevated liver enzymes.
Respiratory: dyspnea, interstitial pneumonitis.
Other: *hot flashes.*

INTERACTIONS

Drug-drug. *Phenytoin, theophylline, vitamin K antagonists:* possible delayed elimination and toxicity. Doses should be modified accordingly.
Drug-lifestyle. *Alcohol use:* may cause alcohol intolerance as evidenced by facial flushing, malaise, and hypotension. Avoid concomitant use.

EFFECTS ON DIAGNOSTIC TESTS

Drug may increase ALT and AST levels.

CONTRAINDICATIONS

Contraindicated in patients with severe hepatic or respiratory disease and hypersensitivity to drug.

NURSING CONSIDERATIONS

• Know that drug is used in combination with surgical castration and should begin on same day or on day after surgery for maximum benefit.
• Know that safety and effectiveness in pediatric patients have not been determined.

• Obtain baseline liver enzymes and periodically, at 3-month intervals, as ordered. Know that drug should be discontinued if transaminase levels exceed three times the upper limit of normal.
• Be aware that a baseline chest X-ray should be obtained before therapy begins. Monitor patient (especially if Asian) for signs of interstitial pneumonitis, and notify doctor if they occur. Obtain chest X-ray, as ordered.

☑ Patient teaching

• Explain purpose of drug, how it is given, and importance of not stopping treatment without consulting doctor.
• Tell patient to report dyspnea or aggravation of preexisting dyspnea immediately.
• Inform patient of risk of developing hepatitis and to report symptoms of nausea, vomiting, abdominal pain, or jaundice to doctor. Tell patient to avoid alcohol.
• Warn patient that visual disturbances, such as a delay in adaptation to darkness, may affect driving at night or through tunnels.

---

tamoxifen citrate
Alpha-Tamoxifen†, Nolvadex, Nolvadex-D†‡, Novo-Tamoxifen†, Tamofen†, Tamone†, Tamoplex†

Pregnancy Risk Category: D

HOW SUPPLIED

Tablets: 10 mg, 20 mg
Tablets (enteric-coated)†: 10 mg, 20 mg

ACTION

Exact antineoplastic action is unknown; acts as an estrogen antagonist.

Route	Onset	Peak	Duration
PO	1-several mo	Unknown	Several wk

INDICATIONS & DOSAGE

Advanced breast cancer in women and men—
Adults: 10 to 20 mg P.O. b.i.d.
Adjunct treatment of breast cancer in women—
Adults: 10 mg P.O. b.i.d. for 5 years.

Reactions may be *common*, uncommon, *life-threatening*, or COMMON AND LIFE-THREATENING.

✱ *NEW INDICATION: Reduction of breast cancer incidence in high risk women—* **Adults:** 20 mg P.O. daily for 5 years.

ADVERSE REACTIONS
CNS: confusion, weakness, sleepiness, headache.
EENT: corneal changes, cataracts, retinopathy.
GI: *nausea, vomiting, diarrhea.*
GU: *vaginal discharge,* vaginal bleeding, *irregular menses, increased BUN, amenorrhea.*
Hematologic: transient fall in WBC or platelet counts, *leukopenia, thrombocytopenia.*
Hepatic: changes in liver enzymes, fatty liver, cholestasis, *hepatic necrosis.*
Skin: *skin changes,* rash.
Other: temporary bone or tumor pain, *hot flashes,* brief exacerbation of pain from osseous metastases, *weight gain or loss, fluid retention, hypercalcemia.*

INTERACTIONS
Drug-drug. *Antacids:* may affect absorption of enteric-coated tablet. Do not use within 2 hours.
Bromocriptine: may elevate tamoxifen levels. Monitor closely.
Coumadin-type anticoagulants: may cause significant increase in anticoagulant effect. Monitor patient, PT, and INR closely.

EFFECTS ON DIAGNOSTIC TESTS
Drug therapy may increase levels of serum calcium, usually in patients with bone metastases. Serum triglycerides, cholesterol, T_4, and hepatic enzymes may be increased. Variations on karyopyknotic index in vaginal smears and various degrees of estrogen effect on Papanicolaou smears have been infrequently seen in postmenopausal patients.

CONTRAINDICATIONS
Contraindicated in patients hypersensitive to drug. Therapy to reduce incidence of breast cancer in high-risk women who require concomitant coumarin-type anticoagulant therapy or in women with history of deep vein thrombosis or pulmonary embolism is also contraindicated.

NURSING CONSIDERATIONS
• Use cautiously in patients with existing leukopenia or thrombocytopenia. Monitor CBC closely, as ordered.
• Monitor serum lipid levels, as ordered, during long-term therapy in patients with preexisting hyperlipidemia.
• Monitor serum calcium levels, as ordered. Drug may compound hypercalcemia related to bone metastases during initiation of therapy.
• Know that drug acts as an "antiestrogen." Best results have been reported in patients with positive estrogen receptors.
• Be aware that adverse reactions are usually minor and well tolerated.

☑ **Patient teaching**
• Tell patient taking enteric-coated tablets (Nolvadex-D) to swallow tablets whole without crushing or chewing. Tell her not to take antacids within 2 hours of dose.
• Reassure patient that acute exacerbation of bone pain during tamoxifen therapy usually indicates drug will produce good response. Use analgesic to relieve pain.
• Strongly encourage female patient who is taking or has taken tamoxifen to have regular gynecologic examinations because of increased risk of uterine cancer associated with its use.
• Encourage female patient to have annual mammograms and breast exams.
• Advise patient to use barrier form of contraception because short-term therapy induces ovulation in premenopausal patients.
• Instruct patient to report vaginal bleeding.
• Caution women of childbearing age to avoid becoming pregnant during therapy and the first 2 months after stopping the drug. Also recommend consulting with doctor before becoming pregnant.
• Advise patient that breast cancer risk assessment tools are available and to discuss her concerns with doctor.

testolactone
Teslac

Controlled Substance Schedule III
Pregnancy Risk Category: C

HOW SUPPLIED
Tablets: 50 mg

ACTION
Exact antineoplastic action is unknown. Appears to inhibit aromatase activity and decrease estrone synthesis.

Route	Onset	Peak	Duration
PO	6-12 wk	Unknown	Unknown

INDICATIONS & DOSAGE
Advanced postmenopausal breast cancer; advanced premenopausal breast cancer in women whose ovarian function has been terminated—
Women: 250 mg P.O. q.i.d.

ADVERSE REACTIONS
CNS: paresthesia, peripheral neuropathy.
CV: increased blood pressure, edema.
GI: nausea, vomiting, diarrhea, anorexia, glossitis.
Skin: alopecia, erythema, nail changes.

INTERACTIONS
Drug-drug. *Oral anticoagulants:* increased pharmacologic effects. Monitor patient, PT, and INR carefully.

EFFECTS ON DIAGNOSTIC TESTS
Drug therapy may increase levels of serum calcium, urinary creatinine, and urinary 17-ketosteroids. Estradiol levels measured by radioimmunoassay may be decreased.

CONTRAINDICATIONS
Contraindicated in patients hypersensitive to drug and in males with breast cancer.

NURSING CONSIDERATIONS
• Monitor fluid and electrolyte levels, especially calcium level.
• Force fluids to aid calcium excretion and encourage exercise to prevent hypercalcemia. Immobilized patients are prone to hypercalcemia.
• Know that higher-than-recommended doses may increase incidence of remission in patients with visceral metastases.

✅ Patient teaching
• Inform patient that therapeutic response isn't immediate. Three months is an adequate trial for drug.
• Tell patient to notify doctor if numbness or tingling occurs in fingers, toes, or face.

toremifene citrate
Fareston

Pregnancy Risk Category: D

HOW SUPPLIED
Tablets: 60 mg

ACTION
Nonsteroidal triphenylethylene that exerts its antitumor effect by competing with estrogen for binding sites in the tumor. This blocks the growth-stimulating effects of endogenous estrogen in the tumor, causing an antiestrogenic effect.

Route	Onset	Peak	Duration
PO	Unknown	3 hr	Unknown

INDICATIONS & DOSAGE
Metastatic breast cancer in postmenopausal women with estrogen-receptor positive or unknown tumors—
Adults: 60 mg P.O. as single daily dose. Treatment is usually continued until disease progression is observed.

ADVERSE REACTIONS
CNS: dizziness, fatigue, depression.
CV: edema, ***thromboembolism, heart failure, MI, pulmonary embolism.***
EENT: visual disturbances, glaucoma, ocular changes (such as dry eyes), *cataracts.*
GI: *nausea,* vomiting.
Other: *hot flashes, sweating, vaginal discharge,* vaginal bleeding, elevated liver function tests, hypercalcemia.

Reactions may be *common,* uncommon, *life-threatening*, or COMMON AND LIFE-THREATENING.

INTERACTIONS
Drug-drug. *Calcium-elevating agents (such as hydrochlorothiazide):* increased risk of hypercalcemia. Monitor calcium levels closely.

Coumadin-like anticoagulants (such as warfarin): prolonged PT and INR times. Monitor PT and INR closely.

Cytochrome P-450 3A4 enzyme inducers (such as carbamazepine, phenobarbital, phenytoin): increased rate of toremifene metabolism. Monitor patient closely.

Cytochrome P-450 3A4-6 enzyme inhibitors (such as erythromycin, ketoconazole): decreased toremifene metabolism. Uncertain clinical relevance.

EFFECTS ON DIAGNOSTIC TESTS
None reported.

CONTRAINDICATIONS
Contraindicated in patients with known hypersensitivity to drug.

NURSING CONSIDERATIONS
● Obtain periodic CBC, calcium levels, and liver function tests.
● Monitor calcium levels closely for first weeks of treatment in patients with bone metastases because of increased risk of hypercalcemia.

☑ **Patient teaching**
● Instruct patient to take drug exactly as prescribed.
● Warn patient not to discontinue therapy without consulting with doctor.
● Inform patient about vaginal bleeding and other adverse effects, and to notify doctor if bleeding occurs.
● Warn patient that a disease flare-up may occur during first weeks of therapy. Reassure her that this does not indicate failure of the treatment.
● Advise patient to report leg or chest pain, severe headache, visual changes, or dyspnea.

asparaginase
bacillus Calmette-Guérin (BCG),
  live intravesical
dacarbazine
docetaxel
etoposide
etoposide phosphate
gemcitabine hydrochloride
irinotecan hydrochloride
mitotane
mitoxantrone hydrochloride
paclitaxel
pegaspargase
porfimer sodium
procarbazine hydrochloride
rituximab
teniposide
topotecan hydrochloride
trastuzumab
tretinoin
vinblastine sulfate
vincristine sulfate
vinorelbine tartrate

COMBINATION PRODUCTS
None.

---

asparaginase
Elspar, Kidrolase†

Pregnancy Risk Category: C

HOW SUPPLIED
Injection: 10,000-unit vial

ACTION
Destroys the amino acid asparagine,
which is needed for protein synthesis in
acute lymphocytic leukemia. This leads to
death of the leukemic cell.

Route	Onset	Peak	Duration
IV	Immediate	Immediate	23-33 days
IM	Unknown	14-24 hr	23-33 days

INDICATIONS & DOSAGE
*Acute lymphocytic leukemia (in combina-
tion with other drugs)—*

Adults and children: 1,000 IU/kg I.V.
daily for 10 days, injected over 10 minutes; or 6,000 IU/m² I.M. at intervals
specified in protocol.
*Sole induction agent for acute lymphocyt-
ic leukemia—*
Adults: 200 IU/kg I.V. daily for 28 days.

ADVERSE REACTIONS
CNS: confusion, drowsiness, depression,
hallucinations, ***intracranial hemorrhage,***
fatigue, ***coma,*** agitation, headache, lethargy, somnolence.
GI: *vomiting, anorexia, nausea,* cramps,
stomatitis.
GU: *azotemia,* ***renal failure,*** glycosuria,
polyuria.
Hematologic: *anemia,* ***hypofibrinogene-
mia,*** depression of other clotting factors,
leukopenia.
Hepatic: elevated AST and ALT levels,
hepatotoxicity.
Skin: *rash, urticaria,* ***hypersensitivity reactions.***
Other: weight loss, HEMORRHAGIC PAN-
CREATITIS, ANAPHYLAXIS, chills, ***death,
fatal hyperthermia,*** fever, *hyperglycemia,*
hyperuricemia, uric acid nephropathy,
hyperammonemia.

INTERACTIONS
Drug-drug. *Methotrexate:* decreased
methotrexate effectiveness. Avoid concomitant use.
Prednisone, vincristine: increased toxicity. Monitor patient closely.

EFFECTS ON DIAGNOSTIC TESTS
Drug therapy alters results of thyroid
function tests by decreasing concentrations of serum thyroxine-binding globulin. Drug may decrease calcium, cholesterol, albumin, and fibrinogen levels.
Drug may increase ALT, AST, alkaline
phosphatase, ammonia, BUN, glucose,
PT, PTT, and uric acid.

CONTRAINDICATIONS
Contraindicated in patients with pancre-

atitis or history of pancreatitis and previous hypersensitivity unless desensitized.

NURSING CONSIDERATIONS
• Use cautiously in patients with preexisting hepatic dysfunction. Drug should be given in hospital setting with close supervision.
• Monitor blood and urine glucose before and during therapy. Watch for signs of hyperglycemia.
• Be aware that allopurinol should be started before therapy begins to help prevent uric acid nephropathy.
Alert: Know that risk of hypersensitivity increases with repeated dosages. An intradermal skin test should be performed before initial dose and when drug is given after an interval of 1 week or more between doses. Give 2 IU asparaginase as intradermal injection, as ordered. Observe site for at least 1 hour for erythema or a wheal, which indicates a positive response. Know that patient with negative skin test may still develop allergic reaction to drug. Desensitization may be required before giving first treatment dose and on retreatment of patient. One IU of drug may be ordered I.V. Dose is then doubled every 10 minutes provided no reaction has occurred, until total amount given equals patient's total dose for that day.
• Know that drug should not be used alone to induce remission unless combination therapy is inappropriate. Not recommended for maintenance therapy.
• For I.M. injection, reconstitute with 2 ml NaCl to the 10,000 unit vial. Refrigerate and use within 8 hours.
• Don't use cloudy solutions.
• If drug contacts skin or mucous membranes, wash with copious amounts of water for at least 15 minutes.
• Keep epinephrine, diphenhydramine, and I.V. corticosteroids available for treating anaphylaxis.
• Monitor CBC and bone marrow function tests, as ordered.
• Obtain serum amylase level determinations, as ordered, to check pancreatic status. If elevated, asparaginase should be discontinued.
• Help prevent occurrence of tumor lysis (which can result in uric acid nephropathy) by increasing fluid intake.
• Know that drug may affect clotting factors, leading to thrombosis or, more commonly, severe bleeding. Monitor patient and bleeding studies closely.
• Because of vomiting, administer parenteral fluids, as ordered, for 24 hours or until oral fluids are tolerated.
• Know that some patients may develop hypersensitivity to asparaginase, derived from cultures of *Escherichia coli. Erwinia* asparaginase, derived from cultures of *Erwinia carotovora,* has been used in these patients without cross-sensitivity.
• Know that drug toxicity is more likely in adults than children.
• Be aware that there are a variety of protocols for use of this drug.

🚫 **I.V. administration**
• Follow institutional policy to reduce risks. Preparation and administration of parenteral form of drug are associated with carcinogenic, mutagenic, and teratogenic risks for personnel.
• Reconstitute with 5 ml of either sterile water for injection or NaCl for injection.
• Give I.V. injection over 30 minutes through a running infusion of 0.9% NaCl solution or D_5W solution.
• Refrigerate unopened dry powder. Reconstituted solution is stable for 8 hours if refrigerated. Use only clear solutions.

☑**Patient teaching**
• Tell patient to watch for signs of infection (fever, sore throat, fatigue) and bleeding (easy bruising, nosebleeds, bleeding gums, melena), and to take temperature daily.
• Stress importance of maintaining an adequate fluid intake to help prevent hyperuricemia. If adverse GI reactions prevent patient from drinking fluids, tell patient to notify doctor.

bacillus Calmette-Guérin (BCG), live intravesical
ImmuCyst†, TheraCys, TICE BCG

Pregnancy Risk Category: C

HOW SUPPLIED
TheraCys
Suspension (freeze-dried) for bladder instillation: 81 mg/vial
TICE BCG
Suspension (freeze-dried) for bladder instillation: about 50 mg/ampule

ACTION
Unknown. Instillation of the live bacterial suspension causes a local inflammatory response. Local infiltration of histiocytes and leukocytes is followed by a decrease in superficial tumors within the bladder.

Route	Onset	Peak	Duration
Intravesical	Unknown	Unknown	Unknown

INDICATIONS & DOSAGE
In situ carcinoma of the urinary bladder (primary and relapsed)—
Adults: three reconstituted and diluted vials, 81 mg, administered intravesically once weekly for 6 weeks (induction), followed by additional treatments at 3, 6, 12, 18, and 24 months (TheraCys); or, one bladder instillation (one ampule suspended in 50 ml of sterile, preservative-free NaCl solution) once weekly for 6 weeks, and then once monthly for 6 to 12 months (TICE BCG).

ADVERSE REACTIONS
GI: *nausea, vomiting, anorexia,* diarrhea.
GU: *dysuria, urinary frequency, hematuria, cystitis, urinary urgency,* nocturia, urinary incontinence, *urinary tract infection,* cramps, pain, decreased bladder capacity, renal toxicity, genital pain.
Hematologic: *anemia, **leukopenia.***
Hepatic: elevated liver enzyme levels.
Other: **hypersensitivity reaction,** *malaise,* fever, chills, myalgia, arthralgia, **disseminated mycobacterial infection,** hypotension.

INTERACTIONS
Drug-drug. *Antibiotics:* may attenuate response to BCG intravesical. Avoid concomitant use.
Bone marrow suppressants, immunosuppressants, radiation therapy: may impair response to BCG intravesical by decreasing the immune response; may also increase the risk of osteomyelitis or disseminated BCG infection. Avoid concomitant use.

EFFECTS ON DIAGNOSTIC TESTS
Tuberculin sensitivity may be rendered positive by BCG intravesical treatment. Determine patient's reactivity to tuberculin before initiating therapy. Drug may cause pyuria and abnormal liver function tests.

CONTRAINDICATIONS
Contraindicated in immunocompromised patients, in those receiving immunosuppressive therapy or asymptomatic carriers with a positive HIV serology, and in those with urinary tract infection, gross hematuria, or fever of unknown origin. If fever is caused by infection, drug should be withheld until patient recovers.

NURSING CONSIDERATIONS
• Determine patient's reactivity to tuberculin before therapy. Tuberculin sensitivity may be rendered positive by BCG intravesical treatment.
• Know that drug should not be handled by caregiver with known immunologic deficiency.
• Be aware that BCG intravesical should not be administered within 7 to 14 days of transurethral resection or biopsy. Fatal disseminated BCG infection has occurred after traumatic catheterization.
• To administer TheraCys, reconstitute only with 3 ml of provided diluent per vial just before use. Do not remove rubber stopper to prepare solution. Use immediately. Add contents of three reconstituted vials to 50 ml of sterile, preservative-free NaCl solution (final volume, 53 ml). Instill a urethral catheter into bladder under aseptic conditions, drain bladder, and then infuse 53 ml of prepared solution by gravity feed. Remove catheter and properly dispose of unused drug.
• To administer TICE BCG, use thermosetting plastic or sterile glass containers and syringes. Draw 1 ml of sterile, preservative-free NaCl solution into a 3-ml syringe. Add to one ampule of drug; gently expel back into ampule three times to ensure thorough mixing. Use immedi-

---

Reactions may be *common,* uncommon, ***life-threatening,*** or COMMON AND LIFE-THREATENING.

ately. Dispense cloudy suspension into top end of a catheter-tipped syringe that contains 49 ml of NaCl solution. Gently rotate syringe. Properly dispose of unused drug.

• Protect drug from exposure to sunlight.

• Handle drug and material used for instillation as infectious material because it contains live, attenuated mycobacteria. Dispose of associated equipment (syringes, catheters, and containers) as biohazardous waste.

• Use strict aseptic technique to administer the drug to minimize trauma to the GU tract and to prevent introducing other contaminants.

• If there is evidence of traumatic catheterization, do not administer drug and alert doctor. Subsequent treatment may resume after 1 week as if no interruption occurred.

• Carefully monitor patient's urinary status because drug causes an inflammatory response in the bladder.

• Closely monitor patient for evidence of systemic BCG infection. BCG infections are rarely detected by positive cultures. Know that therapy should be withheld if systemic infection is suspected (short-term high fever above 103° F [39° C] or persistent fever above 101° F [38° C] for longer than 2 days or with severe malaise). Contact an infectious disease specialist for initiation of fast-acting anti-tuberculosis therapy, as ordered.

• Know that drug is not used as an immunizing agent to prevent cancer or tuberculosis; drug should not be confused with BCG vaccine.

• Keep in mind that drug has the potential to cause hypersensitivity. Manage symptomatically.

• Be aware that patients with a small bladder capacity may experience increased local irritation with the usual dose of BCG intravesical.

• Be prepared to treat bladder irritation symptomatically with phenazopyridine, acetaminophen, and propantheline, as ordered. Systemic hypersensitivity can be treated with diphenhydramine. In order to minimize the risk of systemic infection, some clinicians give isoniazid for 3 days starting on the first day of treatment.

☑ Patient teaching

• Tell patient to retain drug in the bladder for 2 hours after instillation (if possible). For the first hour, have patient lie 15 minutes prone, 15 minutes supine, and 15 minutes on each side; the second hour may be spent in the sitting position.

• Advise patient to sit when voiding.

• Instruct patient to disinfect urine for 6 hours after instillation of drug. Tell him to pour undiluted household bleach (5% sodium hypochlorite solution) in equal volume to voided urine into the toilet and wait 15 minutes before flushing.

• Tell patient to notify doctor if symptoms worsen or if the following symptoms develop: blood in the urine, fever and chills, frequent urge to urinate, painful urination, nausea, vomiting, joint pain, or rash.

Alert: Warn patient that a cough that develops after therapy could indicate a life-threatening BCG infection. Tell him to report it immediately.

• Caution female patient of childbearing age not to become pregnant or breast-feed during drug therapy.

---

dacarbazine (DTIC)
DTIC†, DTIC-Dome

Pregnancy Risk Category: C

HOW SUPPLIED
Injection: 100-mg, 200-mg vials

ACTION
Unknown. Probably cross-links strands of cellular DNA and interferes with RNA transcription, causing an imbalance of growth that leads to cell death. Cell cycle–nonspecific.

Route	Onset	Peak	Duration
IV	Unknown	Unknown	Unknown

INDICATIONS & DOSAGE
Metastatic malignant melanoma—
Adults: 2 to 4.5 mg/kg I.V. daily for 10 days; then repeated q 4 weeks as tolerated. Or 250 mg/m^2 I.V. daily for 5 days, repeated at 3-week intervals.
Hodgkin's disease—
Adults: 150 mg/m^2 I.V. daily (in combi-

nation with other agents) for 5 days, repeated q 4 weeks; or 375 mg/m^2 on first day of a combination regimen, repeated q 15 days.

ADVERSE REACTIONS
GI: *severe nausea and vomiting, anorexia,* stomatitis.
Hematologic: *leukopenia, thrombocytopenia.*
Hepatic: transient increase in liver enzyme levels, *hepatotoxicity* (rare).
Skin: phototoxicity, alopecia, rash, facial flushing.
Other: *flulike syndrome* (fever, malaise; myalgia, beginning 7 days after treatment ends and lasts possibly 7 to 21 days), *anaphylaxis;* severe pain (if I.V. solution infiltrates or if solution is too concentrated); tissue damage; facial paresthesia.

INTERACTIONS
Drug-drug. *Anticoagulants, aspirin:* increased risk of bleeding. Avoid concomitant use.
Bone marrow suppressants: additive toxicity. Monitor closely.
Phenobarbital, phenytoin, other drugs that induce hepatic metabolism: enhanced dacarbazine activation and risk of toxicity. Monitor closely.
Drug-lifestyle. *Sun exposure:* photosensitivity reactions may occur especially during first 2 days of therapy. Take precautions.

EFFECTS ON DIAGNOSTIC TESTS
Drug therapy causes transient increases in serum BUN, ALT, AST, and alkaline phosphatase levels.

CONTRAINDICATIONS
Contraindicated in patients hypersensitive to drug.

NURSING CONSIDERATIONS
• Use cautiously if bone marrow function is impaired.
• To prevent bleeding, avoid all I.M. injections when platelet count is below 100,000/mm^3.
• Anticipate the need for blood transfusions to combat anemia. Patients may receive injections of RBC colony-stimulat-ing factors to promote RBC production and decrease the need for blood transfusions.
• Know that therapeutic effects are often accompanied by toxicity. Monitor CBC and platelet count.
• For Hodgkin's disease, be aware that drug is usually given with bleomycin, vinblastine, and doxorubicin.

◐ I.V. administration
• Administer antiemetics, as ordered, before giving dacarbazine. Nausea and vomiting may sometimes subside after several doses.
• Follow institutional policy to reduce risks. Preparation and administration of parenteral form of drug are associated with carcinogenic, mutagenic, and teratogenic risks for personnel.
• Reconstitute drug using sterile water for injection. Add 9.9 ml to the 100-mg vial or 19.7 ml to the 200-mg vial. The resulting solution will be colorless to clear yellow. For infusion, further dilute by using up to 250 ml of 0.9% NaCl solution or D$_5$W; infuse over 30 minutes.
• May dilute further or slow infusion rate to decrease pain at insertion site.
• Avoid extravasation during infusion. If I.V. solution infiltrates, discontinue immediately, apply ice to area for 24 to 48 hours, and notify doctor.
• Keep in mind that reconstituted solutions are stable for 8 hours at room temperature and normal lighting conditions, or up to 3 days if refrigerated. Diluted solutions are stable for 8 hours at normal room temperature and light, or up to 24 hours if refrigerated. If solutions turn pink, decomposition has occurred; discard drug.
• Discard refrigerated solution after 72 hours and room temperature solution after 8 hours.

☑ Patient teaching
• Tell patient to watch for signs of infection (fever, sore throat, fatigue) and bleeding (easy bruising, nosebleeds, bleeding gums, melena), and to take temperature daily.
• Instruct patient to avoid OTC products containing aspirin.

- Advise patient to avoid sunlight and sunlamps for first 2 days after treatment.
- Reassure patient that flulike syndrome may be treated with mild antipyretics, such as acetaminophen.
- Counsel female patient to avoid pregnancy and breast-feeding during drug therapy.

docetaxel
Taxotere

Pregnancy Risk Category: D

HOW SUPPLIED
Injection: 20 mg, 80 mg, in single-dose vials

ACTION
Disrupts microtubular network in cells essential for mitotic and interphase cellular functions.

Route	Onset	Peak	Duration
IV	Rapid	Unknown	Unknown

INDICATIONS & DOSAGE
Treatment of patients with locally advanced or metastatic breast cancer who have progressed during anthracycline-based therapy or have relapsed during anthracycline-based adjuvant therapy—
Adults: 60 to 100 mg/m^2 I.V. over 1 hour q 3 weeks.
✳ *NEW INDICATION: Treatment of locally advanced or metastatic breast cancer after failure of prior chemotherapy—*
Adults: 60 to 100 mg/m^2 I.V. over 1 hour q 3 weeks.

ADVERSE REACTIONS
CNS: *asthenia,* paresthesia, dysesthesia, pain (including burning sensation), weakness.
CV: *fluid retention,* hypotension.
GI: *stomatitis, nausea, vomiting, diarrhea.*
Hematologic: *anemia,* NEUTROPENIA, FEBRILE NEUTROPENIA, MYELOSUPPRESSION (dose limiting), LEUKOPENIA, THROMBOCYTOPENIA, *septic and nonseptic death.*
Skin: *alopecia,* skin eruptions, desqua-

mation, nail pigmentation alterations, nail pain, flushing, rash, reaction at injection site.
Other: HYPERSENSITIVITY REACTIONS, *infection,* chest tightness, back pain, dyspnea, drug fever, chills, *myalgia,* arthralgia, *increased liver function tests.*

INTERACTIONS
Drug-drug. *Compounds that induce, inhibit, or are metabolized by cytochrome P-450 3A4 (such as cyclosporine, erythromycin, ketoconazole, troleandomycin):* metabolism of docetaxel may be modified by concomitant administration. Use cautiously when administering these agents with docetaxel.

EFFECTS ON DIAGNOSTIC TESTS
Drug may cause increased alkaline phosphatase, ALT, AST, bilirubin; decreased hemoglobin, WBC, platelets.

CONTRAINDICATIONS
Contraindicated in patients with history of severe hypersensitivity to drug or to other formulations containing polysorbate 80 and in those with neutrophil counts below 1,500 cells/mm^3.

NURSING CONSIDERATIONS
- Do not administer docetaxel in patients with bilirubin values above upper limits of normal. Patients with ALT or AST above 1.5 times upper limits of normal, and alkaline phosphatase greater than 2.5 times upper limit of normal, generally should not receive drug.
- Premedicate all patients with oral corticosteroids, such as dexamethasone 16 mg P.O. (8 mg twice daily) daily for 5 days starting 1 day before docetaxel administration, to reduce incidence and severity of fluid retention and hypersensitivity reactions.
- Bone marrow toxicity is the most frequent and dose-limiting toxicity. Frequent blood count monitoring is necessary during therapy.
- Monitor patient closely for hypersensitivity reactions, especially during the first and second infusions.
- Safety and effectiveness in children have not been established.

• Contact of undiluted docetaxel concentrate with polyvinyl chloride equipment or devices is not recommended.

🜄 I.V. administration

• Wear gloves during preparation and administration of docetaxel. If solution contacts skin, wash immediately and thoroughly with soap and water. If drug contacts mucous membranes, they should be flushed thoroughly with water. Mark all waste materials with CHEMOTHERAPY HAZARD labels.

• Prepare and store infusion solutions in bottles (glass or polypropylene) or plastic bags, and administer through polyethylene-lined administration sets. Administer drug as 1-hour infusion; store unopened vials in refrigerator.

• Dilute docetaxel using diluent supplied before administration. Allow drug and diluent to stand at room temperature for 5 minutes before mixing. After adding all the diluent to drug vial, gently rotate vial for about 15 seconds. Allow solution to stand for a few minutes to enable foam to dissipate. All foam need not fully dissipate before proceeding to the next step.

• Prepare docetaxel infusion solution by withdrawing the required amount of premixed solution from the vial and injecting it into 250 ml 0.9% NaCl or D₅W to produce a final concentration of 0.3 to 0.9 mg/ml. Doses exceeding 240 mg require a larger volume of infusion solution so as not to exceed a concentration of 0.9 mg/ml of docetaxel. Mix infusion thoroughly by manual rotation.

• Discard solution if it is not clear or appears to have precipitation.

☑ Patient teaching

• Caution patient of childbearing age to avoid pregnancy or breast-feeding during therapy.

• Warn patient that alopecia occurs in almost 80% of all patients.

• Tell patient to promptly report sore throat, fever, or unusual bruising or bleeding, as well as signs of fluid retention, such as swelling or dyspnea.

---

etoposide (VP-16)
VePesid

etoposide phosphate
Etopophos

Pregnancy Risk Category: D

HOW SUPPLIED
etoposide
Capsules: 50 mg
Injection: 20 mg/ml in 5-ml and 50-ml vials
etoposide phosphate
Injection: 113.6-mg vials equivalent to 100 mg etoposide

ACTION
Unknown. It is thought to damage DNA and inhibit DNA synthesis. Appears to be cell cycle–specific.

Route	Onset	Peak	Duration
PO, IV	Unknown	Unknown	Unknown

INDICATIONS & DOSAGE
Testicular cancer—
Adults: 50 to 100 mg/m² I.V. on 5 consecutive days q 3 to 4 weeks; or 100 mg/m² on days 1, 3, and 5 q 3 to 4 weeks.
Small-cell carcinoma of the lung—
Adults: 35 mg/m²/day I.V. for 4 days; or 50 mg/m²/day I.V. for 5 days. P.O. dosage is two times I.V. dose, rounded to nearest 50 mg.

ADVERSE REACTIONS
CNS: peripheral neuropathy.
CV: hypotension (from too-rapid infusion).
GI: *nausea and vomiting, anorexia, diarrhea,* abdominal pain, *stomatitis.*
Hematologic: anemia, *myelosuppression* (dose-limiting), LEUKOPENIA, THROMBOCYTOPENIA.
Other: *reversible alopecia, anaphylaxis* (rare), phlebitis at injection site (infrequent), rash.

INTERACTIONS
Drug-drug. *Warfarin:* may further prolong PT. Monitor closely.

EFFECTS ON DIAGNOSTIC TESTS
None reported.

CONTRAINDICATIONS
Contraindicated in patients hypersensitive to drug.

NURSING CONSIDERATIONS
• Use cautiously in patients who have had cytotoxic or radiation therapy.
• Obtain baseline blood pressure before starting therapy.
• Anticipate need for antiemetics.
• Have diphenhydramine, hydrocortisone, epinephrine, and emergency equipment available to establish an airway in case anaphylaxis occurs.
• Store capsules in refrigerator.
• Monitor CBC, as ordered. Observe for signs of bone marrow suppression.
• Observe oral cavity for signs of ulceration.
• To prevent bleeding, avoid all I.M. injections when platelet count is below 100,000/mm³.
• Anticipate need for blood transfusion to combat anemia. Patients may receive injections of RBC colony-stimulating factors to promote RBC production and decrease need for blood transfusions.
• Know that etoposide has caused complete remissions in small-cell lung cancer and testicular cancer.
• Be aware that the dose of etoposide phosphate is expressed as etoposide equivalents; 113.6 mg of etoposide phosphate is equivalent to 100 mg of etoposide.

⚫I.V. administration
• Give etoposide by slow I.V. infusion (over at least 30 minutes) to prevent severe hypotension. Etoposide phosphate may be given over 5 to 210 minutes.
• Dilute etoposide for infusion in either D₅W or 0.9% NaCl solution to a concentration of 0.2 or 0.4 mg/ml. Higher concentrations may crystallize. Etoposide phosphate may be given without further dilution or it may be diluted to concentrations as low as 0.1 mg/ml in either D₅W or 0.9% NaCl.
• Know that etoposide diluted to 0.2 mg/ml is stable for 96 hours at room tempera-

ture in plastic or glass unprotected from light; solutions diluted to 0.4 mg/ml are stable for 48 hours under the same conditions. Diluted solutions of etoposide phosphate are stable at room temperature or under refrigeration for 24 hours.
Alert: Monitor blood pressure every 15 minutes during infusion. If systolic pressure falls below 90 mm Hg, stop infusion and notify doctor.
• Follow institutional policy to reduce risks. Preparation and administration of parenteral form of drug are associated with carcinogenic, mutagenic, and teratogenic risks for personnel.

☑Patient teaching
• Tell patient to watch for signs of infection (fever, sore throat, fatigue) and bleeding (easy bruising, nosebleeds, bleeding gums, melena), and to take temperature daily.
• Inform patient of need for frequent blood pressure readings during I.V. administration.
• Caution women of childbearing age to avoid pregnancy or breast-feeding during therapy.

---

gemcitabine hydrochloride
Gemzar

Pregnancy Risk Category: D

HOW SUPPLIED
Powder for injection: 200-mg, 1-g vials

ACTION
Cytotoxic; cell-phase specific; inhibits DNA synthesis and blocks progression of cells through G1/S-phase boundary.

Route	Onset	Peak	Duration
IV	Unknown	Unknown	Unknown

INDICATIONS & DOSAGE
Locally advanced or metastatic adenocarcinoma of the pancreas and those treated previously with fluorouracil—
Adults: 1,000 mg/m² I.V. over 30 minutes once weekly for up to 7 weeks, unless toxicity occurs. Monitor CBC (including differential) and platelet count before giv-

ing each dose. If bone marrow suppression is detected, therapy is adjusted. Give full dose if absolute granulocyte count (AGC) is 1,000/mm³ or more and platelet count is 100,000/mm³ or more. If AGC is 500/mm³ to 999/mm³, or if platelet count is 50,000/mm³ to 99,999/mm³, 75% of dose should be given. Withhold dose if AGC is below 500/mm³ or platelet count is below 50,000/mm³. Treatment course of 7 weeks is followed by 1 week rest. Subsequent dosage cycles consist of 1 infusion weekly for 3 out of 4 consecutive weeks. Dosage adjustments for subsequent cycles are based on AGC and platelet count nadirs and degree of non-hematologic toxicity.

✳ *NEW INDICATION: In combination with cisplatin as first-line treatment of inoperable, locally advanced, or metastatic non-small-cell lung cancer—*
Adults: 4-week schedule: 1,000 mg/m² I.V. over 30 minutes on days 1, 8, and 15 of each 28-day cycle. Cisplatin 100 mg/m² on day 1 after gemcitabine infusion.

3-week schedule: 1,250 mg/m² I.V. over 30 minutes on days 1 and 8 of each 21-day cycle. Cisplatin 100 mg/m² on day 1 after gemcitabine infusion.

ADVERSE REACTIONS
CNS: *somnolence, paresthesia.*
GI: *stomatitis, nausea, vomiting, constipation, diarrhea.*
GU: *proteinuria, hematuria,* elevated BUN and creatinine.
Hematologic: *anemia,* LEUKOPENIA, NEUTROPENIA, THROMBOCYTOPENIA.
Hepatic: *elevated liver enzymes.*
Respiratory: *dyspnea, **bronchospasm.***
Other: *alopecia, pain, fever, rash, flulike symptoms,* HEMORRHAGE, *infection, edema, peripheral edema, **anaphylaxis,*** pain at injection site.

INTERACTIONS
None reported.

EFFECTS ON DIAGNOSTIC TESTS
Drug may increase alkaline phosphatase, ALT, AST, bilirubin, BUN; may decrease hemoglobin, WBC, platelets.

CONTRAINDICATIONS
Contraindicated in patients with hypersensitivity to drug.

NURSING CONSIDERATIONS
• Use cautiously in patients with renal or hepatic impairment.
• Know that drug is not recommended for use in pregnant or breast-feeding patients.
• Monitor patient closely. Expect dosage modification according to toxicity and degree of myelosuppression. Age, gender, and presence of renal impairment may predispose patient to toxicity.
• Know that careful hematologic monitoring, especially of neutrophil and platelet counts, is required.
• Obtain baseline and periodic renal and hepatic laboratory tests, as ordered.
• Know that safety and effectiveness in children have not been determined.

🜊 I.V. administration
• Follow institutional policy to reduce risks. Preparation and administration of parenteral form of drug is associated with mutagenic, teratogenic, and carcinogenic risks for personnel.
• To prepare solution, add 5 ml of 0.9% NaCl injection without preservatives to 200-mg vial or 25 ml of diluent to a 1-g vial. Shake to dissolve. The resulting concentration is 40 mg/ml; reconstitution at greater concentrations is not recommended. Resulting concentration may be further diluted with 0.9% NaCl injection to a concentration as low as 0.1 mg/ml, if needed. Solution should be clear to light straw-colored, and be free of particulate matter. It is stable for 24 hours at room temperature. Do not refrigerate reconstituted drug because crystallization may occur.
• Be aware that prolonging infusion time beyond 60 minutes or administering drug more frequently than once weekly may increase toxicity.

☑ Patient teaching
• Advise patient to watch for signs of infection (fever, sore throat, fatigue) and bleeding (easy bruising, nosebleeds, bleeding gums, melena). Tell patient to take temperature daily.

Reactions may be *common,* uncommon, *life-threatening,* or COMMON AND LIFE-THREATENING.

• Caution women of childbearing age to avoid pregnancy or breast-feeding during therapy.

---

irinotecan hydrochloride
Campto§, Camptosar

Pregnancy Risk Category: D

HOW SUPPLIED
Injection: 100-mg/5-ml vial

ACTION
Irinotecan is a derivative of camptothecin. Camptothecins interact specifically with the enzyme topoisomerase I, which relieves torsional strain in DNA by inducing reversible single-strand breaks. Irinotecan and its active metabolite bind to the topoisomerase I-DNA complex and prevent relegation of these single-strand breaks.

Route	Onset	Peak	Duration
IV	Unknown	1 hr	Unknown

INDICATIONS & DOSAGE
Treatment of metastatic carcinoma of the colon or rectum that has recurred or progressed following fluorouracil (5-FU) therapy—
Adults: initially, 125 mg/m^2 I.V. infusion over 90 minutes. Recommended treatment is 125 mg/m^2 I.V. once weekly for 4 weeks followed by a 2-week rest period. Thereafter, additional courses of treatment may be repeated q 6 weeks (4 weeks on therapy, followed by 2 weeks off therapy). Subsequent doses may be adjusted to a low of 50 mg/m^2 or to a maximum of 150 mg/m^2 in 25- to 50- mg/m^2 increments, based on patient's tolerance. Treatment with additional courses may continue indefinitely in patients who respond favorably and in those whose disease remains stable, provided intolerable toxicity does not occur.

ADVERSE REACTIONS
CNS: *insomnia, dizziness, asthenia, headache,* akathisia.
CV: *vasodilation, edema.*
GI: DIARRHEA, *nausea, vomiting, anorexia, stomatitis, constipation, flatulence,* *dyspepsia, abdominal cramping and pain, abdominal enlargement.*
Hematologic: LEUKOPENIA, *anemia,* NEUTROPENIA.
Metabolic: *weight loss, dehydration, increased alkaline phosphatase, increased AST levels.*
Respiratory: *dyspnea, increased coughing, rhinitis.*
Skin: *alopecia, sweating, rash.*
Other: *fever, pain, back pain, chills, minor infection.*

INTERACTIONS
Drug-drug. *Other antineoplastic agents:* may cause additive adverse effects, such as myelosuppression and diarrhea. Monitor patient closely.
Pelvic or abdominal irradiation: increased risk of severe myelosuppression. Avoid concurrent use of drug with irradiation.

EFFECTS ON DIAGNOSTIC TESTS
Drug may increase alkaline phosphatase and AST levels; may decrease hemoglobin, WBC, and platelet count.

CONTRAINDICATIONS
Contraindicated in patients with hypersensitivity to drug.

NURSING CONSIDERATIONS
• Use cautiously in elderly patients.
• Drug is packaged in a plastic blister to protect against inadvertent breakage and leakage. Inspect vial for damage and visible signs of leakage before removing blister.
• Store vial at room temperature of 59° to 86° F (15° to 30° C), and protect from light.
• Diuretic therapy may be withheld during therapy and periods of active vomiting or diarrhea to decrease risk of dehydration.
• Know that drug can induce severe diarrhea. Diarrhea occurring within 24 hours of administration may be preceded by diaphoresis and abdominal cramping and may be relieved by 0.25 to 1 mg atropine I.V., unless contraindicated. Diarrhea occurring more than 24 hours after administration of irinotecan may be prolonged, leading to dehydration and electrolyte im-

---

balances, and can be life-threatening. Late diarrhea occurring after 24 hours should be treated with loperamide, as ordered. Monitor patient's fluid status and serum electrolytes.

• Temporarily discontinue therapy if neutropenic fever occurs or if absolute neutrophil count drops below 500/mm³. Dosage should be reduced, as ordered, especially if WBC count is below 2,000/mm³, neutrophil is below 1,000/mm³, hemoglobin is below 8 g/dl, or platelet count is below 100,000/mm³.

• Know that routine administration of a colony-stimulating factor is not necessary but may be helpful in patients experiencing significant neutropenia.

• Monitor WBC count with differential, hemoglobin level, and platelet count before each dose of irinotecan.

• Know that safety and effectiveness in children have not been established.

⬛ I.V. administration

• Premedicate patient with antiemetic agents on day of treatment starting at least 30 minutes before administering irinotecan.

• Wear gloves while handling and preparing infusion solutions. If drug contacts skin, wash thoroughly with soap and water. If drug contacts mucous membranes, flush thoroughly with water.

• Know that irinotecan must be diluted in D₅W injection (preferred) or 0.9% NaCl injection before infusion. Final concentration range is 0.12 to 1.1 mg/ml.

• Irinotecan solution is stable for up to 24 hours at room temperature of 77° F (25° C) and in ambient fluorescent lighting. Solutions diluted in D₅W, stored at refrigerated temperatures of 36° to 46° F (2° to 8° C), and protected from light are stable for 48 hours. However, because of possible microbial contamination during dilution, use the admixture within 24 hours if refrigerated or 6 hours if kept at room temperature. Refrigerating admixtures using 0.9% NaCl is not recommended because of a low and sporadic incidence of visible particulate. Do not freeze admixture because drug may precipitate.

• Do not add other drugs to irinotecan infusion.

• Avoid extravasation of drug. If extravasation occurs, flush site with sterile water and apply ice. Notify doctor.

☑ Patient teaching

• Inform patient about risk of diarrhea and how to treat it; tell him to avoid laxatives.

• Tell patient to notify doctor if vomiting occurs, fever or evidence of infection develops, or symptoms of dehydration (fainting, light-headedness, or dizziness) occur following irinotecan administration.

• Warn patient that alopecia may occur.

• Caution women of childbearing age to avoid pregnancy or breast-feeding during therapy.

---

mitotane (o,p′-DDD)
Lysodren

Pregnancy Risk Category: C

HOW SUPPLIED
Tablets (scored): 500 mg

ACTION
Unknown. May suppress function of adrenocortical tissue and hinder extra-adrenal metabolism of cortisol.

Route	Onset	Peak	Duration
PO	2 days-6 wk	3-5 hr	6-7 mo

INDICATIONS & DOSAGE
Inoperable adrenocortical cancer—
Adults: initially, 2 to 6 g P.O. daily in divided doses t.i.d. or q.i.d.; increased to 9 to 10 g P.O. daily, in divided doses t.i.d. or q.i.d. Adjust dosage until maximum tolerated dosage is achieved (varies from 2 to 16 g/day but is usually 9 to 10 g/day).

ADVERSE REACTIONS
CNS: *depression, somnolence, lethargy, vertigo;* brain damage and dysfunction (with long-term, high-dose therapy).
CV: hypertension, orthostatic hypotension.
EENT: visual disturbances, diplopia, lens opacity, toxic retinopathy.
GI: *severe nausea, vomiting, diarrhea, anorexia.*

Reactions may be *common,* uncommon, ***life-threatening,*** or **COMMON AND LIFE-THREATENING.**

GU: hemorrhagic cystitis.
Skin: dermatitis, *maculopapular rash,* flushing.
Other: increased serum cholesterol level, adrenal insufficiency, myalgia, fever, muscle twitching.

INTERACTIONS
Drug-drug. *Corticosteroids:* increased metabolism of corticosteroids requiring higher corticosteroid doses. Monitor carefully.
Warfarin: increased metabolism, which may require higher warfarin doses. Monitor PT and INR closely.

EFFECTS ON DIAGNOSTIC TESTS
Drug therapy may increase concentrations of urinary 17-hydroxycorticosteroid, plasma cortisol, protein-bound iodine, and serum uric acid.

CONTRAINDICATIONS
Contraindicated in patients hypersensitive to drug and in those in shock or who have suffered trauma.

NURSING CONSIDERATIONS
• Use cautiously in patients with hepatic disease.
• To reduce nausea, give antiemetic before mitotane, as ordered.
• Monitor effectiveness according to reduction in pain, weakness, and anorexia.
• Assess and record behavioral and neurologic signs daily. Prolonged therapy has been associated with significant neurologic impairment.
• Be aware that use of corticosteroids may avoid acute adrenocorticoid insufficiency and is usually required. Glucocorticoid dosage should be increased in periods of physiologic stress such as infection or trauma.
• Because drug distributes mostly to body fat, know that obese patients may need higher dosage and may have longer-lasting adverse reactions.
• Keep in mind that an adequate therapeutic trial is at least 3 months, but treatment can continue if clinical benefits are observed.

✓ **Patient teaching**
• Warn ambulatory patient to avoid activities that require alertness and good motor coordination until CNS effects of the drug are known.
• Instruct patient to notify doctor if severe adverse GI or skin reactions occur because dosage adjustment may be needed.
• Counsel women of childbearing age to avoid pregnancy or breast-feeding during therapy.

---

mitoxantrone hydrochloride
Novantrone

Pregnancy Risk Category: D

HOW SUPPLIED
Injection: 2 mg/ml in 10-ml, 12.5-ml, 15-ml vials

ACTION
Not fully understood; probably cell cycle–nonspecific. Reacts with DNA, producing cytotoxic effect.

Route	Onset	Peak	Duration
IV	Unknown	Unknown	Unknown

INDICATIONS & DOSAGE
Combination initial therapy for acute nonlymphocytic leukemia—
Adults: induction begins with 12 mg/m^2 I.V. daily on days 1 to 3, in combination with 100 mg/m^2 daily of cytarabine on days 1 to 7. A second induction may be given if response is not adequate. Maintenance therapy: 12 mg/m^2 on days 1 and 2, in combination with cytarabine on days 1 to 5.
Combination initial therapy for pain related to advanced hormone-refractory prostate cancer—
Adults: 12 to 14 mg/m^2 I.V. infusion over 15 to 30 minutes q 21 days as an adjunct to corticosteroid therapy.

ADVERSE REACTIONS
CNS: *seizures,* headache.
CV: *heart failure, arrhythmias,* tachycardia.
EENT: conjunctivitis.

GI: *bleeding, abdominal pain, diarrhea, nausea, mucositis, vomiting, stomatitis.*
GU: *renal failure.*
Hematologic: *myelosuppression.*
Hepatic: jaundice.
Respiratory: *dyspnea, cough.*
Skin: *alopecia, petechiae, ecchymoses,* local irritation or phlebitis.
Other: hyperuricemia, *sepsis, fungal infections, fever.*

INTERACTIONS
Drug-drug. *Heparin:* physically incompatible. Do not mix together.

EFFECTS ON DIAGNOSTIC TESTS
Drug may increase AST, ALT, bilirubin, and uric acid.

CONTRAINDICATIONS
Contraindicated in patients hypersensitive to mitoxantrone.

NURSING CONSIDERATIONS
• Use cautiously in patients with prior exposure to anthracyclines or other cardiotoxic drugs, prior radiation therapy to the mediastinal area, and preexisting heart disease.
• Be aware that patients with significant myelosuppression should not receive mitoxantrone unless the benefits outweigh the risks.
• Be prepared to administer allopurinol, as ordered. Uric acid nephropathy can be avoided by hydrating the patient before and during therapy.
• Closely monitor hematologic and laboratory chemistry parameters.
• To prevent bleeding, avoid all I.M. injections if platelet count falls below 100,000/mm³.
• Anticipate the need for blood transfusion to combat anemia. Patients may receive injections of RBC colony-stimulating factors to promote RBC production and decrease need for blood transfusions.
• Be aware that left ventricular ejection fraction should be monitored.
• Be prepared to treat infections with antibiotics, as ordered. Patients may receive injections of WBC colony-stimulating factors to promote cell growth and decrease risk for infection.

• If severe nonhematologic toxicity occurs during the first course, know that the second course should be delayed until patient recovers.

◖ **I.V. administration**
• Follow institutional policy to minimize risks. Preparation and administration of parenteral form is associated with mutagenic, teratogenic, and carcinogenic risks to personnel.
• Dilute dose (available as an aqueous solution of 2 mg/ml in volumes of 10, 12.5, and 15 ml) in at least 50 ml of 0.9% NaCl injection or D_5W injection. Administer by direct injection into a free-flowing I.V. line of 0.9% NaCl or D_5W injection over at least 3 minutes, usually 15 to 30 minutes. Mixing with other drugs is not recommended.
• If drug extravasates, discontinue infusion immediately and notify doctor.
• Once vial is penetrated, may store undiluted solution at room temperature for 7 days or 14 days in refrigerator. Do not freeze.

☑ **Patient teaching**
• Inform patient that urine may appear blue-green within 24 hours after administration and some bluish discoloration of the sclera may occur. These effects are not harmful.
• Advise patient to watch for signs of bleeding and infection.
• Caution women of childbearing age to avoid pregnancy during therapy. Also recommend consulting doctor before becoming pregnant.

---

paclitaxel
Taxol

Pregnancy Risk Category: D

HOW SUPPLIED
Injection: 30 mg/5 ml, 100 mg/16.7 ml

ACTION
Prevents depolymerization of cellular microtubules, thus inhibiting the normal reorganization of the microtubule network

---

necessary for mitosis and other vital cellular functions.

Route	Onset	Peak	Duration
IV	Unknown	Unknown	Unknown

INDICATIONS & DOSAGE

Metastatic ovarian cancer after failure of first-line or subsequent chemotherapy—
Adults: 135 mg/m^2 or 175 mg/m^2 I.V. over 3 hours q 3 weeks.
Breast cancer after failure of combination chemotherapy for metastatic disease or relapse within 6 months of adjuvant chemotherapy—
Adults: 175 mg/m^2 I.V. over 3 hours q 3 weeks.
Second-line therapy in patients with AIDS-related Kaposi's sarcoma—
Adults: 135 mg/m^2 I.V. over 3 hours q 3 weeks, or 100 mg/m^2 I.V. over 3 hours q 2 weeks.
Adjust-a-dose: In patients experiencing severe neutropenia (neutrophil count below 500 cells/mm^3 for 1 week or more) or severe peripheral neuropathy, reduce subsequent courses of Taxol by 20%.

ADVERSE REACTIONS

CNS: *peripheral neuropathy.*
CV: *bradycardia, hypotension, abnormal ECG.*
GI: *nausea, vomiting, diarrhea, mucositis.*
Hematologic: NEUTROPENIA, LEUKOPENIA, THROMBOCYTOPENIA, anemia, *bleeding.*
Hepatic: *elevated liver enzyme levels.*
Other: *hypersensitivity reactions (anaphylaxis), alopecia, myalgia, arthralgia, phlebitis, cellulitis at injection site, infections.*

INTERACTIONS

Drug-drug. *Cisplatin:* possible additive myelosuppressive effects. When given together, paclitaxel should be given before cisplatin.
Doxorubicin: parent and metabolite of doxorubicin may be increased when coadministered. Use together cautiously.
Ketoconazole: inhibited paclitaxel metabolism. Use together cautiously.

EFFECTS ON DIAGNOSTIC TESTS

Drug alters hematologic studies because of its suppressive effect on bone marrow. Drug may increase alkaline phosphatase, AST, bilirubin, and triglycerides.

CONTRAINDICATIONS

Contraindicated in patients with hypersensitivity to drug or polyoxyethylated castor oil (a vehicle used in drug solution) and in those with baseline neutrophil counts below 1,500/mm^3 or AIDS-related Kaposi's sarcoma with baseline neutrophil counts below 1,000/mm^3.

NURSING CONSIDERATIONS

• Use cautiously in patients with hepatic impairment.
• Some patients experience peripheral neuropathies, which may be cumulative and dose-related. Severe symptoms may require dose reduction.
• To reduce the incidence or severity of hypersensitivity, anticipate pretreating patient with corticosteroids, such as dexamethasone, and antihistamines, as ordered. Both H$_1$-receptor antagonists, such as diphenhydramine, and H$_2$-receptor antagonists, such as cimetidine or ranitidine, may be used. Severe hypersensitivity reactions have occurred in as many as 2% of patients treated in early clinical trials.
• Frequently monitor blood counts during therapy. Bone marrow toxicity is the most common and dose-limiting toxicity. Packed RBC or platelet transfusions may be necessary in severe cases. Institute bleeding precautions as appropriate.
• Patient may receive injections of RBC colony-stimulating factors to promote RBC production and decrease need for blood transfusions.
• Avoid all I.M. injections when platelet count is below 100,000/mm^3.
• If patient develops significant cardiac conduction abnormalities, initiate appropriate therapy and continuous cardiac monitoring during therapy and subsequent infusions.
• Initiate or repeat doses for Kaposi's sarcoma only if neutrophil count exceeds 1,000 cells/mm^3; patient may also require reduction in dexamethasone premedica-

tion dose and the start of a hematopoietic growth factor.

◘ I.V. administration
• Follow institutional protocol for the safe handling, preparation, and administration of chemotherapeutic drugs. Preparation and administration of parenteral form of drug are associated with carcinogenic, mutagenic, and teratogenic risks for personnel. Mark all waste materials with CHEMOTHERAPY HAZARD labels.
• Dilute concentrate before infusion. Compatible solutions include 0.9% NaCl injection, D₅W, 5% dextrose in 0.9% NaCl injection, and 5% dextrose in Ringer's lactate injection. Dilute to a final concentration of 0.3 to 1.2 mg/ml. Diluted solutions are stable for 24 hours at room temperature.
• Prepare and store infusion solutions in glass containers. The undiluted concentrate shouldn't contact polyvinyl chloride I.V. bags or tubing. Prepared solution may appear hazy. Store diluted solution in glass or polypropylene bottles, or use polypropylene or polyolefin bags. Administer through polyethylene-lined administration sets, and use an in-line 0.22-micron filter.
• Take care to avoid extravasation.
• Continuously monitor patient for 30 minutes after initiating the infusion. Continue close monitoring throughout infusion.

☑ Patient teaching
• Tell patient to watch for signs of infection (fever, sore throat, fatigue) and bleeding (easy bruising, nosebleeds, bleeding gums, melena), and to take temperature daily.
• Teach patient signs and symptoms of peripheral neuropathy, such as a tingling or burning sensation or numbness in the extremities, and advise her to report these symptoms immediately.
• Warn patient that alopecia is common (up to 82% of patients).
• Caution women of childbearing age to avoid becoming pregnant during therapy and to consult with doctor before becoming pregnant.

pegaspargase
(PEG-L-asparaginase)
Oncaspar

Pregnancy Risk Category: C

HOW SUPPLIED
Injection: 750 IU/ml

ACTION
A modified version of the enzyme L-asparaginase that exerts its cytotoxic activity by inactivating the amino acid asparagine. Asparagine is required by tumor cells to synthesize proteins. Because the tumor cells cannot synthesize their own asparagine, protein synthesis and, eventually, synthesis of DNA and RNA is inhibited.

Route	Onset	Peak	Duration
IV, IM	Unknown	Unknown	Unknown

INDICATIONS & DOSAGE
Acute lymphoblastic leukemia (ALL) in patients who require L-asparaginase but have developed hypersensitivity to the native forms of L-asparaginase—
Adults and children with body surface area (BSA) of at least 0.6 m²: 2,500 IU/m² I.M. or I.V. q 14 days.
Children with BSA below 0.6 m²: 82.5 IU/kg I.M. or I.V. q 14 days.

ADVERSE REACTIONS
CNS: *seizures,* headache, paresthesia, *status epilepticus,* somnolence, coma, mental status changes, dizziness, emotional lability, mood changes, parkinsonism, confusion, disorientation, fatigue.
CV: hypotension, tachycardia, chest pain, subacute bacterial endocarditis, hypertension.
EENT: epistaxis.
GI: nausea, vomiting, abdominal pain, anorexia, diarrhea, constipation, indigestion, flatulence, mucositis, mouth tenderness, *pancreatitis (sometimes fulminant and fatal),* increased serum amylase and lipase levels, severe colitis.
GU: increased BUN level, increased creatinine level, increased urinary frequency, hematuria, severe hemorrhagic cystitis, renal dysfunction, *renal failure.*

Reactions may be *common,* uncommon, *life-threatening*, or COMMON AND LIFE-THREATENING.

Hematologic: *thrombosis;* prolonged PT, prolonged PTT, decreased antithrombin III; *disseminated intravascular coagulation;* decreased fibrinogen; hemolytic anemia; *leukopenia; pancytopenia; agranulocytosis; thrombocytopenia;* increased thromboplastin; easy bruising; ecchymoses; *hemorrhage.*

Hepatic: jaundice, abnormal liver function test results, bilirubinemia, increased ALT and AST, ascites, hypoalbuminemia, fatty changes in liver, *liver failure.*

Metabolic: hyperuricemia, hyponatremia, uric acid nephropathy, hypoproteinemia, proteinuria, weight loss, metabolic acidosis, increased blood ammonia level, hyperglycemia, hypoglycemia.

Musculoskeletal: arthralgia, myalgia, musculoskeletal pain, joint stiffness, cramps.

Respiratory: cough, *severe bronchospasm,* upper respiratory tract infection.

Skin: itching, alopecia, fever blister, purpura, hand whiteness, fungal changes, nail whiteness and ridging, erythema simplex, petechial rash, injection pain or reaction, localized edema.

Other: *hypersensitivity reactions,* including *anaphylaxis,* rash, erythema, edema, pain, fever, chills, urticaria, dyspnea, or bronchospasm; pain in extremities; peripheral edema; malaise; night sweats; infection; *sepsis, septic shock.*

INTERACTIONS

Drug-drug. *Aspirin, dipyridamole, heparin, NSAIDs, warfarin:* imbalances in coagulation factors may occur, predisposing the patient to bleeding or thrombosis. Use together cautiously.

Methotrexate: during the period of its inhibition of protein synthesis and cell replication, pegaspargase may interfere with the action of such drugs as methotrexate, which require cell replication for their lethal effects. Monitor for decreased effectiveness.

Protein-bound drugs: depletion of serum proteins by pegaspargase may increase toxicity of other drugs that bind to proteins. Monitor for toxicity. Pegaspargase also may interfere with enzymatic detoxification of other drugs, particularly in the liver. Administer concomitantly with caution.

EFFECTS ON DIAGNOSTIC TESTS

Drug may cause decreased serum glucose, sodium, and albumin; may increase AST, ALT, BUN, creatinine, uric acid, and amylase.

CONTRAINDICATIONS

Contraindicated in patients with pancreatitis or history of pancreatitis; in those who have had significant hemorrhagic events associated with prior L-asparaginase; and in those with previous serious allergic reactions, such as generalized urticaria, bronchospasm, laryngeal edema, hypotension, or other unacceptable adverse reactions to pegaspargase.

NURSING CONSIDERATIONS

● Use cautiously in patients with liver dysfunction and only when clearly indicated in pregnant patients.

● Know that pegaspargase should be used as sole induction agent only when a combined regimen that uses other chemotherapeutic agents is inappropriate because of toxicity or other specific patient-related factors, or in patients refractory to other therapy.

● Be aware that I.M. route is preferred because it has the lowest incidence of hepatotoxicity, coagulopathy, and GI and renal disorders.

● Do not administer if drug has been frozen. Although there may not be a change in the appearance of drug, pegaspargase's activity is destroyed after freezing. Obtain new dose from pharmacist.

● Avoid excessive agitation; do *not* shake. Keep refrigerated at 36° to 46° F (2° to 8° C). Do not use if cloudy or if precipitate is present. Do not use if stored at room temperature for more than 48 hours. Do not freeze. Discard unused portions. Use only one dose per vial; do not reenter vial.

● Drug may be a contact irritant, and solution must be handled and administered with care. Gloves are recommended. Inhalation of vapors and contact with skin or mucous membranes, especially those of the eyes, must be avoided. In case of contact, wash with copious amounts of water for at least 15 minutes.

● When administering I.M., limit volume administered at a single injection site to

2 ml. If volume to be administered is greater than 2 ml, use multiple injection sites.

Alert: Monitor patient closely for hypersensitivity reactions such as life-threatening anaphylaxis, which may occur during therapy, especially in those with known hypersensitivity to the other forms of L-asparaginase. As a routine precaution, keep patient under observation for 1 hour and have resuscitation equipment and other agents necessary to treat anaphylaxis (such as epinephrine, oxygen, and I.V. steroids) readily available. Know that moderate to life-threatening hypersensitivity reactions require discontinuation of L-asparaginase.

• To assess effects of therapy, monitor patient's peripheral blood count and bone marrow, as ordered. A fall in circulating lymphoblasts is often noted after initiating therapy. This may be accompanied by a marked rise in serum uric acid levels.

• Take preventive measures (including adequate hydration) before starting treatment. Hyperuricemia may result from rapid lysis of leukemic cells. Allopurinol may be ordered.

• Obtain frequent serum amylase determinations, as ordered, to detect pancreatitis. Monitor patient's blood glucose during therapy to detect hyperglycemia.

• Monitor patient for liver dysfunction when pegaspargase is used in conjunction with hepatotoxic chemotherapeutic agents.

• Be aware that pegaspargase may affect a number of plasma proteins; therefore, monitoring of fibrinogen, PT, and PTT may be indicated. Question doctor if not ordered.

◖ I.V. administration
• When administering I.V., give over a period of 1 to 2 hours in 100 ml of 0.9% NaCl or D_5W injection through an infusion that is already running.

☑ Patient teaching
• Inform patient of risk of hypersensitivity reactions and importance of alerting the staff immediately if they occur.

• Instruct patient not to take other drugs, including OTC preparations, until approved by doctor because risk of bleeding is higher when pegaspargase is given concomitantly with certain drugs, such as aspirin, or because it may increase the toxicity of other medications.

• Instruct patient to report signs and symptoms of infection (fever, chills, and malaise); drug may have immunosuppressant activity.

• Caution women of childbearing age to avoid pregnancy or breast-feeding during therapy.

---

porfimer sodium
Photofrin

Pregnancy Risk Category: C

HOW SUPPLIED
Injection: 75 mg/vial

ACTION
A photosensitizing drug that damages cancer cells through propagation of radical reactions. Tumor death also occurs through ischemic necrosis secondary to vascular occlusion that appears to be partly mediated by release of thromboxane A_2. Cytotoxic and antitumor actions of porfimer depend on light and oxygen.

Route	Onset	Peak	Duration
IV	Unknown	Unknown	Unknown

INDICATIONS & DOSAGE
Palliative treatment for patients with completely obstructing esophageal cancer or for those with partially obstructing esophageal cancer who cannot be satisfactorily treated with Nd:YAG laser therapy—
Adults: 2 mg/kg I.V. for 3 to 5 minutes (first stage of therapy), followed by illumination with laser light 40 to 50 hours later (second stage). A second laser-light application may be given 96 to 120 hours after injection. A total of three courses (each course consisting of both stages) may be given, separated by at least 30 days.
✷ *NEW INDICATION: Treatment of microinvasive endobronchial non-small cell lung cancer in patients for whom surgery and radiotherapy are not indicated—*

Adults: 2 mg/kg I.V. for 3 to 5 minutes (first stage of therapy), followed by illumination with laser light 40 to 50 hours later (second stage). A second laser-light application may be given 96 to 120 hours after injection. A total of three courses (each course consisting of both stages) may be given, separated by at least 30 days.

ADVERSE REACTIONS
CNS: anxiety, confusion, *insomnia.*
CV: hypotension, hypertension, ***heart failure,*** atrial fibrillation, tachycardia.
EENT: *pharyngitis,* vision problems (diplopia, discomfort, photophobia).
GI: *constipation, abdominal pain, nausea, vomiting,* diarrhea, dyspepsia, dysphagia, eructation, esophageal edema, esophageal tumor bleeding, esophageal stricture, esophagitis, hematemesis, melena, anorexia.
GU: urinary tract infection.
Hematologic: *anemia.*
Respiratory: coughing, *dyspnea, pleural effusion, pneumonia,* respiratory insufficiency, tracheoesophageal fistula.
Skin: *photosensitivity.*
Other: *back or chest pain,* asthenia, substernal or general pain, edema, fever, surgical complication, dehydration, weight loss, candidiasis.

INTERACTIONS
Drug-drug. *Other photosensitizing drugs (griseofulvin, phenothiazines, sulfonamides, sulfonylurea hypoglycemic agents, tetracyclines, thiazide diuretics):* may increase photosensitivity reaction. Use together cautiously.
Drug-lifestyle. *Sun exposure:* photosensitivity reactions may occur. Take precautions.

EFFECTS ON DIAGNOSTIC TESTS
Drug may decrease hematocrit and hemoglobin.

CONTRAINDICATIONS
Contraindicated in patients with porphyria, tracheoesophageal or bronchoesophageal fistula, tumor eroding into major blood vessel, or hypersensitivity to porphyrins.

NURSING CONSIDERATIONS
• Breast-feeding is not recommended during drug therapy because it isn't known if drug is excreted in breast milk.
• Safety and efficacy in children have not been established.
• Before each course of treatment, patient should be evaluated for a tracheoesophageal or bronchoesophageal fistula.
• Don't allow drug to contact eyes or skin during preparation or administration. Protect an exposed person from bright light.
• Know that patient must receive 630-nm wavelength laser-light therapy 40 to 50 hours after porfimer injection for drug to be effective. A second laser-light treatment (but not a second injection) may be given as early as 96 hours or as late as 120 hours after injection. Before a second treatment, the residual tumor should be debrided; be aware that vigorous debridement may cause tumor bleeding. Monitor patient closely.
• Know that inflammation of treatment area may cause substernal chest pain. Notify doctor if this occurs; pain may be sufficiently intense to warrant short-term use of opiate analgesics.
• Monitor CBC regularly to detect anemia. Drug and laser therapy may cause tumor bleeding.

◖ I.V. administration
• Reconstitute each vial of porfimer with 31.8 ml of D_5W solution or 0.9% NaCl solution for injection, resulting in final concentration of 2.5 mg/ml. Shake until dissolved. Do not mix porfimer with other drugs in same solution. Reconstituted drug is opaque. Inspect carefully for particulate and discoloration before administration. Protect reconstituted drug from bright light, and use immediately.
• Administer drug as a single slow I.V. injection over 3 to 5 minutes.
• Take precautions to prevent extravasation at injection site. If it occurs, protect the area from light.

☑ Patient teaching
• Instruct patient to avoid direct sunlight and bright indoor light for 30 days after injection, but tell him to expose skin to ambient indoor light. After 30 days, he

---

should expose a small area of skin (not face) to sunlight for 10 minutes. If he doesn't develop a photosensitivity reaction (erythema, edema, blistering) within 24 hours, he can gradually resume outdoor activities while exercising caution. If photosensitivity occurs, he should avoid sunlight and bright indoor light for 2 weeks before retesting.

• Urge patient traveling to an area with stronger sun to retest his photosensitivity level.

• Warn patient that ultraviolet sunscreens do not protect against photosensitivity.

• Advise patient to wear dark sunglasses with an average white light transmittance of less than 4% when outdoors.

• Caution women of childbearing age to use an effective contraceptive method, avoid pregnancy, and to notify doctor of suspected pregnancy.

---

procarbazine hydrochloride
Matulane, Natulan†

Pregnancy Risk Category: D

HOW SUPPLIED
Capsules: 50 mg

ACTION
Unknown. Thought to inhibit DNA, RNA, and protein synthesis.

Route	Onset	Peak	Duration
PO	Unknown	Unknown	Unknown

INDICATIONS & DOSAGE
Dosage and indications vary. Check treatment protocol with the doctor.
Adjunct treatment of Hodgkin's disease (stages III and IV), other cancers using MOPP (nitrogen mustard, vincristine, procarbazine, prednisone) regimen—
Adults: 2 to 4 mg/kg P.O. daily in single dose or divided doses for first week. Then, 4 to 6 mg/kg/day until WBC count falls below 4,000/mm³ or platelet count falls below 100,000/mm³ or until maximum response obtained. After bone marrow recovers, maintenance dosage of 1 to 2 mg/kg/day resumed. For MOPP regimen, 100 mg/m²/day P.O. for 14 days.

Children: 50 mg/m² P.O. daily for first week; then 100 mg/m² until response or toxicity occurs. Maintenance dosage is 50 mg/m² P.O. daily after bone marrow recovery.

ADVERSE REACTIONS
CNS: nervousness, depression, headache, dizziness, *coma,* insomnia, nightmares, paresthesia, neuropathy, *hallucinations,* confusion, *seizures.*
CV: hypotension, tachycardia, syncope, hypertensive crisis.
EENT: retinal hemorrhage, nystagmus, photophobia.
GI: *nausea, vomiting,* abdominal pain, hematemesis, melena, anorexia, stomatitis, dry mouth, dysphagia, diarrhea, constipation.
GU: hematuria, urinary frequency, nocturia.
Hematologic: *bleeding tendency, thrombocytopenia, leukopenia, anemia,* hemolytic anemia.
Respiratory: *pleural effusion,* cough, pneumonitis.
Skin: reversible alopecia, dermatitis, pruritus, rash, hyperpigmentation, flushing, herpes.
Other: gynecomastia, allergic reaction, *hepatotoxicity.*

INTERACTIONS
Drug-drug. *CNS depressants:* additive depressant effects. Avoid concomitant use.
Digoxin: may decrease serum digoxin levels. Monitor closely.
Drugs high in tyramine, local anesthetics, sympathomimetics, tricyclic antidepressants: possible tremor, palpitations, increased blood pressure. Monitor closely.
Fluoxetine: concurrent use may result in confusion, agitation, restlessness, and GI symptoms. Monitor closely.
Meperidine: concurrent use may result in immediate excitation, sweating, rigidity, and severe hypertension. Monitor closely.
Drug-food. *Caffeine:* concurrent use may result in arrhythmias, severe hypertension. Discourage caffeine intake.
Foods high in tyramine (cheese, Chianti wine): possible tremor, palpitations, increased blood pressure. Monitor closely.

Reactions may be *common*, uncommon, *life-threatening*, or COMMON AND LIFE-THREATENING.

Drug-lifestyle. *Alcohol use:* mild disulfiram-like reaction manifested by flushing, headache, nausea, and hypotension. Warn patient to avoid alcoholic beverages.

EFFECTS ON DIAGNOSTIC TESTS
None reported.

CONTRAINDICATIONS
Contraindicated in patients hypersensitive to drug and in those with inadequate bone marrow reserve as shown by bone marrow aspiration.

NURSING CONSIDERATIONS
• Use cautiously in patients with impaired hepatic or renal function.
• Monitor CBC and platelet counts.
• To prevent bleeding, avoid all I.M. injections when platelet count is below 100,000/mm³.
• Anticipate the need for blood transfusions to combat anemia. Patients may receive injections of RBC colony-stimulating factors to promote RBC production and decrease need for blood transfusions.
• Be prepared to discontinue drug if patient becomes confused or if paresthesia or other neuropathies develop. Notify doctor.

☑ **Patient teaching**
• To decrease nausea and vomiting, advise patient to take drug at bedtime and in divided doses.
• Tell patient to watch for signs of infection (fever, sore throat, fatigue) and bleeding (easy bruising, nosebleeds, bleeding gums, melena), and to take temperature daily.
• Warn patient to avoid alcohol during therapy. Urge him to stop medication and check with doctor immediately if he experiences a disulfiram-like reaction (chest pains, rapid or irregular heartbeat, severe headache, stiff neck).
• Instruct patient to avoid foods high in tyramine, such as wine, cheese, and bananas, and OTC preparations containing sympathomimetics.
• Warn patient to avoid hazardous activities that require alertness and good motor coordination until the CNS effects are known.

• Caution women of childbearing age to avoid becoming pregnant during therapy and to consult with doctor before becoming pregnant.

rituximab
Rituxan

Pregnancy Risk Factor: C

HOW SUPPLIED
Injection: 10 mg/ml; 10 ml, 50 ml single-use, sterile vials

ACTION
A murine/human monoclonal antibody directed against CD20 antigen found on the surface of normal and malignant B-lymphocytes. Binding to this antigen mediates the lysis of the B cells.

Route	Onset	Peak	Duration
IV	Variable	Variable	6-12 mo

INDICATIONS & DOSAGE
B-cell malignant lymphoma with relapsed or refractory low-grade or follicular, CD20 positive disease—
Adults: 375 mg/m² given as I.V. infusion once weekly for four doses (days 1, 8, 15, 22). Initial infusion should be started at 50 mg/hour. If hypersensitivity or infusion-related events do not occur, increase rate 50 mg/hour q 30 minutes, to maximum of 400 mg/hour. Subsequent infusions can be administered at initial rate of 100 mg/hour and increased by increments of 100 mg/hour at 30-minute intervals, to maximum of 400 mg/hour as tolerated.

ADVERSE REACTIONS
CNS: dizziness, *asthenia, headache,* fatigue, paresthesia, malaise, agitation, insomnia, hypesthesia, hypertonia, nervousness.
CV: *hypotension, arrhythmias,* hypertension, peripheral edema, chest pain, tachycardia, postural hypotension, bradycardia.
EENT: sore throat, rhinitis, sinusitis, lacrimation disorder, conjunctivitis.
GI: *nausea,* vomiting, abdominal pain or enlargement, diarrhea, dyspepsia, anorexia, increased LD, taste perversion.

Hematologic: LEUKOPENIA, *thrombocytopenia, neutropenia,* anemia.
Respiratory: *bronchospasm,* dyspnea, cough increase, bronchitis.
Skin: *pruritus, rash,* urticaria, flushing.
Other: ANGIOEDEMA, myalgia, *fever, chills, rigor,* back pain, pain, hyperglycemia, hypercalcemia, pain at injection site, tumor pain.

INTERACTIONS
None reported.

EFFECTS ON DIAGNOSTIC TESTS
None reported.

CONTRAINDICATIONS
Contraindicated in patients with known type I hypersensitivity or anaphylactic reactions to murine proteins or to any component of rituximab.

NURSING CONSIDERATIONS
• Monitor patient closely for signs and symptoms of a hypersensitivity reaction. Have medications such as epinephrine, antihistamine, and corticosteroids available to immediately treat such a reaction. Consider premedicating with acetaminophen and diphenhydramine before each infusion.
• Obtain CBCs at regular intervals and more frequently in patients who develop cytopenias.
• Protect vials from direct sunlight.

◐ I.V. administration
Alert: Drug must be given as I.V. infusion; do not give as an I.V. push or bolus.
• Dilute to a final concentration of 1 to 4 mg/ml in bag of D_5W or 0.9% NaCl. Gently invert bag to mix the solution. Discard unused portion left in vial.
• Monitor patient's blood pressure closely during infusion. If hypotension, bronchospasm, or angioedema occurs, discontinue infusion and restart at a 50% rate reduction when symptoms resolve.
• Discontinue infusion if serious or life-threatening arrhythmias occur. Patients who develop clinically significant arrhythmias should undergo cardiac monitoring during and after subsequent infusions of rituximab.

☑ Patient teaching
• Tell patient to report symptoms during and after infusion.
• Tell patient to watch for signs of infection (fever, sore throat, fatigue) and bleeding (easy bruising, nosebleeds, bleeding gums, melena), and to take temperature daily.

teniposide (VM-26)
Vumon

Pregnancy Risk Category: D

HOW SUPPLIED
Injection: 10 mg/ml

ACTION
A phase-specific cytotoxic drug that acts in the late S or early G_2 phase of the cell cycle, thus preventing cells from entering mitosis.

Route	Onset	Peak	Duration
IV	Unknown	Unknown	Unknown

INDICATIONS & DOSAGE
Refractory childhood acute lymphoblastic leukemia—
Children: optimum dosage hasn't been established. In clinical trials, dosages ranged from 165 to 250 mg/m² I.V. once or twice weekly for 4 to 6 weeks. Usually used in combination with other agents.
Adjust-a-dose: Patients with both Down syndrome and leukemia are at higher risk for myelosuppression. Administer first course of treatment at half the dose.

ADVERSE REACTIONS
CV: hypotension (from rapid infusion).
GI: *nausea, vomiting, mucositis, diarrhea.*
Hematologic: MYELOSUPPRESSION (dose-limiting), LEUKOPENIA, NEUTROPENIA, THROMBOCYTOPENIA, *anemia.*
Other: alopecia (rare), *anaphylaxis* (rare), rash, *infection,* bleeding, *hypersensitivity reactions* (chills, fever, urticaria, tachycardia, *bronchospasm,* dyspnea, hypotension, flushing), *phlebitis and extravasation* (at injection site).

Reactions may be *common,* uncommon, *life-threatening,* or COMMON AND LIFE-THREATENING.

INTERACTIONS

Drug-drug. *Heparin:* physical incompatibility. Don't mix together.

Methotrexate: may increase clearance and intracellular levels of methotrexate. Avoid concurrent use.

Sodium salicylate, sulfamethizole, tolbutamide: may displace teniposide from protein-binding sites and increase toxicity. Do not administer together.

EFFECTS ON DIAGNOSTIC TESTS

Drug therapy may increase blood and urine concentrations of uric acid.

CONTRAINDICATIONS

Contraindicated in patients hypersensitive to drug or to polyoxyethylated castor oil, an injection vehicle.

NURSING CONSIDERATIONS

• Be aware that some clinicians may decide to use drug despite patient's history of hypersensitivity because the therapeutic benefits outweigh its risks. Such patients should be treated with antihistamines and corticosteroids before infusion begins and should be observed continuously for the first hour of infusion and at frequent intervals thereafter.

• Obtain baseline blood counts and renal and hepatic function tests, as ordered.

• Monitor blood pressure before therapy.

• Have on hand diphenhydramine, hydrocortisone, epinephrine, and emergency equipment to establish an airway in case of anaphylaxis.

• Monitor blood counts and renal and hepatic function tests, as ordered.

I.V. administration

• Dilute drug in either D_5W or 0.9% NaCl injection to a final concentration of 0.1, 0.2, 0.4, or 1 mg/ml. Don't agitate vigorously; precipitation of drug may occur. Discard cloudy solutions. Prepare and store drug in glass containers. Infuse over 30 to 60 minutes to prevent hypotension.

• Don't mix with other drugs or solutions.

• Ensure careful placement of I.V. catheter. Extravasation can result in local tissue necrosis or sloughing.

• Occlusion of catheters, including those centrally placed can occur, particularly

during 24 hour infusions at 0.1 to 0.2 mg/ml. Monitor carefully.

• Don't administer through a membrane-type in-line filter because the diluent may dissolve it.

• Monitor blood pressure every 30 minutes during infusion. If systolic blood pressure falls below 90 mm Hg, stop infusion and notify doctor.

• In 0.9% NaCl or D_5W, concentrations of 0.1 to 0.4 mg/ml are chemically stable for at least 24 hours at room or refrigerated temperature in glass containers. In plastic containers, 0.1 mg/ml in 0.9% NaCl is stable for 8 hours at room or refrigerated temperatures. Do not use D_5W and store in plastic containers.

• Follow institutional policy to reduce risks. Preparation and administration of parenteral form of drug are associated with carcinogenic, mutagenic, and teratogenic risks for personnel.

• Use non-DEHP (di[2-ethylhexyl] pthalate) containers and tubing for administration.

☑ Patient teaching

• Tell patient to report signs and symptoms of infection (fever, sore throat, fatigue) and bleeding (easy bruising, nosebleeds, bleeding gums, melena), and to take temperature daily.

• Caution patient of childbearing age to avoid becoming pregnant during therapy and to consult with doctor before becoming pregnant.

topotecan hydrochloride
Hycamtin

Pregnancy Risk Category: D

HOW SUPPLIED

Injection: 4 mg single-dose vial

ACTION

Relieves torsional strain in DNA by inducing reversible single-strand breaks. Binds to the topoisomerase I-DNA complex and prevents relegation of these single-strand breaks. Cytotoxicity of topotecan is thought to be due to double-strand DNA damage produced during DNA synthesis when replication enzymes interact with the ternary complex formed by topotecan, topoisomerase I, and DNA.

Route	Onset	Peak	Duration
IV	Unknown	Unknown	Unknown

INDICATIONS & DOSAGE

Metastatic carcinoma of the ovary after failure of initial or subsequent chemotherapy—
Adults: 1.5 mg/m^2 I.V. infusion given over 30 minutes daily for 5 consecutive days, starting on day 1 of a 21-day cycle. Minimum of four cycles should be given.
Adjust-a-dose: In patients with creatinine clearance of 20 to 39 ml/minute, dosage decreased to 0.75 mg/m^2. If severe neutropenia occurs, dosage decreased by 0.25 mg/m^2 for subsequent courses. Alternatively, if severe neutropenia occurs, granulocyte-colony stimulating factor may be administered following the subsequent course (before resorting to dosage reduction) starting from day 6 of course (24 hours after completion of topotecan administration).

ADVERSE REACTIONS

CNS: *fatigue, asthenia, headache,* paresthesia.
GI: *nausea, vomiting, diarrhea, constipation, abdominal pain, stomatitis, anorexia.*
Hematologic: NEUTROPENIA, LEUKOPENIA, THROMBOCYTOPENIA, *anemia.*
Hepatic: transient elevations of AST, ALT, and bilirubin levels.
Respiratory: *dyspnea.*
Skin: *alopecia.*
Other: *sepsis, fever.*

INTERACTIONS

Drug-drug. *Cisplatin:* increased severity of myelosuppression, if given together. Use both drugs with extreme caution.
Granulocyte-colony stimulating factor: prolonged duration of neutropenia. If granulocyte-colony stimulating factor is to be used, do not start it until day 6 of the course, 24 hours after completion of topotecan treatment.

EFFECTS ON DIAGNOSTIC TESTS

Drug may increase AST, ALT, and bilirubin; may decrease hemoglobin, WBC, and platelets.

CONTRAINDICATIONS

Contraindicated in patients with severe bone marrow depression or hypersensitivity to drug or its components and in pregnant or breast-feeding patients.

NURSING CONSIDERATIONS

Alert: Before administration of first course of therapy, patient must have baseline neutrophil count exceeding 1,500 cells/mm^3 and platelet count above 100,000 cells/mm^3.
● Be aware that topotecan should be prepared under a vertical laminar flow hood while wearing gloves and protective clothing. If drug solution contacts the skin, wash immediately and thoroughly with soap and water. If mucous membranes are affected, flush areas thoroughly with water.
● Know that bone marrow suppression (primarily neutropenia) is the dose-limiting toxicity of topotecan. The nadir occurs at about 11 days. Neutropenia is not cumulative over time.
● Know that duration of thrombocytopenia is about 5 days, with nadir at 15 days. The nadir for anemia is 15 days. Blood or platelet transfusions may be necessary.
● Frequent monitoring of peripheral blood cell counts are necessary. Do not treat patient with subsequent courses of topotecan until neutrophil counts recover to over 1,000 cells/mm^3, platelet counts recover to over 100,000 cells/mm^3, and hemoglobin levels recover to over 9 mg/dl (with transfusion if needed).
● Patient may receive injections of WBC colony-stimulating factors to promote cell growth and decrease risk for infection.
● Be aware that safety and effectiveness in children have not been established.

I.V. administration
● Each 4-mg vial should be reconstituted with 4 ml sterile water for injection. The appropriate volume of reconstituted solution is then diluted in either 0.9% NaCl solution or D$_5$W before administration.
● Because the lyophilized dosage form

Reactions may be *common,* uncommon, *life-threatening,* or COMMON AND LIFE-THREATENING.

contains no antibacterial preservative, use reconstituted product immediately.
• Protect unopened vials of drug from light. Reconstituted vials stored at 68° to 77° F (20° to 25° C) and exposed to ambient lighting are stable for 24 hours.
• Know that inadvertent drug extravasation has been associated with mild local reactions, such as erythema and bruising.

☑ **Patient teaching**
• Instruct patient to promptly report sore throat, fever, chills, or unusual bleeding or bruising.
• Caution women of childbearing age to avoid pregnancy and breast-feeding during therapy.
• Teach patient and family about adverse reactions to expect and need for frequent monitoring of blood counts.

▼ *NEW DRUG*

trastuzumab
Herceptin

Pregnancy Risk Category: B

HOW SUPPLIED
Injection: lyophilized sterile powder containing 440 mg per vial

ACTION
Drug is a recombinant DNA-derived monoclonal antibody that selectively binds to human epidermal growth factor receptor 2 protein (HER2) inhibiting the proliferation of human tumor cells that overexpress HER2.

Route	Onset	Peak	Duration
IV	Unknown	Unknown	Unknown

INDICATIONS & DOSAGE
Single-agent treatment of metastatic breast cancer in patients whose tumors overexpress the HER2 protein and who have received one or more chemotherapy regimens for their metastatic disease, or in combination with paclitaxel for metastatic breast cancer in patients whose tumors overexpress the HER2 protein and who have not received chemotherapy for their metastatic disease—

Adults: initial loading dose 4 mg/kg I.V. over 90 minutes. Maintenance dose is 2 mg/kg I.V. weekly as a 30-minute I.V. infusion if initial loading dose is well tolerated.

ADVERSE REACTIONS
CNS: depression, *dizziness, insomnia,* neuropathy, paresthesia, peripheral neuritis.
CV: *heart failure, peripheral edema,* tachycardia.
EENT: *rhinitis, pharyngitis,* sinusitis.
GI: *anorexia, abdominal pain, diarrhea, nausea, vomiting.*
GU: urinary tract infection.
Hematologic: *leukopenia,* anemia.
Musculoskeletal: arthralgia, *back pain,* bone pain.
Respiratory: *dyspnea, increased cough.*
Skin: acne, herpes simplex, *rash.*
Other: allergic reaction, *asthenia, chills,* edema, *fever, flu syndrome, headache, infection, pain.*

INTERACTIONS
None reported.

EFFECTS ON DIAGNOSTIC TESTS
None reported.

CONTRAINDICATIONS
No known contraindications.

NURSING CONSIDERATIONS
• Use cautiously in patients with preexisting cardiac dysfunction or in those with known hypersensitivity to drug or its components and in the elderly.
• Know that safety and effectiveness in children have not been established.
• Know that before beginning therapy, patient should undergo a thorough baseline cardiac assessment including history and physical examination and appropriate evaluation methods to identify those at risk of developing cardiotoxicity.
• Assess for signs and symptoms of cardiac dysfunction, especially if patient is receiving drug concurrently with anthracyclines and cyclophosphamide.
• Monitor for dyspnea, increased cough, paroxysmal nocturnal dyspnea, peripheral edema, or S_3 gallop. Drug treatment may

be stopped in patients who develop a clinically significant decrease in left ventricular function.

• Monitor patient receiving both drug and chemotherapy closely for cardiac dysfunction or failure, anemia, leukopenia, diarrhea, and infection.

• Know that drug should only be used in patients with metastatic breast cancer whose tumors have HER2 protein overexpression.

• Monitor for first-infusion symptom complex commonly consisting of chills or fever. Treat with acetaminophen, diphenhydramine, and meperidine (with or without reducing the rate of infusion), as ordered. Other signs or symptoms may include nausea, vomiting, pain, rigors, headache, dizziness, dyspnea, hypotension, rash, and asthenia. These symptoms occur infrequently with subsequent infusions.

⚑ I.V. administration

• Do not administer as an I.V. push or bolus.

• Reconstitute each vial with 20 ml of bacteriostatic water for injection, 1.1% benzyl alcohol preserved, as supplied, to yield a multidose solution containing 21 mg/ml. Immediately upon reconstitution, label vial for drug expiration 28 days from date of reconstitution.

Alert: If patient has known hypersensitivity to benzyl alcohol, drug may be reconstituted with sterile water for injection, used immediately and unused portion discarded. Avoid use of other reconstitution diluents.

• Determine dose (mg) of drug needed, based on a loading dose of 4 mg/kg or a maintenance dose of 2 mg/kg. Calculate volume of 21 mg/ml solution and withdraw this amount from vial and add it to an infusion bag containing 250 ml of 0.9% NaCl. Do not use D_5W solution. Gently invert bag to mix solution.

• Do not mix or dilute drug with other drugs.

• Vials of drug are stable at 36° to 46° F (2° to 8° C) before reconstitution. Discard reconstituted solution after 28 days. Do not freeze drug that has been reconstituted. Solution of drug diluted in 0.9% NaCl

for injection should be stored at 36° to 46° F (2° to 8° C) before use, and is stable for up to 24 hours.

☑ Patient teaching

• Tell patient about risk of first dose infusion-associated adverse effects.

• Instruct patient to notify doctor immediately if signs or symptoms of cardiac dysfunction occur, such as shortness of breath, increased cough, or peripheral edema.

• Instruct patient to report adverse effects to doctor.

• Advise breast-feeding women to discontinue breast-feeding during drug therapy and for 6 months after last dose of drug.

---

tretinoin
Vesanoid

Pregnancy Risk Category: D

HOW SUPPLIED
Capsules: 10 mg

ACTION
Unknown.

Route	Onset	Peak	Duration
PO	Unknown	1-2 hr	Unknown

INDICATIONS & DOSAGE
Induction of remission in patients with acute promyelocytic leukemia (APL), French-American-British (FAB) classification M^3 (including M^3 variant), when anthracycline chemotherapy is contraindicated or unsuccessful—
Adults and children 1 year and older: 45 mg/m²/day P.O. in two even doses. Therapy should be discontinued 30 days after complete remission is documented or after 90 days of treatment, whichever occurs first.

ADVERSE REACTIONS
CNS: *headache,* dizziness, *paresthesia, anxiety, insomnia, depression, confusion, cerebral hemorrhage, CVA,* intracranial hypertension, agitation, hallucination, abnormal gait, agnosia, aphasia, asterixis, cerebellar edema, cerebellar disorders,

seizures, coma, CNS depression, dysarthria, encephalopathy, facial paralysis, hemiplegia, hyporeflexia, hypotaxia, no light reflex, neurologic reaction, spinal cord disorder, tremor, leg weakness, unconsciousness, dementia, forgetfulness, somnolence, slow speech.

CV: *chest discomfort,* ARRHYTHMIAS, *hypotension, hypertension, phlebitis, edema,* HEART FAILURE, MI, *pericardial effusions,* impaired myocardial contractility, progressive hypoxemia, enlarged heart, heart murmur, ischemia, myocarditis, pericarditis, secondary cardiomyopathy.

EENT: *earache, ear fullness,* hearing loss, *visual disturbances,* changed visual acuity, visual field defects, *ocular disorders.*

GI: *GI hemorrhage, nausea, vomiting, anorexia, abdominal pain, GI disorders, diarrhea, constipation, dyspepsia, abdominal distention,* hepatosplenomegaly, ulcer.

GU: *renal insufficiency,* dysuria, *acute renal failure,* micturition frequency, renal tubular necrosis, enlarged prostate.

Hematologic: *leukocytosis,* HEMORRHAGE, DISSEMINATED INTRAVASCULAR COAGULATION.

Hepatic: hepatitis, unspecified liver disorder, *hypercholesterolemia, hypertriglyceridemia, elevated liver function studies.*

Respiratory: *pneumonia, upper respiratory tract disorders, dyspnea, respiratory insufficiency, pleural effusion, rales, expiratory wheezing,* lower respiratory tract disorders, pulmonary infiltrates, bronchial asthma, pulmonary edema, laryngeal edema, unspecified pulmonary disease, pulmonary hypertension.

Skin: *flushing, rash, skin and mucous membrane dryness, pruritus, alopecia, increased sweating, skin changes.*

Other: *retinoic acid-APL syndrome* (see Nursing considerations), *septicemia, multiorgan failure,* weakness, fatigue, fever, infections, malaise, shivering, peripheral edema, pain, injection site reactions, myalgia, bone pain, mucositis, flank pain, cellulitis, facial edema, fluid imbalance, pallor, lymph disorder, acidosis, hypothermia, ascites, bone inflammation, *weight gain or loss.*

INTERACTIONS
Drug-drug. *Ketoconazole:* may enhance tretinoin activity when taken together. Use cautiously.

EFFECTS ON DIAGNOSTIC TESTS
None reported.

CONTRAINDICATIONS
Contraindicated in patients with known hypersensitivity to retinoids. Do not give drug to patients who are sensitive to parabens, which are used as preservatives in gelatin capsule.

NURSING CONSIDERATIONS
● Be aware that drug is not recommended for use in pregnant or breast-feeding women.

● Know that because patients with APL are at high risk and can have severe reactions, give drug under supervision of doctor with experience managing such patients and in a facility able to monitor drug tolerance and protect and maintain patient compromised by toxicity.

● Be aware that about 25% of patients in clinical trials experienced Retinoic Acid-APL syndrome, characterized by fever, dyspnea, weight gain, radiographic pulmonary infiltrates, and pleural or pericardial effusions. Notify doctor immediately if these occur because the syndrome has occasionally been accompanied by impaired myocardial contractility and episodic hypotension with or without concomitant leukocytosis. Some patients have died from progressive hypoxemia and multiorgan failure. The syndrome generally occurs during first month of therapy. Prompt treatment with high-dose steroids appears to reduce morbidity and mortality.

● Monitor CBC and platelet counts regularly. Patients with high WBC counts at diagnosis are at increased risk for further, rapid elevations. Rapidly evolving leukocytosis is associated with a higher risk of life-threatening complications.

● Administer drug for induction of remission only. Patients should receive standard consolidation or maintenance regimen after induction therapy.

● Monitor patient (especially child) for

---

pseudotumor cerebri. Early signs and symptoms include papilledema, headache, nausea, vomiting, and visual disturbances. Notify doctor immediately if these occur.

• Monitor cholesterol and triglyceride levels and liver function studies and report abnormalities to doctor.

• Maintain infection control and bleeding precautions, and provide prompt treatment, as ordered.

• Ensure that pregnancy testing and contraception counseling are repeated monthly throughout therapy and for 1 month after completion of therapy.

✅ Patient teaching
• Explain infection control and bleeding precautions. Tell patient to notify doctor of signs and symptoms of infection (fever, sore throat, fatigue) or bleeding (easy bruising, nosebleeds, bleeding gums, melena), and to take temperature daily.

• Inform female patient that a pregnancy test is required 1 week before therapy begins and that therapy will be delayed, if possible, until a negative result is obtained.

• Instruct female patient to use contraception during therapy and for 1 month after completion, despite history of infertility or menopause, unless a hysterectomy has been performed. Tell her to use two methods of contraception simultaneously, unless abstinence is the chosen method, and to notify doctor if pregnancy is suspected.

---

vinblastine sulfate (VLB)
Velban, Velbe†‡, Velsar

Pregnancy Risk Category: D

HOW SUPPLIED
Injection: 10-mg vials (lyophilized powder), 1 mg/ml in 10-ml vials

ACTION
Arrests mitosis in metaphase, blocking cell division.

Route	Onset	Peak	Duration
IV	Unknown	Unknown	Unknown

INDICATIONS & DOSAGE
Breast or testicular cancer, Hodgkin's disease and malignant lymphoma, choriocarcinoma, lymphosarcoma, mycosis fungoides, Kaposi's sarcoma, histiocytosis—
Adults: 3.7 mg/m² I.V. weekly. May increase to maximum dosage of 18.5 mg/m² I.V. weekly according to response. Do not repeat dosage if WBC count is below 4,000/mm³.
Children: initial dose, 2.5 mg/m² I.V. weekly. Dosage increased by 1.25 mg/m² until WBC count is below 3,000/mm³ or tumor response is seen. Maximum dosage is 12.5 mg/m² I.V. weekly.

ADVERSE REACTIONS
CNS: depression, *paresthesia, peripheral neuropathy and neuritis, numbness, loss of deep tendon reflexes, muscle pain and weakness, **seizures**, **CVA**,* headache.
CV: hypertension, ***MI.***
EENT: pharyngitis.
GI: *nausea, vomiting,* ulcer, bleeding, *constipation, ileus, anorexia,* diarrhea, abdominal pain, *stomatitis.*
Hematologic: *anemia,* **leukopenia** (nadir occurs days 4 to 10 and lasts another 7 to 14 days), ***thrombocytopenia.***
Respiratory: ***acute bronchospasm,*** shortness of breath.
Skin: reversible alopecia, vesiculation.
Other: *irritation, phlebitis, weight loss,* cellulitis, necrosis with extravasation, hyperuricemia, uric acid nephropathy.

INTERACTIONS
Drug-drug. *Erythromycin, other drugs that inhibit cytochrome P-450 pathway:* may increase toxicity of vinblastine. Monitor closely.
Mitomycin: increased risk of bronchospasm and shortness of breath. Monitor patient's respiratory status.
Ototoxic drugs: can potentiate loss of hearing. Use concomitantly with extreme caution.
Phenytoin: decreased plasma phenytoin levels. Monitor closely.

EFFECTS ON DIAGNOSTIC TESTS
Drug therapy may increase blood and urine concentrations of uric acid.

Reactions may be *common*, uncommon, ***life-threatening**, or COMMON AND LIFE-THREATENING.

CONTRAINDICATIONS
Contraindicated in patients with severe leukopenia or bacterial infection.

NURSING CONSIDERATIONS
• Use cautiously in patients with hepatic dysfunction.
• To reduce nausea, give antiemetic before drug, as ordered.
• Do not administer into a limb with compromised circulation.
Alert: After administering drug, monitor for development of life-threatening acute bronchospasm. If this occurs, notify doctor immediately. Reaction is most likely to occur in patients who are also receiving mitomycin.
• Monitor patient for stomatitis. Be prepared to stop drug if stomatitis occurs and notify doctor.
• Assess bowel activity. Give laxatives as needed and ordered. May use stool softeners prophylactically.
• Know that dosage should not be repeated more frequently than every 7 days or severe leukopenia will occur.
• Assess for numbness and tingling in hands and feet. Assess gait for early evidence of footdrop.
• Take care to avoid confusing vinblastine with vincristine or vindesine.
• Know that drug is less neurotoxic than vincristine.
• Anticipate a decrease in dosage by 50% if bilirubin levels exceed 3 mg/100 ml.
• Be aware that drugs known to cause urine retention should be discontinued for first few days after vinblastine therapy, particularly in elderly patients.

I.V. administration
• Follow institutional policy to reduce risks. Preparation and administration of parenteral form of drug is associated with carcinogenic, mutagenic, and teratogenic risks for personnel.
Alert: This drug is fatal if given intrathecally; it is for I.V. use only.
• Inject directly into vein or tubing of running I.V. line over 1 minute. Drug is a vesicant; if extravasation occurs, stop infusion immediately and notify doctor. The manufacturer recommends that moderate heat be applied to area of leakage. Local injection of hyaluronidase may help disperse drug, as ordered. Some clinicians prefer to apply ice packs on and off every 2 hours for 24 hours, with local injection of hydrocortisone or 0.9% NaCl.
• Reconstitute 10-mg vial with 10 ml of NaCl injection. This yields 1 mg/ml. Refrigerate reconstituted solution. Protect solution from light and discard after 28 days.

☑ Patient teaching
• Tell patient to report signs and symptoms of infection (fever, sore throat, fatigue) and bleeding (easy bruising, nosebleeds, bleeding gums, melena), and to take temperature daily.
• Warn patient that alopecia may occur, but explain that it's usually reversible.
• Caution women of childbearing age to avoid pregnancy during drug therapy.
• Tell patient that pain in jaw and organ containing tumor may occur.

vincristine sulfate (VCR)
Oncovin, Vincasar PFS

Pregnancy Risk Category: D

HOW SUPPLIED
Injection: 1 mg/ml in 1-ml, 2-ml, 5-ml multiple-dose vials; 1 mg/ml in 1-ml, 2-ml, 5-ml preservative-free vials

ACTION
Arrests mitosis in metaphase, blocking cell division.

Route	Onset	Peak	Duration
IV	Unknown	Unknown	Unknown

INDICATIONS & DOSAGE
Acute lymphoblastic and other leukemias, Hodgkin's disease, malignant lymphoma, neuroblastoma, rhabdomyosarcoma, Wilms' tumor—
Adults: 0.4 to 1.4 mg/m^2 I.V. weekly. Maximum weekly dosage is 2 mg.
Children weighing over 10 kg (22 lb): 1.5 to 2 mg/m^2 I.V. weekly.
Children weighing 10 kg and less or with body surface area below 1 m^2: initially, 0.05 mg/kg I.V. weekly.

ADVERSE REACTIONS

CNS: *peripheral neuropathy,* sensory loss, *loss of deep tendon reflexes, paresthesia, wristdrop and footdrop, seizures, coma,* headache, ataxia, cranial nerve palsies, *jaw pain,* hoarseness, vocal cord paralysis, *muscle weakness and cramps—* some neurotoxicities may be permanent.
CV: hypotension, hypertension.
EENT: visual disturbances, blindness, diplopia, optic and extraocular neuropathy, ptosis.
GI: diarrhea, *constipation, cramps,* ileus that mimics surgical abdomen, paralytic ileus, *nausea, vomiting,* anorexia, dysphagia, *intestinal necrosis, stomatitis.*
GU: urine retention, SIADH, dysuria, acute uric acid neuropathy, polyuria.
Hematologic: anemia, *leukopenia, thrombocytopenia.*
Respiratory: *acute bronchospasm,* dyspnea.
Skin: rash, reversible alopecia.
Other: fever, weight loss, severe local reaction with extravasation, *phlebitis,* cellulitis at injection site, hyponatremia, hyperuricemia, uric acid nephropathy.

INTERACTIONS

Drug-drug. *Asparaginase:* decreased hepatic clearance of vincristine. Concurrent use may also result in additive neurotoxicity. Monitor for toxicity.
Calcium channel blockers: enhanced vincristine accumulation in cells. Monitor closely.
Digoxin: decreased digoxin effects. Monitor serum digoxin level.
Mitomycin: possibly increased frequency of bronchospasm and acute pulmonary reactions. Monitor patient's respiratory status.
Ototoxic drugs: can potentiate loss of hearing. Use concomitantly with extreme caution.
Phenytoin: may reduce phenytoin levels. Monitor closely.

EFFECTS ON DIAGNOSTIC TESTS

Drug therapy may increase blood and urine concentrations of uric acid. Because WBC and platelet counts may decrease, frequently monitor blood counts.

CONTRAINDICATIONS

Contraindicated in patients hypersensitive to drug or in those with the demyelinating form of Charcot-Marie-Tooth syndrome. Do not give to patients who are concurrently receiving radiation therapy through ports that include the liver.

NURSING CONSIDERATIONS

• Use cautiously in patients with hepatic dysfunction, neuromuscular disease, or infection.
• A 50% dose reduction is recommended if direct serum bilirubin level exceeds 3 mg/dl.
• Don't administer 5-mg vials to one patient as a single dose. The 5-mg vials are for multiple-dose use only.
Alert: After administering drug, monitor for development of life-threatening acute bronchospasm. If this occurs, notify doctor immediately. This reaction is most likely to occur in those also receiving mitomycin.
• Monitor for hyperuricemia, especially in patients with leukemia or lymphoma. Maintain hydration and administer allopurinol, as ordered, to prevent uric acid nephropathy. Monitor for toxicity.
• Monitor fluid intake and output. Fluid restriction may be necessary if SIADH develops.
• Because of risk of neurotoxicity, know that drug should not be given more than once weekly. Children are more resistant to neurotoxicity than adults. Neurotoxicity is dose-related and usually reversible.
• Check for depression of Achilles tendon reflex, numbness, tingling, footdrop or wristdrop, difficulty in walking, ataxia, and slapping gait. Also check ability to walk on heels. Support patients when walking.
• Monitor bowel function. Give stool softener or laxative, as ordered, or water before dosing. Constipation may be an early sign of neurotoxicity.
• Take care to avoid confusing vincristine with vinblastine or vindesine.
• Know that all vials (1-mg, 2-mg, 5-mg) contain 1 mg/ml solution and should be refrigerated.
• Discontinue drugs known to cause urine retention, particularly in elderly patients,

for the first few days after vincristine therapy.

Alert: This drug is fatal if given intrathecally; it is for I.V. use only.

▣ I.V. administration
• Follow institutional policy to reduce risks. Preparation and administration of parenteral form of drug is associated with carcinogenic, mutagenic, and teratogenic risks for personnel.
• Inject directly into vein or tubing of running I.V. line slowly over 1 minute. Vincristine is a vesicant; if drug extravasates, stop infusion immediately and notify doctor. Apply heat on and off every 2 hours for 24 hours. Administer 150 units hyaluronidase, as ordered, to area of infiltrate.

☑ Patient teaching
• Tell patient to report signs and symptoms of infection (fever, sore throat, fatigue) and bleeding (easy bruising, nosebleeds, bleeding gums, melena), and to take temperature daily.
• Warn patient that alopecia may occur, but explain that it's usually reversible.
• Caution women of childbearing age to avoid becoming pregnant during therapy and to consult doctor before becoming pregnant.

---

vinorelbine tartrate
Navelbine

Pregnancy Risk Category: D

HOW SUPPLIED
Injection: 10 mg/ml, 50 mg/5 ml

ACTION
A semisynthetic vinca alkaloid that exerts its antineoplastic effect by disrupting microtubule assembly, which, in turn, disrupts spindle formation and prevents mitosis.

Route	Onset	Peak	Duration
IV	Unknown	Unknown	Unknown

INDICATIONS & DOSAGE
Alone or as adjunct therapy with cisplatin for first-line treatment of ambulatory pa-

tients with nonresectable advanced non-small-cell lung cancer (NSCLC); alone or with cisplatin in stage IV of NSCLC; with cisplatin in stage III of NSCLC—
Adults: 30 mg/m² I.V. weekly. In combination treatment, same dosage used along with 120 mg/m² of cisplatin, given on days 1 and 29, then q 6 weeks.

ADVERSE REACTIONS
GI: *nausea, vomiting, anorexia, diarrhea, constipation, stomatitis.*
Hematologic: ***bone marrow suppression (agranulocytosis,*** LEUKOPENIA, ***thrombocytopenia,*** *anemia).*
Hepatic: *abnormal liver function test results, bilirubinemia.*
Respiratory: *dyspnea.*
Skin: *alopecia,* rash, *injection pain or reaction.*
Other: *peripheral neuropathy, asthenia,* jaw pain, *fatigue,* myalgia, SIADH, chest pain, arthralgia, loss of deep tendon reflexes.

INTERACTIONS
Drug-drug. *Cisplatin:* increased risk of bone marrow suppression when used concomitantly with cisplatin. Monitor hematologic status closely.
Mitomycin: may cause pulmonary reactions. Monitor respiratory status closely.

EFFECTS ON DIAGNOSTIC TESTS
Drug may cause increased hepatic enzymes.

CONTRAINDICATIONS
Contraindicated in patients with pretreatment granulocyte counts below 1,000 cells/mm³.

NURSING CONSIDERATIONS
• Use with extreme caution in patients whose bone marrow may have been compromised by previous exposure to radiation therapy or chemotherapy or whose bone marrow is still recovering from chemotherapy.
• Use cautiously in patients with hepatic impairment. Monitor liver enzymes.
• Check patient's granulocyte count before administration. The count should be 1,000 cells/mm³ or more for drug to be

---

administered. Withhold drug and notify doctor if count is less.

Alert: Drug is fatal if given intrathecally; it is for I.V. use only.

• Be aware that dosage adjustments are made according to hematologic toxicity or hepatic insufficiency, whichever results in the lower dosage. Expect dosage reduction of 50% if granulocyte count falls below 1,500 cells/mm³ but is greater than 1,000 cells/mm³. If three consecutive doses are skipped because of agranulocytosis, further vinorelbine therapy should not be given.

• Know that patients may receive injections of WBC colony-stimulating factors to promote cell growth and decrease the risk for infection.

• Know that drug may be a contact irritant, and the solution must be handled and administered with care. Gloves are recommended. Inhalation of vapors and contact with skin or mucous membranes, especially those of the eyes, must be avoided. In case of contact, wash with copious amounts of water for at least 15 minutes.

Alert: Monitor deep tendon reflexes; loss may represent cumulative toxicity.

• Monitor patient closely for hypersensitivity reactions.

• As a guide to the effects of therapy, monitor patient's peripheral blood count and bone marrow, as ordered.

◖I.V. administration

• Know that vinorelbine must be diluted before administration to a concentration of 1.5/ml to 3 mg/ml with D_5W or 0.9% NaCl solution in a syringe. Alternatively, dilute to a concentration of 0.5 mg/ml to 2 mg/ml in an I.V. bag. Administer drug I.V. over 6 to 10 minutes into the side port of a free-flowing I.V. line that is closest to the I.V. bag, followed by flushing with at least 75 to 125 ml of D_5W or 0.9% NaCl solution.

• Avoid extravasation when administering vinorelbine because drug can cause considerable irritation, localized tissue necrosis, and thrombophlebitis. If extravasation occurs, drug administration should be stopped immediately and any remaining dosage portion injected into a different vein.

☑Patient teaching

• Instruct patient not to take other drugs, including OTC preparations, until approved by doctor.

• Tell patient to report signs and symptoms of infection (fever, sore throat, fatigue) and bleeding (easy bruising, nosebleeds, bleeding gums, melena), and to take temperature daily.

• Caution women of childbearing age to avoid becoming pregnant during therapy.

Reactions may be *common*, uncommon, *life-threatening*, or COMMON AND LIFE-THREATENING.

azathioprine
basiliximab
cyclosporine
daclizumab
lymphocyte immune globulin
muromonab-CD3
mycophenolate mofetil
mycophenolate mofetil
   hydrochloride
tacrolimus

COMBINATION PRODUCTS
None.

azathioprine
Imuran, Thioprine‡

Pregnancy Risk Category: D

HOW SUPPLIED
Tablets: 50 mg
Powder for injection: 100 mg

ACTION
Unknown, but thought to cause variable alterations in antibody production.

Route	Onset	Peak	Duration
PO, IV	4-8 wk	1-2 hr	Several days

INDICATIONS & DOSAGE
Immunosuppression in kidney transplantation—
Adults: initially, 3 to 5 mg/kg P.O. or I.V. daily, usually beginning on day of transplantation. Maintained at 1 to 3 mg/kg daily (dosage based on patient response and tolerance).
Adjust-a-dose: In patients with oliguria in the post-transplant period and those with impaired renal function, Imuran is given in lower doses.
Severe, refractory rheumatoid arthritis—
Adults: initially, 1 mg/kg P.O. as a single dose or divided into two doses. If patient response is not satisfactory after 6 to 8 weeks, dosage may be increased by

0.5 mg/kg daily (up to a maximum of 2.5 mg/kg daily) at 4-week intervals.

ADVERSE REACTIONS
GI: *nausea, vomiting, pancreatitis,* steatorrhea, diarrhea, abdominal pain.
Hematologic: LEUKOPENIA, *myelosuppression,* anemia, *pancytopenia,* THROMBOCYTOPENIA, *immunosuppression* (possibly profound).
Hepatic: *hepatotoxicity,* jaundice.
Skin: rash.
Other: arthralgia, alopecia, *infections,* fever, myalgia, *increased risk of neoplasia.*

INTERACTIONS
Drug-drug. *ACE inhibitors:* combination may cause severe leukopenia. Monitor patient closely.
Allopurinol: impaired inactivation of azathioprine. Decrease azathioprine dose to ¼ or ⅓ normal dose.
Co-trimoxazole: Combination may cause leukopenia. Monitor patient closely.
Nondepolarizing neuromuscular blockers: azathioprine may reverse the neuromuscular blockade. Monitor patient closely.
Other myelopoiesis agents: exaggerated leukopenia, especially in renal transplant patients. Monitor patient closely.
Vaccines: decreased immune response. Postpone routine immunization.
Warfarin: azathioprine may decrease action of warfarin. Monitor patient closely.

EFFECTS ON DIAGNOSTIC TESTS
Drug alters CBC and differentiated blood counts, decreases serum uric acid levels, and elevates liver enzyme test results.

CONTRAINDICATIONS
Contraindicated in patients hypersensitive to drug or its components.

NURSING CONSIDERATIONS
• Use cautiously in patients with hepatic or renal dysfunction.

• Administer drug after meals to minimize adverse GI effects.

• To prevent bleeding, avoid all I.M. injections when platelet count is below $100,000/mm^3$.

• Monitor hemoglobin and WBC and platelet counts weekly for 1 month, then twice monthly. Notify doctor if counts drop suddenly or become dangerously low. Drug may need to be temporarily withheld.

• Watch for early signs of hepatotoxicity, such as clay-colored stools, dark urine, pruritus, and yellow skin and sclera; and for increased alkaline phosphatase, bilirubin, AST, and ALT levels.

• Be aware that therapeutic response usually occurs within 8 weeks.

• Keep in mind that the benefits must be weighed against risk with systemic viral infections, such as chickenpox and herpes zoster.

• Be aware that patients with rheumatoid arthritis previously treated with alkylating agents, such as cyclophosphamide, chlorambucil, melphalan, or others may have a prohibitive risk of neoplasia if treated with drug.

• Know that drug should not be used for treating rheumatoid arthritis in pregnant women.

◻ I.V. administration

• Reconstitute 100-mg vial with 10 ml of sterile water for injection. Visually inspect for particles before use. Drug may be administered by direct I.V. injection or further diluted in 0.9% NaCl for injection or D_5W and infused over 30 to 60 minutes. Use only in patients who are unable to tolerate oral medications.

☑ Patient teaching

• Warn patient to report even mild infections (colds, fever, sore throat, and malaise) because drug is a potent immunosuppressant.

• Instruct patient to avoid conception during therapy and for 4 months after stopping therapy.

• Warn patient that some thinning of hair is possible.

• Tell patient taking drug for refractory

rheumatoid arthritis that it may take up to 12 weeks to be effective.

• Advise patient to report unusual bleeding or bruising to doctor.

• Tell patient that drug may be taken with food to decrease nausea.

• Advise patient to use soft toothbrush and perform oral care cautiously.

▼ *NEW DRUG*

basiliximab
Simulect

Pregnancy Risk Category: B

HOW SUPPLIED
Injection: 20-mg vials

ACTION
Binds specifically to and blocks the interleukin-2 receptor alpha-chain on the surface of activated T-lymphocytes. This inhibits interleukin-2 mediated activation of lymphocytes, a critical pathway in the cellular immune response involved in allograft rejection.

Route	Onset	Peak	Duration
IV	Unknown	Immediate	Unknown

INDICATIONS & DOSAGE
Prophylaxis of acute organ rejection in patients receiving renal transplantation when used as part of an immunosuppressive regimen that includes cyclosporine and corticosteroids—
Adults: 20 mg I.V. given within 2 hours before transplant surgery and 20 mg I.V. given 4 days after transplantation.
Children 2 to 15 years: 12 mg/m^2 (up to maximum of 20 mg) I.V. given within 2 hours before transplant surgery and 12 mg/m^2 (up to maximum of 20 mg) I.V. given 4 days after transplantation.

ADVERSE REACTIONS
CNS: agitation, anxiety, *asthenia,* depression, *dizziness, headache,* hypoesthesia, *insomnia,* neuropathy, paresthesia, *tremor.*
CV: angina pectoris, *arrhythmias,* atrial fibrillation, *cardiac failure,* chest pain, abnormal heart sounds, aggravated hyper-

tension, *hypertension,* hypotension, tachycardia.

EENT: abnormal vision, cataract, conjunctivitis, *rhinitis,* sinusitis.

GI: *abdominal pain, candidiasis, constipation, diarrhea, dyspepsia,* esophagitis, enlarged abdomen, flatulence, gastroenteritis, GI disorder, *GI hemorrhage*, gum hyperplasia, melena, *nausea,* ulcerative stomatitis, *vomiting.*

GU: abnormal renal function, albuminuria, bladder disorder, *dysuria,* frequent micturition, genital edema (male), hematuria, *increased nonprotein nitrogen,* oliguria, renal tubular necrosis, surgery, ureteral disorder, *urinary tract infection*, urinary retention, impotence.

Hematologic: *anemia*, hematoma, *hemorrhage*, polycythemia, purpura, *thrombocytopenia*, thrombosis.

Metabolic: *acidosis,* dehydration, diabetes mellitus, fluid overload, hypercalcemia, *hypercholesterolemia, hyperglycemia, hyperkalemia,* hyperlipemia, *hyperuricemia, hypocalcemia, hypokalemia,* hypomagnesemia, *hypophosphatemia,* hypoproteinemia, *weight increase, fever.*

Musculoskeletal: arthralgia, arthropathy, *back pain,* bone fracture, cramps, hernia, *leg pain,* myalgia.

Respiratory: abnormal chest sounds, bronchitis, bronchospasm, *cough, dyspnea, pharyngitis,* pneumonia, pulmonary disorder, *pulmonary edema, upper respiratory tract infection.*

Skin: *acne,* cyst, herpes simplex, herpes zoster, hypertrichosis, pruritus, rash, skin disorder or ulceration, *surgical wound complications.*

Other: accidental trauma, *viral infection, leg or peripheral edema,* fatigue, general edema, infection, *sepsis.*

INTERACTIONS
None reported.

EFFECTS ON DIAGNOSTIC TESTS
None reported.

CONTRAINDICATIONS
Contraindicated in patients with known hypersensitivity to drug or its components.

NURSING CONSIDERATIONS
● Use cautiously and only under the supervision of a doctor qualified and experienced in immunosuppression therapy and management of organ transplantation.
● Use cautiously in elderly patients.
● Anaphylactoid reactions may result following administration of proteins. Be sure that medications for treating severe hypersensitivity reactions are available for immediate use.
● Monitor for electrolyte imbalances and acidosis during drug therapy.
● Monitor patient's intake and output, vital signs, hemoglobin, and hematocrit during therapy.
● Be alert for signs of opportunistic infections during drug therapy.

I.V. administration
● Reconstitute with 5 ml sterile water for injection. Shake vial gently to dissolve powder. Dilute reconstituted solution to volume of 50 ml with normal saline or dextrose 5% for infusion. When mixing solution, gently invert bag to avoid foaming. *Do not shake.*
● Infuse medication over 20 to 30 minutes via a central or peripheral vein. Do not add or infuse other drugs simultaneously through same I.V. line.
● Use reconstituted solution immediately. May be refrigerated at 36° to 46° F (2° to 8° C) for up to 24 hours or at room temperature for 4 hours.

Patient teaching
● Inform patient of potential benefits of therapy and risks associated with immunosuppressive therapy, including a decreased incidence of graft loss or acute rejection.
● Inform women of childbearing age to use effective contraception before beginning therapy and up until 2 months after completion of therapy.
● Instruct patient to report adverse effects immediately.
● Explain that drug is used in conjunction with cyclosporine and corticosteroids.
● Advise patient that immunosuppressive therapy increases risks of developing lymphoproliferative disorders and opportunis-

tic infections. Tell him to report signs of infection promptly.

---

cyclosporine (cyclosporin)
Neoral, Sandimmun‡, Sandimmune

Pregnancy Risk Category: C

HOW SUPPLIED
Oral solution: 100 mg/ml
Injection: 50 mg/ml
Capsules: 25 mg, 50 mg, 100 mg
Capsules for microemulsion: 25 mg, 50 mg

ACTION
Unknown. Thought to inhibit the proliferation and function of T lymphocytes and inhibit production and release of lymphokines.

Route	Onset	Peak	Duration
PO	Unknown	3.5 hr	Unknown
IV	Unknown	Unknown	Unknown

INDICATIONS & DOSAGE
Prophylaxis of organ rejection in kidney, liver, or heart transplantation—
Adults and children: 15 mg/kg P.O. 4 to 12 hours before transplantation and continued daily postoperatively for 1 to 2 weeks. Then dosage reduced by 5% each week to maintenance level of 5 to 10 mg/kg/day. Alternatively, 5 to 6 mg/kg I.V. concentrate 4 to 12 hours before transplantation given as a continuous infusion. Postoperatively, dosage repeated daily until patient can tolerate P.O. forms.
Elderly: dosage adjustment may be necessary.
Severe, active rheumatoid arthritis that has not adequately responded to methotrexate (Neoral only)—
Adults: 2.5 mg/kg/day P.O., taken b.i.d. as a divided dose.
Adjust-a-dose: In patients with adverse effects such as hypertension, elevations in serum creatinine (30% above pretreatment level), or abnormal CBC and liver function tests, decrease dose by 25% to 50%.

ADVERSE REACTIONS
CNS: *tremor, headache, **seizures,** confusion, paresthesia.*
CV: *hypertension.*
EENT: *gum hyperplasia,* oral thrush, sinusitis.
GI: *nausea, vomiting,* diarrhea, abdominal discomfort.
GU: NEPHROTOXICITY.
Hematologic: anemia, ***leukopenia, thrombocytopenia***, hemolytic anemia.
Hepatic: ***hepatotoxicity.***
Skin: acne, flushing.
Other: increased low-density lipoprotein levels, ***infections***, hirsutism, ***anaphylaxis***, gynecomastia.

INTERACTIONS
Drug-drug. *Acyclovir, aminoglycosides, amphotericin B, co-trimoxazole, melphalan, NSAIDs, ranitidine, vancomycin:* increased risk of nephrotoxicity. Avoid concomitant use.
Azathioprine, corticosteroids, cyclophosphamide, verapamil: increased immunosuppression. Monitor closely.
Carbamazepine, isoniazid, phenobarbital, phenytoin, rifabutin, rifampin: possible decreased immunosuppressant effect secondary to low cyclosporine levels. Know that cyclosporine dosage may need to be increased.
Cimetidine, danazol, diltiazem, erythromycin, fluconazole, imipenem-cilastatin, ketoconazole, methylprednisolone, metoclopramide, nicardipine, prednisolone: may increase blood levels of cyclosporine. Monitor for increased toxicity.
Digoxin: cyclosporine may elevate digoxin levels. Monitor patient for toxicity.
Potassium-sparing diuretics: cyclosporine may induce hyperkalemia. Monitor patient closely.
Vaccines: decreased immune response. Postpone routine immunization.
Drug-food. *Grapefruit juice:* slowed metabolism of drug. Avoid concomitant use.

EFFECTS ON DIAGNOSTIC TESTS
Drug therapy may alter CBC and differential blood tests and may increase serum lipid levels. Drug elevation of serum BUN and creatinine and liver function tests may signal nephrotoxicity or hepato-

---

toxicity, increased serum glucose, and anemia.

CONTRAINDICATIONS
Contraindicated in patients hypersensitive to drug or to polyoxyethylated castor oil (found in injectable form). Patients who have rheumatoid arthritis and hypertension, malignancies, or impaired renal function should not receive Neoral.

NURSING CONSIDERATIONS
• Measure oral solution doses carefully in an oral syringe. To increase palatability, the conventional oral solution may be mixed with milk, chocolate milk, or orange juice. Oral cyclosporine solution for emulsion may be mixed with orange or apple juice (avoid grapefruit juice). Solution for emulsion is less palatable when mixed with milk. Use a glass container to mix and have patient drink at once. Do not rinse dosing syringe with water. If syringe requires cleaning, it must be completely dry before reuse.
• Monitor elderly patient for renal impairment and hypotension.
• Know that dosage is typically given once or twice daily.
• Be aware that Neoral has greater bioavailability than Sandimmune form. Less Neoral may be needed to yield the same blood concentration derived from Sandimmune. Switch patients between these two brands using blood concentration monitoring, as ordered.
• Always give cyclosporine concomitantly with adrenal corticosteroids as ordered.
• Monitor cyclosporine blood levels at regular intervals. Absorption of cyclosporine oral solution can be erratic.
• Monitor BUN and serum creatinine levels. Nephrotoxicity may develop 2 to 3 months after transplant surgery, possibly requiring dosage reduction. Notify doctor of signs or symptoms of nephrotoxicity.
• Know that doctor must differentiate between transplanted kidney rejection and cyclosporine-induced nephrotoxicity.

🗂 I.V. administration
• Administer cyclosporine I.V. concentrate at one-third oral dose and dilute before use. Dilute each milliliter of the concentrate in 20 to 100 ml of D_5W or 0.9% NaCl for injection. Dilute immediately before administration; infuse over 2 to 6 hours. I.V. administration is usually reserved for patients who cannot tolerate oral medications. Protect I.V. solution from light.

✓ Patient teaching
• Encourage patient to take drug at same time each day, and teach him how to measure dosage and mask taste of oral solution, if prescribed. Tell him not to take cyclosporine with grapefruit juice.
• Instruct patient to fill glass with water after dose and drink to assure all medication is consumed.
• Advise patient to take drug with meals if nausea occurs.
• Advise patient to take Neoral on an empty stomach.
• Stress that therapy should not be stopped without doctor's approval.
• Advise patient to use mechanical contraceptive measures, such as a diaphragm or condom, while on therapy. Tell female patient not to use oral contraceptives.

▼ *NEW DRUG*

daclizumab
Zenapax

Pregnancy Risk Category: C

HOW SUPPLIED
Injection: 25 mg/5 ml

ACTION
An interleukin (IL)-2 receptor antagonist that inhibits IL-2 binding to prevent IL-2 mediated activation of lymphocytes, a critical pathway in the cellular immune response against allografts. Once in circulation, daclizumab impairs the response of the immune system to antigenic challenges.

Route	Onset	Peak	Duration
IV	Unknown	Unknown	Unknown

INDICATIONS & DOSAGE
Prophylaxis of acute organ rejection in patients receiving renal transplants in

combination with an immunosuppressive regimen that includes cyclosporine and corticosteroids—

Adults: 1 mg/kg I.V. The standard course of therapy is five doses. Administer first dose no more than 24 hours before transplantation; remaining four doses are given at 14-day intervals.

ADVERSE REACTIONS
CNS: tremor, headache, dizziness, insomnia, generalized weakness, prickly sensation, fever, pain, fatigue, depression, anxiety.
CV: tachycardia, hypertension, hypotension, aggravated hypertension, edema, fluid overload, chest pain.
EENT: blurred vision, pharyngitis, rhinitis.
GI: constipation, nausea, diarrhea, vomiting, abdominal pain, dyspepsia, pyrosis, abdominal distention, epigastric pain, flatulence, gastritis, hemorrhoids.
GU: *oliguria,* dysuria, *renal tubular necrosis,* renal damage, urinary retention, hydronephrosis, urinary tract bleeding, urinary tract disorder, renal insufficiency.
Hematologic: lymphocele; platelet, bleeding, and clotting disorders.
Metabolic: diabetes mellitus, dehydration.
Musculoskeletal: musculoskeletal or back pain, arthralgia, myalgia, leg cramps.
Respiratory: dyspnea, coughing, atelectasis, congestion, *hypoxia,* rales, abnormal breath sounds, pleural effusion, pulmonary edema.
Skin: acne, impaired wound healing without infection, pruritus, hirsutism, rash, night sweats, increased sweating.
Other: shivering, extremity edema.

INTERACTIONS
None reported.

EFFECTS ON DIAGNOSTIC TESTS
None reported.

CONTRAINDICATIONS
Contraindicated in patients with known hypersensitivity to drug or its components.

NURSING CONSIDERATIONS
● Use cautiously and only under supervision of a doctor experienced in immunosuppressive therapy and management of organ transplantation.
● Protect undiluted solution from direct light.
● Be aware that drug is used as part of an immunosuppressive regimen that includes corticosteroids and cyclosporine. Monitor for lipoproliferative disorders and opportunistic infections.
● Be aware that anaphylactoid reactions have been reported following the administration of proteins. Medications used in the treatment of anaphylactic reactions should be immediately available.

🔲 I.V. administration
● Do not use drug as direct I.V. injection. Dilute in 50 ml of sterile 0.9% NaCl solution before administration. To avoid foaming, *Do not shake.* Inspect for particulate matter or discoloration before use. If there is evidence of particulate matter or discoloration, do not use.
● Administer over 15 minutes via a central or peripheral line. Do not add or infuse other drugs simultaneously through same I.V. line.
● Drug may be refrigerated at 36° to 46° F (2° to 8° C) for 24 hours and is stable at room temperature for 4 hours. Discard solution if not used within 24 hours.

✅ Patient teaching
● Tell patient to consult doctor before taking other medications during therapy.
● Advise patient to practice infection prevention precautions.
● Inform patient that neither he nor any household member should receive vaccinations unless medically approved.
● Tell patient to report immediately wounds that fail to heal, unusual bruising or bleeding, or fever.
● Advise patient to drink plenty of fluids during drug therapy, and report painful urination, blood in the urine, or decrease in urine amount.
● Instruct women of childbearing age to use effective contraception before beginning therapy and continue until 4 months after completing therapy.

Reactions may be *common,* uncommon, *life-threatening,* or COMMON AND LIFE-THREATENING.

lymphocyte immune globulin (anti-thymocyte globulin [equine], ATG)
Atgam

Pregnancy Risk Category: C

HOW SUPPLIED
Injection: 50 mg of equine IgG/ml in 5-ml ampules

ACTION
Unknown. Inhibits cell-mediated immune responses either by altering T-cell function or eliminating antigen-reactive T cells.

Route	Onset	Peak	Duration
IV	Immediate	5 days	Unknown

INDICATIONS & DOSAGE
Prevention of acute renal allograft rejection—
Adults: 15 mg/kg/day I.V. daily for 14 days, followed by alternate-day dosing for 14 days; first dose should be given within 24 hours of transplantation.
Children: 5 to 25 mg/kg/day I.V. daily for 14 days, followed by alternate-day dosing for 14 days; first dose should be given within 24 hours of transplantation.
Treatment of acute renal allograft rejection—
Adults and children: 10 to 15 mg/kg I.V. daily for 14 days. Additional alternate-day therapy up to a total of 21 doses can be given. Therapy should be initiated when rejection is diagnosed.
Aplastic anemia—
Adults: 10 to 20 mg/kg I.V. daily for 8 to 14 days. Additional alternate-day therapy up to a total of 21 doses can be administered.

ADVERSE REACTIONS
CNS: malaise, *seizures,* headache.
CV: *hypotension, chest pain,* thrombophlebitis, tachycardia, edema, iliac vein obstruction, renal artery stenosis.
EENT: *laryngospasm.*
GI: *nausea, vomiting, diarrhea,* hiccups, epigastric pain, abdominal distention, stomatitis.
Hematologic: LEUKOPENIA, THROMBOCYTOPENIA, hemolysis, *aplastic anemia.*
Hepatic: elevated liver enzyme level.
Respiratory: *dyspnea, pulmonary edema.*
Skin: *rash, pruritus, urticaria.*
Other: *febrile reactions, hypersensitivity reactions, serum sickness, anaphylaxis, infections, arthralgia,* night sweats, lymphadenopathy, hyperglycemia, *chills, myalgia.*

INTERACTIONS
Drug-drug. *Muromonab-CD3:* increased risk of infection. Monitor patient closely.

EFFECTS ON DIAGNOSTIC TESTS
Elevations of hepatic serum enzymes have been reported.

CONTRAINDICATIONS
Contraindicated in patients hypersensitive to drug. An intradermal skin test is recommended at least 1 hour before the first dose. Marked local swelling or erythema larger than 10 mm indicates an increased potential for severe systemic reaction such as anaphylaxis. Severe reactions to the skin test, such as hypotension, tachycardia, dyspnea, generalized rash, or anaphylaxis, usually preclude further administration of drug.

NURSING CONSIDERATIONS
• Use cautiously in patients receiving additional immunosuppressive therapy (such as corticosteroids or azathioprine) because of increased potential for infection.
• Do not dilute ATG concentrate with dextrose solutions or solutions with a low salt concentration because a precipitate may form. The proteins in ATG can be denatured by air. ATG is unstable in acidic solutions.
• Monitor patient for hypotension, respiratory distress, chest, flank, or back pain which may indicate anaphylaxis or hemolysis.
• Keep airway adjuncts and anaphylaxis medications at bedside during administration.
• Monitor for signs of infection.

◙ **I.V. administration**
• Dilute concentrated drug for injection

before administration. Dilute required dose in 250 to 1,000 ml of 0.45% or 0.9% NaCl solution. Final concentration of drug should not exceed 1 mg/ml. When adding ATG to infusion solution, make sure container is inverted so that drug does not contact air inside the container. Gently rotate or swirl container to mix contents; do not shake because this may cause excessive foaming or denature the drug protein. Infuse with an in-line filter with a pore size of 0.2 to 1 micron over no less than 4 hours (most institutions infuse over 4 to 8 hours) into a vascular shunt, arterial venous fistula, or high-flow central vein.
• Do not use solutions that are older than 12 hours, including actual infusion time.
• Refrigerate at 35° to 47° F (2° to 8° C). ATG concentrate is heat-sensitive. Do not freeze. Allow diluted ATG to reach room temperature before infusion.

☑ **Patient teaching**
• Instruct patient to report adverse drug reactions promptly, especially signs of infection (fever, sore throat, fatigue).
• Tell patient to alert nurse immediately if discomfort occurs at I.V. insertion site because drug can cause a chemical phlebitis.
• Advise female patient to avoid pregnancy during drug therapy.

---

muromonab-CD3
Orthoclone OKT₃

Pregnancy Risk Category: C

HOW SUPPLIED
Injection: 1 mg/1 ml in 5-ml ampules

ACTION
Muromonab-CD3 is a murine monoclonal antibody that reacts in the T-lymphocyte membrane with a molecule (CD3) needed for antigen recognition. Drug depletes the blood of $CD3^+$ T cells, which leads to restoration of allograft function and reversal of rejection.

Route	Onset	Peak	Duration
IV	Immediate	Unknown	1 wk

INDICATIONS & DOSAGE
Acute allograft rejection in renal transplant patients; in steroid-resistant hepatic or cardiac allograft rejection—
Adults: 5 mg I.V. bolus once daily for 10 to 14 days.

ADVERSE REACTIONS
CNS: *tremor, headache,* **seizures, encephalopathy, cerebral edema.**
CV: *chest pain, tachycardia,* hypertension, **cardiac arrest,** hypotension, **shock, heart failure.**
EENT: *blindness, blurred vision, tinnitus, otitis media, conjunctivitis.*
GI: *nausea, vomiting, diarrhea.*
GU: oliguria, anuria.
Respiratory: *severe pulmonary edema, dyspnea, wheezing,* **adult respiratory distress syndrome.**
Other: *fever, chills, tremors,* INFECTION, **anaphylaxis,** increased serum creatinine, **cytokine release syndrome** (from flulike symptoms to shock), **aseptic meningitis, risk of neoplasia.**

INTERACTIONS
Drug-drug. *Immunosuppressants:* increased risk of infection. Monitor closely.
Indomethacin: increased muromonab-CD3 levels with encephalopathy and other CNS effects. Monitor patient closely.
Live virus vaccines: may potentiate replication and increase effects of virus vaccine. Monitor patient.

EFFECTS ON DIAGNOSTIC TESTS
Drug may increase BUN and serum creatinine and cause abnormal urine cytology.

CONTRAINDICATIONS
Contraindicated in pregnant and breast-feeding patients. Also contraindicated in patients with hypersensitivity to drug or to other products of murine (mouse) origin; who have antimurine antibody titers of 1:1,000 or more; who have fluid overload, as evidenced by chest X-ray or a weight gain greater than 3% within the week before treatment; or who have history of seizures or are predisposed to seizures.

NURSING CONSIDERATIONS

• Obtain chest X-ray within 24 hours before starting drug treatment, as ordered.
• Assess patient for signs of fluid overload before treatment.
• Keep in mind that treatment should begin in a facility that is equipped and staffed for cardiopulmonary resuscitation and where patient can be monitored closely.
• Be alert that most adverse reactions develop within 30 minutes to 6 hours after first dose.
• Administer an antipyretic, as ordered, before giving drug to help lower incidence of expected pyrexia and chills. Treat fever exceeding 100° F (38° C) with antipyretics before drug administration and evaluate risk for infection.
• Administer corticosteroids, as ordered, before first injection to help decrease incidence of adverse reactions. Methylprednisolone sodium succinate (1 mg/kg) before injection, followed by hydrocortisone sodium succinate (100 mg) 30 minutes after injection, have been recommended to alleviate severity of first-dose reaction.
• Be aware that muromonab-CD3 is a monoclonal antibody preparation. Patients develop antibodies to this preparation that can lead to loss of effectiveness and more severe adverse reactions if a second course of therapy is attempted. Therefore, some clinicians believe that drug should be used for only a single course of treatment.

🖐 **I.V. administration**
• Draw solution into a syringe through a low protein-binding 0.2- or 0.22-micron filter. Discard filter and attach needle for I.V. bolus injection. Give bolus in less than 1 minute.

✅ **Patient teaching**
• Inform patient of expected adverse reactions.
• Reassure patient that reactions will be less severe as treatment progresses.
• Advise female patient to avoid pregnancy during drug therapy.

mycophenolate mofetil
CellCept

mycophenolate mofetil hydrochloride
CellCept Intravenous

Pregnancy Risk Category: C

HOW SUPPLIED
mycophenolate mofetil
Capsules: 250 mg
Tablets: 500 mg
mycophenolate mofetil hydrochloride
Injection: 500 mg/vial

ACTION
Inhibits proliferative response of T- and B-lymphocytes, suppresses antibody formation by B-lymphocytes, and may inhibit recruitment of leukocytes into sites of inflammation and graft rejection.

Route	Onset	Peak	Duration
PO	Unknown	0.5-1.25 hr	7.5-18 hr
IV	Unknown	Unknown	10-17 hr

INDICATIONS & DOSAGE
Prophylaxis of organ rejection in patients receiving allogenic renal transplants—
Adults: 1 g P.O. or I.V. b.i.d. in conjunction with corticosteroids and cyclosporine.
Adjust-a-dose: In patients with severe chronic renal impairment outside of immediate posttransplant period, avoid doses above 1 g b.i.d. If neutropenia develops, interrupt or reduce dosing.
✳ *NEW INDICATION: Prophylaxis of organ rejection in patients receiving allogenic cardiac transplant—*
Adults: 1.5 g P.O. or I.V. b.i.d. in combination with cyclosporine and corticosteroids.

ADVERSE REACTIONS
CNS: *tremor*, insomnia, dizziness, *headache*.
CV: *chest pain, hypertension, edema.*
GI: *diarrhea, constipation, nausea, dyspepsia, vomiting, oral moniliasis, abdominal pain,* **hemorrhage.**

GU: *urinary tract infection, hematuria,* kidney tubular necrosis.
Hematologic: *anemia,* LEUKOPENIA, THROMBOCYTOPENIA, hypochromic anemia, leukocytosis.
Metabolic: *hypercholesterolemia, hypophosphatemia, hypokalemia,* hyperkalemia, hyperglycemia.
Respiratory: *dyspnea, cough, infection,* pharyngitis, bronchitis, pneumonia.
Skin: *acne,* rash.
Other: *pain, fever, infection,* **sepsis,** *asthenia, back pain, peripheral edema.*

INTERACTIONS
Drug-drug. *Acyclovir, ganciclovir, other drugs known to undergo renal tubular secretion:* increased risk of toxicity for both drugs. Monitor patient closely.
Antacids with magnesium and aluminum hydroxides: decreased absorption of mycophenolate. Separate dosages.
Azathioprine: has not been clinically studied. Avoid concomitant use.
Cholestyramine: may interfere with enterohepatic recirculation, reducing mycophenolate bioavailability. Avoid concurrent use.
Oral contraceptives: may affect efficacy of oral contraceptives. Advise patient about alternative methods.

EFFECTS ON DIAGNOSTIC TESTS
None reported.

CONTRAINDICATIONS
Contraindicated in patients with hypersensitivity to drug or its ingredients and to mycophenolic acid.

NURSING CONSIDERATIONS
• Know that drug is not recommended for use during pregnancy (unless benefits outweigh risks to fetus) or in breast-feeding patients.
• Use cautiously in patients with GI disorders.
• Be aware that safety and effectiveness of drug have not been established in children.
• Drug therapy should be started within 24 hours following transplantation. I.V. form is recommended for patients unable to take capsules or tablets.

• Can administer I.V. dosage form for up to 14 days; switch patient to capsules or tablets as soon as oral medications can be tolerated.
• Avoid doses above 1 g b.i.d. after immediate posttransplant period in patients with severe chronic renal impairment.
• Because of potential teratogenic effects, do not open or crush capsule. Avoid inhaling the powder in the capsule or having it contact skin or mucous membranes. If such contact occurs, wash thoroughly with soap and water, and rinse eyes with water.

⬛ **I.V. administration**
• CellCept Intravenous must be reconstituted and diluted to a concentration of 6 mg/ml using 5% dextrose injection.
• Never administer drug by rapid or bolus I.V. injection. Give infusion over at least 2 hours.
• Drug is incompatible with other I.V. solutions.

✅ **Patient teaching**
• Warn patient not to open or crush capsules but to swallow them whole on an empty stomach.
• Stress importance of not interrupting or stopping therapy without first consulting doctor.
• Inform female patient that a pregnancy test is required 1 week before therapy begins.
• Instruct female patient to use contraception during therapy and for 6 weeks after discontinuation, even with a history of infertility, unless a hysterectomy has been performed. Tell her to use two methods of contraception simultaneously, unless abstinence is the chosen method, and to notify doctor immediately of suspected pregnancy.
• Warn patient that there is an increased risk of lymphoma and other malignancies.

---

tacrolimus
Prograf

Pregnancy Risk Category: C

HOW SUPPLIED
Capsules: 1 mg, 5 mg
Injection: 5 mg/ml

ACTION
Precise mechanism unknown. Inhibits T-lymphocyte activation, which results in immunosuppression.

Route	Onset	Peak	Duration
PO, IV	Unknown	1.5-3.5 hr	Unknown

INDICATIONS & DOSAGE
Prophylaxis of organ rejection in allogenic liver or kidney transplants—
Adults: 0.03 to 0.05 mg/kg/day I.V. as a continuous infusion administered no sooner than 6 hours after transplantation. Substitute P.O. therapy as soon as possible, with first oral dose given 8 to 12 hours after discontinuing I.V. infusion. Or, administer P.O. dose within 24 hours of transplantation after renal function has recovered. Recommended initial P.O. dosage for allogenic liver transplants is 0.1 to 0.15 mg/kg/day P.O. in two divided doses q 12 hours. Recommended initial P.O. dosage for allogenic kidney transplants is 0.2 mg/kg/day P.O. in two divided doses q 12 hours. Dosages should be titrated according to clinical response.
Children: initially, 0.03 to 0.05 mg/ kg/ day I.V., followed by 0.15 to 0.2 mg/kg/ day P.O. on a schedule similar to adults, adjusted p.r.n.
Adjust-a-dose: In patients with renal or hepatic impairment, use lowest recommended doses for I.V. and P.O.

ADVERSE REACTIONS
CNS: *headache, tremor, insomnia, paresthesia, delirium,* **coma.**
CV: *hypertension, peripheral edema.*
GI: *diarrhea, nausea, constipation, abnormal liver function test, anorexia, vomiting, abdominal pain.*
GU: *abnormal renal function, increased creatinine or BUN levels, urinary tract infection, oliguria.*
Hematologic: *anemia, leukocytosis,* THROMBOCYTOPENIA.
Metabolic: *hyperkalemia, hypokalemia, hyperglycemia, hypomagnesemia.*

Respiratory: *pleural effusion, atelectasis, dyspnea.*
Skin: *pruritus, rash, alopecia.*
Other: *pain, fever, asthenia, back pain, ascites, photosensitivity,* alopecia, ***anaphylaxis.***

INTERACTIONS
Drug-drug. *Bromocriptine, cimetidine, clarithromycin, clotrimazole, cyclosporine, danazol, diltiazem, erythromycin, fluconazole, itraconazole, ketoconazole, methylprednisolone, metoclopramide, nicardipine, verapamil:* may increase tacrolimus levels. Monitor for adverse effects.
Carbamazepine, phenobarbital, phenytoin, rifabutin, rifampin: may decrease tacrolimus levels. Monitor effectiveness of tacrolimus.
Cyclosporine: increased risk of excess nephrotoxicity. Do not administer together.
Immunosuppressants (except adrenal corticosteroids): may oversuppress immune system. Monitor patient closely, especially during times of stress.
Inducers of cytochrome P-450 enzyme system: may increase tacrolimus metabolism and decrease blood levels. Dosage adjustment may be needed.
Inhibitors of cytochrome P-450 enzyme system (phenobarbital, phenytoin, rifampin): may decrease tacrolimus metabolism and increase blood levels. Dosage adjustment may be needed.
Nephrotoxic drugs (such as aminoglycosides, amphotericin B, cisplatin, cyclosporine): may cause additive or synergistic effects. Monitor closely.
Viral vaccines: may interfere with the immune response to live virus vaccines. Defer routine immunizations.
Drug-food. *Any food:* inhibited drug absorption. Take drug on empty stomach.
Grapefruit juice: increased drug blood levels. Avoid concomitant use.

EFFECTS ON DIAGNOSTIC TESTS
Monitor for hyperglycemia and hyperkalemia.

CONTRAINDICATIONS
Contraindicated in patients with hypersensitivity to drug. I.V. form is contraindi-

cated in patients hypersensitive to castor oil derivatives.

NURSING CONSIDERATIONS

Alert: Know that because of risk of anaphylaxis, injection should be used only in patients who cannot take the oral form.

● Keep epinephrine 1:1,000 and oxygen available to treat anaphylaxis.

● Know that children with normal renal and hepatic function may require higher dosages than adults.

● Also be aware that patients with hepatic or renal dysfunction should receive the lowest dosage possible.

● Expect to administer adrenal corticosteroids concomitantly with drug.

● Monitor patient for signs of neurotoxicity and nephrotoxicity, especially in patients receiving a high dosage or having renal or hepatic dysfunction.

● Monitor patient for signs and symptoms of hyperkalemia, and obtain serum potassium levels regularly, as ordered. Know that potassium-sparing diuretics should be avoided during tacrolimus therapy.

● Monitor patient's blood glucose level regularly, as ordered. Also monitor patient for signs and symptoms of hyperglycemia. Be aware that treatment of hyperglycemia may be necessary. Insulin-dependent posttransplant diabetes may occur; in some cases, it is reversible.

● Be aware that patient receiving drug is at increased risk for infections, lymphomas, and other malignant diseases.

I.V. administration

● Dilute drug with 0.9% NaCl for injection or D_5W injection to a concentration between 0.004 mg/ml and 0.02 mg/ml before use. Store diluted infusion solution for no more than 24 hours in glass or polyethylene containers. Do not store drug in a polyvinyl chloride container because of decreased stability and potential for extraction of phthalates.

● Monitor patient continuously during the first 30 minutes of I.V. administration and frequently thereafter for signs and symptoms of anaphylaxis.

Patient teaching

● Instruct patient to check with doctor before taking other medications during therapy.

● Tell patient to report adverse reactions promptly.

75

Vaccines and toxoids

BCG vaccine
cholera vaccine
diphtheria and tetanus toxoids, adsorbed
diphtheria and tetanus toxoids and acellular pertussis vaccine adsorbed
diphtheria and tetanus toxoids and whole-cell pertussis vaccine
Haemophilus b conjugate vaccines
hepatitis A vaccine, inactivated
hepatitis B vaccine, recombinant
influenza virus vaccine, 1998-1999 trivalent types A & B (purified surface antigen)
influenza virus vaccine, 1998-1999 trivalent types A & B (subvirion or purified subvirion)
influenza virus vaccine, 1998-1999 trivalent types A & B (whole virion)
Japanese encephalitis virus vaccine, inactivated
measles, mumps, and rubella virus vaccine, live
measles and rubella virus vaccine, live attenuated
measles virus vaccine, live attenuated
meningococcal polysaccharide vaccine
mumps virus vaccine, live
plague vaccine
pneumococcal vaccine, polyvalent
poliovirus vaccine, inactivated
poliovirus vaccine, live, oral, trivalent
rabies vaccine, adsorbed
rabies vaccine, human diploid cell
rotavirus vaccine, live, oral, tetravalent
rubella and mumps virus vaccine, live
rubella virus vaccine, live attenuated
tetanus toxoid, adsorbed
tetanus toxoid, fluid

typhoid vaccine, live, oral
typhoid vaccine, parenteral
typhoid Vi polysaccharide vaccine
varicella virus vaccine
yellow fever vaccine

COMBINATION PRODUCTS

AcTHIB/DTP: 10 mcg *Haemophilus* b polyribosylribitol phosphate (PRP) conjugated to 24 mcg tetanus toxoid, 6.7 Lf (limit flocculation) units diphtheria toxoid, 5 Lf units tetanus toxoid, and 4 units whole-cell pertussis vaccine per 0.5 ml.
Comvax: 7.5 mcg *Haemophilus* b PRP, 125 mcg *Neisseria meningitidis* OMPC, and 5 mcg hepatitis B surface antigen per 0.5 ml.
Tetramune: 10 mcg purified *Haemophilus* b saccharide and approximately 25 mcg CRM_{197} protein, 12.5 Lf units inactivated diphtheria, 5 Lf units inactivated tetanus, and 4 protective units pertussis per 0.5 ml.

BCG vaccine
TICE BCG

Pregnancy Risk Category: C

HOW SUPPLIED
Percutaneous vaccine: 1 to 8 x 10^8 colony-forming units (CFU)/vial (Tice strain)

ACTION
A live, attenuated bacterial vaccine prepared from *Mycobacterium bovis* that promotes active immunity to tuberculosis (TB).

Route	Onset	Peak	Duration
Percuta-neous	Unknown	Unknown	Unknown

INDICATIONS & DOSAGE
TB exposure—
Adults and children 1 month and over: 0.2 to 0.3 ml (percutaneous vaccine) ap-

plied to cleaned skin followed by application of multiple-puncture disk.

Infants less than 1 month: dosage reduced by 50% by using 2 ml of sterile water without preservatives when reconstituting.

ADVERSE REACTIONS
Musculoskeletal: osteomyelitis.
Other: lymphadenopathy, allergic reaction, *anaphylaxis.*

INTERACTIONS
Drug-drug. *Immunosuppressants:* may reduce response to BCG vaccine. Avoid if possible.
Isoniazid, rifampin, streptomycin: inhibited multiplication of BCG. Avoid use together.
Steroids: concurrent use may cause systemic infection. Avoid use together.

EFFECTS ON DIAGNOSTIC TESTS
Tuberculin sensitivity may be rendered positive by BCG intravesical treatment. Determine patient's reactivity to tuberculin before initiating therapy.

CONTRAINDICATIONS
Contraindicated in patients with hypogammaglobulinemia, in presence of a positive tuberculin reaction (when meant for use as immunoprophylactic after exposure to TB) in immunosuppressed patients, in those with fresh smallpox vaccinations, in those who have suffered burns, and in patients receiving corticosteroid therapy. Pregnant patients should avoid vaccine. Contraindicated in patients hypersensitive to vaccine.

NURSING CONSIDERATIONS
• Do not inject I.V., S.C., or intradermally.
• Use cautiously in patients with chronic skin disease. Inject in healthy skin only.
• Obtain history of allergies and reaction to immunization.
• Keep epinephrine 1:1,000 available to treat anaphylaxis.
• Do not shake vial after reconstitution. Use within 2 hours.
• Do not administer to febrile individuals unless cause is determined.
• Know that expected lesion forms in 7 to

14 days. Papules reach a maximum diameter of 3 mm, then fade.
• Allow at least 6 to 8 weeks between BCG and live virus vaccines; administer killed virus vaccines 7 days before or 10 days after BCG, as ordered.
• Know that vaccine is of no value as immunoprophylactic in patients with positive tuberculin test.
• Destroy live vaccine by autoclaving or treating with formaldehyde solution before disposal.

☑ Patient teaching
• Advise patient to have tuberculin skin test 2 to 3 months after BCG vaccination.
• Tell patient to report unusual signs and symptoms after vaccination.
• Inform patient to keep site dry for 24 hours and not to expose area to others because live vaccine may infect them.

cholera vaccine

Pregnancy Risk Category: C

HOW SUPPLIED
Injection: suspension of killed *Vibrio cholerae* (each milliliter contains 8 units of Inaba and Ogawa serotypes) in 1.5-ml and 20-ml vials

ACTION
Promotes active immunity to cholera.

Route	Onset	Peak	Duration
IM, SC, Intra-dermal	After 2nd dose	Unknown	3-6 mo

INDICATIONS & DOSAGE
Primary immunization for persons traveling to areas where cholera is endemic or epidemic—
Adults and children over 10 years: two doses of 0.5 ml I.M. or S.C., 1 week to 1 month apart, before traveling in cholera area. Booster is 0.5 ml q 6 months p.r.n.
Adults and children 5 years and older: two doses of 0.2 ml intradermally, 1 week to 1 month apart, and q 6 months p.r.n.
Children 5 to 10 years: 0.3 ml I.M. or

S.C. Boosters of same dose should be given q 6 months, p.r.n.
Children 6 months to 4 years: 0.2 ml I.M. or S.C. Boosters of same dose should be given q 6 months, p.r.n.

ADVERSE REACTIONS
CNS: headache.
Skin: *erythema, swelling, pain, induration* (at injection site).
Other: malaise, fever, ***anaphylaxis.***

INTERACTIONS
Drug-drug. *Plague, typhoid, other vaccines with systemic adverse reactions:* enhanced toxicity. Don't use together.
Yellow fever vaccine: simultaneous administration may interfere with immune response to both vaccines. Administer 3 weeks apart.

EFFECTS ON DIAGNOSTIC TESTS
None reported.

CONTRAINDICATIONS
Contraindicated in those with acute illness or history of severe systemic reaction or allergic response to vaccine.

NURSING CONSIDERATIONS
● Obtain history of allergies and reaction to immunization.
● Keep epinephrine 1:1,000 available to treat anaphylaxis.
● Shake vial vigorously before withdrawing each dose.
● Do not administer I.M. to persons with thrombocytopenia or other coagulation disorders that contraindicate I.M. injection.
● Administer I.M. in deltoid muscle in adults and children over 3 years.
● Keep in mind that I.M. and S.C. routes give higher levels of protection in children less than 5 years of age.
● Know that vaccine is about 50% effective in reducing clinical illness incidence for 3 to 6 months.

☑ Patient teaching
● Advise patient that pain, induration, and swelling are common at the injection site for 24 to 48 hours.

● Tell traveler to avoid food and water that may be contaminated.
● Advise patient that malaise, headache, and mild to moderate fever may persist for 1 to 2 days.

diphtheria and tetanus toxoids, adsorbed

Pregnancy Risk Category: C

HOW SUPPLIED
Available in pediatric (DT) and adult (Td) strengths
Injection (for pediatric use): diphtheria toxoid 6.6 Lf (limit flocculation) units and tetanus toxoid 5 Lf units per 0.5 ml; diphtheria toxoid 7.5 Lf units and tetanus toxoid 7.5 Lf units per 0.5 ml; diphtheria toxoid 10 Lf units and tetanus toxoid 5 Lf units per 0.5 ml; diphtheria toxoid 12.5 Lf units and tetanus toxoid 5 Lf units per 0.5 ml.
Injection (for adult use): diphtheria toxoid 2 Lf units and tetanus toxoid 2 Lf units per 0.5 ml; diphtheria toxoid 2 Lf units and tetanus toxoid 5 Lf units per 0.5 ml.

ACTION
Promotes immunity to diphtheria and tetanus by inducing production of antitoxins.

Route	Onset	Peak	Duration
IM	Unknown	Unknown	10 yr

INDICATIONS & DOSAGE
Primary immunization—
Adults and children 7 years or over: adult strength; 0.5 ml I.M. 4 to 8 weeks apart for two doses and third dose 6 to 12 months after second dose. Booster is 0.5 ml I.M. q 10 years.
Children 1 to 6 years: pediatric strength; 0.5 ml I.M. at least 4 weeks apart for two doses. Give booster dose 6 to 12 months after second injection. If final immunizing dose is given after seventh birthday, use adult strength.
Infants 6 weeks to 1 year: pediatric strength; 0.5 ml I.M. at least 4 weeks apart for three doses. Give booster dose 6 to 12 months after third injection.

---

*Liquid contains alcohol.   **May contain tartrazine.   †Canada   ‡Australia   §U.K.   ◇OTC

ADVERSE REACTIONS
CNS: headache.
CV: tachycardia, hypotension.
Skin: *pain, stinging, edema, erythema, induration* (at injection site); flushing; urticaria; pruritus.
Other: *anaphylaxis,* chills, fever, malaise.

INTERACTIONS
None significant.

EFFECTS ON DIAGNOSTIC TESTS
None reported.

CONTRAINDICATIONS
Contraindicated in patients with hypersensitivity to vaccine or its components that include a mercury derivative, thimerosal.

Also contraindicated in immunosuppressed patients and in those receiving radiation or corticosteroid therapy. Defer vaccination in patients with respiratory illness and during polio outbreaks; also defer use in those with acute illness except during emergency. When polio is a risk, use single antigen. Know that in children under 6 years, use only when diphtheria, tetanus, and pertussis combination is contraindicated because of pertussis component. Do not use DT in patients over 7 years.

NURSING CONSIDERATIONS
• Obtain history of allergies and reaction to immunization.
• Before injection, verify strength (pediatric or adult) of toxoid used.
• Keep epinephrine 1:1,000 available to treat anaphylaxis.
• Give in site not recently used for vaccines or toxoids.
• Know that drug is not used to treat an acute diphtheria infection.
• Document manufacturer, lot number, date of injection, and name, address, and title of person administering the injection on permanent record or log.
• Interruption of recommended dosing schedule does not interfere with final immunity achieved.

☑ **Patient teaching**
• Advise patient that local reactions, such as pain and pruritus, are common at the injection site and a nodule may be present for a few weeks.
• Review primary immunization schedule with patient or parents, and stress importance of compliance with subsequent injections.

diphtheria and tetanus toxoids and whole-cell pertussis vaccine (DPT, DTP)
DTwP, Tri-Immunol

diphtheria and tetanus toxoids and acellular pertussis vaccine
Acel-Imune, DTaP, Tripedia

Pregnancy Risk Category: C

HOW SUPPLIED
whole-cell vaccine
Injection: 6.5 Lf (limit flocculation) units inactivated diphtheria, 5 Lf units inactivated tetanus, and 4 protective units pertussis per 0.5 ml, in 2.5-, 5-, and 7.5-ml vials; 10 Lf units inactivated diphtheria, 5.5 Lf units inactivated tetanus, and 4 protective units pertussis per 0.5 ml in 5-ml vials (DTwP); 12.5 Lf units inactivated diphtheria, 5 Lf units inactivated tetanus, and 4 protective units pertussis per 0.5 ml, in 7.5-ml vials (Tri-Immunol)
acellular vaccine
Injection: 5 Lf units inactivated diphtheria, 5 Lf units inactivated tetanus, and 300 hemagglutinating units of acellular pertussis vaccine per 0.5 ml; 66.7 Lf units inactivated diphtheria, 5 Lf units inactivated tetanus, and 46.8 pertussis antigens per 0.5 ml

ACTION
Promotes active immunity to diphtheria, tetanus, and pertussis (DTP) by inducing production of antitoxins and antibodies.

Route	Onset	Peak	Duration
IM	2 wk after last dose	Unknown	4-6 yr

Reactions may be *common,* uncommon, *life-threatening,* or COMMON AND LIFE-THREATENING.

INDICATIONS & DOSAGE
Primary immunization—
Children 2 months to 7 years: 0.5 ml
I.M. 4 to 8 weeks apart for three doses and
fourth dose after 6 to 12 months. Booster
is 0.5 ml I.M. when starting school unless
fourth dose in series was administered after child's fourth birthday; then, booster is
not necessary at time of school entrance.

ADVERSE REACTIONS
CNS: *seizures, encephalopathy,* peripheral neuropathy, *drowsiness.*
GI: *vomiting, anorexia.*
Skin: *soreness at injection site, redness,*
expected nodule remaining several weeks
at injection site.
Other: *anaphylaxis, shock,* thrombocytopenic purpura, *fever,* hypersensitivity reactions, urticaria.

INTERACTIONS
Drug-drug. *Immunosuppressants:* may
reduce response to DTP vaccine. Avoid if
possible.

EFFECTS ON DIAGNOSTIC TESTS
None reported.

CONTRAINDICATIONS
Contraindicated in patients who developed an immediate anaphylactic reaction
or encephalopathy within 7 days of DTP
dose, in immunosuppressed patients, and in
those on corticosteroid therapy, and in
those with an evolving neurologic condition. Defer vaccination in patients with
acute febrile illness of unknown cause.
Children with preexisting neurologic disorders should not receive pertussis component. Also, children who exhibit neurologic signs after DTP injection shouldn't
receive pertussis component in any succeeding injections. Diphtheria and tetanus
toxoids (called DT) should be given instead. Contraindicated in patients with hypersensitivity to drug or its components.

NURSING CONSIDERATIONS
• Vaccine is not advised for adults or children over 7 years.
• Products containing acellular pertussis
vaccine may now be used for dose in DTP
immunization.

• Obtain history of allergies and reaction
to immunization.
• Keep epinephrine 1:1,000 available to
treat anaphylaxis.
• Shake before using. Refrigerate vaccine.
• Administer only by deep I.M. injection,
preferably in thigh or deltoid muscle.
Don't give S.C.
• Keep in mind that DTP injection may be
given at same time as trivalent oral polio
vaccine.
• Know that acellular vaccine may be associated with a lower incidence of local
pain and fever.

☑ **Patient teaching**
• Make sure parents know the risks and
benefits of this vaccine before it is administered.
• Tell parents to report systemic reactions
promptly; remind them that local reactions are common. Acetaminophen in
age-appropriate dosing will decrease occurrence of post-vaccination fever in children prone to febrile seizure activity.

Haemophilus b conjugate vaccines

Haemophilus b conjugate vaccine, diphtheria CRM$_{197}$ protein conjugate (HbOC)
HibTITER

Haemophilus b conjugate vaccine, diphtheria toxoid conjugate (PRP-D)
ProHIBIT

Haemophilus b conjugate vaccine, meningococcal protein conjugate (PRP-OMP)
PedvaxHIB

Pregnancy Risk Category: C

HOW SUPPLIED
Haemophilus b conjugate vaccine,
diphtheria CRM$_{197}$ protein conjugate
Injection: 10 mcg of purified *Haemophilus* b saccharide and approximately
25 mcg CRM$_{197}$ protein per 0.5 ml

Haemophilus b conjugate vaccine, diphtheria toxoid conjugate
Injection: 25 mcg of *Haemophilus influenzae* type B (HIB) capsular polysaccharide and 18 mcg of diphtheria toxoid protein per 0.5 ml

Haemophilus b conjugate vaccine, meningococcal protein conjugate
Powder for injection: 15 mcg of *Haemophilus* b PRP, 250 mcg *Neisseria meningitidis* OMPC per dose
Injection: 7.5 mcg of *Haemophilus* b PRP and 125 mcg *Neisseria meningitidis* OMPC per 0.5 ml

ACTION
Promotes active immunity to HIB; is a polymer of ribose, ribitol, and phosphate (PRP) and is linked by covalent bonds to highly antigenic substances, enabling the vaccine to promote an immune response in infants.

Route	Onset	Peak	Duration
IM	2 wk after last dose	Unknown	Several yr

INDICATIONS & DOSAGE
Immunization against HIB infection—
Conjugate vaccine, diphtheria CRM$_{197}$ protein conjugate
Infants: 0.5 ml I.M. at age 2 months. Repeated at 4 months and 6 months. Booster dose given at age 15 months.
Previously unvaccinated infants 2 to 6 months: 0.5 ml I.M. Repeated in 2 months and again in 4 months for total of three doses. Booster dose given at age 15 months.
Previously unvaccinated infants 7 to 11 months: 0.5 ml I.M. Repeated in 2 months, for a total of two doses. Booster dose given at age 15 months (but no sooner than 2 months after last vaccination).
Previously unvaccinated infants 12 to 14 months: 0.5 ml I.M. Booster dose given at age 15 months (but no sooner than 2 months after first vaccination).
Previously unvaccinated children 15 months to 71 months: 0.5 ml I.M. Booster dose is not required.
Conjugate vaccine, diphtheria toxoid conjugate
Previously unvaccinated children 15 months to 71 months: 0.5 ml I.M. A booster dose is not required. Not recommended for use in children under 15 months.
Conjugate vaccine, meningococcal protein conjugate
Infants: 0.5 ml I.M. at age 2 months. Repeated at 4 months. Booster dose given at age 12 months.
Previously unvaccinated infants 2 to 6 months: 0.5 ml I.M. Repeated in 2 months. Booster dose given at age 12 months.
Previously unvaccinated infants 7 to 11 months: 0.5 ml I.M. Repeated in 2 months. Booster dose given at 15 months (but no sooner than 2 months after the last vaccination).
Previously unvaccinated infants 12 to 14 months: 0.5 ml I.M. Booster dose given at age 15 months (but no sooner than 2 months after first vaccination).
Previously unvaccinated children 15 months to 71 months: 0.5 ml I.M. Booster dose is not required.
    Premature infants follow same schedule as full-term infants.

ADVERSE REACTIONS
GI: diarrhea, vomiting.
Skin: *erythema, pain* (at injection site).
Other: ***anaphylaxis,*** fever, crying.

INTERACTIONS
Drug-drug. *Immunosuppressants:* may suppress antibody response to HIB vaccine. Defer immunization.

EFFECTS ON DIAGNOSTIC TESTS
None reported.

CONTRAINDICATIONS
Contraindicated in patients with acute illness and hypersensitivity to vaccine or its components.

NURSING CONSIDERATIONS
• Keep epinephrine 1:1,000 available in case of anaphylaxis.
• Don't administer intradermally or I.V. Must administer I.M.
• Administer into anterolateral aspect of the upper thigh in small children. Injections may be made into the deltoid muscle

of larger children if sufficient muscle mass is present.

• Know that vaccine is not routinely administered to adults or children over 5 years unless they are at high risk for infection (including patients with chronic conditions, such as functional asplenia, splenectomy, Hodgkin's disease, or sickle cell anemia).

Alert: Don't administer to febrile children.

• Know that immunization against HIB infection is recommended for children with HIV infections. The usual immunization schedule should be followed in these children.

• Vaccine and DTP may be given simultaneously. A combination product is commercially available.

• Know that diphtheria toxoid conjugate vaccine (ProHIBIT) is not recommended in children under 15 months.

• HIB is an important cause of meningitis in infants and preschool children.

☑ **Patient teaching**

• Warn patient or parents that pain may occur at injection site.

• Tell patient or parents to notify doctor if adverse reactions persist or become severe.

---

hepatitis A vaccine, inactivated
Havrix, Vaqta

Pregnancy Risk Category: C

HOW SUPPLIED
Havrix
Injection: 360 ELISA units (EL.U.)/0.5 ml, 720 EL.U./0.5 ml; 1,440 EL.U./ml
Vaqta
Injection: 25 units/0.5 ml, 50 units/ml

ACTION
Promotes active immunity to hepatitis A virus.

Route	Onset	Peak	Duration
IM	1-15 days	Unknown	6 mo

INDICATIONS & DOSAGE
Active immunization against hepatitis A virus—
Adults: 1,440 EL.U. (Havrix) or 50 units (Vaqta) I.M. as a single dose. For booster dose, 1,440 EL.U. (Havrix) or 50 units (Vaqta) I.M. given 6 to 12 months after initial dose. A booster dose is recommended if prolonged immunity is desired.
Children 2 to 18 years: 720 EL.U. (Havrix) or 25 units (Vaqta) I.M. as a single dose, followed by a booster dose of 720 EL.U. (Havrix) or 25 units (Vaqta) I.M. given 6 to 12 months after initial dose or 360 EL.U. I.M. given 1 month apart and 360 EL.U. I.M. 6 to 12 months after primary course. Booster recommended for prolonged immunity.
Prevention of hepatitis A in patients with chronic liver disease or clotting factor disorders, and in food handlers—
Adults: 1,440 EL.U. (Havrix) I.M. as a single dose. For booster dose, 1,440 EL.U. (Havrix) I.M. given 6 to 12 months after initial dose. A booster dose is recommended if prolonged immunity is desired.
Children 2 to 18 years: 720 EL.U. (Havrix) I.M. as a single dose, followed by a booster dose of 720 EL.U. (Havrix) I.M. given 6 to 12 months after initial dose; or two doses of 360 EL.U. I.M. given 1 month apart and 360 EL.U. I.M. 6 to 12 months after primary course. Booster dose is recommended if prolonged immunity is desired.

ADVERSE REACTIONS
CNS: episode of hypertonia, insomnia, photophobia, vertigo, *headache.*
EENT: pharyngitis.
GI: *anorexia, nausea,* abdominal pain, diarrhea, dysgeusia, vomiting.
Musculoskeletal: arthralgia, myalgia.
Respiratory: other upper respiratory tract infections.
Skin: pruritus, rash, urticaria, *induration, redness, swelling,* hematoma, *injection site soreness.*
Other: *fatigue, fever, malaise,* lymphadenopathy, ***anaphylaxis,*** elevated CK level.

INTERACTIONS
Drug-drug. *Anticoagulants:* increases

---

risk of bleeding. Administer I.M. injections with caution.

EFFECTS ON DIAGNOSTIC TESTS
None reported.

CONTRAINDICATIONS
Contraindicated in patients with hypersensitivity to vaccine's components.

NURSING CONSIDERATIONS
• Use with caution in patients with thrombocytopenia or bleeding disorders and in those who are taking an anticoagulant because bleeding may occur following an I.M. injection.
• As with other vaccines, administration of hepatitis A vaccine should be delayed, if possible, in patient with febrile illness.
• Keep epinephrine 1:1,000 available to treat an anaphylactoid reaction.
• Be aware that if vaccine is administered to immunosuppressed persons or persons receiving immunosuppressants, the expected immune response may not be obtained.
• Know that persons who should receive vaccine include people traveling to or living in areas of high endemicity for hepatitis A (Africa, Asia [except Japan], the Mediterranean basin, Eastern Europe, the Middle East, Central and South America, Mexico, and parts of the Caribbean), military personnel, native peoples of Alaska and the Americas, persons engaging in high-risk sexual activity, and users of illegal injectable drugs. Certain institutional workers, employees of child day-care centers, laboratory workers who handle live hepatitis A virus, and handlers of primate animals also may benefit.
• For I.M. use, shake vial or syringe well before withdrawal. After it has been agitated thoroughly, vaccine is an opaque white suspension. Discard if it appears otherwise. No dilution or reconstitution is necessary.
• Administer as I.M. injection into the deltoid region in adults. It should not be administered in the gluteal region; such injections may result in suboptimal response. Never inject I.V., S.C., or intradermally.

• Delay vaccination in febrile patient, if possible.

☑ **Patient teaching**
• Inform patient that vaccine will not prevent hepatitis caused by other agents or pathogens known to infect the liver.
• Warn patient about local adverse reactions. Tell him to report persistent or severe reactions promptly.
• Alert travelers to the dangers of eating raw or undercooked shellfish or food or drink in countries with poor hygienic conditions.

---

hepatitis B vaccine, recombinant
Engerix-B, Recombivax HB

Pregnancy Risk Category: C

HOW SUPPLIED
Injection: 2.5 mcg hepatitis B surface antigen (HBsAg)/0.5 ml (Recombivax HB, pediatric formulation); 5 mcg HBsAg/0.5 ml (Recombivax HB, adolescent/high-risk infant formulation); 10 mcg HBsAg/0.5 ml (Engerix-B, adolescent/pediatric formulation); 10 mcg HBsAg/ml (Recombivax HB, adult formulation); 20 mcg HBsAg/ml (Engerix-B, adult formulation); 40 mcg HBsAg/ml (Recombivax HB dialysis formulation)

ACTION
Promotes active immunity to hepatitis B.

Route	Onset	Peak	Duration
IM	2 wk after last dose	Unknown	Yrs

INDICATIONS & DOSAGE
Immunization against infection from all known subtypes of hepatitis B virus (HBV); primary preexposure prophylaxis against HBV; or postexposure prophylaxis (when given with hepatitis B immune globulin)—
Engerix-B
Adults: initially, 20 mcg (1-ml adult formulation) is given I.M., followed by a second dose of 20 mcg I.M. 30 days later. A third dose of 20 mcg I.M. is given 30

Reactions may be *common*, uncommon, *life-threatening*, or COMMON AND LIFE-THREATENING.

days after second dose. A fourth dose is given 12 months after initial dose.

Adjust-a-dose: In adults undergoing dialysis or receiving immunosuppressants, initially, 40 mcg I.M. (divided into two 20-mcg doses and administered at different sites). Followed by second dose of 40 mcg I.M. in 30 days, and final dose of 40 mcg I.M. 6 months after initial dose.

Note: Certain populations (neonates born to infected mothers, persons recently exposed to the virus, and travelers to high-risk areas) may receive vaccine on an abbreviated schedule, with initial dose followed by second dose in 1 month, and third dose after 2 months. For prolonged maintenance of protective antibody titers, a booster dose is recommended 12 months after initial dose.

Adolescents 11 to 20 years: initially, 10 mcg (0.5-ml adolescent/pediatric formulation) I.M., followed by second dose of 10 mcg I.M. 30 days later. A third dose of 10 mcg I.M. is given 6 months after the initial dose. Alternatively, 20 mcg (1-ml adult formulation) is given I.M., followed by second dose of 20 mcg I.M. 30 days later. A third dose of 20 mcg I.M. is given 6 months after initial dose.

Neonates and children up to 11 years: initially, 10 mcg (0.5-ml pediatric formulation) I.M., followed by second dose of 10 mcg I.M. 30 days later. A third dose of 10 mcg I.M. is given 6 months after initial dose.

Recombivax HB
Adults: initially, 10 mcg (1-ml adult formulation) I.M., followed by second dose of 10 mcg I.M. 30 days later. A third dose of 10 mcg is given I.M. 6 months after initial dose.

Adjust-a-dose: In adults undergoing dialysis, initially, 40 mcg I.M. (use dialysis formulation, which contains 40 mcg/ml); then second dose of 40 mcg I.M. in 30 days, and final dose of 40 mcg I.M. 6 months after initial dose. A booster or revaccination may be indicated if the anti-HBs level is below 10 mIU/ml 1 to 2 months after third dose.

Children 11 to 19 years: initially, 5 mcg (0.5-ml adolescent/high-risk infant formulation) I.M., followed by second dose of 5 mcg I.M. 30 days later. A third dose

of 5 mcg is given I.M. 6 months after initial dose.

Children 1 to 10 years: initially, 2.5 mcg (0.5-ml pediatric formulation) I.M., followed by second dose of 2.5 mcg I.M. 30 days later. A third dose of 2.5 mcg I.M. is given 6 months after initial dose.

Infants born of HBsAg-negative mothers: initially, 2.5 mcg (0.5-ml pediatric formulation) I.M., followed by second dose of 0.5 mcg 30 days later. A third dose of 0.5 mcg is given I.M. 6 months after initial dose.

Infants born of HBsAg-positive mothers: initially, 5 mcg (0.5-ml adolescent/high-risk infant formulation) I.M., followed by second dose of 5 mcg I.M. 30 days later. A third dose of 5 mcg is given I.M. 6 months after initial dose.

✳ *NEW INDICATION: Chronic hepatitis C infection—*
Engerix-B
Adults: initially, 20 mcg (1-ml adult formulation) is given I.M., followed by a second dose of 20 mcg I.M. 30 days later. A third dose of 20 mcg I.M. is given 6 months after initial dose.

ADVERSE REACTIONS
CNS: headache, dizziness, insomnia, paresthesia, neuropathy.
EENT: pharyngitis.
GI: anorexia, diarrhea.
Musculoskeletal: myalgia, arthralgia.
Skin: local inflammation, *soreness* (at injection site).
Other: *anaphylaxis,* nausea, vomiting, slight fever, transient malaise, flulike symptoms.

INTERACTIONS
Drug-drug. *Immunosuppressants:* inadequate circulating antibody levels. May require larger than usual doses of hepatitis B vaccine (recombinant).

EFFECTS ON DIAGNOSTIC TESTS
None reported.

CONTRAINDICATIONS
Contraindicated in patients hypersensitive to yeast or components of vaccine; recombinant vaccines are derived from yeast cultures.

NURSING CONSIDERATIONS

• Use cautiously in patients with serious, active infections or compromised cardiac or pulmonary status and in those for whom a febrile or systemic reaction could pose a risk.

• Know that the American Academy of Pediatrics recommends hepatitis B vaccination for all neonates and encourages immunization for adolescents when resources allow.

• Although anaphylaxis has not been reported, always keep epinephrine available when giving vaccine to counteract possible reaction.

• Thoroughly agitate vial just before administration to restore suspension.

• Inspect product for particulate matter or discoloration prior to administration. Product should be a slightly opaque white suspension. Discard if appears otherwise.

• Administer vaccine in deltoid muscle for adults and adolescents; for infants and young children, administer in anterolateral aspect of thigh. Never administer I.V.

• Administer S.C. in patients at risk for hemorrhage, such as hemophiliacs. Otherwise, do not use this route; it may lead to an increased incidence or severity of local reactions.

• Keep in mind that certain health care personnel (especially those working with dialysis patients, in blood banks, in emergency medicine, with selected patients and patient contacts, or among populations in which the infection is endemic [Indo-Chinese, native peoples of Alaska, and Haitian refugees]), certain military personnel, morticians and embalmers, sexually active homosexual men, prostitutes, prisoners, and users of illegal injectable drugs are at increased risk for infection and should be considered for vaccine.

• Be aware that recombinant hepatitis B vaccine is not made with human plasma products.

☑ **Patient teaching**

• Warn patient or parents about local adverse reactions. Tell patient to report persistent or severe reactions promptly.

• Review immunization schedule with pa-

tient or parents; stress importance of completing series.

---

influenza virus vaccine, 1998-1999 trivalent types A & B (purified surface antigen)
Fluvirin

influenza virus vaccine, 1998-1999 trivalent types A & B (subvirion or purified subvirion)
Fluogen, Flu-Shield, Fluzone

influenza virus vaccine, 1998-1999 trivalent types A & B (whole virion)
Fluzone

Pregnancy Risk Category: C

HOW SUPPLIED
Injection: each 0.5-ml dose contains 15 mcg HA of A/Johannesburg/82/96 (H_1N1) (A/Bayern/07/95-like [H_1N1]), 15 mcg HA of A/Nanchang/933/95 (H3N2) (A/Wuhan/359/95-like [H3N2]), and 15 mcg HA of B/Harbin/07/94 (B/Beijing/184/93-like)

ACTION
Promotes immunity to influenza by inducing production of antibodies.

Route	Onset	Peak	Duration
IM	2-4 wk	Unknown	Unknown

INDICATIONS & DOSAGE
Influenza prophylaxis—
Adults and children 12 years and older: 0.5 ml whole virus, split virus, or purified split virus I.M. Only one dose is required.
Children 9 to 12 years: 0.5 ml split virus or purified split virus I.M. Only one dose is required.
Children 3 to 8 years: 0.5 ml split virus or purified split virus I.M. Repeated in 4 weeks unless child has been previously vaccinated.
Children 6 to 35 months: 0.25 ml split virus or purified split virus I.M. Repeated

---

in 4 weeks unless child has been previously vaccinated.

ADVERSE REACTIONS
CNS: headache.
Musculoskeletal: myalgia.
Skin: erythema, induration, *soreness at injection site.*
Other: *anaphylaxis,* fever, malaise.

Fever and malaise reactions occur most often in children and in others not exposed to influenza viruses. Severe reactions in adults are rare.

INTERACTIONS
Drug-drug. *Immunosuppressants:* may reduce immune response to vaccine. Monitor patient closely.
Theophylline, warfarin: clearance may be impaired. Monitor patient closely.

EFFECTS ON DIAGNOSTIC TESTS
None reported.

CONTRAINDICATIONS
Contraindicated in patients with hypersensitivity to eggs or components of vaccine including thimerosal. Defer vaccination in patients with acute respiratory or other active infection.

NURSING CONSIDERATIONS
● Use cautiously in patients with history of sulfite allergy.
● Obtain history of allergies, especially to eggs, and reaction to immunization.
● Keep epinephrine 1:1,000 available to treat anaphylaxis.
● Thoroughly agitate vial just before administration to restore suspension.
● Give injections for adults and older children in deltoid muscle; for infants and children under 3 years, give in anterolateral aspect of thigh.
● Ideally, administer vaccinations from October to mid-November because outbreaks of influenza generally don't occur until December. Do not give vaccine too early in season because antibody titers may begin to decline before flu season.
● Know that children 12 years and under should be given their second dose before December, if possible.
● Give vaccines to both children and adults throughout the flu season, even as late as April.
● The American Academy of Pediatrics recommends that influenza vaccine can be administered simultaneously (but at a different site and with a different syringe) with other routine vaccinations in children.
Alert: Do not give influenza vaccine concomitantly or within 3 days after administration of whole cell pertussis vaccine or combined diphtheria/tetanus toxoid/whole cell pertussis vaccine, adsorbed.
● Know that vaccine is considered safe in pregnant patients. Vaccination should not be postponed, regardless of stage of pregnancy, in patients who have high-risk conditions and who will be in the first trimester of pregnancy when flu season begins.
● Keep in mind that immunodeficient patients may receive two doses 1 month apart; however, there is little evidence that booster doses improve immunogenic response to vaccine. Know that chemoprophylaxis with amantadine may be helpful.
● Know that vaccine is strongly recommended for anyone over 6 months; for patients with chronic disease, metabolic disorders, or medical conditions that put them at risk for complications from influenza; for health care workers, especially doctors, nurses, employees of nursing homes, volunteer workers, and other personnel in both hospital and outpatient settings; and for household members who may contact persons at high risk for medical complications of influenza. Also recommended for anyone who wishes to reduce the chance of infection.
● Keep in mind that allergic reactions, which usually occur immediately, are extremely rare.
● Be aware that paralysis associated with Guillain-Barré syndrome is rare and has been associated only with the 1976 vaccine.
● Remember that although there is little information regarding influenza in persons with HIV, it is recommended these patients receive vaccine. Patients with advanced disease may have a low response;

there is no evidence that booster dose will improve the immune response.

☑**Patient teaching**
• Advise patient about risks of vaccination as compared with risk of influenza and its complications.
• Ensure that patient understands that annual vaccination with the current vaccine is necessary because immunity to influenza decreases in the year after the injection.
• Ensure that patient understands vaccine cannot cause influenza. Fever, malaise, and myalgia may begin 6 to 12 hours after vaccination and last 1 to 2 days. Such systemic reactions are not common.
• Advise appropriate acetaminophen dose for fever and ice compresses to injection site to minimize discomfort.

Japanese encephalitis virus vaccine, inactivated
JE-VAX

Pregnancy Risk Category: C

HOW SUPPLIED
Injection: 1-ml, 10-ml vials

ACTION
Provides active immunity against Japanese encephalitis (JE), a mosquito-borne arboviral flavivirus infection that's the main cause of viral encephalitis in Asia.

Route	Onset	Peak	Duration
SC	Unknown	Unknown	2 yr

INDICATIONS & DOSAGE
Active immunization against JE—
Primary immunization schedule
Adults and children 3 years and over: 1 ml S.C. on days 0, 7, and 30.
Children 1 to 3 years: 0.5 ml S.C. on days 0, 7, and 30.
Booster doses
Adults and children 3 years and over: 1 ml S.C., 2 years after last dose.
Children 1 to 3 years: 0.5 ml S.C., 2 years after last dose.

ADVERSE REACTIONS
CNS: *headache, dizziness.*
GI: *nausea, vomiting, abdominal pain.*
Musculoskeletal: *myalgia.*
Respiratory: *respiratory distress.*
Skin: rash, *local tenderness and swelling at injection site.*
Other: *anaphylaxis,* generalized urticaria, *fever, malaise, chills,* angioedema of the face, oropharynx, extremities, or lips.

INTERACTIONS
None significant.

EFFECTS ON DIAGNOSTIC TESTS
None reported.

CONTRAINDICATIONS
Contraindicated in patients hypersensitive to drug or to thimerosal, a preservative, and in patients who exhibited severe adverse reactions, such as generalized urticaria or angioedema, to a prior dose of vaccine. Because vaccine is derived from mouse brain, its use is contraindicated in patients hypersensitive to substances of murine or neural origin.

NURSING CONSIDERATIONS
• Use cautiously in pregnant or breast-feeding patients, elderly patients, and those with history of urticaria after vaccines, drugs, or insect stings. Advanced age may be a risk factor for developing symptomatic illness after JE infection. JE acquired during pregnancy can cause intrauterine infection and fetal death.
• Use vaccine to provide protection against JE in persons planning to travel 1 month or longer or who reside in areas where the virus is endemic. It's not indicated for all persons traveling to or residing in Asia. For most travelers to Asia, the risk for acquiring JE is extremely low. Contact the Centers for Disease Control and Prevention at (404) 332-4555 for current travel advisories.
• Keep epinephrine 1:1,000 and other resuscitation equipment and drugs available to treat anaphylaxis and other adverse reactions.
• To prepare vaccine for injection, use supplied diluent (sterile water for injec-

---

Reactions may be *common*, uncommon, ***life-threatening***, or COMMON AND LIFE-THREATENING.

tion). Add 1.3 ml of diluent to the single-dose vial and 11 ml of diluent to the 10-dose vial. Shake vial thoroughly to ensure dissolution of vaccine. After reconstitution, refrigerate vaccine (36° to 46° F [2° to 8° C]) for up to 8 hours, then discard.

• Follow recommended three-dose schedule for best results. Be aware that when time constraints prohibit use of this schedule, an abbreviated schedule with injections on days 0, 7, and 14 may be used.

• Know that when it isn't possible to follow usual dose schedule, a two-dose regimen with injections on days 0 and 7 may be used. Antibodies will be induced in about 80% of patients with this schedule. A two-dose regimen should not be used unless circumstances are unusual.

• Monitor patient closely for 30 minutes after injection.

• Be aware that reactions to the first dose have occurred a median of 12 hours after injection (88% happened within 3 days). The delay between the second dose and adverse effects was usually longer, with a median of 3 days, and some effects not seen for 2 weeks. Some patients exhibited adverse reactions to the second or third dose, even when the first or second dose was well tolerated.

✅ **Patient teaching**
• Warn patient about possibility of delayed generalized urticaria or delayed angioedema of the extremities, face, oropharynx or (especially) the lips. Generalized urticaria or angioedema may occur within minutes of vaccination. Most reactions occur within 48 hours. However, reactions that may be related to vaccine have occurred as late as 17 days after the injection.

• Because of risk of delayed reactions, advise patient to remain in areas where medical care is available for 10 days after injection. Caution against international travel during this time. Advise patient to seek medical assistance as soon as a reaction appears.

• Encourage patient and parents to report adverse effects after vaccination. Health care providers should report these adverse

effects to the U.S. Department of Health and Human Services Vaccine Adverse Event Reporting System (VAERS). Contact VAERS at (800) 822-7967 for information about the system and reporting forms.

• Teach patient about precautions that may limit exposure to mosquito bites, such as using insect repellents, wearing protective clothing, and avoiding outdoor activities, especially in the evening.

measles, mumps, and rubella virus vaccine, live
M-M-R II

Pregnancy Risk Category: C

HOW SUPPLIED
Injection: single-dose vial containing not less than 1,000 TCID$_{50}$ (tissue culture infective doses) of attenuated measles virus derived from Enders' attenuated Edmonston strain (grown in chick embryo culture), 20,000 TCID$_{50}$ of the Jeryl Lynn (B level) mumps strain (grown in chick embryo culture), and 1,000 TCID$_{50}$ of the Wistar RA 27/3 strain of rubella virus (propagated in human diploid cell culture) per 0.5-ml dose. Multidose vial available to institutions or government agencies.

ACTION
Promotes immunity to measles, mumps, and rubella virus by inducing production of antibodies.

Route	Onset	Peak	Duration
SC	Unknown	Unknown	< 11 yr

INDICATIONS & DOSAGE
Routine immunization—
Adults: one vial S.C. People born after 1957 should receive two doses at least 1 month apart.
Children: one vial S.C. A two-dose schedule is recommended, with the first dose given at 15 months (12 months in high-risk areas) and the second dose given either at 4 to 6 years or at 11 or 12 years.

ADVERSE REACTIONS
GI: diarrhea.
Musculoskeletal: arthritis, arthralgia.
Skin: rash, erythema at injection site.
Other: urticaria, fever, regional lymphadenopathy, *anaphylaxis.*

INTERACTIONS
Drug-drug. *Immune serum globulin, plasma, whole blood:* antibodies in serum may interfere with immune response. Don't use vaccine within 3 to 11 months of these products, depending on dose of antibody or blood given.
Immunosuppressants: may decrease immune response to vaccine. Monitor closely.

EFFECTS ON DIAGNOSTIC TESTS
Vaccine may temporarily decrease response to tuberculin skin testing. If skin test is necessary, administer it either before or simultaneously with vaccine.

CONTRAINDICATIONS
Contraindicated in immunosuppressed patients; in those with cancer, blood dyscrasia, gamma globulin disorders, fever, active untreated tuberculosis, or anaphylactic or anaphylactoid reactions to neomycin or eggs; in those receiving corticosteroid or radiation therapy; and in pregnant patients.

NURSING CONSIDERATIONS
• Obtain history of allergies, especially anaphylactic reactions to antibiotics, or reaction to immunization.
• Keep epinephrine 1:1,000 available to treat anaphylaxis.
• Inject into outer aspect of upper arm. Don't give I.V.
• Use only diluent supplied. Discard 8 hours after reconstituting.
• Refrigerate vaccine; protect from light. Solution may be used if red, pink, or yellow, but must be clear.
• Know that incidence of adverse effects is low (0.5% to 4%).
• Treat fever with antipyretics such as acetaminophen.
• Be aware that presence of maternal antibodies may prevent response in children under 12 months.

• Keep in mind that the Immunization Practices Advisory Committee recommends that colleges and other post–high school educational institutions, as well as medical institutions employing health care providers, obtain documentation of the receipt of two doses of vaccine after age 1 (or other evidence of immunity, such as infection, documented by doctor). Combined measles, mumps, and rubella vaccine is preferred.
Alert: The Centers for Disease Control and Prevention recommends that, during a measles outbreak in a health care facility, susceptible personnel exposed to measles virus (whether or not they received measles vaccine or immunoglobulin) avoid patient contact for days 5 through 21 after such exposure. If they become ill, they should avoid patient contact for at least 7 days after developing rash.

☑ Patient teaching
• Warn parents about adverse reactions associated with vaccine.
• Review immunization schedule with parents, and stress importance of receiving second injection at the appropriate time to maintain immunization.
• Tell female patient of childbearing age to use measures to prevent pregnancy until 3 months after immunization.
• Febrile seizures have rarely occurred in children post-vaccination. Tell parents to treat and promptly report fever, especially in patient with family history of seizures.

measles and rubella virus vaccine, live attenuated
M-R-Vax II

Pregnancy Risk Category: C

HOW SUPPLIED
Injection: single-dose vial containing not less than 1,000 $TCID_{50}$ (tissue culture infective doses) per 0.5 ml of attenuated measles virus derived from Enders' attenuated Edmonston strain (grown in chick embryo culture); 1,000 $TCID_{50}$ of the Wistar RA 27/3 strain of rubella virus

ACTION

Promotes immunity to measles and rubella virus by inducing production of antibodies.

Route	Onset	Peak	Duration
SC	Unknown	Unknown	< 11 yr

INDICATIONS & DOSAGE

Immunization—
Adults and children 15 months and older: 0.5 ml (1,000 units) S.C.

ADVERSE REACTIONS

Musculoskeletal: arthralgia.
Skin: rash, *burning or stinging at injection site.*
Other: fever, lymphadenopathy, ***anaphylaxis.***

INTERACTIONS

Drug-drug. *Immune serum globulin, plasma, whole blood:* antibodies in serum may interfere with immune response. Don't use vaccine within 3 months of transfusion.
Immunosuppressants: may reduce immune response to vaccine. Monitor closely.

EFFECTS ON DIAGNOSTIC TESTS

Vaccine may temporarily decrease response to tuberculin skin testing. If necessary, administer test either before or simultaneously with vaccine.

CONTRAINDICATIONS

Contraindicated in immunosuppressed patients; in those with cancer, blood dyscrasia, gamma globulin disorders, fever, active untreated tuberculosis or anaphylactic or anaphylactoid reactions to eggs or neomycin; in those receiving corticosteroid or radiation therapy; and in pregnant patients.

NURSING CONSIDERATIONS

• Obtain history of allergies, especially anaphylactic reactions to antibiotics.
• Keep epinephrine 1:1,000 available to treat anaphylaxis.
• Use only diluent supplied. Discard 8 hours after reconstituting.

• Inject into outer upper arm. Don't inject I.V.
• Store in refrigerator and protect from light. Reconstituted solution should be clear yellow.
Alert: Vaccine should not be given within 1 month of other live virus vaccines, except oral poliovirus vaccine. Immunization should be deferred in patients with acute illness.
• Allow at least 3 weeks between BCG and rubella vaccines.

☑ **Patient teaching**
• Warn patient or parents about adverse reactions associated with vaccine.
• Caution women of childbearing age to avoid pregnancy until 3 months postimmunization.
• Advise use of antipyretics to control fever.

measles virus vaccine, live attenuated
Attenuvax

Pregnancy Risk Category: C

HOW SUPPLIED

Injection: single-dose vial containing not less than 1,000 TCID$_{50}$ (tissue culture infective doses) of measles virus derived from the more attenuated line of Enders' attenuated Edmonston strain (grown in chick embryo culture). Available in 10- and 50-dose vials.

ACTION

Promotes immunity to measles virus by inducing production of antibodies.

Route	Onset	Peak	Duration
SC	Few days	Unknown	≥ 13 yr

INDICATIONS & DOSAGE

Immunization—
Adults and children age 15 months or over: 0.5 ml (1,000 units) S.C. A two-dose schedule is recommended, with first dose given at 15 months (12 months in high-risk areas) and second dose given at 4 to 6 years or 11 to 12 years.

Measles outbreak control—
Adults: school personnel born in or after 1957 should be revaccinated if they lack evidence of measles immunity. If outbreak is in a medical facility, all workers born in or after 1957 should be revaccinated if they lack evidence of immunity.
Children: if cases occur in children under 1 year, children should be vaccinated as young as 6 months. All students and siblings should be revaccinated if they are without documentation of measles immunity.

ADVERSE REACTIONS

CNS: febrile seizures in susceptible children.
Skin: rash, erythema, swelling, tenderness (at injection site).
Other: anorexia, *leukopenia,* fever, lymphadenopathy, *anaphylaxis.*

INTERACTIONS

Drug-drug. *Immune serum globulin, plasma, whole blood:* antibodies in serum may interfere with immune response. Don't use vaccine for at least 3 months after administration of these products.

EFFECTS ON DIAGNOSTIC TESTS

Vaccine may temporarily decrease response to tuberculin skin test. If skin test is necessary, administer it before, at the same time, or 6 weeks after immunization.

CONTRAINDICATIONS

Contraindicated in immunosuppressed patients; in those with cancer, blood dyscrasia, gamma globulin disorders, fever, active untreated tuberculosis, or anaphylactic or anaphylactoid reactions to neomycin or eggs; in those receiving corticosteroid or radiation therapy; and in pregnant patients.

NURSING CONSIDERATIONS

• Obtain history of allergies, especially anaphylactic reactions to antibiotics, or reaction to immunization. Immunization should be deferred in patients with acute illness or after administration of blood or plasma.

• Keep epinephrine 1:1,000 available to treat anaphylaxis.
• Use only diluent supplied. Discard 8 hours after reconstituting.
• Do not give I.V.
• Know that vaccine may be given with oral poliovirus vaccine.
• Keep in mind that the Immunization Practices Advisory Committee recommends that colleges and other post-high school educational institutions as well as medical institutions employing health care providers obtain documentation of the receipt of two doses of vaccine after 1 year of age (or other evidence of immunity, such as infection, documented by doctor). Combined measles, mumps, and rubella vaccine is preferred.
• Do not give vaccine within 3 months of receiving a blood or plasma transfusion or human immune serum globulin.
Alert: The Centers for Disease Control and Prevention recommends that during a measles outbreak in a health care facility, susceptible personnel exposed to the measles virus (whether or not they received measles vaccine or immune globulin) avoid patient contact for days 5 through 21 after such exposure. If they become ill, they should avoid patient contact for at least 7 days after developing rash.
• Know that if attenuated measles vaccine is administered immediately after exposure to the disease, some protection may be provided. This level of protection is significantly increased if the vaccine is administered even a few days before exposure.

☑ **Patient teaching**
• Warn patient about adverse reactions associated with vaccine.
• Review immunization schedule with patient or parents and stress importance of receiving second injection at appropriate time.
• Stress importance of avoiding pregnancy for 3 months after vaccination. Provide contraception information if necessary.

Reactions may be *common,* uncommon, *life-threatening,* or COMMON AND LIFE-THREATENING.

meningococcal polysaccharide vaccine
Menomune-A/C/Y/W-135

Pregnancy Risk Category: C

HOW SUPPLIED
Injection: 1-dose, 10-dose, and 50-dose vials with vial of diluent

ACTION
Promotes active immunity to meningitis.

Route	Onset	Peak	Duration
SC	Unknown	Unknown	3 yr

INDICATIONS & DOSAGE
Meningococcal meningitis prophylaxis—
Adults and children 2 years and older: 0.5 ml S.C.

ADVERSE REACTIONS
CNS: headache.
Musculoskeletal: muscle cramps.
Skin: *pain, tenderness, erythema, induration* (at injection site).
Other: malaise, chills, fever, *anaphylaxis,* mild lymphadenopathy.

INTERACTIONS
Drug-drug. *Immunosuppressants:* may reduce immune response to vaccine. Monitor closely.

EFFECTS ON DIAGNOSTIC TESTS
None reported.

CONTRAINDICATIONS
Contraindicated during pregnancy and in patients with hypersensitivity to thimerosal or other vaccine components. Defer vaccination in patients with acute illness. Vaccine is not contraindicated in immunocompromised patients.

NURSING CONSIDERATIONS
• Obtain history of allergies and reaction to immunization.
• Keep epinephrine 1:1,000 available to treat anaphylaxis.
• Do not give I.V, I.M., or intradermally.
• Know that vaccine may be given with other immunizations.

• Know that routine vaccination is not recommended. Vaccine should be reserved for individuals at risk such as those who live or are traveling to epidemic or highly endemic areas, household or institutional contacts of meningococcal disease as an adjunct to appropriate antibiotic chemoprophylaxis, medical and laboratory personnel at risk of exposure to meningococcal disease, patients with terminal complement component deficiency, and those with anatomic or functional asplenia.
• Reconstitute only with supplied diluent.
• Be aware that some doctors will revaccinate children if they are at high risk and if they previously received vaccine before 4 years.
• Do not give vaccine within 3 months of receiving a blood or plasma transfusion or human immune serum globulin administration.

☑**Patient teaching**
• Warn patient or parents about adverse reactions associated with vaccine.
• Stress importance of avoiding pregnancy for 3 months after vaccination. Provide contraception information, if necessary.
• Advise correct acetaminophen dose to control fever.

mumps virus vaccine, live
Mumpsvax

Pregnancy Risk Category: C

HOW SUPPLIED
Injection: single-dose vial containing not less than 20,000 $TCID_{50}$ (tissue culture infective doses) of attenuated mumps virus derived from Jeryl Lynn mumps strain (grown in chick embryo culture) per 0.5 ml and vial of diluent; single-dose vial containing not less than 5,000 $TCID_{50}$ (tissue culture infective doses) of the U.S. Reference Mumps Virus in each 0.5 ml†

ACTION
Promotes active immunity to mumps.

Route	Onset	Peak	Duration
SC	Unknown	Unknown	> 15 yr

---

*Liquid contains alcohol.   **May contain tartrazine.   †Canada   ‡Australia   §U.K.   ◇OTC

INDICATIONS & DOSAGE
Immunization—
Adults and children 1 year and older:
0.5 ml (20,000 units) S.C.

Although not recommended in children under 12 months, children vaccinated when under 12 months should be revaccinated.

ADVERSE REACTIONS
CNS: *febrile seizures* (rare).
GI: diarrhea.
Skin: rash, injection-site reaction.
Other: *anaphylaxis, slight fever*, malaise, mild allergic reactions, mild lymphadenopathy.

INTERACTIONS
Drug-drug. *Immune serum globulin, plasma, whole blood:* antibodies in serum may interfere with immune response. Don't use vaccine for at least 3 months after administration of these products.

EFFECTS ON DIAGNOSTIC TESTS
Vaccine may temporarily decrease response to tuberculin skin test. If skin test is necessary, administer it before, at the same time, or 6 weeks after vaccine.

CONTRAINDICATIONS
Contraindicated in immunosuppressed patients; in those with cancer, blood dyscrasia, gamma globulin disorders, fever, untreated active tuberculosis, or anaphylactic or anaphylactoid reactions to neomycin or eggs; in those receiving corticosteroid or radiation therapy; and in pregnant patients.

NURSING CONSIDERATIONS
• Obtain history of allergies, especially anaphylactic reactions to antibiotics, and reaction to immunization. Defer use in patients with acute or febrile illness and for at least 3 months after transfusions or treatment with immune serum globulin.
• Keep epinephrine 1:1,000 available to treat anaphylaxis.
• Use only diluent supplied. Discard 8 hours after reconstituting.
• Do not give I.V.
• Refrigerate and protect from light. Reconstituted solution is clear yellow; do not use if discolored.
• Do not give vaccine less than 1 month before or after immunization with other live virus vaccines; however, trivalent live, oral poliovirus vaccine may be administered simultaneously.
• Administer to asymptomatic HIV-infected children.
• Know that vaccine is not recommended for infants under 12 months because retained maternal mumps antibodies may interfere with immune response.
• Do not use for delayed hypersensitivity (allergy) skin testing. Use mumps skin-test antigen, a killed viral product.

✅ **Patient teaching**
• Warn patient or parents about adverse reactions associated with vaccine.
• Stress importance of avoiding pregnancy for 3 months after vaccination. Provide contraception information if necessary.
• Tell patient to treat fever with antipyretics.

plague vaccine

Pregnancy Risk Category: C

HOW SUPPLIED
Injection: 1.8 to 2.2 billion killed plague bacilli (*Yersinia pestis*)/ml in 20-ml vials

ACTION
Promotes active immunity to plague caused by *Y. pestis*.

Route	Onset	Peak	Duration
IM	Unknown	Unknown	6-12 mo

INDICATIONS & DOSAGE
Primary immunization and booster—
Adults: 1 ml I.M., followed by 0.2 ml in 4 to 12 weeks, then 0.2 ml 5 to 6 months after second dose. Booster is 0.1 to 0.2 ml q 6 months while in plague area. After 3 boosters, use 1- to 2-year booster cycle.
Children: Centers for Disease Control and Prevention does not recommend vaccination because data are insufficient in persons below 18 years.

ADVERSE REACTIONS
CNS: headache.
GI: nausea, vomiting.
Musculoskeletal: arthralgia, myalgia.
Other: malaise, *slight fever, lymphadenopathy,* **anaphylaxis,** leukocytosis, swelling, *induration, erythema at injection site.*

INTERACTIONS
Drug-drug. *Anticoagulants:* increased risk of bleeding. Administer with caution. *Cholera, typhoid vaccine:* increased risk of adverse effects. Don't give at same time.

EFFECTS ON DIAGNOSTIC TESTS
None reported.

CONTRAINDICATIONS
Contraindicated in immunosuppressed or pregnant patients and in those hypersensitive to beef, soy, casein, phenol, sulfite, or formaldehyde. Patients who have had severe local or systemic reactions to plague vaccine should not be revaccinated. Also contraindicated in patients with severe thrombocytopenia or any coagulation disorder that would contraindicate I.M. injections.

NURSING CONSIDERATIONS
• Obtain history of allergies and reaction to immunization. Know that immunization should be deferred in patients with respiratory infection.
• Keep epinephrine 1:1,000 available to treat anaphylaxis.
• Inject into the deltoid area, the preferred site.
• Recommended for all laboratory and field personnel working with *Y. pestis.*

☑ Patient teaching
• Warn patient about adverse reactions associated with vaccine.
• Caution women of childbearing age to notify doctor of suspected pregnancy before administration.
• Tell patient to treat fever with appropriate acetaminophen dose.

---

pneumococcal vaccine, polyvalent
Pneumovax 23, Pnu-Imune 23

Pregnancy Risk Category: C

HOW SUPPLIED
Injection: 25 mcg each of 23 polysaccharide isolates/0.5 ml

ACTION
Promotes active immunity to infections caused by *Streptococcus pneumoniae.*

Route	Onset	Peak	Duration
IM, SC	2-3 wk	Unknown	5 yr

INDICATIONS & DOSAGE
Pneumococcal immunization—
Adults and children 2 years and older: 0.5 ml I.M. or S.C.

ADVERSE REACTIONS
Musculoskeletal: myalgia, arthralgia.
Skin: rash, *soreness at injection site,* severe local reaction associated with revaccination within 3 years.
Other: *anaphylaxis,* slight fever, severe local reaction associated with revaccination within 3 years.

INTERACTIONS
Drug-drug. *Immunosuppressants:* may reduce immune response to vaccine. Monitor closely.

EFFECTS ON DIAGNOSTIC TESTS
None reported.

CONTRAINDICATIONS
Contraindicated in patients with hypersensitivity to drug or its components (phenol) and in those with Hodgkin's disease who have received extensive chemotherapy or nodal irradiation.

NURSING CONSIDERATIONS
• Vaccine is not recommended for children under 2 years.
• Check immunization history to avoid revaccination within 3 years.
• Obtain history of allergies and reaction to immunization. Eggs and egg protein

---

are not used during the manufacture of the vaccine; contains phenol as a preservative.

- Keep epinephrine 1:1,000 available to treat anaphylaxis.
- Inject in deltoid or midlateral thigh. Don't inject I.V or intradermally.
- When splenectomy is being considered, know that vaccine should be given at least 2 weeks before procedure to ensure adequate antibody response. This vaccine may be less effective in splenectomized patients.
- Be aware that this vaccine protects against 23 pneumococcal types, accounting for 90% of pneumococcal disease.
- Know that vaccine may be administered to children 2 years and older to prevent pneumococcal otitis media, although the Centers for Disease Control and Prevention does not recommend otitis media as indicator for this vaccine.
- Vaccine is recommended for all adults over 65 years.
- Be aware that simultaneous administration with influenza virus vaccine is safe and effective.

☑ **Patient teaching**
- Warn patient about adverse reactions associated with vaccine.
- Tell patient to treat fever with mild antipyretics and local site reaction with cold compresses.
- Warn patient with idiopathic thrombocytopenic purpura that there is a possibility of a relapse 2 to 14 days after vaccination.

---

poliovirus vaccine, live, oral, trivalent (TOPV)
Orimune

poliovirus vaccine, inactivated (IPV)
IPOL, Poliovax

Pregnancy Risk Category: C

HOW SUPPLIED
Oral vaccine: mixture of three live viruses (types 1, 2, and 3), grown in monkey kidney tissue culture, in 0.5-ml single-dose Dispettes
Inactivated virus vaccine injection: mixture of three types of poliovirus (types 1, 2, and 3) grown in tissue culture. IPOL uses monkey kidney cultures; Poliovax uses human diploid cell cultures. IPV comes in 0.5-ml prefilled syringes

ACTION
Promotes immunity to poliomyelitis by inducing humoral antibodies and antibodies in the lymphatic tissue.

Route	Onset	Peak	Duration
PO	7-10 days	21 days	Years
SC	Unknown	Unknown	Years

INDICATIONS & DOSAGE
Poliovirus immunization—
Children and nonimmunized adults: 0.5 ml P.O. (TOPV), followed by second dose of 0.5 ml in 6 to 8 weeks. A third 0.5-ml dose is given 6 to 12 months after second dose. A reinforcing dose of 0.5 ml should be given before entry to school.
Infants: 0.5 ml P.O. at 2 months, 4 months, and 18 months.
Poliovirus immunization (IPV) in persons who cannot receive TOPV—
Adults: 0.5 ml S.C., followed by second dose in 4 to 8 weeks. A third dose is given in 6 to 12 months.
Children: 0.5 ml S.C. at 2 months and 4 months. A third dose is given at 15 to 18 months. A reinforcing dose of 0.5 ml S.C. should be given before entry into school.

ADVERSE REACTIONS
GI: decreased appetite.
Skin: erythema, induration, *pain* (at injection site).
Other: *poliomyelitis* (TOPV only), *fever,* sleepiness, crying, hypersensitivity reactions.

INTERACTIONS
Drug-drug. *Immune serum globulin, plasma, whole blood:* antibodies in serum may interfere with immune response. Don't use vaccine within 3 months of transfusion.
Immunosuppressants: may reduce im-

---

mune response to vaccine. Monitor closely.

EFFECTS ON DIAGNOSTIC TESTS
Vaccine may temporarily decrease the response to tuberculin skin test. If skin test is necessary, administer it before, at the same time, or 6 weeks after immunization.

CONTRAINDICATIONS
Oral vaccine is contraindicated in immunosuppressed patients; in those with cancer or immunoglobulin abnormalities; in those receiving radiation, antimetabolite, alkylating agent, or corticosteroid therapy; or in those who have a household contact who fits one of these preceding categories. These patients should receive IPV. Injectable vaccine is contraindicated in patients hypersensitive to neomycin, streptomycin, or polymyxin B.

NURSING CONSIDERATIONS
• Do not use TOPV in siblings of child with known immunodeficiency syndrome; IPV is the preferred form.
• Obtain history of allergies and reaction to immunization.
• Keep TOPV frozen until used. Once thawed, if unopened, may refrigerate up to 30 days; if opened, up to 7 days. Thaw before administration.
• Know that color change of TOPV from pink to yellow has no effect on efficacy of the vaccine. Yellow color is caused by storage at low temperatures.
Alert: Know that parenteral form should be administered to immunodeficient patients or those with altered immune status because they may be at risk for developing the disease if live virus vaccine is administered.
• Have epinephrine 1:1,000 nearby in case of a rapid allergic reaction.
• Oral vaccine should be deferred in patients with vomiting or diarrhea. Both forms of vaccine should be deferred in patients with acute illness.
• Do not administer to neonates under 6 weeks.
• Be aware that the highest risk of poliovirus infection occurs after first dose of oral vaccine.

• Know that adults at high risk for exposure who have completed a primary course may receive another dose.
• Keep in mind that vaccine is not effective in modifying or preventing existing or incubating poliomyelitis.
• Document the manufacturer, lot number, date given, name, address, and title of person administering on permanent patient record or log.

☑ Patient teaching
• Make sure parents know the risks and benefits of this vaccine before it is administered.
• Warn patient or parents about adverse reactions associated with vaccine.

rabies vaccine, adsorbed

Pregnancy Risk Category: C

HOW SUPPLIED
Injection: single dose 1-ml vial

ACTION
Promotes active immunity to rabies.

Route	Onset	Peak	Duration
IM	Unknown	2 wk after 3 doses	Unknown

INDICATIONS & DOSAGE
Preexposure prophylaxis rabies immunization for persons in high-risk groups—
Adults and children: 1 ml I.M. at 0, 7, and 21 or 28 days for total of three injections. Patients at increased risk for rabies should be checked q 6 months and given a booster vaccination, 1 ml I.M, p.r.n., to maintain adequate serum titer (approximately q 2 to 5 years based on antibody titers).
Postexposure rabies prophylaxis—
Adults and children not previously vaccinated against rabies: 20 IU/kg doses of human rabies immune globulin (HRIG) I.M. and five 1-ml injections of rabies vaccine adsorbed I.M. given on days 0, 3, 7, 14, and 28.
Adults and children previously vaccinated against rabies: two 1-ml injections

of rabies vaccine adsorbed I.M. given on days 0 and 3. HRIG should not be given.

ADVERSE REACTIONS
CNS: *headache, dizziness.*
GI: *abdominal pain, nausea.*
Musculoskeletal: *myalgia,* aching of injected muscle.
Skin: *transient pain, erythema, swelling or itching at injection site;* mild inflammatory reaction at injection site.
Other: *slight fever, fatigue,* reaction resembling serum sickness, ***anaphylaxis.***

INTERACTIONS
Drug-drug. *Antimalarial drugs, corticosteroids, immunosuppressants:* decreased response to rabies vaccine. Avoid concomitant use.

EFFECTS ON DIAGNOSTIC TESTS
None reported.

CONTRAINDICATIONS
Contraindicated in patients who have experienced life-threatening allergic reactions to previous injections of vaccine or to components of vaccine, including thimerosal.

NURSING CONSIDERATIONS
• Use with caution in patients with history of non-life-threatening allergic reactions to previous injections of vaccine, in patients with hypersensitivity to monkey-derived proteins, and in children.
• Keep epinephrine 1:1,000 available to treat an anaphylactoid reaction.
• Administer as an I.M. injection into the deltoid region in adults and older children. For younger children, the midanterolateral aspect of the thigh also is acceptable. Know that vaccine is not for use by the intradermal route. Take care not to inject vaccine near a peripheral nerve or into adipose or subcutaneous tissue.
• Know that vaccine is normally a light pink color because of presence of phenol red in the suspension.
Alert: If patient experiences serious adverse reaction to vaccine, report reaction promptly to manufacturer: Michigan Department of Public Health, 517-335-8050

during working hours or 517-335-9030 at other times.
• Don't confuse vaccine with rabies immune globulin. Both drugs may be given in some situations.

☑ **Patient teaching**
• Inform patient about adverse reactions associated with vaccine and importance of alerting doctor so serious adverse reaction can be reported.
• Caution patient not to perform hazardous activities if dizziness occurs.
• Advise proper antipyretic dose for fever.
• Teach proper wound care and signs or symptoms of infection.

rabies vaccine, human diploid cell (HDCV)
Imovax Rabies, Imovax Rabies I.D.

Pregnancy Risk Category: C

HOW SUPPLIED
Intradermal injection: 0.25 IU rabies antigen/dose
I.M. injection: 2.5 IU of rabies antigen/ml, in single-dose vial with diluent

ACTION
Promotes active immunity to rabies.

Route	Onset	Peak	Duration
IM, intra-dermal	1 wk	1-2 mo	> 2 yr

INDICATIONS & DOSAGE
Postexposure antirabies immunization—
Adults and children: five 1-ml doses of HDCV I.M. (for example, in the deltoid region). First dose given as soon as possible after exposure; an additional dose given on each of days 3, 7, 14, and 28 after first dose. If no antibody response after this primary series occurs, a booster dose is recommended.
Preexposure prophylaxis immunization for persons in high-risk groups—
Adults and children: three 1-ml injections administered I.M. First dose given on day 0 (the first day of therapy), second

dose on day 7, and third dose on either day 21 or 28. Alternatively, 0.1 ml intradermally on same dosage schedule.

ADVERSE REACTIONS
CNS: *headache,* dizziness.
GI: *nausea,* abdominal pain, diarrhea.
Musculoskeletal: muscle aches.
Skin: *pain, erythema, swelling, itching* (at injection site).
Other: *fever,* **anaphylaxis,** *serum sickness, fatigue.*

INTERACTIONS
Drug-drug. *Antimalarial drugs, corticosteroids, immunosuppressants:* decreased response to rabies vaccine. Avoid concomitant use.

EFFECTS ON DIAGNOSTIC TESTS
None reported.

CONTRAINDICATIONS
No contraindications reported for persons after exposure. An acute febrile illness contraindicates use of vaccine for persons previously exposed.

NURSING CONSIDERATIONS
• Use cautiously in patients with history of hypersensitivity.
• Keep epinephrine 1:1,000 available to treat anaphylaxis.
• Use vaccine immediately after reconstitution.
Alert: Do not use intradermal route for postexposure rabies vaccination.
• Know that the alternative regimen of 0.1-ml doses is only for preexposure prophylaxis. For postexposure prophylaxis, only use the 1-ml doses.
• Don't confuse vaccine with rabies immune globulin. Both drugs may be given in some situations.
• Be prepared to stop corticosteroid therapy during immunizing period unless therapy is essential for the treatment of other conditions.
• Keep in mind that some patients who receive booster doses experience serum sickness–like hypersensitivity reactions. These reactions usually respond to antihistamines.
• All serious reactions should be reported

to the State Department of Health or the Division of Viral Disease, CDC, (404) 329-3095 (working hours) or (404) 329-8888 at other times.

✅ **Patient teaching**
• Inform patient about adverse reactions associated with vaccine. Tell patient to report persistent or severe reactions to doctor.
• Stress importance of receiving booster, if appropriate for patient.
• Tell patient to treat mild reaction with anti-inflammatory or antipyretic agent at appropriate doses.

▼ *NEW DRUG*

rotavirus vaccine, live, oral, tetravalent
RotaShield

Pregnancy Risk Category: C

HOW SUPPLIED
Oral vaccine: single-dose lyophilized live oral tetravalent rotavirus vaccine containing 4×10^5 PFU total virus which must be diluted with 2.5 ml of provided diluent.

ACTION
Exact mechanism unknown. The live, oral, tetravalent rotavirus vaccine contains 4 live viruses: rhesus rotavirus serotype 3 and three rhesus-human reassortant viruses serotypes 1, 2, and 4. Vaccine induces development of IgG and IgA antibodies against the serotypes it contains.

Route	Onset	Peak	Duration
PO	Unknown	Unknown	1 season (Nov-May) or possibly 2 seasons

INDICATIONS & DOSAGE
Prevention of gastroenteritis caused by the rotavirus serotypes contained in the vaccine—
Infants less than 6 months of age born at least 37 weeks' gestation: 2.5 ml P.O. at 2, 4 and 6 months of age. Alternatively, first dose may be administered as early as

6 weeks of age, with subsequent doses at least 3 weeks apart.

ADVERSE REACTIONS
CNS: *irritability*.
EENT: otitis media, conjunctivitis, pharyngitis, rhinitis.
GI: *decreased appetite,* dyspepsia, gastroenteritis, loose stools.
Respiratory: bronchitis, bronchiolitis, increased cough, pneumonia, asthma.
Skin: rash, eczema.
Other: *fever*, infection, flu syndrome, *decreased activity*.

INTERACTIONS
None reported.

EFFECTS ON DIAGNOSTIC TESTS
Stools excreted during week after vaccination may test positive for rotavirus due to presence of vaccine virus.

CONTRAINDICATIONS
Contraindicated in patients with hypersensitivity to vaccine's components, such as aminoglycoside antibiotics, monosodium glutamate, or amphotericin B. Also contraindicated in immunocompromised persons including those with HIV, combined immunodeficiency hypogammaglobulinemia, agammaglobulinemia, thymic abnormalities, malignancy, leukemia, lymphoma, or other advanced debilitating diseases; immunosuppressed patients; or those with altered immune status such as those who are being treated with systemic corticosteroids, alkylating drugs, antimetabolites, radiation, or other immunosuppressive therapies. Do not give vaccine to children with ongoing diarrhea or vomiting or a moderate to severe febrile illness. Vaccine is not indicated for adults.

NURSING CONSIDERATIONS
• Use with caution in patients with latex allergy. The packaging contains natural rubber.
• Ask parent or guardian about infant's current health and immune status before administration of vaccine. Because of increased incidence of fever, initiation of

vaccine after age 6 months is not currently recommended.
Alert: Vaccine should never be administered parenterally. It is intended for P.O. use only.
• Vaccine may be given with standard childhood vaccines including OPV, HIB, and whole-cell DTP.
• Repeat dosing is not indicated if infant regurgitates vaccine.
• Store lyophilized vaccine and diluent at room temperature below 77° F (25° C). Use only provided diluent for reconstitution. Once reconstituted, solution may appear yellow-orange to purple in color and may contain a fine precipitate. Ideally, vaccine should be administered immediately after reconstitution. However, can delay vaccine administration for up to 1 hour at room temperature (73° to 81° F [23° to 27° C]) or up to 4 hours if refrigerated (36° to 46° F [2° to 8° C]). Discard reconstituted vaccine if it has not been used within these times. Do not freeze.
• Be aware that children receiving vaccine may transmit virus to nonimmunized persons. Avoid contact of vaccinated individuals with immunocompromised persons at high risk for up to 4 weeks. If this is not possible, benefits to recipient should be weighed against possible risk to immunocompromised person.
• Be aware that some clinicians suggest that patients receiving corticosteroids may be safely vaccinated under certain circumstances (such as short-term therapy, alternate-day therapy, or low doses).
• Report suspected adverse events via the Adverse Event Reporting System (VAERS) at 1-800-822-7967.

✅ Patient teaching
• Explain to parent or guardian the importance of completing the immunization series.
• Advise parent or guardian of proper hand-washing technique at time of diaper changes.
• Inform parent or guardian there are no restrictions on infant's consumption of food or liquid, including breast milk, either before or after vaccination.
• Instruct parent or guardian that vaccinated children should not come in contact

with immunocompromised persons for up to 4 weeks.
• Tell parent or guardian to notify doctor if serious adverse reactions occur.

---

rubella and mumps virus vaccine, live
Biavax II

Pregnancy Risk Category: C

HOW SUPPLIED
Injection: single-dose vial containing not less than 1,000 TCID$_{50}$ (tissue culture infective doses) of the Wistar RA 27/3 rubella virus (propagated in human diploid cell culture) and not less than 20,000 TCID$_{50}$ of the Jeryl Lynn mumps strain (grown in chick embryo cell culture)

ACTION
Promotes immunity to rubella and mumps by inducing antibody production.

Route	Onset	Peak	Duration
SC	Unknown	Unknown	10.5 yr

INDICATIONS & DOSAGE
Rubella and mumps immunization—
Adults and children 1 year and older: 0.5 ml S.C.

ADVERSE REACTIONS
GI: diarrhea.
Musculoskeletal: *arthritis, arthralgia.*
Skin: rash, pain, erythema, induration (at injection site).
Other: polyneuritis, thrombocytopenic purpura, urticaria, fever, *anaphylaxis,* lymphadenopathy.

INTERACTIONS
Drug-drug. *Immune serum globulin, plasma, whole blood:* antibodies in serum may interfere with immune response. Don't give vaccine for at least 3 months after use of these products.
Immunosuppressants: may reduce immune response to vaccine. Monitor closely.

EFFECTS ON DIAGNOSTIC TESTS
Vaccine may temporarily decrease response to tuberculin skin test. If skin test is necessary, administer it before, at the same time, or 6 weeks after immunization.

CONTRAINDICATIONS
Contraindicated in pregnant or immunosuppressed patients; in those with cancer, blood dyscrasia, gamma globulin disorders, fever, or active untreated tuberculosis; history of anaphylaxis or anaphylactoid reactions to neomycin or eggs; and in those receiving corticosteroid (except those receiving corticosteroids as replacement therapy) or radiation therapy.

NURSING CONSIDERATIONS
• Obtain history of allergies, especially anaphylactic reaction to antibiotics, and reaction to immunization.
• Keep epinephrine 1:1,000 available to treat anaphylaxis.
• Know that in patients with acute illness and after administration of immune serum globulin, blood, or plasma, vaccination should be deferred.
• Use only diluent supplied. Discard 8 hours after reconstituting.
• Inject into outer upper arm. Don't inject I.V.
• Allow an interval of at least 3 weeks between BCG and rubella vaccines.
• Document drug manufacturer, lot number, date, name, address, and title of person administering dose on permanent record or log.
• Patients born before 1956 are believed to have naturally acquired immunity.

☑ **Patient teaching**
• Inform patient about adverse reactions associated with vaccine.
• Stress importance of avoiding pregnancy for 3 months after vaccination. Provide contraception information if necessary.
• Inform female patients over 12 years of risk of self-limited arthralgia or arthritis occurring 2 to 4 weeks postvaccination.

---

rubella virus vaccine, live attenuated (RA 27/3)
Meruvax II

Pregnancy Risk Category: C

HOW SUPPLIED
Injection: single-dose vial containing not less than 1,000 TCID$_{50}$ (tissue culture infective doses) of the Wistar RA 27/3 strain of rubella virus (propagated in human diploid cell culture)

ACTION
Promotes immunity to rubella by inducing production of antibodies.

Route	Onset	Peak	Duration
SC	2-6 wk	Unknown	> 10 yr

INDICATIONS & DOSAGE
Rubella immunization—
Adults and children 1 year and older: 0.5 ml (1,000 units) S.C.

ADVERSE REACTIONS
CNS: headache.
EENT: sore throat.
Musculoskeletal: arthralgia, arthritis.
Skin: rash, pain, erythema, induration (at injection site).
Other: polyneuritis, thrombocytopenic purpura, urticaria, malaise, fever, *anaphylaxis,* lymphadenopathy.

INTERACTIONS
Drug-drug. *Immune serum globulin, plasma, whole blood:* antibodies in serum may interfere with immune response. Don't use vaccine for at least 3 months after use of these products.
Immunosuppressants: may reduce immune response to vaccine. Monitor closely.

EFFECTS ON DIAGNOSTIC TESTS
Vaccine may temporarily decrease response to tuberculin skin test. If skin test is necessary, administer it before, at the same time, or 6 weeks after immunization.

CONTRAINDICATIONS
Contraindicated in pregnant or immuno-suppressed patients; in those with cancer, blood dyscrasia, gamma globulin disorders, fever, or active untreated tuberculosis; in those with history of hypersensitivity to neomycin; in patients receiving corticosteroids (except those receiving corticosteroids as replacement therapy), and in patients receiving radiation therapy.

NURSING CONSIDERATIONS
• Obtain history of allergies and reaction to immunization.
• Keep epinephrine 1:1,000 available to treat anaphylaxis.
• Immunization should be deferred in patients with acute illness and after administration of human immune serum globulin, blood, or plasma.
• Use only diluent supplied. Discard 8 hours after reconstituting. Protect from light.
• Inject into outer upper arm. Don't inject I.V.
• Document drug manufacturer, lot number, date, name, address, and title of person administering on patient permanent record or permanent log.
• Allow at least 3 weeks between BCG and rubella vaccines.

☑ Patient teaching
• Inform patient about adverse reactions associated with vaccine.
• Stress importance of avoiding pregnancy for 3 months after vaccination. Provide contraception information, if necessary.
• Tell patient to use correct dose of antipyretic medication for treating fever.

tetanus toxoid, adsorbed
tetanus toxoid, fluid

Pregnancy Risk Category: C

HOW SUPPLIED
tetanus toxoid, adsorbed
Injection: 5 to 10 Lf (limit flocculation) units of inactivated tetanus/0.5-ml dose, in 0.5-ml syringes and 5-ml vials
tetanus toxoid, fluid
Injection: 4 to 5 Lf units of inactivated tetanus/0.5-ml dose, in 0.5-ml syringes and 7.5-ml vials

ACTION
Promotes immunity to tetanus by inducing antitoxin production.

Route	Onset	Peak	Duration
IM, SC	2 doses	Unknown	> 10 yr

INDICATIONS & DOSAGE
Primary immunization—
Adults and children 6 years and over:
0.5 ml (adsorbed) I.M. 4 to 8 weeks apart for two doses; then third dose is given 6 to 12 months after second. Alternatively, 0.5 ml (fluid) I.M. or S.C. 4 to 8 weeks apart for three doses; then fourth dose of 0.5 ml 6 to 12 months after third dose.
Children 6 weeks to 6 years: 0.5 ml (adsorbed) I.M. at ages 2, 4, and 6 months. A fourth dose is given at 15 to 18 months. A fifth dose is given at 4 to 6 years, just before entry into school, if indicated.
Booster doses—
Adults: 0.5 ml I.M. at 10-year intervals.

ADVERSE REACTIONS
CNS: headache, *seizures.*
CV: tachycardia, hypotension.
Musculoskeletal: aches, pains.
Skin: erythema, induration, nodule (at injection site), urticaria, pruritus.
Other: slight fever, chills, malaise, flushing, encephalopathy, *anaphylaxis.*

INTERACTIONS
Drug-drug. *Chloramphenicol:* may interfere with response to tetanus toxoid. Monitor for effect.
Immunosuppressants: may reduce immune response to vaccine. Monitor closely.

EFFECTS ON DIAGNOSTIC TESTS
None reported.

CONTRAINDICATIONS
Contraindicated in immunosuppressed patients and in those with immunoglobulin abnormalities or severe hypersensitivity or neurologic reactions to the toxoid or any ingredient in it, such as thimerosal. Also contraindicated in patients with thrombocytopenia or other coagulation disorders that would contraindicate I.M. injection unless the potential benefits outweigh the risks. Vaccination should be deferred in patients with acute illness and during polio outbreaks, except in emergencies.

NURSING CONSIDERATIONS
• Use cautiously (adsorbed form) in infants or children with cerebral damage, neurologic disorders, or history of febrile seizures.
• Obtain history of allergies and reaction to immunization.
• Determine date of last tetanus immunization.
• Keep epinephrine 1:1,000 available to treat anaphylaxis.
• Do not confuse drug with tetanus immune globulin, human. Both drugs may be given in some situations.
• Be aware that adsorbed form produces longer duration of immunity. Fluid form provides quicker booster effect in patients actively immunized previously.
• Document manufacturer, lot number, date, name, address, and title of person administering on permanent record or log.

☑ Patient teaching
• Advise patient to avoid use of hot or cold compresses at injection site; this may increase severity of local reaction.
• Instruct patient to report persistent or severe adverse reactions.
• Advise patient of proper antipyretic dosing for fever reaction.
• Advise patient that a nodule may be present at the injection site for a few weeks.

typhoid vaccine, parenteral

typhoid vaccine, oral
Vivotif Berna Vaccine

Pregnancy Risk Category: C

HOW SUPPLIED
Injection: suspension of killed Ty-2 strain of *Salmonella typhi;* 8 units/ml in 5-ml and 10-ml vials
Capsules (enteric-coated): 2 to 6 x 10^9 colony-forming units of viable *S. typhi* Ty^{21}a and 5 to 50 x 10^9 bacterial cells of nonviable Ty^{21}a2 (four doses of vaccine in a single package)

---

*Liquid contains alcohol.   **May contain tartrazine.   †Canada   ‡Australia   §U.K.   ◊OTC

ACTION
Provides active immunity to typhoid fever.

Route	Onset	Peak	Duration
PO, SC, intradermal	After last dose	Unknown	3-5 yr

INDICATIONS & DOSAGE
Primary immunization—
Adults: one capsule (oral vaccine) on alternate days taken 1 hour before meals for four doses. Protocol repeated as booster q 5 years.
Adults and children over 10 years: 0.5 ml S.C. (injection); repeated in 4 weeks. Protocol repeated as booster q 3 years with either 0.5 ml S.C. or 0.1 ml intradermally.
Children 6 months to 10 years: 0.25 ml S.C. (injection); repeated in 4 weeks. Protocol repeated as booster q 3 years with either 0.25 ml S.C. or 0.1 ml intradermally.

ADVERSE REACTIONS
CNS: headache.
GI: nausea, abdominal cramps, vomiting.
Skin: rash; urticaria; swelling, pain, inflammation (at injection site); induration.
Other: *fever,* malaise, ***anaphylaxis,*** myalgia.

INTERACTIONS
Drug-drug. *Immunosuppressants, phenytoin, sulfonamides:* may impair antibody response. Don't use together. Use with other vaccines could increase adverse effects.

EFFECTS ON DIAGNOSTIC TESTS
None reported.

CONTRAINDICATIONS
Contraindicated in immunosuppressed patients and in those with hypersensitivity to the vaccine or its components. Defer vaccination in patients with acute illness. Use parenteral, inactivated vaccine in HIV-positive patients.

NURSING CONSIDERATIONS
• Obtain history of allergies and reaction to immunization. Keep epinephrine 1:1,000 available to treat anaphylaxis.

• Treat fever with antipyretics.
• Shake thoroughly before withdrawing from vial.
• Refrigerate vaccine at 35.5° to 46.4° F (2° to 8° C).

☑ Patient teaching
• When administering oral vaccine, ensure that patient understands importance of taking all four doses and following the alternate-day regimen.
• Tell patient to take oral vaccine with cold or lukewarm water and not to chew or crush enteric-coated capsules. Capsules should be swallowed immediately.
• Tell patient to take oral vaccine 1 hour before meals.
• Inform patient about adverse reactions associated with vaccine; usually begins within 24 hours and lasts 1 to 2 days.

---

typhoid Vi polysaccharide vaccine
Typhim Vi

Pregnancy Risk Category: C

HOW SUPPLIED
Injection: 0.5-ml syringe, 20-dose vial, 50-dose vial

ACTION
Promotes active immunity to typhoid fever.

Route	Onset	Peak	Duration
IM	2 wk	Unknown	2 yr

INDICATIONS & DOSAGE
Active immunization against typhoid fever—
Adults and children 2 years and older: 0.5 ml I.M. as single dose. Reimmunization q 2 years with 0.5 ml I.M. as single dose, if needed.

ADVERSE REACTIONS
CNS: *headache.*
GI: nausea, vomiting, abdominal cramps.
Skin: *pain, tenderness, induration, erythema* (at injection site); rash, urticaria.
Other: ***anaphylaxis,*** malaise, myalgia, fever.

INTERACTIONS
None significant.

EFFECTS ON DIAGNOSTIC TESTS
None reported.

CONTRAINDICATIONS
Contraindicated in patients with hypersensitivity to vaccine's components. Do not use vaccine to treat patients with typhoid fever or administer to those who are chronic typhoid carriers.

NURSING CONSIDERATIONS
• Use with caution in patients with thrombocytopenia or a bleeding disorder and in those taking an anticoagulant; bleeding may occur following an I.M. injection in these patients.
• As with other vaccines, administration should be delayed, if possible, in patients with febrile illness.
• Although anaphylaxis is rare, keep epinephrine available to treat an anaphylactoid reaction.
• Administer as an I.M. injection into the deltoid region in adults and into the deltoid or vastus lateralis in children. It should not be administered in the gluteal region or areas where there may be a nerve trunk. Never inject I.V.
• Record drug manufacturer, lot number, date, name, address, and title of person administering on patient record or log sheet.

☑ Patient teaching
• Advise patient to take all precautions necessary to avoid contact with or ingestion of contaminated food and water.
• Inform patient that immunization should be given at least 2 weeks prior to expected exposure. Although an optimal reimmunization schedule has not been established, recommended reimmunization consists of a single dose for U.S. travelers every 2 years if exposure to typhoid fever is possible.
• Inform patient about adverse reactions associated with vaccine.

varicella virus vaccine
Varivax

Pregnancy Risk Category: C

HOW SUPPLIED
Injection: single-dose vial containing 1350 plague-forming units (PFU) of Oka/Merck varicella virus (live)

ACTION
Prevents chickenpox by inducing the production of antibodies to varicella-zoster virus.

Route	Onset	Peak	Duration
SC	4-6 wk	Unknown	> 2 yr

INDICATIONS & DOSAGE
Prevention of varicella-zoster (chickenpox) infections—
Adults and children 13 years and over: 0.5-ml S.C. followed by second 0.5-ml dose 4 to 8 weeks later.
Children 1 to 12 years: 0.5 ml S.C.

ADVERSE REACTIONS
Skin: *injection site reactions* (swelling, redness, pain, rash), varicella-like rash.
Other: *anaphylaxis, fever,* herpes zoster.

INTERACTIONS
Drug-drug. *Blood products, immune globulin:* may inactivate vaccine. Defer vaccination for at least 5 months following blood or plasma transfusions or administration of immune globulin or varicella-zoster immune globulin.
Immunosuppressants: risk of severe reactions to live-virus vaccines. Postpone routine vaccination.
Salicylates: Reye's syndrome has been reported after natural varicella infection. Avoid use of salicylates for 6 weeks after varicella immunization.

EFFECTS ON DIAGNOSTIC TESTS
None reported.

CONTRAINDICATIONS
Contraindicated in patients hypersensitive to drug; in those with history of anaphylactoid reaction to neomycin, blood

dyscrasia, leukemia, lymphomas, neoplasms affecting bone marrow or lymphatic system, primary and acquired immunosuppressive states, active untreated tuberculosis, or any febrile respiratory illness or other active febrile infection; and in pregnant patients.

NURSING CONSIDERATIONS
• Vaccine must be stored frozen. Diluent should be stored separately at room temperature or refrigerated.
• To reconstitute vaccine, first withdraw 0.7 ml of diluent into syringe to be used for reconstitution. Inject all diluent in syringe into vial of lyophilized vaccine, and gently agitate to mix thoroughly. Administer immediately after reconstitution. Discard if not used within 30 minutes.
• Have epinephrine available for potential anaphylaxis reaction.
• Vaccine has been safely and effectively used in combination with measles, mumps, and rubella vaccine.
• Document manufacturer, lot number, date, name, address, and title of person administering on patient record or log.
Alert: Know that vaccine contains live, attenuated virus. Vaccinated individuals who develop rash may be able to transmit the virus.

☑ **Patient teaching**
• Inform patient or parents of adverse reactions associated with vaccine.
• Caution female patients of childbearing age to notify doctor of suspected pregnancy before administration.
• Instruct patient to avoid salicylate use 6 weeks after vaccination to prevent Reye's syndrome.
• Tell patient to avoid pregnancy for 3 months after vaccination.
• Inform patient to avoid close contact postinjection with susceptible high-risk individuals (such as pregnant women, immunocompromised persons).

---

yellow fever vaccine
YF-Vax

Pregnancy Risk Category: C

HOW SUPPLIED
Injection: live, attenuated 17D yellow fever virus in 1-, 5-, and 20-dose vials, with diluent; supplied only to centers authorized to issue yellow fever vaccination certificates

ACTION
Provides active immunity to yellow fever.

Route	Onset	Peak	Duration
SC	7-10 days	28 days	> 10 yr

INDICATIONS & DOSAGE
Primary vaccination—
Adults and children 9 months and over: 0.5 ml deep S.C.; booster is 0.5 ml S.C. q 10 years.
Children 6 to 9 months: same dose as above if they are to be exposed to mosquito bites.

ADVERSE REACTIONS
CNS: headache.
Musculoskeletal: myalgia.
Skin: mild swelling, pain at injection site.
Other: *anaphylaxis, fever, malaise.*

INTERACTIONS
Drug-drug. *Cholera vaccine:* concurrent administration may interfere with immune response to both yellow fever and cholera vaccines. Administer 3 weeks apart.
Immunosuppressants: may increase viral replication and the development of infection with yellow fever virus. Defer immunization until immunosuppressant is stopped.

EFFECTS ON DIAGNOSTIC TESTS
None reported.

CONTRAINDICATIONS
Contraindicated in immunosuppressed patients; in those with cancer, gamma globulin deficiency, or hypersensitivity to eggs; or in those receiving corticosteroid or radiation therapy. Also contraindicated during pregnancy and in infants under 6 months, except in high-risk areas.

NURSING CONSIDERATIONS
• Obtain history of allergies, especially to eggs, and reaction to immunization.

• Keep epinephrine 1:1,000 available to treat anaphylaxis.

• Be aware that 8 weeks should pass before administering vaccine in patients who have received blood or plasma transfusions.

• Reconstitute with NaCl injection that contains no preservatives (they inactivate the yellow fever viruses).

• Keep frozen. Don't use unless shipping case contains some dry ice on arrival. Avoid vigorous shaking; carefully swirl mixture until suspension is uniform. Use within 1 hour after reconstituting. Discard remainder.

• Yellow fever vaccine should not be given within 1 month of other live virus vaccines; may be given concurrently with hepatitis B vaccine.

✓ **Patient teaching**

• Inform patient about adverse reactions associated with vaccine.

• Caution female patient of childbearing age to notify doctor of suspected pregnancy before administration.

• Advise patient to avoid being bitten by using sprays, repellents, protective clothing, and screens.

76

Antitoxins and antivenins

black widow spider antivenin
Crotalidae antivenom, polyvalent
diphtheria antitoxin, equine
***Micrurus fulvius* antivenin**

COMBINATION PRODUCTS
None.

---

black widow spider antivenin
Antivenin *(Latrodectus mactans)*

Pregnancy Risk Category: C

HOW SUPPLIED
Injection: combination package—one vial of antivenin (6,000-unit vial), one 2.5-ml vial of diluent (sterile water for injection), and one 1-ml vial of normal equine (horse) serum (1:10 dilution) for sensitivity testing

ACTION
Unknown.

Route	Onset	Peak	Duration
IV	Immediate	Unknown	Unknown
IM	Unknown	2-3 days	Unknown

INDICATIONS & DOSAGE
Black widow spider bite—
Adults and children: 2.5 ml I.M. in anterolateral thigh. Second dose may be needed. In severe cases, antivenin may be given I.V.

Test for sensitivity before giving drug, as ordered; use 0.02 ml of 1:10 antivenin in 0.9% NaCl. Evaluate result in 10 minutes.

For desensitization, use 1:10 and 1:100 dilutions of antivenin in 0.9% NaCl for injection and administer as ordered.

ADVERSE REACTIONS
CNS: *neurotoxicity.*
Other: *hypersensitivity reactions, anaphylaxis,* serum sickness.

INTERACTIONS
Drug-drug. *Antihistamines:* may interfere with sensitivity tests. Avoid concomitant use.

EFFECTS ON DIAGNOSTIC TESTS
None reported.

CONTRAINDICATIONS
Contraindicated in patients hypersensitive to drug or its components (horse serum) when desensitization is not feasible.

NURSING CONSIDERATIONS
• Immobilize patient; splint the bitten limb to prevent spread of venom.
• Obtain history of allergies, especially to horses, and reaction to immunization. Have epinephrine 1:1,000 available in case of anaphylaxis.
• For best results, know that antivenin should be given as soon as possible.
• A skin or conjunctival test should be performed prior to administration.
Alert: Give I.M. dosage in anterolateral thigh so that a tourniquet may be applied if a systemic reaction occurs.
• Watch patient for 2 to 3 days. Venom is neurotoxic and may cause respiratory paralysis and seizures.
• Symptoms usually will subside in 1 to 3 hours.

I.V. administration
• Reconstitute vial of antivenom with 2.5 ml of diluent. Further dilute reconstituted solution in 10 to 50 ml 0.9% NaCl injection and infuse over 15 minutes.
• I.V. administration is the preferred route in severe cases or when patient is in shock or under 12 years old.

Patient teaching
• Explain to patient and family how drug will be administered.
• Instruct patient to report adverse reactions promptly.
• Tell patient that serum sickness can occur 8 to 12 days after administration.

Reactions may be *common*, uncommon, *life-threatening*, or COMMON AND LIFE-THREATENING.

Crotalidae antivenom, polyvalent

Pregnancy Risk Category: C

HOW SUPPLIED
Injection: combination package—one vial of lyophilized serum, one vial of diluent (10 ml of bacteriostatic water for injection), and one 1-ml vial of normal horse serum (diluted 1:10) for sensitivity testing

ACTION
Neutralizes and binds venom of snakes of the species crotalids (pit vipers), including rattlesnakes, water moccasins, and copperheads.

Route	Onset	Peak	Duration
IV	Immediate	Unknown	Unknown

INDICATIONS & DOSAGE
Crotalid (rattlesnake) bites—
Adults and children: initially, 20 to 150 ml I.V., depending on severity of bite and patient response; minimal envenomation: 20 to 40 ml I.V.; moderate envenomation: 50 to 90 ml I.V.; and severe envenomation: 100 to 150 ml I.V. If large amount of venom, more than 150 ml may be given I.V. directly into superficial vein. Subsequent doses based on patient's response; may need another 10 to 50 ml if swelling progresses, if systemic symptoms increase, or if new manifestations appear.

Test for sensitivity before giving drug. Give 0.02 to 0.03 ml of a 1:10 dilution in 0.9% NaCl solution intradermally. Read results after 5 to 10 minutes. Watch carefully for delayed allergic reaction or relapse.

If positive sensitivity test, desensitize as ordered; prepare 1:10 and 1:100 dilutions of antivenom in 0.9% NaCl for injection.

Be aware that children, who have less resistance and less body fluid to dilute venom, may need twice adult dose.

ADVERSE REACTIONS
Musculoskeletal: arthralgia.
Skin: erythema, urticaria.

Other: pain, *hypersensitivity reactions, anaphylaxis, serum sickness,* lymphadenopathy, fever.

INTERACTIONS
Drug-drug. *Antihistamines:* enhanced toxicity of crotaline venoms. Don't use together.

EFFECTS ON DIAGNOSTIC TESTS
None reported.

CONTRAINDICATIONS
Contraindicated in patients hypersensitive to drug or its components.

NURSING CONSIDERATIONS
● Use drug cautiously. Studies indicate that 60% of patients treated with antivenom develop hypersensitivity.
● Immobilize patient immediately. Splint the bitten extremity.
● Obtain history of allergies, especially to horses, and reaction to immunization. Have epinephrine 1:1,000 ready in case of hypersensitivity reaction.
Alert: Type and crossmatch blood as soon as possible; hemolysis from venom prevents accurate crossmatching.
● For best results, administer antivenom as soon as possible.
● Give corticosteroids as prescribed. If a large number of vials are administered, serum sickness may result 5 to 24 days postinfusion.
● Antivenom may be stored without refrigeration for 60 days, but it should not be exposed to temperatures over 98.6° F (over 37° C).

🝊 I.V. administration
● Reconstitute drug by adding 10 ml of supplied diluent. Further dilute to make a 1:1 to 1:10 solution using 0.9% NaCl or 5% dextrose injection. To avoid foaming, do not shake while mixing. Infuse an initial 5 to 10 ml of diluted antivenin over 3 to 5 minutes and observe patient carefully. If no symptoms of immediate systemic reaction occur, infusion may be continued.

☑ Patient teaching
● Explain to patient and family that a test

dose will be given first to check for sensitivity to drug.
• Instruct patient to report adverse reactions promptly.

---

diphtheria antitoxin, equine

Pregnancy Risk Category: C

HOW SUPPLIED
Injection: not less than 500 units/ml in 10,000-unit and 20,000-unit vials

ACTION
Binds with circulating toxin and prevents disease progression.

Route	Onset	Peak	Duration
IV	Immediate	Unknown	Unknown
IM	Unknown	2 days	Unknown

INDICATIONS & DOSAGE
Diphtheria prevention—
Adults and children: 5,000 to 10,000 units I.M.
Diphtheria treatment—
Adults and children: 20,000 to 120,000 units I.M. or slow I.V. Additional doses may be given in 24 hours. I.M. route may be used in mild cases.

ADVERSE REACTIONS
Skin: erythema, urticaria.
Other: pain, *hypersensitivity reactions, anaphylaxis,* serum sickness (urticaria, pruritus, fever, malaise, arthralgia) may occur in 7 to 12 days.

INTERACTIONS
None significant.

EFFECTS ON DIAGNOSTIC TESTS
None reported.

CONTRAINDICATIONS
Contraindicated in patients hypersensitive to drug or its components.

NURSING CONSIDERATIONS
• Obtain history of allergies, especially to horses, and reaction to immunization. Have epinephrine 1:1,000 ready in case of hypersensitivity reaction. Antitoxin

should be used with extreme caution in patients with history of allergic disorders.
• Test for sensitivity before giving drug, as ordered.
Alert: If patient has symptoms of diphtheria (sore throat, fever, tonsillar membrane), therapy should be started immediately, without waiting for culture reports.
• For storage, refrigerate antitoxin at 35.6° to 50° F (2° to 10° C). Before administering, warm to 90° to 95° F (32° to 35° C), never higher.
• Begin appropriate antimicrobial therapy.

I.V. administration
• Dilute appropriate dose in D_5W or 0.9% NaCl solution to achieve a 1:20 dilution.
• Administer the solution by direct infusion at no more than 1 ml/minute.

✔ Patient teaching
• Explain to patient and family that a test dose will be given first to check for sensitivity to drug.
• Tell patient to report adverse reactions promptly.

Micrurus fulvius antivenin

Pregnancy Risk Category: C

HOW SUPPLIED
Injection: combination package with 10 ml of diluent

ACTION
Neutralizes and binds coral snake venom.

Route	Onset	Peak	Duration
IV	Immediate	Unknown	Unknown

INDICATIONS & DOSAGE
Eastern and Texas coral snake bite—
Adults and children: 30 to 50 ml (3 to 5 vials) slow I.V. through running I.V. of 0.9% NaCl solution. First 1 to 2 ml given over 3 to 5 minutes, and signs of allergic reaction watched for. If no signs develop, injection is continued; 100 ml or more may be needed.
    Test for sensitivity before giving drug, as ordered. If sensitivity test is positive, prepare to desensitize as ordered; prepare

1:10 and 1:100 dilutions of antivenin in NaCl for injection.

ADVERSE REACTIONS
Musculoskeletal: arthralgia.
Skin: erythema, urticaria.
Other: pain, *hypersensitivity reactions, anaphylaxis,* fever, lymphadenopathy.

INTERACTIONS
None significant.

EFFECTS ON DIAGNOSTIC TESTS
None reported.

CONTRAINDICATIONS
Contraindicated in patients hypersensitive to drug and its components.

NURSING CONSIDERATIONS
Alert: Drug is not effective for Sonoran or Arizona coral snake bites.
• Immobilize patient and splint bitten limb to prevent spread of venom.
• Obtain accurate patient history of allergies, especially to horses, and reaction to immunization. Make sure epinephrine 1:1,000 is available in case of hypersensitivity reaction.
• Antivenin should be given as soon as possible (before onset of neurotoxic signs); asymptomatic patients should be treated because systemic signs usually develop later.
• Watch patient carefully for 24 hours. Venom is neurotoxic and may cause respiratory paralysis.

I.V. administration
• Reconstitute antivenon powder with the diluent. Further dilute in 0.9% NaCl to achieve a 1:1 to 1:10 dilution. Gently swirl the solution to avoid foaming.
• Infuse initial 1 to 2 ml over 3 to 5 minutes while closely monitoring the patient. If no immediate systemic response occurs, continue infusion at the maximum safe rate for I.V. fluid administration.

Patient teaching
• Explain to patient and family that a test dose will be given first to check for sensitivity to drug.

• Tell patient to report adverse reactions promptly.

---

*Liquid contains alcohol.   **May contain tartrazine.   †Canada   ‡Australia   §U.K.   ◇OTC

77

Immune serums

cytomegalovirus immune
  globulin, intravenous
hepatitis B immune globulin,
  human
immune globulin intramuscular
immune globulin intravenous
rabies immune globulin, human
respiratory syncytial virus
  immune globulin intravenous,
  human
Rh₀(D) immune globulin, human
Rh₀(D) immune globulin intravenous, human
tetanus immune globulin, human
varicella-zoster immune globulin

COMBINATION PRODUCTS
None.

cytomegalovirus immune globulin (human), intravenous (CMV-IGIV)
CytoGam

Pregnancy Risk Category: C

HOW SUPPLIED
Injection: 2.5 g/50 ml†; 1 g/20 ml

ACTION
Provides passive immunity by supplying a relatively high concentration of immuno-globulin (IgG) antibodies against CMV. Increasing these antibody levels in CMV-exposed patients may attenuate or reduce the incidence of serious CMV disease.

Route	Onset	Peak	Duration
IV	Unknown	Unknown	Unknown

INDICATIONS & DOSAGE
To attenuate primary CMV disease in seronegative kidney transplant recipients who receive a kidney from a CMV seropositive donor—
Adults: administered I.V. based on time after transplantation:
  within 72 hours: 150 mg/kg

2 weeks after: 100 mg/kg
4 weeks after: 100 mg/kg
6 weeks after: 100 mg/kg
8 weeks after: 100 mg/kg
12 weeks after: 50 mg/kg
16 weeks after: 50 mg/kg.
  Initial dose given at 15 mg/kg/hour. Increased to 30 mg/kg/hour after 30 minutes if no untoward reactions occur, then to 60 mg/kg/hour after another 30 minutes if no reactions occur. Volume should not exceed 75 ml/hour. Subsequent doses may be given at 15 mg/kg/ hour for 15 minutes, increasing q 15 minutes in a stepwise fashion to 60 mg/kg/hour.

ADVERSE REACTIONS
CV: hypotension.
GI: *nausea, vomiting.*
Musculoskeletal: muscle cramps, *back pain.*
Respiratory: *wheezing.*
Other: *anaphylaxis,* aseptic meningitis syndrome, *flushing, chills,* fever.

INTERACTIONS
Drug-drug. *Live virus vaccines:* may interfere with the immune response to live virus vaccines. Defer vaccination for at least 3 months.

EFFECTS ON DIAGNOSTIC TESTS
None reported.

CONTRAINDICATIONS
Contraindicated in patients with sensitivity to other human Ig preparations or with selective IgA deficiency.

NURSING CONSIDERATIONS
• Monitor patient's vital signs closely pre-infusion, midinfusion, postinfusion, and before and after increases in infusion rate.
Alert: If anaphylaxis or drop in blood pressure occurs, discontinue infusion, notify doctor, and be prepared to administer cardiopulmonary resuscitation and such drugs as diphenhydramine and epinephrine.
• Refrigerate at 36° to 46° F (2° to 8° C).

Reactions may be *common,* uncommon, *life-threatening,* or **COMMON AND LIFE-THREATENING.**

🔵 I.V. administration

• Prepare for administration as follows: Remove tab portion of vial cap and clean rubber stopper with 70% alcohol or equivalent. To avoid foaming, do not shake vial. Inspect vial for clarity and particles.

• If possible, administer through a separate I.V. line, using a constant infusion pump. Filters are unnecessary. If unable to administer through separate line, piggyback into preexisting line of NaCl injection or one of the following dextrose solutions with or without NaCl: $D_{2.5}W$, D_5W, $D_{10}W$, or $D_{20}W$. Do not dilute more than 1:2 with any of the above solutions.

• Begin infusion within 6 hours of entering the vial; finish within 12 hours.

✅ Patient teaching

• Review drug therapy regimen with patient, and stress importance of compliance in follow-up visits.

• Instruct patient to report adverse reactions promptly.

---

hepatitis B immune globulin, human
H-BIG, HyperHep

Pregnancy Risk Category: C

HOW SUPPLIED
Injection: 1-ml, 4-ml, 5-ml vials; 0.5-ml neonatal single-dose syringe

ACTION
Provides passive immunity to hepatitis B.

Route	Onset	Peak	Duration
IM	1-6 days	3-11 days	2 mo

INDICATIONS & DOSAGE
Hepatitis B exposure in high-risk patients—
Adults and children: 0.06 ml/kg I.M. within 7 days after exposure. Dosage repeated 28 days after exposure if patient refuses hepatitis B vaccine.
Neonates born to patients who test positive for hepatitis B surface antigen (HBsAg): 0.5 ml I.M. within 12 hours of birth.

ADVERSE REACTIONS
Skin: urticaria, *pain and tenderness at injection site.*
Other: *anaphylaxis, angioedema.*

INTERACTIONS
Drug-drug. *Live virus vaccines:* may interfere with response to live virus vaccines. Defer routine immunization for 3 months.

EFFECTS ON DIAGNOSTIC TESTS
None reported.

CONTRAINDICATIONS
Contraindicated in patients with history of anaphylactic reactions to immune serum. Administer to patient who has coagulation disorder or thrombocytopenia only if benefit outweighs the risk.

NURSING CONSIDERATIONS
• Obtain history of allergies and reaction to immunizations. Make sure epinephrine 1:1,000 is available.

• Inject into anterolateral aspect of thigh or deltoid muscle areas in older children and adults; inject into anterolateral aspect of thigh for neonates and children under 3 years.

• Inspect for discoloration or particulate matter. Drug is clear, slightly amber, and moderately viscous.

• For postexposure prophylaxis (for example, needle stick, direct contact), know that drug is usually given with hepatitis B vaccine.

• Be aware that this immune globulin provides passive immunity; do not confuse with hepatitis B vaccine. Both drugs may be given at same time. Do not mix in the same syringe.

✅ Patient teaching
• Inform patient that pain and tenderness may occur at injection site.

• Tell patient to report signs of hypersensitivity immediately.

---

immune globulin intramuscular (IGIM, IG, gamma globulin)

immune globulin intravenous (IGIV)

Gamimune N, Gammagard S/D, Gammar-P I.V., Iveegam, Polygam S/D, Sandoglobulin, Venoglobulin-I, Venoglobulin-S

Pregnancy Risk Category: C

HOW SUPPLIED
immune globulin intramuscular
Injection: 2-ml, 10-ml vials
immune globulin intravenous
Injection: 5% and 10% in 10-ml, 50-ml, 100-ml, 250-ml vials (Gamimune N) 5% in 2.5-g, 5-g, 10-g vials; 5%, 10% in 5-g, 10-g, 20-g vials (Venoglobulin-S)
Powder for injection: 50 mg protein/ml in 2.5-g, 5-g, 10-g vials (Gammagard S/D); 2.5-g, 1-g, 5-g vials (Gammar-P IV); 500-mg, 1-g, 2.5-g, 5-g vials (Iveegam); 2.5-g, 5-g, 10-g vials (Polygam S/D); 1-g, 3-g, 6-g, 12-g vials (Sandoglobulin); 500-mg, 2.5-g, 5-g, 10-g vials (Venoglobulin-I)

ACTION
Provides passive immunity by increasing antibody titer. The primary component is immunoglobulin (Ig) G. The mechanism for treating idiopathic thrombocytopenic purpura is unknown.

Route	Onset	Peak	Duration
IV	Immediate	Immediate	Unknown
IM	Unknown	2-5 hr	Unknown

INDICATIONS & DOSAGE
Primary humoral immunodeficiency (IGIV)—
Adults and children: *Gamimune N*—100 to 200 mg/kg I.V. monthly, at rate of 0.01 to 0.02 ml/kg/minute for 30 minutes. If no problems, rate can be slowly increased to maximum rate of 0.08 ml/kg/minute.
  Gammagard S/D—200 to 400 mg/kg I.V. followed by monthly doses of 100 mg/kg. Initiate infusion at 0.5 ml/kg/

hour and increase to maximum of 4 ml/kg/hour. Dose related to patient response.
  Gammar-P IV—200 to 600 mg/kg infused I.V. at 0.01 ml/kg/minute and increased to 0.02 ml/kg/minute after 15 to 30 minutes if no problems, given q 3 to 4 weeks. Maximum infusion rate is 0.06 ml/kg/minute.
  Iveegam—200 mg/kg I.V. monthly. May increase dose to maximum of 800 mg/kg or give more frequently to produce desired effect. Infusion rate is 1 to 2 ml/minute for 5% solution.
  Polygam S/D—initial dose is 200 to 400 mg/kg I.V. at 0.5 ml/kg/hour. increasing to maximum of 4 ml/kg/hour. Subsequent dose is 100 mg/kg I.V. monthly.
  Sandoglobulin—200 mg/kg I.V. monthly. Start initially with 0.5 to 1 ml/minute of 3% solution; gradually increase dose to 2.5 ml/minute after 15 to 30 minutes.
  Venoglobulin-I—initiate I.V. 200 mg/kg monthly at 0.01 to 0.02 ml/kg/minute for 30 minutes, then increase to 0.04 ml/kg/minute or more if no adverse reaction. Dose may be increased to 300 to 400 mg/kg and given more often than once monthly if needed and tolerated.
  Venoglobulin-S—200 mg/kg I.V. monthly. Dose may be increased to 300 to 400 mg/kg and given more often than once monthly if adequate IgG levels have not occurred. Begin infusion at 0.01 to 0.02 ml/kg/minute for 30 minutes, then increase 5% solutions to 0.04 ml/kg/minute and 10% solutions to 0.05 ml/kg/minute if tolerated.
Idiopathic thrombocytopenic purpura (IGIV)—
Adults and children: *Gamimune N*—400 mg/kg 5% solution I.V. for 5 days; or 1,000 mg/kg 10% solution I.V. for 1 to 2 days with maintenance dose of 10% solution at 400 to 1,000 mg/kg I.V. single infusion to maintain 30,000/mm^3 platelet count.
  Sandoglobulin—0.4 g/kg I.V. for 2 to 5 consecutive days.
Bone marrow transplant (IGIV)—
Adults over 20 years: *Gamimune N*—500 mg/kg 5% or 10 % solution I.V. on days 7 and 2 pretransplantation, then weekly until 90 days posttransplant.

Reactions may be *common*, uncommon, ***life-threatening***, or COMMON AND LIFE-THREATENING.

B-cell chronic lymphocytic leukemia (IGIV)—
Adults: 400 mg/kg Gammagard S/D or Polygam S/D I.V. q 3 to 4 weeks.
Hepatitis A exposure (IGIM)—
Adults and children: 0.02 ml/kg I.M. as soon as possible after exposure. Up to 0.1 ml/kg may be administered if prolonged or intense exposure.
Measles exposure (IGIM)—
Adults and children: 0.25 ml/kg I.M. within 6 days postexposure.
Postexposure prophylaxis of measles (IGIM)—
Children: 0.5 ml/kg I.M. within 6 days postexposure (maximum 15 ml).
Chickenpox exposure (IGIM)—
Adults and children: 0.6 to 1.2 ml/kg I.M. as soon as exposed.
Rubella exposure in first trimester pregnancy (IGIM)—
Women: 0.55 ml/kg I.M. as soon as possible postexposure (within 72 hours).
Pediatric HIV infection (IGIV)—
Children: 400 mg/kg Gamimune N I.V. q 28 days, at 0.01 to 0.02 m/kg/minute for 30 minutes and increase to maximum of 0.08 ml/kg/minute.

ADVERSE REACTIONS
CNS: headache, faintness.
GI: nausea, vomiting.
Musculoskeletal: hip pain, chest pain, chest tightness.
Respiratory: dyspnea.
Skin: urticaria; pain, erythema, muscle stiffness (at injection site).
Other: malaise, fever, *anaphylaxis,* chills.

INTERACTIONS
Drug-drug. *Live virus vaccines:* length of time to wait before administering live virus vaccinations varies with dose of immune globulin given. Refer to recommendations by the American Academy of Pediatrics.

EFFECTS ON DIAGNOSTIC TESTS
None reported.

CONTRAINDICATIONS
Contraindicated in patients hypersensitive to drug or its components.

NURSING CONSIDERATIONS
• Obtain history of allergies and reaction to immunizations. Make sure epinephrine 1:1,000 is available in case of anaphylaxis.
• When giving I.M., use gluteal region. Doses over 10 ml should be divided and injected into several muscle sites to reduce pain and discomfort.
• Administer drug soon after reconstitution.
• Know that immune globulin should not be given for prophylaxis against hepatitis A if 6 weeks or more have elapsed since exposure or after onset of clinical illness.

I.V. administration
• Polygam S/D, Gammagard S/D, and Iveegam recommend use of 15-micron in-line filter.
• Know that most adverse effects are related to a rapid infusion rate.

Patient teaching
• Explain to patient and family how drug will be administered.
• Tell patient that local reactions may occur at injection site. Instruct him to notify doctor promptly if adverse reactions persist or become severe.
• Inform patient of possible need to have therapy more than once monthly to maintain appropriate IgG levels.

---

rabies immune globulin, human
Hyperab, Imogam Rabies

Pregnancy Risk Category: C

HOW SUPPLIED
Injection: 150 IU/ml in 2-ml, 10-ml vials

ACTION
Provides passive immunity to rabies.

Route	Onset	Peak	Duration
IM	24 hr	Unknown	Unknown

INDICATIONS & DOSAGE
Rabies exposure—
Adults and children: 20 IU/kg I.M. at time of first dose of rabies vaccine. Half

of dose is used to infiltrate wound area; remainder is given I.M. in a different site.

ADVERSE REACTIONS
Skin: *rash;* pain, redness, induration (at injection site).
Other: slight fever, ***anaphylaxis, angioedema, nephrotic syndrome.***

INTERACTIONS
Drug-drug. *Live virus vaccines (measles, mumps, polio, or rubella):* interferes with response to vaccine. Delay immunization if possible.

EFFECTS ON DIAGNOSTIC TESTS
None reported.

CONTRAINDICATIONS
No known contraindications.

NURSING CONSIDERATIONS
• Use with caution in patients with history of systemic allergic reactions to human immunoglobulin preparations or in patients who are hypersensitive to thimerosal or have immunoglobulin A deficiency.
• Obtain history of animal bites, allergies, and reaction to immunizations. Have epinephrine 1:1,000 available to treat anaphylaxis.
• Ask patient when last tetanus immunization was received; many doctors order a booster at this time.
• Use only with rabies vaccine and immediate local treatment of wound. Do not give rabies vaccine and rabies immune globulin in same syringe or at same site. Administer as soon as possible after exposure or through day 7. After day 8, antibody response to culture vaccine has occurred.
• Don't administer live virus vaccines within 3 months of rabies immune globulin.
• Don't administer more than 5 ml I.M. at one injection site; divide I.M. doses over 5 ml; administer at different sites.
• Administer large volumes (5 ml) in adults only. Use the upper, outer quadrant of the gluteal area.
• Know that this immune serum provides passive immunity. Do not confuse it with rabies vaccine, a suspension of killed microorganisms that confers active immunity. The two drugs are often used together prophylactically after exposure to rabid animals.
• Clean wound thoroughly with soap and water; this is the best prophylaxis against rabies.

✓ Patient teaching
• Inform patient that local reactions may occur at injection site. Instruct him to notify doctor promptly if reactions persist or become severe.
• Tell patient that a tetanus shot also may be necessary.
• Instruct patient in wound care.

---

respiratory syncytial virus immune globulin intravenous, human (RSV-IGIV)
RespiGam

Pregnancy Risk Category: C

HOW SUPPLIED
Injection: 50 mg ±10 mg/ml in 20-ml, 50-ml single-use vial

ACTION
Provides passive immunity to RSV.

Route	Onset	Peak	Duration
IV	Unknown	Unknown	≥ 1 mo

INDICATIONS & DOSAGE
Prevention of serious lower respiratory tract infections caused by RSV in children with bronchopulmonary dysplasia (BPD) or history of premature birth (35 weeks' gestation or less)—
Premature infants and children under 2 years: single infusion monthly. Give 1.5 ml/kg/hour I.V. for 15 minutes; then, if clinical condition allows a higher rate, increase to 3 ml/kg/hour for 15 minutes and then to maximum of 6 ml/kg/hour until infusion ends. Maximum recommended total dosage per monthly infusion is 750 mg/kg.

ADVERSE REACTIONS
CNS: dizziness, anxiety.

Reactions may be *common,* uncommon, ***life-threatening,*** or **COMMON AND LIFE-THREATENING.**

CV: fluid overload, tachycardia, hypertension, palpitations, chest tightness.
GI: vomiting, diarrhea, gastroenteritis, abdominal cramps.
Musculoskeletal: myalgia, arthralgia.
Respiratory: respiratory distress, wheezing, crackles, hypoxia, tachypnea, dyspnea.
Skin: rash, flushing, pruritus, inflammation at injection site.
Other: fever, overdose effect, *hypersensitivity reactions including anaphylaxis, angioneurotic edema.*

INTERACTIONS
Drug-drug. *Live virus vaccines (such as mumps, rubella, and especially measles):* may interfere with response. If such vaccines are given during or within 10 months after RSV-IGIV, be aware that reimmunization is recommended, if appropriate.

EFFECTS ON DIAGNOSTIC TESTS
None reported.

CONTRAINDICATIONS
Contraindicated in patients with history of severe hypersensitivity to drug or other human immunoglobulin and selective immunoglobulin (Ig) A deficiency.

NURSING CONSIDERATIONS
• Know that children with fluid overload should not receive drug.
• Know that first dose should be given before RSV season begins and that subsequent doses should be given monthly throughout the RSV season (approximately November through April) to maintain protection. Children with RSV should continue to receive monthly doses for duration of RSV season.
• Monitor closely for signs of fluid overload. Children with BPD may be more prone to this condition. Report increases in heart rate, respiratory rate, retractions, or crackles. Have a loop diuretic, such as furosemide or bumetanide, available.

▌I.V. administration
• Drug does not contain a preservative. Enter single-use vial only once; do not shake; avoid foaming. Begin infusion

within 6 hours and end within 12 hours after vial is entered. Do not use if solution is turbid. Administer through I.V. line using a constant infusion pump. Predilution of drug before infusion is not recommended. Although filters are not necessary for the infusion, an in-line filter with a pore size larger than 15 microns may be used. Give drug separately from other drugs.
• Adhere to infusion rate guidelines; most adverse reactions may be related to rate used. In especially ill children with BPD, slower rates may be indicated.
• Assess cardiopulmonary status and vital signs before beginning infusion, before each rate increase, and every 30 minutes thereafter until 30 minutes after completion of infusion.
Alert: If patient develops hypotension, anaphylaxis, or severe allergic reaction, stop infusion and administer epinephrine (1:1,000), as ordered. Know that patients with selective IgA deficiency can develop antibodies to IgA and have anaphylactic or allergic reactions to subsequent administration of blood products containing IgA, including RSV-IGIV.

✓Patient teaching
• Explain to parents importance of their child receiving drug monthly throughout RSV season, even if already infected.
• Teach parents how drug is administered and which adverse reactions are associated with administration. Instruct parents to report all adverse reactions promptly.

Rh$_o$(D) immune globulin, human
Gamulin Rh, HypRho-D, HypRho-D Mini-Dose, MICRhoGAM, Mini-Gamulin Rh, RhoGAM

Rh$_o$(D) immune globulin intravenous, human
WinRho SD

Pregnancy Risk Category: C

HOW SUPPLIED
Rh$_o$(D) immune globulin, human
Injection: 300 mcg of Rh$_o$(D) immune

globulin/vial (standard dose); 50 mcg of Rh$_o$(D) immune globulin/vial (microdose)
Rh$_o$ (D) immune globulin I.V., human
Injection: 120 mcg, 300 mcg

ACTION
Suppresses the active antibody response and formation of anti-Rh$_o$(D) antibodies in Rh$_o$(D)-negative, D^u-negative persons exposed to Rh-positive blood. Rh$_o$(D) immune globulin I.V. may form complexes with RBCs blocking platelet destruction in adults who are Rh$_o$(D) antigen-positive. However, mechanism of action is not completely understood.

Route	Onset	Peak	Duration
IV, IM	Unknown	Unknown	Unknown

INDICATIONS & DOSAGE
Rh$_o$(D) immune globulin, human Rh exposure—
Adults (after abortion, miscarriage, ectopic pregnancy; or postpartum): transfusion unit or blood bank determines fetal packed RBC volume entering patient's blood; then one vial I.M. is given if fetal packed RBC volume is less than 15 ml. More than one vial I.M. may be required if large fetomaternal hemorrhage occurs; must be given within 72 hours after delivery or miscarriage.
After abortion or miscarriage to prevent Rh antibody formation—
Adults: consult transfusion unit or blood bank. One microdose vial I.M. will suppress immune reaction to 2.5 ml Rh$_o$ (D)-positive RBCs. Ideally, should be given within 3 hours, but may be given up to 72 hours after abortion or miscarriage.
Rh$_o$ (D) immune globulin I.V., human Rh exposure—
Adults (after abortion, amniocentesis [after 34 weeks' gestation], or any other manipulation late in pregnancy [after 34 weeks' gestation] associated with increased risk of Rh isoimmunization): 120 mcg I.M. or I.V.; must be given within 72 hours after delivery, miscarriage, or manipulation.
Pregnancy—
Adults: 300 mcg (WinRho SD) I.M. or I.V. at 28 weeks' gestation. If adminis-

tered early in the pregnancy, additional doses should be given at 12-week intervals to maintain adequate levels of passively acquired anti-Rh antibodies. Then, within 72 hours of delivery, 120 mcg should be given I.M. or I.V. If 72 hours have elapsed, drug should be given as soon as possible, up to 28 days.
Transfusion accidents—
Adults: 600 mcg I.V. q 8 hours or 1,200 mcg I.M. q 12 hours until total dose administered. Total dose depends on volume of packed red blood cells or whole blood infused. Consult blood bank or transfusion unit at once; must be given within 72 hours.
Immune thrombocytopenic purpura (ITP) in adults who are Rh$_o$(D) antigen-positive—
Adults: initially 50 mcg/kg I.V. If hemoglobin is less than 10 g/dl, reduce initial dose to 25 to 40 mcg/kg. Initial dose may be administered as a single dose or divided into two doses and administered on separate days. Then, 25 to 60 mcg/kg I.V. may be administered, p.r.n., to elevate platelet counts with specific dosage that's determined individually.

ADVERSE REACTIONS
Skin: discomfort at injection site.
Other: *anaphylaxis,* slight fever.

INTERACTIONS
Drug-drug. *Live virus vaccines:* may interfere with response. Delay immunization for 3 months, if possible.

EFFECTS ON DIAGNOSTIC TESTS
None reported.

CONTRAINDICATIONS
Contraindicated in Rh$_o$(D)-positive or D^u-positive patients and those previously immunized to Rh$_o$(D) blood factor. Also contraindicated in patients with anaphylactic or severe systemic reaction to human globulin.

NURSING CONSIDERATIONS
• Use extreme caution when administering drug to patients with immunoglobulin (IgA) deficiency. Because of risk of pa-

---

Reactions may be *common*, uncommon, *life-threatening*, or COMMON AND LIFE-THREATENING.

tient developing IgA antibodies and having an anaphylactic reaction, doctor must weigh the potential benefits of treatment against the potential for hypersensitivity reactions.
• Obtain history of allergies and reaction to immunization. Be sure epinephrine 1:1,000 is available in case of anaphylaxis.
Alert: Immediately after delivery, send a sample of neonate's cord blood to laboratory for typing and crossmatching. Confirm if mother is $Rh_o(D)$-negative and D^u-negative. Administer drug to mother, as ordered, only if infant is $Rh_o(D)$-positive or D^u-positive. Administration must occur within 72 hours of delivery.
• Keep in mind that this immune serum provides passive immunity to patient exposed to $Rh_o(D)$-positive fetal blood during pregnancy and prevents formation of maternal antibodies (active immunity), which would endanger future $Rh_o(D)$-positive pregnancies.
• Know that vaccination with live virus vaccines should be deferred for 3 months after administration of $Rh_o(D)$ immune globulin.
• Know that minidose preparations are recommended for every patient undergoing abortion or miscarriage up to 12 weeks' gestation unless she is $Rh_o(D)$-positive or D^u-positive or has Rh antibodies, or unless the father or fetus is Rh-negative.

I.V. administration
• Reconstitute *only* with 0.9% NaCl solution. Do *not* administer with other products.

☑ Patient teaching
• Explain to patient how drug protects future Rh_o (D)-positive fetuses if used because of pregnancy, or explain to patient drug use in condition indicated.
• Warn patient about adverse reactions associated with drug.
• Assure patient receiving this medication that there is no risk of HIV transmission.

tetanus immune globulin, human
Hyper-Tet

Pregnancy Risk Category: C

HOW SUPPLIED
Injection: 250-unit vial or syringe

ACTION
Provides passive immunity to tetanus.

Route	Onset	Peak	Duration
IM	Unknown	2-3 days	4 wk

INDICATIONS & DOSAGE
Tetanus exposure—
Adults and children: 250 units I.M.
Tetanus treatment—
Adults and children: single doses of 3,000 to 6,000 units I.M. have been used. Optimal dosage schedules have not been established.

ADVERSE REACTIONS
Skin: pain, stiffness, erythema at injection site.
Other: slight fever, *hypersensitivity reactions, anaphylaxis, angioedema,* nephrotic syndrome.

INTERACTIONS
Drug-drug. *Live virus vaccines:* may interfere with response. Defer administration of live virus vaccines for 3 months after administration of tetanus immune globulin.

EFFECTS ON DIAGNOSTIC TESTS
None reported.

CONTRAINDICATIONS
Contraindicated in patients with thrombocytopenia or other coagulation disorders that would contraindicate I.M. injection unless potential benefits outweigh the risks.

NURSING CONSIDERATIONS
• Use cautiously in patients with history of prior systemic allergic reactions following administration of human im-

munoglobulin preparations or those allergic to thimerosal.
• Obtain history of injury, tetanus immunizations, last tetanus toxoid injection, allergies, and reaction to immunizations. Have epinephrine 1:1,000 available to treat hypersensitivity reaction.
• Do not administer I.V. or I.D. Do not administer in the gluteal area.
• Know that tetanus immune globulin is used only if wound is more than 24 hours old or patient has had fewer than two tetanus toxoid injections.
• Thoroughly clean wound and remove all foreign matter.
• Do not confuse this drug with tetanus toxoid. Tetanus immune globulin is not a substitute for tetanus toxoid, which should be given at the same time to produce active immunization. Don't give at same site as toxoid.
• Be aware that antibodies remain at effective levels for about 4 weeks, which is several times the duration of equine antitetanus antibodies. This protects patients for the incubation period of most tetanus cases.
• Do not administer live virus vaccines for 3 months after administering tetanus immune globulin.

☑ **Patient teaching**
• Warn patient about local adverse reactions associated with drug.
• Instruct patient to report serious adverse reactions promptly.
• Advise patient to complete full series of tetanus immunizations.
• Discuss use of acetaminophen for fever reduction and cool compresses at injection site for comfort.

---

varicella-zoster immune globulin (VZIG)

Pregnancy Risk Category: C

HOW SUPPLIED
Injection: 10% to 18% solution of the globulin fraction of human plasma containing 125 units of varicella-zoster virus antibody (volume is about 2.5 ml or less)

ACTION
Provides passive immunity to varicella-zoster virus in immunodeficient patients.

Route	Onset	Peak	Duration
IM	Unknown	Unknown	1 mo

INDICATIONS & DOSAGE
Passive immunization of susceptible immunodeficient patients after exposure to varicella (chickenpox or herpes zoster)—
Adults and children weighing over 40 kg (88 lb): 625 units I.M.
Children weighing 30.1 to 40 kg (66 to 88 lb): 500 units I.M.
Children weighing 20.1 to 30 kg (44 to 66 lb): 375 units I.M.
Children weighing 10.1 to 20 kg (22 to 44 lb): 250 units I.M.
Children weighing up to 10 kg (22 lb): 125 units I.M.

ADVERSE REACTIONS
CNS: headache.
GI: GI distress.
Respiratory: respiratory distress.
Skin: discomfort at injection site, rash.
Other: malaise, *anaphylaxis.*

INTERACTIONS
Drug-drug. *Live virus vaccines:* may interfere with response. Defer vaccination for 3 months after administration of VZIG.

EFFECTS ON DIAGNOSTIC TESTS
None reported.

CONTRAINDICATIONS
Contraindicated in patients with thrombocytopenia or history of severe reaction to human immune serum globulin or thimerosal and during pregnancy.

NURSING CONSIDERATIONS
• Obtain accurate patient history of allergies and reaction to immunization. Make sure epinephrine 1:1,000 is available in case of anaphylaxis.
• For maximum benefit, administer as soon as possible after presumed exposure. May be of benefit when given as late as 96 hours after exposure.
• Administer only by deep I.M. injection

Reactions may be *common,* uncommon, *life-threatening*, or COMMON AND LIFE-THREATENING.

into a large muscle mass such as the gluteal muscle. Never administer I.V.

• Although usually restricted to children under 15 years, be aware that VZIG may be administered to adolescents and adults if necessary.

• VZIG is not recommended for nonimmunosuppressed patients.

• VZIG provides passive immunity; do not confuse with varicella vaccine. Do not use these two drugs in combination.

• Be aware that drug is not commercially distributed and is available only from 20 regional U.S. distribution centers. These centers will distribute to Canada and overseas. Contact the Massachusetts Public Health Biologic Laboratories or The Centers for Disease Control and Prevention for more information.

☑ **Patient teaching**

• Warn patient about local adverse reactions associated with drug.

• Instruct patient to report serious adverse reactions to doctor promptly.

• Discuss use of acetaminophen for fever reduction and cool compresses at injection site for comfort.

78

Biological response modifiers

aldesleukin
epoetin alfa
filgrastim
glatiramer acetate for injection
interferon alfacon-1
interferon alfa-2a, recombinant
interferon alfa-2b, recombinant
interferon beta-1a
interferon beta-1b, recombinant
interferon gamma-1b
levamisole hydrochloride
oprelvekin
sargramostim

COMBINATION PRODUCTS
None.

---

aldesleukin (interleukin-2, IL-2)
Proleukin

Pregnancy Risk Category: C

HOW SUPPLIED
Powder for injection: 22 million IU/vial

ACTION
Unknown, although stimulation of an immunologic host reaction to the tumor may be involved.

Route	Onset	Peak	Duration
IV	4 wk	Unknown	≤ 12 mo

INDICATIONS & DOSAGE
Metastatic renal cell carcinoma—
Adults: 600,000 IU/kg (0.037 mg/kg) I.V. over 15 minutes q 8 hours for 5 days (total of 14 doses). After a 9-day rest, the sequence is repeated for another 14 doses. Repeat courses may be given after a rest period of at least 7 weeks.
✳ *NEW INDICATION: Treatment of metastatic melanoma—*
Adults: 600,000 IU/kg (0.037 mg/kg) I.V. over 15 minutes q 8 hours for total of 14 doses. After 9-day rest, sequence is repeated for another 14 doses. Repeat courses may be given after rest period of at least 7 weeks.
Adjust-a-dose: If toxicity occurs, withhold drug rather than administering a reduced dose. Therapy is continued after evaluation of patient.

ADVERSE REACTIONS
CNS: *headache, mental status changes, dizziness, sensory dysfunction,* special senses disorders, syncope, motor dysfunction, **coma,** fatigue.
CV: *hypotension, sinus tachycardia,* **arrhythmias,** bradycardia, *PVC, premature atrial contractions,* myocardial ischemia, **MI, heart failure, cardiac arrest,** myocarditis, endocarditis, **CVA,** pericardial effusion, *phlebitis,* thrombosis, **capillary leak syndrome (CLS).**
EENT: conjunctivitis.
GI: *nausea, vomiting, diarrhea, stomatitis, anorexia, bleeding,* dyspepsia, constipation.
GU: *oliguria, anuria, proteinuria,* hematuria, dysuria, urine retention, urinary frequency.
Hematologic: *anemia,* THROMBOCYTOPENIA, LEUKOPENIA, *coagulation disorders,* leukocytosis, eosinophilia.
Hepatic: *jaundice;* ascites; hepatomegaly; *elevated bilirubin, serum transaminase, alkaline phosphatase levels.*
Respiratory: *pulmonary congestion, dyspnea, pulmonary edema,* hemoptysis, **respiratory failure, pleural effusion, apnea, pneumothorax,** tachypnea, wheezing.
Skin: *pruritus, erythema, rash, dryness, exfoliative dermatitis,* purpura, alopecia, petechiae, persistent, nonprogressive vitiligo (in melanoma patients).
Other: *elevated BUN and serum creatinine levels; hypomagnesemia; acidosis; hypocalcemia; hypophosphatemia; hypokalemia; hyperuricemia; hypoalbuminemia;* hypoproteinemia; hyponatremia; *hyperkalemia;* arthralgia; myalgia; *fever; chills; abdominal, chest, or back pain; weakness; malaise; edema; infections of

---

Reactions may be *common,* uncommon, *life-threatening,* or COMMON AND LIFE-THREATENING.

catheter tip, urinary tract, or injection site; SEPSIS; *weight gain;* weight loss.

INTERACTIONS
Drug-drug. *Antihypertensives:* increased risk of hypotension. Monitor closely.
Cardiotoxic, hepatotoxic, myelotoxic, or nephrotoxic drugs: enhanced toxicity. Avoid concomitant use.
Corticosteroids: decreased antitumor effectiveness of aldesleukin. Avoid concomitant use.
Psychotropic agents: unpredictable interaction. Because aldesleukin can alter CNS function, use together cautiously.

EFFECTS ON DIAGNOSTIC TESTS
No direct laboratory test interference has been reported. Toxic effects of drug may be seen in decreasing hepatic, renal, and thyroid function tests; abnormal serum electrolytes; or abnormal cardiac or pulmonary function tests.

CONTRAINDICATIONS
Contraindicated in patients with hypersensitivity to drug or its components and in those with abnormal cardiac (thallium) stress test or pulmonary function tests or organ allografts. Retreatment is contraindicated in patients who experience the following adverse effects: pericardial tamponade; disturbances in cardiac rhythm that were uncontrolled or unresponsive to intervention; sustained ventricular tachycardia (five beats or more); chest pain accompanied by ECG changes, indicating MI or angina pectoris; renal dysfunction requiring dialysis for 72 hours or more; coma or toxic psychosis lasting 48 hours or more; seizures that were repetitive or difficult to control; ischemia or perforation of the bowel; GI bleeding requiring surgery.

NURSING CONSIDERATIONS
• Do not use drug unless patient has had definitive tests documenting normal cardiac and pulmonary function. Use with extreme caution in patients with normal test results if they have history of cardiac or pulmonary disease and in patients with history of seizure disorders.
• Use cautiously and with close clinical monitoring because severe adverse effects usually accompany therapy at the recommended dosage.
• Use cautiously in patients who require large volumes of fluid (such as patients with hypercalcemia).
• Know that drug should be administered only in a hospital under direction of a doctor experienced in the use of chemotherapeutic agents. An intensive care facility and intensive care or cardiopulmonary specialist must be available.
• Monitor hematologic tests, including CBC, differential, and platelet counts; serum electrolyte levels; and renal and liver function tests, and obtain chest X-ray before therapy, as ordered. Repeat daily during therapy.
• Treat patients with bacterial infections before therapy, as ordered.
• Be prepared to adjust dosage of other drugs, as ordered, to compensate for renal and hepatic impairment occurring during treatment. Know that dosage is modified by withholding a dose or interrupting therapy rather than by reducing the dose, as ordered.
• Withhold dose and notify doctor if patient develops moderate to severe lethargy or somnolence; continued administration can result in coma.
• Administer packed RBCs or platelets, as ordered. Severe anemia or thrombocytopenia may occur.
Alert: Know that drug has been associated with CLS, a condition caused by loss of vascular tone, in which plasma proteins and fluids escape into the extravascular space. Mean arterial blood pressure begins to drop within 2 to 12 hours of treatment; edema and effusions may be severe, and death can result from hypoperfusion of major organs. Other conditions that accompany CLS include arrhythmias, MI, angina, mental status changes, renal insufficiency, respiratory distress or failure, and GI bleeding or infarction.
• Be aware that therapy is associated with impaired neutrophil function, which can lead to disseminated infection. Many studies employed prophylactic antibiotic therapy with oxacillin, nafcillin, ciprofloxacin, or vancomycin; check protocol and administer antibiotics, as ordered. Monitor for infection.

---

*Liquid contains alcohol.   **May contain tartrazine.   †Canada   ‡Australia   §U.K.   ◊OTC

• Know that patient should be neurologically stable with a negative computed tomography scan for CNS metastases. Drug may exacerbate symptoms in patients with unrecognized or undiagnosed CNS metastases.
• Drug may exacerbate preexisting autoimmune disease.

▸ I.V. administration
• To avoid altering the pharmacologic properties of drug, reconstitute and dilute carefully, and follow manufacturer's recommendations. Do not mix with other drugs or albumin.
• Reconstitute vial containing 22 million IU (1.3 mg) with 1.2 ml of sterile water for injection. *Do not* use bacteriostatic water or 0.9% NaCl for injection; these diluents increase aggregation of drug. Direct the stream at the sides of vial and gently swirl to reconstitute. Do not shake. Reconstituted solution will have a concentration of 18 million IU (1.1 mg)/ml. It should be particle-free and colorless to slightly yellow.
• Add ordered dose of reconstituted drug to 50 ml of D_5W and infuse over 15 minutes. Do not use an in-line filter. Plastic infusion bags are preferred because they provide consistent drug delivery.
• Refrigerate powder for injection or reconstituted solutions. Return drug to room temperature before administering to patients. After reconstitution and dilution, administer within 48 hours.

☑ Patient teaching
• Explain administration schedule to patient and caregivers, and stress importance of compliance.
• Instruct patient to report adverse reactions promptly.

---

epoetin alfa (erythropoietin)
Epogen, Eprex§, Procrit

Pregnancy Risk Category: C

HOW SUPPLIED
Injection: 2,000 units/ml, 3,000 units/ml, 4,000 units/ml, 10,000 units/ml; multidose vials of 10,000 units/ml, 20,000 units/ml

ACTION
Mimics the effects of erythropoietin, a naturally occurring hormone produced by the kidneys. Epoetin alfa is one of the factors controlling the rate of RBC production. It acts on the erythroid tissues in the bone marrow, stimulating mitotic activity of erythroid progenitor cells and early precursor cells. It functions as a growth factor and as a differentiating factor, enhancing rate of RBC production.

Route	Onset	Peak	Duration
IV	1-6 wk	Immediate	Unknown
SC	1-6 wk	5-24 hr	Unknown

INDICATIONS & DOSAGE
Anemia due to reduced production of endogenous erythropoietin caused by end-stage renal disease—
Adults: dosage is individualized. Starting dose is 50 to 100 units/kg I.V. three times weekly. (Nondialysis patients with chronic renal failure or patients receiving continuous peritoneal dialysis may receive the drug by S.C. injection or I.V.) Maintenance dosage is highly individualized.
Adjust-a-dose: Dosage is reduced when target hematocrit level is reached or if the hematocrit rises more than 4 points in any 2-week period. Dosage is increased if hematocrit does not increase by 5 to 6 points after 8 weeks of therapy.
Adjunctive treatment of HIV-infected patients with anemia secondary to zidovudine therapy—
Adults: 100 units/kg I.V. or S.C. three times weekly for 8 weeks or until target hemoglobin level is reached. If response is not satisfactory after 8 weeks, dose may be increased by 50 to 100 units/kg I.V. or S.C. three times weekly. After 4 to 8 weeks, dosage may be further increased in increments of 50 to 100 units/kg three times weekly, up to maximum of 300 units/kg I.V. or S.C. three times weekly.
Anemia secondary to cancer chemotherapy—
Adults: 150 units/kg S.C. three times weekly for 8 weeks or until target hemoglobin level is reached. If response is not satisfactory after 8 weeks, dosage may be

---

increased up to 300 units/kg S.C. three times weekly.

Adjust-a-dose: If hematocrit exceeds 40%, drug should be withheld until hematocrit falls to 36%.

Reduction of need for allogenic blood transfusion in anemic patients scheduled to undergo elective, noncardiac, nonvascular surgery—

Adults: 300 units/kg/day S.C. daily for 10 days before surgery, on day of surgery, and for 4 days after surgery. Alternatively, 600 units/kg S.C. in once-weekly doses (21, 14, and 7 days before surgery), plus one-quarter dose on day of surgery.

ADVERSE REACTIONS
CNS: *headache,* **seizures,** *paresthesia, fatigue,* dizziness.
CV: *hypertension, edema.*
GI: *nausea, vomiting, diarrhea.*
Respiratory: *cough, shortness of breath.*
Skin: *rash, injection site reactions,* urticaria.
Other: increased clotting of arteriovenous grafts, *pyrexia, arthralgia, asthenia.*

INTERACTIONS
None significant.

EFFECTS ON DIAGNOSTIC TESTS
Moderate increases in BUN, uric acid, creatinine, phosphorous, and potassium levels have been reported.

CONTRAINDICATIONS
Contraindicated in patients with uncontrolled hypertension, hypersensitivity to mammalian cell-derived products or albumin (human).

NURSING CONSIDERATIONS
• Use with caution in breast-feeding women.
• Monitor blood pressure before therapy. Up to 80% of patients with chronic renal failure have hypertension. Blood pressure may rise, especially when the hematocrit level is increasing in the early part of therapy.
• When used in HIV-infected patients, be prepared to individualize dosage based on response, as ordered. Dosage recommendations are for patients with endogenous erythropoietin levels of 500 units/L or less and cumulative zidovudine doses of 4.2 g/week or less.
• Be aware that patient treated with epoetin alfa may require additional heparin to prevent clotting during dialysis treatments.
• Monitor blood count, as ordered. Hematocrit level may rise and cause excessive clotting. Renal function, uric acid, and potassium levels may rise.
• Institute diet restrictions or drug therapy to control blood pressure. Reduce dosage in patients who exhibit a rapid rise in hematocrit (more than 4 points in a 2-week period), as ordered, to prevent hypertension.
• Know that patient's response to epoetin alfa depends on amount of endogenous erythropoietin in the plasma. Patients with levels of 500 units/L or more usually have transfusion-dependent anemia and will probably not respond to drug. Those with levels below 500 units/L usually respond well.
• Be aware that patient should receive adequate iron supplementation beginning no later than when epoetin alfa treatment starts and continuing throughout therapy. Also may require vitamin B_{12} and folic acid.

🔃 **I.V. administration**
• Give by direct injection without dilution. Solution contains no preservatives. Discard unused portion. Do not mix with other drugs. Do not shake.

☑ **Patient teaching**
• After injection (usually within 2 hours), inform patient that pain or discomfort in limbs (long bones) and pelvis, and coldness and sweating are not uncommon. Symptoms may persist up to 12 hours and then disappear.
• Advise patient that blood specimens will be drawn weekly for blood counts and that dosage adjustments may be made based on the results.
• Advise patient to avoid driving or operating heavy machinery during initiation of therapy. A relationship between exces-

sively rapid hematocrit rise and seizures may exist.
• Tell patient to monitor blood pressure at home and to adhere to dietary restrictions.
• Instruct patient to check that syringes used to administer medication are in tenths of ml.

filgrastim (granulocyte colony–stimulating factor; G-CSF)
Neupogen

Pregnancy Risk Category: C

HOW SUPPLIED
Injection: 300 mcg/ml

ACTION
A glycoprotein that stimulates proliferation and differentiation of hematopoietic cells. Filgrastim is specific for neutrophils.

Route	Onset	Peak	Duration
IV	5-60 min	24 hr	1-7 days
SC	5-60 min	2-8 hr	1-7 days

INDICATIONS & DOSAGE
To decrease incidence of infection in patients with nonmyeloid malignant disease receiving myelosuppressive antineoplastic agents—
Adults and children: 5 mcg/kg/day I.V. or S.C. as single dose given no sooner than 24 hours after cytotoxic chemotherapy. Doses may be increased in increments of 5 mcg/kg for each chemotherapy cycle depending on duration and severity of the nadir of absolute neutrophil count (ANC).
To decrease incidence of infection in patients with nonmyeloid malignant disease receiving myelosuppressive antineoplastic agents followed by bone marrow transplantation—
Adults and children: 10 mcg/kg/day I.V. infusion of 4 or 24 hours or as a continuous 24-hour S.C. infusion at least 24 hours after cytotoxic chemotherapy and bone marrow infusion. Subsequent dosages adjusted based on neutrophil response.
Adjust-a-dose: In patients with ANC over 1,000/mm³ for 3 consecutive days, reduce

dose to 5 mcg/kg/day; if ANC remains over 1,000/mm³ for 3 more consecutive days, discontinue drug. If ANC decreases to below 1,000/mm³, resume therapy at 5 mcg/kg/day.
Congenital neutropenia—
Adults: 6 mcg/kg S.C. b.i.d. Dosage adjusted based on patient response.
Adjust-a-dose: In patients with a persistently elevated ANC (exceeding 10,000/mm³), reduce dose.
Idiopathic or cyclic neutropenia—
Adults: 5 mcg/kg S.C. daily. Dosage adjusted based on patient response.
Peripheral blood progenitor cell (PBPC) collection and therapy in cancer patients—
Adults: 10 mcg/kg/day S.C. Give 4 days before leukapheresis and continue until last leukapheresis.
Adjust-a-dose: In patients with WBC count over 100,000 mm³, dosage adjustment may be required.

ADVERSE REACTIONS
CNS: headache, weakness.
CV: *MI, arrhythmias,* chest pain.
GI: *nausea, vomiting, diarrhea, mucositis,* stomatitis, constipation.
Hematologic: *thrombocytopenia,* leukocytosis.
Respiratory: dyspnea, cough.
Skin: *alopecia,* rash, cutaneous vasculitis.
Other: *skeletal pain, fever, fatigue, hypersensitivity reactions.*

INTERACTIONS
Drug-drug. *Chemotherapeutic agents:* rapidly dividing myeloid cells are potentially sensitive to cytotoxic agents. Do not use within 24 hours before or after a dose of one of these agents. Use with caution in patients taking lithium.

EFFECTS ON DIAGNOSTIC TESTS
WBC counts may be increased to 100,000/mm³ or more. Transient increases in neutrophils, as well as reversible elevations in uric acid, LD, and alkaline phosphatase levels, have been noted. Transient decreases in blood pressure and increases in serum creatinine and aminotransferase levels have also been reported.

Reactions may be *common,* uncommon, *life-threatening,* or COMMON AND LIFE-THREATENING.

CONTRAINDICATIONS

Contraindicated in patients hypersensitive to proteins derived from *Escherichia coli* or to drug or its components.

NURSING CONSIDERATIONS

• Use with caution in breast-feeding women.
• Obtain baseline CBC and platelet count before therapy, as ordered.
• Once a dose is withdrawn, do not reenter vial. Discard unused portion. Vials are for single-dose use and contain no preservatives.
• Obtain CBC and platelet count two to three times weekly during therapy, as ordered. Patients who receive drug may potentially receive high doses of chemotherapy, which may increase risk of toxicities.
• Be aware that a transiently increased neutrophil count is common 1 or 2 days after initiation of therapy. Give daily for up to 2 weeks or until ANC has returned to 10,000/mm³ after the expected chemotherapy-induced neutrophil nadir, as ordered.

I.V. administration

• Dilute in 50 to 100 ml of D_5W and give by intermittent infusion over 15 to 60 minutes or continuous infusion over 24 hours. If final concentration of drug is 5 to 15 mcg/ml, add albumin at a concentration of 2 mg/ml (0.2%) to minimize binding of drug to plastic containers or tubing. Do not dilute with 0.9% NaCl solution. Dilution to a final concentration of less than 5 mcg/ml is not recommended.

✓ Patient teaching

• If patient is to self-administer drug, teach him how to administer it and how to dispose of used needles, syringes, drug containers, and unused medicine.
• Instruct patient to report persistent or serious adverse reactions promptly.

---

glatiramer acetate for injection (formerly copolymer 1)
Copaxone

Pregnancy Risk Category: B

HOW SUPPLIED

Injection: 20 mg lyophilized glatiramer acetate and 40 mg mannitol, USP, in a single-use 2-ml vial; 1-ml vial of sterile water for injection is included for reconstitution

ACTION

Unknown. Thought to act by modifying immune processes responsible for the pathogenesis of multiple sclerosis.

Route	Onset	Peak	Duration
SC	Unknown	Unknown	Unknown

INDICATIONS & DOSAGE

To reduce the frequency of relapses in patients with relapsing-remitting multiple sclerosis—
Adults: 20 mg S.C. daily.

ADVERSE REACTIONS

CNS: abnormal dreams, agitation, *anxiety, asthenia,* confusion, emotional lability, foot drop, *hypertonia,* migraine, nervousness, nystagmus, speech disorder, stupor, tremor, vertigo.
CV: *chest pain,* hypertension, *palpitations, vasodilation,* syncope, tachycardia.
EENT: ear pain, eye disorder, *rhinitis.*
GI: anorexia, bowel urgency, *diarrhea,* gastroenteritis, GI disorder, *nausea,* oral moniliasis, salivary gland enlargement, tooth caries, ulcerative stomatitis, vomiting.
GU: amenorrhea, dysmenorrhea, hematuria, impotence, menorrhagia, suspicious Papanicolaou smear, *urinary urgency,* vaginal candidiasis, vaginal hemorrhage.
Hematologic: ecchymosis, *lymphadenopathy.*
Metabolic: weight gain.
Respiratory: bronchitis, *dyspnea,* hyperventilation, laryngismus.
Skin: eczema; erythema; herpes simplex and zoster; *pruritus, rash, injection site reaction* or hemorrhage; skin atrophy; skin nodule; *diaphoresis;* urticaria; warts.
Other: *arthralgia, back pain,* bacterial infection, chills, cyst, peripheral and facial edema, fever, *flulike syndrome, infection,* neck pain, *pain.*

INTERACTIONS
None significant.

EFFECTS ON DIAGNOSTIC TESTS
None reported.

CONTRAINDICATIONS
Contraindicated in patients with known hypersensitivity to drug or mannitol.

NURSING CONSIDERATIONS
• Administer drug by S.C. injection only.
• Store drug in refrigerator (36° to 46° F [2° to 8° C]); diluent can be kept at room temperature.
• Lyophilized material and diluent should be swirled gently and allowed to stand at room temperature until completely dissolved; approximately 5 minutes.
• Use immediately after reconstitution because drug does not contain preservatives; discard unused drug. Use diluent provided for reconstitution.
• Immediate postinjection reactions have occurred in 10% of patients with multiple sclerosis; symptoms include flushing, chest pain, palpitations, anxiety, dyspnea, constriction of the throat, and urticaria. These reactions were transient, self-limiting, and did not require specific treatment. Onset may occur several months after initiation of treatment and patients may have more than one episode.
• Approximately 26% of patients experienced at least one episode of transient chest pain, which usually began at least 1 month after treatment began; it was not accompanied by other symptoms and did not appear to be clinically important.
• Because drug can modify immune response, it could interfere with normal immune function. Although evidence is lacking, there has been no evaluation of this risk.
• Drug is antigenic and may lead to induction of unwanted host responses. Systemic study of these effects has not been done.
• It is not known if drug is excreted in breast milk.

☑ **Patient teaching**
• Instruct patient how to reconstitute and self-inject drug. Supervise first self-injection.
• Explain need for aseptic self-injection techniques and warn patient against reuse of needles and syringes. Periodically review proper disposal of needles, syringes, drug containers, and unused medicine.
• Tell patient to notify doctor if pregnancy is being planned, is suspected, or occurs.
• Tell female patient to notify doctor if she is breast-feeding.
• Advise patient not to change drug or dosing schedule or to stop drug without medical approval.
• Tell patient to notify doctor immediately if dizziness, urticaria, diaphoresis, chest pain, difficulty breathing, or severe pain occurs following drug injection.

---

interferon alfacon-1
Infergen

Pregnancy Risk Category: C

HOW SUPPLIED
Injection: 9 mcg/0.3 ml, 15 mcg/0.5 ml vials

ACTION
Type-I interferons induce genetic-mediated biological responses that include antiviral, antiproliferative, and immunomodulatory effects and regulation of cytokine expression.

Route	Onset	Peak	Duration
SC	Unknown	24-36 hr	Unknown

INDICATIONS & DOSAGE
Treatment of chronic hepatitis C viral infection—
Adults: 9 mcg S.C. three times weekly for 24 weeks; for nonresponders or those patients who relapse, 15 mcg S.C. three times weekly for 6 months.
Adjust-a-dose: In patients intolerant to higher doses, dose may be reduced to 7.5 mcg. Do not give doses below 7.5 mcg because decreased efficacy may result.

ADVERSE REACTIONS

CNS: *headache, insomnia, dizziness, paresthesia, amnesia, nervousness, depression, anxiety, emotional lability,* confusion, agitation, ***suicidal ideation.***

CV: hypertension, tachycardia, palpitations.

EENT: *retinal hemorrhages,* loss of visual acuity or visual field, conjunctivitis, tinnitus, ear pain, taste perversion, *pharyngitis, sinusitis, rhinitis,* epistaxis.

GI: *abdominal pain, nausea, diarrhea, anorexia, dyspepsia, vomiting,* constipation, flatulence, toothache, hemorrhoids, decreased saliva.

GU: decreased libido, dysmenorrhea, vaginitis.

Hematologic: *granulocytopenia, **leukopenia, thrombocytopenia,*** ecchymosis, lymphadenopathy, lymphocytosis, increased PT.

Metabolic: hypothyroidism.

Respiratory: *infection, cough, congestion,* dyspnea, bronchitis.

Skin: *alopecia, pruritus, rash,* dry skin; *pain, erythema* (at injection site).

Other: *hypersensitivity reactions,* body pain, flulike symptoms (headache, fatigue, myalgia, fever), malaise.

INTERACTIONS

Drug-drug. *Drugs metabolized by cytochrome P-450:* may alter drug levels. Monitor changes in levels of these drugs. *Myelosuppressive agents:* no studies have been conducted; however, use cautiously with interferon alfacon-1. Monitor CBC and therapeutic or toxic levels of concomitant drugs.

EFFECTS ON DIAGNOSTIC TESTS

Drug may cause decreased hemoglobin, hematocrit, WBC and platelet count, and T_4 serum levels and increased serum triglycerides or thyroid-stimulating hormone (TSH).

CONTRAINDICATIONS

Contraindicated in patients with known hypersensitivity to alpha interferons, to *Escherichia coli*–derived products, or to any component of product. Also contraindicated in patients with history of severe psychiatric disorders, autoimmune hepatitis, or decompensated hepatic disease.

NURSING CONSIDERATIONS

• Use with caution in patients with history of cardiac disease and other autoimmune or endocrine disorders, in those with abnormally low peripheral blood cell counts, or those receiving agents that are known to cause myelosuppression.

• Know that depression and suicidal behavior has been associated with drug.

• The following laboratory tests should be obtained before therapy, 2 weeks after initiation, and periodically during therapy: CBC with platelets, serum creatinine, serum albumin, serum bilirubin, TSH, and T_4.

• Know that at least 48 hours should elapse between doses.

• Store drug in refrigerator at 36° to 46° F (2° to 8° C); do not freeze. Injection may be allowed to reach room temperature just before use. Avoid vigorous shaking. Discard unused portion.

Alert: If hypersensitivity reaction occurs, stop drug immediately and treat as ordered.

✓ Patient teaching

• If drug is to be used at home, instruct patient on appropriate use, dosage, and administration. A patient information leaflet is available. Also instruct patient on proper disposal procedures for needles, syringes, drug containers, and unused medicine.

• Instruct patient not to reuse needles, syringes, or reenter drug vial once initially used.

• Tell patient to discard all syringes and needles in a puncture-resistant container.

• Caution patient to inspect for discoloration and particulate matter in vial prior to use; do not use if either are observed.

• Tell patient that nonnarcotic analgesics and bedtime administration may be used to prevent or lessen the flulike symptoms associated with drug therapy.

• Instruct patient to report symptoms of depression immediately.

interferon alfa-2a, recombinant (rIFN-A)
Roferon-A

Pregnancy Risk Category: C

HOW SUPPLIED
Injection: 3, 6, 9, 36 million IU/single-use vial; 9, 18 million IU/multiple-dose vial
Sterile powder for injection: 18 million IU/vial with diluent

ACTION
Unknown. Appears to involve direct antiproliferative action against tumor cells or viral cells to inhibit replication and modulation of host immune response by enhancing the phagocytic activity of macrophages and by augmenting specific cytotoxicity of lymphocytes for target cells.

Route	Onset	Peak	Duration
IM	Unknown	2-12 hr	Unknown
SC	Unknown	3-12 hr	Unknown

INDICATIONS & DOSAGE
Hairy-cell leukemia—
Adults: for induction, 3 million IU S.C. or I.M. daily for 16 to 24 weeks. For maintenance, 3 million IU S.C. or I.M. three times weekly.
AIDS-related Kaposi's sarcoma—
Adults: for induction, 36 million IU S.C. or I.M. daily for 10 to 12 weeks. For maintenance, 36 million IU S.C. or I.M. three times weekly.
Philadelphia chromosome–positive chronic myelogenous leukemia—
Adults: initially, 3 million IU daily for 3 days; then 6 million IU for 3 days, then 9 million IU for duration of treatment.

ADVERSE REACTIONS
CNS: *dizziness, confusion,* paresthesia, numbness, lethargy, *depression, decreased mental status,* forgetfulness, **coma,** nervousness, insomnia, sedation, apathy, anxiety, irritability, fatigue, vertigo, gait disturbances, incoordination.
CV: hypotension, chest pain, ***arrhythmias,*** palpitations, syncope, ***heart failure,*** hypertension, edema, ***MI.***
EENT: *dryness or inflammation of the*
oropharynx, rhinorrhea, sinusitis, conjunctivitis, earache, eye irritation.
GI: *anorexia, nausea, diarrhea, vomiting,* abdominal fullness, *abdominal pain,* flatulence, constipation, hypermotility, gastric distress, *weight loss,* excessive salivation, *change in taste.*
GU: transient impotence.
Hematologic: *leukopenia, mild thrombocytopenia.*
Hepatic: *hepatitis.*
Respiratory: *cough, dyspnea.*
Skin: *rash,* dryness, pruritus, *partial alopecia,* urticaria, flushing, *inflammation at injection site.*
Other: *flulike syndrome (fever, fatigue, myalgia, headache, chills, arthralgia),* diaphoresis, cyanosis, night sweats, hot flashes.

INTERACTIONS
Drug-drug. *Aminophylline, theophylline:* may reduce theophylline clearance. Monitor serum levels.
Aspirin: increased risk of GI bleeding. Avoid use together.
CNS depressants: enhanced CNS effects. Avoid concomitant use.
Live virus vaccine: increased risk of adverse reactions and decreased antibody response. Don't use together.
Drug-lifestyle. *Alcohol use:* increased risk of GI bleeding. Avoid use during drug therapy.

EFFECTS ON DIAGNOSTIC TESTS
Drug may cause mild and transient changes in blood pressure (hypotension is likely). Interferons may decrease hemoglobin, hematocrit, leukocyte counts, platelets, and neutrophils (dose-related; recovery occurs within several days or weeks after drug withdrawal). Drug may increase PT and PTT (dose-related); ALT, AST, LD, and alkaline phosphatase levels (dose-related; reversible on drug withdrawal); and serum calcium, serum phosphorus, and fasting blood glucose levels; and may affect protein in the urine.

CONTRAINDICATIONS
Contraindicated in patients hypersensitive to drug, murine (mouse) immunoglobulin, or other drug components.

Reactions may be *common,* uncommon, *life-threatening,* or COMMON AND LIFE-THREATENING.

NURSING CONSIDERATIONS
• Use cautiously in patients with severe hepatic or renal function impairment, seizure disorders, compromised CNS function, cardiac disease, or myelosuppression.
• Know that depression and suicidal behavior have been associated with treatment.
• Obtain allergy history. Drug contains phenol as a preservative and serum albumin as a stabilizer.
• Use S.C. administration route in patients whose platelet count is below 50,000/mm^3.
• Administer drug at bedtime to minimize daytime drowsiness.
• Make sure patient is well hydrated, especially during initial stages of treatment.
• At beginning of therapy, assess patient for flulike symptoms, which tend to diminish with continued therapy. Premedicate with acetaminophen to minimize symptoms.
• Monitor for CNS adverse reactions, such as decreased mental status and dizziness, during therapy.
• For patients who develop thrombocytopenia, exercise extreme care in performing invasive procedures; inspect injection site and skin frequently for signs of bruising; limit frequency of I.M. injections; test urine, emesis fluid, stool, and secretions for occult blood.
• Keep in mind that severe adverse reactions may require dosage reduction to one-half or discontinuation of therapy until reactions subside.
• Know that different brands of interferon may not be equivalent and may require different dosage.
Alert: Neurotoxicity and cardiotoxicity are more common in elderly patients, especially those with underlying CNS or cardiac impairment.
• Be aware that use with blood dyscrasia-causing medications, bone marrow suppressant, or radiation therapy may increase bone marrow suppressant effects. Dosage reduction may be required.
• Keep drug refrigerated. Do not freeze.

☑**Patient teaching**
• Advise patient that laboratory tests will be performed before and periodically during therapy. Tests include a CBC with differential, platelet count, blood chemistry and electrolyte studies, liver function tests, and, if he has a preexisting cardiac disorder or advanced stages of cancer, ECG.
• Instruct patient in proper oral hygiene during treatment because the bone marrow suppressant effects of interferon may lead to microbial infection, delayed healing, and gingival bleeding. Drug may also decrease salivary flow.
• Emphasize need to follow doctor's instructions about taking and recording temperature and how and when to take acetaminophen.
• Advise patient to check with doctor for instructions after missing dose.
• Tell patient that drug may cause temporary loss of some hair, which should return when drug is withdrawn.
• If patient will be self-administering drug, teach him how to prepare and administer it and how to dispose of used needles, syringes, containers, and unused medication.
• Instruct patient not to take aspirin or alcohol because concurrent use increases risk of GI bleeding.
• Instruct patient not to change brands of interferon without medical consultation.
• Advise patients against performing tasks that require mental alertness.
• Advise patients to report signs of depression immediately.

interferon alfa-2b, recombinant (IFN-alpha 2)
Intron-A

Pregnancy Risk Category: C

HOW SUPPLIED
Powder for injection: 3, 5, 10, 18, 25, 50 million IU/vial with diluent
Injection: 3, 5 million IU/0.5-ml vial; 1, 10 million IU/1-ml vial; 18 million IU/3.8-ml vial; 25 million IU/3.2-ml vial

ACTION
Unknown. Appears to involve direct antiproliferative action against tumor cells or

viral cells to inhibit replication, and modulation of host immune response by enhancing the phagocytic activity of macrophages and by augmenting specific cytotoxicity of lymphocytes for target cells.

Route	Onset	Peak	Duration
IV	Unknown	15-60 min	4 hr
IM, SC	Unknown	3-12 hr	16 hr

INDICATIONS & DOSAGE

Hairy-cell leukemia—
Adults: 2 million IU/m² I.M. or S.C., three times weekly for 6 months or more.
Condyloma acuminata (genital or venereal warts)—
Adults: 1 million IU for each lesion intralesionally three times weekly for 3 weeks.
AIDS-related Kaposi's sarcoma—
Adults: 30 million IU/m² S.C. or I.M. three times weekly.
Chronic hepatitis B—
Adults: 30 to 35 million IU weekly I.M. or S.C., administered as 5 million IU daily or 10 million IU three times weekly for 16 weeks.
✳ *NEW INDICATION: Chronic hepatitis B—*
Children 1 year and older: 3 million IU/m² S.C. three times weekly for first week, then increase to 6 million IU/m² S.C. three times weekly (maximum is 10 million IU three times weekly) for total of 16 to 24 weeks.
Chronic hepatitis C—
Adults: 3 million IU I.M. or S.C. three times weekly.
Adjunct to surgical treatment in patients with malignant melanoma who are asymptomatic postsurgery but at high risk for systemic recurrence for up to 8 weeks after surgery—
Adults: initially, 20 million IU/m² by I.V. infusion 5 consecutive days weekly for 4 weeks, followed by maintenance dose of 10 million IU/m² S.C. three times weekly for 48 weeks.

ADVERSE REACTIONS

CNS: *dizziness, confusion, paresthesia,* lethargy, *depression, difficulty in thinking or concentrating, insomnia,* anxiety, *fatigue, hypoesthesia, amnesia,* nervousness, *somnolence,* weakness, *malaise.*

CV: hypotension, *chest pain.*
EENT: visual disturbances, hearing disorders, pharyngitis, *nasal congestion, sinusitis,* rhinitis, stye.
GI: *anorexia, nausea, diarrhea, vomiting,* abdominal pain, *dyspepsia,* constipation, loose stools, eructation, *dry mouth,* dysgeusia, stomatitis, gingivitis.
GU: transient impotence, gynecomastia.
Hematologic: *leukopenia,* anemia, *thrombocytopenia.*
Respiratory: *dyspnea, coughing.*
Skin: *rash, dryness, pruritus, alopecia,* candidiasis, flushing, dermatitis.
Other: *flulike symptoms (fever, fatigue, headache, chills, muscle aches), arthralgia, asthenia, rigors, back pain, increased diaphoresis.*

INTERACTIONS

Drug-drug. *Aminophylline, theophylline:* may reduce theophylline clearance. Monitor serum concentrations.
CNS depressants: enhanced CNS effects. Avoid concomitant use.
Live virus vaccines: risk of enhanced adverse reactions to vaccine or decreased antibody response. Postpone immunization.
Zidovudine: may be synergistic adverse effects (higher incidence of neutropenia). Carefully monitor WBC count.

EFFECTS ON DIAGNOSTIC TESTS

Drug may cause mild and transient changes in blood pressure (hypotension is likely). Interferons may decrease hemoglobin, hematocrit, leukocyte counts, platelets, and neutrophils (dose-related; recovery occurs within several days or weeks after drug withdrawal). Drug may increase PT and PTT (dose-related); ALT, AST, LD, and alkaline phosphatase levels (dose-related; reversible on drug withdrawal); and serum calcium, serum phosphorus, and fasting blood glucose levels.

CONTRAINDICATIONS

Contraindicated in patients hypersensitive to drug or its components.

NURSING CONSIDERATIONS

• Use cautiously in patients with history of CV disease, pulmonary disease, diabetes mellitus, coagulation disorders, and severe myelosuppression.

• Use S.C. administration route in patients whose platelet count is below 50,000/mm³.

• Be aware that depression and suicidal behavior has been associated with drug use and patients with preexisting psychotic disorder, especially depression, should not continue treatment with drug therapy.

• Administer drug at bedtime to minimize daytime drowsiness.

• When administering interferon for condylomata acuminata, use only 10-million-IU vial because dilution of other strengths required for intralesional use results in a hypertonic solution. Do not reconstitute 10-million-IU vial with more than 1 ml of diluent. Use tuberculin or similar syringe and 25G to 30G needle. Do not inject too deeply beneath lesion or too superficially. As many as five lesions can be treated at one time. To ease discomfort, administer in evening with acetaminophen.

• Make sure patient is well hydrated, especially during initial treatment.

• At the beginning of treatment, monitor patient for flulike symptoms, which tend to diminish with continued therapy. Premedicate patient with acetaminophen to minimize flulike symptoms.

• Periodically monitor for adverse CNS reactions, such as decreased mental status and dizziness, during therapy.

• For patients who develop thrombocytopenia: exercise extreme care in performing invasive procedures; inspect injection site and skin frequently for signs of bruising; limit frequency of I.M. injections; test urine, emesis fluid, stool, and secretions for occult blood.

• Keep in mind that severe adverse reactions may require dosage reduction to one-half or discontinuation of therapy until reactions subside.

Alert: Be aware that neurotoxicity and cardiotoxicity are more common in elderly patients, especially those with underlying CNS or cardiac impairment.

• Be aware that use with blood dyscrasia–causing medications, bone marrow suppressants, or radiation therapy may increase bone marrow suppressant effects. Dosage reduction may be required.

• In the treatment of condylomata acumi-

nata, keep in mind that maximum response usually occurs 4 to 8 weeks after initiation of therapy. If results are not satisfactory after 12 to 16 weeks, a second course may be instituted. Patients with 6 to 10 condylomata may receive a second course of treatment; patients with more than 10 condylomata may receive additional courses.

I.V. administration

• Infusion solution should be prepared immediately prior to use. Based on desired dose, appropriate vial strength(s) of drug should be reconstituted with diluent provided. Withdraw dose and inject into a 100 ml bag of 0.9% NaCl. Final concentration of drug should be not less than 10 million IU/100 ml. Infuse over 20 minutes.

✓ Patient teaching

• Advise patient to avoid contact with persons with viral illness. The patient is at increased risk for infection during therapy.

• Advise patient that laboratory tests will be performed before and periodically during therapy. Tests include a CBC with differential, platelet count, blood chemistry and electrolyte studies, liver function tests, and, if he has a preexisting cardiac disorder or advanced stages of cancer, ECG.

• Instruct patient in proper oral hygiene during treatment because bone marrow suppressant effects of interferon may lead to microbial infection, delayed healing, and gingival bleeding. Drug may also decrease salivary flow.

• Advise patient to check with doctor for instructions after missing a dose.

• Emphasize need to follow doctor's instructions about taking and recording temperature and how and when to take acetaminophen.

• If patient is to self-administer drug, teach him how to prepare the injection and how to use a disposable syringe. Give him information on drug stability.

• Tell patient drug may cause temporary loss of some hair, which should return after drug is withdrawn.

• Advise patient to notify doctor if signs of depression occur.

---

interferon beta-1a
Avonex

Pregnancy Risk Category: C

HOW SUPPLIED
Lyophilized powder for injection: 33 mcg
(6.6 million IU)

ACTION
Mechanisms by which interferon beta-1a
exerts its actions in multiple sclerosis are
not clearly understood. The biological re-
sponse-modifying properties of the drug
are mediated through its interactions with
specific cell receptors found on the surface of human cells. Binding of these receptors induces the expression of a number of interferon-induced gene products
believed to mediate the biological actions
of interferon beta-1a.

Route	Onset	Peak	Duration
IM	Unknown	3-15 hr	Unknown

INDICATIONS & DOSAGE
*Treatment of relapsing forms of multiple
sclerosis to slow the accumulation of
physical disability and decrease the frequency of clinical exacerbation—*
Adults 18 years and older: 30 mcg I.M.
once weekly.

ADVERSE REACTIONS
CNS: *headache, sleep difficulty, dizzi-
ness,* syncope, suicidal tendency, seizure,
speech disorder, ataxia.
CV: chest pain, vasodilation.
EENT: otitis media, decreased hearing,
sinusitis.
GI: *nausea, diarrhea, dyspepsia,* anorexia, abdominal pain.
GU: ovarian cyst, vaginitis.
Hematologic: anemia, elevated
eosinophil levels, decreased hematocrit.
Musculoskeletal: *muscle ache,* muscle
spasm, arthralgia.
Respiratory: *upper respiratory tract infection,* dyspnea.
Skin: ecchymosis (at injection site), injection site reaction, urticaria, alopecia,
nevus, herpes zoster, herpes simplex.
Other: *flulike symptoms, pain, fever, as-*
thenia, chills, infection, malaise, ***hypersensitivity reaction,*** elevated AST levels.

INTERACTIONS
None reported.

EFFECTS ON DIAGNOSTIC TESTS
Drug may cause increased AST level or
eosinophil count and decreased RBC
count.

CONTRAINDICATIONS
Contraindicated in patients with history
of hypersensitivity to natural or recombinant interferon beta, human albumin, or
other components of the formulation.

NURSING CONSIDERATIONS
• Use cautiously in patients with depression, seizure disorders, or severe cardiac
conditions.
• Be aware that safety and efficacy of interferon beta-1a in chronic progressive
multiple sclerosis or in children under 18
years have not been established.
• Monitor patient closely for depression
and suicidal ideation. It is not known if
these symptoms are related to the underlying neurologic basis of multiple sclerosis or to interferon beta-1a.
• Monitor WBC counts, platelet counts,
and blood chemistries, including liver
function tests.
• To reconstitute drug, inject 1.1 ml of
supplied diluent (sterile water for injection) into vial and gently swirl to dissolve
drug. Do not shake.
• Interferon beta-1a should be used as
soon as possible but may be used within 6
hours after being reconstituted if stored at
36° to 46° F (2° to 8° C).
• It is not known if drug is excreted in
breast milk. Because of potential for serious adverse reactions in breast-fed infants, a decision whether to discontinue
breast-feeding or drug must be made.

☑ Patient teaching
• Teach patient and family member how
to reconstitute drug and administer I.M.
• Caution patient not to change dosage or
schedule of administration. If a dose is
missed, tell him to take it as soon as he remembers. The regular schedule may then

be resumed. Two injections should not be administered within 2 days of each other.

• Instruct patient how to store drug.

• Inform patient that flulike symptoms are not uncommon following initiation of therapy. Acetaminophen 650 mg P.O. may be taken immediately before injection and for an additional 24 hours after each injection, as ordered, to lessen the severity of flulike symptoms.

• Advise patient to report depression, suicidal ideation, or other adverse reactions.

• Instruct patient to keep syringes and needles away from children. Also instruct him not to reuse needles or syringes and to discard them in a syringe-disposal unit.

• Caution female patient of childbearing age not to become pregnant during therapy because of potential of drug to cause spontaneous abortion. If pregnancy occurs, instruct patient to notify doctor immediately and to discontinue drug, as ordered.

• Advise patient to use sunscreen and avoid sun exposure while taking drug because photosensitization may occur.

---

interferon beta-1b, recombinant
Betaferon§, Betaseron

Pregnancy Risk Category: C

HOW SUPPLIED
Powder for injection: 9.6 million IU (0.3 mg)

ACTION
A naturally occurring antiviral and immunoregulatory agent derived from human fibroblasts. It attaches to membrane receptors and causes cellular changes, including increased protein synthesis.

Route	Onset	Peak	Duration
SC	Unknown	1-8 hr	Unknown

INDICATIONS & DOSAGE
To reduce the frequency of exacerbations in patients with relapsing-remitting multiple sclerosis—
Adults: 8 million IU (0.25 mg) S.C. every other day.

ADVERSE REACTIONS
CNS: depression, anxiety, emotional lability, depersonalization, *suicidal tendencies,* confusion, somnolence, *hypertonia, asthenia, migraine, seizures,* headache, dizziness.

CV: palpitations, hypertension, tachycardia, peripheral vascular disorder, *hemorrhage.*

EENT: laryngitis, *sinusitis, conjunctivitis,* abnormal vision.

GI: *diarrhea, constipation, abdominal pain, vomiting.*

GU: *menstrual disorders (bleeding or spotting, early or delayed menses, fewer days of menstrual flow, menorrhagia).*

Hematologic: *decreased WBC and absolute neutrophil counts.*

Respiratory: *dyspnea.*

Skin: *inflammation, pain, necrosis* (at injection site).

Other: *flulike symptoms (fever, chills, malaise, myalgia, diaphoresis), elevated ALT levels, elevated bilirubin levels,* breast pain, *pelvic pain, lymphadenopathy, pain,* generalized edema, *myasthenia, diaphoresis,* alopecia.

INTERACTIONS
None significant.

EFFECTS ON DIAGNOSTIC TESTS
Drug decreases WBC, increases AST and bilirubin, and changes serum glucose.

CONTRAINDICATIONS
Contraindicated in patients hypersensitive to interferon beta or human albumin or formulation components.

NURSING CONSIDERATIONS
• Use cautiously in women of childbearing age. Inconclusive evidence exists about drug's teratogenic effects, but it may be an abortifacient.

• To reconstitute, inject 1.2 ml of the supplied diluent (0.54% NaCl injection) into vial and gently swirl to dissolve drug. Do not shake. Reconstituted solution will contain 8 million IU (0.25 mg)/ml. Discard vials that contain particulate material or discolored solution.

• Inject immediately after preparation.

- Rotate injection sites to minimize local reactions and observe site for necrosis.
- Monitor patient for signs of depression.

☑ **Patient teaching**
- Warn female patient of childbearing age about dangers to fetus. If she becomes pregnant during therapy, tell her to notify doctor and stop taking drug.
- Teach patient how to self-administer S.C. injections, including solution preparation, use of aseptic technique, rotation of injection sites, and equipment disposal. Periodically reevaluate patient's technique.
- Advise patient to take drug at bedtime to minimize the mild flulike symptoms that commonly occur.
- Advise patient to report thoughts of suicidal ideation or depression.
- Tell patient to report signs of necrosis at injection site immediately.

---

interferon gamma-1b
Actimmune

Pregnancy Risk Category: C

HOW SUPPLIED
Injection: 100 mcg (3 million units)/ 0.5-ml vial

ACTION
Acts as an interleukin-type lymphokine. It has potent phagocyte-activating properties and enhances the oxidative metabolism of tissue macrophages.

Route	Onset	Peak	Duration
SC	Unknown	7 hr	Unknown

INDICATIONS & DOSAGE
Chronic granulomatous disease—
Adults with a body surface area (BSA) over 0.5 m²: 50 mcg/m² (1.5 million units/m²) S.C. three times weekly, preferably h.s., and in the deltoid or anterior thigh muscle.
Adults with a BSA 0.5 m² or below: 1.5 mcg/kg S.C. three times weekly.

ADVERSE REACTIONS
CNS: *fatigue,* decreased mental status, gait disturbance, dizziness.
GI: *nausea, vomiting, diarrhea,* abdominal pain.
Hematologic: *neutropenia, thrombocytopenia.*
Metabolic: elevated liver enzyme levels (at high doses).
Skin: *erythema, tenderness* (at injection site); *rash.*
Other: *flulike syndrome* (*headache, fever, chills,* myalgia, arthralgia), weight loss, back pain, proteinuria.

INTERACTIONS
Drug-drug. *Myelosuppressive agents:* possible additive myelosuppression. Monitor closely.
Zidovudine: increased plasma levels of zidovudine. Dosage adjustments are necessary when used concurrently.

EFFECTS ON DIAGNOSTIC TESTS
None reported.

CONTRAINDICATIONS
Contraindicated in patients hypersensitive to drug or to genetically engineered products derived from *Escherichia coli.*

NURSING CONSIDERATIONS
- Use cautiously in patients with cardiac disease, including arrhythmias, ischemia, or heart failure. The flulike syndrome commonly seen at high doses of drug can exacerbate these conditions.
- Use cautiously in patients with compromised CNS function or seizure disorders. CNS adverse reactions that may occur at high doses of drug can exacerbate these conditions.
- Use myelosuppressive agents together with caution.
- Premedicate with acetaminophen to minimize symptoms at the beginning of therapy. Flulike symptoms tend to diminish with continued therapy.
- Before beginning therapy and at 3-month intervals monitor CBC, platelets, renal and hepatic function tests, and urinalysis.
- Discard unused portion. Each vial is for single-dose use only and does not contain a preservative.

☑ **Patient teaching**
• If patient is to self-administer drug, teach him how to administer it and how to dispose of used needles, syringes, containers, and unused medication.
• Instruct patient how to manage flulike symptoms that commonly occur.

---

levamisole hydrochloride
Ergamisol

Pregnancy Risk Category: C

HOW SUPPLIED
Tablets: 50 mg (base)

ACTION
Unknown. Appears to restore depressed immune function and may potentiate the actions of monocytes and macrophages and enhance T-cell responses. Also, inhibits alkaline phosphatase and cholinergic activity.

Route	Onset	Peak	Duration
PO	Unknown	1.5-2 hr	Unknown

INDICATIONS & DOSAGE
Adjuvant treatment of Dukes' stage C colon cancer (with fluorouracil) after surgical resection—
Adults: 50 mg P.O. q 8 hours for 3 days, beginning no sooner than 7 days and no later than 30 days after surgery, provided that patient is out of the hospital, ambulatory, and maintaining normal oral nutrition; has well-healed wounds; and has recovered from postoperative complications. Fluorouracil (450 mg/m²/day I.V.) is given for 5 days with a 3-day course of levamisole starting 21 to 34 days after surgery.
Maintenance dosage is 50 mg P.O. q 8 hours for 3 days q 2 weeks for 1 year. Given in conjunction with fluorouracil maintenance therapy (450 mg/m²/day by rapid I.V. push once weekly, beginning 28 days after the initial 5-day course) for 1 year.
Adjust-a-dose: Dosage modifications are based on hematologic parameters. If WBC count is 2,500 to 3,500/mm³, don't administer fluorouracil as ordered until

WBC count is above 3,500/mm³. When fluorouracil is restarted, reduce dosage by 20%, as ordered. If WBC count stays below 2,500/mm³ for over 10 days after fluorouracil is withdrawn, discontinue levamisole, as ordered. If platelet count is below 100,000/mm³, therapy with both fluorouracil and levamisole should be discontinued.

ADVERSE REACTIONS
CNS: *dizziness, headache, paresthesia, somnolence, depression, nervousness, insomnia, anxiety, fatigue, fever.*
CV: chest pain, edema.
EENT: blurred vision, conjunctivitis, *stomatitis, dysgeusia, altered sense of smell.*
GI: *nausea, diarrhea, vomiting,* anorexia, abdominal pain, constipation, flatulence, dyspepsia.
Hematologic: agranulocytosis, *leukopenia, thrombocytopenia,* anemia.
Skin: dermatitis, exfoliative dermatitis, pruritus, urticaria.
Other: hyperbilirubinemia, rigors, *alopecia, infection,* arthralgia, myalgia.

INTERACTIONS
Drug-drug. *Phenytoin:* plasma levels may be elevated when administered with levamisole and fluorouracil. Monitor phenytoin plasma levels.
Warfarin sodium: may prolong coagulation times if taken together. Warfarin dose may need to be adjusted.
Drug-lifestyle. *Alcohol use:* may precipitate a disulfiram-like reaction. Avoid concomitant use.

EFFECTS ON DIAGNOSTIC TESTS
None reported.

CONTRAINDICATIONS
Contraindicated in patients hypersensitive to drug or its components.

NURSING CONSIDERATIONS
Alert: Use cautiously and with close hematologic monitoring because agranulocytosis, which is sometimes fatal, may occur. Neutropenia is usually reversible when therapy is discontinued.
• Obtain baseline CBC with differential,

---

platelet count, and electrolyte levels, and liver function studies, as ordered, immediately before starting therapy.

• Be aware that if levamisole therapy begins 7 to 20 days after surgery, fluorouracil should be started with the second course of levamisole therapy. It should begin no sooner than 21 days and no later than 34 days after surgery. If levamisole is deferred until 21 to 30 days after surgery, fluorouracil therapy should begin with the first course of levamisole.

• Know that recommended doses should not be exceeded. Higher doses are associated with greater incidence of agranulocytosis.

• Obtain CBC with differential and platelet count at weekly intervals, as ordered, before treatment with fluorouracil. Obtain electrolyte levels and liver function studies every 3 months for 1 year, as ordered.

☑ **Patient teaching**
• Tell patient to promptly report development of stomatitis or diarrhea. If either of these reactions occur during initial course of fluorouracil therapy, drug is discontinued and then weekly fluorouracil therapy is begun 28 days after start of the initial course. If stomatitis or diarrhea develops during the weekly doses of fluorouracil, fluorouracil therapy is deferred until these symptoms subside. Then fluorouracil therapy is started at reduced dosages (decrease dose by 20%).

• Advise patient to immediately report flulike symptoms.

• Advise breast-feeding patient to discontinue nursing during drug therapy.

---

oprelvekin
Neumega

Pregnancy Risk Category: C

HOW SUPPLIED
Injection: 5 mg single-dose vial with diluent

ACTION
A thrombopoietic growth factor that directly stimulates the proliferation of hematopoietic stem cells and megakaryocyte progenitor cells. It also induces megakaryocyte maturation, resulting in increased platelet production.

Route	Onset	Peak	Duration
SC	Unknown	3-5 hr	Unknown

INDICATIONS & DOSAGE
Prevention of severe thrombocytopenia and reduction of need for platelet transfusions following myelosuppressive chemotherapy with nonmyeloid malignancies—
Adults: 50 mcg/kg as a single daily S.C. injection.

ADVERSE REACTIONS
CNS: *asthenia, headache, insomnia, dizziness,* paresthesia.
CV: *tachycardia, palpitations,* ATRIAL FLUTTER OR FIBRILLATION, *syncope.*
EENT: blurred vision, *conjunctival injection,* eye hemorrhage.
GI: *oral candidiasis, nausea, vomiting, diarrhea.*
Respiratory: dyspnea, cough, pharyngitis, pleural effusions.
Skin: *rash,* skin discoloration, exfoliative dermatitis.
Other: dehydration, *edema.*

INTERACTIONS
Drug-drug. *Diuretics, ifosfamide:* severe hypokalemia resulting in death has occurred in patients concomitantly receiving these drugs and oprelvekin. Use with caution.

EFFECTS ON DIAGNOSTIC TESTS
Drug may cause a decrease in hemoglobin concentration and calcium levels because of plasma expansion.

CONTRAINDICATIONS
Contraindicated in patients with history of hypersensitivity to drug or its components.

NURSING CONSIDERATIONS
• Administer S.C. in the abdomen, thigh, hip, or upper arm.
• Dosing should begin 6 to 24 hours following completion of chemotherapy and

---

Reactions may be *common,* uncommon, *life-threatening,* or COMMON AND LIFE-THREATENING.

discontinued at least 2 days before starting the next planned cycle of chemotherapy.
- Each single-dose vial needs to be reconstituted with 1 ml of the supplied diluent. Avoid excessive or vigorous agitation. Discard unused portions.
- Use reconstituted drug within 3 hours.
- Store drug and diluent in the refrigerator until ready to use.
- Use drug cautiously in patients with heart failure because of fluid retention.
- Closely monitor fluid and electrolyte status in patients receiving chronic diuretic therapy.
- Obtain a CBC before chemotherapy and at regular intervals during drug therapy.
- Fluid retention can be severe; monitor closely.

☑ **Patient teaching**
- Instruct patient about appropriate preparation and administration of drug if he is to self-administer at home.
- Tell patient to report adverse effects. Warn him about potential adverse effects.
- Tell patient to keep drug refrigerated and not to reconstitute until before use.
- Advise patient to call doctor immediately if swelling, rapid heart beat, or difficulty breathing occurs.
- Tell patient to report evidence of increased bleeding or bruising.

---

sargramostim
(granulocyte-macrophage colony–stimulating factor; GM-CSF)
Leukine

Pregnancy Risk Category: C

HOW SUPPLIED
Powder for injection: 250 mcg, 500 mcg; liquid: 500 mcg/ml

ACTION
A glycoprotein containing 127 amino acids manufactured by recombinant DNA technology in a yeast expression system. It differs from the natural human granulocyte-macrophage colony–stimulating factor by substitution of leucine for arginine at position 23. The carbohydrate moiety may also be different. Sargramostim induces cellular responses by binding to specific receptors on cell surfaces of target cells.

Route	Onset	Peak	Duration
IV, SC	15 min	2-4 hr	Unknown

INDICATIONS & DOSAGE
Acceleration of hematopoietic reconstitution after autologous bone marrow transplantation in patients with malignant lymphoma or acute lymphoblastic leukemia or during autologous bone marrow transplantation in patients with Hodgkin's disease—
Adults: 250 mcg/m^2 daily for 21 consecutive days given as 2-hour I.V. infusion beginning 2 to 4 hours after bone marrow transplantation.
Bone marrow transplantation failure or engraftment delay—
Adults: 250 mcg/m^2/day for 14 days as 2-hour I.V. infusion. Dose may be repeated after 7 days of no therapy. If engraftment still has not occurred, a third course of 500 mcg/m^2/day I.V. for 14 days may be attempted after another therapy-free 7 days.
Adjust-a-dose: Stimulation of marrow precursors may result in rapid rise of WBC count. If blast cells appear or increase to 10% or more of WBC count or if progression of the underlying disease occurs, discontinue therapy. If absolute neutrophil count is above 20,000/mm^3 or if platelet count is above 50,000/ mm^3, temporarily discontinue drug or reduce dose by 50%.

ADVERSE REACTIONS
CNS: *malaise, CNS disorders, asthenia.*
CV: *blood dyscrasias, edema,* hemorrhage, ***supraventricular arrhythmias,*** pericardial effusion.
GI: *nausea, vomiting, diarrhea, anorexia, hemorrhage, GI disorders, stomatitis.*
GU: *urinary tract disorder,* abnormal kidney function.
Hepatic: *liver damage.*
Respiratory: *dyspnea, lung disorders,* pleural effusion.
Skin: *alopecia, rash.*

Other: *fever, mucous membrane disorder, peripheral edema,* SEPSIS.

INTERACTIONS
Drug-drug. *Corticosteroids, lithium:* may potentiate myeloproliferative effects of sargramostim. Use cautiously together.

EFFECTS ON DIAGNOSTIC TESTS
None reported. Because hematopoiesis is stimulated, effects on CBC and differential blood counts will occur.

CONTRAINDICATIONS
Contraindicated in patients with excessive leukemic myeloid blasts in bone marrow or peripheral blood and in those with hypersensitivity to drug or its components or to yeast-derived products.

NURSING CONSIDERATIONS
• Use cautiously in patients with preexisting cardiac disease, hypoxia, preexisting fluid retention, pulmonary infiltrates, heart failure, or impaired renal or hepatic function because these conditions may be exacerbated.
• Anticipate reducing dose by 50% or temporarily discontinue if severe adverse reactions occur, and notify doctor. Therapy may be resumed when reactions abate. Transient rash and local reactions at injection site may occur; no serious allergic or anaphylactic reactions have been reported.
• Do not administer within 24 hours of last dose of chemotherapy or within 12 hours of last dose of radiotherapy because rapidly dividing progenitor cells may be sensitive to these cytotoxic therapies and drug would be ineffective.
• Monitor CBC with differential, including examination for presence of blast cells biweekly, as ordered.
• Be aware that drug is effective in accelerating myeloid recovery in patients receiving bone marrow that is either unpurged or purged by anti–B cell monoclonal antibodies as compared to patients that receive bone marrow that is chemically purged.
• Be aware that drug may have a limited response in transplant patients who have received extensive radiotherapy or in patients who have received multiple myelotoxic agents.
• Keep in mind that drug can act as a growth factor for any tumor type, particularly myeloid malignant disease.

◖ I.V. administration
• Reconstitute with 1 ml of sterile water for injection. Direct stream of sterile water against side of vial and *gently swirl* contents to minimize foaming. Avoid excessive or vigorous agitation or shaking. Dilute in 0.9% NaCl solution. If final concentration is below 10 mcg/ml, add human albumin at final concentration of 0.1% to NaCl solution *before* adding sargramostim to prevent adsorption to components of the delivery system. For a final concentration of 0.1% human albumin, add 1 mg human albumin/1 ml NaCl (dilute 1 ml of 5% human albumin in 50 ml of NaCl). Administer as soon as possible after mixing and no later than 6 hours after reconstituting.
• Don't add other medications to infusion solution because no data exist regarding solution compatibility and stability.
• Do not use in-line filter for I.V. administration.

☑ Patient teaching
• Review administration schedule with patient and caregivers, and address their concerns.
• Instruct patient to report adverse reactions promptly.

---

bacitracin
chloramphenicol
ciprofloxacin hydrochloride
erythromycin
gentamicin sulfate
natamycin
norfloxacin
ofloxacin 0.3%
polymyxin B sulfate
silver nitrate 1%
sulfacetamide sodium 10%
sulfacetamide sodium 15%
sulfacetamide sodium 30%
tobramycin
vidarabine

COMBINATION PRODUCTS

AK-POLY-BAC: polymyxin B sulfate 10,000 units and bacitracin zinc 500 units.

BLEPHAMIDE STERILE OPHTHALMIC OINTMENT: sulfacetamide sodium 10% and prednisolone acetate 0.2%.

CETAPRED OINTMENT: sulfacetamide sodium 10% and prednisolone acetate 0.25%.

CORTISPORIN OPHTHALMIC OINTMENT: polymyxin B sulfate 10,000 units, bacitracin zinc 400 units, neomycin sulfate 0.35%, and hydrocortisone 1%.

CORTISPORIN OPHTHALMIC SUSPENSION: polymyxin B sulfate 10,000 units, neomycin sulfate 0.35%, and hydrocortisone 1%.

ISOPTO CETAPRED: sulfacetamide sodium 10% and prednisolone acetate 0.25%.

MAXITROL OINTMENT/OPHTHALMIC SUSPENSION: dexamethasone 0.1%, neomycin sulfate 0.35%, and polymyxin B sulfate 10,000 units.

METIMYD OPHTHALMIC OINTMENT/SUSPENSION: sulfacetamide sodium 10% and prednisolone acetate 0.5%.

NEOSPORIN OPHTHALMIC OINTMENT: polymyxin B sulfate 10,000 units, neomycin sulfate 3.5 mg, and bacitracin zinc 400 units/g.

NEOSPORIN OPHTHALMIC SOLUTION: polymyxin B sulfate 10,000 units, neomycin sulfate 1.75 mg, and gramicidin 0.025 mg.

POLYSPORIN OPHTHALMIC OINTMENT: polymyxin B sulfate 10,000 units and bacitracin zinc 500 units.

POLYTRIM OPHTHALMIC: trimethoprim sulfate 1 mg and polymyxin B sulfate 10,000 units/ml.

PRED-G S.O.P.: prednisolone acetate 0.6%, gentamicin sulfate equivalent to gentamicin base 0.3%.

TOBRADEX: dexamethasone 0.1%, tobramycin 0.3%.

VASOCIDIN OPHTHALMIC OINTMENT: sulfacetamide sodium 10% and prednisolone acetate 0.5%.

VASOCIDIN OPHTHALMIC SOLUTION: sulfacetamide sodium 10% and prednisolone phosphate 0.25%.

VASOSULF: sulfacetamide sodium 15% and phenylephrine hydrochloride 0.125%.

bacitracin
AK-Tracin

Pregnancy Risk Category: C

HOW SUPPLIED
Ophthalmic ointment: 500 units/g

ACTION
Inhibits bacterial cell wall synthesis. Bactericidal or bacteriostatic, depending on concentration and infection.

Route	Onset	Peak	Duration
Ophthalmic	Unknown	Unknown	Unknown

INDICATIONS & DOSAGE
Surface bacterial infections involving conjunctiva and cornea—
Adults and children: small amount of ointment applied into conjunctival sac one or more times daily or p.r.n. until favorable response is observed.

---

*Liquid contains alcohol.   **May contain tartrazine.   †Canada   ‡Australia   §U.K.   ◊OTC

ADVERSE REACTIONS
EENT: slowed corneal wound healing, temporary visual haze.
Other: overgrowth of nonsusceptible organisms.

INTERACTIONS
Drug-drug. *Heavy metals (such as silver nitrate):* inactivation of bacitracin. Don't use together.

EFFECTS ON DIAGNOSTIC TESTS
Urinary sediment tests may show increased protein and cast excretion. Serum creatinine and BUN levels may increase during drug therapy.

CONTRAINDICATIONS
Contraindicated in patients with atopy or hypersensitivity to drug.

NURSING CONSIDERATIONS
• Ophthalmic ointment may be stored at room temperature.
• Clean eye area of excessive exudate before application.

☑ **Patient teaching**
• Teach patient how to apply; tell him only a small amount of ointment is needed and that it may cause blurred vision. Advise him to wash hands before and after administering and not to touch tip of tube to eye or surrounding tissue.
• Instruct patient to stop drug and notify doctor of signs of sensitivity (itching lids, swelling, constant burning, or failure to heal).
• Tell patient not to share medication, washcloths, or towels with family members and to notify doctor if anyone develops same symptoms.
• Stress importance of compliance with recommended therapy.
• Advise patient not to allow the tip of the dispenser to touch the eye, eyelid, fingers, or other surfaces.
• Watch for signs and symptoms of super-infection.

chloramphenicol
AK-Chlor, Chloromycetin Ophthalmic, Chloroptic, Chloroptic S.O.P., Chlorsig‡, Dioptic†, Ophthochlor Ophthalmic Solution, Pentamycetin†, Sno-Phenicol§, Sopamycetin†

Pregnancy Risk Category: C

HOW SUPPLIED
Ophthalmic ointment: 1%
Ophthalmic solution: 0.5%
Powder for ophthalmic solution: 25 mg/vial

ACTION
Inhibits protein synthesis. Bacteriostatic or bactericidal, depending on concentration.

Route	Onset	Peak	Duration
Ophthalmic	Unknown	Unknown	Unknown

INDICATIONS & DOSAGE
Surface bacterial infection involving conjunctiva or cornea—
Adults and children: 1 or 2 drops of solution instilled in eye q 3 to 6 hours or more frequently, if necessary. Or, a small amount of ointment applied to lower conjunctival sac q 3 to 6 hours or more frequently, if necessary. Continued for at least 48 hours after eye appears normal.

ADVERSE REACTIONS
EENT: optic atrophy in children, stinging or burning of eye after instillation, blurred vision (with ointment).
Hematologic: *bone marrow hypoplasia* (with prolonged use), *aplastic anemia.*
Skin: dermatitis.
Other: overgrowth of nonsusceptible organisms; *hypersensitivity reactions,* including itching and burning eye, *angioedema.*

INTERACTIONS
None significant.

EFFECTS ON DIAGNOSTIC TESTS
False elevation of urinary PABA levels will result if drug is administered during a

---

bentiromide test for pancreatic function. Drug therapy will cause false-positive results on tests for urine glucose level using cupric sulfate (Clinitest). Platelet, RBC, and WBC counts in the blood and possibly the bone marrow may decrease during drug therapy (from reversible or irreversible bone marrow depression). Hemoglobinuria or lactic acidosis may also occur.

CONTRAINDICATIONS
Contraindicated in patients hypersensitive to drug.

NURSING CONSIDERATIONS
• If chloramphenicol drops are to be given every hour and then tapered, follow order closely to ensure adequate anterior chamber levels.
• Reconstitute powder for ophthalmic solution with supplied diluent. Use 5 ml of diluent to make a 0.5% solution, 10 ml of diluent to make a 0.25% solution, or 15 ml to make a 0.16% solution.
• Store in tightly closed, light-resistant container.
• If patient has more than a superficial infection, anticipate using systemic therapy as well.

☑ Patient teaching
• Teach patient how to instill drops or apply ointment. Advise him to wash hands before and after administering ointment or solution, and warn him not to touch tip of applicator to eye or surrounding tissue.
• Tell patient to clean eye area of excessive exudate before application.
• Instruct patient to apply light finger pressure on lacrimal sac for 1 minute after drops are instilled.
• Tell patient that vision may be blurred for a few minutes after application of ointment.
• Tell patient not to share medication, washcloths, or towels with family members and to notify doctor if anyone develops same symptoms.
• Instruct patient to stop drug and notify doctor of sensitivity (itching lids, swelling, or constant burning).
• Tell patient to notify doctor if no improvement occurs in 3 days.

• Stress importance of compliance with recommended therapy.
• Instruct patient to watch for signs of superinfection.

---

ciprofloxacin hydrochloride
Ciloxan

Pregnancy Risk Category: C

HOW SUPPLIED
Ophthalmic solution: 0.3% (base) in 2.5- and 5-ml containers

ACTION
Inhibits bacterial DNA gyrase, an enzyme necessary for bacterial replication. Bacteriostatic or bactericidal, depending on concentration.

Route	Onset	Peak	Duration
Ophthalmic	Unknown	Unknown	Unknown

INDICATIONS & DOSAGE
Corneal ulcers caused by Pseudomonas aeruginosa, Staphylococcus aureus, S. epidermidis, Streptococcus pneumoniae, *and possibly* Serratia marcescens *and* Streptococcus viridans—
Adults and children over 12 years: 2 drops in affected eye q 15 minutes for first 6 hours; then 2 drops q 30 minutes for remainder of first day. On day 2, 2 drops hourly. On days 3 to 14, 2 drops q 4 hours.
Bacterial conjunctivitis caused by Haemophilus influenzae, S. aureus *and* S. epidermidis *and possibly* Streptococcus pneumoniae—
Adults and children over 12 years: 1 or 2 drops into the conjunctival sac of affected eye q 2 hours while awake for first 2 days. Then 1 or 2 drops q 4 hours while awake for next 5 days.

ADVERSE REACTIONS
EENT: *local burning or discomfort, white crystalline precipitate* (in superficial portion of corneal defect in patients with corneal ulcers), *margin crusting, crystals or scales, foreign body sensation, itching, conjunctival hyperemia,* bad or bitter taste in mouth, corneal staining, al-

lergic reactions, keratopathy, lid edema, tearing, photophobia, decreased vision.
GI: nausea.

INTERACTIONS
None significant.

EFFECTS ON DIAGNOSTIC TESTS
None reported.

CONTRAINDICATIONS
Contraindicated in patients with history of hypersensitivity to ciprofloxacin or other fluoroquinolone antibiotics.

NURSING CONSIDERATIONS
• Be aware that it is unknown if drug is excreted in breast milk after application to eye; however, systemically administered ciprofloxacin has been detected in human milk. Use with caution in breast-feeding patients.
Alert: Discontinue drug at first sign of hypersensitivity reactions, such as rash, and notify doctor. Serious hypersensitivity reactions, including anaphylaxis, have occurred in patients receiving systemic fluoroquinolone therapy.
• Know that a topical overdose may be flushed from the eyes with warm tap water.
• If corneal epithelium is still compromised after 14 days of treatment, continue therapy, as ordered.
• Institute appropriate therapy if superinfection occurs. Prolonged use may result in overgrowth of nonsusceptible organisms, including fungi.

☑ **Patient teaching**
• Tell patient to clean eye area of excessive exudate before instilling.
• Teach patient how to instill drops. Advise him to wash hands before and after administering solution and not to touch tip of dropper to eye or surrounding tissues.
• Instruct patient to apply light finger pressure on lacrimal sac for 1 minute after drops are instilled.
• Tell patient not to share medication, washcloths, or towels with family members and to notify doctor if anyone develops same symptoms.
• Stress importance of compliance with recommended therapy.

---

erythromycin
Ilotycin Ophthalmic Ointment

Pregnancy Risk Category: B

HOW SUPPLIED
Ophthalmic ointment: 0.5%

ACTION
Inhibits protein synthesis. Bacteriostatic, but may be bactericidal in high concentrations or against highly susceptible organisms.

Route	Onset	Peak	Duration
Ophthalmic	Unknown	Unknown	Unknown

INDICATIONS & DOSAGE
Acute and chronic conjunctivitis, other eye infections—
Adults and children: a ribbon of ointment approximately 1 cm long applied directly to infected eye up to six times daily, depending on severity of infection.
Chlamydial ophthalmic infections (trachoma)—
Adults and children: a small amount applied to each eye b.i.d. for 2 months or b.i.d. the first 5 days of each month for 6 months.
Prophylaxis of ophthalmia neonatorum due to Neisseria gonorrhoeae *or* Chlamydia trachomatis—
Neonates: a ribbon of ointment approximately 1 cm long applied in lower conjunctival sac of each eye shortly after birth.

ADVERSE REACTIONS
EENT: slowed corneal wound healing, blurred vision.
Skin: urticaria, dermatitis.
Other: overgrowth of nonsusceptible organisms (with long-term use); hypersensitivity reactions, including itching and burning eyes.

INTERACTIONS
None significant.

EFFECTS ON DIAGNOSTIC TESTS
Drug may interfere with fluorometric determinations of urinary catecholamines.

Reactions may be *common,* uncommon, *life-threatening,* or COMMON AND LIFE-THREATENING.

Liver function test results may become abnormal during drug therapy (rare).

CONTRAINDICATIONS
Contraindicated in patients hypersensitive to drug.

NURSING CONSIDERATIONS
• For prophylaxis of ophthalmia neonatorum, apply ointment no later than 1 hour after birth. Used in neonates born either by vaginal delivery or by cesarean section. Gently massage the eyelids for 1 minute to spread the ointment.
• To be used only when sensitivity studies show it is effective against infecting organisms. Not for use in infections of unknown etiology.
• Use cautiously in breast-feeding women.
• Store at room temperature in tightly closed, light-resistant container.

☑ **Patient teaching**
• Tell patient to clean eye area of excessive exudate before application.
• Teach patient how to apply. Advise him to wash hands before and after administering ointment, and warn him not to touch tip of applicator to eye or surrounding tissue.
• Tell patient that vision may be blurred for a few minutes after application of ointment.
• Advise patient to watch for and report signs of sensitivity (itching lids, redness, swelling, or constant burning).
• Tell patient not to share medication, washcloths, or towels with family members and to notify doctor if anyone develops same symptoms.
• Stress importance of compliance with recommended therapy.

---

gentamicin sulfate
Cidomycin§, Garamycin Ophthalmic, Genoptic, Gentacidin, Gentak, Genticin§, Ocu-Mycin

Pregnancy Risk Category: C

HOW SUPPLIED
Ophthalmic ointment: 0.3% (base)
Ophthalmic solution: 0.3% (base)

ACTION
Unknown. Thought to inhibit protein synthesis and is usually bactericidal.

Route	Onset	Peak	Duration
Ophthalmic	Unknown	Unknown	Unknown

INDICATIONS & DOSAGE
External ocular infections (conjunctivitis, keratoconjunctivitis, corneal ulcers, blepharitis, blepharoconjunctivitis, meibomianitis, and dacryocystitis) caused by susceptible organisms, especially Pseudomonas aeruginosa, Proteus, Klebsiella pneumoniae, Escherichia coli, *and other gram-negative organisms—*
Adults and children: 1 to 2 drops instilled in eye q 4 hours. In severe infections, up to 2 drops q hour. Alternatively, ointment applied to lower conjunctival sac b.i.d. or t.i.d.

ADVERSE REACTIONS
EENT: burning, stinging, or blurred vision (with ointment), transient irritation (from solution), conjunctival hyperemia.
Other: hypersensitivity reactions; overgrowth of nonsusceptible organisms with long-term use.
Systemic absorption from excessive use may cause systemic toxicities.

INTERACTIONS
None significant.

EFFECTS ON DIAGNOSTIC TESTS
Drug-induced nephrotoxicity may elevate BUN, nonprotein nitrogen, or serum creatinine levels and increase urinary excretion of casts.

CONTRAINDICATIONS
Contraindicated in patients hypersensitive to drug.

NURSING CONSIDERATIONS
• Use cautiously in patients with history of sensitivity to aminoglycosides because cross-sensitivity may occur.
• Have culture taken before giving drug. Therapy may begin before culture results are known.
• If ophthalmic gentamicin is given con-

comitantly with systemic gentamicin, monitor serum gentamicin levels.

• Know that solution is not for injection into the conjunctiva or anterior chamber of the eye.

• Store away from heat.

✅**Patient teaching**

• Tell patient to clean eye area of excessive exudate before instilling.

• Teach patient how to instill drops or apply ointment. Advise him to wash hands before and after administering ointment or solution and not to touch tip of dropper or tube to eye or surrounding tissues.

• Instruct patient to apply light finger pressure on lacrimal sac for 1 minute after drops are instilled.

• Instruct patient to stop drug and notify doctor of signs of sensitivity (itching lids, swelling, or constant burning).

• Advise patient not to share medication, washcloths, or towels with family members and to notify doctor if anyone develops same symptoms.

• Tell patient that vision may be blurred for a few minutes after application of ointment.

Alert: Stress importance of following recommended therapy. *Pseudomonas* infections can cause complete vision loss within 24 hours if infection is not controlled.

---

natamycin
Natacyn

Pregnancy Risk Category: C

HOW SUPPLIED
Ophthalmic suspension: 5%

ACTION
Increases fungal cell-membrane permeability.

Route	Onset	Peak	Duration
Ophthalmic	Unknown	Unknown	Unknown

INDICATIONS & DOSAGE
Fungal keratitis—
Adults: initially, 1 drop instilled in conjunctival sac q 1 to 2 hours. After 3 to 4 days, dosage reduced to 1 drop six to eight times daily.

Blepharitis or fungal conjunctivitis—
Adults: 1 drop instilled q 4 to 6 hours.

ADVERSE REACTIONS
EENT: ocular edema, hyperemia, conjunctival chemosis.

INTERACTIONS
None significant.

EFFECTS ON DIAGNOSTIC TESTS
None reported.

CONTRAINDICATIONS
Contraindicated in patients hypersensitive to drug.

NURSING CONSIDERATIONS
• Administer drug as ordered for 14 to 21 days or until active disease subsides. Be prepared to reduce dosage gradually at 4- to 7-day intervals, as ordered, to ensure that organism has been eliminated. If infection does not improve within 7 to 10 days of therapy, clinical and laboratory reevaluation is recommended.

• Shake well before use. Refrigerate or store at room temperature.

• Know that drug is the only antifungal available as ophthalmic preparation.

✅**Patient teaching**

• Tell patient to clean eye area of excessive exudate before application.

• Teach patient how to instill drops. Advise him to wash hands before and after administering solution and not to touch tip of dropper to eye or surrounding tissue.

• Instruct patient to apply light finger pressure on lacrimal sac for 1 minute after drops are instilled.

• Tell patient not to share medication, washcloths, or towels with family members and to notify doctor if anyone develops same symptoms.

• Stress importance of compliance with recommended therapy.

Reactions may be *common,* uncommon, *life-threatening*, or COMMON AND LIFE-THREATENING.

norfloxacin
Chibroxin

Pregnancy Risk Category: C

HOW SUPPLIED
Ophthalmic solution: 0.3% in 5-ml containers

ACTION
Inhibits bacterial DNA gyrase, an enzyme necessary for bacterial replication. Bacteriostatic or bactericidal, depending on concentration.

Route	Onset	Peak	Duration
Ophthalmic	Unknown	Unknown	Unknown

INDICATIONS & DOSAGE
Conjunctivitis caused by susceptible strains of bacteria—
Adults and children 1 year and older: 1 drop in affected eye q.i.d. for up to 7 days. In severe infections, 1 or 2 drops q 2 hours while awake for first 1 to 2 days of treatment.

ADVERSE REACTIONS
EENT: local burning or discomfort, itching, chemosis, photophobia, conjunctival hyperemia, white crystalline precipitates, lid margin crusting, bad or bitter taste in mouth, *hypersensitivity reactions.*
GI: nausea.

INTERACTIONS
Drug-drug. *Cyclosporine, theophylline:* impaired metabolism of these drugs with systemic norfloxacin. It's unknown if ophthalmic norfloxacin will have this effect. Monitor closely.
Oral anticoagulants: enhanced activity with systemic norfloxacin. It's unknown if ophthalmic norfloxacin will have this effect. Monitor closely.
Drug-food. *Caffeine:* impaired metabolism with systemic norfloxacin. It's unknown if ophthalmic norfloxacin will have this effect. Monitor closely.

EFFECTS ON DIAGNOSTIC TESTS
None reported.

CONTRAINDICATIONS
Contraindicated in patients with history of hypersensitivity to norfloxacin or other fluoroquinolone antibiotics. Drug should not be injected into eye.

NURSING CONSIDERATIONS
● Be aware that drug is indicated for treating conjunctivitis when caused by susceptible bacteria. Known susceptible strains include *Acinetobacter calcoaceticus, Aeromonas hydrophila, Haemophilus influenzae, Proteus mirabilis, Serratia marcescens, Staphylococcus aureus, S. epidermidis, S. warnerii,* and *Streptococcus pneumoniae.*
Alert: Discontinue drug at first sign of hypersensitivity, such as rash, and notify doctor. Serious hypersensitivity reactions, including anaphylaxis, have occurred in patients receiving systemic fluoroquinolone therapy.
● Institute appropriate therapy if superinfection occurs. Prolonged use may result in overgrowth of nonsusceptible organisms, including fungi.
● Know that although systemically administered fluoroquinolones have been shown to cause arthropathy in young animals, ophthalmic norfloxacin has not produced this adverse effect.

☑Patient teaching
● Tell patient to clean eye area of excessive exudate before application.
● Teach patient how to instill drops. Advise him to wash hands before and after administering and not to touch the tip of the tube or dropper to eye or surrounding tissue.
● Instruct patient to apply light finger pressure on lacrimal sac for 1 minute after drops are instilled.
● Tell patient not to share medication, washcloths, or towels with family members and to notify doctor if anyone develops same symptoms.
● Stress importance of compliance with recommended therapy.

---

ofloxacin 0.3%
Exocin§, Ocuflox

Pregnancy Risk Category: C

HOW SUPPLIED
Ophthalmic solution: 0.3% in 1-ml, 5-ml, and 10-ml solution

ACTION
Bactericidal; inhibits bacterial DNA gyrase, an enzyme necessary for bacterial replication.

Route	Onset	Peak	Duration
Ophthalmic	Unknown	Unknown	Unknown

INDICATIONS & DOSAGE
Conjunctivitis caused by Staphylococcus aureus, S. epidermidis, Streptococcus pneumoniae, Enterobacter cloacae, Haemophilus influenzae, Proteus mirabilis, Pseudomonas aeruginosa, *and* Propionibacterium acnes—
Adults and children over 1 year: 1 to 2 drops in conjunctival sac q 2 to 4 hours daily, while awake, for first 2 days and then q.i.d. for up to 5 additional days.
Bacterial corneal ulcer caused by S. aureus, S. epidermidis, S. pneumoniae, E. cloacae, H. influenzae, P. mirabilis, P. aeruginosa, Serratia marcescens, *and* P. acnes—
Adults and children older than 1 year: 1 to 2 drops q 30 minutes while awake and 1 to 2 drops 4 to 6 hours after retiring on days 1 and 2. Days 3 to 7, 1 to 2 drops hourly while awake. Days 7 to 9, 1 to 2 drops q.i.d.

ADVERSE REACTIONS
CNS: dizziness (rare).
EENT: *transient ocular burning or discomfort,* stinging, redness, itching, photophobia, lacrimation, eye dryness.

INTERACTIONS
None significant.

EFFECTS ON DIAGNOSTIC TESTS
Drug may increase blood glucose levels.

CONTRAINDICATIONS
Contraindicated in patients with history of hypersensitivity to ofloxacin, to other fluoroquinolones, or to any of components of drug; and in breast-feeding women.

NURSING CONSIDERATIONS
Alert: Know that drug should not be injected into the conjunctiva or introduced directly into the anterior chamber of the eye.
• Be aware that drug should be discontinued if improvement does not occur within 7 days. Prolonged use may result in overgrowth of nonsusceptible organisms, including fungi.

☑ **Patient teaching**
• If an allergic reaction occurs, tell patient to discontinue drug and call doctor. Serious acute hypersensitivity reactions may require emergency treatment.
• Teach patient how to instill drops. Advise him to wash hands before and after instilling solution, and warn him not to touch tip of the dropper to eye or surrounding tissue.
• Advise patient to apply light finger pressure on lacrimal sac for 1 minute after drug instillation.
• Tell patient not to share medication, washcloths, or towels with family members and to notify doctor if anyone develops same symptoms.
• Stress importance of compliance with recommended therapy.
• Warn patient not to use leftover medication for a new eye infection.
• Remind patient to discard drug when no longer needed.

polymyxin B sulfate
Polyfax§

Pregnancy Risk Category: C

HOW SUPPLIED
Ophthalmic sterile powder for solution: 500,000-unit vials to be reconstituted to 20 to 50 ml

---

ACTION
Bactericidal. Alters the osmotic barrier of the bacteria cell membrane.

Route	Onset	Peak	Duration
Ophthalmic	Unknown	Unknown	Unknown

INDICATIONS & DOSAGE
Used alone or in combination with other agents to treat superficial eye infections involving the conjunctiva and cornea resulting from infection with Pseudomonas *or other gram-negative organism—*
Adults and children: 1 to 3 drops of 0.1% to 0.25% (10,000 to 25,000 units/ml) instilled q hour. Interval increased based on patient response; or up to 10,000 units injected subconjunctivally daily.

ADVERSE REACTIONS
EENT: eye irritation, conjunctivitis.
Other: overgrowth of nonsusceptible organisms, hypersensitivity reactions (local burning, itching).

INTERACTIONS
None significant.

EFFECTS ON DIAGNOSTIC TESTS
BUN and serum creatinine levels may increase during drug therapy.

CONTRAINDICATIONS
Contraindicated in patients hypersensitive to drug. Drug is not for injection into the eye or the anterior chamber of the eye.

NURSING CONSIDERATIONS
• Reconstitute carefully to ensure correct drug concentration in solution.
• Know that drug is often used in combination with neomycin sulfate.
• Be aware that drug is one of the most effective antibiotics against gram-negative organisms, especially *Pseudomonas.*
• In severe, life-threatening *Pseudomonas* infections, know that polymyxin B may be used as an ocular irrigant.

☑ **Patient teaching**
• Tell patient to clean eye area of excessive exudate before application.
• Teach patient how to instill drops. Advise him to wash hands before and after administering solution, and warn him not to touch tip of dropper to eye or surrounding tissue.
• Instruct patient to apply light finger pressure on lacrimal sac for 1 minute after drops are instilled.
• Advise patient to watch for and report signs of sensitivity (itching lids, swelling, or constant burning).
• Tell patient not to share medication, washcloths, or towels with family members and to notify doctor if anyone develops same symptoms.
• Stress importance of compliance with recommended therapy.

silver nitrate 1%

Pregnancy Risk Category: C

HOW SUPPLIED
Ophthalmic solution: 1%

ACTION
Causes protein denaturation, which prevents gonorrheal ophthalmia neonatorum. Bacteriostatic, germicidal, astringent, caustic, and escharotic.

Route	Onset	Peak	Duration
Ophthalmic	Unknown	Unknown	Unknown

INDICATIONS & DOSAGE
Prevention of gonorrheal ophthalmia neonatorum—
Neonates: clean eyelids thoroughly; 2 drops of 1% solution instilled into the lower conjunctival sac of each eye at the angle of the nasal bridge and eyes, preferably immediately after delivery but no later than 1 hour after delivery. The eyelids should be separated and elevated to allow the solution to come in contact with the entire conjunctival sac.

ADVERSE REACTIONS
EENT: periorbital edema, redness, temporary staining of lids and surrounding tissue, *conjunctivitis.*

INTERACTIONS

Drug-drug. *Bacitracin:* inactivation of silver nitrate. Don't use together.
Sulfonamides: incompatible with silver preparations. Don't use together.

EFFECTS ON DIAGNOSTIC TESTS

None reported.

CONTRAINDICATIONS

No known contraindications.

NURSING CONSIDERATIONS

• Always wash hands before instilling solution.
• Always clean the eyelids with sterile cotton and sterile water prior to instillation.
• Apply within 1 hour of birth, as ordered. Used in neonates born either by vaginal delivery or by cesarean section.
• Be aware that instillation may be delayed slightly to allow neonate to bond with mother.
• Don't use repeatedly.
• Never use concentrations greater than 1% in the eye.
• If a concentrated solution is accidentally used in eye, promptly irrigate with 0.9% NaCl solution to prevent severe eye irritation or blindness.
• Handle carefully. Solution may stain skin and utensils.
• Know that prophylaxis against gonococcal ophthalmia neonatorum is legally required for neonates in most states. Because of a high incidence of conjunctivitis (more than 90%), many clinicians prefer antibiotic ointments, such as erythromycin, as an alternative.
• Store wax ampules away from light and heat. Do not freeze or use when cold.

☑ **Patient teaching**

• Inform parents of need for drug and explain how it is administered. Answer questions and address their concerns.

sulfacetamide sodium 10%

AK-Sulf, Bleph-10, Cetamide Ophthalmic, OcuSulf-10, Sodium Sulamyd 10% Ophthalmic, Sulf-10 Ophthalmic

sulfacetamide sodium 15%

Isopto Cetamide Ophthalmic, Ocu-Sul-15

sulfacetamide sodium 30%

Ocu-Sul-30, Sodium Sulamyd 30% Ophthalmic

Pregnancy Risk Category: C

HOW SUPPLIED

Ophthalmic ointment: 10%
Ophthalmic solution: 10%, 15%, 30%

ACTION

Bacteriostatic, although may be bactericidal in high concentrations. Prevents uptake of PABA, a metabolite of bacterial folic acid synthesis.

Route	Onset	Peak	Duration
Ophthalmic	Unknown	Unknown	Unknown

INDICATIONS & DOSAGE

Inclusion conjunctivitis, corneal ulcers, chlamydial infection—
Adults and children: 1 to 2 drops of 10% solution instilled into lower conjunctival sac q 2 to 3 hours during day, less often at night; or 1 to 2 drops of 15% solution instilled into lower conjunctival sac q 1 to 2 hours initially. Interval increased as condition responds; or 1 drop of 30% solution instilled into lower conjunctival sac q 2 hours. 1.25 to 2.5 cm 10% ointment applied into conjunctival sac q.i.d. and h.s. Ointment may be used at night along with drops during the day.
Trachoma—
Adults and children: 2 drops of 30% solution instilled into lower conjunctival sac q 2 hours in conjunction with systemic sulfonamide or tetracycline.

ADVERSE REACTIONS

EENT: slowed corneal wound healing (ointment), pain (on instillation of eye-

drops), headache or brow pain, photophobia, periorbital edema.
Other: hypersensitivity reactions (including itching or burning), overgrowth of nonsusceptible organisms, ***Stevens-Johnson syndrome.***

INTERACTIONS
Drug-drug. *Gentamicin (ophthalmic):* in vitro antagonism. Avoid concomitant use. *Local anesthetics (procaine, tetracaine), PABA derivatives:* decreased sulfacetamide sodium action. Wait ½ to 1 hour after instilling anesthetic or PABA derivative before instilling sulfacetamide. *Silver preparations:* precipitate formation. Avoid using together.
Drug-lifestyle. *Sun exposure:* photophobia may occur. Take precautions.

EFFECTS ON DIAGNOSTIC TESTS
None reported.

CONTRAINDICATIONS
Contraindicated in patients hypersensitive to sulfonamides. Drug is not recommended for children under 2 months.

NURSING CONSIDERATIONS
• Be aware that drug is often used with oral tetracycline in treating trachoma and inclusion conjunctivitis.
• Store in tightly closed, light-resistant container away from heat.

☑ Patient teaching
• Tell patient to clean eye area of excessive exudate before instilling.
• Teach patient how to instill drops or apply ointment. Advise him to wash hands before and after administering ointment or solution and not to touch tip of dropper to eye or surrounding tissues.
• Instruct patient to apply light finger pressure on lacrimal sac for 1 minute after drops are instilled.
• Warn patient that eyedrops burn slightly.
• Advise patient to watch for and report signs of sensitivity (itching lids, swelling, or constant burning).
• Tell patient to wait at least 5 minutes before administering other eyedrops.
• Warn patient that solution may stain clothing.

• Tell patient to minimize photophobia by wearing sunglasses and avoiding prolonged exposure to sunlight.
• Advise patient not to use discolored solution.
• Tell patient not to share eye medication, washcloths, or towels with family members and to notify doctor if anyone develops same symptoms.
• Stress importance of compliance with recommended therapy.

---

tobramycin
AKTob, Tobrex

Pregnancy Risk Category: B

HOW SUPPLIED
Ophthalmic ointment: 0.3%
Ophthalmic solution: 0.3%

ACTION
Unknown. Thought to inhibit protein synthesis. Usually bactericidal.

Route	Onset	Peak	Duration
Ophthalmic	Unknown	Unknown	Unknown

INDICATIONS & DOSAGE
External ocular infections caused by susceptible bacteria—
Adults and children: in mild to moderate infections, 1 or 2 drops instilled into the affected eye q 4 hours, or a thin strip (1 cm long) of ointment applied q 8 to 12 hours. In severe infections, 2 drops instilled into the infected eye q 30 to 60 minutes until condition improves; then frequency reduced. Or, a thin strip (1 cm long) of ointment applied q 3 to 4 hours until improvement; then frequency reduced.

ADVERSE REACTIONS
EENT: burning or stinging on instillation, lid itching or swelling, conjunctival erythema, blurred vision (with ointment).
Other: *hypersensitivity reactions,* overgrowth of nonsusceptible organisms.

INTERACTIONS
None significant.

EFFECTS ON DIAGNOSTIC TESTS
Drug may elevate BUN, nonprotein nitrogen, or serum creatinine levels and increase urinary excretion of casts.

CONTRAINDICATIONS
Contraindicated in patients hypersensitive to drug or other aminoglycosides.

NURSING CONSIDERATIONS
• When two different ophthalmic solutions are used, allow at least 5 minutes before instillation.
Alert: Know that tobramycin ophthalmic solution is not for injection.
• If topical ocular tobramycin is administered with systemic tobramycin, carefully monitor serum levels.
• Know that prolonged use may result in overgrowth of nonsusceptible organisms, including fungi.

☑ **Patient teaching**
• Tell patient to clean eye area of excessive exudate before application.
• Teach patient how to instill drops or apply ointment. Advise him to wash hands before and after administering and to avoid touching tip of dropper to eye or surrounding tissue.
• Instruct patient to apply light finger pressure on lacrimal sac for 1 minute after drops are instilled.
• Advise patient to watch for itching lids, swelling, or constant burning. Tell him to discontinue drug and notify doctor if these signs develop.
• Tell patient not to share medication, washcloths, or towels with family members and to notify doctor if anyone develops same symptoms.
• Stress importance of compliance with recommended therapy.

vidarabine
Vira-A

Pregnancy Risk Category: C

HOW SUPPLIED
Ophthalmic ointment: 3% in 3.5-g tube (equivalent to 2.8% vidarabine)

ACTION
Unknown. Thought to interfere with DNA synthesis.

Route	Onset	Peak	Duration
Ophthalmic	Unknown	Unknown	Unknown

INDICATIONS & DOSAGE
Acute keratoconjunctivitis, superficial keratitis, and recurrent epithelial keratitis caused by herpes simplex I and II—
Adults and children: 1 cm of ointment applied into lower conjunctival sac five times daily at 3-hour intervals. If there are no signs of improvement after 7 days, or if complete reepithelialization has not occurred in 21 days, consider other forms of therapy. Some cases may require longer treatment if severe. After reepithelialization has occurred, treat for an additional 5 to 7 days at a reduced dosage (such as b.i.d.) to prevent recurrence.

ADVERSE REACTIONS
EENT: temporary burning, itching, mild irritation, pain, lacrimation, foreign body sensation, conjunctival injection, punctal occlusion, sensitivity, superficial punctate keratitis, photophobia.
Other: *hypersensitivity reactions.*

INTERACTIONS
None significant.

EFFECTS ON DIAGNOSTIC TESTS
None reported.

CONTRAINDICATIONS
Contraindicated in patients hypersensitive to drug.

NURSING CONSIDERATIONS
• Use cautiously and with close monitoring with steroids. Vidarabine therapy should be continued for several days after steroid therapy.
• Be aware that drug is not effective against RNA virus, adenoviral ocular infections, or bacterial, fungal, or chlamydial infections.
• Store in tightly closed, light-resistant container.

Reactions may be *common*, uncommon, *life-threatening*, or COMMON AND LIFE-THREATENING.

✓Patient teaching
• Tell patient to clean eye area of excessive exudate before application.
• Teach patient how to apply. Advise him to wash hands before and after administering ointment and to avoid touching tip of tube to eye or surrounding tissue.
• Instruct patient to apply light finger pressure on lacrimal sac for 1 minute after drops are instilled.
• Explain that the ointment may produce a temporary visual haze.
• Advise patient to watch for signs of sensitivity, such as itching lids, swelling, or constant burning. Tell patient who develops such signs to stop drug and notify doctor immediately.
• Tell patient to minimize photophobia by wearing sunglasses and avoiding prolonged exposure to sunlight.
• Tell patient not to share medication, washcloths, or towels with family members and to notify doctor if anyone develops same symptoms.
• Stress importance of compliance with recommended therapy.

Ophthalmic anti-inflammatory drugs

dexamethasone
dexamethasone sodium
  phosphate
diclofenac sodium 0.1%
fluorometholone
flurbiprofen sodium
ketorolac tromethamine
prednisolone acetate
  (suspension)
prednisolone sodium phosphate
  (solution)
suprofen

COMBINATION PRODUCTS

Corticosteroids for ophthalmic use are commonly combined with antibiotics and sulfonamides. See Chapter 79, Ophthalmic anti-infectives.

---

dexamethasone
Maxidex Ophthalmic Suspension

dexamethasone sodium phosphate
Ak-Dex, Decadron Phosphate Ophthalmic, Maxidex Ophthalmic

Pregnancy Risk Category: C

HOW SUPPLIED
dexamethasone
Ophthalmic suspension: 0.1%
dexamethasone sodium phosphate
Ophthalmic ointment: 0.05%
Ophthalmic solution: 0.1%

ACTION
Unknown. Thought to decrease the infiltration of WBCs at the site of inflammation.

Route	Onset	Peak	Duration
Ophthalmic	Unknown	Unknown	Unknown

INDICATIONS & DOSAGE
Uveitis; iridocyclitis; inflammatory conditions of eyelids, conjunctiva, cornea, anterior segment of globe; corneal injury from chemical or thermal burns, or penetration of foreign bodies; allergic conjunctivitis; suppression of graft rejection after keratoplasty—
Adults and children: 1 to 2 drops of suspension or solution instilled or 1.25 to 2.5 cm of ointment applied into conjunctival sac. In severe disease, drops may be used hourly, tapering to discontinuation as condition improves. In mild conditions, drops may be used up to four to six times daily or ointment applied t.i.d. or q.i.d. As condition improves, dosage tapered to b.i.d., then once daily. Treatment may extend from a few days to several weeks.

ADVERSE REACTIONS
EENT: increased intraocular pressure; thinning of cornea, interference with corneal wound healing, increased susceptibility to viral or fungal corneal infection, corneal ulceration; glaucoma exacerbation, cataracts, defects in visual acuity and visual field, optic nerve damage (with excessive or long-term use); mild blurred vision; burning, stinging, or redness of eyes; watery eyes, discharge, discomfort, ocular pain, foreign body sensation.
Other: systemic effects, adrenal suppression (with excessive or long-term use).

INTERACTIONS
None significant.

EFFECTS ON DIAGNOSTIC TESTS
None reported.

CONTRAINDICATIONS
Contraindicated in patients with acute superficial herpes simplex (dendritic keratitis), vaccinia, varicella, or other fungal or viral diseases of cornea and conjunctiva; ocular tuberculosis; acute, purulent, untreated infections of the eye; or hypersensitivity to any component of the formulation and after uncomplicated removal of a superficial corneal foreign body. Safe use

---

Reactions may be *common*, uncommon, *life-threatening*, or COMMON AND LIFE-THREATENING.

in pregnant and breast-feeding women has not been established.

NURSING CONSIDERATIONS
• Use cautiously in patients with corneal abrasions that may be infected (especially with herpes).
• Use cautiously in patients with glaucoma (any form), because intraocular pressure may increase. Glaucoma medications may need to be increased to compensate.
• Know that drug is not for long-term use.
• Watch for corneal ulceration; may require stopping drug.
• Be aware that corneal viral and fungal infections may be exacerbated by steroid application.

☑ **Patient teaching**
• Tell patient to shake suspension well before use.
• Teach patient how to instill drops or apply ointment. Advise him to wash hands before and after administering ointment or solution, and warn him not to touch tip of dropper to eye or surrounding tissue.
• Tell patient to apply light finger pressure on lacrimal sac for 1 minute after instillation.
• Advise patient that he may use eye pad with ointment.
• Warn patient not to use leftover medication for a new eye inflammation; it may cause serious problems.
Alert: Warn patient to call doctor immediately and to stop drug if visual acuity changes or visual field diminishes.
• Tell patient not to share medication, washcloths, or towels with family members and to notify doctor if anyone develops same symptoms.
• Stress importance of compliance with recommended therapy.

---

diclofenac sodium 0.1%
Voltaren Ophthalmic, Voltarol Ophtha§

Pregnancy Risk Category: B

HOW SUPPLIED
Ophthalmic solution: 0.1%

ACTION
Unknown. Thought to inhibit the enzyme cyclooxygenase, which is essential in the biosynthesis of prostaglandins; prostaglandins may be mediators of certain kinds of intraocular inflammation.

Route	Onset	Peak	Duration
Ophthalmic	Unknown	Unknown	Unknown

INDICATIONS & DOSAGE
Postoperative inflammation following removal of cataract—
Adults: 1 drop in the conjunctival sac q.i.d., beginning 24 hours after surgery and continuing throughout first 2 weeks of postoperative period.
Treatment of photophobia in incisional refractive surgery—
Adults: 1 to 2 drops to operative eye 1 hour before surgery. Within 15 minutes after surgery, instill 1 to 2 drops into operative eye. Then 1 drop q.i.d. beginning 4 to 6 hours after surgery up to 3 days, p.r.n.

ADVERSE REACTIONS
EENT: *transient stinging and burning, increased intraocular pressure, keratitis,* anterior chamber reaction, ocular allergy.
Other: nausea, vomiting, viral infection.

INTERACTIONS
None significant.

EFFECTS ON DIAGNOSTIC TESTS
Drug increases platelet aggregation time but does not affect bleeding time, plasma thrombin clotting time, plasma fibrinogen, or factors V and VII to XII. However, drug may cause increased bleeding of ocular tissues (including hyphemas) in conjunction with ocular surgery.

CONTRAINDICATIONS
Contraindicated in patients with hypersensitivity to any component of drug and in those wearing soft contact lenses. Because of known effects of prostaglandin-inhibiting drugs on the fetal CV system

---

(closure of the ductus arteriosus), avoid use of drug during late pregnancy.

NURSING CONSIDERATIONS
• Use cautiously in patients with hypersensitivity to acetylsalicylic acid, phenylacetic acid derivatives, and other NSAIDs; the potential for cross-sensitivity exists. Also use cautiously in surgical patients with known bleeding tendencies and in those receiving medications that may prolong bleeding time.
• Know that drug may slow or delay healing.
• Most cases of increased intraocular pressure have occurred postoperatively and before drug administration.

☑**Patient teaching**
• Teach patient how to instill drops. Advise him to wash hands before and after instilling solution, and warn him not to touch tip of the dropper to eye or surrounding tissue.
• Advise patient to apply light finger pressure on lacrimal sac for 1 minute after drug instillation.
• Stress importance of compliance with recommended therapy.
• Warn patient not to use leftover medication for a new eye inflammation.
• Remind patient to discard drug when no longer needed.

---

fluorometholone
Flarex, Fluor-Op, FML Forte,
FML Liquifilm Ophthalmic,
FML S.O.P.

Pregnancy Risk Category: C

HOW SUPPLIED
Ophthalmic ointment: 0.1%
Ophthalmic suspension: 0.1%, 0.25%

ACTION
Unknown. Thought to decrease the infiltration of WBCs at inflammation site.

Route	Onset	Peak	Duration
Ophthalmic	Unknown	Unknown	Unknown

INDICATIONS & DOSAGE
Inflammatory and allergic conditions of cornea, conjunctiva, sclera, anterior uvea—
Adults and children: 1 to 2 drops instilled in conjunctival sac b.i.d. to q.i.d. May be given q 2 hours during first 1 to 2 days if needed. Alternatively, 1.25-cm ribbon of ointment applied to conjunctival sac q 4 hours, decreased to once daily to t.i.d. as inflammation subsides.

ADVERSE REACTIONS
EENT: increased intraocular pressure, thinning of cornea, interference with corneal wound healing, corneal ulceration, increased susceptibility to viral or fungal corneal infections; glaucoma exacerbation, discharge, discomfort, ocular pain, foreign body sensation, cataracts, decreased visual acuity, diminished visual field, optic nerve damage (with excessive or long-term use).
Other: systemic effects, adrenal suppression (with excessive or long-term use).

INTERACTIONS
None significant.

EFFECTS ON DIAGNOSTIC TESTS
None reported.

CONTRAINDICATIONS
Contraindicated in patients with vaccinia, varicella, acute superficial herpes simplex (dendritic keratitis), or other fungal or viral eye diseases; ocular tuberculosis; or acute, purulent, untreated eye infections.

NURSING CONSIDERATIONS
• Use cautiously in patients with corneal abrasions that may be contaminated (especially with herpes).
• Safety and efficacy in children under 2 years have not been established.
• Drug is not for long-term use; if used for days, intraocular pressure should be monitored.
• Consult doctor if no improvement after 2 days. Do not discontinue treatment prematurely.
• In chronic conditions, withdraw treat-

---

ment by gradually decreasing frequency of applications.
• Shake well before use.
• Be aware that drug is less likely to cause increased intraocular pressure with long-term use than other ophthalmic anti-inflammatory drugs (except medrysone).
• Store in tightly covered, light-resistant container.

☑ Patient teaching
• Teach patient how to instill drops or apply ointment. Advise him to wash hands before and after administering ointment or solution, and warn him not to touch tip of dropper to eye or surrounding tissue.
• Advise patient to apply light finger pressure on lacrimal sac for 1 minute after instillation.
• Advise patient to call doctor immediately and to stop drug if visual acuity decreases or visual field diminishes.
• Warn patient not to use leftover drug for a new eye inflammation; it may cause serious problems.
• Tell patient not to share medication, washcloths, or towels with family members and to notify doctor if anyone develops same symptoms.

---

flurbiprofen sodium
Ocufen

Pregnancy Risk Category: C

HOW SUPPLIED
Ophthalmic solution: 0.03%

ACTION
Unknown. An NSAID that's thought to inhibit the cyclooxygenase enzyme essential in the biosynthesis of prostaglandins.

Route	Onset	Peak	Duration
Ophthalmic	Unknown	Unknown	Unknown

INDICATIONS & DOSAGE
Inhibition of intraoperative miosis—
Adults: 1 drop instilled into the affected eye approximately q 30 minutes, begin-

ning 2 hours before surgery. A total of 4 drops is given.

ADVERSE REACTIONS
EENT: transient burning and stinging on instillation, ocular irritation.

INTERACTIONS
Drug-drug. *Acetylcholine, carbachol:* may be rendered ineffective. Avoid concomitant use.
Anticoagulants: increased risk of bleeding if significant systemic absorption occurs. Monitor closely.

EFFECTS ON DIAGNOSTIC TESTS
None reported.

CONTRAINDICATIONS
Contraindicated in patients with hypersensitivity to drug. Safe use in pregnant and breast-feeding patients has not been established.

NURSING CONSIDERATIONS
• Use cautiously in patients who may be allergic to aspirin and other NSAIDs.
• Use cautiously in patients with bleeding tendencies and those who are receiving medications that may prolong clotting times.
• Be aware that wound healing may be delayed.

☑ Patient teaching
• Advise patient to alert the doctor immediately if visual acuity decreases or visual field diminishes.
• Urge him to take drug as prescribed.
• Advise patient to report excessive bleeding or bruising.

---

ketorolac tromethamine
Acular

Pregnancy Risk Category: C

HOW SUPPLIED
Ophthalmic solution: 0.5%

ACTION
Unknown. An NSAID thought to inhibit the action of cyclooxygenase, an enzyme

---

responsible for prostaglandin synthesis. Prostaglandins mediate the inflammatory response and also cause miosis.

Route	Onset	Peak	Duration
Ophthalmic	Unknown	Unknown	Unknown

INDICATIONS & DOSAGE
Relief of ocular itching caused by seasonal allergic conjunctivitis—
Adults: 1 drop into the conjunctival sac instilled in each eye q.i.d.
Treatment of postoperative inflammation in patients who have undergone cataract extraction—
Adults: apply 1 drop to the operative eye(s) q.i.d. beginning 24 hours after cataract surgery and continuing through first 2 weeks of postoperative period.

ADVERSE REACTIONS
EENT: *transient stinging and burning on instillation,* superficial keratitis, superficial ocular infections, ocular irritation.
Other: *hypersensitivity reactions.*

INTERACTIONS
None significant.

EFFECTS ON DIAGNOSTIC TESTS
None reported.

CONTRAINDICATIONS
Contraindicated in patients hypersensitive to any component of the formulation and in wearers of soft contact lenses.

NURSING CONSIDERATIONS
• Use cautiously in patients with bleeding disorders or hypersensitivity to other NSAIDs or aspirin.
• Use with caution in breast-feeding women.
• Store drug away from heat in a dark, tightly closed container and protect from freezing.

☑ Patient teaching
• Teach patient how to instill drops. Advise him to wash hands before and after instilling solution, and warn him not to touch tip of dropper to eye or surrounding tissue.
• Advise patient to apply light finger pressure on lacrimal sac for 1 minute after instillation.
• Remind patient to discard drug when it is no longer needed.
• Stress importance of compliance with recommended therapy.
• Tell patient not to administer drug while wearing contact lenses.
• Advise patient to report excessive bleeding or bruising to doctor.

prednisolone acetate (suspension)
Econopred Ophthalmic, Econopred Plus Ophthalmic, Pred Forte, Pred Mild Ophthalmic

prednisolone sodium phosphate (solution)
AK-Pred, Inflamase Forte, Inflamase Mild, Predsol Eye Drops‡

Pregnancy Risk Category: C

HOW SUPPLIED
prednisolone acetate
Ophthalmic suspension: 0.12%, 0.125%, 1%
prednisolone sodium phosphate
Ophthalmic solution: 0.125%, 1%

ACTION
Unknown. Thought to decrease the infiltration of WBCs at site of inflammation.

Route	Onset	Peak	Duration
Ophthalmic	Unknown	Unknown	Unknown

INDICATIONS & DOSAGE
Inflammation of palpebral and bulbar conjunctiva, cornea, and anterior segment of globe—
Adults and children: 1 to 2 drops instilled into eye. In severe conditions, may be used hourly, tapering to discontinuation as inflammation subsides. In mild conditions, may be used b.i.d. to q.i.d.

ADVERSE REACTIONS
EENT: increased intraocular pressure; thinning of cornea, interference with corneal wound healing, increased suscep-

tibility to viral or fungal corneal infection, corneal ulceration; discharge, discomfort, foreign body sensation, glaucoma exacerbation, cataracts, visual acuity and visual field defects, optic nerve damage (with excessive or long-term use).
Other: systemic effects, adrenal suppression (with excessive or long-term use).

INTERACTIONS
None significant.

EFFECTS ON DIAGNOSTIC TESTS
None reported.

CONTRAINDICATIONS
Contraindicated in patients with acute, untreated, purulent ocular infections; acute superficial herpes simplex (dendritic keratitis); vaccinia, varicella, or other viral or fungal eye diseases; or ocular tuberculosis.

NURSING CONSIDERATIONS
• Use cautiously in patients with corneal abrasions that may be contaminated (especially with herpes).
• Shake suspension and check dosage before administering to ensure using the correct strength. Store in tightly covered container.

☑ Patient teaching
• Teach patient how to instill drops. Advise him to wash hands before and after applying, and warn him not to touch tip of dropper to eye or surrounding area.
• Advise patient to apply light finger pressure on lacrimal sac for 1 minute after instillation.
• Tell patient on long-term therapy to have frequent tonometric examinations.
• Warn patient not to use leftover medication for a new eye inflammation because serious problems may occur.
• Tell patient not to share medication, washcloths, or towels with family members and to notify doctor if anyone develops same symptoms.
• Stress importance of compliance with recommended therapy.
• Tell patient to notify doctor if improvement does not occur within several days

or if pain, itching, or swelling of the eye occurs.

suprofen
Profenal

Pregnancy Risk Category: C

HOW SUPPLIED
Ophthalmic solution: 1%

ACTION
Unknown. An NSAID that inhibits action of cyclooxygenase, an enzyme responsible for synthesis of prostaglandins, which mediate inflammatory response and cause miosis.

Route	Onset	Peak	Duration
Ophthalmic	Unknown	Unknown	Unknown

INDICATIONS & DOSAGE
Inhibition of intraoperative miosis—
Adults: 2 drops instilled into the conjunctival sac q 4 hours while awake the day before surgery. On day of surgery, 2 drops instilled 3 hours, 2 hours, and 1 hour before surgery.

ADVERSE REACTIONS
EENT: *transient stinging and burning on instillation,* discomfort, itching, redness, iritis, pain, chemosis, photophobia, irritation, punctate epithelial staining.
Other: hypersensitivity reactions.

INTERACTIONS
Drug-drug. *Acetylcholine, carbachol:* may be ineffective in patients treated with suprofen. Monitor for loss of effect.

EFFECTS ON DIAGNOSTIC TESTS
None reported.

CONTRAINDICATIONS
Contraindicated in patients with epithelial herpes simplex keratitis and hypersensitivity to drug or its ingredients.

NURSING CONSIDERATIONS
• Use cautiously in patients hypersensitive to other NSAIDs or aspirin.

• Use cautiously in patients with bleeding disorders.

Alert: Drug may be absorbed into breast milk following topical ocular administration. Breast-feeding should not be continued during administration.

☑ Patient teaching

• Tell patient to wash hands before and after instilling solution, and not to touch dropper to eye or surrounding tissues.

• Advise patient to apply light finger pressure on lacrimal sac for 1 minute after drops are instilled.

• Instruct patient to store drug away from heat in a dark, tightly closed container and to protect drug from freezing.

• Remind patient to discard drug when it is no longer needed.

acetylcholine chloride
carbachol (intraocular)
carbachol (topical)
demecarium bromide
echothiophate iodide
physostigmine sulfate
pilocarpine
pilocarpine hydrochloride
pilocarpine nitrate

COMBINATION PRODUCTS
E-PILO: epinephrine bitartrate 1% and pilocarpine hydrochloride 1%, 2%, 3%, 4%, or 6%.

acetylcholine chloride
Miochol-E

Pregnancy Risk Category: NR

HOW SUPPLIED
Ophthalmic injection: 1%

ACTION
A cholinergic that causes contraction of the sphincter muscles of the iris, resulting in miosis, and that produces ciliary spasm, deepening of the anterior chamber, and vasodilation of conjunctival vessels of the outflow tract.

Route	Onset	Peak	Duration
Ophthalmic	Seconds	Unknown	10 min

INDICATIONS & DOSAGE
Anterior segment surgery—
Adults and children: before or after securing sutures, doctor gently instills 0.5 to 2 ml into anterior chamber.

ADVERSE REACTIONS
CV: bradycardia, hypotension.
EENT: corneal edema, clouding, decompensation.
Respiratory: breathing difficulties.
Other: flushing, diaphoresis.

INTERACTIONS
None significant.

EFFECTS ON DIAGNOSTIC TESTS
None reported.

CONTRAINDICATIONS
Contraindicated in patients with hypersensitivity to drug or its components.

NURSING CONSIDERATIONS
• Reconstitute immediately before using, shaking vial gently until clear solution is obtained.
• Discard unused solution.
• Don't gas-sterilize vial. Ethylene oxide may produce formic acid. Monitor for hypotension and bradycardia if this occurs.

☑ Patient teaching
• Inform patient about need for drug during surgical procedure, and answer any questions and address concerns.
• Instruct patient to report breathing difficulties immediately.

carbachol (intraocular)
Miostat

carbachol (topical)
Carboptic, Isopto Carbachol

Pregnancy Risk Category: C

HOW SUPPLIED
Intraocular injection: 0.01%
Topical ophthalmic solution: 0.75%, 1.5%, 2.25%, 3%

ACTION
A cholinergic that causes contraction of the sphincter muscles of the iris, resulting in miosis, and that produces ciliary spasm, deepening of the anterior chamber, and vasodilation of conjunctival vessels of the outflow tract.

---

*Liquid contains alcohol.   **May contain tartrazine.   †Canada   ‡Australia   §U.K.   ◇OTC

Route	Onset	Peak	Duration
Ophthalmic	10-20 min	4 hr	8 hr
Intraocular	Unknown	2-5 min	24 hr

INDICATIONS & DOSAGE
To produce pupillary miosis in ocular surgery—
Adults: before or after securing sutures, doctor gently instills 0.5 ml (intraocular form) into anterior chamber.
Open-angle glaucoma—
Adults: 1 to 2 drops instilled (topical form) up to t.i.d.

ADVERSE REACTIONS
CNS: headache, syncope.
CV: *arrhythmias,* hypotension.
EENT: spasm of eye accommodation, conjunctival vasodilation, eye and brow pain, transient stinging and burning, corneal clouding, bullous keratopathy, salivation.
GI: abdominal cramps, diarrhea.
GU: urinary urgency.
Respiratory: asthma.
Other: diaphoresis, flushing.

INTERACTIONS
Drug-drug. *Pilocarpine:* additive effect. Use together cautiously.

EFFECTS ON DIAGNOSTIC TESTS
None reported.

CONTRAINDICATIONS
Contraindicated in patients with hypersensitivity to drug or in those in whom cholinergic effects such as constriction are undesirable (for example, acute iritis, some forms of secondary glaucoma, pupillary block glaucoma, or acute inflammatory disease of the anterior chamber).

NURSING CONSIDERATIONS
• Use cautiously in patients with acute heart failure, bronchial asthma, peptic ulcer, hyperthyroidism, GI spasm, Parkinson's disease, and urinary tract obstruction.
• In case of toxicity, give atropine parenterally as ordered.
• Drug is used in open-angle glaucoma,

especially when patients are resistant or allergic to pilocarpine hydrochloride or nitrate.
Alert: Keep in mind that patients with dark eyes (hazel or brown irises) may require stronger solutions or more frequent instillation because eye pigment may absorb drug.
• If tolerance to drug develops, know that doctor may switch to another miotic for a short time.

☑ Patient teaching
• Teach patient how to instill drug. Advise him to wash hands before and after and to apply light finger pressure on lacrimal sac for 1 minute after drops are instilled. Warn him not to exceed recommended dosage.
• Warn patient to avoid hazardous activities, such as operating machinery or driving, until temporary blurring subsides. Reassure patient that blurred vision usually diminishes with prolonged use.
• Tell glaucoma patient that long-term use may be necessary. Stress compliance. Tell him to remain under medical supervision for periodic tonometric readings.
• Warn patient to use caution during night driving and other hazardous activities in poor light.

---

demecarium bromide
Humorsol

Pregnancy Risk Category: X

HOW SUPPLIED
Ophthalmic solution: 0.125%, 0.25%

ACTION
An anticholinesterase drug that inhibits the enzymatic destruction of acetylcholine by inactivating cholinesterase, leaving acetylcholine free to act on the effector cells of the iridic sphincter and ciliary muscles, causing pupillary constriction and spasm of accommodation.

Route	Onset	Peak	Duration
Ophthalmic	15-60 min	2-24 hr	3-10 days

INDICATIONS & DOSAGE

Acute angle-closure glaucoma after iri-dectomy, primary open-angle glaucoma—
Adults: dosage may range from 1 to 2 drops instilled b.i.d. to 1 to 2 drops instilled twice weekly.

Treatment of convergent strabismus (uncomplicated)—
Adults: 1 drop instilled daily for 2 to 3 weeks, then reduced to 1 drop q 2 days for 3 to 4 weeks. After reevaluation, 1 drop instilled once or twice weekly to once q 2 days based on patient's condition. Reevaluated q 4 to 12 weeks; dosage adjusted p.r.n. Discontinued after 4 months if dosage required is 1 drop q 2 days.

Diagnosis of convergent strabismus—
Adults: 1 drop instilled daily for 2 weeks, then 1 drop q 2 days for 2 to 3 weeks.

ADVERSE REACTIONS

CNS: brow ache, unusual fatigue or weakness, headache.
CV: bradycardia, palpitations.
EENT: retinal detachment, iris cysts, conjunctival thickening, lens opacities, paradoxical increase in intraocular pressure (IOP), *lacrimation,* obstruction of nasolacrimal canals; eye pain, burning, redness, stinging and irritation; twitching eyelids; *blurred vision;* visual disturbances.
GI: nausea, vomiting, diarrhea, abdominal cramps or pain.
GU: loss of bladder control.

INTERACTIONS

Drug-drug. *Anticholinergics, antimyasthenics, other cholinesterase inhibitors:* potential for additive toxicity. Monitor closely.
Epinephrine: additive effect, resulting in better control and lower dosages of both drugs.
Local anesthetics, ophthalmic tetracaine: increased risk of systemic toxicity and prolonged ocular anesthetic effect. Monitor closely.
Ophthalmic adrenocorticoids: increased IOP and decreased antiglaucoma effectiveness. Avoid concomitant use.
Ophthalmic belladonna alkaloids, cyclo-

pentolate: may antagonize miotic effects. Avoid concomitant use.
Succinylcholine: enhanced neuromuscular blockade, possible CV collapse and prolonged respiratory depression or apnea may occur for several weeks or months after demecarium is discontinued. Advise the anesthesiologist that the patient has received demecarium.
Drug-lifestyle. *Carbamate or organophosphate-type insecticides (malathion, parathion):* increased risk of systemic effects through respiratory tract or skin. Warn patients to protect themselves.
Cocaine use: increased risk of cocaine toxicity; anticholinesterase effects may last weeks or months. Avoid concomitant use.

EFFECTS ON DIAGNOSTIC TESTS

None reported.

CONTRAINDICATIONS

Contraindicated in patients with acute angle-closure glaucoma before iridotomy, other forms of glaucoma (except for primary open-angle glaucoma), or hypersensitivity to drug.

NURSING CONSIDERATIONS

● Use with extreme caution, if at all, in patients with history or risk of retinal detachment, marked vagotonia, bronchial asthma, spastic GI conditions, urinary tract obstruction, peptic ulcer, severe bradycardia, hypotension, hypertension, hyperthyroidism, acute cardiac failure, recent MI, epilepsy, marked vasomotor instability, or parkinsonism.
● Monitor vital signs.
● Use with caution in patients with corneal abrasion.
● Administer phenylephrine concurrently, as ordered, to reduce incidence of iris cyst formation.
● If tolerance to drug develops after prolonged use, know that doctor may switch to another miotic for a short time.
● Know that toxicity is cumulative; toxic systemic symptoms may not appear for weeks or months after start of therapy. Atropine sulfate S.C., I.M., or I.V. is antidote of choice.

☑ **Patient teaching**

• Teach patient how to instill demecarium. Advise him to wash hands before and after instilling drug, to avoid touching applicator tip to any surface, and to remove excess solution around eyes with clean tissue and without touching eye. Warn him not to exceed recommended dosage.

• If dose is missed, instruct patient not to double dose. If schedule is every other day, tell patient to instill as soon as possible if remembered same day; if remembered later, tell him not to instill until next day, then skip a day and resume regular schedule. If schedule is once a day, tell patient to instill as soon as possible. If not remembered until next day, tell him to skip missed dose and resume schedule. If schedule is more than once daily, tell patient to instill as soon as possible. If close to time for next dose, tell him to skip missed dose and resume regular schedule.

• Tell patient that regular medical supervision is required to check ocular pressure.

• Advise patient to carry medical identification card at all times during therapy.

• Caution patient to avoid driving, especially at night, until visual side effects subside.

---

echothiophate iodide
(ecothiopate iodide)
Phospholine Iodide

Pregnancy Risk Category: C

HOW SUPPLIED

Ophthalmic powder for solution: for reconstitution to make 0.03%, 0.06%, 0.125%, and 0.25% solutions

ACTION

An anticholinesterase drug that inhibits the enzymatic destruction of acetylcholine by inactivating cholinesterase, leaving acetylcholine free to act on the effector cells of the iridic sphincter and ciliary muscles, causing pupillary constriction and spasm of accommodation.

Route	Onset	Peak	Duration
Ophthalmic	10 min-8 hr	0.5-24 hr	Days-4 wk

INDICATIONS & DOSAGE

Primary open-angle glaucoma, conditions obstructing aqueous outflow—
Adults and children: 1 drop of 0.03% to 0.125% solution instilled into conjunctival sac daily. Maximum dosage is 1 drop b.i.d. Lowest possible dosage used for continuous control of intraocular pressure.
Diagnosis of convergent strabismus—
Adults: 1 drop of 0.125% solution instilled into each eye daily h.s. for 2 to 3 weeks.
Treatment of convergent strabismus—
Adults: initially, 1 drop of 0.125% solution instilled into each eye daily h.s. for 2 to 3 weeks. Dosage decreased to 1 drop of 0.125% solution every other day or 1 drop of 0.06% solution daily. The 0.03% solution may be used instead for some patients.

ADVERSE REACTIONS

CNS: fatigue, muscle weakness, paresthesia, headache.
CV: bradycardia, hypotension.
EENT: ciliary spasm or spasm of eye accommodation, ciliary or circumcorneal injection, nonreversible cataract formation (time- and dose-related), reversible iris cysts, pupillary block, blurred or dimmed vision, eye or brow pain, twitching of eyelids, hyperemia, photophobia, lens opacities, lacrimation, retinal detachment.
GI: diarrhea, nausea, vomiting, abdominal pain, intestinal cramps, salivation.
GU: frequent urination.
Respiratory: *bronchoconstriction.*
Other: diaphoresis, flushing.

INTERACTIONS

Drug-drug. *Anticholinergics, cyclopentolate, ophthalmic belladonna alkaloids (such as atropine):* antagonized miotic effects. Avoid concomitant use.
Local anesthetics, ophthalmic tetracaine: increased rate of systemic toxicity and prolonged ocular anesthesia. Monitor closely.
Ophthalmic adrenocorticoids: increased intraocular pressure and decreased antiglaucoma effectiveness. Avoid concomitant use.
Other cholinesterase inhibitors: possible additive effect causing systemic effects. Monitor patient closely.

Succinylcholine: respiratory and CV collapse. Don't use together.

Systemic anticholinesterase agents for myasthenia gravis, pilocarpine: effects may be additive. Monitor patients for signs of toxicity.

Drug-lifestyle. *Cocaine use:* increased risk of cocaine toxicity. Avoid concomitant use.

Organophosphate insecticides (parathion, malathion): possible additive effect causing systemic effects. Tell at-risk patient to protect himself from exposure.

EFFECTS ON DIAGNOSTIC TESTS
Drug therapy decreases plasma cholinesterase activity.

CONTRAINDICATIONS
Contraindicated in patients with uveal inflammation, acute angle-closure glaucoma before iridectomy, other forms of glaucoma (except for primary open-angle glaucoma), or hypersensitivity to drug or iodine.

NURSING CONSIDERATIONS
• Use with extreme caution, if at all, in patients with seizure disorders, vasomotor instability, parkinsonism, bronchial asthma, spastic GI conditions, urinary tract obstruction, peptic ulcer, severe bradycardia or hypotension, vascular hypertension, MI, or history or risk of retinal detachment.
• Use with caution in patients with corneal abrasion.
• Reconstitute powder, using only diluent provided to avoid contamination. Discard refrigerated, reconstituted solution after 6 months; solution stored at room temperature, after 1 month.
• Stop drug, as ordered, at least 2 weeks preoperatively if succinylcholine is to be used in surgery.
• Know that toxicity is cumulative; toxic systemic symptoms may not appear for weeks or months after start of therapy. Atropine sulfate S.C., I.M., or I.V. is antidote of choice.

☑ **Patient teaching**
• Advise patient to carry medical identification card at all times during therapy.

Drug is potent, long-acting, and irreversible.
• Teach patient how to instill drug. Advise him to wash hands before and after instilling drug, to avoid touching applicator tip to any surface, and to apply light finger pressure on lacrimal sac for 1 minute after instillation.
• Tell patient to instill drug at bedtime because it causes transient blurred vision. Warn him that transient brow pain or dimmed or blurred vision is common at first but usually disappears within 5 to 10 days.
• Warn patient to report salivation, diarrhea, profuse diaphoresis, urinary incontinence, or muscle weakness to the doctor.
• Tell patient to remain under constant medical supervision and not to exceed recommended dosage.
• Advise patient to avoid driving if visual blurring occurs, particularly at night.

---

physostigmine sulfate
Eserine Sulfate

Pregnancy Risk Category: C

HOW SUPPLIED
Ophthalmic ointment: 0.25%

ACTION
Causes contraction of iris sphincter muscles resulting in miosis, and contraction of ciliary muscle, increasing outflow of aqueous humor and decreasing intraocular pressure.

Route	Onset	Peak	Duration
Ophthalmic	10-30 min	Unknown	12-48 hr

INDICATIONS & DOSAGE
Open-angle glaucoma—
Adults and children: apply a thin strip of ointment once daily to t.i.d.

ADVERSE REACTIONS
CNS: headache, weakness.
CV: slow or irregular heartbeat.
EENT: blurred vision, eye pain, burning, redness, stinging, eye irritation, twitching of eyelids, watering of eyes.
GI: nausea, vomiting, diarrhea.

GU: loss of bladder control.
Other: diaphoresis, muscle weakness, shortness of breath.

INTERACTIONS
Drug-drug. *Echothiophate, isofluro-phate:* duration of action may be shortened. Monitor closely.
Ophthalmic belladonna alkaloids: may antagonize miotic actions. Avoid concomitant use.

EFFECTS ON DIAGNOSTIC TESTS
None reported.

CONTRAINDICATIONS
Contraindicated in patients with intolerance to physostigmine, active uveitis, or corneal injury.

NURSING CONSIDERATIONS
• Use with caution in patients with asthma and bradycardia.
• Be aware that ointment may be used at night because of its longer duration of action.
• If tolerance to drug develops, know that doctor may switch to another miotic for a short time.
• Monitor vital signs.

☑ **Patient teaching**
• Warn patient not to exceed recommended dosage.
• Tell patient to avoid driving, particularly at night, if visual blurring occurs.
• Advise patient to carry a medical identification card at all times during therapy.

---

pilocarpine
Ocusert Pilo Ocular System

pilocarpine hydrochloride
Adsorbocarpine, Akarpine, Isopto Carpine, Miocarpine†, Pilocar, Pilogel§, Pilopine HS, Pilopt‡, Piloptic, Pilostat, SnoPilo§

pilocarpine nitrate
Pilagan Liquifilm

Pregnancy Risk Category: C

HOW SUPPLIED
pilocarpine
Extended-release insert: 20 mcg/hour, 40 mcg/hour for 7 days
pilocarpine hydrochloride
Ophthalmic solution: 0.25%, 0.5%, 1%, 2%, 3%, 4%, 5%, 6%, 8%, 10%
Ophthalmic gel: 4%
pilocarpine nitrate
Ophthalmic solution: 1%, 2%, 4%

ACTION
A cholinergic that causes contraction of iris sphincter muscles, resulting in miosis, and that produces ciliary spasm, deepening of the anterior chamber, and vasodilation of conjunctival vessels of the outflow tract.

Route	Onset	Peak	Duration
Ophthalmic	10-30 min	30-85 min	4-8 hr

INDICATIONS & DOSAGE
Primary open-angle glaucoma—
Adults and children: 1 to 2 drops instilled up to q.i.d. or 1-cm ribbon of 4% gel applied h.s. Alternatively, one Ocusert Pilo system (20 or 40 mcg/hour) applied q 7 days.
Emergency treatment of acute angle-closure glaucoma—
Adults and children: 1 drop of 2% solution instilled q 5 to 10 minutes for three to six doses, followed by 1 drop q 1 to 3 hours until pressure is controlled.
Mydriasis caused by mydriatic or cyclo-plegic agents—
Adults and children: 1 drop of 1% solution.

ADVERSE REACTIONS
CV: hypertension, tachycardia, bradycardia, hypotension.
EENT: periorbital or supraorbital headache, *myopia,* ciliary spasm, *blurred vision,* conjunctival irritation, transient stinging and burning, keratitis, lens opacity, retinal detachment, lacrimation, changes in visual field, *brow pain.*
GI: nausea, vomiting, diarrhea, salivation.
Respiratory: *bronchoconstriction, pulmonary edema.*

Reactions may be *common,* uncommon, *life-threatening,* or COMMON AND LIFE-THREATENING.

Other: *hypersensitivity reactions,* diaphoresis.

INTERACTIONS
Drug-drug. *Carbachol, echothiophate:* additive effect. Don't use together.
Cyclopentolate, ophthalmic belladonna alkaloids (such as atropine, scopolamine): decreased pilocarpine antiglaucoma effectiveness and blocked mydriatic effects of these agents. Avoid concomitant use.
Phenylephrine: decreased dilation by phenylephrine. Don't use together.

EFFECTS ON DIAGNOSTIC TESTS
None reported.

CONTRAINDICATIONS
Contraindicated in patients with hypersensitivity to drug or when cholinergic effects such as constriction are undesirable (for example, acute iritis, some forms of secondary glaucoma, pupillary block glaucoma, acute inflammatory disease of the anterior chamber).

NURSING CONSIDERATIONS
• Use cautiously in patients with acute cardiac failure, bronchial asthma, peptic ulcer, hyperthyroidism, GI spasm, urinary tract obstruction, and Parkinson's disease.
• Monitor vital signs.
Alert: Keep in mind that patients with dark eyes (hazel or brown irises) may require stronger solutions or more frequent instillation because eye pigment may absorb drug.

☑ Patient teaching
• Instruct patient to apply gel at bedtime because it will blur vision. Warn him to avoid hazardous activities, such as operating machinery or driving, until temporary blurring subsides.
• Teach patient how to instill pilocarpine. Advise him to wash hands before and after instilling drug and to apply light finger pressure on lacrimal sac for 1 minute after drops are instilled. Warn patient not to touch applicator tip to eye or surrounding tissue.
• If Ocusert Pilo system falls out of the eye during sleep, tell patient to wash

hands, rinse the insert in cool tap water, and reposition it in the eye. Also tell him not to use a deformed insert.
• Warn patient that transient brow pain and myopia are common at first but usually disappear within 10 to 14 days.
• Advise patient to carry a medical identification card at all times during therapy.

atropine sulfate
cyclopentolate hydrochloride
epinephrine hydrochloride
epinephryl borate
homatropine hydrobromide
phenylephrine hydrochloride
scopolamine hydrobromide
tropicamide

COMBINATION PRODUCTS
CYCLOMYDRIL OPHTHALMIC: cyclopentolate hydrochloride 0.2% and phenylephrine hydrochloride 1%.
MUROCOLL-2: scopolamine hydrobromide 0.3% and phenylephrine hydrochloride 10%.
PAREMYD: tropicamide 0.25% and hydroxyamphetamine hydrobromide 1%.
ZINCFRIN ◇ : phenylephrine hydrochloride 0.12% and zinc sulfate 0.25%.

---

atropine sulfate
Atropine-1, Atropisol, Atropt‡,
Isopto Atropine

Pregnancy Risk Category: C

HOW SUPPLIED
Ophthalmic ointment: 1%
Ophthalmic solution: 0.5%, 1%, 2%

ACTION
A potent mydriatic and cycloplegic whose anticholinergic action leaves the pupil under unopposed adrenergic influence, causing it to dilate.

Route	Onset	Peak	Duration
Ophthalmic	Unknown	0.5-3 hr	7-10 days

INDICATIONS & DOSAGE
Acute iritis; uveitis—
Adults: 1 to 2 drops instilled into the eyes up to q.i.d. or small strip of ointment applied to conjunctival sac up to t.i.d.
Children: 1 to 2 drops of 0.5% solution instilled into the eyes up to t.i.d. or small strip of ointment applied to conjunctival sac up to t.i.d.
Cycloplegic refraction—
Adults: 1 to 2 drops of 1% solution instilled 1 hour before refraction.
Children: 1 to 2 drops of 0.5% solution instilled in each eye b.i.d. for 1 to 3 days before eye examination and 1 hour before refraction.

ADVERSE REACTIONS
CNS: confusion, somnolence, headache.
CV: tachycardia.
EENT: ocular congestion with long-term use, conjunctivitis, contact dermatitis of eye, ocular edema, *blurred vision,* eye dryness, photophobia, increased intraocular pressure (IOP), transient stinging and burning, irritation, hyperemia.
GI: dry mouth, abdominal distention in infants.
Skin: dryness.

INTERACTIONS
Drug-lifestyle. *Sun exposure:* photophobia may occur. Take precautions.

EFFECTS ON DIAGNOSTIC TESTS
None reported.

CONTRAINDICATIONS
Contraindicated in patients with glaucoma or hypersensitivity to drug or belladonna alkaloids and in those who have adhesions between the iris and lens. Atropine should not be used during first 3 months of life because of the possible association between cycloplegia produced and development of amblyopia.

NURSING CONSIDERATIONS
• Use cautiously in elderly patients and others in whom increased IOP may be encountered. Excessive use in children or in certain susceptible patients, including those with spastic paralysis, brain damage, or Down syndrome, may produce systemic symptoms of atropine poisoning.
Alert: Treat drops and ointment as poison

Reactions may be *common,* uncommon, *life-threatening,* or COMMON AND LIFE-THREATENING.

(not for internal use); signs of poisoning are disorientation and confusion. Antidote of choice is physostigmine salicylate I.V. or I.M.
• Watch for signs and symptoms of glaucoma: increased intraocular pressure, ocular pain, headache, progressive blurring of vision; notify doctor if they occur.

☑**Patient teaching**
• Teach patient how to instill atropine. Advise to wash hands before and after instilling drug and to apply light finger pressure on lacrimal sac for 1 minute after instillation. Warn patient not to touch tip of dropper or tube to eye or surrounding tissue.
• Warn patient to avoid hazardous activities, such as operating machinery or driving, until temporary blurring subsides.
• Advise patient to ease photophobia by wearing dark glasses.

---

cyclopentolate hydrochloride
AK-Pentolate, Cyclogyl, Mydrilate§, Pentolair

Pregnancy Risk Category: C

HOW SUPPLIED
Ophthalmic solution: 0.5%, 1%, 2%

ACTION
A potent mydriatic and cycloplegic whose anticholinergic action leaves the pupil under unopposed adrenergic influence, causing it to dilate.

Route	Onset	Peak	Duration
Ophthalmic	Rapid	0.5-1.25 hr	0.25-1 day

INDICATIONS & DOSAGE
Diagnostic procedures requiring mydriasis and cycloplegia—
Adults: 1 or 2 drops of 0.5%, 1%, or 2% solution instilled into the eyes followed by 1 or 2 drops in 5 to 10 minutes, if needed.
Children: 1 drop of 0.5%, 1%, or 2% solution instilled into each eye, followed in 5 to 10 minutes with 1 drop 0.5% or 1% solution, if necessary.

ADVERSE REACTIONS
CNS: irritability, confusion, somnolence,

hallucinations, ataxia, *seizures,* behavioral disturbances in children.
CV: tachycardia.
EENT: eye burning on instillation, blurred vision, eye dryness, *photophobia,* ocular congestion, contact dermatitis in eye, conjunctivitis, increased intraocular pressure (IOP), transient stinging and burning, irritation, hyperemia.
GU: urine retention.
Skin: dryness.

INTERACTIONS
Drug-drug. *Carbachol, pilocarpine:* may counteract mydriatic effect. Avoid concomitant use.
Long-acting cholinergic antiglaucoma agents: miotic actions may be inhibited. Avoid concomitant use.
Drug-lifestyle. *Sun exposure:* photophobia may occur. Take precautions.

EFFECTS ON DIAGNOSTIC TESTS
None reported.

CONTRAINDICATIONS
Contraindicated in patients with glaucoma or hypersensitivity to drug or belladonna alkaloids and in those who have adhesions between the iris and lens.

NURSING CONSIDERATIONS
• Use with extreme caution in infants and young children.
• The combination product containing 1% phenylephrine hydrochloride should not be used in infants less than 1 year of age due to risk of precipitating severe hypertension.
• Use cautiously in elderly patients and others where increased IOP may be encountered.
• Know that drug is superior to homatropine hydrobromide, and has a shorter duration of action. Physostigmine is antidote of choice.

☑**Patient teaching**
• Teach patient how to instill drug. Advise him to wash hands before and after instilling drug and to apply light finger pressure on lacrimal sac for 1 minute after drops are instilled. Warn him not to touch tip of

---

dropper to eye or surrounding tissue and that drug will burn when instilled.
• Warn patient to avoid hazardous activities, such as operating machinery or driving, until temporary blurring subsides.
• Advise patient to ease photophobia by wearing dark glasses.

---

epinephrine hydrochloride
Epifrin, Eppy§, Glaucon

epinephryl borate
Epinal, Eppy/N

Pregnancy Risk Category: C

HOW SUPPLIED
epinephrine hydrochloride
Ophthalmic solution: 0.1%, 0.5%, 1%, 2%
epinephryl borate
Ophthalmic solution: 0.5%, 1%

ACTION
An adrenergic that dilates the pupil by contracting the dilator muscle.

Route	Onset	Peak	Duration
Ophthalmic	1 hr	4-8 hr	24 hr

INDICATIONS & DOSAGE
Open-angle glaucoma—
Adults: 1 or 2 drops of 1% or 2% solution once or twice daily. Dosage is adjusted based on tonometric readings.

ADVERSE REACTIONS
CNS: brow ache, headache, light-headedness.
CV: palpitations, tachycardia, ***arrhythmias,*** hypertension.
EENT: corneal or conjunctival pigmentation, corneal edema (with long-term use); follicular hypertrophy; chemosis; conjunctivitis; iritis; hyperemic conjunctiva; maculopapular rash; eye stinging, burning, tearing (on instillation); eye pain; allergic lid reaction; ocular irritation.

INTERACTIONS
Drug-drug. *Antihistamines (dexchlorpheniramine, diphenhydramine), tricyclic antidepressants:* potentiated cardiac effects of epinephrine. Monitor closely.

Beta-adrenergic blockers, osmotic agents, systemic carbonic anhydrase inhibitors, topical miotics: additive lowering of intraocular pressure. Use together cautiously.
Cardiac glycosides: increased risk of arrhythmias. Monitor closely.
Cyclopropane, halogenated hydrocarbons: arrhythmias, tachycardia. Use together cautiously, if at all.
Local or systemic sympathomimetics: additive toxic effects. Avoid concomitant use.
MAO inhibitors: exaggerated adrenergic effects. Adjust dose of epinephrine carefully.

EFFECTS ON DIAGNOSTIC TESTS
Epinephrine therapy alters blood glucose and serum lactic acid levels (both may be increased), increases BUN levels, and interferes with tests for urinary catecholamines.

CONTRAINDICATIONS
Contraindicated in patients with angle-closure glaucoma or when nature of glaucoma has not been established. Also contraindicated in patients with hypersensitivity to drug or sulfites and in those with hypertensive CV disease or coronary artery disease.

NURSING CONSIDERATIONS
• Use cautiously in elderly patients and in those with diabetes mellitus, hypertension, Parkinson's disease, hyperthyroidism, aphakia (eye without lens), cardiac disease, cerebral arteriosclerosis, or bronchial asthma.
• Be aware that drug can also can be injected into anterior chamber to produce rapid mydriasis during cataract removal or can be used to control local bleeding during surgery.
Alert: Don't substitute one salt if another one is ordered; epinephrine salts are not interchangeable.
• Monitor blood pressure and other vital signs.

☑ Patient teaching
• Teach patient how to instill drug. Advise him to wash hands before and after instilling drug and to apply light finger pressure

---

on lacrimal sac for 1 minute after drops are instilled. Warn him not to touch tip of dropper to eye or surrounding tissue.
• Instruct patients to report immediately any decrease in visual acuity.
• Advise patient not to use while wearing soft contact lenses because discoloration of lenses may occur.
• Tell patient not to use darkened solution.

homatropine hydrobromide
AK-Homatropine,
Isopto Homatropine,
Minims Homatropine†

Pregnancy Risk Category: C

HOW SUPPLIED
Ophthalmic solution: 2%, 5%

ACTION
An anticholinergic that leaves the pupil under unopposed adrenergic influence, causing it to dilate.

Route	Onset	Peak	Duration
Ophthalmic	Rapid	40-60 min	1-3 days

INDICATIONS & DOSAGE
Cycloplegic refraction—
Adults and children: 1 to 2 drops instilled into the eyes; if needed, repeated in 5 to 10 minutes for two or three doses.
Uveitis—
Adults and children: 1 to 2 drops instilled into the eyes q 3 to 4 hours.
Note: Use only 2% solution with children.

ADVERSE REACTIONS
CNS: confusion, headache, somnolence.
CV: tachycardia.
EENT: eye irritation, *blurred vision, photophobia,* increased intraocular pressure (IOP), transient stinging and burning, conjunctivitis, vascular congestion, edema.
GI: dry mouth.
Skin: dryness, rash.

INTERACTIONS
Drug-lifestyle. *Sun exposure:* photophobia may occur. Take precautions.

EFFECTS ON DIAGNOSTIC TESTS
None reported.

CONTRAINDICATIONS
Contraindicated in patients with hypersensitivity to drug or other belladonna alkaloids, such as atropine, and in those with glaucoma or who have adhesions between the iris and lens. Use cautiously in the elderly and those with cardiac disease or hypertension.

NURSING CONSIDERATIONS
• Use cautiously in elderly patients and others in whom increased IOP may be encountered.
• In patients with heavily pigmented irises, larger doses may be required.
• Monitor vital signs.
Alert: Be aware that homatropine is similar to atropine but weaker, with a shorter duration of action. May produce symptoms of atropine poisoning, such as severe dryness of mouth or tachycardia.

✓ Patient teaching
• Teach patient how to instill drug. Advise him to wash hands before and after instilling drug and to apply light finger pressure on lacrimal sac for 1 minute after drops are instilled.
• Warn patient not to touch tip of dropper to eye or surrounding tissue.
• Caution patient to avoid hazardous activities, such as operating machinery or driving, until temporary blurring subsides.
• Instruct patient to ease photophobia by wearing dark glasses.
• Advise patient to carry a medical identification card during therapy.

phenylephrine hydrochloride
AK-Dilate, AK-Nefrin
Ophthalmic ◇, Isopto Frin ◇,
Mydfrin, Ocu-Phrin, Phenoptic,
Prefrin Liquifilm ◇, Relief ◇

Pregnancy Risk Category: C

HOW SUPPLIED
Ophthalmic solution: 0.12% ◇, 2.5%, 10%

ACTION

An adrenergic that dilates the pupil by contracting the dilator muscle.

Route	Onset	Peak	Duration
Ophthalmic	Rapid	10-90 min	3-7 hr

INDICATIONS & DOSAGE

Mydriasis without cycloplegia—
Adults and children: 1 drop of 2.5% or 10% solution instilled before examination. May be repeated in 1 hour, if needed.
Mydriasis and vasoconstriction—
Adults and adolescents: 1 drop of 2.5% or 10% solution.
Children: 1 drop of 2.5% solution.
Chronic mydriasis—
Adults and adolescents: 1 drop of 2.5% or 10% solution instilled b.i.d. or t.i.d.
Children: 1 drop of 2.5% solution instilled b.i.d. or t.i.d.
Posterior synechia (adhesion of iris)—
Adults and children: 1 drop of 2.5% or 10% solution. Do not use 10% concentration in infants.

ADVERSE REACTIONS

CNS: brow ache, headache.
CV: *hypertension* (with 10% solution), tachycardia, palpitations, **PVCs, MI.**
EENT: transient eye burning or stinging (on instillation), blurred vision, increased intraocular pressure, keratitis, lacrimation, reactive hyperemia of eye, allergic conjunctivitis, rebound miosis.
Skin: pallor, dermatitis.
Other: trembling, diaphoresis.

INTERACTIONS

Drug-drug. *Beta blockers, MAO inhibitors:* may cause arrhythmias because of increased pressor effect. Use together cautiously.
Guanethidine: increased mydriatic and pressor effects of phenylephrine. Use together cautiously.
Levodopa (systemic): reduced mydriatic effect of phenylephrine. Use together cautiously.
Topically applied atropine, cyclopentolate, homatropine, scopolamine: may increase dilation of pupil. Use together cautiously.
Tricyclic antidepressants: potentiated cardiac effects of epinephrine. Use together cautiously.
Drug-lifestyle. *Sun exposure:* photophobia may occur. Take precautions.

EFFECTS ON DIAGNOSTIC TESTS

Drug may lower intraocular pressure in normal eyes or in open-angle glaucoma; it may also cause false-normal tonometry readings.

CONTRAINDICATIONS

Contraindicated in patients with hypersensitivity to drug or angle-closure glaucoma and in those who wear soft contact lenses.

NURSING CONSIDERATIONS

• Use cautiously in patients with marked hypertension, cardiac disorders, advanced arteriosclerotic changes, type 1 diabetes, or hyperthyroidism; in children of low body weight; and in elderly patients.
• Know that systemic adverse reactions are least likely with 2.5% solution and greatest with 10% solution.

✓Patient teaching

• Teach patient how to instill drug. Advise him to wash hands before and after instilling drug and to apply light finger pressure on lacrimal sac for 1 minute after drops are instilled. Warn him not to touch tip of dropper to eye or surrounding tissue.
• Warn patient not to exceed recommended dosage because systemic effects can result. Monitor blood pressure and pulse rate.
• Advise patient to contact doctor if condition persists longer than 12 hours after discontinuation of the drug.
• Warn patient to avoid hazardous activities, such as operating machinery or driving, until temporary blurring subsides.
• Advise patient to ease photophobia by wearing dark glasses.
• Tell patient not to use brown solutions or solutions that contain precipitate.

scopolamine hydrobromide
Isopto Hyoscine

Pregnancy Risk Category: NR

HOW SUPPLIED
Ophthalmic solution: 0.25%

ACTION
An anticholinergic that leaves the pupil under unopposed adrenergic influence, causing it to dilate.

Route	Onset	Peak	Duration
Ophthalmic	Rapid	15-45 min	< 1 wk

INDICATIONS & DOSAGE
Cycloplegic refraction—
Adults: 1 to 2 drops of 0.25% solution 1 hour before refraction.
Children: 1 drop of 0.25% solution b.i.d. for 2 days before refraction.
Iritis, uveitis—
Adults: 1 to 2 drops of 0.25% solution once daily to q.i.d.
Children: 1 drop of 0.25% solution once daily to q.i.d.

ADVERSE REACTIONS
CNS: confusion, delirium, somnolence, acute psychotic reactions, headache, hallucinations.
CV: tachycardia.
EENT: ocular congestion with prolonged use, conjunctivitis, *blurred vision,* eye dryness, increased intraocular pressure, *photophobia,* transient stinging and burning, edema.
GI: dry mouth.
Skin: dryness, contact dermatitis.

INTERACTIONS
Drug-lifestyle. *Sun exposure:* photophobia may occur. Take precautions.

EFFECTS ON DIAGNOSTIC TESTS
None reported.

CONTRAINDICATIONS
Contraindicated in patients with shallow anterior chamber, angle-closure glaucoma, adhesions (synechia) between the iris and lens, or hypersensitivity to drug and

in children who have previously had a severe systemic reaction to atropine.

NURSING CONSIDERATIONS
• Use with extreme caution (if at all) in infants and small children.
• Use cautiously in patients with cardiac disease and in elderly patients.
• Observe patients closely for adverse CNS effects (such as disorientation and delirium).
• Know that scopolamine may be used in patients sensitive to atropine because it's faster acting and has a shorter duration of action and fewer adverse reactions.

☑ Patient teaching
• Teach patient how to instill drug. Advise him to wash hands before and after instilling drug and to apply light finger pressure on lacrimal sac for 1 minute after drops are instilled. Warn him to avoid touching tip of dropper to eye or surrounding tissue.
• Warn patient to avoid hazardous activities, such as operating machinery or driving, until temporary blurring subsides.
• Advise patient to ease photophobia by wearing dark glasses.
• Instruct patient to carry a medical alert card at all times during therapy.

tropicamide
Mydriacyl, Ocu-Tropic, Opticyl, Tropicacyl

Pregnancy Risk Category: NR

HOW SUPPLIED
Ophthalmic solution: 0.5%, 1%

ACTION
The shortest-acting cycloplegic available, whose anticholinergic action leaves the pupil under unopposed adrenergic influence, causing it to dilate.

Route	Onset	Peak	Duration
Ophthalmic	Rapid	20-40 min	7 hr

INDICATIONS & DOSAGE
Cycloplegic refraction—
Adults: 1 drop of 1% solution; repeated

in 5 minutes. If needed, additional drop in 20 to 30 minutes.

Children: 1 drop of 0.5% or 1% solution; repeated in 5 minutes, if needed.
Fundus examinations—
Adults and children: 1 to 2 drops of 0.5% solution in each eye 15 to 20 minutes before examination; instillation may be repeated q 30 minutes p.r.n. Compress lacrimal sac by digital pressure for 1 to 2 minutes after instillation to avoid excessive systemic absorption.

ADVERSE REACTIONS
CNS: confusion, somnolence, hallucinations, behavioral disturbances in children.
CV: tachycardia.
EENT: *transient eye stinging on instillation,* increased intraocular pressure, hyperemia, irritation, conjunctivitis, edema, *blurred vision, photophobia; dry throat.*
GI: dry mouth.
Skin: dryness.

INTERACTIONS
Drug-lifestyle. *Sun exposure:* photophobia may occur. Take precautions.

EFFECTS ON DIAGNOSTIC TESTS
None reported.

CONTRAINDICATIONS
Contraindicated in patients with shallow anterior chamber, angle-closure glaucoma, or hypersensitivity to drug.

NURSING CONSIDERATIONS
• Use cautiously in elderly patients.
• Wash hands before and after instilling drug and apply light finger pressure on lacrimal sac for 1 minute after drops are instilled. Do not to touch tip of dropper to the eye or surrounding tissue.
• Know that tropicamide's mydriatic effect is greater than its cycloplegic effect.

☑ Patient teaching
• Warn patient that drug causes transient stinging.
• Warn patient to avoid hazardous activities until blurring subsides.
• Advise patient to ease photophobia by wearing dark glasses.

Reactions may be *common,* uncommon, *life-threatening,* or COMMON AND LIFE-THREATENING.

naphazoline hydrochloride
oxymetazoline hydrochloride
tetrahydrozoline hydrochloride

COMBINATION PRODUCTS
VASOCON-A OPHTHALMIC SOLUTION:
naphazoline hydrochloride 0.05% and antazoline phosphate 0.5%.

naphazoline hydrochloride
AK-Con, Albalon Liquifilm,
Allerest ◇, Clear Eyes ◇, Comfort
Eye Drops ◇, Degest 2 ◇, Estivin
II, Nafazair, Naphcon ◇, Naphcon
Forte, Optazine‡, VasoClear ◇,
Vasocon Regular

Pregnancy Risk Category: C

HOW SUPPLIED
Ophthalmic solution: 0.012% ◇,
0.02% ◇, 0.03% ◇, 0.1%

ACTION
Unknown. Thought to cause vasoconstriction by local adrenergic action on the
blood vessels of the conjunctiva.

Route	Onset	Peak	Duration
Ophthalmic	10 min	Unknown	2-6 hr

INDICATIONS & DOSAGE
Ocular congestion, irritation, itching—
Adults: 1 drop of 0.1% solution instilled
q 3 to 4 hours or 1 drop of 0.012% to
0.03% solution up to q.i.d.

ADVERSE REACTIONS
CNS: headache, dizziness, nervousness,
weakness.
EENT: transient eye stinging, pupillary
dilation, eye irritation, photophobia,
blurred vision, increased intraocular pressure, keratitis, lacrimation.
GI: nausea.
Other: diaphoresis.

INTERACTIONS
Drug-drug. *MAO inhibitors, maprotiline,
tricyclic antidepressants:* hypertensive
crisis if naphazoline is systemically absorbed. Use together cautiously.

EFFECTS ON DIAGNOSTIC TESTS
None reported.

CONTRAINDICATIONS
Contraindicated in patients with acute
angle-closure glaucoma or hypersensitivity to drug's ingredients. Use of 0.1% solution is contraindicated in infants and
small children.

NURSING CONSIDERATIONS
• Use cautiously in patients with hyperthyroidism, cardiac disease, hypertension,
or diabetes mellitus.
• Know that drug is most widely used ocular decongestant.
• Store drug in tightly closed container.

☑ **Patient teaching**
• Teach patient how to instill drug. Advise
him to wash hands before and after instilling drug and to apply light finger pressure
on lacrimal sac for 1 minute after drops
are instilled. Warn him not to touch tip of
dropper to eye or surrounding tissue.
• Warn patient not to exceed recommended dosage. Rebound congestion and conjunctivitis may occur with frequent or
prolonged use.
• Tell patient to notify doctor if photophobia, blurred vision, pain, or lid edema develops.
• Instruct patient not to use OTC preparations longer than 72 hours without consulting doctor.

oxymetazoline hydrochloride
OcuClear ◇, Visine L.R. ◇

Pregnancy Risk Category: C

HOW SUPPLIED
Ophthalmic solution: 0.025%

ACTION
A direct-acting sympathomimetic amine that acts on alpha-adrenergic receptors in the arterioles of the conjunctiva to produce vasoconstriction, resulting in decreased conjunctival congestion.

Route	Onset	Peak	Duration
Ophthalmic	5 min	Unknown	6 hr

INDICATIONS & DOSAGE
Relief of eye redness due to minor eye irritations—
Adults and children 6 years and over: 1 to 2 drops in conjunctival sac b.i.d. to q.i.d. (spaced at least 6 hours apart).

ADVERSE REACTIONS
CNS: headache, light-headedness, nervousness, insomnia.
CV: palpitations, tachycardia, irregular heartbeat.
EENT: *transient stinging* (on initial instillation); blurred vision, keratitis, lacrimation, increase in intraocular pressure; reactive hyperemia (with excessive dosage or prolonged use).
Other: trembling.

INTERACTIONS
Drug-drug. *MAO inhibitors, maprotiline, tricyclic antidepressants:* if significant systemic absorption of oxymetazoline occurs, concurrent use may potentiate pressor effect of oxymetazoline. Avoid use together.

EFFECTS ON DIAGNOSTIC TESTS
None reported.

CONTRAINDICATIONS
Contraindicated in patients with angle-closure glaucoma and hypersensitivity to drug or its components.

NURSING CONSIDERATIONS
• Use cautiously in patients with hyperthyroidism, cardiac disease, hypertension, and eye disease, infection, or injury.
• Don't use if solution has become cloudy or changes color.

☑ Patient teaching
• Teach patient how to instill drops. Advise him to wash hands before and after instilling solution, and warn him not to touch tip of dropper to eye or surrounding tissue.
• Instruct patient to apply light finger pressure on lacrimal sac for 1 minute after drug instillation.
• Advise patient to stop drug and see a doctor if eye pain occurs, if vision changes, or if redness or irritation continues, worsens, or lasts for more than 72 hours.

tetrahydrozoline hydrochloride
Collyrium Fresh Eye Drops◇,
Eyesine◇, Murine Plus◇,
Optigene◇, Tetrasine◇,
Visine L.R.◇

Pregnancy Risk Category: C

HOW SUPPLIED
Ophthalmic solution: 0.05%◇

ACTION
Unknown. Thought to cause vasoconstriction by local adrenergic action on the blood vessels of the conjunctiva.

Route	Onset	Peak	Duration
Ophthalmic	Few min	Unknown	1-4 hr

INDICATIONS & DOSAGE
Conjunctival congestion, irritation, and allergic conditions—
Adults and children over 2 years: 1 to 2 drops of 0.05% solution instilled up to q.i.d. or as directed by doctor.

ADVERSE REACTIONS
CNS: headache, drowsiness, insomnia, dizziness, tremor.
CV: *arrhythmias.*
EENT: transient eye stinging, pupillary dilation, increased intraocular pressure, keratitis, lacrimation, eye irritation.

INTERACTIONS
Drug-drug. *Guanethidine, MAO inhibitors, tricyclic antidepressants:* hyper-

tensive crisis if tetrahydrozoline is systemically absorbed. Don't use together.

EFFECTS ON DIAGNOSTIC TESTS
None reported.

CONTRAINDICATIONS
Contraindicated in patients with angle-closure glaucoma, other serious eye diseases, and hypersensitive to drug or its components.

NURSING CONSIDERATIONS
• Use cautiously in patients with hyperthyroidism, heart disease, hypertension, or diabetes mellitus.
• Rebound congestion may occur with frequent or prolonged use.

☑ **Patient teaching**
• Teach patient how to instill drug. Advise him to wash hands before and after instilling drug and to apply light finger pressure on lacrimal sac for 1 minute after drops are instilled. Warn him not to touch tip of dropper to eye or surrounding tissue.
• Warn patient not to exceed recommended dosage.
• Tell patient to stop drug and notify doctor if redness or irritation persists or increases or if no relief occurs within 2 days.
• Warn patient not to share eye medications.

apraclonidine hydrochloride
betaxolol hydrochloride
botulinum toxin type A
brimonidine tartrate
carteolol hydrochloride
dipivefrin
dorzolamide hydrochloride
emedastine difumarate
fluorescein sodium
isosorbide
latanoprost
levobunolol hydrochloride
levocabastine hydrochloride
lodoxamide tromethamine
metipranolol hydrochloride
sodium chloride, hypertonic
timolol maleate

COMBINATION PRODUCTS
FLUORACAINE: fluorescein sodium 0.25% and proparacaine hydrochloride 0.5%.
FLURESS AND FLU-OXINATE: fluorescein sodium 0.25% and benoxinate hydrochloride 0.4%.

---

apraclonidine hydrochloride
Iopidine

Pregnancy Risk Category: C

HOW SUPPLIED
Ophthalmic solution: 0.5%, 1%

ACTION
Unknown; an alpha-adrenergic agonist that reduces intraocular pressure (IOP), possibly by decreasing production of aqueous humor.

Route	Onset	Peak	Duration
Ophthalmic	1 hr	3-5 hr	12 hr

INDICATIONS & DOSAGE
Prevention or control of IOP elevation before and after ocular laser surgery—
Adults: 1 drop of 1% solution instilled 1 hour before initiation of laser surgery on the anterior segment, followed by 1 drop immediately after surgery.
Short-term adjunct therapy in patients who require additional IOP reduction—
Adults: 1 or 2 drops of 0.5% solution instilled into affected eyes t.i.d.

ADVERSE REACTIONS
CNS: insomnia, irritability, dream disturbances, headache, irritability, paresthesia.
CV: bradycardia, vasovagal attack, palpitations, hypotension, orthostatic hypotension.
EENT: upper eyelid elevation, conjunctival blanching and microhemorrhage, mydriasis, eye burning or discomfort, foreign body sensation in eye, eye dryness and *itching, hyperemia,* conjunctivitis, blurred vision, nasal burning or dryness, or increased pharyngeal secretions.
GI: abdominal pain, discomfort, diarrhea, vomiting, taste disturbances, dry mouth.
Skin: pruritus not associated with rash, sweaty palms.
Other: body heat sensation, decreased libido, extremity pain or numbness, allergic response.

INTERACTIONS
Drug-drug. *Beta-adrenergic blockers, topical pilocarpine:* additive effects in lowering IOP. Use together cautiously.

EFFECTS ON DIAGNOSTIC TESTS
None reported.

CONTRAINDICATIONS
Contraindicated in patients hypersensitive to apraclonidine or clonidine or those undergoing concurrent MAO inhibitor therapy.

NURSING CONSIDERATIONS
• Use cautiously in patients with severe cardiac disease including hypertension or history of vasovagal attack.
• Closely monitor patients who tend to develop exaggerated decreases in IOP after drug therapy.

Reactions may be *common,* uncommon, *life-threatening,* or COMMON AND LIFE-THREATENING.

• Observe patient closely for vasovagal attack during laser surgery.
• Closely monitor patient with severe systemic disease, including hypertension, even though drug's systemic effects (altered heart rate and blood pressure) are uncommon after usual dose.

☑ **Patient teaching**
• Teach patient how to instill 0.5% solution. Advise him to wash hands before and after instilling drug and to apply light finger pressure on lacrimal sac for 1 minute after instillation.
• Warn patient not to touch tip of dropper to eye or surrounding tissue.
• Tell patient to separate intervals between each ophthalmic product instillation by at least 5 minutes to avoid washing away the previous dose.
• Encourage patient to comply with the three-times-daily dosage regimen.

---

betaxolol hydrochloride
Betoptic, Betoptic S

Pregnancy Risk Category: C

HOW SUPPLIED
Ophthalmic solution: 0.5%
Ophthalmic suspension: 0.25%

ACTION
Unknown, although as a cardioselective beta blocker it reduces formation and possibly increases outflow of aqueous humor.

Route	Onset	Peak	Duration
Ophthalmic	0.5-1 hr	2 hr	> 12 hr

INDICATIONS & DOSAGE
Chronic open-angle glaucoma and ocular hypertension—
Adults: 1 or 2 drops of 0.5% solution or 0.25% suspension b.i.d.

ADVERSE REACTIONS
CNS: insomnia, *CVA,* depressive neurosis.
CV: *arrhythmias, heart block, heart failure,* palpitations.
EENT: *eye stinging on instillation caus-*

ing brief discomfort, photophobia, erythema, itching, keratitis, occasional tearing.
Respiratory: asthma, *bronchospasm.*

INTERACTIONS
Drug-drug. *Calcium channel blockers:* AV conduction disturbances, ventricular failure, and hypotension if significant systemic absorption occurs. Monitor closely.
Cardiac glycosides: excessive bradycardia. Patient may require ECG monitoring if significant systemic absorption occurs.
Dipivefrin, ophthalmic epinephrine: may produce mydriasis. Use together cautiously.
Inhalation hydrocarbon anesthetics: prolonged severe hypotension if significant systemic absorption occurs. Tell anesthesiologist that patient is receiving ophthalmic betaxolol.
Insulin, oral antidiabetic agents: risk of hypoglycemia or hyperglycemia if significant systemic absorption occurs. May need to adjust dosage of antidiabetic agents.
Phenothiazines: additive hypotensive effects; increased risk of adverse effects if significant systemic absorption occurs. Monitor closely.
Reserpine: excessive beta blockade. Monitor closely.
Systemic beta blockers: additive effects. Monitor closely.
Drug-lifestyle. *Cocaine use:* may inhibit betaxolol's effects. Avoid concomitant use.
Sun exposure: photophobia may occur. Take precautions.

EFFECTS ON DIAGNOSTIC TESTS
None reported.

CONTRAINDICATIONS
Contraindicated in patients with sinus bradycardia, greater-than-first-degree AV block, cardiogenic shock, overt heart failure, or hypersensitivity to drug.

NURSING CONSIDERATIONS
• Use cautiously in patients with restricted pulmonary function, diabetes mellitus, hyperthyroidism, or history of heart failure.
• Keep in mind that some patients may

---

need a few weeks' treatment to stabilize intraocular pressure (IOP)–lowering response. Determine IOP after 4 weeks of treatment.

✓ **Patient teaching**
• Teach patient how to instill drug. Advise him to wash hands before and after instilling drug and to apply light finger pressure on lacrimal sac for 1 minute after instillation. Warn him not to touch tip of dropper to eye or surrounding tissue. He should shake suspension well before instilling.
• Encourage patient to comply with twice-daily dosage regimen.
• Advise patient to ease photophobia by wearing dark glasses.
• Tell patient to remove contact lenses before drug administration.

---

botulinum toxin type A
Botox

Pregnancy Risk Category: C

HOW SUPPLIED
Powder for injection: 100-unit vial

ACTION
A protein that produces a neuromuscular paralysis by binding to acetylcholine receptors on the motor end plate and that may inhibit the release of acetylcholine from presynaptic nerve endings.

Route	Onset	Peak	Duration
Intraocular	1-2 days	1-2 wk	2-6 wk

INDICATIONS & DOSAGE
Strabismus—
Adults and children 12 years and older: injections should be made only by doctors familiar with the technique, which involves surgical exposure of the region as well as electromyographic guidance of the injection needle.

Dosage varies with degree of deviation (lower doses are used for small deviations). For vertical muscles and for horizontal strabismus of less than 20 prism diopters, usual dosage is 1.25 to 2.5 units injected into any one muscle. For horizontal strabismus of 20 to 50 prism diopters, dosage is 2.5 to 5 units into any one muscle. For persistent (over 1 month's duration) palsy of sixth cranial nerve, dosage is 1.25 to 2.5 units into the medial rectus muscle of the eye.

Subsequent injections for recurrent or residual strabismus should not be made until 7 to 14 days after the initial dose and unless substantial function has returned to the injected and adjacent muscles. Dosage may be increased up to twice the initial dose for patients experiencing incomplete paralysis; subsequent doses in patients with adequate response should not be increased. Maximum single dose for any one muscle is 25 units.
Blepharospasm—
Adults: initially, 1.25 to 2.5 units injected into medial and lateral pretarsal orbicularis oculi of the upper lid and into the lateral pretarsal orbicularis oculi of the lower lid. Effects should be apparent within 3 days and peak within 1 to 2 weeks. Dosage may be doubled if inadequate paralysis is achieved; however, exceeding 5 units per site produces no apparent benefit. Each treatment lasts about 3 months and can be repeated indefinitely.

Cumulative dosage should not exceed 200 units in 30 days.

ADVERSE REACTIONS
EENT: *ptosis, vertical deviation* (after treatment of strabismus), *eye irritation, photophobia* (after treatment of blepharospasm), *swelling of eyelid.*
Skin: diffuse rash, ecchymoses.

INTERACTIONS
Drug-drug. *Aminoglycoside antibiotics, other drugs that interfere with neuromuscular transmission:* may potentiate effect of botulinum toxin. Use caution when administered concomitantly.

EFFECTS ON DIAGNOSTIC TESTS
None reported.

CONTRAINDICATIONS
Contraindicated in patients hypersensitive to drug or its components.

NURSING CONSIDERATIONS
• Reconstitute drug with preservative-free 0.9% NaCl solution. The vacuum in the vial should be noticeable when reconstituting. Inject the diluent into the vial gently because severe agitation can denature the protein. Administer within 4 hours of reconstitution.
• Keep in mind reconstituting with 1 ml of 0.9% NaCl solution produces a concentration of 10 units/0.1 ml; adding 2 ml yields 5 units/0.1 ml. Adding more diluent (such as 4 ml to produce 2.5 units/0.1 ml or 8 ml to yield 1.25 units/0.1 ml) or using different injection volumes may also be used to adjust dosage.
• Prepare the injection by drawing slightly more volume than needed into a sterile 1-ml syringe. Expel air bubbles in the barrel of the syringe and attach an electromyographic injection needle (if treating strabismus), such as a 1½″ 27G needle. Expel leftover drug into an appropriate waste container while checking for leakage around the needle. Be sure to use a new needle and syringe for each injection.
Alert: Have epinephrine available in case of an anaphylactic reaction.
• Apply several drops of an ocular decongestant and a topical anesthetic, as ordered, before treating strabismus.
• Freeze at or below 23° F (−5° C).

☑ Patient teaching
• Explain use and administration of drug to patient and family. Answer questions and address concerns.
• Inform patient about adverse reactions associated with drug. Instruct him to report persistent or severe adverse reactions promptly.

---

brimonidine tartrate
Alphagan

Pregnancy Risk Category: B

HOW SUPPLIED
Ophthalmic solution: 0.2%; 5 ml, 10 ml, 15 ml

ACTION
A selective alpha$_2$-adrenergic agonist that reduces aqueous humor production and increases uveoscleral outflow.

Route	Onset	Peak	Duration
Ophthalmic	Unknown	1-4 hr	Unknown

INDICATIONS & DOSAGE
Lowering of intraocular pressure (IOP) in patients with open-angle glaucoma or ocular hypertension—
Adults: 1 drop in affected eye t.i.d., approximately 8 hours apart.

ADVERSE REACTIONS
CNS: anxiety, asthenia, depression, dizziness, *drowsiness, fatigue, headache,* insomnia.
CV: hypertension, palpitations, syncope.
EENT: abnormal vision or taste; blepharitis; *blurring, burning, or stinging;* conjunctival blanching, edema, hemorrhage, discharge, *conjunctival follicles;* corneal staining or erosion; eyelid erythema or eyelid edema; *foreign body sensation;* lid crusting; nasal dryness; *ocular hyperemia, allergic reactions, pruritus,* ache or pain, *dryness,* tearing, or irritation; photophobia.
GI: GI symptoms, *oral dryness.*
Respiratory: upper respiratory symptoms.
Other: muscular pain.

INTERACTIONS
Drug-drug. *Antihypertensives, beta blockers, cardiac glycosides:* may further decrease blood pressure or pulse. Use cautiously.
CNS depressants: may have additive effects. Use cautiously.
Tricyclic antidepressants: may interfere with brimonidine's intraocular pressure-lowering effects. Use cautiously.
Drug-lifestyle. *Alcohol use:* may have additive CNS depressant effect. Use cautiously.

EFFECTS ON DIAGNOSTIC TESTS
None reported.

CONTRAINDICATIONS
Contraindicated in patients with hypersensitivity to drug or benzalkonium chlo-

---

ride and in those receiving MAO inhibitor therapy.

NURSING CONSIDERATIONS
• Use cautiously in patients with CV disease, cerebral or coronary insufficiency, hepatic or renal impairment, depression, Raynaud's phenomenon, orthostatic hypotension, or thromboangiitis obliterans.
• Monitor IOP because loss of effects after first month of therapy may occur.
• It is unknown if drug is excreted in breast milk. Use with caution.

☑ Patient teaching
• Tell patient to wait at least 15 minutes after instilling drug before wearing soft contact lenses.
• Caution patient of potential for decreased mental alertness, fatigue, or drowsiness and to avoid hazardous activities.

carteolol hydrochloride
Ocupress, Teoptic§

Pregnancy Risk Category: C

HOW SUPPLIED
Ophthalmic solution: 1%

ACTION
A nonselective beta-adrenergic blocking agent that reduces intraocular pressure, although the exact mechanism of action has not been demonstrated.

Route	Onset	Peak	Duration
Ophthalmic	Unknown	Unknown	Unknown

INDICATIONS & DOSAGE
Chronic open-angle glaucoma, intraocular hypertension—
Adults: 1 drop in the conjunctival sac of affected eye b.i.d.

ADVERSE REACTIONS
CNS: headache, dizziness, insomnia.
CV: bradycardia, hypotension, *arrhythmias,* palpitations.
EENT: *transient eye irritation, burning, tearing, conjunctival hyperemia, ocular edema,* blurred and cloudy vision, photo-

phobia, decreased night vision, ptosis, blepharoconjunctivitis, abnormal corneal staining, corneal sensitivity, sinusitis, taste perversion.
Respiratory: dyspnea.
Other: asthenia.

INTERACTIONS
Drug-drug. *Catecholamine-depleting agents (such as reserpine), oral beta-adrenergic blockers:* may cause additive effects and the development of hypotension or bradycardia. Monitor patient closely.
Drug-lifestyle. *Sun exposure:* photophobia may occur. Take precautions.

EFFECTS ON DIAGNOSTIC TESTS
None reported.

CONTRAINDICATIONS
Contraindicated in patients with bronchial asthma, severe COPD, sinus bradycardia, second- or third-degree AV block, overt cardiac failure, cardiogenic shock, and hypersensitivity to drug or its components.

NURSING CONSIDERATIONS
• Use with caution in patients with nonallergic bronchospastic disease, diabetes mellitus, hyperthyroidism, hypersensitivity to other beta-adrenergic agents, or decreased pulmonary function and in breast-feeding patients.
• Monitor vital signs.
Alert: Discontinue drug at first sign of cardiac failure and notify doctor.
• Be aware that when drug is used to reduce elevated intraocular pressure in angle-closure glaucoma, it should be used in combination with a miotic and should not be used alone.

☑ Patient teaching
• Tell patient that if more than one topical ophthalmic drug is being used, they should be administered at least 10 minutes apart.
• Teach patient how to instill drops. Advise him to wash hands before and after instilling solution, and warn him not to touch tip of the dropper to eye or surrounding tissue.

• Instruct patient to keep bottle tightly closed when not in use and to protect it from light.
• Tell patient that drug is a beta-adrenergic blocker and, although it is administered topically, it has the potential to be absorbed systemically.
• Advise patient to apply light finger pressure on lacrimal sac for 1 minute after drug instillation to minimize systemic absorption.
• Inform patient that the same types of adverse reactions that can result from beta-adrenergic agents may occur with topical administration. Tell him to discontinue drug and notify doctor immediately if signs or symptoms of serious adverse reactions or hypersensitivity occur.
• Advise patient to ease photophobia by wearing dark glasses.
• Stress importance of compliance with recommended therapy.
• Advise patient to monitor heart rate and blood pressure closely and to report slow heart rate to doctor.

---

dipivefrin
Propine

Pregnancy Risk Category: B

HOW SUPPLIED
Ophthalmic solution: 0.1%

ACTION
A prodrug of epinephrine, dipivefrin is converted to epinephrine in the eye. The liberated epinephrine appears to decrease aqueous production and increase aqueous outflow.

Route	Onset	Peak	Duration
Ophthalmic	0.5 hr	1 hr	> 12 hr

INDICATIONS & DOSAGE
Intraocular pressure (IOP) reduction in chronic open-angle glaucoma—
Adults: for initial glaucoma therapy, 1 drop of 0.1% solution q 12 hours. Dosage adjustments based on patient response as determined by tonometric readings.

ADVERSE REACTIONS
CV: tachycardia, hypertension, ***arrhythmias.***
EENT: eye burning or stinging, conjunctival injection, conjunctivitis, mydriasis, allergic reaction, photophobia, *macular edema.*

INTERACTIONS
Drug-drug. *Cardiac glycosides, inhalation hydrocarbon anesthetics, tricyclic antidepressants:* increased risk of adverse cardiac effects if significant systemic absorption occurs. Monitor closely.
Ophthalmic beta blockers, osmotic agents, systemically administered carbonic anhydrase inhibitors: additive lowering of IOP. Use together cautiously. Monitor for potential adverse effects.
Systemic sympathomimetics: possible additive effects if significant systemic absorption occurs. Monitor closely.

EFFECTS ON DIAGNOSTIC TESTS
None reported.

CONTRAINDICATIONS
Contraindicated in patients with angle-closure glaucoma or hypersensitivity to drug.

NURSING CONSIDERATIONS
• Use cautiously in patients with aphakia or CV disease, history of hypersensitivity to epinephrine, and asthma.
• Monitor patient for hypertension.
• Be aware that drug is commonly used concomitantly with other antiglaucoma drugs.
• Know that drug may have fewer adverse reactions than conventional epinephrine therapy.

☑ Patient teaching
• Teach patient how to instill dipivefrin. Advise him to wash hands before and after instilling drug and to avoid touching tip of dropper to eye or surrounding tissue.
• Instruct patient to report persistent or serious adverse reactions promptly.

---

dorzolamide hydrochloride
Trusopt

Pregnancy Risk Category: C

HOW SUPPLIED
Ophthalmic solution: 2%

ACTION
Inhibits carbonic anhydrase in the ciliary processes of the eye, which decreases aqueous humor secretion, presumably by slowing the formation of bicarbonate ions with a subsequent reduction in sodium and fluid transport. The result is a reduction in intraocular pressure (IOP).

Route	Onset	Peak	Duration
Ophthalmic	Unknown	Unknown	Unknown

INDICATIONS & DOSAGE
Treatment of increased IOP in patients with ocular hypertension or open-angle glaucoma—
Adults: 1 drop in the conjunctival sac of affected eye t.i.d.

ADVERSE REACTIONS
CNS: headache.
EENT: *ocular burning, stinging, or discomfort; superficial punctate keratitis; ocular allergic reaction; blurred vision; lacrimation; dryness; photophobia; bitter taste;* iridocyclitis.
Other: nausea, asthenia, fatigue, rash, urolithiasis.

INTERACTIONS
Drug-drug. *Oral carbonic anhydrase inhibitors:* may cause additive effects. Do not administer concomitantly.

EFFECTS ON DIAGNOSTIC TESTS
None reported.

CONTRAINDICATIONS
Contraindicated in patients hypersensitive to drug or its components.

NURSING CONSIDERATIONS
• Use with caution in patients with hepatic or renal impairment.
• If more than one topical ophthalmic drug is being used, the drugs should be administered at least 10 minutes apart.

☑ **Patient teaching**
• Teach patient how to instill drops. Advise him to wash hands before and after instilling solution, and warn him not to touch tip of the dropper to eye or surrounding tissue.
• Tell patient that drug is a sulfonamide and, although it is administered topically, it can be absorbed systemically. Advise patient to apply light finger pressure on lacrimal sac for 1 minute after drug instillation to minimize systemic absorption.
• Tell patient that same types of adverse reactions that can result from sulfonamides may occur with topical administration. Tell him to discontinue drug and notify doctor immediately if signs or symptoms of serious adverse reactions or hypersensitivity occur.
• Advise patient to discontinue drug and notify doctor if ocular reactions, particularly conjunctivitis and eyelid reactions, occur.
• Tell patient not to wear soft contact lenses while using drug.
• Stress importance of compliance with recommended therapy.

▼ *NEW DRUG*

emedastine difumarate
Emadine

Pregnancy Risk Category: B

HOW SUPPLIED
Ophthalmic solution: 0.05%

ACTION
Emedastine is a selective H_1 receptor antagonist. Inhibition of histamine-stimulated vascular permeability in the conjunctiva occurs following topical ocular administration.

Route	Onset	Peak	Duration
Topical, ophthalmic	Unknown	Unknown	Unknown

INDICATIONS & DOSAGE
Temporary relief of signs and symptoms of allergic conjunctivitis—
Adults and children 3 years and older: 1 drop instilled into affected eye(s) up to q.i.d.

ADVERSE REACTIONS
CNS: *headache,* abnormal dreams, asthenia.
EENT: blurred vision, burning or stinging, corneal infiltrates, corneal staining, discomfort, dry eye, foreign body sensation, hyperemia, keratitis, pruritus, tearing, bad taste, sinusitis, rhinitis.

INTERACTIONS
None reported.

EFFECTS ON DIAGNOSTIC TESTS
None reported.

CONTRAINDICATIONS
Contraindicated in patients with known hypersensitivity to drug or its components.

NURSING CONSIDERATIONS
• Know that the drug is for topical use only and not for injection or oral use.
• Avoid touching the eyelids or surrounding areas with the dropper tip of the bottle.
• Keep the bottle tightly closed when not in use.
• Do not use if the solution has been discolored.
• Know that safety and effectiveness in children under 3 years have not been established.

☑ **Patient teaching**
• Teach patient how to instill eye drops. Wash hands before and after instilling medication. To prevent contaminating the dropper tip and solution, use care not to touch the eyelids or surrounding areas with dropper tip of bottle.
• Tell patient not to wear a contact lens if eye is red.
• Instruct patient not to use drug for contact lens-related irritation.
• Tell patient that solution contains a preservative (benzalkonium chloride) that

may be absorbed by soft contact lenses. If patient wears soft contact lens and his eyes are not red, instruct him to wait at least 10 minutes after instilling drug before inserting a contact lens.

---

fluorescein sodium
AK- Fluor, Fluorescite, Fluor-I-Strip, Fluor-I-Strip-A.T., Ful-Glo ◊ , Funduscein-10, Funduscein-25, Ophthifluor

Pregnancy Risk Category: C

HOW SUPPLIED
Ophthalmic solution: 2%
Ophthalmic strips: 0.6 mg, 1 mg, 9 mg
Parenteral injection: 10%, 25%

ACTION
A water-soluble dye that produces an intense green fluorescence in alkaline solution (pH over 5) or a bright yellow one when viewed under cobalt blue illumination.

Route	Onset	Peak	Duration
IV, ophthalmic	Immediate	Unknown	Unknown

INDICATIONS & DOSAGE
Diagnostic in corneal abrasions and foreign bodies; fitting hard contact lenses; lacrimal patency; fundus photography; applanation tonometry—
Adults and children: 1 or 2 drops of 2% solution followed by irrigation; or strip moistened with sterile water, then conjunctiva or fornix touched with moistened tip, and eye flushed with irrigating solution. Patient should blink several times after application.
Retinal angiography—
Adults: 5 ml of 10% solution (500 mg) or 3 ml of 25% solution (750 mg) rapidly injected into antecubital vein.
Children: 7.5 mg/kg injected rapidly into antecubital vein.

ADVERSE REACTIONS
Topical use:
EENT: eye stinging or burning, yellow tears.

I.V. use:
CNS: headache, dizziness, syncope, *seizures.*
CV: hypotension, *shock, cardiac arrest, thrombophlebitis.*
GI: nausea, vomiting, GI distress.
GU: bright yellow urine (persists for 24 to 36 hours).
Respiratory: transient dyspnea, *bronchospasm.*
Skin: yellow skin discoloration (fades in 6 to 12 hours), pruritus, *hypersensitivity reactions,* including urticaria.
Other: *anaphylaxis,* extravasation at injection site, fever, *angioedema.*

INTERACTIONS
None significant.

EFFECTS ON DIAGNOSTIC TESTS
Bright yellow discoloration of urine may interfere with routine urinalysis.

CONTRAINDICATIONS
Contraindicated in patients with hypersensitivity to drug; do not use with soft contact lenses (lenses may become discolored).

NURSING CONSIDERATIONS
• Use cautiously in patients with history of allergy or bronchial asthma.
• Always use aseptic technique. Easily contaminated by *Pseudomonas aeruginosa.*
• Use topical anesthetic as ordered before instilling to relieve burning and irritation.
• Never instill dye while patients are wearing soft contact lenses; fluorescein will ruin them.
• Be aware that defects appear green under normal light or bright yellow under cobalt blue illumination. Foreign bodies are surrounded by a green ring. Similar lesions of the conjunctiva are delineated in orange-yellow.

⚕ I.V. administration
• Take care to avoid extravasation.
• Inject contents of ampule or prefilled syringe rapidly into the antecubital vein.
• Keep an antihistamine, epinephrine, and oxygen available when giving par-

enterally. Avoid extravasation during injection.

✅ Patient teaching
• Tell patient to report persistent or serious adverse reactions promptly.

---

isosorbide
Ismotic

Pregnancy Risk Category: B

HOW SUPPLIED
Oral solution: 45% (100 g/225 ml) in 220-ml containers

ACTION
Acts as an osmotic agent by promoting redistribution of water and thereby producing diuresis.

Route	Onset	Peak	Duration
PO	0.5 hr	1-1.5 hr	Unknown

INDICATIONS & DOSAGE
Short-term reduction of intraocular pressure (IOP) caused by glaucoma—
Adults: initially, 1.5 g/kg P.O. Usual dosage range is 1 to 3 g/kg b.i.d. to q.i.d., as indicated.

ADVERSE REACTIONS
CNS: vertigo, light-headedness, lethargy, headache, confusion, disorientation, irritability, syncope, dizziness.
GI: gastric discomfort, nausea, vomiting.
Other: hypernatremia, hyperosmolality, thirst.

INTERACTIONS
None significant.

EFFECTS ON DIAGNOSTIC TESTS
None reported.

CONTRAINDICATIONS
Contraindicated in patients with anuria caused by severe renal disease, severe dehydration, acute pulmonary edema, severe cardiac decompensation, and hypersensitivity to drug or its components.

Reactions may be *common,* uncommon, **life-threatening,** or **COMMON AND LIFE-THREATENING.**

NURSING CONSIDERATIONS
• Know that additional doses should be used cautiously, especially in patients with diseases associated with sodium retention, such as heart failure.
• To improve palatability, pour medication over cracked ice and tell patients to sip it.
• Monitor patient closely for 5 to 10 minutes after administration for adverse effects.
• Keep in mind that isosorbide is especially useful for rapid reduction of IOP. May be used to interrupt acute attack of glaucoma before laser surgery.
• In patients with diseases associated with sodium retention, carefully monitor fluid and electrolyte balance.

☑ Patient teaching
• Tell patient that drug may induce thirst.
• Caution patient not to perform hazardous activities if adverse CNS reactions occur.
• Advise patient this is short-term treatment and follow up is necessary.

---

latanoprost
Xalatan

Pregnancy Risk Category: C

HOW SUPPLIED
Ophthalmic solution: 0.005% (50 mcg/ml)

ACTION
Although exact mechanism of drug's ability to lower intraocular pressure (IOP) is unknown, it is believed to involve an increase in the outflow of aqueous humor.

Route	Onset	Peak	Duration
Ophthalmic	2-4 hr	8-12 hr	Unknown

INDICATIONS & DOSAGE
Treatment of increased IOP in patients with ocular hypertension or open-angle glaucoma who are intolerant of other IOP-lowering medications or insufficiently responsive to other IOP-lowering medications—
Adults: 1 drop in the conjunctival sac of affected eye once daily in the evening.

ADVERSE REACTIONS
CV: angina pectoris.
EENT: *blurred vision, burning, stinging,* conjunctival hyperemia, foreign body sensation, itching, increased brown pigmentation of the iris, dry eye, punctate epithelial keratopathy, lid crusting or edema, lid discomfort, excessive tearing, eye pain, photophobia.
Other: upper respiratory tract infection, cold, or flu; muscle, joint, back, or chest pain; rash; allergic skin reaction.

INTERACTIONS
Drug-drug. *Eyedrops containing thimerosal:* precipitation occurs when mixed with latanoprost. If used concomitantly, administer at least 5 minutes apart.

EFFECTS ON DIAGNOSTIC TESTS
None reported.

CONTRAINDICATIONS
Contraindicated in patients with hypersensitivity to drug, benzalkonium chloride, or other ingredients in product.

NURSING CONSIDERATIONS
• Use cautiously when administering to patients with impaired renal or hepatic function.
• Know that drug should not be administered while patients are wearing contact lenses.
• Be aware that more frequent administration than that recommended may decrease the IOP-lowering effects of drug.
• Drug may gradually change eye color, increasing amount of brown pigment in the iris. This change in iris color occurs slowly and may not be noticeable for months or years. Increased pigmentation may be permanent.
• Do not allow tip of dispenser to contact eye or surrounding structures; may cause ocular infections. Be aware that serious damage to the eye and subsequent loss of vision may result from using contaminated solutions.
• Safety and effectiveness in children have not been established.
• It is not known if drug is excreted into breast milk; use caution when administering drug to breast-feeding women.

✓ **Patient teaching**
• Inform patient of potential for change in iris color. Patients receiving treatment in only one eye should be told about risk for increased brown pigmentation in treated eye.
• Teach patient how to instill drops. Advise him to wash his hands before and after instilling solution, and warn him not to touch the dropper or its tip to the eye or surrounding tissue.
• Advise patient to apply light finger pressure on the lacrimal sac for 1 minute after instillation to minimize systemic absorption.
• Instruct patient to report ocular reactions, especially conjunctivitis and lid reactions.
• Tell patient who wears contact lenses to remove them before administering the solution and not to reinsert the lenses until 15 minutes have elapsed.
• Advise patient that if more than one topical ophthalmic drug is being used, the drugs should be administered at least 5 minutes apart.
• If patient develops another ocular condition (such as trauma or infection) or needs ocular surgery, advise him to contact doctor about continued use of the multidose container.
• Stress importance of compliance with recommended therapy.

levobunolol hydrochloride
AKBeta, Betagan

Pregnancy Risk Category: C

HOW SUPPLIED
Ophthalmic solution: 0.25%, 0.5%

ACTION
Unknown. A nonselective beta blocker that is thought to reduce formation and possibly increase outflow of aqueous humor.

Route	Onset	Peak	Duration
Ophthalmic	1 hr	2-6 hr	24 hr

INDICATIONS & DOSAGE
Chronic open-angle glaucoma and ocular hypertension—
Adults: 1 to 2 drops once daily (0.5%) or b.i.d. (0.25%).

ADVERSE REACTIONS
CNS: headache, depression, insomnia, *syncope.*
CV: slight reduction in resting heart rate, *hypotension, bradycardia,* **heart failure.**
EENT: *transient eye stinging and burning,* tearing, erythema, itching, keratitis, corneal punctate staining, photophobia; decreased corneal sensitivity (with long-term use).
GI: nausea.
Respiratory: *asthmatic attacks in patients with history of asthma.*
Skin: urticaria.

INTERACTIONS
Drug-drug. *Dipivefrin, epinephrine, systemically administered carbonic anhydrase inhibitors, topical miotics:* additive lowered intraocular pressure. Use together cautiously.
Metoprolol, propranolol, other oral beta-adrenergic blockers: increased ocular and systemic effects. Use together cautiously.
Reserpine, other catecholamine-depleting drugs: enhanced hypotensive and bradycardiac effects. Monitor closely.
Drug-lifestyle. *Sun exposure:* photophobia may occur. Take precautions.

EFFECTS ON DIAGNOSTIC TESTS
None reported.

CONTRAINDICATIONS
Contraindicated in patients with bronchial asthma, sinus bradycardia, second- or third-degree AV block, cardiac failure, cardiogenic shock, history of bronchial asthma or severe COPD, or hypersensitivity to drug.

NURSING CONSIDERATIONS
• Use cautiously in patients with chronic bronchitis and emphysema, diabetes mellitus, hyperthyroidism, and myasthenia gravis.
• Avoid letting dropper touch patient's eye or surrounding tissue.

Reactions may be *common,* uncommon, *life-threatening,* or COMMON AND LIFE-THREATENING.

• Know that safe use during pregnancy and breast-feeding has not been established.

✅ Patient teaching
• Teach patient how to instill levobunolol. Advise him to wash hands before and after instilling drug and to apply light finger pressure on lacrimal sac for 1 minute after drops are instilled.
• Warn patient not to touch dropper to eye or surrounding tissue.
• Advise elderly patient to report signs and symptoms of dyspnea, chest pain, or heart irregularities to doctor. Drug may be absorbed systemically and produce signs and symptoms of beta blockade.
• Advise patient to carry a medical alert card at all times during therapy.

---

levocabastine hydrochloride
Livostin

Pregnancy Risk Category: C

HOW SUPPLIED
Ophthalmic suspension: 0.05%

ACTION
Selectively blocks ophthalmic H_1 receptors.

Route	Onset	Peak	Duration
Ophthalmic	Unknown	Unknown	Unknown

INDICATIONS & DOSAGE
Temporary relief of seasonal allergic conjunctivitis—
Adults and children 12 years and older: 1 drop q.i.d. for up to 2 weeks.

ADVERSE REACTIONS
CNS: headache, fatigue, somnolence.
EENT: *transient eye discomfort upon instillation (burning, stinging), eye discharge,* dryness, pain, or redness; lacrimation; eyelid edema; visual disturbances; pharyngitis.
GI: dry mouth, nausea.
Respiratory: cough, dyspnea.
Skin: rash.

INTERACTIONS
None significant.

EFFECTS ON DIAGNOSTIC TESTS
None reported.

CONTRAINDICATIONS
Contraindicated in patients hypersensitive to drug or its components and while soft contacts are worn.

NURSING CONSIDERATIONS
• Know that drug is for ophthalmic use only; it should never be injected.

✅ Patient teaching
• Teach patient how to instill levocabastine. Advise him to wash hands before and after instilling drug and to avoid touching tip of dropper to eye or surrounding tissue. He should shake suspension well before instilling.
• Warn patient that he may experience transient discomfort or burning upon instillation. Tell him to contact doctor if pain persists.
• Advise patient not to wear soft contact lenses during therapy.
• Tell patient to store drug at room temperature and to avoid freezing. He should not use a discolored solution.

---

lodoxamide tromethamine
Alomide

Pregnancy Risk Category: B

HOW SUPPLIED
Ophthalmic solution: 0.1%

ACTION
Stabilizes mast cells and prevents the release of inflammation mediators.

Route	Onset	Peak	Duration
Ophthalmic	Unknown	Unknown	Unknown

INDICATIONS & DOSAGE
Vernal conjunctivitis, vernal keratoconjunctivitis, vernal keratitis—
Adults and children 2 years and over: 1 to 2 drops in affected eye q.i.d. for up to 3 months.

ADVERSE REACTIONS
CNS: headache, dizziness, somnolence.
EENT: *transient eye discomfort upon instillation (burning, stinging);* anterior chamber cells; blepharitis; blurred vision; chemosis; corneal erosion, ulcer, or abrasion; crystalline deposits; epitheliopathy; sensation of foreign body, stickiness, or warmth; hyperemia; keratitis; keratopathy; ocular edema, discharge, swelling, fatigue, itching, or allergy; pruritus; scales on eyelids or eyelashes; tearing; dry nose.
GI: nausea, stomach discomfort.
Skin: rash, heat sensation.

INTERACTIONS
None significant.

EFFECTS ON DIAGNOSTIC TESTS
None reported.

CONTRAINDICATIONS
Contraindicated in patients hypersensitive to drug or its components.

NURSING CONSIDERATIONS
• Know that drug is for ophthalmic use only; it should never be injected.
• Check expiration date before using.

☑ **Patient teaching**
• Teach patient how to instill lodoxamide. Advise him to wash hands before and after instilling drug and to avoid touching tip of dropper to eye or surrounding tissue.
• Tell patient to contact doctor if discomfort or burning persists upon instillation.
• Advise patient not to wear soft contact lenses during therapy.

---

metipranolol hydrochloride
OptiPranolol

Pregnancy Risk Category: C

HOW SUPPLIED
Ophthalmic solution: 0.3% in 2-ml, 5-ml, or 10-ml dropper bottles

ACTION
Unknown. A noncardioselective beta-adrenergic blocker that appears to reduce aqueous production and to reduce elevated and normal intraocular pressure (IOP), with or without glaucoma, with little or no effect on pupil size or accommodation. IOP above 24 mm Hg is reduced an average of 20% to 26%.

Route	Onset	Peak	Duration
Ophthalmic	0.5 hr	2 hr	12-24 hr

INDICATIONS & DOSAGE
IOP reduction in ocular conditions, including ocular hypertension and chronic open-angle glaucoma—
Adults: 1 drop into affected eye b.i.d. If IOP is not at a satisfactory level, concomitant therapy to lower it may be instituted.

ADVERSE REACTIONS
CNS: headache, anxiety, dizziness, depression, somnolence, nervousness, asthenia, brow ache.
CV: hypertension, *MI,* atrial fibrillation, angina, palpitation, bradycardia.
EENT: transient local eye discomfort, tearing, conjunctivitis, eyelid dermatitis, blurred vision, blepharitis, abnormal vision, photophobia, eye edema, rhinitis, epistaxis.
GI: nausea.
Respiratory: dyspnea, bronchitis, cough.
Skin: rash.
Other: *hypersensitivity reactions,* myalgia.

INTERACTIONS
Drug-drug. *Calcium channel blockers, cardiac glycosides, quinidine:* increased risk of adverse cardiac effects if significant amount of drug is systemically absorbed. Use together cautiously.
Fentanyl, general anesthetics: excessive hypotension. Monitor closely.
Metoprolol tartrate, propranolol, other oral beta-adrenergic blockers: increased ocular and systemic effects. Use together cautiously.
Reserpine, other catecholamine-depleting drugs: enhanced hypotensive and bradycardia-induced effects. Avoid concurrent use.

Reactions may be *common,* uncommon, *life-threatening,* or COMMON AND LIFE-THREATENING.

EFFECTS ON DIAGNOSTIC TESTS
None reported.

CONTRAINDICATIONS
Contraindicated in patients with bronchial asthma, sinus bradycardia, second- or third-degree AV block, cardiac failure, cardiogenic shock, history of bronchial asthma or severe COPD, and hypersensitivity to drug or its components.

NURSING CONSIDERATIONS
• Use cautiously in patients with nonallergic bronchospasm, chronic bronchitis, emphysema, diabetes mellitus (especially in those subject to spontaneous hypoglycemia), hyperthyroidism, or cerebrovascular insufficiency.
• Anticipate using pilocarpine, other miotics, or systemic carbonic anhydrase inhibitors concomitantly if IOP is not adequately controlled.
• Check expiration date on bottle before use. Do not use if eyedrops have changed color.
• Be aware that a slight increase in outflow facility has been demonstrated with metipranolol. Like other noncardioselective beta-adrenergic blockers, metipranolol does not have significant local anesthetic (membrane-stabilizing) actions or intrinsic sympathomimetic activity.

☑ Patient teaching
• Teach patient how to instill metipranolol. Instruct him to first wash hands thoroughly and then tilt head back or lie down and gaze upward. Tell patient to gently grasp lower eyelid below eyelashes and pull eyelid away from eye to form a pouch. Then have him place dropper directly over eye, avoiding contact with eye or any surface; look up just before applying drop; and look down for several seconds after instillation and slowly release eyelid.
• Tell patient to close eyes gently for 1 to 2 minutes and to apply gentle pressure to inside corner of eye at bridge of nose to retard draining of solution from intended area. Warn him not to rub eye or rinse dropper.
• Advise patient to report signs of dys-

pnea, bradycardia, or chest pain to their doctor.

---

sodium chloride, hypertonic
Adsorbonac, Ak-NaCl ◇, Muro-128 ◇, Muroptic-5 ◇

Pregnancy Risk Category: NR

HOW SUPPLIED
Ophthalmic ointment: 5%
Ophthalmic solution: 2%, 5%

ACTION
An osmotic agent that removes excess fluid from the cornea.

Route	Onset	Peak	Duration
Ophthalmic	Unknown	Unknown	Unknown

INDICATIONS & DOSAGE
Temporary relief of corneal edema—
Adults and children: 1 to 2 drops q 3 to 4 hours, or ¼" (6 mm) of ointment applied q 3 to 4 hours.

ADVERSE REACTIONS
EENT: slight eye stinging.
Other: *hypersensitivity reactions.*

INTERACTIONS
None significant.

EFFECTS ON DIAGNOSTIC TESTS
None reported.

CONTRAINDICATIONS
Contraindicated in patients hypersensitive to drug or its components.

NURSING CONSIDERATIONS
• Know that ophthalmic solution is for topical use only; never inject.
• Check expiration date before using.

☑ Patient teaching
• Teach patient how to instill drug. Advise him to wash hands before and after instilling drug and to apply light finger pressure on lacrimal sac for 1 minute after drops are instilled. Warn patient not to touch dropper to eye or surrounding tissue.

• Tell patient to prevent caking on dropper bottle tip by putting a few drops of sterile irrigation solution inside bottle cap.

• Warn patient that ointment may cause blurred vision.

• If patient experiences severe headache, pain, rapid change in vision, acute redness of eyes, sudden appearance of floating spots, pain on exposure to light, or double vision, tell him to discontinue drug and notify doctor.

• Advise patient to store drug in tightly closed container.

---

timolol maleate
Timoptic, Timoptic-XE

Pregnancy Risk Category: C

HOW SUPPLIED
Ophthalmic solution: 0.25%, 0.5%
Ophthalmic gel: 0.25%, 0.5%

ACTION
Unknown. A beta blocker that is thought to reduce aqueous formation and possibly increase aqueous outflow.

Route	Onset	Peak	Duration
Ophthalmic	0.5 hr	1-2 hr	12-24 hr

INDICATIONS & DOSAGE
Treatment of elevated intraocular pressure (IOP) in patients with ocular hypertension or open-angle glaucoma—
Adults: initially, 1 drop of 0.25% solution in each affected eye b.i.d.; maintenance dosage is 1 drop daily. If no response, 1 drop of 0.5% solution in each affected eye b.i.d. If IOP is controlled, dosage reduced to 1 drop daily. Alternatively, 1 drop of gel in each affected eye once daily.

ADVERSE REACTIONS
CNS: depression, fatigue, dizziness, lethargy, hallucinations, confusion, *syncope.*
CV: slight reduction in resting heart rate, arrhythmia, *CVA, cardiac arrest,* heart block, palpitations, *hypotension, bradycardia, heart failure.*
EENT: minor eye irritation, decreased corneal sensitivity with long-term use,

conjunctivitis, blepharitis, keratitis, visual disturbances, diplopia, ptosis.
Respiratory: *asthmatic attacks in patients with history of asthma.*

INTERACTIONS
Drug-drug. *Calcium channel blockers, cardiac glycosides, quinidine:* increased risk of adverse cardiac effects if significant amounts of timolol are systemically absorbed. Use together cautiously.
Fentanyl, general anesthetics: excessive hypotension. Monitor closely.
Metoprolol tartrate, propranolol, other oral beta-adrenergic blockers: increased ocular and systemic effects. Use together cautiously.
Reserpine, other catecholamine-depleting drugs: enhanced hypotensive and bradycardia-induced effects. Avoid concurrent use.

EFFECTS ON DIAGNOSTIC TESTS
Drug therapy may slightly increase BUN, serum potassium, uric acid, and blood glucose levels and may slightly decrease hemoglobin levels and hematocrit.

CONTRAINDICATIONS
Contraindicated in patients with bronchial asthma, sinus bradycardia, second- or third-degree AV block, cardiac failure, cardiogenic shock, history of bronchial asthma or severe COPD, or hypersensitivity to drug.

NURSING CONSIDERATIONS
• Use cautiously in patients with nonallergic bronchospasm, chronic bronchitis, emphysema, diabetes mellitus, hyperthyroidism, or cerebrovascular insufficiency.

• Administer other ophthalmic agents at least 10 minutes before administering gel form of drug.

• Monitor diabetic patients carefully. Systemic beta-blocking effects can mask some signs of hypoglycemia in diabetic patients.

• Be aware that some patients may need a few weeks' treatment to stabilize pressure-lowering response. Determine IOP after 4 weeks of treatment.

• Know that drug can be used safely in

---

patients with glaucoma who wear conventional hard contact lenses.

☑ Patient teaching
• Teach patient how to instill timolol. Advise him to wash hands before and after instilling drug and to apply light finger-pressure on lacrimal sac for 1 minute after drops are instilled. Warn patient not to touch dropper to eye or surrounding tissue.
• Instruct patient using gel form of drug to invert the container and shake once before each use. Also tell him to administer other ophthalmic agents at least 10 minutes before administering the gel drop.
• Advise patient to monitor pulse rate and report a slow rate to doctor. Drug may be absorbed systemically and produce signs and symptoms of beta blockade.
• Tell patient to report signs of dyspnea or chest pain to doctor.

boric acid
carbamide peroxide
chloramphenicol
triethanolamine polypeptide
    oleate-condensate

COMBINATION PRODUCTS
None.

---

boric acid
Auro-Dri◇, Dri/Ear◇ Ear-Dry◇

Pregnancy Risk Category: NR

HOW SUPPLIED
Otic solution: 2.75% boric acid in iso-propyl alcohol

ACTION
Weak bacteriostatic that inhibits or destroys bacteria in the ear canal; also is a fungistatic agent.

Route	Onset	Peak	Duration
Otic	Unknown	Unknown	Unknown

INDICATIONS & DOSAGE
External ear canal infection—
Adults and children: 3 to 8 drops into ear canal; plug with cotton. Repeated t.i.d. or q.i.d.

ADVERSE REACTIONS
EENT: ear irritation or itching.
Skin: urticaria.
Other: overgrowth of nonsusceptible organisms.

INTERACTIONS
None significant.

EFFECTS ON DIAGNOSTIC TESTS
None reported.

CONTRAINDICATIONS
Contraindicated in patients with a perforated eardrum or excoriated membranes.

NURSING CONSIDERATIONS
• Watch for signs of superinfection.

☑ **Patient teaching**
• Instruct patient or caregiver how to administer drug.
• Warn patient to avoid touching ear with dropper to prevent reinfection.
• Tell patient using cotton plug to always moisten with medication.

---

carbamide peroxide
Auro Ear Drops◇, Debrox◇,
Murine Ear◇

Pregnancy Risk Category: NR

HOW SUPPLIED
Otic solution: 6.5% carbamide in glycerin or glycerin and propylene glycol

ACTION
A ceruminolytic that emulsifies and disperses accumulated cerumen.

Route	Onset	Peak	Duration
Otic	Unknown	Unknown	15-30 min

INDICATIONS & DOSAGE
Impacted cerumen—
Adults and children: 5 to 10 drops into ear canal b.i.d. for up to 4 days. Allow solution to remain in ear canal for several minutes; remove with warm water.

ADVERSE REACTIONS
None reported.

INTERACTIONS
None significant.

EFFECTS ON DIAGNOSTIC TESTS
None reported.

CONTRAINDICATIONS
Contraindicated in patients with a perforated eardrum.

Reactions may be *common*, uncommon, *life-threatening*, or COMMON AND LIFE-THREATENING.

NURSING CONSIDERATIONS
• Use in children under 12 years only under doctor's direction.

✓ Patient teaching
• Instruct patient or caregiver how to administer drug.
• Caution patient that he should avoid touching his ear with dropper to prevent reinfection.
• Instruct patient to flush the ear gently with warm water, using a rubber bulb syringe.
• Advise patient to call doctor if redness, pain, or swelling persists.

---

chloramphenicol
Chloromycetin Otic, Sopamycetin†

Pregnancy Risk Category: NR

HOW SUPPLIED
Otic solution: 0.5%

ACTION
Inhibits or destroys bacteria in the ear canal.

Route	Onset	Peak	Duration
Otic	Unknown	Unknown	Unknown

INDICATIONS & DOSAGE
External ear canal infection—
Adults and children: 2 to 3 drops into ear canal t.i.d.

ADVERSE REACTIONS
EENT: ear itching or burning.
Skin: pruritus, urticaria.
Other: overgrowth of nonsusceptible organisms, burning, bone marrow hypoplasia, *aplastic anemia.*

INTERACTIONS
None significant.

EFFECTS ON DIAGNOSTIC TESTS
RBC, WBC, and platelet counts in the blood, and possibly the bone marrow, may decrease during drug therapy (from reversible to irreversible bone marrow depression). Hemoglobinuria or lactic acidosis may also occur.

CONTRAINDICATIONS
Contraindicated in patients with a perforated eardrum or hypersensitivity to any component of drug.

NURSING CONSIDERATIONS
• Obtain history of use and reactions.
• Watch for signs of superinfection. Avoid prolonged use.
• Reculture persistent drainage.
• Watch for signs of sore throat (early sign of toxicity).

✓ Patient teaching
• Instruct patient or caregiver how to administer drug.
• Warn patient to avoid touching ear with dropper to avoid reinfection.

---

triethanolamine polypeptide oleate-condensate
Cerumenex

Pregnancy Risk Category: NR

HOW SUPPLIED
Otic solution: 10% in 6-ml, 12-ml bottles with droppers

ACTION
A ceruminolytic that emulsifies and disperses accumulated cerumen.

Route	Onset	Peak	Duration
Otic	Unknown	Unknown	15-30 min

INDICATIONS & DOSAGE
Impacted cerumen—
Adults and children: fill ear canal with solution and insert cotton plug. After 15 to 30 minutes, flush with warm water.

ADVERSE REACTIONS
EENT: ear erythema or itching.
Skin: severe eczema.

INTERACTIONS
None significant.

EFFECTS ON DIAGNOSTIC TESTS
None reported.

---

*Liquid contains alcohol.   **May contain tartrazine.   †Canada   ‡Australia   §U.K.   ◊OTC

CONTRAINDICATIONS
Contraindicated in patients with perforated eardrum, otitis media, and otitis externa.

NURSING CONSIDERATIONS
Alert: If hypersensitivity is suspected, anticipate patch test: Place 1 drop of drug on inner forearm; cover with bandage. Read results in 24 hours. If reaction occurs, drug should not be used.

☑ **Patient teaching**
• Teach patient to moisten cotton plug with medication before insertion, leave cotton in place for a maximum of 30 minutes, and flush ear gently with warm water, using a rubber bulb syringe.
• Tell patient not to use drops more often than prescribed.
• Warn patient that drug is for use only in the ears.
• Advise patient to discontinue drug if adverse reactions occur and to contact doctor immediately.
• Tell patient to keep container tightly closed and away from moisture.

beclomethasone dipropionate
budesonide
dexamethasone sodium
    phosphate
ephedrine sulfate
epinephrine hydrochloride
flunisolide
fluticasone propionate
naphazoline hydrochloride
oxymetazoline hydrochloride
phenylephrine hydrochloride
tetrahydrozoline hydrochloride
triamcinolone acetonide
xylometazoline hydrochloride

COMBINATION PRODUCTS
4-WAY FAST ACTING SPRAY ◊ : phenyl-ephrine hydrochloride 0.5%, naphazoline hydrochloride 0.05%, and pyrilamine maleate 0.2%.

---

beclomethasone dipropionate
Beconase, Beconase AQ, Vancenase, Vancenase AQ

Pregnancy Risk Category: C

HOW SUPPLIED
Nasal aerosol: 42 mcg/metered spray, 50 mcg/metered spray‡
Nasal spray: 42 mcg/metered spray, 50 mcg/metered spray‡

ACTION
A corticosteroid that decreases nasal inflammation, mainly by stabilizing leukocyte lysosomal membranes.

Route	Onset	Peak	Duration
Nasal	5-7 days	3 wk	Unknown

INDICATIONS & DOSAGE
Relief of symptoms of seasonal or peren-nial rhinitis; prevention of recurrence of nasal polyps after surgical removal—
Adults and children over 12 years: usual dosage is 1 or 2 sprays in each nostril, b.i.d., t.i.d., or q.i.d.

Children 6 to 12 years: 1 spray into each nostril t.i.d.

ADVERSE REACTIONS
CNS: headache.
EENT: *mild transient nasal burning and stinging,* nasal congestion, sneezing, burning, stinging, dryness, epistaxis, na-sopharyngeal fungal infections.

INTERACTIONS
None significant.

EFFECTS ON DIAGNOSTIC TESTS
None reported.

CONTRAINDICATIONS
Contraindicated in patients with untreated localized infection involving the nasal mucosa or hypersensitivity to drug.

NURSING CONSIDERATIONS
• Use cautiously, if at all, in patients with active or quiescent respiratory tract tubercular infections or untreated fungal, bacterial, or systemic viral or ocular herpes simplex infections. Also use cautiously in patients who have recently had nasal septal ulcers, nasal surgery, or trauma.
• Observe patient for fungal infections.
• Be aware that beclomethasone is not effective for acute exacerbations of rhinitis. Decongestants or antihistamines may be needed.

✓ Patient teaching
• To instill, instruct patient to shake container before use; to blow nose to clear nasal passages; and to tilt head slightly forward and insert nozzle into nostril, pointing away from septum. Tell him to hold the other nostril closed and then to inspire gently and spray. Next, have him shake container again and repeat in other nostril.
• Advise patient to pump nasal spray three or four times before first use, and once or twice before first use each day. The cap and nosepiece of the activator

---

should be cleaned in warm water every day, then allowed to air-dry.

• Advise patient to use drug regularly, as prescribed, because its effectiveness depends on regular use.

• Explain that drug's therapeutic effects, unlike those of decongestants, are not immediate. Most patients achieve benefit within a few days, but some may require 2 to 3 weeks.

• Warn patient not to exceed recommended dosages because of risk of hypothalamic-pituitary-adrenal axis suppression.

• Tell patient to notify doctor if symptoms don't improve within 3 weeks or if nasal irritation persists.

• Teach patient good nasal and oral hygiene.

---

budesonide
Rhinocort

Pregnancy Risk Category: C

HOW SUPPLIED
Nasal spray: 32 mcg/metered spray (7-g canister)

ACTION
Unknown. A corticosteroid that probably decreases nasal inflammation, mainly by inhibiting the activities of specific cells and the mediators involved in the allergic response.

Route	Onset	Peak	Duration
Nasal	Unknown	Unknown	Unknown

INDICATIONS & DOSAGE
Symptoms of seasonal or perennial allergic rhinitis—
Adults and children 6 years and older: 2 sprays in each nostril in the morning and evening or 4 sprays in each nostril in the morning. Maintenance dosage should be the fewest number of sprays needed to control symptoms.

ADVERSE REACTIONS
CNS: nervousness.
EENT: *nasal irritation, epistaxis, pharyngitis,* reduced sense of smell, nasal pain, hoarseness.

GI: bad taste, dry mouth, dyspepsia, nausea.
Respiratory: *cough,* candidiasis, wheezing, dyspnea.
Skin: facial edema, rash, pruritus, contact dermatitis.
Other: myalgia, ***hypersensitivity reactions.***

INTERACTIONS
None significant.

EFFECTS ON DIAGNOSTIC TESTS
None reported.

CONTRAINDICATIONS
Contraindicated in patients hypersensitive to drug or its components and in those who have had recent septal ulcers, nasal surgery, or nasal trauma until total healing has occurred.

NURSING CONSIDERATIONS
• Use cautiously in patients with tuberculous infections; untreated fungal, bacterial, or systemic viral infections; or ocular herpes simplex.

• Systemic effects of steroid therapy may occur if recommended daily dose is increased.

☑ **Patient teaching**
• Tell patient to avoid exposure to chickenpox or measles.

• To instill, instruct patient to shake container before use; to blow nose to clear nasal passages; and to tilt head slightly forward and insert nozzle into nostril, pointing away from septum. Tell him to hold the other nostril closed and then to inspire gently and spray. Next, have him shake container again and repeat in other nostril.

• Instruct patient that product should be used by one person only to prevent the spread of infection.

• Advise patient not to break, incinerate, or store canister in extreme heat; contents under pressure.

• Warn patient not to exceed prescribed dosage or use for long periods of time because of the risk of hypothalamic-pituitary-adrenal axis suppression.

• Tell patient to contact doctor if symp-

Reactions may be *common,* uncommon, *life-threatening*, or **COMMON AND LIFE-THREATENING.**

toms do not improve in 3 weeks or if condition worsens.
• Teach patient good nasal and oral hygiene.
• Tell patients to use drug within 6 months of opening the protective aluminum pouch.

dexamethasone sodium phosphate
Dexacort Phosphate Turbinaire

Pregnancy Risk Category: C

HOW SUPPLIED
Nasal aerosol: 84 mcg/metered spray, 170 doses/12.6-g canister

ACTION
Decreases nasal inflammation, mainly by stabilizing leukocyte lysosomal membranes.

Route	Onset	Peak	Duration
Nasal	Unknown	Unknown	Unknown

INDICATIONS & DOSAGE
Allergic or inflammatory conditions, nasal polyps—
Adults: 2 sprays in each nostril b.i.d. or t.i.d. Maximum dosage is 12 sprays daily.
Children 6 to 12 years: 1 or 2 sprays in each nostril b.i.d. Maximum 8 sprays daily.
  Each spray delivers 0.1 mg dexamethasone sodium phosphate equal to 0.084 mg dexamethasone.

ADVERSE REACTIONS
EENT: nasal irritation, dryness, rebound nasal congestion.
Other: *hypersensitivity reactions,* systemic effects with prolonged use (pituitary-adrenal axis suppression, sodium retention, *heart failure,* hypertension, peptic ulceration, ecchymoses, petechiae, masking of infection).

INTERACTIONS
None significant.

EFFECTS ON DIAGNOSTIC TESTS
None reported.

CONTRAINDICATIONS
Contraindicated in patients with systemic fungal infections, tuberculosis, viral and fungal nasal conditions, ocular herpes simplex, or hypersensitivity to drug and in those who have had recent septal ulcers, nasal surgery, or nasal trauma until total healing has occurred.

NURSING CONSIDERATIONS
• Use cautiously in patients with diabetes mellitus, peptic ulcer, ulcerative colitis, abscess or other pyrogenic infection, diverticulitis, fresh intestinal anastomosis, renal insufficiency, hypertension, osteoporosis, and myasthenia gravis.
• Frequently monitor blood pressure and serum potassium level. Hypertension and hypokalemia can occur with systemic absorption.
• Monitor for fluid retention, which can occur from systemic absorption.
• Be prepared to reduce dosage gradually as nasal condition improves.
• Notify doctor if you suspect underlying bacterial infection that should be controlled with anti-infectives.
• Know that irritation or sensitivity may require stopping drug.

☑ **Patient teaching**
• Tell patient to avoid exposure to chickenpox or measles.
• To instill, instruct patient to shake container before use; to blow nose to clear nasal passages; and to tilt head slightly forward and insert nozzle into nostril, pointing away from septum. Tell him to hold the other nostril closed and then to inspire gently and spray. Next, have him shake container again and repeat in other nostril.
• Teach patient good nasal and oral hygiene.
• Warn patient that product should be used by only one person to prevent spread of infection.
• Warn patient to avoid prolonged use because of risk of hypothalamic-pituitary-adrenal axis suppression.
• Advise patient to contact doctor if he experiences fever, joint or muscle aches, or extreme tiredness.
• When improvement occurs, reduce

---

dosage as ordered by doctor. Discontinue therapy as soon as feasible.
• Advise patient not to break, incinerate, or store canister in extreme heat; contents under pressure.

ephedrine sulfate
Pretz-D ◊ , Vicks Vatronol ◊

Pregnancy Risk Category: NR

HOW SUPPLIED
Nasal solution: 0.5%◊
Nasal spray: 0.25%◊

ACTION
Causes local vasoconstriction of dilated arterioles, reducing blood flow and nasal congestion.

Route	Onset	Peak	Duration
Nasal	Unknown	Unknown	Unknown

INDICATIONS & DOSAGE
Nasal congestion—
Adults and children: 2 to 3 drops of 0.5% solution into each nostril. Use no more frequently than q 4 hours.

ADVERSE REACTIONS
CNS: nervousness, excitation.
CV: *tachycardia.*
EENT: rebound nasal congestion (with long-term or excessive use), mucosal irritation.

INTERACTIONS
Drug-drug. *MAO inhibitors:* hypertensive crisis if ephedrine is absorbed. Don't use together.

EFFECTS ON DIAGNOSTIC TESTS
None reported.

CONTRAINDICATIONS
Contraindicated in patients with angle-closure glaucoma, psychoneurosis, angina pectoris, substantial organic heart disease, CV disease, and hypersensitivity to drug or other sympathomimetics.

NURSING CONSIDERATIONS
• Use cautiously in patients with hyper-thyroidism, hypertension, diabetes mellitus, or prostatic hyperplasia.

☑ Patient teaching
• Teach patient how to instill nose drops or use nasal spray.
• Instruct patient that product should be used by only one person to prevent spread of infection.
• Tell patient not to exceed recommended dosage and to use only when needed.

epinephrine hydrochloride
Adrenalin Chloride

Pregnancy Risk Category: NR

HOW SUPPLIED
Nasal solution: 0.1%

ACTION
Causes local vasoconstriction of dilated arterioles, reducing blood flow and nasal congestion.

Route	Onset	Peak	Duration
Nasal	1 min	Unknown	Unknown

INDICATIONS & DOSAGE
Nasal congestion, local superficial bleeding—
Adults and children 6 years and older: instill 1 or 2 drops of solution.

ADVERSE REACTIONS
CNS: nervousness, excitation.
CV: *tachycardia.*
EENT: rebound nasal congestion, slight sting upon application.

INTERACTIONS
None significant.

EFFECTS ON DIAGNOSTIC TESTS
Drug therapy may increase blood glucose and serum lactic acid levels; increases BUN levels; and interferes with tests for urinary catecholamines.

CONTRAINDICATIONS
Contraindicated in patients with hypersensitivity to drug.

NURSING CONSIDERATIONS
• Use cautiously in patients with hyperthyroidism, coronary artery disease, hypertension, or diabetes mellitus.
• Monitor heart rate.

☑ Patient teaching
• Teach patient how to instill nose drops.
• Instruct patient that product should be used by only one person to prevent spread of infection.
• Tell patient not to exceed recommended dosage and to use only when needed.

---

flunisolide
Nasalide, Rhinalar†, Syntaris§

Pregnancy Risk Category: C

HOW SUPPLIED
Nasal inhalant: 25 mcg/metered spray, 200 doses/bottle‡
Nasal solution: 0.25 mg/ml in pump spray bottle (25 mcg per spray)

ACTION
Decreases nasal inflammation, mainly by stabilizing leukocyte lysosomal membranes by unknown mechanism.

Route	Onset	Peak	Duration
Nasal	Unknown	Unknown	Unknown

INDICATIONS & DOSAGE
Symptoms of seasonal or perennial rhinitis—
Adults: starting dose is 2 sprays (50 mcg) in each nostril b.i.d. Total daily dosage is 200 mcg. If necessary, dosage may be increased to 2 sprays in each nostril t.i.d. Maximum total daily dosage is 8 sprays in each nostril (400 mcg daily).
Children 6 to 14 years: starting dose is 1 spray (25 mcg) in each nostril t.i.d. or 2 sprays (50 mcg) in each nostril b.i.d. Total daily dosage is 150 to 200 mcg. Maximum total daily dosage is 4 sprays in each nostril (200 mcg daily).

ADVERSE REACTIONS
CNS: headache.
EENT: *mild, transient nasal burning and stinging,* nasal congestion, nasopharyngeal fungal infection, burning, stinging, dryness, sneezing, epistaxis, watery eyes.
GI: nausea, vomiting.

INTERACTIONS
None significant.

EFFECTS ON DIAGNOSTIC TESTS
None reported.

CONTRAINDICATIONS
Contraindicated in patients hypersensitive to drug. Also, do not use drug in presence of untreated localized infection involving nasal mucosa.

NURSING CONSIDERATIONS
• Use cautiously, if at all, in patients with active or quiescent respiratory tract tubercular infections or in untreated fungal, bacterial, or systemic viral or ocular herpes simplex infections. Also use cautiously in patients who have recently had nasal septal ulcers, nasal surgery, or nasal trauma.
• Be aware that flunisolide is not effective for acute exacerbations of rhinitis. Decongestants or antihistamines may be needed.

☑ Patient teaching
• Tell patient to avoid exposure to chickenpox or measles.
• To instill, instruct patient to shake the container before using; to blow nose to clear nasal passages; and to tilt head slightly forward and insert nozzle into nostril, pointing away from septum. Tell him to hold the other nostril closed, and then to inspire gently and spray. Have him repeat the above in the other nostril. Tell him to clean nosepiece with warm water if it becomes clogged.
• Explain that drug's therapeutic effects are not immediate. Most achieve benefit within a few days, but some may require 2 to 3 weeks.
• Advise patient to use drug regularly, as prescribed.
• Warn patient not to exceed recommended dosage to avoid hypothalamic-pituitary-adrenal axis suppression.
• Tell him to stop drug and notify doctor

---

*Liquid contains alcohol.   **May contain tartrazine.   †Canada   ‡Australia   §U.K.   ◊OTC

if symptoms don't diminish in 3 weeks or if nasal irritation persists.

fluticasone propionate
Flixonase§, Flonase

Pregnancy Risk Category: C

HOW SUPPLIED
Nasal spray: 50 mcg/metered spray (9-g, 16-g bottles)

ACTION
Decreases nasal inflammation; exact mechanism unknown.

Route	Onset	Peak	Duration
Nasal	Unknown	Unknown	Unknown

INDICATIONS & DOSAGE
Seasonal and perennial allergic rhinitis—
Adults: initially, 2 sprays (100 mcg) in each nostril once daily. Alternatively, 1 spray in each nostril b.i.d. After a few days, dosage may be reduced to 1 spray in each nostril daily. Maximum daily dosage is 2 sprays in each nostril.
Children 12 years and older: initially, 1 spray (50 mcg) in each nostril once daily. If patient doesn't respond or symptoms are severe, increase to 2 sprays in each nostril. Depending on patient's response, may decrease dosage to 1 spray in each nostril daily. Maximum daily dosage is 2 sprays in each nostril.

ADVERSE REACTIONS
CNS: headache.
EENT: epistaxis, nasal burning, blood in nasal mucus, pharyngitis, nasal irritation.

INTERACTIONS
None reported.

EFFECTS ON DIAGNOSTIC TESTS
None reported.

CONTRAINDICATIONS
Contraindicated in patients with hypersensitivity to drug or its component.

NURSING CONSIDERATIONS
• Use cautiously, if at all, in patients with active or quiescent tuberculous infections; glaucoma; untreated fungal, bacterial, or systemic viral infections; or ocular herpes simplex. Also use cautiously in patients already receiving systemic corticosteroids and in breast-feeding women.
• Do not use in patients with recent nasal septal ulcers, nasal surgery, or nasal trauma until healing has occurred.
• Although they rarely occur, monitor for signs of immediate hypersensitivity reactions or contact dermatitis after intranasal administration.

✓ Patient teaching
• Urge patient to read instruction sheet before using drug for first time.
• Explain how to instill drug. Tell patient to shake container gently before use; to blow nose to clear nasal passages; and to tilt head slightly forward and insert nozzle into nostril, pointing away from the septum. Tell him to hold the other nostril closed and then to inspire gently and spray. Next, have patient shake container again and repeat this procedure in the other nostril.
• Stress importance of adhering to a schedule for instillation because drug effectiveness depends on regular use. Caution patient not to exceed recommended dose; doing so may lead to hyperadrenocorticism, hypothalamic-pituitary-adrenal axis suppression, or suppression of growth in children or teenagers.
• Tell patient to notify doctor if symptoms do not improve or condition worsens.
• Warn patient to avoid exposure to chickenpox and measles and, if exposed, to obtain medical advice.
• Instruct patient to watch for and report signs and symptoms of nasal infection.

naphazoline hydrochloride
Privine ◇

Pregnancy Risk Category: NR

HOW SUPPLIED
Nose drops: 0.05% solution
Nasal spray: 0.05% solution

Reactions may be *common,* uncommon, ***life-threatening,*** or **COMMON AND LIFE-THREATENING.**

ACTION
Causes local vasoconstriction of dilated arterioles, reducing blood flow and nasal congestion.

Route	Onset	Peak	Duration
Nasal	10 min	Unknown	2-6 hr

INDICATIONS & DOSAGE
Nasal congestion—
Adults and children 12 years and older: 1 or 2 drops in each nostril at least 6 hours apart. Or, 1 to 2 sprays in each nostril at least 6 hours apart.

Do not give to children under 12 years unless directed by doctor.

ADVERSE REACTIONS
EENT: rebound nasal congestion (with excessive or long-term use), sneezing, stinging, dryness of mucosa.
Other: systemic effects in children (after excessive or long-term use), marked sedation.

INTERACTIONS
None significant.

EFFECTS ON DIAGNOSTIC TESTS
None reported.

CONTRAINDICATIONS
Contraindicated in patients with hypersensitivity to drug.

NURSING CONSIDERATIONS
• Use cautiously in patients with hyperthyroidism, heart disease, hypertension, or diabetes mellitus and in those who have difficulty urinating due to enlargement of the prostate gland.

✓ **Patient teaching**
• Teach patient how to use drug. For nose drops, instruct patient to tilt head back as far as possible, instill drops, then lean head forward while inhaling and to repeat procedure for other nostril. For nasal spray, instruct him to hold spray container and head upright. Tell patient not to shake the container.
• Tell patient that product should be used by only one person to prevent spread of infection.

• Warn patient not to exceed recommended dosage.
• Instruct patient to call doctor if nasal congestion persists after 5 days.

oxymetazoline hydrochloride
Afrin◇, Afrin Children's Strength Nose Drops◇, Allerest 12 Hour Nasal Spray◇, Chlorphed-LA◇, Dristan Long Lasting◇, Drixine Nasal‡, Duramist Plus◇, Duration◇, 4-Way Long Lasting Spray, Genasal Spray◇, Neo-Synephrine 12 Hour◇, Nostrilla◇, NTZ Long Acting Decongestant Nasal Spray◇, Sinarest 12 Hour Nasal◇, Sinex Long-Acting◇, Twice-A-Day Nasal◇

Pregnancy Risk Category: NR

HOW SUPPLIED
Nasal solution: 0.025%◇, 0.05%◇

ACTION
Unknown. Thought to cause local vasoconstriction of dilated arterioles, reducing blood flow and nasal congestion.

Route	Onset	Peak	Duration
Nasal	5-10 min	6 hr	< 12 hr

INDICATIONS & DOSAGE
Nasal congestion—
Adults and children 6 years and older: 2 to 3 drops or sprays of 0.05% solution in each nostril b.i.d.
Children 2 to 5 years: 2 to 3 drops of 0.025% solution in each nostril b.i.d. Use no longer than 3 to 5 days.

ADVERSE REACTIONS
CNS: headache, drowsiness, dizziness, insomnia, possible sedation.
CV: palpitations, *CV collapse,* hypertension.
EENT: rebound nasal congestion or irritation (with excessive or long-term use), dryness of nose and throat, increased nasal discharge, stinging, sneezing.
Other: systemic effects in children (with excessive or long-term use).

---

*Liquid contains alcohol.   **May contain tartrazine.   †Canada   ‡Australia   §U.K.   ◇OTC

INTERACTIONS
None significant.

EFFECTS ON DIAGNOSTIC TESTS
None reported.

CONTRAINDICATIONS
Contraindicated in patients with hypersensitivity to drug.

NURSING CONSIDERATIONS
• Use cautiously in patients with hyperthyroidism, cardiac disease, hypertension, or diabetes mellitus.

☑ **Patient teaching**
• Teach patient how to apply oxymetazoline. Tell him to hold head upright to minimize swallowing of medication, then sniff spray briskly.
• Tell patient that product should be used by only one person to prevent spread of infection.
• Tell patient not to exceed recommended dosage and to use only when needed.
Alert: Warn patient that excessive use may cause bradycardia, hypotension, dizziness, and weakness.

phenylephrine hydrochloride
Alconefrin Nasal Drops 12 ◇,
Alconefrin Nasal Drops 25 ◇,
Alconefrin Nasal Drops 50 ◇,
Doktors ◇, Duration ◇,
Neo-Synephrine ◇, Nostril ◇,
Rhinall ◇, Rhinall-10 Children's
Flavored Nose Drops ◇, Sinex ◇

Pregnancy Risk Category: NR

HOW SUPPLIED
Nasal solution: 0.125%, 0.16%, 0.2%, 0.25%, 0.5%, 1%

ACTION
Causes local vasoconstriction of dilated arterioles, reducing blood flow and nasal congestion.

Route	Onset	Peak	Duration
Nasal	Rapid	Unknown	0.5-4 hr

INDICATIONS & DOSAGE
Nasal congestion—
Adults and children 12 years and over: 2 to 3 drops or 1 to 2 sprays instilled in each nostril q 4 hours, p.r.n. Do not use for more than 3 to 5 days.
Children 6 to 12 years: 2 to 3 drops or 1 to 2 sprays of a 0.25% solution instilled in each nostril q 4 hours, p.r.n.
Children under 6 years: 2 to 3 drops of 0.125% solution q 4 hours, p.r.n.

ADVERSE REACTIONS
CNS: headache, tremor, dizziness, nervousness.
CV: *palpitations, tachycardia, PVCs,* hypertension, pallor.
EENT: transient burning or stinging, dryness of nasal mucosa; rebound nasal congestion (with continued use).
GI: nausea.

INTERACTIONS
None significant.

EFFECTS ON DIAGNOSTIC TESTS
Drug may lower intraocular pressure in normal eyes or in open-angle glaucoma. It may also cause false-normal tonometry readings.

CONTRAINDICATIONS
Contraindicated in patients with hypersensitivity to drug.

NURSING CONSIDERATIONS
• Use cautiously in patients with hyperthyroidism, marked hypertension, type 1 diabetes mellitus, cardiac disease, or advanced arteriosclerotic changes; in children of low body weight; and in elderly patients.

☑ **Patient teaching**
• Teach patient how to apply phenylephrine. Tell him to hold head upright to minimize swallowing of medication, then to sniff spray briskly.
• Inform patient that product should be used by only one person to prevent spread of infection.
• Tell patient not to exceed recommended dosage and to use only when needed.

• Advise patient to contact doctor if symptoms persist beyond 3 days.

---

tetrahydrozoline hydrochloride
Tyzine, Tyzine Pediatric

Pregnancy Risk Category: C

HOW SUPPLIED
Nasal solution: 0.05%, 0.1%

ACTION
Unknown. Thought to cause local vaso-constriction of dilated arterioles, reducing blood flow and nasal congestion.

Route	Onset	Peak	Duration
Nasal	Few min	Unknown	4-8 hr

INDICATIONS & DOSAGE
Nasal congestion—
Adults and children over 6 years: 2 to 4 drops of 0.1% solution or spray into each nostril q 4 to 6 hours, p.r.n.
Children 2 to 6 years: 2 to 3 drops of 0.05% solution into each nostril q 4 to 6 hours, p.r.n.

ADVERSE REACTIONS
EENT: transient burning, stinging; sneezing; rebound nasal congestion (with excessive or long-term use).

INTERACTIONS
None significant.

EFFECTS ON DIAGNOSTIC TESTS
None reported.

CONTRAINDICATIONS
Contraindicated in patients with angle-closure glaucoma, other serious eye diseases, or hypersensitivity to drug and in children under 2 years. The 0.1% solution is contraindicated in children under 6 years.

NURSING CONSIDERATIONS
• Use cautiously in patients with hyperthyroidism, hypertension, and diabetes mellitus.

• Do not use 0.1% solution in children under 6 years.

☑ Patient teaching
• Teach patient how to apply tetrahydrozoline. Tell him to hold head upright to minimize swallowing of medication, then sniff spray briskly.
• Instruct patient that product should be used by only one person to prevent spread of infection.
• Tell patient not to exceed recommended dosage and to use only as needed for 3 to 5 days.

---

triamcinolone acetonide
Nasacort, Nasacort AQ

Pregnancy Risk Category: C

HOW SUPPLIED
Nasal aerosol: 55 mcg/metered spray
Nasal spray pump: 55 mcg/spray

ACTION
Unknown. A glucocorticoid with anti-inflammatory properties.

Route	Onset	Peak	Duration
Nasal	12 hr	3-4 days	Unknown

INDICATIONS & DOSAGE
Relief of symptoms of seasonal or perennial allergic rhinitis—
Adults and children 12 years and older: initially, 2 sprays (110 mcg) in each nostril once daily. Increased p.r.n. up to 440 mcg daily either as once-daily dosage or in divided doses up to q.i.d. After desired effect is obtained, dosage decreased, if possible, to as little as 1 spray (55 mcg) in each nostril daily.
Children 6 to 11 years: initially, 2 sprays in each nostril (220 mcg) once daily.

ADVERSE REACTIONS
EENT: *nasal irritation,* dry mucous membranes, nasal and sinus congestion, irritation, burning, stinging, throat discomfort, sneezing, epistaxis.
Other: *headache.*

---

*Liquid contains alcohol.   **May contain tartrazine.   †Canada   ‡Australia   §U.K.   ◇OTC

INTERACTIONS
None significant.

EFFECTS ON DIAGNOSTIC TESTS
None reported.

CONTRAINDICATIONS
Contraindicated in patients hypersensitive to drug or its components.

NURSING CONSIDERATIONS
• Use with extreme caution, if at all, in patients with active or quiescent tuberculosis infection of respiratory tract and in patients with untreated fungal, bacterial, or systemic viral infection or ocular herpes simplex.
• Use cautiously in patients who are already receiving systemic corticosteroids because of the increased likelihood of hypothalamic-pituitary-adrenal axis suppression compared with a therapeutic dosage of either one alone. Also use cautiously in patients with recent nasal septal ulcers, nasal surgery, or trauma because of the inhibitory effect on wound healing. Also use with caution in breast-feeding patients.
Alert: Be aware that when excessive doses are used, signs and symptoms of hyperadrenocorticism and adrenal axis suppression may occur; drug should be discontinued slowly.

☑ **Patient teaching**
• Urge patient to read the patient-instruction sheet contained in each package before using drug for the first time.
• To instill, instruct patient to shake container before use; to blow nose to clear nasal passages; and to tilt head slightly forward and insert nozzle into nostril, pointing away from the septum. Tell him to hold the other nostril closed and then to inspire gently and spray. Next, have patient shake container and repeat procedure in other nostril.
• Tell patient to discard the canister after 100 actuations.
• Stress importance of using drug on a regular schedule because its effectiveness depends on regular use. However, caution patient not to exceed the dosage prescribed because serious adverse reactions may occur.
• Tell patient to notify doctor if symptoms do not diminish within 2 to 3 weeks or if condition worsens.
• Warn patient to avoid exposure to chickenpox or measles and, if exposed to either, to obtain medical advice.
• Instruct patient to watch for signs and symptoms of nasal infection. If any occur, tell him to notify doctor because drug may need to be discontinued and appropriate local therapy given.
• Advise patient not to break canister, to incinerate canister, or to store canister in extreme heat; contents are under pressure and may explode.

---

xylometazoline hydrochloride
Otrivin ◊

Pregnancy Risk Category: NR

HOW SUPPLIED
Nasal solution: 0.05%, 0.1%

ACTION
Unknown. Thought to cause local vasoconstriction of dilated arterioles, reducing blood flow and nasal congestion.

Route	Onset	Peak	Duration
Nasal	5-10 min	Unknown	5-6 hr

INDICATIONS & DOSAGE
Nasal congestion—
Adults and children 12 years and older: 2 to 3 drops or sprays of 0.1% solution in each nostril q 8 to 10 hours.
Children 2 to 12 years: 2 to 3 drops of 0.05% solution in each nostril q 8 to 10 hours.
Children 6 months to 2 years: 1 drop of 0.05% solution instilled into each nostril q 6 hours, p.r.n.

ADVERSE REACTIONS
EENT: transient burning, stinging; dryness or ulceration of nasal mucosa; sneezing; rebound nasal congestion or irritation (with excessive or long-term use).

Reactions may be *common*, uncommon, *life-threatening*, or COMMON AND LIFE-THREATENING.

INTERACTIONS
None significant.

EFFECTS ON DIAGNOSTIC TESTS
None reported.

CONTRAINDICATIONS
Contraindicated in patients with angle-closure glaucoma or hypersensitivity to drug.

NURSING CONSIDERATIONS
• Use cautiously in patients with hyperthyroidism, cardiac disease, hypertension, diabetes mellitus, and advanced arteriosclerosis.
• Do not use 0.1% solution in children under 6 years.

☑ Patient teaching
• Teach patient how to apply drug. Have patient hold head upright to minimize swallowing of medication, then sniff spray briskly.
• Tell patient that product should be used by only one person.
• Inform patient not to exceed recommended dose and to use only as needed for 3 to 5 days.

acyclovir
amphotericin B
azelaic acid cream
bacitracin
butoconazole nitrate
clindamycin phosphate
clotrimazole
econazole nitrate
erythromycin
gentamicin sulfate
ketoconazole
mafenide acetate
metronidazole (topical)
miconazole nitrate
mupirocin
naftifine hydrochloride
neomycin sulfate
nitrofurazone
nystatin
silver sulfadiazine
sulconazole nitrate
terbinafine hydrochloride
terconazole
tetracycline hydrochloride
tioconazole
tolnaftate

COMBINATION PRODUCTS

BENZAMYCIN: erythromycin 3% and benzoyl peroxide 5%.
LANABIOTIC ◊ : polymyxin B sulfate 5,000 units, neomycin sulfate 5 mg, bacitracin 500 units, and lidocaine 40 mg/g.
LOTRISONE: clotrimazole 1% and betamethasone dipropionate 0.05%.
MYCITRACIN ◊ : polymyxin B sulfate 5,000 units, bacitracin 500 units, and neomycin sulfate 3.5 mg/g.
MYCOLOG II: triamcinolone acetonide 0.1% and nystatin 100,000 units/g.
NEO-CORTEF: hydrocortisone acetate 1% and neomycin sulfate 0.5%.
NEODECADRON: dexamethasone phosphate 0.1% and neomycin sulfate 0.5%.
NEOSPORIN CREAM ◊ : polymyxin B sulfate 10,000 units and neomycin sulfate 5 mg.
NEOSPORIN OINTMENT ◊ : polymyxin B sulfate 5,000 units, bacitracin zinc 400 units, and neomycin sulfate 5 mg/g.
POLYSPORIN OINTMENT ◊ : polymyxin B sulfate 10,000 units and bacitracin zinc 500 units/g.
VIOFORM-HYDROCORTISONE MILD CREAM: iodochlorhydroxyquin 3% and hydrocortisone 0.5%.

---

acyclovir
Acyclo-V‡, Zovirax

Pregnancy Risk Category: C

HOW SUPPLIED
Ointment: 5%

ACTION
Inhibits herpes simplex and varicella-zoster viral DNA synthesis by inhibiting viral DNA polymerase action.

Route	Onset	Peak	Duration
Topical	Unknown	Unknown	Unknown

INDICATIONS & DOSAGE
Initial herpes genitalis; limited, non–life-threatening mucocutaneous herpes simplex virus infections in immunocompromised patients—
Adults: cover all lesions q 3 hours six times daily for 7 days. Although dosage will vary depending on total lesion area, use about a ½″ (1.3 cm) ribbon of ointment on each 4″ (10 cm) square of surface area.

ADVERSE REACTIONS
Skin: *transient burning and stinging, rash,* pruritus, vulvitis; edema, pain (at application site).

INTERACTIONS
None significant.

EFFECTS ON DIAGNOSTIC TESTS
None reported.

CONTRAINDICATIONS

Contraindicated in patients with hypersensitivity or chemical intolerance to drug.

NURSING CONSIDERATIONS

• As ordered, start therapy as early as possible after onset of symptoms.
• Apply with a finger cot or rubber glove to prevent autoinoculation of other body sites and transmission of infection to other persons.
• Be aware that all lesions must be thoroughly covered.
• Know that drug is for cutaneous use only; don't apply to the eye.
• Be aware that drug is not a cure, but it will help with the symptoms.

☑ Patient teaching

• Teach patient that virus transmission can occur during treatment.
• Tell patient that there may be some discomfort with application.
• Emphasize importance of compliance for successful therapy.
• Teach patient that therapy should begin as soon as signs and symptoms appear.
• Tell patient to notify doctor if adverse reactions occur.

---

amphotericin B
Fungizone

Pregnancy Risk Category: B

HOW SUPPLIED

Cream: 3%
Lotion: 3%
Ointment: 3%

ACTION

Usually fungistatic; binds to sterols in the fungal cell membrane, resulting in increased membrane permeability and subsequent cell leakage.

Route	Onset	Peak	Duration
Topical	Unknown	Unknown	Unknown

INDICATIONS & DOSAGE

Cutaneous or mucocutaneous candidal infections—

Adults and children: apply liberally, rubbing in gently, b.i.d. to q.i.d. for 1 to 3 weeks; interdigital lesions and paronychias treated for 2 to 4 weeks, and onychomycoses for several months because relapses are common.

ADVERSE REACTIONS

Skin: possible dryness, contact sensitivity, erythema, burning, pruritus.

INTERACTIONS

None significant.

EFFECTS ON DIAGNOSTIC TESTS

None reported.

CONTRAINDICATIONS

Contraindicated in patients with hypersensitivity to drug or its components.

NURSING CONSIDERATIONS

• Clean area before applying.
• Report local irritation. Cream may dry skin; ointment may irritate if applied to moist, hairy areas.
• Avoid using occlusive dressings.
• Be aware that cream or lotion is preferred for such areas as groin folds, armpits, and neck creases.
• Stop drug if irritation or hypersensitivity occurs, and notify doctor.

☑ Patient teaching

• Tell patient to use drug for full treatment period, even if condition has improved.
• Inform patient that skin may become discolored if amphotericin B is not rubbed in thoroughly; nail lesions may become stained.
• Caution patient against application to eyes.
• Tell patient that fabric discoloration caused by cream or lotion can be removed by washing; discoloration by ointment can be removed by cleaning fluid.
• Instruct patient not to apply occlusive dressing.

---

azelaic acid cream
Azelex, Skinoren§

Pregnancy Risk Category: B

HOW SUPPLIED
Cream: 20%

ACTION
Unknown. May inhibit microbial cellular protein synthesis.

Route	Onset	Peak	Duration
Topical	Unknown	Unknown	Unknown

INDICATIONS & DOSAGE
Mild to moderate inflammatory acne vulgaris—
Adults: apply a thin film and gently but thoroughly massage into affected areas b.i.d., in morning and evening.

ADVERSE REACTIONS
Skin: pruritus, burning, stinging, tingling.

INTERACTIONS
None reported.

EFFECTS ON DIAGNOSTIC TESTS
None reported.

CONTRAINDICATIONS
Contraindicated in patients with hypersensitivity to drug or its components.

NURSING CONSIDERATIONS
• Use with caution in pregnant or breast-feeding patients.
• Monitor patient for early signs of hypopigmentation, especially a patient with dark complexion.
• If sensitivity or severe irritation occurs, notify doctor, who may discontinue drug and order appropriate treatment.
• Avoid use of occlusive dressings.

☑ Patient teaching
• Instruct patient to wash and pat dry affected areas before applying drug and to wash hands well after application. Warn him not to apply occlusive dressings or wrappings to affected areas.
• Warn patient that skin irritation may occur when drug is applied to broken or inflamed skin, usually at start of therapy. Tell him to notify doctor if irritation persists.
• Advise patient to keep drug away from mouth, eyes, and other mucous membranes. If contact occurs, tell him to rinse thoroughly with water and notify doctor if irritation persists.
• Advise patient to report abnormal changes in skin color.
• Urge patient to use drug for the full treatment period.

bacitracin
Baciguent◊, Bacitin†

Pregnancy Risk Category: C

HOW SUPPLIED
Ointment: 500 units/g

ACTION
Bactericidal or bacteriostatic, depending on organism and concentration of drug; inhibits bacterial cell wall synthesis. Effective against gram-positive organisms.

Route	Onset	Peak	Duration
Topical	Unknown	Unknown	Unknown

INDICATIONS & DOSAGE
Topical infections, abrasions, cuts, and minor burns or wounds—
Adults and children: apply thin film one to three times daily, depending on severity of condition. Drug should not be used for more than 1 week.

ADVERSE REACTIONS
Skin: stinging, rashes, other allergic reactions, allergic contact dermatitis; pruritus, burning, swelling of lips or face.
Other: tightness in chest, hypotension.

INTERACTIONS
None significant.

EFFECTS ON DIAGNOSTIC TESTS
Urinary sediment tests may show increased protein and cast excretion. Serum creatinine and BUN levels may increase during therapy.

Reactions may be *common,* uncommon, *life-threatening,* or COMMON AND LIFE-THREATENING.

CONTRAINDICATIONS
Contraindicated in patients with atopy or hypersensitivity to drug.

NURSING CONSIDERATIONS
• Use cautiously in patients with neuromuscular disease or myasthenia gravis.
• Clean area before applying, especially if crusted or suppurative.
• Anticipate alternative treatment for burns that cover more than 20% of body surface, especially if patient suffers from impaired renal function.
• Know that prolonged use may result in overgrowth of nonsusceptible organisms, particularly *Candida* species.
• Know that patients allergic to neomycin may also be sensitive to bacitracin.
• Before applying drug, obtain culture and sensitivity tests, as ordered.

✓ Patient teaching
• Tell patient to stop using drug and notify doctor if no improvement occurs or if condition worsens.
• Instruct patient to report systemic and skin adverse reactions that persist or are severe.
• Tell patient to not use drug for more than 1 week, except on doctor's advice.

---

butoconazole nitrate
Femstat

Pregnancy Risk Category: C

HOW SUPPLIED
Vaginal cream: 2% with applicators supplied

ACTION
Unknown. Thought to control or destroy fungus by disrupting cell membrane permeability, thereby causing osmotic instability.

Route	Onset	Peak	Duration
Intravaginal	Unknown	Unknown	Unknown

INDICATIONS & DOSAGE
Vulvovaginal mycotic infections caused by Candida *species—*
Adults: for nonpregnant patient, 1 applicatorful intravaginally h.s. for 3 days. If needed, treat for another 3 days. For pregnant patient during second or third trimester, 1 applicatorful intravaginally h.s. for 6 days. Only use in pregnant women if absolutely necessary.

ADVERSE REACTIONS
GU: vulvovaginal burning and itching, soreness, discharge, swelling.
Skin: finger itching.

INTERACTIONS
None significant.

EFFECTS ON DIAGNOSTIC TESTS
None reported.

CONTRAINDICATIONS
Contraindicated in patients hypersensitive to drug.

NURSING CONSIDERATIONS
• Use cautiously in breast-feeding women.
• Confirm diagnosis by smears or cultures, as ordered.
• Know that drug use during pregnancy is restricted to the second and third trimesters and only when the potential benefits outweigh the possible risks to the fetus.
• Know that drug may be used with oral contraceptive and antibiotic therapy.

✓ Patient teaching
• Teach patient how to apply drug, and tell her not to use tampons during treatment.
• Advise patient to keep affected area cool and dry, wear loose-fitting cotton clothing, avoid feminine hygiene sprays, wash daily with unscented soap, dry thoroughly with clean towel, and prevent reinfection by wiping perineum from front to back.
• Instruct patient to clean applicator with soap and water after each use.
• Advise patient to use drug for prescribed length of time, even during menses.
• Tell patient that drug should be administered high in the vagina except during pregnancy.
• Advise patient that her sexual partner

should wear a condom during intercourse until treatment is complete. He should consult doctor if penile itching, redness, or discomfort occurs.

• Alert patient that drug base may weaken latex products (such as a condom or diaphragm); concurrent use within 3 days is not recommended as method of birth control.

clindamycin phosphate
Cleocin, Cleocin T

Pregnancy Risk Category: B

HOW SUPPLIED
Gel: 1%
Lotion: 1%
Pledget: 1%
Topical solution: 1%
Vaginal cream: 2%

ACTION
Bacteriostatic or bactericidal, based on drug concentration and susceptibility of organism; suppresses growth of susceptible organisms in sebaceous glands by blocking protein synthesis.

Route	Onset	Peak	Duration
Topical, intravaginal	Unknown	Unknown	Unknown

INDICATIONS & DOSAGE
Inflammatory acne vulgaris—
Adults and adolescents: apply to skin b.i.d., morning and evening.
Bacterial vaginosis—
Adults: 1 applicatorful intravaginally h.s. for 7 consecutive days.

ADVERSE REACTIONS
GI: GI upset, diarrhea, bloody diarrhea, abdominal pain, colitis (including pseudomembranous colitis).
GU: *cervicitis, vaginitis, Candida albicans* overgrowth, *vulvar irritation.*
Skin: *dryness,* rash, *redness,* pruritus, swelling, irritation, contact dermatitis, burning.

INTERACTIONS
Drug-drug. *Erythromycin:* may antago-

nize clindamycin's effect. Separate administration times.
Isotretinoin: potential cumulative dryness, resulting in excessive skin irritation. Use cautiously.
Neuromuscular blocking agents: may enhnace action of neuromuscular blocker. Use cautiously together.
Drug-lifestyle. *Abrasive or medicated soaps or cleansers; acne preparations or other preparations containing peeling agents (benzoyl peroxide, resorcinol, salicylic acid, sulfur, tretinoin); alcohol-containing products (aftershave, cosmetics, perfumed toiletries, shaving creams or lotions); astringent soaps or cosmetics; medicated cosmetics or cover-ups:* potential cumulative dryness, resulting in excessive skin irritation. Use cautiously.

EFFECTS ON DIAGNOSTIC TESTS
Drug therapy may cause abnormal liver function test results in some patients.

CONTRAINDICATIONS
Contraindicated in patients with hypersensitivity to drug or history of ulcerative colitis, regional enteritis, or antibiotic-associated colitis.

NURSING CONSIDERATIONS
• For treating acne, know that drug may be used concurrently with tretinoin or benzoyl peroxide as well as systemic antibiotics.
• Know that drug can cause excessive dryness.
• Monitor elderly patients for systemic effects.

☑ Patient teaching
• Tell patient to wash area with warm water and soap, to rinse and pat dry, and to wait 30 minutes after washing or shaving to apply.
• Warn patient to avoid too-frequent washing of area. Tell him to cover entire affected area but to avoid contact with eyes, nose, mouth, and other areas bearing mucous membranes.
• Tell patient to use only as prescribed.
• Instruct patient to dab, not roll, applicator-tipped bottle. If tip becomes dry, pa-

tient should invert bottle and depress tip several times to moisten.
- Warn patient not to smoke while applying topical solution.
- When used intravaginally, make sure patient knows how to use applicators that come with drug.
- Instruct patient to contact the doctor immediately if diarrhea occurs. Inform patient that antidiarrheal medication may worsen the condition and should only be used as directed by doctor.
- Tell patient to remove pledgets from foil before use.

---

clotrimazole
Canesten†, Femizol-7◊, Gyne-Lotrimin◊, Lotrimin, Mycelex, Mycelex-7◊, Mycelex-G, Mycelex OTC◊

Pregnancy Risk Category: B (C for troches)

HOW SUPPLIED
Troches: 10 mg
Cream: 1%
Topical lotion: 1%
Topical solution: 1%
Vaginal cream: 1%◊
Vaginal tablets: 100 mg◊, 200 mg, 500 mg
Combination pack: vaginal inserts 100 mg and vulvar cream 1%◊

ACTION
Fungistatic but may be fungicidal, depending on concentration. Alters fungal cell wall permeability and produces osmotic instability.

Route	Onset	Peak	Duration
PO	Unknown	Unknown	3 hr
Topical, intravaginal	Unknown	Unknown	Unknown

INDICATIONS & DOSAGE
Superficial fungal infections (tinea corporis, tinea cruris, tinea pedis, or tinea versicolor; candidiasis)—
Adults and children: apply thinly and massage into affected and surrounding area, morning and evening, for 2 to 4

weeks. If no improvement occurs after 4 weeks, patient should be reevaluated.
Vulvovaginal candidiasis—
Adults: two 100-mg vaginal tablets inserted daily h.s. for 7 consecutive days, or one 500-mg vaginal tablet daily h.s. for 1 day; or 1 applicatorful vaginal cream daily h.s. for 7 days.
Oropharyngeal candidiasis treatment—
Adults and children 3 years and older: dissolve troche over 15 to 30 minutes in mouth five times daily for 14 consecutive days.
Prevention of oropharyngeal candidiasis in patients immunocompromised by such conditions as chemotherapy, radiotherapy, or steroid therapy in the treatment of leukemia, solid tumors, or renal transplantation—
Adults and children: dissolve troche over 15 to 30 minutes in mouth t.i.d. for duration of chemotherapy or until steroid is reduced to maintenance levels.

ADVERSE REACTIONS
GI: lower abdominal cramps; nausea, vomiting (with lozenges).
GU: *mild vaginal burning or irritation* (with vaginal use), cramping, urinary frequency.
Skin: blistering, *erythema*, edema, pruritus, burning, stinging, peeling, urticaria, skin fissures, general irritation.
Other: elevated liver function test results.

INTERACTIONS
None significant.

EFFECTS ON DIAGNOSTIC TESTS
Abnormal liver function test results have been reported in patients receiving lozenges.

CONTRAINDICATIONS
Contraindicated in patients hypersensitive to drug. Also contraindicated for ophthalmic use.

NURSING CONSIDERATIONS
- Clean area before applying.
- Watch for and report irritation or sensitivity; discontinue if irritation occurs and notify doctor.
- Know that improvement is usually

---

demonstrated within 1 week; if no improvement occurs in 4 weeks, diagnosis should be reviewed.

• When compliance is a problem, be aware that mild to moderate vaginal candidiasis may be treated with a single 500-mg tablet.

☑ **Patient teaching**
• Reassure patient that hypopigmentation from tinea versicolor will resolve gradually.
• Warn patient not to use occlusive wrappings or dressings.
• Warn patient to avoid drug contact with eyes.
• Ensure that patient understands that frequent or persistent yeast infections may be a symptom of a more serious medical problem such as AIDS.
• Tell patient to refrain from sexual intercourse during treatment.
• Warn patient that topical preparation may stain clothing.
• Emphasize need to continue treatment for full course and to notify doctor if no improvement occurs within 4 weeks.

econazole nitrate
Ecostatin†, Prevaryl§, Spectazole

Pregnancy Risk Category: C

HOW SUPPLIED
Cream: 1%

ACTION
Fungistatic; may be fungicidal, depending on concentration. Alters fungal cell wall permeability and promotes osmotic instability.

Route	Onset	Peak	Duration
Topical	Unknown	Unknown	Unknown

INDICATIONS & DOSAGE
Tinea corporis, tinea cruris, tinea pedis, and tinea versicolor; cutaneous candidiasis—

Adults and children: rub into affected areas once daily for at least 2 weeks.
Cutaneous candidiasis—

Adults and children: rub into affected areas b.i.d.

ADVERSE REACTIONS
Skin: burning, pruritus, stinging, erythema.

INTERACTIONS
None significant.

EFFECTS ON DIAGNOSTIC TESTS
None reported.

CONTRAINDICATIONS
Contraindicated in patients hypersensitive to drug or its components.

NURSING CONSIDERATIONS
• Clean affected area before applying.
• Don't use occlusive dressings.

☑ **Patient teaching**
• Tell patient to use drug for entire treatment period, even if symptoms improve. Instruct him to notify doctor if no improvement occurs after 2 weeks (tinea corporis, tinea cruris, and tinea versicolor) or 4 weeks (tinea pedis).
• Reassure patient that hypopigmentation from tinea versicolor will resolve gradually.
• Tell patient to stop use and call doctor if condition persists or worsens or if irritation occurs.
• Warn patient that drug may stain clothing.
• Tell patient with tinea pedis to change shoes and cotton socks daily.

erythromycin
Akne-mycin, A/T/S, Del-Mycin, Emgel, Erycette, EryDerm, Erygel, Erymax, Ery-Sol†, Erythra-Derm, ETS†, Sans-Acne†, Staticin, T-Stat†

Pregnancy Risk Category: C

HOW SUPPLIED
Ointment: 2%
Topical gel: 2%
Topical solution: 1.5%*, 2%*
Pledgets: 2%

Reactions may be *common,* uncommon, *life-threatening,* or COMMON AND LIFE-THREATENING.

ACTION
Usually bacteriostatic but may be bactericidal in high concentrations or against highly susceptible organisms. Disrupts protein synthesis in susceptible bacteria.

Route	Onset	Peak	Duration
Topical	Unknown	Unknown	Unknown

INDICATIONS & DOSAGE
Inflammatory acne vulgaris—
Adults and children: apply to affected areas b.i.d.

ADVERSE REACTIONS
Skin: sensitivity reactions, erythema, *burning, dryness, pruritus,* irritation, peeling, oily skin.

INTERACTIONS
Drug-drug. *Isotretinoin:* may cause cumulative dryness, resulting in excessive skin irritation. Use cautiously.
Drug-lifestyle. *Abrasive or medicated soaps or cleansers; acne preparations or other preparations containing peeling agents (benzoyl peroxide, resorcinol, salicylic acid, sulfur, tretinoin); alcohol-containing products (aftershave, cosmetics, perfumed toiletries, shaving creams or lotions); astringent soaps or cosmetics; medicated cosmetics or cover-ups:* may cause cumulative dryness, resulting in excessive skin irritation. Use cautiously.

EFFECTS ON DIAGNOSTIC TESTS
Drug may interfere with fluorometric determinations of urinary catecholamines and may cause abnormal liver function test results (rare).

CONTRAINDICATIONS
Contraindicated in patients hypersensitive to drug or its components.

NURSING CONSIDERATIONS
• Wash, rinse, and dry affected areas before application.
• Know that prolonged use may be necessary when treating acne vulgaris; such use may result in overgrowth of nonsusceptible organisms.
• Obtain cultures before beginning therapy.

☑ **Patient teaching**
• Advise patient not to use near eyes, nose, mouth, or other areas bearing mucous membranes and to wash hands after applying.
• Tell patient to stop using drug and notify doctor if no improvement occurs or if condition worsens.
• Advise patient not to share towels or washcloths.
• Instruct patient to use each pledget once, then discard.
• Inform patient to keep product away from heat and open flame.

---

gentamicin sulfate
Garamycin, G-Myticin

Pregnancy Risk Category: C

HOW SUPPLIED
Cream: 0.1%
Ointment: 0.1%

ACTION
A bactericidal agent that disrupts bacterial protein synthesis by binding to ribosomes; however, its exact mechanism is unknown.

Route	Onset	Peak	Duration
Topical	Unknown	Unknown	Unknown

INDICATIONS & DOSAGE
Treatment and prophylaxis of superficial infections and superficial burns of the skin caused by susceptible bacteria—
Adults and children over 1 year: rub in small amount gently t.i.d. or q.i.d., with or without gauze dressing.

ADVERSE REACTIONS
Skin: minor skin irritation, possible photosensitivity, allergic contact dermatitis.

INTERACTIONS
None significant.

EFFECTS ON DIAGNOSTIC TESTS
None reported.

CONTRAINDICATIONS
Contraindicated in patients hypersensitive

to drug and its components or in those who may exhibit cross-sensitivity with other aminoglycosides such as neomycin.

NURSING CONSIDERATIONS
Alert: Avoid use on large skin lesions or over a wide area because of possible systemic toxic effects.
● Know that use should be restricted to selected patients; widespread use may lead to resistant organisms.
● Prolonged use may result in overgrowth of nonsusceptible organisms.

☑ **Patient teaching**
● Tell patient to clean affected area before applying. Have him remove crusts before application for impetigo contagiosa to enhance absorption.
● Instruct patient to store in cool place.
● Tell patient to stop drug and notify doctor immediately if no improvement occurs or if condition worsens.

---

ketoconazole
Nizoral

Pregnancy Risk Category: C

HOW SUPPLIED
Cream: 2%
Shampoo: 2%

ACTION
Unknown. An imidazole that probably inhibits yeast growth by altering the permeability of the cell membrane.

Route	Onset	Peak	Duration
Topical	Unknown	Unknown	Unknown

INDICATIONS & DOSAGE
Tinea corporis, tinea cruris, tinea pedis, and tinea versicolor caused by susceptible organisms; seborrheic dermatitis; cutaneous candidiasis—
Adults: cover affected and immediate surrounding area once daily for at least 2 weeks; for seborrheic dermatitis, apply b.i.d. for 4 weeks. When using shampoo, wet hair, lather, and massage for 1 minute. Rinse and repeat, but leave drug on scalp for 3 minutes before rinsing. Shampoo twice weekly for 4 weeks, with at least 3 days between shampoos and then intermittently p.r.n. to maintain control.

ADVERSE REACTIONS
Skin: severe irritation, pruritus, stinging.

INTERACTIONS
Drug-drug. *Topical corticosteroids:* may cause increased absorption of steroid. Avoid concomitant use.

EFFECTS ON DIAGNOSTIC TESTS
Drug has been reported to cause transient elevations in AST, ALT, and alkaline phosphatase levels. It has also been reported to cause transient alterations in serum cholesterol and triglyceride levels.

CONTRAINDICATIONS
Contraindicated in patients hypersensitive to drug and its components.

NURSING CONSIDERATIONS
● Be aware that most patients show improvement soon after treatment begins.
● Keep in mind that treatment of tinea corporis or tinea cruris should continue for at least 2 weeks to reduce the possibility of recurrence.
● Use cautiously with nursing mothers.
Alert: Product contains sodium sulfite anhydrous, which may cause severe to life-threatening symptoms in asthmatic patients.

☑ **Patient teaching**
● Tell patient to discontinue drug and notify doctor if hypersensitivity reaction occurs.
● Advise patient to check with doctor if condition worsens; drug may have to be discontinued and diagnosis reevaluated.
● Warn patient that shampoo applied to permanent waved hair removes curl.
● Warn patient to avoid medication contact with eyes.

---

mafenide acetate
Sulfamylon

Pregnancy Risk Category: C

HOW SUPPLIED
Cream: 8.5%

ACTION
Unknown, although it is known that it interferes with bacterial cellular metabolism.

Route	Onset	Peak	Duration
Topical	Unknown	Unknown	Unknown

INDICATIONS & DOSAGE
Adjunctive treatment of second- and third-degree burns to prevent infection caused by susceptible organisms (especially Pseudomonas aeruginosa)—
Adults and children: apply $^1/_{16}''$ thickness of cream daily or b.i.d. to clean debrided wounds. Reapply p.r.n. to keep burned area covered.

ADVERSE REACTIONS
Hematologic: eosinophilia, bone marrow depression.
Respiratory: tachypnea.
Skin: pain, *burning sensation,* rash, pruritus, swelling, urticaria, blisters, erythema.
Other: *metabolic acidosis,* facial edema, disseminated intravascular coagulation.

INTERACTIONS
None significant.

EFFECTS ON DIAGNOSTIC TESTS
None reported.

CONTRAINDICATIONS
Contraindicated in patients with hypersensitivity to drug. Cross-sensitivity to other sulfonamides is unknown.

NURSING CONSIDERATIONS
• Use cautiously in patients with acute renal failure, asthma, or known hypersensitivity to drug or sulfonamides.
• Clean area before applying, bathing patient daily, if possible.
• Use sterile gloves and instruments when applying cream to minimize risk of further wound contamination.
• Keep burn areas medicated at all times.
• Know that dressings are not necessary, but if used should be light.
Alert: Closely monitor acid-base balance,

especially in patients with pulmonary and renal dysfunction. If acidosis occurs, discontinue use for 24 to 48 hours and notify doctor.
• Be aware that sometimes it is difficult to distinguish between adverse reactions and effects of severe burn.

☑**Patient teaching**
• Explain purpose of drug and importance of keeping burned areas covered with drug at all times. Tell patient to alert nurse if drug rubs off in any visible area.
• Tell patient to report adverse reactions, especially pain or burning when drug is applied; these symptoms may indicate allergy. Instruct patient to notify doctor if pain is severe or prolonged; treatment may need to be temporarily stopped.

---

metronidazole (topical)
MetroCream, MetroGel,
MetroGel-Vaginal

Pregnancy Risk Category: B

HOW SUPPLIED
Topical cream: 0.75%
Topical gel: 0.75%
Vaginal gel: 0.75%

ACTION
Unknown; may cause bactericidal effect by interacting with bacterial DNA. Active against many anaerobic gram-negative bacilli, anaerobic gram-positive cocci, *Gardnerella vaginalis,* and *Campylobacter fetus.*

Route	Onset	Peak	Duration
Topical	Unknown	Unknown	Unknown
Intravaginal	Unknown	6-12 hr	Unknown

INDICATIONS & DOSAGE
Inflammatory papules and pustules of acne rosacea—
Adults: apply a thin film to affected area b.i.d., morning and evening. Frequency and duration of therapy is adjusted after response is seen.
Bacterial vaginosis—
Adults: 1 applicatorful once or twice dai-

ly for 5 days. For once-daily dosing, administer h.s.

ADVERSE REACTIONS
Topical gel/cream:
EENT: lacrimation (if drug applied around eyes).
Skin: rash, *transient redness, dryness, mild burning, stinging.*
Vaginal form:
CNS: dizziness, light-headedness, headache.
GI: cramps, pain, nausea, diarrhea, constipation, metallic or bad taste in mouth.
GU: *cervicitis, vaginitis.*
Skin: rash, *transient redness, dryness, mild burning, stinging.*
Other: overgrowth of nonsusceptible organisms, decreased appetite.

INTERACTIONS
Drug-drug. *Oral anticoagulants:* may potentiate anticoagulant effect. Monitor patient for potential adverse reactions.
Drug-lifestyle. *Alcohol use:* disulfiram-like reaction may occur. Avoid concomitant use.

EFFECTS ON DIAGNOSTIC TESTS
None reported.

CONTRAINDICATIONS
Contraindicated in patients hypersensitive to drug or its ingredients (such as parabens) and other nitroimidazole derivatives.

NURSING CONSIDERATIONS
• Use cautiously in patients with history or evidence of blood dyscrasia and in those with severe hepatic disease.
• Use vaginal gel cautiously in patients with history of CNS diseases (seizures and peripheral neuropathy are associated with oral form).
• Topical metronidazole therapy has not been linked with adverse effects observed with parenteral or oral metronidazole therapy; however, some drug may be absorbed after topical use.
• Know that vaginal gel should not be used in patients who have taken disulfiram within the past 2 weeks.

• Be aware that oral form has been associated with psychotic reaction.

☑ **Patient teaching**
• Instruct patient to avoid use of topical gel around eyes.
• Advise patient to clean area thoroughly before use, but to wait 15 to 20 minutes after cleaning the skin before applying drug to minimize risk of local irritation. Cosmetics may be used after applying drug.
• If local reactions occur, advise patient to apply drug less frequently or to discontinue its use and contact the doctor.
• Advise patient to avoid sexual intercourse while using vaginal preparation.

miconazole nitrate
Daktarin§, Gyno-Daktarin§, Micatin◇, Monistat-Derm, Monistat 3, Monistat 7◇

Pregnancy Risk Category: B

HOW SUPPLIED
Cream: 2%◇
Powder: 2%◇
Spray: 2%◇
Vaginal cream: 2%◇
Vaginal suppositories: 100 mg◇, 200 mg

ACTION
A fungicidal imidazole that disrupts fungal cell membrane permeability.

Route	Onset	Peak	Duration
Topical, intravaginal	Unknown	Unknown	Unknown

INDICATIONS & DOSAGE
Tinea corporis, tinea cruris, tinea pedis; cutaneous candidiasis (moniliasis); common dermatophyte infections—
Adults and children over 1 year: apply sparingly b.i.d. for 2 to 4 weeks; Powder or spray can be used liberally over affected area.
Tinea versicolor—
Adults and children over 1 year: apply sparingly once daily for 2 weeks.
Vulvovaginal candidiasis—
Adults: 1 applicatorful or 100 mg sup-

pository (Monistat 7) inserted intravaginally h.s. for 7 days; course repeated if necessary. Alternatively, 200 mg suppository (Monistat 3) intravaginally h.s. for 3 days.

ADVERSE REACTIONS
CNS: headache.
GU: pelvic cramps; vulvovaginal burning, pruritus, irritation (with vaginal cream).
Skin: irritation, burning, maceration, allergic contact dermatitis.

INTERACTIONS
None significant.

EFFECTS ON DIAGNOSTIC TESTS
Drug may cause a transient decrease in hematocrit, increase or decrease in platelet count and commonly causes RBC aggregation. Drug also may cause hyponatremia, hyperlipidemia, hypertriglyceridemia, as well as abnormalities in lipoprotein and immunoelectrophoretic patterns, due to the polyoxyl 35 castor oil vehicle.

CONTRAINDICATIONS
Contraindicated in patients hypersensitive to drug or its components.

NURSING CONSIDERATIONS
• Know that concurrent use of intravaginal forms and certain latex products, such as vaginal contraceptive diaphragms, are not recommended because of possible interaction.
• Don't use occlusive dressings.

☑ Patient teaching
• Advise patient that drug is for perineal or intravaginal use only. Keep out of eyes.
• Ensure that patient understands that frequent or persistent yeast infections may be a symptom of a more serious medical problem such as AIDS.
• Tell patient to cautiously insert intravaginal forms high into the vagina with applicator provided.
• Tell patient drug may stain clothing.
• Warn patient to discontinue use if sensitivity or chemical irritation occurs.
• Tell patient to continue using drug for

full treatment period prescribed and to notify doctor if symptoms persist at end of therapy.
• Advise patient to avoid sexual intercourse during vaginal treatment.
• Instruct patient to apply sparingly in skin-fold areas and rub in well to prevent maceration effects.

---

mupirocin
Bactroban

Pregnancy Risk Category: B

HOW SUPPLIED
Ointment: 2%

ACTION
Unknown; thought to inhibit bacterial protein and RNA synthesis.

Route	Onset	Peak	Duration
Topical	Unknown	Unknown	Unknown

INDICATIONS & DOSAGE
Impetigo—
Adults and children: apply to affected areas t.i.d. for 1 to 2 weeks.
Treatment of secondarily infected traumatic skin lesions due to Staphylococcus aureus *and* Streptococcus pyogenes—
Adults and children: apply thin film t.i.d. for 10 days; may cover with gauze dressing if necessary. Reevaluate patient if clinical improvement doesn't occur in 3 to 5 days.

ADVERSE REACTIONS
Skin: burning, pruritus, stinging, rash, pain, erythema.

INTERACTIONS
None significant.

EFFECTS ON DIAGNOSTIC TESTS
None reported.

CONTRAINDICATIONS
Contraindicated in patients hypersensitive to drug or its components.

NURSING CONSIDERATIONS
• Use cautiously in patients with burns or

impaired renal function; may result in serious renal toxicity.
• Be aware that drug is not for ophthalmic or internal use.
• Know that prolonged use may cause overgrowth of nonsusceptible bacteria and fungi.
• Know that local reactions appear to be caused by the polyethylene glycol vehicle.

☑Patient teaching
• Tell patient to notify doctor immediately if no improvement occurs in 3 to 5 days or if condition worsens.
• Warn patient about local adverse reactions associated with drug application.
• Caution patient not to use cosmetics or other skin products on treated area.

---

naftifine hydrochloride
Naftin

Pregnancy Risk Category: B

HOW SUPPLIED
Cream: 1%
Gel: 1%

ACTION
Unknown. A broad-spectrum fungicidal agent that is thought to inhibit sterol biosynthesis in susceptible fungi by blocking the enzyme squalene 2,3 epoxidase.

Route	Onset	Peak	Duration
Topical	Unknown	Unknown	Unknown

INDICATIONS & DOSAGE
Tinea corporis, tinea cruris, and tinea pedis—
Adults: apply cream to affected area once daily; or apply gel b.i.d. in the morning and evening.

ADVERSE REACTIONS
Skin: *burning, stinging,* dryness, pruritus, local irritation, erythema.

INTERACTIONS
None significant.

EFFECTS ON DIAGNOSTIC TESTS
None reported.

CONTRAINDICATIONS
Contraindicated in patients hypersensitive to drug or components.

NURSING CONSIDERATIONS
• Therapy should be reevaluated if no improvement occurs after 4 weeks.
• Keep cream away from mucous membranes. Drug is not for ophthalmic use.

☑Patient teaching
• Tell patient not to use occlusive dressings unless directed otherwise by doctor.
• Instruct patient to wash hands after application.
• Instruct patient to discontinue therapy and notify doctor if irritation or sensitivity develops.

---

neomycin sulfate
Mycifradin†, Myciguent◊

Pregnancy Risk Category: C

HOW SUPPLIED
Cream: 0.5%◊
Ointment: 0.5%◊

ACTION
Unknown. Thought to disrupt bacterial protein synthesis by binding to bacterial ribosomes.

Route	Onset	Peak	Duration
Topical	Unknown	Unknown	Unknown

INDICATIONS & DOSAGE
Prevention or treatment of superficial bacterial infections—
Adults and children: rub fingertip-size dose into affected area once to three times daily.

ADVERSE REACTIONS
Skin: *rash, contact dermatitis,* urticaria.
Other: *nephrotoxicity, ototoxicity,* **neuromuscular blockade.**

INTERACTIONS
None significant.

EFFECTS ON DIAGNOSTIC TESTS
Drug-induced nephrotoxicity may elevate

Reactions may be *common*, uncommon, ***life-threatening***, or COMMON AND LIFE-THREATENING.

levels of BUN, nonprotein nitrogen, or serum creatinine; it may increase urinary excretion of casts, if systemic absorption occurs.

CONTRAINDICATIONS
Contraindicated in patients hypersensitive to drug or its components.

NURSING CONSIDERATIONS
• Use cautiously in patients with extensive dermatologic conditions. Don't use on more than 20% of body surface.
• Don't use more than once daily on burns covering more than 20% of body surface area.
• Be aware that prolonged use may result in overgrowth of nonsusceptible organisms.
• In combination products containing corticosteroids, be aware that use of occlusive dressings increases corticosteroid absorption and the likelihood of systemic effects.
• Keep in mind that enhanced systemic absorption occurs on denuded or abraded areas.
• Watch for signs of hypersensitivity and contact dermatitis.
Alert: Watch for signs of ototoxicity with prolonged or extended use.

☑ Patient teaching
• Tell patient to stop using drug and notify doctor if no improvement occurs or if condition worsens.
• Tell patient to report adverse reactions, especially systemic reactions.
• Instruct patient not to use drug for more than 1 week, unless otherwise directed.

---

nitrofurazone
Furacin

Pregnancy Risk Category: C

HOW SUPPLIED
Cream: 0.2%
Ointment: 0.2% (soluble dressing)
Topical solution: 0.2%

ACTION
Unknown. A broad-spectrum antibiotic that probably inhibits bacterial enzymes involved in carbohydrate metabolism.

Route	Onset	Peak	Duration
Topical	Unknown	Unknown	Unknown

INDICATIONS & DOSAGE
Adjunctive treatment of second- and third-degree burns (especially when resistance to other antibiotics and sulfonamides occurs); prevention of skin allograft rejection—
Adults and children: apply directly to lesion daily or q few days, depending on severity of burn. May also be applied to dressings used to cover affected area.

ADVERSE REACTIONS
Skin: erythema, pruritus, burning, edema, allergic contact dermatitis.

INTERACTIONS
None significant.

EFFECTS ON DIAGNOSTIC TESTS
None reported.

CONTRAINDICATIONS
Contraindicated in patients hypersensitive to drug.

NURSING CONSIDERATIONS
• Use cautiously in patients with known or suspected renal impairment. Monitor serum creatinine levels regularly, as ordered.
• Be aware that flushing dressing with sterile normal saline solution facilitates removal.
• Clean wound, as indicated by doctor, before reapplying dressings.
• Use sterile application technique to prevent further wound contamination.
• When using wet dressing, protect skin around wound with zinc oxide ointment.
• Be aware that dressings impregnated with drug should not be stored for more than 24 hours.
• Be aware that drug may discolor in light but still retains its potency.
• Discard cloudy solutions if warming to 131° to 140° F (55° to 60° C) does not restore clarity.
• Store solution in tight, light-resistant

containers (brown bottles). Avoid exposure to direct light, prolonged heat, and alkaline materials.

✓ **Patient teaching**
• Tell patient to report irritation, sensitization, or infection.
• Explain all procedures to patient.

---

nystatin
Mycostatin, Nadostine†, Nilstat, Nystaform§, Nystan§

Pregnancy Risk Category: NR

HOW SUPPLIED
Cream: 100,000 units/g
Lozenges: 200,000 units
Ointment: 100,000 units/g
Powder: 100,000 units/g
Vaginal tablets: 100,000 units

ACTION
Disrupts integrity of fungal cell wall, promoting osmotic instability.

Route	Onset	Peak	Duration
PO, topical, intravaginal	Unknown	Unknown	Unknown

INDICATIONS & DOSAGE
Cutaneous and mucocutaneous infections caused by Candida albicans—
Adults and children: apply to affected area up to several times daily. Apply cream: b.i.d. or as indicated; powder: b.i.d. or t.i.d.; lozenges: 1 or 2 four to five times daily until 48 hours after oral symptoms subside, but not more than 14 days.
Vulvovaginal candidiasis—
Adults: 1 vaginal tablet daily for 14 days.

ADVERSE REACTIONS
GI: vomiting (vaginal tablets).
Skin: occasional contact dermatitis from preservatives in some forms.

INTERACTIONS
None significant.

EFFECTS ON DIAGNOSTIC TESTS
None reported.

CONTRAINDICATIONS
Contraindicated in patients hypersensitive to drug or its components.

NURSING CONSIDERATIONS
• Do not use occlusive dressings.
• Keep in mind that preparation does not stain skin or mucous membranes.
• Know that cream is recommended for intertriginous areas; powder, for moist areas; ointment, for dry areas.
• Be aware that immunosuppressed patients may tolerate vaginal tablets orally for longer mucous membrane drug exposure.

✓ **Patient teaching**
• Instruct female patient how to administer vaginal tablets, and tell her to continue using the vaginal tablets during her menstrual period.
• Instruct patient to refrigerate tablets.
• Tell patient to use drug for full prescribed period, even if condition improves. Immunosuppressed patients may use drug chronically.
• Warn patient to avoid drug contact with eyes.
• Instruct patient not to use occlusive dressings with skin application.
• Tell patient to dissolve oral lozenges slowly.
• Instruct and stress importance of proper oral hygiene, especially for denture wearers.

---

silver sulfadiazine
Flamazine†, Flint SSD, Silvadene, SSD AF, Thermazene

Pregnancy Risk Category: B

HOW SUPPLIED
Cream: 1%

ACTION
Broad-spectrum sulfonamide that acts on cell membrane and cell wall; bactericidal for many gram-positive and gram-negative organisms.

Route	Onset	Peak	Duration
Topical	Unknown	Unknown	Unknown

Reactions may be *common*, uncommon, *life-threatening*, or COMMON AND LIFE-THREATENING.

INDICATIONS & DOSAGE

Prevention and treatment of wound infection in second- and third-degree burns—
Adults: apply $\frac{1}{16}$" thickness to clean debrided burn wound daily or b.i.d.

ADVERSE REACTIONS

Hematologic: *leukopenia.*
Skin: pain, burning, rash, pruritus, skin necrosis, erythema multiforme, skin discoloration.

INTERACTIONS

Drug-drug. *Topical proteolytic enzymes:* inactivation of enzymes. Do not use together.
Drug-lifestyle. *Sun exposure:* photosensitivity reactions may occur. Take precautions.

EFFECTS ON DIAGNOSTIC TESTS

If used on extensive areas of body surface, systemic absorption may result in a decreased neutrophil count, indicating a reversible leukopenia.

CONTRAINDICATIONS

Contraindicated in premature and full-term neonates during first 2 months of life. Drug may increase possibility of kernicterus. Also contraindicated in patients with hypersensitivity to drug or G6PD deficiency and in pregnant women at or near term.

NURSING CONSIDERATIONS

• Use with caution in patients hypersensitive to sulfonamides.
• Use sterile application technique to prevent wound contamination.
• Use only on affected areas. Keep these areas medicated at all times.
• Bathe patient daily, if possible.
• Inspect patient's skin daily, and note any changes. Notify doctor if burning or excessive pain develops.
• Monitor serum sulfadiazine concentrations and renal function, as ordered, and check urine for sulfa crystals in patients with extensive burns.
• Tell doctor if hepatic or renal dysfunction occurs; drug may need to be stopped.
• Discard darkened cream, which indicates drug is ineffective.

☑ Patient teaching

• Instruct patient to report adverse reactions promptly, especially burning or excessive pain with application.
• Inform patient of need for frequent blood and urine tests to monitor for adverse effects.
• Tell patient that he may develop photosensitivity.

sulconazole nitrate
Exelderm

Pregnancy Risk Category: C

HOW SUPPLIED

Topical solution: 1%
Cream: 1%

ACTION

Unknown. A broad-spectrum antifungal imidazole derivative that inhibits the growth of both fungi and yeast.

Route	Onset	Peak	Duration
Topical	Unknown	Unknown	Unknown

INDICATIONS & DOSAGE

Tinea corporis, tinea cruris, tinea pedis, or tinea versicolor—
Adults: massage a small amount of drug into affected area daily to b.i.d. for 3 weeks. Treat tinea pedis with cream b.i.d. for 4 weeks.

ADVERSE REACTIONS

Skin: pruritus, burning, stinging, redness.

INTERACTIONS

None significant.

EFFECTS ON DIAGNOSTIC TESTS

None reported.

CONTRAINDICATIONS

Contraindicated in patients hypersensitive to drug or its components.

NURSING CONSIDERATIONS

• Use only cream for tinea pedis. Efficacy against tinea pedis has not been proven with the topical solution.
• Know that if no improvement occurs af-

ter 4 weeks, diagnosis should be reconsidered.

✓Patient teaching
• Tell patient to avoid touching the eyes with drug and to wash hands thoroughly after applying.
• Explain necessity of completing full course of therapy to prevent recurrence. Clinical improvement is usually apparent within 1 week, with symptomatic relief within a few days.
• Instruct patient to discontinue drug and contact doctor if irritation develops during treatment.
• Tell patient solution should be kept away from excessive heat and protected from light.

---

terbinafine hydrochloride
Lamisil

Pregnancy Risk Category: B

HOW SUPPLIED
Cream: 1%

ACTION
Fungicidal; selectively inhibits an early step in synthesis of sterols used by fungi for cell wall synthesis.

Route	Onset	Peak	Duration
Topical	Unknown	Unknown	Unknown

INDICATIONS & DOSAGE
Interdigital tinea corporis, tinea cruris, tinea pedis, and plantar tinea pedis—
Adults and children 12 years and older: cover affected area and immediate surrounding area b.i.d. for at least 1 week; use for 2 weeks for plantar tinea pedis.

ADVERSE REACTIONS
Skin: irritation, burning, pruritus, dryness.

INTERACTIONS
None significant.

EFFECTS ON DIAGNOSTIC TESTS
None reported.

CONTRAINDICATIONS
Contraindicated in patients hypersensitive to drug or its components.

NURSING CONSIDERATIONS
• Observe patients for 2 to 6 weeks after therapy is complete to determine whether treatment was successful; review diagnosis if condition persists beyond this observation period.
• Be aware that therapy should not exceed 4 weeks.
• Drug is not intended for oral, ophthalmic, or vaginal use.

✓Patient teaching
• Teach patient proper use of drug. Tell him to use only as directed for full recommended course, even if symptoms disappear, and not to apply near the eyes, mouth, or mucous membranes or to use occlusive dressings unless so directed.
• Tell patient to discontinue drug and contact doctor if irritation or sensitivity develops.

---

terconazole
Terazol 3, Terazol 7

Pregnancy Risk Category: C

HOW SUPPLIED
Vaginal cream: 0.4%, 0.8%
Vaginal suppositories: 80 mg

ACTION
Unknown; may increase fungal cell membrane permeability (*Candida* species only).

Route	Onset	Peak	Duration
Intravaginal	Unknown	Unknown	Unknown

INDICATIONS & DOSAGE
Vulvovaginal candidiasis—
Adults: 1 applicatorful of cream or 1 suppository inserted into vagina h.s.; 0.4% cream used for 7 consecutive days; 0.8% cream or 80-mg suppository for 3 consecutive days. Course repeated, if necessary, after reconfirmation by smear or culture.

ADVERSE REACTIONS
CNS: *headache.*
GI: abdominal pain.
GU: dysmenorrhea, pain of the female genitalia, vulvovaginal burning.
Skin: irritation, *pruritus,* photosensitivity.
Other: fever, chills, body aches.

INTERACTIONS
None significant.

EFFECTS ON DIAGNOSTIC TESTS
None reported.

CONTRAINDICATIONS
Contraindicated in patients with known sensitivity to terconazole or inactive ingredients in drug.

NURSING CONSIDERATIONS
• Keep in mind that therapeutic effect of drug is unaffected by menstruation or oral contraceptive use.

✓ **Patient teaching**
• Advise patient to continue treatment during the menstrual period. However, tell her not to use tampons.
• Tell patient to use for full treatment period prescribed. Explain how to prevent reinfection.
• Instruct patient to discontinue drug if fever, chills, other flulike symptoms, or sensitivity develop, and to notify doctor.
• Caution patient to refrain from sexual intercourse during treatment.
• Tell patient that drug base may react with latex, causing decreased effectiveness of condoms and diaphragms.
• Teach patient to store drug at room temperature.

---

tetracycline hydrochloride
Achromycin, Topicycline

Pregnancy Risk Category: B

HOW SUPPLIED
Ointment: 3%
Topical solution: 2.2 mg/ml

ACTION
Unknown. A broad-spectrum antibiotic that probably disrupts bacterial protein synthesis; usually bacteriostatic.

Route	Onset	Peak	Duration
Topical	Unknown	Unknown	Unknown

INDICATIONS & DOSAGE
Acne vulgaris—
Adults and children over 11 years: rub solution into affected areas b.i.d. until skin is thoroughly covered.
Prevention or treatment of superficial skin infections caused by susceptible bacteria—
Adults: apply to affected area b.i.d. in morning and evening or t.i.d.

ADVERSE REACTIONS
Skin: temporary stinging or burning on application; slight yellowing of treated skin, especially in patients with light complexions; severe dermatitis.

INTERACTIONS
Drug-drug. *Isotretinoin:* may cause cumulative dryness, resulting in excessive skin irritation. Use cautiously.
Drug-lifestyle. *Abrasive or medicated soaps or cleansers; acne preparations or other preparations containing peeling agents (benzoyl peroxide, resorcinol, salicylic acid, sulfur, tretinoin); alcohol-containing products (aftershave, cosmetics, perfumed toiletries, shaving creams or lotions); astringent soaps or cosmetics; medicated cosmetics or cover-ups:* may cause cumulative dryness, resulting in excessive skin irritation. Use cautiously.
Sun exposure: photosensitivity reactions may occur. Take precautions.

EFFECTS ON DIAGNOSTIC TESTS
None reported.

CONTRAINDICATIONS
Contraindicated in patients hypersensitive to drug or its components.

NURSING CONSIDERATIONS
• Use cautiously in patients with hepatic or renal impairment and in breast-feeding women.
• Do not use in patients with sodium bisulfite sensitivity.

• Know that prolonged use may result in overgrowth of nonsusceptible organisms.
• Store drug at room temperature, away from excessive heat.
• Be aware that ointment form should not be used to treat acne vulgaris.

☑ Patient teaching
• Tell patient to wash area before applying.
• Explain that floating plug in bottle of Topicycline—an inert and harmless result of proper reconstitution of the preparation—should not be removed.
• Teach patient how to increase or decrease applicator pressure against skin to control flow rate of solution.
• Instruct patient to apply a generous amount of drug, avoiding eyes, nose, and mouth.
• Inform patient that drug application may cause stinging.
• Tell patient that she may continue normal use of cosmetics.
• Caution patient not to share medication with family members.
• Advise patient to use or discard drug within 2 months.
• Tell patient to stop using drug and to notify doctor if no improvement occurs or if condition worsens.
• Warn patient that drug may stain clothing.
• Tell patient to avoid exposure to sunlight.

---

tioconazole
Vagistat-1

Pregnancy Risk Category: C

HOW SUPPLIED
Vaginal ointment: 6.5%

ACTION
A fungicidal imidazole that alters cell wall permeability.

Route	Onset	Peak	Duration
Intravaginal	Unknown	Unknown	Unknown

INDICATIONS & DOSAGE
Vulvovaginal candidiasis—
Adults: 1 applicatorful (about 4.6 g) inserted intravaginally h.s. one time only.

ADVERSE REACTIONS
GU: *burning, pruritus,* discharge, vaginal pain, dysuria, dyspareunia, vulvar edema, irritation.

INTERACTIONS
None significant.

EFFECTS ON DIAGNOSTIC TESTS
None reported.

CONTRAINDICATIONS
Contraindicated in patients hypersensitive to drug or other imidazole antifungal agents (ketoconazole, miconazole).

NURSING CONSIDERATIONS
• Know that drug is not for use in pregnant women or patients with diabetes mellitus, HIV infection, or AIDS.
• Breast-feeding women should temporarily stop doing so because it is not known if drug is excreted in breast milk.
• Notify doctor if patient reports irritation or sensitivity.
• Be aware that drug should not be used if patient has abdominal pain, high fever, odorous discharge, vomiting, or diarrhea unless directed by doctor.

☑ Patient teaching
• Review proper use of drug with patient. Written instructions for patient are available with product. Tell patient to insert drug high into the vagina.
• To avoid contamination of the ointment, tell patient to open the applicator just before using it.
• Tell patient to use a sanitary napkin to avoid staining her clothing.
• Advise patient to avoid sexual intercourse on the night after insertion, or advise that her partner use a condom to prevent reinfection.
• Emphasize need to complete the full course of therapy, even after symptoms have improved. She should continue using drug during her menstrual period.
• Advise patient to wait 3 days after therapy to resume sexual activity if using a condom or diaphragm, because drug may damage latex or rubber.
• Advise patient to see doctor before self-

Reactions may be *common,* uncommon, *life-threatening,* or COMMON AND LIFE-THREATENING.

medicating if symptoms return within 2 months.

---

tolnaftate
Absorbine Footcare, Aftate for Athlete's Foot ◊, Aftate for Jock Itch ◊, Dr. Scholl's Athlete's Foot Powder ◊, Dr. Scholl's Athlete's Foot ◊, Genaspor ◊, NP-27 ◊, Pitrex, Quinsana Plus, Tinactin ◊, Ting ◊, Zeasorb-AF ◊

Pregnancy Risk Category: C

HOW SUPPLIED
Aerosol liquid: 1% (36% alcohol) ◊
Aerosol powder: 1% (14% alcohol) ◊
Cream: 1% ◊
Gel: 1% ◊
Powder: 1% ◊
Pump spray liquid: 1% (36% alcohol) ◊
Topical solution: 1% ◊

ACTION
Unknown, although drug has been demonstrated to distort the hyphae and stunt mycelial growth in susceptible fungi.

Route	Onset	Peak	Duration
Topical	Unknown	Unknown	Unknown

INDICATIONS & DOSAGE
Superficial fungal infections of the skin; infections due to common pathogenic fungi; tinea pedis, tinea cruris, tinea corporis, and tinea versicolor—
Adults and children: apply ¼" to ½" (6 mm to 1.3 cm) ribbon of cream or 2 to 3 drops of solution to cover area; same amount of cream or 2 to 3 drops of solution to cover toes and interdigital webs of one foot; or gel, powder, or spray to cover affected area. Apply and massage gently into skin b.i.d. for 2 to 6 weeks.

ADVERSE REACTIONS
Skin: possible irritation.

INTERACTIONS
None significant.

EFFECTS ON DIAGNOSTIC TESTS
None reported.

CONTRAINDICATIONS
Contraindicated in patients hypersensitive to drug or its components.

NURSING CONSIDERATIONS
• Be aware that drug is not used to treat fungal infections of hair or nails; tolnaftate is ineffective against these fungi.
• Know that drug is odorless and greaseless; it won't stain or discolor skin, hair, nails, or clothing.
• Know that powder or aerosol may be used inside socks and shoes of persons susceptible to tinea infections.
• Keep in mind that ointments, creams, and liquid are primarily used for treatment; powder and aerosol are adjuncts unless infection is very mild.

✓ Patient teaching
• Teach patient to clean area and dry thoroughly before applying drug.
• Tell patient to continue using for full treatment period prescribed, even if condition has improved. Treatment should continue for at least 2 weeks after symptoms have resolved.
• Advise patient to use only a small quantity of cream or lotion; treated area should not be wet with solution.
• Tell patient to call doctor if no improvement occurs after 10 days.
• Tell patient to discontinue if condition worsens and to check with the doctor.
• Advise patient to wear shoes and cotton socks that fit well, and to change footwear daily.
• Tell patient to keep drug away from eyes.

Scabicides and pediculicides

benzyl benzoate
crotamiton
lindane
permethrin
pyrethrins

COMBINATION PRODUCTS
None.

---

benzyl benzoate
Ascabiol‡

Pregnancy Risk Category: C

HOW SUPPLIED
Lotion: 14% (with benzocaine 2%)‡, 28%
Emulsion: 25%‡

ACTION
Unknown.

Route	Onset	Peak	Duration
Topical	Unknown	Unknown	Unknown

INDICATIONS & DOSAGE
Parasitic infestation (scabies, Phthirus
pubis, Pediculus humanus capitis)—
Adults and children: scrub entire body
with soap and water. Remove scales or
crusts. Apply the undiluted lotion over affected area (include whole body for scabies), except the face and scalp, while still
damp. Be sure to apply around nails. Let
dry. Apply second coat on the most involved areas. Bathe after 24 hours. Treatment may be repeated in 7 to 10 days if
mites appear or new lesions develop.
For hairy area infestation—
Adults and children: apply lotion to area
and remove in 12 to 24 hours. May repeat
application in 1 week.

ADVERSE REACTIONS
Skin: *irritation, pruritus; contact dermatitis* (with repeated applications).

INTERACTIONS
None significant.

EFFECTS ON DIAGNOSTIC TESTS
None reported.

CONTRAINDICATIONS
Contraindicated when skin is raw or inflamed or in patients hypersensitive to
drug.

NURSING CONSIDERATIONS
• Do not apply to face, eyes, mucous
membranes, or urethral meatus. If accidental contact with eyes occurs, flush
with water and notify doctor.
• Apply topical corticosteroids as prescribed if dermatitis develops from
scratching.
• Do not apply to infants' or small children's hands because they put their hands
into their mouths.
• Make sure hospitalized patients are
placed in isolation, with linen-handling
precautions, until treatment is completed.
• Store drug in light-resistant container;
avoid exposure to excessive heat.

☑ Patient teaching
• Teach patient or family member how to
administer drug.
• Tell patient to discontinue drug and to
wash it off skin and notify doctor immediately if skin irritation or hypersensitivity
develops.
• Instruct patient to change and sterilize
(boil, launder, dry clean, or apply very hot
iron) all clothing and bed linens after drug
is washed off.
• Instruct patient to reapply drug if it is
washed off during treatment time.
• After application for lice infestation, tell
patient to use a fine-tooth comb dipped in
white vinegar to remove nits from hairy
areas.
• Tell patient to warn other family members and sexual contacts about infestation.
Sexual contacts should be treated simultaneously.
• Reassure patient that although itching
may continue for several weeks, it will

Reactions may be common, *uncommon,* **life-threatening,** *or* COMMON AND LIFE-THREATENING.

stop; continued itching does not indicate that therapy is ineffective.

crotamiton
Eurax

Pregnancy Risk Category: C

HOW SUPPLIED
Cream: 10%
Lotion: 10%

ACTION
Unknown.

Route	Onset	Peak	Duration
Topical	Unknown	Unknown	Unknown

INDICATIONS & DOSAGE
Parasitic infestation (scabies)—
Adults: scrub entire body with soap and water. Remove scales or crusts. Then apply thin layer of cream over entire body, from chin down (with special attention to folds, creases, interdigital spaces, and genital area). Apply second coat in 24 hours. Wait additional 48 hours, then wash off. Treatment is repeated in 7 to 10 days if mites reappear or new lesions develop.
Itching—
Adults: apply locally, massaging gently in affected area until completely absorbed and repeated p.r.n.

ADVERSE REACTIONS
Skin: *irritation,* allergic skin sensitivity.

INTERACTIONS
None significant.

EFFECTS ON DIAGNOSTIC TESTS
None reported.

CONTRAINDICATIONS
Contraindicated when skin is raw or inflamed and in patients hypersensitive to drug or its components.

NURSING CONSIDERATIONS
• Estimate amount of cream needed per application; most patients have a tendency to overuse scabicides. For most adults, a single tube of cream provides a sufficient amount for two applications.
• Be aware that drug should not be applied to acutely inflamed or raw, weeping areas.
• Apply topical corticosteroids, as prescribed, if dermatitis develops from scratching.
• Make sure hospitalized patients are placed in isolation, with special linen-handling precautions, until treatment is completed.
• Be aware that monthly maintenance treatments may be necessary in long-term care facilities, where infestation is a problem.

✓**Patient teaching**
• Teach patient or family member how to apply drug. Tell patient not to apply to face, eyes, mucous membranes, or urethral meatus. If accidental contact with eyes occurs, tell patient to flush with water and notify doctor.
• Tell patient to discontinue drug and to wash it off skin and notify doctor immediately if skin irritation or hypersensitivity develops.
• Instruct patient to change all clothing and bed linens and launder in the hot cycle of the washing machine or dry clean after drug is washed off of body.
• Instruct patient to reapply drug if it is washed off during treatment time.
• Tell patient to warn other family members and sexual contacts about infestation. Sexual contacts should be treated simultaneously.
• Reassure patient that although itching may continue for several weeks, it will stop; continued itching does not indicate that therapy is ineffective.

lindane
GBH†, G-well, Kwell, Kwellada†, Scabene

Pregnancy Risk Category: B

HOW SUPPLIED
Cream: 1%
Lotion: 1%
Shampoo: 1%

---

*Liquid contains alcohol.   **May contain tartrazine.   †Canada   ‡Australia   §U.K.   ◊OTC

ACTION
Unclear. Appears to inhibit neuronal membrane function in arthropods, causing neuronal hyperactivity, seizures, and death after penetrating the parasite's exoskeleton.

Route	Onset	Peak	Duration
Topical	190 min	Unknown	Unknown

INDICATIONS & DOSAGE
Parasitic infestation (scabies, pediculosis)—

Adults and children: Centers for Disease Control and Prevention recommends avoiding bathing before application on skin. If patient does bathe, let skin dry and cool thoroughly before using. Apply thin layer of cream or lotion over entire skin surface (with special attention to folds, creases, interdigital spaces, and genital area) and rub in thoroughly for scabies, or to hairy areas for pediculosis. After 8 to 12 hours, wash off drug. Repeat process in 1 week if mites appear or new lesions develop.

Apply shampoo undiluted to dry hair and work into lather for 4 to 5 minutes; small amounts of water may enhance formation of lather. Apply 30 ml of shampoo for short hair, 45 ml for medium-length hair, or 60 ml for long hair. Rinse thoroughly and rub dry with towel. Comb with a fine tooth comb.

Elderly: may require a reduced dose because of increased skin absorption.

ADVERSE REACTIONS
CNS: *dizziness, seizures.*
Skin: *irritation* (with repeated use).

INTERACTIONS
Drug-lifestyle. *Oils:* may increase absorption of drug; if oil-based hair products are used, hair must be washed and dried before using lindane.

EFFECTS ON DIAGNOSTIC TESTS
None reported.

CONTRAINDICATIONS
Contraindicated when skin is inflamed or in patients with seizure disorders or hypersensitivity to drug or its components.

Lotion form contraindicated in premature infants.

NURSING CONSIDERATIONS
• Use cautiously in infants, young children, and the elderly who are at greater risk for CNS toxicity.
• Apply topical corticosteroids or administer oral antihistamines, as prescribed, for pruritus.
• Make sure that hospitalized patients are placed in isolation, with special linen-handling precautions, until treatment is completed.
• Know that modest amounts (6% to 13%) are absorbed through intact skin. Absorption is increased if used with creams, oils, or lotions or if applied to face, scalp, axillae, neck, scrotum, or irritated or broken skin.
• Be aware that contact with eyes must be avoided.

☑ **Patient teaching**
• Teach patient or family member how to administer drug. Apply thin layer to cover body only once: 1 oz is used for children less than 6 years and 1 to 2 oz for older children and adults. Drug should not be left on for more than 12 hours and should be removed thoroughly by washing.
• Inform patient that drug can be poisonous when misused. Warn patient not to apply to open areas, acutely inflamed skin, or to face, eyes, mucous membranes, or urethral meatus. If accidental contact with eyes occurs, advise patient to flush with water and notify doctor.
• Tell patient to avoid inhaling vapors.
• Advise patient to wear gloves if applying to another person.
• Tell patient to wash drug off skin and to notify doctor immediately if skin irritation or hypersensitivity develops.
• Discourage repeated use, which can lead to skin irritation, systemic toxicity, or seizures. Advise patient to repeat use only if live lice or nits are found after 1 week.
• Warn patient not to use other creams or oils during treatment due to potential for enhanced absorption.
• Instruct patient to change all clothing and bed linens and launder in hot water or dry clean after drug is washed off of body.

Reactions may be *common*, uncommon, ***life-threatening***, or **COMMON AND LIFE-THREATENING**.

• After application for lice infestation, tell patient to use a fine-tooth comb or tweezers to remove nits from hairy areas.

• Advise patient to use lindane shampoo to clean combs or brushes and to wash them thoroughly afterward. Warn patient not to use lindane in such a way routinely.

• Warn patient that itching may continue for several weeks after effective treatment, especially in scabies.

• Instruct patient to reapply drug if it is washed off during treatment time.

• Tell patient to warn other family members and sexual contacts about infestation. Sexual contacts should be treated simultaneously.

---

permethrin
Elimite, Lyclear§, Nix

Pregnancy Risk Category: B

HOW SUPPLIED
Topical liquid (cream-rinse): 1%
Cream: 5%

ACTION
Acts on the parasites' nerve cells to disrupt the sodium channel current, causing paralysis of the parasite.

Route	Onset	Peak	Duration
Topical	10-15 min	Unknown	10 days

INDICATIONS & DOSAGE
Infestation with Pediculus humanus capitis *(head lice) and its nits—*
Adults and children 2 years and older: use after hair has been washed with shampoo, rinsed with water, and towel-dried. Apply 25 to 50 ml of liquid to saturate the hair and scalp. Allow to remain on hair for 10 minutes before rinsing off with water.
Treatment of Sarcoptes scabiei—
Adults and children 2 months and older: thoroughly massage into the skin from the head to the soles. Infants should be treated on the hairline, neck, scalp, temple, and forehead. Cream should be removed after 8 to 14 hours by washing.

ADVERSE REACTIONS
Skin: pruritus, *burning, stinging,* edema, tingling, numbness or scalp discomfort, mild erythema, scalp rash.

INTERACTIONS
None significant.

EFFECTS ON DIAGNOSTIC TESTS
None reported.

CONTRAINDICATIONS
Contraindicated in patients hypersensitive to pyrethrins, chrysanthemums, or components of drug.

NURSING CONSIDERATIONS
• Be aware that a single treatment is usually all that is necessary. Combing of nits is not required for effectiveness, but drug package supplies a fine-tooth comb for cosmetic use, as desired.

• Retreat for lice, as prescribed, if lice are observed 7 days after the initial application.

☑ Patient teaching
• Explain that treatment may temporarily worsen the symptoms of head lice infestation, such as pruritus, erythema, and edema.

• Tell patient that headgear, comb and brush, scarves, coats, and bed linens should be disinfected by machine washing with hot water and machine drying for at least 20 minutes, using the hot cycle. Nonwashable items should be sealed in a plastic bag for 2 weeks, or sprayed with a product designed to eliminate lice and their nits.

• Warn patient not to use on eyelashes or eyebrows.

• Tell patient to warn other family members and sexual contacts about infestation. Sexual contacts should be treated simultaneously.

---

pyrethrins
A-200, Barc◇, Blue, End Lice, Pronto, Pyrinyl◇, R & C, RID◇, Tisit◇, Triple X◇

Pregnancy Risk Category: C

HOW SUPPLIED
Shampoo: pyrethrins 0.17% and piperonyl butoxide 2%; pyrethrins 0.3% and piperonyl butoxide 3%, pyrethrins 0.33%, and piperonyl butoxide 4%
Topical gel: pyrethrins 0.18% and piperonyl butoxide 2.2%; pyrethrins 0.33% and piperonyl butoxide 3%; pyrethrins 0.3% and piperonyl butoxide 4%
Topical solution: pyrethrins 0.18% and piperonyl butoxide 2%; pyrethrins 0.2%, piperonyl butoxide 2%, and deodorized kerosene 0.8%; pyrethrins 0.3% and piperonyl butoxide 3%

ACTION
Acts as contact poison that disrupts parasites' nervous system, causing paralysis and death of parasite.

Route	Onset	Peak	Duration
Topical	Unknown	Unknown	Unknown

INDICATIONS & DOSAGE
Infestations of head, body, and pubic (crab) lice and their eggs—
Adults and children: apply to hair, scalp, or other infested areas until entirely wet. Allow to remain for 10 minutes but no longer. Wash thoroughly with warm water and soap or shampoo. Remove dead lice and eggs with fine-tooth comb. Treatment repeated, if necessary, in 7 to 10 days to kill newly hatched lice, not to exceed two applications within 24 hours.

ADVERSE REACTIONS
Skin: *irritation* (with repeated use).

INTERACTIONS
None significant.

EFFECTS ON DIAGNOSTIC TESTS
None reported.

CONTRAINDICATIONS
Contraindicated in patients hypersensitive to drug, ragweed, or chrysanthemums.

NURSING CONSIDERATIONS
• Use cautiously in infants and small children.
• Apply topical corticosteroids or oral antihistamines as prescribed if dermatitis develops from scratching.
• Discard container by wrapping in several layers of newspaper.
• Inspect all family members daily for at least 2 weeks for infestation.
• Be aware that drug is not effective against scabies.

✓ Patient teaching
• Instruct patient not to apply to open areas or acutely inflamed skin or to face, eyes, mucous membranes, or urethral meatus. Don't apply to eyebrows or eyelashes. If accidental contact with eyes occurs, advise patient to flush with water and notify doctor.
• Tell patient to discontinue drug and to wash it off skin and notify doctor immediately if skin irritation develops. All preparations contain petroleum distillates.
• Instruct patient to change and sterilize all clothing and bed linens after drug is washed off. Washable items should be disinfected by machine washing in hot water and drying on the hot cycle for at least 20 minutes. Other items can be dry cleaned or sealed in plastic bags for 2 weeks, or treated with products made for this purpose.
• Teach patient to remove dead parasites with a fine-tooth comb.
• Urge patient to warn other family members and sexual contacts about infestation. Sexual contacts should be treated simultaneously.

betamethasone dipropionate
betamethasone valerate
clobetasol propionate
desonide
desoximetasone
dexamethasone
dexamethasone sodium
    phosphate
diflorasone diacetate
fluocinolone acetonide
fluocinonide
flurandrenolide
fluticasone propionate
halcinonide
hydrocortisone
hydrocortisone acetate
hydrocortisone butyrate
hydrocortisone valerate
mometasone furoate
triamcinolone acetonide

COMBINATION PRODUCTS
Corticosteroids for topical use are commonly combined with antibiotics and antifungals. (See Chapter 87, LOCAL ANTI-INFECTIVES.)

---

betamethasone dipropionate
Alphatrex, Diprolene, Diprolene AF, Diprosone, Maxivate

betamethasone valerate
Betacap§, Betatrex, Beta-Val, Betnovate†‡, Valisone

Pregnancy Risk Category: C

HOW SUPPLIED
betamethasone dipropionate
Aerosol: 0.1%
Cream: 0.05%
Lotion: 0.05%
Ointment: 0.05%
betamethasone valerate
Cream: 0.01%, 0.1%
Gel: 0.05%
Lotion: 0.1%
Ointment: 0.1%

ACTION
Unclear. Diffuses across cell membranes to form complexes with specific cytoplasmic receptors. Exhibits anti-inflammatory, antipruritic, vasoconstrictive, and antiproliferative activity. Considered a group III (medium-potency) agent according to vasoconstrictive properties.

Route	Onset	Peak	Duration
Topical	Unknown	Unknown	Unknown

INDICATIONS & DOSAGE
Inflammation and pruritus associated with corticosteroid-responsive dermatoses—
Adults and children over 12 years: clean area; apply cream, ointment, lotion, aerosol spray, or gel sparingly. Dipropionate products are given once or twice daily; valerate products are given once daily to q.i.d. Maximum dosage for Diprolene cream is 45 g/week and 50 ml/week for Diprolene lotion.

ADVERSE REACTIONS
Skin: burning, pruritus, irritation, dryness, erythema, folliculitis, striae, acneiform eruptions, perioral dermatitis, hypopigmentation, hypertrichosis, allergic contact dermatitis; secondary infection, maceration, atrophy, striae, miliaria (with occlusive dressings).
Other: *hypothalamic-pituitary-adrenal axis suppression,* Cushing's syndrome, hyperglycemia, glycosuria (with betamethasone dipropionate).

INTERACTIONS
None significant.

EFFECTS ON DIAGNOSTIC TESTS
None reported.

CONTRAINDICATIONS
Contraindicated in patients hypersensitive to corticosteroids.

---

*Liquid contains alcohol. **May contain tartrazine. †Canada ‡Australia §U.K. ◇OTC

NURSING CONSIDERATIONS
• Gently wash skin before applying. To prevent skin damage, rub medication in gently, leaving a thin coat. When treating hairy sites, part hair and apply directly to lesions.
• Avoid application near eyes, mucous membranes, in ear canal, groin, or axillae.
• Know that because of alcohol content of vehicle, gel preparations may cause mild, transient stinging, especially when used on or near excoriated skin.
• For patients with eczematous dermatitis whose skin may be irritated by adhesive material, hold dressing in place with gauze, elastic bandages, stockings, or stockinette.
• Do not use an occlusive dressing.
• If antifungal agents or antibiotics are used concomitantly without prompt improvement, stop drug until infection is controlled, as ordered.
• Systemic absorption is likely with use of prolonged or extensive body surface treatment. Watch for symptoms.
• Avoid using plastic pants or tight-fitting diapers on treated areas in young children. Children may absorb larger amounts of drug and be more prone to systemic toxicity.
• Continue drug for a few days after lesions clear.
• Know that Diprolene and Diprolene AF may not be substituted generically because other products have different potencies.

☑ **Patient teaching**
• Teach patient how to apply drug; for external use only.
• Tell patient to stop drug and report signs of systemic absorption, skin irritation or ulceration, hypersensitivity, or infection.
• Instruct patient not to use occlusive dressings.
• Discuss personal hygiene measures to reduce chance of infection.

---

clobetasol propionate
Dermovate†, Temovate

Pregnancy Risk Category: C

HOW SUPPLIED
Cream: 0.05%
Gel: 0.05%
Lotion: 0.05%
Ointment: 0.05%

ACTION
Unclear. Diffuses across cell membranes to form complexes with specific cytoplasmic receptors. Exhibits anti-inflammatory, antipruritic, vasoconstrictive, and antiproliferative activity. Considered a group I (very high-potency) agent according to vasoconstrictive properties.

Route	Onset	Peak	Duration
Topical	Unknown	Unknown	Unknown

INDICATIONS & DOSAGE
Inflammation and pruritus associated with corticosteroid-responsive dermatoses—
Adults and children 12 years and older: apply thin layer to affected skin areas b.i.d., in the morning and evening for maximum of 14 days. Total dosage should not exceed 50 g weekly.

ADVERSE REACTIONS
Skin: burning, pruritus, irritation, dryness, erythema, folliculitis, perioral dermatitis, allergic contact dermatitis, hypopigmentation, hypertrichosis, acneiform eruptions.
Other: *hypothalamic-pituitary-adrenal (HPA) axis suppression,* Cushing's syndrome, hyperglycemia, glycosuria.

INTERACTIONS
None significant.

EFFECTS ON DIAGNOSTIC TESTS
None reported.

CONTRAINDICATIONS
Contraindicated in patients with primary scalp infections or hypersensitivity to corticosteroids.

NURSING CONSIDERATIONS
• Gently wash skin before applying. To prevent skin damage, rub medication in gently and completely. When treating hairy sites, part hair and apply directly to lesions.

Reactions may be *common,* uncommon, *life-threatening,* or COMMON AND LIFE-THREATENING.

• Avoid application near eyes or mucous membranes, or in ear canal.

Alert: Don't use occlusive dressings or bandage. Don't cover or wrap treated areas unless directed by doctor.

• If antifungal agents or antibiotics are used concomitantly and there is not prompt improvement, stop corticosteroid drug until infection is controlled, as ordered.

• Discontinue drug and notify doctor if skin infection, striae, or atrophy occurs.

• Know that HPA axis suppression occurs at doses as low as 2 g per day.

☑ **Patient teaching**

• Teach patient how to apply drug and to avoid contact with eye.

• Tell patient to stop drug and report signs of systemic absorption, skin irritation or ulceration, hypersensitivity, or infection.

• Warn patient not to use drug for longer than 14 consecutive days.

desonide
DesOwen, Tridesilon

Pregnancy Risk Category: C

HOW SUPPLIED
Cream: 0.05%
Ointment: 0.05%
Lotion: 0.05%

ACTION
Unclear. Diffuses across cell membranes to form complexes with specific cytoplasmic receptors. Exhibits anti-inflammatory, antipruritic, vasoconstrictive, and antiproliferative activity. Considered a group IV (low-potency) agent according to vasoconstrictive properties.

Route	Onset	Peak	Duration
Topical	Unknown	Unknown	Unknown

INDICATIONS & DOSAGE
Inflammation and pruritus associated with corticosteroid-responsive dermatoses—

Adults: clean area; apply sparingly b.i.d. to q.i.d.

ADVERSE REACTIONS
Skin: burning, pruritus, irritation, dryness, erythema, folliculitis, perioral dermatitis, allergic contact dermatitis, hypertrichosis, hypopigmentation, acneiform eruptions; *maceration of skin, secondary infection, atrophy, striae, miliaria* (with occlusive dressings).

Other: *hypothalamic-pituitary-adrenal axis suppression,* Cushing's syndrome, hyperglycemia, glycosuria.

INTERACTIONS
None significant.

EFFECTS ON DIAGNOSTIC TESTS
None reported.

CONTRAINDICATIONS
Contraindicated in patients hypersensitive to drug.

NURSING CONSIDERATIONS
• Gently wash skin before applying. Rub medication in gently, leaving a thin coat. When treating hairy sites, part hair and apply directly to lesions.

• Avoid application near eyes or mucous membranes, or in ear canal.

• For patients with eczematous dermatitis whose skin may be irritated by adhesive material, hold dressing in place with gauze, stockings, or stockinette.

• Change dressing as ordered. Stop drug and notify doctor if skin infection, striae, or atrophy occurs.

• If an occlusive dressing is ordered and a fever develops, notify doctor and remove dressing.

• If antifungal agents or antibiotics are used concomitantly, stop desonide until infection is controlled, as ordered.

• Systemic absorption is likely with use of occlusive dressings, prolonged treatment, or extensive body surface treatment. Watch for symptoms.

• Avoid using plastic pants or tight-fitting diapers on treated areas in young children. Children may absorb larger amounts of drug and be more prone to systemic toxicity.

• Continue treatment for a few days after lesions clear, as ordered.

✓**Patient teaching**
• Teach patient how to apply drug.
• If an occlusive dressing is ordered, advise patient not to leave dressing in place longer than 12 hours each day, or as ordered, and not to use occlusive dressings on infected or exudative lesions.
• Tell patient to stop drug and report signs of systemic absorption, skin irritation or ulceration, hypersensitivity, or infection.

desoximetasone
Topicort

Pregnancy Risk Category: C

HOW SUPPLIED
Cream: 0.05%, 0.25%
Gel: 0.05%
Ointment: 0.25%

ACTION
Unclear. Diffuses across cell membranes to form complexes with specific cytoplasmic receptors. Exhibits anti-inflammatory, antipruritic, vasoconstrictive, and antiproliferative activity. Considered a group III (medium-potency) agent according to vasoconstrictive properties.

Route	Onset	Peak	Duration
Topical	Unknown	Unknown	Unknown

INDICATIONS & DOSAGE
Inflammation associated with corticosteroid-responsive dermatoses—
Adults and children: clean area; apply sparingly b.i.d.

ADVERSE REACTIONS
Skin: burning, pruritus, irritation, dryness, erythema, folliculitis, hypertrichosis, acneiform eruptions, perioral dermatitis, hypopigmentation, allergic contact dermatitis; *maceration, secondary infection, atrophy, striae, miliaria* (with occlusive dressings).
Other: *hypothalamic-pituitary-adrenal axis suppression,* Cushing's syndrome, hyperglycemia, glycosuria.

INTERACTIONS
None significant.

EFFECTS ON DIAGNOSTIC TESTS
None reported.

CONTRAINDICATIONS
Contraindicated in patients hypersensitive to drug and its components.

NURSING CONSIDERATIONS
• Gently wash skin before applying. To prevent skin damage, rub medication in gently, leaving a thin coat. When treating hairy sites, part hair and apply directly to lesions.
• Avoid application near eyes or mucous membranes, or in ear canal.
• For patients with eczematous dermatitis whose skin may be irritated by adhesive material, hold dressing in place with gauze, elastic bandages, stockings, or stockinette.
• Change dressing as ordered. Stop drug and notify doctor if skin infection, striae, or atrophy occurs.
• If fever develops and an occlusive dressing is in place, notify doctor and remove occlusive dressing.
• If antifungal agents or antibiotics are used concomitantly, stop corticosteroid drug until infection is controlled, as ordered.
• Systemic absorption is likely with use of occlusive dressings, prolonged treatment, or extensive body surface treatment. Watch for symptoms.
• Avoid using plastic pants or tight-fitting diapers on treated areas in young children. Children may absorb larger amounts of drug and be more prone to systemic toxicity.
• Continue drug for a few days after lesions clear, as ordered.
• Gel contains alcohol and may cause burning or irritation in open lesions.

✓**Patient teaching**
• Teach patient how to apply drug.
• If an occlusive dressing is ordered, advise patient not to leave dressing in place longer than 12 hours each day and not to use occlusive dressings on infected or exudative lesions.
• Tell patient to stop drug and report signs of systemic absorption, skin irritation or ulceration, hypersensitivity, or infection.

Reactions may be *common,* uncommon, ***life-threatening,*** or COMMON AND LIFE-THREATENING.

dexamethasone
Aeroseb-Dex, Decaspray

dexamethasone sodium phosphate
Decadron Phosphate

Pregnancy Risk Category: C

HOW SUPPLIED
dexamethasone
Aerosol: 0.01%, 0.04%
dexamethasone sodium phosphate
Cream: 0.1%

ACTION
Unclear. Diffuses across cell membranes to form complexes with specific cytoplasmic receptors. Exhibits anti-inflammatory, antipruritic, vasoconstrictive, and antiproliferative activity. Considered a group IV (low-potency) agent according to vasoconstrictive properties.

Route	Onset	Peak	Duration
Topical	Unknown	Unknown	Unknown

INDICATIONS & DOSAGE
Inflammation associated with corticosteroid-responsive dermatoses—
Adults and children: clean area; apply cream, gel, or aerosol sparingly t.i.d. or q.i.d.

For aerosol use on scalp, shake can well but gently, and apply to dry scalp after shampooing. Hold can upright or inverted and 6″ away from area. Spray while moving container to all affected areas, which should take about 2 seconds. Don't massage medication into scalp or spray forehead or near eyes. When result is obtained, reduce dose gradually and then discontinue.

ADVERSE REACTIONS
Skin: burning, pruritus, irritation, dryness, erythema, folliculitis, hypertrichosis, acneiform eruptions, perioral dermatitis, hypopigmentation, allergic contact dermatitis; *maceration, secondary infection, atrophy, striae, miliaria* (with occlusive dressings).
Other: *hypothalamic-pituitary-adrenal*

axis suppression, Cushing's syndrome, hyperglycemia, glycosuria, and growth and development in children.

INTERACTIONS
None significant.

EFFECTS ON DIAGNOSTIC TESTS
None reported.

CONTRAINDICATIONS
Contraindicated in patients hypersensitive to drug or its components.

NURSING CONSIDERATIONS
• Gently wash skin before applying. To prevent skin damage, rub gel or cream in gently, leaving a thin coat. When treating hairy sites, part hair and apply directly to lesions.
• Avoid application near eyes or mucous membranes, in ear canal, groin, or axillae.
• For patients with eczematous dermatitis whose skin may be irritated by adhesive material, hold dressing in place with gauze, stockings, or stockinette.
• Change dressing as ordered. Stop drug and tell doctor if skin infection, striae, or atrophy occurs.
• If an occlusive dressing has been ordered and a fever develops, notify doctor and remove the dressing.
• When using aerosol around the face, cover patient's eyes and warn against inhalation of spray. Aerosol preparation contains alcohol and may produce irritation or burning in open lesions. To avoid freezing tissues, do not spray longer than 1 to 2 seconds or closer than 6″ (15 cm).
• If antifungal agents or antibiotics are used concomitantly, stop drug until infection is controlled, as ordered.
• Systemic absorption is likely with use of occlusive dressings, prolonged treatment, or extensive body surface treatment. Watch for symptoms.
• Avoid using plastic pants or tight-fitting diapers on treated areas in young children. Children may absorb larger amounts of drug and be more prone to systemic toxicity.
• Continue treatment for a few days after lesions clear, as ordered.

---

*Liquid contains alcohol.   **May contain tartrazine.   †Canada   ‡Australia   §U.K.   ◊OTC

☑ Patient teaching
- Teach patient and family how to apply drug.
- If an occlusive dressing is ordered, advise patient not to leave it in place longer than 12 hours each day and not to use occlusive dressings on infected or exudative lesions.
- Tell patient to stop drug and report signs of systemic absorption, skin irritation or ulceration, hypersensitivity, or infection.
- Tell patient to avoid scratching.

diflorasone diacetate
Florone, Florone E, Maxiflor, Psorcon

Pregnancy Risk Category: C

HOW SUPPLIED
Cream: 0.05%
Ointment: 0.05%

ACTION
Unclear. Diffuses across cell membranes to form complexes with specific cytoplasmic receptors. Exhibits anti-inflammatory, antipruritic, vasoconstrictive, and antiproliferative activity. Considered a group I or II (very high- and high-potency) agent according to vasoconstrictive properties.

Route	Onset	Peak	Duration
Topical	Unknown	Unknown	Unknown

INDICATIONS & DOSAGE
Inflammation and pruritus associated with corticosteroid-responsive dermatoses—
Adults and children: clean area; apply sparingly in thin film. Apply cream b.i.d. to q.i.d. and emollient cream and ointment once daily to t.i.d. Use least amount to achieve effectiveness in children.

ADVERSE REACTIONS
Skin: burning, pruritus, irritation, dryness, erythema, folliculitis, perioral dermatitis, hypertrichosis, hypopigmentation, acneiform eruptions; *maceration, secondary infection, atrophy, striae, miliaria* (with occlusive dressings).

Other: *hypothalamic-pituitary-adrenal axis suppression,* Cushing's syndrome, hyperglycemia, glycosuria; hypertension, osteoporosis (in elderly patients).

INTERACTIONS
None significant.

EFFECTS ON DIAGNOSTIC TESTS
None reported.

CONTRAINDICATIONS
Contraindicated in patients hypersensitive to drug or its components.

NURSING CONSIDERATIONS
- Before applying, gently wash skin. To prevent skin damage, rub medication in gently, leaving a thin coat. When treating hairy sites, part hair and apply directly to lesions. Wear gloves to apply.
- Avoid application near eyes or mucous membranes, in ear canal, axillae, rectal, or groin areas.
- For patients with eczematous dermatitis whose skin may be irritated by adhesive material, hold dressing in place with gauze, elastic bandages, stockings, or stockinette.
- Change dressing as ordered. Stop drug and notify doctor if skin infection, striae, or atrophy occurs.
- If an occlusive dressing has been ordered and a fever develops, notify doctor and remove the dressing.
- If antifungal agents or antibiotics are used concomitantly, stop drug until infection is controlled, as ordered.
- Systemic absorption is likely with use of occlusive dressings, prolonged treatment, or extensive body surface treatment. Watch for symptoms.
- Avoid using plastic pants or tight-fitting diapers on treated areas in young children. Children may absorb larger amounts of drug and be more prone to systemic toxicity.

☑ Patient teaching
- Teach patient how to apply drug.
- Tell patient to wash hands after drug application.
- If an occlusive dressing is ordered, advise patient not to leave it in place longer

than 12 hours each day and not to use occlusive dressings on infected or exudative lesions.
• Tell patient to stop drug and report signs of systemic absorption, skin irritation or ulceration, hypersensitivity, or infection.

fluocinolone acetonide
Derma-Smoothe/FS, Fluonid, Flurosyn, FS Shampoo, Metosyn§, Synalar, Synemol

Pregnancy Risk Category: C

HOW SUPPLIED
Cream: 0.01%, 0.025%, 0.2%
Oil: 0.01%
Ointment: 0.025%
Shampoo: 0.01%
Topical solution: 0.01%

ACTION
Unclear. Diffuses across cell membranes to form complexes with specific cytoplasmic receptors. Exhibits anti-inflammatory, antipruritic, vasoconstrictive, and antiproliferative activity. Considered a group III (medium-potency) agent according to vasoconstrictive properties.

Route	Onset	Peak	Duration
Topical	Unknown	Unknown	Unknown

INDICATIONS & DOSAGE
Inflammation associated with corticosteroid-responsive dermatoses—
Adults and children: clean area; apply cream, ointment, or topical solution sparingly b.i.d. to q.i.d.

ADVERSE REACTIONS
Skin: burning, pruritus, irritation, dryness, erythema, folliculitis, hypertrichosis, hypopigmentation, acneiform eruptions, perioral dermatitis, allergic contact dermatitis; *maceration, secondary infection, atrophy, striae, miliaria* (with occlusive dressings).
Other: *hypothalamic-pituitary-adrenal axis suppression,* Cushing's syndrome, hyperglycemia, glycosuria.

INTERACTIONS
None significant.

EFFECTS ON DIAGNOSTIC TESTS
None reported.

CONTRAINDICATIONS
Contraindicated in patients hypersensitive to drug or its components.

NURSING CONSIDERATIONS
• Gently wash skin before applying. To prevent skin damage, rub medication in gently, leaving a thin coat. When treating hairy sites, part hair and apply directly to lesions.
• Avoid application near eyes or mucous membranes, in axillae, groin, rectal area, or ear canal if ear drum is perforated.
• For patients with eczematous dermatitis whose skin may be irritated by adhesive material, hold dressing in place with gauze, elastic bandages, stockings, or stockinette.
• Change dressing as ordered. Stop drug and notify doctor if skin infection, striae, or atrophy occurs.
• If an occlusive dressing has been ordered and a fever develops, notify doctor and remove dressing.
• If antifungal agents or antibiotics are used concomitantly, stop drug until infection is controlled, as ordered.
• Systemic absorption is likely with use of occlusive dressings, prolonged treatment, or extensive body surface treatment. Watch for symptoms.
• In young children, avoid using plastic pants or tight-fitting diapers on treated areas. Children may absorb larger amounts of drug and be more prone to systemic toxicity.
• Fluonid solution on dry lesions may increase dryness, scaling, or pruritus; on denuded or fissured areas, may produce burning or stinging. If either of these persists and dermatitis has not improved, discontinue use of solution and notify doctor.

✓ Patient teaching
• Teach patient or family how to apply drug using gloves or sterile applicator.
• If an occlusive dressing is ordered, advise patient not to leave it in place longer

---

*Liquid contains alcohol.   **May contain tartrazine.   †Canada   ‡Australia   §U.K.   ◊OTC

than 12 hours each day and not to use occlusive dressings on infected or exudative lesions.

• Tell patient to stop drug and report signs of systemic absorption, skin irritation or ulceration, hypersensitivity, or infection.

---

fluocinonide
Fluonex, Lidex, Lidex-E

Pregnancy Risk Category: C

HOW SUPPLIED
Cream: 0.05%
Gel: 0.05%
Ointment: 0.05%
Topical solution: 0.05%

ACTION
Unclear. Diffuses across cell membranes to form complexes with specific cytoplasmic receptors. Exhibits anti-inflammatory, antipruritic, vasoconstrictive, and antiproliferative activity. Considered a group II (high-potency) agent according to vasoconstrictive properties.

Route	Onset	Peak	Duration
Topical	Unknown	Unknown	Unknown

INDICATIONS & DOSAGE
Inflammation associated with corticosteroid-responsive dermatoses—
Adults and children: clean area; apply cream, gel, ointment, or topical solution sparingly b.i.d. or q.i.d. In children, use lowest dose that promotes healing.

ADVERSE REACTIONS
Skin: burning, pruritus, irritation, dryness, erythema, folliculitis, hypertrichosis, hypopigmentation, acneiform eruptions, perioral dermatitis, allergic contact dermatitis; *maceration, secondary infection, atrophy, striae, miliaria* (with occlusive dressings).
Other: *hypothalamic-pituitary-adrenal axis suppression,* Cushing's syndrome, hyperglycemia, glycosuria.

INTERACTIONS
None significant.

EFFECTS ON DIAGNOSTIC TESTS
None reported.

CONTRAINDICATIONS
Contraindicated in patients hypersensitive to drug or its components.

NURSING CONSIDERATIONS
• Gently wash skin before applying. To prevent skin damage, rub medication in gently, leaving a thin coat. When treating hairy sites, part hair and apply directly to lesion.
• Avoid application near eyes or mucous membranes, or in ear canal.
• For patients with eczematous dermatitis whose skin may be irritated by adhesive material, hold dressing in place with gauze, elastic bandages, stockings, or stockinette.
• Change dressing as ordered. Stop drug and notify doctor if skin infection, striae, or atrophy occurs.
• If an occlusive dressing has been ordered and a fever develops, notify doctor and remove dressing.
• If antifungal agents or antibiotics are used concomitantly, stop drug until infection is controlled, as ordered.
• Systemic absorption is likely with use of occlusive dressings, prolonged treatment, or extensive body surface treatment. Watch for symptoms.
• In young children, avoid using plastic pants or tight-fitting diapers on treated areas. Children may absorb larger amounts of drug and be more prone to systemic toxicity.
• Continue treatment for a few days after lesions clear, as ordered.

✓Patient teaching
• Teach patient and family how to apply drug using gloves, sterile applicator, or with careful hand washing.
• If an occlusive dressing is ordered, advise patient not to leave it in place longer than 12 hours each day and not to use occlusive dressings on infected or exudative lesions.
• Tell patient to stop drug and report signs of systemic absorption, skin irritation or ulceration, hypersensitivity, or infection.

---

flurandrenolide
Cordran, Cordran SP,
Drenison Tape†

Pregnancy Risk Category: C

HOW SUPPLIED
Cream: 0.025%, 0.05%
Lotion: 0.05%
Ointment: 0.025%, 0.05%
Tape: 4 mcg/cm²

ACTION
Unclear. Diffuses across cell membranes to form complexes with specific cytoplasmic receptors. Exhibits anti-inflammatory, antipruritic, vasoconstrictive, and antiproliferative activity. Considered a group III (medium-potency) agent according to vasoconstrictive properties.

Route	Onset	Peak	Duration
Topical	Unknown	Unknown	Unknown

INDICATIONS & DOSAGE
Inflammation and pruritus associated with corticosteroid-responsive dermatoses—

Adults and children: clean area; apply cream, lotion, or ointment sparingly b.i.d. or t.i.d.

Apply Cordran tape q 12 to 24 hours. Before applying tape, clean skin carefully, removing scales, crust, and dried exudate. Let skin dry for 1 hour before applying new tape. Shave or clip hair to allow good contact with skin and comfortable removal. If tape ends loosen prematurely, trim off and replace with fresh tape.

ADVERSE REACTIONS
Skin: burning, pruritus, irritation, dryness, erythema, folliculitis, hypertrichosis, hypopigmentation, acneiform eruptions, allergic contact dermatitis; *maceration, secondary infection, atrophy, striae, miliaria* (with occlusive dressings); purpura, stripping of epidermis, furunculosis (with tape).
Other: *hypothalamic-pituitary-adrenal axis suppression,* Cushing's syndrome, hyperglycemia, glycosuria.

INTERACTIONS
None significant.

EFFECTS ON DIAGNOSTIC TESTS
None reported.

CONTRAINDICATIONS
Contraindicated in patients hypersensitive to drug or its components.

NURSING CONSIDERATIONS
• Gently wash skin before applying. To prevent skin damage, rub medication in gently, leaving a thin coat. When treating hairy sites, part hair and apply directly to lesions.
• Avoid application near eyes or mucous membranes, or in ear canal.
Alert: Know that tape is not advised for exudative lesions or lesions in intertriginous areas. Replace tape q 12 hours or, if well tolerated and adherence is satisfactory, q 24 hours. Do not tear Cordran tape; cut it with scissors. Make sure skin is dry for 1 hour before applying tape.
• For patients with eczematous dermatitis whose skin may be irritated by adhesive material, hold dressing in place with gauze, elastic bandages, stockings, or stockinette.
• Stop drug and tell doctor if skin infection, striae, or atrophy occurs.
• Notify doctor and remove occlusive dressing if fever develops.
• If antifungal agents or antibiotics are used concomitantly, stop drug until infection is controlled, as ordered.
• Systemic absorption is likely with use of occlusive dressings, prolonged treatment, or extensive body surface treatment. Watch for symptoms.
• Avoid using plastic pants or tight-fitting diapers on treated areas in young children. Children may absorb larger amounts of drug and be more prone to systemic toxicity.
• Continue treatment for a few days after lesions clear, as ordered.

☑ **Patient teaching**
• Teach patient or family how to apply drug.
• If an occlusive dressing is ordered, advise patient not to leave it in place longer

than 12 hours each day and not to use occlusive dressings on infected or exudative lesions.

• Tell patient to stop drug and report signs of systemic absorption, skin irritation or ulceration, hypersensitivity, or infection.

---

fluticasone propionate
Cutivate

Pregnancy Risk Category: C

HOW SUPPLIED
Cream: 0.05%
Ointment: 0.005%

ACTION
Exact mechanism unknown. Exhibits anti-inflammatory, antipruritic, and vasoconstrictive activity. Considered a medium-potency agent.

Route	Onset	Peak	Duration
Topical	Rapid	Unknown	10 hr

INDICATIONS & DOSAGE
Inflammatory and pruritic manifestations associated with corticosteroid-responsive dermatoses—
Adults: apply sparingly to affected area b.i.d.; rub in gently and completely.

ADVERSE REACTIONS
CNS: light-headedness.
Skin: hives, burning, hypertrichosis, pruritus, irritation, erythema.
Other: *hypothalamic-pituitary-adrenal axis suppression,* Cushing's syndrome, hyperglycemia, glycosuria.

INTERACTIONS
None significant.

EFFECTS ON DIAGNOSTIC TESTS
None significant.

CONTRAINDICATIONS
Contraindicated in patients with viral, fungal, herpetic, or tubercular skin lesions and hypersensitivity to drug or its components.

NURSING CONSIDERATIONS
• Do not mix drug with other bases or vehicles; this may affect potency.
• Know that safety in children has not been established.
• If adverse reactions occur, doctor may order a less potent agent.
• Discontinue drug if local irritation or systemic infection, absorption, or hypersensitivity occurs, as ordered.
• Know that generally, absorption of corticosteroids is enhanced when applied to inflamed or damaged skin, eyelids, or scrotal area; lowest when applied to intact normal skin, palms of hands, or soles of feet.

☑ Patient teaching
• Teach patient or family member how to apply drug using gloves, sterile applicator, or with careful hand washing if fingers are used.
• Tell patient to avoid prolonged use and contact with eyes. Warn him not to apply around eyes, genitals, axillae, or rectum; on face; or in skin creases.
• Instruct patient to notify doctor if condition persists or worsens or if burning or irritation develops.

---

halcinonide
Halciderm Topical§, Halog, Halog-E

Pregnancy Risk Category: C

HOW SUPPLIED
Cream: 0.025%, 0.1%
Ointment: 0.1%
Topical solution: 0.1%

ACTION
Unclear. Diffuses across cell membranes to form complexes with cytoplasmic receptors. Exhibits anti-inflammatory, antipruritic, vasoconstrictive, antiproliferative activity. Considered a group II (high-potency) agent according to vasoconstrictive properties.

Route	Onset	Peak	Duration
Topical	Unknown	Unknown	Unknown

Reactions may be *common*, uncommon, *life-threatening*, or COMMON AND LIFE-THREATENING.

INDICATIONS & DOSAGE
Inflammation associated with cortico-steroid-responsive dermatoses—
Adults and children: clean area; apply cream, ointment, or topical solution sparingly b.i.d. or t.i.d. Rub cream in gently.

ADVERSE REACTIONS
Skin: burning, pruritus, irritation, dryness, erythema, folliculitis, hypertrichosis, hypopigmentation, acneiform eruptions, allergic contact dermatitis; *maceration, secondary infection, atrophy, striae, miliaria* (with occlusive dressings).
Other: *hypothalamic-pituitary-adrenal axis suppression,* Cushing's syndrome, hyperglycemia, glycosuria.

INTERACTIONS
None significant.

EFFECTS ON DIAGNOSTIC TESTS
None reported.

CONTRAINDICATIONS
Contraindicated in patients hypersensitive to drug or its components.

NURSING CONSIDERATIONS
• Gently wash skin before applying. To prevent skin damage, rub medication in gently, leaving a thin coat. When treating hairy sites, part hair and apply directly to lesions.
• Avoid application near eyes, mucous membranes, in ear canal, axillae, groin, or rectal area.
• Gently rub small amount of cream into lesion until it disappears. Reapply, leaving a thin coating on lesion, and cover with occlusive dressing, if ordered. Apply ointment to lesion and cover with occlusive dressing, if ordered. Do not leave dressing in place longer than 12 hours each day.
• Don't use occlusive dressings on infected or exudative lesions.
• For patients with eczematous dermatitis whose skin may be irritated by adhesive material, hold dressing in place with gauze, stockings, or stockinette.
• Change dressing as ordered. Stop drug and tell doctor if skin infection, striae, or atrophy occurs.
• Be aware that good results have been obtained by applying occlusive dressings in the evening and removing them in the morning, providing 12-hour occlusion. Drug should then be reapplied and no occlusive dressings applied during the day.
• If an occlusive dressing has been ordered and a fever develops, notify doctor and remove dressing.
• If antifungal agents or antibiotics are used concomitantly, stop drug until infection is controlled, as ordered.
• Systemic absorption is especially likely with use of occlusive dressings, prolonged treatment, or extensive body surface treatment. Watch for symptoms.
• Avoid using plastic pants or tight-fitting diapers on treated areas in young children. Children may absorb larger amounts of drug and be more prone to systemic toxicity.
• Continue treatment for a few days after lesions clear, as ordered.

☑ **Patient teaching**
• Teach patient how to apply drug.
• If an occlusive dressing is ordered, advise patient not to leave it in place longer than 12 hours each day and not to use occlusive dressings on infected or exudative lesions.
• Tell patient to stop drug and report signs of systemic absorption, skin irritation or ulceration, hypersensitivity, or infection.

---

hydrocortisone
Acticort 100, Aeroseb-HC, Ala-Cort, Ala-Scalp, Anusol-HC, Bactine Hydrocortisone◇, Carmol-HC, Cetacort, Cort-Dome, Cortef◇, Cortenema, Cortizone-5◇, Cortril, Delacort, Dermacort◇, Dermolate Anti-Itch◇, Dermtex HC, Efcortelan§, Hi-Cor 2.5, Hycort, Hydrocortisyl§, Hydro-Tex, Hytone, LactiCare-HC, Nutracort, Orabase HCA, Penecort, Procort◇, Proctocort, Scalpicin◇, Squibb-HC‡, Synacort, Tegrin-HC◇, Texacort, T/Scalp, Unicort

---

hydrocortisone acetate
Anu-Med HC, CaldeCORT
Anti-Itch, CortaGel Extra
Strength, Cortaid◇, Cortamed†,
Cortef, Corticaine, Corticreme†,
Cortifoam, Dermacort,
Dermol HC, Epifoam, Gynecort,
Hemril-HC, Hydrocortone Acetate,
Lanacort, ProctoCream-HC,
Proctofoam-HC

hydrocortisone butyrate
Locoid

hydrocortisone valerate
Westcort

Pregnancy Risk Category: C

HOW SUPPLIED
hydrocortisone
Aerosol: 0.5%, 1%
Cream: 0.25%◇, 0.5%◇, 1%◇, 2.5%
Enema: 100 mg/60 ml
Gel: 0.5%, 1%
Lotion: 0.125%, 0.25%, 0.5%◇, 1%, 2%, 2.5%
Ointment: 0.5%◇, 1%◇, 2.5%
Pledgets: 0.5%, 1%
Rectal cream: 1%◇
Stick roll-on: 1%
Suppositories: 25 mg
Topical solution: 0.5%, 1%, 2.5%
hydrocortisone acetate
Cream: 0.5%◇, 1%
Lotion: 0.5%◇
Ointment: 0.5%◇, 1%
Paste: 0.5%
Solution: 1%
Suppositories: 10 mg, 25 mg
Rectal foam: 90 mg per application
hydrocortisone butyrate
Cream: 0.1%
Ointment: 0.1%
Solution: 0.1%
hydrocortisone valerate
Cream: 0.2%
Ointment: 0.2%

ACTION
Unknown. Diffuses across cell membranes to form complexes with specific cytoplasmic receptors. Exhibits anti-inflammatory, antipruritic, vasoconstrictive, and antiproliferative activity.

Route	Onset	Peak	Duration
PR, topical	Unknown	Unknown	Unknown

INDICATIONS & DOSAGE
Inflammation and pruritus associated with corticosteroid-responsive dermatoses; adjunctive topical management of seborrheic dermatitis of scalp—
Adults and children: clean area; apply cream, gel, lotion, ointment, or topical solution sparingly daily to q.i.d. Spray aerosol onto affected area daily to q.i.d. until acute phase is controlled; then reduce dosage to one to three times weekly p.r.n. Children should receive the least amount that provides positive results.
Inflammation associated with proctitis—
Adults: 1 applicatorful of rectal foam P.R. daily or b.i.d. for 2 to 3 weeks, then every other day p.r.n; enema is given once nightly for 21 days or until patient improves; may be used for 2 to 3 months if used every other night. Suppositories are inserted b.i.d. for 2 weeks.

ADVERSE REACTIONS
Topical use:
Skin: burning, pruritus, irritation, dryness, erythema, folliculitis, hypertrichosis, hypopigmentation, acneiform eruptions, allergic contact dermatitis; *maceration, secondary infection, atrophy, striae, miliaria* (with occlusive dressings).
Other: *hypothalamic-pituitary-adrenal axis suppression,* Cushing's syndrome, hyperglycemia, glycosuria.
Rectal use:
CNS: *seizures, increased intracranial pressure,* vertigo, headache.
CV: hypertension.
EENT: cataracts, glaucoma.
Endocrine: menstrual irregularities, decreased carbohydrate tolerance.
GI: peptic ulcer, pancreatitis, abdominal distention.
GU: menstrual irregularities.
Metabolic: fluid or electrolyte disturbances—sodium and fluid retention, potassium loss, hypokalemic alkalosis,

---

Reactions may be *common,* uncommon, *life-threatening,* or COMMON AND LIFE-THREATENING.

negative nitrogen balance due to catabolism of protein.

Musculoskeletal: muscle weakness, osteoporosis, necrosis and fractures in bone.

Skin: impaired wound healing, fragile skin, petechiae, erythema, sweating; may suppress skin reaction testing.

INTERACTIONS
None significant.

EFFECTS ON DIAGNOSTIC TESTS
None reported.

CONTRAINDICATIONS
Contraindicated in patients hypersensitive to drug or its components.

NURSING CONSIDERATIONS
• Gently wash skin before applying. To prevent skin damage, rub medication in gently, leaving a thin coat. When treating hairy sites, part hair and apply directly to lesions.
• Avoid application near eyes or mucous membranes, or in ear canal; may be safely used on face, groin, armpits, and under breasts.
• If an occlusive dressing is ordered and a fever develops, notify doctor and remove dressing.
• Change dressing as ordered. Stop drug and tell doctor if skin infection, striae, or atrophy occurs.
• When using aerosol about the face, cover the patient's eyes and warn against inhalation of the spray. Aerosol preparation contains alcohol and may produce irritation or burning in open lesions. Do not spray longer than 3 seconds or closer than 6″ (15 cm) to avoid freezing tissues. If spray is applied to dry scalp after shampooing, there is no need to massage medication into scalp.
• If antifungal agents or antibiotics are used concomitantly, stop corticosteroid drug until infection is controlled, as ordered.
• Systemic absorption is likely with the use of occlusive dressings, prolonged treatment, or extensive body surface treatment. Watch for symptoms.
• Avoid using plastic pants or tight-fitting diapers on treated areas in young children. Children may absorb larger amounts of drug and be more prone to systemic toxicity.
• Continue treatment for a few days after lesions clear, as ordered.

✓ Patient teaching
• Teach patient or family member how to apply drug.
• If an occlusive dressing is ordered, advise patient not to leave it in place longer than 12 hours each day and not to use occlusive dressings on infected or exudative lesions.
• Tell patient to stop drug and report signs of systemic absorption, skin irritation or ulceration, hypersensitivity, infection, or no improvement.
• For enema administration, tell patient to lie on left side and retain fluid for 1 hour.
• Instruct patient to insert suppositories blunt end first after removing foil wrapper.
• For perianal application, instruct patient to place a small amount of drug on a tissue and gently rub it in.
• Tell patient to disassemble applicators or aerosol cap and clean with warm water after each use.

---

mometasone furoate
Elocon

Pregnancy Risk Category: C

HOW SUPPLIED
Cream: 0.1%
Ointment: 0.1%
Lotion: 0.1%

ACTION
Unclear. Diffuses across cell membranes to form complexes with specific cytoplasmic receptors. Exhibits anti-inflammatory, antipruritic, vasoconstrictive, and antiproliferative activity. Considered a group III (medium-potency) agent according to vasoconstrictive properties.

Route	Onset	Peak	Duration
Topical	Unknown	Unknown	Unknown

INDICATIONS & DOSAGE
Inflammation and pruritus associated with corticosteroid-responsive dermatoses—
Adults: apply to affected areas once daily.
Children 2 years and older: apply to affected areas once daily for no more than 3 weeks.

ADVERSE REACTIONS
Skin: burning, erythema, pruritus, atrophy, irritation, acneiform eruptions, hypopigmentation, allergic contact dermatitis.
Other: *hypothalamic-pituitary-adrenal axis suppression,* Cushing's syndrome, hyperglycemia, glycosuria.

INTERACTIONS
None significant.

EFFECTS ON DIAGNOSTIC TESTS
None reported.

CONTRAINDICATIONS
Contraindicated in patients hypersensitive to drug, its components, or other corticosteroids.

NURSING CONSIDERATIONS
• Use cautiously in children 2 years and older.
• Gently wash skin before applying. To prevent skin damage, rub medication in gently, leaving a thin coat. When treating hairy sites, part hair and apply directly to lesions.
• Do not apply near eyes, mucous membranes, in ear canal, axillae, groin, or rectal areas.
Alert: Do not use occlusive dressings with drug. Systemic absorption is likely with use of occlusive dressings, prolonged treatment, or extensive body surface treatment. Watch for symptoms.
• If antimicrobial agents are used concomitantly, stop corticosteroid drug until infection is controlled, as ordered.
• Children may absorb larger amounts of drug and be more prone to systemic toxicity. Avoid using plastic pants or tight-fitting diapers on treated areas in young children. Do not use cream or ointment on the diaper area.

☑ **Patient teaching**
• Teach patient or family member how to apply drug.
• Tell patient to stop drug and report signs of systemic absorption, skin irritation or ulceration, hypersensitivity, infection, or if there is no improvement in 2 weeks.

triamcinolone acetonide
Adcortyl§, Aristocort, Delta-Tritex, Flutex, Kenalog, Kenalone‡, Triacet, Triderm

Pregnancy Risk Category: C

HOW SUPPLIED
Aerosol: 0.2 mg/2-second spray
Cream: 0.02%‡, 0.025%, 0.1%, 0.5%
Lotion: 0.025%, 0.1%
Ointment: 0.02%‡, 0.025%, 0.1%, 0.5%
Paste: 0.1%
Solution: 0.1%

ACTION
Unclear. Diffuses across cell membranes to form complexes with specific cytoplasmic receptors. Exhibits anti-inflammatory, antipruritic, vasoconstrictive, and antiproliferative activity. Considered a group III (medium-potency) agent according to vasoconstrictive properties.

Route	Onset	Peak	Duration
Topical	Several hr	Unknown	≥ 1 wk

INDICATIONS & DOSAGE
Inflammation and pruritus associated with corticosteroid-responsive dermatoses—
Adults and children: clean area; apply aerosol, cream, lotion, or ointment sparingly b.i.d. to q.i.d. Rub in lightly.
Inflammation associated with oral lesions—
Adults and children: apply paste h.s. and, if needed, b.i.d. or t.i.d., preferably after meals. Apply a small amount without rubbing and press to lesion in mouth until a thin film develops.

ADVERSE REACTIONS
Skin: burning, pruritus, irritation, dryness, erythema, folliculitis, hypertri-

chosis, hypopigmentation, acneiform eruptions, perioral dermatitis, allergic contact dermatitis; *maceration, secondary infection, atrophy, striae, miliaria* (with occlusive dressings).

Other: *hypothalamic-pituitary-adrenal axis suppression,* Cushing's syndrome, hyperglycemia, glycosuria, syncope.

INTERACTIONS
None significant.

EFFECTS ON DIAGNOSTIC TESTS
None reported.

CONTRAINDICATIONS
Contraindicated in patients hypersensitive to drug or its components.

NURSING CONSIDERATIONS
• Gently wash skin before applying. To avoid skin damage, rub medication in gently, leaving a thin coat. When treating hairy sites, part hair and apply directly to lesions.
• Don't apply near eyes or in ear canal.
• Change dressing as ordered. Stop drug and tell doctor if skin infection, striae, or atrophy occurs.
• When using aerosol about the face, cover the patient's eyes and warn against inhalation of the spray. Aerosol preparation contains alcohol and may produce irritation or burning in open lesions. Do not spray longer than 3 seconds or closer than 6″ (15 cm) to avoid freezing tissues.
• If antifungal agents or antibiotics are used concomitantly, stop corticosteroids until infection is controlled, as ordered.
• Systemic absorption is likely with the use of occlusive dressings, prolonged treatment, or extensive body surface treatment. Watch for symptoms.
• Avoid using plastic pants or tight-fitting diapers on treated areas in young children. Children may absorb larger amounts of drug and be more prone to systemic toxicity.

☑ Patient teaching
• Teach patient or family member how to apply drug.
• If an occlusive dressing is ordered, advise patient not to leave it in place longer than 12 hours each day and not to use occlusive dressings on infected or exudative lesions.
• Tell patient to stop drug and report signs of systemic absorption, skin irritation or ulceration, hypersensitivity, infection, or no improvement.

---

vitamin A
vitamin B complex
  cyanocobalamin
  folic acid
  hydroxocobalamin
  leucovorin calcium
  niacin
  niacinamide
  pyridoxine hydrochloride
  riboflavin
  thiamine hydrochloride
vitamin C
vitamin D
  cholecalciferol
  ergocalciferol
vitamin D analogue
  paricalcitol
vitamin E
vitamin K analogue
  phytonadione
sodium fluoride
sodium fluoride, topical
trace elements
  chromium
  copper
  iodine
  manganese
  selenium
  zinc

VITAMIN COMBINATION PRODUCTS
B complex vitamins ◊
B complex vitamins with iron ◊
B complex with vitamin C ◊
B vitamin combinations ◊
Calcium and vitamin products ◊
Fluoride with vitamins ◊
Geriatric supplements with multivitamins and minerals ◊
Miscellaneous vitamins and minerals ◊
Multivitamins ◊
Multivitamins and minerals with hormones ◊
Multivitamins with B_{12} ◊
Vitamin A and D combinations ◊

TRACE ELEMENT COMBINATION PRODUCTS
MULTIPLE TRACE ELEMENT PEDIATRIC: zinc sulfate 0.5 mg, copper sulfate 0.1 mg, manganese sulfate 0.03 mg, and chromium chloride 1 mcg per ml.
MULTIPLE TRACE ELEMENT NEONATAL: zinc sulfate 0.5 mg, copper sulfate 0.1 mg, manganese sulfate 0.025 mg, chromium chloride 0.85 mcg.
MULTIPLE TRACE ELEMENT WITH SELENIUM: zinc sulfate 1 mg, copper sulfate 0.4 mg, manganese sulfate 0.1 mg, chromium chloride 4 mcg, and selenious acid 20 mcg.
NEOTRACE-4: zinc sulfate 1.5 mg, copper sulfate 0.1 mg, manganese sulfate 0.025 mg, and chromium chloride 0.85 mcg per ml.
PEDTRACE-4: zinc sulfate 0.5 mg, copper sulfate 0.1 mg, manganese sulfate 0.025 mg, and chromium chloride 0.85 mcg per ml.
PTE-4: zinc sulfate 1 mg, copper sulfate 0.1 mg, manganese sulfate 0.025 mg, and chromium chloride 1 mcg per ml.
PTE-5: zinc sulfate 1 mg, copper sulfate 0.1 mg, manganese sulfate 0.025 mg, chromium chloride 1 mcg, and selenium (as selenious acid) 15 mcg per ml.
TRACE METALS ADDITIVE: zinc chloride 0.8 mg, copper chloride 0.2 mg, manganese chloride 0.16 mg, and chromium chloride 2 mcg per ml.

vitamin A (retinol)
Aquasol A, Del-Vi-A

Pregnancy Risk Category: C

HOW SUPPLIED
Tablets: 10,000 IU
Capsules: 10,000 IU ◊, 25,000 IU, 50,000 IU
Drops: 30 ml with dropper (5,000 IU/ 0.1 ml, 50,000 IU/1 ml)
Injection: 2-ml vials (50,000 IU/ml with 0.5% chlorobutanol, polysorbate 80, buty-

lated hydroxyanisole, and butylated hydroxytoluene)

ACTION
Coenzyme that stimulates retinal function, bone growth, reproduction, and integrity of epithelial and mucosal tissues.

Route	Onset	Peak	Duration
PO	Unknown	3-5 hr	Unknown
IM	Unknown	Unknown	Unknown

INDICATIONS & DOSAGE
RE—
   Note: RDAs have been converted to retinol equivalents (RE). One RE has the activity of 1 mcg all-*trans* retinol, 6 mcg beta carotene.
Neonates and infants to 1 year: 375 mcg RE or 1,250 IU.
Children 1 to 3 years: 400 mcg RE or 1,330 IU.
Children 4 to 6 years: 500 mcg RE or 1,665 IU.
Children 7 to 10 years: 700 mcg RE or 2,330 IU.
Males over 11 years: 1,000 mcg RE or 3,330 IU.
Females over 11 years: 800 mcg RE or 2,665 IU.
Pregnant women: 800 mcg RE or 2,665 IU.
Breast-feeding women (first 6 months): 1,300 mcg RE or 4,330 IU.
Breast-feeding women (second 6 months): 1,200 mcg RE or 4,000 IU.
Severe vitamin A deficiency—
Adults and children over 8 years: 100,000 IU I.M. or 100,000 to 500,000 IU P.O. for 3 days, followed by 50,000 IU I.M. or P.O. for 2 weeks; then 10,000 to 20,000 IU P.O. for 2 months. Follow with adequate dietary nutrition and RE vitamin A supplements.
Children 1 to 8 years: 17,500 to 35,000 IU I.M. daily for 10 days.
Infants under 1 year: 7,500 to 15,000 IU I.M. daily for 10 days.
Maintenance dosage to prevent recurrence of vitamin A deficiency—
Children 1 to 8 years: 5,000 to 10,000 IU P.O. daily for 2 months; then adequate dietary nutrition and RE vitamin A supplements.

ADVERSE REACTIONS
Adverse reactions usually occur only with toxicity.
CNS: irritability, headache, *increased intracranial pressure,* fatigue, lethargy, malaise.
EENT: papilledema, exophthalmos.
GI: anorexia, epigastric pain, vomiting, polydipsia.
GU: hypomenorrhea, polyuria.
Hepatic: jaundice, hepatomegaly, *cirrhosis,* elevated liver enzymes.
Metabolic: slow growth, decalcification, hypercalcemia, periostitis, premature closure of epiphyses, migratory arthralgia, cortical thickening over the radius and tibia.
Skin: alopecia; dry, cracked, scaly skin; pruritus; lip fissures; erythema; inflamed tongue, lips, and gums; massive desquamation; increased pigmentation; night sweats.
Other: splenomegaly, *anaphylactic shock.*

INTERACTIONS
Drug-drug. *Cholestyramine resin, mineral oil:* reduced GI absorption of fat-soluble vitamins. Avoid concomitant use.
Isotretinoin, multivitamins containing vitamin A: increased risk of toxicity. Avoid concomitant use.
Neomycin (oral): decreased vitamin A absorption. Avoid concomitant use.
Oral contraceptives: may increase plasma vitamin A levels. Monitor closely.
Warfarin: increased risk of bleeding. Monitor PT and INR closely.

EFFECTS ON DIAGNOSTIC TESTS
Vitamin A therapy may falsely increase serum cholesterol level readings by interfering with the Zlatkis-Zak reaction. Vitamin A also has been reported to falsely elevate bilirubin determinations with Ehrlich's reagent.

CONTRAINDICATIONS
Contraindicated orally in patients with malabsorption syndrome; if malabsorption is from inadequate bile secretion, oral route may be used with concurrent administration of bile salts (dehydrocholic acid). Also contraindicated in hypervita-

minosis A and hypersensitivity to any ingredient in product. I.V. route contraindicated except for special water-miscible forms intended for infusion with large parenteral volumes. I.V. push of vitamin A of any type also contraindicated (anaphylaxis or anaphylactoid reactions and death have resulted).

NURSING CONSIDERATIONS
• Use cautiously in pregnant patients, avoiding doses exceeding RE.
• Assess patient's vitamin A intake from all sources.
• Know that liquid preparations are available for nasogastric route. Preparation may be mixed with cereal or fruit juice.
• Vitamin may be administered I.M. for malabsorption syndrome or when oral administration is not feasible.
• Know that adequate vitamin A absorption requires suitable dietary protein, fat, vitamin E, and zinc intake and bile secretion; give supplemental salts as ordered. Zinc supplements may be needed in patients receiving long-term total parenteral nutrition.
• Monitor for adverse reactions if dosage is high.
• Acute toxicity has resulted from single doses of 25,000 IU/kg of body weight; 350,000 IU in infants and over 2 million IU in adults have also proved acutely toxic. Doses that do not exceed the RE are usually nontoxic.
• Chronic toxicity in infants (3 to 6 months) has resulted from doses of 18,500 IU daily for 1 to 3 months. In adults, chronic toxicity has resulted from doses of 50,000 IU daily for over 18 months, 500,000 IU daily for 2 months, and 1 million IU daily for 3 days.
• Watch for skin disorders; high dosages may induce chronic toxicity.

✓ Patient teaching
• Tell patient not to take megadoses of vitamins without specific indications to avoid toxicity.
• Stress that prescribed vitamins should not be shared with others.
• Instruct patient to protect drug from light.
• Teach patient about good food sources

of vitamin A such as green vegetables, yellow vegetables, cantaloupe, and liver (note that liver is also high in saturated fat).
• Advise patient that liquid preparation can be mixed with food if desired.

cyanocobalamin (vitamin B₁₂)
Crystamine, Crysti-12, Cyanocobalamin, Cyanoject, Cyomin, Rubesol-1000, Rubramin PC

hydroxocobalamin (vitamin B₁₂)
Hydrobexan, Hydro-Cobex, Hydro-Crysti 12, LA-12

Pregnancy Risk Category: C (if used in doses above the RDA)

HOW SUPPLIED
cyanocobalamin
Tablets: 25 mcg ◊, 50 mcg ◊, 100 mcg ◊, 250 mcg ◊, 500 mcg ◊, 1,000 mcg ◊
Injection: 1,000 mcg/ml
hydroxocobalamin
Injection: 100 mcg, 1,000 mcg/ml

ACTION
Coenzyme that stimulates metabolic functions. Necessary for cell replication, hematopoiesis, and nucleoprotein and myelin synthesis.

Route	Onset	Peak	Duration
PO	Unknown	8-12 hr	Unknown
IM, SC	Unknown	1 hr	Unknown

INDICATIONS & DOSAGE
RDA for cyanocobalamin—
Neonates and infants to 6 months: 0.3 mcg.
Infants 6 months to 1 year: 0.5 mcg.
Children 1 to 3 years: 0.7 mcg.
Children 4 to 6 years: 1 mcg.
Children 7 to 10 years: 1.4 mcg.
Adults and children 11 years and over: 2 mcg.
Pregnant women: 2.2 mcg.
Breast-feeding women: 2.6 mcg.
Vitamin B₁₂ deficiency caused by inade-

quate diet, subtotal gastrectomy, or any other condition, disorder, or disease except malabsorption related to pernicious anemia or other GI disease—
Adults: 30 mcg hydroxocobalamin I.M. daily for 5 to 10 days, depending on severity of deficiency. Maintenance dosage is 100 to 200 mcg I.M. once monthly. For subsequent prophylaxis, advise adequate nutrition and daily RDA vitamin B_{12} supplements.
Children: 1 to 5 mg hydroxocobalamin spread over 2 or more weeks in doses of 100 mcg I.M., depending on severity of deficiency. Maintenance dosage is 30 to 50 mcg/month I.M. For subsequent prophylaxis, advise adequate nutrition and daily RDA vitamin B_{12} supplements.
Pernicious anemia or vitamin B_{12} malabsorption—
Adults: initially, 100 mcg cyanocobalamin I.M. or S.C. daily for 6 to 7 days, then 100 mcg I.M. or S.C. once monthly.
Children: 30 to 50 mcg I.M. or S.C. daily over 2 or more weeks; then 100 mcg I.M. or S.C. monthly for life.
Methylmalonicaciduria—
Neonates: 1,000 mcg cyanocobalamin I.M. daily.
Schilling test flushing dose—
Adults and children: 1,000 mcg hydroxocobalamin I.M. in a single dose.

ADVERSE REACTIONS
CV: peripheral vascular thrombosis, pulmonary edema, heart failure.
GI: transient diarrhea.
Skin: itching, transitory exanthema, urticaria.
Other: *anaphylaxis, anaphylactoid reactions* (with parenteral administration); pain, burning (at S.C. or I.M. injection sites).

INTERACTIONS
Drug-drug. *Aminoglycosides, anticonvulsants, colchicine, extended-release potassium preparations, para-aminosalicylic acid and salts:* malabsorption of vitamin B_{12}. Don't use concomitantly.
Drug-lifestyle. *Alcohol use:* malabsorption of vitamin B_{12}. Don't use concomitantly.

EFFECTS ON DIAGNOSTIC TESTS
Vitamin B_{12} therapy may cause false-positive results for intrinsic factor antibodies, which are present in the blood of half of all patients with pernicious anemia. Methotrexate, pyrimethamine, and most anti-infectives invalidate diagnostic blood assays for vitamin B_{12}.

CONTRAINDICATIONS
Contraindicated in patients hypersensitive to vitamin B_{12} or cobalt and in patients with early Leber's disease.

NURSING CONSIDERATIONS
• Use cautiously in anemic patients with coexisting cardiac, pulmonary, or hypertensive disease; and in patients with severe vitamin B_{12}–dependent deficiencies.
• Use cautiously in premature infants. May contain benzyl alcohol, which may cause a "gasping syndrome."
• Determine reticulocyte count, hematocrit, B_{12}, iron, and folate levels before beginning therapy, as ordered.
• Don't mix parenteral liquids in same syringe with other medications.
• Know that drug is physically incompatible with dextrose solutions, alkaline or strongly acidic solutions, oxidizing or reducing agents, heavy metals, chlorpromazine, phytonadione, prochlorperazine, and other drugs.
• Be aware that hydroxocobalamin is approved for I.M. or deep S.C. use only. Its only advantage over cyanocobalamin is its longer duration.
• Don't give large oral doses of B_{12} routinely; drug is lost through excretion.
• Closely monitor serum potassium levels for first 48 hours. Give potassium supplement, if ordered.
• Be aware that drug may cause false-positive intrinsic factor antibody test.
• Know that infection, tumors, or renal, hepatic, and other debilitating diseases may reduce therapeutic response.
• Keep in mind that deficiencies are more common in strict vegetarians and their breast-fed infants.
• Be aware that B_{12} deficiency may suppress symptoms of polycythemia vera.
• Protect vitamin B_{12} from light. Do not refrigerate or freeze.

✔ **Patient teaching**
- Stress need for patient with pernicious anemia to return for monthly injections. Although total body stores may last 3 to 6 years, anemia will recur if not treated monthly.
- Stress importance of follow-up visits and laboratory studies.
- Teach patient healthy dietary habits.

---

folic acid (vitamin B₉)
Folvite, Novo-Folacid†

Pregnancy Risk Category: A

HOW SUPPLIED
Tablets: 0.4 mg, 0.8 mg, 1 mg
Injection: 10-ml vials (5 mg/ml with 1.5% benzyl alcohol, 5 mg/ml with 1.5% benzyl alcohol and 0.2% EDTA)

ACTION
Stimulates normal erythropoiesis and nucleoprotein synthesis.

Route	Onset	Peak	Duration
PO, IM, SC	Unknown	30-60 min	Unknown

INDICATIONS & DOSAGE
RDA—
Neonates and infants to 6 months: 25 mcg.
Infants 6 months to 1 year: 35 mcg.
Children 1 to 3 years: 50 mcg.
Children 4 to 6 years: 75 mcg.
Children 7 to 10 years: 100 mcg.
Children 11 to 14 years: 150 mcg.
Males 15 years and over: 200 mcg.
Females 15 years and over: 180 mcg.
Pregnant women: 400 mcg.
Breast-feeding women (first 6 months): 280 mcg.
Breast-feeding women (second 6 months): 260 mcg.
Megaloblastic or macrocytic anemia secondary to folic acid or other nutritional deficiency, hepatic disease, alcoholism, intestinal obstruction, excessive hemolysis—
Adults and children over 4 years: 0.4 mg to 1 mg P.O., S.C., or I.M. daily. After anemia secondary to folic acid deficiency is corrected, proper diet and RDA supplements are necessary to prevent recurrence.

Children under 4 years: up to 0.3 mg P.O., S.C., or I.M. daily.
Pregnant and breast-feeding women: 0.8 mg P.O., S.C., or I.M. daily.
Prevention of megaloblastic anemia during pregnancy to prevent fetal damage—
Adults: up to 1 mg P.O., S.C., or I.M. daily throughout pregnancy.
Nutritional supplement—
Adults: 0.1 mg P.O., S.C., or I.M. daily.
Children: 0.05 mg P.O. daily.
To test for folic acid deficiency in patients with megaloblastic anemia without masking pernicious anemia—
Adults and children: 0.1 to 0.2 mg P.O. or I.M. for 10 days while maintaining a diet low in folate and vitamin B₁₂.
Tropical sprue—
Adults: 3 to 15 mg P.O. daily.

ADVERSE REACTIONS
CNS: altered sleep pattern, concentration difficulty, confusion, impaired judgment, irritability, overactivity.
GI: anorexia, nausea, flatulence, bitter taste.
Respiratory: *bronchospasm.*
Skin: allergic reactions (rash, pruritus, erythema).
Other: general malaise.

INTERACTIONS
Drug-drug. *Aminosalicylic acid, chloramphenicol, methotrexate, oral contraceptives, sulfasalazine, trimethoprim:* antagonism of folic acid. Monitor for decreased folic acid effect. Use together cautiously.
Phenytoin: increased anticonvulsant metabolism causing decreased blood levels of the anticonvulsants. Monitor closely.

EFFECTS ON DIAGNOSTIC TESTS
Drug therapy alters serum and RBC folate concentrations; falsely low serum and RBC folate levels may occur with the *Lactobacillus casei* assay in patients receiving anti-infectives, such as tetracycline, which suppress the growth of this organism.

CONTRAINDICATIONS
Contraindicated in patients with undiagnosed anemia because it may mask pernicious anemia. Also contraindicated in those with B₁₂ deficiency.

Reactions may be *common,* uncommon, ***life-threatening,*** or **COMMON AND LIFE-THREATENING.**

NURSING CONSIDERATIONS
• The U.S. Public Health Service recommends use of folic acid during pregnancy to decrease neural tube defects.
• Don't mix with other medications in same syringe for I.M. injections.
• Know that patients with small-bowel resections and intestinal malabsorption may require parenteral administration.
• Protect from light and heat; store at room temperature.

☑**Patient teaching**
• Teach patient about proper nutrition to prevent recurrence of anemia.
• Stress importance of follow-up visits and laboratory studies.
• Teach patient about foods that contain folic acid: liver, oranges, whole wheat, broccoli, brussels sprouts.

---

leucovorin calcium (citrovorum factor, folinic acid)
Wellcovorin

Pregnancy Risk Category: C

HOW SUPPLIED
Tablets: 5 mg, 10 mg, 15 mg, 25 mg
Injection: 1-ml ampule (3 mg/ml with 0.9% benzyl alcohol)
Powder for injection: 50-mg vial, 100-mg vial, 350-mg vial

ACTION
A reduced form of folic acid that is readily converted to other folic acid derivatives.

Route	Onset	Peak	Duration
PO	20-30 min	2-3 hr	3-6 hr
IV	5 min	10 min	3-6 hr
IM	10-20 min	< 1 hr	3-6 hr

INDICATIONS & DOSAGE
Overdose of folic acid antagonist (methotrexate or trimethoprim)—
Adults and children: P.O., I.M., or I.V. dose equivalent to weight of antagonist given.
Leucovorin rescue after high methotrexate dose in treatment of malignant disease—
Adults and children: 10 mg/m² P.O.,

I.M., or I.V. q 6 hours until methotrexate levels fall below 5 × 10⁻⁸ M.
Megaloblastic anemia caused by congenital enzyme deficiency—
Adults and children: 3 to 6 mg I.M., then 1 mg P.O. or I.M. daily for life.
Folate-deficient megaloblastic anemia—
Adults and children: up to 1 mg of leucovorin I.M daily. Duration of treatment depends on hematologic response.
Prevention of hematologic toxicity caused by pyrimethamine or trimethoprim therapy—
Adults and children: 400 mcg to 5 mg I.M. with each dose of the folic acid antagonist.
Treatment of hematologic toxicity caused by pyrimethamine or trimethoprim therapy—
Adults and children: 5 to 15 mg I.M. daily.
Palliative treatment of advanced colorectal cancer—
Adults: 20 mg/m² I.V., followed by fluorouracil 425 mg/m² I.V. or 200 mg/m² I.V. (over a period of 3 minutes or longer) followed by fluorouracil 370 mg/m² daily for 5 consecutive days. Repeated at 4-week intervals for two additional courses; then at intervals of 4 to 5 weeks if tolerated.

ADVERSE REACTIONS
Skin: *hypersensitivity reactions* (urticaria and anaphylactoid reactions).

INTERACTIONS
Drug-drug. *Anticonvulsants:* may decrease effectiveness of these agents. Monitor patient.
Fluorouracil: may enhance fluorouracil toxicity. Dose of fluorouracil may need to be reduced.
Methotrexate: high doses of leucovorin may decrease efficacy of intrathecal methotrexate. Monitor effects.

EFFECTS ON DIAGNOSTIC TESTS
Leucovorin may mask the diagnosis of pernicious anemia.

CONTRAINDICATIONS
Contraindicated in patients with pernicious anemia and other megaloblastic anemias secondary to lack of vitamin B₁₂.

NURSING CONSIDERATIONS
• Know that I.V. route is preferred in patients with GI toxicity when doses are greater than 25 mg.
• Do not confuse leucovorin (folinic acid) with folic acid.
• Follow leucovorin rescue schedule and protocol closely.
• Do not administer leucovorin simultaneously with systemic methotrexate.
• Protect from light and heat; maintain protection and immediately administer reconstituted parenteral drug.

I.V. administration
• When using powder for injection, reconstitute 50-mg vial with 5 ml, 100-mg vial with 10 ml, or 350-mg vial with 17 ml of sterile or bacteriostatic water for injection. When doses are more than 10 mg/m^2 don't use diluents containing benzyl alcohol.
Alert: Don't exceed 160 mg/minute when giving by direct injection.

Patient teaching
• Explain need for drug use to patient and family, and answer any questions or concerns.
• Tell patient to report symptoms of hypersensitivity promptly.

---

niacin
(nicotinic acid, vitamin B$_3$)
Nia-Bid ◊ , Niac, Niacels ◊ ,
Niacor ◊ , Niaspan, Nico-400,
Nicobid ◊ , Nicolar**, Nicotinex,
Slo-Niacin ◊

niacinamide (nicotinamide) ◊

Pregnancy Risk Category: C

HOW SUPPLIED
niacin
Tablets: 25 mg ◊ , 50 mg ◊ , 100 mg ◊ ,
250 mg ◊ , 500 mg
Tablets (timed-release): 250 mg ◊ ,
375 mg ◊ , 500 mg ◊ , 750 mg ◊ ,
1,000 mg ◊
Capsules (timed-release): 125 mg ◊ ,
250 mg ◊ , 300 mg ◊ , 400 mg ◊ , 500 mg
Elixir: 50 mg/5 ml ◊

Injection: 100 mg/ml in 30-ml vials
niacinamide
Tablets: 50 mg ◊ , 100 mg ◊ , 125 mg ◊ ,
250 mg ◊ , 500 mg ◊

ACTION
Niacin and niacinamide stimulate lipid metabolism, tissue respiration, and glycogenolysis; niacin decreases synthesis of low-density lipoproteins and inhibits lipolysis in adipose tissue.

Route	Onset	Peak	Duration
PO	Unknown	45 min	Unknown
IV, IM, SC	Unknown	Unknown	Unknown

INDICATIONS & DOSAGE
RDA—
Neonates and infants to 6 months: 5 mg.
Infants 6 months to 1 year: 6 mg.
Children 1 to 3 years: 9 mg.
Children 4 to 6 years: 12 mg.
Children 7 to 10 years: 13 mg.
Males 11 to 14 years: 17 mg.
Males 15 to 18 years: 20 mg.
Males 19 to 50 years: 19 mg.
Males 51 years and over: 15 mg.
Females 11 to 50 years: 15 mg.
Females 51 years and over: 13 mg.
Pregnant women: 17 mg.
Breast-feeding women: 20 mg.
Pellagra—
Adults: 300 to 500 mg P.O., S.C., I.M., or I.V. daily in divided doses, depending on severity of deficiency.
Children: up to 300 mg P.O. or 100 mg I.V. daily, depending on severity of niacin deficiency.
    After symptoms subside, advise adequate nutrition and RDA supplements to prevent recurrence.
Hartnup disease—
Adults: 50 to 200 mg P.O. daily.
Niacin deficiency—
Adults: up to 100 mg P.O. daily.
Hyperlipidemias, especially with hypercholesterolemia—
Adults: 1 to 2 g P.O. t.i.d. with or after meals, increased at intervals to 6 g daily.

ADVERSE REACTIONS
Most reactions are dose-dependent.
CV: *excessive peripheral vasodilation*

(especially niacin), hypotension, atrial fibrillation, ***arrhythmias.***
GI: *nausea, vomiting, diarrhea,* possible activation of peptic ulceration, epigastric or substernal pain.
Hepatic: elevated liver enzymes, ***hepatic dysfunction.***
Skin: *flushing,* pruritus, dryness, tingling.
Other: hyperglycemia, hyperuricemia, toxic amblyopia.

INTERACTIONS
Drug-drug. *Antihypertensive drugs (ganglionic or sympathetic blockers):* potential additive vasodilating effect, causing orthostatic hypotension. Use together cautiously; also warn patient about orthostatic hypotension.
Lovastatin (statin class): concurrent use may lead to rhabdomyolysis. Avoid concurrent use.
Sulfinpyrazone: uricosuric effects may be decreased by niacin. Avoid concurrent use.

EFFECTS ON DIAGNOSTIC TESTS
Niacin therapy alters fluorometric test results for urine catecholamines and results for urine glucose tests that use cupric sulfate (Benedict's reagent).

CONTRAINDICATIONS
Contraindicated in patients with hepatic dysfunction, active peptic ulcers, severe hypotension, arterial hemorrhage, or hypersensitivity to drug.

NURSING CONSIDERATIONS
• Use cautiously in patients with gallbladder disease, diabetes mellitus, or unstable angina and in patients with a history of liver disease, peptic ulcer, allergy, gout or large alcohol intake.
• Drug may cause dose-related rise in glucose intolerance; blood glucose should be monitored carefully in diabetic patients.
• To minimize adverse GI effects, give niacin with meals.
• Administer aspirin (325 mg P.O. 30 minutes before niacin dose), as ordered, to possibly reduce the flushing response to niacin.
• Timed-release niacin or niacinamide may prevent excessive flushing that occurs with large doses. However, timed-release niacin is linked with hepatic dysfunction, even at very low doses.
• Monitor hepatic function and blood glucose early in therapy, as ordered.

I.V. administration
• Give slow I.V. (no faster than 2 mg/minute). Explain harmlessness of flushing syndrome.

✓ Patient teaching
• Stress that niacin is a potent medication, not just a vitamin, and may cause serious adverse effects. Explain importance of adhering to therapy.
• Tell patient flushing and warmth may subside with continued use and that concurrent use of alcohol may increase flushing.
• Tell patient to take with food to minimize stomach upset.
• Advise patient against self-medicating for hyperlipidemia.

---

pyridoxine hydrochloride (vitamin B₆)
Beesix, Nestrex ◇, Orovite Comploment B₆§ , Rodex

Pregnancy Risk Category: A

HOW SUPPLIED
Tablets: 10 mg ◇ , 25 mg ◇ , 50 mg ◇ , 100 mg ◇ , 200 mg ◇ , 250 mg ◇ , 500 mg ◇
Capsules (timed-release): 100 mg
Capsules: 500 mg
Tablets (timed-release): 100 mg
Injection: 100 mg/ml

ACTION
Acts as a coenzyme that stimulates various metabolic functions, including amino acid metabolism.

Route	Onset	Peak	Duration
PO, IV, IM	Unknown	Unknown	Unknown

INDICATIONS & DOSAGE
RDA—
Neonates and infants to 6 months: 0.3 mg.
Infants 6 months to 1 year: 0.6 mg.

Children 1 to 3 years: 1 mg.
Children 4 to 6 years: 1.1 mg.
Children 7 to 10 years: 1.4 mg.
Males 11 to 14 years: 1.7 mg.
Males 15 years and over: 2 mg.
Females 11 to 14 years: 1.4 mg.
Females 15 to 18 years: 1.5 mg.
Females 19 years and over: 1.6 mg.
Pregnant women: 2.2 mg.
Breast-feeding women: 2.1 mg.
Dietary vitamin B₆ deficiency—
Adults: 10 to 20 mg P.O., I.M., or I.V. daily for 3 weeks, then 2 to 5 mg daily as a supplement to a proper diet.
Seizures related to vitamin B₆ deficiency or dependency—
Adults and children: 100 mg I.M. or I.V. in single dose.
Vitamin B₆–responsive anemias or dependency syndrome (inborn errors of metabolism)—
Adults: up to 600 mg P.O., I.M., or I.V. daily until symptoms subside, then 30 mg daily for life.
Prevention of vitamin B₆ deficiency during drug therapy—
Adults: 10 to 50 mg P.O. daily.
Antidote for isoniazid poisoning—
Adults: 4 g I.V., followed by 1 g I.M. q 30 minutes until the amount of pyridoxine administered equals the amount of isoniazid ingested.

ADVERSE REACTIONS
CNS: paresthesia, unsteady gait, numbness, somnolence, *seizures,* headache.

INTERACTIONS
Drug-drug. *Levodopa:* decreased levodopa effect. Avoid concomitant use.
Phenobarbital, phenytoin: decreased anticonvulsant serum levels, increasing risk of seizures. Avoid concomitant use.
Drug-lifestyle. *Alcohol use:* no conclusive evidence, but incidence of delirium and lactic acidosis was reported after drinking alcohol. Avoid concomitant use.

EFFECTS ON DIAGNOSTIC TESTS
Pyridoxine therapy alters determinations of urobilinogen in the spot test using Ehrlich's reagent, resulting in a false-positive reaction.

CONTRAINDICATIONS
Contraindicated in patients hypersensitive to pyridoxine.

NURSING CONSIDERATIONS
• Not for I.V. use in patients with heart disease.
• Protect from light. Do not use solution if it contains a precipitate, although slight darkening is acceptable.
• When used to treat isoniazid toxicity, expect to also give anticonvulsants.
• If sodium bicarbonate is needed to control acidosis in isoniazid toxicity, don't mix in same syringe with pyridoxine.
• Know that patients taking high doses (2 to 6 g/day) may experience difficulty walking because of diminished proprioceptive and sensory function.
• Carefully monitor the patient's diet. Excessive protein intake increases daily pyridoxine requirements.

▲ I.V. administration
• Inject undiluted drug into I.V. line of a free-flowing compatible solution. Or, infuse diluted drug over prescribed duration for intermittent infusion. Don't use for continuous infusion.

☑ Patient teaching
• Stress importance of compliance and of good nutrition if prescribed for maintenance therapy to prevent recurrence of deficiency. Explain that pyridoxine, in combination therapy with isoniazid, has a specific therapeutic purpose and is not just a vitamin.
• Advise patient taking levodopa alone to avoid multivitamins containing pyridoxine because of decreased levodopa effect.
• Inform patient of injection site burning with drug administration.

---

riboflavin (vitamin B₂)◇

Pregnancy Risk Category: A

HOW SUPPLIED
Tablets: 25 mg ◇, 50 mg ◇, 100 mg ◇
Tablets (sugar-free): 50 mg ◇, 100 mg ◇

Reactions may be *common,* uncommon, *life-threatening,* or COMMON AND LIFE-THREATENING.

ACTION
Converts to two other coenzymes necessary for normal tissue respiration. Necessary for activation of pyridoxine.

Route	Onset	Peak	Duration
PO	Unknown	Unknown	Unknown

INDICATIONS & DOSAGE
RDA—

Neonates and infants to 6 months: 0.4 mg.
Infants 6 months to 1 year: 0.5 mg.
Children 1 to 3 years: 0.8 mg.
Children 4 to 6 years: 1.1 mg.
Children 7 to 10 years: 1.2 mg.
Males 11 to 14 years: 1.5 mg.
Males 15 to 18 years: 1.8 mg.
Males 19 to 50 years: 1.7 mg.
Males 51 years and over: 1.4 mg.
Females 11 to 50 years: 1.3 mg.
Females 51 years and over: 1.2 mg.
Pregnant women: 1.6 mg.
Breast-feeding women (first 6 months): 1.8 mg.
Breast-feeding women (second 6 months): 1.7 mg.
Riboflavin deficiency or adjunct to thiamine treatment for polyneuritis or cheilosis secondary to pellagra—
Adults and children over 12 years: 5 to 25 mg P.O. daily, depending on severity.
Children under 12 years: 3 to 10 mg P.O. daily, depending on severity.
 For maintenance, increase nutritional intake and supplement with vitamin B complex.

ADVERSE REACTIONS
GU: bright yellow urine.

INTERACTIONS
Drug-drug. *Probenecid:* reduced urinary excretion of riboflavin. Avoid concomitant use.
Propantheline, other anticholinergics: decreased rate and extent of absorption. Avoid concomitant use.

EFFECTS ON DIAGNOSTIC TESTS
Drug therapy alters urinalysis based on spectrophotometry or color reactions. Large doses of drug result in bright yellow urine. Riboflavin produces fluorescent substances in urine and plasma, which can falsely elevate fluorometric determinations of catecholamines and urobilinogen.

CONTRAINDICATIONS
No known contraindications.

NURSING CONSIDERATIONS
• Drug may be given I.M. or I.V. as a component of multiple vitamins.
• Know that riboflavin deficiency usually accompanies other vitamin B complex deficiencies and may require multivitamin therapy.
• Protect from air and light.

✔ Patient teaching
• Tell patient to take riboflavin with meals; food increases its absorption.
• Stress proper nutritional habits to prevent recurrence of deficiency.
• Inform patient that riboflavin usually causes bright yellow or orange discoloration of urine.

---

thiamine hydrochloride (vitamin B₁)
Betamin‡, Beta-Sol‡, Biamine

Pregnancy Risk Category: A

HOW SUPPLIED
Tablets: 25 mg ◇, 50 mg ◇, 100 mg ◇, 250 mg ◇, 500 mg
Tablet (enteric-coated): 20 mg
Elixir†: 250 mcg/5 ml
Injection: 100 mg/ml

ACTION
Combines with adenosine triphosphate to form a coenzyme necessary for carbohydrate metabolism.

Route	Onset	Peak	Duration
PO, IV, IM	Unknown	Unknown	Unknown

INDICATIONS & DOSAGE
RDA—

Neonates and infants to 6 months: 0.3 mg.
Infants 6 months to 1 year: 0.4 mg.
Children 1 to 3 years: 0.7 mg.

Children 4 to 6 years: 0.9 mg.
Children 7 to 10 years: 1 mg.
Males 11 to 14 years: 1.3 mg.
Males 15 to 50 years: 1.5 mg.
Males 51 years and older: 1.2 mg.
Females 11 to 50 years: 1.1 mg.
Females 51 years and older: 1 mg.
Pregnant women: 1.5 mg.
Breast-feeding women: 1.6 mg.
Beriberi—
Adults: depending on severity, 10 to
20 mg I.M. t.i.d. for 2 weeks, followed by
dietary correction and multivitamin sup-
plement containing 5 to 10 mg thiamine
daily for 1 month.
Children: depending on severity, 10 to
50 mg I.M. daily for several weeks with
adequate diet.
Wet beriberi with myocardial failure—
Adults and children: 10 to 30 mg I.V.
t.i.d.
Wernicke's encephalopathy—
Adults: initially, 100 mg I.V., followed by
50 to 100 mg I.V. or I.M. daily until patient is consuming a regular balanced diet.

ADVERSE REACTIONS
CNS: restlessness.
CV: *angioedema,* cyanosis, *CV collapse.*
EENT: tightness of throat (allergic reac-
tion).
GI: nausea, *hemorrhage.*
Respiratory: pulmonary edema.
Skin: feeling of warmth, pruritus, urti-
caria, diaphoresis.
Other: weakness; tenderness, induration
(after I.M. administration).

INTERACTIONS
None significant.

EFFECTS ON DIAGNOSTIC TESTS
Thiamine therapy may produce false-
positive results in the phosphotungstate
method for determination of uric acid and
in the urine spot tests with Ehrlich's
reagent for urobilinogen. Large doses of
drug interfere with the Schack and Waxler
spectrophotometric determination of
serum theophylline concentrations.

CONTRAINDICATIONS
Contraindicated in patients hypersensitive
to thiamine products.

NURSING CONSIDERATIONS
• Know that parenteral administration
should be used only when P.O. route is not
feasible.
• Know that thiamine malabsorption is
most likely in alcoholism, cirrhosis, or GI
disease.
• Clinically significant deficiency can occur in approximately 3 weeks of totally
thiamine-free diet.
• Thiamine deficiency usually requires
concurrent treatment for multiple deficiencies.
• Keep in mind that doses larger than
30 mg t.i.d. may not be fully utilized. After tissue saturation with thiamine, it is
excreted in urine as pyrimidine.
• In Wernicke's encephalopathy, administer thiamine before dextrose.

◐ I.V. administration
• Dilute before use.
Alert: Administer large I.V. doses cautiously; give the patient a skin test before
therapy if he has a history of hypersensitivity reactions. Have epinephrine on hand
to treat anaphylaxis.
• Do not use with materials that yield alkaline solutions. Thiamine is unstable in
alkaline solutions.

☑ Patient teaching
• Inform breast-feeding patient that if
beriberi occurs in infant, both she and her
child should be treated with thiamine.
• Stress proper nutritional habits to prevent recurrence of deficiency.
• Instruct patient to protect oral doses
from light.

vitamin C (ascorbic acid)
Ascorbicap ◇, Cebid Timecelles ◇,
Cecon ◇, Cenolate ◇, Cetane ◇,
Cevalin ◇, Cevi-Bid, Ce-Vi-Sol*,
C-Span ◇, Dull-C ◇, Flavorcee ◇,
N'ice w/Vitamin C Drops ◇,
Redoxon†, Vita-C ◇

Pregnancy Risk Category: C

HOW SUPPLIED
Tablets: 25 mg ◇, 50 mg ◇, 100 mg ◇,
250 mg ◇, 500 mg ◇, 1,000 mg ◇

Tablets (chewable): 100 mg◊, 250 mg◊, 500 mg◊, 1,000 mg◊
Tablets (timed-release): 500 mg◊, 1,000 mg◊, 1,500 mg
Capsules (timed-release): 500 mg◊
Crystals: 100 g (4 g/tsp)◊, 500 g (4 g/tsp)◊
Lozenges: 60 mg◊
Oral liquid: 50 ml (35 mg/0.6 ml)*◊
Oral solution: 100 mg/ml◊
Powder: 100 g (4 g/tsp)◊, 500 g (4 g/tsp)◊
Syrup: 500 mg/5 ml◊
Injection: 100 mg/ml; 250 mg/ml; 500 mg/ml

ACTION

Stimulates collagen formation and tissue repair; involved in oxidation-reduction reactions.

Route	Onset	Peak	Duration
PO, IV, IM, SC	Unknown	Unknown	Unknown

INDICATIONS & DOSAGE

RDA—
Neonates and infants to 6 months: 30 mg.
Infants 6 months to 1 year: 35 mg.
Children 1 to 3 years: 40 mg.
Children 4 to 10 years: 45 mg.
Children 11 to 14 years: 50 mg.
Adults and children 15 years and older: 60 mg.
Pregnant women: 70 mg.
Breast-feeding women (first 6 months): 95 mg.
Breast-feeding women (second 6 months): 90 mg.
Frank and subclinical scurvy—
Adults: depending on severity, 300 mg to 1 g P.O., S.C., I.M., or I.V. daily; then 70 to 150 mg daily for maintenance.
Children: depending on severity, 100 to 300 mg P.O., S.C., I.M., or I.V. daily; then at least 30 mg daily for maintenance.
Premature infants: 75 to 100 mg P.O., I.M., I.V., or S.C. daily.
Extensive burns, delayed fracture or wound healing, postoperative wound healing, severe febrile or chronic disease states—
Adults: 300 to 500 mg S.C., I.M., or I.V.

daily for 7 to 10 days. 1 to 2 g daily for extensive burns.
Children: 100 to 200 mg P.O., S.C., I.M., or I.V. daily.
Prevention of vitamin C deficiency in patients with poor nutritional habits or increased requirements—
Adults: 70 to 150 mg P.O., S.C., I.M., or I.V. daily.
Pregnant and breast-feeding women: at least 70 to 150 mg P.O., S.C., I.M., or I.V. daily.
Children: at least 40 mg P.O., S.C., I.M., or I.V. daily.
Infants: at least 35 mg P.O., S.C., I.M., or I.V. daily.
Potentiation of methenamine in urine acidification—
Adults: 4 to 12 g P.O. daily in divided doses.

ADVERSE REACTIONS

CNS: faintness, dizziness (with too-rapid I.V. administration).
GI: diarrhea, heartburn, nausea, vomiting.
GU: acid urine, oxaluria, renal calculi.
Other: discomfort (at injection site).

INTERACTIONS

Drug-drug. *Aspirin (high doses):* increased risk of salicylate toxicity. Monitor patient closely.
Contraceptives, estrogen: increased serum levels of estrogen. Monitor for adverse reactions.
Oral iron supplements: increased iron absorption. Give together.
Warfarin: decreased anticoagulant effect. Monitor closely.
Drug-herb. *Bearberry:* inactivation of bearberry in urine. Monitor for effect.

EFFECTS ON DIAGNOSTIC TESTS

Ascorbic acid is a strong reducing agent; it alters results of tests that are based on oxidation-reduction reactions. Large doses (over 500 mg) may cause false-negative glucose determinations using the glucose oxidase method or false-positive results using the copper reduction method or Benedict's reagent.

Ascorbic acid should not be used for 48 to 72 hours before an amine-dependent test for occult blood in the stool is conducted; a false-negative test may occur. Depending on the reagents used, it may also interact with other diagnostic tests.

CONTRAINDICATIONS
Contraindicated in patients with an allergy to tartrazine or sulfites; contained in some products. Also, large doses are contraindicated during pregnancy.

NURSING CONSIDERATIONS
• When giving for urine acidification, check urine pH to ensure efficacy.
• Protect solution from light, and refrigerate ampules.

I.V. administration
• Infuse cautiously in patients with renal insufficiency.
Alert: Rapid infusion may cause faintness or dizziness.

✔ Patient teaching
• For patient receiving vitamin C I.M., explain that I.M. route may promote better utilization.
• Stress proper nutritional habits to prevent recurrence of deficiency.
• Inform patient that vitamin C is readily absorbed from citrus fruits, tomatoes, potatoes, and leafy vegetables.

---

vitamin D

cholecalciferol (vitamin D₃)
Delta-D ◇ , Vitamin D₃ ◇

ergocalciferol (vitamin D₂)
Calciferol, Deltalin, Drisdol, Radiostol†, Vitamin D

Pregnancy Risk Category: C

HOW SUPPLIED
Tablets: 1.25 mg (50,000 IU)
Capsules: 1.25 mg (50,000 IU)
Oral liquid: 8,000 IU/ml in 60-ml dropper bottle ◇
Injection: 12.5 mg (500,000 IU)/ml

ACTION
Promotes absorption and utilization of calcium and phosphate, helping to regulate calcium homeostasis.

Route	Onset	Peak	Duration
PO, IM	2-14 hr	4-12 hr	2 days-6 mo

INDICATIONS & DOSAGE
RDA for cholecalciferol—
Neonates and infants to 6 months: 300 IU.
Infants 6 months to adults 24 years: 400 IU.
Adults 25 years and over: 200 IU.
Pregnant or breast-feeding women: 400 IU.
Rickets and other vitamin D deficiency diseases; renal osteodystrophy—
Adults: initially, 12,000 IU P.O. or I.M. daily, usually increased based on response up to 500,000 IU daily.
Children: 1,500 to 5,000 IU P.O. or I.M. daily for 2 to 4 weeks, repeated after 2 weeks, if necessary. Alternatively, give single dose of 600,000 IU.

After correction of deficiency, maintenance includes adequate diet and RDA supplements.
Hypoparathyroidism—
Adults and children: 50,000 to 200,000 IU P.O. or I.M. daily, with calcium supplement.
Familial hypophosphatemia—
Adults: 1 to 2 mg P.O. daily with phosphorus supplement, increased in 250- to 500-mcg increments at 3- to 4-month intervals.

ADVERSE REACTIONS
Adverse reactions listed usually occur only in vitamin D toxicity.
CNS: headache, weakness, somnolence, decreased libido, overt psychosis, irritability.
CV: *calcification of soft tissues, including the heart,* hypertension, *arrhythmias.*
EENT: rhinorrhea, conjunctivitis (calcific), photophobia.
GI: anorexia, nausea, vomiting, constipation, dry mouth, metallic taste, polydipsia.
GU: polyuria, albuminuria, hypercalciuria, nocturia, *impaired renal function,* reversible azotemia.
Skin: pruritus.
Other: bone and muscle pain, bone de-

Reactions may be *common*, uncommon, *life-threatening*, or COMMON AND LIFE-THREATENING.

mineralization, weight loss, ***hypercal-cemia,*** hyperthermia.

INTERACTIONS
Drug-drug. *Cardiac glycosides:* increased risk of arrhythmias. Monitor serum calcium levels.

Cholestyramine, colestipol, mineral oil: inhibited GI absorption of oral vitamin D. Space doses. Use together cautiously.

Corticosteroids: antagonized effect of vitamin D. Monitor vitamin D levels closely.

Magnesium-containing antacids: possible hypermagnesemia, especially in patients with chronic renal failure. Monitor serum magnesium levels.

Phenobarbital, phenytoin: increased vitamin D metabolism and decreased effectiveness. Monitor closely.

Thiazide diuretics: may cause hypercalcemia in patients with hypoparathyroidism. Monitor closely.

Verapamil: atrial fibrillation has occurred due to increased calcium. Monitor closely.

EFFECTS ON DIAGNOSTIC TESTS
Ergocalciferol may falsely increase serum cholesterol levels and may elevate AST and ALT levels.

CONTRAINDICATIONS
Contraindicated in patients with hypercalcemia, hypervitaminosis D, malabsorption syndrome, decreased renal function or renal osteodystrophy with hyperphosphatemia.

NURSING CONSIDERATIONS
• Know that ergocalciferol should be given with extreme caution, if at all, to patients with heart disease, renal stones, or arteriosclerosis.

• Use cautiously in cardiac patients, especially those taking cardiac glycosides, as well as in patients with increased sensitivity to these drugs.

• Use I.M. injection of vitamin D dispersed in oil for patients unable to absorb the oral form, as ordered.

Alert: Monitor patient's eating and bowel habits; dry mouth, nausea, vomiting, metallic taste, and constipation may be early signs of toxicity.

• Monitor serum and urine calcium, phos-

phorus, potassium, and urea levels when high therapeutic dosages are used.

• Know that dosages of 60,000 IU/day can cause hypercalcemia. Hypercalcemia may require I.V. hydration and aggressive diuresis.

• Be aware that malabsorption from inadequate bile or hepatic dysfunction may require addition of exogenous bile salts to oral form.

• Patients with hyperphosphatemia require dietary phosphate restrictions and binding agents to avoid metastatic calcifications and renal calculi.

• Be aware that mineral oil interferes with absorption of fat-soluble vitamins.

☑ Patient teaching
• Teach patient that vitamin D is necessary to absorb calcium. Instruct patient to read labels for vitamin D.

• Advise that vitamin D is fat soluble and that mineral oil will interfere with absorption.

• Instruct patient to take only as directed and stress the dangers of excessive doses of fat-soluble vitamins.

• Instruct patient taking vitamin D to restrict intake of magnesium-containing antacids.

▼ *NEW DRUG*

paricalcitol
Zemplar

Pregnancy Risk Category: C

HOW SUPPLIED
Injection: 5 mcg/ml

ACTION
A synthetic vitamin D analogue shown to reduce parathyroid hormone (PTH) levels.

Route	Onset	Peak	Duration
IV	Immediate	Unknown	15 hr

INDICATIONS & DOSAGE
Prevention and treatment of secondary hyperparathyroidism associated with chronic renal failure—
Adults: 0.04 to 0.1 mcg/kg (2.8 to 7 mcg)

I.V. no more frequently than every other day during dialysis. Doses as high as 0.24 mcg/kg (16.8 mcg) have been safely administered. If satisfactory response is not observed, dosage may be increased by 2 to 4 mcg at 2- to 4-week intervals.

ADVERSE REACTIONS
CNS: light-headedness.
CV: palpitation.
GI: dry mouth, GI bleeding, *nausea*, vomiting.
Hepatic: reduced serum total alkaline phosphatase level.
Respiratory: pneumonia.
Other: chills, edema, fever, flu syndrome, malaise, sepsis.

INTERACTIONS
None reported.

EFFECTS ON DIAGNOSTIC TESTS
None reported.

CONTRAINDICATIONS
Contraindicated in patients with evidence of vitamin D toxicity, hypercalcemia, or hypersensitivity to drug or its ingredients.

NURSING CONSIDERATIONS
• Use cautiously in patients taking digitalis compounds. Patients taking digoxin are at greater risk for digitalis toxicity during drug therapy secondary to potential for hypercalcemia.
• Monitor for ECG abnormalities.
• Monitor patient for symptoms of hypercalcemia. Immediately notify doctor if hypercalcemia is suspected.
• Monitor serum calcium and phosphorus levels twice weekly when dose is being adjusted, and then monitor monthly. PTH level should be measured every 3 months during therapy.
• Be aware that as the PTH level is decreased, paricalcitol dose may need to be decreased. Acute overdose of paricalcitol may cause hypercalcemia, which may require emergency attention.
• Be aware that in patients with chronic renal failure, appropriate types of phosphate-binding compounds may be needed to control serum phosphorus levels, but

excessive use of aluminum-containing compounds should be avoided.
• Store drug at room temperature (59° to 86° F [15° to 30° C]).

🔾 I.V. administration
• Drug is only administered as an I.V. bolus. Discard unused portion.
• Inspect drug for particulate matter and discoloration before use.

✅ Patient teaching
• Stress importance of adhering to a dietary regimen of calcium supplementation and phosphorus restriction during drug therapy.
• Caution against use of phosphate or vitamin D–related compounds during drug therapy.
• Explain need for frequent laboratory tests.
• Instruct patient with chronic renal failure to take phosphate-binding compounds as prescribed but to avoid excessive use of aluminum-containing compounds.
• Alert patient to early symptoms of hypercalcemia and vitamin D intoxication, such as weakness, headache, somnolence, nausea, vomiting, dry mouth, constipation, muscle pain, bone pain, and metallic taste.
• Instruct patient to promptly report adverse reactions.
• Remind patient taking digoxin to watch for signs of digitalis toxicity.

---

vitamin E (tocopherol)
Amino-Opti-E ◇, Aquasol E ◇, E-Complex-600 ◇, E-200 I.U. Softgels ◇, E-400 I.U. ◇, E-1000 I.U. Softgels, E-Vitamin Succinate ◇, Vita Plus E Softgels ◇

Pregnancy Risk Category: A

HOW SUPPLIED
Tablets (chewable): 200 IU ◇, 400 IU ◇
Capsules: 100 IU ◇, 200 IU ◇, 400 IU ◇, 500 IU ◇, 600 IU ◇, 1,000 IU ◇, 73.5 mg, 147 mg, 165 mg, 330 mg
Oral solution: 50 mg/ml ◇

ACTION
Unknown. Thought to act as an antioxidant and protect RBC membranes against hemolysis.

Route	Onset	Peak	Duration
PO	Unknown	Unknown	Unknown

INDICATIONS & DOSAGE
RDA—

Note: RDAs for vitamin E have been converted to α-tocopherol equivalents (α-TE). One α-TE equals 1 mg of D-α tocopherol or 1.49 IU.

Neonates and infants to 6 months: 3 α-TE or 4 IU.

Infants 6 months to 1 year: 4 α-TE or 6 IU.

Children 1 to 3 years: 6 α-TE or 9 IU.

Children 4 to 10 years: 7 α-TE or 10 IU.

Males 11 years and over: 10 α-TE or 15 IU.

Females 11 years and over: 8 α-TE or 12 IU.

Pregnant women: 10 α-TE or 15 IU.

Breast-feeding women (first 6 months): 12 α-TE or 18 IU.

Breast-feeding women (second 6 months): 11 α-TE or 16 IU.

Vitamin E deficiency in premature neonates and in patients with impaired fat absorption—

Adults: depending on severity, 60 to 75 IU P.O. daily.

Children: 1 IU/kg daily.

ADVERSE REACTIONS
None reported with recommended dosages. Hypervitaminosis E symptoms include fatigue, weakness, nausea, headache, blurred vision, flatulence, diarrhea.

INTERACTIONS
Drug-drug. *Anticoagulants (oral):* hypoprothrombinemic effects may be increased, possibly causing bleeding. Monitor closely.
Cholestyramine, colestipol, mineral oil: inhibited GI absorption of oral vitamin E. Space doses. Use together cautiously.
Iron: may catalyze oxidation and increase daily requirements. Avoid concurrent use.
Vitamin K: antagonized effects of vitamin K possible with large doses of vitamin E. Avoid concurrent use.

EFFECTS ON DIAGNOSTIC TESTS
None reported.

CONTRAINDICATIONS
No known contraindications.

NURSING CONSIDERATIONS
• Monitor patient with liver or gallbladder disease for response to therapy. Adequate bile is essential for vitamin E absorption.
• Be aware that water-miscible forms are more completely absorbed in GI tract.
• Requirements increase with rise in dietary polyunsaturated acids.
• Do not administer I.V.
• Do not exceed α-TE in pregnancy.

☑ **Patient teaching**
• Tell patient not to crush tablets or open capsules. An oral solution and chewable tablets are commercially available.
• Warn patient against self-medicating with megadoses, which can cause thrombophlebitis. Vitamin is fat soluble and may accumulate.

---

phytonadione (vitamin K₁)
AquaMEPHYTON, Konakion, Mephyton

Pregnancy Risk Category: A

HOW SUPPLIED
Tablets: 5 mg
Injection (aqueous colloidal solution): 2 mg/ml, 10 mg/ml
Injection (aqueous dispersion): 2 mg/ml, 10 mg/ml

ACTION
An antihemorrhagic factor that promotes hepatic formation of active prothrombin.

Route	Onset	Peak	Duration
PO	6-12 hr	Unknown	Unknown
IV, IM, SC	1-2 hr	Unknown	Unknown

INDICATIONS & DOSAGE
RDA—

Neonates and infants to 6 months: 5 mcg.

Infants 6 months to 1 year: 10 mcg.

Children 1 to 3 years: 15 mcg.

Children 4 to 6 years: 20 mcg.
Children 7 to 10 years: 30 mcg.
Children 11 to 14 years: 45 mcg.
Males 15 to 18 years: 65 mcg.
Males 19 to 24 years: 70 mcg.
Males 25 years and older: 80 mcg.
Females 15 to 18 years: 55 mcg.
Females 19 to 24 years: 60 mcg.
Females 25 years and older: 65 mcg
Pregnant or breast-feeding women: 65 mcg.
Hypoprothrombinemia secondary to vitamin K malabsorption, drug therapy, or excessive vitamin A dosage—
Adults: depending on severity, 2.5 to 10 mg P.O., S.C., or I.M. repeated and increased up to 50 mg if necessary.
Infants: 2 mg P.O. or parenterally.
Children: 5 to 10 mg P.O. or parenterally.
Hypoprothrombinemia secondary to effect of oral anticoagulants—
Adults: 2.5 to 10 mg P.O., S.C., or I.M. based on PT, repeated if necessary within 12 to 48 hours after oral dose or within 6 to 8 hours after parenteral dose. In emergency, 10 to 50 mg slow I.V., rate not to exceed 1 mg/minute, repeated q 4 hours, p.r.n.
Prevention of hemorrhagic disease of newborn—
Neonates: 0.5 to 1 mg I.M. within 1 hour after birth.
Treatment of hemorrhagic disease of newborn—
Neonates: 1 mg S.C. or I.M. Higher doses may be necessary if mother has been receiving oral anticoagulants.
Prevention of hypoprothrombinemia related to vitamin K deficiency in long-term parenteral nutrition—
Adults: 5 to 10 mg I.M. weekly.
Children: 2 to 5 mg I.M. weekly.
Prevention of hypoprothrombinemia in infants receiving less than 0.1 mg/L vitamin K in breast milk or milk substitutes—
Infants: 1 mg I.M. monthly.

ADVERSE REACTIONS
CNS: dizziness.
CV: transient hypotension (after I.V. administration), rapid and weak pulse.
Skin: diaphoresis, flushing, erythema.
Other: *anaphylaxis and anaphylactoid reactions* (usually after too-rapid I.V. ad-

ministration); pain, swelling, hematoma (at injection site).

INTERACTIONS
Drug-drug. *Anticoagulants:* temporary resistance to prothrombin-depressing anticoagulants may result, especially when larger doses of phytonadione are used. Monitor closely.
Cholestyramine, mineral oil: inhibited GI absorption of oral vitamin K. Space doses. Use together cautiously.

EFFECTS ON DIAGNOSTIC TESTS
Drug may falsely elevate urine steroid levels.

CONTRAINDICATIONS
Contraindicated in patients with hypersensitivity to drug.

NURSING CONSIDERATIONS
• Check brand name labels for administration route restrictions.
• Effects of I.V. injection are more rapid but shorter-lived than S.C. or I.M. injections.
Alert: I.V. use has resulted in fatalities; use only when other routes of administration are not feasible.
• For I.M. administration in adults and older children, administer in upper outer quadrant of buttocks; for infants, administer in the anterolateral aspect of the thigh or deltoid region.
• Anticipate order of weekly addition of 5 to 10 mg of phytonadione to total parenteral nutrition solutions.
• Monitor PT or INR to determine dosage effectiveness, as ordered.
• If severe bleeding occurs, don't delay other measures, such as fresh frozen plasma or whole blood.
Alert: Watch for signs of flushing, weakness, tachycardia, and hypotension; may progress to shock.
• Be aware that phytonadione therapy for hemorrhagic disease in infants causes fewer adverse reactions than do other vitamin K analogues.

◖ I.V. administration
• Dilute with 0.9% NaCl for injection, D_5W, or D_5W in 0.9% NaCl for injection.

Reactions may be *common,* uncommon, *life-threatening,* or COMMON AND LIFE-THREATENING.

Give I.V. by slow infusion over 2 to 3 hours. Rate shouldn't exceed 1 mg/minute.

• Protect parenteral products from light. Wrap infusion container with aluminum foil.

☑ Patient teaching
• Explain purpose of drug.
• Tell patient to avoid hazardous activities if dizziness occurs.
• Teach patient that drug is fat soluble; it should be taken only as prescribed.
• Teach patient that foods that provide vitamin K include cabbage, cauliflower, kale, spinach, fish, liver, eggs, meats, and dairy products.

---

sodium fluoride
Fluor-A-Day†, Fluoritab, Fluorodex, Fluotic†, Flura, Flura-Drops, Flura-Loz, Karidium, Luride, Luride Lozi-Tabs, Luride-SF Lozi-Tabs, Pediaflor, Pedi-Dent†, Pharmaflur, Pharmaflur df, Pharmaflur 1.1, Phos-Flur

sodium fluoride, topical
ACT ◇, Fluorigard ◇, Fluorinse, Gel-Kam, Gel-Tin ◇, Karigel, Karigel-N, Listermint with Fluoride, Minute-Gel, Point-Two, Prevident, Stop Gel ◇, Thera-Flur, Thera-Flur-N

Pregnancy Risk Category: NR

HOW SUPPLIED
sodium fluoride
Tablets: 1 mg
Tablets (chewable): 0.25 mg, 0.5 mg, 1 mg
Drops: 0.125 mg/drop, 0.25 mg/drop, 0.2 mg/ml, 0.5 mg/ml
Lozenges: 1 mg
sodium fluoride, topical
Gel: 0.1%, 0.5%, 1.23%
Gel drops: 0.5%
Rinse: 0.01% ◇, 0.02% ◇, 0.09%

ACTION
Stabilizes the apatite crystal of bone and teeth. Increases tooth resistance to acid breakdown.

Route	Onset	Peak	Duration
PO	Unknown	30-60 min	Unknown

INDICATIONS & DOSAGE
Prevention of dental caries—
Adults and children over 6 years: 5 to 10 ml of rinse or thin ribbon of gel applied to teeth with toothbrush or mouth trays for at least 1 minute h.s.
Children under 2 years: 0.25 mg P.O. (tablet or drops) daily.
Children 2 to 3 years: 0.5 mg P.O. (tablet or drops) daily.
Children 3 to 13 years: 1 mg P.O. (tablet or lozenge) daily.

ADVERSE REACTIONS
CNS: headache, weakness.
GI: gastric distress.
Skin: hypersensitivity reactions (such as atopic dermatitis, eczema, urticaria).
Other: staining of teeth.

INTERACTIONS
Drug-drug. *Aluminum hydroxide, calcium, iron, magnesium:* may decrease absorption. Separate administration times.
Drug-food. *Dairy products:* incompatibility may occur due to formation of calcium fluoride, which is poorly absorbed. Avoid concomitant use.

EFFECTS ON DIAGNOSTIC TESTS
None reported.

CONTRAINDICATIONS
Contraindicated in patients hypersensitive to fluoride or when intake from drinking water exceeds 0.7 parts per million.

NURSING CONSIDERATIONS
• Administer oral drops undiluted or mixed with fluids or food. Avoid simultaneous ingestion of dairy products.
• Know that chronic toxicity (fluorosis) may result from prolonged use of higher-than-recommended doses.

☑ Patient teaching
• Tell patient that tablets may be dissolved in mouth, chewed, or swallowed whole.

• Advise patient that topical rinses and gels should not be swallowed by children under 3 years, or used if water supply is fluorinated. Most effective when used right after brushing teeth. Tell patient to rinse around and between teeth for 1 minute, then spit out.
• Tell patient not to eat, drink, or rinse mouth for 30 minutes after application.
• Tell patient to dilute drops or rinses in plastic, not glass, containers.
• Advise patient to notify the dentist if tooth mottling occurs.
• Instruct patient not to exceed recommended dose.

---

trace elements
chromium (chromic chloride)
Chroma-Pak, Chromic Chloride

copper (cupric sulfate)
Cupric Sulfate

iodine (sodium iodide)
Iodopen

manganese (manganese chloride, manganese sulfate)

selenium (selenious acid)
Sele-Pak, Selepen

zinc (zinc sulfate)
Zinca-Pak

Pregnancy Risk Category: C

HOW SUPPLIED
chromium
Injection: 4 mcg/ml, 20 mcg/ml
copper
Injection: 0.4 mcg/ml, 2 mg/ml
iodine
Injection: 100 mcg/ml
manganese
Injection: 0.1 mg/ml
selenium
Injection: 40 mcg/ml
zinc
Injection: 1 mg/ml, 5 mg/ml

ACTION
Participates in synthesis and stabilization of proteins and nucleic acids in subcellular and membrane transport systems.

Route	Onset	Peak	Duration
IV	Immediate	Immediate	Unknown

INDICATIONS & DOSAGE
Prevention of individual trace element deficiencies in patients receiving long-term total parenteral nutrition (TPN)—
Chromium—
Adults: 10 to 15 mcg I.V. daily.
Children: 0.14 to 0.20 mcg/kg I.V. daily.
Copper—
Adults: 0.5 to 1.5 mg I.V. daily.
Children: 20 mcg/kg I.V. daily.
Iodine—
Adults: 1 to 2 mcg/kg I.V. daily.
Children: 2 to 3 mcg/kg I.V. daily.
Manganese—
Adults: 0.15 to 0.8 mg I.V. daily.
Children: 2 to 10 mcg/kg I.V. daily.
Selenium—
Adults: 20 to 40 mcg I.V. daily.
Children: 3 mcg/kg I.V. daily.
Zinc—
Adults: 2.5 to 4 mg I.V. daily.
Full-term infants to 5 years: 100 mcg/kg/day.
Neonates under 1,500 g to 3 kg (3.3 to 7 lb): 300 mcg/kg/day.

ADVERSE REACTIONS
None reported when used at recommended dosages except for hypersensitivity to iodides.

INTERACTIONS
None significant.

EFFECTS ON DIAGNOSTIC TESTS
None reported.

CONTRAINDICATIONS
Contraindicated in patients hypersensitive to iodine.

NURSING CONSIDERATIONS
• Check serum levels of trace elements in patients who have received TPN for 2 months or longer, as ordered. Give supplement, if ordered. Report low serum levels of these elements.
• Normal serum levels are 1 to 5 mcg/L

Reactions may be *common,* uncommon, **life-threatening**, or COMMON AND LIFE-THREATENING.

chromium; 80 to 163 mcg/dl copper; 6 to 12 mcg/dl manganese; 0.1 to 0.19 mcg/ml selenium; and 88 to 112 mcg/dl zinc.
• Be aware that solutions of trace elements are compounded by the pharmacist for addition to TPN solutions according to various formulas.

⚡ I.V. administration
• Cautiously infuse diluted solution through a patent I.V. line over the ordered duration.
• Do not administer undiluted due to potential for phlebitis.

✅ Patient teaching
• Explain need for zinc administration to patient and family.
• Tell patient to report signs of hypersensitivity promptly.
• Inform patient and family that trace elements are normally received from dietary intake and when patient begins eating well, supplements will not be necessary.

amino acid infusions, crystalline
amino acid infusions in dextrose
amino acid infusions with
  electrolytes
amino acid infusions with
  electrolytes in dextrose
amino acid infusions for hepatic
  failure
amino acid infusions for high
  metabolic stress
amino acid infusions for renal
  failure
dextrose
fat emulsions
medium-chain triglycerides

COMBINATION PRODUCTS
Various products contain dextrose or invert sugar in combination with electrolytes.

---

amino acid infusions, crystalline
Aminosyn, Aminosyn II,
Aminosyn-PF, FreAmine III,
Novamine, Travasol, TrophAmine

amino acid infusions in dextrose
Aminosyn II with Dextrose

amino acid infusions with electrolytes
Aminosyn with Electrolytes,
Aminosyn II with Electrolytes,
FreAmine III with Electrolytes,
ProcalAmine with Electrolytes,
Travasol with Electrolytes

amino acid infusions with electrolytes in dextrose
Aminosyn II with Electrolytes in
Dextrose

amino acid infusions for hepatic failure
HepatAmine

amino acid infusions for high metabolic stress
Aminosyn-HBC, BranchAmin,
FreAmine HBC

amino acid infusions for renal failure
Aminess, Aminosyn-RF,
NephrAmine, RenAmin

Pregnancy Risk Category: C

HOW SUPPLIED
Injection: 250 ml, 500 ml, 1,000 ml,
2,000 ml containing amino acids in vari-
ous concentrations
amino acid infusions, crystalline
Aminosyn: 3.5%, 5%, 7%, 8.5%, 10%
Aminosyn II: 3.5%, 5%, 7%, 8.5%, 10%,
15%
Aminosyn-PF: 7%, 10%
FreAmine III: 8.5%, 10%
Novamine: 11.4%, 15%
Travasol: 5.5%, 8.5%, 10%
TrophAmine: 6%, 10%
amino acid infusions in dextrose
Aminosyn II: 3.5% in 5% dextrose, 3.5%
in 25% dextrose, 4.25% in 10% dextrose,
4.25% in 20% dextrose, 4.25% in 25%
dextrose, 5% in 25% dextrose
Travasol: 2.75% in 5% dextrose, 2.75% in
10% dextrose, 2.75% in 25% dextrose
Travasol: 4.25% in 5% dextrose, 4.25% in
10% dextrose, 4.25% in 25% dextrose
amino acid infusions with electrolytes
Aminosyn: 3.5%, 7%, 8.5%
Aminosyn II: 3.5%, 7%, 8.5%, 10%
FreAmine III: 3%, 8.5%
ProcalAmine: 3%
Travasol: 3.5%, 5.5%, 8.5%
**amino acid infusions with electrolytes
in dextrose**
Aminosyn II: 3.5% with electrolytes in
5% dextrose, 3.5% with electrolytes in
25% dextrose, 4.25% with electrolytes in
10% dextrose, 4.25% with electrolytes in
20% dextrose, 4.25% with electrolytes in
25% dextrose
Travasol: 2.75% with electrolytes in 5%

Reactions may be *common,* uncommon, *life-threatening,* or COMMON AND LIFE-THREATENING.

dextrose, 2.75% with electrolytes in dextrose, 4.25% with electrolytes in 5% dextrose, 4.25% with electrolytes in 10% dextrose, 4.25% with electrolytes in 25% dextrose

amino acid infusions for hepatic failure
HepatAmine: 8%

amino acid infusions for high metabolic stress
Aminosyn-HBC: 7%
BranchAmin: 4%
FreAmine HBC: 6.9%

amino acid infusions for renal failure
Aminess: 5.2%
Aminosyn-RF: 5.2%
NephrAmine: 5.4%
RenAmin: 6.5%

ACTION

Provides a substrate for protein synthesis or enhances conservation of existing body protein. Formulations for patients with hepatic failure and high metabolic stress contain essential and nonessential amino acids, with high concentrations of the branched chain amino acids isoleucine, leucine, and valine. Formulations for patients with renal failure contain histidine and minimal amounts of essential amino acids; nonessential amino acids are synthesized from excess ammonia in the blood of the uremic patient, thus decreasing azotemia.

Route	Onset	Peak	Duration
IV	Immediate	Immediate	Unknown

INDICATIONS & DOSAGE

Total parenteral nutrition in patients who cannot or will not eat—
Adults: 1 to 1.5 g/kg I.V. daily.
Children weighing under 10 kg (22 lb): 2 to 4 g/kg I.V. daily.
Children weighing over 10 kg: 20 to 25 g I.V. daily for first 10 kg, then 1 to 1.25 g/kg I.V. daily for each kg over 10 kg.
Nutritional support in patients with cirrhosis, hepatitis, and hepatic encephalopathy—
Adults: 80 to 120 g of amino acids (12 to 18 g of nitrogen) I.V. daily of formulation for hepatic failure.

Nutritional support in patients with high metabolic stress—
Adults: 1.5 g/kg I.V. daily of formulation for high metabolic stress.
Nutritional support in patients with renal failure—
Adults: 0.3 to 0.5 g/kg I.V. daily (up to total of 26 g daily). Patients on dialysis may require 1 to 1.2 g/kg daily.

ADVERSE REACTIONS

CV: thrombophlebitis, edema, thrombosis.
GI: nausea.
GU: glycosuria, osmotic diuresis.
Hepatic: elevated liver enzyme levels.
Skin: flushing.
Other: *hypersensitivity reactions,* tissue sloughing at infusion site caused by extravasation, *catheter sepsis, rebound hypoglycemia* (when long-term infusions are abruptly stopped), hyperglycemia, osteoporosis, metabolic acidosis, alkalosis, hypophosphatemia, *hyperosmolar hyperglycemic nonketotic syndrome,* hyperammonemia, electrolyte imbalances, fever, weight gain.

INTERACTIONS

Drug-drug. *Tetracycline:* may reduce the protein-sparing effects of infused amino acids because of its antianabolic activity. Monitor patient.

EFFECTS ON DIAGNOSTIC TESTS
None reported.

CONTRAINDICATIONS

Contraindicated in patients with anuria and in those with inborn errors of amino acid metabolism, such as maple syrup urine disease and isovaleric acidemia.

NURSING CONSIDERATIONS

• Use with extreme caution in children and neonates, especially those with low birth weight.
• Use cautiously in patients with renal insufficiency or failure, cardiac disease, or hepatic impairment.
• Administer cautiously to diabetic patients; insulin may be required to prevent hyperglycemia. Also administer cautiously to patients with cardiac insufficiency;

may cause circulatory overload. Patients with fluid restriction may tolerate only 1 to 2 L.

• Obtain baseline serum electrolytes, glucose, BUN, calcium, and phosphorus levels before therapy, as ordered, and then monitor these levels periodically throughout therapy.

• Know that safe and effective use of parenteral nutrition requires a knowledge of nutrition as well as clinical expertise in the recognition and treatment of potential complications. Frequent evaluation of the patient and laboratory studies are necessary.

• Know that peripheral infusions should be limited to 2.5% amino acids and dextrose 10%. Check infusion site frequently for erythema, inflammation, irritation, tissue sloughing, necrosis, and phlebitis. Change peripheral I.V. sites routinely to prevent irritation and infection. If a subclavian catheter is used, administer solution into the midsuperior vena cava.

• Add vitamins, electrolytes, and trace elements, as ordered.

• Check fractional urine every 6 hours for glycosuria initially, then every 12 to 24 hours in stable patients. Abrupt onset of glycosuria may be an early sign of impending sepsis.

• Assess body temperature every 4 hours; elevation may indicate sepsis or infection.

• Monitor for extraordinary electrolyte losses that may occur during nasogastric suction, vomiting, diarrhea, or drainage from GI fistula.

• Be prepared to individualize dosage to metabolic and clinical response as determined by nitrogen balance and body weight corrected for fluid balance.

• If patient has chills, fever, or other signs of sepsis, replace I.V. tubing and bottle and send them to the laboratory to be cultured.

I.V. administration
• Control infusion rate carefully with infusion pump. If infusion rate falls behind, notify doctor; do not increase the rate to catch up.

Patient teaching
• Explain need for use to patient and family, and answer any questions.
• Tell patient to report adverse reactions promptly.

dextrose (d-glucose)

Pregnancy Risk Category: C

HOW SUPPLIED
Injection: 3-ml ampule (10%); 10 ml (25%); 25 ml (5%); 50 ml (5% and 50% available in vial, ampule, and Bristoject); 70-ml pin-top vial (70% for additive use only); 100 ml (5%); 150 ml (5%); 250 ml (5%, 10%); 500 ml (5%, 10%, 20%, 30%, 40%, 50%, 60%, 70%); 650 ml (38.5%); 1,000 ml (2.5%, 5%, 10%, 20%, 30%, 40%, 50%, 60%, 70%); 2,000 ml (50%, 70%); 25 ml (5%)

ACTION
A simple water-soluble sugar that minimizes glyconeogenesis and promotes anabolism in patients whose oral caloric intake is limited.

Route	Onset	Peak	Duration
IV	Immediate	Immediate	Unknown

INDICATIONS & DOSAGE
Fluid replacement and caloric supplementation in patients who can't maintain adequate oral intake or who are restricted from doing so—
Adults and children: dosage depends on fluid and caloric requirements. Peripheral I.V. infusion of 2.5%, 5%, or 10% solution or central I.V. infusion of 20% solution is used for minimal fluid needs. A 25% solution is used to treat acute hypoglycemia in neonate or older infant. A 50% solution is used to treat insulin-induced hypoglycemia. Solutions of 10%, 20%, 30%, 40%, 50%, 60%, and 70% are diluted in admixtures, usually amino acid solutions, for total parenteral nutrition (TPN) given through a central vein.

ADVERSE REACTIONS
CNS: confusion, *unconsciousness in*

---

hyperosmolar hyperglycemic nonketotic syndrome.
CV: *pulmonary edema, exacerbated hypertension, heart failure* (with fluid overload in susceptible patients); *phlebitis, venous sclerosis,* tissue necrosis (with prolonged or concentrated infusions, especially when administered peripherally).
GU: glycosuria, osmotic diuresis.
Skin: sloughing, tissue necrosis (if extravasation occurs with concentrated solutions).
Other: hyperglycemia, hypervolemia, hypovolemia, dehydration, fever, hyperosmolarity (with rapid infusion of concentrated solution or prolonged infusion); hypoglycemia from rebound hyperinsulinemia (with rapid termination of long-term infusions).

INTERACTIONS
Drug-drug. *Corticosteroids:* may cause salt and water retention and increased potassium excretion. Monitor glucose, sodium, and potassium levels.

EFFECTS ON DIAGNOSTIC TESTS
None reported.

CONTRAINDICATIONS
Contraindicated in patients in diabetic coma while blood glucose remains excessively high. Use of concentrated solutions contraindicated in patients with intracranial or intraspinal hemorrhage, or in dehydrated patients with delirium tremens or in patients with severe dehydration, anuria, hepatic coma, or glucose-galactose malabsorption syndrome.

NURSING CONSIDERATIONS
• Use cautiously in patients with cardiac or pulmonary disease, hypertension, renal insufficiency, urinary obstruction, or hypovolemia.
• Monitor serum glucose levels carefully. Prolonged therapy with D_5W can cause depletion of pancreatic insulin production and secretion.
Alert: Never stop hypertonic solutions abruptly. If necessary, have $D_{10}W$ available to treat hypoglycemia if rebound hyperinsulinemia occurs.
• Use central veins to infuse dextrose so-

lutions with concentrations greater than 10%.
• Take care to prevent extravasation. Check injection site frequently to prevent irritation, tissue sloughing, necrosis, and phlebitis.
• Check vital signs frequently. Report adverse effects promptly.
• Monitor fluid intake, output, and weight carefully, especially patients with renal function impairment.
• Watch closely for signs and symptoms of fluid overload, especially if fluid intake is restricted.

🔵 I.V. administration
• Control infusion rate carefully; maximum rate is 0.5 g/kg/hour. Use infusion pump when administering with amino acids for TPN. Never infuse concentrated solutions rapidly, which may cause hyperglycemia and fluid shift.

✅ Patient teaching
• Explain need for drug to patient and family, and answer any questions.
• Tell patient to report adverse reactions promptly.

fat emulsions
Intralipid 10%, Intralipid 20%, Liposyn II 10%, Liposyn II 20%, Liposyn III 10%, Liposyn III 20%

Pregnancy Risk Category: C

HOW SUPPLIED
Injection: 50 ml (10%, 20%), 100 ml (10%, 20%), 200 ml (10%, 20%), 250 ml (10%, 20%), 500 ml (10%, 20%)

ACTION
Provides neutral triglycerides, predominantly unsaturated fatty acids; acts as a source of calories; and prevents fatty acid deficiency. When substituted for dextrose as a source of calories, fat emulsions decrease carbon dioxide production.

Route	Onset	Peak	Duration
IV	Immediate	Immediate	Unknown

INDICATIONS & DOSAGE

Intralipid:

Source of calories as adjunct to total parenteral nutrition (TPN)—

Adults: 1 ml/minute I.V. for 15 to 30 minutes (10% emulsion); 0.5 ml/minute I.V. for 15 to 30 minutes (20% emulsion). If no adverse reactions occur, rate increased to deliver 500 ml over 4 to 8 hours; total daily dosage should not exceed 3 g/kg.

Children: 0.1 ml/minute for 10 to 15 minutes (10% emulsion), 0.05 ml/minute I.V. for 10 to 15 minutes (20% emulsion). If no adverse reactions occur, rate increased to deliver 1 g/kg over 4 hours; daily dosage should not exceed 3 g/kg. Equals 40% of daily caloric intake; protein-carbohydrate TPN should supply remaining 60%.

Fatty acid deficiency—

Adults and children: 8% to 10% of total caloric intake I.V.

Liposyn:

Prevention of fatty acid deficiency—

Adults: 500 ml (10% emulsion) I.V. twice weekly. Infused initially at rate of 1 ml/minute for 30 minutes. Rate may be increased to, but should not exceed, 500 ml over 4 to 6 hours.

Children: 5 to 10 ml/kg (10% emulsion) I.V. daily. Initially infused at rate of 0.1 ml/minute for 30 minutes. Rate may be increased to, but should not exceed, 100 ml/hour.

ADVERSE REACTIONS

Early reactions to fat overload:

CNS: headache, sleepiness, dizziness.

EENT: pressure over eyes.

GI: nausea, vomiting.

Hematologic: hypercoagulability, ***thrombocytopenia*** in neonates (rare).

Respiratory: dyspnea, cyanosis.

Skin: flushing, diaphoresis.

Other: hyperlipidemia, fever, chest and back pains, ***hypersensitivity reactions,*** irritation at infusion site.

Delayed reactions:

CNS: *focal seizures.*

Hematologic: *thrombocytopenia, leukopenia,* leukocytosis.

Hepatic: transient increases in liver function test values, hepatomegaly.

Other: fever, splenomegaly.

INTERACTIONS

None significant.

EFFECTS ON DIAGNOSTIC TESTS

Abnormally high mean corpuscular hemoglobin and mean corpuscular hemoglobin concentration values may be found in blood samples drawn during or shortly after fat emulsion infusion. Fat emulsions may cause transient abnormalities in liver function and may alter results of serum bilirubin tests (especially in infants).

CONTRAINDICATIONS

Contraindicated in patients with severe egg allergies, hyperlipidemia, lipid nephrosis, or acute pancreatitis accompanied by hyperlipidemia.

NURSING CONSIDERATIONS

• Use cautiously in patients with severe hepatic disease; pulmonary disease; anemia; or blood coagulation disorders, including thrombocytopenia; and in patients at risk for fat embolism.

• Also use cautiously in jaundiced or premature infants.

• Be aware that drug may be mixed with amino acid solution, dextrose, electrolytes, and vitamins in the same I.V. container. Check with pharmacist for acceptable proportions and compatibility information.

• Do not use fat emulsion if it separates or becomes oily.

• Lipids support bacterial growth, so change all I.V. tubing before each infusion. Check injection site daily. Report signs and symptoms of inflammation or infection promptly.

• Watch for adverse reactions, especially during first half of infusion.

• Monitor serum lipid levels closely when the patient is receiving fat emulsion therapy. Lipemia must clear between dosing.

• Monitor hepatic function carefully in long-term therapy.

• Check platelet count frequently in neonates receiving fat emulsions I.V.

• Carefully monitor serum triglycerides and free fatty acids in infants.

• Refrigeration is not necessary.

• Intralipid and Liposyn differ mainly by their fatty acid components.

Reactions may be *common*, uncommon, ***life-threatening***, or **COMMON AND LIFE-THREATENING**.

🔲 I.V. administration
• Avoid rapid infusion, and use an infusion pump to regulate rate.
• Know that an in-line filter with pores of 1.2 microns or larger is sometimes used to remove particulate matter.

✅ Patient teaching
• Explain need for fat emulsion therapy, and answer any questions.
• Tell patient to report adverse reactions promptly.

---

medium-chain triglycerides
MCT ◇

Pregnancy Risk Category: NR

HOW SUPPLIED
Oil: 960 ml (115 calories/15 ml) ◇

ACTION
Source of rapidly hydrolyzable lipid.

Route	Onset	Peak	Duration
PO	Unknown	Unknown	Unknown

INDICATIONS & DOSAGE
Inadequate digestion or absorption of food fats—
Adults: 15 ml P.O. t.i.d. or q.i.d.

ADVERSE REACTIONS
CNS: reversible *coma* in susceptible patients (such as those with advanced hepatic cirrhosis).
GI: *nausea, vomiting, diarrhea, abdominal distention, cramps.*

INTERACTIONS
None significant.

EFFECTS ON DIAGNOSTIC TESTS
None reported.

CONTRAINDICATIONS
No known contraindications.

NURSING CONSIDERATIONS
• Use cautiously in patients with hepatic cirrhosis and complications such as portacaval shunts or tendency to encephalopathy.

• To minimize GI adverse reactions, give smaller, more frequent doses with meals, mixed with salad dressing, or in chilled fruit juice.
• Know that drug is more easily absorbed than long-chain fats; not dependent on bile salts for emulsification.
• Be aware that drug's rapid metabolism provides quick energy.
• Drug provides 7.7 calories/ml and no essential fatty acids.

✅ Patient teaching
• Instruct patient when and how to take drug to minimize GI adverse reactions.
• Tell patient to report persistent or severe adverse reactions promptly.
• Caution patient not to use plastic containers or utensils to give drug.

---

*Liquid contains alcohol.   **May contain tartrazine.   †Canada   ‡Australia   §U.K.   ◇OTC

allopurinol
colchicine
probenecid
sulfinpyrazone

COMBINATION PRODUCTS

COLBENEMID, PROBEN-C, PROBENECID WITH COLCHICINE: probenecid 500 mg and colchicine 0.5 mg.

---

allopurinol
Apo-Allopurinol†, Capurate‡, Lopurin, Purinol†, Zyloprim, Zyloric§

Pregnancy Risk Category: C

HOW SUPPLIED
Tablets (scored): 100 mg, 300 mg
Capsules: 100 mg‡, 300 mg‡

ACTION
Reduces uric acid production by inhibiting the biochemical reactions preceding its formation.

Route	Onset	Peak	Duration
PO	Unknown	0.5-2 hr	1-2 wk

INDICATIONS & DOSAGE
Gout, primary or secondary to hyperuricemia; secondary to diseases such as acute or chronic leukemia, polycythemia vera, multiple myeloma, and psoriasis—
Dosage varies with severity of disease; can be given as single dose or divided, but doses above 300 mg should be divided.
Adults: mild gout, 200 to 300 mg P.O. daily; severe gout with large tophi, 400 to 600 mg P.O. daily. Same dosage for maintenance in secondary hyperuricemia. Maximum dosage is 800 mg/day.
Hyperuricemia secondary to malignancies—
Children under 6 years: 50 mg P.O. t.i.d.
Children 6 to 10 years: 300 mg P.O. daily or divided t.i.d.
Prevention of acute gouty attacks—
Adults: 100 mg P.O. daily; increase at weekly intervals by 100 mg without exceeding maximum dose (800 mg), until serum uric acid falls to 6 mg/dl or less.
Prevention of uric acid nephropathy during cancer chemotherapy—
Adults: 600 to 800 mg P.O. daily for 2 to 3 days, with high fluid intake.
Recurrent calcium oxalate calculi—
Adults: 200 to 300 mg P.O. daily in single or divided doses.
Adjust-a-dose: In renally impaired patients, 200 mg P.O. daily if creatinine clearance is 10 to 20 ml/minute; 100 mg P.O. daily if it is below 10 ml/minute; and 100 mg P.O. more than 24 hours apart if it is below 3 ml/minute.

ADVERSE REACTIONS
CNS: drowsiness, headache, paresthesia, peripheral neuropathy, neuritis.
CV: hypersensitivity vasculitis, necrotizing angiitis.
EENT: epistaxis.
GI: nausea, vomiting, diarrhea, abdominal pain, gastritis, taste loss or perversion, dyspepsia.
GU: *renal failure,* uremia.
Hematologic: *agranulocytosis,* anemia, *aplastic anemia, thrombocytopenia, leukopenia,* leukocytosis, eosinophilia.
Hepatic: increased alkaline phosphatase, AST and ALT levels, *hepatitis, hepatic necrosis,* hepatomegaly, cholestatic jaundice.
Skin: *rash* (usually maculopapular); exfoliative, urticarial, and purpuric lesions; *erythema multiforme;* severe furunculosis of nose; ichthyosis, alopecia, *toxic epidermal necrolysis.*
Other: arthralgia, ecchymoses, fever, myopathy, chills.

INTERACTIONS
Drug-drug. *Amoxicillin, ampicillin, bacampicillin:* increased possibility of rash. Avoid concomitant use.
Anticoagulants (except warfarin): poten-

---

tiation of anticoagulant effect. Dosage adjustments may be necessary.
Antineoplastic agents: increased potential for bone marrow suppression. Monitor patient carefully.
Chlorpropamide: possible increased hypoglycemic effect. Avoid concomitant use.
Diazoxide, diuretics, mecamylamine, pyrazinamide: increased serum uric acid concentration. Adjust dosage of allopurinol.
Ethacrynic acid, thiazide diuretics: increased risk of allopurinol toxicity. Reduce dosage of allopurinol, and closely monitor renal function.
Uricosuric agents: additive effect. May enhance therapy.
Urine-acidifying agents (ammonium chloride, ascorbic acid, potassium or sodium phosphate): may increase possibility of kidney stone formation. Monitor patient carefully.
Xanthines: increased serum theophylline levels. Adjust dosage of theophyllines as needed.
Drug-lifestyle. *Alcohol use:* increased serum uric acid concentration. Avoid alcohol use.

EFFECTS ON DIAGNOSTIC TESTS
None reported.

CONTRAINDICATIONS
Contraindicated in patients with idiopathic hemochromatosis or hypersensitivity to drug.

NURSING CONSIDERATIONS
• Monitor serum uric acid levels to evaluate drug's effectiveness.
• Monitor fluid intake and output; daily urine output of at least 2 L and maintenance of neutral or slightly alkaline urine are desirable.
• Periodically monitor CBC and hepatic and renal function, especially at start of therapy, as ordered.
• Optimal benefits may require 2 to 6 weeks of therapy. Because acute gouty attacks may occur during this time, concurrent use of colchicine may be prescribed prophylactically.

☑ Patient teaching
• To minimize GI adverse reactions, tell patient to take drug with, or immediately after, meals.
• Encourage patient to drink plenty of fluids while taking drug unless otherwise contraindicated.
• Drug may cause drowsiness; tell patient not to drive or perform hazardous tasks requiring mental alertness until CNS effects of drug are known.
• If patient is taking allopurinol for treatment of recurrent calcium oxalate stones, advise him also to reduce his dietary intake of animal protein, sodium, refined sugars, oxalate-rich foods, and calcium.
• Tell patient to discontinue at first sign of rash, which may precede severe hypersensitivity or other adverse reaction. Rash is more common in patients taking diuretics and in those with renal disorders. Tell patient to report all adverse reactions.
• Advise patient to avoid alcohol during therapy.
• Teach patient importance of continuing drug even if asymptomatic.

colchicine
Colgout‡

Pregnancy Risk Category: C (P.O.), D (I.V.)

HOW SUPPLIED
Tablets: 0.5 mg (¹⁄₁₂₀ grain), 0.6 mg (¹⁄₁₀₀ grain) as sugar-coated granules
Injection: 1 mg (¹⁄₆₀ grain)/2 ml

ACTION
Unknown. As antigout agent, apparently decreases WBC motility, phagocytosis, and lactic acid production, decreasing urate crystal deposits and reducing inflammation. As antiosteolytic agent, apparently inhibits mitosis of osteoprogenitor cells and decreases osteoclast activity.

Route	Onset	Peak	Duration
PO	≤ 12 hr	0.5-2 hr	Unknown
IV	6-12 hr	Unknown	Unknown

INDICATIONS & DOSAGE

Prevention of acute gout attacks as prophylactic or maintenance therapy—
Adults: 0.5 or 0.6 mg P.O. daily. Patients who normally have one attack per year or less should receive drug only 1 to 4 days weekly; patients who have more than one attack per year should receive drug daily. In severe cases, 1.5 to 1.95 mg P.O. daily.
Prevention of gout attacks in patients undergoing surgery—
Adults: 0.5 to 0.6 mg P.O. t.i.d. 3 days before and 3 days after surgery.
Acute gout, acute gouty arthritis—
Adults: initially, 0.5 to 1.3 mg P.O., then 0.5 or 0.6 mg q 1 to 2 hours until pain is relieved; nausea, vomiting, or diarrhea ensues; or the maximum dosage of 8 mg is reached. Alternatively, 2 mg I.V., followed by 0.5 mg I.V. q 6 hours if necessary. (Note that some clinicians prefer to give a single I.V. injection of 3 mg.) Total I.V. dosage over 24 hours (one course of treatment) should not exceed 4 mg.

ADVERSE REACTIONS

CNS: peripheral neuritis.
GI: *nausea, vomiting, abdominal pain, diarrhea.*
Hematologic: **aplastic anemia, thrombocytopenia, agranulocytosis** (with long-term use); nonthrombocytopenic purpura.
Hepatic: increased alkaline phosphatase, AST and ALT levels.
Skin: alopecia, urticaria, dermatitis, *hypersensitivity reactions.*
Other: severe local irritation if extravasation occurs, myopathy, reversible azoospermia.

INTERACTIONS

Drug-drug. *Cyclosporine:* increased GI toxicity with concurrent use. Adjust doses if toxicity occurs.
Erythromycin: increased serum colchicine levels. Observe patient; may need to reduce colchicine dosage.
Loop diuretics: may decrease efficacy of colchicine prophylaxis. Avoid concomitant use.
Phenylbutazone: may increase risk of leukopenia or thrombocytopenia. Avoid concomitant use.

Vitamin B₁₂: impaired absorption of oral vitamin B_{12}. Avoid concomitant use.
Drug-lifestyle. *Alcohol use:* may impair efficacy of colchicine prophylaxis. Don't use together.

EFFECTS ON DIAGNOSTIC TESTS

Drug therapy may decrease serum carotene, cholesterol, and thrombocyte values. It may cause false-positive results of urine tests for RBCs or hemoglobin.

CONTRAINDICATIONS

Contraindicated in patients with hypersensitivity to drug and in those with blood dyscrasias or serious CV disease, renal disease, or GI disorders.

NURSING CONSIDERATIONS

• Use cautiously in elderly or debilitated patients and in those with early signs of CV, renal, or GI disease.
• Obtain baseline laboratory studies, including CBC, prior to therapy, as ordered, and then periodically throughout therapy.
Alert: Do not administer I.M. or S.C.; severe local irritation occurs.
• Give with meals to reduce GI effects as maintenance therapy. May be used with uricosuric agents, as ordered.
• Monitor fluid intake and output, and keep output at 2 L daily.
Alert: Know that after a full course of I.V. colchicine (4 mg), no more colchicine should be given by any route for at least 7 days. Colchicine is a toxic drug and fatalities have resulted from overdose.
• The first sign of acute overdose may be GI symptoms, followed by vascular damage, muscle weakness, and ascending paralysis. Delirium and seizures may occur without the patient losing consciousness.
• Discontinue drug as soon as gout pain is relieved or at first sign of GI symptoms, as ordered.

▲ I.V. administration

• Give by slow I.V. push over 2 to 5 minutes. Avoid extravasation because colchicine irritates tissues. Don't dilute colchicine injection with D₅W injection or other fluids that might change pH of colchicine solution. If lower concentration of colchicine injection is needed, dilute with 0.9% NaCl solution or sterile water for injection and give over 2 to 5 minutes by direct injection. Preferably, inject into the tubing of a free-flowing I.V. solution. Don't inject if diluted solution becomes turbid.

☑ **Patient teaching**
• Teach patient how to take drug and tell him to drink extra fluids.
• Tell patient to report adverse reactions, especially signs of acute overdose.
• Advise patient to avoid alcohol while taking drug.
• Tell patient with gout to limit intake of foods high in purine, such as anchovies, liver, sardines, kidneys, sweetbreads, peas, and lentils.

probenecid
Benemid, Benurylt†, Probalan

Pregnancy Risk Category: B

HOW SUPPLIED
Tablets: 500 mg

ACTION
Blocks renal tubular reabsorption of uric acid, increasing excretion, and inhibits active renal tubular secretion of many weak organic acids, such as penicillins and cephalosporins.

Route	Onset	Peak	Duration
PO	Unknown	2-4 hr	Unknown

INDICATIONS & DOSAGE
Adjunct to penicillin therapy—
Adults and children weighing over 50 kg (110 lb): 500 mg P.O. q.i.d.
Children 2 to 14 years or weighing 50 kg or less: initially, 25 mg/kg P.O., then 40 mg/kg/day in divided doses q.i.d.
Gonorrhea—
Adults: 3.5 g ampicillin P.O. with 1 g probenecid P.O. given together; or 1 g probenecid P.O. 30 minutes before dose of 4.8 million units of aqueous penicillin g procaine I.M., injected at two different sites.
Hyperuricemia of gout, gouty arthritis—

Adults: 250 mg P.O. b.i.d. for first week, then 500 mg b.i.d., to maximum of 2 g daily. Maintenance dosage should be reviewed q 6 months and reduced by increments of 500 mg, if indicated.

ADVERSE REACTIONS
CNS: *headache,* dizziness.
GI: anorexia, nausea, vomiting, sore gums.
GU: urinary frequency, renal colic, nephrotic syndrome.
Hematologic: *hemolytic anemia,* anemia, *aplastic anemia.*
Skin: dermatitis, pruritus.
Other: flushing, fever, exacerbation of gout, *hepatic necrosis, hypersensitivity reactions* (including *anaphylaxis,* fever).

INTERACTIONS
Drug-drug. *Acyclovir, cephalosporins, penicillin:* may increase levels of these drugs. Use cautiously.
Indomethacin, ketoprofen, NSAIDS: may enhance toxicity. Avoid concomitant use.
Methotrexate: decreased methotrexate excretion. Lower methotrexate dosage may be required. Serum levels should be determined.
Nitrofurantoin: increased toxicity and reduced effectiveness. Reduce probenecid dose.
Oral antidiabetic agents: enhanced hypoglycemic effect. Monitor blood glucose levels closely. Dosage adjustment may be required.
Salicylates: inhibited uricosuric effect of probenecid, causing urate retention. Do not use together.
Zidovudine: may increase zidovudine levels and toxicity symptoms. Monitor patient.
Drug-lifestyle. *Alcohol use:* increased urate levels. Avoid use.

EFFECTS ON DIAGNOSTIC TESTS
Drug causes false-positive test results for urinary glucose with tests using cupric sulfate reagent (Benedict's reagent, Clinitest, and Fehling's test); perform tests with glucose oxidase reagent (Diastix or Chemstrip uG) instead. Drug also decreases urinary excretion of 17-ketosteroids, bromsulphalein, aminohippuric acid, and

---

iodine-related organic acids, interfering with laboratory procedures.

CONTRAINDICATIONS

Contraindicated in patients with uric acid kidney stones, blood dyscrasias, or hypersensitivity to drug; in acute gout attack; and in children under 2 years.

NURSING CONSIDERATIONS

• Use cautiously in patients with peptic ulcer or renal impairment.
• To minimize GI distress, give drug with milk, food, or antacids. Continued disturbances might indicate need to lower dosage.
• Monitor periodic BUN and renal function tests in long-term therapy.
• Force fluids to maintain minimum daily output of 2 to 3 L. Alkalinize urine with sodium bicarbonate or potassium citrate, as ordered. These measures will prevent hematuria, renal colic, urate stone development, and costovertebral pain.
• Keep in mind that therapy for treatment of gout is not initiated until acute attack subsides. Contains no analgesic or anti-inflammatory agent, and is of no value during acute gout attacks.
• Be aware that drug is suitable for long-term use; no cumulative effects or tolerance reported.
• Drug is ineffective in patients with chronic renal insufficiency (glomerular filtration rate less than 30 ml/minute).
• Drug may increase frequency, severity, and length of acute gout attacks during first 6 to 12 months of therapy. Prophylactic colchicine or another anti-inflammatory agent is given during first 3 to 6 months.

✓ Patient teaching

• Instruct patient and family that, when prescribed as treatment for gout, the drug must be taken regularly, as ordered, or gout attacks might occur.
• Tell patient to visit doctor regularly so that uric acid can be monitored and dosage adjusted, if necessary. Lifelong therapy may be required in patients with hyperuricemia.
• Advise patient with gout to avoid all medications that contain aspirin, which

may precipitate gout. Acetaminophen may be used for pain.
• Instruct patient to drink at least 6 to 8 glasses of water per day.
• Urge patient with gout to avoid alcohol; it increases urate level.
• Tell patient with gout to limit intake of foods high in purine, such as anchovies, liver, sardines, kidneys, sweetbreads, peas, and lentils. Also tell patient to identify and avoid any other foods that may trigger gout attacks.
• Instruct patient to take all medicine as prescribed when given as adjunct to penicillin.

---

sulfinpyrazone
Anturan†, Anturane

Pregnancy Risk Category: C

HOW SUPPLIED
Tablets: 100 mg
Capsules: 200 mg

ACTION
Blocks renal tubular reabsorption of uric acid, increasing excretion, and inhibits platelet aggregation.

Route	Onset	Peak	Duration
PO	Unknown	1-2 hr	4-6 hr

INDICATIONS & DOSAGE
Intermittent or chronic gouty arthritis—
Adults: 200 to 400 mg P.O. b.i.d. first week, then 400 mg P.O. b.i.d. Maximum dosage is 800 mg daily.

ADVERSE REACTIONS
GI: *nausea, dyspepsia,* epigastric pain, reactivation of peptic ulcerations.
Hematologic: *blood dyscrasias* (for example, anemia, *leukopenia, agranulocytosis, thrombocytopenia, aplastic anemia*).
Respiratory: *bronchoconstriction* in patients with aspirin-induced asthma.
Skin: rash.

INTERACTIONS
Drug-drug. *Aspirin, salicylates:* inhibited

---

uricosuric effect of sulfinpyrazone. Do not use together.
Oral anticoagulants: increased anticoagulant effect and risk of bleeding. Use together cautiously.
Oral antidiabetic agents: increased effects. Monitor blood glucose.
Probenecid: inhibited renal excretion of sulfinpyrazone. Use together cautiously.
Theophylline, verapamil: increased clearance. Use cautiously.
Drug-lifestyle. *Alcohol use:* decreased effectiveness. Avoid concomitant use.

EFFECTS ON DIAGNOSTIC TESTS
Drug decreases urinary excretion of aminohippuric acid and phenolsulfonphthalein and may alter renal function test results.

CONTRAINDICATIONS
Contraindicated in patients with hypersensitivity to pyrazole derivatives (including oxyphenbutazone and phenylbutazone), blood dyscrasias, active peptic ulcer, or symptoms of GI inflammation or ulceration.

NURSING CONSIDERATIONS
• Use cautiously in patients with healed peptic ulcer and in pregnant patients.
• Monitor periodic BUN, CBC, and renal function studies during long-term use, as ordered.
• Monitor fluid intake and output closely. Therapy, especially at start, may lead to renal colic and formation of uric acid stones until acid levels are normal (about 6 mg/dl).
• Force fluids to maintain minimum daily output of 2 to 3 L. Alkalinize urine with sodium bicarbonate or other agent, as ordered.
• Be aware that drug contains no analgesic or anti-inflammatory agent and is of no value during acute gout attacks.
• Know that drug may increase frequency, severity, and length of acute gout attacks during first 6 to 12 months of therapy. Prophylactic colchicine or another anti-inflammatory agent is given during first 3 to 6 months.
• Know that lifelong therapy may be required in patients with hyperuricemia.

☑ Patient teaching
• Instruct patient and family that drug must be taken regularly, as ordered, or gout attacks may result.
• Tell patient to visit doctor regularly so blood levels can be monitored and dosage adjusted, if necessary.
• Warn patient with gout not to take any aspirin-containing medications because these may precipitate gout. Acetaminophen may be used for pain.
• Tell patient with gout to avoid foods high in purine, such as anchovies, liver, sardines, kidneys, sweetbreads, peas, and lentils, and to identify and avoid any other foods that may trigger gout attacks.
• Instruct patient to drink at least 10 to 12 glasses of fluid daily.
• Advise patient to avoid alcohol while taking drug.
• Instruct patient to report unusual bleeding or bruising, or flulike symptoms.

chymopapain
fibrinolysin and
    desoxyribonuclease
hyaluronidase

COMBINATION PRODUCTS
None.

---

chymopapain
Chymodiactin

Pregnancy Risk Category: C

HOW SUPPLIED
Powder for injection: 4,000 units/vial;
each unit of chymopapain is also known
as 1 picoKatal (pKat)

ACTION
Hydrolyzes noncollagenous proteins in
the chondromucoprotein of the nucleus
pulposus, lowering pressure within the
disk.

Route	Onset	Peak	Duration
Intradisk	Unknown	Unknown	1 wk

INDICATIONS & DOSAGE
Herniated lumbar disk—
Adults: 2,000 to 4,000 units (pKat)/disk
injected intradiscally. Maximum dosage
for multiple disk herniation is 8,000 units.

ADVERSE REACTIONS
CNS: *subarachnoid and intracerebral
hemorrhage, seizures,* headache, dizziness.
EENT: conjunctivitis, vasomotor rhinitis.
GI: nausea, various GI disturbances.
Musculoskeletal: leg weakness, paresthesia, numbness of legs and toes, *back pain,
stiffness, back spasm, soreness.*
Skin: erythema, rash, pruritic urticaria.
Other: *anaphylaxis, anaphylactoid reaction, angioedema,* paraplegia, acute transverse myelitis.

INTERACTIONS
Drug-drug. *Radiographic contrast media:* potential adverse reactions (increased
risk of neurotoxicity) when injected concomitantly with chymopapain. Avoid concurrent use.

EFFECTS ON DIAGNOSTIC TESTS
None reported.

CONTRAINDICATIONS
Contraindicated in patients with history
of allergy to drug, papaya, or papaya derivatives (such as meat tenderizers); in
those who have previously received an injection of chymopapain; and in those with
severe spondylolisthesis in addition to
spinal stenosis, severe progressing paralysis, or evidence of spinal cord tumor or a
cauda equina lesion.

NURSING CONSIDERATIONS
● Know that a ChymoFAST test can detect hypersensitivity to drug. Giving histamine receptor antagonists before drug
may lessen the severity of anaphylactoid
reactions.
● Be aware that drug should be used only
by physicians qualified and experienced
to perform laminectomy, diskectomy, or
other spinal procedures, and who have received specialized training in chemonu-
cleolysis. It shouldn't be injected in any
region other than the lumbar spine; extremely toxic if injected into the subarachnoid space.
● Do not use bacteriostatic water for injection to reconstitute drug. Use sterile
water. Use within 1 hour after reconstitution. Discard unused drug.
● After wiping stopper with alcohol, allow
to dry before drawing up drug because alcohol inactivates the enzyme.
● Watch very closely for anaphylactoid reaction (0.5% of patients). Reaction may
be immediate or delayed up to 1 hour after injection and may last for minutes to
several hours. Watch for hypotension and
bronchospasm, possibly leading to laryn-

Reactions may be *common*, uncommon, *life-threatening*, or COMMON AND LIFE-THREATENING.

geal edema, arrhythmias, cardiac arrest, coma, and death. Other signs of allergic response include erythema, pilomotor erection, rash, pruritic urticaria, conjunctivitis, vasomotor rhinitis, angioedema, or various GI disturbances.
• Keep an I.V. line open to manage anaphylaxis quickly, if needed. Keep epinephrine and steroids available.

☑ **Patient teaching**
• Instruct patient to anticipate delayed allergic reactions, such as rash, urticaria, or pruritus, which may occur up to 15 days after injection. Patient should report these at once.
• Warn patient that he may experience back pain or involuntary muscle spasm in the lower back for several days after injection. Reassure him that this is common and not chronic.

---

fibrinolysin and desoxyribonuclease
Elase

Pregnancy Risk Category: C

HOW SUPPLIED
Powder for solution: 25 units fibrinolysin and 15,000 units desoxyribonuclease in 30-ml vial
Ointment: 30 units fibrinolysin and 20,000 units desoxyribonuclease in 10-g or 30-g tube (with applicator)

ACTION
Fibrinolysin attacks fibrin of blood clots and fibrinous exudates; desoxyribonuclease attacks DNA. Combined enzymatic action débrides wound surfaces and promotes healing.

Route	Onset	Peak	Duration
Intravaginal, transdermal	Unknown	Unknown	Unknown

INDICATIONS & DOSAGE
Débridement of inflammatory and infected lesions—
Adults and children: ointment applied to lesions daily to t.i.d. for as long as enzyme action is desired. Alternatively, solution prepared from powder applied topically as a liquid, spray, or wet dressing.

For wet-to-dry dressing, mix 1 vial of Elase powder with 10 to 50 ml of 0.9% NaCl solution; saturate strips of fine gauze with solution. Pack ulcerated area with Elase gauze. Let gauze dry in contact with ulcerated lesion for 6 to 8 hours. Remove dried gauze and repeat t.i.d. or q.i.d.
Mild-to-moderate cervicitis or vaginitis—
Adults: 5 g of ointment inserted intravaginally using applicator once daily h.s. for 5 days or until tube is empty.
Irrigation of infected wounds, empyema cavities, abscesses, otorhinolaryngologic wounds, subcutaneous hematomas—
Adults and children: dilute prepared solution and irrigate wound p.r.n., depending on extent and severity.

For solution as irrigating agent, drain cavity and replace Elase q 6 to 10 hours to reduce amount of by-product accumulation and to minimize loss of enzyme activity.

ADVERSE REACTIONS
Other: hyperemia (with high doses), *hypersensitivity reactions.*

INTERACTIONS
None significant.

EFFECTS ON DIAGNOSTIC TESTS
None reported.

CONTRAINDICATIONS
Contraindicated in patients with hypersensitivity to drug or bovine products; it is not for parenteral use.

NURSING CONSIDERATIONS
• Dense, dry eschar is surgically removed before enzymatic débridement. Enzyme must be in constant contact with substrate. Necrotic debris is removed periodically; the enzyme is replenished at least once daily.
• Prepare solution just before use and discard after 24 hours. Refrigerate unused portion.
• Clean and dry the wound; cover with a thin layer of Elase and nonadherent dressing.

• Ensure that aseptic wound-dressing techniques are used and that antibiotic therapy is instituted, as ordered.

• Change patient's dressing up to three times daily. Flush away necrotic debris and then reapply ointment. Be aware that the frequency of application may be more important than the amount of drug used.

✓ Patient teaching
• Explain drug use and administration to patient and family.
• Tell patient to report hypersensitivity reactions promptly.

---

hyaluronidase
Hyalase§, Wydase

Pregnancy Risk Category: C

HOW SUPPLIED
Injection: 150 units/ml in 1-ml, 10-ml vials

ACTION
Hydrolyzes hyaluronic acid, promoting diffusion of fluids in tissues.

Route	Onset	Peak	Duration
SC	Immediate	Unknown	1-2 days

INDICATIONS & DOSAGE
Adjunct to increase absorption and dispersion of other injected drugs—
Adults and children: 150 USP units added to solution containing other drug.
Hypodermoclysis—
Adults and children over 3 years: 150 USP units injected S.C. before clysis or injected into clysis tubing near needle for each 1,000 ml clysis solution.
Excretory urography when contrast medium is given S.C.—
Adults and children: with patient in a prone position, 75 USP units S.C. over each scapula, followed by injection of contrast medium at same sites.

ADVERSE REACTIONS
Skin: allergic reactions (rare).

INTERACTIONS
Drug-drug. *Local anesthetics:* increased potential for toxic local reaction. Use together cautiously.

EFFECTS ON DIAGNOSTIC TESTS
None reported.

CONTRAINDICATIONS
Contraindicated in patients with hypersensitivity to drug.

NURSING CONSIDERATIONS
• Perform a skin test (0.02 ml of solution) for sensitivity. Don't inject into diseased areas. Watch for local reactions (wheal and pseudopods within 5 minutes and persisting, with itching, for 20 to 30 minutes). Erythema alone is *not* considered positive reaction.
• Do not inject into acutely inflamed or cancerous areas.
• Drug not recommended for I.V. use.
• For children, add 15 units to each 100 ml of solution. Drip rate should not exceed 2 ml/minute.
• Don't add to solutions containing epinephrine and heparin.
• For hypodermoclysis, adjust dosage, rate of injection, and type of solution per patient's response, as ordered.
• If solution gets in eyes, flush with water.
• Protect from heat. Don't use cloudy or discolored solution. Store reconstituted solution below 86° F (30° C), and use within 14 days.

✓ Patient teaching
• Explain need for drug to patient and family and describe how drug is given.
• Inform patient about possible adverse skin reactions.

---

carboprost tromethamine
dinoprostone
methylergonovine maleate
oxytocin, synthetic injection
oxytocin, synthetic nasal solution

COMBINATION PRODUCTS
None.

carboprost tromethamine
Hemabate

Pregnancy Risk Category: C

HOW SUPPLIED
Injection: 250 mcg/ml

ACTION
A prostaglandin that produces strong, prompt contractions of uterine smooth muscle, possibly mediated by calcium and cAMP.

Route	Onset	Peak	Duration
IM	Unknown	15-60 min	24 hr

INDICATIONS & DOSAGE
To abort pregnancy between weeks 13 and 20 of gestation—
Adults: initially, 250 mcg deep I.M. Subsequent doses of 250 mcg administered at intervals of 1½ to 3½ hours, depending on uterine response. Dosage may be increased in increments to 500 mcg if contractility is inadequate after several 250-mcg doses. Total dosage should not exceed 12 mg.
Postpartum hemorrhage caused by uterine atony not managed by conventional methods—
Adults: 250 mcg by deep I.M. injection. Repeat doses administered at 15- to 90-minute intervals, as necessary. Maximum total dosage is 2 mg.

ADVERSE REACTIONS
CNS: headache, anxiety, hot flashes, paresthesia, syncope, weakness.
CV: chest pain, *arrhythmias.*
EENT: blurred vision, eye pain.
GI: *vomiting, diarrhea, nausea.*
GU: endometritis, *uterine rupture*, uterine or vaginal pain.
Respiratory: coughing, wheezing.
Skin: flushing, rash.
Other: *fever,* chills, backache, breast tenderness, diaphoresis, leg cramps.

INTERACTIONS
Drug-drug. *Other oxytocics:* may potentiate action. Avoid concomitant use.

EFFECTS ON DIAGNOSTIC TESTS
None reported.

CONTRAINDICATIONS
Contraindicated in patients hypersensitive to drug and in those with acute pelvic inflammatory disease or active cardiac, pulmonary, renal, or hepatic disease.

NURSING CONSIDERATIONS
• Use cautiously in patients with history of asthma; hypotension; hypertension; CV, adrenal, renal, or hepatic disease; anemia; jaundice; diabetes; seizure disorders; or previous uterine surgery.
• Unlike other prostaglandin abortifacients, carboprost is administered by I.M. injection. Injectable form avoids risk of expelling vaginal suppositories, which may occur in the presence of profuse vaginal bleeding.
• Know that carboprost should be used only by trained personnel in a hospital setting.

☑ Patient teaching
• Explain use and administration of drug to patient and family.
• Instruct patient to report adverse reactions promptly.

dinoprostone
Prepidil, Prostin E2

Pregnancy Risk Category: C

HOW SUPPLIED
Vaginal suppositories: 20 mg
Endocervical gel: 0.5 mg per application
(2.5-ml syringe)

ACTION
A prostaglandin that produces strong, prompt contractions of uterine smooth muscle, possibly mediated by calcium and cAMP.

Route	Onset	Peak	Duration
Intravaginal (suppository)	10 min	Unknown	2-6 hr
Intravaginal (gel)	15-30 min	Unknown	Unknown

INDICATIONS & DOSAGE
To abort second-trimester pregnancy; to evacuate uterus in missed abortion, intrauterine fetal deaths up to 28 weeks of gestation, or benign hydatidiform mole (suppository only)—
Adults: 20-mg suppository inserted high into posterior vaginal fornix. Repeated q 3 to 5 hours until abortion is complete.
Ripening of an unfavorable cervix in pregnant patients at or near term (gel only)—
Adults: contents of one syringe administered intravaginally; if cervix remains unfavorable after 6 hours, dosage repeated. No more than 1.5 mg (three applications) should be given within 24-hour period.

ADVERSE REACTIONS
CNS: *headache, dizziness,* anxiety, hot flashes, paresthesia, weakness, syncope.
CV: chest pain, ***arrhythmias.***
EENT: blurred vision, eye pain.
GI: *nausea, vomiting, diarrhea.*
GU: vaginal pain, vaginitis, endometritis.
Respiratory: coughing, dyspnea.
Skin: rash.
Other: *nocturnal leg cramps, fever, shivering, chills,* backache, breast tenderness, diaphoresis, muscle cramps.

INTERACTIONS
Drug-drug. *Other oxytocics:* may potentiate action. Avoid concomitant use.
Drug-lifestyle. *Alcohol use:* inhibited effectiveness of dinoprostone with high doses. Avoid concomitant use.

EFFECTS ON DIAGNOSTIC TESTS
None reported.

CONTRAINDICATIONS
Gel form is contraindicated where prolonged contractions of the uterus are considered inappropriate and in patients with hypersensitivity to prostaglandins or constituents of gel. Also contraindicated in patients with placenta previa or unexplained vaginal bleeding during pregnancy and in whom vaginal delivery is not indicated (that is, because of vasa previa or active herpes genitalia). Suppository form is contraindicated in patients with hypersensitivity to drug, acute pelvic inflammatory disease, and active cardiac, pulmonary, renal, or hepatic disease.

NURSING CONSIDERATIONS
● Use suppository form cautiously in patients with asthma; seizure disorders; anemia; diabetes; hypertension or hypotension; jaundice; CV, renal, or hepatic disease; scarred uterus; cervicitis; or acute vaginitis.
● Use gel form cautiously in patients with asthma or history of asthma, glaucoma or raised intraocular pressure, renal or hepatic dysfunction, and in patients with ruptured membranes.
● Administer only when critical care facilities are available.
● When using gel, warm to room temperature. After administration, patient should remain supine for 10 minutes.
● When used as an abortifacient, be prepared to pretreat patient with an antiemetic and an antidiarrheal agent.
● When used for cervical ripening, have patient lying on her back, with the cervix examined using a speculum. Assist with the insertion: using aseptic technique, catheter provided with the drug is used to administer gel into the cervical canal just below the level of the internal os.
● Be aware that when gel form is used,

Reactions may be *common,* uncommon, ***life-threatening,*** or **COMMON AND LIFE-THREATENING.**

contents of the syringe are used for one patient only. Discard syringe, catheter, and unused drug after administration; do not attempt to administer the small amount of drug remaining in the catheter.

• Treat dinoprostone-induced fever (self-limiting and transient and occurs in approximately 50% of all patients) with water sponging and increased fluid intake, not with aspirin.

• Check vaginal discharge regularly.

• Keep in mind that abortion should be complete within 30 hours when suppository form is used.

• Freeze suppositories at –4° F (–20° C).

☑ **Patient teaching**
• Explain use and administration of drug to patient and family.
• Instruct patient to report adverse reactions promptly.

---

methylergonovine maleate
Methergine

Pregnancy Risk Category: C

HOW SUPPLIED
Tablets: 0.2 mg
Injection: 0.2 mg/ml

ACTION
Increases motor activity of the uterus by direct stimulation of the smooth muscle.

Route	Onset	Peak	Duration
PO	5-10 min	30 min	3 hr
IV	Immediate	Unknown	45 min
IM	2-5 min	Unknown	3 hr

INDICATIONS & DOSAGE
Prevention and treatment of postpartum hemorrhage caused by uterine atony or subinvolution—
Adults: 0.2 mg I.M. q 2 to 4 hours; for excessive uterine bleeding or other emergencies, 0.2 mg I.V. over 1 minute while blood pressure and uterine contractions are monitored. After initial I.M. or I.V. dose, 0.2 mg P.O. q 6 to 8 hours for 2 to 7 days. Dosage decreased if severe cramping occurs.

ADVERSE REACTIONS
CNS: dizziness, headache, *CVA* (with I.V. use), *seizures,* hallucinations.
CV: hypertension, transient chest pain, palpitations, hypotension, thrombophlebitis.
EENT: tinnitus, nasal congestion.
GI: *nausea, vomiting,* diarrhea, foul taste.
GU: hematuria.
Respiratory: dyspnea.
Other: diaphoresis, leg cramps.

INTERACTIONS
Drug-drug. *Dopamine, I.V. oxytocin, regional anesthetics, vasoconstrictors:* excessive vasoconstriction. Use together cautiously.

EFFECTS ON DIAGNOSTIC TESTS
Drug therapy may decrease serum prolactin concentrations.

CONTRAINDICATIONS
Contraindicated in patients with hypertension, toxemia, or sensitivity to ergot preparations, and during pregnancy.

NURSING CONSIDERATIONS
• Use cautiously in patients with sepsis, obliterative vascular disease, hepatic or renal disease, and during last stage of labor.
• Monitor and record blood pressure, pulse rate, and uterine response; report sudden change in vital signs, frequent periods of uterine relaxation, and character and amount of vaginal bleeding.
• Monitor contractions, which may continue 3 hours or more after P.O. or I.M. administration.
• Store tablets in tightly closed, light-resistant containers. Discard if discolored.

🔻 **I.V. administration**
Alert: Keep in mind that drug should not be routinely administered I.V. because of the risk of severe hypertension and CVA. If it must be given by this route, administer slowly over 1 minute with careful blood pressure monitoring. I.V. dose may be diluted to 5 ml with 0.9% NaCl solution before use. Contractions begin immediately after I.V. use and continue for up to 45 minutes.
• Store I.V. solutions below 46.4° F

---

*Liquid contains alcohol.   **May contain tartrazine.   †Canada   ‡Australia   §U.K.   ◊ OTC

(8° C). Daily stock may be kept at room temperature for 60 to 90 days.

✔ Patient teaching
- Explain use and administration of drug to patient and family.
- Instruct patient to report adverse reactions promptly.

---

oxytocin, synthetic injection
Oxytocin, Pitocin

Pregnancy Risk Category: C

HOW SUPPLIED
Injection: 10 units/ml ampule, vial, or tubex

ACTION
Causes potent and selective stimulation of uterine and mammary gland smooth muscle.

Route	Onset	Peak	Duration
IV	Immediate	Unknown	1 hr
IM	3-5 min	Unknown	2-3 hr

INDICATIONS & DOSAGE
Induction or stimulation of labor—
Adults: initially, 1-ml (10 units) ampule in 1,000 ml of D_5W injection or 0.9% NaCl solution I.V. infused at 1 to 2 milliunits/minute. Rate increased in increments not exceeding 1 to 2 milliunits/minute at 15- to 30-minute intervals until normal contraction pattern is established. Rate decreased when labor is firmly established.
Reduction of postpartum bleeding after expulsion of placenta—
Adults: 10 to 40 units added to 1,000 ml of D_5W or 0.9% NaCl solution infused at rate necessary to control bleeding, usually 20 to 40 milliunits/minute. Also, 1 ml (10 units) can be given I.M. after delivery of placenta.
Incomplete or inevitable abortion—
Adults: 10 units of oxytocin I.V. in 500 ml of 0.9% NaCl solution or dextrose 5% in 0.9% NaCl solution. Infuse at rate of 10 to 20 milliunits (20 to 40 drops)/minute.

ADVERSE REACTIONS
Maternal—
CNS: *subarachnoid hemorrhage* (from hypertension); *seizures or coma* (from water intoxication).
CV: hypertension; increased heart rate, systemic venous return, and cardiac output; *arrhythmias.*
GI: nausea, vomiting.
Hematologic: *afibrinogenemia* (may be related to postpartum bleeding).
Other: *hypersensitivity reactions (anaphylaxis),* tetanic uterine contractions, *abruptio placentae,* impaired uterine blood flow, pelvic hematoma, increased uterine motility, *uterine rupture, postpartum hemorrhage.*
Fetal—
CV: bradycardia, *PVC, arrhythmias.*
Respiratory: *anoxia, asphyxia.*
Other: *infant brain damage, low Apgar scores at 5 minutes,* neonatal jaundice, neonatal retinal hemorrhage.

INTERACTIONS
Drug-drug. *Cyclopropane anesthetics:* less pronounced bradycardia and hypotension. Use together cautiously.
Thiopental anesthetics: possible delayed induction. Use together cautiously.
Vasoconstrictors: severe hypertension if oxytocin is given within 3 to 4 hours of vasoconstrictor in patients receiving caudal block anesthetic. Avoid concomitant use.

EFFECTS ON DIAGNOSTIC TESTS
None reported.

CONTRAINDICATIONS
Contraindicated when vaginal delivery is not advised (placenta previa or vasa previa), cephalopelvic disproportion is present, or when delivery requires conversion, as in transverse lie; in fetal distress when delivery isn't imminent, prematurity, and other obstetric emergencies; and in patients with severe toxemia, hypertonic uterine patterns, or hypersensitivity to drug.

NURSING CONSIDERATIONS
- Use with extreme caution during first and second stages of labor because cervical laceration, uterine rupture, and maternal and fetal death have been reported.
- Use with extreme caution, if at all, in patients with history of cervical or uterine surgery (including cesarean section),

---

Reactions may be *common,* uncommon, *life-threatening,* or **COMMON AND LIFE-THREATENING.**

grand multiparity, uterine sepsis, traumatic delivery, or overdistended uterus and in invasive cervical cancer.
• Know that drug is not recommended for routine I.M. use. However, 10 units may be given I.M. after delivery of placenta to control postpartum uterine bleeding.
• Never give oxytocin simultaneously by more than one route.
• Be aware that drug is used to induce or reinforce labor only when pelvis is known to be adequate, when vaginal delivery is indicated, when fetal maturity is assured, and when fetal position is favorable. Should be used only in hospital where critical care facilities and doctor are immediately available.
• Monitor fluid intake and output. Antidiuretic effect may lead to fluid overload, seizures, and coma.
• Monitor and record uterine contractions, heart rate, blood pressure, intrauterine pressure, fetal heart rate, and character of blood loss every 15 minutes.
• Have magnesium sulfate (20% solution) available for relaxation of the myometrium.
• If contractions occur less than 2 minutes apart and if contractions above 50 mm Hg are recorded, or if contractions last 90 seconds or longer, stop infusion, turn the patient on her side, and notify the doctor.
• Oxytocin is not known to present a risk of fetal abnormalities when used as indicated.

I.V. administration
• Dilute drug by adding 10 units to 1 L of 0.9% NaCl, lactated Ringer's, or D₅W solution for induction or stimulation of labor, or by adding 10 units to 500 ml of 0.9% NaCl, lactated Ringer's, or D₅W solution to produce intense uterine contractions and reduce postpartum bleeding.
• Don't give by I.V. bolus injection. Administer by infusion only; give by piggyback infusion so the drug may be discontinued without interrupting the I.V. line. Use an infusion pump.

✓ Patient teaching
• Explain use and administration of drug to patient and family.

• Instruct patient to report adverse reactions promptly.

---

oxytocin, synthetic nasal solution
Syntocinon†

Pregnancy Risk Category: X

HOW SUPPLIED
Nasal solution: 40 units/ml

ACTION
Stimulates smooth muscle to facilitate ejection of milk from breasts.

Route	Onset	Peak	Duration
Intranasal	≤ Few min	Unknown	20 min

INDICATIONS & DOSAGE
Promotion of initial milk ejection—
Adults: 1 spray into one or both nostrils 2 or 3 minutes before breast-feeding or pumping breasts.

ADVERSE REACTIONS
EENT: nasal irritation, rhinorrhea, lacrimation.
Other: uterine bleeding, uterine contractions.

INTERACTIONS
None significant.

EFFECTS ON DIAGNOSTIC TESTS
None reported.

CONTRAINDICATIONS
Contraindicated in patients with hypersensitivity to drug and during pregnancy.

NURSING CONSIDERATIONS
• Inspect nasal cavity for signs of irritation.

✓ Patient teaching
• Teach patient how to administer drug. Instruct her to clear nasal passages first, then hold her head in a vertical position and, holding squeeze bottle upright, eject solution into nostril.
• Inform patient of adverse reactions associated with drug and to notify doctor if severe.

---

*Liquid contains alcohol.   **May contain tartrazine.   †Canada   ‡Australia   §U.K.   ◇ OTC

Spasmolytics

flavoxate hydrochloride
oxybutynin chloride
phenazopyridine hydrochloride

COMBINATION PRODUCTS
None.

---

flavoxate hydrochloride
Urispas

Pregnancy Risk Category: NR

HOW SUPPLIED
Tablets: 100 mg

ACTION
Produces direct spasmolytic effect on smooth muscles of the urinary tract and provides some local anesthesia and analgesia.

Route	Onset	Peak	Duration
PO	Unknown	2 hr	Unknown

INDICATIONS & DOSAGE
Symptomatic relief of dysuria, urinary frequency and urgency, nocturia, incontinence, and suprapubic pain associated with urologic disorders—
Adults and children over 12 years: 100 to 200 mg P.O. t.i.d. to q.i.d. Dosage may be reduced with improvement of symptoms.

ADVERSE REACTIONS
CNS: *confusion* (especially in elderly patients), nervousness, dizziness, headache, drowsiness.
CV: tachycardia, palpitations.
EENT: *blurred vision,* disturbed eye accommodation, increased ocular tension.
GI: dry mouth, nausea, vomiting.
GU: dysuria.
Hematologic: eosinophilia, *leukopenia.*
Skin: urticaria, dermatoses.
Other: fever.

INTERACTIONS
Drug-lifestyle. *Exercise, hot weather:* may precipitate heat stroke. Use cautiously.

EFFECTS ON DIAGNOSTIC TESTS
None reported.

CONTRAINDICATIONS
Contraindicated in patients with pyloric or duodenal obstruction, obstructive intestinal lesions or ileus, achalasia, GI hemorrhage, or obstructive uropathies of lower urinary tract.

NURSING CONSIDERATIONS
• Use cautiously in patients suspected of having glaucoma.
• Know that safety and effectiveness in children 12 years and under is unknown.
• Check history for other drug use before giving drugs with anticholinergic adverse reactions. Such reactions may be intensified by flavoxate.

✓ Patient teaching
• Warn patient to avoid hazardous activities, such as operating machinery or driving, until CNS effects of drug are known.
• Tell patient to contact doctor if adverse reactions occur or if symptoms don't diminish.
• Caution patient that using drug during very hot weather may precipitate fever or heatstroke because it suppresses diaphoresis.

---

oxybutynin chloride
Cystrin§, Ditropan

Pregnancy Risk Category: B

HOW SUPPLIED
Tablets: 5 mg
Syrup: 5 g/5 ml

ACTION
Produces a direct spasmolytic effect and an antimuscarinic (atropine-like) effect on

---

Reactions may be *common*, uncommon, *life-threatening*, or COMMON AND LIFE-THREATENING.

urinary tract smooth muscles, increasing urinary bladder capacity and providing some local anesthesia and mild analgesia.

Route	Onset	Peak	Duration
PO	30-60 min	3-4 hr	6-10 hr

INDICATIONS & DOSAGE
Antispasmodic for uninhibited or reflex neurogenic bladder—
Adults: 5 mg P.O. b.i.d. to t.i.d., to maximum of 5 mg q.i.d.
Children over 5 years: 5 mg P.O. b.i.d., to maximum of 5 mg t.i.d.

ADVERSE REACTIONS
CNS: dizziness, insomnia, restlessness, hallucinations, asthenia.
CV: *palpitations, tachycardia,* vasodilation.
EENT: mydriasis, cycloplegia, decreased lacrimation, amblyopia.
GI: nausea, vomiting, *dry mouth, constipation,* decreased GI motility.
GU: impotence, *urinary hesitancy, urine retention.*
Skin: rash.
Other: decreased diaphoresis, fever, suppression of lactation.

INTERACTIONS
Drug-drug. *Anticholinergics:* increased anticholinergic effects. Use cautiously.
Atenolol, digoxin: increased levels of these drugs. Monitor closely.
CNS depressants: increased CNS effects. Use cautiously.
Haloperidol, levodopa: decreased levels of these drugs. Monitor closely.
Drug-lifestyle. *Alcohol use:* increased CNS effects. Avoid concomitant use.
Exercise, hot weather: may precipitate heat stroke. Use cautiously.

EFFECTS ON DIAGNOSTIC TESTS
None reported.

CONTRAINDICATIONS
Contraindicated in patients with hypersensitivity to drug, myasthenia gravis, GI obstruction, untreated narrow-angle glaucoma, adynamic ileus, megacolon, severe colitis, ulcerative colitis when megacolon is present, or obstructive uropathy; in el-

derly or debilitated patients with intestinal atony; and in hemorrhaging patients with unstable CV status.

NURSING CONSIDERATIONS
● Use cautiously in elderly patients and in patients with autonomic neuropathy, reflux esophagitis, and hepatic or renal disease.
● Before giving oxybutynin, anticipate confirmation of neurogenic bladder by cystometry and rule out partial intestinal obstruction in patients with diarrhea, especially those with colostomy or ileostomy.
● If urinary tract infection is present, administer antibiotics, as ordered.
● Be aware that drug may aggravate symptoms of hyperthyroidism, coronary artery disease, heart failure, arrhythmias, tachycardia, hypertension, or prostatic hyperplasia.
● Periodically prepare patient for cystometry to evaluate response to therapy.

☑ Patient teaching
● Warn patient to avoid hazardous activities, such as operating machinery or driving, until CNS effects of drug are known.
● Caution patient that using oxybutynin during very hot weather may precipitate fever or heatstroke because it suppresses diaphoresis.
● Advise patient to store drug in tightly closed containers at 59° to 86° F (15° to 30° C).
● Advise patient to avoid alcohol while taking drug.

---

phenazopyridine hydrochloride (phenylazo diamino pyridine hydrochloride)
AZO-Standard ◇, Baridium ◇, Eridium ◇, Geridium ◇, Phenazo†, Phenazodine ◇, Prodium ◇, Pyridiate ◇, Pyridium, Pyronium†, Urodine ◇, Urogesic ◇, Viridium ◇

Pregnancy Risk Category: B

HOW SUPPLIED
Tablets: 100 mg ◇, 200 mg

ACTION
Exerts local anesthetic action on urinary mucosa through unknown mechanism.

Route	Onset	Peak	Duration
PO	Unknown	Unknown	Unknown

INDICATIONS & DOSAGE
Pain with urinary tract irritation or infection—
Adults: 200 mg P.O. t.i.d. after meals for 2 days.
Children: 12 mg/kg P.O. daily in three equally divided doses after meals for 2 days.

ADVERSE REACTIONS
CNS: headache.
GI: nausea, GI disturbances.
Hematologic: hemolytic anemia.
Skin: rash, pruritus.
Other: *anaphylactoid reactions,* methemoglobinemia.

INTERACTIONS
None significant.

EFFECTS ON DIAGNOSTIC TESTS
Drug may alter results of Diastix or Chemstrip uG, Acetest, and Ketostix. Clinitest should be used to obtain accurate urine glucose test results. Drug may also interfere with Ehrlich's test for urine urobilinogen; phenolsulfonphthalein excretion tests of kidney function; sulfobromophthalein excretion tests of liver function; and urine tests for protein, steroids, or bilirubin.

CONTRAINDICATIONS
Contraindicated in patients with glomerulonephritis, severe hepatitis, uremia, or renal insufficiency, hypersensitivity to drug, or pyelonephritis during pregnancy.

NURSING CONSIDERATIONS
• Know that when drug is used with an antibacterial agent, therapy should not extend beyond 2 days.

✓ **Patient teaching**
• Advise patient that taking drug with meals may minimize GI distress.
• Caution patient to stop taking drug and to notify doctor immediately if skin or sclera becomes yellow-tinged. These signs may indicate drug accumulation caused by impaired renal excretion.
• Alert patient that drug colors urine red or orange; may stain fabrics or contact lenses.
• Tell diabetic patient that drug may alter Diastix or Chemstrip uG results. He should use Clinitest for accurate urine glucose test results. Also tell patient that drug may interfere with urinary ketone tests (Acetest or Ketostix).
• Advise patient that persistent urinary tract pain should be reported to the doctor and that this drug is not for long-term treatment.

auranofin
aurothioglucose
gold sodium thiomalate

COMBINATION PRODUCTS
None.

---

auranofin
Ridaura

Pregnancy Risk Category: C

HOW SUPPLIED
Capsules: 3 mg

ACTION
Unknown. Anti-inflammatory effects in rheumatoid arthritis are probably caused by inhibition of sulfhydryl systems, which alters cellular metabolism. Auranofin may also alter enzyme function and immune response and suppress phagocytic activity.

Route	Onset	Peak	Duration
PO	Unknown	2 hr	Unknown

INDICATIONS & DOSAGE
Rheumatoid arthritis—
Adults: 6 mg P.O. daily, either as 3 mg b.i.d. or 6 mg once daily. After 6 months, may be increased to 9 mg daily.
Children: initially, 0.1 mg/kg/day. Maintenance dose 0.15 mg/kg/day; maximum dose 0.2 mg/kg/day.

ADVERSE REACTIONS
CNS: confusion, hallucinations, *seizures.*
EENT: conjunctivitis.
GI: *diarrhea, abdominal pain, nausea, stomatitis,* glossitis, anorexia, metallic taste, dyspepsia, flatulence, constipation, dysgeusia, ulcerative colitis.
GU: proteinuria, hematuria, nephrotic syndrome, glomerulonephritis, *acute renal failure.*
Hematologic: *thrombocytopenia* (with or without purpura), *aplastic anemia, agranulocytosis, leukopenia,* eosinophilia, anemia.
Hepatic: jaundice, elevated liver enzymes.
Respiratory: interstitial pneumonitis.
Skin: *rash, pruritus, dermatitis,* exfoliative dermatitis, urticaria, erythema, alopecia.

INTERACTIONS
Drug-drug. *Phenytoin:* may increase phenytoin blood levels. Monitor for toxicity.

EFFECTS ON DIAGNOSTIC TESTS
Serum protein-bound iodine test, especially when done by the chloric acid digestion method, gives false readings during and for several weeks after gold therapy. May enhance tuberculin skin test.

CONTRAINDICATIONS
Contraindicated in patients with history of severe gold toxicity, necrotizing enterocolitis, pulmonary fibrosis, exfoliative dermatitis, bone marrow aplasia, severe hematologic disorders, or history of severe toxicity caused by previous exposure to other heavy metals. Also contraindicated in patients with urticaria, eczema, colitis, severe debilitation, hemorrhagic conditions, or systemic lupus erythematosus, and in patients who have recently received radiation therapy.

NURSING CONSIDERATIONS
• Use cautiously with other drugs that cause blood dyscrasias. Also use cautiously in patients who have preexisting renal, hepatic, or inflammatory bowel disease; rash; or history of bone marrow depression.
• Monitor patient's platelet count monthly. Auranofin should be stopped if platelet count falls below 100,000/mm^3, if hemoglobin drops suddenly, if granulocytes are below 1,500/mm^3, or if leukopenia (WBC count below 4,000/mm^3) or eosinophilia (eosinophils over 75%) is present.

Alert: Monitor patient's urinalysis results monthly. If proteinuria or hematuria is detected, stop drug because it can cause nephrotic syndrome or glomerulonephritis, and notify doctor.
• Monitor liver function tests.

☑ Patient teaching
• Encourage patient to take drug as prescribed.
• Tell patient to continue concomitant drug therapy if prescribed.
• Remind patient to see doctor for monthly platelet counts.
• Suggest patient has regular urinalysis.
• Tell patient to keep taking drug if mild diarrhea occurs but to immediately report blood in stool. Diarrhea is the most common adverse reaction.
• Advise patient to report rash or other skin problems and stop drug until reaction subsides. Pruritus may precede dermatitis; pruritic skin eruptions while patient is receiving auranofin should be considered a reaction until proven otherwise.
• Inform patient that stomatitis may be preceded by a metallic taste, which he should report. Promote careful oral hygiene during therapy.
• Advise patient to report unusual bleeding or bruising.
• Inform patient that beneficial effect may be delayed as long as 3 months. If response is inadequate and maximum dose has been reached, expect doctor to discontinue drug.
• Warn patient not to give drug to others. Auranofin should be prescribed only for selected patients with rheumatoid arthritis.

---

aurothioglucose
Gold-50‡, Solganal

gold sodium thiomalate
Aurolate

Pregnancy Risk Category: C

HOW SUPPLIED
aurothioglucose
Injection (suspension): 50 mg/ml in sesame oil in 10-ml vial

gold sodium thiomalate
Injection: 50 mg/ml with benzyl alcohol

ACTION
Unknown. Anti-inflammatory effects in rheumatoid arthritis are probably caused by inhibition of sulfhydryl systems, which alters cellular metabolism. Gold salts may also alter enzyme function and immune response and suppress phagocytic activity.

Route	Onset	Peak	Duration
IM	Unknown	3-6 hr	Unknown

INDICATIONS & DOSAGE
Rheumatoid arthritis—
aurothioglucose
Adults: initially, 10 mg I.M., followed by 25 mg for second and third doses at weekly intervals. Then, 50 mg weekly until 800 mg to 1 g has been given. If improvement occurs without toxicity, 25 to 50 mg is continued at 3- to 4-week intervals indefinitely.
Children 6 to 12 years: ¼ usual adult dosage. Do not exceed 25 mg per dose.
gold sodium thiomalate
Adults: initially, 10 mg I.M., followed by 25 mg in 1 week. Then, 25 to 50 mg weekly to total dose of 1 g. If improvement occurs without toxicity, 25 to 50 mg q 2 weeks for 2 to 20 weeks; then, 25 to 50 mg q 3 to 4 weeks as maintenance therapy. If relapse occurs, injections are resumed at weekly intervals.
Children: initially, 10 mg I.M., followed by 1 mg/kg I.M. weekly, not to exceed 50 mg for a single injection. Follow adult spacing of doses.

ADVERSE REACTIONS
CNS: confusion, hallucinations, *seizures.*
CV: bradycardia, hypotension.
EENT: corneal gold deposition, corneal ulcers.
GI: *diarrhea,* anorexia, abdominal cramps, nausea, vomiting, ulcerative enterocolitis, *metallic taste, stomatitis.*
GU: albuminuria, proteinuria, nephrotic syndrome, nephritis, acute tubular necrosis, hematuria, *acute renal failure.*
Hematologic: *thrombocytopenia* (with or without purpura), *aplastic anemia,*

Reactions may be *common,* uncommon, *life-threatening,* or COMMON AND LIFE-THREATENING.

agranulocytosis, leukopenia, eosinophilia, anemia.

Hepatic: hepatitis, jaundice, elevated liver function tests.

Skin: photosensitivity, *rash, dermatitis,* erythema, exfoliative dermatitis.

Other: *anaphylaxis, angioedema,* diaphoresis.

INTERACTIONS

Drug-lifestyle. *Sun or ultraviolet light exposure:* photosensitivity reactions may occur. Take precautions.

EFFECTS ON DIAGNOSTIC TESTS

Serum protein-bound iodine test, especially when done by chloric acid digestion method, gives false readings during and for several weeks after therapy.

CONTRAINDICATIONS

Contraindicated in patients with hypersensitivity to drug; in those with history of severe toxicity from previous exposure to gold or other heavy metals, hepatitis, or exfoliative dermatitis; and in patients with severe uncontrollable diabetes, renal disease, hepatic dysfunction, uncontrolled heart failure, systemic lupus erythematosus, colitis, or Sjögren's syndrome. Also contraindicated in patients with urticaria, eczema, hemorrhagic conditions, or severe hematologic disorders and in those who have recently received radiation therapy.

NURSING CONSIDERATIONS

• Use with extreme caution, if at all, in patients with rash, marked hypertension, compromised cerebral or CV circulation, or history of renal or hepatic disease, drug allergies, or blood dyscrasias.

• Give only under constant supervision of doctor thoroughly familiar with drug's toxicities and benefits.

• Give gold salts I.M., as ordered, preferably intragluteally. Drug is pale yellow; don't use if it darkens.

• Immerse aurothioglucose vial in warm water; shake vigorously before injecting.

• When injecting gold sodium thiomalate, have patient lie down for 10 to 20 minutes to minimize hypotension.

• Watch for anaphylactoid reaction for 30 minutes after administration.

Alert: Keep dimercaprol on hand to treat acute toxicity.

• Analyze urine for protein and sediment changes before each injection.

• Monitor CBC, including platelet count, before every second injection.

• Monitor platelet counts if patients develop purpura or ecchymoses.

• Know that gold therapy may alter liver function studies.

• If adverse reactions are mild, some rheumatologists resume gold therapy after 2 to 3 weeks' rest.

☑ Patient teaching

• Inform patient that increased joint pain may occur for 1 to 2 days after injection but usually subsides.

• Advise patient to report rash or skin problems immediately and stop drug until reaction subsides. Pruritus may precede dermatitis; pruritic skin eruptions while patient is receiving gold therapy should be considered a reaction until proven otherwise.

• Instruct patient to report a metallic taste. Promote careful oral hygiene.

• Urge patient to avoid sunlight and artificial ultraviolet light.

• Tell patient that benefits may not appear for 3 to 4 months.

• Stress need for medical follow-up.

97

Miscellaneous antagonists and antidotes

activated charcoal
aminocaproic acid
ammonia, aromatic spirits
deferoxamine mesylate
digoxin immune Fab
dimercaprol
disulfiram
d-penicillamine
edetate calcium disodium
edetate disodium
flumazenil
ipecac syrup
naloxone hydrochloride
naltrexone hydrochloride
pralidoxime chloride
protamine sulfate
sodium polystyrene sulfonate
succimer

(See also Chapter 38, ANTICHOLINERGICS.)
(See also Chapter 40, ADRENERGIC BLOCKERS [SYMPATHOLYTICS].)

COMBINATION PRODUCTS
None.

activated charcoal
Actidose ◊, Actidose-Aqua ◊,
CharcoAid ◊, CharcoCaps ◊,
Liqui-Char ◊

Pregnancy Risk Category: C

HOW SUPPLIED
Tablets: 200 mg‡ ◊, 250 mg ◊,
300 mg‡ ◊
Capsules: 260 mg ◊
Powder: 30 g ◊, 50 g ◊
Oral suspension: 0.625 g/5 ml ◊,
1 g/5 ml ◊, 1.25 g/5 ml ◊

ACTION
An adsorbent that adheres to many drugs and chemicals, inhibiting their absorption from the GI tract.

Route	Onset	Peak	Duration
PO	Immediate	Unknown	Unknown

INDICATIONS & DOSAGE
Flatulence or dyspepsia—
Adults: 600 mg to 5 g P.O. as a single dose or 0.975 g to 3.9 g P.O. t.i.d. after meals.
Poisoning—
Adults and children: initially, 1 to 2 g/kg (30 to 100 g) P.O. or 10 times the amount of poison ingested as a suspension in 120 to 240 ml (4 to 8 oz) of water.

Commonly used for treating poisoning or overdosage with acetaminophen, aspirin, atropine, barbiturates, dextropropoxyphene, digoxin, poisonous mushrooms, oxalic acid, parathion, phenol, phenylpropanolamine, phenytoin, propantheline, propoxyphene, strychnine, or tricyclic antidepressants.

Check with poison control center for use in other types of poisonings or overdoses.

ADVERSE REACTIONS
GI: *black stools,* nausea, constipation, intestinal obstruction.

INTERACTIONS
Drug-drug. *Acetylcysteine, ipecac:* agents inactivated by charcoal. Administer charcoal after vomiting has been induced by ipecac; remove charcoal by nasogastric tube before giving acetylcysteine.

EFFECTS ON DIAGNOSTIC TESTS
None reported.

CONTRAINDICATIONS
No known contraindications.

NURSING CONSIDERATIONS
• Be aware that although there are no contraindications for drug, it is not effective in the treatment of all acute poisonings.
• Give after emesis is complete because activated charcoal absorbs and inactivates syrup of ipecac.
• Mix powder form (most effective) with tap water to form consistency of thick

syrup. Adding a small amount of fruit juice or flavoring will make mix more palatable. Do not mix with ice cream, milk, or sherbet because these will decrease the absorptive capacity of activated charcoal.
• Give by large bore nasogastric tube after lavage if necessary.
• If patient vomits shortly after administration, be prepared to repeat dose.
• Space doses at least 1 hour apart from other drugs if treatment is for indications other than poisoning.
• Follow treatment with stool softener or laxative, as ordered, to prevent constipation unless sorbitol is part of product ingredients.
• Be aware that preparations made with sorbitol have a laxative effect that lessens the risk of severe constipation or fecal impaction.
• Do not use charcoal with sorbitol in fructose-intolerant patients or in children under 1 year.
• Ineffective for poisoning or overdose of cyanide, mineral acids, caustic alkalis, and organic solvents; not very effective with ethanol, lithium, methanol, and iron salts.

☑ **Patient teaching**
• Explain use and administration of drug to patient (if awake) and family.
• Warn patient that stools will be black.

---

aminocaproic acid
Amicar

Pregnancy Risk Category: C

HOW SUPPLIED
Tablets: 500 mg
Syrup: 250 mg/ml
Injection: 250 mg/ml

ACTION
Inhibits plasminogen activator substances and, to a lesser degree, blocks antiplasmin activity by inhibiting fibrinolysis.

Route	Onset	Peak	Duration
PO	1 hr	2 hr	Unknown
IV	1 hr	Unknown	3 hr

INDICATIONS & DOSAGE
Excessive bleeding resulting from hyperfibrinolysis—
Adults: initially, 5 g P.O. or slow I.V. infusion, followed by 1 to 1.25 g hourly until bleeding is controlled. Maximum dosage is 30 g daily.

ADVERSE REACTIONS
CNS: dizziness, malaise, headache, delirium, *seizures*, hallucinations, weakness.
CV: hypotension, bradycardia, *arrhythmias* (with rapid I.V. infusion).
EENT: tinnitus, nasal congestion, conjunctival suffusion.
GI: nausea, cramps, diarrhea.
Hematologic: generalized thrombosis.
Hepatic: increased CK, AST, and ALT levels.
Skin: rash.
Other: myopathy, *acute renal failure.*

INTERACTIONS
Drug-drug. *Estrogens, oral contraceptives:* increased probability of hypercoagulability. Use together cautiously.

EFFECTS ON DIAGNOSTIC TESTS
None reported.

CONTRAINDICATIONS
Contraindicated in patients with hematuria, active intravascular clotting, or presence of disseminated intravascular coagulation, unless heparin is used concomitantly. Injectable form is contraindicated in newborns.

NURSING CONSIDERATIONS
• Use cautiously in patients with cardiac, hepatic, or renal disease.
Alert: Monitor coagulation studies, as ordered, and heart rhythm and blood pressure. Notify doctor of changes immediately.

◖ I.V. administration
• Dilute solution with sterile water for injection, 0.9% NaCl for injection, D_5W, or Ringer's injection. Infuse slowly. Don't give by direct or intermittent injection.

☑ **Patient teaching**
• Explain use and administration of drug to patient and family.
• Instruct patient to report adverse reactions promptly.

ammonia, aromatic spirits ◇

Pregnancy Risk Category: NR

HOW SUPPLIED
Solution: 30 ml ◇, 60 ml ◇, 120 ml ◇; pints ◇; gallons ◇
Inhalant: 0.33 ml ◇, 0.4 ml ◇

ACTION
Irritates the sensory receptors in the nasal membranes, producing reflex stimulation of the respiratory centers.

Route	Onset	Peak	Duration
PO, inhalation	Immediate	Unknown	Unknown

INDICATIONS & DOSAGE
Treatment or prevention of fainting—
Adults and children: 1 broken capsule inhaled until awake or no longer faint; or 2 to 4 ml P.O. diluted in at least 30 ml of water.

ADVERSE REACTIONS
EENT: irritation.

INTERACTIONS
None significant.

EFFECTS ON DIAGNOSTIC TESTS
None reported.

CONTRAINDICATIONS
No known contraindications.

NURSING CONSIDERATIONS
• Avoid inhaling vapors when administering drug.
• Monitor patient closely for response.

☑ **Patient teaching**
• Instruct patient how to use drug.
• Tell patient to store drug in refrigerator.

deferoxamine mesylate
Desferal

Pregnancy Risk Category: C

HOW SUPPLIED
Powder for injection: 500 mg

ACTION
Chelates iron by binding ferric ions.

Route	Onset	Peak	Duration
IV, IM, SC	Unknown	Unknown	Unknown

INDICATIONS & DOSAGE
Adjunctive treatment of acute iron intoxication—
Adults and children: 1 g I.M., followed by 500 mg I.M. for two doses q 4 hours; then 500 mg I.M. q 4 to 12 hours. Maximum dosage is 6 g in 24 hours. Give I.V. by slow infusion (15 mg/kg/hour or less) only in CV collapse.
Chronic iron overload from multiple transfusions—
Adults and children: 500 mg to 1 g I.M. daily and 2 g by slow I.V. infusion in separate solution along with each unit of blood transfused. Maximum dosage is 6 g daily. Alternatively, 20 to 40 mg/kg via S.C. infusion pump daily.

ADVERSE REACTIONS
CV: tachycardia (with long-term use).
EENT: blurred vision, cataracts, hearing loss.
GI: diarrhea, abdominal discomfort (with long-term use).
GU: dysuria (with long-term use).
Other: *hypersensitivity reactions* (cutaneous wheal formation, pruritus, rash, *anaphylaxis*); pain, induration (at injection site); leg cramps, fever; *erythema, urticaria, hypotension, anaphylaxis, severe hypotension* (after too-rapid I.V. administration).

INTERACTIONS
Drug-drug. *Ascorbic acid:* may enhance effects of deferoxamine and increase tissue toxicity of iron. Use together with extreme caution and close monitoring.

EFFECTS ON DIAGNOSTIC TESTS
None reported.

CONTRAINDICATIONS
Contraindicated in patients with severe renal disease, anuria, or primary hemochromatosis.

NURSING CONSIDERATIONS
• Use cautiously in patients with impaired renal function.
• After reconstitution, administer I.M. or add to 0.9% NaCl solution, D_5W, or lactated Ringer's solution and infuse at a rate not exceeding 15 mg/kg hour.
Alert: Have epinephrine 1:1,000 available to treat hypersensitivity reaction.
• Monitor fluid intake and output carefully.

◨ **I.V. administration**
• To reconstitute, add 2 ml of sterile water for injection to each ampule. Make sure drug is completely dissolved. Reconstituted solution is good for 1 week at room temperature. Protect from light.

☑ **Patient teaching**
• Warn patient that urine may be red. Tell him to report persistent or serious adverse reactions promptly.
• Advise patient to have regular eye examinations during long-term therapy because cataract formation has been reported.

---

digoxin immune Fab (ovine)
Digibind

Pregnancy Risk Category: C

HOW SUPPLIED
Injection: 38-mg vial

ACTION
Binds molecules of unbound digoxin and digitoxin, making them unavailable for binding at site of action on cells.

Route	Onset	Peak	Duration
IV	30 min	End of infusion	15-20 hr

INDICATIONS & DOSAGE
Potentially life-threatening digoxin or digitoxin intoxication—
Adults and children: I.V. dosage varies according to amount of digoxin or digitoxin to be neutralized. Each vial binds about 0.5 mg of digoxin or digitoxin. Average dosage is 6 vials (228 mg). However, if toxicity resulted from acute digoxin ingestion and neither a serum digoxin level nor an estimated ingestion amount is known, 20 vials (760 mg) may be needed. See package insert for complete, specific dosage instructions.

ADVERSE REACTIONS
CV: *heart failure* and rapid ventricular rate (both caused by reversal of the cardiac glycoside's therapeutic effects).
Other: *hypersensitivity reactions,* hypokalemia, *anaphylaxis.*

INTERACTIONS
None significant.

EFFECTS ON DIAGNOSTIC TESTS
Therapy alters standard cardiac glycoside determinations by radioimmunoassay procedures. Results may be falsely increased or decreased, depending on separation method used.

CONTRAINDICATIONS
No known contraindications.

NURSING CONSIDERATIONS
• Use cautiously in patients known to be allergic to ovine proteins or those who have previously received antibodies. In these high-risk patients, skin testing is recommended because drug is derived from digoxin-specific antibody fragments obtained from immunized sheep.
• Be aware that drug is used only for life-threatening overdose in patients in anaphylaxis, severe hypotension, or cardiac arrest; with ventricular arrhythmias, such as ventricular tachycardia or fibrillation; with progressive bradycardia, such as severe sinus bradycardia; or with second- or third-degree AV block not responsive to atropine.
• Monitor potassium level closely, as ordered.

---

*Liquid contains alcohol.   **May contain tartrazine.   †Canada   ‡Australia   §U.K.   ◇OTC

• Be aware that in most patients, signs of digitalis toxicity disappear within a few hours.

• Be aware that because drug will interfere with digitalis immunoassay measurements, standard serum digoxin levels will be misleading until drug is cleared from body (about 2 days).

I.V. administration
• Reconstitute 38-mg vial with 4 ml of sterile water for injection. Gently roll vial to dissolve the powder. Reconstituted solution contains 9.5 mg/ml. Drug may be given by direct injection if cardiac arrest seems imminent. Alternatively, dilute with 0.9% NaCl for injection to an appropriate volume and give by intermittent infusion over 30 minutes.

• Infuse drug through a 0.22-micron membrane filter.

• Refrigerate powder for injection. Reconstitute drug immediately before use. Reconstituted solutions may be refrigerated for 4 hours.

Patient teaching
• Explain use and administration of drug to patient and family.
• Instruct patient to report adverse reactions promptly.

---

dimercaprol
BAL in Oil

Pregnancy Risk Category: C

HOW SUPPLIED
Injection: 100 mg/ml

ACTION
Forms complexes with heavy metals to form chelates that are renally excreted.

Route	Onset	Peak	Duration
IM	Unknown	30-60 min	4 hr

INDICATIONS & DOSAGE
Severe arsenic or gold poisoning—
Adults and children: 3 mg/kg deep I.M. q 4 hours for 2 days, then q.i.d. on third day, then b.i.d. for 10 days.

Mild arsenic or gold poisoning—
Adults and children: 2.5 mg/kg deep I.M. q.i.d. for 2 days, then b.i.d. on third day, then once daily for 10 days.
Mercury poisoning—
Adults and children: initially, 5 mg/kg deep I.M., then 2.5 mg/kg daily or b.i.d. for 10 days.
Acute lead encephalopathy or lead level greater than 100 mcg/ml—
Adults and children: 4 mg/kg deep I.M., then q 4 hours with edetate calcium disodium for 2 to 7 days. Use separate sites.

ADVERSE REACTIONS
CNS: headache, paresthesia, muscle pain or weakness, anxiety.
CV: *transient increase in blood pressure* (returns to normal in 2 hours), *tachycardia.*
EENT: blepharospasm, conjunctivitis, lacrimation, rhinorrhea.
GI: *nausea; vomiting; burning sensation in lips, mouth, and throat;* excessive salivation; *abdominal pain.*
Other: *fever* (especially in children); pain or tightness in throat, chest, or hands.

INTERACTIONS
Drug-drug. *Iron:* toxic metal complex formed; concurrent therapy contraindicated. Wait 24 hours after last dimercaprol dose.

EFFECTS ON DIAGNOSTIC TESTS
Drug therapy blocks thyroid uptake of ^{131}I, causing decreased values.

CONTRAINDICATIONS
Contraindicated in patients with hepatic dysfunction (except postarsenical jaundice); iron, cadmium, or selenium poisoning; and in those allergic to peanuts.

NURSING CONSIDERATIONS
• Use cautiously in patients with hypertension, G6PD deficiency, or oliguria.
• Be aware that safe use in pregnancy has not been established and drug should not be used unless judged by doctor to be necessary to treat a life-threatening acute poisoning.
• Don't give I.V.; give by deep I.M. route only.
• Be careful not to let drug come in con-

tact with skin because it may cause a skin reaction.
• Be aware that drug has an unpleasant, garlic-like odor.
• Be aware that solution with slight sediment is usable.
• Use antihistamine, as ordered, to prevent or relieve mild adverse reactions.
• Keep urine alkaline to prevent renal damage.

☑ **Patient teaching**
• Explain use and administration of drug to patient and family.
• Instruct patient to report adverse reactions promptly.

---

disulfiram
Antabuse

Pregnancy Risk Category: C

HOW SUPPLIED
Tablets: 250 mg, 500 mg

ACTION
Blocks oxidation of ethanol at the acetaldehyde stage. Excess acetaldehyde produces a highly unpleasant reaction in the presence of even small amounts of ethanol.

Route	Onset	Peak	Duration
PO	1-2 hr	Unknown	14 days

INDICATIONS & DOSAGE
Adjunct in management of chronic alcoholism—
Adults: 250 to 500 mg P.O. as a single dose in morning for 1 to 2 weeks or in evening if drowsiness occurs. Maintenance dosage is 125 to 500 mg P.O. daily (average dosage 250 mg) until permanent self-control is established. Treatment may continue for months or years.

ADVERSE REACTIONS
CNS: drowsiness, headache, fatigue, delirium, depression, neuritis, peripheral neuritis, polyneuritis, restlessness, psychotic reactions.
EENT: optic neuritis.
GI: metallic or garlic aftertaste.
GU: impotence.
Skin: acneiform or allergic dermatitis, occasional eruptions.
Other: disulfiram reaction (precipitated by ethanol use), which may include flushing, throbbing headache, dyspnea, nausea, copious vomiting, diaphoresis, thirst, chest pain, palpitations, hyperventilation, hypotension, syncope, anxiety, weakness, blurred vision, confusion, arthropathy. Severe disulfiram reaction: *respiratory depression, CV collapse, arrhythmias, MI, acute heart failure, seizures, unconsciousness, or death.*

INTERACTIONS
Drug-drug. *Alfentanil:* prolonged duration of effect. Closely monitor patient.
Anticoagulants: increased anticoagulant effect. Adjust dosage of anticoagulant.
Bacampicillin: may precipitate disulfiram reaction. Don't use concomitantly.
CNS depressants: increased CNS depression. Use together cautiously.
Isoniazid: ataxia or marked change in behavior. Do not use concomitantly.
Metronidazole: psychotic reaction. Do not use concomitantly.
Midazolam: increased plasma levels of midazolam. Use together cautiously.
Paraldehyde: toxic levels of acetaldehyde. Do not use concomitantly.
Phenytoin: increased blood levels of phenytoin. Monitor phenytoin blood levels, and expect doctor to adjust phenytoin dosages.
Tricyclic antidepressants, especially amitriptyline: transient delirium. Closely monitor patient.
Drug-herb. *Guarana:* may increase serum caffeine levels or prolong serum caffeine half-life. Monitor for effect.
Herbal preparations containing alcohol: may precipitate disulfiram reaction. Do use concomitantly. Alcohol reaction may occur as long as 2 weeks after a single disulfiram dose.
Drug-lifestyle. *Alcohol use (all sources, including back-rub preparations, cough syrups, liniments, shaving lotion):* may precipitate disulfiram reaction. Don't use concomitantly. Alcohol reaction may occur as long as 2 weeks after single disulfiram dose; the longer patient remains on drug, the more sensitive he becomes to alcohol.

---

*Liquid contains alcohol.   **May contain tartrazine.   †Canada   ‡Australia   §U.K.   ◇OTC

EFFECTS ON DIAGNOSTIC TESTS
Drug may decrease urinary vanillylmandelic acid excretion and increase urinary concentrations of homovanillic acid. Decrease of radioactive iodine (^{131}I) uptake or protein-bound iodine levels may occur rarely. Serum cholesterol levels may be elevated.

CONTRAINDICATIONS
Contraindicated during alcohol intoxication and within 12 hours of alcohol ingestion; in patients with hypersensitivity to disulfiram or to other thiram derivatives used in pesticides and rubber vulcanization; and in those with psychoses, myocardial disease, or coronary occlusion; and in patients receiving metronidazole, paraldehyde, alcohol, or alcohol-containing preparations.

NURSING CONSIDERATIONS
• Be aware that drug should not be administered during pregnancy.
• Use with extreme caution in patients with diabetes mellitus, hypothyroidism, seizure disorder, cerebral damage, nephritis or hepatic cirrhosis or insufficiency, and with concurrent phenytoin therapy.
• Never administer until the patient has abstained from alcohol for at least 12 hours. Patients should clearly understand consequences of disulfiram therapy and give permission for its use. Use drug only in patients who are cooperative, well motivated, and receiving supportive psychiatric therapy.
• Be aware that complete physical examination and laboratory studies, including CBC, SMA-12, and transaminase level, should precede therapy and be repeated regularly, as ordered.

☑ Patient teaching
Alert: Caution patient's family that disulfiram should never be given to the patient without his knowledge; severe reaction or death could result if patient ingests alcohol.
• Tell patient to wear a medical identification bracelet or carry a card supplied by drug manufacturer identifying him as disulfiram user.
• Mild reactions may occur in sensitive

patient with blood alcohol levels of 5 to 10 mg/100 ml; symptoms are fully developed at 50 mg/100 ml; unconsciousness typically occurs at 125 to 150 mg/100 ml level. Reaction may last from 30 minutes to several hours or as long as alcohol remains in blood.
• Reassure patient that disulfiram-induced adverse reactions (unrelated to concomitant alcohol use), such as drowsiness, fatigue, impotence, headache, peripheral neuritis, and metallic or garlic taste, subside after about 2 weeks of therapy.
• Advise patient not to drink alcoholic beverages or use products containing alcohol, including topical preparations and mouthwash.

---

d-penicillamine
Cuprimine, Depen, D-Penamine‡

Pregnancy Risk Category: D

HOW SUPPLIED
Tablets: 125 mg‡, 250 mg
Capsules: 125 mg, 250 mg

ACTION
Chelates heavy metals and may inhibit collagen formation. Unknown for rheumatoid arthritis.

Route	Onset	Peak	Duration
PO	Unknown	1 hr	Unknown

INDICATIONS & DOSAGE
Wilson's disease—
Adults and children: 250 mg P.O. q.i.d. 30 to 60 minutes before meals. Dosage adjusted to achieve urinary copper excretion of 0.5 to 1 mg daily.
Cystinuria—
Adults: 250 mg to 1 g P.O. q.i.d. before meals. Dosage adjusted to achieve urinary cystine excretion of less than 100 mg daily when renal calculi are present, or 100 to 200 mg daily when no calculi are present. Maximum dosage is 4 g daily.
Children: 30 mg/kg P.O. daily, divided q.i.d. before meals. Dosage adjusted to achieve urinary cystine excretion of less than 100 mg daily when renal calculi are

present, or 100 to 200 mg daily when no calculi are present.
Rheumatoid arthritis—
Adults: initially, 125 to 250 mg P.O. daily, with increases of 125 to 250 mg q 1 to 3 months, if necessary. Maximum dosage is 1.5 g daily.

ADVERSE REACTIONS
EENT: tinnitus, *optic neuritis.*
GI: *anorexia, epigastric pain, nausea, vomiting, diarrhea, loss of or altered taste perception, stomatitis.*
GU: nephrotic syndrome, glomerulonephritis, proteinuria, hematuria.
Hematologic: *leukopenia, eosinophilia, thrombocytopenia, monocytosis, agranulocytosis, aplastic anemia,* lupus-like syndrome.
Hepatic: *hepatotoxicity.*
Skin: alopecia, friability, especially at pressure spots; wrinkling; erythema; urticaria; ecchymoses.
Other: myasthenia gravis syndrome with long-term use, allergic reactions *(rash, pruritus, fever),* arthralgia, lymphadenopathy, or pneumonitis.

INTERACTIONS
Drug-drug. *Antacids, oral iron:* decreased effectiveness of d-penicillamine. Give at least 2 hours apart.
Drug-food. *Any food:* delayed absorption of drug. Administer drug 1 hour before or 3 hours after meals.

EFFECTS ON DIAGNOSTIC TESTS
Drug therapy may cause positive test results for antinuclear antibody with or without clinical systemic lupus erythematosus–like syndrome.

CONTRAINDICATIONS
Contraindicated in breast-feeding patients, during pregnancy with cystinuria present, in patients with penicillamine-related aplastic anemia or granulocytosis, and in those with rheumatoid arthritis and renal insufficiency.

NURSING CONSIDERATIONS
• Use with extreme caution, if at all, in patients with hypersensitivity to penicillin.

• Keep in mind patients should receive supplemental pyridoxine daily.
• If patients have a skin reaction, give antihistamines as prescribed. Handle patients carefully to avoid skin damage.
• Monitor CBC and renal and hepatic function every 2 weeks for the first 6 months, then monthly, as ordered.
• Monitor urinalysis regularly for protein loss.
Alert: Report rash and fever (important signs of toxicity) to doctor immediately.
• Withhold drug and notify doctor if WBC count falls below 3,500/mm^3 or platelet count falls below 100,000/mm^3. A progressive decline in platelet or WBC count in three successive blood tests may necessitate temporary cessation of therapy, even if such counts are within normal limits.

✔ Patient teaching
• Tell patient that therapeutic effect may be delayed up to 3 months in treatment of rheumatoid arthritis.
• Tell patient to take drug on an empty stomach, at least 1 hour before meals, and to maintain adequate fluid intake, especially at night.
• Advise patient to report early signs of granulocytopenia: fever, sore throat, chills, bruising, and prolonged bleeding time.
• Reassure patient that taste impairment usually resolves in 6 weeks without changes in dosage.

---

edetate calcium disodium
Calcium Disodium Versenate, Calcium EDTA

Pregnancy Risk Category: B

HOW SUPPLIED
Injection: 200 mg/ml

ACTION
Forms stable, soluble complexes with metals, particularly lead.

Route	Onset	Peak	Duration
IV, IM	1 hr	24-48 hr	Unknown

INDICATIONS & DOSAGE
Acute lead encephalopathy or blood lead levels above 70 mcg/dl—
Adults and children: 1 to 1.5 g/m^2 I.V. or I.M. daily in two divided doses at 12-hour intervals for 3 to 5 days, usually in conjunction with dimercaprol. A second course may be administered after at least a 2-day drug-free interval.
Lead poisoning without encephalopathy or asymptomatic with blood levels less than 70 mcg/dl—
Children: 1 g/m^2 I.V. or I.M. daily in divided doses for 5 days.

ADVERSE REACTIONS
GU: proteinuria, hematuria; *nephrotoxicity with renal tubular necrosis leading to fatal nephrosis.*
Hepatic: Increased AST and ALT.

INTERACTIONS
Drug-drug. *Zinc insulin:* interferes with action of insulin by binding with zinc. Monitor closely.

EFFECTS ON DIAGNOSTIC TESTS
None reported.

CONTRAINDICATIONS
Contraindicated in patients with anuria, hepatitis, and acute renal disease.

NURSING CONSIDERATIONS
• Use with extreme caution in patients with mild renal disease. Expect dosages to be reduced.
• Add procaine hydrochloride, as ordered, to I.M. solution to minimize pain. Watch for local reactions.
• Because rapid I.V. use may increase intracranial pressure, be aware that I.M. route is preferred for treating lead encephalopathy.
• Be aware that I.M. route is preferred, especially for children and patients with lead encephalopathy.
• Monitor fluid intake and output, urinalysis, BUN level, and ECG daily, as ordered.
• To avoid toxicity, use with dimercaprol, as ordered.
• Do not confuse with edetate disodium, which is used to treat hypercalcemia.

I.V. administration
• Dilute with D$_5$W or 0.9% NaCl for injection to a concentration of 2 to 4 mg/ml. Infuse one-half of the daily dose over 1 hour in asymptomatic patients or 2 hours in symptomatic patients. Give the rest of the infusion at least 12 hours later. Alternatively, give by slow infusion over at least 6 hours.

☑ Patient teaching
• Explain use and administration of drug to patient and family.
• Tell patients with lead encephalopathy to avoid excess fluids.

---

edetate disodium
Disodium EDTA, Disotate, Endrate

Pregnancy Risk Category: C

HOW SUPPLIED
Injection: 150 mg/ml

ACTION
Chelates with metals, such as calcium, to form a stable, soluble complex.

Route	Onset	Peak	Duration
IV	Unknown	Unknown	Unknown

INDICATIONS & DOSAGE
Hypercalcemic crisis—
Adults: 50 mg/kg/day by slow I.V. infusion. Maximum dosage is 3 g/day.
Children: 40 to 70 mg/kg/day by slow I.V. infusion. Maximum dosage is 70 mg/kg/day.

ADVERSE REACTIONS
CNS: circumoral paresthesia, numbness, headache.
CV: hypotension.
EENT: erythema.
GI: nausea, vomiting, diarrhea.
GU: nephrotoxicity with urinary urgency, nocturia, dysuria, polyuria, proteinuria, renal insufficiency, *renal failure, tubular necrosis* (in excessive doses).
Skin: exfoliative dermatitis.
Other: severe hypocalcemia, decreased magnesium, pain at infusion site, thrombophlebitis.

INTERACTIONS
None significant.

EFFECTS ON DIAGNOSTIC TESTS
Drug lowers serum calcium concentrations (when measured by oxalate or other precipitation methods and by colorimetry) and blood glucose concentration in diabetic patients.

CONTRAINDICATIONS
Contraindicated in patients with anuria, known or suspected hypocalcemia, significant renal disease, active or healed tubercular lesions, history of seizures or intracranial lesions, and hypersensitivity to drug.

NURSING CONSIDERATIONS
• Use cautiously in patients with limited cardiac reserve, heart failure, or hypokalemia.
• Keep I.V. calcium available to treat hypocalcemia.
• Keep patients in bed for 15 minutes after infusion to avoid orthostatic hypotension. Monitor blood pressure closely.
• Monitor ECG and renal function tests frequently, as ordered.
• Obtain serum calcium after each dose, as ordered.
• Don't use to treat lead toxicity; be aware that edetate calcium disodium should be used instead.

🔻 I.V. administration
• For adults, dilute drug in 500 ml of D_5W or 0.9% NaCl solution and infuse over 3 or more hours. For children, dilute drug to maximum concentration of 30 mg/ml in D_5W or 0.9% NaCl solution and infuse over 3 or more hours.
• Avoid rapid I.V. infusion; profound hypocalcemia may occur, leading to tetany, seizures, arrhythmias, and respiratory arrest. Not recommended for direct or intermittent injection. Avoid extravasation.
• Record I.V. site used, and avoid repeated use of the same site, which increases likelihood of thrombophlebitis.

✅ Patient teaching
• Explain use and administration of drug to patient and family.

• Instruct patient to report adverse reactions promptly.

---

flumazenil
Anexate§, Romazicon

Pregnancy Risk Category: C

HOW SUPPLIED
Injection: 0.1 mg/ml in 5- and 10-ml multiple-dose vials

ACTION
Benzodiazepine antagonist that competitively inhibits the actions of benzodiazepines on the gamma-aminobutyric acid-benzodiazepine receptor complex.

Route	Onset	Peak	Duration
IV	1-2 min	6-10 min	Variable

INDICATIONS & DOSAGE
Complete or partial reversal of sedative effects of benzodiazepines after anesthesia or short diagnostic procedures (conscious sedation)—
Adults: initially, 0.2 mg I.V. over 15 seconds. If patient does not reach desired level of consciousness after 45 seconds, dose is repeated. Repeated at 1-minute intervals until cumulative dose of 1 mg has been given (initial dose plus four additional doses), if needed. Most patients respond after 0.6 to 1 mg of drug. In case of resedation, dosage may be repeated after 20 minutes; however, no more than 1 mg should be given at any one time and no more than 3 mg/hour.
Suspected benzodiazepine overdose—
Adults: initially, 0.2 mg I.V. over 30 seconds. If patient does not reach desired level of consciousness after 30 seconds, 0.3 mg is administered over 30 seconds. If patient still does not respond adequately, 0.5 mg is administered over 30 seconds; 0.5-mg doses are repeated p.r.n. at 1-minute intervals until cumulative dose of 3 mg has been given. Most patients suffering from benzodiazepine overdose respond to cumulative doses between 1 and 3 mg; rarely, patients who respond partially after 3 mg may require additional doses, up to 5 mg total. If patient does not re-

---

spond in 5 minutes after receiving 5 mg, sedation is unlikely to be caused by benzodiazepines. In case of resedation, dosage may be repeated after 20 minutes; however, no more than 1 mg should be given at any one time and no more than 3 mg/hour.

ADVERSE REACTIONS
CNS: *dizziness, abnormal or blurred vision, headache, **seizures,** agitation,* emotional lability, tremor, insomnia.
CV: *arrhythmias,* cutaneous vasodilation, palpitations.
GI: *nausea, vomiting.*
Respiratory: dyspnea, hyperventilation.
Other: *diaphoresis, pain at injection site.*

INTERACTIONS
Drug-drug. *Antidepressants, drugs that can cause seizures or arrhythmias:* seizures or arrhythmias can develop after effect of benzodiazepine overdose is removed. Flumazenil should not be used in mixed overdose, especially in cases where seizures (from any cause) are likely to occur.

EFFECTS ON DIAGNOSTIC TESTS
None reported.

CONTRAINDICATIONS
Contraindicated in patients hypersensitive to flumazenil or benzodiazepines; in patients who show evidence of serious tricyclic antidepressant overdose; and in those who received benzodiazepines to treat a potentially life-threatening condition (such as status epilepticus).

NURSING CONSIDERATIONS
• Use cautiously in patients at high risk for developing seizures; patients who have recently received multiple doses of a parenteral benzodiazepine; patients displaying some signs of seizure activity; patients who may be at risk for unrecognized benzodiazepine dependence, such as intensive care unit patients; patients with head injury; psychiatric patients; and alcohol-dependent patients.
• Be aware that safety and efficacy in children have not been established.
• Monitor patients closely for resedation that may occur after reversal of benzodi-

azepine effects because flumazenil's duration of action is shorter than that of all benzodiazepines. Duration of monitoring period depends on specific drug being reversed. Monitor closely after long-acting benzodiazepines, such as diazepam, or after high doses of short-acting benzodiazepines, such as 10 mg of midazolam. In most cases, severe resedation is unlikely in patients who fail to show signs of resedation 2 hours after a 1-mg dose of flumazenil.

I.V. administration
• Be sure the airway is secure and patent.
• Administer drug into an I.V. line in a large vein with a free-flowing I.V. solution over 15 to 30 seconds to minimize pain at the injection site. Compatible solutions include D_5W, lactated Ringer's injection, and 0.9% NaCl.
• Avoid extravasation into perivascular tissues.

✓ Patient teaching
• Warn patient not to perform hazardous activities within 24 hours of procedure because of resedation risk.
• Tell patient to avoid alcohol, CNS depressants, and OTC drugs for 24 hours.
• Give family members necessary instructions or provide patient with written instructions. The patient will not recall information given in the postprocedure period; drug does not reverse amnesic effects of benzodiazepines.

---

ipecac syrup

Pregnancy Risk Category: C

HOW SUPPLIED
Syrup*: 70 mg powdered ipecac/ml (contains glycerin 10% and alcohol 1% to 2.5%) ◊

ACTION
Induces vomiting by acting locally on the gastric mucosa and centrally on the chemoreceptor trigger zone.

Route	Onset	Peak	Duration
PO	20-30 min	Unknown	20-25 min

INDICATIONS & DOSAGE
To induce vomiting in poisoning—
Adults and children over 12 years: 15 to 30 ml P.O., followed by 3 to 4 glasses of water.
Children 1 to 12 years: 15 ml P.O., followed by 240 to 480 ml of water. Dose may be repeated in patients older than 1 year if vomiting doesn't occur within 20 minutes. If no vomiting occurs within 30 to 35 minutes after second dose, gastric lavage should be performed.
Children 6 months to 1 year: 5 to 10 ml P.O., followed by 120 to 240 ml of water.

ADVERSE REACTIONS
CNS: depression, *drowsiness.*
CV: *arrhythmias,* bradycardia, hypotension; atrial fibrillation, *fatal myocarditis* (after excessive dose).
GI: *diarrhea.*

INTERACTIONS
Drug-drug. *Activated charcoal:* neutralized emetic effect. Don't give together; may give activated charcoal after vomiting.

EFFECTS ON DIAGNOSTIC TESTS
None reported.

CONTRAINDICATIONS
Contraindicated in semicomatose or unconscious patients, or those with severe inebriation, seizures, anaphylaxis, severe hypotension, or loss of gag reflex.

NURSING CONSIDERATIONS
• Do not administer after ingestion of petroleum products or volatile oils because of potential for dangerous or lethal aspiration. Do not administer after ingestion of caustic substances such as lye because of potential for additional injury to the esophagus and mediastinum.
• Keep in mind that stomach is usually emptied completely; vomitus also may contain some intestinal material.
• If two doses do not induce vomiting, be prepared for gastric lavage.
• Be aware that ipecac syrup usually induces vomiting within 20 to 30 minutes.
• In antiemetic toxicity, be aware that ipecac syrup is usually effective if less

than 1 hour has passed since ingestion of antiemetic.
• Be aware that no systemic toxicity occurs with doses of 1 oz (30 ml) or less.
• Know that ipecac syrup is now commonly abused by bulimics who binge and then purge.

☑ Patient teaching
• Recommend to parents that 1 oz (30 ml) of syrup be available in the home when child becomes 1-year-old for immediate use in case of emergency.
• Instruct parents how to administer drug and what to do in case of accidental poisoning.
• Warn parents not to let child sleep on his back after taking drug. Use a pillow to prop the child on his side.

---

naloxone hydrochloride
Narcan

Pregnancy Risk Category: B

HOW SUPPLIED
Injection: 0.02 mg/ml, 0.4 mg/ml, 1 mg/ml

ACTION
Unknown. Thought to displace previously administered narcotic analgesics from their receptors (competitive antagonism). Has no pharmacologic activity of its own.

Route	Onset	Peak	Duration
IV	1-2 min	5-15 min	Variable
IM, SC	2-5 min	5-15 min	Variable

INDICATIONS & DOSAGE
Known or suspected narcotic-induced respiratory depression, including that caused by pentazocine and propoxyphene—
Adults: 0.4 to 2 mg I.V., S.C., or I.M. repeated q 2 to 3 minutes, p.r.n. If no response is observed after 10 mg has been administered, the diagnosis of narcotic-induced toxicity should be questioned.
Children: 0.01 mg/kg I.V., followed by a second dose of 0.1 mg/kg I.V., if needed. If I.V. route is not available, drug may be administered I.M. or S.C. in divided doses.
Neonates: 0.01 mg/kg I.V., I.M., or S.C.

Dose may be repeated q 2 to 3 minutes p.r.n.

Postoperative narcotic depression—
Adults: 0.1 to 0.2 mg I.V. q 2 to 3 minutes p.r.n. Dosage may be repeated within 1 to 2 hours, if needed.
Children: 0.005 to 0.01 mg I.V. Repeated q 2 to 3 minutes p.r.n.
Neonates (asphyxia neonatorum):
0.01 mg/kg I.V. into umbilical vein. May be repeated q 2 to 3 minutes.

ADVERSE REACTIONS
CV: tachycardia and hypertension with higher-than-recommended doses, hypotension, ***ventricular fibrillation.***
GI: nausea, vomiting (with higher-than-recommended doses).
Other: tremors, withdrawal symptoms (in narcotic-dependent patients with higher-than-recommended doses), diaphoresis, ***seizures, pulmonary edema.***

INTERACTIONS
None reported.

EFFECTS ON DIAGNOSTIC TESTS
None reported.

CONTRAINDICATIONS
Contraindicated in patients with hypersensitivity to drug.

NURSING CONSIDERATIONS
• Use cautiously in patients with cardiac irritability and opiate addiction. Abrupt reversal of opiate-induced CNS depression may result in nausea, vomiting, diaphoresis, tachycardia, CNS excitement, and increased blood pressure.
• Keep in mind that duration of action of the narcotic may exceed that of naloxone and patients may relapse into respiratory depression.
• Be aware that respiratory rate increases within 1 to 2 minutes.
• Be aware that drug is effective only in reversing respiratory depression caused by opiates, not against other drug-induced respiratory depression.
• Be aware that patients who receive naloxone to reverse opioid-induced respiratory depression may exhibit tachypnea.
• Monitor respiratory depth and rate. Be

prepared to provide oxygen, ventilation, and other resuscitation measures.

I.V. administration
• Be prepared to administer continuous I.V. infusion (necessary in many instances to control adverse effects of epidurally administered morphine). If 0.02 mg/ml is not available, be aware that adult concentration (0.4 mg) may be diluted by mixing 0.5 ml with 9.5 ml of sterile water for injection to make neonatal concentration (0.02 mg/ml).

☑ Patient teaching
• Inform family of use and administration of drug.
• Reassure family that patient will be monitored closely until effects of narcotic are alleviated.

---

naltrexone hydrochloride
Nalorex§, ReVia, Trexan

Pregnancy Risk Category: C

HOW SUPPLIED
Tablets: 50 mg

ACTION
Unknown. Probably reversibly blocks the subjective effects of opioids administered I.V. by competitively occupying opiate receptors in the brain.

Route	Onset	Peak	Duration
PO	15-30 min	12 hr	24 hr

INDICATIONS & DOSAGE
Adjunct for maintenance of opioid-free state in detoxified individuals—
Adults: initially, 25 mg P.O. If no withdrawal signs occur within 1 hour, an additional 25 mg is given. Once patient has been started on 50 mg q 24 hours, flexible maintenance schedule may be used. From 50 to 150 mg may be given daily, depending on the schedule prescribed.
Treatment of alcohol dependence—
Adults: 50 mg P.O. once daily.

ADVERSE REACTIONS
CNS: *insomnia, anxiety, nervousness,*

headache, depression, dizziness, fatigue, somnolence, ***suicide ideation.***
GI: *nausea, vomiting,* anorexia, *abdominal pain,* constipation, increased thirst.
GU: delayed ejaculation, decreased potency.
Hepatic: altered liver function test results, ***hepatotoxicity.***
Skin: rash.
Other: *muscle and joint pain,* chills, lymphocytosis.

INTERACTIONS
Drug-drug. *Thioridazine:* increased somnolence and lethargy. Monitor closely.

EFFECTS ON DIAGNOSTIC TESTS
None reported.

CONTRAINDICATIONS
Contraindicated in patients receiving opioid analgesics, in opioid-dependent patients, in patients in acute opioid withdrawal, and in those with positive urine screen for opioids or in acute hepatitis or liver failure. Also contraindicated in patients with hypersensitivity to drug.

NURSING CONSIDERATIONS
• Use cautiously in patients with mild hepatic disease or history of recent hepatic disease.
• Be aware that treatment for opioid dependency shouldn't begin until patients receive naloxone challenge, a provocative test of opioid dependency. If signs of opioid withdrawal persist after naloxone challenge, don't administer naltrexone.
• Keep in mind that patient must be completely free of opioids before taking naltrexone or severe withdrawal symptoms may occur. Patients who have been addicted to short-acting opioids, such as heroin and meperidine, must wait at least 7 days after the last opioid dose before starting naltrexone. Patients who have been addicted to longer-acting opioids, such as methadone, should wait at least 10 days.
• In an emergency, anticipate that patients receiving naltrexone may be given an opioid analgesic, but the dose must be higher than usual to surmount naltrexone's effect.

Monitor for respiratory depression from the opioid; it may be longer and deeper.
• For patients being treated because of history of opioid dependency and who are expected to be noncompliant, be prepared to try a flexible maintenance dosage regimen of 100 mg on Monday and Wednesday and 150 mg on Friday, as ordered.
• Be aware that naltrexone should be used only as part of a comprehensive rehabilitation program.

☑ **Patient teaching**
• Advise patient to carry a medical identification card. Warn him about telling medical personnel that he takes naltrexone.
• Give patient names of nonopioid drugs that he can continue to take for pain, diarrhea, or cough.

pralidoxime chloride (pyridine-2-aldoxime methochloride; 2-PAM chloride)
Protopam Chloride

Pregnancy Risk Category: C

HOW SUPPLIED
Injection: 1 g/20 ml in 20-ml vial without diluent or syringe; 1 g/20 ml in 20-ml vial with diluent, syringe, needle, and alcohol swab (emergency kit); 600 mg/2 ml autoinjector, parenteral

ACTION
Reactivates cholinesterase that has been inactivated by organophosphorus pesticides and related compounds, permitting degradation of accumulated acetylcholine and facilitating normal functioning of neuromuscular junctions.

Route	Onset	Peak	Duration
IV	Unknown	5-15 min	Unknown
IM	Unknown	10-20 min	Unknown
SC	Unknown	Unknown	Unknown

INDICATIONS & DOSAGE
Antidote for organophosphate poisoning—
Adults: 1 to 2 g in 100 ml of 0.9% NaCl solution by I.V. infusion over 15 to 30

minutes. Repeated in 1 hour if muscle weakness persists. Additional doses may be given cautiously. I.M. or S.C. injection may be used if I.V. is not feasible.
Children: 20 to 40 mg/kg I.V., administered as for adults.
Cholinergic crisis in myasthenia gravis—
Adults: 1 to 2 g I.V., followed by 250 mg I.V. q 5 minutes p.r.n.

ADVERSE REACTIONS
CNS: dizziness, headache, drowsiness.
CV: tachycardia.
EENT: blurred vision, diplopia, impaired accommodation.
GI: nausea.
Other: muscular weakness, hyperventilation, mild to moderate pain at injection site, transient elevation of liver enzymes.

INTERACTIONS
None significant.

EFFECTS ON DIAGNOSTIC TESTS
None reported.

CONTRAINDICATIONS
Contraindicated in patients hypersensitive to pralidoxime.

NURSING CONSIDERATIONS
• Use with extreme caution in patients with myasthenia gravis (overdose may trigger myasthenic crisis).
• Initially, remove secretions, maintain patent airway, and institute mechanical ventilation if needed. After dermal exposure to organophosphate, remove patient's clothing and wash his skin and hair with sodium bicarbonate, soap, water, and alcohol as soon as possible. A second washing may be necessary. When washing patient, wear protective gloves and clothes to avoid exposure.
• Draw blood for cholinesterase levels before giving pralidoxime.
• Drug should be used in hospitalized patients only; have respiratory and other supportive measures available. If possible, obtain accurate medical history and chronology of poisoning. Drug should be given as soon as possible after poisoning; treatment is most effective if initiated within 24 hours after exposure.

• To ameliorate muscarinic effects and block accumulation of acetylcholine associated with organophosphate poisoning, give atropine 2 to 4 mg I.V. with pralidoxine if cyanosis is not present, as ordered. (If cyanosis is present, give atropine I.M.) Give atropine every 5 to 6 minutes, as ordered, until signs of atropine toxicity (flushing, tachycardia, dry mouth, blurred vision, excitement, delirium, and hallucinations) appear; atropinization should be maintained for at least 48 hours.
• Observe patient for 48 to 72 hours if poison was ingested. Delayed absorption may occur from lower bowel. It is difficult to distinguish between toxic effects produced by atropine or organophosphate compounds and those resulting from pralidoxime.
• Watch patient with myasthenia gravis treated for overdose of cholinergic drugs for signs of rapid weakening. He can pass quickly from cholinergic crisis to myasthenic crisis and requires more cholinergic drugs to treat myasthenia. Keep edrophonium (Tensilon) available for establishing differential diagnosis.
• Drug is not effective against poisoning due to phosphorus, inorganic phosphates, or organophosphates with no anticholinesterase activity.

🔷 I.V. administration
• Reconstitute by adding 20 ml of sterile water for injection to vial containing 1 g of drug. Further dilute by adding 100 ml of 0.9% NaCl solution. Infuse over 15 to 30 minutes.
• If patient has pulmonary edema, give drug by slow I.V. push over 5 minutes. Do not exceed 200 mg/minute.

✅ Patient teaching
• Explain use and administration of drug to patient and family.
• Tell patient to report adverse effects.
• Caution patient treated for organophosphate poisoning to avoid contact with insecticides for several weeks.

Reactions may be *common*, uncommon, *life-threatening*, or COMMON AND LIFE-THREATENING.

protamine sulfate
Prosulf§

Pregnancy Risk Category: C

HOW SUPPLIED
Injection: 10 mg/ml

ACTION
A heparin antagonist that forms a physiologically inert complex with heparin sodium.

Route	Onset	Peak	Duration
IV	30-60 sec	Unknown	2 hr

INDICATIONS & DOSAGE
Heparin overdose—
Adults: dosage based on venous blood coagulation studies, usually 1 mg for each 90 to 115 units of heparin. Give by slow I.V. injection over 10 minutes in doses not to exceed 50 mg.

ADVERSE REACTIONS
CV: fall in blood pressure, bradycardia, circulatory collapse.
GI: nausea, vomiting.
Respiratory: dyspnea, pulmonary edema, acute pulmonary hypertension.
Other: transitory flushing, feeling of warmth, anaphylaxis, anaphylactoid reactions, lassitude.

INTERACTIONS
None significant.

EFFECTS ON DIAGNOSTIC TESTS
Drug shortens heparin-prolonged PTT.

CONTRAINDICATIONS
Contraindicated in patients with hypersensitivity to drug.

NURSING CONSIDERATIONS
• Be aware that postoperative dose is based on coagulation studies and a repeat prothrombin time 15 minutes after administration is advised.
• Calculate dosage carefully. One mg of protamine neutralizes 90 to 115 units of heparin depending on salt (heparin calci-
um or heparin sodium) and source of heparin (beef or pork).
• Be aware that risk of a hypersensitivity reaction is increased in patients with known hypersensitivity to fish, vasectomized or infertile males, or patients taking protamine-insulin products.
• Monitor patient continually.
• Watch for spontaneous bleeding (heparin "rebound"), especially in dialysis patients and in those who have undergone cardiac surgery.
• Protamine sulfate may act as anticoagulant in very high doses.
• Be aware that I.V. route may cause flushing.

I.V. administration
• Administer slowly by direct I.V. injection. Have emergency equipment available to treat anaphylaxis or severe hypotension.

Patient teaching
• Explain use and administration of drug to patient and family.
• Tell patient to report adverse effects.

sodium polystyrene sulfonate
Kayexalate, SPS

Pregnancy Risk Category: C

HOW SUPPLIED
Powder: 1-lb jar (3.5 g/tsp)
Suspension: 15 g/60 ml*

ACTION
Potassium-removing resin exchanges sodium ions for potassium ions in the intestine: 1 g of sodium polystyrene sulfonate is exchanged for 0.5 to 1 mEq of potassium. The resin is then eliminated. Much of the exchange capacity is used for cations other than potassium (calcium and magnesium) and possibly for fats and proteins.

Route	Onset	Peak	Duration
PO, PR	Unknown	Unknown	Unknown

INDICATIONS & DOSAGE
Hyperkalemia—
Adults: 15 g P.O. daily to q.i.d. in water

or sorbitol (3 to 4 ml/g of resin). Alternatively, mix powder with appropriate medium—aqueous suspension or diet appropriate for renal failure—and instill through a nasogastric (NG) tube.

Or, 30 to 50 g/100 ml of sorbitol q 6 hours as warm emulsion deep into sigmoid colon (20 cm).

Children: 1 g/kg of body weight/dose P.O. or P.R. p.r.n. to correct hyperkalemia.

Oral administration preferred because drug should remain in intestine for at least 30 minutes.

ADVERSE REACTIONS

GI: *constipation,* fecal impaction (in elderly patients), anorexia, gastric irritation, nausea, vomiting, *diarrhea* (with sorbitol emulsions).

Other: hypokalemia, hypocalcemia, sodium retention.

INTERACTIONS

Drug-drug. *Antacids and laxatives (nonabsorbable cation-donating types, including magnesium hydroxide):* systemic alkalosis and reduced potassium exchange capability. Don't use together.

EFFECTS ON DIAGNOSTIC TESTS

Drug therapy may alter serum magnesium and calcium levels.

CONTRAINDICATIONS

Contraindicated in patients with hypokalemia or hypersensitivity to drug.

NURSING CONSIDERATIONS

• Use cautiously in patients with severe heart failure, severe hypertension, or marked edema.

• Don't heat resin; this impairs drug's effect. Mix resin only with water or sorbitol for P.O. administration. *Never* mix with orange juice (high potassium content) to disguise taste.

• Chill oral suspension for greater palatability.

• If sorbitol is given, mix with resin suspension.

• Consider solid form. Resin cookie and candy recipes are available; ask pharmacist or dietitian to supply.

• Be aware that premixed forms are available (SPS and others). If preparing manually, mix polystyrene resin only with water and sorbitol for rectal use. Do not use mineral oil for P.R. administration to prevent impaction; ion exchange requires aqueous medium. Sorbitol content prevents impaction.

• Prepare P.R. dose at room temperature. Stir emulsion gently during administration.

• Use #28 French rubber tube for rectal dose; insert 20 cm into sigmoid colon. Tape tube in place. Or, consider an indwelling urinary catheter with a 30-ml balloon inflated distal to anal sphincter to aid in retention. This is especially helpful for patients with poor sphincter control. Use gravity flow. Drain returns constantly through Y-tube connection. Place patient in knee-chest position or with hips on pillow for a while if back-leakage occurs.

• After P.R. administration, flush tubing with 50 to 100 ml of nonsodium fluid to ensure delivery of all drug. Flush rectum to remove the resin.

• Prevent fecal impaction in elderly patients by administering resin P.R., as ordered. Give cleansing enema before P.R. administration. Have patient retain enema for 6 to 10 hours if possible, but 30 to 60 minutes is acceptable.

• Watch for constipation in oral or ng administration. Use sorbitol (10 to 20 ml of 70% syrup every 2 hours as needed) to produce one or two watery stools daily.

• Monitor serum potassium levels at least once daily. Treatment may result in potassium deficiency and is usually stopped when potassium is reduced to 4 or 5 mEq/L.

• Watch for signs of hypokalemia: irritability, confusion, arrhythmias, ECG changes, severe muscle weakness and sometimes paralysis, and digitalis toxicity in digitalized patients.

• When hyperkalemia is severe, polystyrene resin alone is not adequate in lowering serum potassium. Dextrose 50% with regular insulin I.V. push may also be given.

• Monitor for symptoms of other electrolyte deficiencies (magnesium, calcium) because drug is nonselective. Monitor serum calcium in patients receiving sodi-

um polystyrene therapy for more than 3 days. Supplementary calcium may be needed.
• Watch for sodium overload. Drug contains about 100 mg sodium/g. About one-third of resin's sodium is retained.

☑ Patient teaching
• Explain use and administration of drug to patient.
• Advise patient to report adverse reactions promptly.
• Teach patient about low-potassium diet.

---

succimer
Chemet

Pregnancy Risk Category: C

HOW SUPPLIED
Capsules: 100 mg

ACTION
A chelating agent that forms water-soluble complexes with lead and increases its excretion in urine.

Route	Onset	Peak	Duration
PO	Unknown	1-2 hr	Unknown

INDICATIONS & DOSAGE
Lead poisoning in children with blood lead levels above 45 mcg/dl—
Children: initially, 10 mg/kg or 350 mg/m^2 q 8 hours for 5 days. Dosage rounded as appropriate to nearest 100 mg (see chart). Then, frequency of administration decreased to q 12 hours for an additional 2 weeks of therapy.

Weight in kg (lb)	Dose (mg)
8-15 (17-34)	100
16-23 (35-51)	200
24-34 (52-75)	300
35-44 (76-98)	400
> 45 (> 99)	500

ADVERSE REACTIONS
CNS: *drowsiness, dizziness, sensory motor neuropathy, sleepiness, paresthesia, headache.*
CV: *arrhythmias.*
EENT: plugged ears, cloudy film in eyes, otitis media, watery eyes, sore throat, rhinorrhea, nasal congestion.
GI: *nausea, vomiting, diarrhea, loss of appetite, abdominal cramps, hemorrhoidal symptoms, metallic taste in mouth, loose stools.*
GU: decreased urination, difficult urination, proteinuria.
Hematologic: increased platelet count, intermittent eosinophilia.
Respiratory: cough, head cold.
Skin: papular rash, herpetic rash, mucocutaneous eruptions, pruritus.
Other: *leg, kneecap, back, stomach, rib, or flank pain; flulike symptoms;* candidiasis; *elevated serum AST, ALT, alkaline phosphatase, or cholesterol levels.*

INTERACTIONS
None significant.

EFFECTS ON DIAGNOSTIC TESTS
False-positive results for urinary ketones in tests using nitroprusside reagents (Ketostix) and false decreased levels of serum uric acid and CK have been reported, as well as transient mild elevations of serum transaminase levels.

CONTRAINDICATIONS
Contraindicated in patients with hypersensitivity to drug.

NURSING CONSIDERATIONS
• Use cautiously in patients with compromised renal function.
• Measure severity by initial blood lead level and by rate and degree of rebound of blood lead level. Severity should be used as a guide for more frequent blood lead monitoring.
• Monitor serum transaminase before and at least weekly during therapy. Transient mild elevations of serum transaminases have been observed. Monitor patients with history of hepatic disease.
• Monitor patients at least once weekly for rebound blood lead levels. Elevated levels and associated symptoms may return rapidly after drug is stopped because of redistribution of lead from bone to soft tissues and blood.
• Be aware that course of treatment lasts 19 days. Repeated courses may be neces-

---

sary if indicated by weekly monitoring of blood lead levels.

• Be aware that a minimum of 2 weeks between courses is recommended unless high blood lead levels indicate need for immediate therapy.

• Be aware that false-positive results for ketones in urine using nitroprusside reagents (Ketostix) and falsely decreased levels of serum uric acid and CK have been reported.

• Be aware that concurrent administration of succimer with other chelating agents is not recommended. Patients who have received edetate calcium disodium with or without dimercaprol may use succimer as subsequent therapy after a 4-week interval.

✓ Patient teaching

• Explain use and administration of drug to parents and child. Stress importance of complying with frequently ordered blood tests.

• Tell parents of young child who cannot swallow capsules that capsule can be opened and its contents sprinkled on a small amount of soft food. Alternatively, medicated beads from capsule may be poured on a spoon; follow with flavored beverage.

• Assist parents with identifying and removing sources of lead in child's environment. Chelation therapy is not a substitute for preventing further exposure and should not be used to permit continued exposure.

• Tell patient to notify doctor if rash occurs. Consider possibility of allergic or other mucocutaneous reactions each time drug is used.

alendronate sodium
alprostadil
amifostine
aminoglutethimide
anagrelide hydrochloride
aprotinin
becaplermin
calcipotriene
capsaicin
cisapride
clomiphene citrate
etanercept
finasteride
gallium nitrate
imiglucerase
imiquimod
infliximab
isotretinoin
leflunomide
levocarnitine
levomethadyl acetate
  hydrochloride
mesalamine
mesna
methoxsalen (topical)
minoxidil (topical)
nimodipine
olsalazine sodium
pamidronate disodium
pilocarpine hydrochloride
raloxifene hydrochloride
riluzole
ritodrine hydrochloride
sevelamer hydrochloride
sildenafil citrate
strontium 89 (^{89}SR) chloride
sulfasalazine
tamsulosin hydrochloride
thalidomide
tiludronate disodium
tiopronin
tolterodine tartrate
tretinoin
trilostane

COMBINATION PRODUCTS
None.

---

alendronate sodium
Fosamax

Pregnancy Risk Category: C

HOW SUPPLIED
Tablets: 5 mg, 10 mg, 40 mg

ACTION
Suppresses osteoclast activity on newly formed resorption surfaces, which reduces bone turnover. Bone formation exceeds resorption at remodeling sites, leading to progressive gains in bone mass.

Route	Onset	Peak	Duration
PO	Unknown	Unknown	Unknown

INDICATIONS & DOSAGE
Osteoporosis in postmenopausal women and prevention of fractures—
Adults: 10 mg P.O. daily, taken with water only, at least 30 minutes before first food, beverage, or medication of day.
Paget's disease of bone—
Adults: 40 mg P.O. daily for 6 months, taken with water only, at least 30 minutes before first food, beverage, or medication of day.
Prevention of osteoporosis in postmenopausal women—
Adults: 5 mg P.O. daily, taken with water only, at least 30 minutes before first food, beverage, or medication of day.

ADVERSE REACTIONS
CNS: headache.
GI: abdominal pain, nausea, dyspepsia, constipation, diarrhea, flatulence, acid regurgitation, esophageal ulcer, vomiting, dysphagia, abdominal distention, gastritis, taste perversion.
Other: musculoskeletal pain.

INTERACTIONS
Drug-drug. *Antacids, calcium supplements:* may interfere with drug absorption. Tell patient to wait at least 30 min-

---

utes after taking alendronate before taking other medications.

Aspirin, NSAIDs: increased risk of upper GI adverse reactions with drug doses above 10 mg/day. Monitor patient closely.

Hormone replacement therapy: not recommended for use with alendronate in treating osteoporosis; evidence of effectiveness is lacking.

Ranitidine: increased availability of alendronate. Reduce dosage as needed.

Drug-food. *Any food:* decreased absorption of drug. Administer with full glass of water at least 30 minutes before eating, drinking, or ingesting another drug.

EFFECTS ON DIAGNOSTIC TESTS
None reported.

CONTRAINDICATIONS
Contraindicated in patients with hypocalcemia, abnormalities of the esophagus that delay esophageal emptying, severe renal insufficiency, or hypersensitivity to drug.

NURSING CONSIDERATIONS
• Use cautiously in patients with active upper GI problems (dysphagia, symptomatic esophageal diseases, gastritis, duodenitis, ulcers) or mild to moderate renal insufficiency.

• Hypocalcemia and other disturbances of mineral metabolism (such as vitamin D deficiency) should be corrected before therapy begins.

• When drug is used to treat osteoporosis in postmenopausal women, osteoporosis may be confirmed by findings of low bone mass on diagnostic studies or by history of osteoporotic fracture.

• When used to treat Paget's disease, drug is indicated for patients with alkaline phosphatase level at least two times the upper limit of normal, in those who are symptomatic, and in those at risk for future complications from the disease.

• Monitor patient's serum calcium and phosphate levels throughout therapy, as ordered.

☑ **Patient teaching**
• Stress importance of taking tablet only with a glass (6 to 8 ounces) of plain water

at least 30 minutes before ingesting anything else, including food, beverages, and other medications. Tell patient that waiting longer than 30 minutes will improve absorption.

• Warn patient not to lie down for at least 30 minutes after taking drug to facilitate delivery to stomach and to reduce potential for esophageal irritation.

• Advise patient to report adverse effects immediately, especially difficulty swallowing or chest pain.

• Advise patient to take supplemental calcium and vitamin D if dietary intake is inadequate.

• Tell patient about the benefits of weight-bearing exercises in increasing bone mass. If applicable, explain importance of reducing or eliminating cigarette smoking and alcohol use.

alprostadil
Caverject, Viridal§

Pregnancy Risk Category: X

HOW SUPPLIED
Injections: 5 mcg/ml, 10 mcg/ml, and 20 mcg/ml after reconstitution

ACTION
A prostaglandin derivative that induces erection by relaxing trabecular smooth muscle and dilating cavernosal arteries. This leads to expansion of lacunar spaces and entrapment of blood by compressing venules against the tunica albuginea, a process referred to as the corporal veno-occlusive mechanism.

Route	Onset	Peak	Duration
Intra-cavernous	5-20 min	5-20 min	1-6 hr

INDICATIONS & DOSAGE
Erectile dysfunction due to vasculogenic, psychogenic, or mixed etiology—
Adults: dosages are highly individualized, with initial dose of 2.5 mcg intracavernously. If partial response occurs, second dose of 2.5 mcg is given, then increased further in increments of 5 to 10 mcg until patient achieves erection

(one suitable for intercourse and not exceeding 1 hour's duration). If no response occurs to initial dose, second dose may be increased to 7.5 mcg within 1 hour, then increased further in increments of 5 to 10 mcg until patient achieves suitable erection. Patient must remain in doctor's office until complete detumescence occurs. Procedure should not be repeated for at least 24 hours.

Erectile dysfunction of neurogenic etiology (spinal cord injury)—
Adults: dosages are highly individualized, with initial dose of 1.25 mcg intracavernously. If partial response occurs, second dose of 1.25 mcg is given, followed by an increment of 2.5 mcg, to a dose of 5 mcg, and then in increments of 5 mcg until patient achieves erection (one suitable for intercourse and not exceeding 1 hour's duration). If no response occurs to initial dose, the next higher dose may be given within 1 hour. Patient must remain in doctor's office until complete detumescence occurs. If there is a response, procedure should not be repeated for at least 24 hours.

ADVERSE REACTIONS
CNS: headache, dizziness.
CV: hypertension.
EENT: sinusitis, nasal congestion.
GU: *penile pain;* prolonged erection; penile fibrosis, rash, or edema; penis disorder; prostatic disorder.
Respiratory: upper respiratory infection, flu syndrome, cough.
Other: injection site hematoma or ecchymosis, back pain, localized trauma or pain.

INTERACTIONS
Drug-drug. *Anticoagulants:* increased risk of bleeding from intracavernosal injection site. Monitor patient closely.
Cyclosporine: decreased concentrations of cyclosporine. Monitor closely.
Vasoactive agents: safety and efficacy of concomitant use have not been studied. Avoid concomitant use.

EFFECTS ON DIAGNOSTIC TESTS
None reported.

CONTRAINDICATIONS
Contraindicated in patients hypersensitive to drug and in those with conditions associated with predisposition to priapism (sickle cell anemia or trait, multiple myeloma, leukemia) or penile deformation (angulation, cavernosal fibrosis, Peyronie's disease). Drug also should not be used in men who have penile implants or for whom sexual activity is inadvisable or contraindicated. Drug should not be used by sexual partner of pregnant women unless a condom is used. Drug is not given to women or children.

NURSING CONSIDERATIONS
• Be aware regular follow-up care, with thorough examination of the penis, is strongly recommended to detect signs of penile fibrosis. Drug should be discontinued in patients who develop penile angulation, cavernosal fibrosis, or Peyronie's disease.

✓ Patient teaching
• Teach patient how to prepare and administer drug before he begins treatment at home. Stress importance of reading and following patient instructions in each package insert. Store in refrigerator.
• Tell patient not to shake contents of reconstituted vial, and remind him that vial is designed for single use only. Tell him to discard vial if solution is discolored or contains precipitate.
• Review administration and aseptic technique.
• Inform patient that he can expect an erection 5 to 20 minutes after administration, with a preferable duration of no more than 1 hour. If his erection lasts longer than 6 hours, tell him to seek medical attention immediately.
• Remind patient to take drug as instructed (generally, no more than three times weekly, with at least 24 hours between each use). Warn him not to change dosage without consulting doctor.
• Caution patient to use a condom if there is a chance his sexual partner is pregnant.
• Review possible adverse reactions. Tell patient to inspect his penis daily and to report redness, swelling, tenderness, curva-

ture, priapism, unusual pain, nodules, or hard tissue.
• Urge patient not to reuse or share needles, syringes, or medication.
• Warn patient that drug does not protect against sexually transmitted diseases. Also caution him that bleeding at injection site can increase risk of transmitting blood-borne diseases to his partner.
• Remind patient to keep regular follow-up appointments so doctor can evaluate drug effectiveness and safety.

---

amifostine
Ethyol

Pregnancy Risk Category: C

HOW SUPPLIED
Injection: 500 mg anhydrous base and 500 mg mannitol in 10-ml vial

ACTION
Dephosphorylated by alkaline phosphatase in tissue to a pharmacologically active free thiol metabolite. Free thiol in normal tissues binds and detoxifies reactive metabolites of cisplatin, reducing the toxic effects of cisplatin on renal tissue. Free thiol can also act as a scavenger of free radicals that may be generated in tissues exposed to cisplatin.

Route	Onset	Peak	Duration
IV	5-8 min	Unknown	Unknown

INDICATIONS & DOSAGE
Reduction of the cumulative renal toxicity associated with repeated administration of cisplatin in patients with advanced ovarian cancer or non-small-cell lung cancer—
Adults: 910 mg/m^2 daily as a 15-minute I.V. infusion, starting 30 minutes before chemotherapy. If hypotension occurs and blood pressure doesn't return to normal within 5 minutes after stopping treatment, subsequent cycles should use a dose of 740 mg/m^2.

ADVERSE REACTIONS
CNS: dizziness, somnolence.
CV: *hypotension.*

GI: *nausea, vomiting.*
Other: flushing or feeling of warmth, chills or feeling of coldness, hiccups, sneezing, hypocalcemia, allergic reactions ranging from rash to rigors.

INTERACTIONS
Drug-drug. *Antihypertensive drugs, other drugs that could potentiate hypotension:* may cause profound hypotension. Monitor closely.

EFFECTS ON DIAGNOSTIC TESTS
None reported.

CONTRAINDICATIONS
Contraindicated in patients hypersensitive to aminothiol compounds or mannitol. Amifostine should not be used in patients receiving chemotherapy for potentially curable malignancies (including certain malignancies of germ cell origin), except for patients involved in clinical studies. Also contraindicated in hypotensive or dehydrated patients and in those receiving antihypertensive drugs that can't be stopped during the 24 hours preceding amifostine administration.

NURSING CONSIDERATIONS
• Use cautiously in the elderly and in patients with ischemic heart disease, arrhythmias, heart failure, or history of stroke or transient ischemic attacks.
• Use cautiously in patients in whom the common adverse effects of nausea, vomiting, and hypotension are likely to have serious consequences.
• If possible and if ordered, stop antihypertensive therapy 24 hours preceding amifostine administration.
• Patients receiving amifostine should be adequately hydrated before administration.
• Know that antiemetic medication, including dexamethasone 20 mg I.V. and a serotonin 5HT$_3$ receptor antagonist, should be administered before, and concurrent with, amifostine administration. Additional antiemetics may be needed, based on chemotherapeutic drugs administered.
• Monitor patient's fluid balance if drug

Reactions may be *common*, uncommon, *life-threatening*, or COMMON AND LIFE-THREATENING.

used with highly emetogenic chemotherapy.
• Monitor serum calcium level in patients
at risk for hypocalcemia such as those
with nephrotic syndrome. If necessary,
calcium supplements should be administered, as ordered.
• Safety and effectiveness in children
have not been established.

🖐 I.V. administration

• Reconstitute each single-dose vial with
9.5 ml of sterile 0.9% NaCl injection. Use
of other solutions to reconstitute the drug
is not recommended. Reconstituted solution (500 mg amifostine/10 ml) is chemically stable for 5 hours at room temperature (about 77° F [25° C]) or 24 hours if
refrigerated (35° to 46° F [2° to 8° C]).
• Amifostine can be prepared in polyvinyl
chloride bags in concentrations of 5 to
40 mg/ml and has the same stability as
when drug is reconstituted in a single-use
vial.
• Inspect vial for particulate matter and
discoloration before administration; discard drug if cloudiness or precipitation is
noted.
• Keep patient supine during infusion.
Monitor blood pressure every 5 minutes.
If hypotension occurs and requires interrupting therapy, notify doctor and keep
patient supine with his legs elevated. Then
give an infusion of normal saline solution,
as ordered, using a separate I.V. line. If
blood pressure returns to normal within 5
minutes and patient is asymptomatic, infusion may be restarted so the full dose of
the drug can be given. If the full dose
can't be given, subsequent doses should
be limited to 740 mg/m^2.
• Don't infuse for more than 15 minutes;
a longer infusion has been associated with
a higher incidence of adverse reactions.

☑ Patient teaching

• Instruct patient to remain in a supine position throughout infusion.
• Advise patient not to breast-feed; it is
unknown if drug or its metabolites are excreted in breast milk.

aminoglutethimide
Cytadren, Orimetan§

Pregnancy Risk Category: D

HOW SUPPLIED
Tablets: 250 mg

ACTION
Blocks conversion of cholesterol to delta-
5-pregnenolone in the adrenal cortex, inhibiting the synthesis of adrenal steroids.

Route	Onset	Peak	Duration
PO	Unknown	1.5 hr	1.5-3 days

INDICATIONS & DOSAGE
*Suppression of adrenal function in Cush-
ing's syndrome and adrenal cancer—*
Adults: 250 mg q.i.d. at 6-hour intervals.
Dosage may be increased in increments of
250 mg daily q 1 to 2 weeks to maximum
daily dosage of 2 g.

ADVERSE REACTIONS
CNS: *drowsiness,* headache, dizziness.
CV: hypotension, tachycardia.
GI: *nausea, anorexia,* vomiting.
Hematologic: transient *leukopenia,
agranulocytosis, thrombocytopenia.*
Skin: *morbilliform rash,* hirsutism, pruri-
tus, urticaria.
Other: fever, myalgia, adrenal insuffi-
ciency, masculinization, hypothyroidism.

INTERACTIONS
Drug-drug. *Dexamethasone, medroxyprogesterone:* increased hepatic metabolism of these agents. Monitor patient
closely.
Digoxin: may increase drug clearance.
Monitor closely.
Oral anticoagulants: decreased anticoagulant effect. Monitor PT or INR.
Theophylline: reduced action of theophylline. Monitor patient closely.
Drug-lifestyle. *Alcohol use:* may potentiate effects of aminoglutethimide. Avoid
concomitant use.

EFFECTS ON DIAGNOSTIC TESTS
Drug therapy may decrease plasma cortisol, serum thyroxine, and urinary aldos-

---

terone levels, and may increase serum alkaline phosphatase, AST, and thyroid-stimulating hormone concentrations.

CONTRAINDICATIONS
Contraindicated in patients hypersensitive to drug or to glutethimide.

NURSING CONSIDERATIONS
• Perform baseline hematologic studies, as ordered.
• Blood pressure is to be monitored frequently.
• CBC is to be monitored periodically.
• Be aware that drug may cause adrenal hypofunction, especially under stressful conditions, such as surgery, trauma, or acute illness. Patients may need mineralocorticoid supplements to treat hyponatremia and orthostatic hypotension. Glucocorticoid replacement may also be necessary, especially in patients with breast cancer. Monitor such patients carefully.
• Be aware that drug may cause a decrease in thyroid hormone production. Monitor thyroid function studies.

☑ **Patient teaching**
• Warn patient to watch for signs of infection (fever, sore throat, fatigue) and bleeding (easy bruising, nosebleeds, bleeding gums, melena). Patient should take his temperature daily.
• Warn patient to avoid activities that require alertness and good motor coordination until CNS effects of drug are known.
• Advise patient to stand up slowly to minimize orthostatic hypotension.
• Tell patient to report rash that persists for more than 8 days. Reassure patient that drowsiness, nausea, and loss of appetite usually diminish within 2 weeks after start of aminoglutethimide therapy, but advise him to notify doctor if these symptoms persist.
• Inform patient that masculinizing effects are reversible.

---

anagrelide hydrochloride
Agrylin

Pregnancy Risk Category: C

HOW SUPPLIED
Capsules: 0.5 mg, 1 mg

ACTION
Reduces platelet production, possibly by decreasing megakaryocyte hypermaturation.

Route	Onset	Peak	Duration
PO	Immediate	1 hr	48 hr

INDICATIONS AND DOSAGE
Treatment of patients with essential thrombocythemia to reduce the elevated platelet count and risk of thrombosis and to ameliorate associated symptoms—
Adults: 0.5 mg P.O. q.i.d. or 1 mg P.O. b.i.d. for at least 1 week; then adjust dosage to lowest effective dose required to maintain platelet count below 600,000/mm^3, and ideally to the normal range. Do not increase dosage by more than 0.5 mg/day in any 1 week; do not exceed 10 mg/day or 2.5 mg in a single dose.

ADVERSE REACTIONS
CNS: amnesia, *asthenia*, confusion, depression, *dizziness, headache*, insomnia, migraine, nervousness, pain, paresthesia, somnolence.
CV: *arrhythmias*, angina, *CVA*, chest pain, CV disease, **heart failure, hemorrhage**, hypertension, *palpitations*, orthostatic hypotension, vasodilatation, syncope, tachycardia.
EENT: abnormal vision, amblyopia, diplopia, epistaxis, rhinitis, sinusitis, tinnitus, visual field abnormality.
GI: *abdominal pain*, aphthous stomatitis, constipation, *diarrhea*, dyspepsia, eructation, *flatulence*, GI distress, **GI hemorrhage**, gastritis, melena, *nausea*, vomiting.
GU: dysuria, hematuria.
Hematologic: anemia, ecchymosis, lymphadenoma, **thrombocytopenia**.
Musculoskeletal: arthralgia, back pain, leg cramps, myalgia, neck pain.
Respiratory: asthma, bronchitis, *dyspnea*, pneumonia, respiratory disease.
Skin: alopecia, photosensitivity, pruritus, rash, skin disease, urticaria.
Other: anorexia, chills, dehydration, *edema*, fever, flulike symptoms, malaise.

Reactions may be *common*, uncommon, *life-threatening*, or COMMON AND LIFE-THREATENING.

INTERACTIONS
Drug-drug. *Sucralfate:* may interfere with anagrelide absorption. Monitor closely.
Drug-food. *All food:* may decrease bioavailability. Drug is to be taken 1 hour before or 2 hours after eating.

EFFECTS ON DIAGNOSTIC TESTS
None reported.

CONTRAINDICATIONS
No known contraindications.

NURSING CONSIDERATIONS
• Use with caution in patients with CV disease because drug may cause vasodilation, tachycardia, palpitations, and heart failure.
• Use with caution in patients with serum creatinine over 2 mg/dl and in those with liver function tests exceeding 1.5 times the upper normal limits.
• During the first 2 weeks of treatment, monitor blood counts and liver and renal function tests.
• Because it is not known if drug is excreted in breast milk, use caution when administering drug to breast-feeding women.

☑ Patient teaching
• Instruct patient to report increased bleeding, bruising, or cardiac symptoms.
• Instruct female patients of childbearing age to use contraception while on anagrelide hydrochloride therapy.

---

aprotinin
Trasylol

Pregnancy Risk Category: B

HOW SUPPLIED
Injection: 10,000 KIU (kallikrein inactivator units)/ml (1.4 mg/ml) in 100-ml and 200-ml vials.

ACTION
A naturally occurring protease inhibitor that acts as a systemic hemostatic agent, decreasing bleeding and turnover of coagulation factors. It inhibits fibrinolysis by affecting kallikrein and plasmin, prevents triggering of the contact phase of the coagulation pathway, and increases the resistance of platelets to damage from mechanical injury and high plasmin levels that occur during cardiopulmonary bypass.

Route	Onset	Peak	Duration
IV	Unknown	Unknown	Unknown

INDICATIONS & DOSAGE
To reduce blood loss or the need for transfusion in patients undergoing coronary artery bypass grafts—
Adults: start with 10,000 units (1 ml) I.V. test dose at least 10 minutes before the loading dose. If no allergic reaction is evident, anesthesia may be induced while the loading dose of 2 million units is given I.V. slowly over 20 to 30 minutes. When loading dose is complete, sternotomy may be performed. Before bypass is initiated, the cardiopulmonary bypass circuit is primed with 2 million units of the drug by replacing an aliquot of the priming fluid with drug. A continuous infusion at a rate of 500,000 units/hour is then given I.V. until patient leaves the operating room. This is known as *regimen A.* Alternatively, a second regimen known as *regimen B* may be given, which is half the dosage of *regimen A* (except for test dose).

ADVERSE REACTIONS
CV: *cardiac arrest, heart failure, ventricular tachycardia, MI, heart block, atrial fibrillation, atrial flutter,* hypotension, supraventricular tachycardia.
GU: *nephrotoxicity, renal failure.*
Respiratory: pneumonia, respiratory disorder, apnea, asthma, dyspnea.
Other: *hypersensitivity reactions, anaphylaxis,* fever, *shock,* sepsis.

INTERACTIONS
Drug-drug. *Captopril:* decreased hypotensive effects. Monitor patient closely.

EFFECTS ON DIAGNOSTIC TESTS
Because aprotinin inhibits contact activation of the intrinsic clotting system, drug therapy prolongs the results of coagulation assays that depend on contact activa-

---

tion, including the PTT and celite activation clotting time assays.

Aprotinin has resulted in elevated serum creatinine levels postoperatively. Aprotinin may alter liver function studies.

CONTRAINDICATIONS
Contraindicated in patients hypersensitive to beef because drug is prepared from bovine lung.

NURSING CONSIDERATIONS
Alert: Use drug cautiously and monitor patients closely for hypersensitivity reaction. Patients may experience anaphylaxis after the full therapeutic dose even if they remained asymptomatic after the test dose. If symptoms of hypersensitivity occur (skin eruptions, itching, dyspnea, nausea, tachycardia), discontinue infusion immediately, make doctor aware, and provide supportive treatment.

• Obtain history of possible allergies. Patients with a history of allergies to drugs or other substances may be at higher risk of developing an allergic reaction to aprotinin.

• To avoid hypotension, make sure patient is supine when loading dose is given. Monitor blood pressure.

• Monitor laboratory studies, including liver function tests, as ordered. Aprotinin will prolong activated clotting time and PTT. It may increase CK and transaminase levels and may falsely prolong whole blood clotting times when determined by surface activation methods, such as the Hemachron method.

• Monitor patient for increased serum creatinine levels and other signs of nephrotoxicity. If nephrotoxicity occurs, it is usually mild and reversible.

• Store between 36° and 77° F (2° and 25° C). Protect drug from freezing.

🖐 I.V. administration
• Keep in mind that aprotinin is incompatible with amino acids, corticosteroids, fat emulsions, heparin, and tetracyclines. Don't add any drugs to the I.V. container and use a separate I.V. line.

• Be prepared to administer a test dose. Test dose is particularly important in patients who have previously received the drug because they have a higher risk of anaphylaxis. In such patients, pretreat with an antihistamine, as ordered.

• Administer all doses through a central line.

✅ Patient teaching
• Explain use and administration of drug to patient and family.
• Reassure patient and family that he will be monitored continuously throughout drug administration for adverse reactions.

▼ *NEW DRUG*

becaplermin
Regranex Gel

Pregnancy Risk Category: C

HOW SUPPLIED
Gel: 100 mcg/g in tubes of 2 g, 7.5 g, 15 g

ACTION
Drug is thought to promote chemotactic recruitment and proliferation of cells involved in wound repair and formation of new granulation tissue.

Route	Onset	Peak	Duration
Topical	Unknown	Unknown	Unknown

INDICATIONS & DOSAGE
Treatment of lower extremity diabetic neuropathic ulcers that extend into the subcutaneous tissue or beyond and have adequate blood supply—
Adults: apply daily in ¹⁄₁₆″ even thickness to entire surface of wound. The following table will calculate the length of gel to apply in inches (or centimeters) which is dependent on wound size and tube size:

Tube size	(inches)	(cm)
2 g	Ulcer length × ulcer width × 1.3	(Ulcer length × ulcer width) ÷ 2
7.5, 15 g	Ulcer length × ulcer width × 0.6	(Ulcer length × ulcer width) ÷ 4

ADVERSE REACTIONS
Skin: erythematous rash.
Other: cellulitis, infection, osteomyelitis.

Reactions may be *common,* uncommon, *life-threatening,* or COMMON AND LIFE-THREATENING.

INTERACTIONS
None significant.

EFFECTS ON DIAGNOSTIC TESTS
None reported.

CONTRAINDICATIONS
Contraindicated in patients with known hypersensitivity drug or its components (such as parabens or m-cresol) and in those patients with known neoplasms at application site.

NURSING CONSIDERATIONS
• Use cautiously in breast-feeding women.
• Be aware that drug increases incidence of complete healing of diabetic ulcers when used as an adjunct to good ulcer care practices, which include initial sharp debridement, infection control, and pressure relief.
• Know that treatment efficacy has not been evaluated for diabetic neuropathic ulcers that do not extend through the dermis into subcutaneous tissue or for ischemic diabetic ulcers.
• Drug should not be used in wounds that close by primary intention.
• To apply drug, calculate length of gel by measuring the ulcer's greatest length and width and use dosage formula. Squeeze the calculated length of gel to apply onto a clean measuring surface, such as waxed paper. Use a cotton swab or other application aid to transfer and spread drug over the entire ulcer area in a ¹⁄₁₆″-thick continuous layer. Place a saline-moistened dressing over the site and leave in place for approximately 12 hours. After 12 hours, remove dressing and rinse away residual gel with normal saline or water, and apply a fresh moist dressing, without becaplermin, for rest of day.
• Monitor wound size and healing; recalculate amount of drug to be applied at least once weekly. If ulcer does not decrease in size by about one-third after 10 weeks, or if complete healing has not occurred within 20 weeks, treatment should be reassessed.
• Monitor for application site reactions. Sensitization, or irritation caused by parabens or m-cresol, should be considered.

• Drug is for external use only.
• Safety and effectiveness in children younger than 16 years have not been established.

☑ **Patient teaching**
• Instruct patient to wash hands thoroughly before applying gel.
• Advise patient not to touch tip of tube against ulcer or any other surfaces.
• Instruct patient on proper procedure for wound care including applying gel and changing dressings.
• Stress need to keep area covered with a wet dressing at all times.
• Tell patient to store drug in the refrigerator (36° to 46° F [2° to 8° C]).
• Instruct patient not to use drug after expiration date.

---

calcipotriene
Dovonex

Pregnancy Risk Category: C

HOW SUPPLIED
Ointment: 0.005%
Cream: 0.005%
Solution: 0.005%

ACTION
A synthetic vitamin D_3 analogue that regulates the development and production of skin cells.

Route	Onset	Peak	Duration
Topical	Unknown	Unknown	Unknown

INDICATIONS & DOSAGE
Moderate plaque psoriasis—
Adults: apply a thin layer to the affected area b.i.d. Rub in gently and completely.

ADVERSE REACTIONS
Skin: *burning, pruritus, irritation,* atrophy, dermatitis, dry skin, erythema, folliculitis, hyperpigmentation, peeling, rash, worsening of psoriasis.
Other: hypercalcemia.

INTERACTIONS
None significant.

EFFECTS ON DIAGNOSTIC TESTS
None reported.

CONTRAINDICATIONS
Contraindicated for use on the face and in patients with hypercalcemia, evidence of vitamin D toxicity, or hypersensitivity to drug or its components,.

NURSING CONSIDERATIONS
• Use cautiously in breast-feeding patients.
• Use cautiously in elderly patients; they may experience more severe adverse skin reactions.

✓ **Patient teaching**
• Advise patients to apply only a thin layer of ointment. Transient elevations of serum calcium can occur, especially when applied excessively.
• Advise patient not to use drug on face, in eyes, orally, or vaginally. Tell him to wash his hands after applying ointment.
• Tell patient to discontinue drug and call doctor if drug irritates lesions or surrounding, uninvolved skin.

---

capsaicin
Axsain ◇, Capzacin-P, Zostrix ◇, Zostrix-HP

Pregnancy Risk Category: NR

HOW SUPPLIED
Cream: 0.025% ◇ (Zostrix ◇), 0.075% ◇ (Axsain ◇)

ACTION
Unknown. May increase the release of substance P, a principal neurotransmitter for pain, from peripheral type C sensory fibers to central neurons.

Route	Onset	Peak	Duration
Topical	Unknown	Unknown	Unknown

INDICATIONS & DOSAGE
Temporary relief of pain after herpes zoster infections; neuralgias, such as postoperative pain and painful diabetic
neuropathy; pain associated with osteoarthritis or rheumatoid arthritis—
Adults and children over 2 years: apply to affected areas not more than q.i.d.

ADVERSE REACTIONS
Respiratory: cough, irritation.
Skin: redness, *stinging or burning on application.*

INTERACTIONS
None significant.

EFFECTS ON DIAGNOSTIC TESTS
None reported.

CONTRAINDICATIONS
Contraindicated in patients hypersensitive to drug.

NURSING CONSIDERATIONS
• Be aware drug is for external use only.

✓ **Patient teaching**
• Warn patient to avoid getting drug in eyes or on broken skin.
• Advise patient not to bandage area tightly after applying drug.
• Tell patient to wash hands after applying drug.
• Inform patient that transient burning or stinging is usually evident at initial therapy but decreases with cautious use. This effect persists in patients who use drug less often than three times daily.
• Tell patient who is self-medicating with capsaicin to contact doctor if symptoms persist beyond 2 to 4 weeks or resolve and shortly reappear.

---

cisapride
Propulsid

Pregnancy Risk Category: C

HOW SUPPLIED
Tablets: 10 mg, 20 mg
Suspension: 1 mg/ml

ACTION
Stimulates serotonin-4 (5-HT$_4$) receptors, enhancing the release of acetylcholine at

---

the myenteric plexus and increasing GI motility.

Route	Onset	Peak	Duration
PO	30-60 min	1-2 hr	Unknown

INDICATIONS & DOSAGE
Symptoms of nocturnal heartburn caused by gastroesophageal reflux disease that do not respond adequately to lifestyle modifications, antacids, and gastric acid-reducing agents—
Adults: initially, 10 mg P.O. q.i.d. 15 minutes before meals and h.s. If response is inadequate, increase to 20 mg q.i.d.

ADVERSE REACTIONS
CNS: *headache,* insomnia, anxiety, nervousness.
EENT: rhinitis, sinusitis, abnormal vision.
GI: *diarrhea, abdominal pain,* nausea, constipation, flatulence, dyspepsia.
GU: frequency, urinary tract infection, vaginitis.
Respiratory: cough, upper respiratory tract infections.
Skin: rash, pruritus.
Other: pain, fever, viral infections, arthralgia.

INTERACTIONS
Drug-drug. *Antiarrhythmics (class IA and III), astemizole, bepridil, phenothiazines, sertindole, sparfloxacin, terodiline, tetracyclic antidepressants, tricyclic antidepressants:* increased likelihood of QT interval prolongation. Avoid concomitant use.
Anticholinergics: decreased effectiveness of cisapride. Avoid concomitant use.
Anticoagulants: may increase clotting times. Monitor closely.
Benzodiazepines: enhanced sedation. Avoid concomitant use.
Cimetidine, ranitidine: increased absorption of these agents; cimetidine increases cisapride levels. Use together cautiously.
Clarithromycin, erythromycin, fluconazole, indinavir, itraconazole, ketoconazole, miconazole, nefazodone, ritonavir, troleandomycin: increased cisapride levels, which may cause ventricular arrhythmias. Concomitant use is contraindicated.
Drug-lifestyle. *Alcohol use:* enhanced sedation. Avoid concomitant use.

EFFECTS ON DIAGNOSTIC TESTS
None reported.

CONTRAINDICATIONS
Contraindicated in patients hypersensitive to drug. Also contraindicated in patients for whom increased GI motility may be harmful, such as those with mechanical obstruction, hemorrhage, or perforation of the GI tract. Concurrent use with macrolides, antifungals, protease inhibitors, and nefazodone is contraindicated. Also contraindicated for patients with history of prolonged QT intervals, ventricular arrhythmia, ischemic heart disease, congestive heart failure, renal failure, respiratory failure, and uncorrected electrolyte disorders such as hypokalemia or hypomagnesemia.

NURSING CONSIDERATIONS
• Use cautiously in breast-feeding patients because small amounts of drug are excreted in breast milk.
• Protect 20-mg tablets from light; protect all products from moisture.

☑**Patient teaching**
• Remind patient to avoid alcohol and sedatives while using drug.
• Advise patient to report immediately adverse effects.

---

clomiphene citrate
Clomid, Milophene, Serophene

Pregnancy Risk Category: X

HOW SUPPLIED
Tablets: 50 mg

ACTION
Unknown. Appears to stimulate release of pituitary gonadotropins, follicle-stimulating hormone, and luteinizing hormone. This results in maturation of the ovarian follicle, ovulation, and development of the corpus luteum.

Route	Onset	Peak	Duration
PO	Unknown	Unknown	Unknown

INDICATIONS & DOSAGE
To induce ovulation—
Adults: 50 mg P.O. daily for 5 days starting on day 5 of menstrual cycle (first day of menstrual flow is day 1) if bleeding occurs, or at any time if patient has not had recent uterine bleeding. If ovulation does not occur, may increase dose to 100 mg P.O. daily for 5 days as soon as 30 days after previous course. Repeated until conception occurs or until three courses of therapy are completed.

ADVERSE REACTIONS
CNS: headache, restlessness, insomnia, dizziness, light-headedness, depression, fatigue.
EENT: blurred vision, diplopia, scotoma, photophobia.
GI: nausea, vomiting, bloating, distention, weight gain.
GU: urinary frequency and polyuria; abnormal uterine bleeding; *ovarian enlargement* and cyst formation, which regress spontaneously when drug is stopped.
Skin: reversible alopecia, urticaria, rash, dermatitis.
Other: *hot flashes, breast discomfort.*

INTERACTIONS
None significant.

EFFECTS ON DIAGNOSTIC TESTS
Drug therapy may increase levels of serum thyronine, thyroxine-binding globulin, and sex hormone-binding globulin. It may also increase sulfobromophthalein retention and follicle-stimulating hormone and luteinizing hormone secretion.

CONTRAINDICATIONS
Contraindicated during pregnancy and in patients with undiagnosed abnormal genital bleeding, ovarian cyst not due to polycystic ovarian syndrome, hepatic disease or dysfunction, uncontrolled thyroid or adrenal dysfunction, or presence of organic intracranial lesion (such as a pituitary tumor). Also contraindicated in liver disease.

NURSING CONSIDERATIONS
• Be aware that patient must be monitored closely because of potentially serious adverse reactions.

☑ **Patient teaching**
• Tell patient there is risk of multiple births with drug, which increases with higher doses.
• Teach patient to take and chart basal body temperature to ascertain whether ovulation has occurred.
• Reassure patient that ovulation generally occurs after first course of therapy. If pregnancy does not occur, course of therapy may be repeated twice.
• Advise patient to stop drug and contact doctor immediately if pregnancy is suspected because drug may have teratogenic effect.
Alert: Advise patient to stop drug and contact the doctor immediately if abdominal symptoms or pain occur because these may indicate ovarian enlargement or ovarian cyst. Also tell patient to immediately notify doctor if signs of impending visual toxicity occur, such as blurred vision, diplopia, scotoma, or photophobia.
• Warn patient to avoid hazardous activities, such as driving or operating machinery, until CNS effects are known. Drug may cause dizziness or visual disturbances.

▼ *NEW DRUG*

etanercept
Enbrel

Pregnancy Risk Category: B

HOW SUPPLIED
Injection: 25 mg single-use vial

ACTION
Binds specifically to tumor necrosis factor (TNF) and blocks its action with cell surface TNF receptors, reducing inflammatory and immune responses found in rheumatoid arthritis.

Route	Onset	Peak	Duration
SC	Unknown	72 hr	Unknown

INDICATIONS & DOSAGE
Reduction in signs and symptoms of moderately to severely active rheumatoid arthritis in patients with demonstrated inadequate response to one or more

---

Reactions may be *common*, uncommon, *life-threatening*, or COMMON AND LIFE-THREATENING.

disease-modifying antirheumatic drugs in combination with methotrexate in patients who do not respond adequately to methotrexate alone—
Adults: 25 mg S.C. twice weekly.

ADVERSE REACTIONS
CNS: asthenia, *headache,* dizziness.
EENT: *rhinitis,* pharyngitis, sinusitis.
GI: abdominal pain, dyspepsia.
Respiratory: *upper respiratory tract infections,* cough, respiratory disorder.
Skin: *injection site reaction,* rash.
Other: *infections,* malignancies.

INTERACTIONS
None reported.

EFFECTS ON DIAGNOSTIC TESTS
None reported.

CONTRAINDICATIONS
Contraindicated in patients with sepsis and hypersensitivity to drug or its components.

NURSING CONSIDERATIONS
• Be aware that anti-TNF therapies, including etanercept, may affect defenses against infection. Notify doctor and discontinue therapy, as ordered, if serious infection occurs.
Alert: Live vaccines should not be given concurrently during drug therapy.
• Be aware that juvenile rheumatoid arthritis patients should, if possible, be brought up-to-date with all immunizations in compliance with current immunization guidelines prior to initiating treatment. Etanercept 0.4 mg/kg (maximum of 25 mg) S.C. twice weekly for 3 months has been used in children ages 4 to 17 years with juvenile rheumatoid arthritis.
• Reconstitute aseptically with 1 ml of supplied sterile bacteriostatic water for injection, USP (0.9% benzyl alcohol). Do not filter reconstituted solution during preparation or administration. Inject diluent slowly into vial. Minimize foaming by gently swirling during dissolution rather than shaking. Dissolution takes less than 5 minutes.

• Visually inspect the solution for particulate matter and discoloration before use. Reconstituted solution should be clear and colorless. Do not use if solution is discolored, cloudy, or if particulate matter remains.
• Do not add other medications or diluents to reconstituted solution.
• Use reconstituted solution as soon as possible; may be refrigerated in vial for up to 6 hours at 36° to 46° F (2° to 8° C).
• Injection sites should be at least 1" apart; areas where skin is tender, bruised, red, or hard should never be used. Recommended sites include the thigh, abdomen, or upper arm. Rotate sites regularly.
• Be aware that patient may develop positive ANA or positive anti-double-stranded DNA antibodies measured by radioimmunoassay and *Crithidia lucilae* assay.
• Safety and effectiveness have not been studied in children under than 4 years.
• Know that the needle cover of the diluent syringe contains dry natural rubber (latex) and should not be handled by persons sensitive to latex.

☑ **Patient teaching**
• Instruct patient who will be self-administering about mixing and injection techniques including rotation of injection sites.
• Instruct patient to use a puncture-resistant container for disposal of needles and syringes.
• Tell patient injection site reactions generally occur with first month of therapy and decrease thereafter.
• Inform patient of importance of avoiding live vaccine administration while receiving drug. Stress importance of alerting doctor or other health care providers of drug use.
• Instruct patient to promptly report signs and symptoms of infection to doctor.
• Advise breast-feeding patient to discontinue nursing during drug therapy.

finasteride
Propecia, Proscar

Pregnancy Risk Category: X

HOW SUPPLIED
Tablets: 1 mg, 5 mg

ACTION
Competitively inhibits steroid 5 alpha-reductase, an enzyme responsible for formation of the potent androgen 5 alpha-dihydrotestosterone (DHT) from testosterone. Because DHT influences development of the prostate gland, decreasing levels of this hormone in adult males should relieve the symptoms associated with BPH.

Route	Onset	Peak	Duration
PO	Unknown	1-2 hr	24 hr

INDICATIONS & DOSAGE
Propecia
Treatment of male pattern hair loss (androgenetic alopecia) in men only—
Adult males: 1 mg P.O. daily.
Proscar
Symptomatic BPH—
Adults: 5 mg P.O. daily.
✳ *NEW INDICATION: Reduce risk of acute urine retention and need for surgery including transurethral resection of prostate and prostatectomy—*
Adults: 5 mg P.O. daily.

ADVERSE REACTIONS
GU: impotence, decreased volume of ejaculate.
Other: decreased libido.

INTERACTIONS
None reported.

EFFECTS ON DIAGNOSTIC TESTS
Finasteride will decrease levels of prostate-specific antigen (PSA) even in prostate cancer. This does not indicate a beneficial effect.

CONTRAINDICATIONS
Contraindicated in patients hypersensitive to drug. Be aware that although drug is not used in women, manufacturer indicates pregnancy as a contraindication.

NURSING CONSIDERATIONS
• Before therapy, be aware that patient should be evaluated for conditions that mimic BPH, including hypotonic bladder; prostate cancer, infection, or stricture; or relevant neurologic conditions.
• Anticipate baseline and periodic digital rectal examinations. Although drug decreases serum PSA levels, even in prostate cancer, in clinical trials it didn't appear to decrease rate of prostate cancer detection.
• Carefully monitor patients who have a large residual urine volume or severely diminished urine flow. Be aware these patients may not be candidates for drug therapy.
• Carefully evaluate sustained increases in serum PSA levels, which could indicate noncompliance with therapy.
• Be aware that although drug's elimination rate is decreased in elderly patients, dosage adjustments aren't necessary.
• Because it's impossible to identify which patients will respond to finasteride, be aware a minimum of 6 months of therapy may be necessary.
• Keep in mind that long-term effects on complications of BPH, including acute urinary obstruction and incidence of surgery, are unknown.

☑ Patient teaching
• Warn female patient who is or may become pregnant not to handle crushed tablets because of risk of adverse effects on a male fetus.
• Inform patient that 3 months or more of daily use is generally necessary in order to see benefits when treating for hair loss.
• Caution patient whose sexual partner is or may become pregnant to discontinue drug or take precautions to avoid exposing her to his semen.
• Reassure patient that drug may decrease volume of ejaculate but doesn't appear to impair normal sexual function. However, impotence and decreased libido have occurred in less than 4% of patients.

---

gallium nitrate
Ganite

Pregnancy Risk Category: C

HOW SUPPLIED
Injection: 25 mg/ml

ACTION
Unknown. Appears to reduce hypercalcemia by inhibiting resorption of bone and reducing bone turnover in patients with increased bone turnover.

Route	Onset	Peak	Duration
IV	Unknown	Unknown	6 days

INDICATIONS & DOSAGE
Symptomatic, unresponsive hypercalcemia caused by cancer—
Adults: 200 mg/m^2 as a continuous I.V. infusion daily for 5 consecutive days or until serum calcium is normal. Lower doses (100 mg/m^2) may be given to patients with mild hypercalcemia.

ADVERSE REACTIONS
CNS: lethargy, confusion, paresthesia.
CV: tachycardia, lower extremity edema, decreased mean systolic and diastolic blood pressures.
EENT: visual or hearing impairment, acute optic neuritis.
GI: nausea and vomiting, diarrhea, constipation.
GU: *acute renal failure, increased BUN and creatinine levels.*
Hematologic: anemia, *leukopenia.*
Respiratory: dyspnea, crackles and rhonchi, pulmonary infiltrates, pleural effusion.
Skin: rash.
Other: *hypophosphatemia, hypocalcemia, decreased serum bicarbonate,* fever, hypothermia.

INTERACTIONS
Drug-drug. *Nephrotoxic drugs (such as aminoglycosides or amphotericin B):* increased risk of nephrotoxicity. Avoid concomitant use.

EFFECTS ON DIAGNOSTIC TESTS
None reported.

CONTRAINDICATIONS
Contraindicated in patients with severe renal impairment (serum creatinine over 2.5 mg/ml).

NURSING CONSIDERATIONS
• Make sure that patient is adequately hydrated, either with oral fluids or I.V. NaCl solution, as ordered, before using drug. Establish adequate urine flow (2 L/day) before treatment. Diuretic therapy is not recommended before correction of hypovolemia. Avoid overhydration, especially in patients with decreased CV function.
• Monitor BUN and serum creatinine levels, as ordered, during therapy. Discontinue drug if serum creatinine rises above 2.5 mg/dl and notify doctor.
• Carefully monitor fluid intake and output and renal function, as ordered. Short-term therapy with I.V. calcium may also be needed. Overdosage is usually treated with vigorous hydration, sometimes with diuretics, for 2 to 3 days.
• In patients who require treatment with a potentially nephrotoxic drug, such as an aminoglycoside, be prepared to discontinue gallium nitrate therapy and continue hydration for several days after administration of the nephrotoxic drug, as ordered. Monitor renal function closely.
• Monitor serum calcium levels, as ordered, and assess patients for signs of hypocalcemia, including a positive Chvostek's sign. If hypocalcemia occurs, discontinue drug and notify doctor. Treatment of hypocalcemia may be required.
• Be aware that transient hypophosphatemia is common. Patients may require oral phosphorus supplements.

I.V. administration
• Dilute daily dose in 1 L of 0.9% NaCl for injection or D$_5$W. Discard unused portion (drug contains no preservatives).
• Be aware rapid I.V. infusion or dosage over 200 mg/m^2 may increase risk of nephrotoxicity or cause nausea and vomiting. Accepted practice is administration over 24 hours.

☑ Patient teaching
• Stress importance of forcing fluids as directed throughout therapy.
• Advise patient to report hearing or vision problems. In early clinical trials, a few patients experienced hearing loss and optic neuritis after high-dose gallium ni-

---

*Liquid contains alcohol.   **May contain tartrazine.   †Canada   ‡Australia   §U.K.   ◇OTC

trate therapy when combined with investigational antineoplastic agents.

imiglucerase
Cerezyme

Pregnancy Risk Category: C

HOW SUPPLIED
Injection: 200 units/vial

ACTION
Catalyzes the hydrolysis of glucocerebroside to glucose and ceramide (part of the normal degradation pathway for lipids) and thus prevents the sequelae of Gaucher's disease, which normally occur as a result of the accumulation of glucocerebroside.

Route	Onset	Peak	Duration
IV	Unknown	1 hr	Unknown

INDICATIONS & DOSAGE
Long-term endogenous enzyme (glucosylceramidase) replacement therapy in confirmed type I Gaucher's disease—
Adults and children: dosage individualized; initially, 2.5 to 60 U/kg I.V. administered over 1 to 2 hours. Frequency of dosing typically is once q 2 weeks, but may range from three times weekly to once monthly, depending on severity of disease. Dosage may be reduced for maintenance therapy, at intervals of 3 to 6 months, while response parameters are carefully monitored.

ADVERSE REACTIONS
CNS: headache, dizziness.
CV: mild hypotension.
GI: nausea, abdominal discomfort.
GU: decreased urinary frequency.
Skin: pruritus, rash.
Other: *hypersensitivity reactions.*

INTERACTIONS
None significant.

EFFECTS ON DIAGNOSTIC TESTS
None reported.

CONTRAINDICATIONS
Contraindicated in patients with a hypersensitivity to drug.

NURSING CONSIDERATIONS
• Use with caution in patients who have previously been treated with alglucerase and who have developed antibody to alglucerase or exhibited symptoms of hypersensitivity to alglucerase.
• Monitor response parameters for doctor to determine lowest effective dosage.

I.V. administration
• Reconstitute each vial with 5.1 ml of sterile water for injection USP. Inspect solution for particulate matter and discoloration before use; if either is present, do not use. Withdraw 5 ml (amount in vial after reconstitution is 5.3 ml) of the reconstituted solution and dilute solution further with 0.9% NaCl solution to a final volume of 100 to 200 ml. Because drug is preservative-free, use immediately. Administer by I.V. infusion over 1 to 2 hours.
• Be aware when diluted to 50 ml, drug has been shown to be stable for up to 24 hours when stored at 36° to 46° F (2° to 8° C).

Patient teaching
• Explain use and administration of drug to patient and family. Stress importance of compliance with administration schedule.
• Tell patient to report persistent or severe adverse reactions promptly.

imiquimod
Aldara

Pregnancy Risk Category: B

HOW SUPPLIED
Cream: 5% in single-use packets containing 250 mg

ACTION
Immune response modifier; exact mechanism of action in treating genital or perianal warts is unknown. Drug has no direct antiviral activity.

Route	Onset	Peak	Duration
Topical	Unknown	Unknown	Unknown

INDICATIONS & DOSAGE
Treatment of external genital and perianal warts—

Adults: apply thin layer to affected area three times weekly before normal sleeping hours. Rub in until no longer visible. Leave on skin for 6 to 10 hours. Following treatment period, cream should be removed by washing treated area with mild soap and water. Continue until there is total clearance of the genital or perianal warts or for a maximum of 16 weeks.

ADVERSE REACTIONS
CNS: headache.
Skin: local itching, burning, pain, soreness, erythema, ulceration, edema, erosion, induration, flaking, excoriation.
Other: flulike symptoms, myalgia.

INTERACTIONS
None reported.

EFFECTS ON DIAGNOSTIC TESTS
None reported.

CONTRAINDICATIONS
No known contraindications.

NURSING CONSIDERATIONS
• Safety in breast-feeding patients is unknown. Safety and efficacy in patients under 18 years have not been established.
• Be aware drug is not recommended for treatment of urethral, intravaginal, cervical, rectal, or intra-anal human papilloma viral disease.
• Do not use until genital or perianal tissue is healed from previous drug or surgical treatment.
• Be aware it is common for patient to experience local skin reactions at site of application or surrounding areas. Use non-occlusive dressings such as cotton gauze or cotton undergarments in the management of skin reactions. Patient's discomfort or severity of the local skin reaction may require a rest period of several days. Resume treatment once reaction subsides.
• Be aware drug is not a cure; new warts may develop during therapy.

☑**Patient teaching**
• Advise patient that effect of cream on

transmission of genital or perianal warts is unknown. New warts may develop during therapy; drug is not a cure.
• Tell patient to use cream only as directed and to avoid contact with eyes.
• Tell patient to wash hands before and after applying cream.
• Advise patient to apply cream in a thin layer over affected area and rub in until cream is no longer visible. Advise patient to avoid excessive use of cream. Tell patient not to occlude area after applying cream and to wash with mild soap and water 6 to 10 hours following application of cream.
• Advise patient that mild local skin reactions such as erythema, erosion, excoriation, flaking, and edema at site of application or surrounding areas are common. Tell patient that most skin reactions are mild to moderate. Advise him to report severe skin reactions promptly.
• Instruct uncircumcised male patient being treated for warts under the foreskin to retract the foreskin and clean the area daily.
• Advise patient that drug can weaken condoms and vaginal diaphragms and that concomitant use is not recommended.
• Advise patient to avoid sexual contact while cream is on the skin.

▼ *NEW DRUG*

infliximab
Remicade

Pregnancy Risk Category: C

HOW SUPPLIED
Injection: 100-mg vial

ACTION
Drug is a monoclonal antibody which binds to human tumor necrosis factor (TNF)-alpha to neutralize its activity and inhibit its binding with receptors reducing the infiltration of inflammatory cells and TNF-alpha production in inflamed areas of the intestine.

Route	Onset	Peak	Duration
IV	Unknown	Unknown	Unknown

INDICATIONS & DOSAGE
Reduction of signs and symptoms in patients with moderately to severely active Crohn's disease with inadequate response to conventional therapy—
Adults: 5 mg/kg single I.V. infusion over a period of not less than 2 hours.
Reduction in the number of draining enterocutaneous fistulas in patients with fistulizing Crohn's disease—
Adults: 5 mg/kg I.V. infused over a period of not less than 2 hours. Additional doses of 5 mg/kg should be given at 2 and 6 weeks after initial infusion.

ADVERSE REACTIONS
CNS: *headache, fatigue,* dizziness, malaise, insomnia.
CV: hypertension, hypotension, tachycardia, chest pain.
EENT: pharyngitis, rhinitis, sinusitis, conjunctivitis, toothache.
GI: *nausea, abdominal pain,* vomiting, constipation, dyspepsia, flatulence, intestinal obstruction, oral pain, ulcerative stomatitis.
GU: dysuria, increased micturition frequency.
Hematologic: anemia, hematoma, ecchymosis.
Hepatic: elevated liver enzymes.
Musculoskeletal: myalgia, arthralgia, arthritis, back pain.
Respiratory: *upper respiratory tract infections,* bronchitis, coughing, dyspnea, flu syndrome, respiratory tract allergic reaction.
Skin: rash, pruritus, moniliasis, acne, alopecia, eczema, erythema, erythematous rash, maculopapular rash, papular rash, dry skin, increased sweating, urticaria.
Other: *fever,* chills, pain, peripheral edema, hot flashes, abscess, flushing.

INTERACTIONS
None significant.

EFFECTS ON DIAGNOSTIC TESTS
None reported.

CONTRAINDICATIONS
Contraindicated in patients with hypersensitivity to murine proteins or other components of drug.

NURSING CONSIDERATIONS
• Use cautiously in the elderly.
• Monitor for infusion-related reactions such as fever, chills, pruritus, urticaria, dyspnea, hypotension, hypertension, and chest pain. If an infusion reaction occurs, discontinue drug, notify doctor, and be prepared to give acetaminophen, antihistamines, corticosteroids, and epinephrine, as ordered.
• Monitor for development of lymphomas and infection. Patients with long duration of Crohn's disease and chronic exposure to immunosuppressant therapies are more prone to develop lymphomas and infections.
• Know that drug may affect normal immune responses. Patient may develop autoimmune antibodies and lupus-like syndrome; drug therapy should be discontinued. Symptoms can be expected to resolve.
• Be aware some patients test positive for ANA antibodies. Some have developed a lupus-like syndrome that resolved after drug was discontinued.

◪ I.V. administration
• Know that drug is incompatible with plasticized polyvinyl chloride equipment or devices; prepare only in glass infusion bottles or polypropylene or polyolefin infusion bags; administer through polyethylene-lined administration sets with an in-line, sterile, nonpyrogenic, low-protein-binding filter (pore size of 1.2 mm or less).
• Know that vials do not contain antibacterial preservatives; reconstituted dose should be used immediately. Reconstitute with 10 ml sterile water for injection, using a syringe with a 21G or smaller needle. Do not shake; gently swirl to dissolve powder. Solution should be colorless to light yellow and opalescent and may develop a few translucent particles. Do not use if other particles or discoloration are present.
• Dilute total volume of reconstituted dose to 250 ml with 0.9% NaCl injection. Infusion concentration range is 0.4 to

---

Reactions may be *common,* uncommon, ***life-threatening,*** or COMMON AND LIFE-THREATENING.

4 mg/ml. Infusion should begin within 3 hours of preparation and must be administered over a period of not less than 2 hours.
• Be aware that drug should not be infused concomitantly in same I.V. line with other agents.

✓ **Patient teaching**
• Tell patient about infusion-reaction symptoms and instruct him to report them if they occur.
• Inform patient of postinfusion side effects and instruct him to report them promptly.
• Inform breast-feeding patient to stop if therapy is to be administered.

---

isotretinoin
Accutane, Roaccutane‡

Pregnancy Risk Category: X

HOW SUPPLIED
Capsules: 10 mg, 20 mg, 40 mg

ACTION
Unknown. Thought to normalize keratinization, reversibly decrease size of sebaceous glands, and alter composition of sebum to a less viscous form that is less likely to cause follicular plugging.

Route	Onset	Peak	Duration
PO	Unknown	3 hr	Unknown

INDICATIONS & DOSAGE
Severe recalcitrant nodular acne unresponsive to conventional therapy—
Adults and adolescents: 0.5 to 2 mg/kg P.O. daily in two divided doses for 15 to 20 weeks.

ADVERSE REACTIONS
CNS: headache, fatigue, *pseudotumor cerebri* (benign intracranial hypertension).
EENT: *conjunctivitis,* corneal deposits, dry eyes, visual disturbances, *epistaxis, dry nose.*
GI: nonspecific GI symptoms, *nausea, vomiting,* anorexia, *abdominal pain, dry mouth,* gum bleeding and inflammation.

Hematologic: anemia, elevated platelet count.
Hepatic: elevated AST, ALT, and alkaline phosphatase levels.
Skin: *cheilosis, rash, dry skin, facial skin desquamation,* peeling of palms and toes, *petechiae, nail brittleness,* thinning of hair, skin infection, photosensitivity, *cheilitis, pruritus, fragility.*
Other: *hypertriglyceridemia, musculoskeletal pain (skeletal hyperostosis), drying of mucous membranes,* hyperglycemia.

INTERACTIONS
Drug-drug. *Carbamazepine:* decreased carbamazepine levels. Monitor levels.
Tetracyclines: increased risk of pseudotumor cerebri. Avoid concomitant use.
Vitamin A, products containing vitamin A: increased toxic effects of isotretinoin. Don't use together without the doctor's permission.
Drug-food. *Any food:* enhanced absorption of drug. Administer drug with milk, a meal, or shortly after a meal.
Drug-lifestyle. *Alcohol use:* increased risk of hypertriglyceridemia. Avoid concomitant use.
Sun exposure: increased photosensitivity reactions. Avoid prolonged or unprotected exposure to sun.

EFFECTS ON DIAGNOSTIC TESTS
Physiologic effects of drug may alter liver function tests, blood counts, and blood glucose, uric acid, cholesterol, and triglyceride levels. May cause elevation of erythrocyte sedimentation rate.

CONTRAINDICATIONS
Contraindicated in women of childbearing age unless patient has had a negative serum pregnancy test within 2 weeks before beginning therapy; will begin drug therapy on second or third day of next menstrual period; and will comply with stringent contraceptive measures for 1 month before therapy, during therapy, and for at least 1 month after therapy. Also contraindicated in patients hypersensitive to parabens, which are used as preservatives, vitamin A, or other retinoids.

---

*Liquid contains alcohol.   **May contain tartrazine.   †Canada   ‡Australia   §U.K.   ◇OTC

NURSING CONSIDERATIONS

• Monitor baseline serum lipid studies and liver function tests before therapy and at regular intervals.

• Monitor blood glucose level regularly and CK levels in patients who participate in vigorous physical activity, as ordered.

• Be aware most adverse reactions appear to be dose-related, occurring at dosages greater than 1 mg/kg daily. They are generally reversible when therapy is discontinued or dosage is reduced.

Alert: Be aware that patient who experiences headache, nausea and vomiting, or visual disturbances should be screened for papilledema. Signs and symptoms of pseudotumor cerebri require immediate discontinuation of therapy and prompt neurologic intervention. Also, be aware that severe fetal abnormalities may occur if used during pregnancy.

• Anticipate a second course of therapy, if needed, not to start for at least 8 weeks after completion of first course because improvement may continue after withdrawal of drug.

✓Patient teaching

• Advise patient to take drug with or shortly after meals to facilitate absorption.

• Tell patient to immediately report visual disturbances and bone, muscle, or joint pain.

• Warn patient that contact lenses may feel uncomfortable during isotretinoin therapy.

• Warn patient against using abrasives, medicated soaps and cleansers, acne preparations containing peeling agents, and topical alcohol preparations (including cosmetics, after shave, cologne) because these agents cause cumulative irritation or excessive drying of skin.

• Tell patient to avoid prolonged sun exposure and to use sunblock. Drug may have additive effect if used with other agents that cause photosensitivity.

• Advise patient of childbearing age to use two reliable forms of contraception simultaneously, unless abstinence is the chosen method of birth control, for 1 month before, during, and 1 month after treatment.

• Advise patient not to donate blood during or for 30 days after therapy; severe fetal abnormalities may occur if a pregnant patient receives blood containing isotretinoin.

▼ NEW DRUG

leflunomide
Arava

Pregnancy Risk Category: X

HOW SUPPLIED
Tablets: 10 mg, 20 mg, 100 mg

ACTION
Immunomodulatory agent that inhibits dihydroorotate dehydrogenase, an enzyme involved in pyrimidine synthesis, and has antiproliferative activity and anti-inflammatory effects.

Route	Onset	Peak	Duration
PO	Unknown	6-12 hr	Unknown

INDICATIONS & DOSAGE
Treatment of active rheumatoid arthritis to reduce signs and symptoms and to retard structural damage as evidenced by X-ray erosions and joint space narrowing—
Adults: 100 mg P.O. q 24 hours for 3 days, followed by 20 mg (maximum daily dose) P.O. q 24 hours. Dose may be decreased to 10 mg daily if higher dose is not well-tolerated.

ADVERSE REACTIONS
CNS: asthenia, dizziness, headache, paresthesia, malaise, migraine, sleep disorder, vertigo, neuritis, anxiety, depression, insomnia, neuralgia.
CV: angina pectoris, *hypertension*, chest pain, palpitation, tachycardia, vasculitis, vasodilation, varicose vein, peripheral edema.
EENT: pharyngitis, rhinitis, sinusitis, epistaxis, mouth ulcer, oral candidiasis, enlarged salivary glands, stomatitis, tooth disorder, dry mouth, blurred vision,

---

Reactions may be *common,* uncommon, *life-threatening,* or COMMON AND LIFE-THREATENING.

cataract, conjunctivitis, eye disorder, gingivitis, taste perversion.

GI: anorexia, *diarrhea,* dyspepsia, gastroenteritis, nausea, abdominal pain, vomiting, cholelithiasis, colitis, constipation, esophagitis, flatulence, gastritis, melena.

GU: urinary tract infection, albuminuria, cystitis, dysuria, hematuria, menstrual disorder, pelvic pain, vaginal candidiasis, prostate disorder, urinary frequency.

Hematologic: anemia, ecchymosis, hyperlipidemia.

Hepatic: elevated liver enzymes.

Metabolic: diabetes mellitus, fever, hyperglycemia, hyperthyroidism, hypokalemia.

Musculoskeletal: arthrosis, back pain, bursitis, muscle cramps, myalgia, bone necrosis, bone pain, arthralgia, leg cramps, joint disorder, neck pain, synovitis, tendon rupture, tenosynovitis.

Respiratory: bronchitis, increased cough, pneumonia, *respiratory infection,* asthma, dyspnea, lung disorder.

Skin: *alopecia,* eczema, pruritus, *rash,* dry skin, acne, contact dermatitis, fungal dermatitis, hair discoloration, hematoma, herpes simplex, herpes zoster, nail disorder, skin nodule, subcutaneous nodule, maculopapular rash, skin disorder, skin discoloration, skin ulcer.

Other: allergic reaction, flu syndrome, injury or accident, pain, weight loss, abscess, cyst, hernia, increased sweating, increased CK.

INTERACTIONS

Drug-drug. *Charcoal, cholestyramine:* decreased plasma concentrations of leflunomide. Sometimes used for this effect in overdose.

Methotrexate, other hepatotoxic drugs: increased risk of hepatotoxicity. Monitor liver enzymes as ordered.

NSAIDs (diclofenac, ibuprofen): increased levels of NSAIDs. Clinical significance is unknown.

Rifampin: increased active leflunomide metabolite level. Use caution with concomitant use.

Tolbutamide: increased levels of tolbutamide. Clinical significance is unknown.

EFFECTS ON DIAGNOSTIC TESTS
None reported.

CONTRAINDICATIONS
Contraindicated in patients with known hypersensitivity to drug or its components and in women who are or may become pregnant or who are breast feeding. Drug is not recommended for patients with hepatic insufficiency, hepatitis B or C, severe immunodeficiency, bone marrow dysplasia, or severe uncontrolled infections. Vaccination with live vaccines is not recommended. The long half-life of drug should be considered when contemplating administration of a live vaccine after stopping drug treatment. Drug is not recommended for use in patients under 18 years and in men attempting to father a child.

NURSING CONSIDERATIONS
• Use cautiously in patients with renal insufficiency.

Alert: Know that drug can cause fetal harm when administered to pregnant women; it is recommended that women planning to become pregnant discontinue leflunomide therapy and consult doctor. It is recommended that men planning to father a child discontinue drug therapy and follow recommended leflunomide removal protocol (cholestyramine 8 g, P.O. three times daily for 11 days).

• Be aware of that the risk of malignancy, particularly lymphoproliferative disorders, is increased with the use of some immunosuppression medications, including leflunomide.

• Monitor liver enzymes (ALT and AST) before starting therapy and monthly thereafter until stable. Frequency can then be decreased based on clinical situation.

✓ Patient teaching
• Explain need and frequency of required blood tests and monitoring.

• Instruct patient to use birth control during course of treatment and until it has been determined that drug is no longer active.

• Warn patient that if signs or symptoms of pregnancy occurs (such as late menses

---

or breast tenderness), to immediately notify doctor.

• Advise breast-feeding patient to discontinue breast-feeding during drug therapy.

• Inform patient that aspirin, other NSAIDs, and low-dose corticosteroids may be continued during treatment. However, combined use of drug with antimalarials, intramuscular or oral gold, penicillamine, azathioprine, or methotrexate has not been adequately studied.

---

levocarnitine (L-carnitine)
Carnitor, VitaCarn

Pregnancy Risk Category: B

HOW SUPPLIED
Tablets: 330 mg
Capsules: 250 mg ◊
Oral liquid: 100 mg/ml
Injection: 1 g/5 ml

ACTION
Facilitates transport of long chain fatty acids into cellular mitochondria. The fatty acids are then used to produce energy.

Route	Onset	Peak	Duration
PO, IV	Unknown	Unknown	Unknown

INDICATIONS & DOSAGE
Primary and secondary systemic carnitine deficiency—
Adults: 990 mg P.O. b.i.d. or t.i.d. Alternatively, 10 to 30 ml (1 to 3 g) of oral liquid daily.
Children: 50 to 100 mg/kg/day P.O. in divided doses.

All dosages depend on clinical response. Higher dosages may be given. However, for children, maximum dosage is 3 g/day.
Acute and chronic treatment of secondary carnitine deficiency—
Adults: 50 mg/kg I.V. slowly over 2 to 3 minutes q 3 to 4 hours.

ADVERSE REACTIONS
GI: *nausea, vomiting, cramps, diarrhea.*
Other: *body odor.*

INTERACTIONS
Drug-drug. *D,L-carnitine (sold as vitamin B_T):* inhibition of levocarnitine and possible deficiency. Avoid concomitant use.
Valproic acid: increased requirement for carnitine. Adjust dosage as ordered.
Drug-food. *Any food:* decreased GI upset. Dissolve drug in drink or liquid food or take with meals.

EFFECTS ON DIAGNOSTIC TESTS
None reported.

CONTRAINDICATIONS
No known contraindications.

NURSING CONSIDERATIONS
• Give enteral liquid alone or dissolved in drinks or liquid food.
• Use entire or partial contents of containers of liquid immediately after opening; discard any unused contents.
• Monitor patient's tolerance during first week of therapy and after increasing dosage, as ordered.
• Monitor blood chemistry results and plasma carnitine concentrations periodically, as ordered, as well as vital signs and patient's overall clinical condition.

I.V. administration
• Be aware that a loading dose often is given to patients with severe metabolic crisis, followed by an equivalent dose over the following 24 hours.
• Drug is compatible when mixed in solutions of 0.9% NaCl or lactated Ringer's in concentrations ranging from 250 mg/500 ml to 4,200 mg/500 ml.
• Store mixed infusions at room temperature (77° F [25° C]) for up to 24 hours in polyvinyl chloride plastic bags.
• Do not refrigerate solution.

Patient teaching
• Tell patient to consume oral liquid slowly to minimize GI distress. If GI intolerance persists, dosage may have to be reduced.
• Warn patient to avoid "vitamin B_T." This will interact with drug and render it ineffective.
• Caution patient not to share drug with

Reactions may be *common,* uncommon, *life-threatening,* or COMMON AND LIFE-THREATENING.

others. Some people have used it to improve athletic performance.
• Warn patient about possible body odor.
• Space doses evenly every 3 to 4 hours and give drug with or after meals, if possible.

---

levomethadyl acetate hydrochloride
Orlaam

Controlled Substance Schedule II
Pregnancy Risk Category: C

HOW SUPPLIED
Oral solution: 10 mg/ml

ACTION
A synthetic opiate agonist structurally similar to methadone that suppresses symptoms of withdrawal in opiate-tolerant persons by cross-substituting for opiate agonists. Long-term administration may produce sufficient tolerance to block the euphoric effects of opiate agonists.

Route	Onset	Peak	Duration
PO	Unknown	1.5-4 hr	48-72 hr

INDICATIONS & DOSAGE
Opiate addiction—
Adults: dosage is highly individualized. Initially, 20 to 40 mg q 48 to 72 hours. Subsequent doses increased in increments of 5 to 10 mg at 48- to 72-hour intervals until steady state is reached, usually within 1 to 2 weeks. Most patients are stable on 60 to 90 mg three times weekly.

ADVERSE REACTIONS
CNS: drowsiness, sedation.
CV: bradycardia, edema, prolonged QT interval.
EENT: blurred vision, rhinitis.
GI: *dry mouth, abdominal pain, diarrhea, constipation, nausea, vomiting.*
GU: *impotence, difficulty with ejaculation.*
Respiratory: *cough.*
Skin: *rash, diaphoresis.*
Other: yawning, arthralgia, asthenia, back pain, chills, flulike syndrome, malaise, abstinence syndrome with sudden withdrawal.

INTERACTIONS
Drug-drug. *Carbamazepine, phenobarbital, phenytoin, rifampin:* increased hepatic enzyme activity; may increase levomethadyl's peak activity or shorten its duration of action. Monitor closely for withdrawal symptoms.
Cimetidine, erythromycin, ketoconazole: decreased hepatic enzyme activity; may decrease levomethadyl's peak activity or prolong its duration of action. Monitor closely.
Naloxone, pentazocine, other opioid agonist-antagonists: may precipitate abstinence syndrome. Don't use together.
Drug-lifestyle. *Alcohol use:* increased CNS effects. Avoid concomitant use.

EFFECTS ON DIAGNOSTIC TESTS
None reported.

CONTRAINDICATIONS
Contraindicated in patients hypersensitive to drug.

NURSING CONSIDERATIONS
• Use cautiously in patients with cardiac conduction defects or with hepatic or renal failure.
• Be aware that levomethadyl is to be used only by certain licensed and approved clinics. There are no recognized clinical uses for the drug outside of addiction treatment programs. Levomethadyl may only be dispensed by treatment programs approved by the FDA, Drug Enforcement Agency, and designated state authority. By law, take-home doses are forbidden. Also by law, oral solutions must be diluted before being administered to the patient. The diluent should be a different color than the one used to dilute the methadone oral solution in the same clinic setting.
• If administering to women of childbearing age, anticipate monthly pregnancy tests. Patients should be switched to methadone if pregnancy occurs.
Alert: Be aware drug should never be administered on a daily basis because of risk of fatal overdose.

---

*Liquid contains alcohol.   **May contain tartrazine.   †Canada   ‡Australia   §U.K.   ◊OTC

• Be aware most patients can tolerate the 72-hour interval between weekly regimens. If withdrawal is a problem during the 72-hour interval, be prepared to increase the preceding dose or switch to an alternate-day schedule as ordered. Never give levomethadyl on 2 consecutive days; instead, give small supplemental doses of methadone. Consider risk of drug diversion before giving patients take-home methadone.

• When used to replace methadone, the suggested initial dose is 1.2 to 1.3 times the daily methadone dose three times weekly, not to exceed 120 mg. Adjust dosage according to clinical response, as ordered. The crossover to methadone should be done in a single dose rather than decreasing doses of methadone and increasing doses of levomethadyl.

✔ Patient teaching
• Advise patient not to engage in hazardous activities, such as driving or operating heavy machinery, until CNS effects are known.
• Advise patient to avoid alcohol while taking drug.
• Explain how drug is administered, and review administration schedule with patient and family.
• Inform female patient of need for monthly pregnancy tests. Advise patient to avoid pregnancy, but if pregnancy is suspected to call doctor immediately because drug will need to be discontinued.
• Advise female patient of childbearing age to use contraception during drug therapy.

---

mesalamine
Asacol, Mesasal, Pentasa,
Rowasa, Salofalk

Pregnancy Risk Category: B

HOW SUPPLIED
Tablets (delayed-release): 400 mg
Capsules (controlled-release): 250 mg
Rectal suspension: 4 g/60 ml
Suppositories: 500 mg

ACTION
Unknown. An active metabolite of sulfasalazine; probably acts topically by inhibiting prostaglandin production in the colon. Exact mechanism is unknown.

Route	Onset	Peak	Duration
PO, PR	Unknown	3-12 hr	Unknown

INDICATIONS & DOSAGE
Active mild-to-moderate distal ulcerative colitis, proctitis, or proctosigmoiditis—
Adults: 800 mg P.O. (tablets) t.i.d. for total dose of 2.4 g/day for 6 weeks; 1 g P.O. (capsules) q.i.d. for total dose of 4 g up to 8 weeks; 500 mg P.R. (suppository) b.i.d., or 4 g as a retention enema once daily (preferably h.s.). Rectal dosage form should be retained overnight (for about 8 hours). Usual course of therapy for rectal form is 3 to 6 weeks.

ADVERSE REACTIONS
CNS: headache, dizziness, fatigue, malaise, asthenia, chills.
GI: abdominal pain, cramps, discomfort, flatulence, diarrhea, rectal pain, bloating, nausea, *pancolitis,* vomiting, constipation, eructation.
Respiratory: wheezing.
Skin: itching, rash, urticaria, hair loss.
Other: *anaphylaxis* (rare), fever, arthralgia, chest pain, myalgia, back pain, hypertonia.

INTERACTIONS
Drug-drug. *Lactulose:* may impair release of delayed or extended-release preparations. Monitor closely.
Omeprazole: increased absorption of mesalamine. Monitor closely.

EFFECTS ON DIAGNOSTIC TESTS
None reported.

CONTRAINDICATIONS
Contraindicated in patients hypersensitive to drug, its components, or salicylates.

NURSING CONSIDERATIONS
• Use cautiously in patients with renal impairment. Problems have not been documented, but nephrotoxic potential from absorbed mesalamine exists.

• Monitor periodic renal function studies in patients on long-term therapy, as ordered.

• Because it contains potassium metabisulfite, keep in mind that mesalamine may cause hypersensitivity reactions in patients sensitive to sulfites.

✓ Patient teaching

• Instruct patient to carefully follow instructions supplied with medication and to swallow tablets whole.

• Advise patient to discontinue drug if he experiences a fever or rash. Patient intolerant of sulfasalazine may also be hypersensitive to mesalamine.

• Teach patient about proper use of retention enema.

mesna
Mesnex, Uromitexan§

Pregnancy Risk Category: B

HOW SUPPLIED
Injection: 100 mg/ml

ACTION
Prevents ifosfamide-induced hemorrhagic cystitis by reacting with urotoxic ifosfamide metabolites.

Route	Onset	Peak	Duration
IV	Unknown	Unknown	Unknown

INDICATIONS & DOSAGE
Prophylaxis of hemorrhagic cystitis in patients receiving ifosfamide—
Adults: dosage varies with amount of ifosfamide administered; calculated as 20% (w/w) of the ifosfamide dose at time of ifosfamide administration. Usual dosage is 240 mg/m² as an I.V. bolus with administration of ifosfamide; repeated at 4 and 8 hours after administration of ifosfamide.

ADVERSE REACTIONS
CNS: *headache, fatigue.*
GI: *soft stools, nausea, vomiting, diarrhea, dysgeusia.*
Other: *limb pain, hypotension, allergy.*
   Note: Because mesna is used concomi-

tantly with ifosfamide and other chemotherapeutic agents, it is difficult to determine adverse reactions attributable solely to mesna.

INTERACTIONS
None significant.

EFFECTS ON DIAGNOSTIC TESTS
Mesna may produce a false-positive test for urinary ketones. A red-violet color will return to violet with the addition of acetic acid.

CONTRAINDICATIONS
Contraindicated in patients hypersensitive to mesna or thiol-containing compounds.

NURSING CONSIDERATIONS
• Monitor urine samples for hematuria daily. Monitor BUN, creatinine, and intake or output.

• Be aware mesna is not effective in preventing hematuria from other causes (such as thrombocytopenia).

• Although formulated to prevent hemorrhagic cystitis from ifosfamide, be aware that drug will not protect against other toxicities associated with ifosfamide therapy.

⚡ I.V. administration
• Prepare I.V. solution by diluting commercially available ampules with D₅W solution, dextrose 5% and 0.9% NaCl for injection, 0.9% NaCl for injection, or lactated Ringer's solution to obtain a final solution of 20 mg mesna/ml.

• Diluted solutions are stable for 24 hours at room temperature, but it is recommended that they be refrigerated and used within 6 hours. After opening ampule, discard any unused drug.

• Mesna I.V. is incompatible with cisplatin; do not mix them.

✓ Patient teaching
• Explain to patient and family or other caregiver need for drug and how it is administered.

• Instruct patient to report persistent or severe adverse reactions.

• Advise patient to promptly report blood in urine.

---

*Liquid contains alcohol.   **May contain tartrazine.   †Canada   ‡Australia   §U.K.   ◊OTC

methoxsalen (topical)
Oxsoralen

Pregnancy Risk Category: C

HOW SUPPLIED
Lotion: 1%

ACTION
Unknown. May enhance melanogenesis, either directly or secondarily, to an inflammatory process.

Route	Onset	Peak	Duration
Topical	Unknown	Unknown	Unknown

INDICATIONS & DOSAGE
To induce repigmentation in vitiligo; psoriasis—
Adults and children over 12 years: lotion applied to small, well-defined vitiliginous lesions. For optimum effect, lotion should be applied about 1 to 2 hours before exposure to ultraviolet light. The treated area may be exposed to ultraviolet light for a limited time.

After exposure, wash lesions with soap and water, and protect area with sunblock. Manufacturer recommends weekly treatment.

ADVERSE REACTIONS
Skin: edema, erythema, painful blistering, burning, peeling, pruritus.

INTERACTIONS
Drug-drug. *Photosensitizing agents:* may increase methoxsalen toxicity. Don't use together.
Drug-lifestyle. *Sun exposure:* increased photosensitivity reactions. Avoid prolonged or unprotected sun exposure.

EFFECTS ON DIAGNOSTIC TESTS
Abnormal liver function test results have been reported, but exact relationship is unknown.

CONTRAINDICATIONS
Contraindicated in patients sensitive to psoralen compounds and in those with diseases associated with photosensitivity (such as porphyria, acute lupus erythematosus, xeroderma, or hydromorphic and polymorphic light eruptions). Also contraindicated in patients with melanoma, invasive squamous cell carcinoma, and aphakia.

NURSING CONSIDERATIONS
• Use cautiously in patients with familial history of sunlight allergy, GI diseases, or chronic infection.
• Be prepared to regulate therapy carefully. Overdosage or overexposure to light can cause serious burning or blistering.
• Protect patient's eyes and lips during light exposure treatments.
• Obtain monthly liver function tests for patients with vitiligo (especially at beginning of therapy), as ordered.

✔ Patient teaching
• Tell patient to avoid excessive sunlight and ultraviolet light during therapy and wear protective clothing and sunscreen.
• Inform patient of need for monthly blood tests, and stress importance of compliance to test schedule.

minoxidil (topical)
Rogaine

Pregnancy Risk Category: C

HOW SUPPLIED
Topical solution: 2%

ACTION
Unknown. Stimulates hair growth, possibly by dilating arterial microcapillaries around hair follicles.

Route	Onset	Peak	Duration
Topical	Unknown	Unknown	Unknown

INDICATIONS & DOSAGE
Androgenetic alopecia—
Adults: 1 ml of 2% solution applied to affected area b.i.d. Maximum daily dosage is 2 ml.

ADVERSE REACTIONS
CNS: headache, dizziness, faintness, light-headedness.
CV: edema, chest pain, hypertension, hy-

potension, palpitations, increased or decreased pulse rate.
EENT: sinusitis.
GI: diarrhea, nausea, vomiting.
GU: urinary tract infection, renal calculi, urethritis.
Respiratory: bronchitis, upper respiratory infection.
Skin: *irritant dermatitis,* allergic contact dermatitis, eczema, hypertrichosis, *local erythema, pruritus, dry skin or scalp, flaking,* alopecia, exacerbation of hair loss.
Other: back pain, tendinitis, edema, weight gain.

INTERACTIONS
Drug-drug. *Petrolatum, topical corticosteroids, topical retinoids, or other drugs that may enhance skin absorption:* increased risk of systemic effects of minoxidil. Do not apply minoxidil with other drugs.

EFFECTS ON DIAGNOSTIC TESTS
None reported.

CONTRAINDICATIONS
Contraindicated in patients hypersensitive to drug or components of the solution.

NURSING CONSIDERATIONS
• Use cautiously in patients over 50 years old and in those with cardiac, renal, or hepatic disease.
• Be aware patients need to have normal, healthy scalps before beginning therapy, because absorption of drug through irritated skin may cause adverse systemic effects.
• Be aware that treatment is most likely to succeed in patients with balding area smaller than 4″ (10 cm) that developed within the past 10 years.

☑ **Patient teaching**
• Teach patient how to apply topical minoxidil. Hair and scalp should be thoroughly dry before application, and drug should not be applied to any other body areas. Tell patient not to use drug on irritated or sunburned scalp or with any other medication on scalp. Tell him to thoroughly wash hands after application.

• Warn patient to avoid inhaling any spray or mist from drug. He should avoid spraying around eyes because solution contains alcohol and may be irritating.
• Teach patient to monitor pulse rate and body weight.
• Advise patient of need for medical follow-ups 1 month after therapy starts and every 6 months thereafter.
• Advise patient that therapy will be prolonged and will continue for at least 4 months before clinical effects appear and that drug must be used daily for optimal results. About 40% of patients will see moderate to dense hair growth.
• Tell patient that discontinuing drug may result in loss of new hair growth. New hair growth is usually fine and may be colorless, but will resemble existing hair after continued treatment.

nimodipine
Nimotop

Pregnancy Risk Category: C

HOW SUPPLIED
Capsules: 30 mg

ACTION
Inhibits calcium ion influx across cardiac and smooth muscle cells, decreasing myocardial contractility and oxygen demand, and dilates coronary and cerebral arteries and arterioles.

Route	Onset	Peak	Duration
PO	Unknown	1 hr	Unknown

INDICATIONS & DOSAGE
Improvement of neurologic deficits in patients after subarachnoid hemorrhage from ruptured congenital aneurysms—
Adults: 60 mg P.O. q 4 hours for 21 days. Therapy begun within 96 hours after subarachnoid hemorrhage.
Adjust-a-dose: In patients with hepatic failure, 30 mg P.O. q 4 hours for 21 days.

ADVERSE REACTIONS
CNS: headache, psychic disturbances.
CV: decreased blood pressure, flushing, edema, tachycardia.

GI: nausea, diarrhea, abdominal discomfort.
Respiratory: dyspnea.
Skin: dermatitis, rash.
Other: muscle cramps.

INTERACTIONS
Drug-drug. *Antihypertensives:* possible enhanced hypotensive effect. Monitor patient closely.
Calcium channel blockers: possible enhanced CV effects. Monitor patient closely.
Cimetidine: increased nimodipine bioavailability. Monitor closely.

EFFECTS ON DIAGNOSTIC TESTS
None reported.

CONTRAINDICATIONS
No known contraindications.

NURSING CONSIDERATIONS
• Use cautiously in patients with hepatic failure.
• Be aware nimodipine should be reserved for patients who are in good neurologic condition (for example, Hunt and Hess grades I to III).
• Monitor blood pressure and heart rate in all patients, especially at start of therapy.
• If capsule cannot be swallowed, make a hole in each end of the capsule with an 18G needle, and extract the contents into a syringe. Empty the syringe into patient's nasogastric tube. Flush tube with 30 ml of 0.9% NaCl solution.

☑ **Patient teaching**
• Explain use of drug, and review administration schedule with patient and family. Stress importance of compliance for maximum drug effectiveness.
• Instruct patient to report persistent or severe adverse reactions promptly.

---

olsalazine sodium
Dipentum

Pregnancy Risk Category: C

HOW SUPPLIED
Capsules: 250 mg

ACTION
Unknown. After oral administration, converts to 5-aminosalicylic acid (5-ASA or mesalamine) in the colon, where it has a local anti-inflammatory effect.

Route	Onset	Peak	Duration
PO	Unknown	1 hr	Unknown

INDICATIONS & DOSAGE
Maintenance of remission of ulcerative colitis in patients intolerant of sulfasalazine—
Adults: 500 mg P.O. b.i.d. with meals.

ADVERSE REACTIONS
CNS: headache, depression, vertigo, dizziness, fatigue.
GI: *diarrhea*, nausea, *abdominal pain*, dyspepsia, bloating, anorexia.
Skin: rash, itching.
Other: arthralgia.

INTERACTIONS
Drug-drug. *Anticoagulants, coumarin derivatives:* prolonged PT or INR. Monitor bleeding studies.
Drug-food. *Any food:* decreased GI irritation. Administer drug with food.

EFFECTS ON DIAGNOSTIC TESTS
None reported.

CONTRAINDICATIONS
Contraindicated in patients hypersensitive to salicylates.

NURSING CONSIDERATIONS
• Use cautiously in patients with preexisting renal disease. Although problems have not been reported with this drug, the possibility of renal tubular damage from absorbed mesalamine or its metabolites must be considered.
• Regularly monitor BUN and creatinine levels and urinalysis in patients with preexisting renal disease, as ordered.
• Be aware that in clinical trials, 17% of all patients reported diarrhea during therapy. Although diarrhea appears dose-related, it is difficult to distinguish from worsening of disease symptoms. Exacerbation of disease has been noted with similar drugs.

Reactions may be *common*, uncommon, *life-threatening*, or COMMON AND LIFE-THREATENING.

☑ **Patient teaching**
• Teach patient to take drug in evenly divided doses and with food to minimize adverse GI reactions.
• Instruct patient to report persistent or severe adverse reactions promptly.

---

pamidronate disodium
Aredia

Pregnancy Risk Category: C

HOW SUPPLIED
Injection: 30-mg, 60-mg, 90-mg vials

ACTION
An antihypercalcemic agent that inhibits resorption of bone. Adsorbs to hydroxyapatite crystals in bone and may directly block dissolution of calcium phosphate. Blocks mature osteoclast formation. Drug apparently doesn't inhibit bone formation or mineralization.

Route	Onset	Peak	Duration
IV	Unknown	Unknown	Unknown

INDICATIONS & DOSAGE
Moderate to severe hypercalcemia associated with cancer (with or without bone metastases)—
Adults: dosage depends on severity of hypercalcemia. Serum calcium levels should be corrected for serum albumin. Corrected serum calcium (CCa) is calculated using this formula:

$$CCa = serum\ calcium + 0.8\ (4-serum\ albumin)$$
$$(mg/dl) \quad (mg/dl) \quad\quad (g/dl)$$

Patients with moderate hypercalcemia (CCa levels of 12 to 13.5 mg/dl) may receive 60 to 90 mg by I.V. infusion over 4 hours for 60-mg dose and over 24 hours for 90-mg dose. Patients with severe hypercalcemia (CCa levels over 13.5 mg/dl) may receive 90 mg by I.V. infusion over 24 hours. A minimum of 7 days should elapse before retreatment to allow for full response to initial dose.
Moderate to severe Paget's disease—
Adults: 30 mg I.V. as a 4-hour infusion on 3 consecutive days for total dose of 90 mg. Cycle repeated, p.r.n.

Osteolytic bone metastases of breast cancer in combination with standard antineoplastic therapy—
Adults: 90 mg I.V. infusion over 2 to 4 hours q 3 to 4 weeks.

ADVERSE REACTIONS
CNS: *seizures, fatigue,* somnolence.
CV: *atrial fibrillation,* syncope, tachycardia, *hypertension.*
GI: *abdominal pain,* anorexia, constipation, nausea, vomiting, *GI hemorrhage.*
Hematologic: *leukopenia, thrombocytopenia,* anemia.
Other: *hypophosphatemia, hypokalemia, hypomagnesemia, hypocalcemia, fever,* infusion-site reaction.

INTERACTIONS
None significant.

EFFECTS ON DIAGNOSTIC TESTS
None reported.

CONTRAINDICATIONS
Contraindicated in patients hypersensitive to drug or other bisphosphonates, such as etidronate.

NURSING CONSIDERATIONS
• Use with extreme caution, and consider risks versus benefits in patients with renal impairment.
• Assess hydration status before treatment. Be aware drug should be used only after patients have been vigorously hydrated with 0.9% NaCl solution. In patients with mild-to-moderate hypercalcemia, hydration alone may be sufficient.
• Because drug can cause electrolyte disturbances, carefully monitor serum electrolytes, especially calcium, phosphate, and magnesium, as ordered. Short-term administration of calcium may be necessary in patients with severe hypocalcemia. Also monitor creatinine level, CBC and differential count, and hematocrit and hemoglobin levels, as ordered.
• Carefully monitor patients with preexisting anemia, leukopenia, or thrombocytopenia during first 2 weeks of therapy.
• Monitor patient's temperature. In clinical trials, 27% of patients experienced an

---

elevation of 1.8° F (1° C) for 24 to 48 hours after therapy.
• Solution is stable for 24 hours at room temperature.

🔲 I.V. administration
• Reconstitute vial with 10 ml of sterile water for injection. After drug is completely dissolved, add to 1,000 ml of 0.45% or 0.9% NaCl for injection or D₅W. Do not mix with infusion solutions that contain calcium, such as Ringer's injection or lactated Ringer's injection. Visually inspect for precipitate before administering.
• Give only by I.V. infusion. Animal studies have shown evidence of nephropathy when drug is given as a bolus.

✅ Patient teaching
• Explain use and administration of drug to patient and family.
• Instruct patient to report adverse reactions promptly.

---

pilocarpine hydrochloride
Salagen

Pregnancy Risk Category: C

HOW SUPPLIED
Tablets: 5 mg

ACTION
A cholinergic parasympathomimetic agent that increases secretion of salivary glands, eliminating dryness.

Route	Onset	Peak	Duration
PO	20 min	1 hr	3-5 hr

INDICATIONS & DOSAGE
Treatment of xerostomia from salivary gland hypofunction caused by radiotherapy for cancer of head and neck—
Adults: 5 mg P.O. t.i.d.; may be increased to 10 mg P.O. t.i.d., p.r.n.
✳ NEW INDICATION: *Treatment of symptoms of dry mouth in patients with Sjögren's syndrome—*
Adults: 5 mg P.O. q.i.d.

ADVERSE REACTIONS
CNS: *dizziness, headache,* tremor.
CV: hypertension, tachycardia.
EENT: *rhinitis,* lacrimation, amblyopia, pharyngitis, voice alteration, conjunctivitis, epistaxis, *sinusitis, abnormal vision.*
GI: *nausea,* dyspepsia, diarrhea, abdominal pain, vomiting, dysphagia, taste perversion.
GU: *urinary frequency.*
Skin: *flushing,* rash, pruritus.
Other: *sweating, chills, asthenia,* edema, myalgia.

INTERACTIONS
Drug-drug. *Beta-adrenergic antagonists:* may increase risk of conduction disturbances. Use together cautiously.
Drugs with anticholinergic effects: may antagonize anticholinergic effects. Use together cautiously.
Drugs with parasympathomimetic effects: may result in additive pharmacologic effects. Monitor patient closely.

EFFECTS ON DIAGNOSTIC TESTS
None reported.

CONTRAINDICATIONS
Contraindicated in patients with uncontrolled asthma or hypersensitivity to pilocarpine and when meiosis is undesirable, such as in acute iritis or narrow-angle glaucoma.

NURSING CONSIDERATIONS
• Use cautiously in patients with CV disease, controlled asthma, chronic bronchitis, chronic obstructive pulmonary disease, cholelithiasis, biliary tract disease, nephrolithiasis, or cognitive or psychiatric disturbances.
• Drug should not be used in breast-feeding women.
• Safety and efficacy in children have not been established.
• Because retinal detachment has been reported with pilocarpine use in patients with retinal disease, examine the patient's fundus carefully before therapy begins.
• Monitor patient for signs of toxicity: headache, visual disturbance, lacrimation, sweating, respiratory distress, GI spasm, nausea, vomiting, diarrhea, atrioventricular

---

block, tachycardia, bradycardia, hypotension, hypertension, shock, mental confusion, arrhythmia, and tremors. Immediately notify doctor of suspected toxicity.

☑ **Patient teaching**
• Warn patient that driving ability may be impaired by drug-induced visual disturbances, especially at night.
• Advise patient to drink plenty of fluids to prevent dehydration.
• Inform elderly patients with Sjögren's syndrome that they may be especially prone to urinary frequency, diarrhea, and dizziness.

▼ *NEW DRUG*

raloxifene hydrochloride
Evista

Pregnancy Risk Category: X

HOW SUPPLIED
Tablets: 60 mg

ACTION
Selective estrogen receptor modulator that reduces resorption of bone and decreases overall bone turnover. These effects on bone are manifested as reductions in serum and urine levels of bone turnover markers and increases in bone mineral density.

Route	Onset	Peak	Duration
PO	Unknown	Unknown	24 hr

INDICATIONS & DOSAGE
Prevention of osteoporosis in postmenopausal women—
Adults: 60 mg P.O. once daily.

ADVERSE REACTIONS
CNS: depression, insomnia, migraine.
CV: *hot flashes,* chest pain.
EENT: *sinusitis,* pharyngitis, laryngitis.
GI: nausea, dyspepsia, vomiting, flatulence, GI disorder, gastroenteritis, abdominal pain.
GU: vaginitis, urinary tract infection, cystitis, leukorrhea, endometrial disorder, vaginal bleeding.
Metabolic: weight gain, fever.

Musculoskeletal: *arthralgia,* myalgia, arthritis, leg cramps, breast pain.
Respiratory: increased cough, pneumonia.
Skin: rash, sweating.
Other: *infection, flu syndrome,* peripheral edema.

INTERACTIONS
Drug-drug. *Cholestyramine:* causes a significant reduction in absorption of raloxifene. Avoid concomitant use.
Highly protein-bound drugs (such as clofibrate, diazepam, diazoxide, ibuprofen, indomethacin, naproxen): may interfere with binding sites. Use with caution.
Warfarin: may cause a decrease in PT. Monitor PT and INR closely.

EFFECTS ON DIAGNOSTIC TESTS
None reported.

CONTRAINDICATIONS
Contraindicated in pregnant women or those planning pregnancy, breast-feeding patients, or children. Also contraindicated in women hypersensitive to drug or its constituents, or with past history or currently active venous thromboembolic events including deep vein thrombosis, pulmonary embolism, and retinal vein thrombosis.

NURSING CONSIDERATIONS
• Use cautiously in patients with severe hepatic impairment.
• Monitor for signs of blood clots. The greatest risk for thromboembolic events (deep vein thrombosis, pulmonary embolism, retinal vein thrombosis) occurs during first 4 months of treatment.
• Be aware that drug should be discontinued at least 72 hours before prolonged immobilization and resumed only after patient is fully mobilized.
• Report unexplained uterine bleeding since endometrial proliferation has not been associated with drug use.
• Monitor for breast abnormalities that occur during treatment. Be aware that no association between breast enlargement, breast pain, or an increased risk of breast cancer has been shown.
• Know that the following laboratory

changes may occur: increased apolipoprotein A; reduced serum total cholesterol; low-density lipoprotein cholesterol; fibrinogen; apolipoprotein B and lipoprotein (a); modest increases in hormone-binding globulin concentrations; small decreases in serum total calcium, inorganic phosphate, total protein, albumin, and platelet count.

• Safety and efficacy have not been evaluated in men.

• Be aware that the effect on bone mineral density beyond 2 years of drug treatment is not known.

• Concomitant use of raloxifene with hormone replacement therapy or systemic estrogen has not been evaluated and, therefore, is not recommended.

☑ **Patient teaching**
• Advise patient to avoid long periods of restricted movement (such as during traveling) because of an increased risk of venous thromboembolic events.

• Inform patient that hot flashes or flushing may occur and that raloxifene does not aid in reducing them.

• Instruct patient to exercise other bone loss prevention measures including supplemental calcium and vitamin D if dietary intake is inadequate, weight-bearing exercises, and discontinuing alcohol consumption and smoking.

• Tell patient that drug may be taken without regard for food.

• Advise patient to report unexplained uterine bleeding or breast abnormalities during treatment.

• Explain adverse effects and instruct patient to read the patient package insert before starting therapy and to reread each time the prescription is renewed.

---

riluzole
Rilutek

Pregnancy Risk Category: C

HOW SUPPLIED
Tablets: 50 mg

ACTION
May protect motor neurons from excito-toxic effects of glutamate by inhibiting glutamate release, inactivating some sodium channels, and interfering with transmitter binding.

Route	Onset	Peak	Duration
PO	Unknown	Unknown	Unknown

INDICATIONS & DOSAGE
Amyotrophic lateral sclerosis—
Adults: 50 mg P.O. q 12 hours, taken on empty stomach.

ADVERSE REACTIONS
CNS: headache, aggravation reaction, *asthenia,* hypertonia, depression, dizziness, insomnia, malaise, somnolence, vertigo, circumoral paresthesia.
CV: hypertension, tachycardia, palpitation, orthostatic hypotension.
EENT: rhinitis, sinusitis.
GI: abdominal pain, *nausea,* vomiting, dyspepsia, anorexia, diarrhea, flatulence, stomatitis, tooth disorder, dry mouth, oral candidiasis.
GU: urinary tract infection, dysuria.
Respiratory: *decreased lung function,* increased cough.
Skin: pruritus, eczema, alopecia, exfoliative dermatitis.
Other: back pain, phlebitis, weight loss, peripheral edema, arthralgia.

INTERACTIONS
Drug-drug. *Allopurinol, methyldopa, sulfasalazine:* increased risk of hepatotoxicity. Monitor patient closely.
Inducers of CYP 1A2 (omeprazole, rifampin): may increase riluzole elimination. Monitor closely.
Potential inhibitors of CYP 1A2 (amitriptyline, caffeine, phenacetin, quinolones, theophylline): may decrease riluzole elimination. Monitor closely.
Drug-food. *Any food:* decreased bioavailability. Administer 1 hour before or 2 hours after meals.
Charbroiled foods: may increase riluzole elimination. Avoid concomitant use.
Drug-lifestyle. *Alcohol use:* may increase risk of hepatotoxicity. Avoid excessive use.
Smoking: may increase riluzole elimination. Avoid contact.

EFFECTS ON DIAGNOSTIC TESTS
None reported.

CONTRAINDICATIONS
Contraindicated in patients with history of severe hypersensitivity to drug or its components.

NURSING CONSIDERATIONS
• Use cautiously in patients with hepatic or renal dysfunction, in elderly patients, females, and Japanese patients (who may have a lower metabolic capacity to eliminate drug than do males and Caucasians, respectively).
• Be aware that elevations in baseline liver function studies (especially bilirubin) preclude drug use. Liver function studies should be done periodically during therapy, as ordered. In many patients, drug may increase serum aminotransferase; if level exceeds five times upper limit of normal or if clinical jaundice develops, notify doctor.
• Give drug at least 1 hour before or 2 hours after a meal to avoid decreased bioavailability.

☑**Patient teaching**
• Tell patient to take drug at same time each day. If a dose is missed, tell him to take next tablet when planned.
• Instruct patient to take on an empty stomach to facilitate full dose absorption.
• Instruct patient to report fever to doctor, who may order a WBC count.
• Warn patient to avoid hazardous activities until CNS effects of drug are known and to limit alcohol use while taking drug.
• Tell patient to store drug at room temperature, protected from bright light, and to keep it out of children's reach.

ritodrine hydrochloride
Yutopar, Yutopar S.R.†

Pregnancy Risk Category: B

HOW SUPPLIED
Tablets†: 10 mg
Capsules (extended-release)†: 40 mg
Injection: 10 mg/ml, 15 mg/ml

Injection for I.V. infusion: 0.3 mg/ml (150 mg in 500 ml D_5W)

ACTION
Beta-receptor agonist that stimulates the beta$_2$-adrenergic receptors in uterine smooth muscle, inhibiting contractility.

Route	Onset	Peak	Duration
PO	30-60 min	30-60 min	Unknown
IV	5 min	60 min	Unknown

INDICATIONS & DOSAGE
Preterm labor—
Adults: usual initial dose is 0.05 mg/minute I.V., gradually increased by 0.05 mg/minute q 10 minutes until desired result is obtained or until maternal heart rate reaches 130 beats/minute. Effective dosage usually ranges from 0.15 to 0.35 mg/minute.

ADVERSE REACTIONS
CNS: nervousness, anxiety, *headaches, tremors,* emotional upset, malaise.
CV: dose-related alterations in blood pressure, palpitations, *pulmonary edema, tachycardia.*
GI: *nausea, vomiting.*
Hematologic: *leukopenia, agranulocytosis.*
Other: *erythema, hyperglycemia,* hypokalemia, *anaphylactic shock.*

INTERACTIONS
Drug-drug. Atropine: may potentiate systemic hypertension. Monitor blood pressure.
Beta-adrenergic blockers: may inhibit ritodrine's action. Avoid concurrent use.
Corticosteroids: may produce pulmonary edema in mother. Monitor patient closely.
Diazoxide, inhalation anesthetics, magnesium sulfate, meperidine: potentiated adverse cardiac effects, arrhythmias, and hypotension. Monitor patient closely.
Sympathomimetics: additive sympathomimetic effects. Use together cautiously.

EFFECTS ON DIAGNOSTIC TESTS
I.V. administration of ritodrine elevates the plasma insulin and glucose levels and decreases plasma potassium concentra-

tions (values usually return to normal within 24 hours after drug is stopped).

CONTRAINDICATIONS

Contraindicated in pregnant women before 20th week of pregnancy and in women with antepartum hemorrhage, eclampsia and severe preeclampsia, intrauterine fetal death, chorioamnionitis, maternal cardiac disease, pulmonary hypertension, maternal hyperthyroidism, or uncontrolled maternal diabetes mellitus. Also contraindicated in patients hypersensitive to drug or with preexisting maternal medical conditions that would seriously be affected by the known pharmacologic properties of drug, such as hypovolemia, pheochromocytoma, or uncontrolled hypertension.

NURSING CONSIDERATIONS

• Use cautiously in patients with a sulfite sensitivity.
Alert: Because CV responses are common and more pronounced during I.V. administration, closely monitor CV effects—including maternal pulse rate and blood pressure, and fetal heart rate. Maternal tachycardia of over 140 beats/minute or persistent respiratory rate of over 20 breaths/minute may be a sign of impending pulmonary edema. Discontinue drug if pulmonary edema develops and notify doctor.
• Monitor blood glucose concentrations during infusion, especially in diabetic mother.
• Monitor amount of fluids administered I.V. to prevent circulatory overload.
• Keep patient in left lateral position to minimize risks of hypotension.

I.V. administration

• Dilute 150 mg in 500 ml D₅W to yield a concentration of 0.3 mg/ml.
• In patients whose condition contraindicates dextrose, dilute drug in 0.9% NaCl, Ringer's, or lactated Ringer's solution to avoid risk of pulmonary edema.
• Don't use ritodrine I.V. if solution is discolored or contains precipitates.
• I.V. infusion should be continued for 12 hours after contractions have stopped. Recurrence of preterm labor may be treated with repeated infusion of ritodrine.

☑ Patient teaching

• Explain use and administration of drug and how it is administered.
• Instruct patient to report adverse reactions promptly.

▼ *NEW DRUG*

sevelamer hydrochloride
Renagel

Pregnancy Risk Category: C

HOW SUPPLIED
Capsules: 403 mg

ACTION
A phosphate binder that inhibits intestinal phosphate absorption and decreases serum phosphorus concentrations.

Route	Onset	Peak	Duration
PO	Unknown	Unknown	Unknown

INDICATIONS & DOSAGE
Reduction of serum phosphorus in patients with endstage renal disease —
Adults: initially, two to four capsules P.O. t.i.d. with meals, depending on severity of hyperphosphatemia. Gradually adjust dose based on serum phosphorus level with goal of lowering serum phosphorus to 6 mg/dl or less. If serum phosphorus level is 9 mg/dl or greater, four capsules P.O., t.i.d. with meals; for serum phosphorus level between 7.5 and 9 mg/dl, three capsules P.O. t.i.d. with meals. For serum phosphorus level between 6 and 7.5 mg/dl, two capsules P.O. t.i.d. with meals.

ADVERSE REACTIONS
CNS: *headache, pain.*
CV: hypertension, *hypotension, **thrombosis.***
GI: *vomiting,* nausea, constipation, *diarrhea,* flatulence, *dyspepsia.*
Respiratory: increased cough.
Other: *infection.*

INTERACTIONS
None significant.

EFFECTS ON DIAGNOSTIC TESTS
None reported.

CONTRAINDICATIONS
Contraindicated in patients with hypophosphatemia, bowel obstruction, or known hypersensitivity to drug or its components.

NURSING CONSIDERATIONS
• Use cautiously in patients with dysphagia, swallowing disorders, severe GI motility disorders, or major GI tract surgery.
• Monitor serum calcium, bicarbonate, and chloride levels, as ordered.
• Monitor for symptoms of thrombosis (numbness or tingling of extremities, chest pain, shortness of breath) and notify doctor.
• Be aware that although no known drug interactions have been studied, the possibility exists that sevelamer would bind to concomitantly administered drugs and decrease their bioavailability. Administer other medications 1 hour before or 3 hours after sevelamer.
• Do not crush or break capsules and only administer with meals.

☑ **Patient teaching**
• Instruct patient to take with meals and adhere to prescribed diet.
• Inform patient that capsules must be taken whole because the contents expand in water; caution patient not to open or chew the capsules.
• Instruct patient to take other medications as directed, but they must be taken either 1 hour before or 3 hours after sevelamer.
• Inform patient about common adverse effects and instruct him to report them immediately. Teach patient signs and symptoms of thrombosis (numbness, tingling extremities, chest pain, changes in level of consciousness).

▼ *NEW DRUG*

sildenafil citrate
Viagra

Pregnancy Risk Category: B

HOW SUPPLIED
Tablets: 25 mg, 50 mg, 100 mg

ACTION
Drug has no direct relaxant effect on isolated human corpus cavernosum, but enhances effect of nitric oxide (NO) by inhibiting phosphodiesterase type 5 (PDE5), which is responsible for degradation of cyclic guanosine monophosphate (cGMP) in the corpus cavernosum. When sexual stimulation causes local release of NO, inhibition of PDE5 by sildenafil causes increased levels of cGMP in the corpus cavernosum, resulting in smooth muscle relaxation and inflow of blood to the corpus cavernosum.

Route	Onset	Peak	Duration
PO	Unknown	0.5-2 hr	4 hr

INDICATIONS & DOSAGE
Treatment of erectile dysfunction—
Adults under 65 years: 50 mg P.O. p.r.n., approximately 1 hour before sexual activity. Dosage range is 25 mg to 100 mg based on effectiveness and toleration. Maximum one dose daily.
Elderly (65 years and older): 25 mg P.O. p.r.n., approximately 1 hour before sexual activity. Dose may be adjusted based on patient response. Maximum one dose daily.
Adjust-a-dose: For adults with hepatic or severe renal impairment: 25 mg P.O., approximately 1 hour before sexual activity. Dose may be adjusted based on patient response. Maximum one dose daily.

ADVERSE REACTIONS
CNS: anxiety, *headache*, dizziness, *seizure*, somnolence, vertigo.
CV: myocardial infarction, sudden cardiac death, ventricular arrhythmias, cerebrovascular hemorrhage, transient ischemic attack, hypertension, flushing.
EENT: diplopia, temporary vision loss, decreased vision, ocular redness or bloodshot appearance, ocular burning, ocular swelling, ocular pressure, increased intraocular pressure, retinal vascular disease, retinal bleeding, vitreous detachment or traction, paramacular edema, abnormal vision (photophobia, color-tinged vision, blurred vision).

GI: *dyspepsia,* diarrhea.
GU: hematuria, prolonged erection, priapism, urinary tract infection.
Musculoskeletal: arthralgia, back pain.
Respiratory: respiratory tract infection.
Skin: rash.
Other: flulike syndrome.

INTERACTIONS
Drug-drug. *Beta blockers, loop and potassium-sparing diuretics:* increased blood levels of major metabolite of sildenafil, N-desmethyl sildenafil. Clinical significance of these interactions is not known.
CYP3A4 inducers, rifampin: reduced sildenafil plasma levels. Monitor effect.
Hepatic isoenzyme inhibitors (such as cimetidine, erythromycin, ketoconazole, itraconazole): may reduce clearance of sildenafil. Avoid concomitant use.
Nitrates: sildenafil enhances hypotensive effects. Do not use together.
Drug-food. *High-fat meal:* reduced rate of absorption and decreased peak serum concentrations. Separate administration time from meals.

EFFECTS ON DIAGNOSTIC TESTS
None reported.

CONTRAINDICATIONS
Contraindicated with concomitant use of organic nitrates at any frequency and in any form, in patients with underlying CV disease or known hypersensitivity to drug or its components.

NURSING CONSIDERATIONS
• Use cautiously in patients 65 years or older; those with hepatic or severe renal impairment; those who have suffered an MI, stroke, or life-threatening arrhythmias within the last 6 months; those who have history of cardiac failure, coronary artery disease, uncontrolled high or low blood pressure, anatomic deformation of the penis (such as angulation, cavernosal fibrosis, or Peyronie's disease); those who have conditions that may predispose them to priapism (such as sickle cell anemia, multiple myeloma, leukemia); or those who have retinitis pigmentosa, bleeding disorders, or active peptic ulcer disease.

Alert: Increased cardiac risk. Systemic vasodilatory properties of sildenafil cause transient decreases in supine blood pressure and cardiac output (approximately 2 hours after ingestion). This, plus the potential cardiac risk of sexual activity, increases risk for patients with underlying CV disease.
Alert: Serious CV events, including MI, sudden cardiac death, ventricular arrhythmias, cerebrovascular hemorrhage, transient ischemic attack, and hypertension have been reported in temporal association with drug use. Most, but not all, of these patients had preexisting CV risk factors. Many of these events occurred during or shortly after sexual activity; a few occurred shortly after use of drug without sexual activity; and others occurred hours to days after drug use and sexual activity.
• Be aware that there is no indication for use of drug in newborns, children, or women.

✓ Patient teaching
• Advise patient that drug should not be regularly or intermittently used with nitrates.
• Advise patient of potential cardiac risk of sexual activity, especially in the presence of preexisting CV risk factors. Instruct patient to notify doctor of symptoms such as angina pectoris, dizziness, or nausea on initiation of sexual activity, and to refrain from further activity.
• Warn patient that erections lasting more than 4 hours and priapism (painful erections longer than 6 hours in duration) can occur and should be reported immediately. Penile tissue damage and permanent loss of potency may result if priapism is not treated immediately.
• Inform patient that drug does not offer protection against sexually transmitted diseases; protective measures such as condoms should be used.
• Instruct patient to take drug 30 minutes to 4 hours before sexual activity; maximum benefit can be expected less than 2 hours after ingestion.
• Advise patient that drug is most rapidly absorbed if taken on an empty stomach.
• Inform patient that impairment of color

Reactions may be *common,* uncommon, *life-threatening,* or COMMON AND LIFE-THREATENING.

discrimination (blue/green) may occur and to avoid hazardous activities that rely on color discrimination.
• Instruct patient to notify doctor of visual changes.
• Advise patient that drug is effective only in presence of sexual stimulation.
• Caution patient to take drug only as prescribed.

---

strontium 89 (⁸⁹Sr) chloride
Metastron

Pregnancy Risk Category: D

HOW SUPPLIED
Injection: 4 millicuries (mCi)/10 ml

ACTION
Acts as a calcium analogue that is actively taken up by bone, particularly in areas of active osteogenesis, such as metastatic bone tumors. Drug locally irradiates tissue with beta radiation.

Route	Onset	Peak	Duration
IV	Within hr	7-20 days	4-12 mo

INDICATIONS & DOSAGE
Relief of bone pain in patients with painful metastatic lesions—
Adults: 4 mCi by slow I.V. injection over 1 to 2 minutes.

ADVERSE REACTIONS
CV: cutaneous flushing (with rapid injection).
Hematologic: bone marrow suppression.
Other: transient increase in pain ("flare" reaction).

INTERACTIONS
Drug-drug. *Calcium supplements:* decreased effectiveness of ⁸⁹Sr. Discontinue calcium supplements about 2 weeks before ⁸⁹Sr administration.
Cytotoxic agents: additive bone marrow suppression. Monitor closely.

EFFECTS ON DIAGNOSTIC TESTS
None reported.

CONTRAINDICATIONS
No known contraindications.

NURSING CONSIDERATIONS
• Use cautiously in patients with platelet counts below 60,000/mm³ or WBC counts below 2,400/mm³.
Alert: Follow institutional safety measures to minimize radiation exposure. Urinary excretion of radiation is greatest during first 2 days after administration.
• Consider placing an indwelling urinary catheter in incontinent patients to minimize contamination of the environment with radiation.
• Frequently assess degree of pain relief after administration of drug. During first week, a transient increase in pain may necessitate a dosage increase in concomitantly administered analgesics. Pain relief from ⁸⁹Sr usually occurs after 2 to 3 weeks. In clinical trials, over 75% of patients received substantial pain relief, allowing a reduction or elimination of opioid analgesics.
• Because drug is a potential carcinogen, be aware use should be restricted to patients with documented metastatic bone cancer.
• Because of delayed onset of pain relief, be aware that drug should not be used in patients with a short life expectancy.

I.V. administration
• Measure dose by suitable radioactivity calibration system immediately prior to use.
• Store vial and contents inside the lead transportation container at room temperature (59° to 77° F [15° to 25° C]).

✓ Patient teaching
• Teach patient proper radiation precautions; during first few days of treatment, patient should flush toilet twice, wipe spilled urine with tissue that is subsequently flushed, and immediately launder linens soiled with blood or urine. Tell patient to wash hands after using toilet. Make sure patient understands that drug has a low level of radioactivity and that he will pose no risk to family members.
• Inform patient that there may be an increase in pain for 2 to 3 days after admin-

---

istration, followed by diminishing pain after 1 to 2 weeks.
• Advise female patient of childbearing age to avoid becoming pregnant while taking drug.

sulfasalazine (salazosulfapyridine, sulphasalazine)
Azulfidine, Azulfidine EN-Tabs, PMS-Sulfasalazine E.C.†, Salazopyrin†‡, Salazopyrin EN-Tabs†‡

Pregnancy Risk Category: B

HOW SUPPLIED
Tablets: 500 mg with or without enteric coating

ACTION
Unknown.

Route	Onset	Peak	Duration
PO	Unknown	3-12 hr	Unknown

INDICATIONS & DOSAGE
Mild-to-moderate ulcerative colitis, adjunctive therapy in severe ulcerative colitis, Crohn's disease—
Adults: initially, 3 to 4 g P.O. daily in evenly divided doses; usual maintenance dosage is 2 g P.O. daily in divided doses q 6 hours. Dosage may be started with 1 to 2 g, with a gradual increase in dosage to minimize adverse effects.
Children over 2 years: initially, 40 to 60 mg/kg P.O. daily, divided into three to six doses; then 30 mg/kg daily in four doses. Dosage may be started at lower dose if GI intolerance occurs.
Rheumatoid arthritis in patients who have responded inadequately to salicylates or NSAIDs—
Adults: 2 g P.O. daily in evenly divided doses. Dosage may be started at 0.5 to 1 g daily to reduce possible GI intolerance.

ADVERSE REACTIONS
CNS: headache, depression, *seizures,* hallucinations.
GI: *nausea, vomiting, diarrhea,* abdominal pain, anorexia, stomatitis.
GU: *toxic nephrosis with oliguria and anuria,* crystalluria, hematuria, oligospermia, infertility.
Hematologic: *agranulocytosis,* aplastic anemia, megaloblastic anemia, ***thrombocytopenia, leukopenia,*** hemolytic anemia.
Hepatic: elevated liver function tests, jaundice, *hepatotoxicity.*
Skin: *erythema multiforme (Stevens-Johnson syndrome), generalized skin eruption,* epidermal necrolysis, *exfoliative dermatitis,* photosensitivity, urticaria, pruritus.
Other: *hypersensitivity reactions (serum sickness, drug fever, **anaphylaxis**).*

INTERACTIONS
Drug-drug. *Antibiotics:* may alter action of sulfasalazine by altering internal flora. Monitor closely.
Digoxin: may reduce absorption of digoxin. Monitor closely.
Folic acid: absorption may be decreased. No intervention necessary.
Iron: lowered blood concentrations of sulfasalazine caused by iron chelation. Monitor closely.
Oral anticoagulants: increased anticoagulant effect. Monitor for bleeding.
Oral antidiabetic agents: increased hypoglycemic effect. Monitor blood glucose levels.
Oral contraceptives: decreased contraceptive effectiveness and increased risk of breakthrough bleeding. Suggest a nonhormonal form of contraception.

EFFECTS ON DIAGNOSTIC TESTS
Drug alters results of urine glucose tests that use cupric sulfate (Benedict's reagent or Clinitest).

CONTRAINDICATIONS
Contraindicated in patients with porphyria, intestinal and urinary obstruction, or hypersensitivity to drug or its metabolites and in infants under 2 years.

NURSING CONSIDERATIONS
• Use cautiously and in reduced dosages in patients with impaired hepatic or renal function, severe allergy, bronchial asthma, and G6PD deficiency.
• Although therapeutic response in rheu-

matoid arthritis has been noted as soon as 4 weeks after starting therapy, it may take 12 weeks of therapy before some patients show benefit.

• Be aware that drug colors alkaline urine orange-yellow.

• Administer with food to decrease GI irritation.

Alert: Discontinue immediately if patient shows signs and symptoms of hypersensitivity, and notify doctor.

☑ **Patient teaching**

• Instruct patient to take drug after food intake and to space doses evenly.

• Warn patient to avoid ultraviolet light.

• Advise patient that drug may produce an orange-yellow discoloration of the skin and urine.

• Instruct patient to notify doctor immediately if discoloration of skin or urine occurs.

• Advise patient to make sure fluid intake is adequate.

---

tamsulosin hydrochloride
Flomax

Pregnancy Risk Category: B

HOW SUPPLIED
Capsules: 0.4 mg

ACTION
Selectively blocks alpha-receptors in the prostate, leading to relaxation of smooth muscles in the bladder neck and prostate, improving urine flow and reduction in symptoms of BPH.

Route	Onset	Peak	Duration
PO	Unknown	4-5 hr	9-15 hr

INDICATIONS AND DOSAGE
Treatment of BPH—
Adults: 0.4 mg P.O. once daily, administered 30 minutes after same meal each day. If no response after 2 to 4 weeks, dose may be increased to 0.8 mg P.O. once daily.

ADVERSE REACTIONS
CNS: asthenia, *dizziness, headache,* insomnia, somnolence, syncope, vertigo.
CV: chest pain, orthostatic hypotension.
EENT: amblyopia, pharyngitis, *rhinitis,* sinusitis.
GI: diarrhea, nausea, tooth disorder.
GU: abnormal ejaculation, decreased libido.
Respiratory: increased cough.
Other: back pain, *infection.*

INTERACTIONS
Drug-drug. *Alpha-adrenergic blocking agents:* may interact with tamsulosin. Avoid concomitant use.
Cimetidine: decreased clearance of tamsulosin. Use with caution.

EFFECTS ON DIAGNOSTIC TESTS
None reported.

CONTRAINDICATIONS
Contraindicated in patients with hypersensitivity to drug or its components.

NURSING CONSIDERATIONS
• Monitor patient for decreases in blood pressure.

• Symptoms of BPH and carcinoma of the prostate are similar; rule out carcinoma prior to therapy initiation.

• If treatment is interrupted for several days or more, restart therapy at one capsule daily.

☑ **Patient teaching**

• Instruct patient not to crush, chew, or open capsules.

• Tell patient to get up slowly from chair or bed during initiation of therapy and to avoid situations where injury could occur due to syncope. Advise him that drug may cause a sudden drop in blood pressure, especially after the first dose or when changing doses.

• Instruct patient not to drive or perform hazardous tasks for 12 hours following the initial dose or changes in dose until response can be monitored.

• Tell patient to take drug approximately 30 minutes following same meal each day.

▼ NEW DRUG

thalidomide
Thalomid

Pregnancy Risk Category: X

HOW SUPPLIED
Capsules: 50 mg

ACTION
An immunomodulatory agent whose mechanism of action in patients with erythema nodosum leprosum (ENL) is not fully understood.

Route	Onset	Peak	Duration
PO	Unknown	3-6 hr	Unknown

INDICATIONS & DOSAGE
Acute treatment of cutaneous manifestations of moderate-to-severe ENL—
Adults: 100 to 300 mg P.O. daily h.s.
Note: if patient weighs less than 50 kg (110 lb), start dosing at the lower end of range.
Maintenance therapy for prevention and suppression of the cutaneous manifestations of ENL recurrence—
Adults: up to 400 mg P.O. daily h.s. or in divided doses.

ADVERSE REACTIONS
CNS: *asthenia, drowsiness, somnolence, dizziness,* peripheral neuropathy, *headache,* agitation, insomnia, malaise, nervousness, *paresthesia,* tremor, vertigo.
CV: orthostatic hypotension, bradycardia, peripheral edema.
EENT: dry mouth, oral candidiasis, pharyngitis, sinusitis.
GI: abdominal pain, anorexia, constipation, *diarrhea,* flatulence, *nausea.*
GU: albuminuria, *hematuria,* impotence.
Hematologic: ***neutropenia, increased HIV viral load,*** anemia, *lymphadenopathy,* LEUKOPENIA.
Hepatic: abnormal liver function tests, increased AST.
Musculoskeletal: back pain, neck pain, neck rigidity.
Skin: acne, fungal dermatitis, nail disorder, pruritus, *rash,* **maculopapular rash,** *sweating.*

Other: ***human teratogenicity, hypersensitivity reactions,*** facial edema, hyperlipidemia, lymphadenopathy, fever, chills, accidental injury, infection, pain.

INTERACTIONS
Drug-drug. *Barbiturates, chlorpromazine, reserpine:* enhanced sedative activity. Use with caution together.
Medications associated with peripheral neuropathy: increased risk of peripheral neuropathy. Use cautiously together.
Drug-food. *Any food:* decreased absorption of drug. Take 1 hour after meals.
Drug-lifestyle. *Alcohol use:* increased sedation. Avoid concomitant use.

EFFECTS ON DIAGNOSTIC TESTS
Drug may cause neutropenia and increased HIV viral load.

CONTRAINDICATIONS
Contraindicated in patients hypersensitive to drug or its components; in pregnant women and those capable of becoming pregnant, except when alternative therapies are inappropriate and patient meets all conditions listed in the System for Thalidomide Education and Prescribing Safety (S.T.E.P.S.) program.

NURSING CONSIDERATIONS
Alert: Thalidomide must only be administered in compliance with all of the terms outlined in the S.T.E.P.S. program; may only be prescribed by doctors registered with the S.T.E.P.S. program; and may only be dispensed by pharmacists registered with the S.T.E.P.S. program.
• Be aware that all sexually mature patients (male or female) capable of reproduction must meet rigid S.T.E.P.S. program requirements including: ability to understand and carry out instructions; ability and willingness to comply with mandatory contraceptive measures (concomitant use of at least 2 highly effective means of contraception); and a written acknowledgment of understanding of all warnings concerning the hazards of fetal exposure to thalidomide and the risk of contraception failure.
• Know that sexually mature women who have not undergone a hysterectomy or

who have not been postmenopausal for at least 24 consecutive months (that is, who have had menses at some time in the preceding 24 consecutive months) are considered to be women of childbearing potential even with history of infertility.

• Perform mandatory pregnancy test within 24 hours before thalidomide therapy for women of childbearing potential, then weekly during first month of therapy, then monthly for women with regular menstrual cycles. If menstrual cycles are irregular, pregnancy testing continues every 2 weeks during therapy. Retesting is performed if menstrual changes occurs, including missed menses.

• Report immediately suspected fetal exposure to FDA via MedWATCH at 1-800-FDA-1088, and to manufacturer.

• Know that corticosteroids may be administered concomitantly in patients with moderate-to-severe neuritis associated with severe ENL reaction. Corticosteroids can be tapered and discontinued when neuritis improves.

• Be aware that patient with history of requiring prolonged treatment to prevent recurrence of cutaneous ENL or who experiences flare during tapering, should use minimum effective dose. Tapering should be attempted every 3 to 6 months at a dose reduction rate of 50 mg every 2 to 4 weeks.

• Perform WBC and differential before initiating therapy and periodically thereafter, as ordered. Patients with an absolute neutrophil count falling below 750/mm^3 while on treatment should be reevaluated.

• Monitor patient for signs and symptoms of neuropathy at least once monthly during first 3 months of drug therapy, then periodically. If symptoms occur (such as numbness, tingling, or pain in hands or feet), immediately notify doctor.

✓ **Patient teaching**

• Warn patient of dangers of fetal exposure to any amount of thalidomide. Ascertain that S.T.E.P.S. program protocol has been fully followed and is understood by patient.

• Reinforce that blood and sperm donations are prohibited while taking thalidomide.

• Explain that at least two highly reliable

means of contraception must be used simultaneously and continuously from at least 1 month before thalidomide therapy until 1 month following completion of therapy.

• Instruct patient to report signs or symptoms of pregnancy immediately without regard to probability or improbability of pregnancy.

• Inform women with childbearing potential of mandatory pregnancy testing schedule.

• Inform patient that if pregnancy occurs, drug must be discontinued immediately.

• Caution patient that it is not known whether drug is present in ejaculate of males receiving drug, and that males receiving thalidomide must always use a latex condom when engaging in sexual activity with women of childbearing potential.

• Advise patient to read package insert carefully.

• Tell female patient if she is taking drugs that reduce hormonal contraceptive agents (such as HIV-protease inhibitors, griseofulvin, rifampin, rifabutin, phenytoin, carbamazepine), she must use two other effective means of contraception.

• Tell breast-feeding patient to discontinue this practice during therapy.

• Stress importance of storing drug out of reach of children or others who may mistakenly take drug, and that drug should be stored at room temperature and protected from light.

• Instruct patient to take drug only as prescribed.

• Caution patient against sharing drug with others, including those who also have a thalidomide prescription.

• Caution patient concerning potential for dizziness and orthostatic hypotension; instruct patient to change position slowly when rising.

• Inform patient that drug frequently causes drowsiness and somnolence. Advise patient to avoid hazardous activities and the use of alcohol or other medications that might cause drowsiness.

• Tell patient to take drug at bedtime with a glass of water, at least 1 hour after the evening meal.

• Teach patient signs and symptoms of

---

peripheral neuropathy and to report their occurrence immediately.
• Tell patient hypersensitivity reactions have occurred and to notify doctor if erythematous macular rash, fever, tachycardia, and hypotension, as well as any other adverse reactions occur.

tiludronate disodium
Skelid

Pregnancy Risk Category: C

HOW SUPPLIED
Tablets: 240 mg (equivalent of 200 mg of tiludronic acid)

ACTION
Bisphosphonate analogue that is thought to suppress bone resorption by reducing osteoclastic activity.

Route	Onset	Peak	Duration
PO	Unknown	2 hr	Unknown

INDICATIONS & DOSAGE
Paget's disease of bone in patients who have serum alkaline phosphatase level at least twice the upper limit of normal, who are symptomatic, or who are at risk for future complications of their disease—
Adults: 400 mg P.O. once daily for 3 months, taken with a full glass of plain water (6 to 8 oz) 2 hours before or after meals.

ADVERSE REACTIONS
CNS: anxiety, dizziness, headache, insomnia, involuntary muscle contractions, paresthesia, somnolence, vertigo.
CV: chest pain, hypertension.
EENT: cataracts, conjunctivitis, glaucoma, pharyngitis, rhinitis, sinusitis.
Endocrine: hyperparathyroidism.
GI: anorexia, constipation, diarrhea, dyspepsia, flatulence, gastritis, nausea, vomiting, dry mouth, tooth disorder.
Metabolic: vitamin D deficiency.
Musculoskeletal: arthralgia, arthrosis, back pain, *whole body pain.*
Respiratory: bronchitis, coughing.
Skin: pruritus, rash.
Other: edema, sweating, infection.

INTERACTIONS
Drug-drug. *Aluminum antacids, calcium supplements, magnesium antacids:* may dramatically reduce bioavailability of tiludronate. Do not administer within 1 hour of each other.
Aspirin: may decrease bioavailability of tiludronate. Do not administer within 2 hours of drug.
Indomethacin: may increase bioavailability of tiludronate. Use cautiously; drug should not be taken within 2 hours of indomethacin.
Drug-food. *Any food:* delayed drug absorption. Do not give within 2 hours of meals.
Beverages other than plain water: may reduce drug absorption. Do not give with drug.

EFFECTS ON DIAGNOSTIC TESTS
None reported.

CONTRAINDICATIONS
Contraindicated in patients with severe renal failure (creatinine clearance below 30 ml/minute) or known hypersensitivity to drug or its components.

NURSING CONSIDERATIONS
• Use cautiously in patients with upper GI disease such as dysphagia, esophagitis, esophageal ulcer, or gastric ulcer.
• Be aware hypocalcemia and other disturbances of mineral metabolism (such as vitamin D deficiency) should be corrected before initiating therapy.
• Administer drug for 3 months to assess response.
• It is not known if drug is excreted in breast milk. Use caution when administering drug to breast-feeding women.

☑ Patient teaching
• Tell patient to take drug with 6 to 8 oz (180 to 240 ml) of plain water.
• Instruct patient that drug should not be taken within 2 hours of food.
• Advise patient to maintain adequate vitamin D and calcium intake.
• Advise patient not to take calcium supplements, aspirin, or indomethacin within 2 hours of taking drug.
• Tell patient that aluminum- and magne-

sium-containing antacids can be taken 2 hours after taking drug.

---

tiopronin
Thiola

Pregnancy Risk Category: C

HOW SUPPLIED
Tablets: 100 mg

ACTION
Forms a water-soluble chemical complex with cysteine in the urine, increasing cysteine solubility and preventing formation of urinary cysteine stones.

Route	Onset	Peak	Duration
PO	Rapid	Unknown	< 10 hr

INDICATIONS & DOSAGE
Prevention of urinary cysteine stone formation in patients with severe homozygous cysteinuria unresponsive to or intolerant of other therapies—
Adults: 800 mg P.O. daily, divided t.i.d.
Children: initially, 15 mg/kg P.O. daily, divided t.i.d. Maintenance dosage may be individualized.

ADVERSE REACTIONS
GI: hypogeusia.
Skin: rash, pruritus, wrinkling, friability.
Other: drug fever, lupus erythematosus–like reaction.

INTERACTIONS
Drug-food. *Any food:* delayed absorption of drug. Administer 30 minutes before or 2 hours after meals.

EFFECTS ON DIAGNOSTIC TESTS
None reported.

CONTRAINDICATIONS
Contraindicated in patients with history of agranulocytosis, aplastic anemia, or thrombocytopenia, and in pregnant and breast-feeding patients.

NURSING CONSIDERATIONS
• Institute conservative measures to treat cysteinuria before tiopronin is adminis-tered. Patients should drink at least 3 L of fluid daily, including at least two 8-oz glasses of water at each meal and at bedtime. Urine output should be at least 3 L daily, and urine pH should be 6.5 to 7. Excessive alkalization may precipitate calcium stones. Urine pH should not exceed 7.
• Monitor CBC, platelet counts, hemoglobin, serum albumin, liver function tests, 24-hour urine protein, and routine urinalysis at 3- to 6-month intervals during treatment, as ordered.
• Frequently monitor urine cysteine during first 6 months of treatment to identify optimal dosage level and then at least every 6 months, as ordered.
• Inspect skin for rash. Generalized rash with mild pruritus that develops may be controlled with antihistamines and will disappear after stopping drug. A rash accompanied by intense pruritus may appear on the trunk after 6 months of therapy. This rash disappears slowly after stopping drug.
• Drug fever may develop, especially during first month of therapy. Expect drug to be stopped until fever subsides and to be restarted at lower dosages.
• Be aware dosage is usually adjusted to keep urine cysteine levels below 250 mg/L.
• Be aware about two-thirds of patients who cannot tolerate penicillamine will tolerate tiopronin.

☑ Patient teaching
• Tell patient to take tiopronin at least 1 hour before or 2 hours after meals.
• Advise patient to have annual abdominal X-ray to assess for presence of stones.
• Tell patient to report signs or symptoms of hematologic abnormalities, including fever, sore throat, bleeding or bruising, and chills.
• Inform patient of importance of maintaining adequate fluid intake.

▼ *NEW DRUG*

---

tolterodine tartrate
Detrol

Pregnancy Risk Category: C

HOW SUPPLIED
Tablets: 1 mg, 2 mg

ACTION
Tolterodine is a competitive muscarinic receptor antagonist. Both urinary bladder contraction and salivation are mediated via cholinergic muscarinic receptors.

Route	Onset	Peak	Duration
PO	Unknown	1-2 hr	Unknown

INDICATIONS & DOSAGE
Treatment of patients with overactive bladder with symptoms of urinary frequency, urgency, or urge incontinence—
Adults: 2 mg P.O. b.i.d. Dose may be lowered to 1 mg P.O. b.i.d. based on patient response and tolerance.
Adjust-a-dose: In adults with significantly reduced hepatic function or in those who are currently taking drug that inhibits cytochrome P-450 3A4 isoenzyme system, 1 mg P.O. b.i.d.

ADVERSE REACTIONS
CNS: *dry mouth,* fatigue, paresthesia, vertigo, dizziness, *headache,* nervousness, somnolence.
CV: hypertension, chest pain.
EENT: abnormal vision (accommodation), xerophthalmia, pharyngitis, rhinitis, sinusitis.
GI: abdominal pain, constipation, diarrhea, dyspepsia, flatulence, nausea, vomiting.
GU: dysuria, micturition frequency, urine retention, urinary tract infection.
Musculoskeletal: arthralgia, back pain.
Respiratory: bronchitis, coughing, upper respiratory infection.
Skin: pruritus, rash, erythema, dry skin.
Other: flulike symptoms, falls, fungal infection, infection, weight gain.

INTERACTIONS
Drug-drug. *Antifungal agents (itraconazole, ketoconazole, miconazole), cytochrome P-450 3A4 inhibitors (such as macrolide antibiotics—clarithromycin, erythromycin):* effects have not been studied. However, tolterodine doses above 1 mg b.i.d. should not be given concurrently.

EFFECTS ON DIAGNOSTIC TESTS
None reported.

CONTRAINDICATIONS
Contraindicated in patients with urine or gastric retention, uncontrolled narrow-angle glaucoma, or hypersensitivity to drug or its ingredients.

NURSING CONSIDERATIONS
• Use with caution in patients with significant bladder outflow obstruction, GI obstructive disorders (such as pyloric stenosis), controlled narrow-angle glaucoma, and hepatic or renal impairment.
• Assess baseline bladder function and monitor therapeutic effects.
• Safety and effectiveness in children have not been established.

☑ Patient teaching
• Tell patient that sugarless gum, hard candy, or saliva substitute may help relieve dry mouth.
• Advise patient to avoid driving or other potentially hazardous activities until visual effects of drug are known.
• Advise breast-feeding patient to stop this practice while on drug therapy.
• Instruct patient to immediately report signs of infection, urine retention, or GI problems.

---

tretinoin (retinoic acid, vitamin A acid)
Renova, Retin-A, StieVA-A†

Pregnancy Risk Category: C

HOW SUPPLIED
Cream: 0.025%, 0.05%, 0.1%
Gel: 0.01%, 0.025%
Solution: 0.05%

ACTION
Inhibits comedones by increasing epidermal cell mitosis and turnover.

Route	Onset	Peak	Duration
Topical	Unknown	Unknown	Unknown

INDICATIONS & DOSAGE
Acne vulgaris—

Adults and children: clean affected area and lightly apply once daily h.s.
Adjunct therapy to skin care and sun avoidance program—
Adults: apply to affected area once daily h.s.

ADVERSE REACTIONS
Skin: *feeling of warmth, slight stinging, local erythema, peeling,* chapping, swelling, blistering, crusting, temporary hyperpigmentation or hypopigmentation.

INTERACTIONS
Drug-drug. *Topical agents containing sulfur, resorcinol, or salicylic acid:* increased risk of skin irritation. Don't use together.
Topical minoxidil or photosensitizing medications: increased risk of skin irritation. Don't use together.
Drug-lifestyle. *Abrasive cleansers, medicated cosmetics, skin preparations containing alcohol:* increased risk of skin irritation. Don't use together.
Sun exposure: increased photosensitivity reactions. Avoid prolonged or unprotected exposure to sun.

EFFECTS ON DIAGNOSTIC TESTS
None reported.

CONTRAINDICATIONS
Contraindicated in patients hypersensitive to any tretinoin component.

NURSING CONSIDERATIONS
• Use cautiously in patients with eczema.
• Be aware relapses generally occur within 3 to 6 weeks after therapy is stopped.

☑ Patient teaching
• Instruct patient to clean area thoroughly before application and to avoid getting drug in eyes, mouth, or mucous membranes.
• Tell patient to wash face with mild soap no more than two or three times daily. Warn against using strong or medicated cosmetics, soaps, or other skin cleansers. Also advise patient to avoid topical products containing alcohol, astringents, spices, and lime because they may interfere with drug.

• Advise patient not to discontinue drug if transient exacerbation of inflammatory lesions occurs. If severe local irritation develops, advise patient to discontinue temporarily and notify doctor. Dosage will be readjusted when application is resumed. Some redness and scaling are normal reactions.
• Warn patient that he may experience increased sensitivity to wind or cold temperatures.
• Instruct patient to minimize exposure to sunlight or ultraviolet rays during treatment. If he becomes sunburned, he should delay therapy until sunburn subsides. Tell patient who can't avoid exposure to sunlight to use SPF-15 sunblock and to wear protective clothing.
• Warn patient that he may have a temporary increase in lesions, which will improve in 2 to 3 weeks.

---

trilostane
Modrastane, Modrenal§

Pregnancy Risk Category: X

HOW SUPPLIED
Capsules: 30 mg, 60 mg

ACTION
Reversibly lowers elevated circulating levels of glucocorticoids by inhibiting the enzyme system essential for their production in the adrenal gland.

Route	Onset	Peak	Duration
PO	Unknown	Unknown	Unknown

INDICATIONS & DOSAGE
Adrenocortical hyperfunction in Cushing's syndrome—
Adults: 30 mg P.O. q.i.d. initially. May be increased at intervals of 3 to 4 days to maximum of 480 mg/day. Most patients respond to doses below 360 mg/day.

ADVERSE REACTIONS
CNS: headache, dizziness, light-headedness.
CV: *orthostatic hypotension.*
EENT: burning of nasal membranes.
GI: *diarrhea, upset stomach,* nausea, flat-

ulence, cramps, bloating, burning of oral membranes.
Skin: flushing, rash.
Other: fever, fatigue, hot flashes, muscle aches, hyperkalemia.

INTERACTIONS
Drug-drug. *Aminoglutethimide, mitotane:* may cause severe adrenocortical hypofunction. Monitor patient closely.
Loop diuretics, thiazides: decreased potassium loss because trilostane inhibits aldosterone production. Monitor for effects.

EFFECTS ON DIAGNOSTIC TESTS
None reported.

CONTRAINDICATIONS
Contraindicated in patients with severe renal or hepatic disease.

NURSING CONSIDERATIONS
• Use cautiously in patients receiving drugs that suppress adrenal function.
• Monitor blood pressure regularly.
• Be aware that drug may prevent normal response to physiologically stressful situations. Therefore, patients who develop a severe illness or need surgery may need to have drug temporarily discontinued. Supplemental corticosteroids may be necessary.

✓ Patient teaching
• Explain that drug does not cure underlying disease.
• Tell patient to seek medical attention if stressful situation arises.

Appendices
and Index

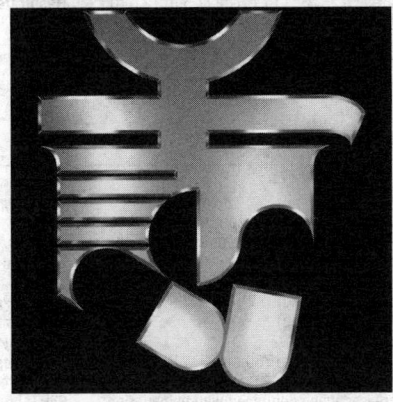

Selected local and topical anesthetics

DRUG, INDICATIONS, DOSAGE	ADVERSE REACTIONS

Local

bupivacaine hydrochloride
(Marcain‡, Marcaine, Sensorcaine)
Dosages given are for the drug without epinephrine and for adults.
Volume listed below refers to the total volume of anesthetic given,
sometimes in incremental doses of 2 to 6 ml.
Epidural block—
0.25% solution: 10 to 20 ml (25 to 50 mg)
0.5% solution: 10 to 20 ml (50 to 100 mg)
0.75% solution: 10 to 20 ml (75 to 150 mg), single-dose only
Caudal block—
0.25% solution: 15 to 30 ml (37.5 to 75 mg)
0.5% solution: 15 to 30 ml (75 to 150 mg)
Spinal block—
0.75% solution (in dextrose 8.25%): 1 to 1.6 ml (7.5 to 12 mg)
Peripheral nerve block—
0.25% solution: 5 ml (12.5 mg)
0.5% solution: 5 ml (25 mg)

Skin: dermatologic reactions.
Other: *anaphylactoid reactions,
anaphylaxis,* edema, *status
asthmaticus.*
Systemic effects from high blood
levels of the drug—
CNS: anxiety, nervousness,
seizures followed by drowsiness.
CV: *arrhythmias, bradycardia,
cardiac arrest,* hypotension,
myocardial depression.
EENT: blurred vision, tinnitus.
GI: nausea, vomiting.
Respiratory: *respiratory arrest.*

---

chloroprocaine hydrochloride
(Nesacaine, Nesacaine-MPF)
Dosages given are for the drug without epinephrine and for adults.
Volume listed below refers to the total volume of anesthetic given,
sometimes in incremental doses of 2 to 6 ml.
Infiltration and nerve block—
1% solution: 3 to 20 ml (30 to 200 mg)
2% solution: 2 to 40 ml (40 to 800 mg)
Caudal and epidural block—
2% to 3% solution: 15 to 25 ml (300 to 750 mg)
  May be repeated with smaller doses q 40 to 50 minutes. Dose
and interval may be increased when combined with epinephrine.
Maximum adult dosage is 800 mg; when combined with epinephrine, maximum dosage is 1 g.

Skin: dermatologic reactions.
Other: *anaphylactoid reactions,
anaphylaxis,* edema, *status asth-
maticus.*
Systemic effects from high blood
levels of the drug—
CNS: anxiety, nervousness,
seizures followed by drowsiness.
CV: *arrhythmias,* bradycardia, *car-
diac arrest,* hypotension, myocar-
dial depression.
EENT: blurred vision, tinnitus.
GI: nausea, vomiting.
Respiratory: *respiratory arrest.*

---

etidocaine hydrochloride
(Duranest, Duranest-MPF)
Dosages given are for the drug without epinephrine and for adults.
  Dose limit is 4 mg/kg or 300 mg per injection. When combined
with epinephrine, dose limit is 5.5 mg/kg or 400 mg per injection.
May be repeated q 2 to 3 hours.
Peripheral nerve block—
1% solution: 5 to 40 ml (50 to 400 mg)
*Central neural block (lower limbs, cesarean section, lumbar,
epidural)—*
1% solution: 10 to 30 ml (100 to 300 mg)
Transvaginal block—
1% solution: 5 to 20 ml (50 to 200 mg)
Caudal block—
1% solution: 10 to 30 ml (100 to 300 mg)

Skin: dermatologic reactions.
Other: *anaphylactoid reactions,
anaphylaxis,* edema, *status
asthmaticus.*
Systemic effects from high blood
levels of the drug—
CNS: anxiety, apprehension, nervousness, *seizures* followed by
drowsiness.
CV: *arrhythmias,* bradycardia,
cardiac arrest, hypotension,
myocardial depression.
EENT: blurred vision, tinnitus.
GI: nausea, vomiting.
Respiratory: *respiratory arrest.*

Reactions may be *common,* uncommon, *life-threatening,* or COMMON AND LIFE-THREATENING.

INTERACTIONS

NURSING CONSIDERATIONS

Beta-adrenergic blockers: enhanced sympathomimetic effects when used with bupivacaine and epinephrine. Use with caution.
Butyrophenones, phenothiazines: may reduce or reverse pressor effect of epinephrine. Monitor patient.
Chloroprocaine: may lessen bupivacaine's action. Don't use together.
CNS depressants: may cause additive CNS effects. Reduce dosage of CNS depressants.
Cyclic antidepressants, MAO inhibitors: severe, sustained hypertension when used with bupivacaine and epinephrine. Use with extreme caution.
Enflurane, halothane, isoflurane, related drugs: arrhythmias when used with bupivacaine and epinephrine. Use with extreme caution.

• Contraindicated in children under 12 years, for spinal or topical anesthesia or paracervical block, and in patients with known history of hypersensitivity reactions to local anesthetics of the amide type.
• Some solutions contain sulfites and should be avoided in patients with sulfite hypersensitivity.
• Should not be used for I.V. regional anesthesia (Bier block, Bier's local anesthesia).
• Don't use 0.75% solution for obstetric surgery; lower concentrations are effective and less hazardous.
• Use cautiously in debilitated, elderly, or acutely ill patients and in patients with severe hepatic disease or drug allergies.
• Use solutions with epinephrine cautiously in patients with CV disorders and in body areas with limited blood supply (ears, nose, fingers, toes).
• Keep resuscitation equipment and drugs available.
• Don't use solution with preservatives for caudal or epidural block.
• Discard partially used vials without preservatives.
• Check solution for particles.
• Protect solutions containing epinephrine from light.

Bupivacaine: chloroprocaine may lessen bupivacaine's action. Monitor for effect.
CNS depressants: may cause additive CNS effects. Reduce dosage of CNS depressants.
Sulfonamides: chloroprocaine inhibits the action of sulfonamides. Do not use in conditions in which a sulfonamide drug is required.

• Contraindicated in patients with hypersensitivity to procaine, tetracaine, or other PABA derivatives and for spinal or topical anesthesia. Epidural and caudal blocks are contraindicated in patients with CNS disease.
• Use cautiously in debilitated, elderly, or acutely ill patients; in children; and in patients with drug allergies, paracervical block, or CV disease.
• Keep resuscitation equipment and drugs available.
• Don't use solution with preservatives for caudal or epidural block.
• Don't use discolored solution.
• Check solution for particles.
• Discard partially used vials without preservatives.

Cyclic antidepressants, MAO inhibitors, phenothiazines: severe, sustained hypertension or hypotension with etidocaine and epinephrine. Use with extreme caution.
Enflurane, halothane, isoflurane, related drugs: arrhythmias when used with etidocaine and epinephrine. Use with extreme caution.
CNS depressants: may cause additive CNS effects. Reduce dosage of CNS depressants.

• Contraindicated in patients with inflammation or infection in puncture region, septicemia, severe hypertension, spinal deformities, or neurologic disorders; in children under 14 years; and for spinal anesthesia.
• Contraindicated in patients with known history of hypersensitivity to local anesthetics of the amide type.
• Some solutions contain sulfites and should be avoided in patients with sulfite hypersensitivity.
• Use cautiously in debilitated, elderly, or acutely ill patients; in patients with severe shock, heart block, general drug allergies, or hepatic and renal disease; and as epidural block in obstetric patients.
• Use solutions with epinephrine cautiously in patients with CV disease and in body areas with limited blood supply (ears, nose, fingers, toes).
• Don't use solution with preservatives for caudal or epidural block; check solution for particles.
• Keep resuscitation equipment and drugs available.

(continued)

---

*Liquid contains alcohol.   **May contain tartrazine.   †Canada only.   ‡Australia only.   ◇OTC.

Selected local and topical anesthetics (continued)

DRUG, INDICATIONS, DOSAGE	ADVERSE REACTIONS

Local (continued)

lidocaine hydrochloride
[lignocaine hydrochloride]
(Dilocaine, Lidoject-1, Lidoject-2, Nervocaine, Xylocaine)
Dosages given are for drug without epinephrine and for adults. Volume listed below refers to total volume of anesthetic given, sometimes in incremental doses of 2 to 6 ml.
For anesthesia other than spinal—
Maximum single dose is 4.5 mg/kg or 300 mg. With epinephrine, maximum dose is 7 mg/kg or 500 mg.
Caudal (obstetric) or epidural (thoracic) block—
1% solution: 20 to 30 ml (200 to 300 mg)
Epidural (lumbar anesthesia) block—
1% solution: 25 to 30 ml (250 to 300 mg)
1.5% solution: 15 to 20 ml (225 to 300 mg)
2% solution: 10 to 15 ml (200 to 300 mg)
Spinal surgical anesthesia—
5% (with 7.5% dextrose): 1.5 to 2 ml (75 to 100 mg)
Caudal (surgery) block—
1.5% solution: 15 to 20 ml (225 to 300 mg)

Skin: dermatologic reactions.
Other: *anaphylactoid reactions, anaphylaxis,* edema, *status asthmaticus.*
Systemic effects from high blood levels of the drug—
CNS: anxiety, nervousness, *seizures* followed by drowsiness.
CV: *arrhythmias,* bradycardia, *cardiac arrest,* myocardial depression, hypotension.
EENT: blurred vision, tinnitus.
GI: nausea, vomiting.
Respiratory: *respiratory arrest.*

---

procaine hydrochloride
(Novocain)
Spinal anesthesia—
Adults: initial dose should not exceed 1 g. Before using, dilute 10% solution with 0.9% NaCl injection, sterile distilled water, or CSF. For hyperbaric technique, use dextrose solution.
Perineum: 0.5 ml of 10% solution (50 mg) and 0.5 ml diluent injected at the L4 interspace
Perineum and lower extremities: 1 ml of 10% solution (100 mg) and 1 ml diluent injected at the L3 or L4 interspace
Up to costal margin: 2 ml of 10% solution (200 mg) and 1 ml diluent injected at the L2, L3, or L4 interspace
Peripheral nerve block—
1% solution: 50 ml (500 mg)
2% solution: 25 ml (500 mg)
Infiltration—
350 to 600 mg in 0.25% to 0.5% solution. Maximum initial dose is 1 g.

Skin: dermatologic reactions.
Other: *anaphylactoid reactions, anaphylaxis,* edema, *status asthmaticus.*
Systemic effects from high blood levels of the drug—
CNS: anxiety, nervousness, *seizures* followed by drowsiness.
CV: *arrhythmias,* bradycardia, *cardiac arrest.* hypotension, myocardial depression.
EENT: blurred vision, tinnitus.
GI: nausea, vomiting.
Respiratory: *respiratory arrest.*

---

ropivacaine hydrochloride
(Naropin)
Avoid rapid injection of large volume of local anesthetic and use incremental doses. Use smallest dose and concentration required to produce desired result.
Lumbar epidural block in surgery—
0.5% solution: 15 to 30 ml (75 to 150 mg)
0.75% solution: 15 to 25 ml (119 to 188 mg)
1.0% solution: 15 to 20 ml (150 to 200 mg)
Lumbar epidural block for cesarean section—
0.5% solution: 20 to 30 ml (100 to 150 mg)
Thoracic epidural administration to establish block for postoperative pain relief—
0.5% solution: 5 to 15 ml (25 to 75 mg)
Major nerve block (brachial plexus)—
0.5 % solution: 35 to 50 ml (175 to 250 mg)
Field block (minor nerve blocks and infiltration)—
0.5% solution: 1 to 10 ml (5 to 200 mg)

CNS: anxiety, dizziness, headache, hypoesthesia, pain, paresthesia.
CV: bradycardia, chest pain, hypotension, hypertension, tachycardia.
GI: nausea, vomiting.
GU: oliguria, urine retention.
Hematologic: anemia.
Skin: pruritus.
Other: back pain, fever, chills, postoperative complications, rigors.
*Neonatal—*vomiting, jaundice, tachypnea, respiratory distress.
Fetal— bradycardia, fever, tachycardia, distress.

Reactions may be *common,* uncommon, *life-threatening,* or COMMON AND LIFE-THREATENING.

INTERACTIONS

NURSING CONSIDERATIONS

Beta-adrenergic blockers: enhanced sympathomimetic effects. Don't use with lidocaine and epinephrine.
Butyrophenones, phenothiazines: may reduce or reverse the pressor effect of epinephrine. Monitor patient.
CNS depressants: may cause additive CNS effects. Reduce dosage of CNS depressants.
Cyclic antidepressants, MAO inhibitors: severe, sustained hypertension when used with lidocaine and epinephrine. Use with extreme caution.
Enflurane, halothane, isoflurane, related drugs: arrhythmias when used with lidocaine and epinephrine. Use with extreme caution.

- Contraindicated in patients with inflammation or infection in puncture region, septicemia, severe hypertension, spinal deformities, and neurologic disorders.
- Also contraindicated in patients with known history of hypersensitivity to local anesthetics of the amide type.
- Use cautiously in debilitated, elderly, or acutely ill patients; in patients with severe shock, heart block, or general drug allergies; in obstetric patients; and for paracervical block.
- Dose and interval are increased with epinephrine.
- Use solutions with epinephrine cautiously in patients with CV disorders and in body areas with limited blood supply (ears, nose, fingers, toes).
- Don't use solution with preservatives for spinal, epidural, or caudal block.
- Keep resuscitation equipment and drugs available.
- Discard partially used vials without preservatives.
- Check solution for particles.

CNS depressants: may cause additive CNS effects. Reduce dosage of CNS depressants.
Echothiophate iodide: reduced hydrolysis of procaine. Use together cautiously.
Succinylcholine: prolonged neuromuscular blockade. Use cautiously together.
Sulfonamides: procaine inhibits the action of sulfonamides. Do not use in conditions in which a sulfonamide drug is required.

- Contraindicated in patients with traumatized urethras and in those with hypersensitivity to chloroprocaine, tetracaine, or other PABA derivatives.
- Also contraindicated in obstetric patients with cephalopelvic disproportion, placenta previa, abruptio placentae, floating fetal head, and intrauterine manipulation.
- Use cautiously in hyperexcitable patients; in those with CNS disease, infection at puncture site, shock, profound anemia, cachexia, sepsis, hypertension, hypotension, GI hemorrhage, bowel perforation or strangulation, peritonitis, cardiac decompensation, massive pleural effusion, or increased intra-abdominal pressure; and in obstetric patients.
- Keep resuscitation equipment and drugs available.
- Use preservative-free solution for epidural block.
- Discard partially used vials without preservatives.

Amide-type anesthetics: additive effects if given with ropivacaine. Use with caution.
CNS depressants: may cause additive CNS effects. Reduce dosage of CNS depressants.
Fluvoxamine, imipramine, theophylline, verapamil: may interact with ropivacaine. Use with caution.

- Contraindicated in patients with known hypersensitivity to drug or local anesthetics of amide type.
- Use cautiously (especially when giving repeat doses) in debilitated, elderly, acutely ill, or breast-feeding patients and in patients with hypotension, hypovolemia, impaired CV function, heart block, or hepatic disease.
- Do not inject drug rapidly.
- Aspiration for blood should be done before all doses to avoid intravascular or subarachnoid injection.
- Drug should only be used by personnel familiar with use of drug. Have emergency equipment and personnel available.
- Do not use in emergency situations.
- Drug should not be used for the production of obstetric paracervical block anesthesia, retrobulbar block, or spinal anesthesia (subarachnoid block).
- Should not be used for I.V. regional anesthesia (Bier block).
(continued)

---

*Liquid contains alcohol.   **May contain tartrazine.   †Canada only.   ‡Australia only.   ◇OTC.

Selected local and topical anesthetics (continued)

DRUG, INDICATIONS, DOSAGE	ADVERSE REACTIONS

Local (continued)

ropivacaine hydrochloride (continued)
Lumbar epidural block in labor—
Initially, 0.2% solution: 10 to 20 ml (20 to 40 mg); then 6 to 14
ml/hour (12 to 28 mg/hour) as continuous infusion or 10 to 15
ml/hour (20 to 30 mg/hour) as incremental "top-up" injections
Lumbar epidural block in postoperative pain management—
0.2% solution: 6 to 10 ml/hour (12 to 20 mg/hour) as continuous
infusion
Thoracic epidural block in postoperative pain management—
0.2% solution: 4 to 8 ml/hour (8 to 16 mg/hour) as continuous infusion
Infiltration (minor nerve block) in postoperative pain management—
0.2% solution: 1 to 100 ml (2 to 200 mg)
0.5% solution: 1 to 40 ml (5 to 200 mg)

---

tetracaine hydrochloride
(Pontocaine)
Dosage for adults varies according to extent of block.
Low spinal (saddle) block in vaginal delivery—
2 to 5 mg as hyperbaric solution (in 10% dextrose)
Perineum and lower extremities: 5 to 10 mg
Up to costal margin: 15 to 20 mg

Skin: dermatologic reactions.
Other: *anaphylactoid reactions,
anaphylaxis,* edema, *status
asthmaticus.*
Systemic effects from high
blood levels of the drug—
CNS: anxiety, nervousness,
seizures followed by drowsiness.
CV: *arrhythmias,* bradycardia,
cardiac arrest, hypotension,
myocardial depression.
EENT: blurred vision, tinnitus.
GI: nausea, vomiting.
Respiratory: *respiratory arrest.*

Topical

proparacaine hydrochloride
(AK-Taine, Alcaine, Ophthaine, Ophthetic)
Anesthesia for tonometry, gonioscopy—
Adults and children: 1 or 2 drops of 0.5% solution instilled in eye
just before procedure.
Anesthesia for cataract extraction, glaucoma surgery—
Adults and children: 1 or 2 drops of 0.5% solution instilled in eye q
5 to 10 minutes for five to seven doses.
Removal of foreign bodies or sutures—
Adults and children: 1 or 2 drops 2 to 3 minutes before procedure
or q 5 to 10 minutes for one to three doses.

EENT: conjunctival redness,
transient eye pain.
Other: hypersensitivity reactions.

---

tetracaine
(Pontocaine Solution)
tetracaine hydrochloride
(Pontocaine)
*Anesthesia for tonometry, gonioscopy; removal of corneal foreign
bodies, suture removal from cornea; other diagnostic and minor
surgical procedures—*
Adults and children: 1 to 2 drops of 0.5% or 1%† in eye just before
procedure.

EENT: transient stinging in eye
30 seconds after initial instillation, epithelial damage in excessive or long-term use.
Other: sensitization with repeated use (allergic skin rash, urticaria).

Reactions may be *common*, uncommon, *life-threatening*, or COMMON AND LIFE-THREATENING.

INTERACTIONS	NURSING CONSIDERATIONS
	• Use an adequate test dose (3 to 5 ml of short-acting local anesthetic solution containing epinephrine) before induction of complete block. • Be aware that restlessness, anxiety, incoherent speech, light-headedness, numbness and tingling of mouth and lips, metallic taste, tinnitus, dizziness, blurred vision, tremors, twitching, depression, or drowsiness may be early warning signs or symptoms of CNS toxicity. • Do not use in ophthalmic surgery.
CNS depressants: may cause additive CNS effects. Reduce dosage of CNS depressants. *Sulfonamides:* tetracaine inhibits the action of sulfonamides. Do not use in conditions in which a sulfonamide drug is required.	• Safety and efficacy in children have not been established. • Contraindicated in patients with infection at injection site, CNS disease, or hypersensitivity to procaine or related agents. • Saddle block is contraindicated in patients with cephalopelvic disproportion, placenta previa, abruptio placentae, intrauterine manipulation, and floating fetal head. • Use cautiously in patients with shock, profound anemia, cachexia, hypertension, hypotension, peritonitis, cardiac decompensation, massive pleural effusion, increased intracranial pressure, and infection. • Keep resuscitation equipment and drugs available. • When CSF is added to powdered drug or drug solution during spinal anesthesia, solution may be cloudy. Don't use discolored or crystallized solutions. • Protect from light; store in refrigerator.
None significant.	• Contraindicated in patients with hypersensitivity to ester-type local anesthetics, PABA or its derivatives, or to other ingredients in these preparations. • Use cautiously in patients with cardiac disease and hyperthyroidism. • Not for long-term use; may delay wound healing. • Warn patients not to rub or touch eye while cornea is anesthetized. • Warn patients with corneal abrasion that pain is relieved only temporarily. • Don't use discolored solution. • Store in tightly closed container. Refrigerate opened containers. • Check solution for particles.
Cholinesterase inhibitors: prolonged ocular anesthesia and increased risk of toxicity. Use with caution. *Sulfonamides:* interference with sulfonamide antibacterial activity. Wait 30 minutes after anesthesia before instilling sulfonamide.	• Contraindicated in patients with hypersensitivity to drug or similar drugs (such as ester-type local anesthetics), PABA or its derivatives, or other ingredients in these preparations. • Avoid long-term use. • Does not dilate the pupil, paralyze accommodation, or increase intraocular pressure. • Don't use discolored solution. Keep container tightly closed. • Warn patient not to touch or rub eye while cornea is anesthetized.

*Liquid contains alcohol.   **May contain tartrazine.   †Canada only.   ‡Australia only.   ◇OTC.

Cancer chemotherapy: Acronyms and protocols

Combination chemotherapy is well established for treatment of cancer. The chart below lists commonly used acronyms and protocols, including standard dosages for specific cancers.

ACRONYM & INDICATION	DRUG		DOSAGE
	Generic name	Trade name	
ABVD (Hodgkin's disease)	doxorubicin	Adriamycin	25 mg/m^2 I.V., days 1 and 15
	bleomycin	Blenoxane	10 U/m^2 I.V., days 1 and 15
	vinblastine	Velban	6 mg/m^2 I.V., days 1 and 15
	dacarbazine	DTIC-Dome	350 to 375 mg/m^2 I.V., days 1 and 15 *Repeat cycle q 28 days.*
AC (Bony sarcoma)	doxorubicin	Adriamycin	75 to 90 mg/m^2 (total dose) by 96-hour continuous I.V. infusion
	cisplatin	Platinol	90 to 120 mg/m^2 intra-arterial. or I.V., day 6 *Repeat cycle q 28 days.*
AC (Breast cancer)	doxorubicin	Adriamycin	60 mg/m^2 I.V., day 1
	cyclophosphamide	Cytoxan	400 to 600 mg/m^2 I.V., day 1 *Repeat cycle q 21 days.*
ACE (CAE) (Small-cell lung cancer)	doxorubicin	Adriamycin	45 mg/m^2 I.V., day 1
	cyclophosphamide	Cytoxan	1,000 mg/m^2 I.V., day 1
	etoposide (VP-16)	VePesid	50 mg/m^2 I.V., days 1 to 5 *Repeat cycle q 21 days.*
AP (Endometrial cancer)	doxorubicin	Adriamycin	50 to 60 mg/m^2 I.V., day 1
	cisplatin	Platinol	50 to 60 mg/m^2 I.V., day 1 *Repeat cycle q 21 days.*
BEP (Testicular cancer)	bleomycin	Blenoxane	30 U I.V., days 2, 9, and 16
	etoposide (VP-16)	VePesid	100 mg/m^2, days 1 to 5
	cisplatin	Platinol	20 mg/m^2 I.V., days 1 to 5 *Repeat cycle q 21 days.*
CAF (FAC) (Breast cancer)	cyclophosphamide	Cytoxan	100 mg/m^2 P.O., days 1 to 14
	doxorubicin	Adriamycin	30 mg/m^2 I.V., days 1 (and day 8, optional)
	fluorouracil (5-FU)	Adrucil	400 to 500 mg/m^2 I.V., days 1 and 8 *Repeat cycle q 28 days.*
or	cyclophosphamide	Cytoxan	500 mg/m^2 I.V., day 1
	doxorubicin	Adriamycin	50 mg/m^2 I.V., day 1
	fluorouracil (5-FU)	Adrucil	500 mg/m^2 I.V., day 1 *Repeat cycle q 21 days.*
CAP (Non-small-cell lung cancer)	cyclophosphamide	Cytoxan	400 mg/m^2 I.V., day 1
	doxorubicin	Adriamycin	40 mg/m^2 I.V., day 1
	cisplatin	Platinol	60 mg/m^2 I.V., day 1 *Repeat cycle q 28 days.*

ACRONYM & INDICATION	DRUG		DOSAGE
	Generic name	Trade name	
CAV (VAC) (Small-cell lung cancer)	cyclophosphamide	Cytoxan	750 to 1,000 mg/m² I.V., day 1
	doxorubicin	Adriamycin	40 to 50 mg/m² I.V., day 1
	vincristine	Oncovin	1.4 mg/m² (2 mg maximum) I.V., day 1 *Repeat cycle q 21 days.*
CC (Ovarian cancer, epithelial)	carboplatin	Paraplatin	300 mg/m² I.V., day 1
	cyclophosphamide	Cytoxan	600 mg/m² I.V., day 1 *Repeat cycle q 28 days.*
CF (Head and neck cancer)	cisplatin	Platinol	100 mg/m² I.V., day 1
	fluorouracil (5-FU)	Adrucil	1,000 mg/m² daily by continuous I.V. infusion, days 1 to 5 *Repeat cycle q 21 to 28 days.*
or	carboplatin	Paraplatin	400 mg/m² I.V., day 1
	fluorouracil (5-FU)	Adrucil	1,000 mg/m² daily by continuous I.V. infusion, days 1 to 5 *Repeat cycle q 21 to 28 days.*
CFM (CNF, FNC) (Breast cancer)	cyclophosphamide	Cytoxan	500 mg/m² I.V., day 1
	fluorouracil (5-FU)	Adrucil	500 mg/m² I.V., day 1
	mitoxantrone	Novantrone	10 mg/m² I.V., day 1 *Repeat cycle q 21 days.*
CHOP (Malignant lymphoma)	cyclophosphamide	Cytoxan	750 mg/m² I.V., day 1
	doxorubicin	Adriamycin	50 mg/m² I.V., day 1
	vincristine	Oncovin	1.4 mg/m² (2 mg maximum) I.V., day 1
	prednisone	Deltasone	100 mg P.O., days 1 to 5 *Repeat cycle q 21 days.*
CHOP-Bleo (Malignant lymphoma)	cyclophosphamide	Cytoxan	750 mg/m² I.V., day 1
	doxorubicin	Adriamycin	50 mg/m² I.V., day 1
	vincristine	Oncovin	2 mg I.V., days 1 and 5
	prednisone	Deltasone	100 mg P.O., days 1 to 5
	bleomycin	Blenoxane	15 U I.V., days 1 and 5 *Repeat cycle q 14 to 21 days.*
CISCA (Genitourinary cancer)	cisplatin	Platinol	70 to 100 mg/m² I.V., day 2
	cyclophosphamide	Cytoxan	650 mg/m² I.V., day 1
	doxorubicin	Adriamycin	50 mg/m² I.V., day 1 *Repeat cycle q 21 to 28 days.*
CMF (Breast cancer)	cyclophosphamide	Cytoxan	100 mg/m² P.O., days 1 to 14, or 400 to 600 mg/m² I.V., day 1
	methotrexate	Folex	40 mg/m² I.V., days 1 and 8
	fluorouracil (5-FU)	Adrucil	400 to 600 mg/m² I.V., days 1 and 8 *Repeat cycle q 28 days.*
COP (Malignant lymphoma)	cyclophosphamide	Cytoxan	750 to 1,000 mg/m² I.V., day 1
	vincristine	Oncovin	1.4 mg/m² (2 mg maximum) I.V., day 1
	prednisone	Deltasone	60 mg/m² P.O., days 1 to 5 *Repeat cycle q 21 days.*

(continued)

Cancer chemotherapy: Acronyms and protocols (continued)

ACRONYM & INDICATION	DRUG		DOSAGE
	Generic name	Trade name	
COPP (Hodgkin's disease and malignant lymphoma)	cyclophosphamide	Cytoxan	500 to 650 mg/m^2 I.V., days 1 and 8
	vincristine	Oncovin	1.4 mg/m^2 (2 mg maximum) I.V., days 1 and 8
	procarbazine	Matulane	100 mg/m^2 P.O., days 1 to 10 or 1 to 14
	prednisone	Deltasone	40 mg/m^2 P.O., days 1 to 14 *Repeat cycle q 28 days.*
CP (Ovarian cancer)	cyclophosphamide	Cytoxan	600 to 1,000 mg/m^2 I.V., day 1
	cisplatin	Platinol	50 to 100 mg/m^2 I.V., day 1 *Repeat cycle q 21 days.*
CVP (Leukemia—CLL)	cyclophosphamide	Cytoxan	400 mg/m^2 P.O., days 1 to 5
	vincristine	Oncovin	1.4 mg/m^2 (2 mg maximum) I.V., day 1
	prednisone	Deltasone	100 mg/m^2 P.O., days 1 to 5 *Repeat cycle q 21 days.*
CVPP (Hodgkin's disease)	lomustine (CCNU)	CeeNU	75 mg/m^2 P.O., day 1
	vinblastine	Velban	4 mg/m^2 I.V., days 1 and 8
	procarbazine	Matulane	100 mg/m^2 P.O., days 1 to 14
	prednisone	Deltasone	30 mg/m^2 P.O., days 1 to 14 (cycles 1 and 4 only) *Repeat cycle q 28 days.*
CYVADIC (Soft-tissue sarcoma)	cyclophosphamide	Cytoxan	500 to 600 mg/m^2 I.V., day 1
	vincristine	Oncovin	1.4 mg/m^2 (2 mg maximum) I.V., days 1 and 5
	doxorubicin	Adriamycin	50 mg/m^2 I.V., day 1
	dacarbazine	DTIC-Dome	250 mg/m^2 I.V., days 1 to 5 *Repeat cycle q 21 days.*
DCBT (Dartmouth regimen) (Melanoma)	dacarbazine	DTIC-Dome	220 mg/m^2 I.V., days 1 to 3, days 22 to 24
	cisplatin	Platinol	25 mg/m^2 I.V., days 1 to 3, days 22 to 24
	carmustine (BCNU)	BiCNU	150 mg/m^2 I.V., day 1
	tamoxifen	Nolvadex	10 mg P.O. b.i.d., starting day 4
DVP (Leukemia—ALL, adult induction)	daunorubicin	Cerubidine	45 mg/m^2 I.V., days 1 to 3 and day 14
	vincristine	Oncovin	2 mg I.V., days 1, 8, 15, and 22
	prednisone	Deltasone	45 mg/m^2 P.O., for 28 to 35 days
EP (Small-cell or non-small-cell lung cancer)	cisplatin	Platinol	75 to 100 mg/m^2 I.V., day 1
	etoposide (VP-16)	VePesid	75 to 100 mg/m^2 I.V., days 1 to 3 *Repeat cycle q 21 to 28 days.*
FAC (CAF) (Breast cancer)	fluorouracil (5-FU)	Adrucil	500 mg/m^2 I.V., days 1 and 8
	doxorubicin	Adriamycin	50 mg/m^2 I.V., day 1
	cyclophosphamide	Cytoxan	500 mg/m^2 I.V., day 1 *Repeat cycle q 21 days.*
FAM (Adenocarcinoma, gastric cancer)	fluorouracil (5-FU)	Adrucil	600 mg/m^2 I.V., days 1, 8, 29, and 36
	doxorubicin	Adriamycin	30 mg/m^2 I.V., days 1 and 29
	mitomycin	Mutamycin	10 mg/m^2 I.V., day 1 *Repeat cycle q 8 weeks.*

ACRONYM & INDICATION	DRUG		DOSAGE
	Generic name	Trade name	
F-CL (Colorectal cancer)	fluorouracil (5-FU)	Adrucil	600 mg/m² I.V., 1 hour after initiating leucovorin infusion weekly for 6 weeks
	leucovorin calcium	Wellcovorin	500 mg/m² over 2 hours weekly for 6 weeks *Repeat cycle after 2-week break.*
or	fluorouracil (5-FU)	Adrucil	370 to 400 mg/m² I.V., days 1 to 5, following leucovorin
	leucovorin calcium	Wellcovorin	200 mg/m² daily I.V., days 1 to 5 *Repeat cycle q 28 to 35 days.*
or	fluorouracil (5-FU)	Adrucil	425 mg/m² I.V., days 1 to 5, following leucovorin
	leucovorin calcium	Wellcovorin	20 mg/m² I.V., days 1 to 5 *Repeat q 28 to 35 days.*
5 + 2 (Leukemia— AML, induction)	cytarabine (ara-C)	Cytosar-U	100 to 200 mg/m² by continuous I.V. infusion, days 1 to 5
	daunorubicin	Cerubidine	45 mg/m² I.V., days 1 and 2
FL (Prostate cancer)	flutamide	Eulexin	250 mg P.O. t.i.d.
	leuprolide acetate	Lupron	1 mg S.C. daily
or	flutamide	Eulexin	250 mg P.O. t.i.d.
	leuprolide acetate	Lupron Depot	7.5 mg I.M. q 28 days *Repeat cycle q 28 days.*
FLe (Colorectal cancer)	levamisole	Ergamisol	50 mg P.O. q 8 hours for days 1 to 3, repeated q 2 weeks for 1 year
	fluorouracil (5-FU)	Adrucil	450 mg/m² I.V. for days 1 to 5 and day 28; weekly thereafter for 48 weeks
FZ (Genitourinary, prostate cancer)	flutamide	Eulexin	250 P.O. q 8 hours
	goserelin acetate	Zoladex	3.6 mg implant S.C. q 28 days
HDMTX (high-dose methotrexate) (Bony sarcoma)	methotrexate	Folex	8 to 12 g/m² I.V. weekly for 2 to 12 weeks
	leucovorin calcium	Wellcovorin	15 to 25 mg/m² I.V. or P.O. q 6 hours for 10 doses, beginning 24 hours after methotrexate dose (serum methotrexate levels must be monitored) *Repeat cycle q 7 days for 2 to 4 weeks.*
MACOP-B (Malignant lymphoma)	methotrexate	Folex	400 mg/m² I.V., weeks 2, 6, and 10
	leucovorin calcium	Wellcovorin	15 mg/m² P.O. q 6 hours for six doses, beginning 24 hours after methotrexate dose
	doxorubicin	Adriamycin	50 mg/m² I.V., weeks 1, 3, 5, 7, 9, and 11
	cyclophosphamide	Cytoxan	350 mg/m² I.V., weeks 1, 3, 5, 7, 9, and 11
	vincristine	Oncovin	1.4 mg/m² (2 mg maximum) I.V., weeks 2, 4, 6, 8, 10, and 12
	bleomycin	Blenoxane	10 U/m² I.V., weeks 4, 8, and 12
	prednisone	Deltasone	75 mg P.O. daily for 12 weeks; taper dose over last 2 weeks *Repeat cycle as indicated in protocol.*

(continued)

Cancer chemotherapy: Acronyms and protocols (continued)

ACRONYM & INDICATION	DRUG		DOSAGE
	Generic name	Trade name	
MAID (Soft-tissue sarcoma)	mesna	MESNEX	Uroprotection 1.5 to 2.5 g/m²/day by continuous I.V. infusion, days 1 to 3
	doxorubicin	Adriamycin	15 to 20 mg/m² by continuous I.V. infusion, days 1 to 3
	ifosfamide	Ifex	1.5 to 2.5 g/m² I.V., days 1 to 3
	dacarbazine	DTIC-Dome	250 to 300 mg/m² by continuous I.V. infusion days 1 to 3 *Repeat cycle q 28 days.*
MBC (Head and neck cancer)	methotrexate	Folex	40 mg/m² I.V., days 1 and 15
	bleomycin	Blenoxane	10 U/m² I.M. or I.V., days 1, 8, and 15
	cisplatin	Platinol	50 mg/m² I.V., day 4 *Repeat cycle q 21 days.*
MC (Leukemia— AML, induction)	mitoxantrone	Novantrone	12 mg/m² I.V. daily, days 1 to 3
	cytarabine (ara-C)	Cytosar-U	100 to 200 mg/m² daily by continuous I.V. infusion, days 1 to 7 *Repeat cycle q 28 days.*
MICE (ICE) (Non-small-cell lung cancer)	mesna	MESNEX	Dosage is 20% of ifosfamide dose given I.V. immediately before and at 4 and 8 hours after ifosfamide infusion
	ifosfamide	Ifex	2,000 mg/m² I.V., days 1 to 3
	carboplatin	Paraplatin	300 to 350 mg/m² I.V., day 1
	etoposide (VP-16)	VePesid	60 to 100 mg/m² I.V., days 1 to 3 *Repeat cycle q 28 days.*
MOPP (Hodgkin's disease)	mechlorethamine (nitrogen mustard)	Mustargen	6 mg/m² I.V., days 1 and 8
	vincristine	Oncovin	1.4 mg/m² (2 mg maximum) I.V., days 1 and 8
	procarbazine	Matulane	100 mg/m² P.O., days 1 to 14
	prednisone	Deltasone	40 mg/m² P.O., days 1 to 14 *Repeat cycle q 28 days.*
MOPP (ABV hybrid) (Hodgkin's disease)	mechlorethamine (nitrogen mustard)	Mustagen	6 mg/m² I.V., day 1
	vincristine	Oncovin	1.4 mg/m² I.V., day 1 (2 mg maximum)
	procarbazine	Matulane	100 mg/m² P.O., days 1 to 7
	prednisone	Deltasone	40 mg/m² P.O., days 1 to 14
	doxorubicin	Adriamycin	35 mg/m² I.V., day 8
	bleomycin	Blenoxane	10 U/m² I.V., day 8
	vinblastine	Velban	6 mg/m² I.V., day 8 *Repeat cycle q 28 days.*

ACRONYM & INDICATION	DRUG		DOSAGE
	Generic name	Trade name	
MP (Multiple myeloma)	melphalan (L-phenylalanine mustard)	Alkeran	8 to 10 mg/m² P.O., days 1 to 4
	prednisone	Deltasone	40 to 60 mg/m² P.O., days 1 to 7 *Repeat cycle q 28 to 42 days.*
MVAC (Genitourinary cancer)	methotrexate	Folex	30 mg/m² I.V., days 1, 15, and 22
	vinblastine	Velban	3 mg/m² I.V., days 2, 15, and 22
	doxorubicin	Adriamycin	30 mg/m² I.V., day 2
	cisplatin	Platinol	70 mg/m² I.V., day 2 *Repeat cycle q 28 days.*
MVPP (Hodgkin's-disease)	mechlorethamine (nitrogen mustard)	Mustargen	6 mg/m² I.V., days 1 and 8
	vinblastine	Velban	6 mg/m² I.V., days 1 and 8
	procarbazine	Matulane	100 mg/m² P.O., days 1 to 14
	prednisone	Deltasone	40 mg/m² P.O., days 1 to 14 *Repeat cycle q 4 to 6 weeks.*
PCV (Brain tumors)	procarbazine	Matulane	60 mg/m² P.O., days 8 to 21
	lomustine (CCNU)	CeeNu	110 mg/m² P.O., day 1
	vincristine	Oncovin	1.4 mg/m² (2 mg maximum) I.V., days 8 and 29 *Repeat cycle q 6 to 8 weeks.*
ProMACE (Malignant lymphoma)	prednisone	Deltasone	60 mg/m² P.O., days 1 to 14
	methotrexate	Folex	1.5 g/m² I.V., day 14
	leucovorin calcium	Wellcovorin	50 mg/m² I.V. q 6 hours for five to six doses, beginning 24 hours after methotrexate dose
	doxorubicin	Adriamycin	25 mg/m² I.V., days 1 and 8
	cyclophosphamide	Cytoxan	650 mg/m² I.V., days 1 and 8
	etoposide (VP-16)	VePesid	120 mg/m² I.V., days 1 and 8
ProMACE/ cytaBOM (Malignant lymphoma)	cyclophosphamide	Cytoxan	650 mg/m² I.V., day 1
	doxorubicin	Adriamycin	25 mg/m² I.V., day 1
	etoposide (VP-16)	VePesid	120 mg/m² I.V., day 1
	prednisone	Deltasone	60 mg/m² P.O., days 1 to 14
	cytarabine (ara-C)	Cytosar-U	300 mg/m² I.V., day 8
	bleomycin	Blenoxane	5 U/m² I.V., day 8
	vincristine	Oncovin	1.4 mg/m² (2 mg maximum) I.V., day 8
	methotrexate	Folex	120 mg/m² I.V., day 8
	leucovorin calcium	Wellcovorin	25 mg/m² P.O. q 6 hours for six doses beginning 24 hours after methotrexate dose *Repeat cycle q 21 to 28 days.*

(continued)

Cancer chemotherapy: Acronyms and protocols (continued)

ACRONYM & INDICATION	DRUG		DOSAGE
	Generic name	Trade name	
7 + 3 (A + D) (Leukemia—AML, induction)	cytarabine (ara-C)	Cytosar-U	100 or 200 mg/m²/day by continuous I.V. infusion, days 1 to 7
	daunorubicin	Cerubidine	45 mg/m² I.V., days 1 to 3
VAC Standard (Soft-tissue sarcoma)	vincristine	Oncovin	2 mg/m² (2 mg/week maximum) I.V. weekly for 12 weeks
	dactinomycin (actinomycin D)	Cosmegen	0.015 mg/kg/day (0.5 mg/day maximum) continuous I.V. infusion, days 1 to 5 q 3 months
	cyclophosphamide	Cytoxan	2.5 mg/kg daily P.O. for 2 years
VAD (Multiple myeloma)	vincristine	Oncovin	0.4 mg by continuous I.V. infusion, days 1 to 4
	doxorubicin	Adriamycin	9 to 10 mg/m² by continuous I.V. infusion, days 1 to 4
	dexamethasone	Decadron	40 mg P.O. on days 1 to 4, 9 to 12, and 17 to 20 *Repeat cycle q 4 to 5 weeks.*
VBP (Genitourinary, testicular cancer)	vinblastine	Velban	46 mg/m² I.V., days 1 and 2
	bleomycin	Blenoxane	30 U I.V., days 1, 8, 15, and (optional) 22
	cisplatin	Platinol	20 mg/m² I.V., days 1 to 5 *Repeat cycle q 21 to 28 days.*
VC (Non-small-cell lung cancer)	vinorelbine	Navelbine	30 mg/m² I.V. weekly
	cisplatin	Platinol	120 mg/m² I.V., days 1 and 29 *Repeat cycle q 6 weeks.*
VDP (Malignant melanoma)	vinblastine	Velban	5 mg/m² I.V., days 1 and 2
	dacarbazine	DTIC-Dome	150 mg/m² I.V., days 1 to 5
	cisplatin	Platinol	75 mg/m² I.V., day 5 *Repeat cycle q 21 to 28 days.*
VIP (Genitourinary, testicular cancer)	vinblastine	Velban	0.11 mg/kg I.V., days 1 and 2
	ifosfamide	Ifex	1.2 g/m²/day continuous I.V. infusion, days 1 to 5
	cisplatin	Platinol	20 mg/m² I.V. over 1 hour, days 1 to 5
	mesna	MESNEX	400 mg I.V. 15 minutes before ifosfamide day 1; then 1.2 g daily by continuous I.V. infusion, days 1 to 5 *Repeat cycle q 21 days.*
or	etoposide (VP-16)	VePesid	75 mg/m² I.V., days 1 to 5
	ifosfamide	Ifex	1.2 g/m²/day continuous I.V. infusion, days 1 to 5
	cisplatin	Platinol	20 mg/m², days 1 to 5
	mesna	MESNEX	400 mg I.V. 15 minutes before ifosfamide day 1; then 1.2 g daily by continuous I.V. infusion, days 1 to 5 *Repeat cycle q 21 days.*

Table of equivalents

Metric system equivalents

Metric weight

1 kilogram (kg or Kg)	=	1,000 grams (g or gm)
1 gram	=	1,000 milligrams (mg)
1 milligram	=	1,000 micrograms (µg or mcg)
0.6 g	=	600 mg
0.3 g	=	300 mg
0.1 g	=	100 mg
0.06 g	=	60 mg
0.03 g	=	30 mg
0.015 g	=	15 mg
0.001 g	=	1 mg

Metric volume

1 liter (l or L)	=	1,000 milliliters (ml)*
1 milliliter	=	1,000 microliters (µl)

Household / **Metric**

1 teaspoon (tsp)	=	5 ml
1 tablespoon (T or tbs)	=	15 ml
2 tablespoons	=	30 ml
1 measuring cupful	=	240 ml
1 pint (pt)	=	473 ml
1 quart (qt)	=	946 ml
1 gallon (gal)	=	3,785 ml

Temperature conversions

FAHRENHEIT DEGREES	CENTIGRADE DEGREES	FAHRENHEIT DEGREES	CENTIGRADE DEGREES	FAHRENHEIT DEGREES	CENTIGRADE DEGREES
106.0	41.1	100.6	38.1	95.2	35.1
105.8	41.0	100.4	38.0	95.0	35.0
105.6	40.9	100.2	37.9	94.8	34.9
105.4	40.8	100.0	37.8	94.6	34.8
105.2	40.7	99.8	37.7	94.4	34.7
105.0	40.6	99.6	37.6	94.2	34.6
104.8	40.4	99.4	37.4	94.0	34.4
104.6	40.3	99.2	37.3	93.8	34.3
104.4	40.2	99.0	37.2	93.6	34.2
104.2	40.1	98.8	37.1	93.4	34.1
104.0	40.0	98.6	37.0	93.2	34.0
103.8	39.9	98.4	36.9	93.0	33.9
103.6	39.8	98.2	36.8	92.8	33.8
103.4	39.7	98.0	36.7	92.6	33.7
103.2	39.6	97.8	36.5	92.4	33.6
103.0	39.4	97.6	36.4	92.2	33.4
102.8	39.3	97.4	36.3	92.0	33.3
102.6	39.2	97.2	36.2	91.8	33.2
102.4	39.1	97.0	36.1	91.6	33.1
102.2	39.0	96.8	36.0	91.4	33.0
102.0	38.9	96.6	35.9	91.2	32.9
101.8	38.8	96.4	35.8	91.0	32.8
101.6	38.7	96.2	35.7	90.8	32.7
101.4	38.6	96.0	35.6	90.6	32.6
101.2	38.4	95.8	35.4	90.4	32.4
101.0	38.3	95.6	35.3	90.2	32.3
100.8	38.2	95.4	35.2	90.0	32.2

Weight conversions

1 oz = 30 g	1 lb = 453.6 g	2.2 lb = 1 kg

*1 ml = 1 cubic centimeter (cc); however, ml is the preferred measurement term today.

Diagnostic skin tests

DRUG, INDICATIONS, DOSAGE

coccidioidin
BioCox, Spherulin

Suspected coccidioidomycosis—
Adults and children: 0.1 ml of 1:100 dilution I.D. into flexor surface of forearm. In persons nonreactive to this form, test is repeated using 1:10 dilution. Use 1:1,000 or 1:10,000 dilution if erythema nodosum is evident.

histoplasmin
Histolyn-CYL, Histoplasmin Diluted

To differentiate histoplasmosis from coccidioidomycosis, tuberculosis, sarcoidosis, and other mycotic or bacterial infections—
Adults and children: 0.1 ml into flexor surface of forearm.

mumps skin test antigen
MSTA

For detection of delayed hypersensitivity to mumps antigens and assessment of cell-mediated immunity—
Adults and children: 0.1 ml I.D. into flexor surface of forearm.

tuberculin purified protein derivative (PPD, Mantoux, TST)
Aplisol, PPD-Stabilized Solution (Mantoux test), Selavo-PPD Solution, Tubersol

Diagnosis of tuberculosis—
Adults and children: initially, 1 tuberculin unit (TU; for patients suspected of being highly sensitized) or 5 TU (for patients not expected to be highly sensitized) I.D. into flexor surface of forearm. If negative, patient is retested with 250 TU.

tuberculosis multiple-puncture tests
Aplitest (dried purified protein derivative [PPD]), Mono-Vacc Test (liquid Old Tuberculin [OT]), Tine Test (dried OT, dried PPD)

Screening for tuberculosis—
Adults and children: clean skin thoroughly with alcohol and allow to dry; make skin taut on flexor surface of forearm and press points firmly into selected site. Hold device at injection site for about 3 seconds to ensure depositing of dried tuberculin B in tissue lymph.

ADVERSE REACTIONS	SPECIAL CONSIDERATIONS
Other: hypersensitivity reactions (vesiculation, ulceration, necrosis), ***anaphylaxis,*** Arthus reaction.	• Pregnancy Risk Category: C. • Contraindicated in patients with hypersensitivity to thimerosal or erythema nodosum. • Read test at 24 and 48 hours.
Skin: urticaria, ulceration, vesiculation, or necrosis in highly sensitive patients. **Other:** angioedema, ***anaphylaxis***.	• Pregnancy Risk Category: C. • Contraindicated in patients known to be positive reactors. • Read test within 48 to 72 hours. • For cell-mediated immunity in conjunction with other antigens, reaction should be examined in 24 to 48 hours.
Other: hypersensitivity reactions (vesiculation, ulceration), ***anaphylaxis,*** Arthus reaction.	• Pregnancy Risk Category: C. • Contraindicated in patients with hypersensitivity to eggs, egg products, or thimerosal. • Read test at 48 and 72 hours.
Skin: pruritus, vesiculation. **Other:** hypersensitivity reactions, ***anaphylaxis,*** Arthus reaction, pain, ulceration, necrosis.	• Pregnancy Risk Category: C. • Contraindicated in known tuberculin-positive reactors; severe reactions may occur. • Read test within 48 to 72 hours. If repeat test using 250 TU shows no response, patient is nonreactive. • An individual who does not show a positive reaction to 1 TU or 5 TU on the first test may be retested with 5 TU, and if negative, with 250 TU. Repeat testing should be done on the other forearm. The 250 TU should not be used for the initial injection.
Other: hypersensitivity reactions (vesiculation, ulceration, necrosis), ***anaphylaxis***.	• Pregnancy Risk Category: C. • Contraindicated in known tuberculin-positive reactors. • Read test within 48 to 72 hours. Verify questionable or positive reactions with the Mantoux test.

Reactions may be *common,* uncommon, ***life-threatening****,* or COMMON AND LIFE-THREATENING.

Selected drugs used for conscious sedation

Defined as the induction of a minimally depressed level of consciousness (LOC), conscious sedation is used during certain short medical procedures to relieve pain and anxiety, produce a hypnotic state, or cause short-term amnesia (or to achieve a combination of these effects). Over the last decade, conscious sedation has gained widespread popularity and is now performed in gastroenterology, radiology, pulmonology, and cardiac catheterization suites as well as in critical care settings.

Required safeguards
Conscious sedation must take place in a controlled environment with emergency resuscitative equipment readily available. During the procedure, the patient must be able to maintain a patent airway independently and respond appropriately to physical or verbal commands. To avoid deep sedation and cardiopulmonary depression, the patient receives the sedative agents in doses titrated to decrease his LOC only to the point of slurred speech and nystagmus.

DRUG	DOSAGE
fentanyl citrate (Sublimaze) Opioid agonist; 100 times more potent than morphine sulfate. Analgesic activity of 100 mcg is equivalent to 10 mg morphine or 75 mg meperidine.	*Adults:* 0.5 to 1 mcg/kg I.V. titrated in 25-mcg increments over several minutes. *Elderly or debilitated patients with renal or hepatic disease:* Individualize and reduce dosage.
midazolam (Versed) Ultrashort-acting, water-soluble benzodiazepine with amnestic, anxiolytic, sedative, and anticonvulsant properties	*Healthy adults:* 0.5 mg I.V. over a 2-minute period. Initial dose should not exceed 2.5 mg. Some patients may respond to as little as 0.5 to 1 mg. *Adults 60 years or older or debilitated patients with decreased pulmonary reserve:* Incremental 0.25- to 0.5-mg doses administered over a 2-minute period. Wait several minutes to evaluate pharmacologic effect before administering additional sedative doses.
propofol (Diprivan) Sedative-hypnotic; produces rapid hypnosis through nonspecific cortical depression; also possesses intrinsic antiemetic properties; has no analgesic properties.	*Adults:* 10-mg incremental doses administered I.V. to augment effects of benzodiazepines and opioids. *Elderly or debilitated patients:* Reduce dosage.

Drug options

Drugs used for conscious sedation include analgesics, hypnotics, and amnesia-inducing medications. Nurses who administer these agents first must demonstrate an understanding of their pharmacology, familiarity with facility policy, and knowledge of and clinical competency in preprocedure patient assessment, procedural monitoring parameters (including electrocardiography, blood pressure, pulse oximetry, and LOC), airway management, postprocedure monitoring, and discharge criteria.

The chart shown on these pages gives general dosing guidelines and key nursing considerations for the drugs most commonly used to produce conscious sedation in adults. Administered alone or in combination, these agents produce varying levels of sedation and commonly have potent synergistic effects.

KEY CONSIDERATIONS

- Be alert for bradycardia, hypotension, apnea, respiratory depression, and chest wall rigidity.
- Know that drug may cause nausea and vomiting.
- Drug is contraindicated in patients with elevated intracranial pressure or head trauma.
- If overdose occurs, patent airway must be maintained and respiratory and CV support provided.
- Use naloxone (Narcan), as ordered, to reverse respiratory and CV depressant effects. Low doses (1 to 4 mcg/kg) have been used to reverse respiratory depression associated with conscious sedation procedures. Patient may require additional doses (0.1 to 0.2 mg) based on total dosage and time elapsed since last narcotic dose.

- Individualize doses and titrate to achieve desired effect.
- Know that bolus administration is not recommended for conscious sedation procedures.
- Be aware that drug is potent respiratory depressant, particularly when combined with opioids.
- Know that hypotension and bradycardia may occur in patients premedicated with a narcotic.
- Excessive doses or development of hypoxia may lead to agitation, involuntary movement, hyperactivity, and combativeness.
- For pharmacologic reversal of sedative effects, administer flumazenil (Romazicon). Reversal dosage is individualized; generally, 0.2 mg is given I.V. over 15 seconds. May repeat dose to achieve desired effect; however, don't exceed 3 mg in any 1-hour period.

- To avoid deep sedation or general anesthesia, use extreme caution when administering drug. Give incremental doses slowly over several minutes and allow adequate circulation time to assess full pharmacologic effect.
- Stay alert for dose-dependent respiratory depression, which may lead to apnea.
- Remember that drug potentiates CNS and cardiopulmonary depressant effects of concomitantly administered narcotics and sedatives.
- If overdose occurs, patent airway must be maintained and respiratory and CV support provided.

Estimating surface area in children

Pediatric drug dosages should be calculated on the basis of body surface area or body weight. If your pediatric patient is of average size, find his weight and corresponding surface area in the box. Otherwise, to use the nomogram, lay a straightedge on the correct height and weight points for your patient, and observe the point where it intersects on the surface area scale. *Note:* Don't use drug dosages based on body surface area in premature or full-term newborns. Instead, use body weight.

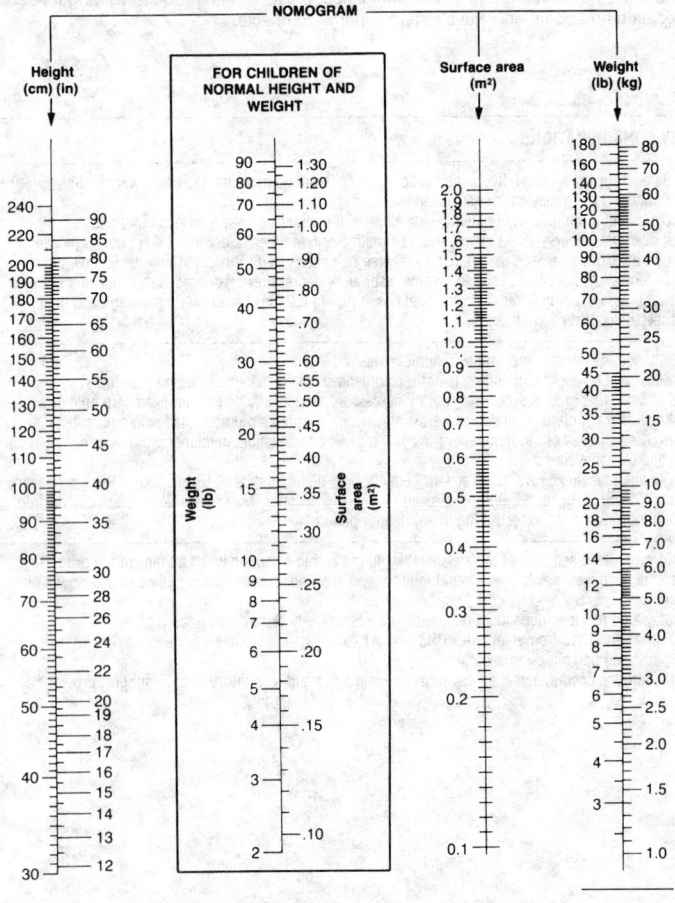

Behrman, R.E., et al. *Nelson Textbook of Pediatrics,* 15th edition.1996. Courtesy W.B.Saunders Co., Philadelphia.

Drug imprint codes

When administering medications, you may come across some pills that are not recognizable by sight. A reliable method for identifying these pills is to check the drug's imprint code found on the tablet or capsule.

Below are drug imprint codes and descriptions for some of the most commonly prescribed tablets and capsules. Column 1 lists the drug code in numeric and alphabetical order. Column 2 describes the pill's shape, color, type (tablet or capsule), and additional characteristics (C = coated; S = scored). Column 3 lists the generic drug name, trade name, manufacturer, strength, and class.

CODE	COLOR AND SHAPE	DRUG, FORM, THERAPEUTIC CLASS
25	round orange tablet, S	levothyroxine (Synthroid/Knoll), 25 mcg, thyroid hormone replacement
25 W 701	shield-shaped peach tablet, S	venlafaxine (Effexor/Wyeth-Ayerst), 25 mg, antidepressant
37.5 W 781	shield-shaped peach tablet, S	venlafaxine (Effexor/Wyeth-Ayerst), 37.5 mg, antidepressant
50	round white tablet, S	levothyroxine (Synthroid/Knoll), 50 mcg, thyroid hormone replacement
50 W 703	shield-shaped peach tablet, S	venlafaxine (Effexor/Wyeth-Ayerst), 50 mg, antidepressant
51 51	oblong pink tablet, S	metoprolol (Lopressor/Novartis), 50 mg, antihypertensive
54 543	round white tablet	acetaminophen/oxycodone (Roxicet/Roxane), 325 mg/5 mg, analgesic
71 71	oblong blue tablet, S	metoprolol (Lopressor/Novartis), 100 mg, antihypertensive
75 W 704	shield-shaped peach tablet, S	venlafaxine (Effexor/Wyeth-Ayerst), 75 mg, antidepressant
93 50	round white tablet, S	acetaminophen/codeine (Teva), 300 mg/15 mg, analgesic
93 152	coral/scarlet capsule	acetaminophen/codeine (Teva), 300 mg/30 mg, analgesic
93 172	brown/gray capsule	acetaminophen/codeine (Teva), 300 mg/60 mg, analgesic
93 490	oblong white tablet, C	acetaminophen/propoxyphene (Teva), 650 mg/100 mg, analgesic
93 541	gray/orange capsule	cephalexin (Teva), 250 mg, antibiotic
93 543	orange capsule	cephalexin (Teva), 500 mg, antibiotic
100	round yellow tablet, S	levothyroxine (Synthroid/Knoll),100 mcg, thyroid hormone replacement
100 W 705	shield-shaped peach tablet, S	venlafaxine (Effexor/Wyeth-Ayerst), 100 mg, antidepressant
150	round blue tablet, S	levothyroxine (Synthroid/Knoll), 150 mcg, thyroid hormone replacement

(continued)

S = scored   C = coated

Drug imprint codes (continued)

CODE	COLOR AND SHAPE	DRUG, FORM, THERAPEUTIC CLASS
200	round pink tablet, S	levothyroxine(Synthroid/Knoll), 200 mcg, thyroid hormone replacement
458 CLARITIN	round white tablet	loratadine (Claritin/Schering), 10 mg, antihistamine
884 MILES 30	round pink tablet	nifedipine (Adalat CC/Bayer), 30 mg, antihypertensive
885 MILES 60	round salmon tablet	nifedipine (Adalat CC/Bayer), 60 mg, antihypertensive
886 MILES 90	round dark red tablet	nifedipine (Adalat CC/Bayer), 90 mg, antihypertensive
3170	blue/gray capsule	loracarbef (Lorabid/Lilly), 200 mg, antibiotic
5513	round white tablet	carisoprodol (Schein), 350 mg, muscle relaxant
A 49	round white tablet, S	atenolol (Lederle), 50 mg, antihypertensive
A 71	round white tablet	atenolol (Lederle), 100 mg, antihypertensive
A KT KT	oval yellow tablet, C	clarithromycin (Biaxin/Abbott), 250 mg, antibiotic
ALTACE 2.5 HOECHST	orange capsule	ramipril (Altace/Hoechst Marion Roussel), 2.5 mg, antihypertensive
ALTACE 5 HOECHST	red capsule	ramipril (Altace/Hoechst Marion Roussel), 5 mg, antihypertensive
ALTACE 10 HOECHST	blue capsule	ramipril (Altace/Hoechst Marion Roussel), 10 mg, antihypertensive
AMB 5 5401	capsule-shaped pink tablet, C	zolpidem (Ambien/Searle), 5 mg, sedative
AMB 10 5421	capsule-shaped white tablet, C	zolpidem (Ambien/Searle), 10 mg, sedative
A MO	round white tablet; C, S	metoprolol (Toprol-XL/Astra), 50 mg, antihypertensive
AMOXIL 250	pink chewable tablet	amoxicillin (Amoxil/SK Beecham), 250 mg, antibiotic
AMOXIL 250	blue/pink capsule	amoxicillin (Amoxil/SK Beecham), 250 mg, antibiotic
AMOXIL 500	blue/pink capsule	amoxicillin (Amoxil/SK Beecham), 500 mg, antibiotic
A MS	round white tablet; C, S	metoprolol (Toprol-XL/Astra), 100 mg, antihypertensive
A MY	oval white tablet; C, S	metoprolol (Toprol-XL/Astra), 200 mg, antihypertensive
AUGMENTIN 250/125	oval white tablet	amoxicillin/clavulanic acid (Augmentin/SK Beecham), 250 mg/125 mg, antibiotic
AUGMENTIN 500/125	oval white tablet	amoxicillin/clavulanic acid (Augmentin/SK Beecham), 500 mg/125 mg, antibiotic
AUGMENTIN 875 SB	capsule-shaped white tablet	amoxicillin/clavulanic acid (Augmentin/SK Beecham), 875 mg/125 mg, antibiotic
B 11	round light green tablet	ethinyl estradiol/levonorgestrel (Tri-Levlen/Berlex), placebo, oral contraceptive
B 95	round brown tablet	ethinyl estradiol/levonorgestrel (Tri-Levlen/Berlex), 0.030 mg/0.05 mg, oral contraceptive

S = scored   C = coated

CODE	COLOR AND SHAPE	DRUG, FORM, THERAPEUTIC CLASS
B 96	round white tablet	ethinyl estradiol/levonorgestrel (Tri-Levlen/Berlex), 0.040 mg/0.075 mg, oral contraceptive
B 97	round light yellow tablet	ethinyl estradiol/levonorgestrel (Tri-Levlen/Berlex), 0.030 mg/0.125 mg, oral contraceptive
BARR 514	gray/orange capsule	cephalexin (Barr), 250 mg, antibiotic
BARR 515	orange capsule	cephalexin (Barr), 500 mg, antibiotic
BARR 545	capsule-shaped orange tablet	cephalexin (Barr), 250 mg, antibiotic
BARR 546	capsule-shaped dark orange tablet	cephalexin (Barr), 500 mg, antibiotic
BIOCRAFT 01	caramel/buff capsule	amoxicillin (Teva), 250 mg, antibiotic
BIOCRAFT 03	buff capsule	amoxicillin (Teva), 500 mg, antibiotic
BIOCRAFT 33	oval white tablet, S	sulfamethoxazole/trimethoprim (Teva), 800 mg/160 mg, antibiotic
BIOCRAFT 115	gray/orange capsule	cephalexin (Teva), 250 mg, antibiotic
BIOCRAFT 117	orange capsule	cephalexin (Teva), 500 mg, antibiotic
BL 32	round white tablet, S	sulfamethoxazole/trimethoprim (Teva), 400 mg/80 mg, antibiotic
BMS 7720 250	oval light orange tablet, C	cefprozil (Cefzil/Bristol-Myers Squibb), 250 mg, antibiotic
BMS 7721 500	oval white tablet, C	cefprozil (Cefzil/Bristol-Myers Squibb), 500 mg, antibiotic
BRISTOL 7278	pink/maroon capsule	amoxicillin (Apothecon), 250 mg, antibiotic
BRISTOL 7279	pink/maroon capsule	amoxicillin (Apothecon), 500 mg, antibiotic
BUSPAR MJ 5	ovoid-rectangular white tablet, S	buspirone (BuSpar/Bristol-Myers Squibb), 5 mg, antianxiety
BUSPAR MJ 10	ovoid-rectangular white tablet, S	buspirone (BuSpar/Bristol-Myers Squibb), 10 mg, antianxiety
C	oval white tablet, S	medroxyprogesterone (Cycrin/ESI Lederle), 2.5 mg, progestin
CALAN SR 120	oval light pink tablet, C	verapamil (Calan SR/Searle), 120 mg, antihypertensive
CALAN SR 180	oval pink , C	verapamil (Calan SR/Searle), 180 mg, antihypertensive
CALAN SR 240	capsule-shaped green tablet; C, S	verapamil (Calan SR/Searle), 240 mg, antihypertensive
CAPOTEN 12.5	oval white tablet, S	captopril (Capoten/Bristol-Myers Squibb), 12.5 mg, antihypertensive
CAPOTEN 25	rounded square white tablet, S	captopril (Capoten/Bristol-Myers Squibb), 25 mg, antihypertensive
CAPOTEN 50	oval white tablet	captopril (Capoten/Bristol-Myers Squibb), 50 mg, antihypertensive

(continued)

S = scored   C = coated

Drug imprint codes (continued)

CODE	COLOR AND SHAPE	DRUG, FORM, THERAPEUTIC CLASS
CAPOTEN 100	oval white tablet	captopril (Capoten/Bristol-Myers Squibb), 100 mg, antihypertensive
CARDIZEM CD 120MG	turquoise capsule	diltiazem (Cardizem CD/Hoechst Marion Roussel), 120 mg, antihypertensive
CARDIZEM CD 180MG	turquoise/blue capsule	diltiazem (Cardizem CD/Hoechst Marion Roussel), 180 mg, antihypertensive
CARDIZEM CD 240MG	blue capsule	diltiazem (Cardizem CD/Hoechst Marion Roussel), 240 mg, antihypertensive
CARDIZEM CD 300MG	gray blue capsule	diltiazem (Cardizem CD/Hoechst Marion Roussel), 300 mg, antihypertensive
CARDURA	oval white tablet	doxazosin (Cardura/Pfizer), 1 mg, antihypertensive
CARDURA	oval yellow tablet	doxazosin (Cardura/Pfizer), 2 mg, antihypertensive
CARDURA	oval orange tablet	doxazosin (Cardura/Pfizer), 4 mg, antihypertensive
CARDURA	oval green tablet	doxazosin (Cardura/Pfizer), 8 mg, antihypertensive
CEFACLOR 250 4760 ZENITH	purple capsule	cefaclor (Zenith), 250 mg, antibiotic
CEFACLOR 500 4761 ZENITH	white/gray capsule	cefaclor (Zenith), 500 mg, antibiotic
CLARITIN-D 24 HOUR	round white tablet	loratadine/pseudoephedrine (Claritin-D/Schering), 5 mg/120 mg, antihistamine/decongestant
CIBA 3	round pale green tablet, S	methylphenidate (Ritalin/Novartis), 10 mg, psychotherapeutic
CIBA 7	round yellow tablet	methylphenidate (Ritalin/Novartis), 5 mg, psychotherapeutic
CIBA 34	round pale yellow tablet, S	methylphenidate (Ritalin/Novartis), 20 mg, psychotherapeutic
CIPRO 250	round white tablet	ciprofloxacin (Cipro/Bayer), 250 mg, antibiotic
CIPRO 500	capsule-shaped light white tablet, C	ciprofloxacin (Cipro/Bayer), 500 mg, antibiotic
CIPRO 750	capsule-shaped light white tablet, C	ciprofloxacin (Cipro/Bayer), 750 mg, antibiotic
COTRIM 93 93	round white tablet, S	trimethoprim/sulfamethoxazole (Cotrim/Teva), 80 mg/400 mg, antibiotic
COTRIM DS 93 93	oval white tablet, S	trimethoprim/sulfamethoxazole (Cotrim DS/Teva), 160 mg/800 mg, antibiotic
COUMADIN 1 DUPONT	round red tablet, S	warfarin (Coumadin/DuPont), 1 mg, anticoagulant
COUMADIN 2 DUPONT	round lavender tablet, S	warfarin (Coumadin/DuPont), 2 mg, anticoagulant
COUMADIN 2.5 DUPONT	round green tablet, S	warfarin (Coumadin/DuPont), 2.5 mg, anticoagulant

S = scored   C = coated

CODE	COLOR AND SHAPE	DRUG, FORM, THERAPEUTIC CLASS
COUMADIN 4 DUPONT	round blue tablet, S	warfarin (Coumadin/Dupont), 4 mg, anticoagulant
COUMADIN 5 DUPONT	round peach tablet, S	warfarin (Coumadin/DuPont), 5 mg, anticoagulant
COUMADIN 7.5 DUPONT	round yellow tablet, S	warfarin (Coumadin/DuPont), 7.5 mg, anticoagulant
COUMADIN 10 DUPONT	round white tablet, S	warfarin (Coumadin/DuPont), 10 mg, anticoagulant
CYCRIN	oval light purple tablet, S	medroxyprogesterone (Cycrin/ESI Lederle), 5 mg, progestin
CYCRIN	oval peach tablet, S	medroxyprogesterone (Cycrin/ESI Lederle), 10 mg, progestin
DAN 5442 DAN	round white tablet, S	prednisone (Geneva), 10 mg, anti-inflammatory
DAN 5443 DAN	round peach tablet, S	prednisone (Danbury), 20 mg, anti-inflammatory
DAN 5490 DAN	round white tablet, S	prednisone (Schein), 50 mg, anti-inflammatory
DAYPRO 1381	capsule-shaped white tablet; C, S	oxaprozin (Daypro/Searle), 600 mg, anti-inflammatory
DELTASONE 10	round white tablet, S	prednisone (Deltasone/Pharmacia & Upjohn), 10 mg, anti-inflammatory
DELTASONE 20	round peach tablet	prednisone (Deltasone/Pharmacia & Upjohn), 20 mg, anti-inflammatory
DELTASONE 50	round off-white tablet	prednisone (Deltasone/Pharmacia & Upjohn), 50 mg, anti-inflammatory
DEPAKOTE SPRINKLE 125 MG THIS END UP	white/blue capsule	divalproex (Depakote Sprinkle/Abbott), 125 mg, anticonvulsant
DIFLUCAN 50	trapezoid pink tablet	fluconazole (Diflucan/Pfizer), 50 mg, antifungal
DIFLUCAN 100	trapezoid pink tablet	fluconazole (Diflucan/Pfizer), 100 mg, antifungal
DIFLUCAN 200	trapezoid pink tablet	fluconazole (Diflucan/Pfizer), 200 mg, antifungal
DILACOR XR 120 MG RPR	gold/white capsule	diltiazem (Dilacor XR/Watson), 120 mg, antihypertensive
DILACOR XR 180 mg RPR	orange/white capsule	diltiazem (Dilacor XR/Watson), 180 mg, antihypertensive
DILACOR XR 240 MG RPR 0252	brown/white capsule	diltiazem (Dilacor XR/Watson), 240 mg, antihypertensive
DISTA 3104 Prozac 10 mg	green/green capsule	fluoxetine (Prozac/Dista), 10 mg, antidepressant
DISTA 3105 Prozac 20 mg	green/white capsule	fluoxetine (Prozac/Dista), 20 mg, antidepressant
DP 25 LEVOXYL	oval orange tablet	levothyroxine (Levoxyl/Daniels), 25 mcg, thyroid hormone replacement

(continued)

S = scored   C = coated

Drug imprint codes (continued)

CODE	COLOR AND SHAPE	DRUG, FORM, THERAPEUTIC CLASS
DP 50 LEVOXYL	oval white tablet	levothyroxine (Levoxyl/Daniels), 50 mcg, thyroid hormone replacement
DP 100 LEVOXYL	oval yellow tablet	levothyroxine (Levoxyl/Daniels), 100 mcg, thyroid hormone replacement
DP 150 LEVOXYL	oval blue tablet	levothyroxine (Levoxyl/Daniels), 150 mcg, thyroid hormone replacement
DP 200 LEVOXYL	oval pink tablet	levothyroxine (Levoxyl/Daniels), 200 mcg, thyroid hormone replacement
DP 301	oval white tablet, S	methylprednisolone (Duramed), 4 mg, anti-inflammatory
DYAZIDE SB	red/white capsule	triamterene/hydrochlorothiazide (Dyazide/SK Beecham), 37.5 mg/25 mg, antihypertensive
E 647	yellow capsule	phentermine (Eon Labs), 30 mg, anorexant
EC	rectangular pink tablet	erythromycin base (Ery-Tab/Abbott), 250 mg, antibiotic
ED	oval pink tablet	erythromycin base (Ery-Tab/Abbott), 500 mg, antibiotic
EH	rectangular white tablet	erythromycin base (Ery-Tab/Abbott), 333 mg, antibiotic
ES	round pink tablet, C	erythromycin stearate (Erythrocin/Abbott), 250 mg, antibiotic
ET	oval pink tablet, C	erythromycin stearate (Erythrocin/Abbott), 500 mg, antibiotic
FLOXIN 200	pale gold tablet, C	ofloxacin (Floxin/Ortho-McNeill), 200 mg, antibiotic
FLOXIN 300	pale white tablet, C	ofloxacin (Floxin/Ortho-McNeill), 300 mg, antibiotic
FLOXIN 400	pale gold tablet, C	ofloxacin (Floxin/Ortho-McNeill), 400 mg, antibiotic
FOSAMAX MRK 212	triangular white tablet	alendronate (Fosamax/Merck), 40 mg, antiosteoporotic
FOSAMAX MRK 936	round white tablet	alendronate (Fosamax/Merck), 10 mg, antiosteoporotic
G 0556	round peach tablet	hydrochlorothiazide (Zenith), 25 mg, antihypertensive
G 800	capsule-shaped white tablet, C	ibuprofen (Greenstone), 800 mg, anti-inflammatory
G 3719	oval white tablet, S	alprazolam (Greenstone), 0.25 mg, antianxiety
G 3720	oval peach tablet, S	alprazolam (Greenstone), 0.5 mg, antianxiety
G 3721	oval blue tablet, S	alprazolam (Greenstone), 1 mg, antianxiety
G 3722	oval white tablet, S	alprazolam (Greenstone), 2 mg, antianxiety
G 3725	round white tablet, S	glyburide (Greenstone), 1.25 mg, antidiabetic
G 3726	round pink tablet, S	glyburide (Greenstone), 2.5 mg, antidiabetic
G 3727	round blue tablet, S	glyburide (Greenstone), 5 mg, antidiabetic
G 3740	round orange tablet, S	medroxyprogesterone (Greenstone), 2.5 mg, progestin
G 3741	hexagonal white tablet, S	medroxyprogesterone (Greenstone), 5 mg, progestin

S = scored   C = coated

CODE	COLOR AND SHAPE	DRUG, FORM, THERAPEUTIC CLASS
G 3742	round white tablet, S	medroxyprogesterone (Greenstone), 10 mg, progestin
GG 172	round yellow tablet, S	triamterene/hydrochlorothiazide (Geneva), 75 mg/50 mg, antihypertensive
GG 263	round white tablet; C, S	atenolol (Geneva), 50 mg, antihypertensive
GG 264	round white tablet, C	atenolol (Geneva), 100 mg, antihypertensive
GG 580	red capsule	triamterene/hydrochlorothiazide (Geneva), 50 mg/25 mg, antihypertensive
GG 606	white capsule	triamterene/hydrochlorothiazide (Geneva), 37.5 mg/25 mg, antihypertensive
GL 500	cylindrical white tablet, C	metformin (Glucophage/Bristol-Myers Squibb), 500 mg, antidiabetic
GL 850	cylindrical white tablet, C	metformin (Glucophage/Bristol-Myers Squibb), 850 mg, antidiabetic
GLAXO 387	capsule-shaped light blue tablet, C	cefuroxime axetil (Ceftin/Glaxo Wellcome), 250 mg, antibiotic
GLAXO 394	capsule-shaped dark blue tablet, C	cefuroxime axetil (Ceftin/Glaxo Wellcome), 500 mg, antibiotic
GLAXO 395	capule-shaped white tablet, C	cefuroxime axetil (Ceftin/Glaxo Wellcome), 125 mg, antibiotic
GLUCOTROL XL 5	round white tablet	glipizide (Glucotrol XL/Pfizer), 5 mg, antidiabetic
GLUCOTROL XL 10	round white tablet	glipizide (Glucotrol XL/Pfizer), 10 mg, antidiabetic
GLYBUR 364 364	round blue tablet	glyburide (Copley), 5 mg, antidiabetic
GLYBUR 433 433	round pink tablet, S	glyburide (Copley), 2.5 mg, antidiabetic
GLYBUR 477 477	round white tablet, S	glyburide (Copley), 1.25 mg, antidiabetic
GLYNASE 1.5 PT PT	oval white tablet, S	glyburide (Glynase PresTab/Pharmacia & Upjohn), 1.5 mg, antidiabetic
GLYNASE 3 PT PT	oval blue tablet, S	glyburide (Glynase PresTab/Pharmacia & Upjohn), 3 mg, antidiabetic
GLYNASE 6 PT PT	oval yellow tablet, S	glyburide (Glynase PresTab/Pharmacia & Upjohn), 6 mg, antidiabetic
HH	gray capsule	terazosin (Hytrin/Abbott), 1 mg, antihypertensive
HK	red capsule	terazosin (Hytrin/Abbott), 5 mg, antihypertensive
HN	blue capsule	terazosin (Hytrin/Abbott), 10 mg, antihypertensive
HY	yellow capsule	terazosin (Hytrin/Abbott), 2 mg, antihypertensive
I25	round white tablet, C	sumatriptan (Imitrex/Glaxo Wellcome), 25 mg, antimigraine
IBU 600	oval white tablet, C	ibuprofen (Boots), 600 mg, anti-inflammatory

(continued)

S = scored   C = coated

Drug imprint codes (continued)

CODE	COLOR AND SHAPE	DRUG, FORM, THERAPEUTIC CLASS
IBU 800	oval white tablet, C	ibuprofen (Boots), 800 mg, anti-inflammatory
IMDUR 60 MG	oval yellow tablet, S	isosorbide mononitrate (Imdur/Key), 60 mg, antianginal
IMITREX 50	capsule-shaped white tablet, C	sumatriptan (Imitrex/Glaxo Wellcome), 50 mg, antimigraine
JANSSEN P 10	round white tablet, S	cisapride (Propulsid/Janssen), 10 mg, GI stimulant
JANSSEN P 20	oval blue tablet	cisapride (Propulsid/Janssen), 20 mg, GI stimulant
JANSSEN R 1	oval white tablet, S	risperidone (Risperdal/Janssen), 1 mg, antipsychotic
JANSSEN R 2	oval orange tablet	risperidone (Risperdal/Janssen), 2 mg, antipsychotic
JANSSEN R 3	oval yellow tablet	risperidone (Risperdal/Janssen), 3 mg, antipsychotic
JANSSEN R 4	oval green tablet	risperidone (Risperdal/Janssen), 4 mg, antipsychotic
K DUR 20	oblong white tablet, S	potassium chloride (K-Dur/Key), 20 mEq, potassium supplement
KL	oval yellow tablet, C	clarithromycin (Biaxin/Abbott), 500 mg, antibiotic
KLONOPIN ROCHE 05	round orange tablet	clonazepam (Klonopin/Roche), 0.5 mg, anticonvulsant
KLONOPIN ROCHE 1	round blue tablet	clonazepam (Klonopin/Roche), 1 mg, anticonvulsant
KLONOPIN ROCHE 2	round white tablet	clonazepam (Klonopin/Roche), 2 mg, anticonvulsant
KLOR-CON 8	round blue tablet, C	potassium chloride (Klor-Con/Upsher-Smith), 8 mEq, potassium supplement
KLOR-CON 10	round yellow tablet, C	potassium chloride (Klor-Con/Upsher-Smith), 10 mEq, potassium supplement
LANOXIN T9A	round green tablet, S	digoxin (Lanoxin/Glaxo Wellcome), 0.5 mg, antiarrhythmic
LANOXIN X3A	round white tablet, S	digoxin (Lanoxin/Glaxo Wellcome), 0.25 mg, antiarrhythmic
LANOXIN Y3B	round yellow tablet, S	digoxin (Lanoxin/Glaxo Wellcome), 0.125 mg, antiarrhythmic
LASIX HOECHST	oval white tablet	furosemide (Lasix/Hoechst Marion Roussel), 20 mg, diuretic
LASIX 40 HOECHST	round white, S	furosemide (Lasix/Hoechst Marion Roussel), 40 mg, diuretic
LASIX 80 HOECHST	round white, S	furosemide (Lasix/Hoechst Marion Roussel), 80 mg, diuretic
LEDERLE V6 VERELAN 360 MG	purple/yellow capsule	verapamil (Verelan/Lederle), 360 mg, antihypertensive
LEDERLE V7 VERELAN 180 MG	gray/yellow capsule	verapamil (Verelan/Lederle), 180 mg, antihypertensive

S = scored   C = coated

CODE	COLOR AND SHAPE	DRUG, FORM, THERAPEUTIC CLASS
LEDERLE V8 VERELAN 120 MG	yellow capsule	verapamil (Verelan/Lederle), 120 mg, antihypertensive
LEDERLE V9 VERELAN 240 MG	blue/yellow capsule	verapamil (Verelan/Lederle), 240 mg, antihypertensive
LESCOL 20 S	brown/light brown capsule	fluvastatin (Lescol/Novartis), 20 mg, antihyperlipidemic
LESCOL 40 S	brown/gold capsule	fluvastatin (Lescol/Novartis), 40 mg, antihyperlipidemic
LILLY 3144 Axid 150 mg	yellow capsule	nizatidine (Axid/Lilly), 150 mg, antiulcer
LILLY 3145 Axid 300 mg	yellow/brown capsule	nizatidine (Axid/Lilly), 300 mg, antiulcer
LILLY DARVOCET-N 50	oval orange tablet	propoxyphene/acetaminophen (Darvocet-N 50/Lilly), 50 mg/325 mg, analgesic
LILLY DARVOCET-N 100	oval orange tablet	propoxyphene/acetaminophen (Darvocet-N 100/Lilly), 100 mg/650 mg, analgesic
LL HEART B12	round yellow tablet	hydrochlorothiazide/bisoprolol (Ziac/Lederle), 6.25 mg/2.5 mg, antihypertensive
LL HEART B13	round pink tablet	hydrochlorothiazide/bisoprolol (Ziac/Lederle), 6.25 mg/5 mg, antihypertensive
LL HEART B14	round white tablet	hydrochlorothiazide/bisoprolol (Ziac/Lederle), 6.25 mg/10 mg, antihypertensive
LODINE 200	two-tone gray capsule with red bands	etodolac (Lodine/Wyeth-Ayerst), 200 mg, anti-inflammatory
LODINE 300	light gray capsule with red bands	etodolac (Lodine/Wyeth-Ayerst), 300 mg, anti-inflammatory
LODINE 400	oval yellow-orange tablet, C	etodolac (Lodine/Wyeth-Ayerst), 400 mg, anti-inflammatory
LOTENSIN 5	round yellow tablet	benazepril (Lotensin/Novartis), 5 mg, antihypertensive
LOTENSIN 10	round tan tablet	benazepril (Lotensin/Novartis), 10 mg, antihypertensive
LOTENSIN 20	round light pink tablet	benazepril (Lotensin/Novartis), 20 mg, antihypertensive
LOTENSIN 40	round pink tablet	benazepril (Lotensin/Novartis), 40 mg, antihypertensive
M 32	round pink tablet, S	metoprolol (Mylan), 50 mg, antihypertensive
M 37	round purple tablet	amitriptyline (Mylan), 75 mg, antidepressant
M 47	round blue tablet; C, S	metoprolol (Mylan), 100 mg, antihypertensive
M 53	five-sided green tablet, C	cimetidine (Mylan), 200 mg, antiulcer

(continued)

S = scored   C = coated

Drug imprint codes *(continued)*

CODE	COLOR AND SHAPE	DRUG, FORM, THERAPEUTIC CLASS
M 77	round white tablet, C	amitriptyline (Mylan), 10 mg, antidepressant
M 241	round white tablet, S	atenolol (Mylan), 50 mg, antihypertensive
M 321	round white tablet	lorazepam (Mylan), 0.5 mg, antianxiety
M 537	round blue tablet, C	naproxen (Mylan), 275 mg, anti-inflammatory
M 751	round orange tablet, C	cyclobenzaprine (Mylan), 10 mg, muscle relaxant
M 757	round white tablet	atenolol (Mylan), 100 mg, antihypertensive
MACROBID	black/yellow capsule	nitrofurantoin (Macrobid/Procter & Gamble), 100 mg, antibiotic
MCNEIL 659	capsule-shaped white tablet, C	tramadol (Ultram/Ortho-McNeil), 50 mg, analgesic
MD 530	round green-blue tablet, S	methylphenidate (MD Pharm), 10 mg, psychotherapeutic
MD 531	round yellow tablet	methylphenidate (MD Pharm), 5 mg, psychotherapeutic
MEVACOR 730 MSD	octagonal peach tablet	lovastatin (Mevacor/Merck), 10 mg, antihyperlipidemic
MEVACOR 731 MSD	octagonal blue tablet	lovastatin (Mevacor/Merck), 20 mg, antihyperlipidemic
MEVACOR 732 MSD	octagonal green tablet	lovastatin (Mevacor/Merck), 40 mg, antihyperlipidemic
MJ 021	round white tablet	estradiol (Estrace/Bristol-Myers Squibb), 0.5 mg, estrogen replacement
MJ 755	round lavender tablet	estradiol (Estrace/Bristol-Myers Squibb), 1 mg, estrogen replacement
MJ 756	round turquoise tablet	estradiol (Estrace/Bristol-Meyers Squibb), 2 mg, estrogen replacement
MONOPRIL 10 BMS	diamond-shaped white tablet, S	fosinopril (Monopril/Bristol-Meyers Squibb), 10 mg, antihypertensive
MONOPRIL 20 BMS	oval white tablet	fosinopril (Monopril/Bristol-Meyers Squibb), 20 mg, antihypertensive
MONOPRIL 40 BMS	hexagonal white tablet	fosinopril (Monopril/Bristol-Meyers Squibb), 40 mg, antihypertensive
MRK 951	teardrop-shaped light green tablet	losartan (Cozaar/Merck), 25 mg, antihypertensive
MRK 952	teardrop-shaped green tablet	losartan (Cozaar/Merck), 50 mg, antihypertensive
MSD 963	U-shaped beige tablet, C	famotidine (Pepcid/Merck), 20 mg, antiulcer
MSD 964	U-shaped light brown tablet, C	famotidine (Pepcid/Merck), 40 mg, antiulcer
MYLAN 130	capsule-shaped reddish orange tablet, C	propoxyphene/acetaminophen (Mylan), 65 mg/650 mg, analgesic

S = scored   C = coated

CODE	COLOR AND SHAPE	DRUG, FORM, THERAPEUTIC CLASS
MYLAN 152	round white tablet, S	clonidine (Mylan), 0.1 mg, antihypertensive
MYLAN 185	round white tablet, S	clonidine (Mylan), 0.2 mg, antihypertensive
MYLAN 199	round white tablet, S	clonidine (Mylan), 0.3 mg, antihypertensive
MYLAN 216 40	round white tablet, S	furosemide (Mylan), 40 mg, diuretic
MYLAN 232 80	round white tablet, S	furosemide (Mylan), 80 mg, diuretic
MYLAN 271	round white tablet, S	diazepam (Mylan), 2 mg, antianxiety
MYLAN 345	round orange tablet, S	diazepam (Mylan), 5 mg, antianxiety
MYLAN 457	round white tablet, S	lorazepam (Mylan), 1 mg, antianxiety
MYLAN 477	round green tablet, S	diazepam (Mylan), 10 mg, antianxiety
MYLAN 521	capsule-shaped white tablet	propoxyphene/acetaminophen (Mylan), 100 mg/650 mg, analgesic
MYLAN 733	oval light blue tablet, C	naproxen (Mylan), 550 mg, anti-inflammatory
MYLAN 777	round white tablets, S	lorazepam (Mylan), 2 mg, antianxiety
MYLAN 4010	peach capsule	temazepam (Mylan), 15 mg, sedative
MYLAN 5050	yellow capsule	temazepam (Mylan), 30 mg, sedative
MYLAN 7250	pink/white capsule	cefaclor (Mylan), 250 mg, antibiotic
MYLAN 7500	pink/gray capsules	cefaclor (Mylan), 500 mg, antibiotic
MYLAN A	round white tablet, S	alprazolam (Mylan), 0.25 mg, antianxiety
MYLAN A1	round blue tablet, S	alprazolam (Mylan), 1 mg, antianxiety
MYLAN A3	round peach tablet, S	alprazolam (Mylan), 0.5 mg, antianxiety
MYLAN A4	round white tablet, S	alprazolam (Mylan), 2 mg, antianxiety
MYLAN G1	round white tablets, S	glipizide (Mylan), 5 mg, antidiabetic
MYLAN G2	round white tablets, S	glipizide (Mylan), 10 mg, antidiabetic
NORVASC 2.5	diamond-shaped white tablet	amlodipine (Norvasc/Pfizer), 2.5 mg, antihypertensive
NORVASC 5	ocatogon-shaped white tablet	amlodipine (Norvasc/Pfizer), 5 mg, antihypertensive
NORVASC 10	round white tablet	amlodipine (Norvasc/Pfizer), 10 mg, antihypertensive
NR	oval peach tablet	divalproex (Depakote/Abbott), 250 mg, anticonvulsant
NS	oval lavender tablet	divalproex (Depakote/Abbott), 500 mg, anticonvulsant
NT	oval salmon tablet	divalproex (Depakote/Abbott), 125 mg, anticonvulsant
ORTHO 75	round light peach tablet	ethinyl estradiol/norethindrone (Ortho-Novum 7/7/7/Ortho-McNeil), 35 mcg/0.75 mg, oral contraceptive

(continued)

S = scored   C = coated

Drug imprint codes (continued)

CODE	COLOR AND SHAPE	DRUG, FORM, THERAPEUTIC CLASS
ORTHO 135	round peach tablet	ethinyl estradiol/norethindrone (Ortho-Novum 7/7/7/Ortho-McNeil), 35 mcg/1 mg, oral contraceptive
ORTHO 180	round white tablet	ethinyl estradiol/norgestimate (Ortho Tri-Cyclen/Ortho-McNeil), 35 mcg/0.18 mg, oral contraceptive
ORTHO 215	round light blue tablet	ethinyl estradiol/norgestimate (Ortho Tri-Cyclen/Ortho-McNeil), 35 mcg/0.215 mg, oral contraceptive
ORTHO 250	round blue tablet	ethinyl estradiol/norgestimate (Ortho Cyclen/Ortho-McNeil), 35 mcg/0.25 mg, oral contraceptive
ORTHO 535	round white tablet	ethinyl estradiol/norethindrone (Ortho-Novum 7/7/7/Ortho-McNeil), 35 mcg/0.5 mg, oral contraceptive
ORTHO D 150	round orange tablet	ethinyl estradiol/desogestrel (Ortho-Cept/Ortho-McNeil), 30 mcg/0.15mg, oral contraceptive
ORUVAIL 100	pink/dark green capsule	ketoprofen (Oruvail/Wyeth-Ayerst),100 mg, anti-inflammatory
ORUVAIL 150	pink/light green capsule	ketoprofen (Oruvail/Wyeth-Ayerst),150 mg, anti-inflammatory
ORUVAIL 200	pink/white capsule	ketoprofen (Oruvail/Wyeth-Ayerst),200 mg, anti-inflammatory agent
P 57	round white tablet, S	lorazepam (Purpac), 0.5 mg, antianxiety
P 59	round white tablet, S	lorazepam (Purpac), 1 mg, antianxiety
PAR 161 300	round white tablet	ibuprofen (Par), 300 mg, anti-inflammatory
PAR 467	capsule-shaped white tablet, C	ibuprofen (Par), 400 mg, anti-inflammatory
PAR 468	capsule-shaped white tablet, C	ibuprofen (Par), 600 mg, anti-inflammatory
PAXIL 10	oval yellow tablet, C	paroxetine (Paxil/SK Beecham), 10 mg, antidepressant
PAXIL 20	oval pink tablet; C, S	paroxetine (Paxil/SK Beecham), 20 mg, antidepressant
PAXIL 30	oval blue tablet, C	paroxetine (Paxil/SK Beecham), 30 mg, antidepressant
PAXIL 40	oval green tablet, C	paroxetine (Paxil/SK Beecham), 40 mg, antidepressant
P-D 362	orange-banded white capsule	phenytoin sodium (Dilantin Kapseals/Parke-Davis), 100 mg, anticonvulsant
P-D 365	pink-banded white capsule	phenytoin sodium (Dilantin Kapseals/Parke-Davis), 30 mg, anticonvulsant
P-D 532 20	round brown tablet, C antihypertensive	quinapril (Accupril/Parke-Davis), 20 mg,
P-D 535 40	oval brown tablet, C	quinapril (Accupril/Parke-Davis), 40 mg, antihypertensive

S = scored   C = coated

CODE	COLOR AND SHAPE	DRUG, FORM, THERAPEUTIC CLASS
P-D 916	round green tablet	ethinyl estradiol/norethindrone (Loestrin [Fe]/Parke-Davis), 30 mcg/1.5 mg, oral contraceptive
PFIZER 305	red capsule	azithromycin (Zithromax/Pfizer), 250 mg, antibiotic
PFIZER 308	oval white tablet	azithromycin (Zithromax/Pfizer), 600 mg, antibiotic
PFIZER 550	round off-rectangular white tablet, C	cetirizine (Zyrtec/Pfizer), 5 mg, antihistamine
PFIZER 551	round off-rectangular white tablet, C	cetirizine (Zyrtec/Pfizer), 10 mg, antihistamine
PPP 784 DURICEFF 500	red/white capsule	cefadroxil (Duricef/Bristol-Myers Squibb), 500 mg, antibiotic
PPP 785	oval white tablet, S	cefadroxil (Duricef/Bristol-Myers Squibb), 1000 mg, antibiotic
PRAVACHOL 10	rectangular pink tablet	pravastatin (Pravachol/Bristol-Myers Squibb), 10 mg, antihyperlipidemic
PRAVACHOL 20	rectangular yellow tablet	pravastatin (Pravachol/Bristol-Myers Squibb), 20 mg, antihyperlipidemic
PRAVACHOL 40	rectangular green tablet	pravastatin (Pravachol/Bristol-Myers Squibb), 40 mg, antihyperlipidemic
PREMARIN 0.3 mg	oval green tablet, C	conjugated estrogens (Premarin/Wyeth-Ayerst), 0.3 mg, estrogen replacement
PREMARIN 0.625 mg	oval red tablet, C	conjugated estrogens (Premarin/Wyeth-Ayerst), 0.625 mg, estrogen replacement
PREMARIN 0.9 mg	oval pink tablet, C	conjugated estrogens (Premarin/Wyeth-Ayerst), 0.9 mg, estrogen replacement
PREMARIN 1.25 mg	oval yellow tablet, C	conjugated estrogens (Premarin/Wyeth-Ayerst), 1.25 mg, estrogen replacement
PREMARIN 2.5 mg	oval purple tablet, C	conjugated estrogens (Premarin/Wyeth-Ayerst), 2.5 mg, estrogen replacement
PREMPRO	oval peach tablet, C	conjugated estrogens/medroxyprogesterone (Prempro/Wyeth-Ayerst), 0.625 mg/2.5 mg, estrogen replacement
PRILOSEC 10 606	apricot/amethyst capsule	omeprazole (Prilosec/Astra Merck), 10 mg, antiulcer
PRILOSEC 20 742	amethyst capsule	omeprazole (Prilosec/Astra Merck), 20 mg, antiulcer
PRINIVIL 207 MSD	shield-shaped peach tablet	lisinopril (Prinivil/Merck), 20 mg, antihypertensive
PRINIVIL 237 MSD	shield-shaped red tablet	lisinopril (Prinivil/Merck), 40 mg, antihypertensive
PROCARDIA 265 XL 30	round rose-pink tablet, C	nifedipine (Procardia XL/Pfizer), 30 mg, antihypertensive
PROCARDIA 266 XL 60	round rose-pink tablet, C	nifedipine (Procardia XL/Pfizer), 60 mg, antihypertensive

(continued)

S = scored   C = coated

Drug imprint codes *(continued)*

CODE	COLOR AND SHAPE	DRUG, FORM, THERAPEUTIC CLASS
PROCARDIA XL 90	round rose-pink tablet, C	nifedipine (Procardia XL/Pfizer), 90 mg, antihypertensive
PROPACET	oblong white tablet, C	propoxyphene/acetaminophen (Propacet/Teva), 100 mg /650 mg, analgesic
PROVERA 2.5	oval white tablet, S	medroxyprogesterone (Provera/Pharmacia & Upjohn), 2.5 mg, progestin
PROVERA 5	hexagonal white tablet, S	medroxyprogesterone (Provera/Pharmacia & Upjohn), 5 mg, progestin
PROVERA 10	round white tablet, S	medroxyprogesterone (Provera/Pharmacia & Upjohn), 10 mg, progestin
R 001 3	round white tablet, S	acetaminophen/codeine (Purepac), 300 mg/30 mg, analgesic
R 003 4	round white tablet, S	acetaminophen/codeine (Purepac), 300 mg/60 mg, analgesic
R 027	round white tablet, S	alprazolam (Purepac), 0.25 mg, antianxiety
R 029	round peach tablet, S	alprazolam (Purepac), 0.5 mg, antianxiety
R 031	round blue tablet, S	alprazolam (Purepac), 1.0 mg, antianxiety
R 063	round white tablet, S	lorazepam (Purepac), 2 mg, antianxiety
RELAFEN 500	oval white tablet, C	nabumetone (Relafen/SK Beecham), 500 mg, anti-inflammatory
RELAFEN 750	oval beige tablet, C	nabumetone (Relafen/SK Beecham), 750 mg, anti-inflammatory
RUGBY 3367	blue capsule	dicyclomine (Rugby), 10 mg, antispasmodic
RUGBY 3377	round blue tablet	dicyclomine (Rugby), 20 mg, antispasmodic
SEARLE 151	round white tablet	ethinyl estradiol/ethynodiol diacetate (Demulen 1/35/Searle), 35 mcg/1 mg, oral contraceptive
SGP 1/35	round pale blue tablet	ethinyl estradiol/norethindrone (Genora 1/35/Rugby), 35 mcg/1 mg, oral contraceptive
SQUIBB 181	orange/gray capsule	cephalexin (Apothecon), 250 mg, antibiotic
SQUIBB 239	orange capsule	cephalexin (Apothecon), 500 mg, antibiotic
SQUIBB 603	oblong pink tablet, C	tetracycline (Sumycin/Apothecon), 500 mg, antibiotic
SQUIBB 648	round white tablet, C	penicillin V potassium (Veetids 500/Apothecon), 500 mg, antibiotic
SQUIBB 663	pink tablet, C	tetracycline (Sumycin/Apothecon), 250 mg, antibiotic
SQUIBB 684	round peach tablet, C	penicillin V potassium (Veetids 250/ Apothecon), 250 mg, antibiotic
SQUIBB 971	red/gray capsule	ampicillin (Principen/Apothecon), 250 mg, antibiotic
SQUIBB 974	red/gray capsule	ampicillin (Principen/Apothecon), 500 mg, antibiotic
SUPRAX 200 LL	white tablet; C, S	cefixime (Suprax/Lederle), 200 mg, antibiotic

S = scored   C = coated

CODE	COLOR AND SHAPE	DRUG, FORM, THERAPEUTIC CLASS
SUPRAX 400 LL	white tablet; C, S	cefixime (Suprax/ Lederle), 400 mg, antibiotic
TAP PREVACID 15	sphere pink/green capsule	lansoprazole (Prevacid/TAP), 15 mg, antiulcer
TAP PREVACID 30	sphere pink/black capsule	lansoprazole (Prevacid/TAP), 30 mg, antiulcer
TEGRETOL 27	capsule-shaped pink tablet, S	carbamazepin (Tegretol/Novartis), 200 mg, anticonvulsant
TEGRETOL 52	round pink and red speckled tablet, S	carbamazepin (Tegretol/Novartis), 100 mg, anticonvulsant
TENORMIN 101	round white tablet	atenolol (Tenormin/Zeneca), 100 mg, antihypertensive
TENORMIN 105	round white tablet	atenolol (Tenormin/Zeneca), 50 mg, antihypertensive
TR 5/ORGANON	round white tablet	ethinyl estradiol/desogestrel (Desogen/Organon), 30 mcg/0.15 mg, oral contraceptive
TRENTAL	oblong pink tablet, S	pentoxifylline (Trental/Hoechst Marion Roussel), 400 mg, hemorheologic
VASOTEC 14 MSD	barrel-shaped yellow tablet, S	enalapril (Vasotec/Merck), 2.5 mg, antihypertensive
VASOTEC 712 MSD	barrel-shaped white tablet, S	enalapril (Vasotec/Merck), 5 mg, antihypertensive
VASOTEC 713 MSD	barrel-shaped salmon tablet	enalapril (Vasotec/Merck), 10 mg, antihypertensive
VASOTEC 714 MSD	barrel-shaped peach tablet	enalapril (Vasotec/Merck), 20 mg, antihypertensive
W 641	round brown tablet	ethinyl estradiol/levonorgestrel (Triphasil/Wyeth-Ayerst), 30 mcg/0.05 mg, oral contraceptive
W 642	round white tablet	ethinyl estradiol/levonorgestrel (Triphasil/Wyeth-Ayerst), 40 mcg/0.075 mg, oral contraceptive
W 643	round light yellow tablet	ethinyl estradiol/levonorgestrel (Triphasil/Wyeth-Ayerst), 30 mcg/0.125 mg, oral contraceptive
W 650	round light green tablet	ethinyl estradiol/levonorgestrel (Triphasil/Wyeth-Ayerst), placebo, oral contraceptive
WATSON 540	oval blue tablet, S	hydrocodone/acetaminophen (Watson), 10 mg/500 mg, analgesic
WC 084	oval white tablet, C	gemfibrozil (Warner Chilcott), 600 mg, antihyperlipidemic
WELLCOME ZOVIRAX 200	blue capsule	acyclovir (Zovirax/Glaxo Wellcome), 200 mg, antiviral
WYETH 78	round white tablet	ethinyl estradiol/norgestrel (Lo/Ovral/Wyeth-Ayerst), 30 mcg/0.3 mg, oral contraceptive
XANAX 0.25	oval white tablet, S	alprazolam (Xanax/Pharmacia & Upjohn), 0.25 mg, antianxiety

(continued)

S = scored   C = coated

Drug imprint codes (continued)

CODE	COLOR AND SHAPE	DRUG, FORM, THERAPEUTIC CLASS
XANAX 0.5	oval peach tablet, S	alprazolam (Xanax/Pharmacia & Upjohn), 0.5 mg, antianxiety
XANAX 1.0	oval lavender tablet, S	alprazolam (Xanax/Pharmacia & Upjohn), 1 mg, antianxiety
XANAX 2	oblong white tablet, S	alprazolam (Xanax/Pharmacia & Upjohn), 2 mg, antianxiety
Z 2984	light blue/white capsule	doxycycline (Zenith), 50 mg, antibiotic
Z 2985	light blue capsule	doxycycline (Zenith), 100 mg, antibiotic
Z 4280	capsule-shaped white tablet; C, S	verapamil (Verapamil SR/Zenith), 240 mg, antihypertensive
Z 4286	oval white tablet; C, S	verapamil (Verapamil SR/Zenith), 180 mg, antihypertensive
ZANTAC 150 GLAXO	beige capsule	ranitidine (Zantac/Glaxo Wellcome), 150 mg, antiulcer
ZANTAC 150 GLAXO	five-sided peach tablet, C	ranitidine (Zantac/Glaxo Wellcome), 150 mg, antiulcer
ZANTAC 300 GLAXO	capsule-shaped yellow tablet, C	ranitidine (Zantac/Glaxo Wellcome), 300 mg, antiulcer
ZANTAC 300 GLAXO	beige capsule	ranitidine (Zantac/Glaxo Wellcome), 300 mg, antiulcer
ZESTRIL 20 132	round red tablet	lisinopril (Zestril/Zeneca), 20 mg, antihypertensive
ZESTRIL 40 134	round yellow tablet	lisinopril (Zestril/Zeneca), 40 mg, antihypertensive
ZOCOR 726 MSD	shield-shaped buff tablet	simvastatin (Zocor/Merck), 5 mg, antihyperlipidemic
ZOCOR 735 MSD	shield-shaped peach tablet	simvastatin (Zocor/Merck), 10 mg, antihyperlipidemic
ZOCOR 740 MSD	shield-shaped tan tablet	simvastatin (Zocor/Merck), 20 mg, antihyperlipidemic
ZOCOR 749 MSD	shield-shaped red tablet	simvastatin (Zocor/Merck), 40 mg, antihyperlipidemic
ZOLOFT 50 MG	capsule-shaped light blue tablet; C, S	sertraline (Zoloft/Pfizer), 50 mg, antidepressant
ZOLOFT 100 MG	capsule-shaped light yellow tablet; C, S	sertraline (Zoloft/Pfizer), 100 mg, antidepressant
ZOVIRAX 400	shield-shaped white tablet	acyclovir (Zovirax/Glaxo Wellcome), 400 mg, antiviral
ZOVIRAX 800	oval blue tablet	acyclovir (Zovirax/Glaxo Wellcome), 800 mg, antiviral

S = scored   C = coated

Cultural aspects of drug therapy

Nearly every nurse will at some time care for patients from culturally diverse backgrounds. A patient's beliefs and customs may affect many aspects of therapy, including medication administration. Understanding your patient's cultural background can help you prevent drug interactions with food or folk medicines as well as interpret his reactions to symptoms and response to prescribed therapies. The chart below describes traditional food practices, symptom management, and folk remedies of selected cultural groups in the United States. However, keep in mind that not every member of a given cultural group necessarily follows traditional practices.

CULTURAL GROUP	FOOD PRACTICES	SYMPTOM MANAGEMENT	HOME OR FOLK REMEDIES
American Indian (Native American)	• Usually eat three meals per day, with a light breakfast; however, number of meals may vary with activity. • Food sharing is common. • May believe that blessed food contains no harmful substances. • Traditional indigenous diet of lean game and seasonal fruits and vegetables may improve health.	• Typically express pain as discomfort or "not feeling right"; may express it indirectly through trusted family member or visitor. • May describe dyspnea as "the air is not right," or "the air is heavy." • Commonly recognize depression; screening tests are useful.	• Use herbs and roots for common illness, such as coughs, diarrhea, and stomach problems. • Some members use sweat lodges for purification ritual. • May use spiritual healing and healers. Health care providers should coordinate care with spiritual healers.
Arab	• Usually eat three meals a day, with main meal in midafternoon. • Many Moslems avoid pork, ham, or foods cooked in or prepared with alcohol. • Generally avoid cold beverages in morning and iced beverages when sick. • Typically don't eat raw fish and prefer well-done meat. • Don't eat hot and cold foods simultaneously. • Acceptance of coffee, tea, or sweets indicates acceptance and trust.	• Express pain freely, especially in presence of family. May fear pain. • May panic when experiencing dyspnea or pain. • May be embarrassed by nausea and vomiting • May not acknowledge depression because emotional health is considered a family matter. • May hesitate to discuss constipation or diarrhea because of modesty. May become distressed if bowel movement doesn't occur at specified time. May use laxatives.	• Generally respect and seek Western medicine. • May use amulets (charms and prayers), sweating, rituals, prayer, and balanced diet as home remedies. • May use hot chicken soup, herbal teas, camphor ointments, and enemas as folk remedies. • May believe that "evil eye" influences illness.
Black/African American	• Usually eat three meals per day, with large meal in late afternoon (especially on Sundays after church). • Some religions (Islamic and Seventh Day Ad-	• Typically express pain openly. • May avoid pain medications out of fear of addiction. • For nausea and vomiting, may prefer non-	• May treat colds with teas, herbs, and warm chest compresses. • May place cotton balls in nose to protect against cold winds. *(continued)*

Cultural aspects of drug therapy (continued)

CULTURAL GROUP	FOOD PRACTICES	SYMPTOM MANAGEMENT	HOME OR FOLK REMEDIES
Black/African American (continued)	ventists) forbid consumption of pork. • Fresh fruits, cooked greens, or yellow and red vegetables may be recommended for blood or circulation problems.	pharmacologic remedies, such as ginger ale, soda crackers, and tea.	• May seek advice from folk or faith healers. • May use magic or voodoo after first seeking advice from family members.
Chinese	• Usually eat three meals per day, with largest meal at dinner. • Typically try to balance *yin* (cold) and *yang* (hot) foods to avoid illness. May perceive illness as result of excess of *yin* foods (commonly treated with *yang* foods, and vice versa). • Family members may bring special foods to hospitalized patient to treat illness. • Typically don't put ice in drinks in belief that cold drinks cause imbalance in body.	• May not express pain openly; health care providers may need to rely on nonverbal cues. • May believe dyspnea results from excess of *yin;* may treat with hot soups or broths or warm clothes. • May believe nausea, vomiting, constipation, and diarrhea result from excess *yang;* may treat with fruits and vegetables. • May view depression and mental illness as shameful and refrain from discussing these topics.	• Use ginseng root for common ailments, such as anemia, colic, depression, impotence, indigestion, and rheumatism. • Use other remedies, including deer antlers, to strengthen bones and treat impotence; use turtle shells to remove gallstones and stimulate weak kidneys. • May rely on home remedies for minor illnesses and consult professional Chinese practitioners for herbs and acupuncture.
Colombian	• Usually eat three meals per day, with largest meal at lunch. • Usually prefer hot drinks in morning. • Catholics may avoid meat on Fridays, especially during Lent.	• Females may express pain more openly than males. • May fear addiction to pain medication and sleeping pills. • May react to dyspnea with anxiety. • May be embarrassed by nausea and vomiting; will accept medication to control symptoms. Typically report loose stools as diarrhea. • Reluctant to discuss depression openly.	• Typically try herbal teas before consulting medical professional. • May self-medicate with remedies from Colombian pharmacies because most remedies can be bought without prescription. (Pharmacies in Colombia generally are main source of health care.)
Cuban	• Usually eat three meals per day, with largest meal at lunch. • Don't drink water when eating fish.	• Express pain openly. Males may be less tolerant of pain than females. • Fear addiction to narcotics and prefer to be weaned from them quickly. • Typically ignore depression because it's	• Rely on herbal medicines to treat minor illnesses. • Usually seek Western medical care first, but may turn to Santaria, an African voodoo-like religion, as last resort.

CULTURAL GROUP	FOOD PRACTICES	SYMPTOM MANAGEMENT	HOME OR FOLK REMEDIES
Cuban *(continued)*		considered a mark on family.	• May try spiritual healers, amulets, and prayers to cure illnesses and maintain health.
Filipino	• Usually eat three meals per day, with snacks in between. • Some Filipinos are lactose-intolerant and have problems digesting wheat bread. • Catholics avoid meat on Fridays, especially during Lent. • Typically avoid extremely cold or acidic foods first thing in morning. Prefer rice porridge, or other soft, warm food when sick. • Don't put ice in drinks.	• Generally don't express pain; some have high pain threshold. • Fear addiction to narcotics. • May react to dyspnea with panic. • Rarely acknowledge depression because of shame. • Feel shamed by nausea and vomiting; may accept medication. • Dislike I.M. injections; prefer P.O. or I.V. administration routes.	• May use herbal remedies before seeking medical advice. • Rely on Western medical care while in hospital. • May seek healers to exorcise spirits or ghosts out of belief that physical ailments are caused by supernatural.
Japanese	• Usually eat three meals per day, with snacks in between. • Many Japanese are lactose- and alcohol-intolerant. • Believe that some food combinations (eel and pickled plums, watermelon and crab, and cherries and milk) cause illness. • Prefer rice porridge with pickled vegetables when sick and hot tea for stomach ailments.	• Generally don't express pain; some have high pain threshold. • May be stoic and not ask for medication. • May fear addiction (especially older Japanese) and may refuse medication. • May be embarrassed by nausea and vomiting. Prefer to try own remedies before taking medications. • Rarely acknowledge depression because of shame; may delay seeking professional help.	• Older Japanese may not respond to illness until advanced and may use herbal remedies to try to cure ailments. Younger Japanese tend to rely more on Western medicine. • May use combination of Western and nontraditional treatments.
Korean	• Don't always eat three meals per day; largest meal at dinner. May have frequent snacks; usually eat until satisfied. • Many Koreans are lactose-intolerant and avoid milk and cheese. • May relate cold foods and beverages with imbalances or cause of illness. • Believe that some soups have therapeutic value.	• May moan or use exaggerated statements to express pain. However, many Koreans (particularly males) are stoic. • Fear addiction and thus use pain medication infrequently. Prefer P.O. or I.V. administration routes. View I.M. injections as invasive. • May react to dyspnea with anxiety and faster breathing. Typically refuse supplemental oxygen.	• Herbal treatments widely used. Typically drink ginseng tea. • May use spiritual healers to drive out evil spirits. • May consult herbal medicine doctor for herbs, acupuncture, and other traditional remedies. *(continued)*

Cultural aspects of drug therapy (continued)

CULTURAL GROUP	FOOD PRACTICES	SYMPTOM MANAGEMENT	HOME OR FOLK REMEDIES
Korean (continued)	• May use onions, garlic, and spices to clear sinuses.	• May hesitate to use antidepressants. • May refuse antinausea medication.	
Mexican	• Usually eat three meals per day, with lunch and dinner larger than breakfast. • Belief in humoral theory is basis for most food prohibitions. Consider certain illnesses hot or cold states; treat with foods that complement those states. • Avoid processed foods because of mistrust. Catholics may avoid meat on Fridays, especially during Lent. • Use chicken soup and herbal teas to speed recovery. Use chamomile tonic to treat gastric upset, especially colic in newborn.	• Generally don't express pain; health care providers may need to rely on nonverbal cues. • Males more stoic than females; view expression of pain as sign of weakness. • Use of supplemental oxygen for dyspnea may cause feeling that something is wrong. • Typically believe vomiting and diarrhea are necessary to purge illness; may refuse medication to control these symptoms, posing risk for dehydration. • Commonly respond to stress with depression, but hesitate to discuss depression out of belief that doing so indicates weakness.	• View herbs as key part of home remedies. Take herbs as broths or teas. • May consult traditional Mexican healers (curanderas), who use blend of folk remedies and spiritualism to correct imbalances. • May not be willing to disclose use of folk remedies with Western medicine practitioner. • Believe that some illnesses are unique to their culture and can't be explained by medicine.
Puerto Rican	• Usually eat three meals per day, with full breakfast and tradition of coffee breaks in mid-morning and midafternoon. • Avoid red meat and chicken on certain religious occasions, but may eat fish. • Prohibit certain foods during pregnancy and postpartum. • Use honey, lemon, and rum mixture as expectorant and antitussive. • Use milk, fruit juice, and malt beverages (mixed with egg yolk and sugar) to treat chronic or terminal illness.	• Express pain openly and loudly. • Prefer P.O. or I.V. pain administration routes. • Attempt to relieve dyspnea by fanning or blowing on patient. Believe that tea from alligator's tail and plant leaf improves or heals dyspnea-related illnesses, such as asthma and heart failure. • View depression as suffering from "nerves." Family history of mental illness carries shame.	• Use more than 100 herbal teas to treat illness and promote health. • Typically apply mixture of fresh urine and mud to treat insect bites or eye illnesses. • Treat body aches, colds, pneumonia, and flu with camphor, eucalyptus oil, menthol, or leaves from mint, orange, and lemon trees. • May use folk remedies before or along with Western medicine. • Have many specific remedies for variety of illnesses.

CULTURAL GROUP	FOOD PRACTICES	SYMPTOM MANAGEMENT	HOME OR FOLK REMEDIES
Russian	• Usually eat three meals per day, with largest meal at lunch. • Some Jewish and Molokan Russians avoid pork and various shellfish. • Prefer hot soups, such as borscht, chicken, or rice soups, when ill. May treat illness with light, bland foods, such as oatmeal, boiled chicken, ground meat patties, potatoes, fresh fruit, vegetables, and plain yogurt.	• May not express pain; some Russians have high pain threshold. May not ask for pain medication. • May avoid morphine because of fear of developing pneumonia and becoming addicted. • May believe that large amounts of medication can poison body. • May respond to dyspnea with anxiety because of language barrier. • May refuse routine medications to treat nausea.	• Use herbal teas, tea with honey and lemon, and hot soups. • May try such remedies as rubbing with camphor oil and mixtures of oils and ointments, enemas, light exercise in sunlight and fresh air, mud and steam baths, and leech therapy. • Usually treat themselves before consulting medical professional. • May try cupping to treat respiratory illnesses. May wear amber necklace to treat thyroid problems.
Salvadoran	• Usually eat three meals per day, with largest meal at lunch (which may be followed by traditional nap, or siesta). • Avoid cold foods during strenuous activities. Believe ice cream and iced beverages cause stomach pain. • View certain illnesses as hot or cold states and treat them with foods that complement that state. • May avoid raw fruits and vegetables in belief that they cause illness.	• Believe pain is necessary part of life; express pain openly through moaning and crying. • May react to dyspnea with anxiety; view need for oxygen as sign of increased gravity of illness. • May attribute depression to real event, such as death or illness. May suffer posttraumatic stress disorder after catastrophic event. • May take laxatives to "purge" stomach.	• Generally use herbal teas. • Believe that pure water, lemon, and eggs have special protective and healing properties. • Rely heavily on nonprescription medications. • May rely on such remedies as amulets: rosary beads, statues, herb bag bundles, and red earrings. Attribute illnesses to outside sources, such as evil eye, witch's curse, ghosts, bad winds, or forces entering body.
Vietnamese	• Usually eat three meals per day, with larger meals at lunch and dinner. • Avoid very cold drinks • May be lactose-intolerant and avoid dairy products in belief that they cause bowel irritation. • Avoid shellfish for 3 to 6 months after surgery. • Prefer rice porridge, clear broth with vegetables, and rice when sick.	• Generally don't express pain; may not ask for pain medication because of stoic nature and fear of addiction and adverse effects. • May respond to dyspnea with anxiety and hyperventilation. • Reluctant to acknowledge depression; may not seek treatment until condition is acute. • Treat nausea and vomiting with home reme-	• Use herbal remedies and teas, spiritual practice, and acupuncture. • May rely on other treatments, include cupping, coin rubbing, pinching skin, and inhaling aromatic oils. Coin rubbing may leave blue-red mark on skin, which may be mistaken as sign of child abuse. • May believe traditional folk healers can exorcise spirits.

(continued)

Cultural aspects of drug therapy (continued)

CULTURAL GROUP	FOOD PRACTICES	SYMPTOM MANAGEMENT	HOME OR FOLK REMEDIES
Vietnamese (continued)		dies first, but may accept medications after many episodes of vomiting.	• Typically believe in both folk medicine and Western medicine.
West Indian	• Usually eat three meals per day, with largest at lunch; eat snacks in between. • Typically avoid meat on Fridays during Lent for religious reasons, but will eat fish. • Some follow Moslem or Hindu traditions and avoid pork or beef. • Treat illness with soups and broths made from animal organs; use liver to combat anemia. • Family may bring special meals to hospital.	• View pain as onset of illness. • Fear addiction and harm from prescription medications; may discontinue these when symptoms disappear. Health care providers should emphasize importance of completing full medication course. • View dyspnea as serious and accept treatment for it. • May acknowledge depression only as "feeling under the weather" and consider it a sign of weakness.	• Drink herbal teas, or "bush teas," to prevent, control, and cure most illnesses. • Consider home remedies an integral part of health care. Each illness is assigned a plant, root, flower, leaf, or bark for treatment. • Reliance on home remedies may cause patients to delay seeking Western medicine until advanced disease stage.

Data from *Culture & Nursing Care: A Pocket Guide,* by Lipson, Dibble, and Minarik. UCSF Nursing Press. © 1996.

Dialyzable drugs

The amount of a drug removed by dialysis differs among patients and depends on several factors, including the patient's condition, drug's properties, length of dialysis and dialysate used, rate of blood flow or dwell time, and purpose of dialysis. The chart below indicates the effect of hemodialysis on selected drugs.

DRUG	REDUCED BY HEMODIALYSIS	DRUG	REDUCED BY HEMODIALYSIS
acetaminophen	Yes (may not influence toxicity)	ceftazidime	Yes
		ceftizoxime	Yes
acyclovir	Yes	ceftriaxone	No
allopurinol	Yes	cefuroxime	Yes
alprazolam	No	cephalexin	Yes
amikacin	Yes	cephalothin	Yes
aminoglutethimide	Yes	cephapirin	Yes
amiodarone	No	cephradine	Yes
amitriptyline	No	chloral hydrate	Yes
amoxicillin	Yes	chlorambucil	No
amoxicillin/clavulanate potassium	Yes	chloramphenicol	Yes
		chlordiazepoxide	No
amphotericin B	No	chloroquine	No
ampicillin	Yes	chlorpheniramine	No
ampicillin/clavulanate potassium	Yes	chlorpromazine	No
		chlorthalidone	No
aspirin	Yes	cimetidine	Yes
atenolol	Yes	ciprofloxacin	Yes (only slightly [20%])
azathioprine	Yes		
aztreonam	Yes	cisplatin	No
bretylium	Yes	clindamycin	No
captopril	Yes	clofibrate	No
carbamazepine	No	clonazepam	No
carbenicillin	Yes	clonidine	No
carmustine	No	clorazepate	No
cefaclor	Yes	cloxacillin	No
cefadroxil	Yes	codeine	No
cefamandole	Yes	colchicine	No
cefazolin	Yes	cortisone	No
cefonicid	Yes (only slightly [20%])	co-trimoxazole	Yes
		cyclophosphamide	Yes
cefoperazone	Yes	diazepam	No
cefotaxime	Yes	diazoxide	No
cefotetan	Yes (only slightly [20%])	diclofenac	No
cefoxitin	Yes		

(continued)

Dialyzable drugs (continued)

DRUG	REDUCED BY HEMODIALYSIS	DRUG	REDUCED BY HEMODIALYSIS
dicloxacillin	No	ibuprofen	No
digoxin	No	imipenem/cilastatin	Yes
diltiazem	No	imipramine	No
diphenhydramine	No	indomethacin	No
dipyridamole	No	insulin	No
disopyramide	Yes	isoniazid	Yes
doxazosin	No	isosorbide	No
doxepin	No	isradipine	No
doxorubicin	No	kanamycin	Yes
doxycycline	No	ketoconazole	No
enalapril	Yes	ketoprofen	Yes
erythromycin	Yes (only slightly [20%])	labetalol	No
		lidocaine	No
ethacrynic acid	No	lithium	Yes
ethambutol	Yes (only slightly [20%])	lomustine	No
		lorazepam	No
ethchlorvynol	Yes	mechlorethamine	No
ethosuximide	Yes	mefenamic acid	No
famotidine	No	meperidine	No
fenoprofen	No	mercaptopurine	Yes
flecainide	No	methadone	No
fluconazole	Yes	methicillin	No
flucytosine	Yes	methotrexate	Yes
fluorouracil	Yes	methyldopa	Yes
fluoxetine	No	methylprednisolone	No
flurazepam	No	metoclopramide	No
fosinopril	No	metolazone	No
furosemide	No	metoprolol	No
ganciclovir	Yes	metronidazole	Yes
gentamicin	Yes	mexiletine	Yes
glipizide	No	mezlocillin	Yes
glutethimide	Yes	miconazole	No
glyburide	No	midazolam	No
guanfacine	No	minocycline	No
haloperidol	No	minoxidil	Yes
heparin	No	misoprostal	No
hydralazine	No	morphine	No
hydrochlorothiazide	No	nadolol	Yes
hydroxyzine	No		

DRUG	REDUCED BY HEMODIALYSIS	DRUG	REDUCED BY HEMODIALYSIS
nafcillin	No	propoxyphene	No
naproxen	No	propranolol	No
netilmicin	Yes	protriptyline	No
nifedipine	No	quinidine	Yes
nitroglycerin	No	ranitidine	Yes
nitroprusside	Yes	rifampin	No
nizatidine	No	streptomycin	Yes
norfloxacin	No	sucralfate	No
nortriptyline	No	sulbactam	Yes
omeprazole	No	sulfamethoxazole	Yes
oxacillin	No	sulindac	No
oxazepam	No	temazepam	No
penicillin G	Yes	theophylline	Yes
pentamidine	No	ticarcillin	Yes
pentazocine	Yes	timolol	No
phenobarbital	Yes	tobramycin	Yes
phenylbutazone	No	tocainide	Yes
phenytoin	No	tolbutamide	No
piperacillin	Yes	trazodone	No
piroxicam	No	triazolam	No
prazepam	No	trimethoprim	Yes
prazosin	No	valproic acid	No
prednisone	No	vancomycin	No
primidone	Yes	verapamil	No
procainamide	Yes	warfarin	No

Therapeutic drug monitoring guidelines

DRUG	LABORATORY TEST MONITORED	THERAPEUTIC RANGES OF TEST
aminoglycoside antibiotics (amikacin, gentamicin, tobramycin)	Serum amikacin peak trough Serum gentamicin/tobramycin peak trough Serum creatinine	20 to 25 mcg/ml 5 to 10 mcg/ml 4 to 8 mcg/ml 1 to 2 mcg/ml 0.6 to 1.3 mg/dl
amphotericin B	Serum creatinine BUN Serum electrolytes (especially potassium and magnesium) Liver function tests CBC with differential and platelets	0.6 to 1.3 mg/dl 7 to 18 mg/dl Potassium: 3.5 to 5 mEq/L Magnesium: 1.7 to 2.1 mEq/L Sodium: 135 to 145 mEq/L Chloride: 98 to 106 mEq/L * *****
antibiotics	WBC with differential Cultures and sensitivities	*****
biguanides (metformin)	Serum creatinine Fasting serum glucose Glycosolated hemoglobin CBC	0.6 to 1.3 mg/dl 65 to 110 mg/dl 5.5 to 8.5% of total hemoglobin *****
clozapine	WBC with differential	*****
digoxin	Serum digoxin Serum electrolytes (especially potassium, magnesium, and calcium) Serum creatinine	0.5 to 2 ng/ml Potassium: 3.5 to 5 mEq/L Magnesium: 1.7 to 2.1 mEq/L Sodium: 135 to 145 mEq/L Chloride: 98 to 106 mEq/L Calcium: 8.6 to 10 mg/dl 0.6 to 1.3 mg/dl
diuretics	Serum electrolytes Serum creatinine BUN Uric acid Fasting serum glucose	Potassium: 3.5 to 5 mEq/L Magnesium: 1.7 to 2.1 mEq/L Sodium: 135 to 145 mEq/L Chloride: 98 to 106 mEq/L Calcium: 8.6 to 10 mg/dl 0.6 to 1.3 mg/dl 7 to 18 mg/dl 2 to 7 mg/dl 65 to 110 mg/dl
erythropoietin	Hematocrit	Female: 36% to 48% Male: 42% to 52%
ethosuximide	Serum ethosuximide	40 to 75 mcg/ml
gemfibrozil	Serum lipids	Total cholesterol: < 200 mg/dl LDL: < 130 mg/dl HDL: female: 40 to 85 mg/dl male: 37 to 70 mg/dl Triglycerides: 40 to 160 mg/dl

Note: ***** For those areas marked with asterisks, the following values can be used:

Hemoglobin: Female: 12 to 16 g/dl
  Male: 14 to 18 g/dl
Hematocrit: Female: 37% to 48%
  Male: 42% to 52%
RBCs: 4 to 5.5 x 10⁶/mm³
WBCs: 5 to 10 x 10³/mm³

Differential: Neutrophils: 45% to 74%
  Bands: 0% to 4%
  Lymphocytes: 16% to 45%
  Monocytes: 4% to 10%
  Eosinophils: 0% to 7%
  Basophils: 0% to 2%

MONITORING GUIDELINES

Wait until the administration of the third dose to check drug levels. Obtain blood for peak level 30 minutes after I.V. infusion or 60 minutes after I.M. administration. For trough levels, draw blood just before next dose. Notify doctor of drug levels so that dosage may be adjusted accordingly. Recheck after three doses. Montior serum creatinine, BUN, and urine output for signs of decreasing renal function.

Monitor serum creatinine, BUN, and serum electrolytes at least weekly during therapy. Blood counts and liver function tests should also be monitored regularly during therapy.

Specimen cultures and sensitivities will determine the causative agent of the infection and the best treatment. Monitor WBC with differential weekly during therapy.

Check renal function and hematologic parameters before initiation of therapy and at least annually thereafter. In the presence of impaired renal function, metformin may cause lactic acidosis and should not be used. Monitor response to therapy with periodic evaluations of fasting glucose and glycosolated hemoglobin. Home glucose monitoring by the patient can also be very useful.

Obtain WBC with differential before initiating therapy, weekly during therapy, and 4 weeks after discontinuation.

Serum digoxin levels should be checked at least 12 hours after the administration of the last dose, preferably 24 hours after the last dose. For monitoring maintenance therapy, levels should be checked at least 1 to 2 weeks after the initiation or a change of therapy. Adjustments in therapy should be made based on entire clinical picture, not solely on drug levels. Electrolytes and renal function should also be checked periodically during therapy.

Baseline and periodic determinations of serum electrolytes, serum calcium, BUN, uric acid, and serum glucose should be performed to monitor fluid and electrolyte balance.

With the initiation of therapy and after any dosage change, monitor the hematocrit twice weekly for 2 to 6 weeks until stabilized in the target range and a maintenance dose determined. The hematocrit should be monitored at regular intervals thereafter.

Check level 10 to 13 days after initiation or change in therapy.

Therapy is usually withdrawn after 3 months if response is not adequate. Patient must be fasting to measure triglycerides.

(continued)

* For those areas marked with one asterisk, the following values can be used:

ALT: 7 to 56 U/L
AST: 5 to 40 U/L
Alkaline phosphotase: 17 to 142 U/L
LD: 60 to 220 U/L
GGTP: < 40 U/L
Total bilirubin: 0.2 to 1 mg/dl

Therapeutic drug monitoring guidelines *(continued)*

DRUG	LABORATORY TEST MONITORED	THERAPEUTIC RANGES OF TEST
heparin	Activated partial thromboplastin time (APTT)	1.5 to 2 times control
HMG-CoA reductase inhibitors (fluvastatin, lovastatin, pravastatin, simvastatin)	Serum lipids	Total cholesterol: < 200 mg/dl LDL: < 130 mg/dl HDL: female: 40 to 85 mg/dl 　　　male: 37 to 70 mg/dl Triglycerides: 40 to 160 mg/dl
	Liver function tests	*
insulin	Fasting serum glucose Glycosylated hemoglobin	65 to 110 mg/dl 5.5% to 8.5% of total hemoglobin
lithium	Serum lithium Serum creatinine CBC Serum electrolytes (especially potassium and sodium)	0.8 to 1.2 mEq/L 0.6 to 1.3 mg/dl ***** Potassium: 3.5 to 5 mEq/L Magnesium: 1.7 to 2.1 mEq/L Sodium: 135 to 145 mEq/L Chloride: 98 to 106 mEq/L
	Fasting serum glucose Thyroid function tests	65 to 110 mg/dl TSH: 0.2 to 5.4 microU/mL T_3: 80 to 200 ng/dl T_4: 5.4 to 11.5 mcg/dl
methotrexate	Serum methotrexate	Normal elimination: 　< 10 micromol 24 hours post dose 　< 1 micromol 48 hours post dose 　< 0.2 micromol 72 hours post dose
	CBC with differential Platelet count Liver function tests Serum creatinine	***** 140 to 400 x 10^3/mm³ * 0.6 to 1.3 mg/dl
phenytoin	Serum phenytoin CBC	10 to 20 mcg/ml *****
potassium chloride	Serum potassium	3.5 to 5 mEq/L
procainamide	Serum procainamide Serum N-acetylprocainamide CBC	4 to 8 mcg/ml (procainamide) 5 to 30 mcg/ml (combined procainamide and NAPA) *****
quinidine	Serum quinidine CBC Liver function tests Serum creatinine Serum electrolytes (especially potassium)	2 to 6 mcg/ml ***** * 0.6 to 1.3 mg/dl Potassium: 3.5 to 5 mEq/L Magnesium: 1.7 to 2.1 mEq/L Sodium: 135 to 145 mEq/L Chloride: 98 to 106 mEq/L

Note: ***** For those areas marked with asterisks, the following values can be used:

Hemoglobin: Female: 12 to 16 g/dl
　Male: 14 to 18 g/dl
Hematocrit: Female: 37% to 48%
　Male: 42% to 52%
RBCs: 4 to 5.5 x 10^6/mm³
WBCs: 5 to 10 x 10^3/mm³

Differential: Neutrophils: 45% to 74%
　Bands: 0% to 4%
　Lymphocytes: 16% to 45%
　Monocytes: 4% to 10%
　Eosinophils: 0% to 7%
　Basophils: 0% to 2%

MONITORING GUIDELINES

When given by continuous I.V. infusion, check APTT every 4 hours in the early stages of therapy. When given by deep S.C. injection, check APTT 4 to 6 hours after injection.

Know that liver function tests should be determined at baseline, 6 to 12 weeks after the initiation of therapy or any increase in dose, and periodically thereafter. If adequate response is not achieved within 6 weeks, a change in therapy should be considered.

Monitor response to therapy with evaluations of serum glucose and glycosolated hemoglobin. Glycosolated hemoglobin is a good measure of long-term control. Home glucose monitoring by the patient is also useful for measuring compliance and response.

Determination of lithium blood concentration is crucial to the safe use of the drug. Obtain serum lithium levels immediately before next dose. Levels should be monitored twice weekly until stable. Once at steady state, levels may be obtained weekly; when the patient is on the appropriate maintenance dose, levels may be monitored every 2 to 3 months. Monitor serum creatinine, CBC, serum electrolytes, fasting serum glucose, and thyroid function tests, as ordered, before the initiation of therapy and periodically during therapy.

Monitor methotrexate levels according to dosing protocol. CBC with differential and platelet, liver, and renal function tests should be monitored more frequently during initial or changing dosing and times when methotrexate levels may be elevated (such as in dehydration).

Monitor serum phenytoin levels immediately before next dose, 2 to 4 weeks after initiation of therapy or dosage adjustment. Obtain a CBC at baseline and monthly early in therapy. Notify doctor if toxic effects appear at therapeutic levels. The measured level should be adjusted for hypoalbuminemia or renal impairment, which can increase free drug levels.

Check level weekly after initiation of oral replacement therapy until stable, and every 3 to 6 months thereafter.

Measure procainamide levels 6 to 12 hours after the start of a continuous infusion, or immediately prior to the next oral dose. Combined (procainamide and NAPA) levels can be used as an index of toxicity when renal impairment exists. CBC should be obtained periodically during longer-term therapy.

Obtain levels immediately before next oral dose, 30 to 35 hours after initiation of therapy or dosage change. Obtain periodic blood counts, liver and kidney function tests, and serum electrolytes.

(continued)

* For those areas marked with one asterisk, the following values can be used:

ALT: 7 to 56 U/L
AST: 5 to 40 U/L
Alkaline phosphotase: 17 to 142 U/L
LD: 60 to 220 U/L
GGTP: < 40 U/L
Total bilirubin: 0.2 to 1 mg/dl

Therapeutic drug monitoring guidelines (continued)

DRUG	LABORATORY TEST MONITORED	THERAPEUTIC RANGES OF TEST
sulfonylureas	Fasting serum glucose Glycosylated hemoglobin	65 to 110 mg/dl 5.8% to 8.5% of total hemoglobin
theophylline	Serum theophylline	10 to 20 mcg/ml
thyroid hormone	Thyroid function tests	TSH: 0.2 to 5.4 microU/ml T_3: 80 to 200 ng/dl T_4: 5.4 to 11.5 mcg/dl
vancomycin	Serum vancomycin	20 to 40 mcg/ml (peak) 5 to 10 mcg/ml (trough)
	Serum creatinine	0.6 to 1.3 mg/dl
warfarin	INR	For acute MI, atrial fibrillation, treatment of pulmonary embolism, prevention of systemic embolism, tissue heart valves, valvular heart disease, or prophylaxis or treatment of venous thrombosis: 2 to 3 For mechanical prosthetic valves or recurrent systemic embolism: 3 to 4.5

Note: ***** For those areas marked with asterisks, the following values can be used:

Hemoglobin: Female: 12 to 16 g/dl
  Male: 14 to 18 g/dl
Hematocrit: Female: 37% to 48%
  Male: 42% to 52%
RBCs: 4 to 5.5 x 10^6/mm^3
WBCs: 5 to 10 x 10^3/mm^3

Differential: Neutrophils: 45% to 74%
  Bands: 0% to 4%
  Lymphocytes: 16% to 45%
  Monocytes: 4% to 10%
  Eosinophils: 0% to 7%
  Basophils: 0% to 2%

MONITORING GUIDELINES

Monitor response to therapy with periodic evaluations of fasting glucose and glycosolated hemoglobin. Home glucose monitoring by the patient is a good measure of compliance and response.

Obtain serum quinidine levels immediately before next dose of sustained-release oral product, at least 2 days after initiation or change of therapy.

Monitor thyroid function tests every 2 to 3 weeks until appropriate maintenance dose is determined.

Serum vancomycin levels may be checked with the third dose administered (at the earliest). Peak levels should be drawn ½ hour after the completion of an I.V. infusion. Trough levels should be drawn immediately before the administration of the next dose. Renal function can be used to adjust dosing and intervals.

Obtain daily INR beginning 3 days after initiation of therapy, continue until therapeutic goal is achieved, monitor periodically thereafter. Also check levels 7 days after any change in warfarin dose or concomitant, potentially interacting therapy.

* For those areas marked with one asterisk, the following values can be used:

ALT: 7 to 56 U/L
AST: 5 to 40 U/L
Alkaline phosphotase: 17 to 142 U/L
LD: 60 to 220 U/L
GGTP: < 40 U/L
Total bilirubin: 0.2 to 1 mg/dl

ACKNOWLEDGMENTS

We would like to thank the following companies for granting us permission to include their drugs in the full-color photoguide.

Abbott Laboratories
Biaxin®
Depakote®
Depakote® Sprinkle
E.E.S.®
Ery-Tab®
Erythrocin Stearate Filmtab®
Erythromycin Base Filmtab®
Hytrin®
PCE®

Astra Pharmaceuticals
Prilosec®
Toprol XL®

Bayer Corporation
Adalat CC®
Cipro®

Bristol-Myers Squibb Company
BuSpar®
Capoten®
Cefzil®
cephalexin
Duricef®
Estrace®
Glucophage®
Pravachol®
Sumycin®
Trimox®
Veetids®

DuPont Pharmaceuticals Company
Coumadin®
Sinemet®
Sinemet® CR

Endo Pharmaceuticals, Inc.
Percocet®

Ethex Corporation
potassium chloride

Forest Pharmaceuticals, Inc.
Lorcet® 10/650

Glaxo Wellcome, Inc.
Ceftin®
Lanoxin®
Zantac®
Zantac® EFFERdose®
Zovirax®

Hoechst Marion Roussel
Allegra®
Altace®
Carafate®
Cardizem®
Cardizem® CD
DiaBeta®
Lasix®
Trental®

Janssen Pharmaceutica, Inc.
Hismanal®
Propulsid®
Risperdal®

Jones Pharma
Levoxyl®

Knoll Pharmaceutical Company
E-Mycin®
ibuprofen
Synthroid®
Vicodin®
Vicodin ES®

Eli Lilly and Company
Axid®
Ceclor®
Darvocet-N® 100
Lorabid®
Prozac®

McNeil PPC, Inc.
Motrin®

Medeva Pharmaceuticals
methylphenidate hydrochloride

Merck & Co., Inc.
Cozaar®
Fosamax®
Mevacor®
Pepcid®
Prinivil®
Vasotec®
Zocor®

Mylan Pharmaceuticals, Inc.
amitriptyline hydrochloride
cimetidine
cyclobenzaprine hydrochloride
doxepin hydrochloride
furosemide
glipizide
naproxen
propoxyphene napsylate with acetaminophen

Novartis Pharmaceuticals Corporation
Fiorinal® with Codeine
Lotensin®
Pamelor®

**Novopharm USA, Inc., Division of
Novopharm Limited**
amoxicillin trihydrate

Ortho-McNeil Pharmaceutical
Floxin®
Tylenol® with Codeine No. 3
Ultram®

Pfizer, Inc.
Cardura®
Diflucan®
Glucotrol®
Glucotrol XL®
Norvasc®
Procardia XL®
Zithromax®
Zoloft®
Zyrtec®

Pharmacia & Upjohn Company
Deltasone®
Glynase®
Micronase®
Provera®
Xanax®

Proctor and Gamble Pharmaceuticals, Inc.
Macrobid®

**Rhône-Poulenc Rorer Pharmaceuticals,
Inc.**
Dilacor XR®
Slo-bid™ Gyrocaps®

Roche Laboratories, Inc.
Bumex®
Klonopin®
Naprosyn®
Ticlid®
Toradol®
Valium®

Roxane Laboratories, Inc.
Roxicet ™

Schein Pharmaceutical, Inc.
nortriptyline hydrochloride

**Schering-Plough
Corporation**
Claritin®
K-Dur®
Theo-Dur®

Schwarz Pharma
Verelan®

G.D. Searle & Company
Ambien®
Calan®
Daypro®

SmithKline Beecham Pharmaceuticals
Amoxil®
Augmentin®
Compazine®
Coreg®
Dyazide®
Paxil®
Relafen®
Tagamet®

Tap Pharmaceuticals, Inc.
Prevacid®

Warner-Lambert Company
Accupril®
Dilantin® Infatabs®
Dilantin® Kapseals®
Lipitor®
Lopid®
Nitrostat®

Watson Laboratories, Inc.
hydrocodone bitartrate and acetaminophen

Wyeth-Ayerst Laboratories
atenolol
Ativan®
Cordarone®
Effexor®
Inderal®
Lodine®
Micro-K Extencaps®
Oruvail®
Premarin®

Zeneca Pharmaceuticals
Nolvadex®
Tenormin®
Zestril®

Zenith Goldline Pharmaceuticals
verapamil hydrochloride

Index

t refers to a table; **boldface** refers to full-color photographs

t refers to a table; **boldface** refers to full-color photographs

---

t refers to a table; **boldface** refers to full-color photographs

t refers to a table; **boldface** refers to full-color photographs

t refers to a table; **boldface** refers to full-color photographs

t refers to a table; **boldface** refers to full-color photographs

t refers to a table; **boldface** refers to full-color photographs

---

t refers to a table; **boldface** refers to full-color photographs

---

t refers to a table; **boldface** refers to full-color photographs

t refers to a table; **boldface** refers to full-color photographs

---

t refers to a table; **boldface** refers to full-color photographs

---

t refers to a table; **boldface** refers to full-color photographs

---

t refers to a table; **boldface** refers to full-color photographs

---

t refers to a table; **boldface** refers to full-color photographs

---

t refers to a table; **boldface** refers to full-color photographs